KT-548-139

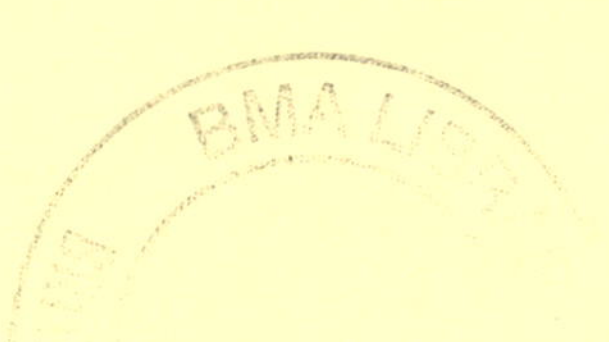
BMA LIB

WITHDRAWN
FROM LIBRARY
BRITISH MEDICAL ASSOCIATION
0849327

VASCULAR MEDICINE

A Companion to Braunwald's Heart Disease

VASCULAR MEDICINE

A Companion to Braunwald's Heart Disease

Mark A. Creager, MD
Professor of Medicine
Harvard Medical School
Simon C. Fireman Scholar in Cardiovascular Medicine
Director, Vascular Center
Brigham and Women's Hospital
Boston, Massachusetts

Victor J. Dzau, MD
James B. Duke Professor of Medicine
Chancellor
Duke University
President and CEO
Duke University Medical Center
Durham, North Carolina

Joseph Loscalzo, MD, PhD
Hersey Professor of the Theory and Practice of Medicine
Harvard Medical School
Chairman, Department of Medicine
Physician-in-Chief
Brigham and Women's Hospital
Boston, Massachusetts

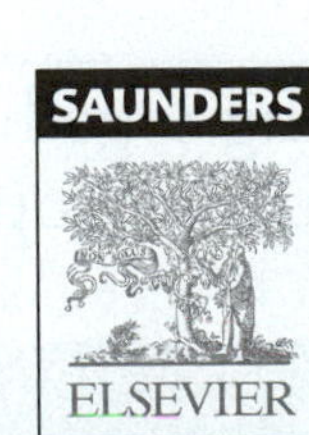

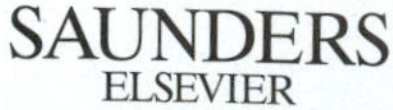

1600 John F. Kennedy Blvd.
Ste 1800
Philadelphia, PA 19103-2899

VASCULAR MEDICINE: A COMPANION TO BRAUNWALD'S HEART DISEASE ISBN-13: 978-0-7216-0284-4
ISBN-10: 0-7216-0284-3

Notice

Knowledge and best practice in this field are constantly changing. As new research and experience broaden our knowledge, changes in practice, treatment, and drug therapy may become necessary or appropriate. Readers are advised to check the most current information provided (i) on procedures featured or (ii) by the manufacturer of each product to be administered, to verify the recommended dose or formula, the method and duration of administration, and contraindications. It is the responsibility of the practitioner, relying on their own experience and knowledge of the patient, to make diagnoses, to determine dosages and the best treatment for each individual patient, and to take all appropriate safety precautions. To the fullest extent of the law, neither the Publisher nor the Editors assume any liability for any injury and/or damage to persons or property arising out of or related to any use of the material contained in this book.

The Publisher

Library of Congress Cataloging-in-Publication Data

Vascular medicine: a companion to Braunwald's heart disease/[edited by] Mark A. Creager, Victor Dzau, Joseph Loscalzo. — 1st ed.
p. ; cm.
Companion v. to: Braunwald's heart disease / [edited by] Douglas P. Zipes ... [et al.]. 7th ed. c2005.
Includes bibliographical references.
ISBN-13: 978-0-7216-0284-4 ISBN-10: 0-7216-0284-3
1. Blood-vessels—Diseases. I. Creager, Mark A. II. Dzau, Victor J. III. Loscalzo, Joseph. IV. Braunwald's heart disease.
[DNLM: 1. Vascular Diseases—diagnosis. 2. Vascular Diseases—therapy.
WG 500 V3322 2006
RC691.V3837 2006
616.1'3—dc22

2005042924

Acquisitions Editor: Susan Pioli
Publishing Services Manager: Frank Polizzano
Project Manager: Jeff Gunning
Design Direction: Karen O'Keefe-Owens

ISBN-13: 978-0-7216-0284-4
ISBN-10: 0-7216-0284-3

Printed in the United States of America

Last digit is the print number: 9 8 7 6 5 4 3 2

We dedicate this book to our wives, Shelly, Ruth, and Anita, and to our children, Michael and Alyssa Creager, Jacqueline and Merissa Dzau, and Julia Giordano and Alex Loscalzo.

CONTRIBUTORS

Amjad AlMahameed, MD
Associate Staff, Cardiovascular Medicine, Cleveland Clinic Foundation, Cleveland, Ohio
Pernio (Chilblains)

Jack E. Ansell, MD
Professor of Medicine, Boston University School of Medicine; Vice Chairman for Clinical Affairs, Department of Medicine, Boston Medical Center, Boston, Massachusetts
Venous Thrombosis

Melinda Aquino, MD
Vascular Fellow, Department of Vascular Surgery, Boston Medical Center, Boston, Massachusetts
Vascular Trauma

John Aruny, MD
Assistant Professor, Department of Radiology and Surgery, Yale University School of Medicine; Chief, Interventional Radiology, Department of Diagnostic Imaging, Yale-New Haven Hospital, New Haven, Connecticut
Lower Extremity Ulceration

Juan Ayerdi, MD
Assistant Professor of Surgery, Wake Forest University School of Medicine; Staff Physician, Department of General Surgery, Wake Forest University Baptist Medical Center, Winston-Salem, North Carolina
Surgical Management of Atherosclerotic Renal Artery Disease

Joshua A. Beckman, MD, MS
Assistant Professor of Medicine, Harvard Medical School; Associate Attending, Cardiovascular Division, Brigham and Women's Hospital, Boston, Massachusetts
The History and Physical Examination; Vascular Laboratory Testing; Peripheral Arterial Disease: Clinical Evaluation; Pathophysiology, Epidemiology, and Prognosis [Aortic Aneurysm]; Clinical Evaluation [Aortic Aneurysm]

Jill J. F. Belch, MBChB, MDHons, FRCP
Head, Institute for Cardiovascular Research, University of Dundee; Professor of Vascular Medicine, Department of Medicine and Clinical Therapeutics, Ninewells Hospital and Medical School, Dundee, Scotland
Pathophysiology of Critical Limb Ischemia

Michael Belkin, MD
Associate Professor of Surgery, Harvard Medical School; Chief, Division of Vascular and Endovascular Surgery, Brigham and Women's Hospital, Boston, Massachusetts
Reconstructive Surgery [Peripheral Arterial Disease]

Bradford C. Berk, MD, PhD
Professor and Chairman, Department of Medicine, and Director, Cardiovascular Research Institute, University of Rochester Medical School; Physician-in-Chief and Attending Physician, Department of Medicine, Strong Memorial Hospital, Rochester, New York
Vascular Smooth Muscle

Francine Blei, MD
Associate Professor, Department of Pediatrics and Surgery (Plastic), New York University School of Medicine; Medical Director, Vascular Anomalies Program, Institute for Reconstructive Plastic Surgery and Stephen D. Hassenfeld Children's Center, NYU Medical Center, New York, New York
Peripheral Vascular Anomalies and Vascular Tumors

Peter Blume, DPM
Assistant Clinical Professor of Surgery, Orthopaedics and Rehabilitation, Yale University School of Medicine; Director of Limb Preservation, Department of Orthopaedics and Rehabilitation, Yale-New Haven Hospital, New Haven, Connecticut
Lower Extremity Ulceration

Eric P. Brass, MD, PhD
Professor of Medicine, David Geffen School of Medicine at UCLA, Los Angeles; Staff Physician, Harbor-UCLA Medical Center, Torrance, California
Pathophysiology of Intermittent Claudication

Allen P. Burke, MD
Staff Pathologist, Department of Cardiovascular Pathology, Armed Forces Institute of Pathology, Washington, DC
Congenital Malformations of the Vasculature

Louis R. Caplan, MD
Senior Neurologist, Beth Israel Deaconess Medical Center, Boston, Massachusetts
Cerebrovascular Disease: Clinical Presentation and Diagnosis

Maria C. Cid, MD
Associate Professor, Department of Medicine, University of Barcelona Medical School; Senior Specialist, Department of Internal Medicine, Hospital Clinic, Barcelona, Spain
Giant Cell Arteritis

Jay D. Coffman, MD
Professor of Medicine, Division of Vascular Medicine, Boston University School of Medicine; Staff Physician, Boston Medical Center, Boston, Massachusetts
Raynaud's Phenomenon; Acrocyanosis

John P. Cooke, MD, PhD
Professor of Medicine, Division of Cardiovascular Medicine, Stanford University School of Medicine; Staff Physician, Stanford Hospital and Clinics, Stanford, California
Diseases of the Lymphatic Circulation

Mark A. Creager, MD
Professor of Medicine, Harvard Medical School; Simon C. Fireman Scholar in Cardiovascular Medicine; Director, Vascular Center, Brigham and Women's Hospital, Boston, Massachusetts
The History and Physical Examination; Vascular Laboratory Testing; Peripheral Arterial Disease: Clinical Evaluation; Medical Treatment of Peripheral Arterial Disease; Clinical Evaluation [Aortic Aneurysm]; Raynaud's Phenomenon

Michael H. Criqui, MD, MPH
Professor, Department of Family and Preventive Medicine; Professor, Department of Medicine, University of California, San Diego, School of Medicine, La Jolla, California
The Epidemiology of Peripheral Arterial Disease

Jack L. Cronenwett, MD
Professor of Surgery, Dartmouth Medical School; Chief, Section of Vascular Surgery, Dartmouth-Hitchcock Medical Center, Lebanon, New Hampshire
Surgical Treatment of Abdominal Aortic Aneurysms

Mark D.P. Davis, MB, MRCPI, MD
Professor of Dermatology, Mayo Medical School; Consultant, Department of Dermatology, Rochester Methodist Hospital, Saint Mary's Hospital, and Mayo Clinic, Rochester, Minnesota
Erythromelalgia

Gregory J. del Zoppo, MD
Associate Professor, Department of Molecular and Experimental Medicine, The Scripps Research Institute; Member, Division of Hematology/Medical Oncology, Department of Medicine, The Scripps Clinic and Green Hospital, La Jolla, California
Antithrombotic Approaches in Cerebrovascular Disease

Magruder C. Donaldson, MD
Associate Professor of Surgery, Harvard Medical School; Surgeon, Department of Surgery, Brigham and Women's Hospital, Boston, Massachusetts
Varicose Veins; Venous Insufficiency

Matthew J. Eagleton, MD
Staff, Department of Vascular Surgery, Cleveland Clinic Foundation; Assistant Professor, Cleveland Clinic Lerner College of Medicine at Case Western Reserve University, Cleveland, Ohio
Endovascular Therapy; [Aortic Dissection]; Endovascular Grafts [Aortic Aneurysms]

Matthew S. Edwards, MD
Assistant Professor of Surgery, Wake Forest University School of Medicine; Staff Surgeon, Department of General Surgery, Wake Forest University Baptist Medical Center, Winston-Salem, North Carolina
Surgical Management of Atherosclerotic Renal Artery Disease

Jonathan E.E. Fisher, MD
Zena and Michael A. Wiener Cardiovascular Institute, Mount Sinai School of Medicine, New York, New York
Renal Artery Stenosis: Clinical Evaluation

Thomas G. Flohr, PhD
Director of CT Physics and Application Engineering, Computed Tomography Division, Siemens Medical Solutions, Forchheim, Germany
CT Angiography

Jane E. Freedman, MD
Associate Professor, Department of Medicine and Pharmacology, Boston University School of Medicine; Staff Physician, Department of Medicine, Boston Medical Center, Boston, Massachusetts
Thrombosis

Julie A. Freischlag, MD
Chair, Department of Surgery, Johns Hopkins Medical Institution, Baltimore, Maryland
Vascular Compression Syndromes

David R. Fulton, MD
Chief, Cardiology Outpatient Services, Department of Cardiology, Children's Hospital; Associate Professor of Pediatrics, Harvard Medical School, Boston, Massachusetts
Kawasaki Disease

Marie Gerhard-Herman, MD, MMSc
Assistant Professor of Medicine, Department of Cardiology, Harvard Medical School; Medical Director, Vascular Diagnostic Laboratory, Cardiovascular Division, Brigham and Women's Hospital, Boston, Massachusetts
Vascular Laboratory Testing

Mary E. Giswold, MD
General Surgeon, St. Joseph Hospital, Denver, Colorado
Treatment [Visceral Ischemia]

Samuel Z. Goldhaber, MD
Professor of Medicine, Harvard Medical School; Staff Cardiologist, Cardiovascular Division, Brigham and Women's Hospital, Boston, Massachusetts
Pulmonary Embolism

Irwin Goldstein, MD
Director, Institute for Sexual Medicine, Boston University School of Medicine; Director, Center for Sexual Medicine, Boston Medical Center, Boston, Massachusetts; Editor-in-Chief, *The Journal of Sexual Medicine*
Erectile Dysfunction

Heather L. Gornik, MD
Associate Staff Physician, Sections of Clinical Cardiology and Vascular Medicine, Cleveland Clinic Foundation, Cleveland, Ohio
Medical Treatment of Peripheral Arterial Disease

Christopher H. Gram, MD
Vascular Surgery Fellow, Boston University School of Medicine and Boston Medical Center, Boston, Massachusetts
Vascular Trauma

Edwin C. Gravereaux, MD
Instructor in Surgery and Medicine, Harvard Medical School; Director of Endovascular Surgery, Division of Vascular Surgery; Associate Physician, Division of Interventional Cardiovascular Medicine, Brigham and Women's Hospital, Boston, Massachusetts
Varicose Veins; Venous Insufficiency

Jonathan L. Halperin, MD
Robert and Harriet Heilbrunn Professor of Medicine (Cardiology), Mount Sinai School of Medicine; Director, Cardiology Clinical Services, Zena and Michael A. Wiener Cardiovascular Institute, Marie-Josee and Henry R. Kravis Center for Cardiovascular Health, Mount Sinai Medical Center, New York, New York
Raynaud's Phenomenon

Kimberley J. Hansen, MD
Professor of Surgery, Head, Section on Vascular Surgery, Division of Surgical Sciences, Wake Forest University School of Medicine, Winston-Salem, North Carolina
Surgical Management of Atherosclerotic Renal Artery Disease

George Hanzel, MD
Co-Director, Percutaneous Valve Program, Division of Cardiology, William Beaumont Hospital, Royal Oak, Michigan
Treatment of Renal Artery Stenosis

William R. Hiatt, MD
Novartis Foundation Professor of Cardiovascular Research, Department of Medicine, University of Colorado School of Medicine; President, Colorado Prevention Center, Denver, Colorado
Pathophysiology of Intermittent Claudication

Robert W. Hobson II, MD
Professor of Surgery, Department of Surgery, UMDNJ–New Jersey Medical School; Director, Department of Surgery, St. Michael's Medical Center, Newark, New Jersey; Principal Investigator, CREST Study
Cerebrovascular Disease: Carotid Endarterectomy

Gary S. Hoffman, MD, MS
Harold C. Scott Chair and Professor of Medicine, Department of Rheumatic and Immunologic Diseases, Cleveland Clinic Lerner College of Medicine at Case Western Reserve University, Cleveland, Ohio
Takayasu's Arteritis

Sriram S. Iyer, MD
Associate Chairman, Department of Interventional Cardiology, Lenox Hill Heart and Vascular Institute of New York, Lenox Hill Hospital, New York, New York
Carotid Artery Stenting

Laura B. Kane, MD
Fellow, Department of Pulmonary and Critical Care Medicine, Boston University School of Medicine and Boston Medical Center, Boston, Massachusetts
Pulmonary Arterial Hypertension

Andrew Kang, MD
Goodman Professor of Medicine, Department of Medicine, Division of Rheumatology, University of Tennessee Health Science Center College of Medicine, Memphis, Tennessee
Connective Tissues of the Subendothelium

William B. Kannel, MD, MPH
Professor of Medicine and Public Health, Framingham Heart Study, Boston University School of Medicine, Boston, Massachusetts
Epidemiology of Cerebrovascular Disease

Tara Karamlou, MD
Research Fellow and Surgery Resident, Department of Cardiothoracic Surgery, Oregon Health and Science University School of Medicine; Staff Surgeon, Department of General Surgery, Veterans Hospital (VA) and Medical Center, Portland, Oregon
Epidemiology and Pathophysiology [Visceral Ischemia]

Noel N. Kim, PhD
Research Assistant Professor, Department of Urology, Boston University School of Medicine; Assistant Director, Laboratory for Sexual Medicine Research, Institute for Sexual Medicine, Boston, Massachusetts
Erectile Dysfunction

Elizabeth S. Klings, MD
Assistant Professor of Medicine, The Pulmonary Center, Department of Medicine, Boston University School of Medicine, Boston, Massachusetts
Secondary Pulmonary Hypertension

Itzhak Kronzon, MD, FACC, FASE
Professor of Medicine, New York University School of Medicine; Director, Non-Invasive Cardiology, Department of Medicine/Cardiology, New York University Medical Center, New York, New York
Atheroembolism

Nils Kucher, MD
Staff Interventional Cardiologist, Department of Medicine, Cardiovascular Division, University Hospital, Zurich, Switzerland
Pulmonary Embolism

Everett Y. Lam, MD
Vascular Surgeon, Kaiser Permanente San Jose Medical Center, San Jose, California
Clinical Evaluation [Visceral Ischemia]

Gregory J. Landry, MD
Associate Professor of Surgery, Division of Vascular Surgery, Oregon Health and Science University School of Medicine, Portland, Oregon
Epidemiology and Pathophysiology [Visceral Ischemia]

Scott A. LeMaire, MD
Assistant Professor, Michael E. DeBakey Department of Surgery, Division of Cardiothoracic Surgery, Baylor College of Medicine; Attending Surgeon, Cardiovascular Surgery Service, Texas Heart Institute at St. Luke's Hospital, Houston, Texas
Surgical Therapy [Aortic Dissection]

Lilach O. Lerman, MD, PhD
Professor of Medicine, Division of Nephrology and Hypertension, Mayo Medical School and Mayo Graduate School of Medicine, Rochester, Minnesota
Renal Artery Disease: Pathophysiology

Peter Libby, MD
Mallinckrodt Professor of Medicine, Harvard Medical School; Chief, Cardiovascular Medicine, Brigham and Women's Hospital, Boston, Massachusetts
Atherosclerosis; Pathophysiology of Vasculitis

Martin J. Lipton, MD, FACR, FRCP, FACC
Professor, Department of Radiology, Harvard Medical School; Attending, Brigham and Women's Hospital, Boston, Massachusetts; Professor Emeritus, Department of Radiology and Medicine (Cardiology), University of Chicago Pritzker School of Medicine, Chicago, Illinois
Magnetic Resonance Imaging; CT Angiography

Joseph Loscalzo, MD, PhD
Hersey Professor of the Theory and Practice of Medicine, Harvard Medical School; Chairman, Department of Medicine, Physician-in-Chief, Brigham and Women's Hospital, Boston, Massachusetts
Normal Mechanisms of Hemostasis; Thrombosis; Pulmonary Arterial Hypertension; Secondary Pulmonary Hypertension

Herbert I. Machleder, MD
Professor Emeritus, Division of Vascular Surgery, David Geffen School of Medicine at UCLA; UCLA Medical Center, Gonda (Goldschmied) Vascular Center, Los Angeles, California
Vascular Compression Syndromes

Kathleen Maksimowicz-McKinnon, DO
Fellow, Department of Rheumatic and Immunologic Disease, Cleveland Clinic Foundation, Cleveland, Ohio
Takayasu's Arteritis

Jess Mandel, MD
Associate Professor of Medicine and Assistant Dean, University of Iowa Roy J. and Lucille A. Carver College of Medicine; Director, Pulmonary Hypertension Program, University of Iowa Hospitals and Clinics, Iowa City, Iowa
Pulmonary Veno-occlusive Disease

Matthew T. Menard, MD
Instructor in Surgery, Harvard Medical School; Associate Surgeon and Co-Director of Endovascular Surgery, Division of Vascular and Endovascular Surgery, Brigham and Women's Hospital, Boston, Massachusetts
Reconstructive Surgery [Peripheral Arterial Disease]

James O. Menzoian, MD, FACS
Professor of Surgery, University of Connecticut School of Medicine; Vascular Surgeon and Medical Director, Collaborative Center for Clinical Improvement, University of Connecticut Health Center, Farmington, Connecticut
Vascular Trauma

Peter A. Merkel, MD, MPH
Associate Professor of Medicine, Section of Rheumatology, Department of Medicine, Director, Boston University Vasculitis Center, Boston University School of Medicine, Boston, Massachusetts
Overview of Vasculitis; Giant Cell Arteritis

Virginia M. Miller, PhD
Professor of Surgery and Physiology, Mayo Medical School; Consultant, Department of Surgery, Mayo Clinic Rochester, Rochester, Minnesota
Vascular Pharmacology

Gregory L. Moneta, MD
Professor of Surgery and Chief, Division of Vascular Surgery, Oregon Health and Science University School of Medicine; Staff Surgeon, Department of Vascular Surgery, University Hospital and Department of Veterans Affairs Hospital, Portland, Oregon
Epidemiology and Pathophysiology [Visceral Ischemia]; Clinical Evaluation [Visceral Ischemia]; Treatment [Visceral Ischemia]

Ricardo Munarriz, MD
Assistant Professor, Department of Urology, Boston University School of Medicine; Staff Physician, Institute for Sexual Medicine, Boston Medical Center, Boston, Massachusetts
Erectile Dysfunction

Jane W. Newburger, MD, MPH
Professor of Pediatrics, Harvard Medical School; Associate Cardiologist-in-Chief, Children's Hospital Boston, Boston, Massachusetts
Kawasaki Disease

John Ninomiya, PhD, MSc
Department of Family and Preventive Medicine, University of California, San Diego, School of Medicine, San Diego, California
The Epidemiology of Peripheral Arterial Disease

Patrick O'Gara, MD
Associate Professor of Medicine, Harvard Medical School; Director, Clinical Cardiology, and Vice Chairman, Department of Medicine, Brigham and Women's Hospital, Boston, Massachusetts
Pathophysiology, Clinical Evaluation, and Medical Management [Aortic Dissection]

Jeffrey W. Olin, DO
Professor of Medicine, Mount Sinai School of Medicine; Director, Vascular Medicine, Zena and Michael A. Wiener Cardiovascular Institute, Marie-Josee and Henry R. Kravis Center for Cardiovascular Health, Mount Sinai Medical Center, New York, New York
Renal Artery Stenosis: Clinical Evaluation; Thromboangiitis Obliterans (Buerger's Disease); Pernio (Chilblains)

Stephen T. O'Rourke, PhD
Associate Professor, Department of Pharmaceutical Sciences, North Dakota State University College of Pharmacy, Fargo, North Dakota
Vascular Pharmacology

Kenneth Ouriel, MD, FACS, FACC
Professor, Department of Surgery, Cleveland Clinic Lerner College of Medicine at Case Western Reserve University; Chairman, Department of Vascular Surgery, Cleveland Clinic, Cleveland, Ohio
Acute Arterial Occlusion

Jacek Paszkowiak, MD
Resident, Department of Surgery, Yale–New Haven Hospital, New Haven, and St. Mary's Hospital, Waterbury, Connecticut
Lower Extremity Ulceration

Dean Patterson, MBChB, MRCP, MD
University of Dundee, The Institute of Cardiovascular Research, Ninewells Hospital and Medical School, Dundee, United Kingdom
Pathophysiology of Critical Limb Ischemia

Joseph D. Raffetto, MD
Assistant Professor of Surgery, Boston University School of Medicine; Attending Staff, Department of Surgery, Boston Medical Center, Boston, and Veterans Affairs Boston Healthcare System, West Roxbury, Massachusetts
Vascular Trauma

Rajendra Raghow, PhD
Professor, Department of Pharmacology, Pediatrics and Biomedical Engineering; Senior Research Career Scientist, University of Tennessee Health Science Center, Memphis, Tennessee
Connective Tissues of the Subendothelium

David A. Rigberg, MD
Assistant Professor of Surgery, Division of Vascular Surgery, UCLA Medical Center, Gonda (Goldschmied) Vascular Center, Los Angeles; Section Chief, Vascular Surgery, Santa Monica Hospital, Santa Monica, California
Vascular Compression Syndromes

Stanley G. Rockson, MD
Associate Professor of Medicine, Stanford University School of Medicine; Chief of Consultative Cardiology; Director, Center for Lymphatic and Venous Disorders, Division of Cardiovascular Medicine, Stanford Hospital and Clinics, Stanford, California
Diseases of the Lymphatic Circulation

Thom W. Rooke, MD
John and Posy Krehbiel Professor in Vascular Medicine and Professor of Medicine, Mayo Medical School; Director, Section of Vascular Medicine, Mayo Clinic, Rochester, Minnesota
Erythromelalgia

Gary S. Roubin, MD, PhD
Clinical Professor of Medicine, New York University School of Medicine, New York; Chairman, Department of Interventional Cardiology; Director of Cardiovascular Interventional Laboratories, Lenox Hill Hospital, New York, New York
Carotid Artery Stenting

Frederick L. Ruberg, MD
Fellow, Department of Medicine, Division of Cardiology, Boston Medical Center; Whitaker Cardiovascular Institute, Boston University School of Medicine, Boston, Massachusetts
Normal Mechanisms of Hemostasis

Eva M. Rzucidlo, MD
Assistant Professor, Department of Surgery, Dartmouth Medical School; Staff Surgeon, Department of Surgery, Dartmouth-Hitchcock Medical Center, Lebanon, New Hampshire
Surgical Treatment of Abdominal Aortic Aneurysms

Robert D. Safian, MD, FACC
Director, Cardiac and Vascular Intervention, Division of Cardiology, William Beaumont Hospital, Royal Oak, Minnesota
Treatment of Renal Artery Stenosis

U. Joseph Schoepf, MD
Associate Professor and Director, CT Research and Development, Department of Radiology, Medical University of South Carolina College of Medicine, Charleston, South Carolina
CT Angiography

Jerome Seyer, PhD
Formerly Professor, Department of Physiological Sciences, Eastern Virginia Medical School, Norfolk; Senior Research Chemist, Hampton VA Medical Center, Hampton, Virginia
Connective Tissues of the Subendothelium

Piotr Sobieszczyk, MD
Instructor in Medicine, Harvard Medical School; Cardiovascular Division, Brigham and Women's Hospital, Boston, Massachusetts
Magnetic Resonance Imaging

Sunita D. Srivastava, MD
Assistant Professor of Surgery and Radiology, Sections of Vascular Surgery and Interventional Radiology, University of Michigan Medical School, Ann Arbor, Michigan
Endovascular Therapy [Aortic Dissection]; Endovascular Grafts [Aortic Aneurysms]

Michael Stanton-Hicks, MBBS, MD, FRCA
Professor and Vice-Chairman, Division of Anesthesiology, Cleveland Clinic Lerner College of Medicine at Case Western Reserve University, Cleveland, Ohio
Complex Regional Pain Syndrome

Bauer E. Sumpio, MD, PhD
Professor of Surgery and Radiology and Chief, Vascular Surgery Section, Yale University School of Medicine; Chief, Vascular Surgery Services, Yale–New Haven Hospital; Director, Endovascular Center, Yale–New Haven Medical Center, New Haven, Connecticut
Lower Extremity Ulceration

Allen J. Taylor, MD
Director, Cardiology Service, Walter Reed Army Medical Center, Washington, DC
Congenital Malformations of the Vasculature

Lloyd M. Taylor, Jr., MD
Professor of Surgery, Division of Vascular Surgery, Oregon Health and Science University School of Medicine, Portland, Oregon
Epidemiology and Pathophysiology [Visceral Ischemia]

Stephen C. Textor, MD
Professor of Medicine, Mayo Clinic College of Medicine; Vice-Chair and Consultant, Division of Nephrology and Hypertension, Mayo Clinic, Rochester, Minnesota
Renal Artery Disease: Pathophysiology

Robert W. Thompson, MD
Professor of Surgery, Radiology, and Cell Biology and Physiology, Department of Surgery, Section of Vascular Surgery, Washington University in St. Louis School of Medicine; Attending Surgeon, Barnes-Jewish Hospital of St. Louis, St. Louis, Missouri
Surgical Therapy [Aortic Dissection]

James N. Topper, MD, PhD
General Partner, Frazier Healthcare Ventures, Palo Alto; Clinical Assistant Professor, Department of Medicine, Division of Cardiovascular Medicine, Stanford University School of Medicine, Stanford, California
The Endothelium

Abdul M. Traish, MBA, PhD
Professor of Biochemistry and Urology, Department of Biochemistry, Boston University School of Medicine, Boston, Massachusetts
Erectile Dysfunction

Paul A. Tunick, MD
Professor of Medicine, Department of Medicine, Cardiology Division, New York University School of Medicine, New York, New York
Atheroembolism

Gilbert R. Upchurch Jr., MD
Associate Professor of Surgery, University of Michigan Medical School; Attending Surgeon, Vascular Surgery Section, University of Michigan Health System and Veterans Administration Hospital, Ann Arbor, Michigan
Endovascular Therapy [Aortic Dissection]; Endovascular Grafts [Aortic Aneurysms]

R. James Valentine, MD
Frank H. Kidd, Jr., Professor and Vice Chairman, Department of Surgery, UT Southwestern Medical School; Attending Staff, Department of Surgery, Zale Lipsky University Hospital, Parkland Memorial Hospital, St. Paul Medical Center, and Veterans Administration Medical Center; Courtesy Staff, Clinical Department of Surgery, Children's Medical Center at Dallas, Dallas, Texas
Vascular Infection

Paul M. Vanhoutte, MD, PhD, DHC
Professor, Department of Pharmacology, Li Ka Chin Faculty of Medicine, University of Hong Kong, Hong Kong, China
Vascular Pharmacology

Renu Virmani, MD
Chairman, Department of Cardiovascular Pathology, Armed Forces Institute of Pathology, Washington, DC
Congenital Malformations of the Vasculature

Jiri J. Vitek, MD, PhD
Interventional Neuroradiologist, Department of Medicine/Radiology/Cardiology, Lenox Hill Heart and Vascular Institute of New York, Lenox Hill Hospital, New York, New York
Carotid Artery Stenting

Scott M. Wasserman, MD
Global Development Leader, Amgen Inc., Thousand Oaks; Instructor in Cardiovascular Medicine, Stanford University School of Medicine, Stanford, California
The Endothelium

Giora Weisz, MD
Assistant Professor of Clinical Medicine, Co-Director, Clinical Services, Center for Interventional Vascular Therapy, Columbia University Medical Center; Cardiovascular Research Foundation, New York, New York
Carotid Artery Stenting

M. Burress Welborn, MD
Staff Surgeon, Vascular Surgery Section, Huntsville Hospital, Huntsville, Alabama
Vascular Infection

Christopher J. White, MD
Chairman, Department of Cardiology, Ochsner Clinic Foundation, New Orleans, Louisiana
Peripheral Arterial Angiography; Catheter-Based Intervention [Peripheral Arterial Disease]

David B. Wilson, MD
Vascular Surgery Fellow, Michigan Vascular Center, Flint, Michigan
Surgical Management of Atherosclerotic Renal Artery Disease

Philip A. Wolf, MD
Professor of Neurology, Boston University School of Medicine, Boston, Massachusetts
Epidemiology of Cerebrovascular Disease

E. Kent Yucel, MD, FACR
Chief Radiology Services, Boston VA Healthcare Systems, West Roxbury Division, West Roxbury, Massachusetts
Magnetic Resonance Imaging

FOREWORD

With the aging of the population and the greatly increasing prevalence of diabetes mellitus, extracoronary vascular disease is a serious and rapidly growing health problem. Clinical manifestations of compromised blood flow in all arterial beds, including those of the extremities, kidneys, central nervous system, viscera, and lungs, are common, and the management of these problems often presents an immense challenge to the clinician. Diseases of vessels of all sizes are responsible for the clinical manifestations, ranging from annoyances and discomfort to life-threatening emergencies.

Fortunately, our understanding of the underlying pathobiology of these conditions and of their diagnosis—using both clinical and modern imaging techniques—is advancing rapidly and on many fronts. Simultaneously, treatment of vascular diseases is becoming much more effective. Catheter-based, surgical, and pharmacologic interventions each are making important strides. Since vascular diseases affect a large number of organ systems and are managed by a variety of therapeutic approaches, treatment is not within the domain of a single specialty. Medical vascular specialists, vascular surgeons, radiologists, interventionalists, urologists, neurologists, neurosurgeons, and experts in coagulation are just some of those who contribute to the care of these patients. There are few fields in medicine in which the knowledge and skills of so many experts are needed for the provision of effective care.

Because the totality of important knowledge about vascular diseases has increased so enormously in the past decade, there is a pressing need for a treatise that is at once scholarly and thorough and at the same time up to date and practical. Drs. Creager, Dzau, and Loscalzo have combined their formidable talents and experiences in vascular diseases to provide a book that fills this important void. Working with a group of talented authors, they have provided a volume that is both broad and deep, and which will be immensely useful to clinicians, investigators, and trainees who focus on these important conditions. I predict that *Vascular Medicine* will become the "bible" in its field, and I am especially proud that it takes its place as a Companion to *Braunwald's Heart Disease, A Textbook of Cardiovascular Medicine.*

Eugene Braunwald, MD
Boston, Massachusetts

PREFACE

Vascular diseases constitute some of the most common causes of disability and death in Western society. Approximately 25 million persons in the United States are affected by clinically significant sequelae of atherosclerosis and thrombosis. Many others suffer discomfort and disabling consequences of vasospasm, vasculitis, chronic venous insufficiency, and lymphedema. Recent discoveries in the field of vascular biology have enhanced our understanding of vascular diseases. Technological achievements in vascular imaging, novel medical therapies, and advances in endovascular interventions provide an impetus for an integrative view of the vascular system and vascular diseases. Vascular medicine is an important and dynamic medical discipline, well poised to facilitate the transfer of information acquired at the bench to the bedside of patients with vascular diseases.

Accordingly, this textbook has been written to integrate a contemporary understanding of vascular biology with a detailed and thorough review of clinical vascular diseases. The book is organized into major sections that include important precepts in vascular biology, principles of the evaluation of the vascular system, and detailed discussions of common, as well as unusual, vascular diseases. The authors of each of the chapters are recognized experts in their fields. The tenets of vascular biology are provided in the first section of the book, which includes chapters on vascular endothelium, smooth muscle, connective tissue and matrix, hemostasis, and vascular pharmacology. The next section, on blood vessel pathobiology, includes chapters on atherosclerosis, vasculitis, and thrombosis. The section on principles of vascular evaluation provides tools for the approach to the patient with vascular disease, beginning with the history and physical examination, and comprises illustrated chapters on noninvasive vascular tests, magnetic resonance imaging, computed tomographic angiography, and conventional contrast angiography. The sections that follow cover major vascular diseases, including peripheral arterial disease, renal artery disease, mesenteric vascular disease, cerebral vascular disease, aortic diseases, vasculogenic erectile dysfunction, vasculitis, acute limb ischemia, vasospasm, venous thromboembolism, chronic venous disorders, pulmonary hypertension, and lymphatic disorders. Many of the sections have individual chapters that elaborate on the epidemiology, pathophysiology, and medical, endovascular, and surgical management of specific vascular diseases. Other chapters are devoted to uncommon vascular diseases, including thromboangiitis obliterans, acrocyanosis, erythromelalgia, and pernio. The final section of the book includes chapters on other important vascular diseases, including ulcers, infection, trauma, compression syndrome, congenital vascular malformations, and neoplasms. All of the clinical chapters include recent developments in diagnosis and treatment.

This textbook will be useful for vascular medicine physicians, as well as for all clinicians who care for patients with vascular diseases, including internists, cardiologists, vascular surgeons, and interventional radiologists. We anticipate that it will serve as an important resource for medical students and trainees. The information is presented in a manner that will enable readers to understand the relevant concepts of vascular biology and to use these concepts in a rational approach to the broad range of vascular diseases that confront them frequently in their daily practice. The vasculature is an organ system in its own right, and we believe that the approach presented in this textbook will place physicians in a better position to evaluate patients with a broad and complex range of vascular diseases and to implement important diagnostic and therapeutic strategies in the care of these patients.

Mark A. Creager
Victor J. Dzau
Joseph Loscalzo

ACKNOWLEDGMENTS

We are extremely grateful for the editorial assistance provided by Stephanie Tribuna and Joanne Normandin.

CONTENTS

Color plates follow frontmatter.

SECTION 8
Cerebrovascular Disease

SECTION 9
Aortic Dissection

SECTION 10
Aortic Aneurysms

SECTION 11
Vasculitis

SECTION 12
Acute Limb Ischemia

SECTION 13
Vasospasm and Other Related Vascular Diseases

SECTION 14
Venous Thromboembolic Disease

SECTION 15
Chronic Venous Disorders

SECTION 16
Pulmonary Hypertension

■ SECTION 17
Lymphatic Disorders

■ SECTION 18
Miscellaneous

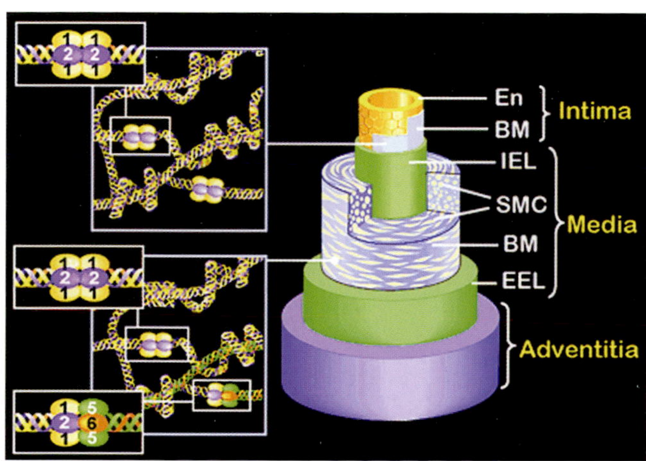

COLOR PLATE 3-8. Localization of the α1·α2· and α1·α2·α5·α6 networks of type IV collagen in vascular basement membranes (BMs). A schematic diagram of a large artery (aorta) depicts its multilayered structure (*right*). The endothelial cells (En) rest on a subendothelial BM, which contains the α1·α2(IV) collagen network (*right*). The smooth muscle cells (SMCs) in the media are surrounded by smooth muscle BM and are sandwiched between an internal and an external elastic lamina (IEL and EEL, respectively). The α1·α2· and α1·α2·α5·α6 networks of type IV collagen coexist in smooth muscle BM (*right*). (From Borza DB, Bondar O, Ninomiya Y, et al: The NC1 domain of collagen IV encodes a novel network composed of the alpha 1, alpha 2, alpha 5, and alpha 6 chains in smooth muscle basement membranes. J Biol Chem 276[30]:28532, 2001.)

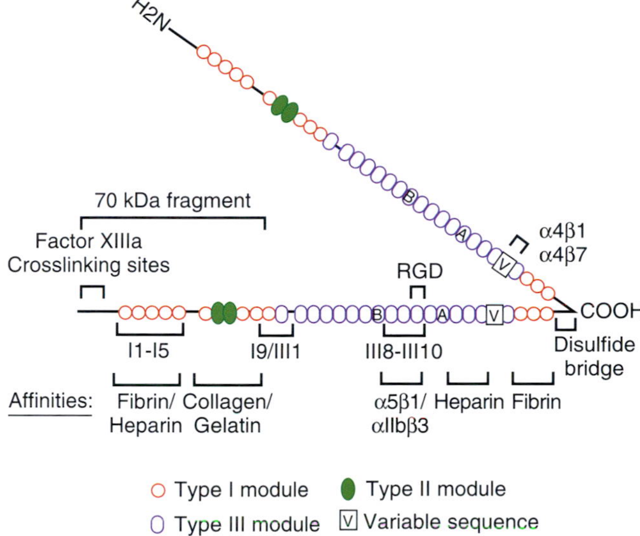

COLOR PLATE 3-12. Schematic diagram of modular structure of FN dimer. Two subunits are shown, with amino termini to the left and carboxyl termini to the right. Regions implicated in adhesion and assembly are shown (discussed in the text). Variably spliced ED-A (A) and ED-B (B) modules and variable sequence (V) are shown as being present in both subunits, whereas in vivo all combinations of dimers exist. (From Magnusson MK, Mosher DF: Fibronectin: Structure, assembly, and cardiovascular implications. Arterioscler Thromb Vasc Biol 18[9]:1363, 1998.)

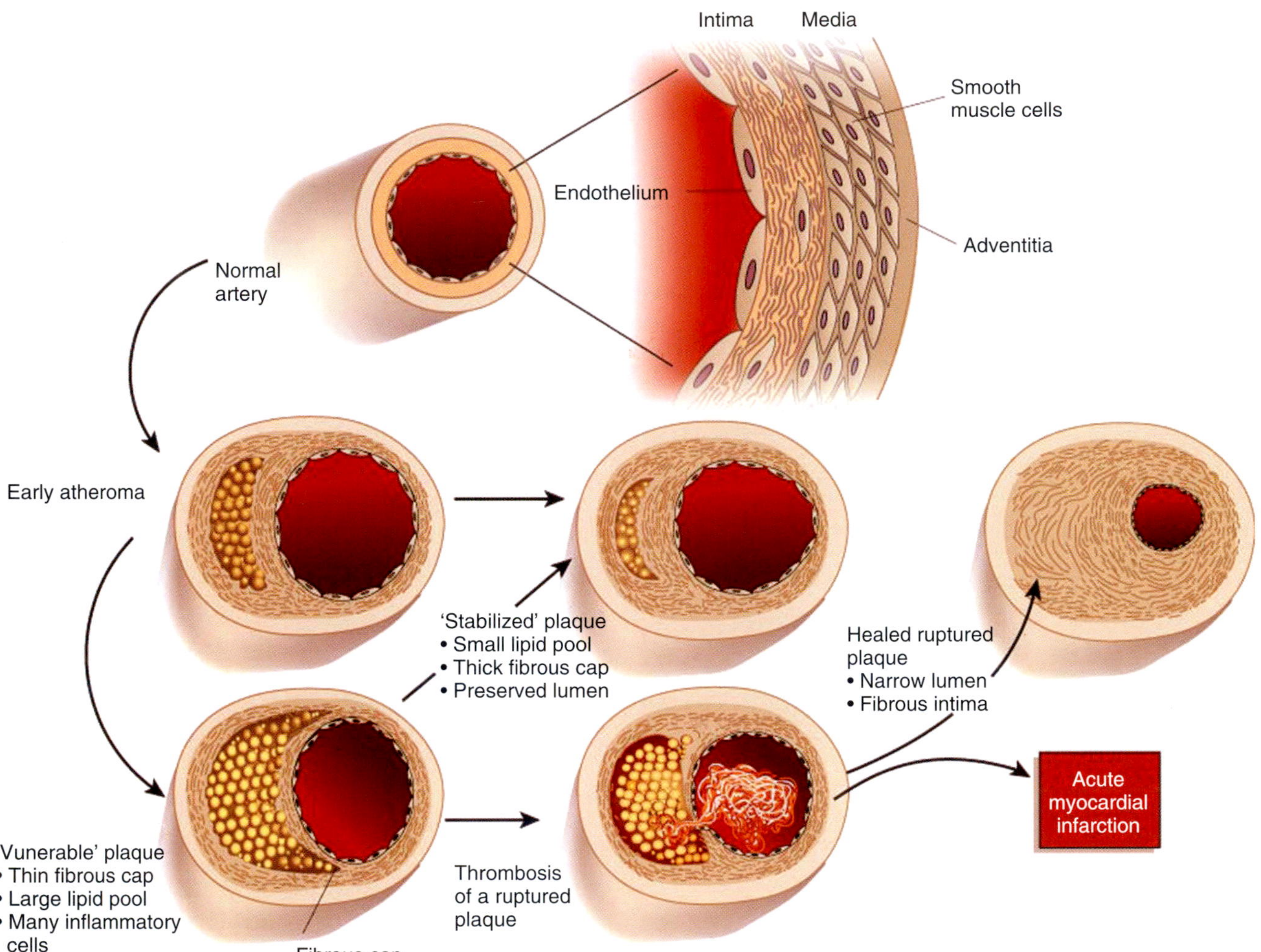

COLOR PLATE 6-5. Schematic of the life history of an atheroma. The normal human coronary artery has a typical trilaminar structure. The endothelial cells in contact with the blood in the arterial lumen rest on a basement membrane. The intimal layer in adult humans generally contains a small amount of smooth muscle cells scattered within the intimal extracellular matrix. The internal elastic lamina forms the barrier between the tunica intima and the underlying tunica media. The media consists of multiple layers of smooth muscle cells, much more tightly packed than in the diffusely thickened intima, and embedded in a matrix rich in elastin as well as collagen. In early atherogenesis, recruitment of inflammatory cells and the accumulation of lipids leads to formation of a lipid-rich core, as the artery enlarges in an outward, abluminal direction to accommodate the expansion of the intima. If inflammatory conditions prevail and risk factors such as dyslipidemia persist, the lipid core can grow, and proteinases secreted by the activated leukocytes can degrade extracellular matrix, whereas proinflammatory cytokines such as interferon-gamma can limit the synthesis of new collagen. These changes can thin the fibrous cap and render it friable and susceptible to rupture.

When the plaque ruptures, blood coming in contact with the tissue factor in the plaque coagulates; platelets activated by thrombin generated from the coagulation cascade, as well as by contact with collagen in the intimal compartment, instigate thrombus formation. If the thrombus occludes the vessel persistently, an acute myocardial infarction can result (the dusky blue area in the anterior wall of the left ventricle, (*lower right*). The thrombus may eventually resorb due to endogenous or therapeutic thrombolysis. However, a wound-healing response triggered by thrombin generated during blood coagulation can stimulate smooth muscle proliferation. Platelet-derived growth factor (PDGF) released from activated platelets stimulates smooth muscle cell migration.

Transforming growth factor-beta (TFG-β), also released from activated platelets, stimulates interstitial collagen production. This increased migration, proliferation, and extracellular matrix synthesis by smooth muscle cells thickens the fibrous cap and causes further expansion of the intima, often now in an inward direction constricting the lumen. Such stenotic lesions produced by the luminal encroachment of the fibrosed plaque may restrict flow, particularly under situations of increased cardiac demand, leading to ischemia, commonly provoking symptoms such as *angina pectoris*. Such advanced stenotic plaques, being more fibrous, may prove less susceptible to rupture and renewed thrombosis. Lipid lowering can reduce lipid content and calm the intimal inflammatory response, yielding a more stable plaque with a thick fibrous cap and a preserved lumen (*center*). (Reproduced with permission from Libby P: Inflammation in atherosclerosis. Nature 420:868, 2002.)

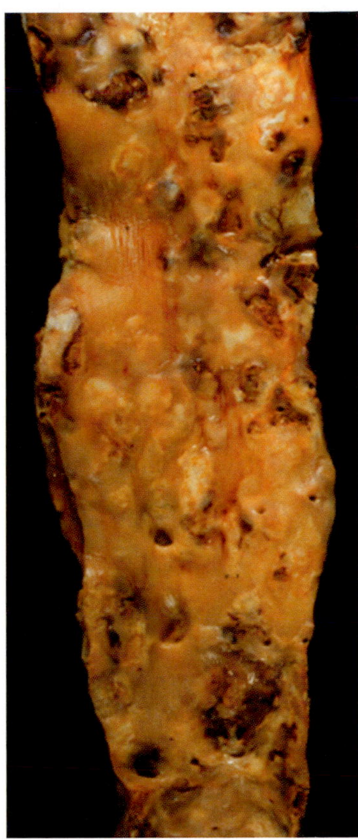

COLOR PLATE 6-6. Widespread atheromatous involvement of the abdominal aorta in a patient with atherosclerosis. Note the variety of atheromata in different stages of evolution within a few centimeters of one another. There are ulcerated plaques, raised lesions, and fatty streaks, among other types of lesions demonstrated in this example.

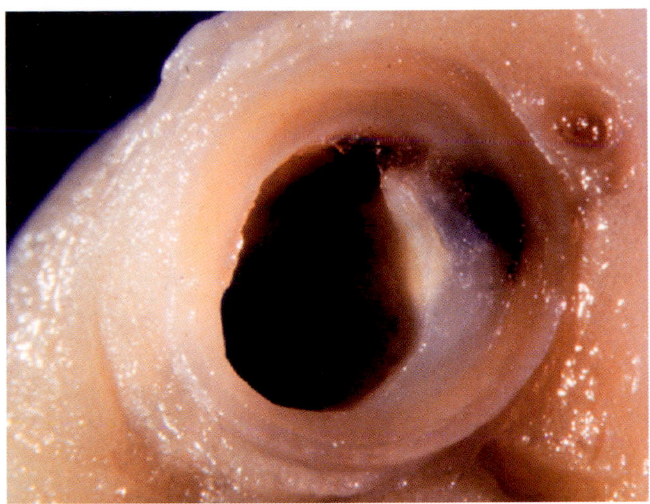

A

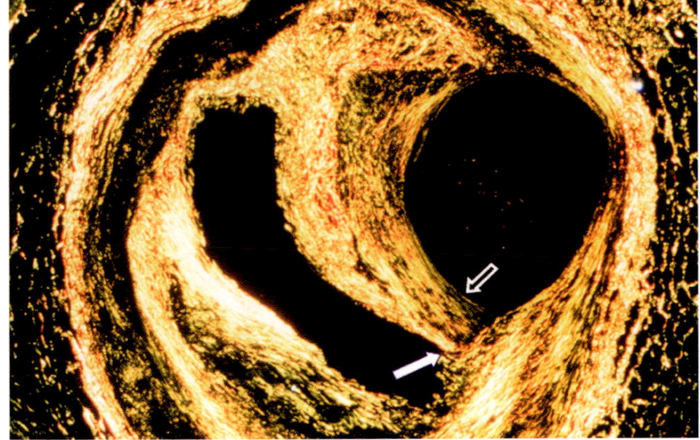

B

COLOR PLATE 6-7. Hemorrhage, thrombosis, and plaque healing as a mechanism of atheroma progression. **A,** Photograph of a coronary artery with a plaque rupture that has led to an intraplaque hematoma without an occlusive thrombus. As explained in the text, thrombin and platelet products such as platelet-derived growth factor (PDGF) and transforming growth factor-beta (TGF-β) elaborated locally at the site of microthrombosis and hematoma formation can stimulate fibrosis. **B,** This Sirius-red-stained preparation of a cross-section of a coronary artery shows an area of plaque rupture (*solid arrow*) that healed to cause further accretion of a layer of collagen (*open arrow*) and luminal encroachment. This example illustrates the "archaeology" of the atherosclerotic plaque: distant plaque rupture followed by healing and fibrosis with progression of the lesion to stenosis. Note that the arterial lumen at the time of the original plaque rupture would not have shown a critical narrowing. (These figures were kindly provided by the late Prof. Michael J. Davies.)

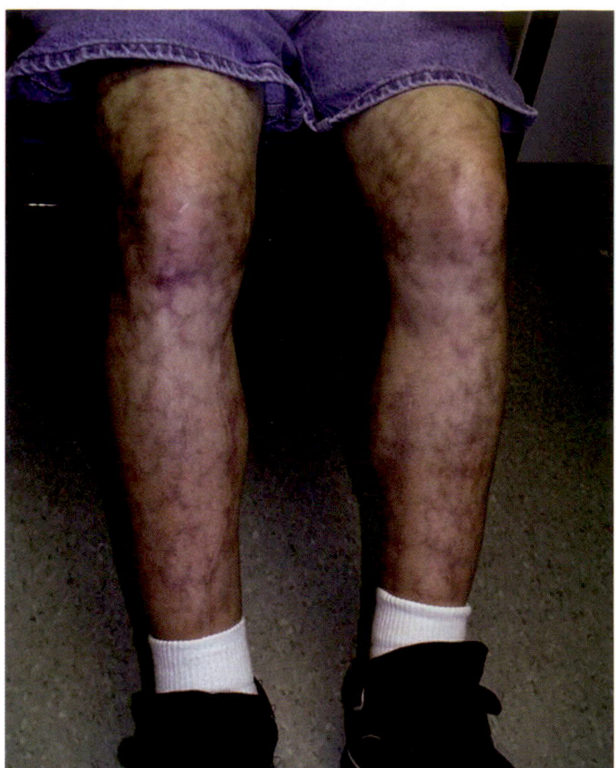

COLOR PLATE 9-7. Livedo reticularis. This patient was referred to a vascular specialist for livedo reticularis. Note the lace-like pattern of superficial skin vessels surrounding a clear area. This patient reported these findings were chronic and without symptoms. Secondary causes were excluded and a diagnosis of idiopathic livedo reticularis was made.

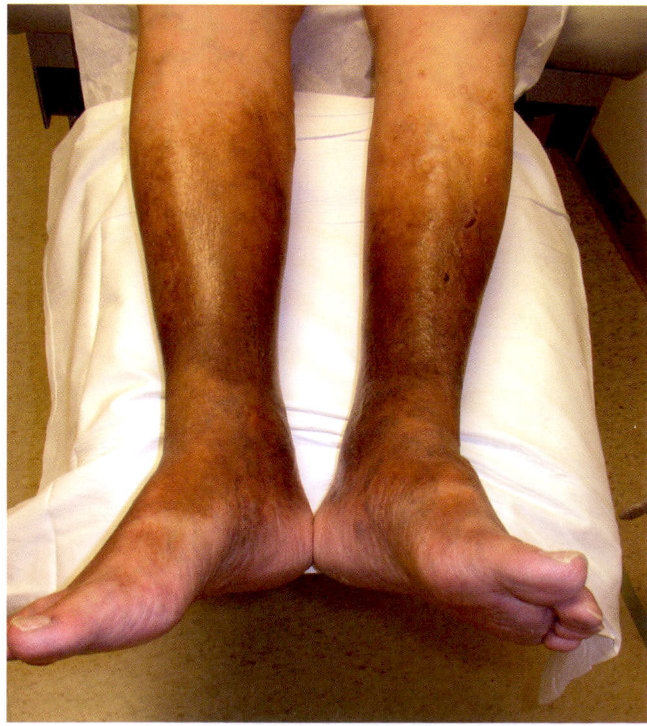

COLOR PLATE 9-8. The skin changes of chronic venous insufficiency. Chronic venous insufficiency and edema result in the deposition of hemosiderin causing the darkening and toughening of the skin giving the calf a brawny appearance. Note the small, superficial venous ulcers mid-calf above the shin.

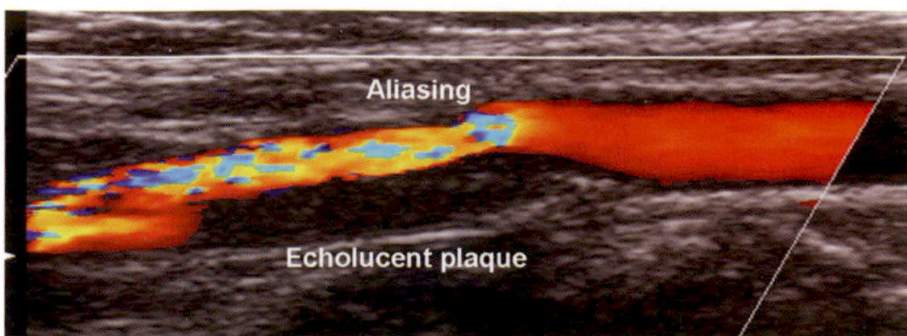

COLOR PLATE 10-6. Aliasing at the site of arterial stenosis. There is an abrupt change as the velocity exceeds the Nyquist limits. An echolucent (dark) plaque is evident at the site of stenosis.

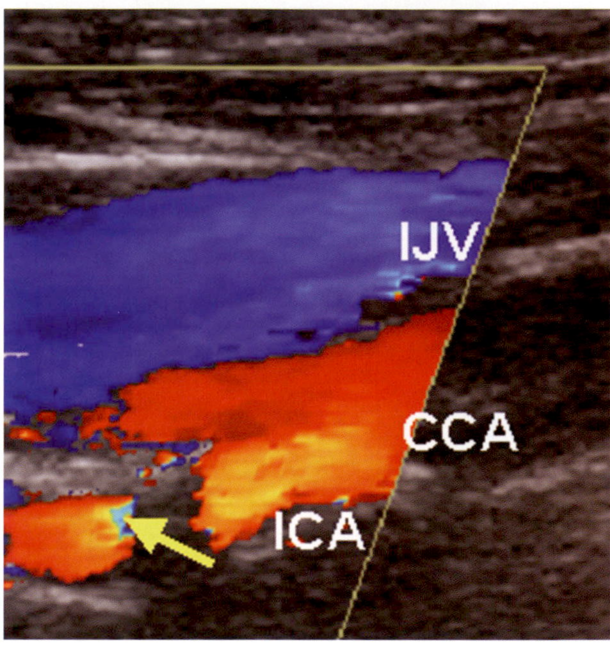

COLOR PLATE 10-7. Carotid bifurcation. A calcified lesion obscures the color Doppler signal in the proximal internal carotid artery (ICA). The presence of aliasing distal to the calcification artifact (*arrow*) is helpful in identifying possible stenosis with the pulsed-wave Doppler sample volume. The transducer should be rocked side to-side in this situation in an attempt to see the flow in the region of calcification. CCA, common carotid artery; IJV, internal jugular vein.

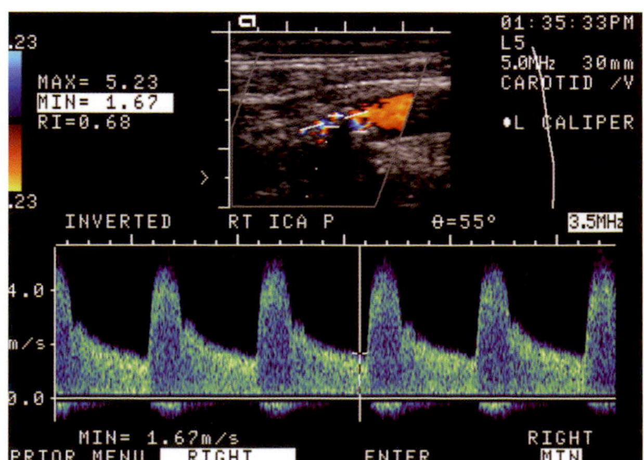

COLOR PLATE 10-10. Internal carotid artery stenosis. The pulsed-wave sample volume is placed at the site of aliasing. The peak-systolic velocity is elevated to 523 cm/sec. The end-diastolic velocity is elevated to 167 cm/sec. There is marked spectral broadening. The waveform resembles that in Fig. 10-9C, except that the "temporal tap" is not reflected in the diastolic portion of the waveform.

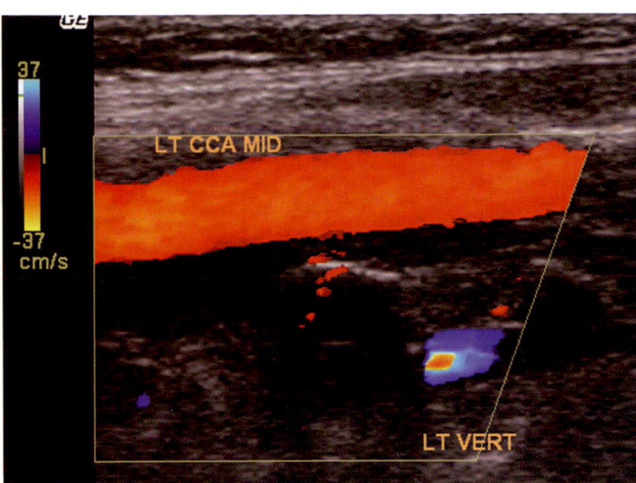

COLOR PLATE 10-12. Color Doppler of the CCA and vertebral arteries demonstrating antegrade carotid flow and retrograde vertebral flow. CCA, common carotid artery.

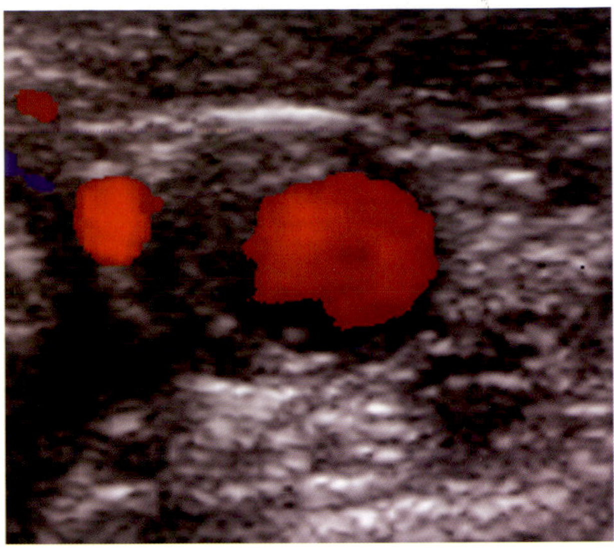

COLOR PLATE 10-15. Transverse view of the internal carotid artery origin with atherosclerotic plaque of mixed echogenicity evident in the left half of the vessel.

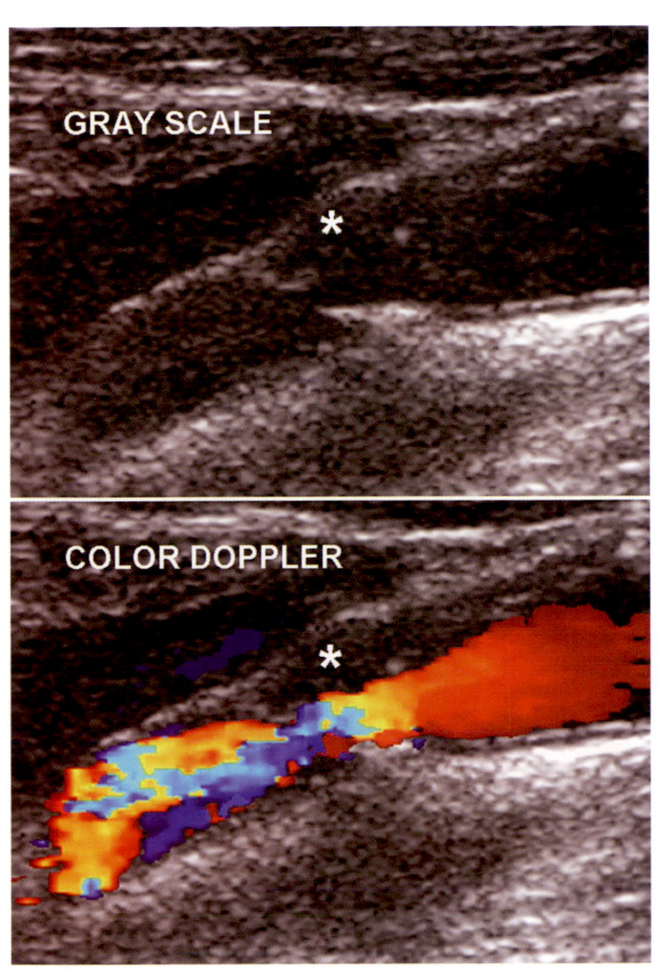

COLOR PLATE 10-14. Echolucent plaque is indicated (*asterisk*) in the gray-scale and Doppler image of this internal carotid artery.

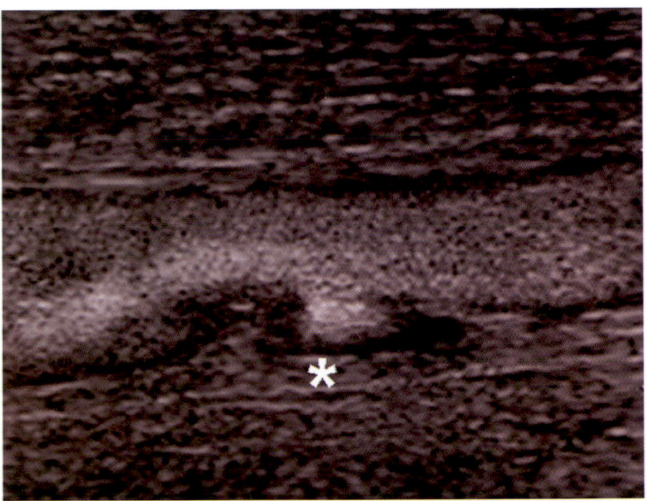

A

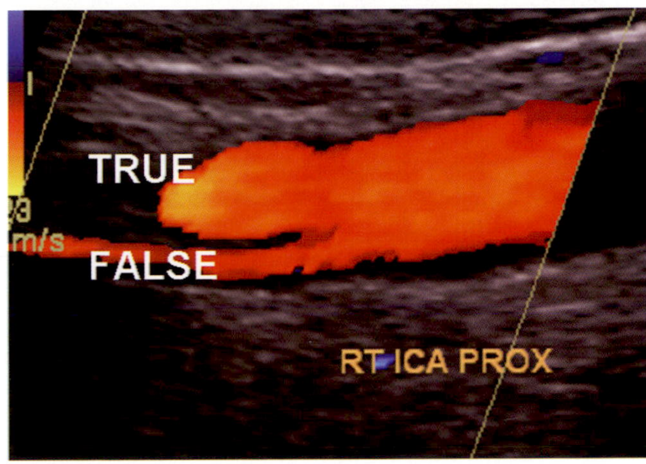

B

COLOR PLATE 10-16. Arterial wall characteristics. **A,** Ulceration of atherosclerotic plaque in the common carotid artery. Contrast is evident within an echolucent plaque (*asterisk*). **B,** Dissection of the internal carotid artery (ICA) with flow evident in both the true and false lumina.

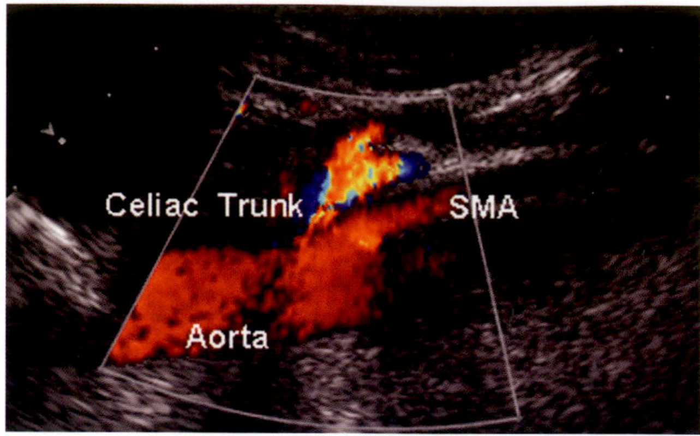

COLOR PLATE 10-19. Proximity of the origin of the celiac trunk (bifurcating into hepatic and splenic arteries) and the origin of the superior mesenteric artery (SMA).

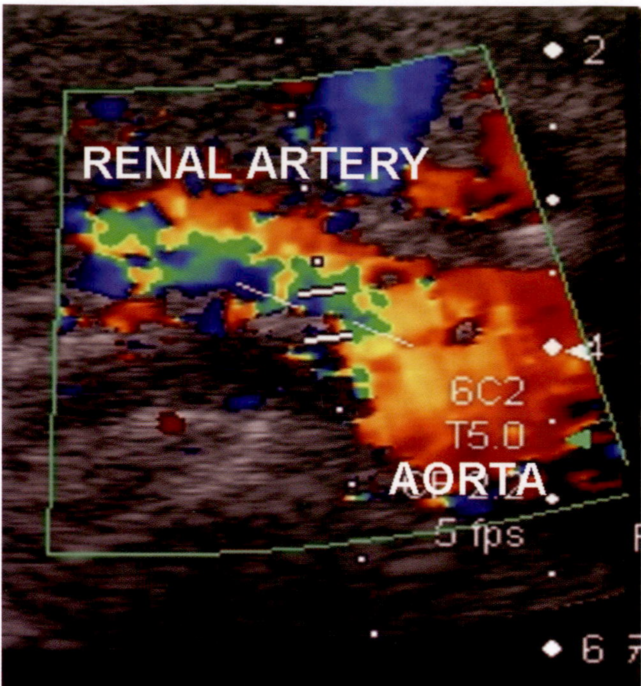

COLOR PLATE 10-23. Transverse Doppler image of the origin of the right renal artery. Turbulent flow is evident in the renal artery origin, suggesting the presence of atherosclerotic plaque and the possibility of stenosis.

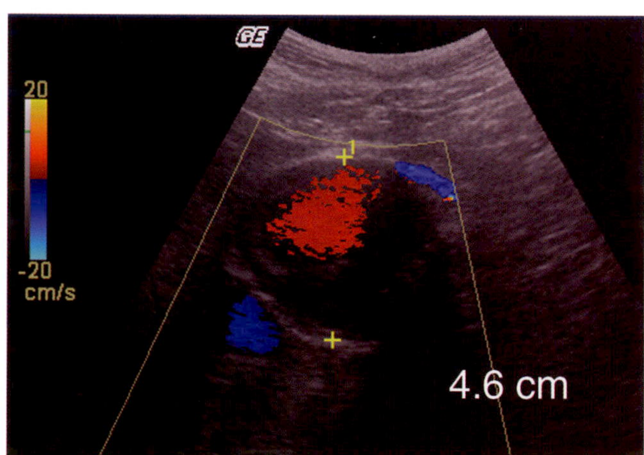

COLOR PLATE 10-21. Transverse image of the abdominal aorta with a diameter of 4.6 cm indicating aneurysm. The dropout of acoustic echoes in the right lower corner of this image is due to bowel gas.

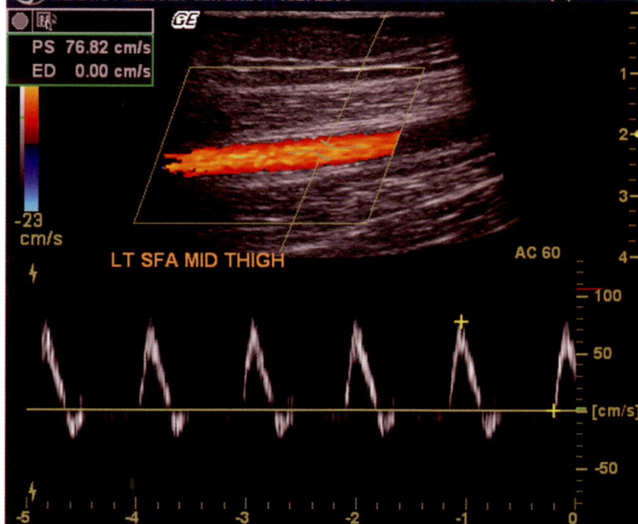

COLOR PLATE 10-24. Duplex ultrasound of a superficial femoral artery (SFA) stent. Laminar flow is evident in the Doppler image. The peak systolic velocity of 76 cm/sec is within normal limits.

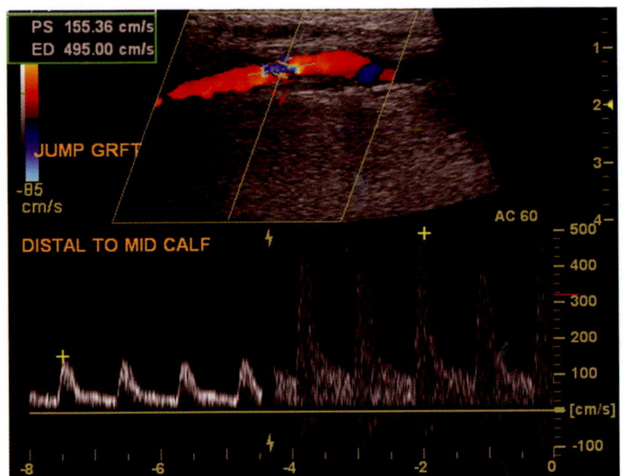

COLOR PLATE 10-26. Duplex ultrasound of peripheral bypass graft. The proximal velocity is 155 cm/sec and increases to 495 cm/sec at the site of stenosis. Aliasing of the Doppler is also evident at the site of stenosis.

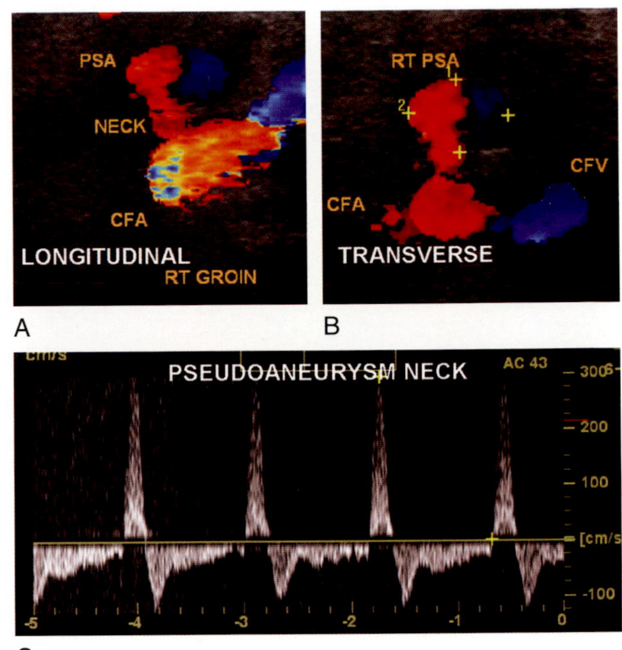

COLOR PLATE 10-27. Doppler evaluations of a pseudoaneurysm (PSA). The "yin-yang" appearance of the PSA cavity is evident in the longitudinal (**A**) and transverse (**B**) images. Whereas the artery lengthens in the longitudinal image, the contained rupture sac of the PSA retains its saccular shape. Pulsed Doppler placed in the neck of the pseudoaneurysm demonstrates the pathognomonic "to-and-fro" pattern of bidirectional flow into and out of the contained rupture (**C**).

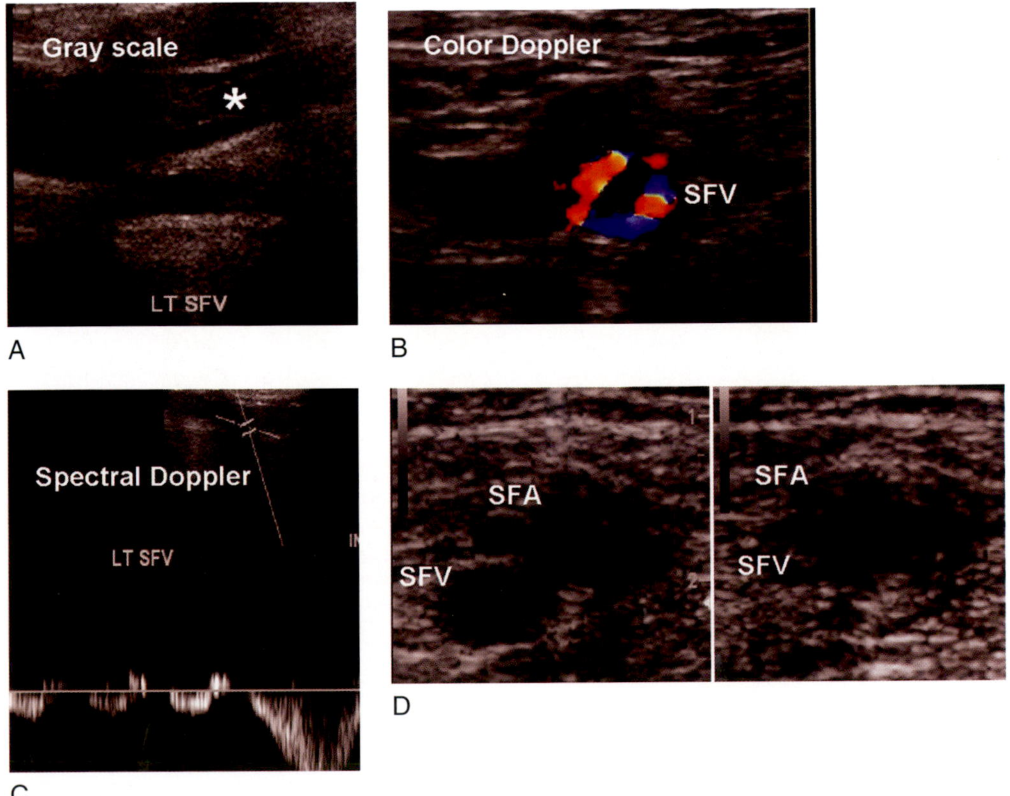

COLOR PLATE 10-32. Ultrasound evaluation of the femoral vein thrombosis. **A,** Gray imaging with echogenic material (*asterisk*) seen within the lumen of the superficial femoral vein (SFV). **B,** Doppler in the superficial femoral vein shows a flow void within the lumen. **C,** Spectral Doppler demonstrates diminished flow with respirophasic variation. **D,** Superficial femoral artery (SFA) and vein without (*left*) and with (*right*) compression; the vein is only partially obliterated due to thrombus.

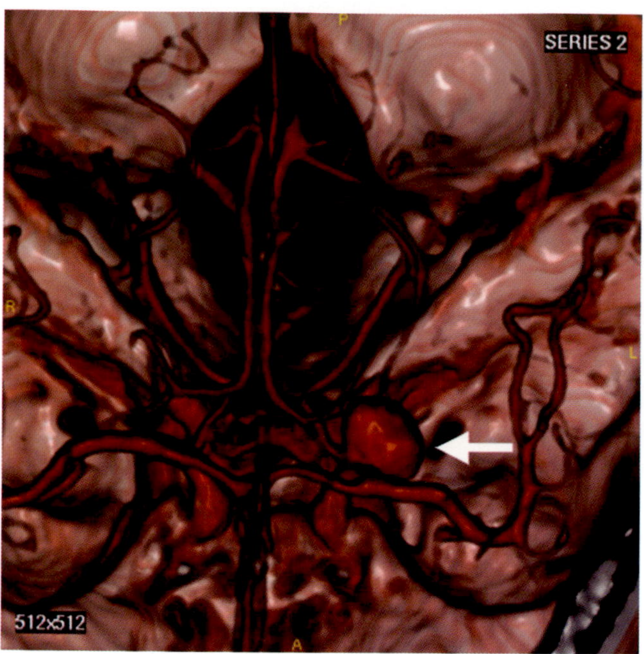

COLOR PLATE 12-7. Aneurysm (*arrow*) of the left internal carotid artery seen craniofrontally with a 4-slice CT scanner. Colored volume rendering technique. The shape and location of the aneurysm and the spatial relationship with its feeding vessel is intuitively visualized.

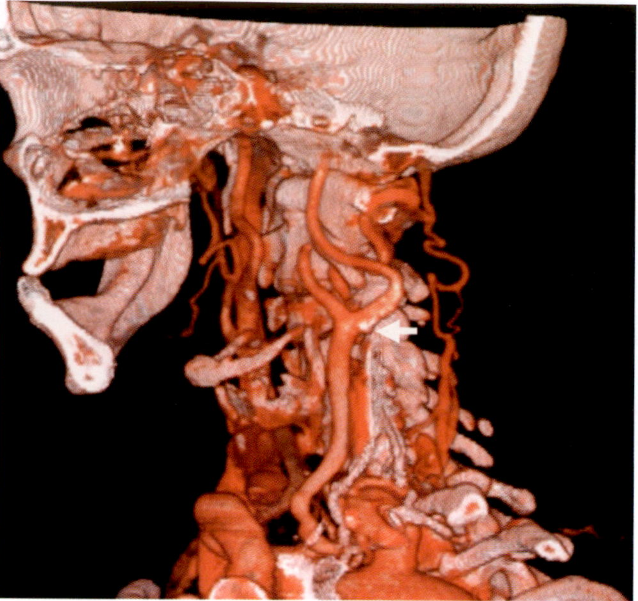

COLOR PLATE 12-8. Multislice CT angiography of the carotid arteries with a 4-slice CT scanner. Nonstenotic calcified plaques in the left internal carotid artery near the bifurcation. Characterization of atherosclerotic lesions by means of visualization of calcium (*arrow*) is a significant advantage of CT over competing imaging modalities. The speed of multislice CT allows scanning of the entire length of the carotids with 1-mm spatial resolution along the z-axis without significant venous enhancement that would get in the way of 3-D post-processing. Colored volume rendering technique.

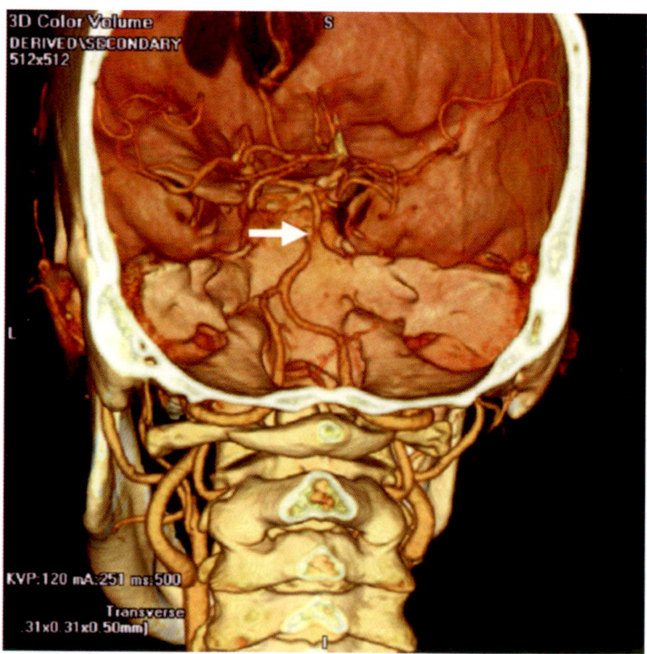

COLOR PLATE 12-9. Stenosis of the basilar artery (*arrow*) is shown with a 16-slice CT scanner. Colored volume rendering technique.

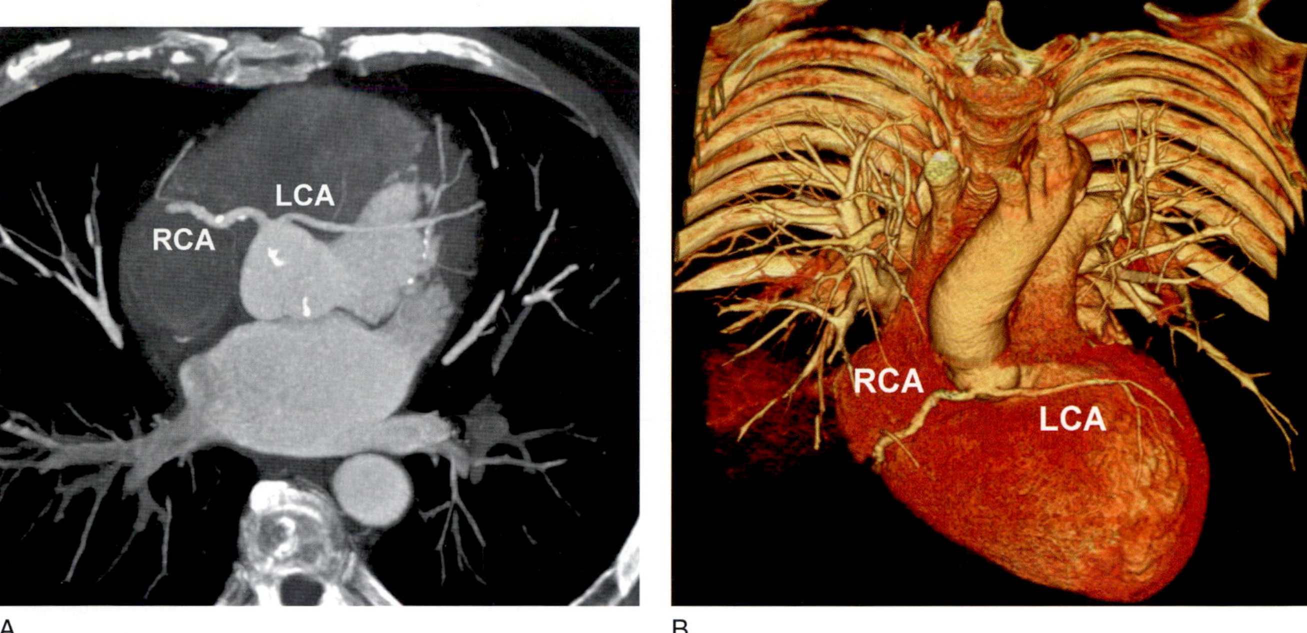

COLOR PLATE 12-12. A 42-year-old man with anomalous origin and course of the left coronary artery (LCA). Retrospectively ECG-gated 16-slice CT coronary angiography displayed as axial maximum intensity projection **(A)** and colored volume rendering **(B)**. The vessel originates medial to the origin of the right coronary artery (RCA) and crosses the median line before giving off branches supplying the left side of the myocardium.

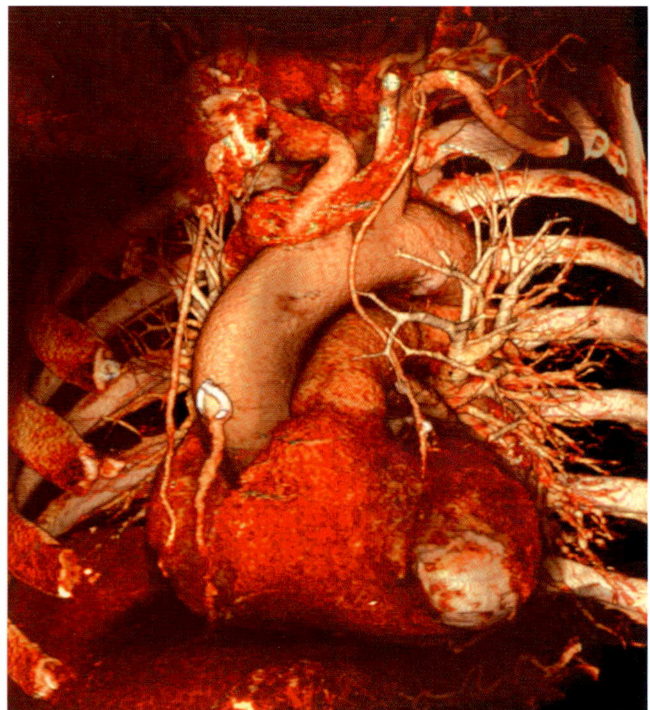

COLOR PLATE 12-13. Patient with left internal mammary artery (LIMA) bypass graft to the left anterior descending (LAD) coronary artery and saphenous bypass graft to the right coronary artery. Note calcified aneurysm in the apex of the left ventricle as sequelae of ischemic heart disease. Colored 3-D volume-rendered display enables visualization of native and graft vessels in their relationship to surrounding thoracic anatomy.

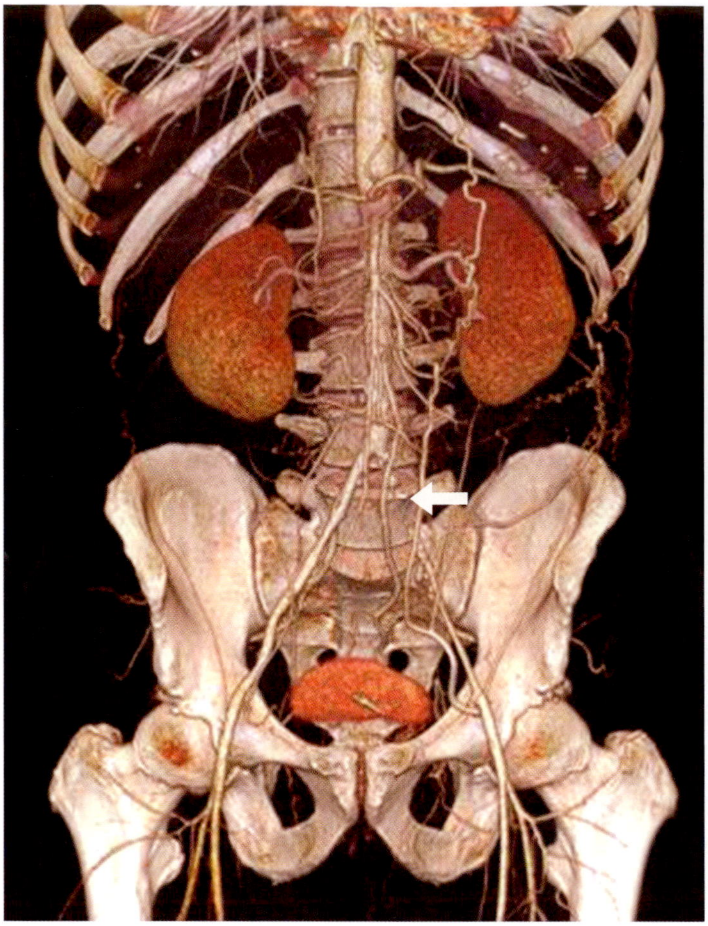

A 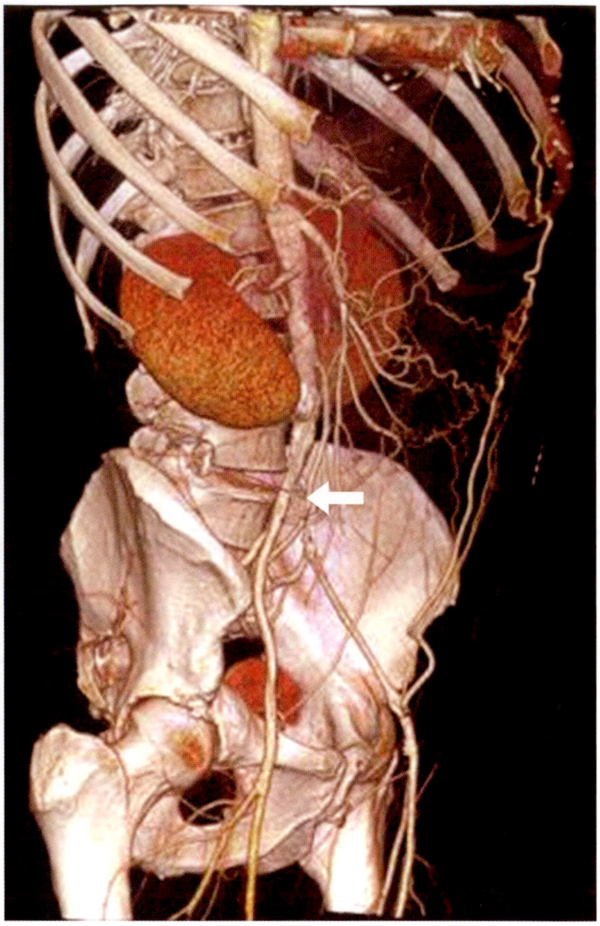 B

COLOR PLATE 12-16. Case study illustrating the clinical performance of 16-slice CT: patient with occlusion (*arrow*) of the left common iliac artery, scanned with 16 × 0.75 mm collimation. Frontal **(A)** and oblique **(B)** views.

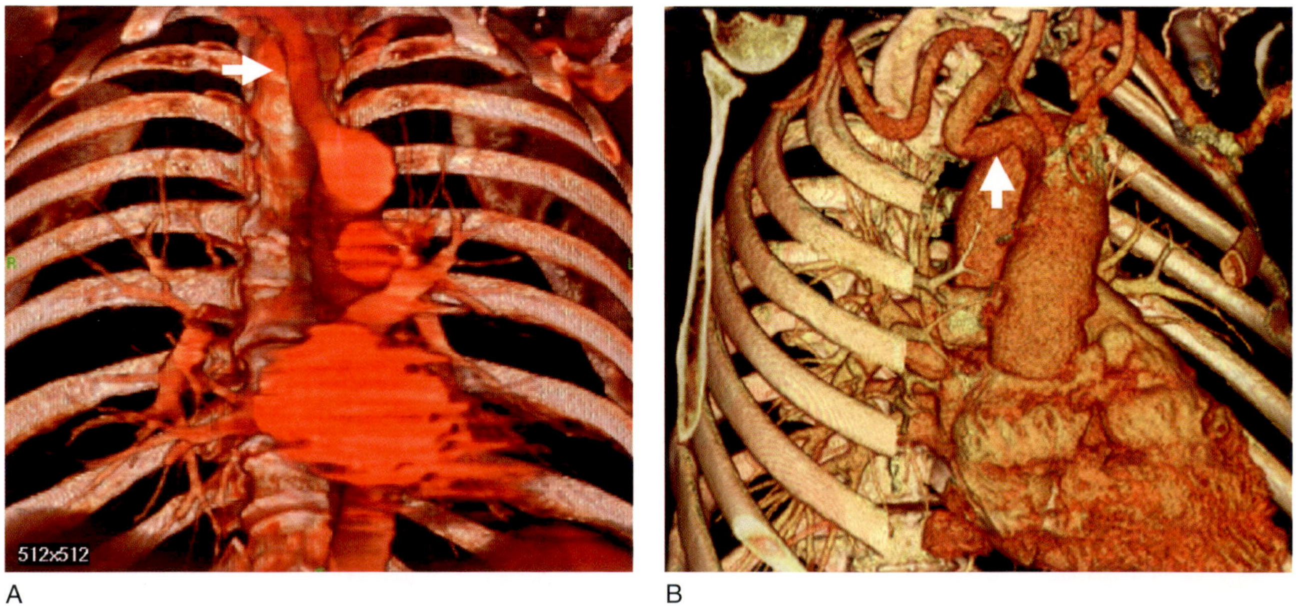

A B

COLOR PLATE 12-17. Two patients with aberrant right subclavian arteries (*arrow*). **A,** A 4-slice MSCT study with 4 × 1 mm collimation and 29-second total scan time and **B,** 16-slice CT acquisition with 16 × 0.75 mm collimation and 7-second total scan time. Note substantially improved spatial resolution and image quality with high-resolution 16-slice CT, despite significantly shorter scan time.

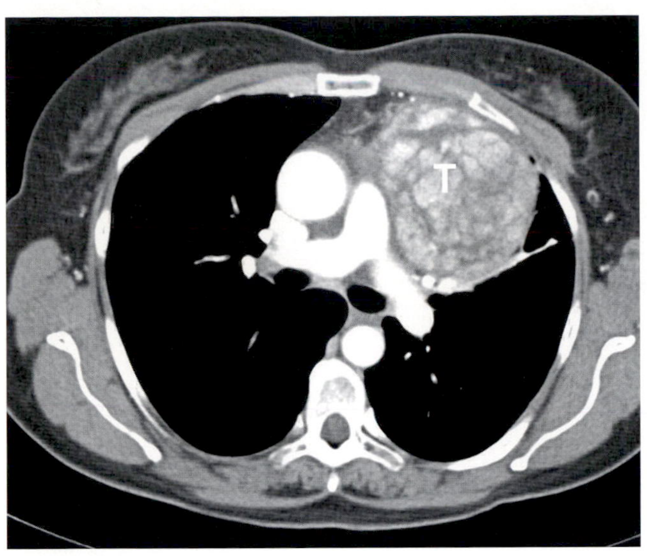

A

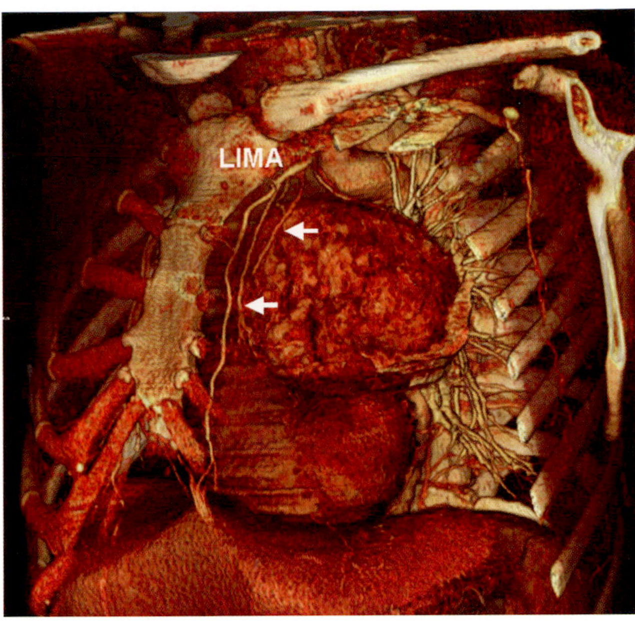

B

COLOR PLATE 12-18. Invasive thymoma. **A,** Contrast-enhanced axial image shows an intensely enhancing nodular mediastinal tumor (T) with adjacent atelectasis. **B,** Color enhanced 3-D volume-rendered image effectively shows enlarged left internal mammary artery (LIMA) and tumor neovasculature (*arrows*). Preoperative information on the vascular supply of the tumor was invaluable in surgical planning. The extent of the vessels was not demonstrated on the axial images.

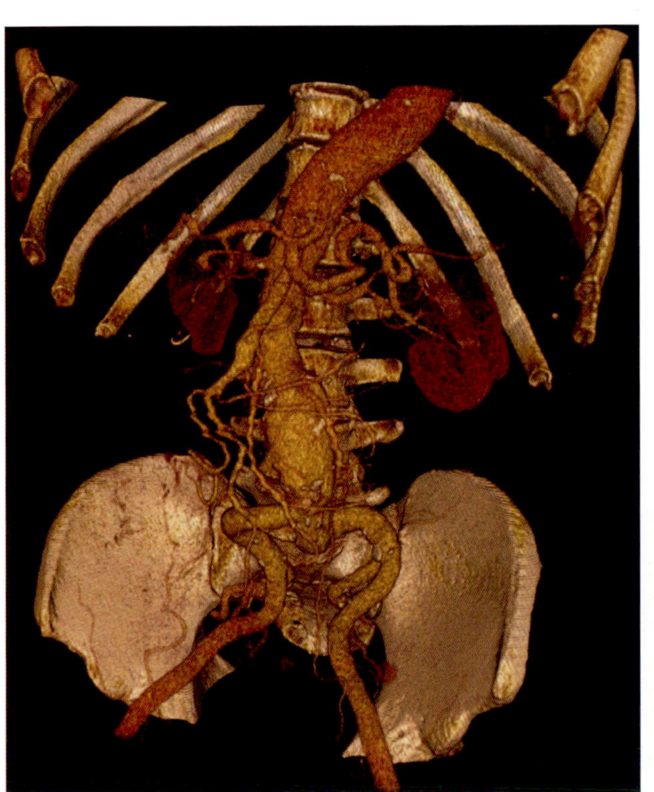

A

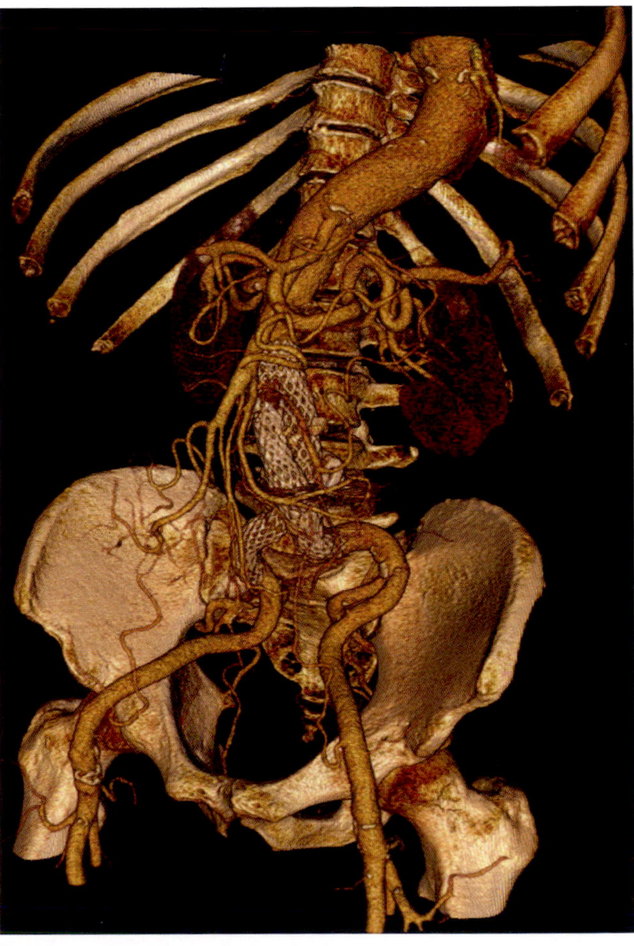

B

COLOR PLATE 12-20. A 62-year-old man with abdominal aortic aneurysm before **(A)** and after **(B)** placement of an aortic stent. The patient underwent contrast-enhanced CT for preinterventional evaluation of the abdominal aorta and the aneurysm and for therapeutic planning **(A)**. After successful placement of the stent, the CT scan demonstrates effective exclusion of the aneurysm and restitution of the aortic lumen **(B)**.

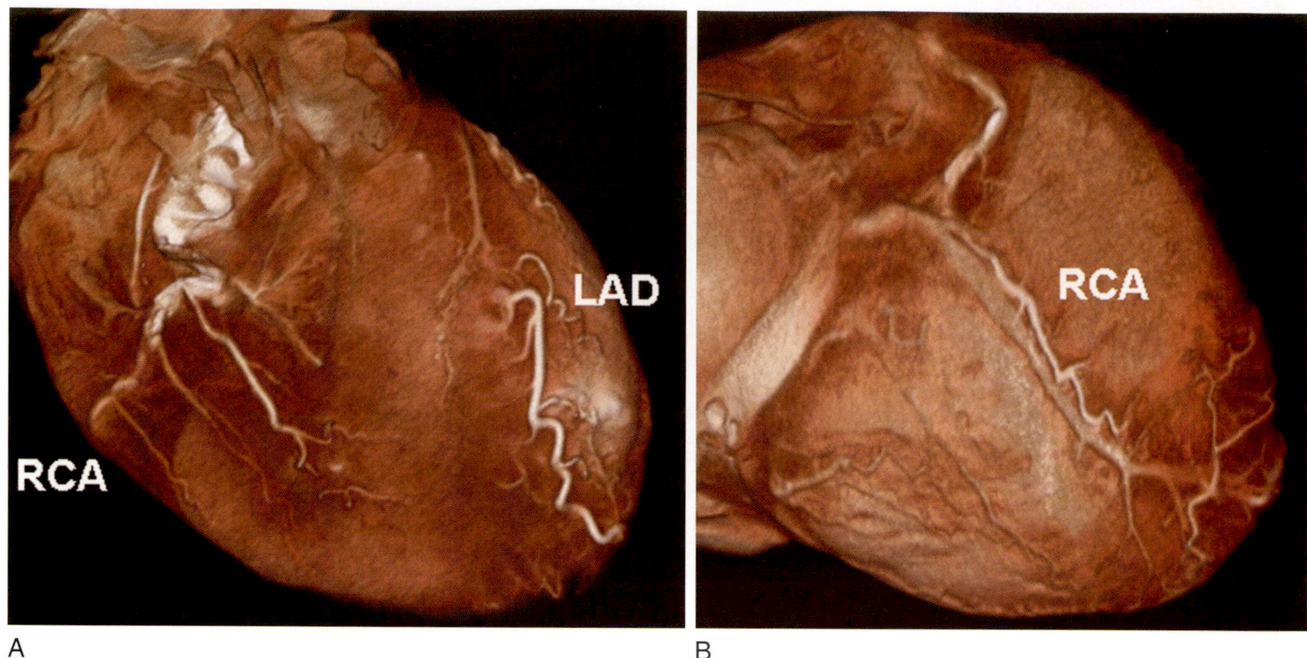

COLOR PLATE 12-25. Flat panel CT volume acquisition of a stationary human cadaveric heart specimen. Display in colored volume rendering technique seen from anterior **(A)** and inferior **(B)** projections. Coronary arteries filled with iodinated contrast media. Isotropic in-plane and through-plane resolution of 0.25 mm enables visualization of small caliber marginal branches of the partially calcified right (RCA) and left anterior descending (LAD) coronary arteries.

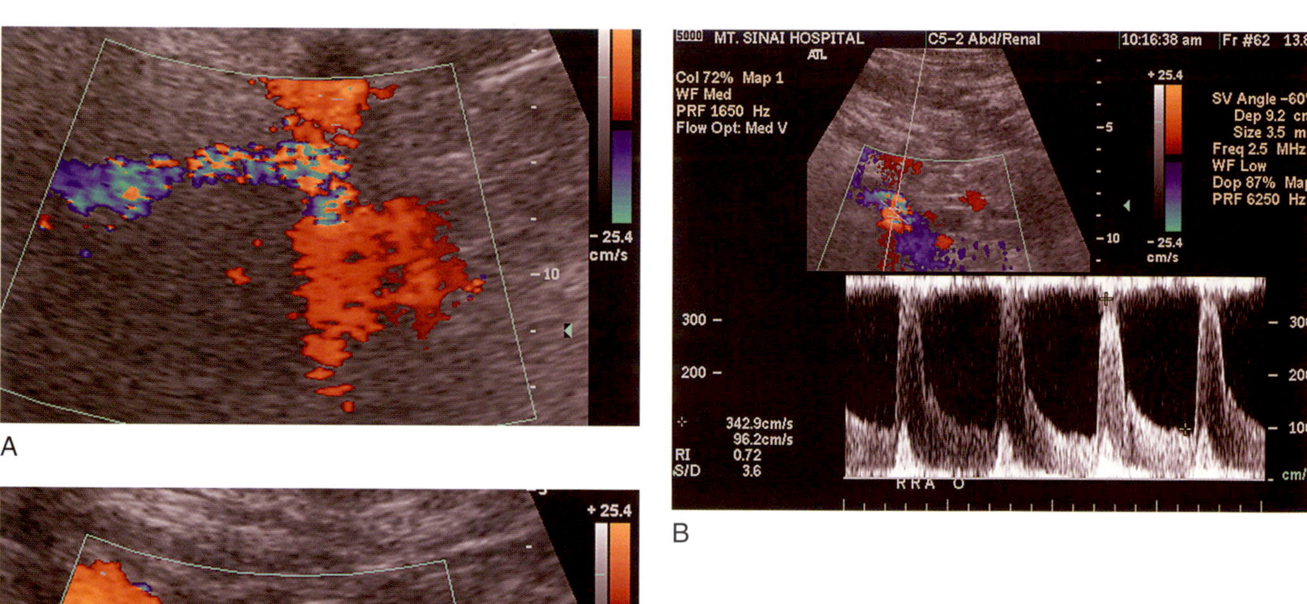

COLOR PLATE 22-4. A, Color duplex ultrasound of the renal artery from the anterior approach. The right renal artery takes off at approximately the ten-o'clock position. Note the color mosaic pattern indicative of turbulence. **B,** The peak systolic velocity was 343 cm/sec indicative of a 60% to 99% stenosis. **C,** The left renal artery arises at about the four-o'clock position and there is no turbulence to flow in this example. The color is blue because blood is flowing away from the transducer.

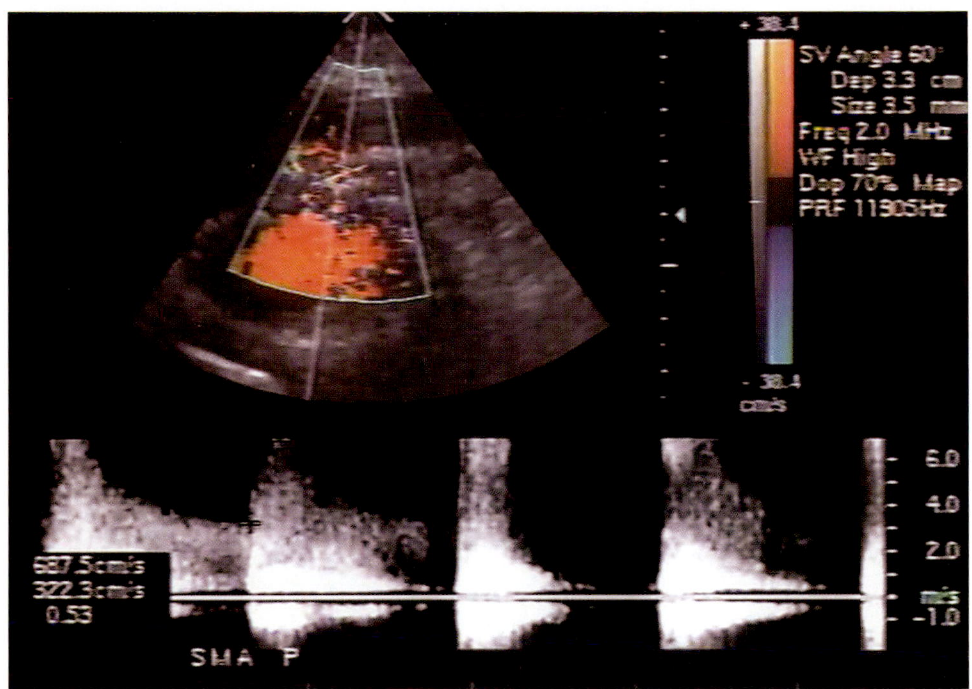

COLOR PLATE 26-7. Duplex ultrasonography of the superior mesenteric artery (SMA) with a peak systolic velocity of 687 cm/sec signifying ≥ 70% stenosis of the SMA.

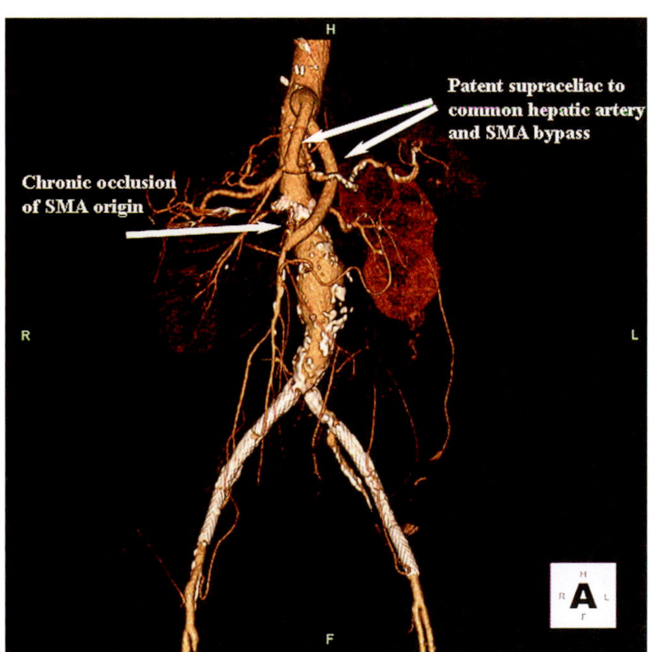

COLOR PLATE 26-8. CT angiogram demonstrating a patent supraceliac aorta to common hepatic artery and superior mesenteric artery (SMA) bypass. The proximal SMA is occluded.

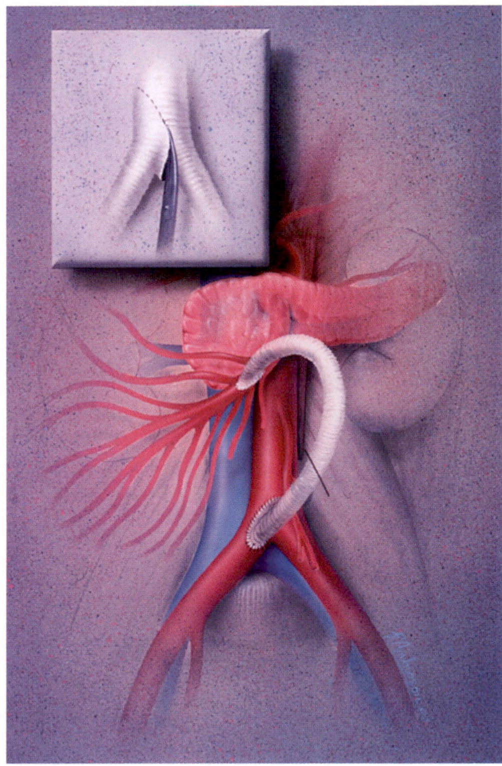

COLOR PLATE 27-1. Artist's depiction of the technique of infrarenal aorta to superior mesenteric artery bypass. The graft is fashioned using one limb of a bifurcated graft.

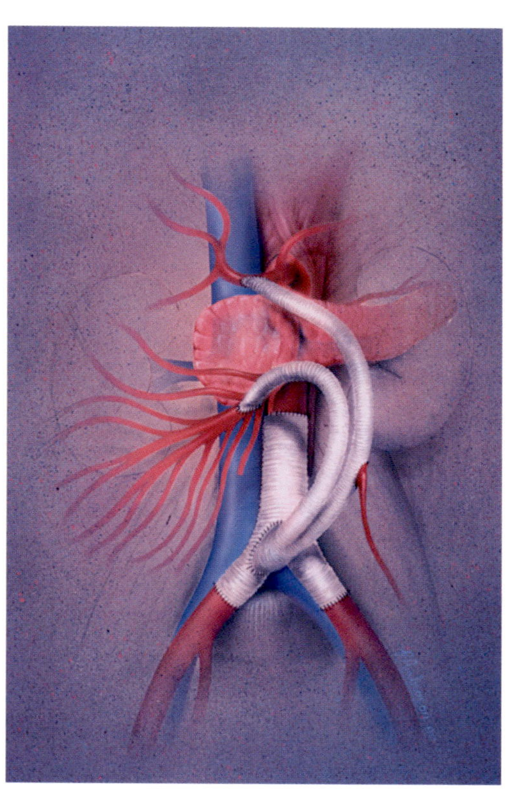

COLOR PLATE 27-2. Artist's depiction of a retrograde mesenteric bypass to the celiac and superior mesenteric artery with reimplantation of the inferior mesenteric artery.

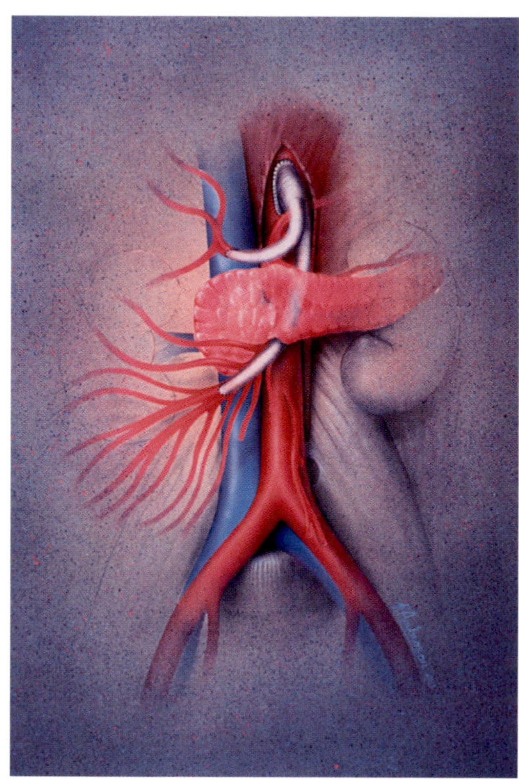

COLOR PLATE 27-4. Artist's depiction of the technique of antegrade bypass from the supraceliac aorta to the celiac and superior mesenteric arteries.

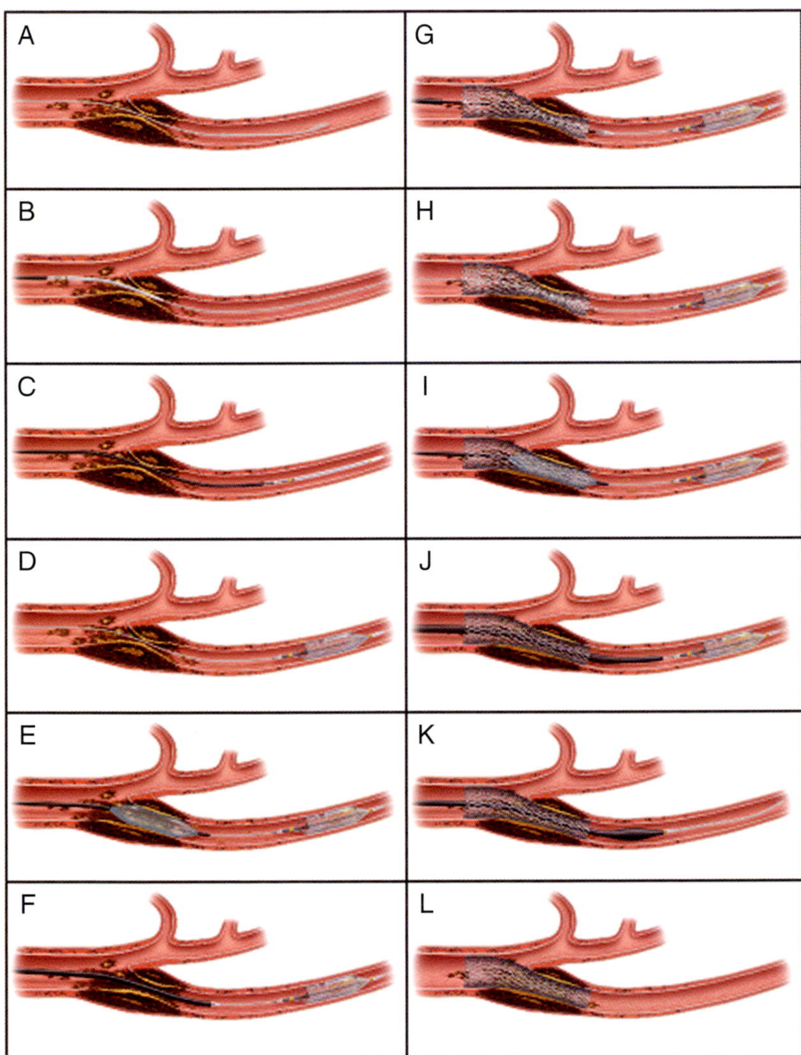

COLOR PLATE 32-7. Carotid artery stenting technique using a filter for distal protection. **A,** After placement of a guiding catheter in the common carotid artery, the lesion is crossed with a guidewire. **B** and **C,** Specially designed filter guidewire. The lesion is crossed with the distal protection filter delivery catheter, which can be advanced easily over the guidewire by means of a rapid-exchange system (**D**), opening the filter (**E**). Balloon predilatation before stent placement (**F**), positioning of the stent (**G**), deployment of self-expanding stent (**H**). The self-expanding stent is deployed, but the vessel still is stenosed (**I**). Balloon postdilatation after stent placement allows further dilatation of the stenosed segment (**J**). Advancement of the retrieval catheter (**K**) and retrieval of the filter that contains the embolic debris into the retrieval catheter (**L**). Stent is fully deployed with good apposition to the vessel wall.

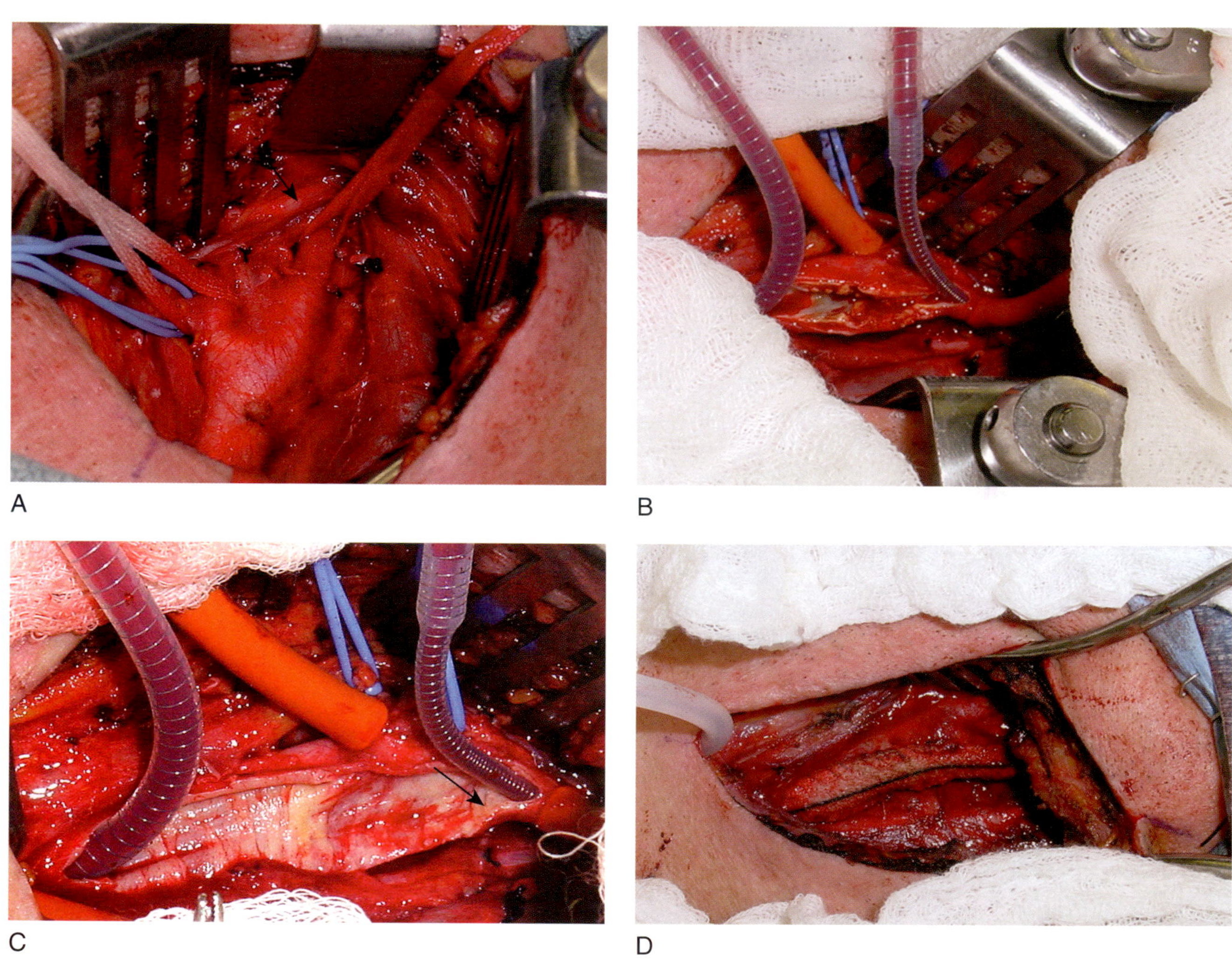

COLOR PLATE 33-3. **A,** Exposure of the carotid bifurcation. The hypoglossal nerve (*arrow*) is seen superiorly crossing the internal carotid artery. **B,** An arteriotomy has been made exposing an ulcerative plaque and shunt placement. **C,** The operative site illustrates the fine tapering of the distal plaque (*arrow*) removed from the internal carotid artery. **D,** Patch angioplasty using Dacron.

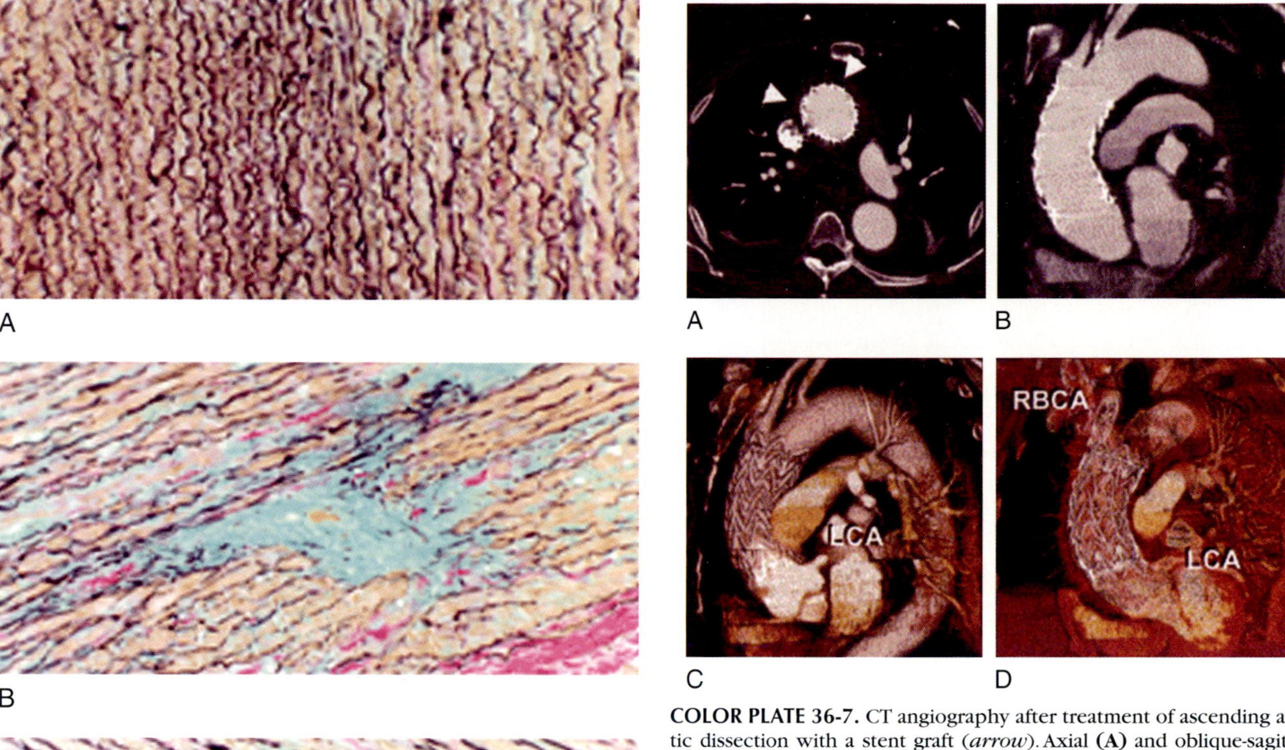

COLOR PLATE 34-2. Cystic medial degeneration. Representative cross sections of a control ascending aorta **(A)**, an aortic aneurysm associated with Marfan's syndrome **(B)**, and an aneurysm associated with bicuspid aortic valve **(C)**, stained with Alcian blue and Verhoeff van Gieson (magnification ×250). In the control aorta, the elastic lamellae form dense, parallel sheets. In the Marfan and bicuspid aortic valve specimens, there are areas of elastic lamellar degradation and fragmentation with variable accumulation of mucoid substances. No inflammatory cells are present. (From Nataatmadja M, West M, West J, et al: Abnormal extracellular matrix protein transport associated with increased apoptosis of vascular smooth muscle cells in Marfan syndrome and bicuspid aortic valve thoracic aortic aneurysm. Circulation 108:II-329, 2003.)

COLOR PLATE 36-7. CT angiography after treatment of ascending aortic dissection with a stent graft (*arrow*). Axial **(A)** and oblique-sagittal **(B)** CT images confirm coverage of intimal tear with aortic stent graft. Volume-rendered views **(C, D)** show relationship of stent graft to left coronary artery (*LCA*) and right brachiocephalic artery (*RBCA*). (From Ihnken K, Sze D, Dake MD, et al: Successful treatment of a Stanford type A dissection by percutaneous placement of a covered stent graft in the ascending aorta. J Thorac Cardiovasc Surg 127:1809, 2004.)

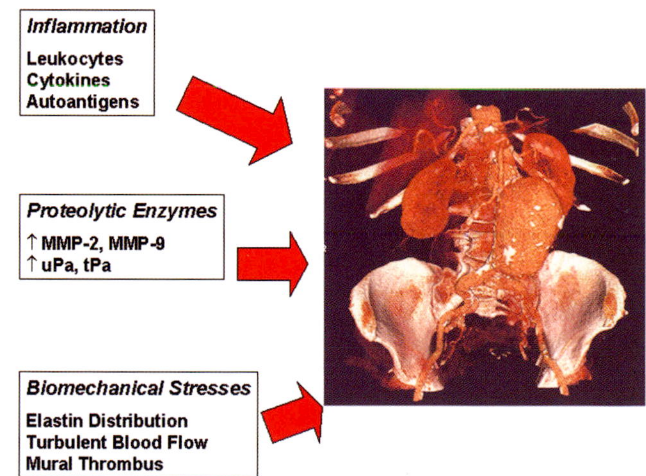

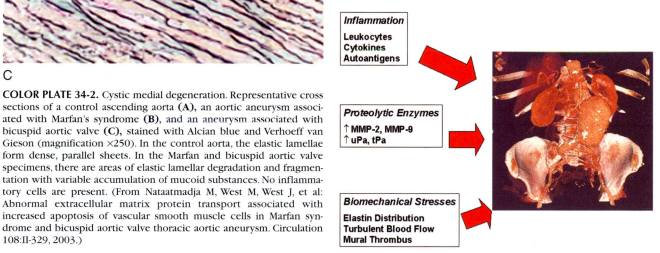

COLOR PLATE 37-2. Three pathophysiologic mechanisms best characterize the process of aneurysm formation. Aortic aneurysm specimens reveal an increase in leukocyte infiltration, cytokine concentration, and leukocyte adhesion molecules. Both elastin-related and collagen-related autoantigens have been identified and may participate in the initiation of the process. Once the process has begun, proteolytic enzymes, particularly matrix metalloproteinases-2 and -9, increase in concentration and break down elastin and collagen. Increases in enzyme coactivators, such as urokinase plasminogen activator (uPa) and tissue plasminogen activator (tPa), further augment matrix breakdown. This increase in proteolysis is not accompanied by a change in inhibitors of this process, yielding a degenerative environment. Finally, the abdominal aorta is predisposed to aneurysm formation because of its relative lack of elastin and vascular smooth muscle compared with the thoracic aorta and adverse blood flow patterns. (Volumetric rendering CT image of the abdominal aortic aneurysm used with permission of Joseph Schoepf, MD.)

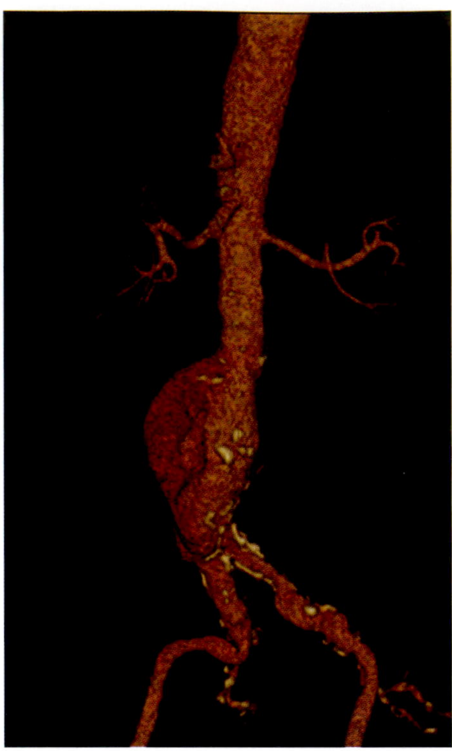

COLOR PLATE 38-5. Three-dimensional reconstruction of an abdominal aortic aneurysm from a multidetector computed tomographic angiographic scan. Note the infrarenal location of the aneurysm, the vascular calcification in white, and the tortuosity of the iliac arteries.

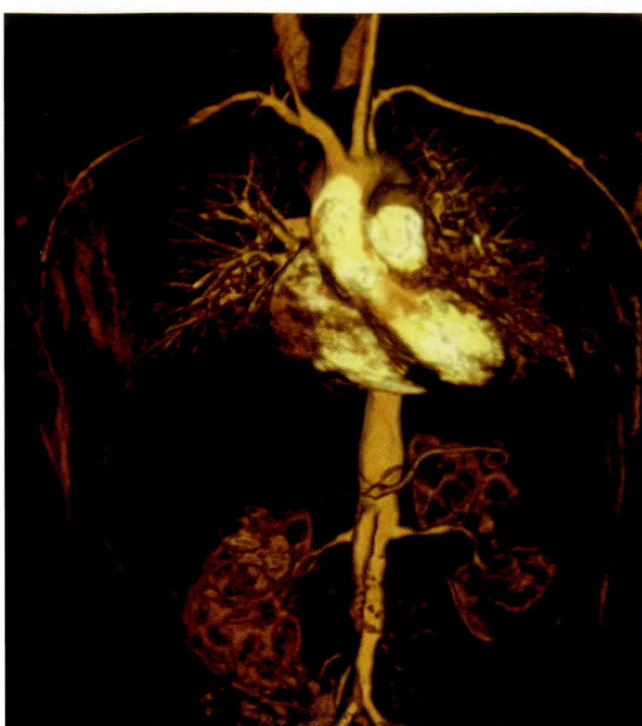

COLOR PLATE 41-1. Large vessel vasculitis with stenotic lesions of abdominal aorta and the left subclavian, left carotid, and bilateral renal arteries as imaged using three-dimensional, dynamic, gadolinium-enhanced MRA.

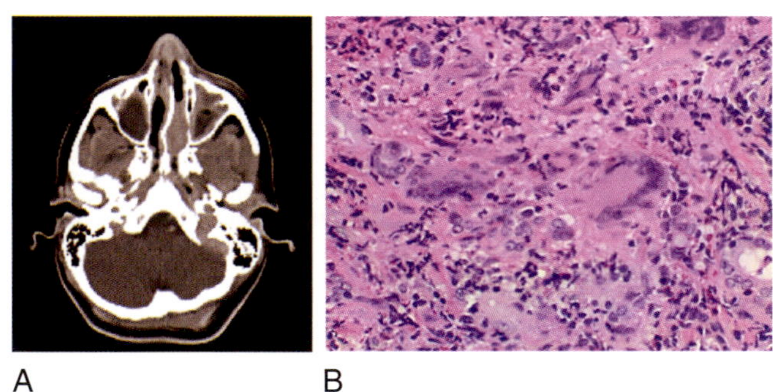

COLOR PLATE 41-3. Severe sinusitis in a patient with Wegener's granulomatosis. **A,** CT scan during an acute flare of disease. **B,** H&E stain of a sinus biopsy from this patient demonstrating characteristic inflammation, including a giant cell.

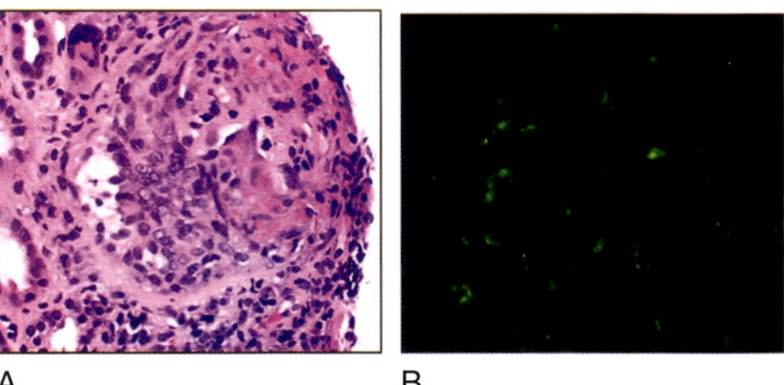

COLOR PLATE 41-5. Renal biopsy in a patient with Wegener's granulomatosis (same patient as in Fig. 41-4) with rapidly progressive glomerulonephritis. **A,** (H&E stain) demonstrates marked glomerular destruction as well as a multinucleated giant cell *(upper left)*. **B,** demonstrates the characteristic "pauci-immune" immunofluorescent staining seen in Wegener's granulomatosis and microscopic polyangiitis.

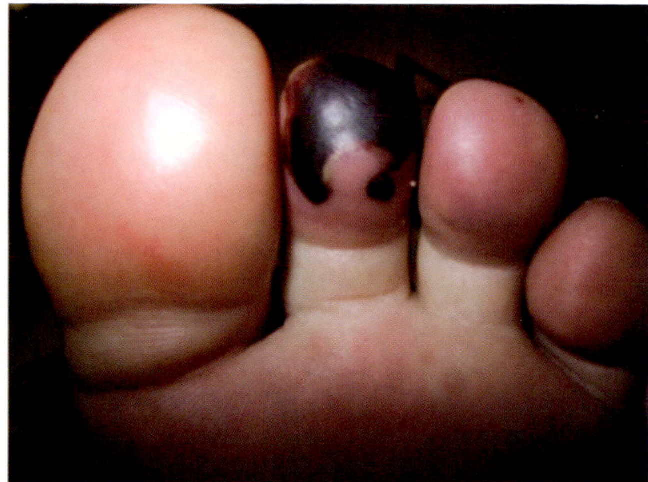

A

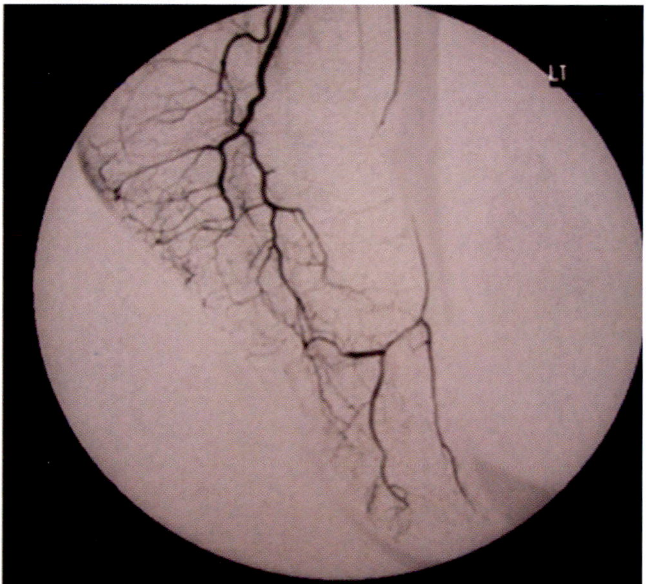

B

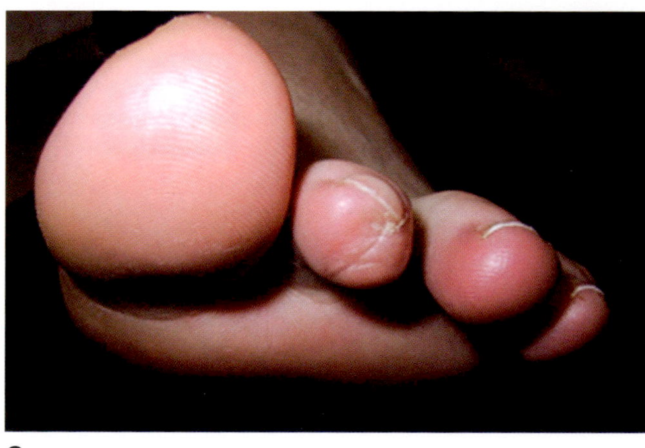

C

COLOR PLATE 41-6. Gangrenous toe in a patient with Wegener's granulomatosis. **A,** Gangrenous left fourth toe pretreatment. **B,** Conventional angiogram of left foot at time of gangrene seen in **A** demonstrating marked stenosis/occlusion of dorsal pedal artery and runoff. **C,** Same toe months after initiation of glucocorticoids and cyclophosphamide. Only minimal tissue loss resulted, and toe is now well perfused.

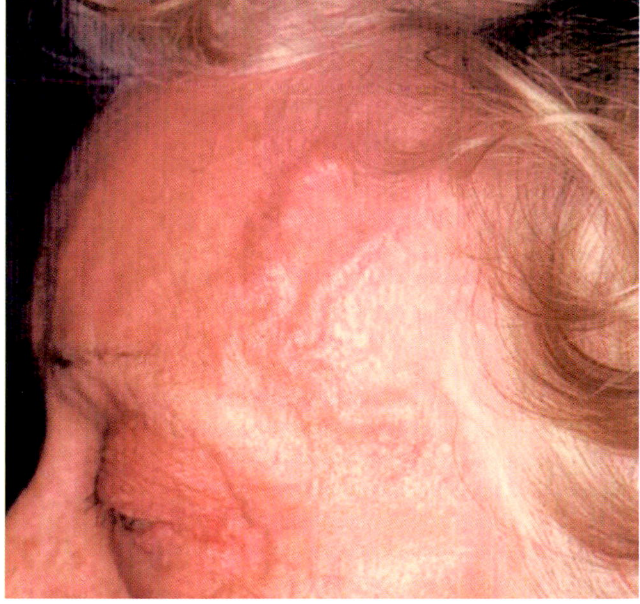

COLOR PLATE 43-1. Enlarged, hardened, and pulseless temporal and frontal arteries in a patient with giant cell arteritis.

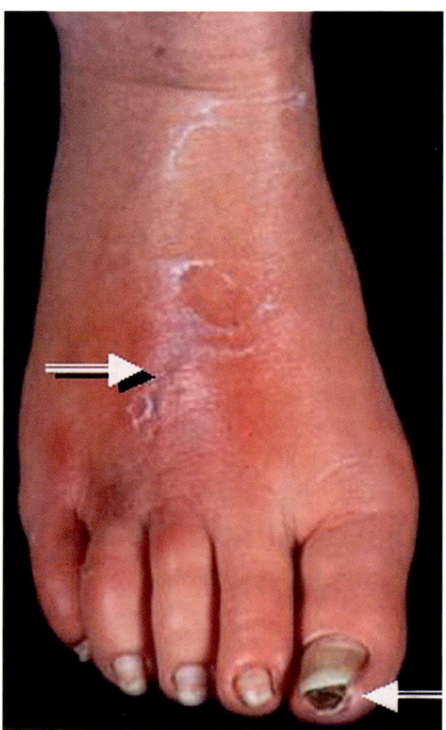

COLOR PLATE 44-7. Ischemic ulcer (*arrow*) on the distal great toe in a young man with Buerger's disease. Note the area of superficial thrombophlebitis on the dorsum of the right foot (*arrow*). (Reproduced with permission from Olin JW, Lie JT: Current Management of Hypertension and Vascular Disease. In Cooke JP, Frohlich ED (eds): Thromboangiitis Obliterans (Buerger's Disease). St Louis, Mosby-Yearbook, 1992, p 65.)

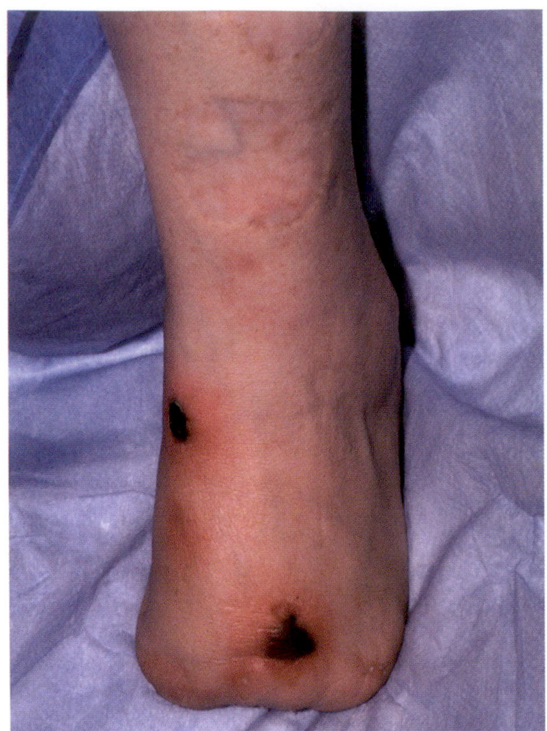

COLOR PLATE 44-12. This patient underwent a transmetatarsal amputation in the past. He continued to smoke and has developed several areas of ischemic ulceration on the foot.

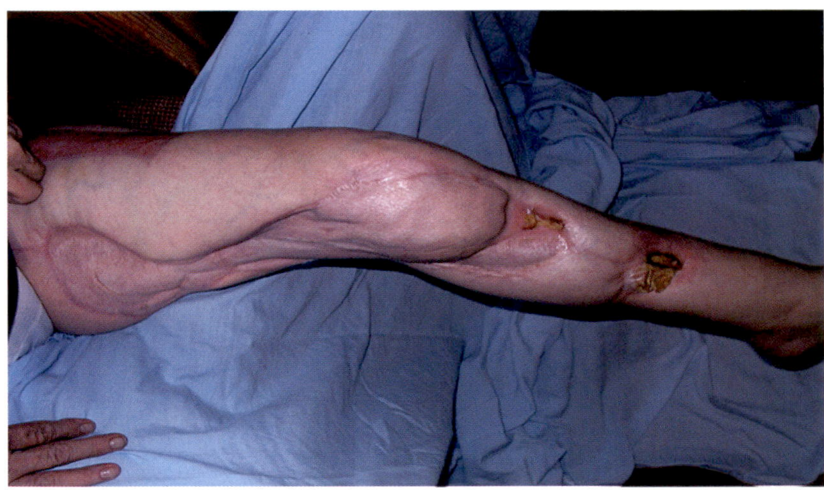

COLOR PLATE 46-2. Extensive fasciotomies, skin grafts, and free flaps after successful recanalization of the iliac and femoral arteries with thrombolysis.

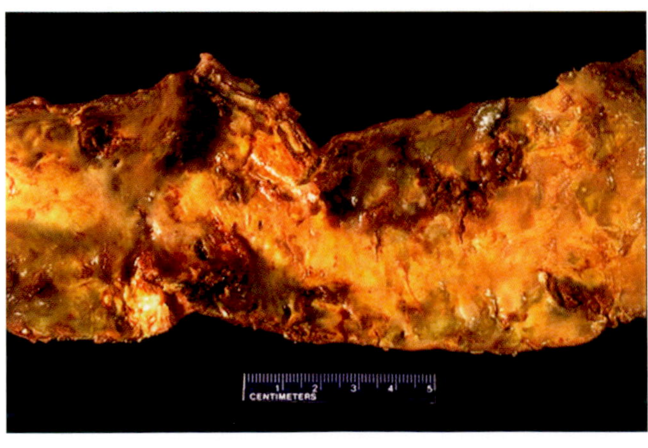

COLOR PLATE 47-1. Severely atherosclerotic aorta. Note the ulcerated plaques and superimposed thrombi. (From the University of Utah WebPath and Edward C. Klatt, MD, professor and academic administrator, Florida State University College of Medicine.)

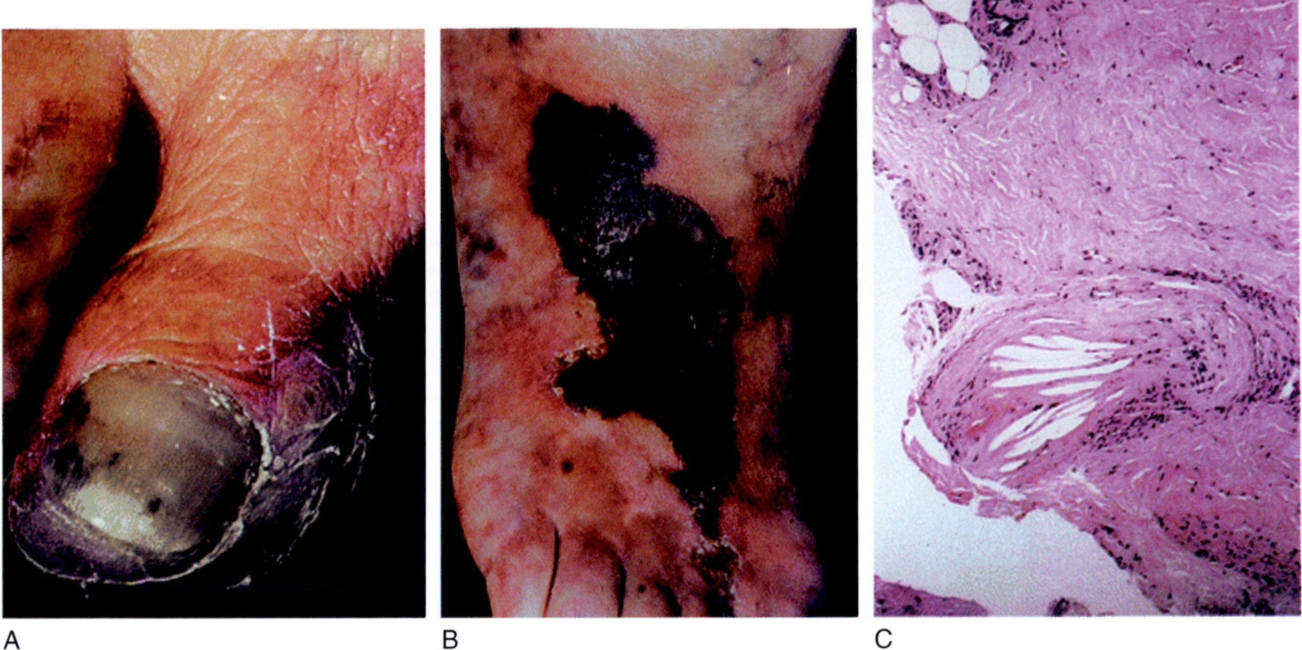

COLOR PLATE 47-2. Peripheral lesions. **A,** Blue toe. **B,** Necrotic skin ulcer. **C,** Cholesterol clefts in small artery from biopsy of lesion. (From Schanz S, Metzler G, Metzger S, et al: Cholesterol embolism: An often unrecognized cause of leg ulcers. Br J Dermatol 146:1107, 2002.).

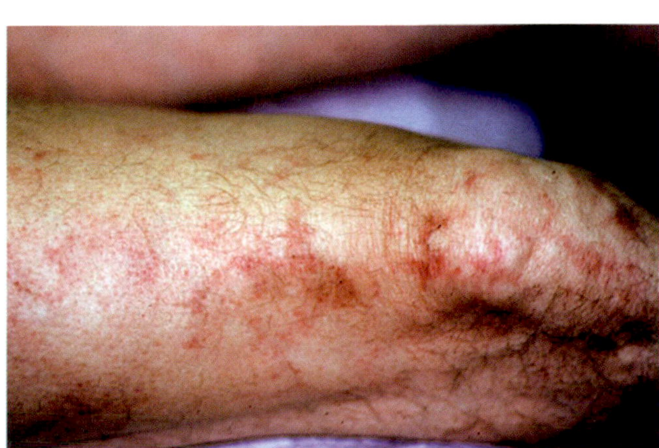

COLOR PLATE 47-3. Livedo reticularis. (Copyright-protected material used with permission of the author and the University of Iowa's Virtual Hospital, *www.vh.org*.)

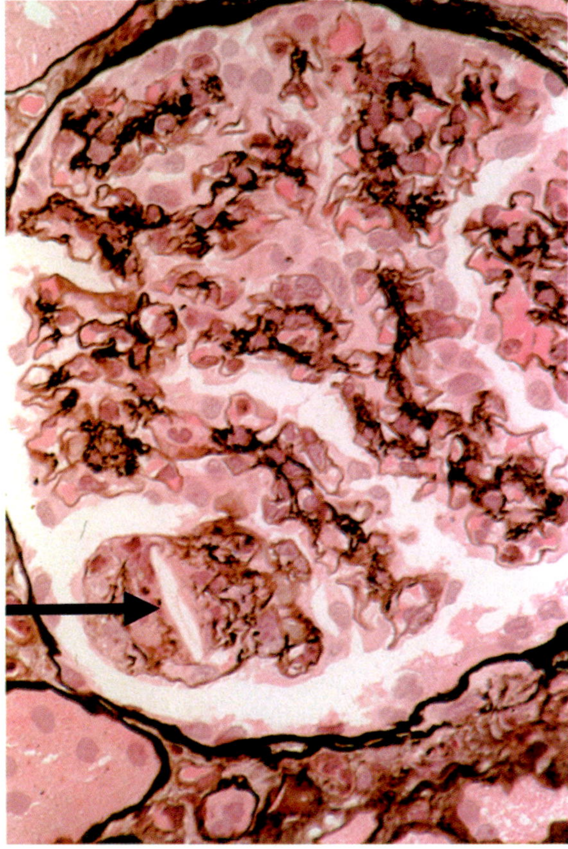

COLOR PLATE 47-4. Empty cholesterol cleft (*arrow*) in a glomerulus of a patient with cholesterol crystal embolization. (Courtesy Gloria Gallo, MD, Department of Pathology, New York University School of Medicine.)

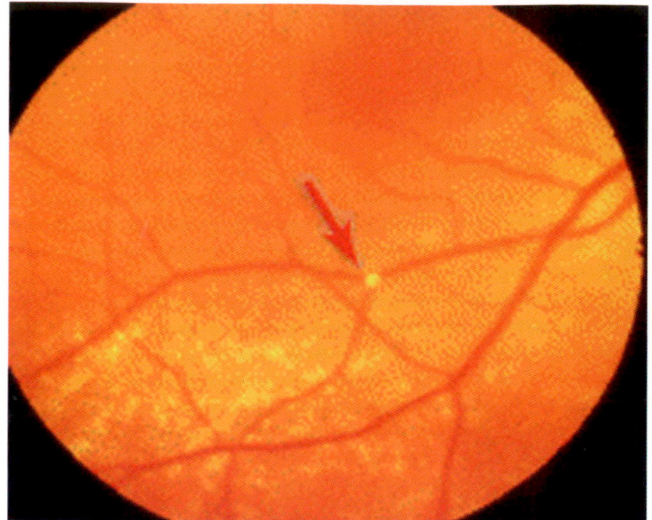

COLOR PLATE 47-5. Retina with Hollenhorst plaque (*arrow*). (From the Washington Academy of Eye Physicians and Surgeons, Kory Diement, executive director.)

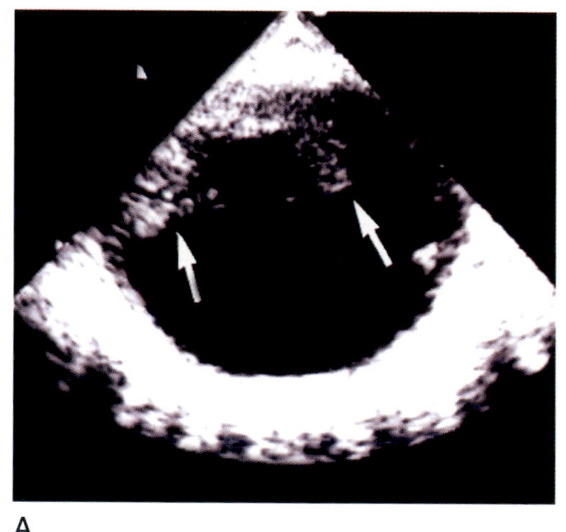

A

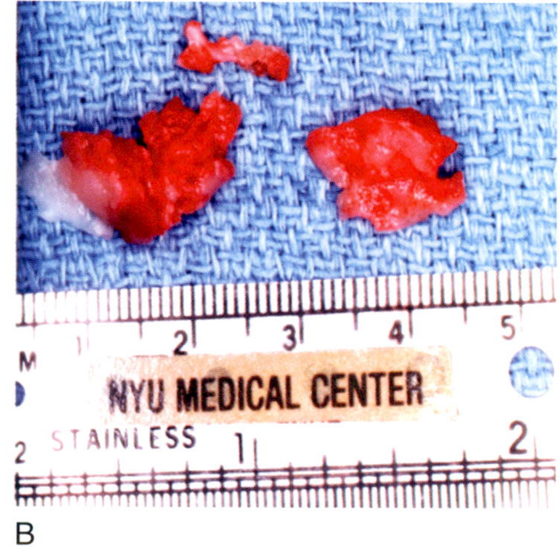

B

COLOR PLATE 47-7. A, Transesophageal echocardiogram of the distal aortic arch with two mobile clots present (*arrows*). **B,** Clots removed from the aorta seen in echo on left. (From Tunick PA, Lackner H, Katz ES, et al: Multiple emboli from a large aortic arch thrombus in a patient with thrombotic diathesis. Am Heart J 124:239, 1992.)

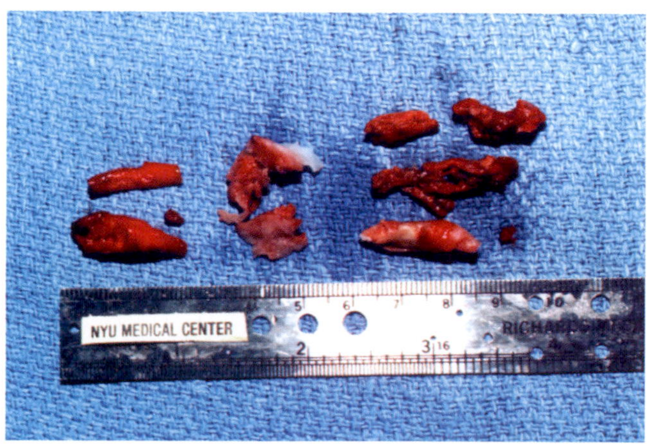

COLOR PLATE 47-8. Clots removed from the femoral artery of the same patient seen in the aorta in Figure 47-7.

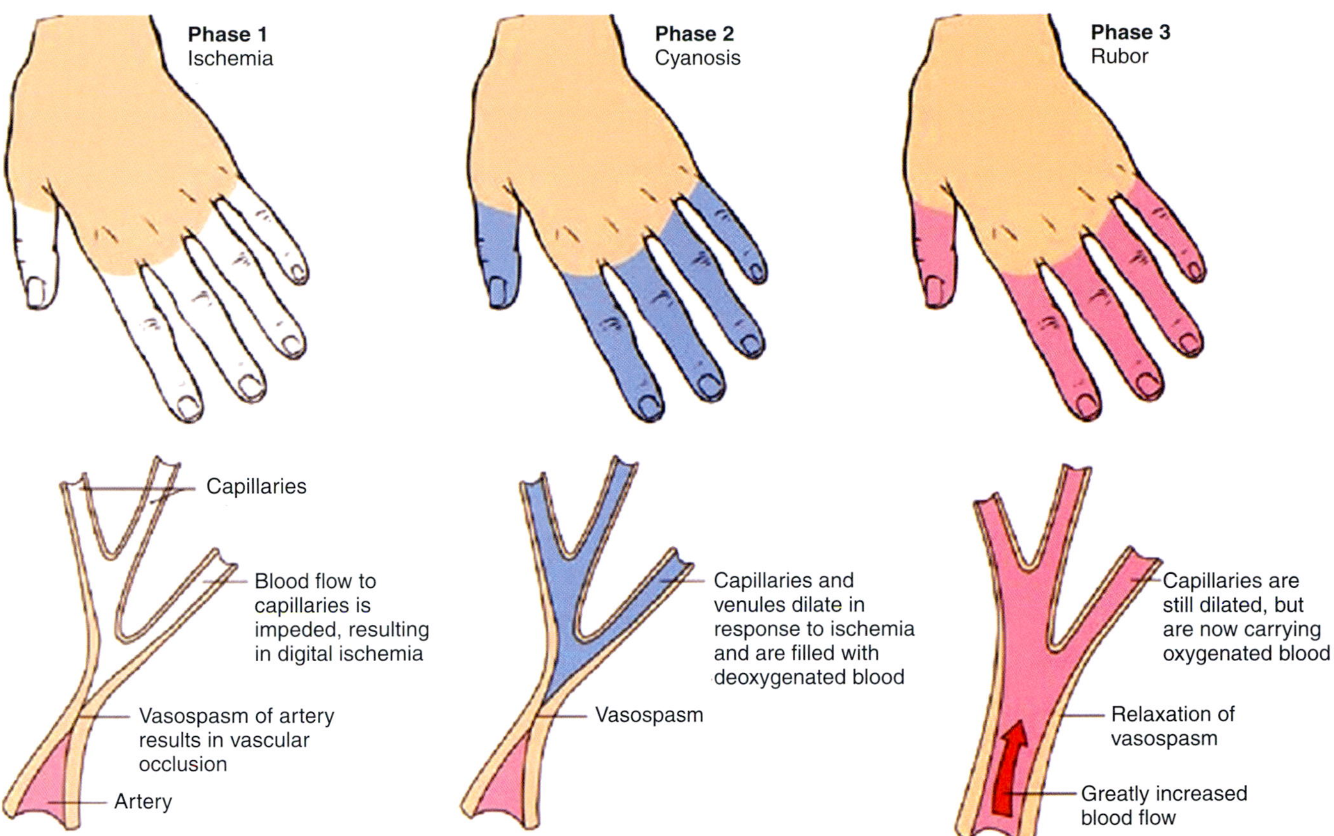
Phase 1
Ischemia
Phase 2
Cyanosis
Phase 3
Rubor
Capillaries
Blood flow to capillaries is impeded, resulting in digital ischemia
Vasospasm of artery results in vascular occlusion
Artery
Capillaries and venules dilate in response to ischemia and are filled with deoxygenated blood
Vasospasm
Capillaries are still dilated, but are now carrying oxygenated blood
Relaxation of vasospasm
Greatly increased blood flow

COLOR PLATE 48-2. Raynaud's phenomenon may have three color phases: blanching, cyanosis, and rubor. (From Creager MA: Raynaud's phenomenon. Med Illus 1983;2:84.)

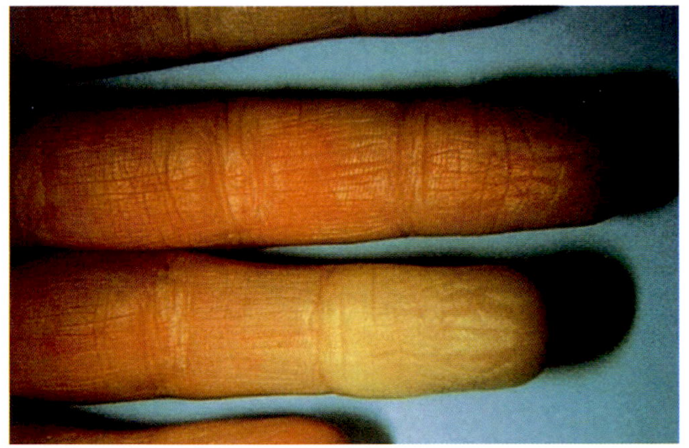

COLOR PLATE 48-3. Raynaud's phenomenon presenting as blanching of one finger.

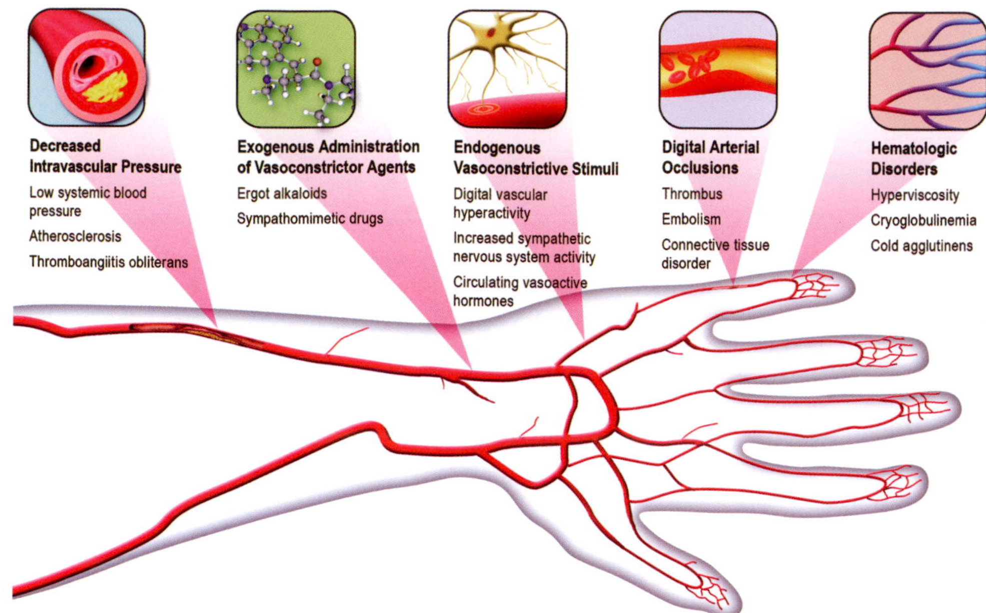

COLORE PLATE 48-4. Pathophysiology of digital vasospasm. Digital vasospasm may occur as a consequence of vasoconstrictive stimuli, decreased intravascular pressure, or both. Mechanisms that contribute to exercise vasoconstriction include local vascular hypersensitivity to vasoactive stimuli (e.g., increased α-adrenoceptor sensitivity); sympathetic efferent activity; and local or circulating vasoactive hormones such as angiotensin II, endothelin-1, serotonin, or thromboxane A_2. Low blood pressure, even in a healthy young person, may predispose to Raynaud's phenomenon when the person encounters vasoconstrictive stimuli. Pathologic conditions that may decrease intravascular pressure include arterial occlusion in proximal arteries (e.g., atherosclerosis), digital vascular occlusion (e.g., scleroderma), or hyperviscosity.

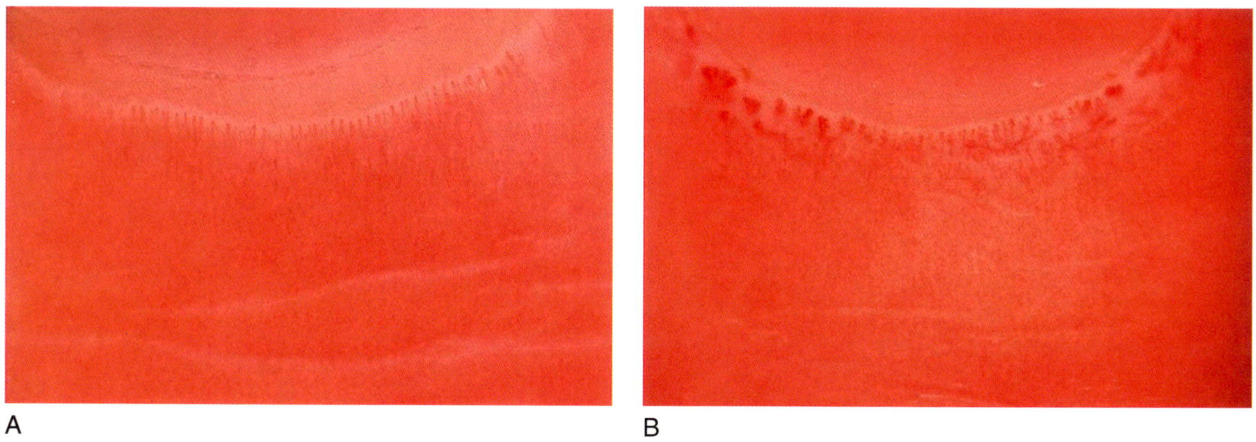

COLOR PLATE 48-7. Nailfold capillary microscopy is performed using a magnifying glass, ophthalmoscope, or compound microscope (magnification, ×10) to view the clean nailfold covered with immersion oil. Normally **(A)**, the superficial capillaries are regularly spaced hairpin loops. **B**, Results of this test are abnormal in patients with connective tissue disorders. Avascular areas and enlarged and deformed capillary loops are present in the nailfold of this patient with scleroderma. Disorganized nailfold capillaries associated with avascular areas and hemorrhage are present in patients with dermatomyositis and polymyositis (magnification, ×10). (Courtesy H. Maricq, MD.)

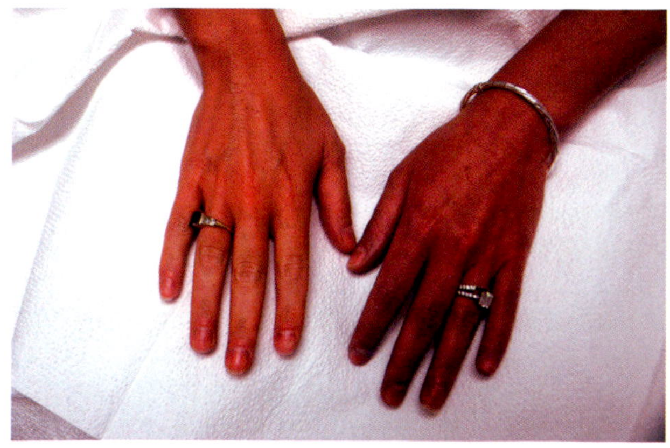

COLOR PLATE 49-1. Acrocyanosis of the left hand is evident in this 36-year-old, otherwise healthy woman.

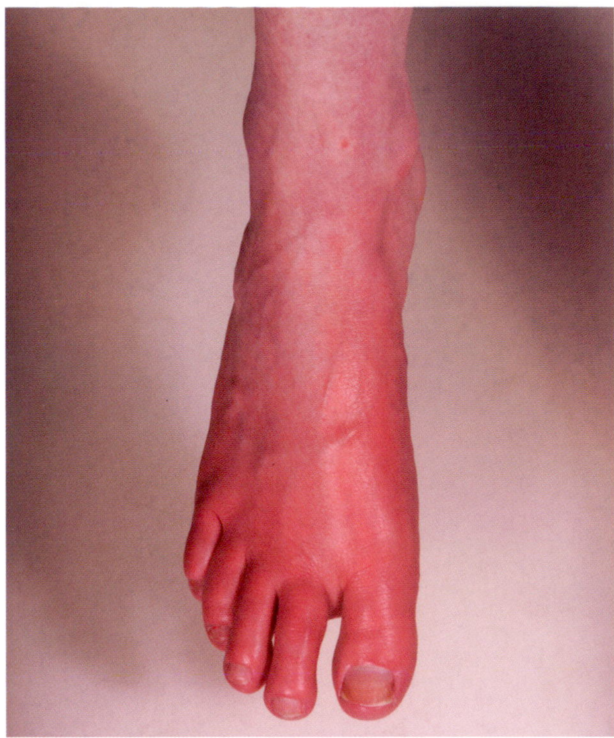

A

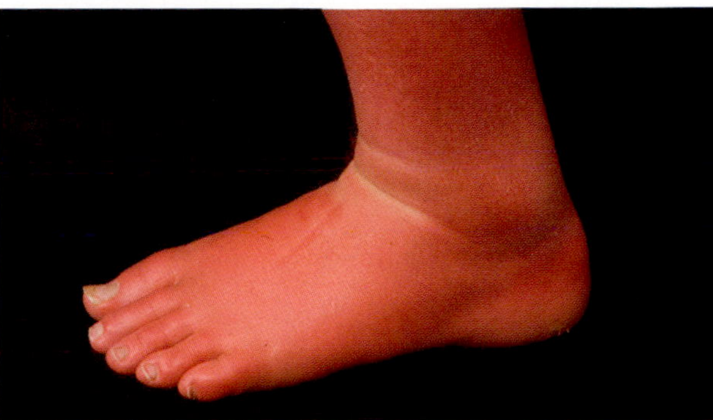

B

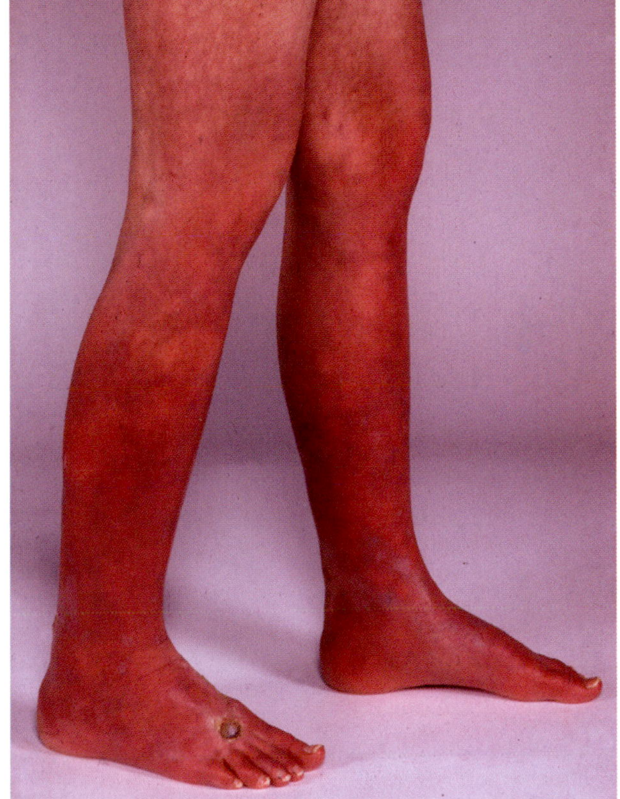

C

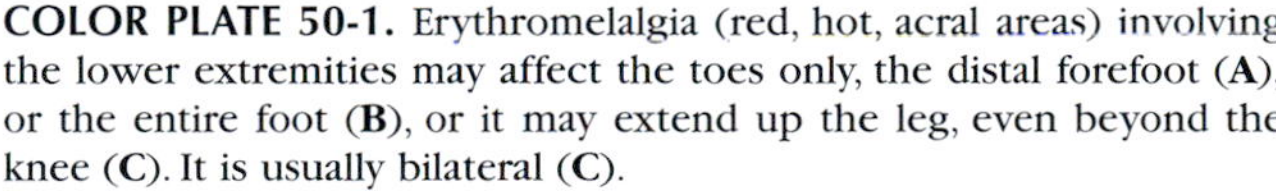

COLOR PLATE 50-1. Erythromelalgia (red, hot, acral areas) involving the lower extremities may affect the toes only, the distal forefoot (**A**), or the entire foot (**B**), or it may extend up the leg, even beyond the knee (**C**). It is usually bilateral (**C**).

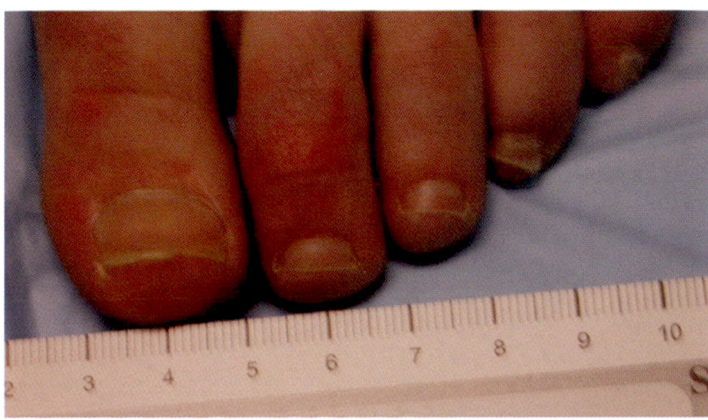

COLOR PLATE 51-1. Early manifestation of pernio demonstrating erythema on the dorsum of the phalanges of the toes. At this stage the affected extremities often itch and burn.

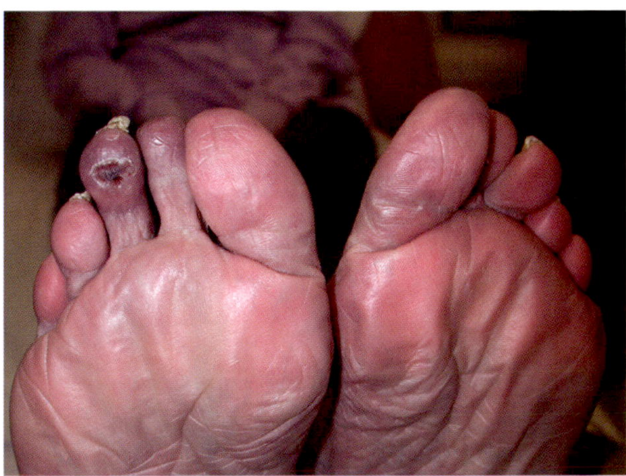

COLOR PLATE 51-2. Advanced stage of pernio. The toes are cyanotic, and there is a shallow ulcer on the right third toe. This stage of pernio is often quite painful and may be mistaken for atheromatous embolization in the elderly patient.

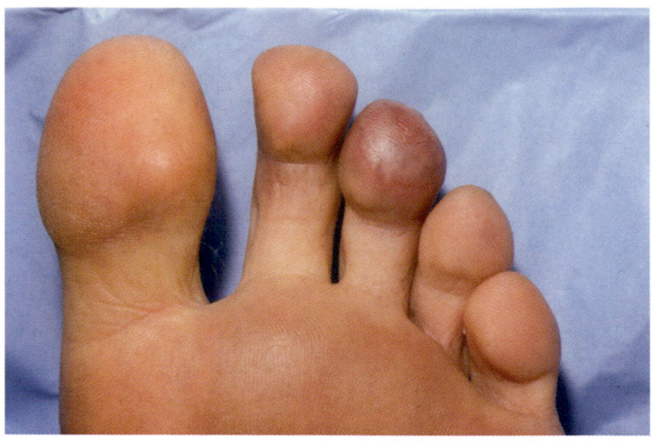

COLOR PLATE 51-3. Typical appearance of pernio. Note swelling and brownish yellow appearance of the left third toe. Flaking, itching, burning, and pain are common in pernio.

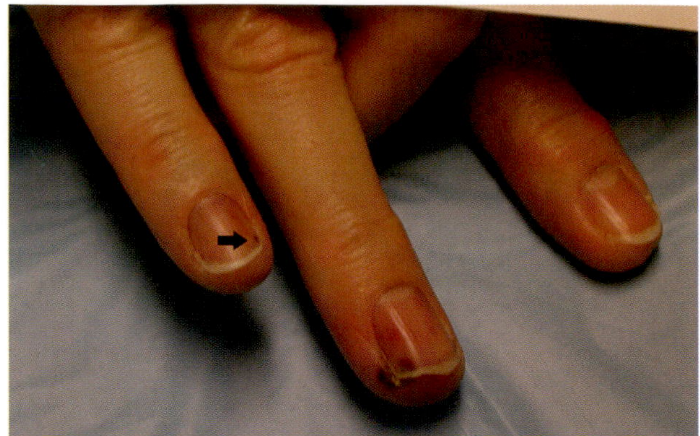

COLOR PLATE 51-4. Pernio of the fourth and fifth (*arrow*) fingers of the right hand in a woman exposed to a cold, wet climate. Note the presence of superficial digital infarcts.

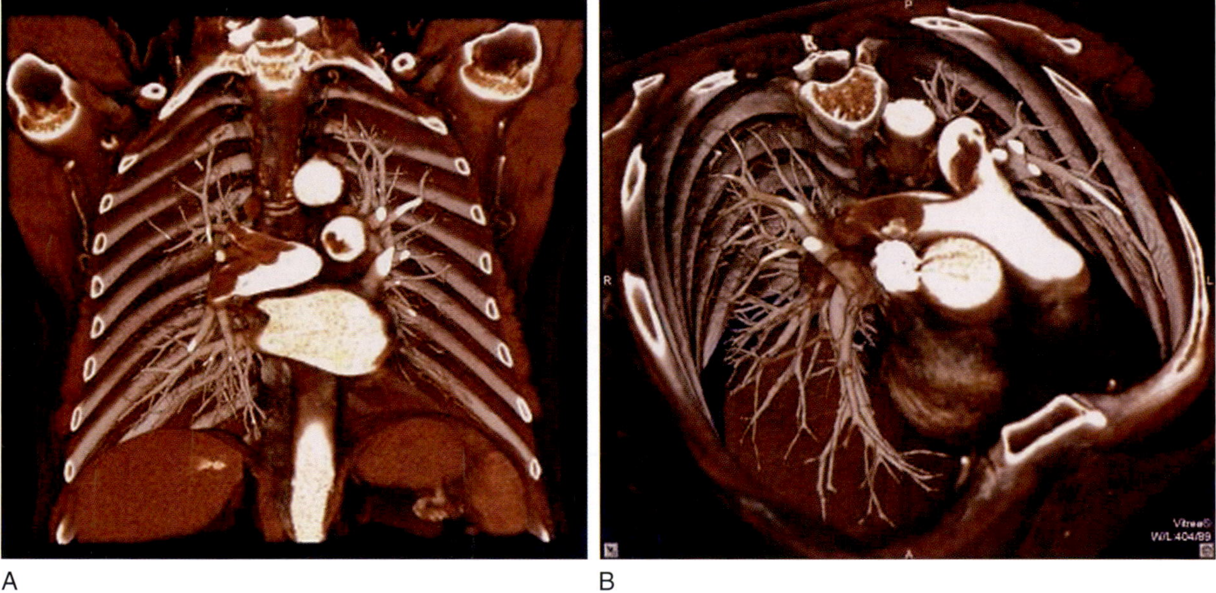

COLOR PLATE 54-5. Contrast-enhanced multislice CT in a 72-year-old man with acute central pulmonary embolism showing a "saddle embolus." Colored volume rendering technique seen from an anterior-cranial **(A)** and anterior **(B)** perspective allows intuitive visualization of location and extent of embolism. (Figures kindly provided by Joseph Schoepf, MD, Department of Radiology, Brigham and Women's Hospital, Boston.)

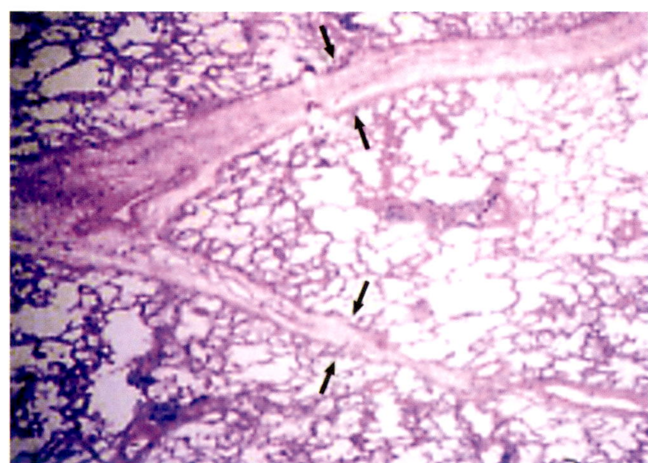

COLOR PLATE 58-1. Histopathology of pulmonary veno-occlusive disease. Longitudinal section of lobular septa (*arrows*), which are widened by interstitial edema and fibrosis (hematoxylin & eosin, ×4).[7]

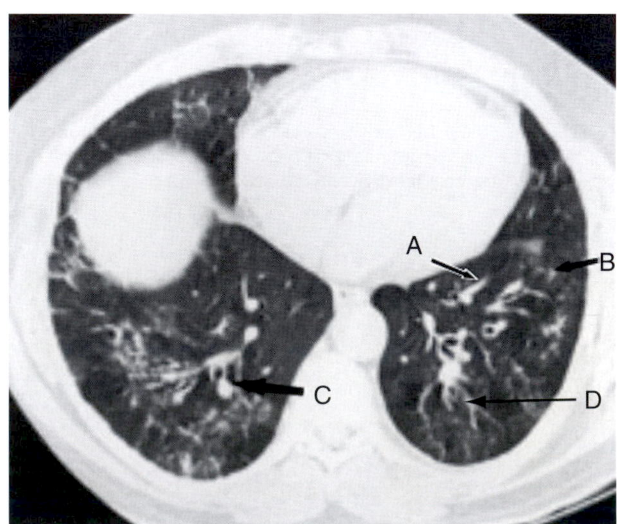

COLOR PLATE 58-2. CT scan of a patient with pulmonary veno-occlusive disease demonstrating numerous thickened septal lines **(D)** and patchy foci of ground glass attenuation **(B)**. The arteries are enlarged **(C)**, whereas the pulmonary veins appear of normal caliber **(A)**.[7]

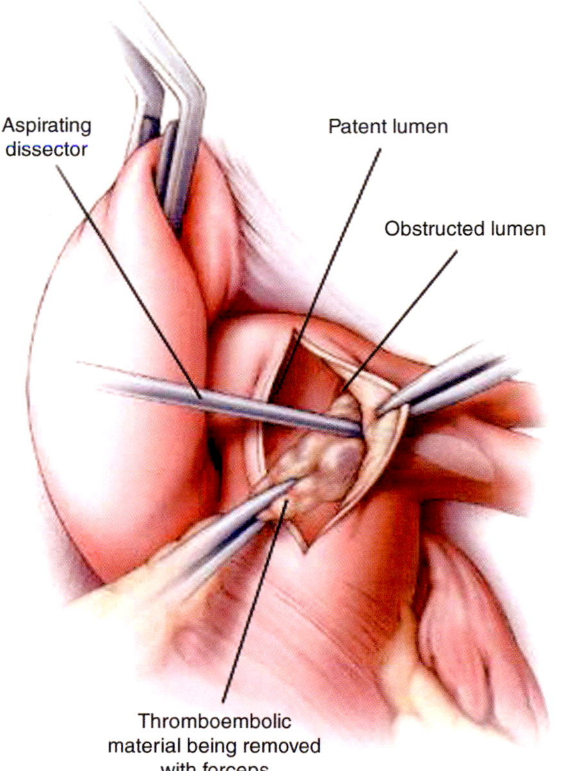

COLOR PLATE 58-5. Intraluminal view of the pulmonary artery during thromboendarterectomy. The thromboembolic material is grasped with a forceps and circumferentially dissected from the vessel wall by an aspirating dissector. The process is repeated until all the material has been removed and the patency of the vessel restored. (From Castro O, Hoque M, Brown BD: Pulmonary hypertension in sickle cell disease: Cardiac catheterization results and survival. Blood 101:1257, 2003.)

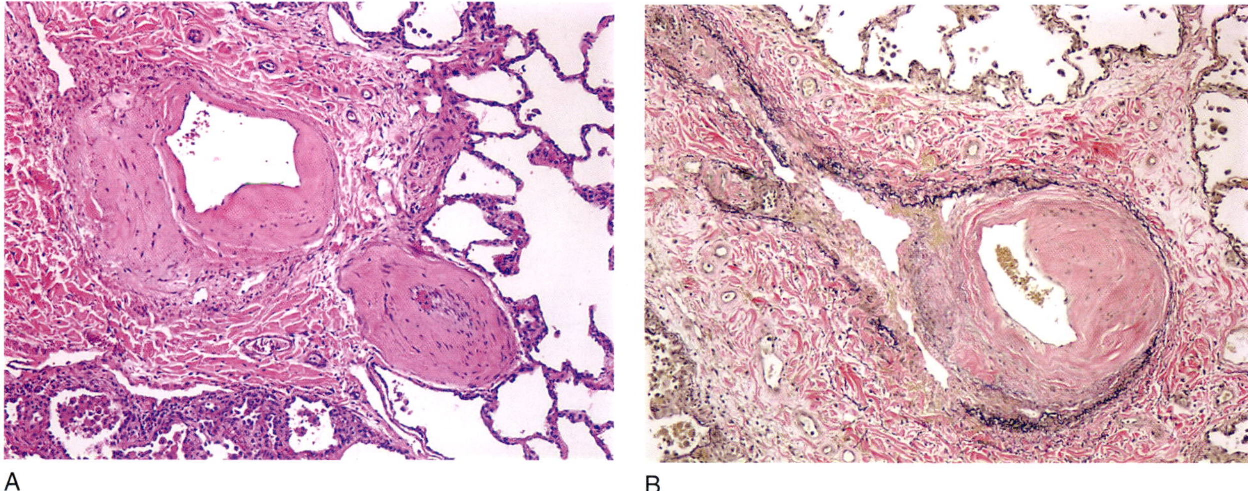

COLOR PLATE 59-1. High magnification (original magnification ×100) photomicrograph showing venous sclerosis and occlusion in pulmonary veno-occlusive disease. **A,** hematoxylin & eosin stain. **B,** Verhoeff Van Gieson stain. There is marked luminal narrowing resulting from sclerosis of the intima. (Courtesy Jeffrey L. Myers, MD.)

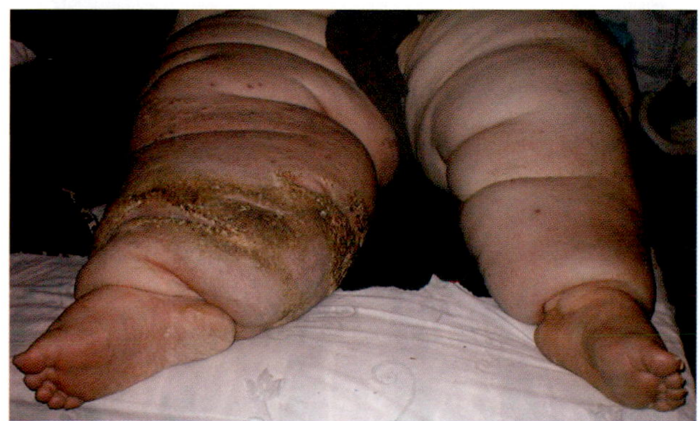

COLOR PLATE 60-4. Profound cutaneous and subdermal changes in chronic lower extremity lymphedema.

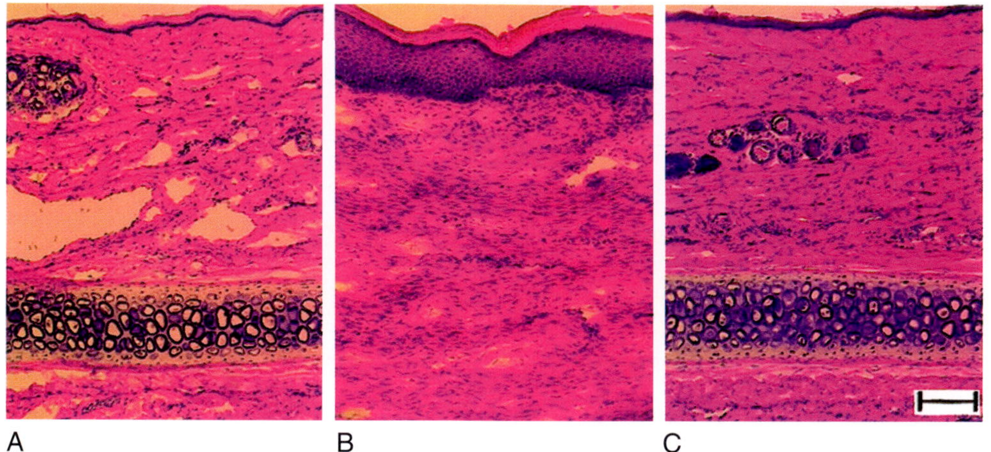

COLOR PLATE 60-7. Postmortem histology (H&E stained frozen sections) of rabbit skin after recombinant human VEGF-C therapy (**A**) and in untreated lymphedema (saline control) (**B**). Histology of a normal skin specimen (**C**) is provided for comparison. The thickening of the dermal and epidermal structures in untreated lymphedema is so profound that, in contrast to both normal and VEGF-C–treated specimens, visualization of the subdermal cartilage within the microscopic field is rendered impossible. All three panels were photographed at the same magnification (scale = 100 μm). (From Szuba A, Skobe M, Karkkainen MJ, et al: Therapeutic lymphangiogenesis with human recombinant VEGF-C. FASEB J 16:1985, 2002.)

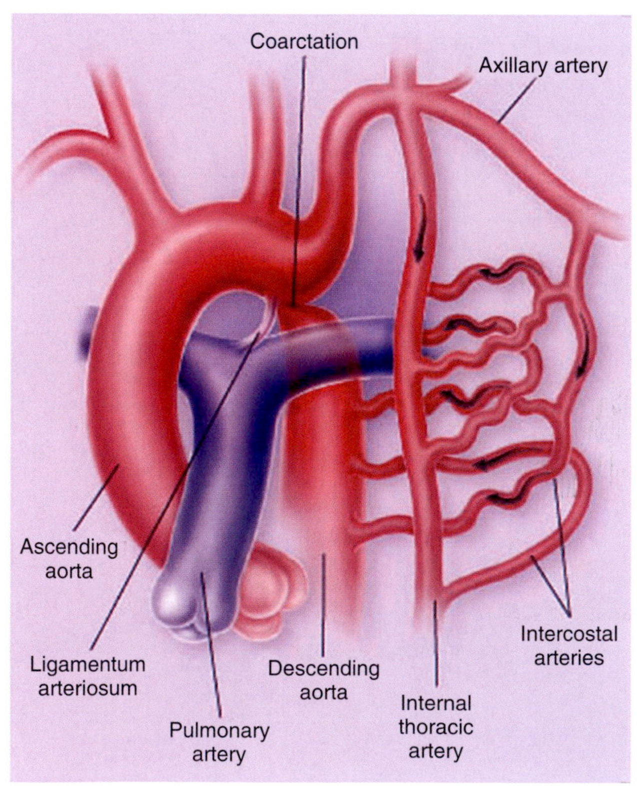

COLOR PLATE 65-5. Coarctation of the aorta. Coarctation causes severe obstruction of blood flow in the descending thoracic aorta. The descending aorta and its branches are perfused by collateral channels from the axillary and internal thoracic arteries through the intercostal arteries (*arrows*). (From Brickner ME: Congenital heart disease in adults. N Engl Med 342:256, 2000.)

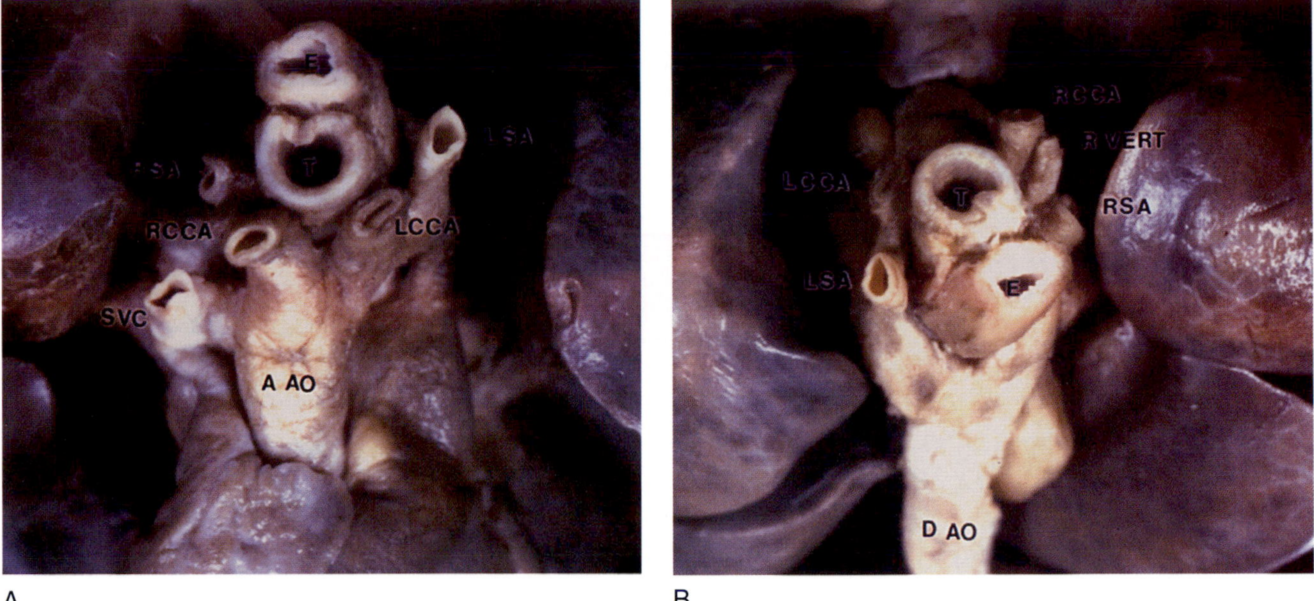

COLOR PLATE 65-8. A, Double aortic arch, anterior/cranial view. The ascending aorta bifurcates into an anterior left branch, supplying the left common carotid artery and the left subclavian artery, and a posterior right branch, supplying the right common carotid and right subclavian arteries. **B,** Double aortic arch, posterior/cranial view. The continuation of the aorta viewed from behind demonstrates the anterior left branch wrapping around the trachea and esophagus, as well as the right posterior branch emerging from under the esophagus. The distal aorta continues as a centrally located structure. A AO, ascending aorta; D AO, descending aorta; E, esophagus; LCCA, left common carotid artery; LSA, left subclavian artery; RCCA, right common carotid artery; RSA, right subclavian artery; Rvert, right vertebral artery; SVC, superior vena cava; T, trachea.

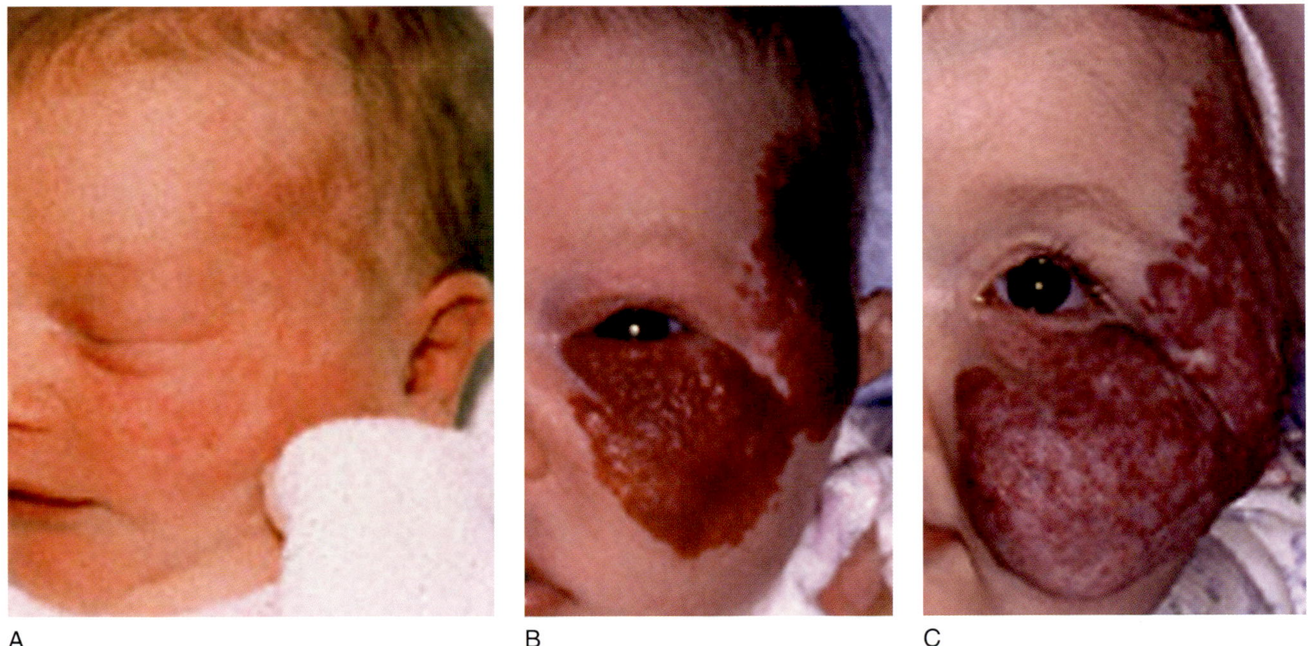

COLOR PLATE 66-1. A-C, Sequential photos of infant who developed aggressive, proliferative hemangioma with ophthalmologic as well as cosmetic issues. In early phases (*left photograph*), this lesion is not easily differentiated from a capillary malformation.

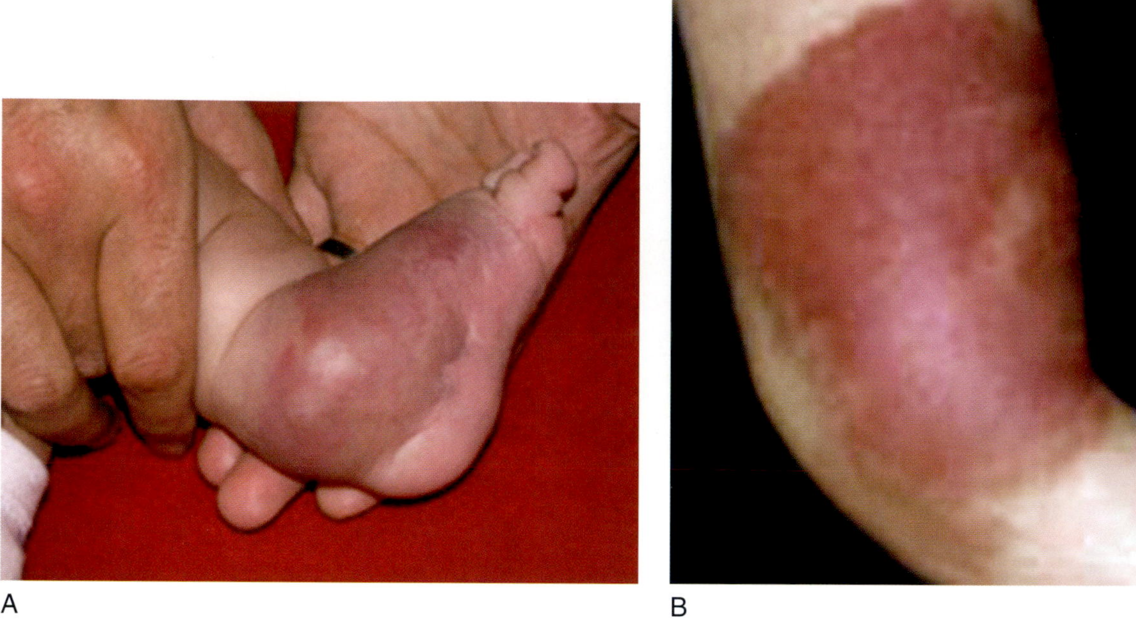

COLOR PLATE 66-2. Kaposiform hemangioendothelioma presenting as soft tissue at birth (**A**), swelling, and leathery mass (**B**). Both patients developed lymphedema and leg-length discrepancy. Patient on left (**A**) had mild Kasabach-Merritt phenomenon.

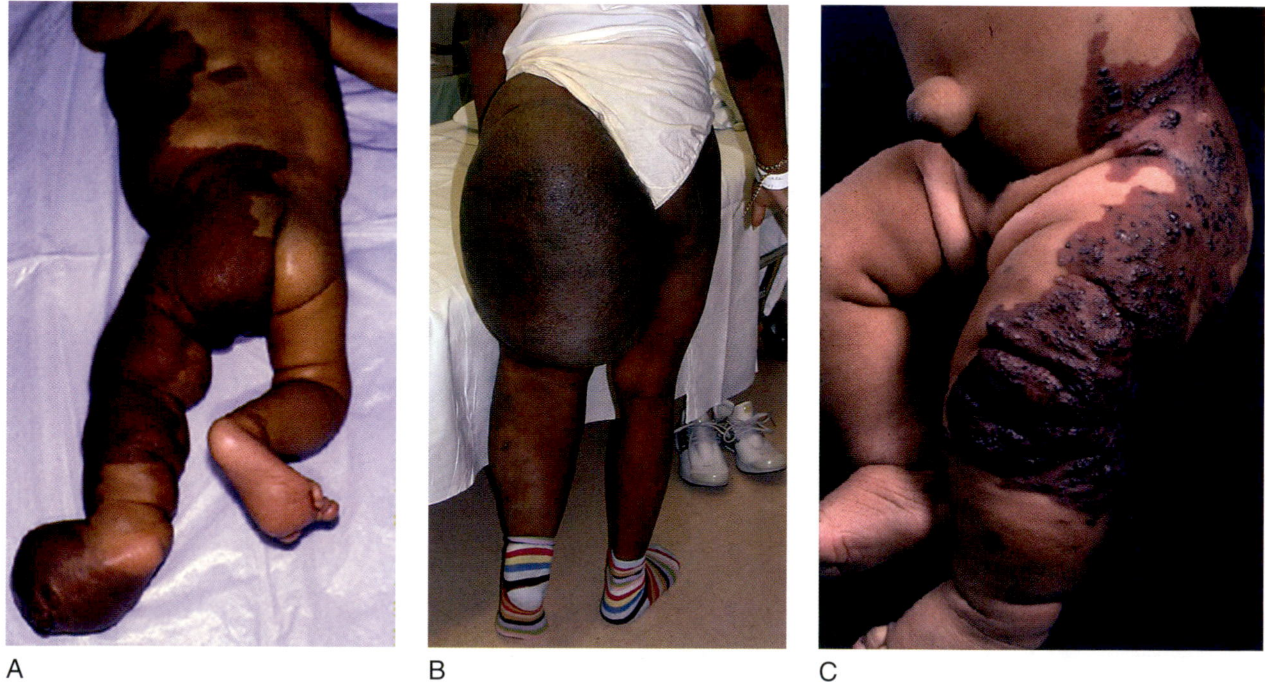

COLOR PLATE 66-6. A, Patient with Klippel-Trénaunay vascular malformation syndrome, complicated by leg-length discrepancy, asymmetric foot size requiring custom orthotics, lymphopenia, and frequent septic episodes due to abnormal lymphatic communications. **B,** Patient with Klippel-Trénaunay syndrome with associated gigantism, lymphatic dysfunction, frequent infections, gastrointestinal bleeding, severe pain, and thromboses within lesions. **C,** Patient with Klippel-Trénaunay vascular malformation syndrome, with cutaneous capillary malformation and blebs prone to bleeding.

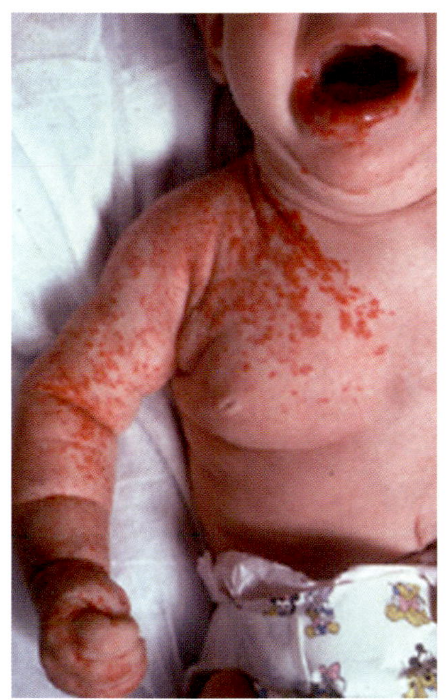

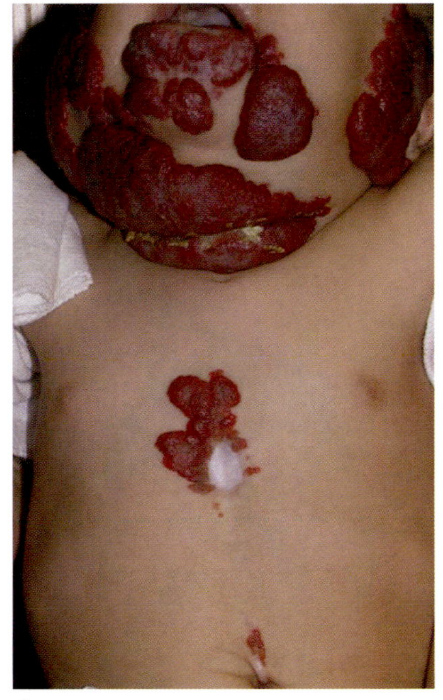

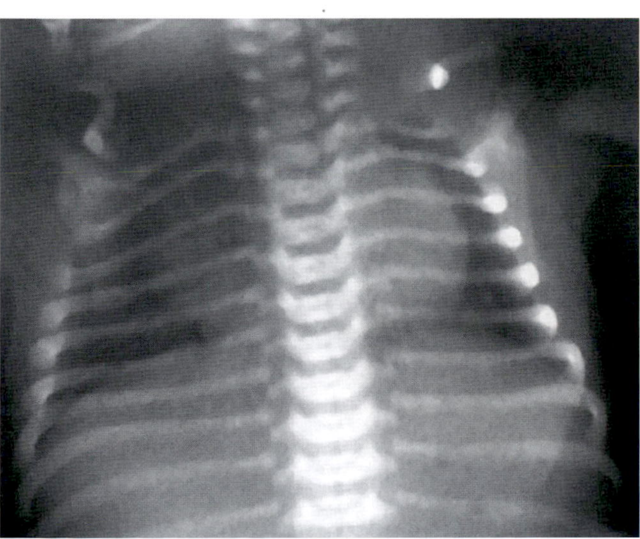

COLOR PLATE 66-8. Patient with PHACES syndrome and supraumbilical mid-abdominal raphe (vertical scar above umbilicus) (**A**) and absence of sternum as demonstrated on chest radiograph (**B**). Patient with hemangioma in "beard" distribution, sternal anomaly and supraumbilical midabdominal raphe (**C**).

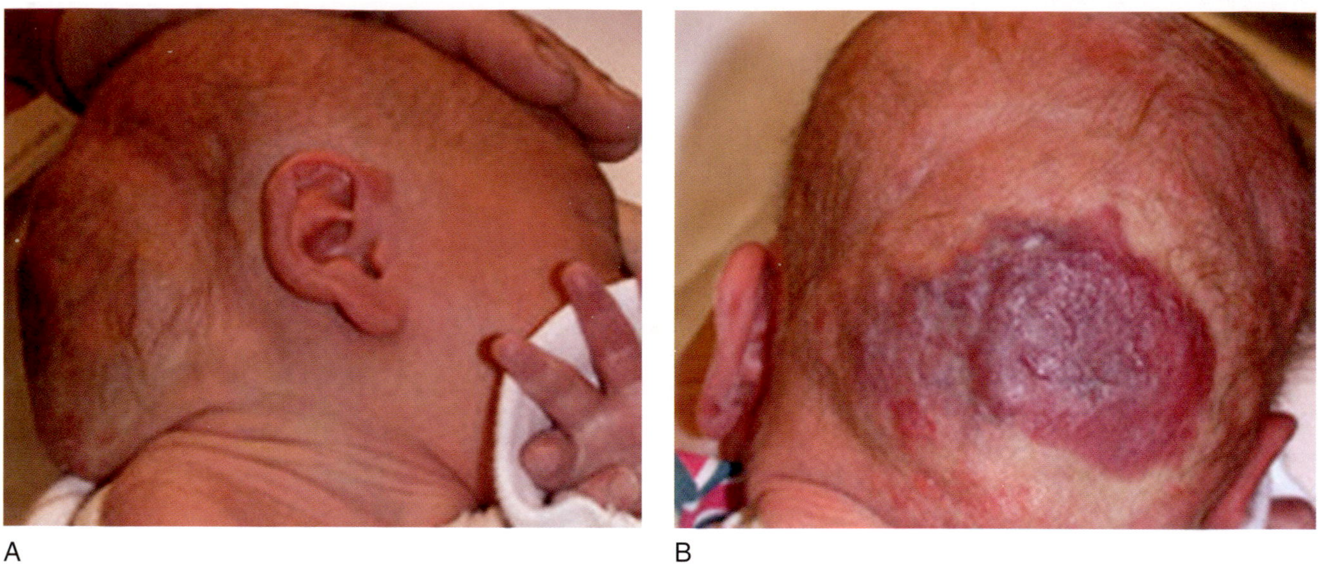

A B

COLOR PLATE 66-9. Vascular lesion of scalp detected in utero caused high-output failure in the fetus, necessitating prenatal treatment with maternal digoxin. Postnatally, the mass had arterial flow and behaved clinically as a rapidly involuting congenital hemangioma (RICH).

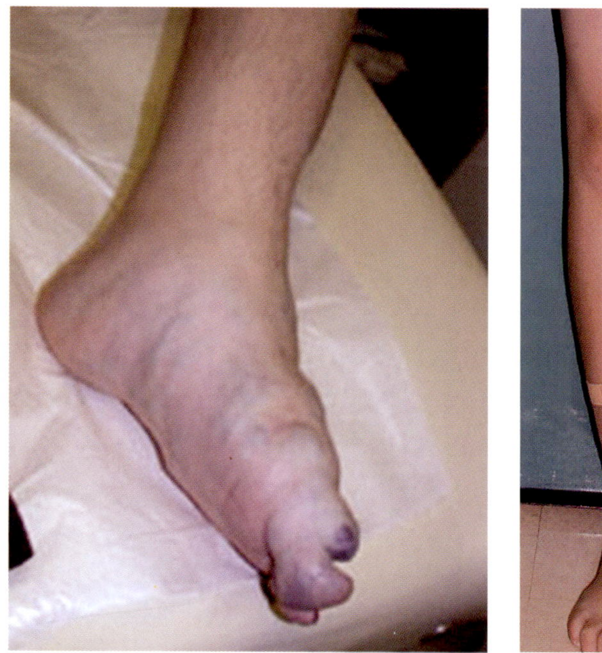

A

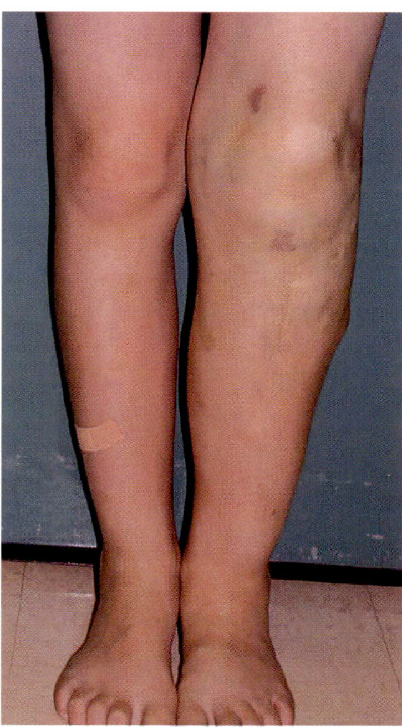

B

COLOR PLATE 66-10. Two patients with venous vascular malformations (**A** and **B**) causing foot (**A**) and knee (**B**) pain.

chapter 1

The Endothelium

Scott M. Wasserman
James N. Topper

The blood vessel wall is composed of endothelial cells, smooth muscle cells, connective tissue (elastic and collagen fibers), and extracellular matrix (Fig. 1-1). The relative amount of these different components in the vessel wall varies greatly throughout the vasculature depending on the vessel size, location, and function. For example, large, elastic arteries, such as the aorta and common iliac arteries contain elastin and collagen fibers that are synthesized by smooth muscle cells. This elastic connective tissue helps these vessels receive blood under high pressure from the left ventricle and transmit it in a continuous fashion to the medium-sized distributing arteries. Meanwhile, capillaries are composed almost exclusively of endothelial cells and basement membrane because their primary functions are those of macromolecular transport and diffusion. Despite these variations in the cellular constituents of the vessel wall, the endothelium is common to every segment of the vascular tree.

The endothelium serves as the innermost lining of all blood vessels (see Fig. 1-1). It is the largest "organ" in the body weighing approximately 1.0 to 1.8 kilograms, containing approximately 1×10^{13} cells, and representing a surface area roughly equivalent to 6 to 8 tennis courts.[1-3] In general, the endothelium is a continuous simple monolayer that is the primary cellular component of the tunica intima. On their luminal surface, endothelial cells are directly exposed to the pulsatile flow of circulating blood elements and macromolecules, whereas on their abluminal surface they interact with the basement membrane and the underlying cells. In addition to acting as a physical anatomic boundary, the endothelium serves as a biologic interface, actively transducing biochemical and biomechanical signals between these two compartments.

Over the last half century, our understanding of the endothelium and its role in vascular disease has changed dramatically (Table 1-1). It was not long ago that the endothelium was believed to be an inert, homogeneous, passive container for blood. Studies examining the microscopic characteristics of the endothelium, its interaction with components of the immune system, and its secretion of products involved in the modulation of vascular tone, permeability, and hemostasis challenged the "passive container" model of the endothelium and increased our understanding of its active role in vascular health and disease.[4-9] Advances in cell and molecular biology and the continued work of pathologists, vascular biologists, and cardiologists have led to the working concept of the endothelium as a dynamic, plastic interface interacting with its local and systemic environments to mediate phenotypic changes that maintain vascular homeostasis or result in disease.[3,10-12] This chapter will introduce key concepts in the biology of the endothelium and its role in vascular diseases.

COMMON VITAL FUNCTIONS OF THE NORMAL ENDOTHELIUM

The endothelium is a heterogeneous organ composed of endothelial cell populations that subserve the needs and rigors of their local environments (see Fig. 1-1).[3,13-17] Despite this heterogeneity, virtually all endothelial cells perform multiple, common vital functions (see Table 1-1).

Thromboresistant Container for Blood and Hemostasis

First and foremost, the endothelium is a non-thrombogenic container for blood that actively maintains the fluidity of blood and, thus, permits the delivery of essential elements and nutrients to the body (Fig. 1-2). The quiescent, normal endothelium promotes fibrinolysis, whereas it inhibits platelet aggregation and clotting cascade activation. These actions are achieved by the production of cell surface-associated anticoagulant factors, such as thrombomodulin, tissue factor pathway inhibitor (TFPI), protein C, and heparan sulfate proteoglycans (HSPG); and the active synthesis and secretion of soluble factors, such as prostacyclin (PGI_2), nitric oxide (NO), tissue-type plasminogen activator (tPA), and CD39. These molecules can modulate both the coagulation cascade and platelet activation. For example, both thrombomodulin and protein C play critical roles in modulating the coagulation cascade, and genetic deficiencies of the latter are associated with thrombosis. CD39 is a secreted ecto-ADPase, capable of degrading ADP, an important mediator of platelet activation and aggregation. Together, these various factors actively maintain an antithrombotic environment on the endothelial surface.

Conversely, the endothelium is poised to achieve hemostasis rapidly via controlled, localized mechanisms in the setting of acute vascular trauma or injury. This action is

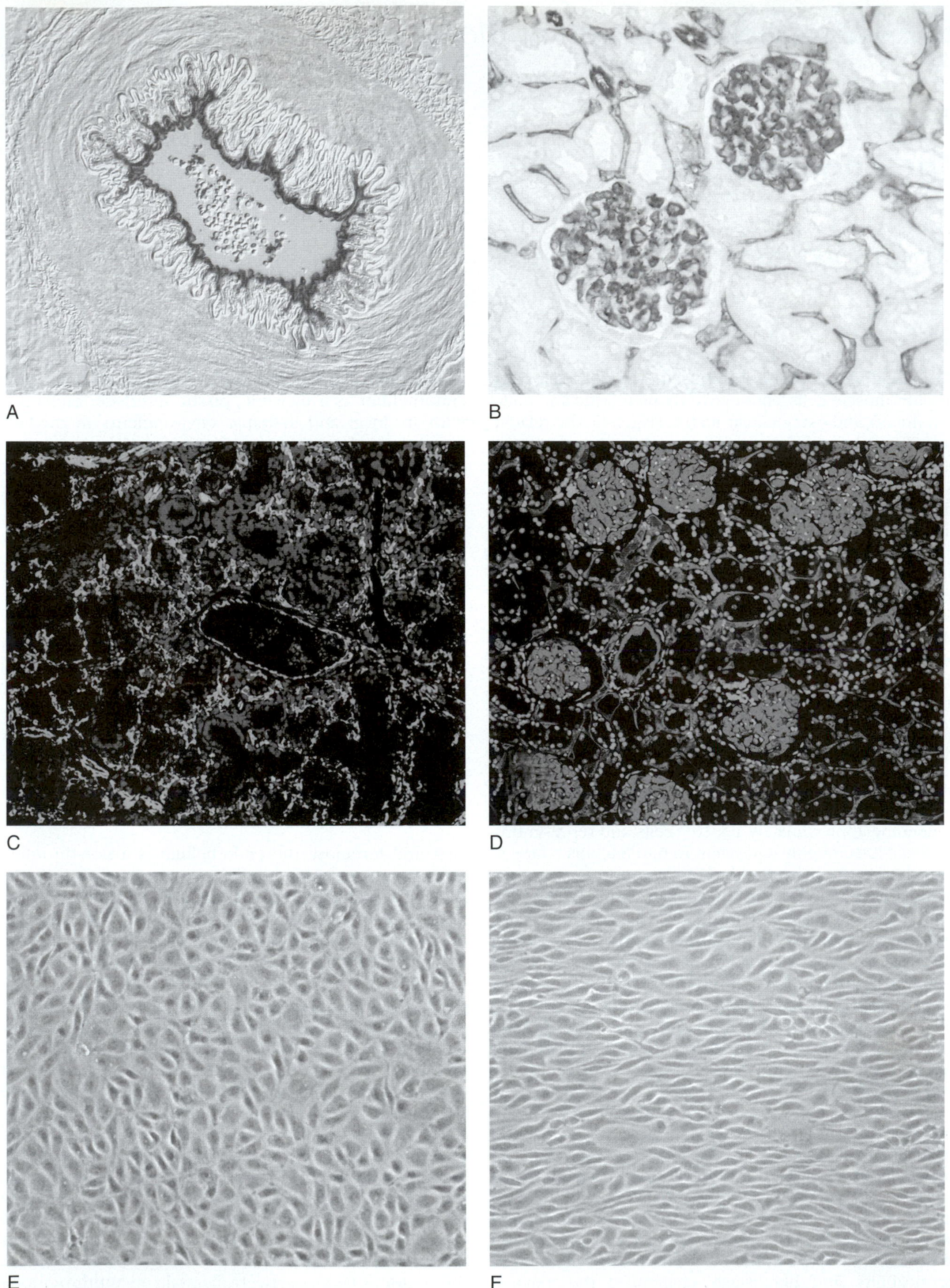

FIGURE 1-1. The vascular endothelium in vivo and in vitro. Light, fluorescence, and phase microscopy of endothelial cells in the macrovasculature, the microvasculature, and culture. Specific-staining of the endothelial monolayer (**A, B, C, D**) using immunohistochemistry (**A, B**) and fluorescence in situ hybridizations (**C, D**). **A** represents a muscular artery. **B** and **D** are sections of the kidney. **C** is lung tissue. **E** and **F** are phase micrographs of cultured endothelial cells in no flow and flow environments, respectively. Note the alignment of the endothelial cells in the directions of flow (*left to right*) in **F**. (Courtesy of Laszlo G, Komuves, Ph.D. and Ruey-Bing Yang, Ph.D.)

TABLE 1-1 COMMON VITAL FUNCTIONS OF THE ENDOTHELIUM

- Maintenance of a blood-compatible container
- Regulation of hemostasis and thrombosis
- Generation of selective permeability barrier
- Regulation of vascular tone
- Regulation of inflammation
- Regulation of vascular growth and remodeling
- Sense, integrate, and respond to biochemical and biomechanical environments

accomplished by the regulated synthesis and release of prothrombotic species, such as tissue factor and von Willebrand factor (vWF). Tissue factor, an integral membrane glycoprotein involved in activating the extrinsic pathway of the coagulation cascade, is not expressed by normal endothelial cells, but it is expressed by activated endothelial cells and subendothelial cellular species, such as fibroblasts and smooth muscle cells.[18-20] Thus, injury or activation of the endothelium by trauma (e.g., balloon angioplasty) or inflammatory mediators (e.g., bacterial lipopolysaccharide [LPS]) can expose the subendothelial stores of tissue factor to blood, or can induce the rapid expression of tissue factor on the surface of endothelial cells.[21-23] The large polymeric glycoprotein vWF is synthesized by platelets and

ANTITHROMBOTIC ◄——► PROTHROMBOTIC

Endothelial Cells

ANTICOAGULANT	PROCOAGULANT
ATIII/HSPG Thrombomodulin/protein C TFPI	Thrombin receptor Protein C receptor Tissue factor Coagulation factor binding sites
FIBRINOLYTIC tPA uPA	ANTIFIBRINOLYTIC PAI-1
PLATELET INHIBITION NO Carbon monoxide Prostacyclin ADPase (CD 39)	PLATELET ACTIVATION vWF PAF

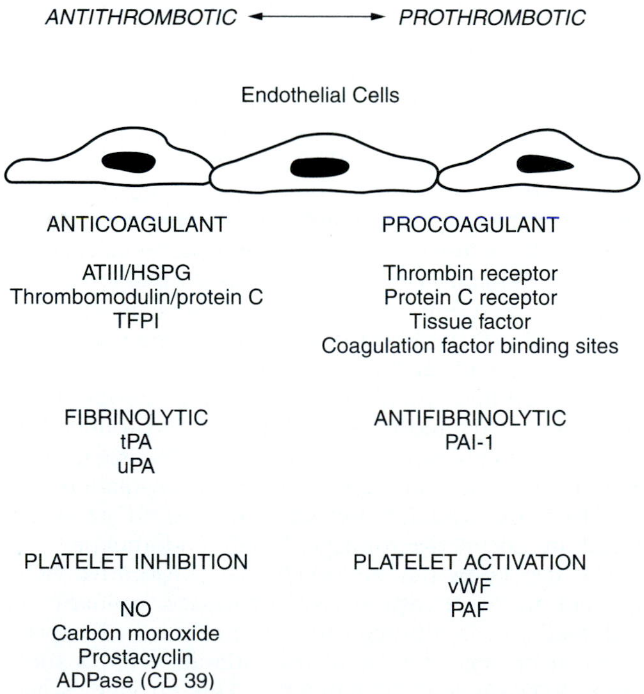

FIGURE 1-2. The endothelial hemostatic balance. Schematic diagram of the endothelial mechanisms maintaining a nonthrombogenic surface or achieving hemostasis through the production of factors implicated in coagulation, fibrinolysis, and platelet inhibitions/activation. ATIII, antithrombin III; HSPG, heparan sulfate proteoglycan; NO, nitric oxide; PAI-1, plasminogen activator inhibitor-1; PAF, platelet activating factor; TFPI, tissue factor pathway inhibitor; tPA, tissue-type plasminogen activator; uPA, urokinase-type plasminogen activator; vWF, von Willebrand factor.

endothelial cells.[24-26] In endothelial cells, vWF is stored in rod-shaped granules called Weibel-Palade bodies, which are unique to endothelial cells.[27-29] This stored pool of vWF can be quickly mobilized to the endothelial surface at sites of vascular injury and by various soluble mediators such as histamine and thrombin. This release of vWF promotes platelet adhesion and formation of the hemostatic plug. Thus, compartmentalization of the pro- and antithrombotic functions of the endothelium allows for the maintenance of blood fluidity and the physiologic hemostatic response to vascular injury. This tightly regulated balance is crucial to proper endothelial function.

Selective Permeability Barrier and Transport

As an anatomic boundary between the intra- and extravascular spaces, the endothelium acts as a selective permeability barrier to regulate the transport of water, solutes, and macromolecules through the synthesis and maintenance of specialized intercellular junctions, as well as via transcellular pathways involving vesicles, channels, and transporters.[30] The selectivity of the endothelial barrier function varies throughout the vasculature and this regional specialization is dependent on the endothelial structure, as well as the characteristics (i.e., size, charge, metabolic processing needs) of the solute to be transported.

At the macrostructural level, the endothelium can be continuous, discontinuous, or fenestrated.[3,31] Continuous endothelium is the most common type of endothelium, and is found lining the endocardium and the lumina of arteries, veins, arterioles, venules, and capillaries of skin, connective tissue, muscle, lung, retina, spinal cord, brain, and mesentery. In general, it is the most selectively permeable type of endothelial monolayer. Except for solutes that can diffuse passively across the plasma membrane, the transport of species across continuous endothelial monolayers requires the use of specialized structures, such as plasmalemmal vesicles and tight junctions. Fenestrated endothelium is observed in the exchange vessels of synovia, glomeruli, ascending vasa recta and peritubular capillaries of the kidney, endocrine and exocrine glands, intestinal villi, and choroid plexus of the brain. This type of endothelial monolayer has transcellular, round openings (i.e., fenestrae) that are 50 to 80 nm in diameter that facilitate secretion, filtration, and absorption, and contribute to making this endothelial monolayer more permeable to water, ions, and small solutes.[31-34] Discontinuous endothelial monolayers are located in the bone marrow, spleen, and liver sinusoids. This type of endothelium permits extensive cellular trafficking between intercellular gaps.

At the microstructural level, endothelial permeability is regulated by intercellular junctions, vesicles, channels/transporters, surface glycocalyx, and cell surface receptors.[3,31,35] Paracellular transport across the endothelium, which is generally restricted to small molecules on the order of 1 to 4 nm in diameter, is largely dictated by the intercellular junction.[36] There are three main types of intercellular junction complexes in the endothelium: gap, tight, and adherens type junctions.[35,37] Gap and tight junctions are found in endothelial cells lining large vessels and arterioles. As their name implies, gap junctions create channels between neighboring endothelial cells to permit intercellular communications.[38] These structures are unique because the two halves of the structure, called hemichannels, are contributed by adjacent endothelial cells, or between endothelial cells and neighboring vascular smooth muscle cells or pericytes.[39-41] Tight junctions are composed of proteins, such as claudin family members, junctional adhesion molecules (JAMs), ZO-family members, and occludin.[35,42,43] These complexes seal any gap between adjacent endothelial cells and, thus, prevent unregulated paracellular exchange and maintain cell polarity. Adherens type junctions are common to all endothelial cells and are made of integral membrane proteins of the calcium-dependent cadherin family, such as E-cadherin and VE-cadherin, as well as the catenin family (α, β, γ).[35,44-46] As omnipresent complexes in endothelial cells, adherens junctions strengthen cell to cell connections and participate in signal transduction.[30] The selectivity/tightness of the intercellular junctional complex is regulated by a variety of soluble factors, such as bradykinin, thrombin, cytokines, and oxidants.[47]

Transcellular exchange of solutes and soluble factors is mediated by plasmalemmal vesicles, channels/transporters, cell surface receptors, and surface glycocalyx, although the precise contribution of the individual mechanisms is controversial.[48-50] Intracellular plasmalemmal vesicles, such as caveolae, are spherical or flask-shaped plasma membrane invaginations approximately 70 nm in diameter.[4,34,43] These membrane-associated vesicles exist by themselves, in clusters, or in chains, and have been implicated in mechanotransduction, signal transduction, and endocytosis/transcytosis of macromolecules that include iron and cholesterol.[4,47,51-53] The transendothelial channel network includes tubule-lined pores, 50 to 70 nm diameter fenestrae with diaphragms, and specialized solute transporters/channels, such as Na-K-Cl cotransporters or water channels.[49,54-60] These structures can be transcellular or can involve systems of luminal and abluminal channels that shuttle molecules from the intravascular to extravascular space and vice versa. Similarly, cell-surface receptors can participate in receptor-mediated endocytosis. The expression of all of these structures varies among the vascular beds and reflects their environmental purpose.

Regulation of Vascular Tone

It was initially believed that only vascular smooth muscle cells (SMC) regulated vascular tone exclusively through ligand-receptor interactions and input from the sympathetic and parasympathetic divisions of the autonomic nervous system. Now, it is appreciated that the endothelium plays an important role in the regulation of blood flow and blood pressure by generating and secreting vasoregulatory substances (Fig. 1-3). In 1975, Gimbrone and Alexander discovered that cultured human umbilical vein endothelial cells (HUVEC) secreted prostaglandin and they hypothesized that the endothelium produced this molecule to regulate vascular tone, vessel permeability, and platelet-dependent thrombosis.[7] Five years later, while studying the vasomotor response of rabbit thoracic aorta sections to acetylcholine, Furchgott and Zawadzki noted the dependence of vasodilation on an intact endothelial monolayer.[61] They proposed the existence of an endothelium-derived relaxing factor (EDRF), which turned out to be nitric oxide (NO) and/or related nitroso-containing compounds.[62-64] Further elucidation of the endothelium-dependent vasoregulatory mechanism has demonstrated that vascular tone is maintained by the regulated secretion of vasodilators, such as NO and prostacyclin (PGI_2), and vasoconstrictors, such as angiotensin II and endothelin-1 (see Fig. 1-3).

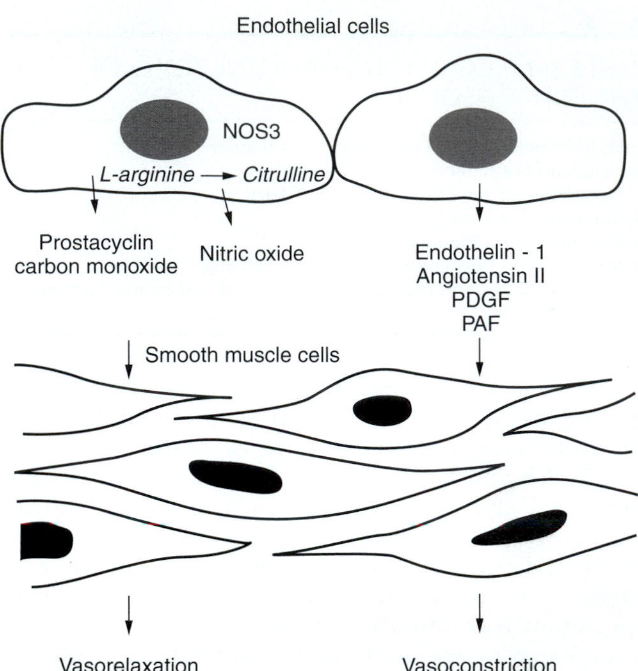

FIGURE 1-3. Endothelial regulation of vascular tone. Schematic diagram of the vasoactive mediators produced by the endothelium. These soluble factors diffuse to the smooth muscle cells where they result in vasodilation or vasoconstriction. NO, nitric oxide; NOS3, nitric oxide synthase 3; PAF, platelet-activating factor; PDGF, platelet-derived growth factor.

Endothelium-dependent vasodilation is mediated primarily by NO and prostacyclin.[65] NO is produced by three structurally similar NO synthase (NOS) isoenzymes that demonstrate different patterns of regulation and tend to be expressed in distinct tissues (NOS1, neuronal; NOS2, monocyte-macrophage; NOS3, endothelium).[66-68] NOS3, also known as endothelial or constitutive NOS, appears to be "constitutively" expressed primarily in endothelial cells, although the level of its gene expression can be regulated by diverse stimuli, such as shear stress, hypoxia, and cytokines.[69-72] This enzyme is also regulated post-transcriptionally by phosphorylation, acylation, palmitoylation, myristoylation, interprotein interactions, and cellular compartmentalization in specialized organelles (i.e., caveolae).[73] It catalyzes the conversion of L-arginine to L-citrulline generating NO as a by-product. Release of NO from endothelial cells is mediated by numerous agonists, including acetylcholine, thrombin, and vasopressin, as well as biomechanical factors such as shear stress.[31,74] It is very soluble and capable of paracrine effects via diffusion; however, the effects of NO are limited by its lability and proclivity to undergo quenching by heme-containing compounds (e.g., hemoglobin).[74] Endothelium-derived NO has three important paracrine effectors: SMC, platelets, and leukocytes. SMC relaxation and, thus, vasodilation are mediated by NO-induced increases in SMC cyclic guanosine monophosphate (cGMP). Interestingly, more chronic exposure to NO can modulate the proliferative and migratory states of vascular SMC.[31,68] Platelet activation, adhesion, and aggregation are also inhibited by endothelial-derived NO.[3,31] These actions occur through the apparent inhibition of platelet activation pathways that, ultimately, prevent changes in glycoprotein $\alpha_{IIb}\beta_3$ (GP IIb-IIIa) conformation that are necessary for fibrinogen binding.[75] Leukocyte adhesion and activation are inhibited by NO.[76] Thus, in addition to serving as a key regulator of vascular tone, NO appears to play a broader role in the maintenance of vessel wall homeostasis.

Prostacyclin, also known as PGI_2, is a vasodilatory eicosanoid generated by the enzyme cyclooxygenase via arachidonic acid metabolism in the endothelium.[77,78] Like NO, PGI_2 has vascular biologic roles that extend beyond simple vasodilation. Both SMC and platelets have receptors for PGI_2.[79-83] In SMC, PGI_2 causes a potent vasodilatory response, whereas in platelets it appears to inhibit aggregation, but does not have a significant effect on adhesion.[77,84]

Endothelin-1 (ET-1), angiotensin II, platelet-derived growth factor (PDGF), and platelet activating factor (PAF) are all endothelium-derived or -metabolized paracrine factors that contribute to physiologic vasoconstriction (see Fig. 1-3). ET-1 is a 21 amino acid peptide with potent vasoconstrictor properties that is processed from a large precursor polypeptide (preproendothelin-1).[85,86] It is a member of a family of three genes, and is the member that is found primarily in endothelial cells.[87] Since ET-1 is not stored in granules, its endothelial production is driven by transcription of the preproendothelin-1 gene in response to stimuli that include hypoxia, transforming growth factor β (TGFβ), and shear stress.[88-96] Once synthesized, processed, and released, ET-1 acts as a vasoconstrictor agent by binding to endothelin receptors on the vascular smooth muscle cells of the media. Thus, the endothelium is capable of generating both potent vasodilators and vasoconstrictors, and the balance of these effectors plays a critical role in the maintenance of vascular tone.

Inflammatory and Immunologic Functions

The endothelium acts as both an immunosurveillance and immunomodulatory organ. It is constantly exposed to blood-borne or tissue-based pathogens (i.e., bacterial or viral products), inflammatory cells (i.e., monocytes/macrophages, neutrophils, lymphocytes), and pathophysiologic stimuli (i.e., advanced glycosylation end products, inflammatory cytokines, chemokines, non-uniform flow patterns, oxidant stresses). Under normal physiologic conditions, the endothelium actively maintains an anti-inflammatory phenotype; however, following exposure to proinflammatory stimuli, such as those listed above, the endothelium mounts a regulated immunoinflammatory response to contain the injury and restore homeostasis.

In its effort to preserve an anti-inflammatory phenotype, the endothelium is capable of generating anti-inflammatory cytokines, harnessing the protective effects of soluble factors, and activating cytoprotective genes, such as oxidoreductases. One of the best-characterized cytokines with anti-inflammatory properties is TGFβ_1. TGFβ_1 is a member of three structurally-related TGFβ signaling ligands that bind specific cell-surface receptors to activate intracellular effectors called Smad proteins. Endothelial cells synthesize and secrete TGFβ_1 in response to environmental stimuli ranging from shear stress to growth factors.[97,98] In endothelial cells, TGFβ_1 has been implicated in mitigating cytokine production (i.e., MCP1, IL8), expression of cytokine receptors (i.e., TNF receptor) and leukocyte adherence.[99] Some of these anti-inflammatory effects are mediated by Smad protein-regulated inhibition of the proinflammatory nuclear factor kappa B (NFκB) pathway.[100] The importance of this anti-inflammatory cytokine in endothelial biology is highlighted by the TGF$_1$ knockout mouse, which dies in utero or perinatally, due to marked, unchecked vascular inflammation.[101] Other circulating or paracrine factors, such as high-density lipoprotein, IL4, IL10, IL13, and IL1 receptor antagonist, have been implicated in mitigating endothelial inflammatory responses.[99] In addition, the endothelium is capable of activating gene transcription to produce an array of cytoprotective proteins. These protective genes include NFκB inhibitory genes, such as Bcl-2 and TNFα-induced protein 3 (A20), and a large number of oxidoreductases, such as heme oxygenase-1, NOS3, Cu/Zn superoxide dismutase, and glucose-6-phosphate dehydrogenase.[97,99]

Equally important to its anti-inflammatory actions is the fact that, once activated, the endothelium can rapidly promote an inflammatory process. This process relies on a variety of chemokines (chemoattractant cytokines) and chemokine receptors/presenters that regulate the interaction between leukocytes and endothelial cells.[102] Chemokines released by a variety of cell types, including platelets, leukocytes, and endothelial cells, can generate a chemoattractant gradient for cellular homing. Chemokine receptors, expressed on the luminal or abluminal surfaces of the endothelium, can bind their specific chemokines and transport them to the contralateral surface, if needed, for presentation to an effector cell.[102] Endothelial cells have been demonstrated to express a number of chemokine receptors, such as CXCR4, CCR2, and CCR8. The polysaccharide glycosaminoglycans, such as heparan sulfate, coat the endothelial surface in the form of proteoglycans and can also serve as chemokine presenters.[102] These polyanions are believed to bind the basic chemokines via electrostatic interactions. The chemokine presenter/receptor-ligand interactions activate cellular signaling pathways that promote and regulate endothelial-leukocyte interactions; however, homing of leukocytes to tissues is directly mediated by endothelial expression of a variety of cell-surface adhesion molecules (Fig. 1-4).

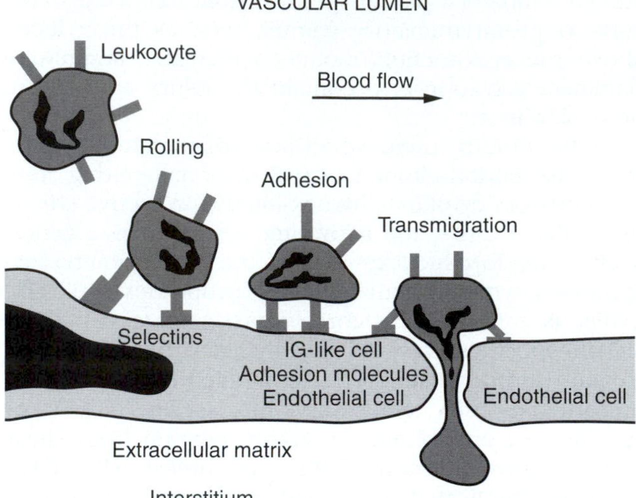

FIGURE 1-4. Endothelial-leukocyte interactions. Schematic diagram of the recruitment of circulating leukocytes by activated endothelium using the regulated expression of cell adhesion molecules on the endothelial surface. The selectins, P-selectin and E-selectin, mediate the initial endothelial interaction with leukocytes. Once the leukocytes stop rolling, they adhere to the endothelial cells via the immunoglobulin-like (IG-like) cell adhesion molecules, such as ICAM-1 and VCAM-1. This is followed by diapedesis which is mediated, in part, by PECAM-1 (CD31). Cytokines and chemokines (not shown in this diagram) play an important role in regulating this process.

Endothelial cells are capable of expressing two main types of cell-surface adhesion molecules that govern endothelial-leukocyte interaction: selectins and immunoglobulin superfamily molecules.[31,103] The lectin-like molecules, E-selectin and P-selectin, are both expressed on the surface of endothelial cells in response to inflammatory stimuli, although their expression patterns vary. Both of these selectins mediate leukocyte rolling by binding specific sialyl-Lewis X type ligands on the leukocyte (see Fig. 1-4). P-selectin is stored in the Weibel-Palade bodies of the endothelium and is rapidly mobilized to the endothelial surface in response to inflammatory stimuli. In contrast, E-selectin requires transcriptional activation and de novo protein synthesis for its expression. The immunoglobulin-like adhesion molecules expressed on endothelial cells include ICAM-1, ICAM-2, PECAM-1 (CD31), and VCAM-1.[103] The expression of both ICAM-2 and PECAM-1 is constitutive in endothelial cells. ICAM-1 exhibits a heterogeneous pattern of endothelial expression across a variety of tissues and its expression can be increased in response to cytokines. VCAM-1 demonstrates low to no expression in normal endothelium; however, injurious stimuli, such as cytokines, hyperlipidemia, or non-uniform shear stresses, can markedly upregulate its endothelial expression.

As part of its anti-inflammatory phenotype, the normal endothelial surface is non-adhesive, allowing leukocytes to remain in the circulation. In response to inflammatory stimuli, the endothelium becomes rapidly activated and begins to use the chemokines and molecules described above in an orchestrated process that actively recruits leukocytes and facilitates their rolling, attachment, and diapedesis to underlying tissue (see Fig. 1-4).[103] The expression of the selectins, P-selectin and E-selectin, by the activated endothelium initiates the process of leukocyte rolling, tethering, and attachment. Tethering results in the release of chemokines and more stable adhesion of leukocytes to the endothelium by VCAM-1 and ICAM-1. Firm attachment leads to a series of changes in both endothelial cells and leukocytes that permits the transendothelial migration of the leukocyte into the subendothelial space. This process is dependent on a variety of molecular interactions. One that is particularly critical to the diapedesis of leukocytes through the endothelial monolayer is the homotypic interaction between PECAM-1 on the endothelial surface and PECAM-1 on the leukocyte surface. To regulate the immunoinflammatory process, this leukocyte recruitment cascade is actively downregulated by mechanisms that are less well understood. These mechanisms seem to limit the inflammatory response, ultimately restoring or maintaining a non-adhesive endothelial surface, and, thus, preventing maladaptive or pathologic activation of the endothelium.

Vascular Growth and Remodeling

Vascular growth and remodeling are carefully regulated physiologic and pathophysiologic processes. The endothelium plays an important role in the processes of vasculogenesis (i.e., in situ development of vessels from angioblasts), angiogenesis (i.e., sprouting of new capillaries from existing vessels), and the remodeling of existing vessels.[104-106] Vasculogenesis and the majority of physiologic angiogenesis occur during development. In the adult vasculature, the normal vessel wall undergoes very little cellular proliferation except during physiological processes—such as wound healing or menses. Much of this vascular quiescence appears to be mediated by the endothelium. Perturbation of the endothelial monolayer by biochemical factors (i.e., oxidized lipoproteins, cytokines) or biomechanical forces (i.e., non-uniform shear stresses, balloon angioplasty) can injure or activate the endothelium and disrupt this antiproliferative state leading to endothelial cell loss or denudation and subsequent intimal hyperplasia. This process is seen in restenosis following vascular manipulations, such as percutaneous coronary intervention (PCI).

In response to changing physiologic and pathophysiologic conditions, the vessel wall undergoes chronic adaptive changes (i.e., remodeling) that are dependent on a functional vascular endothelium. For example, in response to chronically elevated levels of blood flow (i.e., as seen in the setting of an arteriovenous shunt/fistula), the vessel wall will grow and expand. These adaptive changes will not occur in the absence of a functional endothelium. In addition to flow, vascular growth and remodeling can also be modulated by hypoxia. Because normal endothelium is generally a quiescent organ, the presence of growth, mitogenic, or angiogenic factors, as well as endothelial expression of their respective receptors, is required to stimulate and regulate endothelial migration and proliferation. Stimuli such as hypoxia or flow can activate a genetic program in endothelial cells necessary for these processes.

These molecular mechanisms involve the regulated expression of proangiogenic soluble factors, such as VEGF, basic fibroblast growth factor (bFGF), platelet-derived growth factor (PDGF), and insulin-like growth factor 1 (IGF1); and negative growth regulators, such as TGFβ and angiostatin.[31] In addition to these ligand receptor-based processes, the expression and activity of a number of proteases, such as urokinase-type plasminogen activator (uPA) and matrix metalloproteases (MMPs), and their respective inhibitors, plasminogen activator inhibitor-1 (PAI-1) and tissue inhibitors of matrix metalloproteases (TIMPs), are also regulated by these stimuli, and result in the degradation of the basement membrane and extracellular matrix creating a path for endothelial cell migration. Interestingly, there is also increasing evidence that circulating cells of endothelial origin (likely derived from bone marrow) may participate in reseeding denuded vascular segments and contribute to new vessel formation.[106] Thus, a regulated balance of vascular growth-promoting and -inhibiting products permits the endothelium to maintain vascular quiescence while being poised to form new vessels and remodel old vessels in response to physiologic and pathophysiologic stimuli.

Sensory and Transducing Organ

The endothelium acts as biosensor and transducer to sense its local and systemic milieu, and then modulate its various functions to adapt to these environmental changes (Fig. 1-5). Endothelial cells function as important tissue response regulators through expression of cell surface receptors for various cytokines (e.g., TNFα, IL1, TGFβ), growth factors, and hormones (e.g., basic FGF, VEGF, insulin), as well as bacterial products, (e.g., Gram-negative endotoxins and related binding proteins). These ligand-receptor interactions are coupled to intracellular second messenger systems that result in gene transcription and the de novo production of biological effectors. Many of these effectors permit the endothelium to perform its common functions or adapt these functional properties to their unique environments. Throughout the circulatory system, the endothelium is sensing and responding to the local physiologic and/or pathophysiologic milieu; it transmits these responses from the luminal surface of capillaries directly to the interstitium of adjacent tissues (e.g., myocardium), or from the intimal lining into the walls of larger vessels (e.g., coronary arteries). This sensing and transducing function extends beyond classic humoral stimuli to the biotransduction of distinct types of mechanical forces generated by pulsatile blood flow, such as transmural pressure, fluid shear stresses, and circumferential wall stress. The ability of the endothelium to undergo local or systemic "activation" in response to such stimuli, with resultant dramatic changes in functional status (i.e., phenotypic modulation), is an important aspect of its biology and pathobiology (see Fig. 1-5). Originally described in the setting of MHC-II histocompatibility antigen upregulation by T-lymphocyte products, and then extended to the induction of procoagulant tissue factor activity and endothelial-leukocyte adhesion molecules by bacterial LPS and inflammatory cytokines, the phenomenon of "endothelial activation" in response to biochemical stimuli and/or biomechanical forces has become an important paradigm for endothelial phenotypic modulation and its role in vascular health and disease.[74]

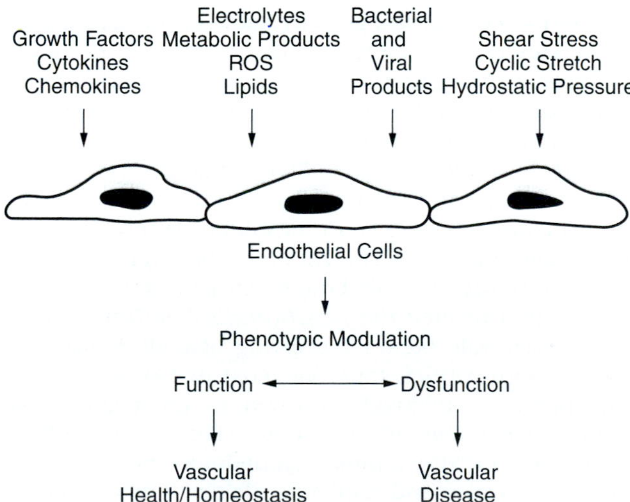

FIGURE 1-5. Modulation of endothelial phenotype by local and systemic environmental factors. The endothelial monolayer is constantly subjected to local and systemic factors, which can affect its metabolic, rheologic, and immunologic functions. Alteration of endothelial phenotype can lead to two types of responses: those that permit the endothelium to maintain its functionality and homeostasis, and those that lead to loss of endothelial functionality and the initiation of vascular disease. ROS, reactive oxygen species.

ENVIRONMENTAL IMPACT ON ENDOTHELIAL PHENOTYPE

Endothelial Heterogeneity

During development, cells are committed to the endothelial phenotype from a lineage known as hemangioblasts. As these differentiated endothelial cells migrate and mature within their various tissues, they retain many of the common vital functions described earlier (see Table 1-1). The adult endothelium, however, also demonstrates regional differences in terms of structure and function among the various vascular beds and tissues. It is believed that local environmental signals contribute to modulating the endothelial phenotype. This concept of endothelial heterogeneity is termed "regional specialization" and is a function of unique environments throughout the body.

Maintenance of Blood Fluidity

The endothelium has a vast repertoire of biologic effectors to maintain a nonthrombogenic interface, yet there are differences in their expression in small versus large vessels, as well as in different tissue beds. For example, the overall amount and proportions of surface glycosaminoglycans, which have been implicated in selective permeability, hemostatic balance, and immune function, differ depending on vessel size. Human aortic endothelial cells (HAEC) and HUVEC both synthesize mainly heparan sulfate; however, HUVEC produce more dermatan and chondroitin sulfate than HAEC.[107] Another in vitro study demonstrated that fat pad microvascular endothelial cells generated 5- to 10-fold more heparan sulfate than those from the aorta.[16,108] Tissue factor pathway inhibitor (TFPI) is expressed in the endothelium of venules and capillaries, but is not found in large vessels.[109] The expression of vWF is higher in veins than in arteries, and is absent in the small arterioles, capillaries, and sinusoidal endothelial cells of the liver.[16,31] Tissue-specific expression of proteins involved in the fibrinolytic balance has been demonstrated: PAI-1 expression is highest in the aorta, uPA expression is highest in the kidney, and tPA expression is highest in the brain and heart.[16] Endothelial production of tPA is observed in the bronchial, but not pulmonary circulations.[110] These regional differences in the expression of these pro-/anti-thrombotic/fibrinolytic factors suggest that the endothelial cells of these various vascular beds are uniquely adapted to balance the maintenance of blood fluidity and hemostasis in their respective environments.

Selective Permeability

The macro- and micro-structural elements of the endothelium vary throughout the vasculature resulting in permeability differences in distinct vascular beds. Two strikingly different vascular beds are those of the brain and the glomerulus of the kidney. The blood-brain barrier was originally described more than a century ago when it was noted that dyes injected into the vasculature rapidly accumulated in all tissues except the brain.[111] Conversely, dyes injected into the cerebrospinal fluid stained neural tissue, but did not cross freely into the cerebral blood supply. A specialized endothelial monolayer makes up the blood-brain barrier. Its selective permeability is mediated, in large part, by tight junctions with high electrical resistance and few fenestrations or pinocytotic vesicles, in addition to specialized molecular transport systems.[111-123] The endothelium lining the blood-brain barrier is continuous, except in the choroid plexus where it is fenestrated. Functionally, it isolates blood elements from neural tissue, metabolizes blood- or brain-borne species, and selectively transports molecules into or out of the cerebrospinal fluid. Induction of this specialized endothelium is mediated in part by neighboring astrocytic glia.[124,125]

The glomerulus of the kidney, which filters out circulating waste and assists in the maintenance of proper electrolyte balance, is composed of a fenestrated endothelium, which allows efficient filtration of ions, solutes, and water while preventing the loss of plasma proteins. Additionally, the luminal surface of these capillary endothelial cells and their fenestrae are covered by glycocalyx composed of both glycoproteins and sulfated proteoglycans, which are also believed to contribute to the ultrafiltration of plasma.[126-128] These distinct endothelial monolayers are examples of how the endothelium adapts its permeability and selectivity properties to subserve the overall function of its unique environment.

Regulation of Vascular Tone

Although vascular SMCs are responsible for altering the vasomotor tone of the vessel wall, this process is regulated in part through the release of endothelium-derived vasoactive mediators, such as NO (see Fig 1-3). Generation of NO by the endothelium is rapidly modulated via alterations in NOS3 activity and/or availability of substrate, cofactors, and inhibitors; and chronically affected by the rate of NOS3 synthesis and/or posttranslational changes. Interestingly, arterial expression of NOS3 appears to be higher than venous expression—as evidenced by the increased NOS3 expression in porcine epicardial arterioles compared with venules.[16] Within the arterial tree, there is further regional heterogeneity in NOS3 expression; increased expression of NOS3 is seen in the coronary arteries and aorta compared with the brachial and carotid arteries.[129,130] Meanwhile, alterations in NOS3 expression and activity have been observed between porcine epicardial conduit arteries and resistance arteries.[131] As mentioned, the "activity" of this system is not uniform across the vasculature. The sensitivity to flow-mediated vasodilation, a surrogate marker for NO generation/bioavailability, differs among the various types of vessels and vascular beds. Resistance vessels rely on flow-mediated vasodilation to maintain vascular tone, whereas the conduit vessels are less dependent on this process. Small arteries and arterioles of the brain autoregulate their diameters in response to changes in systemic arterial pressure in an effort to maintain constant cerebral blood flow. Similarly, resistance vessels of the myocardium are able to regulate regional blood flow in response to alterations in local metabolic requirements. Both of these processes are, in part, dependent on the endothelial NOS systems of these unique vascular beds.

Regulation of Vascular Growth and Remodeling

As described earlier, the growth status of the vasculature is maintained by a careful balance of growth inhibitors and promoters. Under normal physiologic conditions, adult tissues do not form new blood vessels. However, the endothelium of the endometrium is uniquely adapted to undergo physiologic angiogenesis during menses. During the menstrual cycle, the vessels of the endometrium undergo an orchestrated pattern of vessel growth and regression. The endometrium consists of two parts, a basal section called the *basalis* and a more superficial section termed the *functionalis*. The *basalis* contains an arteriole plexus consisting of endothelial cells covered with a thick muscular coat of SMCs. This vascular plexus is relatively resistant to the proliferative changes that occur during menses. The *functionalis* is situated below the luminal epithelium and is fed by smaller arteriolar and capillary plexuses with little or no SMC coating, respectively.[132] This section undergoes tremendous vessel growth and proliferation under the influence of estrogen and progesterone. Subsequently, in the absence of a productive implantation event, these newly formed vessels rapidly disappear, a process involving widespread apoptosis. The temporal and spatial distribution of VEGF plays a role in the vascular growth and degradation of the *functionalis*.[133] Interestingly, the proliferative response of endothelial cells not in contact with mesenchymal cells (i.e., SMC or pericytes) has been shown to be more sensitive to changing levels of VEGF than endothelial cells with established connections. This environmental component may account for the proliferative response of the *functionalis* endothelium in the presence of VEGF and the apoptosis induced by the withdrawal of VEGF.[132]

Endothelial Dysfunction and Vascular Disease

The previous section provided examples of how common endothelial functions are adapted to their unique vascular beds to perform site-specific functions. At times, however, environmental stimuli can lead to maladaptive phenotypical changes of the endothelium resulting in the initiation and progression of vascular diseases (see Fig. 1-5). When confronted with pathophysiologic stimuli, the endothelium modulates its phenotype and becomes activated. Endothelial activation can consist of augmented adhesiveness to blood leukocytes; increased permeability to plasma proteins; and an altered balance in the generation of vasoactive species, pro- and antithrombotic substances, and vessel growth stimulators and inhibitors. These actions of the activated endothelium can be appropriate—leading to physiologic adaptation or they can be inappropriate—resulting in pathophysiologic maladaptation. In the former situation, the endothelial response can be conceptualized as reacting to and containing the inciting stimulus, and working toward the reinstitution of a quiescent, homeostatic state. The ultimate outcome is that the functional status of the endothelium remains intact and continues to promote vascular health. In pathophysiologic maladaptation, the activated endothelial phenotype propagates responses that are detrimental to the host and lead to more chronic changes in endothelial structure and function that do not permit the reinstitution of vascular homeostasis. This maladaptive response, termed endothelial dysfunction, contributes to the pathobiologic changes implicated in a variety of vascular diseases (see Fig. 1-5). The role of endothelial dysfunction in a number of vascular disease processes is outlined below.

Thrombosis

Generation of a thrombus within the vessel lumen is a process that occurs on the endothelial surface at a site of vascular injury. The injurious stimuli leading to thrombosis can be due to chronic processes, such as progressive plaque-eroding atherosclerosis; or acute processes, such as infection/sepsis, vascular compromise, or the mechanical trauma associated with vascular procedures (see Chapter 9). Both acute and chronic mechanisms of vascular injury result in thrombosis via activation of the coagulation cascade and platelets. Normal, healthy endothelium maintains a nonthrombogenic surface, but pathophysiologic stimuli, such as reactive oxygen species (ROS), inflammatory cytokines, and non-uniform shear stresses, tip the hemostatic balance in favor of thrombosis by activating the endothelium and contributing to endothelial dysfunction (see Fig. 1-2). For example, tissue factor expression and activity are usually undetectable in normal endothelial cells; however, endothelial cells activated by mechanical forces or soluble factors, such as thrombin or inflammatory cytokines (e.g., TNFα, IL1, LPS), express tissue factor.[134-136] Meanwhile, dysfunctional endothelium generates less NO which has potent platelet inhibitory properties. In addition to endothelial activation and dysfunction, denudation or disruption of the endothelial monolayer can expose subendothelial prothrombotic substances, such as tissue factor, vWF, and collagen, to platelets and clotting factors. Loss of endothelial monolayer integrity is seen in regions of atherosclerotic plaque as well as acutely following many vascular interventions.

Sepsis

Sepsis is a pathologic syndrome initiated and propagated by the response of the host to infection. Circulating microorganisms, their products (e.g., LPS), and soluble factors generated by the host (e.g., TNFα, IL1, complement) can have dramatic effects on endothelial phenotype. At the structural level, endothelial cells can manifest cytoplasmic swelling and fragmentation, nuclear vacuolization, and detachment; however, the functional consequences of sepsis on the endothelium are even more dramatic. These include increased permeability, the generation of a procoagulant phenotype, augmented leukocyte adhesion and trafficking, changes in vasomotor tone, and apoptosis.[137-139] Alterations in the selective permeability barrier of the endothelium are due, in part, to the disruption of the endothelial monolayer from apoptosis/cell loss and changes in the composition of intercellular junctions. Early in sepsis, there is activation of the coagulation cascade and platelets, as well as a shift of endothelial phenotype toward a procoagulant surface. This activated endothelium demonstrates increased expression of PAI1, tissue factor, and possibly procoagulant microparticles; and decreased production of surface heparan sulfate, thrombomodulin, and tPA.[139,140] Losses of antithrombin III and TFPI, and the inability to activate protein C are also believed to contribute to this procoagulant state. The activated endothelial monolayer also expresses an array of cell-surface adhesion molecules that include members of the selectin family, P-selectin and E-selectin, and of the immunoglobulin-like receptors, ICAM-1 and VCAM-1. These species can mediate inappropriate and maladaptive activation and recruitment of inflammatory leukocytes, a phenomenon believed to be an important contributor to the pathophysiology of the sepsis syndrome. The balance of endothelium-derived vasoconstrictor and vasodilator substances is also altered in sepsis. Endothelium-dependent vasodilation is impaired, and animal models of sepsis suggest that this may be due to endothelial downregulation of NOS3 or an alteration in its activity leading to a decrement in NO production.[137] Sepsis and its associated inflammatory mediators have been linked to the induction of endothelial apoptosis.[138,139,141] Recently, a novel therapy consisting of activated protein C has been demonstrated to improve mortality in this devastating syndrome.[142] It appears that this therapy works, at least in part, via the modulation of endothelial dysfunction and apoptosis.[138,141] Thus, endothelial dysfunction, in terms of both structure and function, is a critical component of the sepsis syndrome.

Vasculitis

The primary systemic vasculitides (see Chapter 7) are grouped according to the size of the affected vessel. For example, the large vessel type of vasculitis includes Takayasu's arteritis, which affects the aorta and its major branches, whereas the small vessel type includes Wegener's granulomatosis, which primarily affects the kidneys and lungs. These heterogeneous disease processes are united in their aberrant immunoinflammatory targeting of the vessel wall. In these disease processes, the endothelium serves as both a target as well as an amplifier-mediator of the inflammatory reaction. In fact, some conditions such as systemic lupus erythematosus are associated with the development of anti-endothelial antibodies.[143] Immune-complex deposition, neutrophil-mediated injury, and complement-mediated lysis/damage alter endothelial phenotype.[144,145] Some endothelial cells are irretrievably damaged and undergo apoptosis, whereas the surviving endothelial cells become activated and express adhesion molecules that recruit neutrophils. The activated endothelial cells can produce an array of cytokines, growth factors, and chemokines that include IL1, IL6, IL8, MCP1, RANTES, and colony-stimulating factors. These mediators promulgate the inflammatory milieu. The end product of the aberrant inflammatory response can include vessel occlusion, collateral angiogenesis, and abnormal vessel remodeling.

Atherosclerosis

Atherosclerosis (see Chapter 6) is a progressive disease of the medium- and large-sized arteries characterized by accumulation of lipid within the vessel wall that eventually can lead to ischemia and/or infarction of the heart, brain, or extremities. This chronic inflammatory and thrombotic process is characterized by initial endothelial dysfunction as evidenced by the early subendothelial accumulation of lipid and infiltration of T lymphocytes and monocyte-derived macrophages (i.e., the fatty streak).[146] A variety of environmental factors contribute to the initiation of this process. These include the well-characterized cardiovascular risk factors diabetes mellitus, smoking, hyperlipidemia, and hypertension—all of which can induce endothelial dysfunction. Despite the presence of these systemic risk factors, early atherosclerotic lesions typically develop at vessel bifurcations, branch points, and curvatures where the arterial geometries generate localized regions of complex, non-uniform blood flow.[147,148] This strikingly non-random distribution of early atherosclerotic lesions has led investigators to examine the effect of hemodynamic forces on endothelial phenotype. From these studies, it is clear that distinct biomechanical forces can modulate endothelial structure and function, and play an important role in the development of atherosclerosis. In addition to its central role in the initiation of early atherosclerosis, the endothelium also plays an important role in the progression of the disease. Continued recruitment of inflammatory cells to established lesions, the inability to generate NO, and the production of prothrombotic species are all believed to contribute to plaque progression, maturation, and, eventually, clinical sequelae such as tissue ischemia. These pathologic processes are mediated by activated and, subsequently, dysfunctional endothelial cells.

Tumor Angiogenesis

As described previously, the endothelium lining the adult vascular tree is usually quiescent, except under conditions of physiological angiogenesis. Endothelial quiescence is maintained by tilting the balance of pro- and anti-angiogenic factors in favor of inhibition of vessel growth/angiogenesis. In tumor angiogenesis, this regulated balance is upset and favors activators of vessel growth/angiogenesis, such as angiopoietin-1, VEGF-A, and placental growth factor.[149] Tumor vessels, such as those seen in neovascularization associated with diabetic retinopathy, are poorly organized, tortuous, and dilated vascular networks that lack well-defined artery-vein structure and hierarchic branching patterns. The ultrastructural elements of tumor endothelium are also abnormal. At some sites, layers of endothelial cells are observed, whereas at others, the endothelial monolayer is discontinuous. Tumor vessel leakiness, which leads to hemorrhage and loss of plasma proteins, is believed to be due to excessive amounts of VEGF (initially named vascular permeability factor), but may also reflect the lack of monolayer integrity. The phenotype of tumor endothelium is also heterogeneous in terms of the expression of endothelial markers, such as PECAM-1 and adhesion molecules.[150] Some of this endothelial mosaicism may be due to microenvironments within the tumor that vary in their cellular and biochemical milieus. Currently, there are a number of exciting cancer therapies that attempt to shift the angiogenic balance back toward endothelial quiescence.[149]

EMERGING CONCEPTS IN ENDOTHELIAL BIOLOGY

Functional Assessment of Endothelium In Vivo

NO-Mediated Vasodilation

In vivo, endothelium-dependent vasodilation can be used as a measure of endothelial NO generation and NO bioavailability, both of which are believed to be important in vascular health and homeostasis. In this assay, the ability of a resistance artery to dilate appropriately in response to biophysic stimuli, such as shear stresses, and pharmacologic substances, such as acetylcholine, bradykinin, or serotonin, is determined. Under normal circumstances, infusion of acetylcholine will result in the release of NO from healthy endothelium and, subsequently, lead to SMC relaxation and vasodilation. In a diseased artery where the bioavailability of NO is diminished—due to the inability of the endothelium to produce it or to the presence of soluble quenchers (i.e., ROS)—paradoxic vasoconstriction or blunted vasodilation is observed following acetylcholine infusion.

In 1986, Ludmer and colleagues performed the first in vivo assessment of endothelial function/dysfunction in human subjects.[151] In their study, intracoronary infusion of nitroglycerin and graded doses of acetylcholine were administered to a series of patients with either angiographically diseased or normal vessels. Quantitative angiography was performed to determine endothelial-dependent and -independent vasomotion. Their results demonstrated normal vasodilatory responses in the angiographically smooth vessels, whereas paradoxic epicardial vasoconstriction was seen in the patients with evidence of coronary atherosclerosis—both minor and advanced. Over time, the techniques for assessing endothelial-dependent vasodilation have become less invasive and have been extended to the peripheral arterial circulation. Imaging of the brachial artery with high-resolution vascular ultrasound (flow-mediated dilation) or strain-gauge forearm plethysmography (forearm blood flow) in response to reactive hyperemia (generated by the release of a blood pressure cuff tourniquet) is now commonly used as a methodology for assessing endothelial function and NO-bioavailability in vivo.[152,153]

The observations of impaired endothelium-dependent vasomotion and endothelial dysfunction in patients with clinically apparent atherosclerosis have been extended to include patients with cardiovascular risk factors in the absence of overt atherosclerosis.[153,154] Evidence is accumulating that impaired endothelium-dependent vasomotor responses can serve as prognostic indicators for atherosclerotic risk.[152-154] These studies have also shown that therapies beneficial to patients with coronary artery disease, such as angiotensin-converting enzyme inhibitors and 3-hydroxy-3-methylglutaryl coenzyme A reductase inhibitors (statins), can reverse these aberrant responses and treat endothelial dysfunction.

Detection of Endothelial Products

Once activated, endothelial cells can express a variety of cell adhesion molecules and prothrombotic or antithrombotic substances. Some of these species dissociate from the endothelial cell surface and enter the circulation. Studies in humans and animals have observed the presence of elevated circulating levels of many of these cell adhesion molecules and thrombotic factors in the setting of pathologic conditions, such as cardiac transplantation, dyslipidemia, vasculitis, pulmonary fibrosis, and atherosclerosis.[155-160] For example, elevated amounts of soluble ICAM-1 (sICAM), vWF, and soluble thrombomodulin have been detected in patients with underlying atherosclerosis of the heart, brain, and peripheral vasculature.[160-163] Interestingly, treatment with statins has been shown to diminish the levels of some of the circulating adhesion molecules.[164] It has been postulated that these circulating endothelial products can serve as surrogate markers of inflammation, endothelial activation, or endothelial dysfunction; however, their significance, in terms of their roles in pathogenesis and/or prognosis of vascular diseases, remains unclear.[158,161,165,166]

Circulating Endothelial Cells

Although the presence of endothelial cells in the circulation has been appreciated for 30 years, there has been recent interest in understanding the biology of circulating endothelial cells (CEC) owing to their potential roles as diagnostic markers of endothelial function, prognostic indictors of cardiovascular risk, and an emerging therapeutic option for ischemic arterial disease and hemophilia.[143,167-169] Circulating endothelial cells can arise from the vessel wall and/or the bone marrow. The true origin of these cells is the subject of continued debate because the phenotype varies depending on the isolation-culture protocol and the nature of the defining cellular and molecular markers used. Nevertheless, it is likely that both vessel wall- and bone marrow-derived CEC comprise the circulating endothelial cell pool. CEC derived from the vessel wall demonstrate a mature phenotype that is relatively growth quiescent and expresses endothelial markers that include VE-cadherin, vWF, and CD146.[143] One study evaluating the phenotype of CEC in patients who underwent bone marrow transplantation found that vessel wall-derived CEC were more represented in fresh blood than those derived from bone marrow.[167] Bone marrow-derived CEC are synonymous with endothelial progenitor cells (EPC). These undifferentiated, immature cells in the adult bone marrow originate from hemangioblasts and express stem-cell markers, CD34 and/or CD133. In culture, these EPC express mature endothelial markers, such as VE-cadherin and vWF.[143]

In a healthy adult, there are 2 to 5 CEC per milliliter of peripheral blood.[167] This number is markedly increased in disease processes that result in endothelial injury and activation. These include acute coronary syndromes, diabetes, sickle cell crisis, and active systemic lupus erythematosus.[143] A recent study by Hill and colleagues evaluated the number of CEC and endothelium-dependent/endothelium-independent vasomotor functions in a group of patients with cardiovascular risk factors, but no overt cardiovascular disease.[169] They found that CEC number correlated inversely with the patient's cumulative cardiovascular risk and directly with their flow-mediated vasodilation; thus, in contrast to the above studies, they found that a lower number of CEC was associated with higher cardiovascular risk. Interestingly, the CEC from high-risk individuals were also more senescent than those from low-risk patients. It is plausible that the acute pathologic processes associated with higher levels of CEC have a much different intravascular milieu than that observed in the setting of long-term cardiovascular risk factors. Indeed, there is evidence to suggest that the decrease in CEC observed by Hill and colleagues may be a consequence of either increased total cholesterol (which, in addition to increased cumulative cardiovascular risk and decreased flow-mediated brachial reactivity, strongly correlated with decreased CEC) or insufficient bioactive NO.[169-171]

CEC may have a number of therapeutic uses. Based on animal models of angiogenesis, it appears that EPC contribute to new vessel formation, making up approximately 10% of the new endothelial cells.[143,172] These cells may also have the ability to reconstitute important deficiencies, such as clotting factor defects, and, thus, have potential wide therapeutic implications.[168] Further molecular characterization of these cells will enhance our understanding of CEC biology and may lead to novel diagnostic, prognostic, and therapeutic modalities.

Molecular Phenotype of Endothelial Cells

The genome-wide characterization of the gene expression profile(s) of endothelial cells has been facilitated by the completion of the human genome project, advances in molecular biology, and the emergence of new technologies, such as DNA microarrays. Recent studies have examined the transcriptional profiles of cultured endothelial and non-endothelial cell types in an effort to define the molecular signature of the endothelium in vivo.[173-175] These studies have identified numerous endothelial-enriched genes whose expression has been validated in the endothelium in vivo. Determination of the transcriptional profile of the endothelium has potentially wide-spanning implications for our understanding of vascular development (i.e., vessel patterning, differentiation), vascular homeostasis, and the diagnostic, prognostic, and therapeutic options for patients with cardiovascular diseases. As the biology underlying these gene lists is further delineated, we will gain more insight into the molecular mechanisms that are essential to the maintenance of endothelial phenotypes in vivo.

Conclusions

The vascular endothelium comprises a dynamic, multifunctional interface between blood and all of the tissues in the body. Among its most essential functions are the regulation of vascular permeability, thrombosis and hemostasis, inflammation, and vascular tone. These functions are modulated in response to both the local and systemic milieus. This adaptation accounts for its extensive regional specialization/heterogeneity within the vasculature, as well as its role in the maintenance of vascular homeostasis or the initiation/propagation of vascular diseases. Endothelial adaptation/activation occurs in the setting of physiologic and pathophysiologic stimuli, and can lead to phenotypical changes that maintain homeostasis and endothelial function or that result in pathologic alterations and endothelial dysfunction. Advances in our ability to measure endothelial function in vivo and to define endothelial phenotypes at the molecular level will enhance our understanding of endothelial phenotypic modulation in vivo and promise to yield new prognostic and therapeutic options for patients with vascular disease.

REFERENCES

1. Augustin HG, Kozian DH, Johnson RC: Differentiation of endothelial cells: Analysis of the constitutive and activated endothelial cell phenotypes. Bioessays 16:901, 1994.
2. Henderson AH: St Cyres lecture. Endothelium in control. Br Heart J 65:116, 1991.
3. Cines DB, Pollak ES, Buck CA, et al: Endothelial cells in physiology and in the pathophysiology of vascular disorders. Blood 91:3527, 1998.
4. Palade GE: Fine structures of blood capillaries. J Appl Physics 24:1424, 1953.
5. Fishman AP: Endothelium: A distributed organ of diverse capabilities. Ann N Y Acad Sci 401:1, 1982.
6. Fishman AP, Pietra GG: Permeability of pulmonary vascular endothelium. CIBA Found Symp:29, 1976.
7. Gimbrone MA, Jr, Alexander RW: Angiotensin II stimulation of prostaglandin production in cultured human vascular endothelium. Science 189:219, 1975.
8. Gimbrone MA, Jr: Endothelial dysfunction and atherosclerosis. J Card Surg 4:180, 1989.
9. Biegelsen ES, Loscalzo J: Endothelial function and atherosclerosis. Coron Artery Dis 10:241, 1999.
10. Gimbrone MA, Jr, Cotran RS, Folkman J: Human vascular endothelial cells in culture: Growth and DNA synthesis. J Cell Biol 60:673, 1974.
11. Jaffe EA, Nachman RL, Becker CG, et al: Culture of human endothelial cells derived from umbilical veins: Identification by morphologic and immunologic criteria. J Clin Invest 52:2745, 1973.
12. Lewis LJ, Hoak JC, Maca RD, et al: Replication of human endothelial cells in culture. Science 181:453, 1973.
13. Page C, Rose M, Yacoub M, et al: Antigenic heterogeneity of vascular endothelium. Am J Pathol 141:673, 1992.
14. Gerritsen ME: Functional heterogeneity of vascular endothelial cells. Biochem Pharmacol 36:2701, 1987.
15. Rajotte D, Arap W, Hagedorn M, et al: Molecular heterogeneity of the vascular endothelium revealed by in vivo phage display. J Clin Invest 102:430, 1998.
16. Aird WC: Endothelial cell heterogeneity. Crit Care Med 31:S221, 2003.
17. Lim YC, Garcia-Cardena G, Allport JR, et al: Heterogeneity of endothelial cells from different organ sites in T-cell subset recruitment. Am J Pathol 162:1591, 2003.
18. Broze GJ, Jr: Tissue factor pathway inhibitor and the revised theory of coagulation. Annu Rev Med 46:103, 1995.
19. Maynard JR, Dreyer BE, Stemerman MB, et al: Tissue-factor coagulant activity of cultured human endothelial and smooth muscle cells and fibroblasts. Blood 50:387, 1977.
20. Drake TA, Morrissey JH, Edgington TS: Selective cellular expression of tissue factor in human tissues: Implications for disorders of hemostasis and thrombosis. Am J Pathol 134:1087, 1989.
21. Wilcox JN, Smith KM, Schwartz SM, et al: Localization of tissue factor in the normal vessel wall and in the atherosclerotic plaque. Proc Natl Acad Sci U S A 86:2839, 1989.
22. Toomey JR, Kratzer KE, Lasky NM, et al: Targeted disruption of the murine tissue factor gene results in embryonic lethality. Blood 88:1583, 1996.
23. Osterud B: Tissue factor: A complex biological role. Thromb Haemost 78:755, 1997.
24. Wagner DD, Olmsted JB, Marder VJ: Immunolocalization of von Willebrand protein in Weibel-Palade bodies of human endothelial cells. J Cell Biol 95:355, 1982.
25. Wagner DD, Marder VJ: Biosynthesis of von Willebrand protein by human endothelial cells: Processing steps and their intracellular localization. J Cell Biol 99:2123, 1984.
26. Sporn LA, Chavin SI, Marder VJ, et al: Biosynthesis of von Willebrand protein by human megakaryocytes. J Clin Invest 76:1102, 1985.
27. Wiebel ER, Palade GE: New cytoplasmic components in arterial endothelia. J Cell Biol 23:101, 1964.
28. Fuchs A, Weibel ER: [Morphometric study of the distribution of a specific cytoplasmatic organoid in the rat's endothelial cells]. Z Zellforsch Mikrosk Anat 73:1, 1966.
29. Wagner DD: The Weibel-Palade body: The storage granule for von Willebrand factor and P-selectin. Thromb Haemost 70:105, 1993.
30. Dejana E: Endothelial adherens junctions: Implications in the control of vascular permeability and angiogenesis. J Clin Invest 98:1949, 1996.
31. Gerritsen ME: Physiological functions of normal endothelial cells. In Loscalzo J, Creager MA, Dzau VJ (eds): Vascular Medicine. New York, Little, Brown, 1996, p 3.
32. Renkin EM: Multiple pathways of capillary permeability. Circ Res 41:735, 1977.

33. Stan RV, Kubitza M, Palade GE: PV-1 is a component of the fenestral and stomatal diaphragms in fenestrated endothelia. Proc Natl Acad Sci U S A 96:13203, 1999.
34. Palade GE, Simionescu M, Simionescu N: Structural aspects of the permeability of the microvascular endothelium. Acta Physiol Scand Suppl 463:11, 1979.
35. Schnittler HJ: Structural and functional aspects of intercellular junctions in vascular endothelium. Basic Res Cardiol 93 Suppl 3:30, 1998.
36. Tedgui A: Endothelial permeability under physiological and pathological conditions. Prostaglandins Leukot Essent Fatty Acids 54:27, 1996.
37. Dejana E, Corada M, Lampugnani MG: Endothelial cell-to-cell junctions. Faseb J 9:910, 1995.
38. Simionescu M, Simionescu N, Palade GE: Segmental differentiations of cell junctions in the vascular endothelium: Arteries and veins. J Cell Biol 68:705, 1976.
39. Larson DM, Haudenschild CC, Beyer EC: Gap junction messenger RNA expression by vascular wall cells. Circ Res 66:1074, 1990.
40. Larson DM, Sheridan JD: Intercellular junctions and transfer of small molecules in primary vascular endothelial cultures. J Cell Biol 92:183, 1982.
41. Goodenough DA, Paul DL: Beyond the gap: Functions of unpaired connexon channels. Nat Rev Mol Cell Biol 4:285, 2003.
42. Alexander JS, Elrod JW: Extracellular matrix, junctional integrity and matrix metalloproteinase interactions in endothelial permeability regulation. J Anat 200:561, 2002.
43. Firth JA: Endothelial barriers: From hypothetical pores to membrane proteins. J Anat 200:541, 2002.
44. Lampugnani MG, Resnati M, Raiteri M, et al: A novel endothelial-specific membrane protein is a marker of cell-cell contacts. J Cell Biol 118:1511, 1992.
45. Lampugnani MG, Caveda L, Breviario F, et al: Endothelial cell-to-cell junctions: Structural characteristics and functional role in the regulation of vascular permeability and leukocyte extravasation. Baillieres Clin Haematol 6:539, 1993.
46. Lampugnani MG, Corada M, Caveda L, et al: The molecular organization of endothelial cell to cell junctions: Differential association of plakoglobin, beta-catenin, and alpha-catenin with vascular endothelial cadherin (VE-cadherin). J Cell Biol 129:203, 1995.
47. Stevens T, Rosenberg R, Aird W, et al: NHLBI workshop report: Endothelial cell phenotypes in heart, lung, and blood diseases. Am J Physiol Cell Physiol 281:C1422, 2001.
48. Rippe B, Rosengren BI, Carlsson O, et al: Transendothelial transport: The vesicle controversy. J Vasc Res 39:375, 2002.
49. Bendayan M: Morphological and cytochemical aspects of capillary permeability. Microsc Res Tech 57:327, 2002.
50. Michel CC: Transport of macromolecules through microvascular walls. Cardiovasc Res 32:644, 1996.
51. Bruns RR, Palade GE: Studies on blood capillaries. I. General organization of blood capillaries in muscle. J Cell Biol 37:244, 1968.
52. Stan RV: Structure and function of endothelial caveolae. Microsc Res Tech 57:350, 2002.
53. Simionescu M, Gafencu A, Antohe F: Transcytosis of plasma macromolecules in endothelial cells: A cell biological survey. Microsc Res Tech 57:269, 2002.
54. O'Donnell ME: Endothelial cell sodium-potassium-chloride cotransport: Evidence of regulation by Ca2+ and protein kinase C. J Biol Chem 266:11559, 1991.
55. Lau YT: Sodium transport in endothelial cells: A brief review. Chin J Physiol 38:139, 1995.
56. O'Donnell ME, Martinez A, Sun D: Endothelial Na-K-Cl cotransport regulation by tonicity and hormones: Phosphorylation of cotransport protein. Am J Physiol 269:C1513, 1995.
57. Topper JN, Wasserman SM, Anderson KR, et al: Expression of the bumetanide-sensitive Na-K-Cl cotransporter BSC2 is differentially regulated by fluid mechanical and inflammatory cytokine stimuli in vascular endothelium. J Clin Invest 99:2941, 1997.
58. Yerby TR, Vibat CR, Sun D, et al: Molecular characterization of the Na-K-Cl cotransporter of bovine aortic endothelial cells. Am J Physiol 273:C188, 1997.
59. Verkman AS: Aquaporin water channels and endothelial cell function. J Anat 200:617, 2002.
60. Milici AJ, L'Hernault N, Palade GE: Surface densities of diaphragmed fenestrae and transendothelial channels in different murine capillary beds. Circ Res 56:709, 1985.
61. Furchgott RF, Zawadzki JV: The obligatory role of endothelial cells in the relaxation of arterial smooth muscle by acetylcholine. Nature 288:373, 1980.
62. Palmer RM, Ferrige AG, Moncada S: Nitric oxide release accounts for the biological activity of endothelium-derived relaxing factor. Nature 327:524, 1987.
63. Ignarro LJ, Buga GM, Wood KS, et al: Endothelium-derived relaxing factor produced and released from artery and vein is nitric oxide. Proc Natl Acad Sci U S A 84:9265, 1987.
64. Fleming I, Busse R: Signal transduction of eNOS activation. Cardiovasc Res 43:532, 1999.
65. Vanhoutte PM, Scott-Burden T: The endothelium in health and disease. Tex Heart Inst J 21:62, 1994.
66. Marletta MA: Nitric oxide synthase structure and mechanism. J Biol Chem 268:12231, 1993.
67. Welch G, Loscalzo J: Nitric oxide and the cardiovascular system. J Card Surg 9:361, 1994.
68. Loscalzo J, Welch G: Nitric oxide and its role in the cardiovascular system. Prog Cardiovasc Dis 38:87, 1995.
69. Ranjan V, Xiao Z, Diamond SL: Constitutive NOS expression in cultured endothelial cells is elevated by fluid shear stress. Am J Physiol 269:H550, 1995.
70. Topper JN, Cai J, Falb D, et al: Identification of vascular endothelial genes differentially responsive to fluid mechanical stimuli: Cyclooxygenase-2, manganese superoxide dismutase, and endothelial cell nitric oxide synthase are selectively up-regulated by steady laminar shear stress. Proc Natl Acad Sci U S A 93:10417, 1996.
71. Arnet UA, McMillan A, Dinerman JL, et al: Regulation of endothelial nitric-oxide synthase during hypoxia. J Biol Chem 271:15069, 1996.
72. Saura M, Zaragoza C, Cao W, et al: Smad2 mediates transforming growth factor-beta induction of endothelial nitric oxide synthase expression. Circ Res 91:806, 2002.
73. Govers R, Rabelink TJ: Cellular regulation of endothelial nitric oxide synthase. Am J Physiol Renal Physiol 280:F193, 2001.
74. Gimbrone MA, Topper JN: Biology of the vessel wall: Endothelium. In Chien KR (ed): Molecular Basis of Heart Diseases. Troy, Mich, Harcourt Brace, 1998, p 331.
75. Michelson AD, Benoit SE, Furman MI, et al: Effects of nitric oxide/EDRF on platelet surface glycoproteins. Am J Physiol 270:H1640, 1996.
76. De Caterina R, Libby P, Peng HB, et al: Nitric oxide decreases cytokine-induced endothelial activation: Nitric oxide selectively reduces endothelial expression of adhesion molecules and proinflammatory cytokines. J Clin Invest 96:60, 1995.
77. Marcus AJ, Broekman MJ, Weksler BB, et al: Interactions between stimulated platelets and endothelial cells in vitro. Philos Trans R Soc Lond B Biol Sci 294:343, 1981.
78. Marcus AJ, Weksler BB, Jaffe EA: Enzymatic conversion of prostaglandin endoperoxide H2 and arachidonic acid to prostacyclin by cultured human endothelial cells. J Biol Chem 253:7138, 1978.
79. Oliva D, Nicosia S: PGI2-receptors and molecular mechanisms in platelets and vasculature: State of the art. Pharmacol Res Commun 19:735, 1987.
80. Miller OV, Gorman RR: Evidence for distinct prostaglandin I2 and D2 receptors in human platelets. J Pharmacol Exp Ther 210:134, 1979.
81. Schillinger E, Prior G: Prostaglandin I2 receptors in a particulate fraction of platelets of various species. Biochem Pharmacol 29:2297, 1980.
82. Majerus PW: Arachidonate metabolism in vascular disorders. J Clin Invest 72:1521, 1983.
83. Coleman RA, Smith WL, Narumiya S: International union of pharmacology classification of prostanoid receptors: Properties, distribution, and structure of the receptors and their subtypes. Pharmacol Rev 46:205, 1994.
84. Curwen KD, Gimbrone MA, Jr, Handin RI: In vitro studies of thromboresistance: The role of prostacyclin (PGI2) in platelet adhesion to cultured normal and virally transformed human vascular endothelial cells. Lab Invest 42:366, 1980.
85. Yanagisawa M, Kurihara H, Kimura S, et al: A novel potent vasoconstrictor peptide produced by vascular endothelial cells. Nature 332:411, 1988.
86. Inoue A, Yanagisawa M, Takuwa Y, et al: The human preproendothelin-1 gene: Complete nucleotide sequence and regulation of expression. J Biol Chem 264:14954, 1989.

87. Inoue A, Yanagisawa M, Kimura S, et al: The human endothelin family: Three structurally and pharmacologically distinct isopeptides predicted by three separate genes. Proc Natl Acad Sci U S A 86:2863, 1989.
88. Yoshizumi M, Kurihara H, Sugiyama T, et al: Hemodynamic shear stress stimulates endothelin production by cultured endothelial cells. Biochem Biophys Res Commun 161:859, 1989.
89. Malek AM, Greene AL, Izumo S: Regulation of endothelin 1 gene by fluid shear stress is transcriptionally mediated and independent of protein kinase C and cAMP. Proc Natl Acad Sci U S A 90:5999, 1993.
90. Shinoki N, Kawasaki T, Minamino N, et al: Shear stress downregulates gene transcription and production of adrenomedullin in human aortic endothelial cells. J Cell Biochem 71:109, 1998.
91. Masatsugu K, Itoh H, Chun TH, et al: Physiologic shear stress suppresses endothelin-converting enzyme-1 expression in vascular endothelial cells. J Cardiovasc Pharmacol 31:S42, 1998.
92. Harrison VJ, Ziegler T, Bouzourene K, et al: Endothelin-1 and endothelin-converting enzyme-1 gene regulation by shear stress and flow-induced pressure. J Cardiovasc Pharmacol 31 Suppl 1: S38, 1998.
93. Le Brun G, Aubin P, Soliman H, et al: Upregulation of endothelin 1 and its precursor by IL-1beta, TNF-alpha, and TGF-beta in the PC3 human prostate cancer cell line. Cytokine 11:157, 1999.
94. Morawietz H, Talanow R, Szibor M, et al: Regulation of the endothelin system by shear stress in human endothelial cells. J Physiol 525 Pt 3:761, 2000.
95. Gonzalez W, Chen Z, Damon DH: Transforming growth factor-beta regulation of endothelin expression in rat vascular cell and organ cultures. J Cardiovasc Pharmacol 37:219, 2001.
96. Lee SD, Lee DS, Chun YG, et al: Transforming growth factor-beta1 induces endothelin-1 in a bovine pulmonary artery endothelial cell line and rat lungs via cAMP. Pulm Pharmacol Ther 13:257, 2000.
97. Wasserman SM, Mehraban F, Komuves LG, et al: Gene expression profile of human endothelial cells exposed to sustained fluid shear stress. Physiol Genomics 12:13, 2002.
98. Cucina A, Sterpetti AV, Borrelli V, et al: Shear stress induces transforming growth factor-beta 1 release by endothelial cells. Surgery 123:212, 1998.
99. Tedgui A, Mallat Z: Anti-inflammatory mechanisms in the vascular wall. Circ Res 88:877, 2001.
100. DiChiara MR, Kiely JM, Gimbrone MA, Jr, et al: Inhibition of E-selectin gene expression by transforming growth factor beta in endothelial cells involves coactivator integration of Smad and nuclear factor kappaB-mediated signals. J Exp Med 192:695, 2000.
101. Shull MM, Ormsby I, Kier AB, et al: Targeted disruption of the mouse transforming growth factor-beta 1 gene results in multifocal inflammatory disease. Nature 359:693, 1992.
102. Middleton J, Patterson AM, Gardner L, et al: Leukocyte extravasation: Chemokine transport and presentation by the endothelium. Blood 100:3853, 2002.
103. Krieglstein CF, Granger DN: Adhesion molecules and their role in vascular disease. Am J Hypertens 14:S44, 2001.
104. Schaper W, Ito WD: Molecular mechanisms of coronary collateral vessel growth. Circ Res 79:911, 1996.
105. Zakrzewicz A, Secomb TW, Pries AR: Angioadaptation: Keeping the vascular system in shape. News Physiol Sci 17:197, 2002.
106. Luttun A, Carmeliet P: De novo vasculogenesis in the heart. Cardiovasc Res 58:378, 2003.
107. Oohira A, Wight TN, Bornstein P: Sulfated proteoglycans synthesized by vascular endothelial cells in culture. J Biol Chem 258:2014, 1983.
108. Kojima T, Leone CW, Marchildon GA, et al: Isolation and characterization of heparan sulfate proteoglycans produced by cloned rat microvascular endothelial cells. J Biol Chem 267:4859, 1992.
109. Werling RW, Zacharski LR, Kisiel W, et al: Distribution of tissue factor pathway inhibitor in normal and malignant human tissues. Thromb Haemost 69:366, 1993.
110. Levin EG, Santell L, Osborn KG: The expression of endothelial tissue plasminogen activator in vivo: A function defined by vessel size and anatomic location. J Cell Sci 110:139, 1997.
111. Risau W, Wolburg H: Development of the blood-brain barrier. Trends Neurosci 13:174, 1990.
112. Reese TS, Karnovsky MJ: Fine structural localization of a blood-brain barrier to exogenous peroxidase. J Cell Biol 34:207, 1967.
113. Brightman MW, Reese TS: Junctions between intimately apposed cell membranes in the vertebrate brain. J Cell Biol 40:648, 1969.
114. Crone C, Olesen SP: Electrical resistance of brain microvascular endothelium. Brain Res 241:49, 1982.
115. Nagy Z, Peters H, Huttner I: Fracture faces of cell junctions in cerebral endothelium during normal and hyperosmotic conditions. Lab Invest 50:313, 1984.
116. Banks WA, Kastin AJ, Broadwell RD: Passage of cytokines across the blood-brain barrier. Neuroimmunomodulation 2:241, 1995.
117. Broadwell RD: Endothelial cell biology and the enigma of transcytosis through the blood-brain barrier. Adv Exp Med Biol 331:137, 1993.
118. Broadwell RD: Transcytosis of macromolecules through the blood-brain barrier: A cell biological perspective and critical appraisal. Acta Neuropathol (Berl) 79:117, 1989.
119. Keep RF, Xiang J, Betz AL: Potassium transport at the blood-brain and blood-CSF barriers. Adv Exp Med Biol 331:43, 1993.
120. Betz AL: An overview of the multiple functions of the blood-brain barrier. NIDA Res Monogr 120:54, 1992.
121. Goldstein GW, Betz AL: The blood-brain barrier. Sci Am 255:74, 1986.
122. Betz AL, Goldstein GW: Specialized properties and solute transport in brain capillaries. Annu Rev Physiol 48:241, 1986.
123. Betz AL, Gilboe DD, Drewes LR: The characteristics of glucose transport across the blood brain barrier and its relation to cerebral glucose metabolism. Adv Exp Med Biol 69:133, 1976.
124. Abbott NJ: Astrocyte-endothelial interactions and blood-brain barrier permeability. J Anat 200:629, 2002.
125. Chishty M, Reichel A, Begley DJ, et al: Glial induction of blood-brain barrier-like l-system amino acid transport in the ECV304 cell line. Glia 39:99, 2002.
126. Deen WM, Lazzara MJ, Myers BD: Structural determinants of glomerular permeability. Am J Physiol Renal Physiol 281:F579, 2001.
127. Simionescu M, Simionescu N: Functions of the endothelial cell surface. Annu Rev Physiol 48:279, 1986.
128. Rostgaard J, Qvortrup K: Electron microscopic demonstrations of filamentous molecular sieve plugs in capillary fenestrae. Microvasc Res 53:1, 1997.
129. Fulton D, Papapetropoulos A, Zhang X, et al: Quantification of eNOS mRNA in the canine cardiac vasculature by competitive PCR. Am J Physiol Heart Circ Physiol 278:H658, 2000.
130. Wang J, Felux D, VandeBerg J, et al: Discordance of endothelial nitric oxide synthase in the arterial wall and its circulating products in baboons: Interactions with redox metabolism. Eur J Clin Invest 33:288, 2003.
131. Xu XP, Liu Y, Tanner MA, et al: Differences in nitric oxide production in porcine resistance arteries and epicardial conduit coronary arteries. J Cell Physiol 168:539, 1996.
132. Smith SK: Regulation of angiogenesis in the endometrium. Trends Endocrinol and Metab 12:147, 2001.
133. Gargett CE, Rogers PA: Human endometrial angiogenesis. Reproduction 121:181, 2001.
134. Herbert JM, Savi P, Laplace MC, et al: IL-4 inhibits LPS-, IL-1 beta- and TNF alpha-induced expression of tissue factor in endothelial cells and monocytes. FEBS Lett 310:31, 1992.
135. Bartha K, Brisson C, Archipoff G, et al: Thrombin regulates tissue factor and thrombomodulin mRNA levels and activities in human saphenous vein endothelial cells by distinct mechanisms. J Biol Chem 268:421, 1993.
136. Grabowski EF, Zuckerman DB, Nemerson Y: The functional expression of tissue factor by fibroblasts and endothelial cells under flow conditions. Blood 81:3265, 1993.
137. Vallet B, Wiel E: Endothelial cell dysfunction and coagulation. Crit Care Med 29:S36, 2001.
138. Joyce DE, Gelbert L, Ciaccia A, et al: Gene expression profile of antithrombotic protein C defines new mechanisms modulating inflammation and apoptosis. J Biol Chem 276:11199, 2001.
139. Aird WC: The role of the endothelium in severe sepsis and multiple organ dysfunction syndrome. Blood 101:3765, 2003.
140. Hack CE, Zeerleder S: The endothelium in sepsis: Source of and a target for inflammation. Crit Care Med 29:S21, 2001.
141. Cheng T, Dong L, Griffin JH, et al: Activated protein C blocks p53-mediated apoptosis in ischemic human brain endothelium and is neuroprotective. Nat Med 9:338, 2003.

142. Warren HS, Suffredini AF, Eichacker PQ, et al: Risks and benefits of activated protein C treatment for severe sepsis. N Engl J Med 347:1027, 2002.
143. Segal MS, Bihorac A, Koc M: Circulating endothelial cells: Tea leaves for renal disease. Am J Physiol Renal Physiol 283:F11, 2002.
144. Savage CO: The evolving pathogenesis of systemic vasculitis. Clin Med 2:458, 2002.
145. Cid MC: Endothelial cell biology, perivascular inflammation, and vasculitis. Cleve Clin J Med 69:SII45, 2002.
146. Ross R: Atherosclerosis: An inflammatory disease. N Engl J Med 340:115, 1999.
147. Zarins CK, Giddens DP, Bharadvaj BK, et al: Carotid bifurcation atherosclerosis: Quantitative correlation of plaque localization with flow velocity profiles and wall shear stress. Circ Res 53:502, 1983.
148. Gimbrone MA, Jr: Vascular endothelium, hemodynamic forces, and atherogenesis. Am J Pathol 155:1, 1999.
149. Bergers G, Benjamin LE: Tumorigenesis and the angiogenic switch. Nat Rev Cancer 3:401, 2003.
150. Jain RK: Molecular regulation of vessel maturation. Nat Med 9:685, 2003.
151. Ludmer PL, Selwyn AP, Shook TL, et al: Paradoxical vasoconstriction induced by acetylcholine in atherosclerotic coronary arteries. N Engl J Med 315:1046, 1986.
152. Behrendt D, Ganz P: Endothelial function: From vascular biology to clinical applications. Am J Cardiol 90:L40, 2002.
153. Kuvin JT, Karas RH: Clinical utility of endothelial function testing: Ready for prime time? Circulation 107:3243, 2003.
154. Bonetti PO, Lerman LO, Lerman A: Endothelial dysfunction: A marker of atherosclerotic risk. Arterioscler Thromb Vasc Biol 23:168, 2003.
155. Hackman A, Abe Y, Insull W, Jr, et al: Levels of soluble cell adhesion molecules in patients with dyslipidemia. Circulation 93:1334, 1996.
156. Blann AD, Seigneur M, Steiner M, et al: Circulating ICAM-1 and VCAM-1 in peripheral artery disease and hypercholesterolaemia: Relationship to the location of atherosclerotic disease, smoking, and in the prediction of adverse events. Thromb Haemost 79:1080, 1998.
157. Blann AD, McCollum CN, Steiner M, et al: Circulating adhesion molecules in inflammatory and atherosclerotic vascular disease. Immunol Today 16:251, 1995.
158. Malik I, Danesh J, Whincup P, et al: Soluble adhesion molecules and prediction of coronary heart disease: A prospective study and meta-analysis. The Lancet 358:971, 2001.
159. Shijubo N, Imai K, Aoki S, et al: Circulating intercellular adhesion molecule-1 (ICAM-1) antigen in sera of patients with idiopathic pulmonary fibrosis. Clin Exp Immunol 89:58, 1992.
160. Blann AD, Lip GY, McCollum CN: Changes in von Willebrand factor and soluble ICAM, but not soluble VCAM, soluble E-selectin or soluble thrombomodulin, reflect the natural history of the progression of atherosclerosis. Atherosclerosis 165:389, 2002.
161. Blann AD, Amiral J, McCollum CN: Prognostic value of increased soluble thrombomodulin and increased soluble E-selectin in ischaemic heart disease. Eur J Haematol 59:115, 1997.
162. Blann A, Kumar P, Krupinski J, et al: Soluble intercelluar adhesion molecule-1, E-selectin, vascular cell adhesion molecule-1 and von Willebrand factor in stroke. Blood Coagul Fibrinolysis 10:277, 1999.
163. Blann AD, Farrell A, Picton A, et al: Relationship between endothelial cell markers and arterial stenosis in peripheral and carotid artery disease. Thromb Res 97:209, 2000.
164. Seljeflot I, Tonstad S, Hjermann I, et al: Reduced expression of endothelial cell markers after 1 year treatment with simvastatin and atorvastatin in patients with coronary heart disease. Atherosclerosis 162:179, 2002.
165. Blann AD, McCollum CN: Circulating endothelial cell/leukocyte adhesion molecules in atherosclerosis. Thromb Haemost 72:151, 1994.
166. Blann AD, Seigneur M, Steiner M, et al: Circulating endothelial cell markers in peripheral vascular disease: Relationship to the location and extent of atherosclerotic disease. Eur J Clin Invest 27:916, 1997.
167. Lin Y, Weisdorf DJ, Solovey A, et al: Origins of circulating endothelial cells and endothelial outgrowth from blood. J Clin Invest 105:71, 2000.
168. Lin Y, Chang L, Solovey A, et al: Use of blood outgrowth endothelial cells for gene therapy for hemophilia a. Blood 99:457, 2002.
169. Hill JM, Zalos G, Halcox JPJ, et al: Circulating endothelial progenitor cells, vascular function, and cardiovascular risk. N Engl J Med 348:593, 2003.
170. Vasa M, Fichtlscherer S, Aicher A, et al: Number and migratory activity of circulating endothelial progenitor cells inversely correlate with risk factors for coronary artery disease. Circ Res 89:E1-7, 2001.
171. Aicher A, Heeschen C, Mildner-Rihm C, et al: Essential role of endothelial nitric oxide synthase for mobilization of stem and progenitor cells. Nat Med 9:1370, 2003.
172. Asahara T, Murohara T, Sullivan A, et al: Isolation of putative progenitor endothelial cells for angiogenesis. Science 275:964, 1997.
173. Yang R-B, Tomlinson JE, Conley PB, et al: Molecular profile of human endothelium revealed by large-scale expression profiling analyses. Physiologist 45:76, 2002.
174. Tomlinson JE, Topper JN: New insights into endothelial diversity. Curr Atheroscler Rep 5:223, 2003.
175. Ho M, Yang E, Matcuk G, et al: Identification of endothelial cell genes by combined database mining and microarray analysis. Physiol Genomics 13:249, 2003.

■ ■ ■ chapter 2

Vascular Smooth Muscle

Bradford C. Berk

In this chapter the biology of vascular smooth muscle cells (VSMC) will be discussed. Because recent studies of VSMC development provide important information about the mechanisms responsible for the differentiation of VSMC precursors and organization of blood vessels, developmental biology will provide the basis for the first portion of the chapter. Next the functions of VSMC as regulators of vascular tone and pressure will be examined. Finally, the role of VSMC in structural adaptations of vessels, especially as they pertain to pathogenic conditions such as wound repair, hypertension, and atherosclerosis, will be discussed.

WHAT IS A VASCULAR SMOOTH MUSCLE CELL?

VSMC were first identified by their appearance (elongated, bipolar, containing actin-myosin fibers anchored to dense bodies, and arrangement in palisading rows) and location (in the tunica media and neointima after injury); however, it quickly became clear that cells with differing morphologies could also appear in the same location. Are these VSMC? Do they function as VSMC? The answer to the first question is being addressed by use of differentiation markers of protein and gene expression. There are many markers of differentiated VSMC that reflect activation of a genetic program that in aggregate is characteristic of VSMC. The most classic markers of differentiated VSMC are contractile proteins. Unfortunately, after phenotypic modulation, many of these markers are no longer expressed, and thus, particularly in neointima, it is not always possible to use them to identify VSMC.

The answer to the second question is also difficult because VSMC have many functions other than contraction, including matrix production, immune regulation, and cytokine production. It has become clear that "normal" VSMC are functionally heterogeneous. Several mechanisms could explain this heterogeneity. (1) As described subsequently, the sources of precursor cells that generate VSMC differ during development. Thus, there may be embryonic cells (progenitors) left from development similar to those isolated from fetal animals.[1] For example, Schwartz and colleagues[2] have shown that proliferating VSMC isolated from the aorta express unique cytochrome P-450 enzymes that are typical of embryonic VSMC. Alternatively, circulating bone marrow-derived cells may differentiate into VSMC.[3-8] (2) There may be two types of VSMC—one that can undergo a dedifferentiation process to proliferate recapitulating development (a resident stem cell); and another that is terminally differentiated and, therefore, able to migrate but not to proliferate. These two types could be genetically determined or a consequence of environmental modification. For example, inflammatory cells or oxidized low-density lipoproteins may stimulate expression of growth factor receptors in VSMC, which could then lead to growth factor-dependent proliferation. Because VSMC are sources of many autocrine growth factors, they may be constantly exposed to potential mitogens. (3) There may be heterogeneity within the vessel wall that modifies the local environment. Here I cite three examples: (a) Variations in hemodynamic forces may cause local gradients in nutrients (e.g., increased residence time of oxidized lipids) or local metabolic requirements (e.g., increased energy metabolism or altered cytoskeleton arrangements).[9-11] Hemodynamic forces are sensed by the vessel; data show that EC production and release of growth factors are regulated by shear stress.[10-12] (b) Variation in matrix composition may be important, as illustrated by the fact that fibronectin is believed to be growth promoting and laminin to be growth inhibiting.[13,14] (c) Variations in uptake of circulating cells (e.g., leukocytes) or circulating substances (e.g., low-density lipoprotein) may create different local environments. In summary, it is useful to think of VSMC as pluripotent cells able to serve many functions in the vessel wall. The plasticity of VSMC is likely a result of differing origin and ability to undergo phenotypic modulation in response to environmental cues.

DEVELOPMENT AND DIFFERENTIATION OF VASCULAR SMOOTH MUSCLE

Blood Vessel Formation: Role of VSMC

The embryonic processes of vessel formation, growth, and remodeling provide important insights into mechanisms that regulate VSMC function in the adult (Fig. 2-1). The process of blood vessel formation in the embryo is termed vasculogenesis and initially involves the differentiation of angioblasts into endothelial cells (EC) that assemble into a primitive vascular network. Subsequently, growth and remodeling of the network occur to yield mature vasculature. In the adult, three processes can be used to form new vessels (1) vasculogenesis (rarely); (2) angiogenesis; and (3) arteriogenesis. Angiogenesis is the growth of new vessels from existing vessels, and it usually involves budding and then branching of EC-lined tubes from existing vessels. Arteriogenesis has frequently been termed *collateral vessel growth* and refers to enlargement of small arterioles into larger vessels.

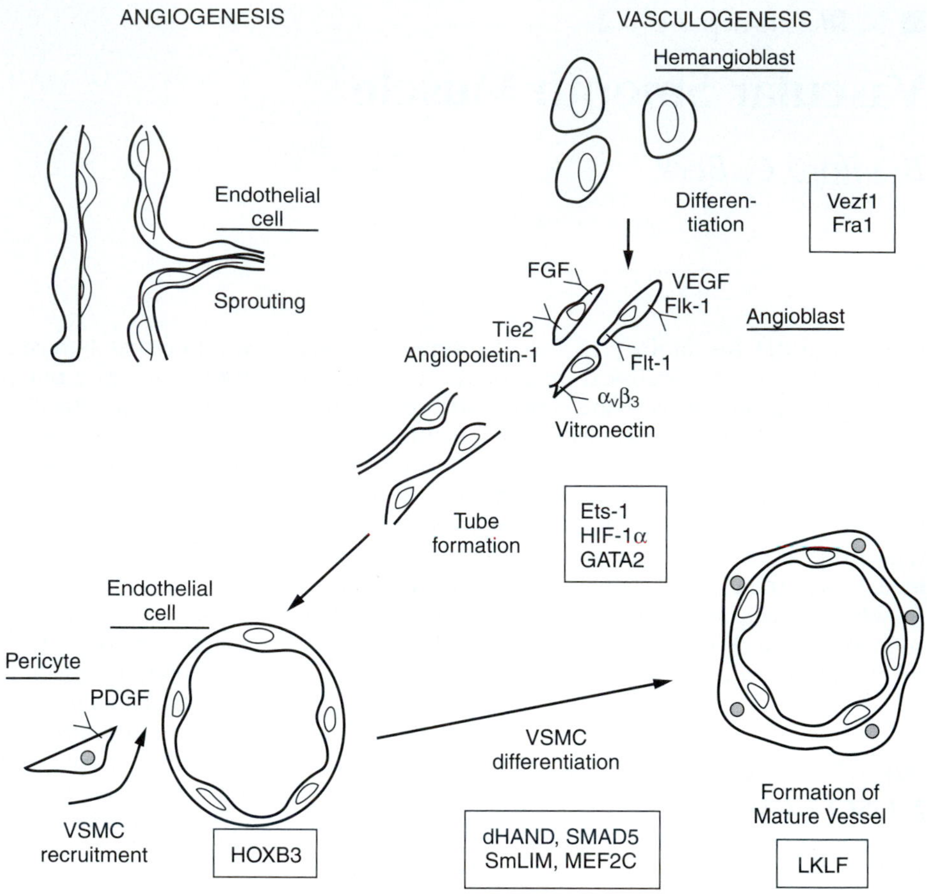

FIGURE 2-1. A model for vasculogenesis and angiogenesis. Cell types are underlined, transcription factors relevant to each stage are shown in boxes, and growth factors and their receptors are shown next to the cells. PDGF, platelet-derived growth factor; VSMC, vascular smooth muscle cells. (From Oettgen P: Transcriptional regulation of vascular development. Circ Res 89:380, 2001.)

Because these processes have been extensively reviewed,[15-17] this section will focus primarily on VSMC developmental features, especially as they relate to vessel heterogeneity and patterning, VSMC differentiation, and vascular remodeling.

An important concept in VSMC biology is phenotypic modulation, which referred originally to the morphologic change in VSMC from contractile (many actin-myosin fibers) to synthetic (many endoplasmic reticulum and Golgi).[18] This term is now used to define VSMC biochemically (based on protein and gene expression) that are changing their function in response to environmental stimuli. Phenotypic modulation is particularly useful to explain the diversity and heterogeneity of VSMC because it has become clear that VSMC serve multiple roles besides contraction and maintenance of tone. Many stimuli have been shown to promote phenotypic modulation (Table 2-1), and these same factors are important in vascular development and the response of VSMC to injury and disease.

The process by which VSMC contribute to vessel formation may be divided into three stages (1) recruitment and growth; (2) differentiation; and (3) remodeling (see Fig. 2-1)[19] For each stage, a specific set of signal events mediates the proper spatio-temporal coordination that results in formation of different types of vessels (e.g., arteries and veins) with unique properties. The concepts of lineage determination and differentiation are important to understand VSMC function during vessel formation. Lineage determination refers to the progenitor cells that give rise to differentiated cells that appear to be VSMC on the basis of morphology, gene expression, and function. Markers for lineage serve to identify VSMC to the exclusion of other cell types, whereas markers for differentiation serve to characterize the extent to which a given cell type resembles a mature, contractile VSMC. Clearly, the two markers overlap under many circumstances because contractile protein markers characterize both lineage and differentiation. Differentiation markers[20] include α-actin, SM22α (a calponin-like protein), telokin (a gene contained within the myosin light chain kinase gene), smoothelin (a cytoskeletal protein), and smooth muscle myosin heavy chain (MHC). It is important to note that many VSMC may not express all normal VSMC markers as part of a disease process or response to injury. Importantly, many VSMC differentation markers are expressed by other cells. For example, α-actin is a classic VSMC differentiation marker because it is the first known protein expressed during VSMC development,[16] and it is highly expressed in a selective manner in adult VSMC; however, α-actin is also expressed by skeletal and cardiac muscle during development, in fibroblasts during wound repair, and in EC during vascular remodeling. Another important concept is the distinction of differentiation from proliferation. Although it is true that many cell types "dedifferentiate" to proliferate, it is possible for VSMC to proliferate while they differentiate (as measured by VSMC-specific markers).

TABLE 2-1 FACTORS THAT INFLUENCE VSMC PHENOTYPE AND GROWTH

Factors	Specific Mediators
Cellular	Endothelial cells
	Inflammatory cells
	Nerves
	VSMC
Mechanical force	Hemodynamic forces
	Wall-stress strain
	Shear stress
Extracellular matrix	Matrix proteins (collagen, fibronectin, vitronectin, HSPGs, perlecan, biglycan)
	Integrin-mediated interactions
	Matrix turnover (MMPs, uPA, tPA, TIMPs)
Hormones (paracrine and autocrine)	Growth factors: TKR ligands (EGF, FGF, PDGF)
	Growth factors: GPCR ligands (angiotensin II, endothelin-1, norepinephrine, thrombin)
	Lipid mediators (LPA, sphingosine, lipoproteins)
	Other factors: TGF-β, SOXF (cyclophilins, heat shock proteins)
	Inflammatory mediators (LPS, ROS, interleukins, MCP-1, eotaxin)
Small molecules	Oxygen tension
	Reactive oxygen and nitrogen species
	Chemicals (glucose, advanced glycosylation end products)

EGF, epidermal growth factor; FGF, fibroblast growth factor; GPCR, G protein-coupled receptor; HSPG, heparan sulfate proteoglycan; LPA, lysophosphatidic acid; LPS, lipopolysaccharide; MCP-1, monocyte chemotactic peptide-1; MMPs, matrix metalloprotease; PDGF, platelet-derived growth factor; ROS, reactive oxygen species; TIMPs, tissue inhibitor of metalloproteinases; TKR, tyrosine kinase receptor; uPA, urokinase; VSMC, vascular smooth muscle cell.

Blood Vessel Formation: VSMC Recruitment and Growth

The first cell responsible for the formation of the primordial blood vessel tube is the EC (see Fig. 2-1).[15-17,19,21] Once the primitive EC tubes are formed, the endothelium secretes factors that lead to the recruitment and/or induction of primordial smooth muscle, a process termed vascular myogenesis. Several recent reviews have carefully documented the current state of knowledge regarding the differentiation and growth of VSMC to form the tunica media.[15-17] This process may occur by (1) angiopoietin-1-mediated production of VSMC inducing factor(s) by EC that causes differentiation from mesoderm; (2) angiopoietin-1 induced differentiation of EC, bone marrow precursors, or macrophages into VSMC (transdifferentiation)[22]; (3) transformation of epicardial cells to form the coronary VSMC[16,23]; and (4) differentiation of the mesoectoderm of the neural crest into VSMC.[24,25] It is clear from these examples that VSMC have a complex origin depending on their location within the vasculature. For example, VSMC of coronary veins are derived from atrial myocardium, whereas VSMC of coronary arteries are derived from epicardium.[26] This distinction suggests that individual growth factors and their receptors will have different effects on VSMC growth and differentiation in specific vascular beds.

Factors that act as chemoattractants for VSMC recruitment include platelet-derived growth factor (PDGF)-BB and VEGF. Studies in mice lacking PDGF-BB and PDGFR-β[27] suggest that PDGFR-β–expressing VSMC progenitors form around certain vessels by a process independent of PDGF-BB. These cells then undergo angiogenic sprouting and vessel enlargement in a process that is both PDGF-BB-dependent and -independent depending on tissue context. The growth factors secreted by embryonic EC that stimulate VSMC proliferation remain to be identified. It is possible that VSMC themselves, on interacting with embryonic EC, activate autocrine and paracrine pathways that lead to VSMC growth. Important roles for TGF-β1 and endoglin (an endothelial TGF-β receptor family member) have been established in that they stimulate VSMC differentiation and extracellular matrix deposition, strengthening EC-VSMC interactions.[28,29] Endothelin-1 appears to have an important role in migration and differentiation of VSMC from neural crest cells.[30] Other growth factors with important roles in VSMC recruitment and growth include tissue factor, HBEGF, and the ephrin-Eph receptor system.[17,31,32]

Several transcription factors appear to be important in VSMC recruitment and growth in the developing vessel. HOX genes are powerful regulators of pattern formation, as evidenced by the homeotic mutations (i.e., mutations in which one normal body part is substituted for another normal body part, as in *Antennapedia*). Several members of the HOX clusters are expressed in the cardiovascular system during embryogenesis, including *HOXA5*, *HOXA11*, *HOXB1*, *HOXB7*, and *HOXC9*.[33,34] Of these, *HOXB7* and *HOXC9* are expressed at markedly higher levels in embryonic VSMC compared with adult VSMC, suggesting a role in the proliferation and remodeling that occur during embryogenesis.[34] In addition, overexpression of *HOXB7* in C3H10T1/2 cells results in increased proliferation, induction of a VSMC-like morphology, and expression of VSMC markers. These observations suggest a role for *HOXB7* and perhaps *HOXC9* in vascular remodeling and VSMC proliferation. Functional evidence for involvement of HOX genes in vasculogenesis includes the finding that transgenic mice with null mutations of the *HOXA3* gene die shortly after birth, suffering from defects such as heart-wall malformations, persistent patent ductus arteriosus, and aortic stenosis.[35] Another important HOX-like gene is *Gax* (also known as *Mox-2*), which encodes a homeodomain-containing transcription factor whose expression has multiple effects on vascular phenotype.[34] *Gax* controls the migration of VSMC toward chemotactic growth factors through its ability to alter integrin expression.[36] In VSMC, *Gax* expression is downregulated rapidly by mitogens such as those contained in serum, PDGF, and angiotensin II. *Gax* expression induces G0/G1 cell-cycle arrest and upregulates p21 expression accounting for its antiproliferative activity. These data suggest that *Gax* may function to coordinate vascular cell growth and motility through its ability to regulate integrin expression in a cell cycle-dependent manner.

Blood Vessel Formation: VSMC Differentiation

As described earlier, VSMC differentiation occurs simultaneously with VSMC proliferation such that candidate mediators include many VSMC growth factors (see Table 2-1).[37] Important factors that stimulate VSMC differentiation from mesoderm include PDGF and TGF-β.[16,38] TGF-β is particularly important through its effects on the MADS-box factors, such as SMAD5 and MEF2C.[39,40] There is much information now regarding the transcription factors involved in VSMC differentiation.[19] VSMC differentiation involves transcriptional events mediated by the serum response factor (SRF); *Prx-1* and *Prx-2*; *CRP2/SmLIM*; and members of the *HOX*, *MEF2*, and *GATA* families among many others (Fig. 2-2).[9,34,40] A particularly important role for MADS (MDM1, agamous, deficiens, SRF) domain-containing proteins (MEF2C, SMAD5, and SRF) and their accessory binding factors (coactivators and corepressors) has recently been established.[40] SRF is required for specification of muscle lineages from early mesoderm. Transcriptional control that restricts gene expression to SMC is mediated by a conserved *cis*-regulatory element termed a CarG box (CC[A/T]$_6$GG). The CarG box binds SRF, which acts as a multifunctional protein to bind DNA and to assemble accessory cofactors. Among the SRF-dependent coactivators, recent data suggest that myocardin is a potent mediator of VSMC differentiation.[40-42] Myocardin expression is limited to cardiac and VSMC lineages in developing mouse embryos and is also expressed in adult VSMC. It is likely that myocardin-related transcription factors (MRTFs) also play a role in the maintenance of VSMC differentiation. Current data show that decreasing myocardin function reduces expression of VSMC-specific genes such as SM22α, SM α-actin, and SM-MHC. In addition to myocardin and MRTFs, SRF also interacts with the NK class homeodomain proteins including Nkx2.5, Nkx3.1, and Nkx3.2. Other factors that interact with the SRF-MADS domain include GATA6, Phox1, homeodomain-only protein (HOP), the LIM domain-containing cysteine-rich proteins Crp1 and Crp2, and chromatin organizing factors (HMGI[Y] and SSRP1). In addition to the SRF family, other well-studied transcription factors include dHAND and SmLIM. The phenotype of dHAND null mice suggests an important role for this transcription factor in EC-VSMC interactions as VSMC recruitment is normal, but differentiation fails to occur.[43] The diversity of these binding factors provides the signaling complexity necessary to create vessel heterogeneity and spatio-temporal patterning discussed subsequently.

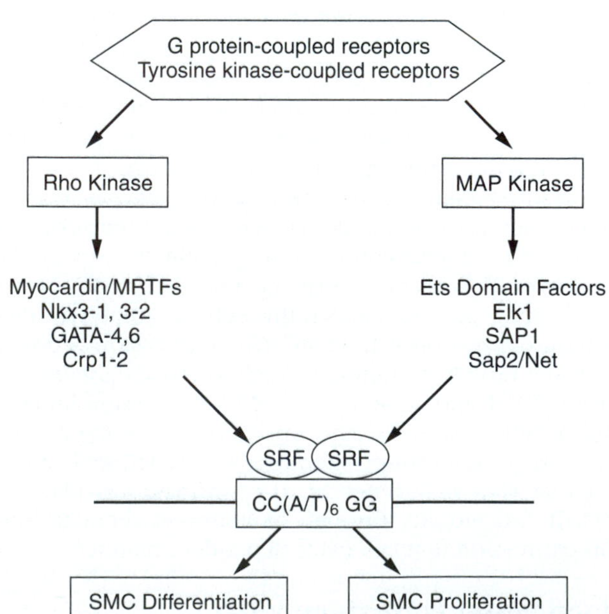

FIGURE 2-2. A model for regulation of SRF transcription by G protein-coupled receptor and tyrosine kinase-coupled receptor signal transduction. CC(A/T)$_6$GG represents the CarG box. SMC, smooth muscle cells; SRF, serum response factor.

The SRF accessory proteins are themselves regulated by phosphorylation by several kinases which are activated by classic VSMC growth factors that bind to both tyrosine kinase receptors and G protein-coupled receptors (see Fig. 2-2 and Table 2-1). Important roles for Rho kinase and MAP kinases (BMK1 [or ERK5], ERK1/2, p38 and JNK) have been elucidated. For example, the BMK1 knockout mouse has a vascular phenotype similar to the MEF2C knockout mouse, which is partially explained by the knowledge that MEF2C is a key BMK1 substrate.[44] A significant coincidence is the important role for these same kinases in contraction, growth, and migration, which likely reflects the fact that many of the same ligand-receptor combinations that are critical for VSMC differentiation play a functional role in the adult vessel.

Blood Vessel Formation: Remodeling

Remodeling during development includes both changes in existing vessels (increases or decreases in size), as well as formation of additional blood vessels (angiogenesis). Both processes involve growth factors and, importantly, physical forces. Among the growth factors are many angiogenic factors, such as vascular endothelial growth factor (VEGF). Physical forces, notably the initiation of blood flow, may have important effects on stimulating the primitive vessel to remodel especially via regulation of nitric oxide production. Angiogenesis is largely driven by hypoxia which activates transcription factors and stimulates expression of angiogenic factors. As one example, the hypoxia-inducible factor (HIF)-1α is a transcription factor that is highly regulated by hypoxia and by proteolysis leading to expression of VEGF and tissue factor.[45] Similar to SRF, HIF-1α interacts with adapter proteins (p300 and CREB-binding protein) to form a protein/DNA complex on angiogenic genes. Induction of HIF-1α by hypoxia is mediated by the phosphatidylinositol 3-kinase (PI3K) and by ERK1/2. HIF-1α is also rapidly regulated by proteolysis following ubiquitination mediated by the von Hippel-Lindau tumor-suppressor protein.

Many other transcription factors are involved in remodeling based on knockout mouse studies. Aortic arch abnormalities, as an example of defective remodeling, have been demonstrated in knockout mice that include MFH-1, dHAND or Msx1, Pax-3, Prx1, retinoic receptors, the neurofibromatosis type-p1 gene product, Wnt-1, connexin 43, and endothelin-1. An important class of regulators are the Kruppel-like family of zinc finger transcription factors. Mice deficient in LKLF, a family member, exhibit multiple vascular defects with a decreased number of differentiated VSMC and pericytes. A similar phenotype was observed in mice expressing a mutant ephrin B2 receptor, suggesting that ephrin B2 signaling may activate LKLF during vessel remodeling. In summary, it is clear that multiple cell-cell, transcriptional, and growth factor-related events participate in the process by which VSMC create the vascular media; many of these same processes occur in the adult during arteriogenesis and angiogenesis.

Veins Versus Arteries and Macrocirculation Versus Microcirculation

The most obvious functional heterogeneity in the vascular tree is the difference in function of arteries compared with veins. For example, veins are nearly immune to atherosclerosis, whereas conduit arteries (especially coronary arteries) are exquisitely sensitive to the pathologic process. Much has been learned regarding the characteristics of VSMC in arteries compared with veins.[17,31,32] Although the precise mechanisms responsible for the tissue boundaries and morphologic patterning that create arteries, capillaries, and veins remain unknown, several concepts are clear (Fig. 2-3).[46] Soluble and matrix-bound stimuli drive cells to migrate and provide the proper spatio-temporal information to cells that are not fully differentiated. These cells then encounter positional stimuli that provide information regarding the proper topographic patterns by restricting cell and tissue interactions. Three well-studied molecules[17,31,32] that have been shown to participate in these processes include: (1) soluble mediators such as semaphorins and netrins; (2) membrane-bound proteins such as the ephrin-Eph receptor system; and (3) extracellular matrix proteins. Most important for understanding the tissue boundaries responsible for arteries versus veins are the ephrins and Eph receptors that mediate cell-cell adhesion (or disruption of adherence) restricting cell intermingling and establishing (and maintaining) tissue boundaries. Wang and colleagues[32] showed that ephrin-B2, an Eph family transmembrane ligand, marks arterial, but not venous, EC from the onset of angiogenesis. Conversely, Eph-B4, a receptor for ephrin-B2, marks veins but not arteries. Ephrin-B2 knockout mice display defects in both arteries and veins in the capillary networks. These results provide evidence that differences between arteries and veins are, in part, genetically determined, and suggest that reciprocal signaling between these two types of vessels is crucial for morphogenesis of the capillary bed. In addition, many of the factors listed in Table 2-1 mediate differences between arteries and veins, including transcription factors, growth factors, and matrix. For example, SM22-α is uniquely expressed in arteries, suggesting that the transcription factors that regulate SM22-α promoter activity are only active in arteries.[47] Thus, much of the biology described above for SRF and myocardin function likely differs between arteries and veins.

In addition to differences in arteries and veins, there are clear examples of diversity in VSMC origin such as the arterial pole in the developing heart.[46] The great vessels connected to the heart contain VSMC with diverse embryologic origins because the mesenchymal precursor cells arise from both local and distant sources.[46] Primary among these are neural crest cells that migrate from the neural folds to the pharyngeal arches where they separate each arch artery and aortic sac from the pharyngeal ectoderm. In contrast, neural crest cells do not contribute to the venous pole.

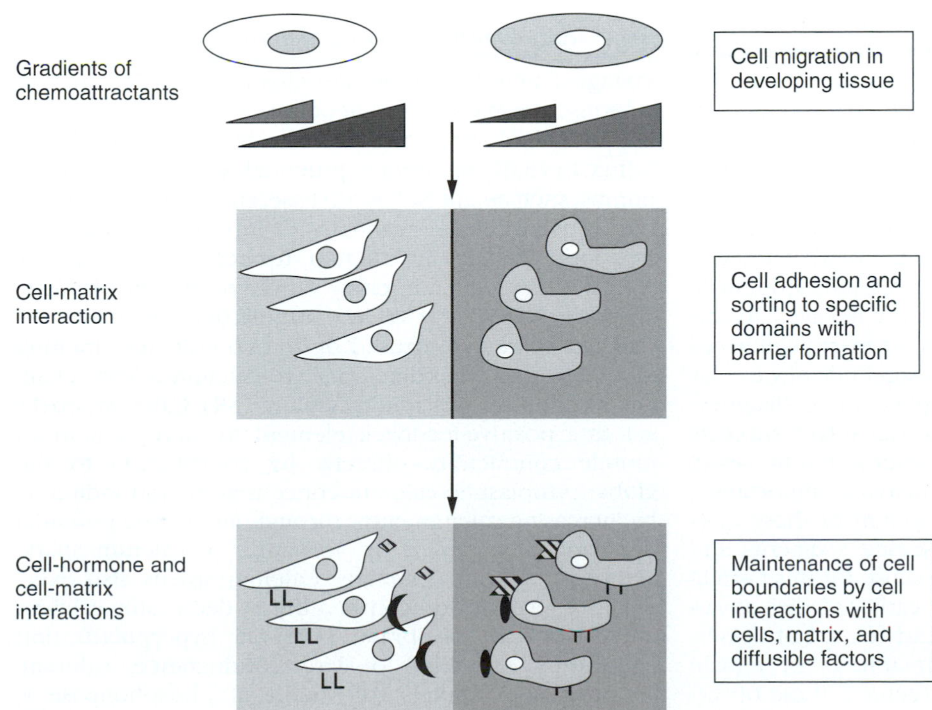

FIGURE 2-3. Mechanisms for formation of tissue boundaries and morphologic patterning of veins, capillaries, and arteries on the basis of soluble and matrix-bound stimuli. In the bottom panel, the *cross-hatched diamonds* and *rhomboids* represent soluble ligands and their receptors; the *solid ovals* and *crescents* represent heterophilic interacting ligands and receptors, such as the ephrin-Eph receptors, and the "feet" represent integrins that interact with matrix. (From Ausoni S, Sartore S: Cell lineages and tissue boundaries in cardiac arterial and venous poles: Developmental patterns, animal models, and implications for congenital vascular diseases. Arterioscler Thromb Vasc Biol 21:312, 2001.)

Another dramatic difference in the vascular tree is the unique nature of the microcirculation. As an example, the extracellular matrix protein fibulin-2 is synthesized by the VSMC precursor cells of developing aortic arch vessels that originate from neural crest cells.[48] Epicardial cells produce fibulin-2 on their migration over the myocardial surface, and its expression persists throughout coronary vasculogenesis and angiogenesis. Fibulin-2 is produced by the EC of coronary arteries and veins but not by the capillary EC in the myocardium. Thus, fibulin-2 not only uniquely marks the transformed mesenchymal cells during mouse embryonic cardiovascular development, but also indicates vascular EC of coronary arteries and veins in postnatal life.

Progenitor Cells: Bone Marrow and in Situ

It is clear that progenitor cells are the source of VSMC in the developing vessel during vasculogenesis, but in the adult, the source for new VSMC required for wound repair or remodeling remains unclear.[3-7] Three mechanisms seem likely to contribute to "new" VSMC in adult vessels: phenotypic modulation of preexisting VSMC, circulating bone marrow-derived VSMC progenitor cells, and vessel resident VSMC progenitor cells. Phenotypic modulation appears well supported as a mechanism by which a contractile VSMC changes its pattern of gene expression to allow it to assume a phenotype that is able to migrate and proliferate. Based on studies of neointima formation after balloon injury of a vessel, this process appears to recapitulate many of the events that likely occur in human restenosis. Indeed, when VSMC from arteries are placed in tissue culture, the process of phenotypic modulation ensues to permit proliferation.

Recent studies suggest a potential role for circulating progenitor cells in both neointima formation after vascular injury and in atherosclerosis.[3-7] In one study, mice were lethally irradiated and their bone marrow reconstituted with cells from a ROSA26 mouse that ubiquitously expresses β-galactosidase to permit lineage tracing by the presence of LacZ.[49] On severe injury of the femoral artery, the authors showed at 4 weeks that approximately 60% of the neointima cells and approximately 45% of the media cells expressed LacZ, indicating that bone-marrow–derived cells contributed to vessel repair after injury. A similar result was obtained by Han and colleagues, who used bone marrow reconstitution from male donors into female recipients to identify lineage.[7] In this study, the relative contribution of bone-marrow–derived cells appeared to correlate with the magnitude of vascular injury and repair. More recently, Caplice and colleagues[8] used sex-mismatched bone-marrow transplant subjects to show that VSMC throughout the atherosclerotic vessel wall can derive from donor bone marrow. Importantly, they demonstrated extensive recruitment of these cells in diseased compared with nondiseased segments and excluded cell-cell fusion events as a cause for this enrichment. The results of Caplice support earlier studies of vascular remodeling in mismatched heart transplant vessels (Y-chromosome-positive cells in recipients of female hearts). In transplanted hearts, between 6%[50] and 60%[51] of new vessel growth appeared to derive from the bone marrow. These data suggest that bone-marrow–derived cells contribute importantly to the VSMC response to injury and disease.

FUNCTIONS OF VASCULAR SMOOTH MUSCLE CELLS

Contraction and Maintenance of Tone

The key functional role of VSMC in many vessels (especially arterioles) is to maintain tone. In resistance arterioles, this is a major task, requiring energy expenditure 24 hours every day all year long. The need to maintain contraction continuously is the result of efficient energy use. This chapter will focus on the intracellular mechanisms responsible for VSMC contraction (Fig. 2-4), because many aspects of contraction induced by specific hormones and agonists will be covered in the chapter on vascular pharmacology (Chapter 5).

The second messenger that triggers contraction is a rise in intracellular calcium. The rise is usually the result of both calcium influx through plasma membrane channels and calcium release from intracellular stores. Following several signal events discussed subsequently, an increase in the activity of myosin light chain kinase (MLCK) and/or decrease in the activity of myosin light chain phosphatase (MLCP) results in increased MLC phosphorylation and increased myosin ATPase activity. Importantly, there are mechanisms that alter the sensitivity of this pathway to calcium termed *calcium sensitization*. In addition to calcium-dependent events, there are calcium-independent events, many of which are mediated by the Rho kinase pathway. Relaxation is mediated by multiple mechanisms that promote calcium efflux, calcium sequestration, and dephosphorylation of MLC.

Regulation of Intracellular Calcium

Voltage-dependent L-type Ca^{2+} channels (VDCC) open in response to membrane depolarization, indicating the importance of membrane potential in regulating calcium influx. In VSMC, membrane potential is regulated by both pumps, such as the Na^+, K^+-ATPase, and channels, such as the Ca^{2+}-sensitive K^+ channels.[52-54] It is important to note that local changes in calcium, termed *calcium sparks* activated by calcium entry through dihydropyridine-sensitive VDCC are a key regulatory mechanism.[55] Calcium sparks are caused by the coordinated opening of a cluster of ryanodine-sensitive calcium release channels in the sarcoplasmic reticulum (SR). Calcium sparks act as a positive-feedback element to increase smooth muscle contractility—directly by contributing to the global cytoplasmic calcium concentration and indirectly by increasing calcium entry through membrane potential depolarization caused by activation of calcium spark-activated chloride channels. Calcium sparks also exert negative feedback on contractility by decreasing calcium entry through membrane potential hyperpolarization caused by activation of large-conductance, calcium-sensitive K^+ channels. Activation of phospholipase C (PLC) and inositol 1,4,5-trisphosphate (IP_3) formation

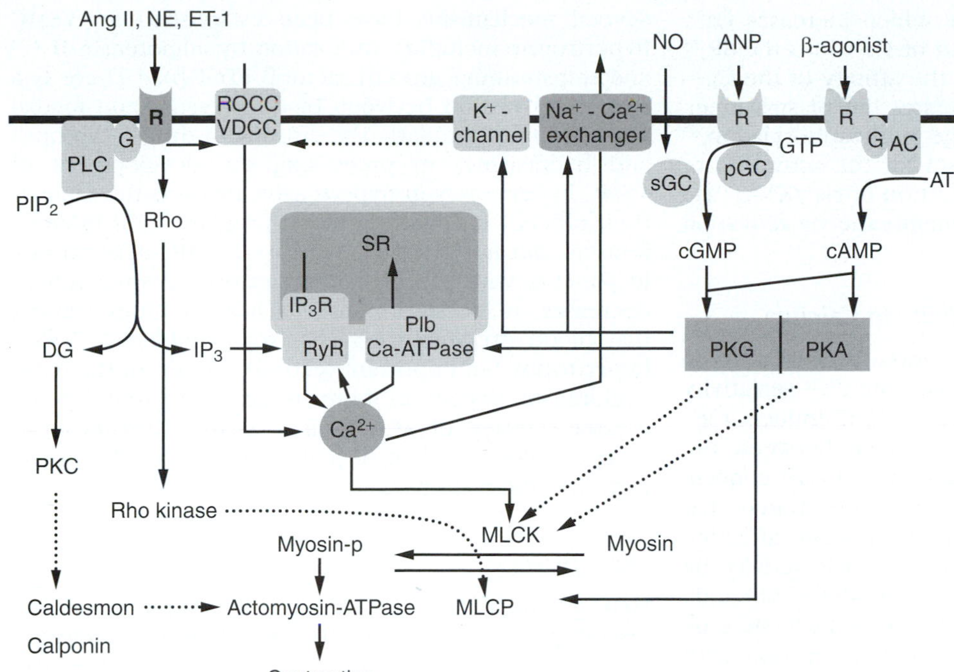

FIGURE 2-4. Regulation of VSMC tone and intracellular calcium. On *left side* are shown vasoconstrictor pathways that increase calcium and stimulate myosin phosphorylation. Regulation of myosin phosphorylation is via activation of MLCK and/or inhibition of MLCP. On the *right side* are shown vasodilator pathways that lower calcium and inhibit myosin phosphorylation. MLCP, myosin light chain phosphatase; MLCK, myosin light chain kinase.

are early key steps in hormone-stimulated increases in intracellular Ca^{2+} in VSMC. G-Protein-activated PLC catalyzes the hydrolysis of phosphatidylinositol 4, 5-biphosphates (PIP_2) to generate diacylglycerol (DAG) and IP_3, leading to the activation of PKC and the mobilization of intracellular Ca^{2+}. IP_3 generated by activation of PLC binds to its receptor present in the SR membrane; the IP_3 receptor is a channel protein that opens when bound to IP_3. Opening the IP_3 receptor channel permits Ca^{2+} efflux into the cytoplasm, increasing intracellular Ca^{2+}.

The contractile force of VSMC is primarily dependent on the status of MLC phosphorylation, which is regulated by the balance of MLCK and MLCP activities. MLCK is activated in a Ca^{2+} and calmodulin-dependent manner; and activation of MLCK leads to phosphorylation of MLC, increased MLC ATPase activity, and contraction. In contrast, activation of MLCP produces relaxation of VSMC. MLCP is a trimer composed of a 110 kD regulatory myosin-binding subunit (MBS), a 37 kD catalytic subunit (PP1c), and a 20-kD protein of uncertain function (M20). Phosphorylation of the MBS as described below is a key mechanism for regulation of MLCP.

Among calcium-independent pathways, Rho kinase is an important mediator of contraction via its effects on MLCP. The activity of the small GTPase RhoA is stimulated by guanosine exchange factors (GEF) and inhibited by GTPase-activating proteins (GAP). Activation of Rho kinase has been implicated in mediating many vasoconstrictor-elicited effects, such as angiotensin II-induced vascular contraction[56] and VSMC hypertrophy.[57] An important recent finding is that NO inactivates RhoA in a cGMP/PKG-dependent manner.[58] Specifically PKG was found to inhibit Rho kinase by phosphorylation and inactivation of RhoA, which is critical for RhoA-induced Ca^{2+} sensitization in VSMC (see Fig. 2-4).[58] For example, phosphorylation of the MBS regulatory subunit of MLCP by Rho kinase at threonine 695 leads to inhibition of MLCP activity, inducing Ca^{2+} sensitization of the contractile apparatus.[58,59] In contrast, PKG inactivation of RhoA/Rho kinase increases MLCP activity and inhibits vascular contraction.[58,59]

Intracellular Ca^{2+} Sequestration and PKG Action

Nitric oxide (NO) lowers intracellular Ca^{2+} in VSMC both by direct effects and by increasing intracellular cGMP and activating PKG. Both exogenous NO and native EDRF can directly activate Ca^{2+}-dependent K^+ channels in cell-free membrane patches without requiring cGMP. In addition, Cohen and colleagues showed that the initial, rapid decrease in intracellular Ca^{2+} caused by NO in VSMC was due to uptake of Ca^{2+} by SERCA into intracellular stores.[60] They further proposed that the refilling of the stores inhibited store-operated Ca^{2+} influx through non-L-type Ca^{2+} conducting ion channels and that this maintained the intracellular Ca^{2+} at a low level facilitating relaxation. Increases in cGMP and activation of PKG by NO could regulate Ca^{2+} in at least five different ways (see Fig. 2-4): (1) downregulating IP_3 formation; (2) decreasing Ca^{2+} mobilization through the IP_3 receptor; (3) promoting Ca^{2+} sequestration in the SR; (4) reducing Ca^{2+} influx; and (5) increasing Ca^{2+} efflux. The two most important sites for PKG regulation appear to be the IP_3 receptor and phospholamban. PKG phosphorylates the IP_3 receptor reducing channel activity and decreasing Ca^{2+} concentration.[61] Recently, a protein termed the IP_3 receptor-associated cGMP kinase substrate (IRAG) has been identified[62] that appears to be required for NO/PKG-dependent regulation of IP_3-induced Ca^{2+} release. PKG increases uptake of Ca^{2+} into the SR via activation of the SR Ca^{2+}-pumping ATPase (Ca^{2+}-ATPase).[63] The activity of the Ca^{2+}-ATPase in SR is regulated by the protein phospholamban.[64] In VSMC, PKG phosphorylates phospholamban, which increases Ca^{2+}-ATPase activity and sequestration of Ca^{2+} into the SR,[65] probably due to the increase in the affinity of the Ca^{2+}-ATPase for Ca^{2+}.[66] PKG Iα stimulates the plasma membrane Ca^{2+}-ATPase without change in phosphorylation,[67] suggesting an indirect mechanism for the activation of the Ca^{2+}-ATPase, perhaps via activation of Na^+/K^+-ATPase or hyperpolarization of the cell membrane via activation of K^+ channels.[68]

Regulation of Contractile Sensitivity to Calcium

In addition to its effects to lower intracellular Ca^{2+} concentration, NO/cGMP also decreases the Ca^{2+} sensitivity of contractile proteins. For example, cGMP induces Ca^{2+} desensitization by altering the balance between the activities of MLCK and MLCP at a constant Ca^{2+} concentration (see Fig. 2-4). Studies have demonstrated that cGMP/PKG induces MLCP activity without affecting MLCK activity.[69] PKG may increase MLCP activity by phosphorylation of the MBS subunit of MLCP.[70] In addition, it is known that PKG Iα is targeted to the VSMC contractile apparatus by a leucine zipper interaction with the MBS subunit of MLCP. Uncoupling of the PKG Iα-MBS interaction prevents cGMP-dependent dephosphorylation of MLC, demonstrating that this interaction is essential to the regulation of VSMC tone.[71] Finally, as described above, PKG phosphorylation of RhoA activates MLCP and promotes VSMC relaxation.

VSMC Functions in Wound Repair: Focus on Growth

VSMC Growth Responses

Growth factors have been isolated and characterized by their ability to stimulate growth of cultured cells. This research approach has caused us to think of growth factors as circulating factors that are released by platelets during injury (e.g., PDGF) or generated from circulating prohormones (e.g., angiotensin I to angiotensin II, prothrombin to thrombin); however, this simple concept may be the exception rather than the rule. In fact, temporal and spatial expressions of growth factors and their receptors are dynamically regulated locally within the vessel wall. Newer molecular techniques, as well as the availability of antibodies to specific vascular growth factors, have helped define the growth factors that are important in vessel growth.[37]

One of the distinguishing features of VSMC is the plasticity of their growth responses. VSMC respond in three ways to alterations in their environment: hyperplasia, hypertrophy, and apoptosis. In diseases such as chronic hypertension, all three responses may be observed in different-sized vessels or even within the same vessel. Although VSMC plasticity offers an advantage in terms of its adaptability, this process may be pathologic in humans. In particular, although hypertrophy is reversible, hyperplasia and apoptosis are not.

Hypertrophy

Hypertrophy is defined as an increase in cell size without cell division (and usually without DNA synthesis). Several mechanisms have been established for VSMC hypertrophy, including stimulation by angiotensin II[72,73] and transforming growth factor-β (TGF-β).[74] There is a strong correlation between blood pressure and medial VSMC content. Similarly, the efficacy of drugs (captopril and hydralazine) in preventing the development of VSMC hypertrophy in hypertensive rats was the same as their efficacy in lowering blood pressure.[75] Of interest, losartan, but not atenolol, decreased VSMC hypertrophy in patients with essential hypertension, despite similar decreases in blood pressure.[76] These findings suggest that blood pressure itself is a key regulator of VSMC hypertrophy, but important secondary roles for the renin angiotensin system in humans are suggested by the greater efficacy of ACE inhibitors and angiotensin II receptor blockers than of β-blockers in modulating the hypertrophic responses.

Hyperplasia

Hyperplasia of VSMC is a dominant component of the disease process in human atherosclerosis, hypertension, and restenosis. In many of these diseases, there is also medial atrophy (due both to necrosis and apoptosis) associated with loss of VSMC. Thus, if cell death precedes VSMC growth, hyperplasia could be viewed as an adaptive change; however, the reverse appears to be true: VSMC proliferation precedes medial atrophy. Hyperplasia is a slow process in chronic human disease. In rats, aortic VSMC growth is 0.01% per day[77]; in hypertensive models, this increases to a maximum of 1% per day. Simple calculations indicate that if this rate persisted, an arteriole of 30 μm in diameter would occlude in 40 days, based on a medial thickness of 20 μm and cell diameter of 5 μm. This result implies that only a certain percentage of cells may be able to replicate (VSMC heterogeneity) or that there must be only brief periods of proliferation (e.g., environmental stimuli) followed by inhibition of cell growth. Both processes appear to occur and contribute to the proliferation of VSMC in hypertension and restenosis. Alternatively, there may be programmed cell death of some proliferating cells, a process termed *apoptosis*.[78] It has recently been shown that there is increased apoptosis of VSMC in atherosclerosis—suggesting that when cells enter the cell cycle to proliferate, they are also more prone to undergo cell death.

Apoptosis

Apoptosis has been defined as cell death without inflammation and is a key mechanism for tissue repair and remodeling. The significance of apoptosis in atherosclerosis depends on the stage of plaque development and on cell localization and the cell types involved.[37,79,80] Both macrophages and VSMC undergo apoptosis in atherosclerotic plaques. Apoptosis of macrophages is mainly present in regions associated with high rates of DNA synthesis. In contrast, VSMC apoptosis is mainly present in less cellular regions and is not associated with DNA synthesis. Moreover, recent data indicate that VSMC may be killed by activated macrophages. The loss of the VSMC can be detrimental for plaque stability because most of the interstitial collagen fibers, which are important for the tensile strength of the fibrous cap, are produced by VSMC. Apoptotic cells that are not scavenged in the plaque activate thrombin, which could further induce intraplaque thrombosis. One can then conclude that apoptosis in primary atherosclerosis is detrimental because it could lead to plaque rupture and thrombosis.

VSMC Growth Mechanisms

Growth Factors

More than 100 molecules have been shown to promote VSMC growth.[37] These molecules fall into several classes: peptides that bind to G protein-coupled receptors (e.g., angiotensin II, norepinephrine, thrombin); tyrosine kinase-coupled receptors (e.g., EGF, PDGF); cytokine receptors (e.g., toll receptors, CD40 ligand); and integrins (fibronectin, vitronectin). Although regulation of VSMC growth by these molecules is complex, some generalizations are useful. G protein-coupled receptors promote growth of VSMC in disease-specific states such as hypertension and atherosclerosis. Growth regulation is mediated in part by increases in receptor expression and in part by alterations in downstream signaling pathways that activate cell cycle entry. Particularly important is the process of transactivation in which G protein-coupled receptors stimulate tyrosine kinases that activate tyrosine kinase-coupled receptors by promoting dimerization. In addition, G protein-coupled receptors may activate matrix metalloproteases that cleave cell- and matrix-bound prohormones, thereby yielding endogenous ligands such as EGF. Tyrosine kinase-coupled receptors play important roles in both cell proliferation and cell migration. Expression of tyrosine kinase receptors in VSMC is normally very low, but during VSMC dedifferentiation receptor expression increases. This altered expression makes VSMC hyperresponsive to both tyrosine kinase receptor ligands (e.g., EGF and PDGF) and G protein-coupled receptor ligands (e.g., angiotensin II, endothelin, and thrombin via transactivation). In addition to peptides, there are a number of environmental factors such as oxygen tension, reactive oxygen species (ROS), pressure, stretch, and strain that influence VSMC growth.

Hypoxia

Hypoxia has been reported to cause two direct and distinct effects on VSMC growth.[81] Exposure to very low O_2 tension induces production of IL-1α, whereas exposure to moderately low O_2 tension induces VSMC proliferation, independent of IL-1. Levels of IL-1α and IL-1β mRNA increased in VSMC after 48 hours' incubation in low O_2 compared with levels in normoxic cells. Both IL-1α and IL-1β decreased on subsequent reoxygenation. Levels of cell-associated IL-1α also increased progressively after 48 hours in low O_2; however, detectable IL-1α was not released from the cells in the media.

Reactive Oxygen Species

Recent evidence suggests an important role for reactive oxygen species (ROS, which include O_2^-, H_2O_2, and OH^-) in the control of VSMC proliferation, both in vitro and in vivo.[82,83] ROS increase cell proliferation, mediate hormone-induced hypertrophy, and under certain conditions induce apoptosis.[83] ROS directly stimulate VSMC growth and also act as second messengers for classic G protein-coupled and tyrosine kinase-coupled growth receptors. Direct effects of ROS to stimulate VSMC growth are mediated by activation of signal transduction events, increased expression and secretion of growth factors, and transactivation of tyrosine kinase-coupled receptors.[84] H_2O_2 is an important VSMC growth factor based on its stimulation of autocrine growth factors, protein kinases (e.g., MAP kinases), DNA synthesis, and cell number.[85] Growth factors regulated by H_2O_2 include bFGF,[86] IGF-1,[87] VEGF,[88] HB-EGF,[89] cyclophilin A,[90] and HSP90.[90] The relative roles of H_2O_2-induced growth factors in vivo remain to be defined.

The role of ROS as second messengers for more classic VSMC growth factors has become well established.[83] VSMC growth factors that use intracellular ROS as mediators include angiotensin II, insulin, IL-1, EGF, PDGF, and TGF-β. Three lines of evidence support the concept that ROS act as autocrine mediators for growth factors (1) PDGF and angiotensin II increase ROS production in VSMC.[91,92] (2) Most of the O_2^- generated in VSMC appears to be produced by the intracellular NAD(P)H oxidase, which includes a novel p91 homolog termed Nox1.[92,93] (3) Signal transduction by PDGF is inhibited when cells are transduced with superoxide dismutase or catalase, or after treatment with antioxidants.[91] Sundaresan and colleagues[91] showed that PDGF transiently increased H_2O_2, which was required for PDGF-induced tyrosine phosphorylation and ERK1/2 activation. The increase in H_2O_2 could be blunted by increasing the intracellular concentration of the scavenging enzyme catalase or by the chemical antioxidant *N*-acetylcysteine. The response of VSMC to PDGF, which included tyrosine phosphorylation, mitogen-activated protein kinase stimulation, DNA synthesis, and chemotaxis, was inhibited when the growth factor-stimulated rise in H_2O_2 concentration was blocked.[91] Transactivation of tyrosine kinase-coupled receptors as a mechanism of action for H_2O_2 was first described by Rao.[94] Specifically, he showed that H_2O_2 stimulated tyrosine phosphorylation of several proteins, including the EGF receptor in VSMC. ROS have now been shown to activate many intracellular kinases including protein kinase C,[95] ERK1/2,[85] and many tyrosine kinases.[94] Thus, ROS (and H_2O_2 in particular) act as intracellular autocrine growth mediators for VSMC in response to both G protein- and tyrosine kinase-coupled receptors.

Mechanical Forces: Stretch, Pressure, and Shear Stress

VSMC in the vessel wall are continuously exposed to mechanical forces that modulate function. In addition to regulating vessel tone, these physical forces modulate vessel architecture by changing VSMC gene expression. Strain may be a very specific stimulus as shown by Feng and colleagues[96] who observed (using a microarray with 5000 genes) that only 3 transcripts were induced greater than 2.5-fold: cyclooxygenase-1, tenascin-C, and plasminogen activator inhibitor-1. Downregulated transcripts included matrix metalloprotease-1 (MMP-1) and thrombomodulin. An early study[97] showed that exposure to mechanical strain increased the basal rate of VSMC DNA synthesis by threefold and increased cell number by 40% compared with cells grown on stationary rubber plates. Strain appeared to induce the production of an autocrine growth factor(s) because conditioned medium from cells subjected to strain induced a fourfold increase in DNA synthesis in control cells. Western blots of medium conditioned on the cells subjected to strain indicate that the cells secrete both PDGF-A and PDGF-B in response to strain. Increased production of angiotensin II and increased cell responsiveness to angiotensin II also occur with mechanical strain.[98] Using a similar model, Standley and colleagues[99] showed that cyclic stretch increased IGF-I secretion from stretched cells by 20- to 30-fold, and stretch-induced increases in growth were completely blocked by addition of anti-IGF-I antibody. Stretching VSMC also increases collagen synthesis that was shown to be due to the actions of angiotensin II and TGF-β.[100] Increased pressure has been suggested to stimulate both IGF and PDGF expression.[101,102] It has been suggested that pressure maintains a differentiated phenotype in culture[103] as shown by continued expression of high-molecular-weight caldesmon and filamin in the organ cultures of pressurized and stretched vessels. In vivo, increased pressure due to aortic coarctation was associated with enhanced IGF-1 expression.[101] In general, it appears that pressure stimulates fewer autocrine growth mechanisms that strain. Although VSMC are not usually exposed to fluid shear stress, after vascular injury the developing neointima lacks an endothelium and is exposed to blood flow. Shear stress has been shown to regulate TGF-β expression[104] and PDGF receptor phosphorylation.[105] Exposure of VSMC to fluid flow for 24 hours inhibited proliferation significantly in association with increased expression of TGF-β and tissue-type plasminogen activator.[104]

Extracellular Matrix Composition and Matrix Dissolution

Matrix is important in determining cell growth and shape. The best characterized interaction between VSMC and matrix is mediated by integrins (cell receptors) and their ligands (extracellular matrix proteins). Examples include the interactions of the $\alpha_v\beta_3$ integrin heterodimer with vitronectin and the $\alpha_5\beta_1$ heterodimer with fibronectin. Integrin interactions with their ligands stimulate many signal transduction events that are required for cell growth and survival. Numerous examples exist for matrix effects on VSMC growth responses. When VSMC were cultured on plastic, angiotensin II induced only a 1.6-fold increase in DNA synthesis, but when cultured on fibronectin- or type I collagen-coated plastic, the response to angiotensin II was enhanced from two- to fourfold.[98] In addition, angiotensin II is able to alter the matrix expressed by VSMC. Osteopontin is a matrix molecule whose expression is dramatically increased by angiotensin II.[106] Osteopontin has been shown to exert important effects on VSMC growth, and arterial injury induced large increases in osteopontin by VSMC.[106,107] There are many other matrix molecules whose expression has been shown to be regulated by VSMC growth factors including fibronectin, vitronectin, and type I collagen.

The nature of matrix assembly (fibrils versus monomers) is also critically important for VSMC growth. bFGF has been shown to exert powerful effects on assembly of type I collagen fibers,[108] which may have important implications for VSMC growth because VSMC are arrested in the G1 phase of the cell cycle on polymerized type I collagen fibrils, whereas monomer collagen supports SMC proliferation.[109] Specifically, fibrillar collagen regulates early integrin signaling that may lead to upregulation of cdk2 inhibitors and inhibition of VSMC proliferation.[109]

It should be noted that VSMC have several inducible matrix metalloproteinases (MMPs) that may regulate the nature of the matrix.[110] For example, VSMC stimulated with interleukin-1 or TNF-α synthesized de novo 92-kD gelatinase, interstitial collagenase, and stromelysin. Together, the constitutive and cytokine-induced enzymes can digest all the major components of the vascular matrix. In summary, extracellular matrix and the receptors for these proteins represent an important regulatory mechanism that modulates the nature of the VSMC growth response.

Inflammation—ROS

Inflammation with accumulation of activated mononuclear cells has been proposed to play a role in plaque disruption through the elaboration of proteases, such as matrix-degrading metalloproteinases and other proteases, inhibition of function and/or survival, or promotion of apoptosis of matrix synthesizing VSMC. Inflammation may also contribute to thrombosis after plaque disruption by providing a source for tissue factor in the plaque. Inflammation in the plaque may result from accumulation of modified lipids, oxidant and hemodynamic stress, and infective agents. VSMC, themselves, may play a role in inflammation by secreting cytokines that attract inflammatory cells such as MCP-1, and cytokines that regulate the inflammatory response such as heat shock proteins, CD40 ligand, and cyclophilins.[111-113] A key feature of inflammation induced by VSMC is the production of ROS mediated by NAD(P)H oxidase. This growth factor-responsive enzyme appears to be a key mediator for gene expression and inflammatory effects of VSMC.[114]

Injury and Neointima Formation: Vascular Remodeling

In response to arterial injury many mechanical and hormonal events are stimulated that promote VSMC growth (Fig. 2-5). Both VSMC proliferation and migration contribute to neointima formation. Separating the relative contributions of individual growth factors to these two VSMC functions is not simple. In general, PDGF is involved primarily in chemotaxis, not in proliferation.[115] Important roles in cell proliferation have been proposed for angiotensin II[116] and TGF-β but not for bFGF.[117]

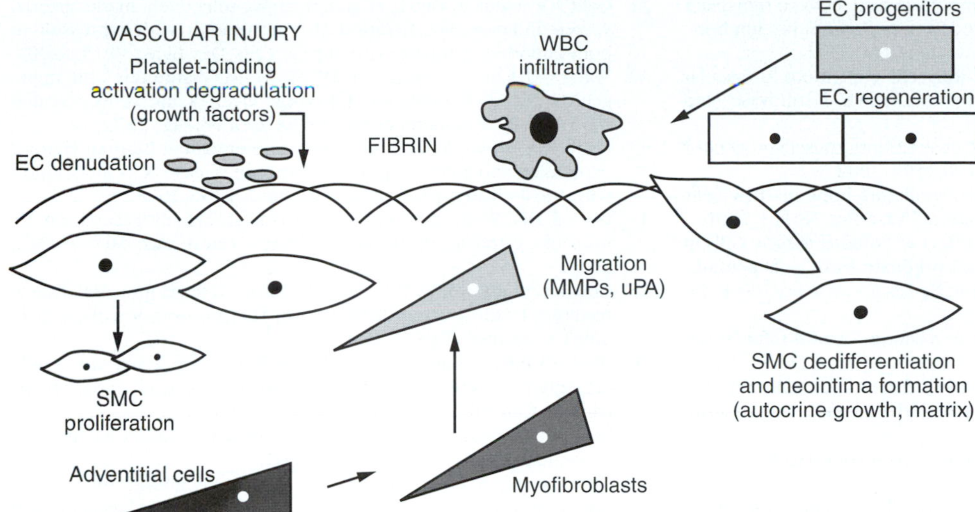

FIGURE 2-5. Vascular injury stimulates multiple cellular processes. EC, endothelial cells; SMC, smooth muscle cell.

In contrast, growth arrest genes, such as gax, are downregulated in the injured vessel,[118] except for Gas6.[119] Key roles for cell-mediated matrix dissolution and expression of MMPs and plasminogen activators (especially uPA) have been shown. In addition, it is likely that there are significant contributions of progenitor cells as well as transdifferentiation (adventitial cells to myofibroblasts) and VSMC dedifferentiation.

Vascular remodeling (Fig. 2-6) is a physiologic response to alterations in flow, pressure, and diseases (e.g., atherosclerosis). Remodeling involves changes in VSMC growth and migration, as well as alterations in vessel matrix.[120] Remodeling may be classified (as proposed by Mulvany) based on the nature of changes in vessel diameter (inward or outward) and by changes in mass (increased = hypertrophic, decreased = atrophic, no change = eutrophic).[120] As an example "eutrophic outward" remodeling would be an increase in lumen diameter without change in amount or characteristics of the vessel (measured by the area contained within the internal elastic lamina [IEL])—such as may occur with increased flow and atherosclerosis. In contrast "hypertrophic inward" remodeling would be defined as a decrease in lumen diameter with increased wall thickness—such as may occur with increased pressure.

In response to changes in blood flow, remodeling appears to be fundamentally dependent on the presence of an intact endothelium as shown by Langille and Kohler.[121,122] During inward remodeling, there is a coordination of increased VSMC apoptosis and decreased VSMC proliferation to effect the decrease in vessel wall mass that occurs.[123] An important role for monocytes has been elucidated in remodeling, especially in response to ischemia such as occurs after occlusion of a supply artery.[124] In response to increased pressure, remodeling appears to be due to activation of autocrine mechanisms that stimulate VSMC growth and changes in vessel wall matrix.[125-127] Remodeling also occurs in atherosclerosis. Although many atherosclerotic vessels show VSMC hyperplasia and formation of a neointima, in many vessels there is actually outward vessel remodeling, a process termed the Glagov phenomenon.[128]

In summary, the plasticity and diversity of VSMC enable these cells to respond to multiple environmental stimuli. Many aspects of wound repair and vascular remodeling recapitulate development. Thus, we may anticipate vascular bed specific responses to pathologic conditions on the basis of VSMC diversity that arises during development.

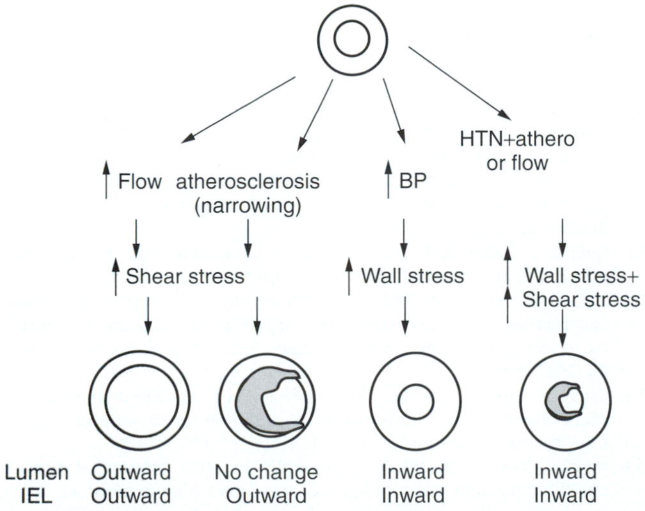

FIGURE 2-6. Vascular remodeling. In response to changes in flow, pressure, and pathologic states, vessels remodel to normalize shear stress and wall stress. Athero, atherosclerosis; BP, blood pressure; HTN, hypertension.

REFERENCES

1. Schwartz SM, Reidy MR, Clowes A: Kinetics of atherosclerosis: A stem cell model. Ann NY Acad Sci 454:292, 1985.
2. Majesky MW, Giachelli CM, Reidy MA, et al: Rat carotid neointimal smooth muscle cells reexpress a developmentally regulated mRNA phenotype during repair of arterial injury. Circ Res 71:759, 1992.
3. Asahara T, Masuda H, Takahashi T, et al: Bone marrow origin of endothelial progenitor cells responsible for postnatal vasculogenesis in physiological and pathological neovascularization. Circ Res 85:221, 1999.

4. Hu Y, Davison F, Ludewig B, et al: Smooth muscle cells in transplant atherosclerotic lesions are originated from recipients, but not bone marrow progenitor cells. Circulation 106:1834, 2002.
5. Sata M: Circulating vascular progenitor cells contribute to vascular repair, remodeling, and lesion formation. Trends Cardiovasc Med 13:249, 2003.
6. Simper D, Stalboerger PG, Panetta CJ, et al: Smooth muscle progenitor cells in human blood. Circulation 106:1199, 2002.
7. Han CI, Campbell GR, Campbell JH: Circulating bone marrow cells can contribute to neointimal formation. J Vasc Res 38:113, 2001.
8. Caplice NM, Bunch TJ, Stalboerger PG, et al: Smooth muscle cells in human coronary atherosclerosis can originate from cells administered at marrow transplantation. Proc Natl Acad Sci U S A 100:4754, 2003.
9. Ku DN, Giddens DP: Pulsatile flow in a model carotid bifurcation. Arteriosclerosis 3:31, 1983.
10. Davies PF: Endothelial cells, hemodynamic forces, and the localization of atherosclerosis. In: Ryan US (ed): Endothelial Cells. Boca Raton, Fla, CRC Press; 1988, p 123.
11. Davies PF: How do vascular endothelial cells respond to flow? NIPS 4:22, 1989.
12. Mitsumata M, Fishel RS, Nerem RN, et al: Fluid shear stress stimulates platelet-derived growth factor expression in endothelial cells. Am J Physiol 265:H3, 1993.
13. Saouaf R, Takasaki I, Eastman E, et al: Fibronectin biosynthesis in the rat aorta in vitro: Changes due to experimental hypertension. J Clin Invest 88:1182, 1991.
14. Takasaki I, Chobanian AV, Sarzani P, et al: Effects of hypertension on fibronectin expression in the rat aorta. J Biol Chem 265:21935, 1990.
15. Carmeliet P: Mechanisms of angiogenesis and arteriogenesis. Nat Med 6:389, 2000.
16. Hungerford JE, Little CD: Developmental biology of the vascular smooth muscle cell: Building a multilayered vessel wall. J Vasc Res 36:2, 1999.
17. Yancopoulos GD, Davis S, Gale NW, et al: Vascular-specific growth factors and blood vessel formation. Nature 407:242, 2000.
18. Campbell-Chamley JH, Campbell GR: What controls smooth muscle phenotype. Atherosclerosis 40:347, 1981.
19. Oettgen P: Transcriptional regulation of vascular development. Circ Res 89:380, 2001.
20. Owens GK: Molecular control of vascular smooth muscle cell differentiation. Acta Physiol Scand 164:623, 1998.
21. Carmeliet P, Moons L, Dewerchin M, et al: Insights in vessel development and vascular disorders using targeted inactivation and transfer of vascular endothelial growth factor, the tissue factor receptor, and the plasminogen system. Ann N Y Acad Sci 811:191, 1997.
22. DeRuiter MC, Poelmann RE, VanMunsteren JC, et al: Embryonic endothelial cells transdifferentiate into mesenchymal cells expressing smooth muscle actins in vivo and in vitro. Circ Res 80:444, 1997.
23. Vrancken Peeters MP, Gittenberger-de Groot AC, Mentink MM, et al: Smooth muscle cells and fibroblasts of the coronary arteries derive from epithelial-mesenchymal transformation of the epicardium. Anat Embryol (Berl) 199:367, 1999.
24. Rosenquist TH, Beall AC: Elastogenic cells in the developing cardiovascular system: Smooth muscle, nonmuscle, and cardiac neural crest. Ann N Y Acad Sci 588:106, 1990.
25. Bergwerff M, Verberne ME, DeRuiter MC, et al: Neural crest cell contribution to the developing circulatory system: Implications for vascular morphology? Circ Res 82:221, 1998.
26. Dettman RW, Denetclaw W, Jr, Ordahl CP, et al: Common epicardial origin of coronary vascular smooth muscle, perivascular fibroblasts, and intermyocardial fibroblasts in the avian heart. Dev Biol 193:169, 1998.
27. Hellstrom M, Kalen M, Lindahl P, et al: Role of PDGF-B and PDGFR-beta in recruitment of vascular smooth muscle cells and pericytes during embryonic blood vessel formation in the mouse. Development 126:3047, 1999.
28. Dickson MC, Martin JS, Cousins FM, et al: Defective haematopoiesis and vasculogenesis in transforming growth factor-beta 1 knockout mice. Development 121:1845, 1995.
29. Li DY, Brooke B, Davis EC, et al: Elastin is an essential determinant of arterial morphogenesis. Nature 393:276, 1998.
30. Yanagisawa H, Hammer RE, Richardson JA, et al: Role of endothelin-1/endothelin-A receptor-mediated signaling pathway in the aortic arch patterning in mice. J Clin Invest 102:22, 1998.
31. Gale NW, Baluk P, Pan L, et al: Ephrin-B2 selectively marks arterial vessels and neovascularization sites in the adult, with expression in both endothelial and smooth-muscle cells. Dev Biol 230:151, 2001.
32. Wang HU, Chen ZF, Anderson DJ: Molecular distinction and angiogenic interaction between embryonic arteries and veins revealed by ephrin-B2 and its receptor Eph-B4. Cell 93:741, 1998.
33. Firulli AB, Miano JM, Bi W, et al: Myocyte enhancer binding factor-2 expression and activity in vascular smooth muscle cells: Association with the activated phenotype. Circ Res 78:196, 1996.
34. Gorski DH, Walsh K: Control of vascular cell differentiation by homeobox transcription factors. Trends Cardiovasc Med 13:213, 2003.
35. Chisaka O, Capecchi MR: Regionally restricted developmental defects resulting from targeted disruption of the mouse homeobox gene hox-1.5. Nature 350:473, 1991.
36. Witzenbichler B, Kureishi Y, Luo Z, et al: Regulation of smooth muscle cell migration and integrin expression by the Gax transcription factor. J Clin Invest 104:1469, 1999.
37. Berk BC: Vascular smooth muscle growth: Autocrine growth mechanisms. Physiol Rev 81:999, 2001.
38. Gittenberger-de Groot AC, DeRuiter MC, et al: Smooth muscle cell origin and its relation to heterogeneity in development and disease. Arterioscler Thromb Vasc Biol 19:1589, 1999.
39. Lin Q, Lu J, Yanagisawa H, et al: Requirement of the MADS-box transcription factor MEF2C for vascular development. Development 125:4565, 1998.
40. Miano JM: Serum response factor: Toggling between disparate programs of gene expression. J Mol Cell Cardiol 35:577, 2003.
41. Wang Z, Wang DZ, Pipes GC, et al: Myocardin is a master regulator of smooth muscle gene expression. Proc Natl Acad Sci U S A 100:7129, 2003.
42. Li S, Wang DZ, Wang Z, et al: The serum response factor coactivator myocardin is required for vascular smooth muscle development. Proc Natl Acad Sci U S A 100:9366, 2003.
43. Yamagishi H, Olson EN, Srivastava D: The basic helix-loop-helix transcription factor, dHAND, is required for vascular development. J Clin Invest 105:261, 2000.
44. Kato Y, Kravchenko VV, Tapping RI, et al: BMK1/ERK5 regulates serum-induced early gene expression through transcription factor MEF2C. Embo J 16:7054, 1997.
45. Carmeliet P, Dor Y, Herbert JM, et al: Role of HIF-1alpha in hypoxia-mediated apoptosis, cell proliferation and tumour angiogenesis. Nature 394:485, 1998.
46. Ausoni S, Sartore S: Cell lineages and tissue boundaries in cardiac arterial and venous poles: Developmental patterns, animal models, and implications for congenital vascular diseases. Arterioscler Thromb Vasc Biol 21:312, 2001.
47. Moessler H, Mericskay M, Li Z, et al: The SM 22 promoter directs tissue-specific expression in arterial but not in venous or visceral smooth muscle cells in transgenic mice. Development 122:2415, 1996.
48. Tsuda T, Wang H, Timpl R, et al: Fibulin-2 expression marks transformed mesenchymal cells in developing cardiac valves, aortic arch vessels, and coronary vessels. Dev Dyn 222:89, 2001.
49. Sata M, Saiura A, Kunisato A, et al: Hematopoietic stem cells differentiate into vascular cells that participate in the pathogenesis of atherosclerosis. Nat Med 8:403, 2002.
50. Glaser R, Lu MM, Narula N, et al: Smooth muscle cells, but not myocytes, of host origin in transplanted human hearts. Circulation 106:17, 2002.
51. Quaini F, Urbanek K, Beltrami AP, et al: Chimerism of the transplanted heart. N Engl J Med 346:5, 2002.
52. Archer SL, Huang JM, Hampl V, et al: Nitric oxide and cGMP cause vasorelaxation by activation of a charybdotoxin-sensitive K channel by cGMP-dependent protein kinase. Proc Natl Acad Sci U S A 91:7583, 1994.
53. Carrier GO, Fuchs LC, Winecoff AP, et al: Nitrovasodilators relax mesenteric microvessels by cGMP-induced stimulation of Ca-activated K channels. Am J Physiol 273:H76, 1997.
54. Swayze RD, Braun AP: A catalytically inactive mutant of type I cGMP-dependent protein kinase prevents enhancement of large conductance, calcium-sensitive K+ channels by sodium nitroprusside and cGMP. J Biol Chem 276:19729, 2001.
55. Jaggar JH, Porter VA, Lederer WJ, et al: Calcium sparks in smooth muscle. Am J Physiol Cell Physiol 278:C235, 2000.

56. Matrougui K, Tanko LB, Loufrani L, et al: Involvement of Rho-kinase and the actin filament network in angiotensin II-induced contraction and extracellular signal-regulated kinase activity in intact rat mesenteric resistance arteries. Arterioscler Thromb Vasc Biol 21:1288, 2001.
57. Yamakawa T, Tanaka S, Numaguchi K, et al: Involvement of Rho-kinase in angiotensin II-induced hypertrophy of rat vascular smooth muscle cells. Hypertension 35:313, 2000.
58. Sauzeau V, Le Jeune H, Cario-Toumaniantz C, et al: Cyclic GMP-dependent protein kinase signaling pathway inhibits RhoA-induced Ca^{2+} sensitization of contraction in vascular smooth muscle. J Biol Chem 275:21722, 2000.
59. Sandu OA, Ito M, Begum N: Selected contribution: Insulin utilizes NO/cGMP pathway to activate myosin phosphatase via Rho inhibition in vascular smooth muscle. J Appl Physiol 91:1475, 2001.
60. Cohen RA, Weisbrod RM, Gericke M, et al: Mechanism of nitric oxide-induced vasodilatation: Refilling of intracellular stores by sarcoplasmic reticulum Ca^{2+} ATPase and inhibition of store-operated Ca^{2+} influx. Circ Res 84:210, 1999.
61. Komalavilas P, Lincoln TM: Phosphorylation of the inositol 1,4, 5-trisphosphate receptor. Cyclic GMP-dependent protein kinase mediates cAMP and cGMP dependent phosphorylation in the intact rat aorta. J Biol Chem 271:21933, 1996.
62. Schlossmann J, Ammendola A, Ashman K, et al: Regulation of intracellular calcium by a signalling complex of IRAG, IP3 receptor and cGMP kinase Iβ. Nature 404:197, 2000.
63. Andriantsitohaina R, Lagaud GJ, Andre A, et al: Effects of cGMP on calcium handling in ATP-stimulated rat resistance arteries. Am J Physiol 268:H1223, 1995.
64. Horowitz A, Menice CB, Laporte R, et al: Mechanisms of smooth muscle contraction. Physiol Rev 76:967, 1996.
65. Cornwell TL, Pryzwansky KB, Wyatt TA, et al: Regulation of sarcoplasmic reticulum protein phosphorylation by localized cyclic GMP-dependent protein kinase in vascular smooth muscle cells. Mol Pharmacol 40:923, 1991.
66. Raeymaekers L, Hofmann F, Casteels R: Cyclic GMP-dependent protein kinase phosphorylates phospholamban in isolated sarcoplasmic reticulum from cardiac and smooth muscle. Biochem J 252:269, 1988.
67. Yoshida Y, Toyosato A, Islam MO, et al: Stimulation of plasma membrane Ca^{2+} -pump ATPase of vascular smooth muscle by cGMP-dependent protein kinase: Functional reconstitution with purified proteins. Mol Cell Biochem 190:157, 1999.
68. Tamaoki J, Tagaya E, Nishimura K, et al: Role of Na+ - K+ ATPase in cyclic GMP-mediated relaxation of canine pulmonary artery smooth muscle cells. Br J Pharmacol 122:112, 1997.
69. Lee MR, Li L, Kitazawa T: Cyclic GMP causes Ca^{2+} desensitization in vascular smooth muscle by activating the myosin light chain phosphatase. J Biol Chem 272:5063, 1997.
70. Carvajal JA, Germain AM, Huidobro-Toro JP, et al: Molecular mechanism of cGMP-mediated smooth muscle relaxation. J Cell Physiol 184:409, 2000.
71. Surks HK, Mochizuki N, Kasai Y, et al: Regulation of myosin phosphatase by a specific interaction with cGMP-dependent protein kinase I alpha. Science 286:1583, 1999.
72. Geisterfer AAT, Peach MJ, Owens GK: Angiotensin II induces hypertrophy, not hyperplasia, of cultured rat aortic smooth muscle cells. Circ Res 62:749, 1988.
73. Berk BC, Vallega G, Muslin AJ, et al: Spontaneously hypertensive rat vascular smooth muscle cells in culture exhibit increased growth and Na+/H+ exchange. J Clin Invest 83:822, 1989.
74. Stouffer GA, Owens GK: Angiotensin II-induced mitogenesis of spontaneously hypertensive rat-derived cultured smooth muscle cells is dependent on autocrine production of transforming growth factor-beta. Circ Res 70:820, 1992.
75. Owens GK: Influence of blood pressure on development of aortic medial smooth muscle hypertrophy in spontaneously hypertensive rats. Hypertension 9:178, 1987.
76. Schiffrin EL, Park JB, Intengan HD, et al: Correction of arterial structure and endothelial dysfunction in human essential hypertension by the angiotensin receptor antagonist losartan. Circulation 101:1653, 2000.
77. Thomas WA, Lee KT, Kim DN: Cell population kinetics in atherogenesis: Cell births and losses in intimal cell mass-derived lesions in the abdominal aorta of swine. Ann NY Acad Sci 454:305, 1985.
78. Bennett MR, Evan GI, Schwartz SM: Apoptosis of human vascular smooth muscle cells derived from normal vessels and coronary atherosclerotic plaques. J Clin Invest 95:2266, 1995.
79. Kockx MM, Knaapen MW: The role of apoptosis in vascular disease. J Pathol 190:267, 2000.
80. Rossig L, Dimmeler S, Zeiher AM: Apoptosis in the vascular wall and atherosclerosis. Basic Res Cardiol 96:11, 2001.
81. Cooper AL, Beasley D: Hypoxia stimulates proliferation and interleukin-1alpha production in human vascular smooth muscle cells. Am J Physiol 277:H1326, 1999.
82. Alexander RW: Theodore Cooper Memorial Lecture. Hypertension and the pathogenesis of atherosclerosis. Oxidative stress and the mediation of arterial inflammatory response: A new perspective. Hypertension 25:155, 1995.
83. Griendling KK, Ushio-Fukai M: Redox control of vascular smooth muscle proliferation. J Lab Clin Med 132:9, 1998.
84. Rao GN, Berk BC: Active oxygen species stimulate vascular smooth muscle cell growth and proto-oncogene expression. Circ Res 70:593, 1992.
85. Baas AS, Berk BC: Differential activation of mitogen-activated protein kinases by H2O2 and O2 in vascular smooth muscle cells. Circ Res 77:29, 1995.
86. Herbert JM, Bono F, Savi P: The mitogenic effect of H2O2 for vascular smooth muscle cells is mediated by an increase of the affinity of basic fibroblast growth factor for its receptor. FEBS Lett 395:43, 1996.
87. Delafontaine P, Ku L: Reactive oxygen species stimulate insulin-like growth factor I synthesis in vascular smooth muscle cells. Cardiovasc Res 33:216, 1997.
88. Ruef J, Hu ZY, Yin LY, et al: Induction of vascular endothelial growth factor in balloon-injured baboon arteries: A novel role for reactive oxygen species in atherosclerosis. Circ Res 81:24, 1997.
89. Kayanoki Y, Higashiyama S, Suzuki K, et al: The requirement of both intracellular reactive oxygen species and intracellular calcium elevation for the induction of heparin-binding EGF-like growth factor in vascular endothelial cells and smooth muscle cells. Biochem Biophys Res Commun 259:50, 1999.
90. Liao D-F, Jin Z-G, Baas AS, et al: Purification and identification of secreted oxidative stress-induced factors from vascular smooth muscle cells. J Biol Chem 275:189, 2000.
91. Sundaresan M, Yu ZX, Ferrans VJ, et al: Requirement for generation of H2O2 for platelet-derived growth factor signal transduction. Science 270:296, 1995.
92. Griendling KK, Minieri CA, Ollerenshaw JD, et al: Angiotensin II stimulates NADH and NADPH oxidase activation in cultured vascular smooth muscle cells. Circ Res 74:1141, 1994.
93. Suh YA, Arnold RS, Lassegue B, et al: Cell transformation by the superoxide-generating oxidase Mox1. Nature 401:79, 1999.
94. Rao GN: Hydrogen peroxide induces complex formation of SHC-Grb2-SOS with receptor tyrosine kinase and activates Ras and extracellular signal-regulated protein kinases group of mitogen-activated protein kinases. Oncogene 13:713, 1996.
95. Rao GN, Lassegue B, Griendling KK, et al: Hydrogen peroxide-induced c-fos expression is mediated by arachidonic acid release: Role of protein kinase C. Nucl Acids Res 21:1259, 1993.
96. Feng Y, Yang JH, Huang H, et al: Transcriptional profile of mechanically induced genes in human vascular smooth muscle cells. Circ Res 85:1118, 1999.
97. Wilson E, Mai Q, Sudhir K, et al: Mechanical strain induces growth of vascular smooth muscle cells via autocrine action of PDGF. J Cell Biol 123:741, 1993.
98. Sudhir K, Wilson E, Chatterjee K, et al: Mechanical strain and collagen potentiate mitogenic activity of angiotensin II in rat vascular smooth muscle cells. J Clin Invest 92:3003, 1993.
99. Standley PR, Obards TJ, Martina CL: Cyclic stretch regulates autocrine IGF-I in vascular smooth muscle cells: Implications in vascular hyperplasia. Am J Physiol 276:E697, 1999.
100. Li Q, Muragaki Y, Hatamura I, et al: Stretch-induced collagen synthesis in cultured smooth muscle cells from rabbit aortic media and a possible involvement of angiotensin II and transforming growth factor-beta. J Vasc Res 35:93, 1998.
101. Fath KA, Alexander RW, Delafontaine P: Abdominal coarctation increases insulin-like growth factor I mRNA levels in rat aorta. Circ Res 72:271, 1993.

102. Negoro N, Kanayama Y, Haraguchi M, et al: Blood pressure regulates platelet-derived growth factor A-chain gene expression in vascular smooth muscle cells in vivo: An autocrine mechanism promoting hypertensive vascular hypertrophy. J Clin Invest 95:1140, 1995.
103. Birukov KG, Bardy N, Lehoux S, et al: Intraluminal pressure is essential for the maintenance of smooth muscle caldesmon and filamin content in aortic organ culture. Arterioscler Thromb Vasc Biol 18:922, 1998.
104. Ueba H, Kawakami M, Yaginuma T: Shear stress as an inhibitor of vascular smooth muscle cell proliferation: Role of transforming growth factor-beta 1 and tissue-type plasminogen activator. Arterioscler Thromb Vasc Biol 17:1512, 1997.
105. Hu Y, Bock G, Wick G, et al: Activation of PDGF receptor alpha in vascular smooth muscle cells by mechanical stress. FASEB J 12:1135, 1998.
106. deBlois D, Lombardi DM, Su EJ, et al: Angiotensin II induction of osteopontin expression and DNA replication in rat arteries. Hypertension 28:1055, 1996.
107. Ashizawa N, Graf K, Do YS, et al: Osteopontin is produced by rat cardiac fibroblasts and mediates AII-induced DNA synthesis and collagen gel contraction. J Clin Invest 98:2218, 1996.
108. Pickering JG, Ford CM, Tang B, et al: Coordinated effects of fibroblast growth factor-2 on expression of fibrillar collagens, matrix metalloproteinases, and tissue inhibitors of matrix metalloproteinases by human vascular smooth muscle cells: Evidence for repressed collagen production and activated degradative capacity. Arterioscler Thromb Vasc Biol 17:475, 1997.
109. Koyama H, Raines EW, Bornfeldt KE, et al: Fibrillar collagen inhibits arterial smooth muscle proliferation through regulation of Cdk2 inhibitors. Cell 87:1069, 1996.
110. Galis ZS, Khatri JJ: Matrix metalloproteinases in vascular remodeling and atherogenesis: The good, the bad, and the ugly. Circ Res 90:251, 2002.
111. Kol A, Bourcier T, Lichtman AH, et al: Chlamydial and human heat shock protein 60s activate human vascular endothelium, smooth muscle cells, and macrophages. J Clin Invest 103:571, 1999.
112. Libby P: Inflammation in atherosclerosis. Nature 420:868, 2002.
113. Mach F, Schonbeck U, Sukhova GK, et al: Functional CD40 ligand is expressed on human vascular endothelial cells, smooth muscle cells, and macrophages: Implications for CD40-CD40 ligand signaling in atherosclerosis. Proc Natl Acad Sci U S A 94:1931, 1997.
114. Griendling KK, Sorescu D, Ushio-Fukai M: NAD(P)H oxidase: Role in cardiovascular biology and disease. Circ Res 86:494, 2000.
115. Reidy MA, Fingerle J, Lindner V: Factors controlling the development of arterial lesions after injury. Circulation 86:III43, 1992.
116. Powell JS, Clozel JP, Muller RK, et al: Inhibitors of angiotensin-converting enzyme prevent myointimal proliferation after vascular injury. Science 245:186, 1989.
117. Olson NE, Chao S, Lindner V, et al: Intimal smooth muscle cell proliferation after balloon catheter injury: The role of basic fibroblast growth factor. Am J Pathol 140:1017, 1992.
118. Weir L, Chen D, Pastore C, et al: Expression of gax, a growth arrest homeobox gene, is rapidly down-regulated in the rat carotid artery during the proliferative response to balloon injury. J Biol Chem 270:5457, 1995.
119. Melaragno MG, Wuthrich DA, Poppa V, et al: Increased expression of Axl tyrosine kinase after vascular injury and regulation by G protein-coupled receptor agonists in rats. Circ Res 83:697, 1998.
120. Mulvany MJ, Baumbach GL, Aalkjaer C, et al: Vascular remodeling. Hypertension 28:505, 1996.
121. Langille BL, O'Donnell F: Reductions in arterial diameter produced by chronic decreases in blood flow are endothelium-dependent. Science 231:405, 1986.
122. Kohler TR, Kirkman TR, Kraiss LW, et al: Increased blood flow inhibits neointimal hyperplasia in endothelialized vascular grafts. Circ Res 69:1557, 1991.
123. Cho A, Mitchell L, Koopmans D, et al: Effects of changes in blood flow rate on cell death and cell proliferation in carotid arteries of immature rabbits. Circ Res 81:328, 1997.
124. Schaper W, Ito WD: Molecular mechanisms of coronary collateral vessel growth. Circ Res 79:911, 1996.
125. Mulvany MJ, Hansen PK, Aalkjaer C: Direct evidence that the greater contractility of resistance vessels in spontaneously hypertensive rats is associated with a narrower lumen, a thicker media, and a greater number of smooth muscle cell layers. Circ Res 43:854, 1978.
126. Mulvany MJ, Baadrup U, Gundersen HJG: Evidence for hyperplasia in mesenteric resistance vessels of spontaneously hypertensive rats using a three-dimensional dissector. Circ Res 57:794, 1985.
127. Heagerty AM, Aalkjaer C, Bund SJ, et al: Small artery structure in hypertension: Dual processes of remodeling and growth. Hypertension 21:391, 1993.
128. Glagov S, Weisenberg E, Zarins CK, et al: Compensatory enlargement of human atherosclerotic coronary arteries. N Engl J Med 316:1371, 1987.

chapter 3

Connective Tissues of the Subendothelium

Rajendra Raghow
Jerome Seyer
Andrew Kang

GENERAL CHARACTERISTICS AND COMPOSITION

The development of subendothelial connective tissue that provides mechanical strength and elasticity to the blood vessel and maintains its structural integrity was a crucial event in the evolution of multicellular organisms. Like all connective tissues, the subendothelium comprises cells and extracellular matrix (ECM), which consists of fibrillar and amorphous components. The fibrillar macromolecules, consisting mainly of collagen and elastin, are enmeshed within the amorphous acidic-glycosaminoglycans, a number of glycoproteins such as fibronectin (FN) and laminin, and other less well-characterized ECM molecules.

More than two dozen genetically distinct types of collagen, comprising 38 unique α chains, have been identified in various mammalian connective tissues (Table 3-1). Based on their supramolecular organization (Fig. 3-1), collagens may be categorized as (1) fibrillar collagens represented by types I, II, III, V, and VI; (2) fibril-associated collagens with interrupted triple helices (FACIT)—such as IX, XII, XIV, XVI, XIX and XX collagens; (3) collagens capable of forming hexagonal network such as VIII and X; (4) basement membrane (BM) collagens, mainly comprising various IV collagens; (5) collagens that assemble into beaded filaments such as type VI; (6) BM anchoring fiber-forming collagens such as VII; (7) collagens with membrane-spanning domains such as types XIII and XVII collagens; and (8) a family of collagens represented by types XV and XVIII collagens. It is noteworthy, however, that in light of the intrinsic heterogeneity of the supramolecular organization of various collagens in vivo, this classification is somewhat limited. Furthermore, there are additional -Gly-X-Y-repeat-containing proteins in the genome that have been characterized only at the cDNA and genomic levels, and their analyses at the protein level will undoubtedly modify the current classification scheme. Although several collagens that include I, III, IV, V, VI, VIII, XII, XIV, XV, XVI, XVIII and XIX are found in blood vessels, type I and type III collagens are the major collagens in the blood vessel wall.[1-4] Type IV collagen, represented by six homologous α chains (α1 to α6), is found exclusively in the BM.[5] Type V collagen appears with type I and type III in striated fibrils but in some tissues is present as V/XI hybrids. Type V collagen in the form of α1(V) and α4(V) heterotrimer is mainly found in Schwann cells.[6] Type VI collagen was initially isolated from the aortic intima[7]; type VIII collagen was originally isolated from endothelial cells but is ubiquitously expressed.[8] Collagen types XIII and XVII are transmembrane collagens; whereas the former is found in many tissues, the latter is mainly restricted to hemidesmosomes of the skin and is involved in bullous pemphigoid. Type VII collagen forms the anchoring fibrils that link BM to the anchoring plaques of type IV collagen and laminin. A number of recently discovered noncollagenous domains of various collagens may be involved in more subtle and sophisticated functions in addition to their roles as adhesive molecules. Thus, a 22 kDa C-terminal fragment of XVII collagen, named endostatin, is a potent inhibitor of angiogenesis and tumor growth; similarly, type XV collagen contains an endostatin analog with antiangiogenic properties.[9,10] Presumably, these noncollagenous domains are released in vivo by proteinases under a variety of pathophysiologic conditions.[11]

VARIATIONS IN THE VASCULATURE

The vascular system consists of a massive network of tubular channels that carry blood throughout the body. The walls of these channels are considered specialized connective tissues, with collagen and elastin as their major structural protein constituents. The size and composition of individual blood vessels vary with their specific functional requirements. The major arteries that carry blood directly from the heart must be relatively thick and elastic and, therefore, their walls contain a relatively large amount of elastin, which allows for elastic expansion and contraction in response to contractions of the heart. In this fashion, the large arteries contribute to a more continuous blood flow.

The smaller arteries are more rigid and contain a larger proportion of collagen. Their function is to regulate blood flow into the tissue. This regulation is achieved by the contractile activity of smooth muscle cells, which control the size of the vessel lumen based on the required blood flow.

The capillary contains only one layer of endothelial cells with an underlying BM. This thin-walled tube permits a rapid exchange of water, nutrients, and metabolic products between blood and interstitial fluids. Capillaries deliver blood to the venous system at reduced pressure. Thus, the venules have thinner walls, less dense connective tissue, and a larger lumen than their arterial counterparts. They have far fewer smooth muscle cells and are equipped with valves to prevent reversal of blood flow due to hydrostatic forces.

TABLE 3-1 COLLAGEN TYPES AND THE LOCATION OF THEIR GENES ON HUMAN CHROMOSOMES

Type	Constituent α Chains	Gene	Chromosome	Occurrence
I	α1(I)	*COL1A1*	17q21.3-q22	Most connective tissues, especially in dermis, bone, tendon, ligament
	α2(I)	COL1A2	7q21.3-q22	
II	α1(II)	*COL2A1*	12q13-q14	Cartilage, vitreous humor, cornea
III	α1(III)	*COL3A1*	2q24.3-q31	Tissues containing collagen I except absent in bone and tendon
IV	α1(IV)	*COL4A1*	13q34	Basement membranes (BM)
	α2(IV)	*COL4A2*	13q34	
	α3(IV)	*COL4A3*	2q35-q37	
	α4(IV)	*COL4A4*	2q35-q37	
	α5(IV)	*COL4A5*	Xq22	
	α6(IV)	*COL4A6*	Xq22	
V	α1(V)	*COL5A1*	9q34.2-q34.3	Tissues containing collagen I
	α2(V)	*COL5A2*	2q24.3-q31	
	α3(V)	*COL5A3*	19p13.2	
	α4(V)	*COL5A4*		Nervous system
VI	α1(VI)	*COL6A1*	21q22.3	Most connective tissues
	α2(VI)	*COL6A2*	21q22.3	
	α3(VI)	*COL6A3*	2q37	
VII	α1(VII)	*COL7A1*	3p21	Anchoring fibrils
VIII	α1(VIII)	*COL8A1*	3q12-q13.1	Many tissues
	α2(VIII)	*COL8A2*	1p32.3-p34.3	
IX	α1(IX)	*COL9A1*	6q12-q14	Tissues containing collagen II
	α2(IX)	*COL9A2*	1p32	
	α3(IX)	*COL9A3*	20q13.3	
X	α1(X)	*COL10A1*	6q21-q22	Hypertrophic cartilage
XI	α1(XI)	*COL11A1*	1p21	Tissues containing collagen II
	α2(XI)	*COL11A2*	6p21.2	
	α3(XI)	*COL11A3*	12q13-q14	
XII	α1(XII)	*COL12A1*	6q12-q13	Tissues containing collagen I
XIII	α1(XIII)	*COL13A1*	10q22	Many tissues
XIV	α1(XIV)	*COL14A1*	8q23	Tissues containing collagen I
XV	α1(XV)	*COL15A1*	9q21-q22	Many tissues in the BM zone
XVI	α1(XVI)	*COL16A1*	1p34-p35	Many tissues
XVII	α1(XVII)	*COL17A1*	10q24.3	Skin hemidesmosomes
XVIII	α1(XVIII)	*COL18A1*	21q22.3	Many tissues in the BM zone
XIX	α1(XIX)	*COL19A1*	6q12-q14	Many tissues in the BM zone
XXI	α1(XXI)	*COL21A1*	6p11.2-p12.3	Fetal tissues and blood vessels

Adapted from Myllyharju J, Kivirikko KI: Collagens and collagen-related diseases. Ann Med 33(1):7, 2001.

The walls of the large elastic arteries contain three identifiable tissue layers. The tunica intima, the innermost layer, contains a single layer of polygonal endothelial cells joined by gap junctions. This cell layer rests on a BM, which in turn is supported by a network of elastic fibers in a fenestrated plate called the internal elastic lamina. The tunica media, which represents the bulk of the vessel wall, contains few elastic fibers but a large number of smooth muscle cells, their long axes perpendicular to the lumen axis.[12] The extracellular space contains collagen fibers in a continuous sheath adjacent to the elastic fibers. Fibers contain a variable mixture of types I, III, and V collagens. Smooth muscle cells synthesize types I, III, V, VI, XII, and XIV collagen. The outermost sheet of elastin, the external elastic lamina, separates the medial and adventitial layers. The adventitia consists primarily of collagen fibers with elastin, nerves, fibroblasts, and vasa vasorum (vascular network that serves the outer portion of the wall of arteries that are too thick for diffusion of nutrients and O_2 from intima).

The walls of smaller arteries are intermediate in size. The tunica intima is relatively thin, as is the medial layer. The tunica adventitia is usually much thicker than those of large arteries, with more densely packed collagen fibers arranged longitudinally along the vessel axis. Arterioles have simple walls. Smooth muscle cells surround the endothelial layer, and the adventitia is smaller and more pliable than that in larger arteries.[1] The capillaries adjoining the arterioles are surrounded by a few smooth muscle cells that control the amount of blood passing through them. The walls of arterial and venous capillaries consist of flat endothelial cells surrounded by a BM, to which are attached pericapillary cells called *pericytes*. These cells form a discontinuous sheath of reticulum fibers that are primarily type III collagen.[12]

The walls of venules in the venous system contain a reticular network of collagen fibers derived from type III collagen along with smaller quantities of type I collagen fibers. As the vessel size increases, the relative proportions of type I collagen, smooth muscle cells, and elastic fibers also increase. The larger veins contain paired semilunar flaps, which consist of collagen fiber bundles covered by a layer of endothelial cells.

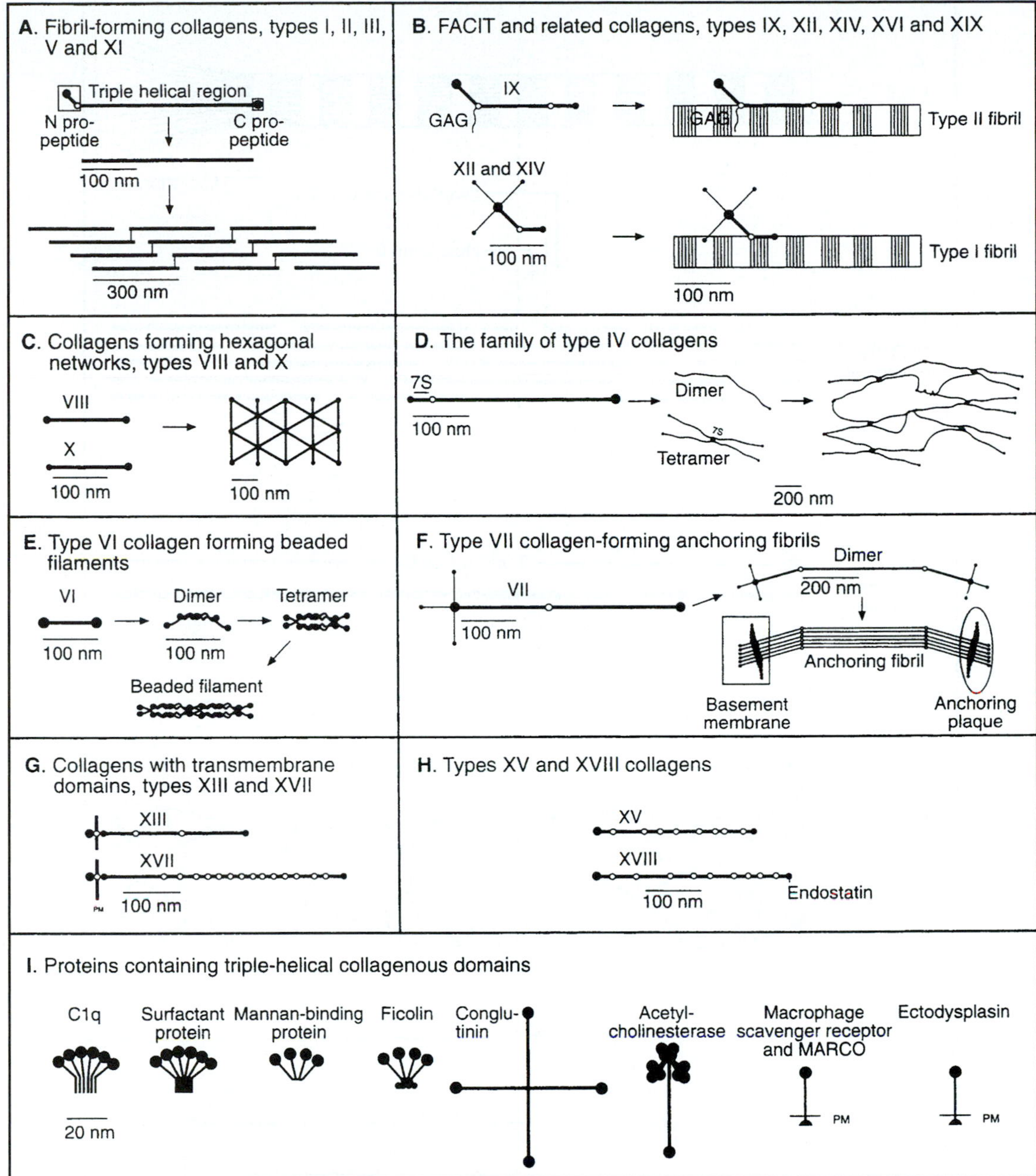

FIGURE 3-1. Schematic representation of various members of the collagen superfamily and their known supramolecular assemblies. The letters refer to the families described in the text. The supramolecular assemblies of families G and H have not been elucidated and, hence, are not shown. At present, there are complete cDNA sequences for four additional collagen α chains that are not shown. These encode a fibril-forming collagen-like chain, two FACIT collagen-like chains, and a collagen XIII-like chain (Personal communication, Koch M, Gordon M, Burgeson RE, 2000). Some of the members of family I are also not shown. The *closed circles* indicate N- and C-terminal noncollagenous domains, whereas *open circles* indicate noncollagenous domains interrupting the collagen triple helix. GAG, glycosaminoglycan; PM, plasma membrane. (From Myllyharju J, Kivirikko KI: Collagens and collagen-related diseases. Ann Med 33(1):7, 2001).

THE CHEMISTRY AND STRUCTURE OF COLLAGENS

Collagens are the major constituents of the ECM of the vasculature. In addition to being critical in maintaining the structural integrity of the vascular bed, collagens are involved in cell attachment, chemotaxis, platelet aggregation, and filtration barrier function in BMs. Collagens are characterized by -Gly-X-Y repeating structures that allow triple helix formation in at least part of their structure. Collagens undergo extensive posttranslational modifications that are essential to impart mechanical strength to their tertiary and quaternary organization.

The Collagen Molecule

The collagen molecule, the basic unit of collagen fibers, has an asymmetric, rod-like structure composed of three polypeptide chains, called α chains. Because of

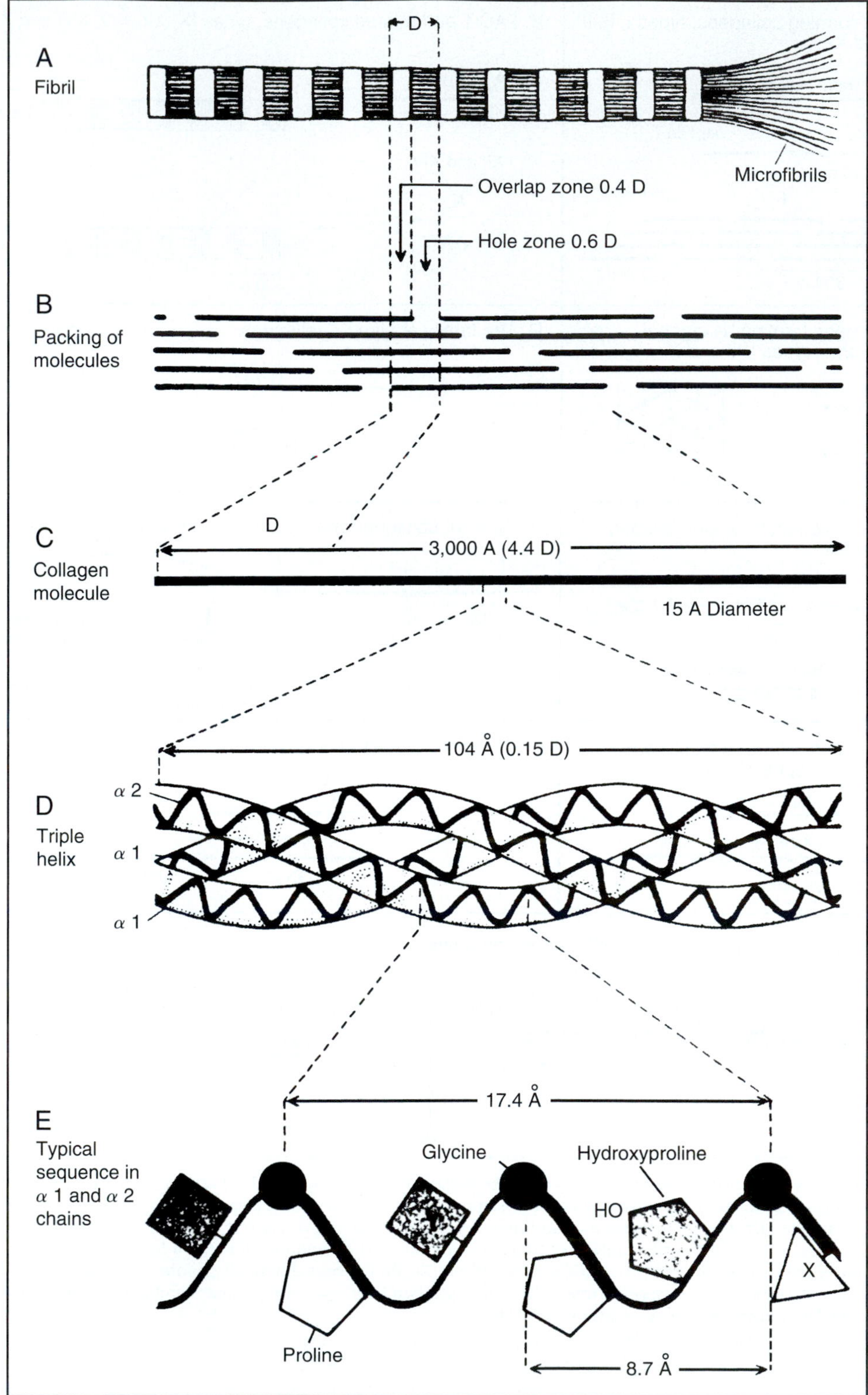

FIGURE 3-2. Diagrammatic representation of the collagen triple-helical structure. **A,** A large fibril of collagen exhibiting a dense packing of microfibrils with characteristic cross-striations and a regular repeat period (D) of approximately 69 nm and **(B)** a 2-D representation of the packing arrangement of the collagen molecule in the microfibril. **C,** The collagen molecule consists of three α chains in a rigid rod, 300 nm in length and 1.5 nanometers in diameter with a 4.4-D spacing. **D,** The three α chains are in the left-handed helix with approximately three residues per turn. **E,** Glycine occurs at every third position and is mandatory. The X and Y positions in the GLY-X-Y triplet can be any amino acid, but proline and hydroxyproline each occur approximately 10% of the time in the X and Y positions, respectively. (From Prockop DJ, Guzman NA: Collagen diseases and the biosynthesis of collagen. Hosp Pract 12:61, 1977.)

the -Gly-X-Y repeating units and the high content of proline and hydroxyproline and their stereochemistry, each α chain forms a helical structure (minor helix) shown in Figure 3-2. Three α chains then wind around a common axis to form a right-handed triple helix. Owing to the complexity of the different collagens in blood vessels, they will be discussed in three groups: group 1 collagens have an α chain size with an approximate molecular mass of 95 kDa and a helical domain of approximately 300 nm in length (types I, III, and V) and group 2 collagens have an α chain size greater than 95 kDa with helical regions that are interrupted by short nonhelical segments (types IV and VII collagens). Group 3 collagens have triple helical domains of less than 95 kDa but have large globular domains. As in the case of the group 2 collagens, the globular end pieces remain with the original chain in the extracellular matrix. In contrast to the collagens of group 1, which shed their globular end pieces when they are incorporated into the ECM, collagen types VI, VII, VIII, XII, XIII, XIV, XV, XVI, XVII, XVIII, and XIX (group 3) retain their noncollagenous domains. In most cases, the globular domains may have vital functions with respect to tissue architecture.[11] The remaining collagens, types II, IX, X, and XI, are excluded from this discussion because they are not found in the vascular connective tissue.

Group 1 molecules consist of an uninterrupted triple-helical domain of approximately 300 nm (see Fig. 3-2). The type I collagen α chains contain 338 Gly-X-Y repeats or 1014 amino acid residues each. There are 341 triplets, or 1023 amino acid residues in type III α chains. The genomic DNAs that encode collagen chains may have evolved by duplication and rearrangement from a primordial gene of 54 base pairs. At both the NH_2 and COOH ends of each α chain are short segments of nonhelical sequences of approximately 15 to 20 residues, referred to as telopeptides. Clearly, type I and type III collagens are quantitatively the major collagens in the blood vessel and together form the striated fibrils. Type V collagen also contains a 300-nm uninterrupted helical domain containing much longer telopeptide domains that may function to regulate striated fibril formation.

Collagen types IV and VII contain interruptions in their triple-helical domain, generally 5 to 20 amino acids in length. The nonhelical segments of these collagens are flexible, thus allowing the formation of a network of crisscrossing molecules. In addition to end-to-end associations, the helical domains of these collagens intertwine to form supercoiled structures in the BMs (see Fig. 3-1). The type IV collagens, which are found exclusively in BM structures, are the best characterized of this group and are represented by a family of six homologous α chains (α1 to α6). The chains assemble into supramolecular structures (see Fig. 3-7) that vary in chain composition from one tissue to another. As shown in Figure 3-8, the subendothelial BM contains predominantly α1 (IV) and α2 (IV) collagen networks.

In contrast, in the medial layer of the blood vessels the BMs of the smooth muscle cells contain two distinct networks made up of type IV collagen. Thus, supramolecular meshworks of α1(IV) and α2(IV) chains as well as those formed by α1(IV), α2(IV), α5(IV) and α6(IV) chains can be readily isolated (see Fig. 3-8). These macromolecular structures are assembled by stoichiometric associations among the 7S modules (head-to-head association) and the NC1 domains (tail-to-tail association) of various α chains of type IV collagen.[13] The precise structural determinants of the supramolecular assemblies remain to be defined.[13]

The type VII collagen molecule is distinguished by its extraordinary length, nearly 467 nm, in which all but a very small portion is triple helix. Type VII forms anchoring fibrils that link BMs to anchoring plaques of type IV collagen and laminin in the underlying extracellular matrix. The triple-helical segment of type VII collagen contains 1530 amino acids in the -Gly-X-Y repeats that are interrupted at 19 sites. In contrast to type IV collagen, the globular domains of the type VI collagen chains, which flank the 336-residue triple-helical regions, are quite large. Type VI monomers contain three distinct α chains, αl[VI], α2[VI], and α3[VI], with molecular weights of 150, 140, and 300 kDa, respectively. Each chain has regions similar to the type A repeats found in the von Willebrand factor (vWF). The α3[VI] collagen chain is much larger because it contains 11 repeats of type A domain of vWF. It also has a 73 amino acid-long segment homologous to platelet glycoprotein lb. This region in the COOH-terminus is also flanked by a type III repeat of FN and a Kunitz-type proteinase inhibitor. The type III domain suggests a role of type VI collagen in cell adhesion and type I collagen binding. Several α2(VI) and α3[VI] chain variants are generated by alternate splicing of the repetitive, noncollagenous domains.[2,3,8]

Another member of the mixed collagen group, type VIII collagen, was originally described as a product of endothelial cells. Type VIII collagen is located in the subendothelium and in the media of small cardiac arteries. It has also been characterized from sheet-like structures found in Descemet membrane that separates the corneal epithelial cells from the corneal stroma, and consists of stacks of collagen lattices made up of type VIII collagen.

In situ hybridization and immunohistologic localization studies reveal that type VIII collagen is a minor component of healthy arteries; however, during plaque formation, enhanced production of type VIII collagen is believed to contribute to remodeling of the newly growing intima in response to atherogenic stimuli.[4] Type VIII collagen is also found in the medial and adventitial layers and in the atherosclerotic intima indicating that smooth muscle cells and infiltrating inflammatory cells may be the main source of its biosynthesis during atherogenesis. Thus, the primary function of type VIII collagen appears to be the maintenance of vessel wall integrity because of its ability to form a 3-D meshwork analogous to the Descemet membrane in the cornea. Its subendothelial accumulation is consistent with its involvement in endothelial cell differentiation, angiogenesis, monocyte infiltration, and thrombosis; and its cellular and ECM distribution also implies that type VIII collagen may be intimately involved in vascular repair and stabilization.[4]

The so called FACIT collagens, such as types XIV and XVI, participate in the process of fibril formation and are believed to regulate the diameter of the collagen fibers.[2,3]

Type XVI collagen is produced by smooth muscle cells, and type XIV is located in the medial layer of the placental vessels.[14,15] Types IV, XV, XVIII, and XIX collagen are also important elements of vascular BMs. It should be mentioned that although a specific function for type IV collagen as a general scaffold of the BM is well established (see earlier), the roles of other collagens are somewhat uncertain. There are indications that some of the minor collagens may become more important during repair and regeneration of the damaged vasculature.[4]

Structure and Properties of Interstitial (Type I and Type III) Collagens

Because of their similarities, type I and type III collagens are discussed together here. The type I collagen molecule is a heterotrimer of two identical α chains, αl(I), and a different α chain, α2(I), and has the chain structure $[\alpha 1(I)]_2$ α2(I). The type III collagen molecule is a homotrimer of three identical α chains and has the chain structure $[\alpha 1(III)]_3$. The helical domain of the α chain contains a repeating triplet sequence of $[\text{Gly-X-Y}]_n$ where X and Y may be any amino acid but are most frequently proline or hydroxyproline. The imino acid residues in the Y position are nearly always hydroxylated (4-hydroxyproline). The stereochemical configuration of the imino acids forces the α chains to assume a left-handed helical structure. Glycine, which occurs at every third residue in the helical domain, is critical because it contains no bulky side chain and will occupy the center position within the triple helix. Substitution of Gly for any other amino acid is not tolerated because of the space restriction.

The triple helix is stabilized by interchain hydrogen bonding contributed by hydroxyproline. Thus, the collagen molecule is a long cylindrical rod with the dimensions of 1.5 nm × 300 nm (see Fig. 3-2). Under physiologic conditions of ionic strength, pH, and temperature, collagen molecules are not soluble and spontaneously aggregate into striated fibrils similar to those seen in tissues. The fibril formation occurs by lateral aggregation of the collagen molecules, in which each neighboring row of molecules is displaced along its long axis by a distance of 68 nm. In addition, within the same row, there is a gap, or "hole," of approximately 40 nm between the end of one molecule and the beginning of the next (see Figs. 3-1 and 3-2). The short nonhelical telopeptides at the NH_2 and COOH ends of each α chain are located in the gap or hole zone of the fibril and are, therefore, accessible to enzymes that regulate collagen crosslinking (see the subsection "Extracellular Maturation").

METABOLISM OF COLLAGEN

Biosynthesis of Collagen

The collagen chains are synthesized as prepro-α chains from which the hydrophobic leader sequence is removed prior to secretion, and the pro-α chains are secreted into the extracellular space. The pro-αl(I) chain contains an NH_2 propeptide and a COOH propeptide. The NH_2 propeptide (pN) consists of a 139-residue sequence that precedes a 17-residue sequence of nonhelical telopeptide. This is followed by a 1014 amino acids-long Gly-X-Y helical sequence attached to a 26 residues-long nonhelical COOH telopeptide followed by the COOH propeptide (pC), which is a 262-residue nonhelical sequence. The structures of pro-α2(I) and pro-αl(III) chains are similar except for minor variations in the number of amino acid residues.[2,3]

The genomic organization and chromosomal locations for various collagen-encoding genes have been studied. In humans, the majority of the 39 genes are dispersed on at least 15 chromosomes (see Table 3-1), however, unlike the majority of the collagen genes, the six homologous α-chains of type IV collagen are encoded by genes that are located in pairs with head-to-head orientation on chromosomes 13 (COL4A1 and COL4A2), 2 (COL4A3 and COL4A4), and the X chromosome (COL4A5 and COL4A6). Interestingly, the promoters of these pairs of type IV collagens overlap—suggesting a coordinate regulation of the gene pairs. The precise molecular mechanisms of this regulation, however, remain incompletely known.[2-4]

Distinct genes encode various α chains of collagens (see Table 3-1). The molecular events for procollagen synthesis (transcription and splicing of precursor RNA, leading to mRNA formation) are essentially identical to other eukaryotic systems. Regulation at the level of transcription and mRNA turnover appears to be involved in the coordinated synthesis of two pro-α1(I) chains per pro-α2(I) chain. Most cells that produce type I collagen also produce type III collagen in variable amounts, depending on the specific type of tissue, the age, and the physiological and pathological situations. Regulation of interstitial collagen biosynthesis has been extensively studied both in physiologic and pathologic settings, in vivo and in vitro.[16,17]

Regulation of pro-α1(I) and pro-α2(I) collagen genes has been extensively studied using a variety of in vitro and in vivo methods, and a number of key *cis*-acting elements and transcription factors that bind to these sequences have been delineated in these genes. The regulatory sequences of collagen genes are modularly organized on either side of the transcription start point (TSP) and may encompass 100-150 kb of DNA, depending on the specific gene and the assays used to study transcriptional regulation. Thus, interactions among these modules (some located in the introns) determine the tissue-specific and inducible promoter activation. The promoters of all known collagen genes contain TATA boxes, located 25 to 35 bp upstream of the TSP. The existence of several conserved sequence elements around the TSP and in the first intron in type I collagen genes has been established. The binding sites for CAAT-binding factor, CBF, Sp1, Sp3, Ap1, and NFkB and a number of orientation-dependent enhancer elements have also been documented.[16,17]

Interstitial collagens found in the subendothelial ECM as well as BM collagens are regulated in response to a variety of physiologic and pathophysiologic stimuli. These include inflammatory stimuli, cytokines such as TGF-β, TNF-α, various interleukins, and nuclear hormones (e.g., glucocorticoids, estrogen, androgen, and retinoids). Distinct *cis*-acting elements that bind Sp1-4, jun-fos, and related factors with Ap1, NF-1-binding sites, and Smads have been demonstrated to mediate collagen gene expression in response to unique cytokines/growth factors/hormones. The emerging theme from these studies is that collagen gene expression is mediated by combinatorial associations among the various *cis*- and *trans*-acting factors.[16,17]

Following translation, pre-procollagens undergo post-translational modifications that include cleavage of signal peptides, hydroxylation of proline and lysine residues, addition of various sugar residues, association of the COOH-terminal propeptides, and formation of interchain and intrachain disulfide bonds.[1,2] Four-proline hydroxylation is carried out by the ubiquitous enzyme 4-prolyl hydroxylase, inhibition of which results in the synthesis of an underhydroxylated procollagen. Underhydroxylated procollagen, as in vitamin C deficiency, is secreted at a greatly reduced rate and is considerably less stable than normal collagen and undergoes rapid degradation. A second enzyme, lysyl hydroxylase, catalyzes the hydroxylation of lysine, requires the same cofactors as prolyl hydroxylase, and reacts only with a lysine residue in the Y position of the Gly-X-Y triplets. Hydroxylation of lysine residues that eventually become involved in crosslink formation imparts significantly greater stability to the crosslink. Deficiency of lysine hydroxylase is associated with skeletal deformities, tissue fragility, and vascular malformations.[2,3] A third hydroxylation reaction involves the formation of 3-hydroxyproline by the action of a prolyl hydroxylase, which is distinct from the prolyl 4-hydroxylase. Only one proline residue is hydroxylated in the αl(I) collagen chain, none in the type III collagen chain, and one to four residues in type IV collagen chains. In every case so far identified, the proline residue must be in the X position.

Several collagens undergo glycosylation; both galactose and glucose residues are attached to some hydroxylysine residues during pre-procollagen biosynthesis. The enzyme UDP-galactose:hydroxylysine galactosyltransferase adds a galactose residue to the hydroxyl group of hydroxylysine. The UDP glucose: galactosylhydroxylysine glucosyltransferase then transfers a glucose residue to some of the hydroxylysine-linked galactose residues. Both enzymes require a divalent cation, and they act in sequence such that galactose is added first, with glucose added only to galactose. Glycosylation occurs during nascent chain synthesis and before the formation of triple helices.[2] Only two of seven hydroxylysine residues of α1(I), α2(I), and αl(III) contain the disaccharide, however, all—or nearly all—the hydroxylysine in other collagens are glycosylated. Glycosylation of specific hydroxylysine that later becomes involved in collagen crosslinking imparts greater stability to the crosslink.

The assembly of procollagen chains into triple-helical molecules is directed by the COOH-terminal propeptide with the formation of interchain disulfide bonds. There is a high degree of structural conservation including the disulfide bonds, within the propeptide of collagens from different species,[2] suggesting the importance of these regions in directing triple-helix formation. Following its triple-helical assembly, the procollagen molecule is secreted into the extracellular space by an incompletely known mechanism.[18] Once secreted, however, the NH_2 and COOH propeptides are proteolytically removed by the actions of N- and C-specific peptidases to yield the collagen molecule. Whether different procollagens require specific peptidases to remove their NH_2 or COOH terminal propeptides is currently unknown. The fragments of the propeptides can specifically suppress procollagen biosynthesis by fibroblasts by means of feedback inhibition of procollagen mRNA translation.[19,20]

Extracellular Maturation

During the extracellular collagen fibril formation, an enzyme, lysyl or hydroxylysyl oxidase, catalyzes the oxidative deamination of specific lysine or hydroxylysine residues in the NH_2- or COOH-terminal telopeptides (Fig. 3-3) to yield allysine and hydroxyallysine, respectively.[21] These reactive aldehydes, being located in the hole zone of the fibril, are free to react with the ε-amino group of lysine or hydroxylysine residues on adjacent chains to form a Schiff base, which can rearrange to a ketoimine via Amadori rearrangement, to yield a more stable interchain crosslink (Fig. 3-4). With time, two ketoimine structures condense to form a trivalent crosslink, 3-hydroxy-pyridinium. At any given time, all three crosslinkages may be found in a specific connective tissue, despite the fact that they are not in equilibrium with each other.[22]

A second basic type of crosslink compound found in collagen originates from the condensation of two aldehydes in allysine or hydroxyallysine on adjacent chains with the formation of a dehydrated aldol condensate (Fig. 3-5). This aldol condensate has a free aldehyde that could react with other ε-amino groups of lysine or histidine to form, potentially, the tri- and tetrafunctional crosslinks, dehydrohydroxymerodesmosine, aldolhistidine,

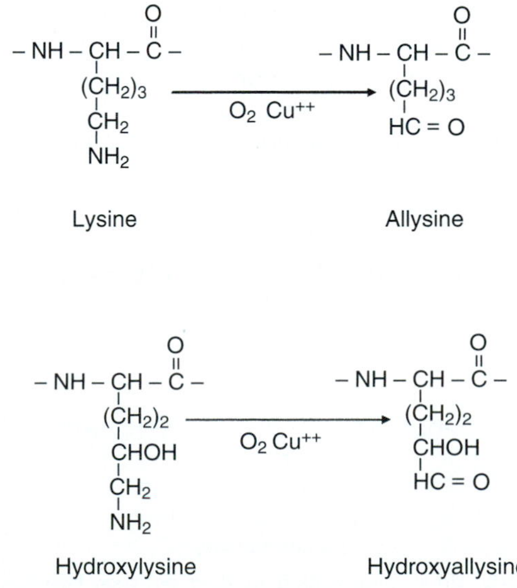

FIGURE 3-3. Reactions catalyzed by peptidyl lysine oxidase.

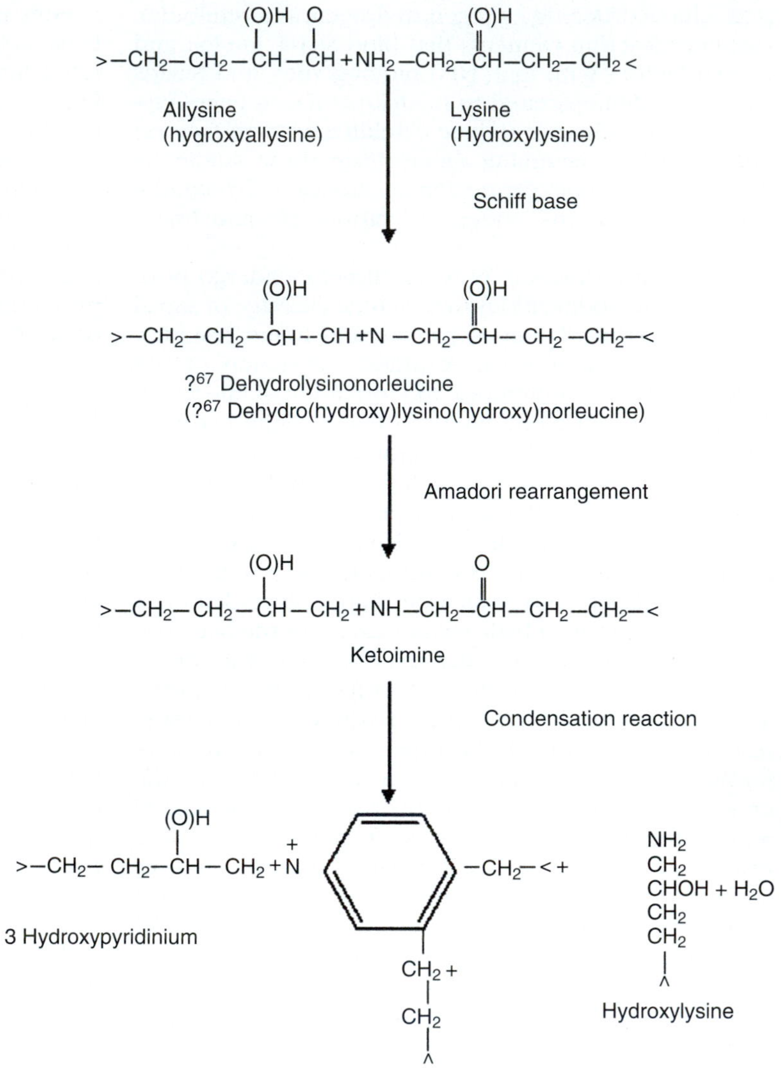

(O)H O (O)H

>–CH_2–CH_2–CH–CH + NH_2–CH_2–CH–CH_2–CH_2<

Allysine (hydroxyallysine) Lysine (Hydroxylysine)

Schiff base

(O)H (O)H

>–CH_2–CH_2–CH--CH +N –CH_2–CH– CH_2 –CH_2–<

?[67] Dehydrolysinonorleucine
(?[67] Dehydro(hydroxy)lysino(hydroxy)norleucine)

Amadori rearrangement

(O)H O

>–CH_2–CH_2–CH–CH_2+ NH–CH_2–CH–CH_2–CH_2–<

Ketoimine

Condensation reaction

(O)H

>–CH_2– CH_2–CH–CH_2+N –CH_2–< +

3 Hydroxypyridinium

CH_2+
CH_2

NH_2
CH_2
CHOH + H_2O
CH_2
CH_2

Hydroxylysine

FIGURE 3-4. Aldamine crosslinks of collagen. Natural reduction of the double bond between N and C of the dehydro compounds apparently does not occur in collagen. In elastin, both dehydrolysinonorleucine and its reduced form lysinonorleucine are found. Hydroxylysine-containing crosslinks in collagen are stabilized by the formation of ketoimine structures by Amadori rearrangement. The proposed condensation of the two ketoimine structures yields a hydroxypyridinium residue and free hydroxylysine.

and histidinohydroxymerodesmosine, which link three or four collagen chains.[23]

Once the aldehydes of allysine and hydroxyallysine are formed, subsequent aldamine and aldol condensation reactions proceed spontaneously but slowly in the tissue. The crosslinking results in an enormous complex of macromolecules, covalently linked, and gives rise to the high tensile strength and insolubility of the collagen fibrils.

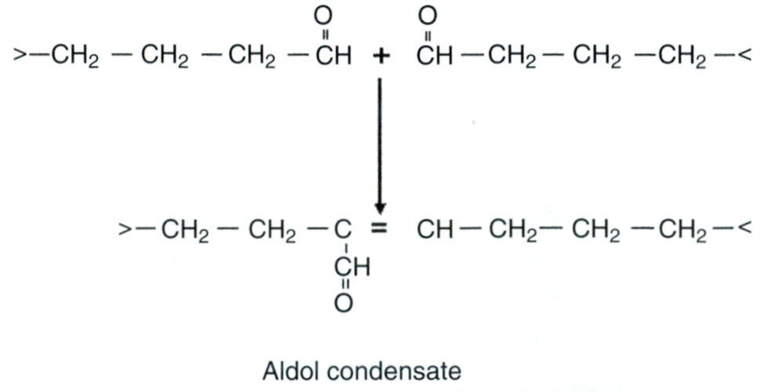

O O

>–CH_2 – CH_2 – CH_2 – CH + CH – CH_2– CH_2 – CH_2 –<

>– CH_2 – CH_2 – C = CH – CH_2– CH_2 – CH_2 –<

CH

O

Aldol condensate

FIGURE 3-5. Aldol condensation product between two residues of allysine. This crosslink is found in both collagen and elastin.

These reactions depend on the high degree of organization imparted by the specific aggregation of collagen molecules in the fibril itself. The particular stagger of the collagen molecules in the fibrils allows nonhelical allysine or hydroxyallysine in the NH_2 and COOH telopeptides to form a crosslink at potentially four areas in the helical domain of the adjacent collagen molecules (see Fig. 3-2).

Turnover of Collagen

The metabolic turnover of interstitial collagen in the intact tissues is extremely low, unlike a very rapid breakdown and synthesis of collagen that takes place during tissue remodeling. The fibrillar collagens in the native state are resistant to the action of general proteases, although they are readily degraded by a wide variety of proteases once the molecules are denatured or the helical structures are disrupted. In contrast, the FACIT collagens (types IX, XII, and XIV) and others containing noncollagenous domains within their helices (e.g., type VI collagen) may be more susceptible to proteases. After cleavage of the nonhelical segments, the short triple-helical domains denature at 37°C, and become susceptible to nonspecific proteases, such as gelatinases and stromelysin. A specific class of proteinases, the matrix metalloproteinases (MMPs) degrade collagens in vivo and in vitro.[24,25] MMPs cleave the native collagen molecule at a single position within the triple helix (between residues 775 and 776) and the resulting collagen fragments denature spontaneously at body temperature and pH, and become highly susceptible to the actions of many proteases.

Metalloproteinases

The matrix metalloproteinases (MMPs) constitute a superfamily of homologous enzymes; there are 22 known homologues found in humans to date (Table 3-2). The individual MMPs are named according to a sequential numerical nomenclature and may be grouped according to their modular organization.[24,25] All MMPs, except MMP7, MMP23, and MMP26, possess a hemopexin/vitronectin-like domain that is connected to the catalytic domain by a short linker (Fig. 3-6). The hemopexin domain influences binding of MMPs to tissue inhibitors of metalloproteinases (TIMPs) as well as to the substrates. The substrate specificity of various MMPs is dictated by their catalytic domains in concert with a number of additional sequences removed from the catalytic site of the molecule. MMPs degrade a plethora of proteins that include other proteinases, protease inhibitors, chemotactic molecules, growth factors, cell adhesion molecules, and nearly all constituents of the ECM. This confounding multitude of targets has presumably evolved to subserve many important pathophysiologic processes.

All MMPs are synthesized as pre-proenzymes. Although most MMPs are secreted, at least six discovered thus far contain transmembrane domains (e.g., MT-MMPs) and are associated with plasma membranes on the cell surface. The "pro" domain functions to maintain MMPs in latent conformations and its removal causes the activation of the catalytic domain, which requires Zn^{++} for its enzymatic activity. Although in vitro enzymology

TABLE 3-2 CHARACTERISTICS OF MMP FAMILY MEMBERS

MMP	Common Name	Substrate**	Expression
MMP-1	Collagenase-1	CN types I, II, III, V, VII, VIII, and X, aggrecan, gelatin, and serpins	Fibroblasts, keratinocytes, epithelial and endothelial cells, osteoblasts, macrophages
MMP-2	Gelatinase A	CN types I, IV, V, VII, and X, gelatin, elastin, FN, LN, nidogen, active MMP-9 and active MMP-13	Fibroblasts, macrophages, and platelets
MMP-3	Stromelysin-1	CN types II, IV, IX, X, and XI, LN, nidogen, FN, proteoglycan, aggrecan, elastin, gelatin, proMMP-1, proMMP-8, and proMMP-9	Fibroblasts, epithelial cells, macrophages, vascular smooth muscle cells, and endothelial cells
MMP-7	Matrilysin	CN type IV, elastin, proteoglycan and gelatin	Macrophages, mesangial cells, and epithelial cells
MMP-8	Collagenase-2	CN types I, II, III, and V	PMN, chondrocytes, fibroblasts, and endothelial cells
MMP-9	Gelatinase B	CN type IV, gelatin, aggrecan, LN, and nidogen	Macrophages, endothelial cells, megakaryocytes, neutrophils and eosinophils
MMP-10	Stromelysin-2	CN type IV, LN, nidogen, FN, proteoglycan, and gelatin	Fibroblasts, epithelial cells, keratinocytes, and T lymphocytes
MMP-11	Stromelysin-3	LN, α1-proteinase inhibitor, and α1-antitrypsin	Epithelial cells and fibroblasts
MMP-12	Macrophage Elastase	Elastin	Macrophages
MMP-13	Collagenase-3	CN types I, II, III, IV, V, IX, X, and XI, gelatin, LN, tenascin, aggrecan, and FN	Fibroblasts and osteocytes
MMP-14	MT1-MMP	CN types I, II, and III, gelatin, FN, LN, VN, aggrecan, nidogen, tenascin, perlecan, proMMP-2, proMMP-13, and proteoglycan	Fibroblasts, epithelial cells, macrophages, and osteoclasts
MMP-15	MT2-MMP	CN types I, II, and III, proMMP-2, proMMP-13, gelatin, FN, LN, nidogen, tenascin, perlecan, VN, and aggrecan	Macrophages and fibroblasts
MMP-16	MT3-MMP	CN types I and III, FN, LN, aggrecan, perlecan, gelatin, casein, VN, proMMP-2 and proMMP-13	Placenta and vascular smooth muscle cells
MMP-17	MT4-MMP	FN, fibrin, and gelatin	Brain, reproductive tissues, and leukocytes
MMP-20	Enamelysin	Amelogenin, aggrecan, and cartilage oligomeric matrix protein (COMP)	Odontoblastic cells
MMP-23			Reproductive tissue
MMP-24	MT5-MMP	ProMMP-2 and proMMP-13	Brain
MMP-25	MT6-MMP	ProMMP-2	Neutrophils

CN, collagen; FG, fibrinogen; FN, fibronectin; LN, laminin; VN, vitronectin.

Adapted from Nagase H, Woessner JF, Jr: Matrix metalloproteinases. J Biol Chem 274(31):21491, 1999; Sternlicht MD, Werb Z: How matrix metalloproteinases regulate cell behavior. Annu Rev Cell Dev Biol 17:463, 2001.

A) Minimal Domain MMPs (MMP7/matrilysin, MMP26/endometase)

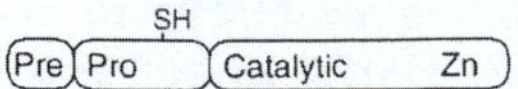

B) Simple Hemopexin Domain-Containing MMPs
(MMP1/collagenase-1, MMP8/collagenase-2, MMP13/collagenase-3, MMP18/collagenase-4, MMP3/stromelysin-1, MMP10/stromelysin-2, MMP27, MMP12/metalloelastase, MMP19/RASI-1, MMP20/enamelysin, MMP22/CMMP)

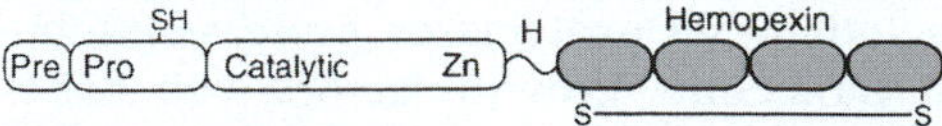

C) Gelatin-binding MMPs (MMP2/gelatinase A, MMP9/gelatinase B)

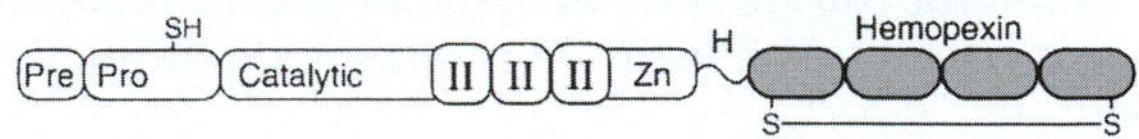

D) Furin-activated Secreted MMPs (MMP11/stromelysin-3, MMP28/epilysin)

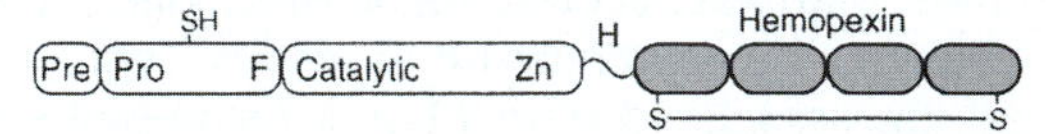

E) Transmembrane MMPs
(MMP14/MT1-MMP, MMP15/MT2-MMP, MMP16/MT3-MMP, MMP24/MT5-MMP)

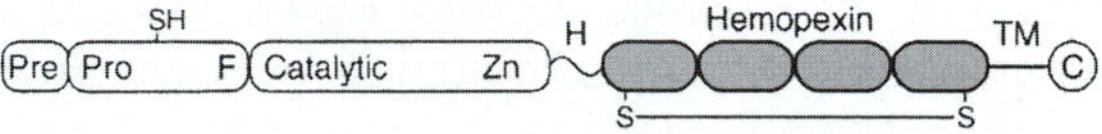

F) GPI-linked MMPs (MMP17/MT4-MMP, MMP25/MT6-MMP)

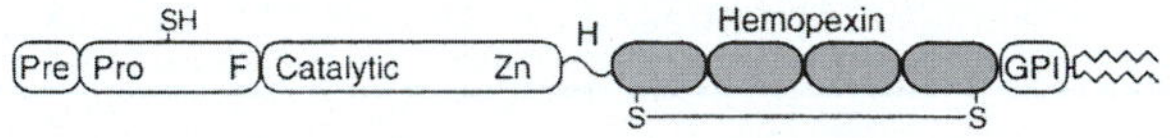

G) Vitronectin-like Insert Linker-less MMPs (MMP21/XMMP)

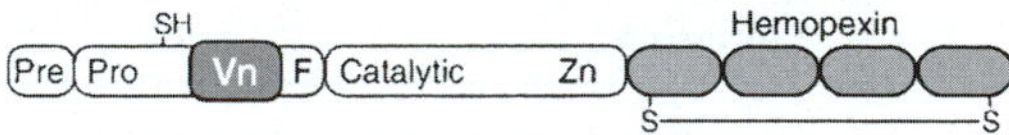

H) Cysteine/Proline-Rich IL-1 Receptor-like Domain MMPs (MMP23)

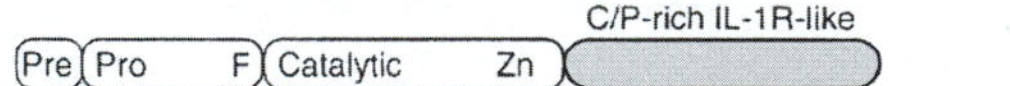

FIGURE 3-6. Domain structure of the MMPs. The hemopexin/vitronectin-like domain contains four repeats with the first and last linked by a disulfide bond. C, cytoplasmic tail; C/P, cysteine/proline; F, furin-susceptible site; GPI, glycophosphatidyl inositol-anchoring domain; H, hinge region; IL-IR, interleukin-1 receptor; Pre, signal sequence; Pro, propeptide with a free zinc-ligating thiol (SH) group; TM, transmembrane domain; II, collagen-binding fibronectin type II inserts; Zn, zinc-binding site. (From the Annual Review of Cell and Developmental Biology, vol 17, 2001, www.annualreviews.org.)

has identified numerous substrates for various MMPs (see Table 3-2), the precise identities of their in vivo targets of degradation remain largely elusive. Several potential in vivo targets of MMPs may be associated with ECM of the subendothelial connective tissues. For example, MMP1 (collagenase 1) readily degrades collagen types I, II, and III, whereas MMP-8 (collagenase 2) digests types I, III, IV, V, VII, X, and XI collagen. Similarly MMP2 (gelatinase A) degrades types I, III, IV, V, VII, X, and XI collagens, whereas gelatinase B (MMP9) digests collagen types IV, V, XI, and XIV preferentially. MMP13 (collagenase 3) is also capable of degrading collagens that are prevalent in the subendothelial connective tissue (types I, III, VI, IX, and XIV). Many collagenous and noncollagenous ECM components are readily degraded by stromelysin-1 (MMP3) and stromelysin-2 (MMP10), whereas stromelysin-3 (MMP11) does not degrade known collagens but readily breaks down laminin. MMPs are also capable of digesting a number of other constituents of ECM, such as FN and elastin, and a variety of additional cell- and ECM-associated molecules. The processing of ECM-bound pro-TGFβ and pro-TNFα may be facilitated by the actions of some MMPs.

Numerous studies have been aimed at elucidating the underlying mechanisms by which MMPs discriminate their in vivo targets and two major regulatory themes to explain the exquisite specificity of various MMPs have emerged from these studies. First, the synthesis and localization of various pro-MMPs and their specific TIMPs are highly regulated. Both autocrine and paracrine factors regulate the rates of mRNA transcription, turnover, intracellular and extracellular processing and deposition, and activation of the catalytic domains of various MMPs. The second key regulatory attribute of a particular pro-MMP resides in the modular organization of its functional domains. For example, the presence of three cysteine-rich repeats, akin to type II repeats found in FN (see later) in gelatinase A and gelatinase B, determines their affinity and specificity toward elastin and collagen.[25-27] The structure of various pro-MMPs also dictates their ability to be regulated by TIMPs; these inhibitors reversibly bind to MMPs in a 1:1 stoichiometry and inhibit enzymatic activity. TIMPs are represented by four homologous proteins (TIMP1 to 4) of 20 to 29 kDa in size that specifically interact with various MMPs.[25,28] For example, whereas only TIMP3 potently inhibits MMP9, both TIMP2 and TIMP3 inhibit MTI-MMP. In contrast, TIMP1 is a very poor inhibitor of MT3-MMP but a potent inhibitor of MMP3. In addition to inhibiting the activities of various MMPs, TIMPs are also involved in the regulation of other cellular activities that include apoptosis[29,30] and cell growth and differentiation.[28]

Concerted actions of various MMPs and their TIMPs regulate key events in the formation of blood vessels in the developing embryo, and the processes of neovasculogenesis and angiogenesis in the adult in response to injury and regeneration (Table 3-3). The formation of new blood vessels from existing vessels is dependent on extensive turnover of the subendothelial ECM. This process enables migration of blood vessel-associated cells, liberation of sequestered angiogenic factors, and exposure of cryptic, cell-regulatory domains found in the intact ECM macromolecules. Therefore, a crucial balance between MMPs and TIMPs is essential for ensuring the maturation of newly formed blood vessels and ongoing maintenance of their structural integrity. This phenomenon is especially critical during the early development of solid tumors that depends on the emergence of new blood vessels before they assume an invasive, metastatic phenotype.[31] MMP2 binds to the $a_v\beta_3$ integrin and promotes angiogenesis and tumor growth.[32] In contrast, transmembrane MMP, MT1-MMP, cleaves $a_v\beta_3$ integrin and enhances its affinity for its ligands containing arginine-glycine-aspartic acid (RGD) sequences.

LESS ABUNDANT COLLAGENS FOUND IN THE SUBENDOTHELIAL ECM

In addition to the interstitial collagens (types I, III, and V), other types of collagens are present in much smaller quantities and are, therefore, referred to as *minor collagens.*

TABLE 3-3 THE EFFECT OF MATRIX TURNOVER ON VASCULAR PATHOLOGIES*

	Model	Effects
Aneurysm	MMP-3 -/-/ApoE -/-	↓ Aneurysm
	MMP-9 -/-	↓ Aneurysm
	MMP-12 -/-	↔ Aneurysm
	Broad-range MMP inhibitor LDLR -/-	↓ Aneurysm
	TIMP-1 -/-ApoE-/-	↑ Aneurysm
	TIMP-1 ↑ rat	↓ Aneurysm
Neo-intima formation	MMP-9 ↑ rat	↑ SMC migration ↓ matrix content ↑ Luminal diameter
	Broad-range MMP inhibitor	↓ Early and ↔ late neo-intima formation
	LDLR -/- Doxycycline, MMP inhibition rat	↓ Neo-intima formation
	TIMP-1 ↑ human vein	↓ Neo-intima formation
	TIMP-2 ↑ human vein	↓ Neo-intima formation
	TIMP-3 ↑ human and pig vein	↓ Neo-intima formation
	MMP-9 -/-, mouse carotid ligation	↓ Intimal hyperplasia, ↑ collagen content
Remodeling	MMP-12 ↑	↓ Luminal diameter
	MMP inhibitor pig	↓ Constrictive remodeling
Atherosclerosis	MMP-1 ↑/ApoE -/-	↓ Plaque size ↓ collagen content
	MMP-3 -/-/ApoE -/-	↓ Plaque size ↑ collagen content
	MMP-3 ↓ human, promoter polymorphism	↑ Plaque progression
	MMP-9 ↑ human, promoter polymorphism	↑ Triple vessel disease
	MMP-9 ↑ human promoter polymorphism	↔ Coronary artery stenosis
	Broad-range MMP inhibitor LDL -/-	↔ Plaque size
	TIMP-1 -/-/ApoE -/-	↓ Plaque size ↑ lipid core content
	TIMP-1 -/-/ApoE -/-	↔ Plaque size, medial rupture, micro-aneurysms
	TIMP-1 ↑/ApoE -/-	↓ Plaque size ↑ collagen content
	TGFβ inhibition ApoE -/-	↑ Plaque vulnerability, intraplaque hemorrhage

-/-, knockout or homozygous-deficient mice; +/+, transgenic overexpressing mice; ↑, upregulated or increased; ↓, downregulated or decreased; Apo, apolipoprotein; LDLR, LDL receptor; MMP, matrix metalloproteinase; SMC, smooth muscle cell; TGF, transforming growth factor; TIMP, tissue inhibitor of matrix metalloproteinase.

Adapted from Heeneman S, Cleutjens JP, Faber BC, et al: The dynamic extracellular matrix: Intervention strategies during heart failure and atherosclerosis. J Pathol 2003:516, 2003.

Although accurate in a quantitative sense, the term is not appropriate in a biologic sense because there is nothing functionally minor about these collagens.

Network Forming and Basement Membrane Collagens

As shown in Figure 3-2, this group includes type IV collagens (α1 to α6 chains) and collagen types VIII and X. The type IV collagens are molecules with helical domains—each greater than 95,000 kDa—with nonhelical segments interspersed within the helical domains. Rather than a quarter-stagger, side-by-side alignment of the individual molecules, as in the interstitial collagens, type IV collagen forms supramolecular structures by end-to-end associations stabilized by both lysine-derived crosslinks and interchain disulfide bonds (Fig. 3-7).

The six α chains of type IV collagen have now been identified (see Fig. 3-7); each α chain contains approximately 1700 amino acid residues.[5] Unlike fibrillar collagens, the amino and carboxyl propeptides of type IV collagen remain as integral parts of the molecules when deposited in the tissue. The NH_2 terminus, or 7S domain, of the αl(IV) chain contains a nonhelical segment of 20 amino acid residues followed by a helical segment of 108 amino acid residues and a nonhelical 13-residue segment (see Fig. 3-7). Twelve α chains from four molecules are crosslinked within the 7S region.[33,34] The COOH-terminal NC1 domain contains 229 amino acids, is nonhelical, and has many cysteine residues. Surprisingly, greater homology exists between these COOH-nonhelical propeptide regions of αl(IV) and interstitial collagen than any other segment.[5] The globular domains of the NH_2 terminus (7S segment) and the COOH terminus (NC1) participate in the intermolecular crosslinks. The triple-helical domain between the two globular ends is 330 nm long and contains 21 interruptions in the Gly-X-Y triplet sequence; these interruptions impart a high degree of flexibility. Four triple-helical molecules are joined at their amino terminal globular ends to form a 7S region, whereas two carboxyl globular domains are joined to form the NC1 region.[33] Surprisingly, there is little homology between the αl(IV) and α2(IV) chains. As demonstrated recently,[13] two other molecular species, $[\alpha3(IV)1]_2$ α4(IV) and $[\alpha5(IV)1]_2$ α6(IV), are present together with the predominant dimer of α1(IV) and α2(IV) chains.

The random combination of the six (α1 to α6) chains of type IV collagen can theoretically form 56 different triple-helical isoforms, that may assemble into supramolecular networks by further associations among the different protomers, however, it appears that these associations are not totally random (Fig. 3-8). For example, in the aorta only three major networks of type IV collagen (α1-α2; α3-α4-α5, and α1-α2-α5-α6) could be detected.

The genomic structure of the type IV collagen genes is unusual.[5] The αl(IV) and α2(IV) collagen genes are paired head to head on the same chromosome and are transcribed in opposite directions. The α3 and α4 and

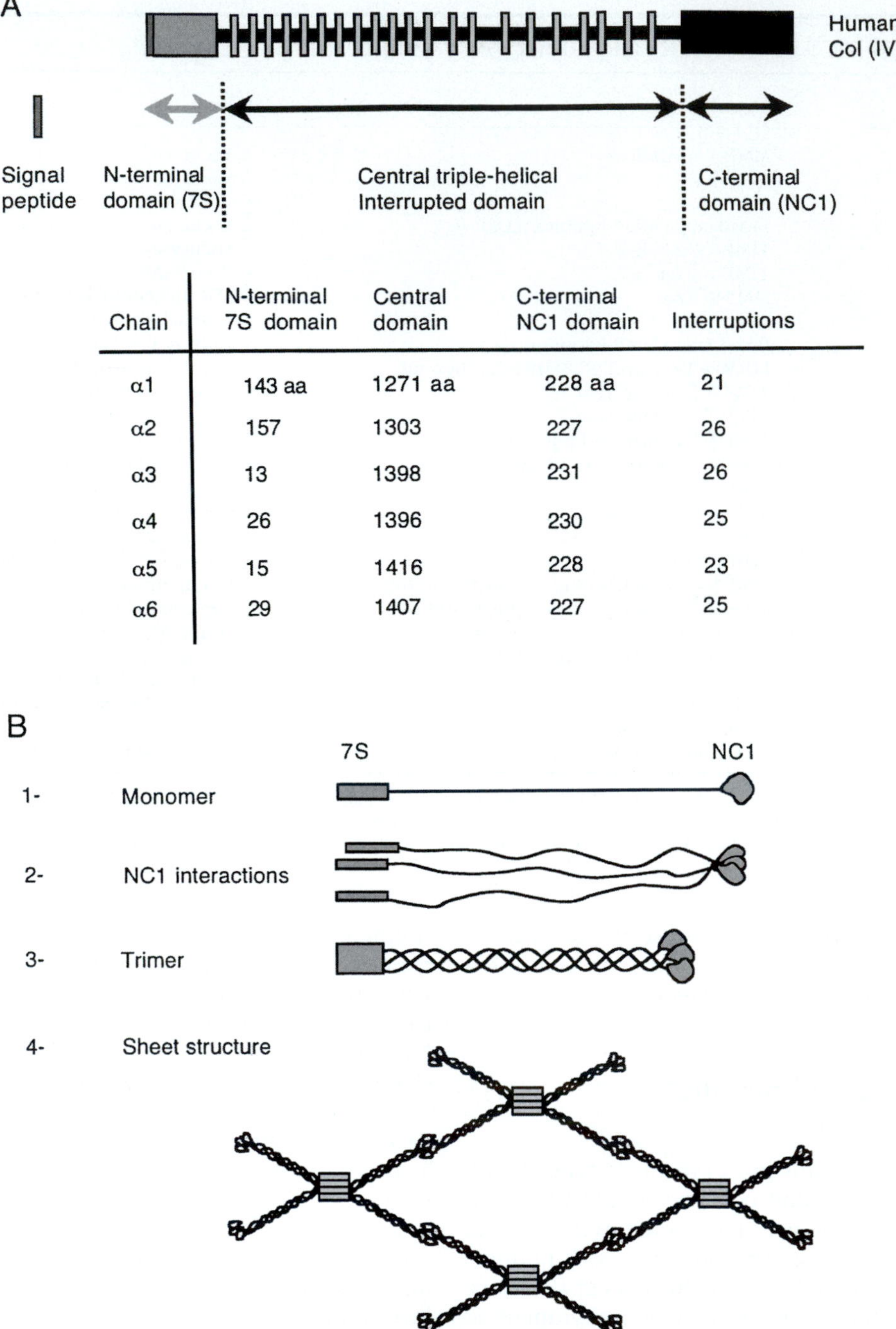

Chain	N-terminal 7S domain	Central domain	C-terminal NC1 domain	Interruptions
α1	143 aa	1271 aa	228 aa	21
α2	157	1303	227	26
α3	13	1398	231	26
α4	26	1396	230	25
α5	15	1416	228	23
α6	29	1407	227	25

FIGURE 3-7. A, Linear structure of human collagen IV α chains. Six different genes encode collagen IV α chains; each polypeptide is composed of three distinct domains: a cysteine-rich N terminal 7S domain, a central triple-helical domain with multiple small interruptions (*boxes*) and a globular C-terminal noncollagenous NC1 domain. The NC1 and central triple-helical domains are of an equivalent size, whereas the 7S domains are shorter in the cases of α3, α4, α5, and α6 compared with α1 and α2. On the basis of sequence homology, these different chains can be divided in two groups, the α1-like (α1, α2, α5) and the α2-like (α2, α4, α6). **B,** Assembly of collagen IV α chains. The assembly of trimers is dependent first on the association of the NC1 domains, then on the triple-helical structure forms and 7S domains in a spider-shaped structure; the two trimers interact head to head through their NC1 domains, forming a sheet structure. Several trimers can also lace together along their triple-helical domain, thickening the structure. (From Company of Biologists, Ltd., Ortega N, Werb Z: New functional roles for non-collagenous domains of basement membrane collagens. J Cell Sci 115:4201, 2002.)

the α5 and α6 are similarly arranged except they are located on two different chromosomes. The type IV collagen genes are very large and complex—the αl and α5 genes exceeding 100 kilobases in size. The mechanisms of transcriptional and posttranscriptional regulation of α1 to α6 (IV) collagen genes are incompletely known.[2]

Microfibrillar Collagen, Type VI

Type VI collagen, is a highly unusual collagen consisting of collagenous and noncollagenous domains that assemble into beaded filaments.[7,35] Type VI collagen microfibrils have been located in the vascular subendothelium.[35-37]

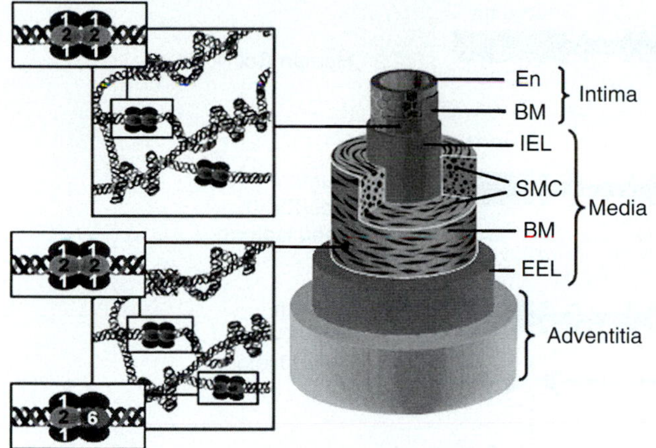

FIGURE 3-8. (See also Color Plate 3-8.) Localization of the α1·α2· and α1·α2·α5·α6 networks of type IV collagen in vascular basement membranes (BMs). A schematic diagram of a large artery (aorta) depicts its multilayered structure (*right*). The endothelial cells (En) rest on a subendothelial BM, which contains the α1·α2(IV) collagen network (*right*). The smooth muscle cells (SMCs) in the media are surrounded by smooth muscle BM and are sandwiched between an internal and an external elastic lamina (IEL and EEL, respectively). The α1·α2· and α1·α2·α5·α6 networks of type IV collagen coexist in smooth muscle BM (*right*). (From Borza DB, Bondar O, Ninomiya Y, et al: The NC1 domain of collagen IV encodes a novel network composed of the alpha 1, alpha 2, alpha 5, and alpha 6 chains in smooth muscle basement membranes. J Biol Chem 276[30]:28532, 2001.)

Type VI collagen microfibrils exhibit unique adhesive properties to other ECM components, such as other collagens, heparin, and vWF, and may be involved in the adhesion of platelets and smooth muscle cells. In the medial layer, type VI collagen facilitates interaction between smooth muscle cells and elastin by bridging the elastic fibers and cells.[38]

The type VI collagen molecule is a 400-kDa triple-helical molecule that contains globular domains of about 150 kDa each at both its NH_2 and COOH ends (see Fig. 3-1). The intact molecule has been difficult to isolate owing to its exquisite sensitivity to nonspecific proteases. Its molecular structure consists of a heterotrimer of three different α chains, α1, α2 and α3 (VI), encoded by unique genes. Several α2 (VI) and α3 (VI) chain variants, generated by alternate splicing of mRNAs, have also been documented.[2,3]

The aggregates that type VI collagen forms are relatively unusual; the triple-helical monomeric units form dimers in an antiparallel fashion. These staggered aggregates contain 75-nm overlap regions held together in a supratwist by disulfide bonds. Tetramers are formed from dimers and held together by disulfide bonds in the scissors-like regions (see Fig. 3-1).

Types XV and XVIII collagens, identified as chondroitin sulfate and heparan sulfate proteoglycans, respectively, comprise a unique subfamily of collagens (see Table 3-1). As shown in Figure 3-9, these two collagens have distinct structures, with central triple helical domains interrupted several times and noncollagenous fragments on their NH_2 and COOH termini.[39] Degradation of type XV and type XVIII collagens by various MMPs generates biologically active fragments capable of regulating motility, angiogenesis, and branching morphogenesis in vitro and in vivo.[11]

The Facit Collagens

The types IX, XII, XIV, XVI, and XIX collagens are another subfamily of collagens that do not form fibrils themselves but associate with other fibril-forming collagens. The type IX collagen, the prototype of this group, represents the group of collagens collectively named FACIT (fibril-associated collagens with interrupted triple helices) collagens. Their structures may be divided into triple-helical (COL) and nontriple-helical (NC) domains. The triple-helical domain nearest the COOH terminus (COL-1) associates with collagen fibrils of type II (cartilage) and type I and type III in noncartilagenous tissues.

Type IX collagen consists of three α chains, [αl(IX) α2(IX) α3(IX)], whereas type XII and type XIV collagens are homotrimers, $[\alpha\ (XII)]_3$ and $[\alpha l(XIV)]_3$. The second noncollagenous domain of type IX collagen often contains a proteoglycan, a single glycosaminoglycan (GAG) side chain that is covalently attached to the collagen molecule (see Fig. 3-1). Type XII and type XIV collagens show structural similarities to type IX collagen and, likewise, contain a GAG chain. Among the FACIT collagens, XVI and XIX are associated with vessels, but by no means are restricted to the vasculature. As in other locations, their primary function in the subendothelial connective tissue has not been defined with precision.[2-4]

THE ELASTIC FIBER

To perform their physiologic function, blood vessels are endowed with a high degree of distensibility, including the ability to deform to large extensions with small forces. The subendothelial ECM and ECM of the arterial media are responsible for the known resilience of the vessels to repeated cycles of deformity and passive recoil during diastole and systole, respectively. This apparent elasticity and resilience of blood vessels is primarily provided by a macromolecular structure that consists of elastin and associated molecules and is referred to as the elastic fiber. The large arteries contain as much as 50% elastin by dry weight, and the elastin-enriched fiber has mechanical properties that are similar to rubber (i.e., the degree of elongation without irreversible changes per unit force applied to unit cross-sectional areas is high).

The organization of the elastic fibers has been studied by ultrastructural, biochemical, and genetic approaches, and a number of key insights have been gathered in recent years. The insoluble elastic fiber is a complex structure made up of elastin and nonelastin molecules. The elastic fibers are generated in the developing organs in the embryo by deposition of tropoelastin, the soluble precursor of the crosslinked, mature elastin, on a template of fibrillin-rich microfibers. The crosslinked elastin produced during late fetal and postnatal development generally lasts the lifetime of the organism. The core of the mature elastic fiber is made up of laterally packed filaments of crosslinked elastin and an outer mantle of fibrillin and associated molecules.[8,40] Microfibers composed of

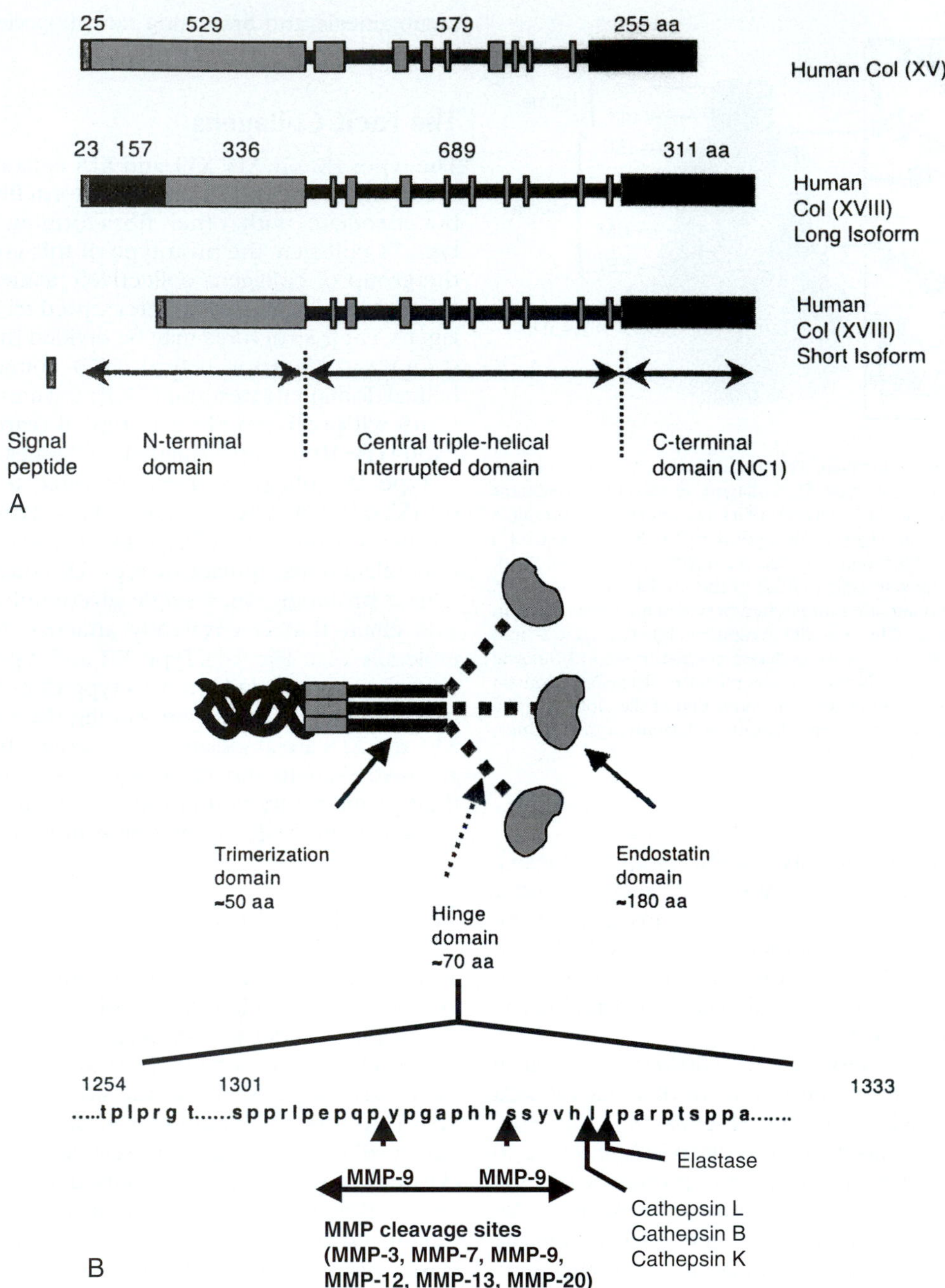

FIGURE 3-9. **A,** Linear structure of human collagen XV and XVIII α1 chains. The α1 chains of collagen XV and XVIII are structurally homologous; they define a new collagen subfamily, the multiplexin family, on the basis of their central triple-helical domain with multiple long interruptions. They are also characterized by a long noncollagenous N-terminal domain-containing thrombospondin sequence motif with two splicing variants in human collagen XVIII and long noncollagenous globular C-terminal domain or NC1 domain. **B,** Functional subdomains of human NC1 (XVIII) and protease cleavage sites. The NC1 domain contains three functionally different subdomains: these domains consist of an N terminal noncovalent trimerization domain necessary for the association of trimers; a hinge domain containing multiple sites that are sensitive to different proteases; and an endostatin globular domain covering a fragment of 20 kDa with antiangiogenic and antibranching morphogenesis activities. Numerous enzymes can generate fragments containing endostatin. Cathepsin L and elastase are the most efficient, but in contrast to MMP cleavage leading to accumulation of endostatin, cathepsins L and B degrade the molecule (cleavage sites are indicated according to the data published by Ferreras.[39]) (From Company of Biologists, Ltd., Ortega N, Werb Z: New functional roles for non-collagenous domains of basement collagens. J Cell Sci 115:4201, 2002.)

fibrillin are found in jellyfish and invertebrates, and the evolution of elastin seems to have occurred more recently to facilitate the development of a high pressure, closed circulatory system of the higher vertebrates.[8,41,42]

Fibrillin is the major constituent of microfibers that form loosely packed parallel bundles in the tissues (Fig. 3-10). X-ray studies and mechanical testing of microfibril bundles indicate that calcium ions influence load deformation but are not needed for elasticity. Tropoelastin and other microfibril-associated molecules determine the biomechanical properties of the microfibrils (see Fig. 3-10). Fibrillins are represented by three homologous proteins,

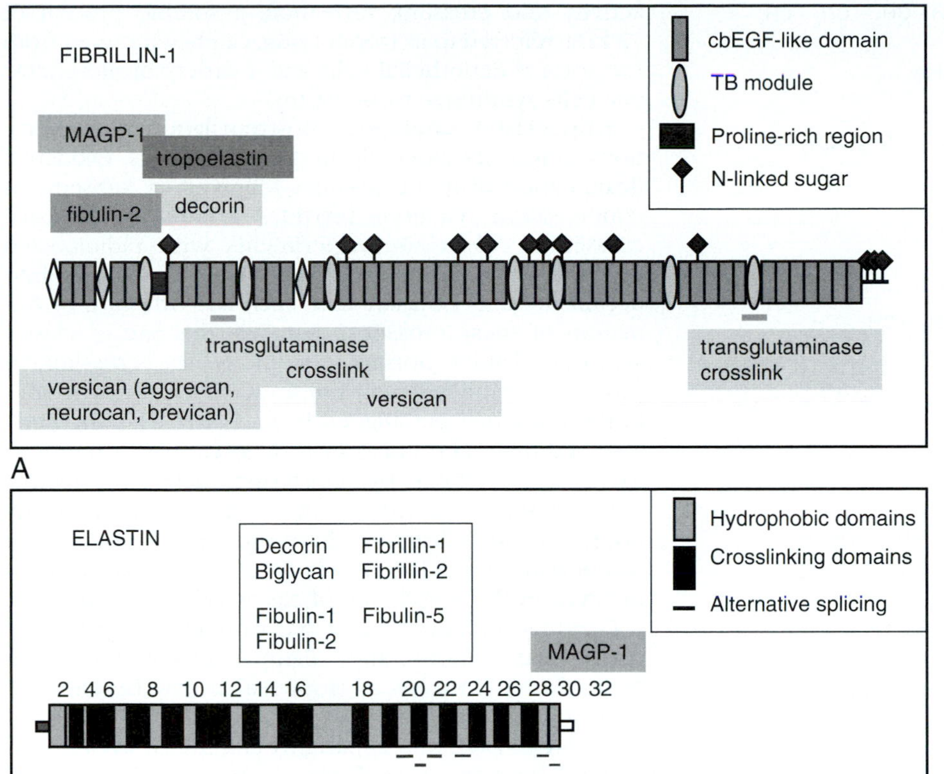

FIGURE 3-10. Domain structures of fibrillin-1 and elastin, showing molecular interaction sites identified in vitro. **A,** Fibrillin-1 has 47 cbEGF-like domains, interspersed with TB modules. A proline-rich region is toward the N terminus. *N*-glycosylation sites are indicated. **B,** Elastin contains alternating hydrophobic and crosslinking domains. The C terminus has two cysteines and a negatively charged pocket. (From Company of Biologists, Ltd., Kielty CM, Sherratt MJ, and Shuttleworth, CA: Elastic fibres. J Cell Sci 115: 2817, 2002.)

fibrillin-1, fibrillin-2, and fibrillin-3. Fibrillins are approximately 350 kDa glycoproteins that contain multiple subdomains that interact with other macromolecules (see Fig. 3-10). The fibrillin superfamily also includes the four latent TGFβ-binding proteins, LTBP1, 2, 3, and 4. Although LTBPs are highly homologous proteins with multiple EGF-repeats, the four LTBPs may serve unique functions in vivo. LTBP1, 3, and 4 may be involved in targeting the latent TGFβ to various specialized ECM. LTBP2 does not bind TGFβ and is highly expressed in response to arterial injury. The microfibril-associated glycoproteins, MAGP-1 and MAGP-2, are also believed to impart structural integrity to the microfibrils.[43,44] Additionally, proteoglycans, such as biglycan, decorin, and versican, also associate with the microfibrils and are believed to facilitate their incorporation into the surrounding ECM.[8,41]

ELASTIN

Elastin is the principal ECM protein of the vascular ECM comprising the amorphous elastic fiber. The elastic fiber assembly is believed to occur by deposition of tropoelastin on a preformed microfibrillar template, produced by a cell-regulated reaction that does not depend on the presence of tropoelastin. Tropoelastin is the soluble monomer of elastin encoded by a single gene on human chromosome 7q.11.23. Elastin is one of the most apolar and insoluble proteins in nature, which is evident from its amino acid composition (330 glycine, 128 proline, 174 alanine, 177 valine, and 52 leucine per 1000 residues). The glycine and proline content of elastin is similar to collagen, but elastin contains no hydroxyproline or hydroxylysine, and very small amounts of polar amino acids.

Elucidation of the molecular organization of elastin has been difficult because of its relative insolubility when extracted from tissues. Therefore, little is known about how newly synthesized and secreted tropoelastin monomer is converted into an "elastomeric polymer." The tropoelastin is characterized by a series of tandem repeats, with each repeated segment including a lysine-rich crosslinking domain followed by a hydrophobic motif. In vitro elastin undergoes a process of ordered self-aggregation caused by specific interactions of the individual hydrophobic domains and it is believed that the protein has an intrinsic ability to organize into polymeric structures. In vivo, tropoelastin probably interacts with microfibrils prior to aggregation and becomes crosslinked by lysyl oxidase.[8]

Elastin Crosslink

As in collagen crosslinking, the first step in the elastin crosslink formation is the oxidative deamination of the ε-amino group of lysine following polypeptide chain synthesis. In fact, the same lysyl oxidase reacts with both collagens and elastin. Because no hydroxylysine is present in elastin, only the allysine aldehyde becomes involved.[45] In contrast to collagen, however, reduction of the double bonds in the elastin crosslink occurs spontaneously by an unknown mechanism, and the quantity of lysine involved in crosslinking is much larger in elastin than in collagen. As shown in Figure 3-11, four basic types of crosslink compounds have been identified in elastin: dehydrolysinonorleucine and its reduced form, lysinonorleucine;

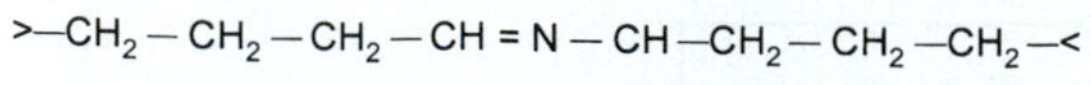

>—CH_2—CH_2—CH_2—CH = N—CH—CH_2—CH_2—CH_2—<

Dehydrolysinonorleucine

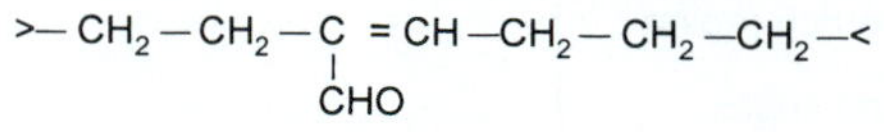

>—CH_2—CH_2—C = CH—CH_2—CH_2—CH_2—<
CHO

Allysinealdol

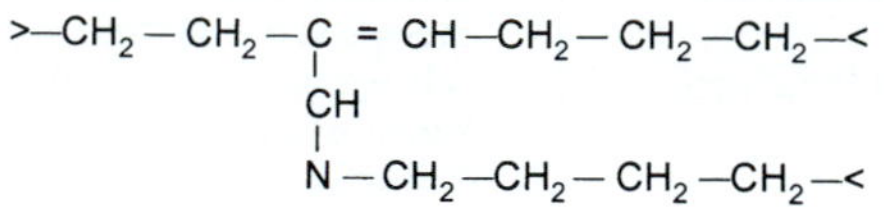

>—CH_2—CH_2—C = CH—CH_2—CH_2—CH_2—<
CH
N—CH_2—CH_2—CH_2—CH_2—<

Dehydromerodesmosine

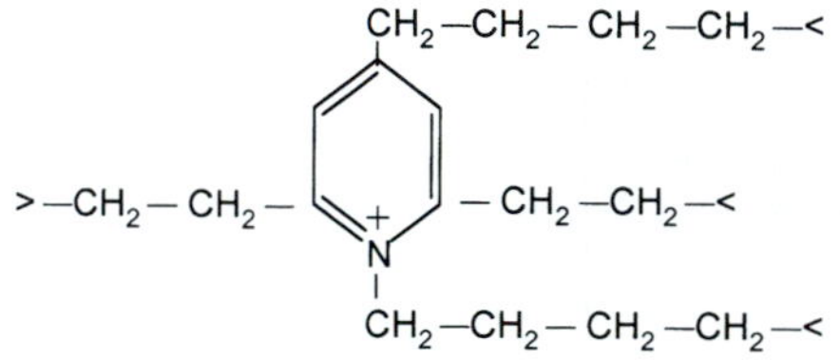

CH_2—CH_2—CH_2—CH_2—<
>—CH_2—CH_2— + —CH_2—CH_2—<
N
CH_2—CH_2—CH_2—CH_2—<

Desmosine

—CH_2—CH_2—<
>—CH_2—CH_2— + —CH_2—CH_2—CH_2—<
N
CH_2—CH_2—CH_2—CH_2—<

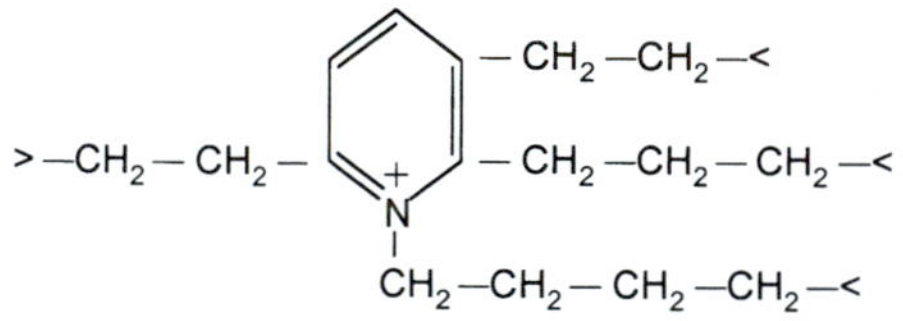

Isodesmosine

FIGURE 3-11. The structures of crosslinks found in elastin. The desmosine and isodesmosine represent final products of the lysine-derived crosslinks.

the aldol condensation product of two residues of allysine; dehydromerodesmosine and its reduced form, merodesmosine; and desmosine and isodesmosine.[46] Biosynthetically, all of the crosslinks are derived from lysyl residues through allysine.[47] The mechanism of formation of the aldol condensate and dehydrolysinonorleucine in elastin is identical to that described for collagen. The origin of dehydromerodesmosine appears to be through the aldamine-bond formation between lysine and the aldol condensate. The pathway for the formation of desmosine has not been well characterized. Crosslinking in elastin occurs frequently, not only between peptide chains but also within the same polypeptide chain, producing intrapolypeptide chain kinks.

Elastin Precursor, Tropoelastin

Soluble precursors of elastin are not found in extracts of normal tissue. This provides a clue as to the rapid formation of mature, highly crosslinked elastin fibers and the low rate of synthesis. In experimental conditions, such as copper deficiency or lathyrism induced by β-aminopropionitrile administration, which inhibit lysyl oxidase activity and crosslink formation, a soluble protein of 72 kDa, referred to as tropoelastin, can be extracted from the aorta.[48] Endothelial cells and a variety of mesenchymal cells synthesize tropoelastin.

Tropoelastin undergoes posttranslational modifications before its assembly into elastin fibers. Oxidative deamination of lysine residues followed by subsequent condensation reactions provides a family of unusual crosslinks. Pulse-chase experiments with radiolabeled lysine indicate rapid incorporation of the labels into desmosine and isodesmosine such that the rate of formation of these crosslinks parallels the rate of elastin synthesis. Under normal conditions, the crosslinking process is highly efficient but how the crosslinking sites in the monomer get aligned is unclear. It has long been assumed that microfibrils provide a scaffold or template for elastin assembly by registering their crosslinkable lysines. Using an in vitro model system of elastin assembly, Kozel and colleagues[49] have shown that a domain of tropoelastin, encoded by exons 29 to 36, is critically involved in the association of elastin with microfibrils.

Genomic organization of the tropoelastin gene indicates that functionally distinct crosslinking and hydrophobic domains of tropoelastin may be encoded by distinct exons. Short segments rich in alanine and lysine are clustered to apparently delimit the crosslinked region. These amino acids are clustered in the α-helical configuration of tropoelastin, and each begins with tyrosine followed by Ala-Ala-Lys or Ala-Ala-Ala-Lys. In humans, several distinct tropoelastin polypeptides may be generated by alternative splicing. Space-filling atomic models indicate that lysines separated by two or three alanyl residues in α-helical conformation protrude on the same side of the helix. Hence, the sequence Lys-Ala-Ala-Lys allows the formation of dehydrolysinonorleucine, whereas the sequence Lys-Ala-Ala-Ala-Lys accommodates either aldol condensation or dehydrolysinonorleucine formation. Condensation of the two intrachain crosslinks could result in the formation of the interchain desmosine crosslinks.[50] The alanine- and lysine-rich crosslinking segments are separated by large hydrophobic segments of 6 to 8 kDa, which are in a β-spiral structure with elastomeric properties. Within the hydrophobic segments, a repeating pentapeptide (Pro-Gly-Val-Gly-Val) is present. A collagen-like sequence (Gly-Val-Pro-Gly) occurs quite frequently, which would explain the limited susceptibility of tropoelastin to bacterial collagenase (Pro-Gly-X-Y). The sequence Gly-X-Pro-Gly is recognized by the collagen enzyme prolyl hydroxylase.[51]

Elastin Metabolism and Vascular Homeostasis

The half-life of elastin in normal humans has been estimated in years. Urine excretion of desmosine is normally 40 to 50 μg, which is equivalent to the turnover of 1% of the total body elastin per year. Elastin fibers may be degraded by a number of MMPs, present in latent forms under normal physiologic conditions but activated following vessel wall injury.[52] Cells within the vessel wall produce and secrete MMPs and atherosclerotic lesions secrete enhanced rates of elastin-degrading enzymes.

The MMPs from neutrophils or macrophages are believed to degrade the elastin-rich ECM in inflamed tissues. The hereditary defect in the circulating elastase inhibitors is associated with a progressive destruction of the elastin-rich alveolar wall, resulting in premature emphysema. Furthermore, experimental instillation of elastase into the lungs of animals causes destruction of the lung similar to that seen in patients with the α-1 proteinase inhibitor deficiency.

A direct link between occlusive vascular diseases and perturbation in the organization of the elastic fibers in the vessels has also been established.[41] Mutations in elastin gene are associated with supravalvular aortic stenosis (SVAS) and Williams-Beuren syndrome (WBS), pediatric disorders characterized by hemodynamic stress and loss of elasticity.[53] Furthermore, haploinsufficiency of elastin resulting from aberrant degradation of mutated protein in humans or ablation of elastin gene in transgenic mice caused intimal hyperplasia and thickened arteries.[54-56] Apparently, the vascular smooth muscle cells (VSMC), the primary producers of elastin, organized more cell layers to compensate for the lost elasticity and biomechanical support in the developing blood vessels of the elastin haploinsufficient patients and transgenic mice. Elastin knockout mice die prematurely due to arterial occlusion caused by endothelial cell and VSMC hyperplasia.[41]

Vascular smooth muscle cells from SVAS patients, WBS patients, and elastin-/- mice show increased rates of proliferation, chemotactic migration and reduced rates of elastin synthesis in vitro.[54-56] Exogenous supplementation of recombinant tropoelastin and α elastin to these cultures reversed their phenotype. The elastin-rich ECM serves as an autocrine regulator of VSMC; Karnik and colleagues[57] inserted elastin-coated stents in a porcine coronary injury model of restenosis and found that the intimal thickness and arterial stenosis were significantly reduced. Although the identities of the specific receptors mediating elastin VSMC interactions and the signaling mechanisms underlying vascular remodeling remain obscure,[58] restoring elastin to an injured arterial wall is known to reduce obstructive vascular pathology.[59,60] The inhibitors of MMPs have been shown to prevent degradation of elastic fibers after vascular injury and to ameliorate neointimal thickening.[52]

FIBRONECTIN

Fibronectin is the best characterized of an increasing number of adhesive glycoproteins that have been identified in the ECM.[61,62] It provides a crucial substrate for cell migration during embryogenesis and postinflammatory wound healing. Fibronectin exists in a soluble protomeric state in blood plasma and in an insoluble supramolecular form in the ECM; the latter acts as a potent adhesive molecule. Interestingly, several proteolytic fragments of FN can also promote chemotactic migration and activate signaling that is mediated via integrins.[61-65] Fibronectin is especially abundant in the ECM of the developing embryo and in regenerating tissues, where it signals via heterodimeric transmembrane integrin receptors.[66]

Fibronectin Structure

The soluble FN exists as a disulfide-linked dimer of 450 kDa in plasma. Each subunit is a mosaic of several repeating modules: 12 type I modules, 2 type II modules, 15 to 17 type III modules (depending on the alternative splicing), and a variable sequence that is not homologous to other parts of FN (Fig. 3-12). The primary amino acid sequence of FN is extremely well conserved across species; there is a 71% amino acid identity between *Xenopus* and rat.[67] Fibronectin has a striking series of repeating polypeptide sequences, encoded by similarly organized exons of the gene indicating that the FN gene evolved from a primordial gene by duplications, followed by evolutionary modifications of these sequences to subserve various functions.[68] A high degree of interspecific homology in specific functional domains of FN corroborates the evolutionary origin of FN. For example, a 97% identity between bovine and human FN occurs in the 29 kDa amino-terminal domain. Similarly, the amino-terminal region of the collagen-binding domain contains a 90% homology.[61,69]

Functional Domains of Fibronectin

Fibronectin can be viewed as a multifunctional molecule with a series of specialized modules (see Fig. 3-12). For example, specific proteotytic cleavage of FN generates subfragments with binding affinity for the specific ligands. The domain organization has been further

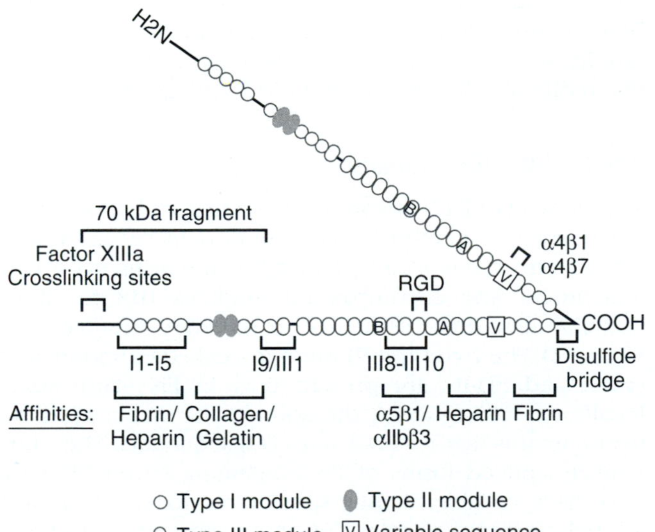

FIGURE 3-12. (See also Color Plate 3-12.) Schematic diagram of modular structure of FN dimer. Two subunits are shown, with amino termini to the left and carboxyl termini to the right. Regions implicated in adhesion and assembly are shown (discussed in the text). Variably spliced ED-A (A) and ED-B (B) modules and variable sequence (V) are shown as being present in both subunits, whereas in vivo all combinations of dimers exist. (From Magnusson MK, Mosher DF: Fibronectin: Structure, assembly, and cardiovascular implications. Arterioscler Thromb Vasc Biol 18[9]:1363, 1998.)

confirmed via competitive inhibition of FN to various ligands and cell surface receptors by specific FN peptide fragments.[65]

The Aminoterminal Domain

The aminoterminal 70 kDa fragment of FN binds to a surprisingly large number of ECM ligands that include collagen, gelatin, fibrin, and heparin. The NH_2 terminal domain also specifically binds several gram-positive bacteria such as *Staphylococcus aureus, Streptococcus pyogenes,* and *Streptococcus pneumoniae.* A number of FN binding molecules, referred to as MSCRAMMs (microbial surface components recognizing adhesive matrix molecules) have been isolated from Group A *Streptococcus* species.[70,71] These include lipoteichoic acid, M-proteins, and several other bacterial adhesins. Fibronectin-binding bacterial proteins, anchored in the bacterial cell wall bind to FN and enhance opsonization and phagocytosis.[70] Gram-negative bacteria do not bind to FN. The amino terminal domain of FN is also the primary site for covalent crosslinking of FN to fibrin through the action of the transglutaminases. Presumably, FN bound to the fibrin in the clot provides a temporary adhesive matrix that serves as a scaffold for cell growth and wound healing.

The Collagen-Binding Domain

The collagen-binding domain of FN is enriched in disulfide bonds that are essential for collagen-binding activity.[72,73] In addition to several types of collagen, the first component of complement, Clq, which contains a collagen-like structure, also has an affinity for FN.[74] Surprisingly, denatured collagen (gelatin) has a much greater affinity for FN than does native collagen and this observation has allowed the discovery of several FN binding sites along the collagen, including the greatest affinity site located in the precise region of type I collagen molecule cleaved by interstitial collagenases.

The Cell-Binding Domain

The domains of FN involved in binding to cell surfaces have received extraordinary attention in recent years. Fibronectin binds to $a_5\beta_1$ and $a_{II}b\beta_3$ integrins via a cell attachment site encompassing modules III8 to III10, containing an RGD sequence in the III10 module (see Fig. 3-12). The two type III modules, called extradomains (ED-A and ED-B), are present only in FN synthesized locally by various cells; the soluble FN synthesized by liver contains neither ED-A nor ED-B sequences. The alternatively spliced forms of FN containing either ED-A or ED-B have variable binding specificities for integrins and are believed to play roles during developmental histogenesis, and wound healing and regeneration.[62,66] Binding of FN to integrins initiates intracellular signals with extensive crosstalk with growth factor-initiated signals, leading to adhesion and proliferation of numerous cell types.[66]

Incorporation of monomeric FN into an ECM-incorporated state is a cell-mediated process. The 70 kDa aminoterminal domain of soluble FN binds to cell surface and is converted into disulfide-linked multimers. This multimerization of FN occurs at specialized surfaces of many cells, including smooth muscle cells and fibroblasts and needs the coordinated action of integrins and LAMMs, large apparent molecular mass molecules.[62,75] Most of the activity that directs FN incorporation into ECM is located in the 70 kDa region, particularly within modules I1 to I5 and I9/III1 (see Fig. 3-12). Integrins $a_5\beta_1$, $a_{IIb}\beta_3$, or $a_v\beta_3$ can polymerize FN indicating that integrin-assisted binding and assembly of FN matrix are somewhat redundant.[62]

The Heparin-Binding Domain

The heparin-binding domain of FN is clearly devoid of carbohydrates and several polyanionic macromolecules (e.g., heparin, heparan sulfate, dextran sulfate, and DNA) compete with each other for binding to the FN, suggesting that they all share the same binding site.[68] The binding is specific because other polyanionic macromolecules, such as chondroitin sulfates and dermatan sulfate, do not bind to FN. The binding of some macromolecules to one of the FN domains apparently influences the binding of other macromolecules. Addition of polyanionic GAGs, such as heparan sulfate or hyaluronic acid, to FN-coated gelatin-Sepharose enhances the stability of FN-gelatin binding. Similarly, gelatin-coated beads can be agglutinated by the addition of FN and GAGs. Fibronectin causes precipitation of type I or type III collagen in solution only in the presence of heparin. Such cooperative binding of various modules of FN enhances interaction of FN, collagen, and GAGs and may facilitate the formation of an insoluble matrix in vivo. Similarly, the addition of heparin to a solution of fibrinogen and FN causes precipitation at low temperatures indicating that the trimolecular complex may be a more physiologic state of these complexes.

The Fibrin-Binding Domains and Clotting

The carboxyl terminal 70 kDa fragment of FN binds weakly to fibrin. The human FN molecule also contains a fibrin-binding domain at the carboxyl end of each chain. The well organized architecture of the vascular wall and their cellular elements are occasionally perturbed due to vascular injury, atherosclerosis, restenosis and hypertension and FN-ECM plays a central role during these processes. Following injury, clot formation serves a dual function to restore vascular integrity and to provide a provisional matrix during the initial phases of tissue remodeling and regeneration.[61,62,69,76] During the final step of clotting, factor XIIIa crosslinks not only fibrin to itself but also crosslinks fibrin and FN that allows migration of inflammatory and reparative cells to the site of injury. Fibroblasts become myofibroblasts after coming in contact with fibrin-FN matrix and continue the regenerative process and lay down more permanent ECM. Somewhat similar events are believed to occur in the atherosclerotic lesions, where VSMC acquire a proliferative and highly synthetic phenotype, and move into the subendothelial lesion. Increased expression of ED-A and ED-B domain-containing FN is often associated with such a transformation of VSMC. How ED-A or ED-B contribute to the development of atherosclerotic plaques remains speculative.

Functional Relationships among Domains

The functional characteristics of multiple FN domains suggest that simultaneous interactions of FN with other components of ECM may indeed be essential for its physiological role.[62] Thus, the repeating globular domains of FN interact with cell surface integrin receptors. The circulating plasma FN promotes adhesion and spreading of platelets, chemotaxis of circulating cells to the fibrin clot and exposed collagen, and nonimmune opsonization for phagocytic cells by binding to cell debris. Potentially, some of the modules capable of binding to various cell and ECM constituents may be cryptic and only unraveled as a result of proteolysis during tissue injury and remodeling. Crosstalk between FN and growth factor/cytokine-mediated signals modulates activity of many cell types during repair and regeneration, and in the anchorage-independent growth of cancer cells.

LAMININ

Laminins are a diverse superfamily of glycoproteins that, along with type IV collagen, nidogen, and proteoglycans, constitute the structural scaffold of the BMs. Since its discovery as a cross-shaped heterotrimeric protein made up of α, β and γ polypeptide chains held together with disulfide bonds, a large number of cDNAs encoding homologous polypeptides with characteristic laminin-specific organization have been described (Fig. 3-13). At present five distinct α chains, three β chains and three γ chains have been biochemically characterized.[77-79] At least three laminin chains (α2, α3, and γ3) may also be generated by alternative splicing. Although it is theoretically possible to assemble more than 40 different laminin isoforms, the

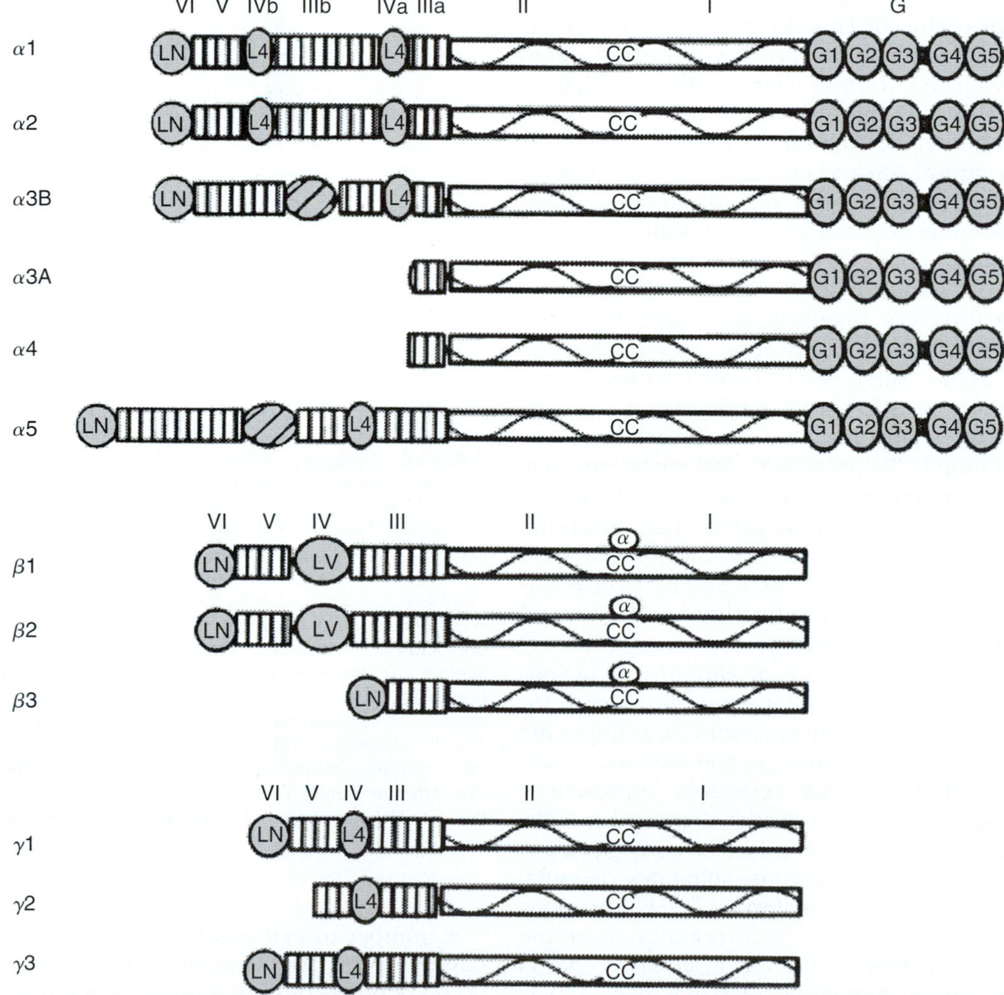

FIGURE 3-13. Structural motifs of laminin subunits. The α, β, and γ chain subunits of laminins are each polypeptides with tandem arrays of globular and rod-like motifs. The N terminal (LN, Domain VI) and internal short arm globular (L4, domain IV) modules are indicated by ovals. The rod-like epidermal growth factor (EGF) repeats are shown as vertical rectangles. The coiled-coil (cc) forming domains are shown as horizontal rectangles containing a wavy line. They mediate heterotrimeric assembly. The C terminal G-repeat modules are indicated as circles. (From Colognato H, Yurchenco PD: Form and function: The laminin family of heterotrimers. Dev Dyn 218[2]:213, 2000. Reprinted by permission of Wiley-Liss, Inc., a subsidiary of John Wiley & Sons, Inc.)

heterotrimeric assembly of α, β, and γ polypeptides appears to be nonrandom, presumably owing to the constrains intrinsic to the formation of a biologically functional trimer of laminin. Twelve distinct isoforms of mammalian laminins are currently known.

Different laminin isoforms show tissue-specific expression and deposition and are believed to play unique functions in vivo. For example, laminin 1 ($\alpha_1\beta_1\gamma_1$), the most ancient and best-studied laminin, is synthesized abundantly during embryogenesis, whereas laminin 2 ($\alpha_2\beta_1\gamma_1$) is found in the BMs surrounding myocytes and cardiac muscle. Similarly, laminin 8 ($\alpha_4\beta_1\gamma_1$) and laminin 10 ($\alpha_5\beta_1\gamma_1$) are considered to be the primary laminins of the vasculature. The α, β, and γ chains of laminin are characterized by amino acid sequences repeated in tandem that give rise to globular, rod-like (containing EGF-specific motifs) and coiled-coil subdomains. The EGF-like repeated region of the laminin chains interacts with ECM protein nidogen, that serves as a link between type IV collagen and laminin. The assembly of the coiled-coil domain is determined by binding of heptad motifs such that each laminin is formed by a combination of one α, one β, and one γ chain.[80] The globular domains of the COOH-terminal region of laminin α chains serve as ligands for $\alpha_6\beta_1$, $\alpha_6\beta_4$ and $\alpha_7\beta_1$ integrins, whereas the amino terminal module (LN) of the α chain interacts with $\alpha_1\beta_1$ and $\alpha_2\beta_1$ integrins (see Figs. 3-13 and 3-14).

In vivo functions of laminin isoforms have been deduced from careful cell and molecular biologic studies and from observing the phenotypes of transgenic mice carrying a congenital deletion in one or both alleles of a particular laminin chain.[79] Generally, such mice are either embryonal lethal or die soon after birth due to major complications of organogenesis such as severe muscular dystrophy or peripheral nerve defects. Although the architectural role of laminin in the formation of the BMs is well known, laminin also appears to regulate an astonishing variety of cellular functions. Thus, intact laminin or its proteolytic fragments, and synthetic peptides derived from various laminin chains, can modulate adhesion, migration, and phenotypic differentiation of many cell types. Laminin and its fragments are known to promote tumor cell growth and metastasis and enhance angiogenesis by modulating protease and growth-related gene expression of the target cells.[81,82] This rather confounding variety of laminin on various cellular processes has prompted a concerted search for receptors for laminin and more than 20 cell-specific receptors have been documented in the past few years. The potential laminin-binding receptors represent a remarkable variety of macromolecules that include $\alpha_1\beta_1$, $\alpha_2\beta_1$, $\alpha_6\beta_1$, $\alpha_6\beta_4$ and $\alpha_7\beta_1$ integrins, α-dystroglycan, a 32/67 kDa protein, proteoglycans sulfatides, gangliosides, lectins and galactosyltransferases.[79,81,83] The polymerization of laminin and its incorporation into the BMs is a receptor-mediated process, a situation that is rather reminiscent of supramolecular assembly of FN. Binding of laminin to cell surface receptors facilitates both multimerization and its incorporation into a cortical network that induces receptor ligation leading to profound reorganization of the cytoskeleton and cell shape.[78,79]

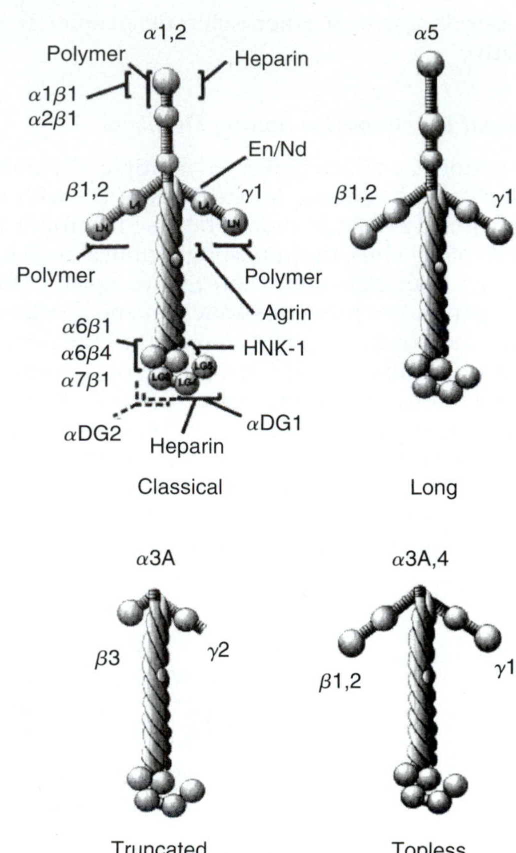

FIGURE 3-14. Laminin heterotrimer morphologies and functions. Each laminin is a heterotrimer composed of α, β, and γ chains joined together in parallel in a coiled coil. Although most trimeric combinations are allowed, the γ2 chain and β3 chains are found only in association with each other and with the α3 chain. Splice variants of α3B have not yet been isolated and characterized; however, it can be predicted that they can form associations with either β1/β2-γ1 and β3-γ2 dimers (*not shown*). Mapping studies have led to the identification of α1β1 and α2β1 integrin binding sites in the α-LN domain and to α6β1, α6β4, and α7β1 integrin binding sites in the proximal region of G domain, probably LG1 and/or LG2. Polymerization (self-assembly) sites have been assigned to the LN domains, possibly requiring the participation of more distal domains. The nidogen/entactin binding site lies within α1(III)-repeat 4. A calcium binding site for polymerization is assigned to γ1-LN. Heparin binding sites are found in the α chain in both G domain (major) and the N terminal LN domain (minor). Alpha-dystroglycan (αDG) binds to fragment E3 of laminin, corresponding to G4/G5 in laminin-1. Agrin binds to the coiled coil through a conformation-dependent interaction mediated largely through the γ1 chain. In laminin-2, receptor interactions seem to be similar with several exceptions. First, there are quantitative differences in integrin binding, with a greater contribution from the α3β1 integrin. Second, dystroglycan is found to bind both G1-3 and G4-5. Few sites have been mapped in other laminins. (From Colognato H, Yurchenco PD: Form and function: The laminin family of heterotrimers. Dev Dyn 218[2]:213, 2000. Reprinted by permission of Wiley-Liss, Inc., a subsidiary of John Wiley & Sons, Inc.)

A number of cell regulatory reactions can also be elicited by proteolytic fragments of laminin chains or synthetic peptides designed from the sequence of the native laminins. For example, two laminin-specific peptides, Tyr-Ile-Gly-Ser-Arg (amino acids 828 to 933 of β1 chain) and Ser-Ile-Lys-Val-Ala-Val (amino acids 2099 to 2104 located on the α1 chain of laminin), can promote melanoma cell growth, angiogenesis, and malignancy.[73,81]

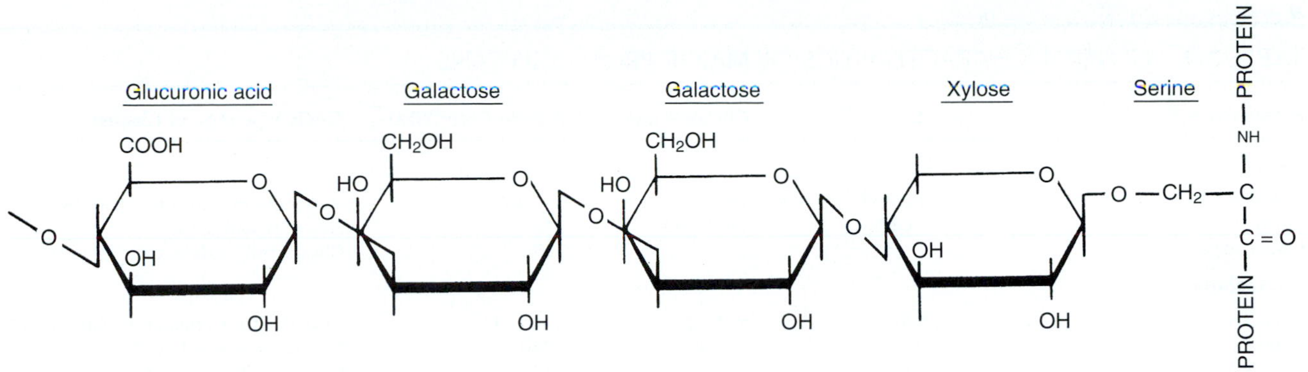

FIGURE 3-15. Oligosaccharide linkage between glycosaminoglycans and protein core.(From Silber JE: Structure and metabolism of proteoglycans and glycosaminoglycans. J Invest Dermatol 79:31, 1982. Copyright by Williams & Wilkins.)

Although there are discrepancies between in vitro and in vivo observations, it is evident that the receptor and ECM-binding properties of laminins are encoded within different heterotrimer subunits as well as in various sequence motifs located on different subunits. Thus, the myriad biologic functions such as cell attachment, neurite outgrowth, angiogenesis, tumor invasion, and metastasis may be specified by different isoforms of laminin that may vary with respect to tissue distribution and developmental expression.

GLYCOSAMINOGLYCANS

The main constituents of the amorphous ground substance in the extracellular, interfibrillar milieu are GAGs that are composed of repeating disaccharide units in which one of the sugars is always an amino sugar such as *N*-acetylglucosamine or *N*-acetylgalactosamine. The second sugar of the disaccharide unit of GAG is usually a uronic acid (e.g., glucuronic acid or iduronic acid). Because there are sulfate or carboxyl groups on most of their sugars, GAGs are negatively charged. The four major groups of GAGs are distinguished based on the types of bonds between the sugars and the number of sulfate groups and their locations; these are hyaluronan, chondroitin sulfate and dermatan sulfate, heparan sulfate, and keratan sulfate. Most of the GAGs are covalently bound to a specific core protein. The exception is hyaluronan, which is an extremely long polysaccharide chain (containing up to 25,000 nonsulfated disaccharide units) that in most cases exists alone in the tissue. The covalently bound GAG core protein complexes, called proteoglycans, comprise a superfamily that currently consists of about 30 members.[84-87]

Structure and Distribution of Glycosaminoglycans

Seven GAGs have been identified and characterized: hyaluronic acid (HA), chondroitin 4- and chondroitin 6-sulfates (CS), dermatan sulfate (DS), heparan sulfate (HS), heparin, and keratan sulfate (KS).[87] GAGs are unbranched polymers of repeating disaccharide units, of which one sugar is invariably a glucosamine or a galactosamine, and the other is either a glucuronic or an L-iduronic acid in all cases except KS, which contains a galactose in the place of the hexuronic acid. Hexosamine is, as a rule, *N*-acetylated except in HS, where it may be *N*-sulfated. The structures of the repeating units of GAGs are presented in Figure 3-15. These polyanions are highly charged because of the presence of sulfate groups, carboxyl groups—or both—along the chains.

The uronic-acid linkage in chondroitin sulfates and the hyaluronate is β1,3, whereas it is α1,3 in DS because of the presence of L-iduronic acid in the latter as the hexuronyl group. The hexosaminidic linkage in all of these is β1,4. The disaccharide unit of KS is β-galactosyl (1,4)-*N*-acetylglucosamine. It is polymerized by a β1, 3 glucosaminidic bond. The structure of HS contains some disaccharide units composed of D-glucosamine and D-glucuronic acid and others of D-glucosamine and L-iduronic acid. Unlike other GAGs, the uronyl linkage is α1-4 rather than β1-3, and the hexosaminidic linkage is α1-4 rather than β1-4. The glucosamine residues are partly *N*-sulfated as well as O-sulfated. HS is closely related structurally to the anticoagulant heparin (synthesized and stored by mast cells) which contains a higher content of sulfate than does HS. The GAG chains are linear polymers of disaccharide units (15 to 5000) with molecular weights ranging from several thousand to several million daltons. All hexosamine residues are *N*-substituted with either acetyl or sulfate groups. In addition, most GAGs have ester O-sulfate on one or both sugars of the disaccharide unit.

Proteoglycans

Proteoglycans are a complex and diverse group of macromolecules. Because it is beyond the scope of this text to review all the proteoglycans, we will provide a brief outline of their salient structure and function. Except for HA, they all contain a protein core to which the GAG chains are attached.[85,87,88] As shown in Table 3-4, proteoglycans may be classified into (1) BM proteoglycans, (2) hyalectans, and (3) small leucine-rich proteoglycans.[85]

Basement Membrane Proteoglycans

Perlecan, agrin, and bamacan are usually present in the vascular and epithelial BMs of the mammalian tissues.

TABLE 3-4 GENERAL CHARACTERISTICS OF MAJOR PROTEOGLYCANS

Proteoglycan**	Gene	Chromosome	Protein Core (kDa)	GAGs Type (No. of Chains)
BM Type				
Perlecan	HSPG2	1p36	400-467	Heparan/chondroitin sulfate (3)
Agrin	AGRN	1p32-pter	250	Heparan sulfate (3)
Bamacan			138	Chondroitin sulfate (3)
Hyalectans				
Versican	CSPG2	5q13.2	265-370	Chondroitin/dermatan sulfate (10-30)
Aggrecan	AGC1	15q26	~220	Chondroitin sulfate (~100)
Neurocan	NCAN		~136	Chondroitin sulfate (3-7)
Brevican	BCAN	1q25-q31	~100	Chondroitin sulfate (1-3)
SLRPs				
Decorin	DCN	12q23	40	Dermatan/chondroitin sulfate (1)
Biglycan	BGN	X128	40	Dermatan/chondroitin sulfate (2)
Fibromodulin	FMOD	1q32	42	Keratan sulfate (2-3)
Lumican	LIM	12q21.3-22	38	Keratan sulfate (3-4)
Keratocan			38	Keratan sulfate (3-5)
PRELP	PRELP	1q32	44	Keratan sulfate (2-3)
Osteoadherin			42	Keratan sulfate
Epiphycan	ESPG3	12q21	35	Dermatan/chondroitin
Osteoglycin	OG		35	Keratan sulfate

Adapted from Iozzo RW: Matrix proteoglycans: From molecular design to cellular function. Ann Rev Biochem 67:609, 1998.
BM, basement membrane; GAGs, glycosaminoglycans; SLRPs, small leucine-rich proteoglycans.

Whereas the three GAG chains of perlecan and agrin are primarily heparin and chondroitin sulfate, bamacan contains 3 GAGs with only chondroitin sulfate. BM proteoglycans contain 4 or 5 domains that are made up of a mosaic of sequence motifs with homologies to molecules involved in a variety of cell functions. Thus, 5 modules of perlecan contain homologues of LDL receptor, α1 chain of laminin, EGF-like domains, and a SEA subdomain, consisting of homologous sequences from a sperm protein, enterokinase, and agrin (Fig. 3-16). Perlecan also contains 21 immunoglobulin-like (IgG) motifs that are missing in agrin and bamacan. The sequences that constitute the 4 domains of agrin and 5 domains of bamacan are analogous to those seen in perlecan but are uniquely organized in the two proteoglycans (see Fig. 3-16). Agrin is a major proteoglycan of the neuromuscular junction BMs. Bamacan is found more widely but is specifically enriched in Reichert's membrane.

Although proteoglycans are essential for the structural integrity of the BMs, they also subserve additional cell regulatory functions. For example, expression of perlecan appears early in the primordial heart and in major blood vessels and its expression is particularly strong in the developing BMs of highly vascularized organs such as liver, kidney, and pancreas. Perlecan is believed to regulate smooth muscle cell proliferation via fibroblast growth factor-2 (FGF-2) signaling. During aortic morphogenesis, there is an inverse correlation between perlecan expression and smooth muscle proliferation in rat. Heparan sulfate GAGs of perlecan associate with FGF-2 and serve as a reservoir of this growth factor in the walls of the blood vessels. Perlecan also regulates the behavior of neoplastically transformed cells and promotes metastasis.[85]

Agrin is a major proteoglycan of the BMs of nerve-muscle junctional synapses. Although the 4-domain structure of agrin, with 3 heparan sulfate-rich GAG chains, resembles perlecan, there are critical structural differences between perlecan and agrin (see Fig. 3-16). The amino terminus of agrin is required for binding to laminin-1 as well as for secretion of the newly synthesized agrin. Agrin is essential to aggregate the acetylcholine receptors at the neuromuscular synapse and facilitates synaptogenesis during neuromuscular junction development.

Although originally isolated from Reichert's membrane, CS-rich bamacan is found in variable amounts in most BMs. The mechanism of bamacan polymerization and its incorporation into BMs, and how bamacan regulates cellular functions remain incompletely understood.

Hyaluronan and Lectin-Binding Proteoglycans

Four distinct proteoglycans, named versican, aggrecan, neurocan, and brevican, constitute a family of molecules with homologous structural organization and similar biologic functions.[85] These proteoglycans share a tripartite organization; the amino and carboxyl terminal domains of these proteoglycans interact with hyaluronan and lectins, respectively. For this reason, these four proteoglycans are collectively called hyalectans (see Table 3-4). The central domain of hyalectans contains variable numbers of GAG chains, composed of chondroitin/dermatan sulfate (e.g., versican) or predominantly chondroitin sulfate—as is the case for aggrecan, neurocan, and brevican (see Table 3-4).

Versican may be considered a prototype of the hyalectan family. Versican and other hyalectans are believed to noncovalently connect lectin-containing proteins on the cell surface with hyaluronan in the intercellular space. Usually hyaluronan is bound to its transmembrane

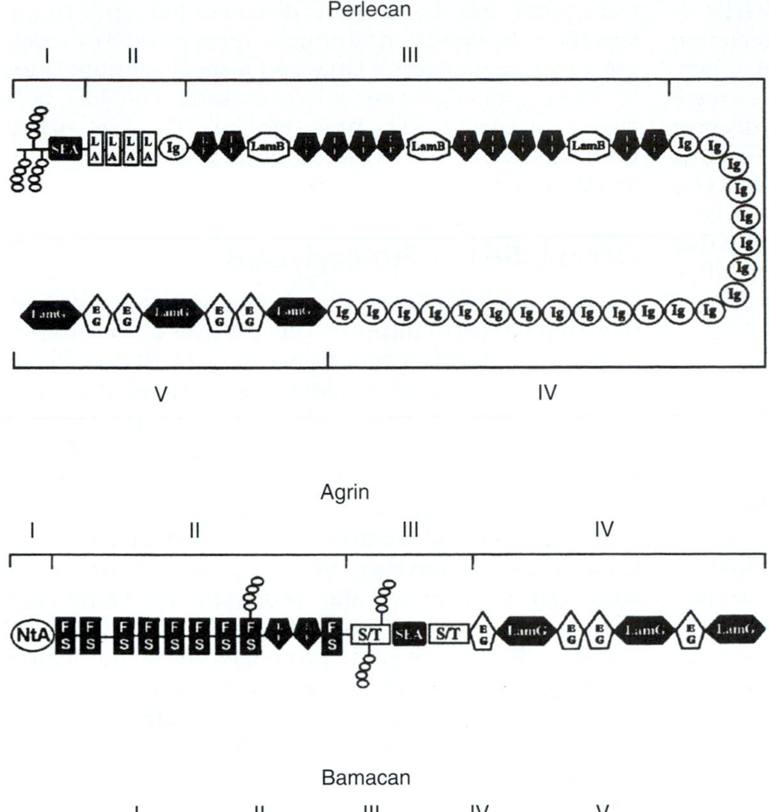

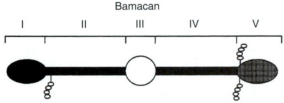

FIGURE 3-16. Schematic representation of three major proteoglycans found in basement membranes. The roman numerals indicate the proposed domains. The symbols and designations of individual protein modules for perlecan and agrin are according to Bork and Patthy[24] with minor modifications: EG, EGF-like; FS, follistatin-like; Ig, immunoglobulin-like repeat typically found in N-CAM; LA, LDL receptor class A module; LamG, first identified as the G domain on long arm of the α chain of laminin-1; LE, laminin-1; NtA, N-terminal domain that binds laminins; SEA, a module first identified in sperm protein, enterokinase, and agrin; S/T, serine/threonine rich. The glycosaminoglycan side chains are designated by strings of small circles. (From Iozzo, RV: Matrix proteoglycans: From molecular design to cellular function. Annu Rev Biochem 67:609, 1998.)

cell surface receptor (CD44) and it has been hypothesized that versican may be involved in stabilizing large, supramolecular structures assembled at the plasma membranes.

Aggrecan typically contains approximately 100 CS- and approximately 30 KS-enriched GAGs that are covalently linked to about a 220-kDa core protein (see Table 3-4). As the most abundant constituent of the cartilage ECM, aggrecan is found in giant aggregates with link proteins and hyaluronan, and occupies a large hydrodynamic volume (2×10^{-12} cm^3) that may be equivalent to a bacterium.[88] The lectin modules of both versican and aggrecan can interact with simple sugars found in glycoproteins; this binding is calcium dependent.[89] In addition to its structural role in the cartilage ECM, aggrecan modulates chondrogenesis. Defective cartilage and shortened limb development have been demonstrated in mice and chickens that contain mutated aggrecan genes.[90,91]

A neurocan-specific cDNA was first isolated from rat brain and the core-protein sequence encoded by this cDNA was reminiscent of the tripartite organization seen in other hyalectans. The most abundant proteoglycan of this class in the brain is brevican,[92] which is synthesized in the brain as a secreted, full-length molecule as well as a truncated form lacking the COOH-terminal domain. The short form of brevican is attached to plasma membrane via a GPI anchor.[85,92,93] Hyalectans interact with hyaluronan and tenascin in the neuronal tissue.[92]

Small Leucine-Rich Proteoglycans (SLRPs)

Nine known members of this family of proteoglycans, characterized by central leucine-rich domains and dermatan sulfate/keratan sulfate GAG chains, are currently known.[85] Based on their primary structures and evolutionary relationships, this family of proteoglycans may be further divided into three subclasses (see Table 3-4). The members of the SLRP family have been implicated in diverse functions that include regulation of growth factor accessibility (e.g., TGFβ) and control of collagen fibrillogenesis.[85] The presence of decorin, fibromodulin, or lumican retards collagen fibrillogenesis in vitro.[94-97] A reciprocal relationship between the amount of decorin and rate of collagen fibril growth in the developing tendon of chicken was also demonstrated.[98] The abnormal collagen fibril formation and reduced tensile strength of the skin seen in decorin knockout mice support a functional role for decorin in proper collagen fibrillogenesis.[94]

Decorin, a prototype of the SLRP, is organized into four discernible domains. Core protein of decorin binds TGFβ-1, -2 and -3 with high affinity. Because TGFβ:decorin complex is unable to signal intracellularly, decorin is believed to facilitate deposition of inactive TGFβs at specific tissue locations. Perturbation of this interaction and activation of TGFβs may occur in response to inflammatory reactions. Decorin itself has been shown to regulate cell proliferation and ectopic expression of decorin could suppress the growth of cancer cells.[85] Vascular endothelial cells undergoing cord formation in vitro synthesize decorin, whereas proliferating endothelial cells showed enhanced synthesis of biglycan—indicating that these two structurally similar SLRPs may regulate endothelial cell phenotype in an opposite manner.

Biosynthesis of Proteoglycans

The biosynthesis of all proteoglycans appears to occur through a similar pathway, and the rate-limiting step appears to be the synthesis of the core protein.[85,87,99] The core protein is synthesized on a ribosomal template, and the sugar chains are assembled posttranslationally, one sugar at a time, starting with the linkage of xylose to serine in a specific part of the core protein molecule. Sulfation occurs after the appropriate monosaccharide has been linked to the growing GAG chain. Proteoglycan synthesis begins in the late endoplasmic reticulum and the Golgi with the addition of xylose by xylosyltransferase to the hydroxyl group of serine in the protein core.[100] The transfer of galactose from uridine diphosphate galactose (UDPgalactose) to xylose depends on galactosyl transferase. The second galactose residue is also transferred via UDPgalactose to galactosyl-xylose by a distinct galactosyl transferase. This is followed by the addition of the first glucuronic acid moiety by the action of UDP glucuronic acid transferase. Growth of the GAG chain, then, occurs by alternating transfer of hexosamine and uronic acid residues from their respective UDP derivatives by the action of specific transferases. Thus, the UDP derivatives of *N*-acetylglucosamine and glucuronic acid are precursors for HA, heparin, and HS; whereas *N*-acetylgalactosamine and glucuronic acid are precursors for CS and DS. After addition of the first hexosamine, elongation occurs by the same *N*-acetylhexosaminyltransferase and glucuronosyltransferase, regardless of which chain is being synthesized. The respective chains are variably modified by pathway-specific epimerization and sulfation reactions to yield iduronic acid and sulfation.

Sulfation occurs by direct transfer of the sulfate group from 3-phosphoribosyl phosphoadenosine-5 phosphoribosyl phosphosulfate to the appropriate site on the GAG by a nonspecific sulfotransferase. Sulfation may occur during synthesis or on finished chains. Because no partial sulfation occurs, it is believed that the GAG may become attached to the particulate-bound sulfotransferase and glycosyl transferase and are completely sulfated before release. Heparin and HS contain an *N*-sulfate that is unique because all others are in an O-sulfate linkage. The synthesis of this *N*-sulfate linkage proceeds through the *N*-acetylglucosamine addition to the GAG chain, deacetylation, and replacement of the acetyl group by sulfate. Iduronic-acid formation in heparin, HS, and DS takes place after polysaccharide synthesis by epimerization of glucuronic acid. Variation in the size of the proteoglycan monomers has been well documented and tissue-specific subpopulations are now recognized. For example, cartilage contains a large and a small subpopulation of KS-CS proteoglycans, whereas aorta contains both large and small CS-DS proteoglycans. The size of the proteoglycan, in many cases, appears to be related to the length of the core protein.[101]

Degradation of Proteoglycans

Compared with collagen and elastin, proteoglycans have more rapid rates of turnover. The half-lives of various proteoglycans in younger animals may be 2 to 10 days,[102] and somewhat longer in older tissues. Degradation of the proteoglycans involves proteolysis of the core protein by a number of proteases, including some MMPs (see Table 3-2), breakdown of the sugar chain, and desulfation of the sugars. The dramatic loss of cartilage matrix that results from experimental intravenous injection of papain illustrates the importance of the protein core to the structural integrity of the proteoglycan. Fibroblasts, macrophages, and neutrophils produce a variety of enzymes that can degrade proteoglycans at the neutral pH. Degradation of the sugar chains occurs mainly in lysosomes.[103] Perhaps the best-characterized GAG-degrading enzyme is testicular hyaluronidase, which is an endo-*N*-acetyl-β-hexosaminidase that degrades HA, CS, and DS to oligosaccharides. A similar enzyme has been demonstrated in the liver, skin, and synovium. Other glycosidases are required to complete the breakdown of the oligosaccharides to monosaccharides. Lysosomes contain glucuronidase and *N*-acetylhexosaminidases; these exoenzymes remove the terminal glucuronic acid and hexosamine residues, respectively. Lysosomes also contain β-xylosidase, β-galactosidase, and α-iduronidase, which are required to complete the breakdown. Lysosomal sulfatases are responsible for the removal of the sulfate groups from the oligosaccharides. Inherited defects in the activity of various GAG-degrading enzymes cause mucopolysaccharidoses, characterized by faulty catabolism of one or another type of GAGs.[104]

The Subendothelial ECM as a Regulator of Cell Signaling

The dominant function of the subendothelial ECM is to endow the blood vessels with the ability to undergo repeated cycles of extension and passive recoil throughout the life of the organism. The structural contributions of ECM have engaged the attention of scientists ever since their ubiquitous presence in the tissues was discovered; however, an equally pivotal role of ECM in regulating cell behavior has recently been unraveled. Various constituents of ECM can also modulate the survival, adhesion, motility, proliferation and differentiation of many cells. Following is a brief outline of how the integrated reactions of ECM via its biomechanical function and cell-specific signaling regulate the development and homeostasis of the blood vessels.

The fibrillar components of the vascular ECM, (e.g., collagens, laminin, elastin, and FN) and the nonfibrillar proteoglycans and GAGs are in direct contact with the platelets, endothelial cells, and smooth muscle cells at least some of the time under physiologic conditions. The cells of the blood vessels engage in an ongoing and dynamic adhesive interaction with their ECM to ensure anchorage-dependent survival and growth. When this essential property of normal epithelial, endothelial, and smooth muscle cells is lost, these cells acquire anchorage-independent growth potential, a hallmark of neoplastic transformation and tumorigenesis.

ECM and Integrin Signaling

The dynamic interactions between the cells of the vascular bed and their ECM have been studied extensively and a number of key insights have emerged from these observations. Both the fibrillar and nonfibrillar components of ECM interact with a superfamily of cell-surface receptors called integrins—so named because they integrate extracellular signals and the intracellular cytoskeletal network. Integrins are heterodimeric transmembrane proteins composed of α and β subunits. The integrin superfamily in vertebrates is composed of 18 α-unique chains and 8 β chains.[105,106] Based on their ligand selectivities, cell-specific expression and signaling properties, at least 24 distinct integrins have been described from the mammalian tissues. Various integrins are believed to subserve unique physiologic and pathologic functions in vivo as is superbly illustrated from the studies of transgenic mice that lack one or both alleles of a given α or β integrin gene.[107,108] For example, a lack of preimplantation development was observed in the β1-/- mice, whereas major postimplantation defects were seen in the embryos that lacked either α4, β8, or αv integrins, whereas, α3-/-, α6-/-, α8-1- and β4-/- mice succumbed to perinatal death. A number of integrins may play an even more tissue-restricted role; αIIb-, β3- or α2-deficient mice were defective in hemostasis, whereas angiogenic defects were observed in mice lacking a functional α1 or β3 integrin gene.

ECM-liganded integrins not only transduce the usual "outside-in" signals but the signals may also be generated by "inside-out" mechanisms induced by conformational changes of the cytoplasmic tails.[109-112] Due to their ability to transduce highly localized, discrete signals that bidirectionally link the ECM with the intracellular cytoskeletal networks, integrins may be considered as "bidirectional, allosteric signaling machines."[61] Thus, integrins lie at a unique intersection of cellular mechanics, cytoskeletal networks, and signals that regulate cell behavior and phenotype.[112] Integrins also engage in extensive crosstalk with several growth factors, cytokines, and hormones; such an integrated signaling greatly expands the functional repertoire and strength of the integrin-mediated signals.[66,111] The coordination of integrin and growth factor-mediated signals involves receptor transactivation, mutually-regulated expression, and compartmentalization of receptors facilitated via reorganization of the cytoskeleton.

The mitogenic signals from growth factor/cytokine-liganded transmembrane receptors and integrin-initiated signals converge on the canonical Ras-Raf-MEK-ERK kinase signaling pathway.[113] Both ECM-engaged integrins and activated growth factor receptors rapidly activate Ras that sequentially leads to the activation of the mitogen-activated protein (MAP) kinases Raf, MEK and, ultimately, ERK1 and ERK2 (Fig. 3-17). When cells unattached to ECM (lacking integrin signals) are treated with mitogen, platelet-derived growth factor (PDGF), they elicit weak ERK1 and ERK2 activation. However, this weak and transient activation of ERKs is strengthened greatly if cells are also provided with adhesion-mediated signals. Integrin-engagement also enhances the nuclear translocation of ERK. A pivotal element in this signaling pathway is the recruitment of Src to the focal adhesion

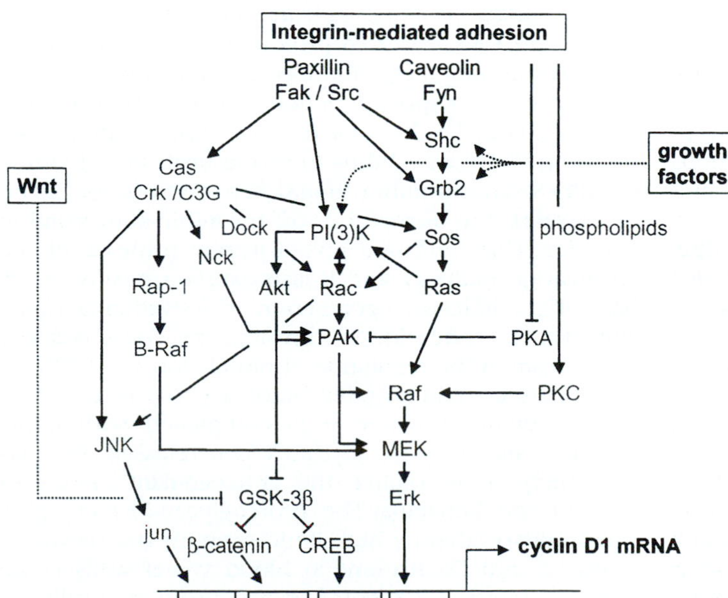

FIGURE 3-17. Cyclin D1 transcription—a point of convergence of signaling by Wnt, mitogens, and the extracellular membrane (ECM). Integrin-mediated cell adhesion to ECM components such as fibronectin stimulates multiple signal transduction cascades. Together with growth factor and Wnt signaling, the ECM controls transcriptional activity of the cyclin D1 gene in this manner. See text for details. (From Danen EH, Yamada KM: FN, integrins, and growth control. J Cell Physiol 189[1]:1, 2001.

kinase (FAK), which was originally identified as protein that was rapidly phosphorylated v-Src by tyrosine kinase in response to ECM-integrin interaction.[114,115] In common with sodium-proton antiporter and protein kinase C (PKC), FAK could also be phosphorylated and activated by a number of mitogenic growth factors, thus bolstering the paradigm of crosstalk between integrins and mitogenic cytokines.[66,109-112]

The activated FAK in turn recruits Fyn to caveolin in the plasma membrane that activates the Shc pathway[66,111] affecting the activity of a number of key proteins involved in the regulation of motility, cell cycle, and differentiation. Cell adhesion to various constituents of ECM, such as FN, leads to rapid activation of the Rho family small GTPases, Cdc 42, and Rac that leads to changes in cell shape and stimulation of transcription of D1 cyclin, a pivotal regulator of cell cycle. Concomitant activation of Rac and Rho pathway also inhibits the accumulation of p21 and p27, the two key inhibitors of cell cycle. Through a coordinated action of these pathways, integrin-modulated signals regulate mitogenesis (see Fig. 3-17). The integrin-mediated signal transduction pathways crosstalk with signals that are downstream of Ras/Rho GTPases and P13-kinase-PKB/Akt kinases.[66] Aberrant signaling caused by constitutive activation of these pathways leads to dramatic changes in the growth factor- and anchorage-independent proliferation of many cells.

Although supramolecular organization of ECM is essential for its structural role, a large number of biologically active subfragments have been identified from many ECM macromolecules in recent years. The BM collagen types IV, XV, and XVIII, possess both triple-helical and noncollagenous domains.[11] Because degradation of BM occurs during many physiologic and pathologic processes, potentially specific subfragments of BM collagens with unique biologic and physical characteristics could be generated by the actions of various degradative enzymes. A number of noncollagenous fragments of type IV collagen promote chemotaxis and adhesion of normal endothelial cells and several cancer cell lines, and induce phosphorylation of FAK and P13 kinase. In contrast, a noncollagenous peptide from α3 (IV) collagen (amino acids 56 to 139) caused apoptosis of endothelial cells. Similarly, a soluble endostatin-like fragment from XV collagen reduced growth of tumor cells and FGF-2-induced migration of endothelial cells, whereas a noncollagenous endostatin trimer inhibited angiogenesis in vitro and in vivo.[11,116]

Specific subfragments of laminin that modulate adhesion, motility, and invasion of many cell types have also been documented.[81] Laminin subfragments bind to specific cell surface receptors and modulate angiogenesis and tumor invasion owing to their ability to induce MMPs. Thus, just like some subfragments of BM collagens, the laminin peptides also bind to various integrins and initiate signaling. Several subfragments of FN also recognize specific integrin receptors and some of these peptides serve as FN mimetics in adhesion and migration assays.[63,65,117] Even more significantly, Livant and colleagues demonstrated that an FN mimetic, Pro-His-Ser-Arg-Asn, activated cell invasion and accelerated wound healing, whereas a site-specifically modified version of the same peptide had the opposite effect.[118,119] These elegant studies challenge the conventional view of how ECM modulates wound healing and metastasis in vivo.

The elastin-rich matrix is a negative modulator of vascular smooth muscle cells (VSMCs). The disruption of elastic matrix organization by genetic mutations or inflammation disrupts these signals. Although the bona fide elastin receptor remains unknown, it has been suggested that the degradation products of elastin regulate proliferation of VSMC via a pertussis toxin-sensitive G-protein-coupled receptor and L-type calcium channels; these two signals converge on a number of key proteins involved in mitogenesis (e.g., cyclins, Rb, and c-*fos*). The identity of the elastin receptor involved in the VSMC proliferation is also unknown, but it is certainly not an integrin.[41]

Proteoglycans, GAGs, and Regulation of Cell Behavior

Like the fibrillar constituents of ECM, proteoglycans and free GAGs are also involved in many biologic functions, in addition to their architectural role in the ECM.[85,120-122] Proteoglycans and GAGs bind growth factors and cytokines and their receptors may serve as "sinks" for several growth factors and thus limit their actions in a discrete cell-specific manner.

An important observation made in 1991[123,124] indicated that heparan sulfate was essential for FGF to efficiently interact with its receptors. Since the initial findings, additional growth factors and signaling morphogens have been shown to use a similar mechanism for their activities. For example, EGF-like growth factor, hepatocyte growth factor, and members of the Wnt and hedgehog family of secreted morphogens coordinate their activities with proteoglycans and GAGs.[121,122] The soluble GAGs such as HS also can modulate the actions of a number of chemokines; heparin-inhibited intracellular influx of calcium, respiratory burst, and chemotactic responses of eosinophils to CCL11, CCL24, and CCL13, that correlated with their affinities for heparin. Although the cell surface proteoglycans may not be needed for signaling via CCR3, they can profoundly modulate chemokine actions and allergy-induced inflammation by other mechanisms.[125] Exposure of dermal microvascular endothelial cells to DS, but not to HS or CS, initiated NFkB signaling.[126] Heparin binds to serine protease inhibitors (SERPINS), antithrombin III and heparin cofactor II, and accelerates the formation of thrombin-antithrombin complex. Thrombin is a pivotal serine protease of the coagulation pathway and it also exerts a positive feedback effect on its own generation by activating factors V and VIII. The inhibition of thrombin by GAGs is a key mechanism in the regulation of blood clotting.[127-130]

Platelets contain platelet factor 4 (PF4) in the cytoplasmic granules where it is complexed with chondroitin 4 sulfate proteoglycan. When released, PF4 has the ability to neutralize the anticoagulant effects of heparin and heparans. The proteoglycan-PF4 complex can be dissociated by high ionic strength and by GAGs. Thus, HS and DS present in blood vessel walls could serve to control the complex's deposition locally by dissociating PF4 from proteoglycan-PF4 complex.

GAGs from blood vessels such as the aorta also bind low-density lipoproteins (LDLs) and very low-density lipoproteins (VLDLs) .The binding occurs more strongly with iduronic-acid-containing GAGs (HS, DS, and heparin) and is mediated by interactions between the apoproteins of LDL and VLDL and the anionic groups of the GAG chains.[131] Dermatan sulfate-proteoglycan isolated from arterial walls binds LDL, suggesting a possible role in the formation of atherosclerotic lesions. The HS and DS proteoglycans on the endothelial-cell surface can bind lipoprotein lipase,[132,133] which is the primary extrahepatic enzyme that hydrolyzes the circulating plasma triglycerides of VLDL and chylomicrons. The enzyme is synthesized by adipocytes, and is secreted and transported to the vascular compartment, where it binds to the luminal surface of the endothelial cell.[134] Treatment of endothelial cells with trypsin or pronase, which would degrade the HS proteoglycan greatly reduces binding of lipoprotein lipase. Similarly, treatment of endothelial cells with platelet endoglucuronidase to degrade HS chains, inhibits the binding of lipoprotein lipase almost completely.[135] The bound enzyme can be readily released in circulation by heparin. The possible physiologic significance of these observations remains to be explored further.

ECM-Platelet Interaction

Following disruption of the endothelial surface, platelets adhere to the exposed subendothelium and aggregate, releasing several biologically active substances, including adenosine diphosphate and thromboxane A_2, which promote thrombus formation at the site of the injury. The identity and nature of the specific molecules on the platelet membrane and the subendothelium have been extensively studied. The first step in the hemostatic cascade is interaction of platelets with the exposed ECM at the injured vessel. The subendothelial component responsible for platelet adhesion and aggregation is collagen.[136] Fibrils derived from purified types I, II, and III collagen can induce platelet aggregation in vitro. Besides glycoprotein 16 (GP16) and $\alpha II_b\beta_3$ integrin on platelets, which indirectly bind to platelets via vWF, a number of other collagen receptors have been described. These include the $\alpha_2\beta_1$ integrin and the GPVI, platelet protein belonging to the IgG superfamily of receptors. Collagens bind directly or indirectly to at least two platelet integrins, $\alpha_2\beta_1$ and $\alpha_{IIb}\beta_3$, respectively. Fibrillar collagens, types I and III, are the major components of the vascular ECM. The monomeric type I/III collagens interact selectively to $\alpha_2\beta_1$ in suspension. Small triple helical synthetic collagen peptides can also potently activate platelets.[137] The platelet protein GPVI was identified as a major signaling receptor for collagen; the human GPVI, contains two Ig-C2-like extracellular domains bridged with disulfide bonds, a mucin-like stalk, a transmembrane motif, and a small 51-amino acid cytoplasmic tail. The transmembrane and intracellular fragments of human GPVI may interact with distinct proteins that include Fc receptor γ chain and SH3-containing tyrosine kinases Fyn and Lyn.[138-141] The adhesion of platelets to collagen seems to occur only if the integrin has been activated by "inside-out" signals coordinated by GPVI, and ADP and thromboxane A_2. Thus, platelet GPVI FcRγ chain is a crucial molecular complex involved in the tethering, aggregation, and degranulation of platelets prior to thrombus formation on collagen substrates.[136]

A number of other platelet-specific receptors that bind types I and III collagen have been described by Chiang and colleagues.[142,143] A novel 68 kDa type III collagen binding receptor was also described.[144,145] GPV may also serve as a collagen receptor because GPV-/- mice elicit defective hemostasis.[146,147] However, precise contributions of various receptors on the platelets remain to be rigorously tested.[136]

Perspectives

A brief review of the distribution and potential functions of various constituents of ECM in the vasculature indicates that these macromolecular aggregates are crucial to the structural and functional integrity of the vascular system. The distinct vascular pathologies associated with spontaneous or induced mutations in various macromolecules of the vascular ECM strongly support this view. For example, the fragility of the vessels seen in the Ehlers-Danlos syndrome (EDS) type IV, the dissecting aortic aneurysms that characterize Marfan's syndrome, and the characteristic arterial defects seen in SVAS, are caused by mutations in type III collagen, fibrillin-1, and elastin genes, respectively.[148] Fibers made of types I and III collagen are the primary source of the tensile strength of the vessel wall and a spectrum of recessive mutations in type III collagen gene is associated with EDS type IV. In contrast, the congenital narrowing of the large arteries results from haplo-insufficiency of the elastin gene consistent with a key role of elastin in regulating both the integrity of the vessel wall and the phenotype of the endothelial and smooth muscle cells. Similarly, weakening and spontaneous rupture of the vessels seen in Marfan syndrome patients result from mutations in the fibrillin-1 gene. A direct role of FN, laminin, and various integrins in the development of the vessels has clearly emerged from gene knockout studies in mice. Although numerous observations indicating a pivotal role of ECM in the homeostatic regulation of vasculature in experimental animals remain to be extended to human vascular pathologies, it may be concluded that the ECM macromolecules dynamically regulate the development and functional integrity of the vasculature. Elucidating the molecular mechanisms by which the subendothelial ECM participates in an astounding array of biologic responses; how to exploit these mechanisms for novel diagnoses and therapeutic interventions will continue to challenge us for many years.

REFERENCES

1. Fleishmajer R, Olsen B, Kuhn K: Structure, molecular biology, and pathology of collagens. Ann N Y Acad Sci 580:1, 1990.
2. Prockop DJ, Kivirikko KI: Collagens: Molecular biology, diseases, and potentials for therapy. Annu Rev Biochem 64:403, 1995.
3. Myllyharju J, Kivirikko KI: Collagens and collagen-related diseases. Ann Med 33:7, 2001.

4. Plenz GA, Deng MC, Robenek H, et al: Vascular collagens: Spotlight on the role of type VIII collagen in atherogenesis. Atherosclerosis 166:1, 2003.
5. Hudson BG, Reeders ST, Tryggvason K: Type IV collagen: Structure, gene organization, and role in human diseases. Molecular basis of Goodpasture and Alport syndromes and diffuse leiomyomatosis. J Biol Chem 268:26033, 1993.
6. Chernousov MA, Rothblum K, Tyler WA, et al: Schwann cells synthesize type V collagen that contains a novel alpha 4 chain. Molecular cloning, biochemical characterization, and high affinity heparin binding of alpha 4(V) collagen. J Biol Chem 275:28208, 2000.
7. Chung E, Rhodes K, Miller EJ: Isolation of three collagenous components of probable basement membrane origin from several tissues. Biochem Biophys Res Commun 71:1167, 1976.
8. Kielty CM, Grant ME: The collagen family: Structure, assembly and organization in the extracellular matrix. In Royce PM, Steimann B (eds): Connective Tissue and its Heritable Disorders (2nd ed). New York, Wiley & Sons, 2002, p 159.
9. O'Reilly MS, Boehm T, Shing Y, et al: Endostatin: An endogenous inhibitor of angiogenesis and tumor growth. Cell 88:277, 1997.
10. Sasaki T, Larsson H, Tisi D, et al: Endostatins derived from collagens XV and XVIII differ in structural and binding properties, tissue distribution and anti-angiogenic activity. J Mol Biol 301:1179, 2000.
11. Ortega N, Werb Z: New functional roles for non-collagenous domains of basement membrane collagens. J Cell Sci 115:4201, 2002.
12. Madri JA, Dreyer B, Pitlick FA, et al: The collagenous components of the subendothelium: Correlation of structure and function. Lab Invest 43:303, 1980.
13. Borza DB, Bondar O, Ninomiya Y, et al: The NC1 domain of collagen IV encodes a novel network composed of the alpha 1, alpha 2, alpha 5, and alpha 6 chains in smooth muscle basement membranes. J Biol Chem 276:28532, 2001.
14. Grassel S, Timpl R, Tan EM, et al: Biosynthesis and processing of type XVI collagen in human fibroblasts and smooth muscle cells. Eur J Biochem 242:576, 1996.
15. Graf R, Matejevic D, Schuppan D, et al: Molecular anatomy of the perivascular sheath in human placental stem villi: The contractile apparatus and its association to the extracellular matrix. Cell Tissue Res 290:601, 1997.
16. Wang Q, Raghow R: Molecular mechanisms of regulation of type collagen biosynthesis. Proc Indian Acad Sci 111:185, 1999.
17. Bornstein P: Regulation of expression of the alpha 1 (I) collagen gene: A critical appraisal of the role of the first intron. Matrix Biol 15:3, 1996.
18. Birk DE, Trelstad RL: Fibroblasts create compartments in the extracellular space where collagen polymerizes into fibrils and fibrils associate into bundles. Ann N Y Acad Sci 460:258, 1985.
19. Bornstein P, Horlein D, McPherson J: Regulation of collagen synthesis, myelofibrosis and the biology of connective tissue. Prog Clin Biol Res 154:61, 1984.
20. Aycock RS, Raghow R, Stricklin GP, et al: Post-transcriptional inhibition of collagen and fibronectin synthesis by a synthetic homolog of a portion of the carboxyl-terminal propeptide of human type I collagen. J Biol Chem 261:14355, 1986.
21. Tanzer M: Cross-linking (of collagen). In Ramachandran GN, Reddi AH (eds): Biochemistry of Collagen. New York, Plenum, 1976, p 192.
22. Fujimoto D, Moriguchi T, Ishida T, et al: The structure of pyridinoline: A collagen crosslink. Biochem Biophys Res Commun 84:52, 1978.
23. Bernstein PH, Mechanic GL: A natural histidine-based imminium cross-link in collagen and its location. J Biol Chem 255:10414, 1980.
24. Nagase H, Woessner JF, Jr: Matrix metalloproteinases. J Biol Chem 274:21491, 1999.
25. Sternlicht MD, Werb Z: How matrix metalloproteinases regulate cell behavior. Annu Rev Cell Dev Biol 17:463, 2001.
26. Murphy G, Nguyen Q, Cockett MI, et al: Assessment of the role of the fibronectin-like domain of gelatinase A by analysis of a deletion mutant. J Biol Chem 269:6632, 1994.
27. Shipley JM, Doyle GA, Fliszar CJ, et al: The structural basis for the elastolytic activity of the 92-kDa and 72-kDa gelatinases: Role of the fibronectin type II-like repeats. J Biol Chem 271:4335, 1996.
28. Woessner JF, Jr, Nagase H: Matrix Metalloproteinases and TIMPs. New York, Oxford University Press, 2002, p 238.
29. Smith MR, Kung H, Durum SK, et al: TIMP-3 induces cell death by stabilizing TNF-alpha receptors on the surface of human colon carcinoma cells. Cytokine 9:770, 1997.
30. Ahonen M, Baker AH, Kahari VM: Adenovirus-mediated gene delivery of tissue inhibitor of metalloproteinases-3 inhibits invasion and induces apoptosis in melanoma cells. Cancer Res 58:2310, 1998.
31. Ruoslahti E: Specialization of tumour vasculature. Nat Rev Cancer 2:83, 2002.
32. Silletti S, Kessler T, Goldberg J, et al: Disruption of matrix metalloproteinase 2 binding to integrin alpha v beta 3 by an organic molecule inhibits angiogenesis and tumor growth in vivo. Proc Natl Acad Sci U S A 98:119, 2001.
33. Timpl R, Oberbaumer I, von der Mark H, et al: Structure and biology of the globular domain of basement membrane type IV collagen. Ann N Y Acad Sci 460:58, 1985.
34. Timpl R, Brown JC: Supramolecular assembly of basement membranes. Bioessays 18:123, 1996.
35. Fauvel-Lafeve F: Microfibrils from the arterial subendothelium. Int Rev Cytol 188:1, 1999.
36. Wu XX, Gordon RE, Glanville RW, et al: Morphological relationships of von Willebrand factor, type VI collagen, and fibrillin in human vascular subendothelium. Am J Pathol 149:283, 1996.
37. Kuo HJ, Keene DR, Glanville RW: The macromolecular structure of type-VI collagen: Formation and stability of filaments. Eur J Biochem 232:364, 1995.
38. Dingemans KP, Teeling P, Lagendijk JH, et al: Extracellular matrix of the human aortic media: An ultrastructural histochemical and immunohistochemical study of the adult aortic media. Anat Rec 258:1, 2000.
39. Ferreras M, Felbor U, Lenhard T, et al: Generation and degradation of human endostatin proteins by various proteinases. FEBS Lett 486:247, 2000.
40. Mecham RP, Davis EC: Elastic fiber structure and assembly. In Yurchenco PD, Birk DE, Mecham RP (eds): Extracellular Matrix Assembly and Structure. New York, Academic Press, 1994, p 281.
41. Brooke BS, Bayes-Genis A, Li DY: New insights into elastin and vascular disease. Trends Cardiovasc Med 13:176, 2003.
42. Faury G: Function-structure relationship of elastic arteries in evolution: From microfibrils to elastin and elastic fibres. Pathol Biol (Paris) 49:310, 2001.
43. Trask BC, Trask TM, Broekelmann T, et al: The microfibrillar proteins MAGP-1 and fibrillin-1 form a ternary complex with the chondroitin sulfate proteoglycan decorin. Mol Biol Cell 11:1499, 2000.
44. Trask TM, Trask BC, Ritty TM, et al: Interaction of tropoelastin with the amino-terminal domains of fibrillin-1 and fibrillin-2 suggests a role for the fibrillins in elastic fiber assembly. J Biol Chem 275:24400, 2000.
45. Siegel RC: Lysyl oxidase. Int Rev Connect Tissue Res 8:73, 1979.
46. Partridge SM, Elsden DF, Thomas J, et al: Biosynthesis of the desmosine and isodesmosine cross-bridges in elastin. Biochem J 93:30C, 1964.
47. Miller EJ, Martin GR, Piez KA: The utilization of lysine in the biosynthesis of elastin crosslinks. Biochem Biophys Res Commun 17:248, 1964.
48. Bashir MM, Indik Z, Yeh H, et al: Characterization of the complete human elastin gene: Delineation of unusual features in the 5′-flanking region. J Biol Chem 264:8887, 1989.
49. Kozel BA, Wachi H, Davis EC, et al: Domains in tropoelastin that mediate elastin deposition in vitro and in vivo. J Biol Chem 278:18491, 2003.
50. Foster JA, Rubin L, Kagan HM, et al: Isolation and characterization of cross-linked peptides from elastin. J Biol Chem 249:6191, 1974.
51. Indik Z, Yeh H, Ornstein-Goldstein N, et al: Structure of the elastin gene and alternative splicing of elastin mRNA: Implications for human disease. Am J Med Genet 34:81, 1989.
52. Galis ZS, Khatri JJ: Matrix metalloproteinases in vascular remodeling and atherogenesis: The good, the bad, and the ugly. Circ Res 90:251, 2002.
53. Brooke BS, Bays-Gerris A, Li DY: New insights into elastin and vascular disease. Trends Cardiovasc Med 13:176, 2003.
54. Li DY, Brooke B, Davis EC, et al: Elastin is an essential determinant of arterial morphogenesis. Nature 393:276, 1998.

55. Li DY, Faury G, Taylor DG, et al: Novel arterial pathology in mice and humans hemizygous for elastin. J Clin Invest 102:1783, 1998.
56. Urban Z, Riazi S, Seidl TL, et al: Connection between elastin haploinsufficiency and increased cell proliferation in patients with supravalvular aortic stenosis and Williams-Beuren syndrome. Am J Hum Genet 71:30, 2002.
57. Karnik SK, Brooke BS, Bayes-Genis A, et al: A critical role for elastin signaling in vascular morphogenesis and disease. Development 130:411, 2003.
58. Raines EW: The extracellular matrix can regulate vascular cell migration, proliferation, and survival: Relationships to vascular disease. Int J Exp Pathol 81:173, 2000.
59. Waugh JM, Li-Hawkins J, Yuksel E, et al: Therapeutic elastase inhibition by alpha-1-antitrypsin gene transfer limits neointima formation in normal rabbits. J Vasc Interv Radiol 12:1203, 2001.
60. Zaidi SH, You XM, Ciura S, et al: Overexpression of the serine elastase inhibitor elafin protects transgenic mice from hypoxic pulmonary hypertension. Circulation 105:516, 2002.
61. Hynes RO: Fibronectins. New York, Springer, 1990, p 546.
62. Magnusson MK, Mosher DF: Fibronectin: Structure, assembly, and cardiovascular implications. Arterioscler Thromb Vasc Biol 18:1363, 1998.
63. Yamada KM, Danen EH: Integrin signaling. In Gutkind JS (ed): Signaling Networks and Cell Cycle Control: The Molecular Basis of Cancer and Other Disease. Humana Press, Totowa, NJ, 2000, p 1.
64. Hynes RO: Integrins: Versatility, modulation, and signaling in cell adhesion. Cell 69:11, 1992.
65. Yamada KM: Fibronectin peptides in cell migration and wound repair. J Clin Invest 105:1507, 2000.
66. Danen EH, Yamada KM: Fibronectin, integrins, and growth control. J Cell Physiol 189:1, 2001.
67. DeSimone DW: Adhesion and matrix in vertebrate development. Curr Opin Cell Biol 6:747, 1994.
68. Ginsberg MH, Loftus JC, Plow EF: Cytoadhesins, integrins, and platelets. Thromb Haemost 59:1, 1988.
69. Mosher D: Fibronectin. In: Mosher DF (ed): Fibronectins: Biology of extracellular matrix. San Diego, Academic Press, 1989, p 530.
70. Bisno AL, Brito MO, Collins CM: Molecular basis of group A streptococcal virulence. Lancet Infect Dis 3:191, 2003.
71. Schwarz-Linek U, Plevin MJ, Pickford AR, et al: Binding of a peptide from a *Streptococcus dysgalactiae* MSCRAMM to the *N*-terminal F1 module pair of human fibronectin involves both modules. FEBS Lett 497:137, 2001.
72. Klebe RJ: Isolation of a collagen-dependent cell attachment factor. Nature 250:248, 1974.
73. Kleinman HK, Klebe RJ, Martin GR: Role of collagenous matrices in the adhesion and growth of cells. J Cell Biol 88:473, 1981.
74. Engvall E, Ruoslahti E, Miller EJ: Affinity of fibronectin to collagens of different genetic types and to fibrinogen. J Exp Med 147: 1584, 1978.
75. Wierzbicka-Patynowski I, Schwarzbauer JE: The ins and outs of fibronectin matrix assembly. J Cell Sci 116:3269, 2003.
76. Raghow R: The role of extracellular matrix in postinflammatory wound healing and fibrosis. FASEB J 8:823, 1994.
77. Aumailley M, Pesch M, Tunggal L, et al: Altered synthesis of laminin 1 and absence of basement membrane component deposition in (beta)1 integrin-deficient embryoid bodies. J Cell Sci 113 Pt 2:259, 2000.
78. Aumailley M, Smyth N: The role of laminins in basement membrane function. J Anat 193 (Pt 1):1, 1998.
79. Colognato H, Yurchenco PD: Form and function: The laminin family of heterotrimers. Dev Dyn 218:213, 2000.
80. Beck K, Dixon TW, Engel J, et al: Ionic interactions in the coiled-coil domain of laminin determine the specificity of chain assembly. J Mol Biol 231:311, 1993.
81. Engbring JA, Kleinman HK: The basement membrane matrix in malignancy. J Pathol 200:465, 2003.
82. Kleinman HK, Koblinski J, Lee S, et al: Role of basement membrane in tumor growth and metastasis. Surg Oncol Clin N Am 10:329, 2001.
83. Powell SK, Kleinman HK: Neuronal laminins and their cellular receptors. Int J Biochem Cell Biol 29:401, 1997.
84. Bernfield M, Kokenyesi R, Kato M, et al: Biology of the syndecans: A family of transmembrane heparan sulfate proteoglycans. Annu Rev Cell Biol 8:365, 1992.
85. Iozzo RV: Matrix proteoglycans: From molecular design to cellular function. Annu Rev Biochem 67:609, 1998.
86. Iozzo RV: The family of the small leucine-rich proteoglycans: Key regulators of matrix assembly and cellular growth. Crit Rev Biochem Mol Biol 32:141, 1997.
87. Kjellen L, Lindahl U: Proteoglycans: Structures and interactions. Annu Rev Biochem 60:443, 1991.
88. Roughley PJ, Lee ER: Cartilage proteoglycans: Structure and potential functions. Microsc Res Tech 28:385, 1994.
89. Drickamer K: A conserved disulphide bond in sialyltransferases. Glycobiology 3:2, 1993.
90. Li H, Schwartz NB, Vertel BM: cDNA cloning of chick cartilage chondroitin sulfate (aggrecan) core protein and identification of a stop codon in the aggrecan gene associated with the chondrodystrophy, nanomelia. J Biol Chem 268:23504, 1993.
91. Watanabe H, Kimata K, Line S, et al: Mouse cartilage matrix deficiency (cmd) caused by a 7 bp deletion in the aggrecan gene. Nat Genet 7:154, 1994.
92. Yamaguchi Y: Lecticans: Organizers of the brain extracellular matrix. Cell Mol Life Sci 57:276, 2000.
93. Seidenbecher CI, Richter K, Rauch U, et al: Brevican: A chondroitin sulfate proteoglycan of rat brain, occurs as secreted and cell surface glycosylphosphatidylinositol-anchored isoforms. J Biol Chem 270:27206, 1995.
94. Danielson KG, Baribault H, Holmes DF, et al: Targeted disruption of decorin leads to abnormal collagen fibril morphology and skin fragility. J Cell Biol 136:729, 1997.
95. Vogel KG, Paulsson M, Heinegard D: Specific inhibition of type I and type II collagen fibrillogenesis by the small proteoglycan of tendon. Biochem J 223:587, 1984.
96. Hedbom E, Heinegard D: Binding of fibromodulin and decorin to separate sites on fibrillar collagens. J Biol Chem 268:27307, 1993.
97. Nurminskaya MV, Birk DE: Differential expression of fibromodulin mRNA associated with tendon fibril growth: Isolation and characterization of a chicken fibromodulin cDNA. Biochem J 317 (Pt 3):785, 1996.
98. Birk DE, Nurminskaya MV, Zycband EI: Collagen fibrillogenesis in situ: Fibril segments undergo post-depositional modifications resulting in linear and lateral growth during matrix development. Dev Dyn 202:229, 1995.
99. Lindahl U, Kusche-Gullberg M, Kjellen L: Regulated diversity of heparan sulfate. J Biol Chem 273:24979, 1998.
100. Ruoslahti E: Structure and biology of proteoglycans. Annu Rev Cell Biol 4:229, 1988.
101. Fellini SA, Kimura JH, Hascall VC: Polydispersity of proteoglycans synthesized by chondrocytes from the Swarm rat chondrosarcoma. J Biol Chem 256:7883, 1981.
102. Schiller S, Mathews MB, Cifonelli JA, et al: The metabolism of mucopolysaccharides in animals. III. Further studies on skin utilizing C14-glucose, C14-acetate, and S35-sodium sulfate. J Biol Chem 218:139, 1956.
103. Truppe W, Kresse H: Uptake of proteoglycans and sulfated glycosaminoglycans by cultured skin fibroblasts. Eur J Biochem 85:351, 1978.
104. Fluharty AL: The mucopolysaccharidoses: A synergism between clinical and basic investigation. J Invest Dermatol 79 Suppl 1:38s, 1982.
105. van der Flier A, Sonnenberg A: Function and interactions of integrins. Cell Tissue Res 305:285, 2001.
106. Hemler ME: Integrins. In Kreis T, Vale R (eds): Guidebook to the Extracellular Matrix, Anchor and Adhesion Proteins, Oxford University Press, 1999, p 196.
107. Hynes RO: Targeted mutations in cell adhesion genes: What have we learned from them? Dev Biol 180:402, 1996.
108. Hynes RO, Zhao Q: The evolution of cell adhesion. J Cell Biol 150:F89, 2000.
109. Hynes RO: A reevaluation of integrins as regulators of angiogenesis. Nat Med 8:918, 2002.
110. Hynes RO: Integrins: Bidirectional, allosteric signaling machines. Cell 110:673, 2002.
111. Miranti CK, Brugge JS: Sensing the environment: A historical perspective on integrin signal transduction. Nat Cell Biol 4:E83, 2002.
112. Schwartz MA, Ginsberg MH: Networks and crosstalk: Integrin signaling spreads. Nat Cell Biol 4:E65, 2002.

113. Schaeffer HJ, Weber MJ: Mitogen-activated protein kinases: Specific messages from ubiquitous messengers. Mol Cell Biol 19:2435, 1999.
114. Hanks SK, Calalb MB, Harper MC, et al: Focal adhesion protein-tyrosine kinase phosphorylated in response to cell attachment to fibronectin. Proc Natl Acad Sci U S A 89:8487, 1992.
115. Kanner SB, Reynolds AB, Parsons JT: Immunoaffinity purification of tyrosine-phosphorylated cellular proteins. J Immunol Methods 120:115, 1989.
116. Shichiri M, Hirata Y: Antiangiogenesis signals by endostatin. FASEB J 15:1044, 2001.
117. Giancotti FG, Ruoslahti E: Integrin signaling. Science 285:1028, 1999.
118. Livant DL, Brabec RK, Kurachi K, et al: The PHSRN sequence induces extracellular matrix invasion and accelerates wound healing in obese diabetic mice. J Clin Invest 105:1537, 2000.
119. Livant DL, Brabec RK, Pienta KJ, et al: Anti-invasive, antitumorigenic, and antimetastatic activities of the PHSCN sequence in prostate carcinoma. Cancer Res 60:309, 2000.
120. Bosman FT, Stamenkovic I: Functional structure and composition of the extracellular matrix. J Pathol 200:423, 2003.
121. Lander AD, Selleck SB: The elusive functions of proteoglycans: In vivo veritas. J Cell Biol 148:227, 2000.
122. Skandalis SS, Theocharis AD, Papageorgakopoulou N, et al: Glycosaminoglycans in early chick embryo. Int J Dev Biol 47:311, 2003.
123. Rapraeger AC, Krufka A, Olwin BB: Requirement of heparan sulfate for bFGF-mediated fibroblast growth and myoblast differentiation. Science 252:1705, 1991.
124. Yayon A, Klagsbrun M, Esko JD, et al: Cell surface, heparin-like molecules are required for binding of basic fibroblast growth factor to its high affinity receptor. Cell 64:841, 1991.
125. Culley FJ, Fadlon EJ, Kirchem A, et al: Proteoglycans are potent modulators of the biological responses of eosinophils to chemokines. Eur J Immunol 33:1302, 2003
126. Penc SF, Pomahac B, Eriksson E, et al: Dermatan sulfate activates nuclear factor-kappa b and induces endothelial and circulating intercellular adhesion molecule-1. J Clin Invest 103:1329, 1999.
127. Carrell RW, Huntington JA, Mushunje A, et al: The conformational basis of thrombosis. Thromb Haemost 86:14, 2001.
128. Casu B: Structural features and binding properties of chondroitin sulfates, dermatan sulfate, and heparan sulfate. Semin Thromb Hemost 17:9, 1991.
129. Furie B, Furie BC: Molecular and cellular biology of blood coagulation. N Engl J Med 326:800, 1992.
130. Warkentin TE, Greinacher A: Heparin-induced thrombocytopenia and cardiac surgery. Ann Thorac Surg 76:638, 2003.
131. Iverius P: Possible role of the glycosaminoglycans in the genesis of atherosclerosis. In Atherogenesis: Initiating factors, Ciba Foundation Symposium 12, 1973. Associated Scientific Publishers, Amsterdam, p 185.
132. Cheng CF, Oosta GM, Bensadoun A, et al: Binding of lipoprotein lipase to endothelial cells in culture. J Biol Chem 256:12893, 1981.
133. Shimada K, Gill PJ, Silbert JE, et al: Involvement of cell surface heparin sulfate in the binding of lipoprotein lipase to cultured bovine endothelial cells. J Clin Invest 68:995, 1981.
134. Nilsson-Ehle P, Garfinkel AS, Schotz MC: Lipolytic enzymes and plasma lipoprotein metabolism. Annu Rev Biochem 49:667, 1980.
135. Madri JA, Stenn KS: Aortic endothelial cell migration. I. Matrix requirements and composition. Am J Pathol 106:180, 1982.
136. Nieswandt B, Watson SP: Platelet-collagen interaction: Is GPVI the central receptor? Blood 102:449, 2003.
137. Morton LF, Hargreaves PG, Farndale RW, et al: Integrin alpha 2 beta 1-independent activation of platelets by simple collagen-like peptides: Collagen tertiary (triple-helical) and quaternary (polymeric) structures are sufficient alone for alpha 2 beta 1-independent platelet reactivity. Biochem J 306:337, 1995.
138. Zheng XF, Podell S, Sefton BM, et al: The sequence of chicken c-yes and p61c-yes. Oncogene 4:99, 1989.
139. Berlanga O, Tulasne D, Bori T, et al: The Fc receptor gamma-chain is necessary and sufficient to initiate signaling through glycoprotein VI in transfected cells by the snake C-type lectin, convulxin. Eur J Biochem 269:2951, 2002.
140. Suzuki-Inoue K, Tulasne D, Shen Y, et al: Association of Fyn and Lyn with the proline-rich domain of glycoprotein VI regulates intracellular signaling. J Biol Chem 277:21561, 2002.
141. Andrews DA, Yang L, Low PS: Phorbol ester stimulates a protein kinase C-mediated agatoxin-TK-sensitive calcium permeability pathway in human red blood cells. Blood 100:3392, 2002.
142. Chiang TM, Cole F, Woo-Rasberry V: Cloning, characterization, and functional studies of a 47-kDa platelet receptor for type III collagen. J Biol Chem 277:34896, 2002.
143. Chiang TM, Rinaldy A, Kang AH: Cloning, characterization, and functional studies of a nonintegrin platelet receptor for type I collagen. J Clin Invest 100:514, 1997.
144. Monnet E, Depraetere H, Legrand C, et al: A monoclonal antibody to platelet type III collagen-binding protein (TIIICBP) binds to blood and vascular cells, and inhibits platelet vessel-wall interactions. Thromb Haemost 86:694, 2001.
145. Monnet E, Fauvel-Lafeve F: A new platelet receptor specific to type III collagen. Type III collagen-binding protein. J Biol Chem 275:10912, 2000.
146. Moog S, Mangin P, Lenain N, et al: Platelet glycoprotein V binds to collagen and participates in platelet adhesion and aggregation. Blood 98:1038, 2001.
147. Ni H, Ramakrishnan V, Ruggeri ZM, et al: Increased thrombogenesis and embolus formation in mice lacking glycoprotein V. Blood 98:368, 2001.
148. Arteaga-Solis E, Gayraud B, Ramirez F: Elastic and collagenous networks in vascular diseases. Cell Struct Funct 25:69, 2000.

■ ■ ■ chapter 4

Normal Mechanisms of Hemostasis

Frederick L. Ruberg
Joseph Loscalzo

MECHANISMS OF HEMOSTASIS

The hemostatic system is an exquisitely regulated concert of circulating and endothelium-derived factors that has evolved to arrest the flow of blood at the site of vascular injury. Concurrent complementary processes share key regulatory proteins and serve to initiate and stabilize the nascent clot, limit its expansion, and foster its dissolution. This carefully balanced interplay affords swift and efficient hemostasis at the site of injury; however, dysregulation of this adaptive process results in pathological hemostasis or thrombosis. Occurring in the setting of an atherosclerotic plaque, atherothrombosis is the primary mechanism of morbidity and mortality in cardiovascular disease. Loss of function or deficiency of important regulatory factors or platelet surface proteins can result in bleeding diatheses. This chapter outlines the normal mechanisms of hemostasis with attention afforded to platelet function, the coagulation cascade, and fibrinolysis and their regulatory determinants in an effort to provide a context for the thrombotic and hemorrhagic disorders to be discussed in later chapters.

ENDOTHELIAL FUNCTION AND PLATELET ACTIVATION

The intimal surface of blood vessels to which circulating blood is exposed consists of endothelial cells that participate in the regulation of vascular tone, potentiate inflammatory responses, and present to circulating blood a thrombo-resistant surface that facilitates laminar flow. Quiescent and normally functioning endothelial cells produce potent inhibitors of inflammation and platelet activation, including prostacyclin and nitric oxide, and do not express proteins that activate the inflammatory or coagulation processes. Disruption of the endothelial cell barrier function occurs with direct injury from trauma, exposure to injurious substances, or by chronic inflammatory processes, such as atherosclerosis or vasculitis. Loss of normal endothelial cell function exposes intensely thrombogenic molecules to circulating blood, including tissue factor, von Willebrand factor (vWF), and subendothelial collagen.

Following endothelial activation or disruption, circulating platelets localize and adhere to the site of injury forming the initial or primary ("white") thrombus. Circulating platelets are quiescent and do not adhere to normal endothelium until exposed to activating substances, such as thromboxane A_2, adenosine diphosphate (ADP), thrombin, or serotonin, or by the binding of vWF (Fig. 4-1).[1] Platelet activation is also directly inhibited by endothelium-derived substances, the two most important being endothelium-derived nitric oxide (NO•) and prostacyclin (PGI_2) (Table 4-1). NO• is produced constitutively by the endothelial isoform of nitric oxide synthase (eNOS) through the metabolism of L-arginine to L-citrulline, using tetrahydrobiopterin (BH_4), flavins, NADPH, calcium/calmodulin, and heme as essential cofactors. NO• plays a critical role in the regulation of smooth muscle contraction in the vessel media and, hence, vascular tone. NO• also directly inhibits platelet activation, adhesion, and aggregation through its stimulation of platelet guanylyl cyclase and subsequent increase in cyclic guanosine-monophosphate (cGMP) concentration, as well as through the inhibition of platelet phosphoinositol-3-kinase (PI-3 kinase).[2] PGI_2 is an eicosanoid (prostaglandin) synthesized from endothelial arachidonic acid that inhibits platelet activation and aggregation (but not adhesion) through its stimulation of adenylyl cyclase and subsequent increase in platelet cyclic adenosine-monophosphate (cAMP). PGI_2 is antagonized by the potent platelet activator thromboxane A_2 (TXA_2), which is produced by platelet

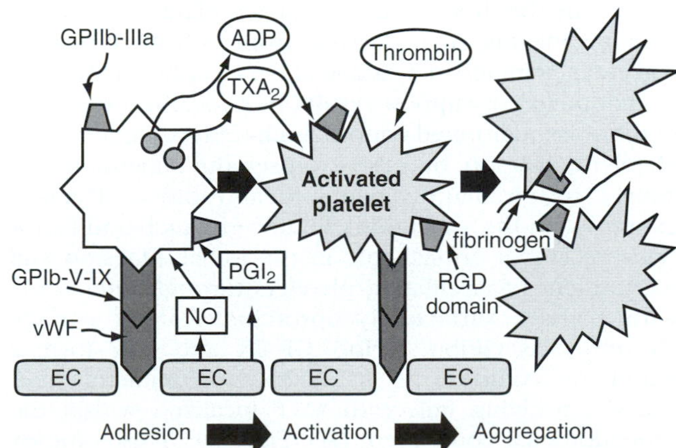

FIGURE 4-1. Platelet adhesion, activation and aggregation in normal hemostasis. Platelet adhesion is mediated by interactions between vascular wall expressed von Willebrand Factor (vWF) and platelet surface GP Ib-V-IX. Platelet activation occurs via vWF binding, and exposure to agonists including thrombin, adenosine diphosphate (ADP), and thromboxane A2 (TXA_2)—the latter two released from platelet granules. Activation causes a calcium-mediated conformational change in GPIIb/IIIa allowing fibrinogen binding and aggregation.

TABLE 4-1 PRINCIPAL REGULATORY MOLECULES PARTICIPATING IN NORMAL HEMOSTASIS

Prohemostatic	Function
Endothelium-Derived	
Plasminogen activator inhibitor-1 (PAI-1)	Inhibits activity of t-PA
Tissue factor (TF)	Binds factor VIIa to activate factor X to Xa
von Willebrand Factor (vWF)	Binds platelet glycoproteins Ib-V-IX (adhesion) and activates platelets
Circulating	
α_2-antiplasmin	Serine protease inhibitor, specifically binds and inhibits plasmin
Thrombin	Converts fibrinogen to fibrin, activates platelets and factors V, VIII, and XIII. Also binds thrombomodulin and other protease-activated receptors on cell surfaces
Thrombin-activatable fibrinolysis inhibitor (TAFI)	Cleaves terminal lysine from fibrin, thus interfering with plasminogen binding
Antihemostatic	**Function**
Endothelium-Derived	
Ecto-ADPase/CD39	Metabolizes platelet activator ADP to AMP
Heparan sulfate	Accelerates function of antithrombin III
Nitric oxide (NO•)	Elicits vasodilation and inhibits platelet adhesion, activation and aggregation
Prostacyclin (PGI_2)	Inhibits platelet activation and aggregation
Thrombomodulin	Binds thrombin and activates protein C and TAFI
Tissue plasminogen activator (t-PA)	Activates plasminogen to plasmin. May mediate mechanisms of inflammation and cell migration through annexin binding
Urokinase plasminogen activator (u-PA)	Activates plasminogen to plasmin. May mediate mechanisms of inflammation and cell migration through u-PAR binding
Circulating	
Antithrombin III	Serine protease inhibitor, binds thrombin and factors IXa and Xa
Protein C	Protease that cleaves factors Va and VIIIa, as well as PAI-1. May be involved in endothelial cell signaling via surface receptor binding
Protein S	Binds thrombomodulin and protein C to liberate activated protein C
Tissue factor pathway inhibitor (TFPI)	Binds and inhibits factor VIIa-TF complex

cyclooxygenase (COX1).[3] Irreversible acetylation of platelet COX1 at serine 529 by aspirin is responsible for the drug's selective antiplatelet effect. Platelet activation is also inhibited by the endothelial ecto-ADPase (CD-39), an enzyme that impairs ADP-mediated platelet activation by metabolizing ADP derived from activated platelet secretory granules to 5′-adenosine-monophosphate.[4]

Endothelial disruption results in a localized decrease in the aforementioned endothelium-derived inhibitors of platelet activation, but also exposes the subendothelial matrix to circulating platelets and blood. Densely expressed in the subendothelium, von Willebrand factor (vWF) serves a critical role in the initial adhesion and recruitment of circulating platelets through interaction with platelet surface glycoproteins. Platelet surface glycoproteins GPIbα, GPIbβ, GP IX, and GPV form a tetrameric complex (in a 2:2:2:1 stoichiometry) that forms a bridging link with vWF localized within the subendothelial component (see Fig. 4-1).[5] This complex firmly adheres the platelet to the site of injury, and resists disruption by shear stress or turbulent blood flow. Binding of vWF occurs specifically through the GPIbα component, a molecule that also contains a binding site for thrombin, facilitating activation of the adherent platelet.[6] Activation results in TXA_2 production and release of platelet-dense granules (containing ADP), thereby promoting activation and recruitment of other platelets in the growing hemostatic plug. The integral role of vWF in the hemostatic process is exemplified by the hemorrhagic complications suffered by patients who have qualitative or quantitative deficiencies of vWF (von Willebrand's disease) or lack the platelet glycoproteins to bind vWF (e.g., Bernard-Soulier syndrome).[7,8]

Platelet activation promotes a calcium-dependent conformational change in another critical platelet surface glycoprotein, GPIIb-IIIa. GPIIb-IIIa is a dimeric cell adhesion molecule of the integrin family composed of single alpha (α_{IIb}) and beta (β_3) subunits. Following activation, a conformational change in the extracellular domain of GPIIb-IIIa occurs resulting in the exposure of an RGD binding motif (Arg-Gly-Asp) that has a high affinity for fibrinogen, vWF, and fibronectin.[9] Fibrinogen, an important circulating clotting factor and the direct precursor of fibrin, then serves as a bridging molecule to crosslink other activated platelets, thereby fostering aggregation. The integral role of GPIIb-IIIa in primary hemostasis is clearly demonstrated by Glanzmann thrombasthenia—a rare, autosomal recessive disorder characterized by a congenital absence or dysfunction of GPIIb-IIIa that is marked by recurrent episodes of spontaneous mucocutaneous bleeding.[10] Pharmacologic inhibition of GPIIb-IIIa by various intravenous drugs is now widely embraced as of salutary benefit in the treatment of atherothrombosis and as adjuvant therapy to percutaneous coronary interventions.[11] Following aggregation, this relatively delicate platelet thrombus is then anchored by an intervening meshwork of fibrin, red blood cells, and circulating factors, ultimately produced by coincident activation of the coagulation cascade.

COAGULATION CASCADE AND THE FORMATION OF FIBRIN

Endothelial cell disruption or injury exposes circulating blood to proteins that activate the coagulation cascade, which ultimately produces the insoluble fibrin that forms the substance of the secondary clot. The coagulation cascade is an ordered, but complex, interdependent series of enzymatic reactions (proteolytic cleavages) dependent on circulating inactive plasma proteins (proenzyme clotting factors), endothelium-expressed proteins, calcium, and phospholipid. Clotting factors are biologically inactive under normal circumstances, but serve as enzyme precursors (zymogens) that are converted to an active enzyme with serine protease activity. The active form of a factor then catalyzes subsequent zymogen-protease reactions in a cascade of activation that ultimately produces the most important protease, thrombin. Thrombin plays a multifaceted, pivotal role in hemostasis serving to activate and recruit platelets, accelerate coagulation, and crosslink fibrin; however, it also slows its own generation (see later), and thereby limits the propagation of the developing thrombus.[12] Direct inhibitors of thrombin such as hirudin, hirudin analogs, or ximelagatran, are potent anticoagulants that are developing an expanding role in the practice of vascular medicine.[13,14] In addition, thrombin interacts with G-protein-linked cell-surface receptors (protease-activated receptors or PARs) on various different cell types, including platelets and endothelial cells, to initiate intracellular signaling cascades that can modulate inflammatory and proliferative responses.[15] Thus, participant proteins in the coagulation cascade can modulate not only hemostasis, but mechanisms of inflammation, repair, and regeneration, as well.

Thrombin is generated from the proteolytic cleavage of its inactive precursor prothrombin through the catalytic activity of activated factor X (Xa) (Fig. 4-2). This process releases byproduct prothrombin-fragment molecules F1 and F2, often used as serum markers of thrombin formation.[16] The activity of Xa is accelerated in the presence of factor Va (the active form of factor V), calcium, and a negatively charged phospholipid surface adeptly provided by activated platelets. The factor Va-Xa complex (prothrombinase) is 300,000-fold more catalytically active than factor Xa alone in the generation of thrombin. Positively charged calcium forms a noncovalent association between the gamma-carboxyglutamate residues found in factors Xa and prothrombin and the negatively charged phospholipid surface.[12] Gamma-carboxylation of prothrombin, factor VII, factor IX, factor X, and the anticoagulant proteins C and S, is a vitamin K-dependent posttranslational modification that is inhibited by coumarin derivatives. In this manner, thrombin

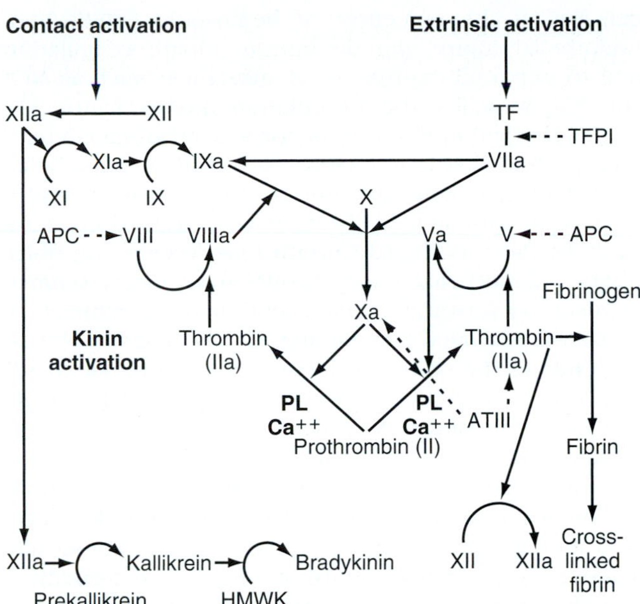

FIGURE 4-2. Normal mechanisms of the coagulation cascade. The coagulation cascade is a complicated yet carefully regulated interdependent series of enzymatic reactions that ultimately produce the fibrin clot. Initiation can occur via tissue factor (TF) release (extrinsic pathway) or contact activation of factor XII (intrinsic pathway). Thrombin formation by factor Xa occurs in the presence of calcium (Ca^{++}) and a negatively charged phospholipid (PL) surface. Contact factor XIIa also activates the kinin system ultimately resulting in the conversion of high-molecular-weight kininogen (HMWK) to bradykinin.

generation is enhanced locally, at the site of injury and platelet deposition. Factor Va is itself generated by the cleavage of factor V by thrombin, thus providing a positive-feedback mechanism of amplification. The production of thrombin by factor Xa has been previously termed the "final common pathway" of the coagulation cascade, a term in view of the prior conception that two distinct upstream pathways could result in factor X activation. The concept of the *extrinsic*, or tissue factor-dependent, and *intrinsic*, or contact-dependent, activation of factor X was conceived following the development of in vitro plasma tests of fibrin formation (see Fig. 4-2). The prothrombin time (PT) relies on the addition of an extrinsic substance (tissue factor or thromboplastin) to facilitate activation of the coagulation cascade, whereas the activated partial thromboplastin time (aPTT) simply presents a foreign surface to plasma to initiate coagulation (contact activation).[17] It is now accepted that the former pathway involving tissue factor is predominantly responsible for in vivo hemostasis and thrombosis, whereas the latter contact pathway participates in an accessory role. The observation that a congenital absence of contact pathway factors results in few clinical bleeding complications has substantiated this conclusion. In addition, clear links between the pathways (such as activation of factor IX by tissue factor—factor VII) make this classic distinction less relevant than previously believed.

Because of its localization at the interface between circulating blood and the vessel wall, as well as its normal expression of antithrombotic substances, the endothelial cell lies at the epicenter of hemostatic equilibrium. Endothelial injury and disruption initiate coagulation due to impaired expression of substances such as NO• and PGI_2, as well as the presentation of tissue factor (TF) to the circulation.[18] Tissue factor is a membrane-bound glycoprotein that is inducibly expressed by endothelial cells and macrophages under conditions of injury (a process inhibited by NO•); it is expressed constitutively by subendothelial smooth muscle cells and fibroblasts.[19] Endothelial injury results from direct trauma; exposure to activators, such as endotoxin, inflammatory mediators, activated complement, or immune complexes. TF binds to the *activated* form of circulating factor VII (VIIa) to form a protein-protein complex that directly activates both factors X and IX. Factor VIIa exists in the plasma at a concentration of approximately 10 nmol/liter or 1% to 2% of the total factor VII concentration. Although synthesized by the liver, its source of low-level activation is controversial. Factor VIIa itself is biologically inactive as a protease until bound to TF, forming a complex that increases its catalytic activity for its active substrate factor X by four orders of magnitude. The factor VIIa-TF-X-IX complex, or extrinsic factor Xase or tenase, produces both Xa and IXa. Factor Xa then activates prothrombin to thrombin locally as detailed earlier.[12]

Thrombin, in addition to activating both platelets and factor V, also activates factor VIII. Factor VIII circulates in the blood noncovalently associated to vWF. Factor VIIIa then serves as an accelerating cofactor for factor IXa (produced from the TF-VIIa complex), which also serves to activate factor X to Xa (the intrinsic tenase complex, so-termed because factor Xa formation does not *directly* involve tissue factor), and, hence, yield thrombin. This latter reaction using factors IXa and VIIIa is the predominant activator of factor X, being 50-fold more efficient at factor X activation than the direct TF-VIIa complex.[12] The congenital absence of factor VIII (hemophilia A) or factor IX (hemophilia B), therefore, results in severe bleeding diatheses due to the markedly reduced generation factor Xa. Factor X activation occurs through both tenase mechanisms on a phospholipid surface in the presence of calcium, as factors VII, IX, and X have γ-carboxyglutamate residues. Through the different mechanisms that lead to factor X activation, the two arms of the coagulation cascade unite. Functionality of the extrinsic pathway and the final common pathway of coagulation can be specifically determined by the prothrombin time (PT) test in which tissue factor is added to a plasma sample, thereby directly activating the extrinsic cascade and forming factors Xa and thrombin. In this way, deficiencies or abnormalities in factors II, V, VII, X, and/or fibrinogen can be detected. Because functionality of factors II, VII, and X, is vitamin K dependent, the efficacy of anticoagulation by coumarin derivatives is also assessed by this test.[17]

Factor IXa can also be formed by activation of the intrinsic or contact system, thus providing an alternative means by which factor Xa can be generated (although, as previously mentioned, of less physiologic relevance). Although less relevant to coagulation, the contact system is emerging as an important effector in the simultaneous processes of inflammation and fibrinolysis. The intrinsic pathway can be initiated through contact autoactivation of factor XII (Hageman factor) in vitro by exposure of plasma to foreign, negatively charged surfaces, including glass or kaolin, or in vivo on exposure to negatively charged subendothelial collagen.[20] Activated factor XII participates in the coagulation cascade through the subsequent activation of factors XI and then IX. In addition, the zymogen prekallikrein is converted to the enzyme kallikrein following proteolytic cleavage by factor XIIa, a reaction requiring the essential cofactor high-molecular-weight kininogen (HMWK). Prekallikrein can also autoactivate itself on the endothelial cell surface in the presence of HWMK. Kallikrein then cleaves HMWK to the inflammatory mediator bradykinin, a potent vasodilator and mediator of vascular permeability. Through the subsequent generation of bradykinin, factor XIIa, therefore, participates in mechanisms of inflammation, complement activation, the regulation of vascular tone, and fibrinolysis.[21] Bradykinin stimulates endothelial cell expression of NO• and the fibrinolytic effector, tissue-type plasminogen activator (t-PA).[22] Because factor XIIa can also be generated by the activity of the fibrinolytic enzyme plasmin, a self-amplifying link between the concurrent processes that foster clot development and dissolution can be established. The activated partial thromboplastin time (aPTT) test is used to assess the functionality of the factors associated with intrinsic pathway activation (as well as the final common pathway, although it is a less sensitive test than the PT for the abnormalities of factors II, V, X, and fibrinogen). The aPTT uses foreign substances such as glass or silicates to activate factor XII, and is, therefore, sensitive to abnormalities in factors XII, XI, IX, and VIII, as well as to the inhibitory action of unfractionated heparin.[17]

The generation of fibrin from circulating fibrinogen is the principal role of thrombin in regard to the propagation of the developing clot (see Fig. 4-2). Soluble fibrin monomer is formed by the proteolytic cleavage of the Aα and Bβ chains of fibrinogen by thrombin, releasing the byproduct fibrinopeptides A and B.[23] Cleavage of fibrinogen triggers a conformational change that results in a fibrin molecule that exposes polymerization sites. Fibrin then polymerizes in end-to-end and staggered side-to-side noncovalent associations, trapping platelets, red blood cells, and plasma proteins in an insoluble meshwork that becomes the secondary clot, known as *red thrombus*. Covalent crosslinked associations between glutamyl and lysyl residues of the γ chain of fibrin are catalyzed by factor XIII, a protransglutaminase that itself is activated by thrombin.[24] Although a kinetically slow reaction, fibrin crosslinks stabilize the developing thrombus and provide protection from both shear stress and fibrinolysis. Formation of fibrin crosslinks mask binding sites for molecules that initiate fibrinolysis (t-PA), and, hence, can provide a mechanism for the autoregulation of the clot's formation and destruction.

The exquisitely regulated process of hemostasis concurrently slows the development of the propagating clot while it is developing. Two important circulating plasma proteins participate primarily in the attenuation of coagulation (see Table 4-1). Antithrombin III (ATIII) is a serine protease inhibitor that binds and inactivates factors IXa, Xa, and thrombin.[25] The activity of ATIII is increased 2000-fold when bound to endothelium-expressed heparan sulfate, a surface glycosaminoglycan that is believed to be the physiologic analog for intravenous unfractionated heparin.[26] In addition, circulating tissue factor pathway inhibitor (TFPI) can inhibit the extrinsic tenase (TF-VIIa-IX-X) complex. TFPI is a multivalent protease inhibitor that is structurally composed of three Kunitz-type domains allowing for the binding and inactivation of both factor Xa and the TF-factor VIIa complex. Because TFPI can inhibit the generation of both factors Xa and IXa, its role as a therapeutic anticoagulant is currently being evaluated.[27] TFPI-2 has a similar domain structure to TFPI; however, it is expressed predominantly in human placental tissues and is a more potent inhibitor of factor Xa than the TF-factor VIIa complex.[28]

Once generated, thrombin plays an essential role in its own attenuation through the generation of activated protein C (APC). Thrombomodulin, a membrane-bound glycoprotein expressed on the endothelial cell surface, binds thrombin in a quaternary complex with circulating plasma proteins C and S to produce APC. APC then binds and proteolytically cleaves factors Va and VIIIa, thereby significantly slowing the generation of factors Xa and thrombin. APC also inactivates plasminogen activator inhibitor-1 (PAI-1) and, hence, promotes fibrinolysis (see later).[29] A single nucleotide polymorphism (G1691A or the Leiden mutation) within the factor V gene results in the substitution of a glutamine for an arginine at position 506 of the protein, and confers resistance to APC-mediated degradation.[30] Although this mutation has been associated with an increased risk of venous thromboembolism, its association with atherothrombosis remains inconclusive.[31,32] APC, like thrombin, also seems to represent a link between the complementary pathways of inflammation and hemostasis through interactions with its endothelial cell receptor (EPCR) and, perhaps, other protease-activated receptors.[29] The pharmacologic application of recombinant activated protein C (drotrecogin alpha) in the treatment of septic shock underscores the perceived multifaceted role of this protease; however, its benefit in sepsis likely derives from a reduction in microvascular thrombosis.

FIBRINOLYSIS

Hemostatic balance is also predicated on the concurrent activation of an analogous protease system that fosters clot dissolution. Components of the fibrinolytic system share numerous similarities with their procoagulant counterparts, including serine protease activity, the use of circulating proenzyme (zymogen) proteins, an integrated system of lysis inhibition, and the central role of the endothelial cell in initiation. Homology exists among the various activators of the fibrinolytic system, an observation that has yielded numerous pharmacologic substitutes for these endogenous molecules. Indeed, therapeutic application of fibrinolytic drugs to thrombotic processes, such as myocardial infarction, stroke, and pulmonary embolism, has become a standard of care in the management of these vascular diseases.

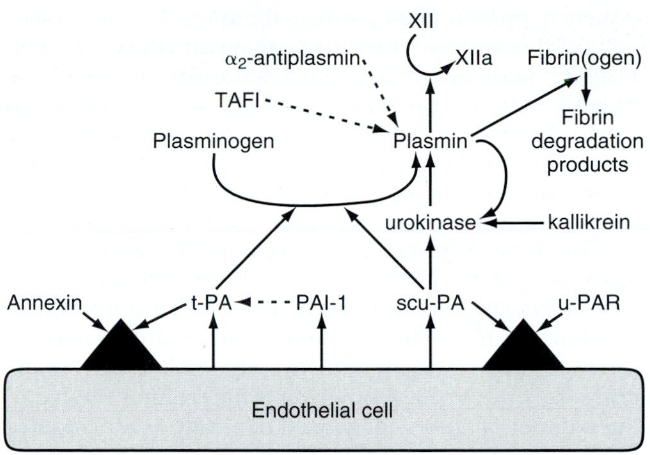

FIGURE 4-3. Normal mechanisms of the fibrinolytic system. Fibrinolysis occurs with the cleavage of fibrin to fibrin degradation products by the enzyme plasmin. Plasmin is activated by the endothelium-derived molecules: tissue plasminogen activator (t-PA) or urokinase plasminogen activator (scu-PA). scu-PA is converted to urokinase by plasmin and kallikrein. Plasmin also activates factor XIIa and can cleave t-PA and plasminogen. Binding of t-PA and u-PA to surface receptors annexin and u-PAR modulate the activity of these proteases. Plasmin activity is inhibited by α_2-antiplasmin and thrombin-activatable fibrinolysis inhibitor (TAFI), whereas t-PA is inhibited by plasminogen activator inhibitor-1 (PAI-1).

Fibrinolysis occurs through the action of the serine protease enzyme plasmin, activated from its circulating zymogen plasminogen by two critical proteins: t-PA and urokinase-type plasminogen activator (u-PA) (Fig. 4-3) (see Table 4-1).[33] Native plasminogen (Glu-plasminogen) is synthesized by the liver as a single-chain molecule, whereas t-PA and u-PA are endothelium-derived proteins. Within the aminoterminal portion of plasminogen, t-PA and u-PA, resides a specific molecular domain termed a *kringle*. Kringles are approximately 80 amino acid residues in length, and through the forces exerted by three specific disulfide linkages, have a unique folded structure that affords a high-affinity homotypic binding site capable of associating with plasminogen, fibrinogen, and fibrin.[34] Plasminogen itself contains 5 kringle domains, whereas t-PA contains two, and u-PA contains one. The marked homology of the kringles among these molecules suggests significant genetic conservation specifically among lysine binding sites.

As kringles bind fibrinogen and fibrin, circulating plasminogen and endothelium-derived t-PA are incorporated into the developing thrombus as it is formed, a feature affording significant clot localization and specificity. Plasminogen is converted to plasmin through proteolytic cleavage by t-PA and u-PA between Arg_{560} and Val_{561}, producing the active double-chain molecule. Plasminogen can also be cleaved at position 77 of the aminoterminus of the molecule, forming a product termed *Lys-plasminogen* that has a higher affinity for fibrin than its uncleaved counterpart.[35] The proteolytic reaction occurs in the presence of plasmin, but also on binding of plasminogen to various proteins (specifically annexins) expressed on the endothelial cell surface.[36] Three amino acid residues on the B chain of plasmin compose the active site of the molecule: His_{602}, Asp_{645}, Ser_{740}. Although remote in sequence, protein folding brings these residues into proximity in the tertiary structure, forming an active site with serine protease activity. Once activated, plasmin can cleave any protein with an accessible Arg-Lys bond, although it has a high affinity for fibrin. Plasmin can also cleave Glu-plasminogen to Lys-plasminogen; activate contact pathway factor XII; and inactivate factors V and VIII, complement, and hormones—including adrenocorticotropic hormone (ACTH), human placental lactogen (HPL), and growth hormone (GH).[37] Plasmin cleaves fibrin into differently sized degradation or split products (FDP). Gamma-chain crosslinks in fibrin are resistant to plasmin degradation, however, thus releasing a host of crosslinked FDP of differing sizes, the smallest of which is the D-dimer fragment. The D-dimer is now widely used clinically as a marker of acute or chronic thrombosis, and has an established role in the diagnosis of venous thromboembolism and disseminated intravascular coagulopathy (DIC).[16]

Tissue-type plasminogen activator (t-PA) is a single-chain protein of molecular weight 72-kDa that is constitutively synthesized by a number of different tissues, the most relevant being the endothelium.[38] Of the two endogenous activators of plasminogen, t-PA is the most important physiologically in both normal hemostasis and thrombosis. Under normal circumstances, the concentration of t-PA in plasma is approximately 5 ng/ml; however, under conditions of mechanical or biochemical endothelial injury, the endothelial cell can upregulate t-PA expression, thereby creating local increases in concentration. The aforementioned kringle domains shared among t-PA and plasminogen allow fibrinogen and fibrin binding and, hence, incorporation into a developing clot. Without binding and protection from plasma proteases, the half-life of t-PA is approximately 4 minutes. Intact recombinant t-PA (alteplase) and derivative agents that maintain the integrity of the kringle domain(s) with various truncations (reteplase) or amino acid substitutions (tenecteplase) are now the most widely used agents for the thrombolytic therapy of acute arterial or venous thrombosis.[39]

In addition to the two kringles, the structure of t-PA from the aminoterminus inward also has a defined "finger" region at residues 5 to 40 (similar to that of fibronectin) and an epidermal growth factor (EGF)-like domain from residues 51 to 87 similar to those found in u-PA, protein C, and factors IX and X. One or both of these domains in the aminoterminus likely affords t-PA the ability to associate with endothelial cell surface proteins, specifically a t-PA receptor similar to annexin II and platelet glycoproteins.[36] Interactions between endothelium-derived proteins, such as matrix metalloproteinases (MMPs) and elements of the fibrinolytic system may also affect hemostatic control.[40] Thus, like thrombin, plasminogen and t-PA can be bound to the endothelial cell surface, a process by which local control (both plasmin formation, acceleration, and retardation) is exerted by the endothelial cell in response to its milieu.

t-PA can itself be proteolytically cleaved by plasmin, specifically at the Arg_{275}-Ile_{276} site, forming a two-chain entity. The A or heavier chain contains the aminoterminus finger, EGF, and kringle domains, and, hence, fibrinogen avidity; whereas the B chain contains the active proteolytic site of the molecule composed of residues His_{325}, Asp_{374}, and Ser_{481}.[41] Both forms of t-PA, the one- and two-chain entities, can activate plasminogen; however, in the absence of fibrinogen, the two-chain form appears to have greater catalytic efficiency.[42] Both can also cleave other molecules in addition to fibrin, including prorenin, fibronectin, and fibrinogen. The elegant interaction between clot-bound plasminogen, fibrin, and t-PA affords specificity and localized enhancement of the fibrinolytic process.

In contrast to t-PA, urokinase-type plasminogen activator (u-PA) is an endothelium-derived molecule first isolated from human urine that exists as two major species: high-molecular-weight (HMW) u-PA with a mass of 54-kDa and low-molecular-weight (LMW) u-PA with a mass of 33-kDa.[43] Both are similarly efficacious in plasminogen activation, with the HMW species being the native form and the LMW species resulting from autodigestion or proteolysis by urinary or plasma proteases. Like t-PA, u-PA activates plasminogen by cleavage of the Arg_{560}-Val_{561} bond to create plasmin. Unlike t-PA, however, u-PA does not bind fibrin and, as such, can activate only endothelial-bound or circulating plasminogen and not clot-bound plasminogen.[43] Urokinase is synthesized as a single chain precursor molecule (scu-PA) expressed by endothelial cells and is activated to a two-chain active molecule by hydrolysis by plasmin or kallikrein (see Fig. 4-3).[44] However, in the presence of insoluble fibrin, scu-PA itself is a potent plasminogen activator without further modification, and can mediate activation only of clot-bound plasminogen without direct fibrin binding. Similar to t-PA, a specific receptor for u-PA (u-PAR) has been identified that fosters u-PA-plasminogen interactions and accelerates plasmin formation.[45] Endothelial cell binding to u-PAR is felt to be of significant physiologic relevance for the function of u-PA. In addition, u-PA synthesized by leukocytes can bind to u-PAR on the surface of endothelial and other inflammatory cells. Through u-PAR interactions, u-PA may also act proteolytically on other molecules, such as matrix proteins or other proteases, thereby potentially participating in diverse biologic processes, including cell migration rather than fibrinolysis alone.[46,47]

Streptokinase (SK) is a plasminogen activator isolated from β-hemolytic streptococci that is a 45- to 50-kDa single chain glycoprotein. Although it does not participate in normal hemostasis, SK is important historically as a therapeutic agent in the treatment of acute thrombosis. Unlike t-PA and u-PA, SK is not an enzyme and must complex with plasminogen to form an active molecule that then can cleave both complexed and free plasminogen to plasmin.[48] Because it is a foreign substance, an immune response is initiated with formation of antistreptokinase antibodies coincident with evidence of systemic inflammation on SK administration. Because of this problem with immunity and the current availability of recombinant forms of t-PA, SK is now rarely used. Another synthetic variant of SK previously used therapeutically to initiate fibrinolysis is acylated Lys-plasminogen-streptokinase activator complex (anistreplase or APSAC). APSAC is simply a 1:1 stoichiometric inert complex of SK and plasminogen with protection of the active proteolytic site by acylation. When introduced into the aqueous phase at neutral pH (i.e., plasma), deacylation occurs by first-order kinetics yielding an active molecule capable of free and clot-bound plasminogen activation. For reasons similar to SK, APSAC is no longer used in the treatment of thrombosis.[48]

An intricate and tightly regulated system of fibrinolytic pathway inhibition has also evolved in a fashion analogous to regulation of the coagulation cascade, using both circulating and endothelium-derived inhibitors that are responsive to local and systemic factors (see Table 4-1). Most circulating specific and nonspecific inhibitors act through serine protease inhibition (serpin), thus affecting not only plasmin, but also other serine proteases, including the effectors involved in coagulation. A 67-kDa single-chain glycoprotein termed α_2-antiplasmin retains specificity for plasmin, and can rapidly inactivate the enzyme. α_2-antiplasmin also can be crosslinked to fibrin by factor XIII_a, perhaps allowing for additional local modulation of fibrinolytic activity at the level of the developing clot.[49] Nonspecific inhibitors of plasmin are also found in plasma, albeit of less physiologic importance than α_2-antiplasmin; these include α_2-macroglobulin, α_1-antitrypsin, C1-esterase inhibitor, and antithrombin III.

Another important circulating inhibitor of the fibrinolytic pathway that is not a member of the serpin family is thrombin-activatable fibrinolysis inhibitor (TAFI), a glycoprotein also known as carboxypeptidase B, U, or R. Carboxypeptidases are enzymes that cleave the carboxyterminal peptide bond of proteins. Synthesized in the liver, TAFI exists in plasma at a concentration of 50 to 150 nM. TAFI is, itself, a protease that cleaves the carboxyterminal lysine from fibrin, thereby interfering with plasminogen binding and, hence, slowing clot-specific fibrinolysis. As its name suggests, TAFI is activated by the thrombin-thrombomodulin complex.[50]

Endothelium-derived specific inhibitors of t-PA/u-PA are critically important to the regulation of these enzymes (see Table 4-1). By far, the most important of these substances is plasminogen activator inhibitor-1 (PAI-1). PAI-1 is a 48-kDa serine protease inhibitor inducibly expressed by endothelial cells (or activated platelets) following exposure to a diverse number of substances, including thrombin; inflammatory mediators, such as TNFα; growth factors, such as IGF-1 and TGF-β; lipids, such as lipoprotein(a) and fatty acids; insulin; angiotensin II; and endotoxin.[51] The half-life of PAI-1 following release from the endothelial cell is approximately 30 minutes; however, binding to vitronectin can stabilize the molecule and increases its longevity. PAI-1 can also bind to fibrin, and, when bound, retain its inhibitory effect on plasminogen activators. This effect, however, is attenuated in the presence of polymerized, crosslinked fibrin, perhaps because of the impaired access of PAI-1 to the catalytic domain of t-PA. Platelet release of PAI-1 following stimulation by thrombin is important in preventing the premature dissolution of a nascent clot. The importance of PAI-1 and vascular disease cannot be understated, as recent investigations have associated elevated levels of PAI-1 with atherothrombosis, and, specifically, with oxidant stress of endothelial cells, perhaps related to pathological perturbations of the renin-angiotensin-aldosterone system. Particularly among diabetic patients with hyperlipidemia (the metabolic syndrome), dysfunction of PAI-1 appears of unique importance.[51]

The contribution of angiotensin II to the development of atherosclerosis and the potentiation of atherothrombotic events has been the subject of extensive recent investigation. Angiotensin II has been shown to induce PAI-1 expression both in endothelial cells and vascular smooth muscle cells.[52] Angiotensin converting enzyme (ACE) inhibitors are potent antihypertensives that inhibit the conversion of angiotensin I to angiotensin II, but also inhibit the degradation of bradykinin by ACE. ACE inhibitors have been demonstrated to reduce PAI-1 levels and activity in vivo, likely through direct effects on endothelial cell PAI-1 expression, but also may potentiate bradykinin-induced t-PA expression. In this manner, ACE inhibitor therapy may improve mortality among patients following coronary atherothrombotic events through the restoration of a favorable hemostatic balance.[53] These observations are likely mediated through modulations in endothelial cell oxido-reductive balance that are improved by ACE inhibition, as angiotensin II stimulates the cellular enzyme NAD(P)H oxidase (likely the principal source of endothelial cell reactive oxygen species) to produce the potent oxidant superoxide ($^\bullet O_2^-$).[54]

Of much less importance in the homeostatic mechanism of hemostasis, PAI-2 has been isolated from human placental tissue, specifically keratinocytes and macrophages, and likely participates in placental cell invasion of the uterine myometrium.[28] PAI-3, also known as protein C inhibitor, is a nonspecific serpin that inhibits not only t-PA/u-PA, but also thrombin, factor Xa, factor XIa, and the thrombin-thrombomodulin complex, thereby inhibiting activated protein C and TAFI. PAI-3 is expressed primarily in the liver, but also in the testes, kidney, and pancreas; its physiologic mechanism relevant to hemostasis remains unclear, as knockout studies in mice have not detected abnormalities in the regulation of coagulation or fibrinolysis. Although perhaps not relevant to coagulation, the observation that male PAI-3 null mice are infertile suggests a role in spermatogenesis or testicular development.[55]

THROMBOSIS

Dysregulation of hemostasis occurring through the potentiation of coagulation or inhibition of fibrinolysis results in thrombosis, the pathologic deposition of clots within the venous or arterial systems. Discussed in detail in future chapters in this text, thrombotic events resulting in subtotal or total vascular occlusion are the proximate causes of infarction (myocardial or cerebral), ischemia (peripheral arterial disease), and venous thromboembolism that comprise the vast majority of morbid and mortal complications in vascular disease. An understanding of the causes and treatments of thrombosis is predicated on a thorough knowledge of the mechanisms of hemostasis detailed earlier.

In atherothrombosis, the pathophysiology of the development and destabilization of the atherosclerotic plaque contributes to the hemostatic imbalance that promotes dysfunctional clotting. Now best conceived as a process of chronic inflammation, the development of the atheroma occurs in the setting of prothrombotic, inflammatory mediators expressed by inflammatory cells, such as macrophages and T-cell lymphocytes, that invade the subendothelium.[56] This process results fundamentally in endothelial cell dysfunction, likely based on a perturbation in the oxido-reductive balance of the endothelial cell milieu—resulting in (but not limited to) reduced bioactivity of nitric oxide and prostacyclin and increased expression of PAI-1 and tissue factor. Rupture of the fibrous cap of the atheroma exposes the circulating blood, especially platelets, to the lesion core where tissue factor, von Willebrand factor, and PAI-1 are highly expressed.[57] These events are believed to contribute to platelet adhesion and activation, while concurrently activating the coagulation cascade and inhibiting the thrombo-protective arm of fibrinolysis. In addition, abnormalities in expression level or function of any of the effectors in the hemostatic pathway can promote thrombosis in the proper setting. For example, myocardial infarction has been associated with elevated circulating levels of fibrinogen and PAI-1, and decreased t-PA/PAI-1 ratios.[51] Other lines of investigation have associated genetic polymorphisms with varying levels of increased risk for atherothrombotic events, including the 4G/5G polymorphism of PAI-1 and the Leu33Pro or PL^{A2} mutation of platelet glycoprotein IIIa (or β3 integrin subunit).[58,59] Evidence of dysfunction in atherosclerosis of the renin-angiotensin-aldosterone system (elevated levels of angiotensin II) has been associated with prothrombotic endothelial cell pathology, including decreased nitric oxide availability, induction of endothelial cell oxidases (such as NAD(P)H oxidase), and increased expression of PAI-1 as detailed earlier.

Other genetic polymorphisms have been associated definitively with venous thrombosis but not atherothrombosis, an observation suggesting that while sharing the same hemostatic pathways, different initiating or propagating pathophysiologic mechanisms underlie thrombotic events in different vascular beds. For example, the Leiden mutation in the factor V gene (G1691A) and the G20210A mutation in the prothrombin gene have both been conclusively associated with venous thrombosis but not atherothrombosis. It appears that venous thrombosis relies more on blood stasis and is disproportionately affected by coagulation protein function—a distinction from the platelet-mediated, inflammatory milieu of atherothrombosis.[60]

The complicated and interdependent pathways of coagulation, fibrinolysis, inflammation, and neurohormonal activation comprise the mosaic of effectors, inhibitors, and modulators that contribute to hemostasis. Ongoing investigation, although likely revealing yet other layers of complexity in regulation and further obfuscating the process of hemostasis, will also provide therapeutic targets that may interrupt the cascade of molecular events that ultimately results in thrombosis.

REFERENCES

1. Kroll MS, Sullivan R: Mechanisms of platelet activation. In Loscalzo J, Schafer AI, (eds): Thrombosis and Hemorrhage, 3rd ed. Philadelphia, Williams and Wilkins, 2003, p 187.
2. Pigazzi A, Heydrick S, Folli F, et al: Nitric oxide inhibits thrombin receptor-activating peptide-induced phosphoinositide 3-kinase activity in human platelets. J Biol Chem 274:14368, 1999.
3. Loscalzo J: Endothelial injury, vasoconstriction, and its prevention. Tex Heart Inst J 22:180, 1995.
4. Gayle RB, III, Maliszewski CR, Gimpel SD, et al: Inhibition of platelet function by recombinant soluble ecto-ADPase/CD39. J Clin Invest 101:1851, 1998.
5. Berndt MC, Shen Y, Dopheide SM, et al: The vascular biology of the glycoprotein Ib-IX-V complex. Thromb Haemost 86:178, 2001.
6. Savage B, Cattaneo M, Ruggeri ZM: Mechanisms of platelet aggregation. Curr Opin Hematol 8:270, 2001.
7. Kunishima S, Kamiya T, Saito H: Genetic abnormalities of Bernard-Soulier syndrome. Int J Hematol 76:319, 2002.
8. Sadler JE: Von Willebrand disease type 1: A diagnosis in search of a disease. Blood 101:2089, 2003.
9. Bennett JS: Platelet-fibrinogen interactions. Ann N Y Acad Sci 936:340, 2001.
10. Bellucci S, Caen J: Molecular basis of Glanzmann's thrombasthenia and current strategies in treatment. Blood Rev 16:193, 2002.
11. Bhatt DL, Topol EJ: Scientific and therapeutic advances in antiplatelet therapy. Nat Rev Drug Discov 2:15, 2003.
12. Mann KG, Butenas S, Brummel K: The dynamics of thrombin formation. Arterioscler Thromb Vasc Biol 23:17, 2003.
13. Connolly SJ: Preventing stroke in patients with atrial fibrillation: Current treatments and new concepts. Am Heart J 145:418, 2003.
14. Eikelboom J, White H, Yusuf S: The evolving role of direct thrombin inhibitors in acute coronary syndromes. J Am Coll Cardiol 41:70S, 2003.
15. Sambrano GR, Weiss EJ, Zheng YW, et al: Role of thrombin signalling in platelets in haemostasis and thrombosis. Nature 413:74, 2001.
16. Horan JT, Francis CW: Fibrin degradation products, fibrin monomer and soluble fibrin in disseminated intravascular coagulation. Semin Thromb Hemost 27:657, 2001.
17. Bajaj SP, Joist JH: New insights into how blood clots: Implications for the use of APTT and PT as coagulation screening tests and in monitoring of anticoagulant therapy. Semin Thromb Hemost 25:407, 1999.
18. Cines DB, Pollak ES, Buck CA, et al: Endothelial cells in physiology and in the pathophysiology of vascular disorders. Blood 91:3527, 1998.
19. Wilcox JN, Smith KM, Schwartz SM, et al: Localization of tissue factor in the normal vessel wall and in the atherosclerotic plaque. Proc Natl Acad Sci USA 86:2839, 1989.
20. Kitchens CS: The contact system. Arch Pathol Lab Med 126:1382, 2002.
21. Skidgel RA, Alhenc-Gelas F, Campbell WB: Prologue: Kinins and related systems: New life for old discoveries. Am J Physiol Heart Circ Physiol 284:H1886, 2003.
22. Schmaier AH: Plasma kallikrein/kinin system: A revised hypothesis for its activation and its physiologic contributions. Curr Opin Hematol 7:261, 2000.
23. Mosesson MW, Siebenlist KR, Meh DA: The structure and biological features of fibrinogen and fibrin. Ann N Y Acad Sci 936:11, 2001.
24. Ariens RA, Lai TS, Weisel JW, et al: Role of factor XIII in fibrin clot formation and effects of genetic polymorphisms. Blood 100:743, 2002.
25. Jesty J, Lorenz A, Rodriguez J, et al: Initiation of the tissue factor pathway of coagulation in the presence of heparin: Control by antithrombin III and tissue factor pathway inhibitor. Blood 87:2301, 1996.
26. Weitz JI: Heparan sulfate: Antithrombotic or not? J Clin Invest 111:952, 2003.
27. Kato H: Regulation of functions of vascular wall cells by tissue factor pathway inhibitor: Basic and clinical aspects. Arterioscler Thromb Vasc Biol 22:539, 2002.
28. Lanir N, Aharon A, Brenner B: Procoagulant and anticoagulant mechanisms in human placenta. Semin Thromb Hemost 29:175, 2003.
29. Rezaie AR: Exosite-dependent regulation of the protein C anticoagulant pathway. Trends Cardiovasc Med 13:8, 2003.
30. Bertina RM, Koeleman BP, Koster T, et al: Mutation in blood coagulation factor V associated with resistance to activated protein C. Nature 369:64, 1994.
31. Ridker PM, Hennekens CH, Lindpaintner K, et al: Mutation in the gene coding for coagulation factor V and the risk of myocardial

infarction, stroke, and venous thrombosis in apparently healthy men. N Engl J Med 332:912, 1995.
32. Atherosclerosis, Thrombosis, and Vascular Biology Italian Study Group. No evidence of association between prothrombotic gene polymorphisms and the development of acute myocardial infarction at a young age. Circulation 107:1117, 2003.
33. Lijnen HR: Elements of the fibrinolytic system. Ann N Y Acad Sci 936:226, 2001.
34. Castellino FJ, McCance SG: The kringle domains of human plasminogen. Ciba Found Symp 212:46; discussion 60, 1997.
35. Miles LA, Castellino FJ, Gong Y: Critical role for conversion of glu-plasminogen to lys-plasminogen for optimal stimulation of plasminogen activation on cell surfaces. Trends Cardiovasc Med 13:21, 2003.
36. Kim J, Hajjar KA: Annexin II: A plasminogen-plasminogen activator co-receptor. Front Biosci 7:d341, 2002.
37. Russell J, Sherwood L, Kowalski K, et al: Recombinant hormones from fragments of human growth hormone and human placental lactogen. J Biol Chem 256:296, 1981.
38. Kooistra T, Schrauwen Y, Arts J, et al: Regulation of endothelial cell t-PA synthesis and release. Int J Hematol 59:233, 1994.
39. Smalling RW: Molecular biology of plasminogen activators: What are the clinical implications of drug design? Am J Cardiol 78:2, 1996.
40. Lijnen HR. Extracellular proteolysis in the development and progression of atherosclerosis. Biochem Soc Trans 30:163, 2002.
41. van Zonneveld AJ, Veerman H, MacDonald ME, et al: Structure and function of human tissue-type plasminogen activator (t-PA). J Cell Biochem 32:169, 1986.
42. Nieuwenhuizen W: Fibrin-mediated plasminogen activation. Ann N Y Acad Sci 936:237, 2001.
43. Rijken DC, Sakharov DV: Basic principles in thrombolysis: Regulatory role of plasminogen. Thromb Res 103:S41, 2001.
44. Colman RW: Role of the light chain of high molecular weight kininogen in adhesion, cell-associated proteolysis and angiogenesis. Biol Chem 382:65, 2001.
45. Blasi F, Carmeliet P: uPAR: A versatile signalling orchestrator. Nat Rev Mol Cell Biol 3:932, 2002.
46. Chavakis T, Kanse SM, May AE, et al: Haemostatic factors occupy new territory: The role of the urokinase receptor system and kininogen in inflammation. Biochem Soc Trans 30:168, 2002.
47. Kjoller L: The urokinase plasminogen activator receptor in the regulation of the actin cytoskeleton and cell motility. Biol Chem 383:5, 2002.
48. Bell WR: Present-day thrombolytic therapy: Therapeutic agents—pharmacokinetics and pharmacodynamics. Rev Cardiovasc Med 3 Suppl 2:S34, 2002.
49. Lee KN, Lee CS, Tae WC, et al: Crosslinking of alpha 2-antiplasmin to fibrin. Ann N Y Acad Sci 936:335, 2001.
50. Zhao L, Buckman B, Seto M, et al: Mutations in the substrate binding site of thrombin-activatable fibrinolysis inhibitor (TAFI) alter its substrate specificity. J Biol Chem 278:32359, 2003.
51. Kohler HP, Grant PJ: Plasminogen-activator inhibitor type 1 and coronary artery disease. N Engl J Med 342:1792, 2000.
52. Vaughan DE: Angiotensin and vascular fibrinolytic balance. Am J Hypertens 15:3S, 2002.
53. Vaughan DE: Angiotensin, fibrinolysis, and vascular homeostasis. Am J Cardiol 87:18C, 2001.
54. Lassegue B, Clempus RE: Vascular NAD(P)H oxidases: Specific features, expression, and regulation. Am J Physiol Regul Integr Comp Physiol 285:R277, 2003.
55. Meijers JC, Marquart JA, Bertina RM, et al: Protein C inhibitor (plasminogen activator inhibitor-3) and the risk of venous thrombosis. Br J Haematol 118:604, 2002.
56. Libby P, Ridker PM, Maseri A: Inflammation and atherosclerosis. Circulation 105:1135, 2002.
57. Ruberg FL, Leopold JA, Loscalzo J: Atherothrombosis: Plaque instability and thrombogenesis. Prog Cardiovasc Dis 44:381, 2002.
58. Goldschmidt-Clermont PJ, Cooke GE, Eaton GM, et al: PlA2: A variant of GPIIIa implicated in coronary thromboembolic complications. J Am Coll Cardiol 36:90, 2000.
59. Yamada Y, Izawa H, Ichihara S, et al: Prediction of the risk of myocardial infarction from polymorphisms in candidate genes. N Engl J Med 347:1916, 2002.
60. Ruberg FL, Loscalzo J: Prothrombotic determinants of coronary atherothrombosis. Vasc Med 7:289, 2002.

chapter 5

Vascular Pharmacology

Stephen T. O'Rourke
Paul M. Vanhoutte
Virginia M. Miller

Preceding chapters discussed in detail components of the blood vessel wall as separate entities in terms of their anatomical features and biochemical, molecular, and genetic characteristics. However, because pharmacologic interventions have the potential to affect all components of the vascular wall, this chapter will reconstruct these components into an integrated system. To do so, salient features of these components will be reviewed from the standpoint of a control system consisting of an effector (vascular smooth muscle) and regulatory mechanisms (autonomic innervation and endothelium). Within each section, major categories of pharmacologic compounds (ion channel agents, enzyme inhibitors, and receptor antagonists) will be discussed relative to their effects on each component. This chapter is meant to provide an overview of the pharmacologic regulation of blood vessel diameter (Tables 5-1 and 5-2) rather than a comprehensive catalog of vasoactive compounds. For additional details regarding specific pharmacologic agents, the interested reader is referred to the International Union of Pharmacology web site (www.IUPHAR.org) and to references listed within each section of this chapter. Most of the pharmacological agents discussed within the context of vascular pharmacology will also affect functions of blood elements, that is, platelets and leukocytes. Because each of these elements will be covered in detail in subsequent chapters, they will not be addressed here.

Over the last 10 years, there has been an explosion of information regarding molecular mechanisms of cellular processes and classification of receptors and their subtypes. This information has yet to be translated into new pharmaceuticals for the detection, prevention, and treatment of cardiovascular diseases. However, with the advent of genomics and the potential in the future for individualized treatment, possibilities for development of new treatment modalities still shine. The final section will present concepts of how genetic sex, genetic polymorphism, and hormonal milieu influence vascular function differentially across the life span.

THE EFFECTOR SYSTEM: VASCULAR SMOOTH MUSCLE

The degree of contraction of vascular smooth muscle changes the diameter and tension of the blood vessel wall. In the aorta and large arteries, this change is reflected as changes in compliance, whereas in arterioles, the change affects blood flow to specific organs through changes in resistance. Together, changes in compliance and resistance affect blood pressure and the afterload of the heart. Changes in diameter of the small arteries and arterioles determine the blood flow to the individual tissues, provided the arterial blood pressure is adequate. In the veins, contractions of the smooth muscle affect the capacity of the cardiovascular system and the filling pressure or preload of the heart. Changes in diameter of cutaneous arteries and veins contribute not only to total vascular resistance and capacity, but also contribute to control of body temperature through heat loss via the skin.

Mechanisms of Contraction

Actin and myosin are the major contractile proteins in vascular smooth muscle. Regulation of myosin phosphorylation is the final common pathway, which affects the degree of interaction between actin and myosin and, therefore, the degree of contraction.[1,2] A rise in the level of free calcium ions in the cytoplasm of vascular smooth muscle cells is the major trigger for contraction. Cytoplasmic concentrations of calcium greater than 10^{-7}M initiate the contractile process. However, transporters for Ca^{2+} located on closely opposed cellular and intracellular membranes (sarcoplasmic reticulum, mitochondria, nucleus) provide the structure for targeted changes in intracellular Ca^{2+}. This "linked Ca^{2+} transport" results in site- and time-specific changes in Ca^{2+} without diffusion into the "bulk" intracellular cytosol.[3,4] In brief, see Figure 5-1; for details see Chapter 2. To initiate contraction, intracellular free calcium binds to calmodulin, the complex of which then binds to the catalytic subunit of myosin light chain kinase. This activated enzyme phosphorylates myosin light chain, with cross-bridge linkage to actin, resulting in a conformational change of the actin-myosin subunit (shortening of the smooth muscle cell, i.e., contraction) and hydrolysis of adenosine triphosphate (ATP). Dephosphorylation of myosin light chain by myosin light chain phosphatase results in relaxation. Thus, the level of myosin phosphorylation, and, hence, the contractile state of vascular smooth muscle, is governed by the balance between the activity of myosin light chain kinase and myosin light chain phosphatase.[1]

Several actin binding proteins may possibly regulate cross-bridge formation: tropomyosin, caldesmon, calponin, and smooth muscle-specific protein, 22 kDa protein (SM22). In general, these proteins regulate actomyosin

TABLE 5-1 SUMMARY OF CLASSIFICATION OF DRUGS, SITE OF ACTION, AND EFFECTS ON VASCULAR SMOOTH MUSCLE

Drug	Site of Action	Physiologic Consequence
Ion Channel Agents		
Iberiotoxin Charybdotoxin	Inhibit BKCa channels	Contraction
Apamin	Inhibits SKCa channels	Contraction
Glibenclamide (glyburide)	Inhibits K_{ATP} channels	Contraction
Tetraethylammonium, Tetrabuytlammonium	Nonselective inhibitors of calcium-activated K channels	Contraction
4-Aminopyridine	Nonselective K_v channel blocker	Contraction
NS 1619/NS 1608	Open BK_{Ca} channels	Relaxation
Diazoxide Minoxidil sulfate Cromakalim Pinancidil Nicorandil	Open K_{ATP} channels	Relaxation
Dihydropyridines (e.g., amlodipine, nifedipine, nimodipine, nitrendipine) Phenylalkylamine (e.g., verapamil) Benzothiazepines (e.g., diltiazem)	Inhibit Ca^{2+} Influx	Relaxation
Enzyme Inhibitors/Activators		
Ouabain	Inhibits Na^+-K^+-ATPase	Contraction
Pargyline Tranylcypromine	Inhibits monoamine oxidase	Contraction
Aplysinopsin-type indole alkaloid	Selective inhibitor of nNOS	Contraction
Guanabenzene	Selective and irreversible inhibitor or neuronal nNOS	Contraction
Aminoguanidine	Inhibitor of iNOS	Contraction
N^G mono-methyl-L-arginine (L-NMMA) Nitro-L-arginine (L-NAME)	Inhibitors of eNOS	Contraction
Methylene blue, ODQ	Inhibitors of soluble guanylyl cyclase	Contraction
Fasudil, hydroxy fasudil	Inhibitor of Rho kinase	Relaxation
Papaverine Dipyridamole Methylxanthines	Nonselective inhibitors of phosphodiesterase	Relaxation
Sildenafil Tadalafil Vardenafil	Selective inhibition of PDE5	Relaxation
Nitroglycerin, isosorbide dinitrate, isosorbide mononitrate, sodium nitroprusside, SIN-1	NO donors; activate soluble guanylyl cyclase	Relaxation
Statins (simvastatin, lovastatin, pravastatin)	Inhibits 3-hydroxy-3-methylguanyl (HMG) Co-A reductase	Pleiotropic effects related to isoprenylation of Rho and RHS proteins

NE, norepinephrine; NO donors, nitric oxide donors; ODQ, 1H-[1,2,4]oxadiazolo[4,3-α]quinoxalin-1.

ATPase activity. However, controversy exists as to their role in the physiologic regulation of smooth muscle contraction.[5]

Increases in cytoplasmic Ca^{2+} concentration, which activates the contractile process in vascular smooth muscle cells, can be due to an increased permeability of the cell membrane for extracellular calcium (i.e., calcium influx) or to mobilization of Ca^{2+} from cellular stores (e.g., sarcoplasmic reticulum and mitochondria). The source of the activator ion differs depending on the anatomical origin of the vascular smooth muscle, the contractile stimulus, or the experimental conditions to which the tissues are exposed (Fig. 5-2).

At rest, the plasma membrane of vascular smooth muscle cells is relatively impermeable to Ca^{2+}. On activation, however, Ca^{2+} channels in the plasma membrane are opened, thereby allowing Ca^{2+} to flow down its concentration gradient into the cell. Two types of calcium channels have been proposed: potential, or voltage-operated channels, which are regulated by changes in membrane potential, and receptor-operated channels, which are governed by ligand-receptor interactions. Modulation of these channels by various pharmacologic agents affects the contractile capability of vascular smooth muscle.[1-3]

As stated, Ca^{2+} release and uptake from intracellular organelles results in targeted or site-specific fluctuations in intracellular Ca^{2+}. Indeed, in the absence of extracellular calcium, certain agonists (e.g., norepinephrine) can evoke contractions in some blood vessels. Although a small component of Ca^{2+} release may derive from the

TABLE 5-2 SUMMARY OF DRUGS, SITE OF ACTION, AND EFFECTS ON ADRENERGIC NERVE ENDINGS

Drug	Site of Action	Physiologic Consequence
Tetrodotoxin	Blocks sodium channels	Inhibits release of NE from adrenergic nerve endings
Pargyline Tranylcypromine	Inhibits monoamine oxidase	Increases NE content in adrenergic nerve endings; augments NE contraction
6-Hydroxydopamine	Taken up by biogenic amine pump	Destroys adrenergic nerve terminals
Guanethidine	Taken up by neuronal NE transport mechanism; stored in vesicles	Depletes NE from storage vesicles
Bretylium tosylate	Competes for NE transport mechanism	Inhibits NE release
Tyramine Amphetamine Ephedrine	Taken up by neuronal NE transport mechanism; stored in vesicles	Displaces NE from storage vesicles; contraction
Reserpine	Binds to storage vesicles	Depletes NE from storage vesicles
Cocaine, tricyclic antidepressants	Inhibits neuronal NE transport mechanism	Potentiates response to NE
Hydrocortisone	Inhibits extraneuronal NE transport mechanism	Potentiates response to NE
ARL-67 156	Inhibits NTPDase	Potentiates exocytotic release of NE
SolCD39	Recombinant NTPDase	Attenuates exocytotic release of NE

NE, norepinephrine.

inner plasmalemmal surface, it is apparent that the major component originates from the sarcoplasmic reticulum.

Agonist-induced release of small amounts of Ca^{2+} from the inner plasmalemmal surface results in transient increases in the concentration of Ca^{2+} near the superficial sarcoplasmic reticulum. This small increase in Ca^{2+} concentration may initiate the release of Ca^{2+} from the latter itself by a process known as Ca^{2+}-induced Ca^{2+} release. Nerve-like Ca^{2+} oscillations and Ca^{2+} sparks result from release and uptake of Ca^{2+} from intracellular organelles.[2,3]

Another potential pathway mediating intracellular Ca^{2+} release involves the breakdown of membrane phospholipids following agonist-receptor interactions. The initial event following binding of agonists to specific plasma membrane receptors is the activation of phospholipase C, which catalyzes the breakdown of inositol phospholipids. The action of phospholipase C on phosphatidylinositol 4,5-bisphosphate results in the formation of 1,2-diacylglycerol and inositol 1,4,5-trisphosphate, which is responsible for a rapid mobilization of intracellular Ca^{2+} by activating Ca^{2+} efflux from the sarcoplasmic reticulum.

Vascular smooth muscle contraction is dependent not only on the concentration of cytoplasmic calcium ions, but also on the sensitivity of the contractile apparatus to calcium. Indeed, smooth muscle contraction can occur without a change in cytoplasmic calcium levels, a phenomenon known as *calcium sensitization*.[2,6] The major mechanism underlying calcium sensitization is phosphorylation of myosin light chain phosphatase, which inactivates the enzyme and leads to an increase in the

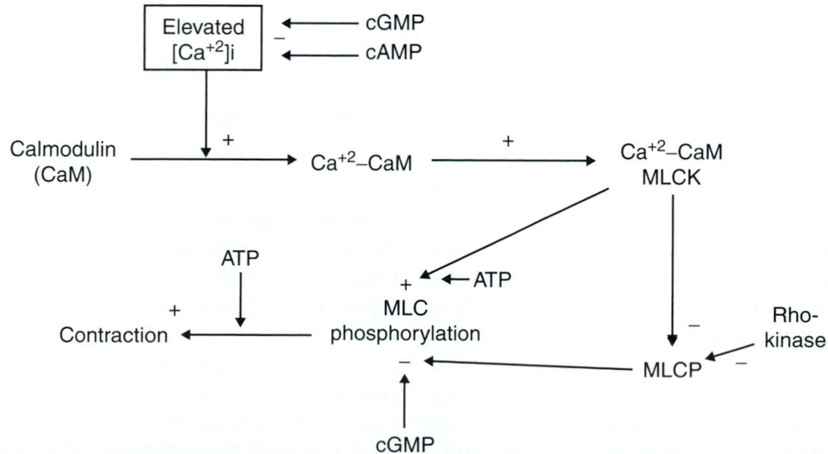

FIGURE 5-1. Schematic of regulation of myosin activation in smooth muscle cells. Activation of the smooth muscle cell increases intracellular calcium which binds calmodulin necessary for activation of myosin light chain kinase (MLCK). MLCK causes phosphorylation of myosin light chains which allows binding to actin. The resulting conformational change initiates contraction. Relaxation is caused by dephosphorylation of myosin light chain. Dephosphorylation of myosin light chain is stimulated by the enzyme myosin light chain phosphatase (MLCP), and by cyclic GMP. Stimulation of some receptors on cell membrane, in addition to activating calcium calmodulin and MLCK leading to contraction, activate Rho kinase, an enzyme which inhibits MLCP. Inhibition of MLCP allows myosin light chain to be phosphorylated during low concentrations of intracellular calcium. Thus, the ratio of MLCK to MLCP activity is the major determinant of calcium sensitivity for the myosin fibers.

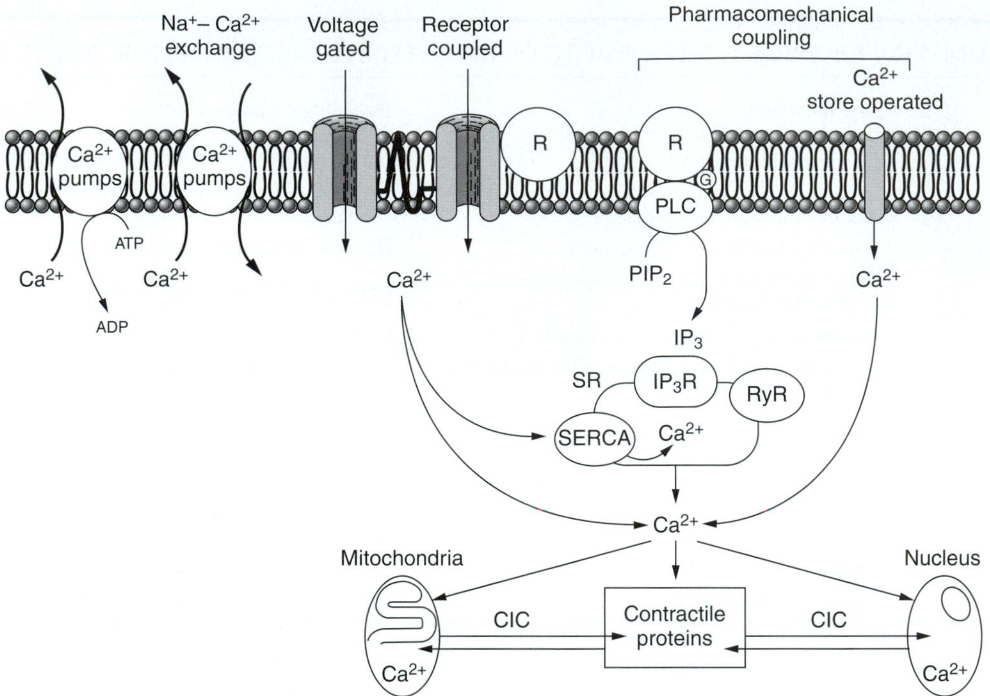

FIGURE 5-2. Schematic of mechanisms which control calcium in smooth muscle cells. At rest, the concentration of calcium in the cell is buffered by the SR. As calcium enters from the extracellular space as a result of the opening of excitable calcium channels and a putative "leak" channel, it is taken up by the SR. Through activation of inositol (1,4,)-triphosphate receptors (IP_3R) and ryanodine (RyR) receptors, calcium in the SR is recycled to the sodium calcium exchanger on the membrane surface. This exchange represents a superficial calcium buffer. Intracellular calcium is also extruded by plasmalemmal calcium-ATP pumps. Following agonist stimulation, calcium is released from the SR through stimulation of the IP_3R receptors. Depolarization of the membrane also opens voltage-gated calcium channels on the plasmalemma. Accumulation of sodium in the extracellular space reverses the sodium calcium exchanger to deliver calcium to the SR through activation of calcium ATPase activity (SERCA). Calcium actively cycles between the IP_3R receptors and SERCA. CIC, calcium induced calcium release; G, guanidine nucleotide regulatory protein; PLC, phospholipase C; PIP_2, phosphatidyl inositol 4,5-bisphosphate; R, receptor; SR, sarcoplasmic reticulum.

phosphorylated (i.e., activated) form of myosin light chain. Agonist-mediated calcium sensitization occurs via activation of the RhoA/RhoA-kinase pathway. Agonists acting on specific G-protein-coupled receptors activate the small GTPase, RhoA, which is a member of the Ras superfamily of monomeric GTPases. Like most GTPases, RhoA cycles between the inactive cytoplasmic GDP-bound form and the active membrane-associated form in which the bound nucleotide is GTP. The downstream effector of RhoA-GTP is a serine/threonine kinase, RhoA kinase, which contains a RhoA-binding domain. Activated RhoA-kinase phosphorylates the regulatory subunit of myosin light chain phosphatase, thereby inhibiting phosphatase activity. In addition to RhoA, arachidonic acid may also mediate calcium sensitization in smooth muscle. Arachidonic acid, released in response to certain agonists, can activate RhoA-kinase directly and thereby inhibit myosin light chain phosphatase activity. Activation of the RhoA/RhoA-kinase pathway contributes to maintaining the tonic phase of agonist-induced contraction of the smooth muscle (see Fig. 5-1). Many vasoconstrictor signaling molecules (e.g., serotonin, endothelin, angiotensin II) induce smooth muscle contraction by both calcium-dependent activation of myosin light chain kinase and by calcium sensitization.

Each of these pathways then represents a potential target for pharmacologic intervention to sustain and or reduce contraction. Direct relaxation of vascular smooth muscle may occur by one or more of the following mechanisms: (1) hyperpolarization of the smooth muscle cell membrane; (2) inhibition of Ca^{2+} entry; (3) increased cytoplasmic concentration of cyclic nucleotides 3′,5′-adenosine monophosphate (cAMP) and/or cyclic 3′,5′-guanosine monophosphate (cGMP); and (4) inhibition of Rho-kinase.

Mechanisms of Relaxation

Hyperpolarization

In most blood vessels, the membrane potential of the smooth muscle cells and the level of vascular tone are coupled tightly. Because calcium entry via voltage-dependent calcium channels plays a pivotal role in the contraction, changes in membrane potential that lead to opening or closure of these channels will have important effects on the contractile activity of vascular smooth muscle. Thus, regulation of smooth muscle membrane potential is a major mechanism underlying vasodilation and vasoconstriction. Hyperpolarization causes relaxation, which results from closure of voltage-dependent calcium channels and decreased entry of extracellular calcium needed to initiate and sustain contraction; depolarization has the opposite effect. Activation of either Na^+,K^+-ATPase or K^+ channels in the plasma membrane causes hyperpolarization of vascular smooth muscle cells.[7-10]

Na^+,K^+-ATPase

Sodium, potassium-adenosine triphosphatase (Na^+,K^+-ATPase) is responsible for the electrogenic pumping of Na^+ and K^+. This enzyme is localized in the cell membrane and contributes to the resting membrane potential of vascular smooth muscle cells. Three Na^+ are transported out of the cell in exchange for two K^+ pumped in per molecule of ATP hydrolyzed. Stimulation of Na^+,K^+-ATPase leads to hyperpolarization of vascular smooth muscle cells; endothelium-derived hyperpolarizing factor (EDHF), as discussed later in this chapter, may produce relaxation by this mechanism. Alternatively, cardiac glycosides such as ouabain produce contraction of isolated blood vessels due, in part, to inhibition of Na^+,K^+-ATPase.

K^+ Channel

Increased membrane K^+ permeability via specific K^+ channels serves to stabilize the cell membrane because the outward movement of K^+ shifts the membrane potential toward more negative values. K^+ channels play an important role in setting the resting membrane potential in vascular smooth muscle cells, and may contribute to the actions of endogenous vasoactive substances. In general, those mediators that activate K^+ channels cause hyperpolarization and vasodilation, whereas those that inhibit K^+ channels may cause depolarization and vasoconstriction. Although K^+ channels are also present on other cell types within the blood vessel wall (e.g., endothelial cells and perivascular nerves) the following discussion will be limited to those that have been consistently identified in smooth muscle cells from several vascular beds, and contribute directly to the regulation of vasomotor tone.

Four major types of K^+ channels are present in vascular smooth muscle cells. These include (1) calcium-activated K^+ channels ($K_{Ca^{++}}$); (2) voltage-dependent K^+ channels (Kv); (3) inward rectifier K^+ channels (Kir); and (4) ATP-sensitive K^+ channels (K_{ATP}). The distribution of K^+ channel types, as well as their activity, varies with blood vessel size and location.

Large-conductance, calcium-activated K^+ channels (BK_{Ca}), so named because of the high amplitude unitary K^+ currents associated with their open state, are present in smooth muscle cells from most vascular beds. BK_{Ca} channel activity increases in response to both depolarization and increased levels of cytoplasmic calcium. In many blood vessels, BK_{Ca} channels contribute to the resting membrane potential of the smooth muscle. By opening in response to stimuli that cause depolarization or increased intracellular calcium, these channels may also play an important physiologic role in providing a negative-feedback system to prevent excessive vasoconstriction. Indeed, when applied to isolated arteries from several species, inhibitors of BK_{Ca} channels, such as iberiotoxin and charybdotoxin, evoke contractions under resting conditions and augment the response to endogenous vasoconstrictors, such as norepinephrine and angiotensin II. Conversely, synthetic BK_{Ca} channel openers, such as NS 1619 and NS 1608, cause relaxation of vascular smooth muscle and vasodilation. The expression of BK_{Ca} channels is upregulated in certain pathologic conditions, including arterial hypertension.

K_v channels are widely distributed in the vasculature. These channels are voltage dependent and are activated by membrane depolarization. Like BK_{Ca} channels, K_v channels contribute to setting the resting membrane potential and may limit the response to vasoconstrictors. Consistent with this role are the observations that 4-aminopyridine, a relatively nonselective K_v channel blocker, causes smooth muscle contraction in numerous vascular beds (e.g., coronary, cerebral, renal, pulmonary, and skeletal) and potentiates contractile responses to KCl. Altered expression and function of K_v channels may contribute to hypoxic pulmonary vasoconstriction and primary pulmonary hypertension.

K_{ir} channels are also voltage-dependent K channels, but unlike BK_{Ca} and K_v channels, potassium currents through K_{ir} channels show inward rectification in vascular smooth muscle. Such currents are increased at more negative membrane potentials and decreased by membrane depolarization. The expression of K_{ir} channels is greater in small resistance-sized arteries than in larger conduit arteries, but their physiologic role is uncertain. K_{ir} channels may contribute to resting membrane potential in small arteries (e.g., cerebral, coronary) and play a secondary role in the response to certain vasoactive mediators. Vasoconstrictors that cause membrane depolarization tend to decrease K_{ir} channel activity and lead to further membrane potential depolarization, whereas those vasodilators that cause membrane hyperpolarization will tend to increase K_{ir} channel activity and lead to additional membrane hyperpolarization. K_{ir} channel activity is also increased directly by modest increases in extracellular K^+ (5 to 15 mM). This function may account for the observation that K^+ exiting endothelial cells via K_{Ca} channels may act as an endothelium-derived factor that causes hyperpolarization and relaxation of vascular smooth muscle. Activation of K_{ir} channels may also underlie the vasodilator effect of K^+ released locally from active tissues, such as neurons and cardiac myocytes, and serve to link blood flow in small arteries with metabolic demand by mediating vasodilation in response to a rise in external K^+.

K_{ATP} channels are present throughout the cardiovascular system, including vascular smooth muscle cells. Functional K_{ATP} channels show little voltage sensitivity and are composed of two distinct moieties: a membrane-spanning pore, and a sulfonylurea receptor. Binding of sulfonylureas, such as glibenclamide (glyburide), to the sulfonylurea receptor inhibits channel opening. A characteristic feature of these channels is their inhibition by physiologic levels of intracellular ATP and activation by intracellular ADP. As such, K_{ATP} channels may adjust cell membrane potential according to changes in cellular metabolic state. The contribution of K_{ATP} channels to the control of vascular smooth muscle membrane potential varies depending on the vessel and physiologic conditions. In most blood vessels, the activity of K_{ATP} channels is low under normal metabolic conditions and, therefore, has little role in establishing the resting membrane potential. In resistance-sized arteries, K_{ATP} channels may be open and contribute to membrane potential under resting conditions because exposure to glibenclamide causes concentration-dependent smooth muscle contractions. Activation of K_{ATP} channels may play a pivotal role in the vasodilator response to hypoxia observed in the coronary, skeletal muscle, and cerebral circulation.

Of the various K^+ channel types found in vascular smooth muscle, K_{ATP} channels serve as the primary molecular target for most of the K^+ channel activators and inhibitors currently developed for clinical use. Indeed, sulfonylureas, such as glibenclamide and tolbutamide, are widely used in the treatment of diabetes. These drugs selectively block K_{ATP} channels in pancreatic beta cells, and thereby stimulate insulin release. They also inhibit vascular responses to a number of pharmacologic agents that increase membrane K^+ conductance (i.e., net efflux of K^+ from the cell). These agents, termed K^+ channel openers, produce vasodilation by activating K_{ATP} channels and hyperpolarizing vascular smooth muscle cells.

Because of their vasodilator effects, there is great interest in developing K^+ channel openers for the treatment of vascular disorders that involve enhanced vascular contractility, such as hypertension, angina, and cerebrovascular disease. In addition, K^+ channel openers have become important pharmacologic tools in elucidating the role of K^+ channels in controlling blood vessel diameter.

The K_{ATP} channel openers are a chemically diverse group including cromakalim, pinacidil, and nicorandil; nicorandil has nitrovasodilator properties as well (see later). Moreover, the vasodilator effects of the antihypertensive drugs, diazoxide and minoxidil sulfate, are due to the opening of K_{ATP} channels in vascular smooth muscle cells. In addition to these synthetic agents, adenosine, EDHF, and certain neuropeptides (e.g., calcitonin gene-related peptide [CGRP], vasoactive intestinal polypeptide [VIP]) may also act as endogenous K_{ATP} channel openers and, thus, play a role in regulating vasomotor tone.

In isolated vascular preparations, the K_{ATP} channel openers inhibit spontaneous tone, as well as contractions evoked by vasoconstrictors such as norepinephrine, angiotensin II, and serotonin. Unlike some vasodilators, such as acetylcholine, the inhibitory effects of the K_{ATP} channel openers are not dependent on the presence of an intact endothelium. The K_{ATP} channel openers have in common three general characteristics in isolated tissues. First, K^+ channel openers induce an outward K^+ current, resulting in hyperpolarization of the cell membrane and a net efflux of $^{42}K^+$ or $^{86}Rb^+$. Second, K_{ATP} channel openers cause relaxation of preparations contracted with low (<30 mM) but not high (>50 mM) concentrations of KCl. This behavior would be expected of substances that act simply by opening K^+ channels because in the presence of high external K^+ concentrations, the actual membrane potential approaches the Nernst equilibrium potential for K^+, thereby reducing the achievable degree of hyperpolarization. Under these conditions (i.e., high external K^+ concentrations), the Nernst potential may be more positive than the threshold potential needed to interfere with calcium handling by the cell, thus abolishing the ability of the K^+-channel openers to interfere with these processes. Third, the mechanical and electrophysiologic effects of the K_{ATP} channel openers can be antagonized by sulfonylureas, such as glibenclamide and tolbutamide.

K_{ATP} channel openers probably act indirectly as Ca^{2+} channel antagonists. They increase membrane permeability to K^+ causing hyperpolarization, which in turn inhibits Ca^{2+} entry through voltage-dependent calcium channels and relaxation (i.e., vasodilation) ensues. However, it is clear from several studies that the inhibitory effects of the K_{ATP} channel openers cannot be explained solely by the indirect closure of voltage-dependent calcium channels. Other proposed mechanisms include (1) interference with refilling of intracellular Ca^{2+} stores; (2) inhibition of the synthesis of phosphoinositides; and (3) decreased Ca^{2+} sensitivity of the contractile elements in vascular smooth muscle cells.

Inhibition of Calcium Entry

In light of the importance of Ca^{2+} in vascular smooth muscle contraction, it is not surprising that compounds have been designed for interfering with the entry of calcium through specific channels in the cell membrane. These so-called calcium antagonists inhibit contractions induced by a wide variety of agents, but they differ in their ability to interfere with the function of vascular smooth muscle from different anatomic origins or under different experimental conditions.

The organic calcium antagonists (e.g., amlodipine, diltiazem, flunarizine, nifedipine, nimodipine, and verapamil) inhibit smooth muscle contraction by blocking stimulated (receptor activation or membrane depolarization) calcium influx (see Fig. 5-2). For example, in the presence of diltiazem, flunarizine, or nifedipine, the inhibition of potassium-stimulated unidirectional calcium influx in various vascular smooth muscle preparations is highly correlated with the inhibition of potassium-induced contraction. In concentrations considered to correspond to therapeutic doses, the organic calcium antagonists do not (1) inhibit intracellular calcium release induced by specific agonists (cellular mobilization); (2) reduce passive calcium entry (calcium leak); or (3) stimulate calcium extrusion mechanisms (Ca^{2+}-ATPase and Na^+/Ca^{2+} exchange).

Although the organic calcium antagonists can be subdivided into several distinct classes based on their chemical structures, in general their pharmacologic selectivity and potency suggest that specific sites exist for these compounds. The molecular and biochemical nature of these sites can be identified with radiolabeled compounds (e.g., [^{3}H]-flunarizine, [^{3}H]-nitrendipine, [^{3}H]-nimodipine) in vascular and nonvascular preparations. The binding of [^{3}H]-nitrendipine (and other labeled compounds) to isolated cell membranes from smooth muscle satisfies the requirements for specific receptor binding (i.e., high affinity, saturation, stereoselectivity, and pharmacologic specificity that correlates with functional response). The binding sites for the structurally dissimilar calcium antagonists are not identical, but they do interact. This helps explain how the various classes of calcium antagonists can act in a similar fashion functionally but still have specific sites of action. Data from binding, as well as functional studies, suggest that the synthetic calcium antagonists probably do not interact with the site at which inorganic cations, such as lanthanum, bind to block calcium entry. It is more likely that the various calcium-entry blockers specifically bind to other components within the calcium channel, thus causing their inactivation.

In certain vascular preparations, most notably the portal-mesenteric vein of various species and the human coronary artery, spontaneous rhythmic (myogenic) contractions can be observed under control conditions. This myogenic activity depends on the availability of extracellular calcium and is proposed to result from spatially restricted membrane currents and release of Ca^{2+} from the sarcolemma following depolarization of the cell membrane. Calcium antagonists inhibit the myogenic activity of portal-mesenteric veins with varying potencies, with the dihydropyridines (e.g., nifedipine) being the most potent. Because myogenic tone in the arterioles also depends on the entry of extracellular calcium, it is not surprising that the calcium antagonists that are the most potent in inhibiting the myogenic activity of portal-mesenteric veins cause the greatest reduction in peripheral vascular resistance in the intact organism and, hence, are the most likely candidates for use as antihypertensive agents.

Depolarization of the vascular smooth muscle cell membrane, for example, by increasing the extracellular K^+ concentration, opens potential-operated calcium channels and accelerates the entry of extracellular calcium (see Fig. 5-2). Contractions of isolated blood vessels caused by potassium depolarization can be inhibited by all available calcium-entry blockers. In general, for a given calcium-entry blocker (e.g., diltiazem), the sensitivity of the K^+-induced contraction is relatively constant throughout the vasculature. However, the potency of the various agents varies widely; the agents are ranked here from most to least potent: dihydropyridines, phenylalkylamines, and benzothiazepines. The time of onset and the duration of the inhibitory effect of the calcium antagonists on potassium-induced contractions in given blood vessels also vary widely, reflecting the differing pharmacokinetic properties of these substances.

Other factors influencing the ability of calcium-entry blockers to inhibit the contractile response in various blood vessels (see Fig. 5-2) include the ability of a given vasoconstrictor agonist to induce membrane depolarization (and thereby activate the potential-operated channels, which are more sensitive to calcium-entry blockade) or to cause release of intracellularly bound calcium (which is insensitive to calcium-entry blockers).

Regulation of Cyclic Nucleotides

cAMP

Stimulation of a number of plasma membrane receptors (e.g., β-adrenergic receptors, adenosine receptors, prostacyclin receptors) promotes the conversion of intracellular ATP to cAMP by the enzyme adenylyl cyclase.[1] Adenylyl cyclase is coupled to the plasma membrane receptor by a guanine nucleotide-binding protein. Within the cell, cAMP binds to and activates cAMP-dependent protein kinase. The activated protein kinase catalyzes phosphorylation of specific enzymes, thereby stimulating or inhibiting their activities. In vascular smooth muscle, increasing the cytoplasmic concentration of cAMP accelerates the removal of Ca^{2+} from the cytoplasm. This cAMP-mediated decrease in cytoplasmic Ca^{2+} probably accounts for the relaxation of vascular smooth muscle by β-adrenergic receptor agonists (e.g., epinephrine, isoproterenol) and prostaglandins (e.g., prostacyclin).

Intracellular cAMP is metabolized rapidly by cyclic nucleotide phosphodiesterase. Thus, inhibitors of phosphodiesterase increase cytoplasmic cAMP levels. Inhibitors of phosphodiesterase, such as papaverine, dipyridamole, and methylxanthines (e.g., theophylline), most likely relax vascular smooth muscle by this mechanism.

Cyclic GMP

Cyclic GMP (cGMP) is formed by the action of guanylyl cyclase on guanosine triphosphate, and its effects are mediated by cGMP-dependent protein kinase. The activation of guanylyl cyclase and the subsequent elevation of cGMP in vascular smooth muscle cells are associated with relaxation. Cyclic GMP-mediated relaxation of vascular smooth muscle occurs via several mechanisms.[11] Increased accumulation of cGMP occurs with dephosphorylation of the myosin light chain. Possible calcium-specific effects include the inhibition of sarcolemmal calcium channels to inhibit Ca^{2+} influx or the activation of sarcolemmal calcium-extrusion pumps, both secondary to activation of cGMP-dependent protein kinase. The intracellular liberation of calcium may be impaired following inhibition of phosphatidylinositol hydrolysis, and the intracellular sequestration or binding of calcium may be increased. Nitrovasodilators, including endogenously produced nitric oxide (NO; see Nitrergic Nerves and Endothelium) and NO donors, including organic nitrates, such as nitroglycerin, isosorbide dinitrate, and isosorbide mononitrate, the inorganic compound sodium nitroprusside, and SIN-1, the active metabolite of molsidomine, initiate relaxation through increases in cGMP. Treatment with these agents produces dilation of both arteries and veins, resulting in decreased peripheral vascular resistance and venous return, which subsequently leads to reductions in cardiac workload and blood pressure.

In addition to activating guanylyl cyclase, an alternative approach to increasing cGMP is to inhibit degradation of the cyclic nucleotide. Cyclic GMP is hydrolyzed to an inactive form, 5′-GMP, by phosphodiesterase (PDE) enzymes. PDE5 is highly specific for cGMP hydrolysis and is the major cGMP-hydrolyzing isoform expressed in vascular smooth muscle cells. Inhibition of PDE5 results in increased intracellular accumulation of cGMP and relaxation of smooth muscle. Sildenafil, tadalafil, and vardenafil are selective PDE5 inhibitors that are used in the treatment of erectile dysfunction. In the corpora cavernosa, relaxation of the smooth muscle in arterioles and sinusoids occurs in response to NO released from endothelial cells and nitrergic nerves. Sildenafil and related agents inhibit PDE hydrolytic activity, thus causing increased cGMP accumulation in response to NO and thus facilitating erection. PDE5 inhibitors also have shown promise in the treatment of pulmonary hypertension.[12]

As expected from their mechanism of action, PDE5 inhibitors are most effective when the guanylyl cyclase/cGMP signaling pathway is activated. These agents have only a modest blood pressure-lowering effect under normal conditions, but a potentially dangerous drug interaction may occur when combined with nitroglycerin and other NO donors. Thus, concurrent use of PDE5 inhibitors and NO donors may cause excessive accumulation of cGMP and a sudden, potentially life-threatening drop in blood pressure.

Inhibition of Ras Superfamily Isoprenylation

As discussed, agonist-mediated calcium sensitization occurs via activation of the RhoA/RhoA-kinase pathway.[2,6] These small proteins of the Ras superfamily require posttranslational isoprenylation by intermediates of the cholesterol biosynthetic pathway to form covalent attachment to subcellular and cellular membranes. Originally developed as lipid-lowering drugs by interfering with cholesterol biosynthesis in the liver, a group of 3-hydroxy-3-methylglutaryl (HMG)-CoA reductase inhibitors, statins, depending on the lipid solubility of the drug, affect isoprenylation of Rho and Ras proteins in smooth muscle and endothelial cells as well.[13]

Inhibition of isoprenoid synthesis by statins reduces growth-factor induced retinoblastoma (Rb)-protein hyperphosphorylation and cyclin-dependent kinases required for gene transcription and cell proliferation.[14] This pleiotropic effect of the statins is being taken advantage of in drug-eluting stents to reduce restenosis of coronary arteries following angioplasty.[15]

Statins reduce blood pressure in humans using the drug to treat hyperlipidemia. However, it is unclear at this time if the hypotensive actions are due to direct effects on the vascular smooth muscle or on production of endothelium-derived relaxing factors (see Endothelium for details).

CONTROL SYSTEMS

Vascular smooth muscle, the effector of the vascular system, is anatomically situated between two control systems: autonomic neurons, which enter the medial smooth muscle from the adventitia of the blood vessel and the endothelium, which lines the surface of medial smooth muscle adjacent to the blood vessel lumen. Autonomic neurons, which represent the effector branch of a reflex arch, affect change in vascular tone in response to baro- and chemoreceptors within the aortic arch and carotid arteries and thermoreceptors in the skin. These reflexes are rapid and can be modulated by input from central processes that facilitate cardiovascular performance in response to visual, auditory, tactile, and olfactory stimuli, and mental/emotional processes, such as pleasure, fear, and so on. Regulation by the endothelium, on the other hand, is not associated with reflex sensor-effector mechanisms in the traditional sense. Rather, endothelial cells act as both sensors of the local physical and chemical environment (i.e., laminar shear and tangential stress, oxygen tension and concentration of cytokines and hormones in the blood) and effectors through release of endothelium-derived factors. Unlike the control offered by the autonomic neurons related to central command in response to external stimuli, the endothelium provides sensing of the local environment. Both systems can affect the threshold and gain of the intracellular pathways controlling contraction of the vascular smooth muscle. The relative contribution of each regulatory system varies depending on the anatomical origin of the blood vessel. These systems are phyllogenetically conserved. Under pathologic conditions, such as endothelial dysfunction in atherosclerosis or denervation associated with organ transplantation, feedback between the systems is disrupted and one or the other may predominate. Each system will be discussed in detail subsequently.

Autonomic Innervation

Sympathetic Nerves

The sympathetic (adrenergic) nerves are the dominant pathway for the nervous and reflex control of the vasculature. The sympathetic outflow to peripheral blood vessels originates in neurons located in the lateral parts of the reticular formation in the bulbar area of the brain stem, the vasomotor center. The activity of the vasomotor center is governed by the solitary tract nucleus, which relays information from arterial and cardiopulmonary mechanoreceptors (baroreceptors) and other afferents. The axons from neurons of the vasomotor center form the bulbospinal tract and descend in the intermediolateral column to the preganglionic neurons of the spinal cord, located in the anterolateral column. The neurons of the bulbospinal tract consist of both excitatory and inhibitory fibers, which innervate the preganglionic sympathetic cell bodies. The interplay between these pressor and depressor neurons determines the sympathetic outflow to the periphery. Preganglionic cholinergic neurons interconnect with postganglionic adrenergic neurons in the sympathetic ganglia. The postganglionic adrenergic neurons innervate the heart and the peripheral blood vessels (Fig. 5-3).

With the exception of the umbilical and placental vasculature, blood vessels contain smooth muscle cells that are innervated by postganglionic sympathetic nerves. The density of innervation varies widely, however, and may reflect the contribution of individual vascular beds to centrally controlled responses. The postganglionic sympathetic nerve terminals form a network of unmyelinated slender processes that widen at regular intervals into varicosities. Thus, a single nerve fiber forms many synapses en passant over groups of smooth muscle cells. Varicosities are in close apposition to the smooth muscle cells they innervate; there is a minimal distance of 50 nm between the two types of cells, but in certain blood vessels, this junctional cleft is much larger. In most arteries, the nerves are restricted to the adventitial medial border; in veins, they usually penetrate into the media. Both in animals and in humans, the density of adrenergic innervation of the blood vessels decreases progressively with age.[16,17]

Synthesis, Storage, and Release of Neurotransmitter

In the periphery, catecholamines, such as norepinephrine and epinephrine, are stored and released from

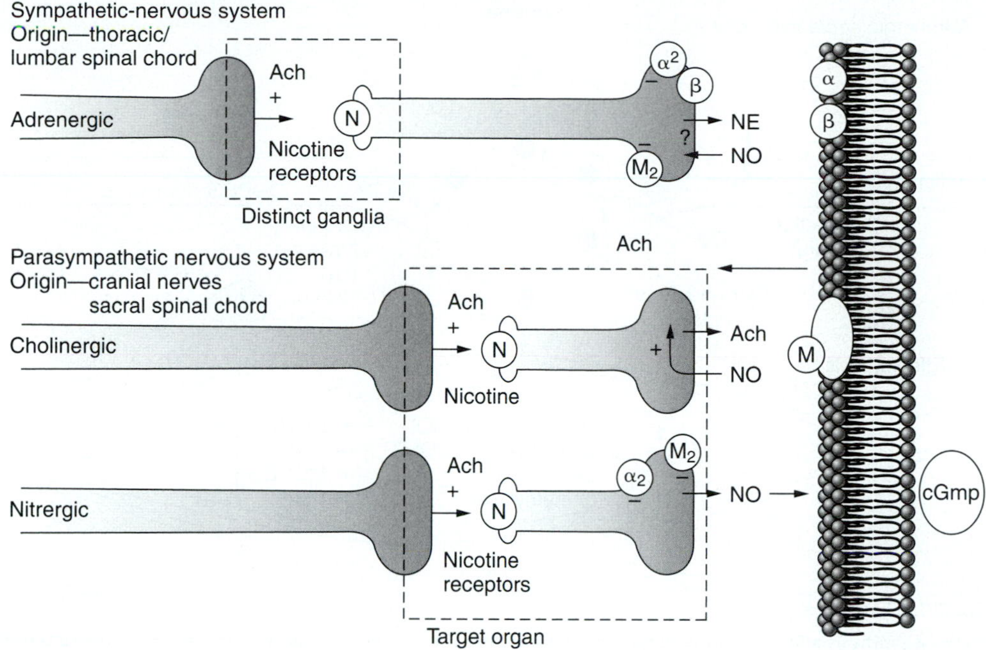

FIGURE 5-3. Schematic classification of neuronal pathways within the autonomic nervous system. There are two main classifications of efferent fibers within the autonomic nervous system: sympathetic and parasympathetic nerves, which are defined by the transmitter released at the postganglionic nerve terminal. The primary transmitter released from the sympathetic, postganglionic fiber is norepinephrine (noradrenaline), and thus, these fibers are called adrenergic fibers. The parasympathetic nervous system is subdivided into those fibers that secrete acetylcholine at the postganglionic terminal, and thus are called cholinergic neurons, and those that secrete nitric oxide, the nitrergic neurons. Another distinction between the sympathetic and parasympathetic systems is the termination of the preganglionic fiber (*outlined by dotted lines*). The preganglionic fiber of the sympathetic nervous system synapses on neurons forming distinct ganglia somewhat distant from the target organ, whereas the preganglionic fiber of the parasympathetic nervous system is quite long—terminating on neurons forming ganglia located on the target tissue. The neurotransmitter of preganglionic fibers of both the sympathetic and parasympathetic systems is acetylcholine which stimulates nicotinic receptors on the postganglionic fiber. The transmitter released from neuronal fibers can bind to receptors on the target organ. In addition, released transmitter can bind to receptors on the neuronal terminal affecting further local release of neurotransmitter (see Fig. 5-5). +, indicates stimulation; – indicates inhibition; Ach, acetylcholine; α, alpha$_2$-adrenergic receptors, a subclass of α-adrenergic receptors; β, β-adrenergic receptors; cGMP, cyclic guanylase monophosphate; M, muscarinic receptors, a subclass of muscarinic receptors; N, nicotinic receptor; NE, norepinephrine; NO, nitric oxide.

two primary sites. Postganglionic adrenergic neurons are the major source of norepinephrine, whereas epinephrine is released predominantly into the bloodstream from the adrenal medulla.

Postganglionic adrenergic neurons actively take up tyrosine from the extracellular fluid and transform it to dopamine by successive enzymatic reactions in the neuronal cytoplasm. Dopamine is then incorporated into the storage vesicles, where it is converted to norepinephrine by the enzyme dopamine-β-hydroxylase, which is present in both the membrane and the content of the vesicles (Fig. 5-4). Increases in the concentration of norepinephrine in the neuronal cytoplasm exert an end-product inhibition (negative feedback) on the enzyme tyrosine hydroxylase, which is the rate-limiting step in the synthesis of the neurotransmitter. Increased activity of the adrenergic neuron or depletion of the catecholamine stores, on the other hand, stimulates the activity of the enzyme.

Most of the norepinephrine, whether synthesized or taken up from the extracellular space, is held in the storage vesicles as a complex with proteins, of which chromogranin A is the most important. The storage of adrenergic transmitter is reflected by the electron-dense core of the storage vesicles. The norepinephrine content of the blood vessel wall varies with the degree of innervation and decreases with age and after sympathectomy, reserpine treatment, and inhibition of tyrosine hydroxylase and dopamine β-hydroxylase.[17]

Norepinephrine stored in the adrenergic-nerve endings may be released by three different mechanisms (1) leakage of the neurotransmitter to the neuronal cytoplasm and toward the extracellular space; (2) pharmacologic displacement by other substances such as tyramine, amphetamine, or ephedrine, which have a higher affinity for the storage proteins in the vesicles (indirect sympathomimetic effect); or (3) exocytotic release initiated by action potentials generated in the ganglionic cell body (see Fig. 5-4).

The exocytotic emptying of the vesicles creates the concentration gradient of norepinephrine between the nerve terminal and the innervated smooth muscle cells; this is the driving force for the diffusion of the adrenergic transmitter and, thus, for the activation of the effector tissue. When norepinephrine reaches the smooth muscle cells, it binds to and activates adrenoceptors on the cell membrane.

Norepinephrine release can be impaired by several pharmacologic agents.[18] The adrenolytic agent, 6-hydroxydopamine, exerts its effect by destroying

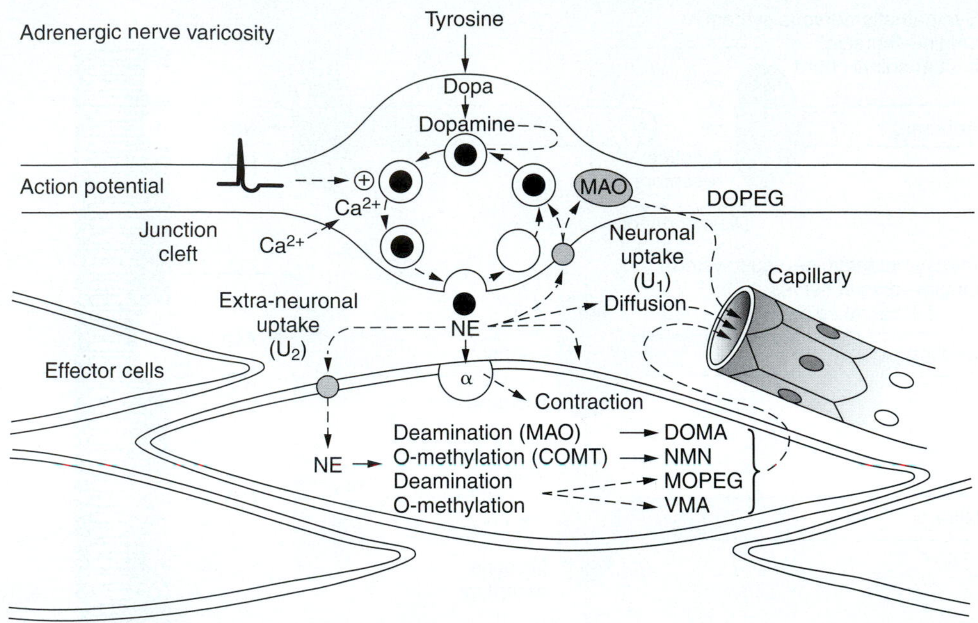

FIGURE 5-4. Schematic of synthesis and disposition of norepinephrine from the sympathetic (adrenergic nerve) nerve varicosity. Norepinephrine is synthesized by tyrosine hydroxylase to dopamine, which is taken up into vesicles and converted to norepinephrine by dopamine β-hydroxylase. The nerve impulse activates the entry of calcium ions into the adrenergic nerve varicosity. This causes norepinephrine containing vesicles to migrate and fuse to the neuronal surface, then rupture and release norepinephrine into the junctional cleft. Norepinephrine released into the cleft activates α-adrenergic receptors on the smooth muscle or is removed (1) by uptake into the nerve ending (U_1) where part of it is enzymatically degraded by neuronal monoamine oxidase (MOA) to 3,4-dihydroxyphenylethyleneglycol (DOPEG), but most is recycled by the storage vesicles; (2) by uptake by effector cells (U_2) and enzymatic degradation by the enzyme monoamine (MAO) and catechol-O-methyltransferase (COMT) to 3,4-hydroxymandelic acid (DOMA), normetanephrine (NMN), 3-methoxy,4-dihydroxy phenyl glycol (MOPEG), and 3-methoxy,4-hydroxymandelic acid (VMA); and (3) by diffusion into the capillaries. The metabolites of norepinephrine are inactive and diffuse to the extracellular fluid and the capillaries.

adrenergic-nerve endings. This effect depends on uptake of 6-hydroxydopamine by the biogenic amine pump located in the plasma membrane of adrenergic nerve endings. Guanethidine is taken up into adrenergic nerve endings by the same mechanism responsible for transport of norepinephrine. It accumulates in and displaces norepinephrine from intraneuronal storage granules, thereby depleting norepinephrine stores. Guanethidine may also produce local blockade of membrane electrical activity in nerve endings. Bretylium tosylate is structurally similar to guanethidine and also inhibits norepinephrine release from adrenergic nerve terminals (Fig. 5-5).

The puffer fish poison, tetrodotoxin, selectively blocks sodium channels in nervous tissue, thereby inhibiting the inward sodium current. By suppressing the generation of action potentials, tetrodotoxin inhibits the release of norepinephrine from adrenergic nerve endings.

Secretory activity of the adrenergic-nerve ending can be modulated by substances released into the junctional cleft during the exocytotic process and by other substances present in the junctional cleft (see Prejunctional Regulation of Transmitter Release).

Disposition of the Released Transmitter

Norepinephrine is removed from the junctional cleft (see Fig. 5-4) by several mechanisms (1) uptake by the neuronal cell membrane (uptake 1) and subsequent storage or intraneuronal deamination by the enzyme monoamine oxidase; (2) overflow to the extracellular space—where part of the liberated neurotransmitter leaves the junctional cleft by diffusion and may overflow into the capillaries to constitute the most important fraction of circulating norepinephrine; (3) nonspecific binding to collagen structures and uptake by nonmuscle cells (e.g., fat cells); and (4) extraneuronal uptake by vascular smooth muscle cells (uptake 2) and subsequent enzymatic degradation.

Neuronal Uptake The cell membrane of the adrenergic neuron can take up norepinephrine and a number of other substances that can interact with adrenergic sites. This is an active process mediated by a carrier linked to Na^+,K^+ ATPase. This uptake operates only when the neuronal cell membrane is polarized. Thus, neuronal uptake normally plays a small role in determining the effector-response amplitude to sympathetic-nerve stimulation. Because this system recaptures norepinephrine near the nerve endings or the blood, it is particularly important when the media are innervated throughout and when the blood vessel wall is relatively thin, for example, in the case of densely innervated veins. By contrast, arteries, where the innervation is limited to the adventitial medial border, do not easily recapture circulating catecholamines. Inhibition of neuronal uptake can prolong contraction and delay the onset of relaxations. Common inhibitors of neuronal uptake include cocaine and most antidepressant drugs (see Fig. 5-5).

A portion of the norepinephrine taken up by the adrenergic nerve terminal is enzymatically destroyed by

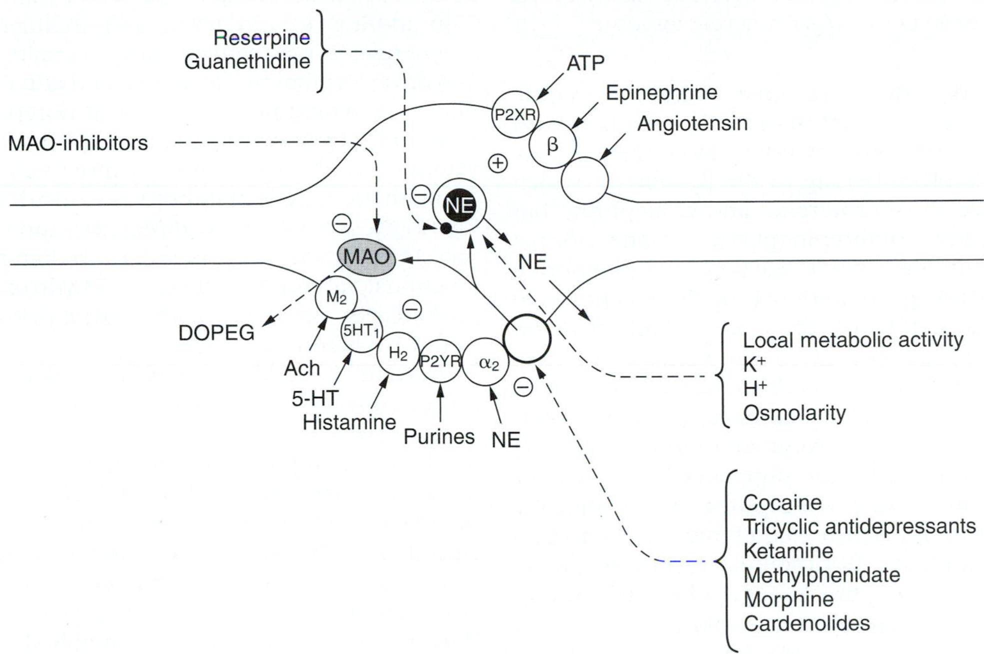

FIGURE 5-5. Schematic of prejunctional modulation of neurotransmitter release. Release of norepinephrine (NE) can be regulated as a result of stimulation of specific receptors on the adrenergic nerve terminal. For example, stimulation of receptors for acetylcholine (Ach), 5-hydroxytryptamine (5-HT), histamine, purines, prostanoids, and norepinephrine can inhibit release of neurotransmitter, whereas vasoactive substances, such as epinephrine and angiotensin II, activate receptors that increase the output of norepinephrine. Pharmacologic agents such as cocaine and tricyclic antidepressants inhibit uptake of NE, whereas metabolites of smooth muscle activity such as potassium ions, acidosis, and changes in osmolarity of the intracellular fluid inhibit release of NE from vesicles in the nerve terminal (see text for further details). +, indicates stimulation; –, indicates inhibition; DOPEG, 3,4-dihydroxyphenylethyleneglycol; MAO, monoamine oxidase inhibitors.

intraneuronal monoamine oxidase (see Fig. 5-4). Inhibitors of monoamine oxidase (such as pargyline and tranylcypromine) may augment the overflow of intact transmitter, thereby causing a moderate augmentation of the contractile response.

Extraneuronal Uptake Vascular smooth muscle cells possess an active carrier process for the uptake of norepinephrine. The extraneuronal uptake of norepinephrine is followed by enzymatic inactivation of the amine by catechol-O-methyltransferase, monoamine oxidase, or both. Certain steroids (hydrocortisone and 17β-estradiol) can inhibit extraneuronal uptake. Inhibitors of extraneuronal uptake can sometimes, but not always, augment the contractile responses to exogenous norepinephrine.[19]

The relative importance of the different pathways for the disposition of released norepinephrine varies from blood vessel to blood vessel and depends on factors such as density of adrenergic innervation, anatomic arrangement of adrenergic-nerve terminals within the vessel wall, presence of nonspecific binding sites and uptake by nonvascular cells, and the width of the junctional cleft. If the junctional cleft is narrow, neuronal uptake plays a prominent role. If it is wide, overflow to the capillaries and extraneuronal uptake become more important.

Postjunctional Activation of Vascular Smooth Muscle

Norepinephrine and epinephrine produce their physiologic effects by activating α- and β-adrenergic receptors (or adrenoceptors) on target tissues. Based on pharmacologic and molecular studies, these receptors can be further subdivided into α_1, α_2, β_1, β_2, and β_3 subtypes. Moreover, three distinct subtypes of α_1- and α_2-adrenoceptors have also been identified. These are designated α_{1A}, α_{1B}, α_{1D}, and α_{2A}, α_{2B}, and α_{2C} (see also the NC-IUPHAR Receptor Database at (www.iuphar.org). Studies on blood vessels from different species and origins indicate that each of the known adrenoceptor subtypes is present on one or more of the major cell types within the blood vessel wall (i.e., adrenergic nerve endings, vascular smooth muscle, or endothelial cells). Numerous selective adrenoceptor agonists and antagonists are used clinically for vascular indications. Most of these agents are highly selective for either α_1-, α_2-, β_1-, or β_2-adrenoceptors; therapeutic use of drugs with selectivity for the individual subtypes of α_1- and α_2-adrenoceptors or β_3-adrenoceptors remains limited.

α-Adrenoceptors In most blood vessels innervated by sympathetic neurons, norepinephrine activates postjunctional α-adrenoceptors. This process, by increasing the cytoplasmic Ca^{2+} concentration, triggers the contractile process, thus causing contraction and vasoconstriction. Not all postjunctional vascular α-adrenoceptors belong to the same subtype. Most large arteries, when studied in vitro, respond with contraction to selective α_1-adrenergic agonists (such as phenylephrine) but are relatively insensitive to selective α_2-adrenergic agonists (e.g., clonidine, tramazoline, BHT-920, UK 14,304). Contraction of most arteries to norepinephrine is competitively antagonized by specific α_1- but not by specific α_2-adrenergic antagonists. However, smaller arteries, arterioles and certain veins, respond to selective α_2-adrenergic agonists.

β-Adrenoceptors Most vascular smooth muscle responds to β-adrenergic activation with relaxation. With the exception of the coronary artery in certain species, the receptors involved belong to the β_2-subtype, which is more sensitive to isoproterenol and epinephrine but relatively insensitive to norepinephrine.[20] Under normal physiologic conditions, nerve-released norepinephrine primarily activates postjunctional α-adrenoceptors in most blood vessels. However, the concomitant activation of postjunctional β-adrenoceptors may attenuate the vasoconstrictor response to sympathetic-nerve stimulation. Alpha-adrenergic blockade may unmask a β-adrenoceptor-mediated dilator effect of exogenous norepinephrine, whereas β-adrenergic blockade augments the constrictor effect of the adrenergic transmitter. Neurogenically induced relaxation of vascular smooth muscle due to activation of postjunctional β-adrenergic receptors, in the absence of α-adrenergic blockade, is observed only in certain facial veins and in coronary arteries.

Prejunctional Regulation of Transmitter Release

The adrenergic neuronal membrane senses the concentration of transmitter present in the junctional cleft by means of α-adrenoreceptors on the sympathetic nerve endings (prejunctional or presynaptic α-adrenoceptors) (see Fig. 5-5). Receptors that exert a negative feedback on the exocytotic process belong to the α_2-adrenergic subtype and are sensitive to α_2-adrenergic agonists, of which clonidine is the prototype.[18,21] If these receptors are activated on a background of sympathetic-nerve stimulation, the release of norepinephrine is decreased. Inhibitory prejunctional α_2-adrenoceptors are present in a number of isolated blood vessels from various species, including humans. In experimental hypertension, prejunctional inhibition of adrenergic neurotransmission becomes less effective as arterial pressure rises; thus, a defect in prejunctional modulation of adrenergic neurotransmission may contribute to the development of high blood pressure.

Exogenous acetylcholine exerts a potent prejunctional inhibitory effect on the exocytotic release of norepinephrine in a wide variety of systemic arteries and veins from different species, including humans, through activation of muscarinic receptors on the nerve terminal (see Fig. 5-3). Thus, vagal nerve stimulation inhibits the release of norepinephrine in the heart and in the gastric circulation (see Parasympathetic Innervation). Both exogenous and endogenous acetylcholines inhibit the release of norepinephrine in coronary arteries.[22]

The inhibitory effect of acetylcholine is due to activation of muscarinic receptors, which presumably causes hyperpolarization of the adrenergic nerve endings. The prejunctional muscarinic receptor located on adrenergic nerve endings has been characterized as an M_2 receptor. In higher concentrations, acetylcholine can activate nicotinic receptors on adrenergic postsynaptic fibers; nicotine itself can facilitate or initiate the release of adrenergic neurotransmitter in the blood vessel wall.

In addition to adrenergic and cholinergic receptors, adrenergic nerve endings also contain receptors for 5-hydroxytryptamine, histamine and adenosine, the stimulation of which inhibit release of norepinephrine. This action of 5-hydroxytryptamine explains best the observations that the monoamine causes vasodilation when sympathetic tone is high but vasoconstriction when it is low: in the latter case, the direct activation of the smooth muscle by 5-hydroxytryptamine predominates. The prejunctional inhibitory action of 5-hydroxytryptamine is mediated by receptors with pharmacologic similarities to the 5-HT_1-serotonergic subtype.

In arteries isolated from experimental animals, histamine causes relaxation of the smooth muscle during sympathetic-nerve activation, which is paralleled by a decreased overflow of norepinephrine. In addition, histamine reduces release of transmitter evoked by high K^+ but not its displacement evoked by tyramine. Thus, it has been concluded that histamine causes prejunctional inhibition of adrenergic neurotransmission. Effects of histamine during sympathetic-nerve stimulation can be mimicked by H_2-receptor agonists; they are inhibited by H_2-receptor antagonists but not by H_1-receptor-blocking drugs. Thus, the prejunctional inhibiting effect of histamine is caused by activation of H_2 receptors on the neuronal cell membrane.

The prejunctional effect of histamine probably contributes to the vasodilator properties it has in certain vascular beds and, in particular, helps explain why the vasodilator effect it causes is prolonged: the direct dilator effect of histamine on the vascular smooth muscle cells is unopposed by norepinephrine released from sympathetic nerve endings.

Chemical byproducts of smooth and skeletal muscle contractions (adenosine, H^+, and changes in osmolarity) in the extracellular space will also reduce release of norepinephrine from adrenergic nerve endings (see Fig. 5-5). Therefore, under conditions of sustained sympathetic neuronal stimulation to vascular smooth muscle, relaxation and subsequent decreases in vascular resistance result because of combined inhibitory mechanisms that reduce release of transmitter. Vasodilation under conditions of sustained adrenergic stimulation is called functional sympatholysis.

In addition to adenosine being released as a byproduct of skeletal muscle contraction, adenosine triphosphate (ATP) is stored in synaptic vesicles with norepinephrine and is released simultaneously with the adrenergic transmitter. ATP can affect adrenergic transmission through two mechanisms. First, ATP can bind to purinergic receptors (P2XR) on the synaptic terminal and increase exocytotic release of adrenergic transmitter, forming a positive feedback. However, ATP can also bind to P2YR, purinergic G-protein-coupled receptors, which inhibit exocytotic release of norepinephrine, forming a negative feedback regulatory mechanism. ATP is metabolized by the membrane associated ectoenzyme, nucleotidase hydrolyzing enzymes (ecto-ATPase and NTPDase-1 or ecto-ADPase/CD39). Therefore, receptor-mediated effects of ATP on adrenergic synaptic activity depend on the relative concentration of ATP within the synapse as regulated by NTPDase-1 activity. Indeed, the NTPDase-1 inhibitor, ARL-67156 (6-N,N-diethethyl-β-γ-dibromomethylene-D-adenosine-5′-triphosphate) increases the concentration of norepinephrine in the synaptic terminal, whereas the recombinant form of the enzyme, solCD39, reduces exocytotic release of norepinephrine.[23]

β-Adrenergic agonists, in particular, isoproterenol and epinephrine, can augment the evoked release of norepinephrine in the blood vessel wall by activating prejunctional β-adrenoceptors (see Fig. 5-5). This prejunctional β-adrenergic facilitation is more pronounced in human than in animal blood vessels. Cardioselective β-receptor antagonists are less effective in blocking prejunctional excitatory β-receptors than are nonselective agents.[20]

In at least some hypertensive individuals, plasma epinephrine levels are increased. It has been postulated that the primary abnormality in essential hypertension might be an increased adrenal secretion of epinephrine, which in turn, by facilitation of junctional norepinephrine release, might contribute to the development of essential hypertension. Whether the prejunctional β-adrenoceptors, indeed, play a role under normal conditions and, in particular, in essential hypertension, is still uncertain. If they do, β-adrenergic antagonists also may act at this site and cause a decrease in neurotransmitter release, which could help to explain their antihypertensive properties.

Parasympathetic Innervation

Neurons of the parasympathetic system are carried with the cranial nerves and exit the sacral spinal cord. The transmitter for both the pre- and postgangiolinic fibers is acetylcholine (see Fig. 5-3). Postganglionic cholinergic nerves innervate several blood vessels—including nasal mucosa, retina, coronary arteries, icterus clitoris, and corpora cavernosa. Acetylcholine is not present in significant amounts in plasma, however, which suggests that the effects of acetylcholine would be very localized. In addition to neurons, acetylcholine is synthesized in endothelial cells, epithelial cells, and leukocytes.

Acetylcholine is synthesized enzymatically by choline acetyltransferase (ChAT) from choline, which is transported into the nerve by a transporter. Synthesis is regulated by availability of choline and acetyl coenzyme A and by activity of ChAT. Activity, binding to plasma membranes and interaction of ChAT with other proteins is regulated by posttranslational phosphorlyation.[24-26]

The transmitter is accumulated into synaptic vesicles by a 12-transmembrane domain protein transporter (vesicular acetylcholine transporter, VAChT). Phosphorylation of VAChT represents one mechanism that regulates storage and release of acetylcholine. NO facilitates release of acetylcholine through presynaptic potentiation.[27]

Tissue responses to acetylcholine are mediated by activation of muscarinic or nicotinic receptors. Nicotinic receptors are found predominantly in autonomic ganglia and skeletal muscle. Muscarinic receptors are found on vascular smooth muscle, adrenergic nerve endings, and endothelial cells. Five genes have been sequenced that encode muscarinic acetylcholine receptors: M_1, M_2, M_3, M_4, and M_5.

Non-Adrenergic Non-Cholinergic (NANC) Nerves

This general category of innervation to the vasculature was developed in the 1970s and used to describe innervation that could not be attributed to either adrenergic or cholinergic neurotransmitters. Transmitters in this category include NO, substance P, vasoactive intestinal peptide (VIP), calcitonin gene-related peptide (CGRP), and ATP.[16]

Nitrergic Nerves

In general, vasodilation caused by either electrical nerve stimulation or nicotine that is abolished by tetrodotoxin, methylene blue, or an inhibitor of soluble guanylyl cyclase but not by ganglionic blockade, antagonists of CGRP or removal of the endothelium is attributed to neuronal release of NO.[28]

Synthesis and Mechanism of Action Unlike transmitters of adrenergic and cholinergic neurons, NO is not stored in granules of the axon terminal but rather is synthesized in response to action potential-induced Ca^{++} entry into the nerve terminal. NO is synthesized enzymatically by the neuronal isoform of NO synthase (nNOS). As is required for other isoforms of the enzyme (see also sections on Endothelium), L-arginine, the substrate for NOS is taken up from the extracellular space through the cation amino acid transporter system (system y^+). NOS requires calmodulin and tetrahydrobiopterin for optimal activity. L-citrulline is a byproduct of NO production and can be converted to L-arginine intracellularly. NO released from the nerve terminal diffuses to the underlying smooth muscle and causes relaxation through activation of guanylyl cyclase and formation of cyclic GMP (see Regulation of Cyclic Nucleotides).

Pharmacologic Regulation of Neuronally Derived Nitric Oxide As with other neurotransmitters, regulation of enzymatic production of NO will depend on substrate (L-arginine) availability and cofactors required by the enzyme—such as tetrahydrobiopterin. In addition, oxygen free radicals, such as superoxide and hydroxyl radicals, will interact with NO to reduce its biologic availability, and inactivation of endogenous superoxide dismutase depresses responses to neurogenic NO.[29] Inactivation of NO by oxygen-derived free radicals, in particular because of the formation of peroxy nitrite, may contribute to vascular damage related to ischemia and lipid peroxidation. Some herbal extracts, for example ginsenosides, and hormones, like 17β-estradiol, exert antioxidant effects and may increase the bioavailability of NO, regardless of the source of production (nerve or endothelium, see later).

An analog of L-arginine selective for a specific isoform of NOS is an area of pharmacologic investigation. However, endogenous guanidino-methylated derivatives of L-arginine, which are not isoform specific, are emerging as endogenous risk factors for cardiovascular disease. In particular, N^G, N^G-dimethyl-L-arginine (asymmetrical dimethlylarginine, ADMA) which ranges from 0.5 to 1 μmol/L in plasma of normal human volunteers increases to 2 to 10 μmol/L in patients with cardiovascular disease, such as hypertension, diabetes mellitus, preeclampsia, or hypercholesterolemia. The usefulness of compounds that suppress synthesis or actions of ADMA or accelerate its breakdown, such as dimethlylarginine dimethylaminohydrolase or alanine:glyoxylate aminotransferase-2, remain to be explored in the prevention or treatment of cardiovascular disease.[30]

Compounds selective for inhibiting nNOS include aplysinopsin-type indole alkaloid, isolated from marine sponge, and Ni^{++} act as selective and reversible inhibitors of nNOS. Guanabenz is an irreversible inhibitor of nNOS. In terms of the systemic circulation, neuronally released NO is associated with vasodilation. Therefore, the therapeutic usefulness of specific nNOS inhibitors may be limited to situations of hyperdynamic circulation characterized by extremely low blood pressure and vascular resistance—as would occur with cirrhosis of the liver.

Distribution By immunoreactivity, NOS-containing fibers have been identified in afferent sensory nerves, preganglionic parasympathetic and sympathetic nerves, and postganglionic parasympathetic nerves. For intracranial structures, preganglionic fibers of nitrergic nerves originate in the superior salivatory nucleus and track with the greater petrosal nerve to synapse in the pterygopalatine ganglion. Postganglionic nitrergic fibers synapse onto cerebral and ocular arteries. Other cranial structures innervated by nitrergic nerves in some species include the nasal vasculature, the tongue, and superficial temporal arteries. The contribution of perivascular nitrergic neurons to the etiology of spontaneous migraine and cerebrovasospasm remains to be determined.[31,32]

In the heart, immunoreactivity for nitrergic fibers is observed in the adventitia of epicardial coronary arteries. However, how these neurons participate in regulation of coronary arterial tone remains to be determined. Nitrergic nerves to the heart are derived from the nodose ganglia and may facilitate vagally induced bradycardia by presynaptic potentiation.[33,34]

Immunoreactive nitrergic networks are associated also with pulmonary arteries and veins, mesenteric arteries, posterior caval vein, hepatic arteries, arcuate and interlobal renal arteries, and preglomerular afferent arterioles. In these tissues, neuronally released NO inhibits contraction of the smooth muscle directly, but in some tissues indirect inhibition of adrenergic neurotransmission by presynaptic inhibition is also possible.

Nitrergic neurons also innervate the reproductive tract of females and males.[34,35] Parasympathetic, nitrergic immunoreactive neurons originate from the pelvic paracervical ganglia and innervate the uterine artery. Pregnancy and estrogen treatments augment the activity of calcium-dependent NOS activity in uterine arteries. Whether this represents specific regulation of nNOS or other NOS isoforms remains to be determined. nNOS is regulated post-transcriptionally and exhibits multiple splice variations, but how these factors contribute to regulation of uterine blood flow is uncertain. However, PDE5 inhibitors increase uterine blood flow in patients undergoing in vitro fertilization. Nitrergic fibers are found in clitoral vasculature but the use of L-arginine supplementation, and PDE5 inhibitors to treat sexual arousal disorders in women have not been efficacious.

In human males, NOS immunoreactive nerve plexes are present in the adventitia of penile arteries and cavernosal tissue.[28] Stimulation of lumbosacral parasympathetic and lumbosacral somatic nerves and release of NO dilates penile arteries and the corpora cavernosa. Increased blood flow and increased capacitance of the cavernosum compresses the penile veins, thus decreasing outflow. The resulting increased intravenous pressure causes penile erection. As NO mediates relaxation by increasing tissue content of cGMP, drugs that inhibit hydrolysis of cGMP by 5′-GMP phosphodiesterase (PDE5) have been successful in correcting erectile dysfunction for some individuals. Inhibitory nitrergic nerves also facilitate erection through prejunctional inhibition of excitatory, adrenergic nerves innervating penile arteries by neurons originating from thoracolumbar sympathetic tracts.

The number of NOS-immunoreactive fibers in penile tissue varies with age, hormonal status, and some pathologic conditions such as diabetes. In rats, androgen receptors are present on neurons of the pelvic ganglia innervating the corpora cavernosa. As might be expected, castration or administration of androgen antagonists decreases erection in these animals. The relationship of androgen status to penile erection has not been established in humans. In addition, genetic variants of nNOS and infertility in men or women have not been defined.

Other physiologic responses attributed to nitrergic-derived NO include vasodilation of the skin following stimulation of cholinergic nerves, stimulation of axon reflexes by focal heating of the skin, and sympathetic cholinergic vasodilation of small arteries in skeletal muscle.[36] Exercise will increase blood flow to contracting fast-twitch skeletal muscle and upregulation of nNOS. However, whether nNOS is localized only to nerves or is associated with skeletal muscle is controversial.

Peptigergic Nerves

Neurons releasing substance P, vasoactive intestinal peptide (VIP), and calcitonin gene-related peptide (CGRP) are detected in some cerebral and human epicardial coronary arteries and veins.[16] However, functional significance of these fibers remains to be determined.

Substance P Substance P is widely distributed in sensory nerve endings localized to the adventitia of large and small blood vessels. It is a potent vasodilator, although in high doses the peptide causes constriction of some blood vessels. The relaxation elicited by substance P is endothelium dependent (see later), which raises the possibility that endothelial cells may contribute to the vasodilation that accompanies axon reflexes.[37]

Vasoactive Intestinal Peptide Vasoactive intestinal polypeptide (VIP) is present in postganglionic cholinergic neurons innervating many tissues. It also is a potent vasodilator and contributes to the atropine-resistant vasodilation observed during parasympathetic-nerve stimulation. In some blood vessels, relaxations induced by VIP may be endothelium dependent.

Calcitonin Gene-Related Peptide Calcitonin gene-related peptide (CGRP) is localized in sensory neurons, often together with substance P, and has strong vasodilator properties.[28] It is present in perivascular nerves of the brain and several peripheral organs including the heart. Depending on the vascular bed, CGRP causes relaxation either through direct action on the vascular smooth muscle or through an endothelium-dependent mechanism. Additionally, CGRP may inhibit neurogenic vasoconstriction via a prejunctional effect on adrenergic neurons. The relaxant effects of CGRP appear to be closely linked to K^+-channel activation and to increased production of cAMP within vascular smooth muscle.

Interaction of Nitrergic Neurons with Sympathetic and Cholinergic Parasympathetic Neurons

Release of acetylcholine from presynaptic fibers of both the sympathetic and parasympathetic neurons stimulate nicotinic receptors on the postganglionic fiber. Therefore, nicotine facilitates adrenergic and/or cholinergic neurotransmission through stimulation of post-synaptic fibers. Nicotine will also stimulate release of NO from nitrergic nerves, which colocalize with peripheral parasympathetic fibers.[28]

Functionally, the predominant postganglionic transmitter of nerves to cerebral arteries and the corpora cavernosa, which are described classically as parasympathetic nerves, is NO. Therefore, it is proposed that the parasympathetic autonomic system be defined or divided based on the transmitter of the postganglionic fibers as either "cholinergic" or "nitrergic" for acetylcholine and NO, respectively (see Fig. 5-3).[28]

In general, postsynaptic actions of nitrergic and sympathetic transmitters are functional antagonists, with the former causing vasodilation and the latter, if α-adrenergic receptors dominate on the smooth muscle, contraction. Prejunctionally at the nerve terminal, there is no evidence that activation of β-adrenergic receptors affect NO released from perivascular nerves. In addition, for reasons yet to be determined, inhibition of release of neuronally derived NO by selective α_2-receptor agonists seem to be artery and species specific. Whether or not neuronally derived NO inhibits synaptic release of norepinephrine remains controversial.[28,33]

In contrast to conflicting evidence for presynaptic interactions between adrenergic and nitrergic fibers, acetylcholine inhibits release of NO from nitrergic fibers through activation of M_2 muscarinic-receptors. Direct application of acetylcholine dose-dependently inhibits NO-mediated neurogenic relaxations in cerebral arteries. Because physostigmine inhibits catabolism of acetylcholine by acetylcholinesterase, these observations suggest that endogenous neuronally released acetylcholine may act similarly under physiologic conditions. Alternatively, atropine and selective M_2 antagonists also augment neuronally mediated NO relaxations, suggesting that activation of M_2 receptors is required for muscarinic prejunctional inhibition of neuronal release of NO (see Fig. 5-3).[28]

Endothelium

The endothelium is the layer of squamous epithelial cells that is in direct contact with the blood. As such, the endothelium is ideally situated to perform a number of important functions. These include: (1) acting as a diffusion barrier between substances in the blood and the tissues; (2) regulating hemostasis and cellular immunogenic processes; (3) sensing mechanical shear and tangential stresses; and (4) activating, inactivating, or producing several vasoactive substances that can affect the underlying vascular smooth muscle cells. Detailed mechanisms of these processes are presented in other parts of this textbook (see Chapters 1, 4, and 8). Hence, the present discussion will focus mainly on the pharmacologic characterization of endothelium-derived factors. These factors impact not only on the thrombogenicity of the blood, the activation of blood elements, and the tone of the underlying smooth muscle, but also on the production of extracellular matrix—as well as the differentiation and the proliferation of vascular smooth muscle cells.

Activation and Inactivation of Circulating Substances

Endothelial cells, in particular those of the pulmonary vasculature, have many metabolic functions. Pulmonary endothelial cells take up norepinephrine and 5-hydroxytryptamine (5HT, serotonin) and subsequently degrade them via monoamine oxidase or catechol-O-methyltransferase; uptake is the rate-limiting step in this process. The pharmacologic evidence available suggests that the uptake sites for norepinephrine and 5-hydroxytryptamine are distinct; epinephrine, dopamine, and isoproterenol are not taken up. Studies with cultured animal aortic endothelial cells demonstrate that, although these cells contain monoamine oxidase, they do not possess the amine-transport process present in the lung.

Estrogens are degraded in target tissues like the endothelium through sulfatase, sulfotransferase and 17β-hydroxysteroid dehydrogenase. Metabolites of estradiol, such as the catechol estrogens, compete with norepinephrine for binding to catechol-O-methyltransferase. Therefore, circulating levels of 17β-estradiol and its metabolites can affect clearance of adrenergic neurotransmitter as well as synthesis of other endothelium-derived factors as will be detailed in other sections.[38,39]

Angiotensin 1, encephalins, and bradykinin are substrates for converting enzyme (angiotensin converting enzyme [ACE]/kininase II) that is located at the luminal surface.[40] Products of this enzymatic conversion are angiotensin II and peptide fragments of bradykinin and encephalins. Inhibitors of angiotensin converting enzyme prevent formation of angiotensin II and inhibit degradation of bradykinin. Each of these actions could facilitate relaxation of vascular smooth muscle, the former by decreasing stimulation of contractile effects of angiotensin II, the latter by increasing bradykinin stimulated release of relaxing factors from the endothelium (see Endothelium-Derived Relaxing Factors).

Endothelial cells also possess specific mechanisms for the uptake and release of ATP, adenosine diphosphate (ADP), and AMP. Membrane-associated ectoenzymes regulate purine availability (ecto-ATPase hydrolyzes ATP to ADP; ecto-ADPase/CD30 metabolizes ADP to AMP).[41] ATP released from dense granules of platelets facilitates aggregation and interaction of platelets with leukocytes and endothelial cells, thus facilitating formation of occlusive thrombi. Therefore, the nucleotide hydrolyzing enzyme family (NTPDase-1) represents a potential target for drug development both for affecting platelet aggregation and adrenergic neurotransmission (see Presynaptic Inhibition).[23] Modulation of ACE and NTPDase-1 by sex steroids may contribute to sex differences in the development of various cardiovascular pathologies such as hypertension and thrombotic disorders.[42,43] Circulating prostaglandins of the E and F series are also extensively metabolized by the pulmonary endothelium; prostaglandin A and prostacyclin are not metabolized in vivo.

In certain blood vessels, endothelial cells contain the enzyme choline acetyltransferase and can produce acetylcholine, which then may act as an autocrine and paracrine substance.[37] Likewise, shear stress or hypoxia may cause the endothelial production of other vasoactive substances including adenosine triphosphate (ATP), serotonin, substance P, vasopressin, bradykinin, and/or histamine.[44]

Thus, endothelial cells can influence the amounts of vasoactive substances reaching vascular smooth muscle by activation, inactivation, and production. Furthermore, the ability of the endothelium to alter the concentration of various vasoactive agents that affect blood platelet and leukocyte function may also be important in hemostasis, thrombosis, and immunogenicity.[45]

Endothelium-Derived Vasoactive Factors

Endothelium-derived factors can be classified by their action of causing either vasodilation or vasoconstriction. However, as more becomes known about the cellular mechanisms of these compounds, it is clear that their functions are not singular. That is, endothelium-derived factors which cause vasodilation may also inhibit platelet activation, leukocyte rolling and adhesion, and cell proliferation; and the opposite applies for factors previously classified as vasoconstrictor substances. However, for the sake of simplicity, these factors will be classified and discussed based on the ability to relax or contract the underlying vascular smooth muscle.

Endothelium-Derived Relaxing Factors

The evidence for an obligatory role of arterial endothelial cells in the responses of smooth muscle was provided by Furchgott and Zawadzki in 1980, when they demonstrated that arteries denuded of endothelium failed to relax when exposed to acetylcholine.[46] The arterial endothelium also accounts, at least in part, for the relaxation of smooth muscle caused by α_2-adrenergic agonists, ADP, ATP, bradykinin, histamine, oxytocin, substance P, thrombin, and vasopressin. These substances are believed to interact with specific receptors on endothelial cells to stimulate the release of one or more endothelium-derived relaxing factors (EDRFs). By comparison, agents such as adenosine, isoproterenol, and nitrates, as a rule, do not depend on the endothelium for their effect but act directly on the smooth muscle. EDRFs are classified by their chemical structure or by the physiologic response they initiate (i.e., endothelium-derived hyperpolarizing factor or EDHF).

Nitric Oxide The labile diffusible mediator of endothelium-dependent relaxations initiated by acetylcholine is NO. NO is formed from the guanidino-nitrogen terminal of L-arginine, by an enzyme called NO synthase (NOS). There are three isoforms of the enzyme: NOS I, II, and III—commonly referred to as neuronal (nNOS), inducible (iNOS) and endothelial (eNOS), respectively. The enzyme present in endothelial cells is the III isoform. This isoform has a molecular mass of 135 kDa. Even though eNOS is considered to be a constitutively expressed form of NOS, its expression is regulated. For example, 17β-estradiol through activation of estrogen receptor α increases transcription of the eNOS gene. In addition, statin drugs with high lipid solubility (simvastatin and lovastatin as compared with pravastatin) increase stability of eNOS mRNA through inhibition of Rho and Rho kinase. Therefore, quantity of eNOS protein in endothelial cells is influenced by transcriptional and posttranscriptional biochemical pathways.[47-51]

Enzyme Activity and Release of NO Activity of eNOS is regulated through allosteric association with intracellular proteins and posttranslational modification of the protein by myristolylation, glycosylation, and phosphorylation (Fig. 5-6). Initial discoveries identified that constitutive activity of eNOS required binding to calmodulin and that the activity was regulated by concentration of the intracellular Ca^{2+}. eNOS also requires reduced nicotine-amide-adenine-dinucleotide phosphate (NADPH) and 5,6,7,8-tetra-hydrobiopterin(BH_4) for optimal activity. In addition, activity of eNOS is characterized by dynamic multiprotein signaling complexes that not only regulate subcellular targeting of the enzyme to microdomains within endothelial cells, such as caveolae, but also affect calcium sensitivity of the enzyme. For example, *N*-myristolyation does not affect eNOS activity in cell lysate but is required for NO release stimulated by calcium ionophore in intact cells. A 90-kDa tyrosine-phosphorylated protein, heat shock protein 90 (hsp90), coprecipitates with eNOS. Stimuli that increase release of NO, such as shear stress, histamine, vascular endothelial growth factor (VEGF), and 17β-estradiol increase the association of eNOS with hsp90. Association of eNOS with hsp90 may act as an allosteric modulator to stabilize the activated conformation of the enzyme.[52,53]

Contrary to binding of eNOS to hsp90, binding of eNOS to caveolin-1 or -3 inhibits enzyme activity. Caveolin-1, eNOS, and hsp90 coprecipitate in the same complex. Binding of calmodulin to eNOS reduces binding of eNOS to caveolin, thus increasing eNOS activity. It is not known

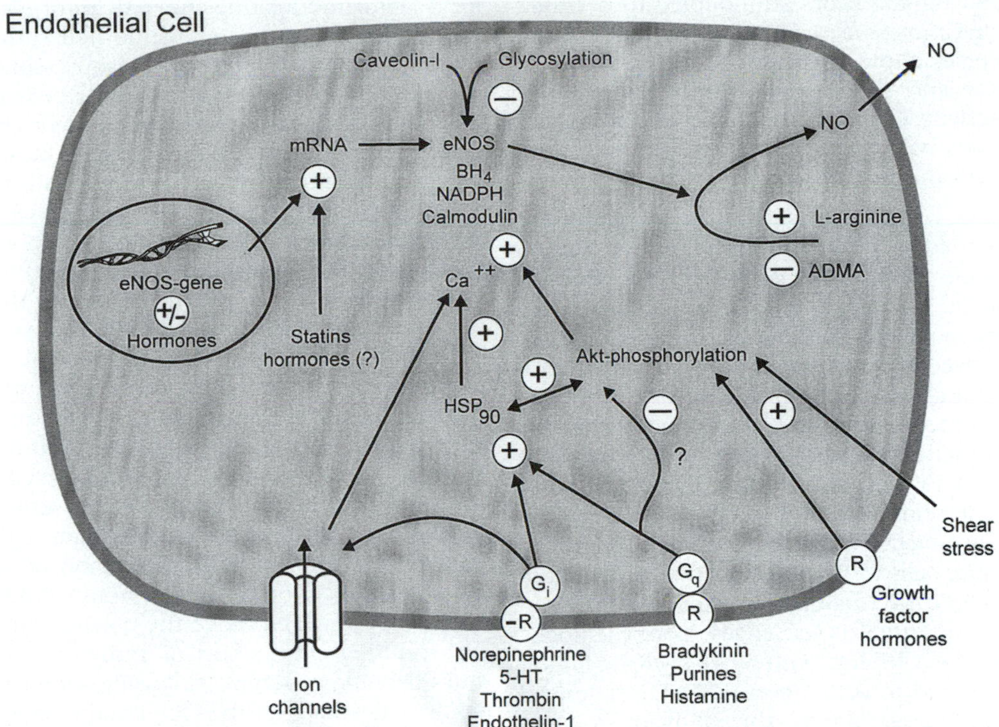

FIGURE 5-6. Schematic of possible mechanisms by which production of nitric oxide is regulated in endothelial cells. Nitric oxide is produced through enzymatic conversion of L-arginine by nitric oxide synthase (endothelial or type III, eNOS). The transcription of this enzyme is regulated genomically by hormones and growth factors. Stability of eNOS mRNA is modulated by statins and hormones. eNOS enzyme activity requires calcium, calmodulin, nicotinamide adenine dinucleotide phosphate (NADPH), and 5,6,7,8-tetra-hydrobiopterine (BH_4). Enzyme activity is regulated by complexing to these proteins in microdomains of the endothelial cell. Association with this complex of heat shock protein 90 (HSP 90) increases enzyme activity. Stimulation of specific receptors on the endothelial surface (R) complexed with guanine nucleotide regulatory proteins, which are sensitive to pertussis toxin (G_i) or insensitive to pertussis toxin (G_q), activate intracellular pathways that modulate eNOS activity posttranslationally through heat shock protein 90 or AKT-phosphorylation. Association of eNOS with caveolin-1 or glycosylation of the enzyme reduces activity. A metabolite of L-arginine, asymmetric dimethyl arginine (ADMA) decreases production of nitric oxide through competitive binding to eNOS. Thus, this endogenous amine may be a risk factor for the development of cardiovascular disease. +, indicates stimulation; –, indicates inhibition; ?, indicates those pathways in which the regulation is unknown.

if calmodulin results in a physical displacement of eNOS from caveolin or only a change in conformation without translocation away from caveolin. Increases in caveolin-1 in experimental models of cirrhosis decrease basal and stimulate release of NO. If a similar condition exists in humans, this may explain, in part, increased portal pressures associated with the disease.

Alternating phosphorylation and glycosylation of serine-1177 of eNOS results in opposite posttranslational modification of enzyme activity. Phosphorylation of serine-1177 by protein kinase Akt/PKB increases NO production, whereas glycosylation of serine-1177 through activity of β-O-linked-*N*-acetylglucosaminyl transferase decreases NO production. Protein kinase Akt is activated by 3-phosphorylated inositol lipids generated by phosphatidylinositol 3-kinase. Cytokines like VEGF and IGF-1 increase release of NO through this mechanism. Estrogen also increases Akt-phosphorylation of eNOS and may represent a mechanism by which the hormone exerts a rapid, nongenomic release of NO from endothelial cells. The Akt pathway is also involved in flow mediated release of NO. Calcium sensitivity of Akt-phosphorylated eNOS is about 15 times that of unphosphorylated enzyme, thus enabling enzyme activity at low levels of intracellular calcium. Hyperglycemia, on the other hand, causes increases in glycosylation of eNOS, which may represent one mechanism causing diabetic-associated vasculopathy.[53]

NO synthase can be inhibited competitively by exogenous L-arginine analogs—of which the prototype is N^G-monomethyl-L-arginine (L-NMMA), which have permitted the exploration of the role of NO in vivo. A circulating, endogenous inhibitor of NOS, asymmetric dimethylarginine (ADMA), is being examined in association with risk for development of cardiovascular disease.[54,55]

Several neurohumoral substances augment the release of NO by activating specific endothelial receptors (see Fig. 5-6). They include circulating hormones (e.g., catecholamines [stimulating α_2-adrenoceptors], 17β-estradiol, vasopressin and oxytocin [V_1-receptors], endothelin 1 [ET_B-receptors], and possibly angiotensin II [AT_2-receptors]), platelet products (serotonin [$5HT_{1D}$-receptors] and adenine nucleotides [P_{2Y}-receptors]), products of coagulation (thrombin) and autacoids produced by the blood vessel wall itself, for example, histamine and bradykinin (B_2 receptors). The cell membrane receptors for these different endogenous substances are coupled to the activity of endothelial NO synthase by different G-proteins. Thus, thrombin-receptors, $5HT_{1D}$-receptors, α_2-adrenoceptors, and ET_B-receptors are coupled to pertussis toxin-sensitive G_i-proteins, whereas

B_2 receptors and P_{2Y}-receptors are coupled to pertussis toxin-insensitive G_q-proteins or other membrane-binding mechanisms. For example, the intracellular domain 4 of the B_2 receptor and the angiotensin II R1 receptor inhibit eNOS activity. Therefore, polymorphisms in these receptor subtypes will affect NO release through post-translational mechanisms (see Fig. 5-6).[53,56-58]

Actions of NO NO is a freely diffusible gas. Its half-life under physiologic conditions is but a few seconds because it is avidly scavenged by superoxide anions and heme-containing molecules, in particular, oxyhemoglobin. Endothelium-derived NO acts directly on the endothelial cells themselves, and diffuses both in luminal and abluminal directions. In the endothelial cells, it inhibits the production of endothelium-derived hyperpolarizing factor(s) (EDHF) as well as that of endothelin-1, the oxidation of low-density lipoproteins (LDL) to oxy LDL, and the expression of adhesion molecules that permit the adhesion of platelets and white cells to the endothelium. At the interface with the blood, NO cannot penetrate deeply into the bloodstream because it is scavenged by oxyhemoglobin. However, it acts in synergy with prostacyclin to inhibit platelet activation, and, thus, the release of platelet-derived substances including serotonin, thromboxane A_2, and platelet-derived growth factor (PDGF). In the underlying vascular smooth muscle, endothelium-derived NO inhibits the contractile process and cell proliferation. The cellular actions of NO (and of NO donors—such as the nitrovasodilators) are due mainly to activation of soluble guanylyl cyclase (see Smooth Muscle Relaxation).[54,59]

The cyclic GMP-mediated effects of NO, which contribute to endothelium-dependent relaxations and to the regulation of vascular tone include: (1) stimulating Na^+-K^+ ATP-ase and opening of ATP-dependent K^+ channels (K_{ATP}) causing hyperpolarization of the cell membrane; (2) inhibiting Ca^{2+}-channels, stimulating plasma membrane associated calcium ATP-ase and reducing calcium release from the sarcoplasmic reticulum—these actions jointly reduce the intracellular Ca^{2+} concentration; (3) inhibiting phospholipase C and reducing the amount of stimulatory phosphoinositides; and (4) phosphorylating proteins accelerating the relaxation process and inhibiting Rho-kinase causing reduced interaction of the contractile proteins. In addition, NO can open certain Ca^{2+}-dependent K^+-channels, and accelerate K^+ efflux directly, thus hyperpolarizing the cell membrane of the vascular smooth muscle cells.

Indirect actions of NO include: (1) inhibiting phosphodiesterase II which is responsible for the breakdown of cyclic AMP, potentiating the relaxations caused by adenosine, prostacyclin, and β-adrenergic agonists; (2) inhibiting renin release and the production of angiotensin II; (3) inhibiting the production of endothelin-1; and (4) scavenging of superoxide anions and other radicals that underlie endothelium-dependent contractions (see later). These indirect actions all help to explain the vasoconstrictor responses and the increase in arterial blood pressure observed in vivo with inhibitors of NO synthase.

Physiologic Role The increased release of NO in response to shear stress explains flow-dependent vasodilation in vivo, and probably is the single most important local factor modulating the activity of eNOS, as well as the hallmark of proper endothelial function.[60] The effects of catecholamines and vasopressin on endothelial cells in certain, but not all, vascular beds (coronary and cerebral circulation, respectively) favor the preferential distribution of blood flow to those tissues. The release of NO by angiotensin II and endothelin-1 present in the blood may blunt exaggerated responses to those two powerful vasoconstrictor peptides. The stimulated production of NO by histamine and substance P underlies the local vasodilation and the redness of the skin (*rubor*) during allergic reactions and axon reflexes, respectively. The effect of bradykinin on endothelial B_2-kinin receptors sustains the secretion of exocrine glands, but also contributes to the responses to shear stress (which activates a local kinin-generating system both in animal and human blood vessels). The endothelial response to thrombin and platelet products is essential for the protective role played by the endothelium against unwanted platelet aggregation and coagulation of blood. Indeed, platelet aggregation causes serotonin and ADP release, as well as local activation of the coagulation process with the resulting production of thrombin. Serotonin, ADP, and thrombin synergize to locally stimulate the production of NO which diffuses toward the underlying smooth muscle. The resulting dilation helps to disperse the microaggregate. The diffusion of NO toward the lumen, in further synergy with prostacyclin, inhibits the adhesion and aggregation of platelets, eliminating the imminent danger of vascular occlusion.

Inducible NO Synthase Besides the constitutive eNOS, vascular cells may express an inducible form (NOS II) in response to endotoxin and cytokines, which will evoke a long-lasting release of large amounts of NO, resulting in cytotoxic activities. Activated endothelial cells express a cytosolic enzyme, of 150-kDa molecular mass, independent of Ca^{++}-calmodulin with characteristics similar to those of cytokine-activated macrophages. This form of NO synthase can also be induced in vascular smooth muscle cells and produces large amounts of NO for prolonged periods of time during immunologic and inflammatory reactions. Such events may play a role in the irreversible phase of septic shock, which is characterized by peripheral vascular paralysis.

Chronic Modulation Several chronic factors can upregulate the release or the bioavailability of NO. These include chronic exposure to estrogens, chronic increases in blood flow, exercise training and intake of ω_2-unsaturated fatty acids, and red wine polyphenols or other antioxidants (vitamins C and E). From the pharmacologic point of view, the sex steroids, in particular estrogens, are the most important. Indeed, 17β-estradiol increases the efficacy of the NO-cyclic GMP pathway. First, the hormone possesses antioxidant properties, and, like other antioxidants, augments the bioavailability of NO through scavenging of oxygen-derived free radicals. In addition, 17β-estradiol may increase eNOS through nongenomic stimulation of surface estrogen receptors (most likely estrogen receptor α or ERS 1) in caveolae. It remains controversial whether or not changes in intracellular calcium are required for this signaling cascade and whether or not other signaling mechanisms, such as heat shock protein 90, mitogen-activated protein kinase, and cyclic AMP contribute to the estrogenic regulation of NO (see Fig. 5-6). The gene for eNOS (NOS III) also contains partial sequences for estrogen receptors. Therefore, prolonged treatment or exposure of endothelial cells to estrogen increases both the mRNA expression and the protein amount for NOS III. Changes in NO observed in experimental animals and humans with sexual development, ovariectomy, or menopause and estrogen treatment probably reflect these combined effects of estrogen at the membrane and cytoplasmic (nongenomic) and nuclear (genomic) sites. Disruption in regulation of NO by ERS 1 may account for development of cardiovascular disease in individuals with polymorphisms in this estrogen receptor.[53,61,62]

Endothelium-Dependent Hyperpolarizations In 1982, De Mey and coworkers compared endothelium-dependent relaxations induced by acetylcholine, thrombin, and arachidonic acid in isolated femoral arteries.[63] This comparison prompted the conclusion that the functional coupling between endothelial cells and the underlying vascular smooth muscle involves at least three different pathways. One pathway does not involve the metabolism of arachidonic acid and obviously is the production of NO by eNOS (see earlier). Another pathway depends on the activity of cyclooxygenase and most likely involves the release of prostacyclin. The inquiry into the alternative route initiated the quest and debate to identify a third factor, which became endothelium-derived hyperpolarizing factor (EDHF).

An obvious first question was whether or not NO, and/or prostacyclin, could explain endothelium-dependent hyperpolarizations. There is no doubt that NO and NO donors, as well as prostacyclin, can cause hyperpolarizations and/or repolarizations in certain arterial smooth muscle cells. However, in the majority of arteries, NO, unlike acetylcholine and/or bradykinin, does not cause hyperpolarization. Under most circumstances, inhibitors of eNOS (and other agents interfering with the L-arginine-NO pathway) and of cyclooxygenase do not prevent endothelium-dependent hyperpolarizations. Endothelium-dependent hyperpolarization must involve the opening of a K^+-conductance as it is prevented by increasing the extracellular K^+ concentration and by nonselective K^+ channel blockers such as tetraethylammonium and tetrabutylammonium. In those cases where NO and prostacyclin cause hyperpolarizations of vascular smooth muscle, these are usually prevented by blockers of ATP-dependent K^+ channels, such as sulfonylureas. This is not the case for endothelium-dependent hyperpolarizations caused by acetylcholine, bradykinin, or substance P. The combination of apamin (an inhibitor of small conductance calcium-activated potassium channels) plus charybdotoxin (a nonspecific inhibitor of calcium-activated potassium channels) prevents the occurrence of endothelium-dependent hyperpolarizations, without affecting hyperpolarization caused by NO, NO donors, or prostacyclin. Not only is it difficult to regard NO as EDHF, but it is more and more likely that NO exerts a tonic negative influence on the release of EDHF, and that blockade or absence of eNOS favors the contribution of endothelium-dependent relaxations mediated by EDHF. Likewise, prostacyclin also cannot be regarded as EDHF, which does not preclude the prostanoid from acting as an alternative relaxing factor when the release of NO and that of EDHF are impaired. The term "EDHF- mediated response" should be restricted to endothelium-dependent hyperpolarizations that cannot be explained by the release of either NO or prostacyclin. Although theoretically it should be used only when the cell membrane potential is actually recorded in the smooth muscle of the vascular preparation studied, it seems reasonable to attribute to endothelium-dependent hyperpolarization the component of endothelium-dependent relaxations that resists full blockade of eNOS and cyclooxygenase. The exact nature of EDHF remains speculative. Among the more recent candidates to explain endothelium-dependent hyperpolarizations are gap junctions, epoxyeicosatrienoic acids (EETs), potassium ions, and hydrogen peroxide (Fig. 5-7).[64-67]

The physiologic role of EDHFs in mediating vasodilation is unclear at this time. Indirect evidence suggests that in the forearm, the increases in blood flow caused by bradykinin and substance P involve a non-NO, non–prostanoid-mediated mechanism that depends on potassium channel activation. Until truly selective inhibitors of EDHF-mediated responses become available for in vivo studies, we will not know whether endothelium-dependent hyperpolarizations are an epiphenomenon or truly contribute to endothelium-dependent vasodilations in the intact organism, and which one(s) of the possible mediators is (are) involved. Data obtained in experiments from isolated blood vessels suggest that EDHF may be more important in smaller resistance vessels than in large arteries. This may explain why animals deficient for connexion-40 (one of the gap junction proteins) are hypertensive. Changes in expression of another gap junction protein, connexin-43, by estrogen also modifies EDHF-mediated responses. Therefore, estrogen may enhance vasodilation through expression of membrane K^+-channels.

Prostacyclin Prostacyclin, a product of cyclooxygenase, is formed primarily in endothelial cells, and causes relaxation of most vascular smooth muscle by activating adenylyl cyclase and augmenting the level of cyclic 3′,5′-adenosine monophosphate (cyclic AMP). In most mammalian arteries, the contribution of prostacyclin to endothelium-dependent relaxations is minor to judge from the limited effect of cyclooxygenase-inhibitors on these responses. However, prostacyclin acts synergistically with NO to inhibit platelet aggregation.

Endothelium-Dependent Contractions

Soon after the pivotal discovery of endothelium-dependent relaxations, De Mey and Vanhoutte (1982)[68] reported that in veins, under given circumstances, the endothelial cells cause contractions, rather than relaxations of the underlying vascular smooth muscle cells. These endothelium-dependent contractions were attributed to the production of a diffusible factor(s), termed *endothelium-derived contracting factor* (EDCF). Endothelium-dependent contractions can be caused by withdrawal of relaxing factors or

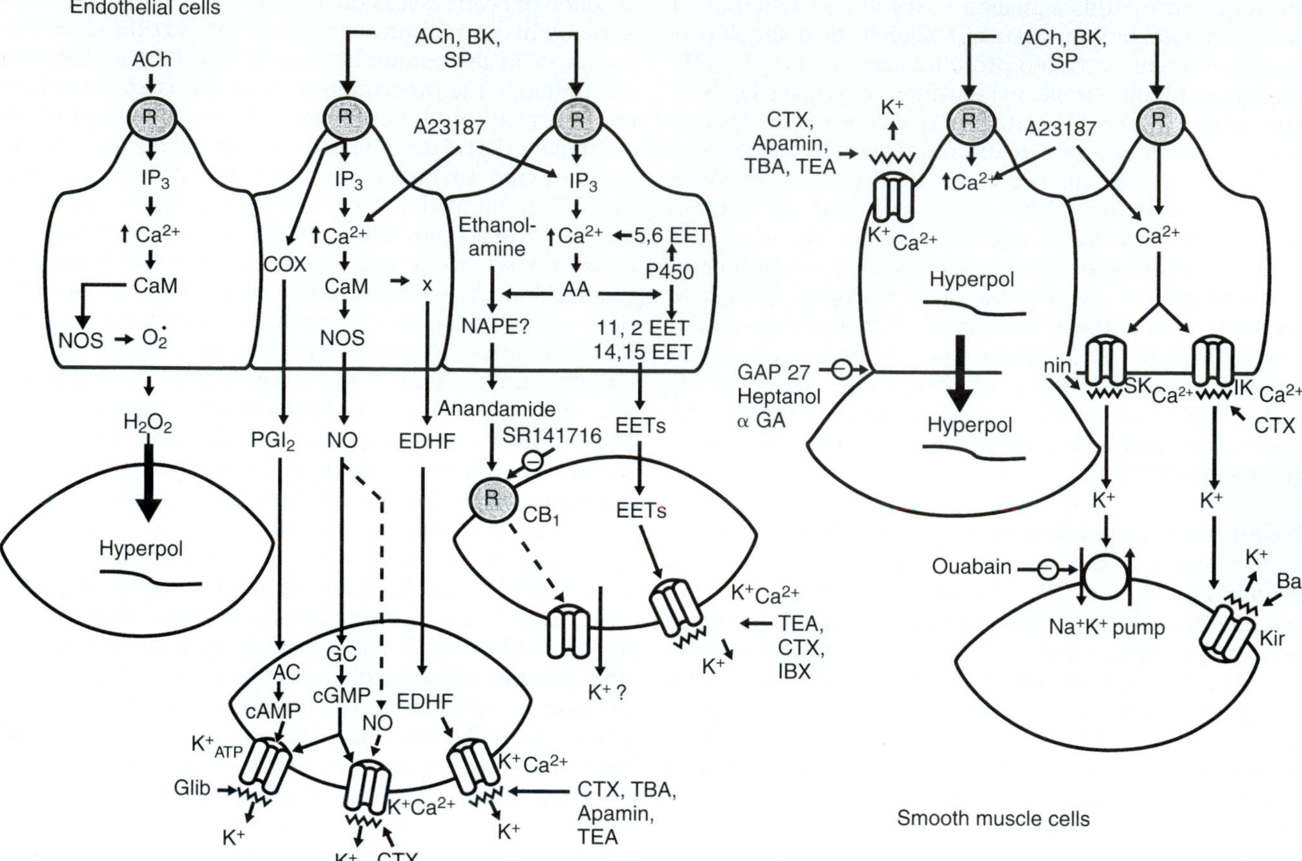

FIGURE 5-7. Schematic of mechanisms leading to endothelium-dependent hyperpolarization. Substances such as acetylcholine (ACh), bradykinin (BK), and substance P (SP), through the activation of M_3-muscarinic, B_2-bradykinin, and NK_1-neurokinin receptor subtypes, respectively, and agents that increase intracellular calcium, such as the calcium ionophore A23187, release endothelium-derived hyperpolarizing factors. SR141716 is an antagonist of the cannabinoid CB_1 receptor subtype (CB_1). Glibenclamide (Glib) is a selective inhibitor of ATP-sensitive potassium channels (K^+_{ATP}). Tetraethylammonium (TEA) and tetrabutylammonium (TBA) are nonspecific inhibitors of potassium channels when used at high concentrations (>5 mM), whereas at lower concentrations (1 to 3 mM) these drugs are selective for calcium-activated potassium channels ($K^+_{Ca^{2+}}$). Iberiotoxin (IBX) is a specific inhibitor of large conductance $K^+_{Ca^{2+}}$. Charybdotoxin (CTX) is an inhibitor of large conductance $K^+_{Ca^{2+}}$, intermediate conductance $K^+_{Ca^{2+}}$ ($IK_{Ca^{2+}}$), and voltage-dependent potassium channels. Apamin is a specific inhibitor of small conductance $K^+_{Ca^{2+}}$ ($SK_{Ca^{2+}}$). Barium (Ba^{2+}), in the micromolar range, is a specific inhibitor of the inward rectifier potassium channel (K_{ir}). GAP 27 (an eleven-amino acid peptide possessing conserved sequence homology to a portion of the second extracellular loop of connexin), 18[α]-glycyrrhetinic acid ([α]GA), and heptanol are gap junction uncouplers. CaM, calmodulin; COX, cyclooxygenase; EET, epoxyeicosatrienoic acid; IP_3, inositol trisphosphate; GC, guanylate cyclase; Hyperpol, hyperpolarization; NAPE, *N*-acylphosphatidylethanolamine; NOS, NO synthase; $O_2^{\cdot}$, superoxide anions; PGI_2, prostacyclin; P450, cytochrome P450 monooxygenase; R, receptor; X, putative EDHF synthase. (Reprinted with permission from Vanhoutte, PM: Endothelium-derived free radicals: For worse and for better. J Clin Invest, 107:23, 2001).

through production of specific factors activating receptors on vascular smooth muscle.

Withdrawal of the Release of NO If the vascular smooth muscle of a blood vessel possesses spontaneous (myogenic) tone, or is exposed to vasoconstrictor signals (e.g., sympathetic nerve activity), a sudden withdrawal of the basal release of NO evokes acute endothelium-dependent contractions in isolated blood vessels, or acute increases in peripheral resistance and/or arterial blood pressure in the intact organism. In vivo, the response is due in part to the withdrawal of the inhibitory effect of NO on the production of the vasoconstrictor peptides angiotensin II (via inhibition of renin release) and endothelin-1, rather than that of its direct relaxing effect on the smooth muscle cells. A decreased basal release of NO also probably explains the endothelium-dependent contractions caused by anoxia, particularly in arteries previously exposed to ischemia-reperfusion injury. In the intact organism, besides hypoxia, they may be induced by a sudden surge in the production of the endogenous inhibitors of NOS, asymmetric dimethyl arginine (ADMA).

Cyclooxygenase-Dependent Endothelium-Dependent Contractions The first observations demonstrating the phenomenon of endothelium-dependent contractions were made in isolated veins.[68] In these preparations, arachidonic acid and thrombin, which are endothelium-dependent dilators in isolated arteries, potentiated, in an endothelium-dependent fashion, contractions evoked by α_1-adrenergic agonists. In quiescent cerebral arteries, acetylcholine, a potent endothelium-dependent dilator in most other arteries, evokes pronounced endothelium-dependent contractions. In both arteries and veins, endothelium-dependent contractions are prevented by incubation with inhibitors of cyclooxygenase. Thus, product(s) of cyclooxygenase (COX) must play a key role in EDCF-mediated responses. At least in animal blood vessels, preferential inhibitors of COX-1 rather than those of COX-2 prevent endothelium-dependent contractions to acetylcholine. Dazoxiben (an inhibitor of thromboxane synthase) does not significantly affect indomethacin-sensitive endothelium-dependent contractions to acetylcholine, ruling out a major contribution of thromboxane A_2. However, the response is prevented by endoperoxide/thromboxane (TP)-receptor antagonists, implying that an endogenous agonist at TP-receptors, other than thromboxane A_2, mediates the response. Endoperoxides, the precursors of thromboxane A_2, which are formed by cyclooxygenase and also activate TP-receptors, are the likely alternative candidates. In arteries where it induces endothelium-dependent contractions, acetylcholine, indeed, causes an augmented release of endoperoxides. The activation of TP-receptors on the vascular smooth muscle cells is the final event leading to endothelium-dependent contractions.[69]

Endothelium-dependent contractions are not seen in isolated blood vessels incubated in calcium-free solutions. The calcium ionophore A23187 causes endothelium-dependent contractions of preparations where acetylcholine does so. These observations imply that an increase in intracellular concentration of Ca^{2+} is the initiating step leading to EDCF-mediated responses. Oxygen-derived free radicals also play a key role in the phenomenon. Indeed, endothelium-contractions are prevented by intracellular and sometimes even by extracellular scavengers of superoxide anions. By contrast, a background production of oxygen-derived free radicals potentiates EDCF-mediated responses.

The most likely hypothesis to explain the occurrence of cyclooxygenase-dependent, endothelium-dependent contractions is as follows: in certain arteries acetylcholine activates muscarinic receptors on the endothelial cell membrane, resulting in an increased intracellular concentration of calcium, which has two consequences. The activity of eNOS is augmented, and NO diffuses to the underlying arterial smooth muscle, where it stimulates soluble guanylyl cyclase to produce more cyclic GMP. The increased intracellular calcium concentration also stimulates the production by the endothelial cells of superoxide anions, from an undefined source. Depending on the amount of NO, which scavenges superoxide anions, more or less superoxide anions, or its derivatives, can diffuse outside the endothelial cells. The intracellular, but maybe also extracellular, superoxide anions activate COX1 to transform arachidonic acid into endoperoxides. The latter cross the intercellular space and stimulate the TP-receptors of the vascular smooth muscle. Thus, both an augmented activity of COX1 and a sufficient responsiveness of the TP-receptors are required for the occurrence of endothelium-dependent contractions. A reduction in the release or the bioavailability of NO augments the amplitude of the endothelium-dependent contractions, as does an increased production of oxygen-derived free radicals. By contrast, scavenging or depleting superoxide anions depresses the response.

The stimulation of TP-receptors leads to an increase in intracellular calcium concentration in the vascular smooth muscle cells, and thus to activation of the contractile process. TP-receptor activation also has a permissive role for the action of other growth-promoting substances. It is unknown if, at the interface between the endothelial cells and the blood, EDCF acts on TP-receptors of the platelets to potentiate their aggregation.

In large cerebral arteries, acute distention causes endothelium-dependent contractions. It is likely that this type of response could participate in autoregulatory adjustments of the diameter in response to sudden surges in arterial blood pressure. However, in most other cases, endothelium-dependent contractions are a pathologic occurrence. Endothelium-dependent contractions to acetylcholine appear in arteries of estrogen-deprived female animals, presumably as a consequence of the reduced production of NO.

Endothelin In addition to metabolites of arachidonic acid, which contract vascular smooth muscle, endothelial cells produce a potent vasoconstrictor, endothelin (ET). The ET family consists of three vasoconstrictor peptides, termed ET-1, ET-2, and ET-3—but ET-1 is the only member of the family to be synthesized by endothelial cells. Because there are no known endothelial storage sites for ET, the peptide is apparently produced on demand with the messenger RNA (mRNA) for its production being rapidly inactivated. Factors that induce mRNA production and release of ET include thrombin, arginine-vasopressin, angiotensin II, epinephrine, prolonged (12 to 24 hours) hypoxia, the calcium ionophore A23187, phorbol esters, and shear stress. ET is synthesized by endothelial cells initially as a 203-residue peptide named pre-proendothelin. After subsequent processing, it becomes the 39-amino acid termed big endothelin (proendothelin). Big endothelin is transformed by ET-converting enzyme (ECE) to the 21-amino acid peptide ET. Stimulation of angiotensin-1 receptors on the endothelial surface by angiotensin II will enhance the conversion of big endothelin-1 to endothelin-1. Therefore, inhibition of ACE decreases vascular resistance because of decreased stimulation of angiotensin II-mediated contraction of the vascular smooth muscle, but also indirectly through inhibition of production of ET-1 in endothelial cells. Statins also inhibit production of ET-1 by inhibiting transcription and mRNA expression for pre-proendothelin by a mechanism mediated by Rho proteins.[70,71]

ET-1 binds to a single class of sites consisting of two receptor subtypes: ET_A or ET_B. Distribution of these receptors varies with the anatomic origin of the blood vessel (systemic or pulmonary; artery or vein). Stimulation of endothelin receptors on endothelial cells releases endothelium-derived relaxing factors, and alternatively endothelium-derived NO inhibits stimulated release of ET. Under basal conditions, an intact endothelium reduces the contractile response to ET; this could be due both to basal release of NO and EDHF because NO released by the endothelium inhibits the constrictor response to the peptide.

On vascular smooth muscle, stimulation of ET-receptors causes a rise in intracellular calcium and initiates contraction. The available evidence suggests that ET-1 activates the phosphoinositide cascade to generate inositol triphosphate, which releases calcium from intracellular stores. The entry of extracellular calcium is not required for contraction to ET-1 in all blood vessels; this most likely reflects the heterogeneity in extracellular calcium requirements of vascular smooth muscle from different sites.

Infusion of ET-1 in vivo induces a transient vasodilation, which likely is due to the release of vasodilator prostaglandins (e.g., prostacyclin), of endothelium-derived NO, and of EDHF. The depressor response to ET-1 is followed by a sustained and long-lasting increase in blood pressure resulting from an increase in peripheral vascular resistance that is best explained by the direct constrictor effect of the peptide on vascular smooth muscle. Endothelin is a more potent constrictor of arterioles than large arteries and a more potent constrictor of veins than arteries.

The slow onset and prolonged action of ET-1, coupled with its relatively slow rate of production (requiring de novo protein synthesis), suggests that the peptide is more likely to contribute to physiologic mid- or long-term regulation rather than to contribute to moment-to-moment changes in vascular tone. In addition, alterations in regulation of ET-1 may participate in a variety of cardiovascular disorders because circulating blood levels of ET in patients are increased in several disease states, including hypertension, heart failure, acute myocardial infarction, and ischemic heart disease. Both ET_A- (e.g., darusentan, sitaxsentan) and ET_B- (e.g., BQ-788) selective receptor antagonists, as well as nonselective antagonists (e.g., bosentan, tezosentan), have been developed during the past decade but it remains unclear whether receptor subtype selective antagonists or nonselective receptor antagonists will provide the most therapeutic benefits. Overall, the clinical benefits of ET receptor antagonists have been very modest. The only proved efficacy has been with the use of bosentan in the short-term treatment of patients with pulmonary arterial hypertension.[72-78]

NEUROHUMORAL MEDIATORS OF VASCULAR TONE

In addition to pharmacologic compounds released from nerve endings and the endothelium, other substances derived as byproducts of energy metabolism or synthesized in nonvascular tissues, such as blood elements or the liver, affect vascular tone. These substances may affect vascular tone directly through activation of receptors on vascular smooth muscle or indirectly by modulating release of neurotransmitter or endothelium-derived factors. Those of major clinical relevance are discussed in this section.

Amines

5-Hydroxytryptamine (5-HT, Serotonin)

With the exception of some areas of the cerebral circulation, most blood vessels are not innervated by serotonergic neurons. Most of the circulating serotonin originates in the enterochromaffin cells of the gastrointestinal tract that synthesize and release it into the portal circulation. Serotonin is inactivated by the liver or by endothelial cells (mainly in the lungs); the remaining part is taken up and stored by the platelets. As a consequence, very little, if any, serotonin is present in the plasma. Hence, levels of serotonin sufficient to affect the blood vessel wall probably occur only at sites of endothelial damage where platelet aggregation occurs. Serotonin causes both vasoconstriction and vasodilation by interacting with receptors located on vascular smooth muscle cells, endothelial cells, or adrenergic nerve endings (Fig. 5-8). In most systemic arterial smooth muscle, serotonin induces contractions that are antagonized by $5HT_{2A}$-antagonists such as ketanserin and sarpogrelate.[79] In cerebral and coronary arteries, serotonin-induced contractions may be mediated by activation of $5\text{-}HT_1$ receptors.

In addition to its direct contractile effects on vascular smooth muscle, serotonin amplifies the effects of other vasoconstrictor agonists such as histamine, angiotensin II, prostaglandin F_{2a}, and norepinephrine. In vascular smooth muscle endowed with $5\text{-}HT_{2A}$-serotonergic receptors, this action of serotonin is antagonized by ketanserin.

The release of norepinephrine from adrenergic nerve varicosities can be inhibited by serotonin. This action of the monoamine explains why it causes vasodilation when sympathetic tone is high but vasoconstriction when it is low; in the latter case, the direct activation of the smooth muscle by serotonin predominates. The prejunctional inhibitory action of serotonin is mediated by receptors with pharmacological similarities to the $5\text{-}HT_1$-serotonergic subtype.

At high concentrations, serotonin can act as an indirect sympathomimetic amine by displacing norepinephrine from sympathetic nerve endings—an effect that can be blocked by inhibitors of neuronal uptake. In some arteries, serotonin produces endothelium-dependent relaxations. These are due mainly to the release of NO.

The endothelium-dependent relaxation evoked by serotonin is inhibited by the $5\text{-}HT_{1D}$-antagonists, indicating that the endothelial receptors involved belong to the $5\text{-}HT_{1D}$ subtype. These receptors are coupled to the release of NO by G_i-proteins. The demonstration of endothelium-dependent effects of serotonin is complicated by the direct activation of the smooth muscle that it causes.

Aggregating platelets release enough serotonin to affect smooth muscle cells, adrenergic nerves, and endothelium. However, serotonin plays a role in disease only if exaggerated amounts of it are released, if the removal of the monoamine from the plasma is deficient, or if the vascular wall is hyperresponsive to its constrictor effect. The latter occurs mainly when the endothelial cells are mechanically removed or become dysfunctional.

Augmented vascular responsiveness to serotonin appears to characterize the blood vessel wall chronically exposed to an abnormally high blood pressure. The potent contractile effect of serotonin may contribute to vasospastic disorders, in arteries covered with regenerated endothelium, and in atherosclerotic arteries.

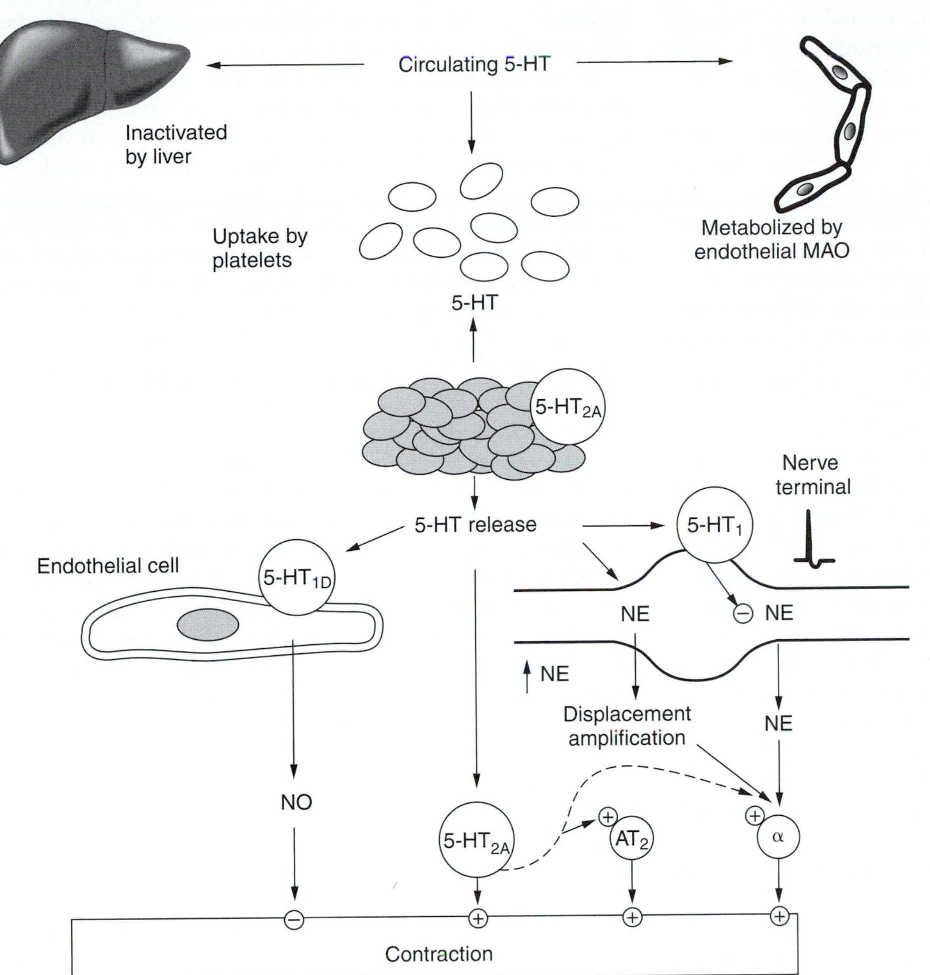

FIGURE 5-8. Schematic of metabolism and actions of serotonin (5-HT). Serotonin is metabolized by the liver and endothelial cells and taken up by platelets. When released from platelets, it can bind to receptors on adrenergic nerve terminals, endothelial cells, and vascular smooth muscle cells. The direct action of 5-HT on endothelial cells is to initiate release of endothelium-derived nitric oxide (NO). Under normal physiologic conditions, stimulation of serotonin receptors on the adrenergic terminal will inhibit the release of norepinephrine. However, under pathophysiologic situations, such as hypertension, 5-HT facilitates the release of NE as well as displaces it from vesicles in the nerve terminal. On vascular smooth muscle cells, 5-HT causes contraction and potentiates contractions caused by stimulation of α-adrenergic receptors and angiotensin receptors. 5-HT receptor subclasses: 5-HT_{2A}, 5-HT_{1D}; MAO, monoamine oxidase; NE, norepinephrine.

Histamine

Histamine is stored primarily in mast cells and basophils. In large arteries and veins, histamine is also stored in a non-mast cell pool, presumably the smooth muscle cells. Based on the relative potencies of several antagonists, two classes of histamine receptors are known to exist: H_1- and H_2-histamine receptors.[80]

Functional histamine receptors are present in vascular smooth muscle, adrenergic nerve endings, and endothelial cells. The predominant effect of histamine in humans is to reduce peripheral vascular resistance and lower systemic blood pressure. Depending on the blood vessel, species, and concentration, however, histamine can elicit either contraction or relaxation by virtue of its direct effect on vascular smooth muscle. Contractions are mediated by H_1-receptors, because they are attenuated by H_1-receptor antagonists; in some blood vessels, contractions are reversed to relaxations by such antagonists. These relaxations are inhibited by H_2-receptor antagonists. Thus, H_1 and H_2-receptors are present in the vascular wall. The contractions are initiated by H_1 receptors, and the relaxation is mediated by H_2 receptors on vascular smooth muscle. However, relaxations can also be due to activation of H_1-receptors on the endothelium. Such endothelium-dependent relaxations to histamine are mediated by prostacyclin or NO (or both) released from the endothelial cells. In most cases, combined treatment with H_1- and H_2-receptor antagonists abolishes relaxations to histamine. Classical histamine-receptor antagonists, such as mepyramine and diphenhydramine, are selective for H_1-histamine receptors. H_2-histamine receptor antagonists include metiamide, cimetidine, and ranitidine. Histamine is an important mediator of the vasodilation accompanying inflammatory reactions, presumably because of its combined action on smooth muscle, adrenergic nerves, and endothelial cells.[81]

C-Reactive Protein (CRP)

CRP is a highly conserved pentraxin protein (five noncovalently associated protomers arranged symmetrically around a central core). CRP is classified as an "acute phase" protein or first-line defense molecule against pathogenic organisms as it binds to phosphocholine of bacterial and fungal membranes and activates the complement system. CRP also stimulates phagocytic cells that remove apoptotic and necrotic cells, thus contributing to healing of injured tissue. Production of CRP from the liver is stimulated by cytokines associated with nonspecific tissue injury such as interleukin-1B, interleukin-6, and tumor necrosis factor.[82]

Whether or not concentrations of CRP differ between males and females or increases with age is unresolved, with some studies showing trends for increases with age and higher values in females than in males. Oral conjugated equine estrogen—but not estradiol patches or the selective estrogen receptor modulator raloxifene—increases CRP.[83-85]

As a component of the "acute phase response" associated with infection, inflammation, and tissue damage, measurement of CRP in the general clinical setting is used to diagnose new disease, monitor chronic inflammatory disease, or screen for unknown infections and malignancies.[83] Atherosclerosis has long been identified as an inflammatory disease. Therefore, it is not surprising that CRP is emerging as a potential risk factor for cardiovascular disease.[86] Although significant statistical correlation exists between plasma CRP and adverse cardiovascular events, a clear cause-and-effect relationship between elevated CRP levels alone and cardiovascular disease has not been established. Indeed, few studies have attempted to define how CRP affects vascular smooth muscle or endothelial function. One theory is that CRP binds to modified LDL within atherosclerotic plaques. Because CRP is an acute phase reactant, activation of thrombosis and complement would result. CRP applied to endothelial cells in culture decreases expression of eNOS. Acute application of commercially available CRP to isolated rings of human internal mammary artery causes dose- and endothelium-independent relaxations.[87] Therefore, CRP exerts direct hyperpolarizing effects on the smooth muscle as well as perhaps more chronic effects on eNOS in endothelial cells. However, these responses may be due to sodium azide contaminating the commercially available product.[88]

Guidelines or reference standards for interpretation of plasma CRP, as they might be applied to predicting cardiovascular risk, are beginning to emerge—especially to guide intensity of risk reduction in individuals with high lipids or metabolic syndrome in women.[89] However, whether or not CRP may be considered one of a group or list of inflammation-associated cytokines that affect endothelium-dependent responses[90] remains to be seen.

Peptides

Vasopressin

The neurohypophyseal peptide vasopressin promotes water reabsorption by the kidney, vasoconstriction in most peripheral vascular beds, and dilation of large cerebral arteries. Vasopressin exerts its peripheral effects by activating two subtypes of receptors (1) V_1-vasopressinergic receptors located in the blood vessel wall; and (2) V_2-vasopressinergic receptors in the renal tubules. The V_2-vasopressinergic receptors are closely linked to adenylyl cyclase formation, which increases the water permeability of the luminal membrane in the distal portions of the nephron. V_2 receptors are also present on digital arteries where they cause vasodilation by an endothelium-dependent, NO-dependent mechanism.

Receptors for vasopressin in systemic vascular smooth muscle mediate vasoconstriction by increasing cytosolic Ca^{2+} concentration. Besides its direct vasoconstrictor effects, vasopressin also interacts with pre- and postjunctional adrenergic sites to facilitate both the indirect and direct effects of adrenergic agonists.

In cerebral arteries, vasopressin induces an endothelium-dependent relaxation. These relaxations can be prevented by the V_1-vasopressinergic antagonist $d(CH_2)_5Tyr(Me)AVP$, suggesting that effects of the neuropeptide are mediated by activation of V_1-vasopressinergic receptors on endothelial cells. Inhibitors of cyclooxygenase and lipoxygenase do not affect the inhibitory effect of vasopressin, which rules out a major role of prostacyclin in the phenomenon. The endothelium-dependent relaxations of the basilar artery to vasopressin are prevented by inhibitors of Na^+,K^+-ATPase; it is unknown whether the inhibition of Na,K-ATPase affects the endothelial or smooth muscle cells of the basilar artery.

The differential effects of vasopressin on cerebral and peripheral arteries (vasodilation and vasoconstriction, respectively) favor the redistribution of blood from the periphery to the cerebral circulation during hemorrhage and shock. Considerable experimental work has identified differences in responses to vasopressin between blood vessels derived from male and female animals. However, the relationship between these differences and regulation of vascular function or development of cardiovascular disease in humans is unclear.

Angiotensin II

The renin-angiotensin system regulates blood pressure, water, and electrolyte balance. The primary mediator of this system is the octapeptide angiotensin II. Besides stimulating the synthesis and secretion of aldosterone by the adrenal cortex, angiotensin II is also a potent vasoconstrictor. The synthesis of angiotensin II is initiated when the enzyme renin, which is secreted from the kidney, acts on angiotensinogen in the plasma to release the decapeptide angiotensin I. This decapeptide has minimal pharmacologic activity. Angiotensin I is cleaved by angiotensin-converting enzyme (ACE) to generate angiotensin II. ACE is present in endothelial cells and is downregulated transcriptionally by 17β estradiol. The octapeptide, in turn, may be further cleaved by aminopeptidase to form angiotensin III. Although angiotensin I and angiotensin III are pharmacologically active, they are considerably less potent than angiotensin II. The conversion of angiotensinogen to angiotensin I by renin is the rate limiting step in the biosynthesis of angiotensin II. Inhibitors of angiotensin-converting enzyme, such as captopril and enalapril, inhibit the biosynthesis of angiotensin II, thus limiting the amount of octapeptide available for receptor activation.

Angiotensin II causes contraction of most arterial and arteriolar smooth muscle cells and of certain venous smooth muscle cells. It also augments the vasoconstrictor responses to sympathetic-nerve stimulation by enhancing local synthesis of norepinephrine, inhibiting neuronal uptake of catecholamines, and facilitating the exocytotic release of norepinephrine. The stimulation of adrenergic neurotransmission caused by the octapeptide, combined with the activation of central angiotensin-receptor sites and the facilitation of transmission at the sympathetic ganglia, can augment the amount of norepinephrine present in the vicinity of the vascular effector cells.

The development of angiotensin receptor antagonists has been a major focus since the discovery of the renin-angiotensin system. Initially, a number of angiotensin II-receptor antagonists were synthesized by modifying the amino acid composition of the octapeptide. Saralasin is the best studied of these antagonists. It is a weak partial agonist that behaves as a competitive antagonist at angiotensin II receptors. Like all peptides, these agents suffer from poor oral bioavailability, thus limiting their clinical usefulness. More recently, several potent, orally active nonpeptide receptor antagonists, such as losartan, valsartan, and candesartan have been developed. These newer, so-called *angiotensin receptor blockers* (ARBs) are highly selective for the angiotensin II type-1 receptor. As with the ACE inhibitors, ARBs are widely used in treating several cardiovascular disorders, including hypertension and congestive heart failure.[91-94]

In contrast to its direct vasoconstrictor effect, angiotensin II can induce endothelium-dependent relaxation of renal and cerebral arteries; this effect is apparently mediated by the production of prostacyclin.

To judge from animal data, renovascular hypertension may be accompanied by an augmented responsiveness to angiotensin II at a time when the resistance vessels respond normally to other vasoconstrictor agonists, particularly catecholamines. Thus, angiotensin-receptor antagonists and converting-enzyme inhibitors lower blood pressure in certain forms of hypertension. Numerous studies have examined associations among angiotensin II receptor polymorphisms and cardiovascular disease. However, none has provided consistent relationships.

Bradykinin

The physiologic role of bradykinin is not well understood, but it has long been associated with the secretion of exocrine glands and with defense and repair responses, particularly inflammatory reactions.[40] Bradykinin is a nonapeptide formed in plasma and other biologic fluids by cleavage of precursors known as kininogens. The cleavage of kininogens is affected by enzymes, referred to as *kallikreins*, produced by the liver and by the exocrine glands. The synthesis of bradykinin is activated by Hageman factor when blood comes into contact with negatively charged surfaces, such as glass or collagen, which is readily exposed by tissue damage. Bradykinin is inactivated by the same enzyme responsible for the conversion of angiotensin I to angiotensin II, namely, angiotensin-converting enzyme (ACE) and by neutral endopeptidase.[95] Therefore, the new class of "vasopeptidase" inhibitors with combined inhibition of ACE and NEP enhance vasorelaxation through inhibition of contractile actions of angiotensin II and enhanced biologic vasodilatory activity of bradykinin. Such inhibitors, however, do not possess a safety profile compatible with clinical use.[96-99]

The biologic actions of bradykinin are mediated by specific receptors on the cell surface. Based on the order of potency of a series of structurally related peptides, at least two different receptors for bradykinin may exist.[100] These receptors have been designated B_1- and B_2-bradykinin receptors. Bradykinin is a potent vasodilator in vivo. Depending on their anatomical origin and species, however, isolated blood vessels may relax, contract, or show no response at all to bradykinin. Contractions to bradykinin are most prominent in veins. The stimulatory action of bradykinin on vascular smooth muscle is independent of the endothelium and may be mediated by both B_1 and B_2 receptors.

Relaxation of vascular smooth muscle by bradykinin appears to be an indirect effect mediated by the release of other vasoactive substances. Bradykinin-induced relaxations of cat and rabbit arteries are independent of the endothelium. These relaxations are suppressed by inhibitors of cyclooxygenase, suggesting that vasodilator prostaglandins, such as PGE_2 and prostacyclin, may play a role in mediating the response to bradykinin in these blood vessels.

Bradykinin depresses the response of isolated arteries to electrical stimulation of the adrenergic nerves; a similar depression is reported in the perfused kidney during sympathetic-nerve activation. In isolated pulmonary arteries, bradykinin reduces the overflow of norepinephrine evoked by electrical impulses. The decrease of the vasoconstrictor response in the kidney and the reduction of the overflow of transmitter in the pulmonary artery are accompanied by an augmented production of prostaglandin-like material, as shown by modulation of these effects by inhibitors of prostaglandin synthesis. Thus, the prejunctional inhibitory effect exerted by bradykinin in blood vessels apparently is secondary to the enhanced biosynthesis of prostanoids that it causes.

In canine and human blood vessels, the relaxation elicited by bradykinin is endothelium dependent. This response is due to the activation of B_2-bradykinin receptors coupled to the release of both NO and EDHF. That the endothelium-dependent response to bradykinin contributes to the local regulation of blood flow is no longer a matter of debate. Thus, potentiation of the endothelium-dependent effects of endogenous bradykinin contributes to the beneficial therapeutic effect of ACE inhibitors. It is likely that the augmented release of NO caused by ACE inhibitors explains, in part, the protective effects of these agents on the cardiovascular system, whereas the potentiated endothelium-dependent hyperpolarizations underlie the reduction in peripheral resistance and in arterial blood pressure. These endothelial effects of ACE inhibitors are of particular importance in patients with low renin.

Atrial (ANP), Brain-Type (BNP), C (CNP), and D (DNP)-Type Natriuretic Peptides

The natriuretic peptides are a family of structurally related but genetically distinct peptides.[101] Atrial natriuretic peptide (ANP—formally ANF) was the first peptide of this family to be described and, as the name implies, was identified in granules in the atria. Subsequently, it was discovered to also be secreted by endothelial cells. ANP is a 28-amino acid peptide with a 17-amino acid ring structure formed by a disulfide bond. C-type natriuretic peptide is a 22-amino acid peptide that, like ANP, has a 17-amino acid ring but lacks a COOH-terminal amino acid on its ring structure. CNP is also produced by endothelial cells.

BNP is a 32-amino acid polypeptide first isolated from brain tissue but is also produced by cardiac tissue. DNP is a 38-amino acid peptide first isolated from venom of the green mamba (*Dendroaspis angusticeps*). DNP can be measured in human blood and is elevated with congestive heart failure and causes relaxation of isolated arteries.[102-104]

Both ANP and BNP are released from arterial and cardiac myocytes, respectively, in response to increased stretch resulting from high filling pressure, high arterial pressure, or cardiac dilation. Physiologic actions of ANP and BNP act to reduce the adverse stimulus of stretch by causing arterio- and venodilation, reduction in blood volume through natriuresis, and suppression of secretions of renin and aldosterone. Therefore, the cause and effect relationship between stretch and release of ANP and BNP is established through basic science experiments and represents a classical physiologic negative-feedback regulatory system.

There are three classes of natriuretic peptide receptors (NPR): -A, -B, and -C. NPR-A is found on endothelial cells; whereas both NPR-A and -B are found on vascular smooth muscle. NPR-C is an intracellular clearance receptor found in both endothelial and vascular smooth muscle. This receptor is required for internalization and degradation of the peptides.

NPR receptors are transmembrane receptors that contain as part of their intracellular domain particulate guanylate cyclase. Therefore, relaxations are mediated, in part, through increases in cGMP as are relaxations to NO. CNP activates potassium channels causing membrane hyperpolarization. Therefore, CNP may represent another class of endothelium-derived hyperpolarizing factors (see earlier). Production of CNP, like NO, is also regulated by shear stress.

The natriuretic peptides act as both paracrine and autocrine regulators of vascular tone because the peptides are produced by the endothelium as well as from cardiac sources. The natriuretic peptides are catabolized by a metalloproteinase on the endothelial surface called *neutral endopeptidase* (NEP). NEP is not selective for the natriuretic peptides and will also inactivate bradykinin.

In general, the natriuretic peptides cause relaxation of vascular smooth muscle but the potency varies depending on the peptide and the anatomic origin of the blood vessel. DNP recognized NPR-A and -C but not -B. Particular vascular pathologies have not been associated with CNP. However, both BNP and DNP increase with congestive heart failure in humans.

VASCULAR PHARMACOGENOMICS

Differences in response to pharmacologic agents between males and females and among humans of different races have been documented for more than 75 years. The emergence of the era of genomics provides an opportunity to better understand sex and racial differences in the presentation of disease and to better target therapeutic and preventive strategies to individuals.[62,105-107]

The sexually dimorphic pair of chromosomes, the sex chromosomes, or the XX or XY chromosomes, influences the incidence of cardiovascular disease, such that cardiovascular disease begins at younger ages in men whereas the incidence of cardiovascular disease increases in women after menopause. In males the XY chromosomes act as a homologous pair with the X chromosome being donated from the mother; in females, the XX chromosomes act as a pair with females having two copies of the X chromosome in each somatic cell, one of which is inactivated. Responses to testosterone are influenced in part by the X chromosome because the gene for the androgen receptor is located on the X chromosome. In terms of cardiovascular disease, the Y chromosome is associated with development of hypertension in males, a response that is modulated by the presence of testosterone.[108]

Unlike the androgen receptor, receptors for estrogen are located on autosomes: estrogen receptor α (ESR1) on chromosome 6 and estrogen receptor β (ESR2) on chromosome 14. Estrogen receptors are present on endothelium and smooth muscle cells throughout the vasculature of both men and women. There have not been systematic studies to evaluate the relative distribution of either receptor on endothelium compared with vascular smooth muscle. However, when mRNA for estrogen receptors was compared from homogenates of whole blood vessels, estrogen receptor β was the predominant receptor and mRNA for estrogen receptor β was greater in blood vessels from females compared with males. No data are available regarding distribution of androgen receptors throughout the vasculature of men and women.[109]

Androgen or estrogen through ligation of their receptors, activate transcription of genes for receptors and proteins which affect regulation and function of vascular smooth muscle (as has been discussed in other sections of this chapter) including α-adrenoceptors receptors; angiotensin II (AT) receptors; endothelin (ET) receptors; endoperoxide-thromboxane (TP) receptors; ion channels and enzymes affecting production of angiotensin, endothelin-1, NO, and prostacyclin.[47,62]

Some polymorphisms in ERS1 are associated with changes in production of NO, synthesis of high density lipoproteins and C-reactive protein, decreases in angiogenesis, and increases in proliferative response to vascular injury.[109-111] Polymorphisms in ERS2 have been associated with changes in protein synthesis, regulation of cell cycle, production of the inducible form of NO synthase related to inflammation and development of hypertension.

In addition to ligand-dependent activation of gene transcription, sex steroids also stimulate membrane receptors and cytosolic enzymes independent of gene transcription by mechanisms classified as nongenomic actions of the hormones. Unlike genomic actions of hormones, which are expressed over hours or days, nongenomic actions of hormones are observed within minutes. Although the physiologic significance of nongenomic actions of hormones on the vasculature is debated, it is possible to consider nongenomic effects as modulating the threshold or cellular milieu on which responses of subsequent agonists, for example—those that affect intracellular calcium or production of NO (see Nitric Oxide), or genomic actions are expressed (see Figs. 5-6 and 5-9).

Because production of sex-specific steroids varies across the life span (childhood to puberty to adulthood), receptors, enzymes, and other cellular processes regulated by the hormones will also vary. Although this association is obvious, it is often not considered in design of clinical trials testing new pharmacologic agents or in prescribing practices for cardiovascular therapies. Such influences should be considered in developing prevention strategies for cardiovascular disease in adolescent boys compared with girls, women during their reproductive years, women transitioning to menopause with associated loss of ovarian hormones, and loss of testosterone in aging men.

There is considerable interest in defining genetic polymorphisms for both receptors and enzymes associated with neurotransmission and humoral modulators of vascular function (see Table 5-3).[106,112] Polymorphisms in potassium channels (i.e., human ether a-go-go related gene, HERG) are associated with drug-induced long QT syndrome and torsades de pointes, which is more prevalent in women than in men. This observation may relate to estrogenic modulation of potassium channel expression. Genetic variation in coagulation factors, estrogen receptors and lipids also contribute to increased risks for thrombotic disease and hyperlipidemia.

Enzymes required for drug metabolism by methylation, acetylation and oxidation will affect dosing efficacy for individuals.[113] Of particular importance for drugs used to treat cardiovascular diseases is methylation by cytochrome P450 enzymes (Table 5-4). Some of these enzymes show different metabolizing activity in males than in females. However, much additional work is required to understand

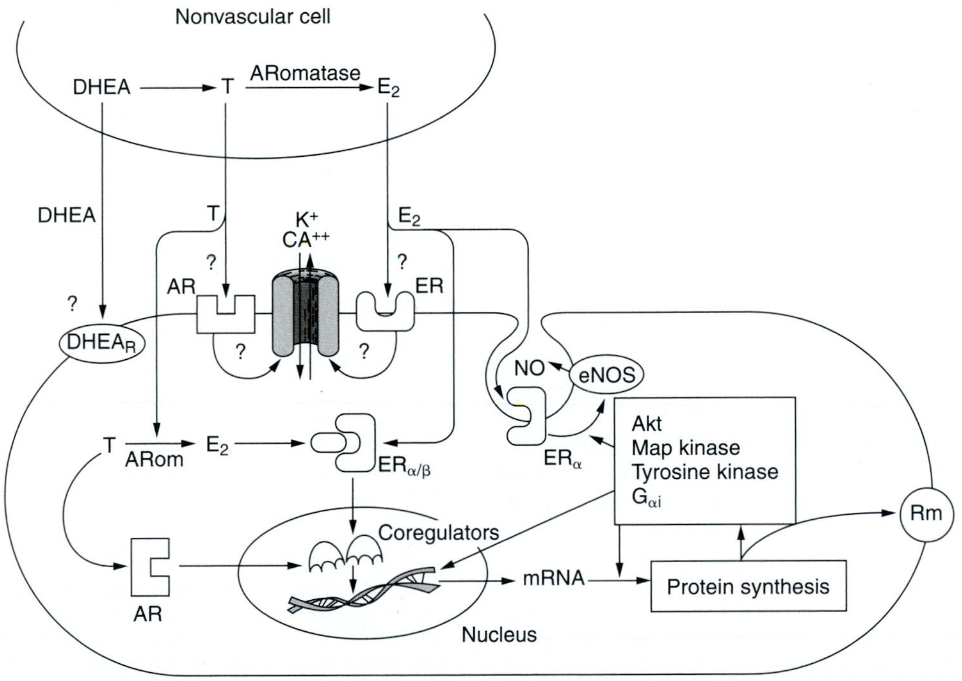

FIGURE 5-9. Schematic representation of possible mechanisms by which sex steroid hormones could affect vascular function. Testosterone and 17β-estradiol are synthesized in extravascular tissue. Whether DHEA, the precursor to testosterone, activates a membrane receptor, is controversial. Testosterone can be aromatized to 17β-estradiol in extravascular or vascular tissue. Both androgen and estrogen receptors are present in vascular tissue. However, little is known about their regulation in cells of the vascular wall or how they might interact to regulate nongenomic or genomic pathways that participate in development of atherosclerosis—including regulation of vascular tone, adhesion of macrophages, aggregation of platelets, cellular apoptosis, differentiation or proliferation. Therefore, expression of an atherosclerotic phenotype associated with a particular polymorphism in, for example, estrogen receptor α may depend on the type of initiating stimulus or combination of stimuli (endothelial denudation, lipid peroxidation, infection), coregulators needed for receptor activation, duration of stimulus and/or hormone exposure, genetic sex and hormonal status. Although this schematic depicts actions of steroids in endothelial cells, similar mechanisms are likely to be present in smooth muscle cells, macrophages and platelet-precursors, megakaryocytes. Akt, a serine-threonine kinase important for regulation of several cellular processes; AR, androgen receptor; Arom, aromatase; DHEA, dihydroepiandrosterone; $DHEA_R$, dihydroepiandrosterone receptor; E_2, 17β-estradiol; ER, estrogen receptor α or β; eNOS, endothelial nitric oxide synthase; G_{ai}, guanine nucleotide regulator protein subunit that inhibits guanylyl cyclase; NO, nitric oxide; Rm, membrane receptor; ?, denotes unknown interactions or pathways needing additional research (Reprinted with permission from Miller VM, Tindall DJ, Liu PY: Of mice, men, and hormones. Arterioscler Thromb Vasc Biol 24:995, 2004.).

TABLE 5-3 GENETIC POLYMORPHISMS, VASCULAR PHARMACOLOGY, AND DISEASE

Gene	Polymorphism or Allele	Implication in Cardiovascular Disease
α-Adrenergic receptors		
α1A	Arg492Cys	None
α2b	Glu9/Gl712	Increased risk for coronary events for homozygous deletion
α2c	A2cDcl322-325	Ethnic differences in the development of hypertension; risk of heart failure
Angiotensin-converting enzyme (ACE)	Insertion/deletion in intron 16	The D allele or the DD genotype is associated with increased risk for atherosclerotic disease, heart failure, and response to ACE inhibitors
Angiotensin II type 1 receptor	1166A>C Ala-Cys	Increased risk for pregnancy-induced hypertension; increased ANP and response to AII
β1-Adrenergic receptor (ADRβ1)	Ser49Gly	Increased resting heart rate and idiopathic dilated cardiomyopathy
	Arg389Gly	Acts synergistically with α1c-adrenergic receptor to increase risk of heart failure in blacks. Higher levels of baseline and isoproterenol-stimulated adenylyl cyclase activity
β2-Adrenergic receptor (ADRβ2)	Arg16Gly	Increased agonist mediated desensitization of β-2 receptors; family history of hypertension; risk of obesity
	Glu27Gln	Higher maximal response to isoproterenol; hypertension in whites with type 2 diabetes
	Thr164IIe	Decreased affinity for agonist and worse outcome for congestive heart failure
B2-Bradykinin receptor	Cys-58Thr; Cys- 412Gly; Thr21Met	Increased risk for hypertension in some ethnic populations
Endothelial nitric oxide synthase (eNOS)	Nucleotide repeats in intron 4 and 13′; Glu298Asp;	Increased risk for cardiovascular events including myocardial infarction and venous thrombosis. It is controversial as to whether modifications in this gene are associated with hypertension, which may be related to ethnic origin
	Thr-785Cys	Early coronary artery disease

Alleles are designated using a three-letter code for amino acids followed by the codon location. For example, Arg492Cys indicates that the arginine at codon 492 is considered the original and cystine is the mutated form.

Derived from Schaefer BM, Caracciolo V, Frishman WH, Charney P: Gender, ethnicity and genetics in cardiovascular disease: Part 1: Basic principles. Heart Dis 5:129, 2003.

how sex and sex-specific hormones influence drug metabolism.

Although large-scale clinical trials enable generalizations to be made regarding drug efficacy and dosing, physicians treat individuals. The generalizability of results will depend on the number of diverse individuals (sex/gender and ethnicity) participating in these trials. Results from trials conducted in ethnically homogeneous populations may not apply to more diverse populations around the world. Pharmacologic management of cardiovascular disease in the future may become tailored to individual genetic profile, age, and lifestyle characteristics—such as food/drug interactions.

TABLE 5-4 METABOLISM OF VASCULAR DRUGS BY CYTOCHROME P450

Cytochrome	Drug
CYP3A4	**ACE inhibitors** (losartan); **calcium channel blockers** (amlodipine, diltiazem, felodipine, lercanidipine, nicardipine, nifedipine, nimodipine, nisoldipine, nitrendipine, verapamil); **HMG-CoA inhibitors–statins** (atorvastatin, lovastatin, pravastatin, simvastatin)
CYP2D6	**Beta blockers** (propranolol, S-metoprolol)
CYP2C9	**ACE inhibitors** (losartan); **HMG-CoA inhibitor** (fluvastatin)

Derived from Schaefer BM, Caracciolo V, Frishman WH, Charney P: Gender, ethnicity and genetics in cardiovascular disease: Part 1: Basic principles. Heart Dis 5:129, 2003.

REFERENCES

1. Somlyo AP, Wu X, Walker LA, et al: Pharmacomechanical coupling: The role of calcium, G-proteins, kinases and phosphatases. Rev Physiol Biochem Pharmacol 134:201, 1999.
2. Somlyo AP, Somlyo AV: Ca^{2+} sensitivity of smooth muscle and non-muscle myosin II: Modulated by G proteins, kinases, and myosin phosphatase. Physiol Rev 83:1325, 2003.
3. Poburko D, Kuo KH, Dai J, et al: Organellar junctions promote targeted Ca^{2+} signaling in smooth muscle: Why two membranes are better than one. Trends Pharmacol Sci 25:8, 2004.
4. Smani T, Zakharov SI, Csutora P, et al: A novel mechanism for the store-operated calcium influx pathway. Nat Cell Biol 6:113, 2004.
5. Morgan KG, Gangopadhyay SS: Signal transduction in smooth muscle. Invited review: Cross-bridge regulation by thin filament-associated proteins. J Appl Physiol 91:953, 2001.
6. Sakurada S, Takuwa N, Sugimoto N, et al: Ca^{2+}-dependent activation of Rho and Rho kinase in membrane depolarization-induced and receptor stimulation-induced vascular smooth muscle contraction. Circ Res 93:548, 2003.
7. Amberg GC, Bonev AD, Rossow CF, et al: Modulation of the molecular composition of large conductance, Ca(2+) activated K(+) channels in vascular smooth muscle during hypertension. J Clin Invest 112:717, 2003.
8. Cox RH, Rusch NJ: New expression profiles of voltage-gated ion channels in arteries exposed to high blood pressure. Microcirculation 9:243, 2002.
9. Nelson MT, Quayle JM: Physiological roles and properties of potassium channels in arterial smooth muscle. Am J Physiol 268:C799, 1995.

10. Quayle JM, Nelson MT, Standen NB: ATP-sensitive and inwardly rectifying potassium channels in smooth muscle. Physiol Rev 77:1165, 1997.
11. Munzel T, Feil R, Mulsch A, et al: Physiology and pathophysiology of vascular signaling controlled by cyclic guanosine 3′,5′-cyclic monophosphate-dependent protein kinase. Circulation 108:2172, 2003.
12. Reffelmann T, Kloner RA: Therapeutic potential of phosphodiesterase 5 inhibition for cardiovascular disease. Circulation 108:239, 2003.
13. Wu LNY, Sauer GR, Genge BR, et al: Effects of analogues of inorganic phosphate and sodium ion on mineralization of matrix vesicles isolated from growth plate cartilage of normal rapidly growing chickens. J Inorganic Biochem 94:221, 2003.
14. Kamemura K, Hart GW: Dynamic interplay between O-glycosylation and O-phosphorylation of nucleocytoplasmic proteins: A new paradigm for metabolic control of signal transduction and transcription. Prog Nucl Acid Res Mol Biol 73:107, 2003.
15. Wolfrum S, Jensen KS, Liao JK: Endothelium-dependent effects of statins. Arterioscler Thromb Vasc Biol 23:729, 2003.
16. Burnstock G: Changing face of autonomic and sensory nerves in circulation. In Edvinsson L, Uddmans R (Eds): Vascular Innervation and Receptor Mechanisms. New Perspectives 1, Academic Press, 1993, p 1.
17. Moore A, Mangoni AA, Lyons D, et al: The cardiovascular system in the ageing patient. J Clin Pharmacol 56:254, 2003.
18. Langer SZ: Presynaptic regulation of the release of catecholamines. Pharmacol Rev 32:337, 1980.
19. Zacharia LC, Jackson EK, Gillespie DG, et al: Catecholamines abrogate antimitogenic effects of 2-hydroxyestradiol on human aortic vascular smooth muscle cells. Arterioscler Thromb Vasc Biol 21:1745, 2001.
20. Toda N: Vasodilating beta-adrenoceptor blockers as cardiovascular therapeutics. Pharmacol Ther 100:215, 2003.
21. Vanhoutte PM, Verbeuren TJ, Webb RC: Local modulation of the adrenergic neuroeffector interaction in the blood vessel wall. Physiol Rev 61:151, 1981.
22. Recordati G: A thermodynamic model of the sympathetic and parasympathetic nervous systems. Auton Neurosci 103:1, 2003.
23. Marcus AJ, Broekman MJ, Drosopoulos JHF, et al: Heterologous cell-cell interactions: Thromboregulation, cerebroprotection and cardioprotection by CD39 (NTPDase-1). J Thromb Haemos 1:2497, 2003.
24. Dobransky T, Rylett RJ: Functional regulation of choline acetyltransferase by phosphorylation. Neurochem Res 28:537, 2003.
25. Parsons SM, Prior C, Marshall IG: Acetylcholine transport, storage, and release. Int Rev Neurobiol 35:279, 1993.
26. Prado MAM, Reis RAM, Prado VF, et al: Regulation of acetylcholine synthesis and storage. Neurochem Int 41:291, 2002.
27. Parsons SM: Transport mechanisms in acetylcholine and monoamine storage. FASEB J 14:2423, 2000.
28. Toda N, Okamura T: The pharmacology of nitric oxide in the peripheral nervous system of blood vessels. Pharmacol Rev 55:271, 2003.
29. Gibson A, Lilley E: Superoxide anions, free-radical scavengers, and nitrergic neurotransmission. Gen Pharmacol 28:489, 1997.
30. Kielstein JT, Impraim B, Simmel S, et al: Cardiovascular effects of systemic nitric oxide synthase inhibition with asymmetrical dimethylarginine in humans. Circulation 109:172, 2004.
31. Vincent SR, Kimura H: Histochemical mapping of nitric oxide synthase in the rat brain. Neuroscience 46:755, 1992.
32. Wessler I, Kilbinger H, Bittinger F, et al: The non-neuronal cholinergic system in humans: Expression, function and pathophysiology. Life Sci 72:2055, 2003.
33. Herring N, Danson EJF, Paterson DJ: Cholinergic control of heart rate by nitric oxide is site specific. News Physiol Sci 17:202, 2002.
34. Vincent SR: Histochemistry of nitric oxide synthase in the peripheral nervous system. In Toda N, Moncada S, Furchgott R Higgs EA (eds): Nitric Oxide and the Peripheral Nervous System. London, Portland Press, 2000, p 1.
35. Berman JR, Goldstein I: Female sexual dysfunction. Urol Clin North Am 28:405, 2001.
36. Minson CT, Berry LT, Joyner MJ: Nitric oxide and neurally mediated regulation of skin blood flow during local heating. J Appl Physiol 91:1619, 2001.
37. Milner P, Ralevic V, Hopwood AM, et al: Ultrastructural localization of substance P and choline acetyl transferase in endothelial cells of rat coronary artery and release of substance P and acetylcholine during hypoxia. Experientia 45:121, 1989.
38. Hamlet MA, Rorie DK, Tyce GM: Effects of estradiol on release and disposition of norepinephrine from nerve endings. Am J Physiol 239:H450, 1980.
39. Dubey RK, Jackson EK, Gillespie DG, et al: Catecholamines block the antimitogenic effect of estradiol on human coronary artery smooth muscle cells. J Clin Endocrinol Metab 89:3922, 2004.
40. Skidgel RA, Alhenc-Gelas F, Campbell WB: Regulation of cardiovascular signaling by kinins and products of similar converting enzyme systems. Prologue: Kinins and related systems. New life for old discoveries. Am J Physiol Heart Circ Physiol 284:H1886, 2003.
41. Meghji P, Burnstock G: Inhibition of extracellular ATP degradation in endothelial cells. Life Sci 57:763, 1995.
42. Faas MM, Bakker WW, Klok PA, et al: Modulation of glomerular ECTO-ADPase expression by oestradiol: A histochemical study. Thromb Haemost 77:767, 1997.
43. Gallagher PE, Li P, Lenhart JR, et al: Estrogen regulation of angiotensin-converting enzyme mRNA. Hypertension 33:323, 1999.
44. Lincoln J, Loesch A, Burnstock G: Localization of vasopressin, serotonin and angiotensin II in endothelial cells of the renal and mesenteric arteries of the rat. Cell Tissue Res 259:341, 1990.
45. Widlansky ME, Gokce N, Keaney JF, Jr, et al: The clinical implications of endothelial dysfunction. J Am Coll Cardiol 42:1149, 2003.
46. Furchgott RF, Zawadski J: The obligatory role of endothelium cells in the relaxation of arterial smooth muscle by acetylcholine. Nature 288:373, 1980.
47. Komesaroff PA, Sudhir K: Estrogens and human cardiovascular physiology. Reprod Fertil Dev 13:261, 2001.
48. Li H, Wallerath T, Forstermann U: Physiological mechanisms regulating the expression of endothelial-type NO synthase. Nitric Oxide 7:132, 2002.
49. Shimokawa H: Rho-kinase as a novel therapeutic target in treatment of cardiovascular diseases. J Cardiovasc Pharm 39:319, 2002.
50. Trochu JN, Mital S, Zhang X, et al: Preservation of NO production by statins in the treatment of heart failure. Cardiovasc Res 60:250, 2003.
51. Vallance P: Nitric oxide: Therapeutic opportunities. Fundam Clin Pharmacol 17:1, 2003.
52. Alderton WK, Cooper CH, Knowles RG: Nitric oxide synthases: Structure, function and inhibition. Biochem J 357:593, 2001.
53. Fulton D, Gratton J-P, Sessa WC: Post-translational control of endothelial nitric oxide synthase: Why isn't calcium/calmodulin enough? J Pharmacol Exp Ther 299:818, 2001.
54. Ignarro LJ, Napoli C, Loscalzo J: Nitric oxide donors and cardiovascular agents modulating the bioactivity of nitric oxide: An overview. Circ Res 90:21, 2002.
55. Salerno L, Sorrenti V, Di Giacomo C, et al: Progress in the development of selective nitric oxide synthase (NOS) inhibitors. Curr Pharm Des 8:177, 2002.
56. Kalinowski L, Dobrucki LW, Szczepanska-Konkel M, et al: Third-generation beta-blockers stimulate nitric oxide release from endothelial cells through ATP efflux: A novel mechanism for antihypertensive action. Circulation 107:2747, 2003.
57. Tabrizchi R: Amiodipine and endothelial nitric oxide synthase activity. Cardiovasc Res 59:807, 2003.
58. Venema RC: Post-translational mechanisms of endothelial nitric oxide synthase regulation by bradykinin. Int Immunopharmacol 2:1755, 2002.
59. Napoli C, Ignarro LJ: Nitric oxide-releasing drugs. Ann Rev Pharmacol Toxicol 43:97, 2003.
60. Busse R, Fleming I: Regulation of endothelium-derived vasoactive autacoid production by hemodynamic forces. Trends Pharma Sci 24:24, 2003.
61. Li H, Wallerath T, Munzel T, et al: Regulation of endothelial-type NO synthase expression in pathophysiology and in response to drugs. Nitric Oxide 7:149, 2002.
62. Liu PY, Death AK, Handelsman DJ: Androgens and cardiovascular disease. Endocr Rev 24:313, 2003.
63. DeMey JG, Claeys M, Vanhoutte PM: Endothelium-dependent inhibitory effects of acetylcholine, adenosine triphosphate, thrombin and arachidonic acid in the canine femoral artery. J Pharmacol Exp Ther 222:166, 1982.
64. Archer SL, Gragasin FS, Wu X, et al: Endothelium-derived hyperpolarizing factor in human internal mammary artery is 11,12-epoxyeicosatrienoic acid and causes relaxation by activating smooth muscle BK(Ca) channels. Circulation 107:769, 2003.

65. Bussemaker E, Popp R, Binder J, et al: Characterization of the endothelium-derived hyperpolarizing factor (EDHF) response in the human interlobar artery. Kidney Int 63:1749, 2003.
66. Matoba T, Shimokawa H, Nakashima M, et al: Hydrogen peroxide is an endothelium-derived hyperpolarizing factor in mice. J Clin Invest 106:1521, 2000.
67. Morikawa K, Shimokawa H, Matoba T, et al: Pivotal role of Cu, Zn-superoxide dismutase in endothelium-dependent hyperpolarization. J Clin Invest 112:1871, 2003.
68. DeMey JG, Vanhoutte PM: Heterogeneous behavior of the canine arterial and venous wall. Circ Res 51:439, 1982.
69. Belhassen L, Pelle G, Dubois-Rande JL, et al: Improved endothelial function by the thromboxane A2 receptor antagonist S 18886 in patients with coronary artery disease treated with aspirin. J Am Coll Cardiol 41:1198, 2003.
70. Masaki T: Historical review: Endothelin. Trends Pharm Sci 25:219, 2004.
71. Noori A, Kabbani S: Endothelins and coronary vascular biology. Coron Artery Dis 14:491, 2003.
72. Barton M, Traupe T, Haudenschild CC: Endothelin, hypercholesterolemia and atherosclerosis. Coron Artery Dis 14:477, 2003.
73. Nakov R, Pfarr E, Eberle S: HEAT Investigators: Darusentan: An effective endothelin A receptor antagonist for treatment of hypertension. Am J Hypertens 15:583, 2002.
74. O'Callaghan D, Gaine SP: Bosentan: A novel agent for the treatment of pulmonary arterial hypertension. Int J Clin Prac 58:69, 2004.
75. Boerrigter G, Burnett L: Endothelin in neurohormonal activation in heart failure. Coron Artery Dis 14:495, 2003.
76. Galie N, Manes A, Branzi A: The endothelin system in pulmonary arterial hypertension. Cardiovasc Res 61:227, 2004.
77. VanBuren P: Endothelin in cardiovascular disease. Coron Artery Dis 14:475, 2003.
78. Rich S, McLaughlin VV: Endothelin receptor blockers in cardiovascular disease. Circulation 108:2184, 2003.
79. Sanders-Bush E, Fentress H, Hazelwood L: Serotonin 5-HT_2 receptors: Molecular and genomic diversity. Molec Interv 3:319, 2003.
80. Repka-Ramirez MS, Baraniuk JN: Histamine in health and disease. Clin Allergy Immunol 17:1, 2002.
81. Toda N: Heterogeneous responses to histamine in blood vessels. In Vanhoutte PM (ed): Vasodilatation: Vascular Smooth Muscle, Peptides, Autonomic Nerves, and Endothelium. New York, Raven, 1988, p 531.
82. Volanakis JE: Human C-reactive protein: Expression, structure, and function. Mol Immunol 38:189, 2001.
83. Macy EM, Hayes TE, Tracy RP: Variability in the measurement of C-reactive protein in healthy subjects: Implications for reference intervals and epidemiological applications. Clin Chem 43:52, 1997.
84. McConnell JP, Branum EL, Ballman KV, et al: Gender differences in C-reactive protein concentrations—Confirmation with two sensitive methods. Clin Chem Lab Med 40:56, 2002.
85. Ockene IS, Matthews CE, Rifai N, et al: Variability and classification accuracy of serial high-sensitivity C-reactive protein measurements in healthy adults. Clin Chem 47:444, 2001.
86. Ridker PM: Clinical application of C-reactive protein for cardiovascular disease detection and prevention. Circulation 107:363, 2003.
87. Sternik L, Samee S, Schaff HV, et al: C-reactive protein relaxes human vessels in vitro. Arterioscler Thromb Vasc Biol 22:1865, 2002.
88. van den Berg CW, Taylor KE, Lang D: C-reactive protein-induced in vitro vasorelaxation is an artefact caused by the presence of sodium azide in commercial preparations. Arterioscler Thromb Vasc Biol 24:e168, 2004.
89. Pearson TA, Mensah GA, Alexander RW, et al: Markers of inflammation and cardiovascular disease: Application to clinical and public health practice. A statement for healthcare professionals from the Centers for Disease Control and Prevention and the American Heart Association. Circulation 107:499, 2003.
90. Iversen PO, Nicolaysen A, Kvernebo K, et al: Human cytokines modulate arterial vascular tone via endothelial receptors. Pflugers Archiv—Eur J Physiol 439:93, 1999.
91. Azizi M, Menard J: Combined blockade of the renin-angiotensin system with angiotensin-converting enzyme inhibitors and angiotensin II type 1 receptor antagonists. Circulation 109:2492, 2004.
92. Zaman MA, Oparil S, Calhoun DA: Drugs targeting the renin-angiotensin-aldosterone system. Nat Rev Drug Discov 1:621, 2002.
93. Schiffrin EL: Vascular and cardiac benefits of angiotensin receptor blockers. Am J Med 113:409, 2002.
94. de Gasparo M, Catt KJ, Inagami T, et al: The angiotensin II receptors. Pharmacol Rev 52:415, 2000.
95. Mombouli JV, Vanhoutte PM: Endothelial dysfunction: From physiology to therapy. J Mol Cell Cardiol 31:61, 1999.
96. Tabrizchi R: Dual ACE and neutral endopeptidase inhibitors: Novel therapy for patients with cardiovascular disorders. Drugs 63:2185, 2003.
97. Quaschning T, Galle J, Wanner C: Vasopeptidase inhibition: A new treatment approach for endothelial dysfunction. Kidney Int 63:S54, 2003.
98. Yamamoto K, Burnett JC, Jr, Bermudez EA, et al: Clinical criteria and biochemical markers for the detection of systolic dysfunction. J Cardiac Fail 6:194, 2000.
99. Shapiro BP, Chen HH, Burnett JC, Jr., et al: Use of plasma brain natriuretic peptide concentration to aid in the diagnosis of heart failure. Mayo Clin Proc 78:481, 2003.
100. Tom B, Dendorfer A, Danser AH: Bradykinin, angiotensin-(1-7), and ACE inhibitors: How do they interact? Int J Biochem Cell Biol 35:792, 2003.
101. D'Souza SP, Davis M, Baxter GF: Autocrine and paracrine actions of natriuretic peptides in the heart. Pharmacol Ther 101:113, 2004.
102. Collins E, Bracamonte MP, Burnett JC, Jr, et al: Mechanism of relaxations to D-type natriuretic peptide (DNP) in canine coronary arteries. J Cardiovasc Pharmacol 35:614, 2000.
103. Best, P.J., Burnett JC, Wilson SH, et al: Dendroaspis natriuretic peptide relaxes isolated human arteries and veins. Cardiovasc Res 55:375, 2002.
104. Richards AM, Lainchbury JG, Nicholls MG, et al: Dendroaspis natriuretic peptide: Endogenous or dubious? Lancet 359:5, 2002.
105. Pham TV, Rosen MR: Sex-differences in electrophysiology of the heart and cardiac arrhythmias. In Bittar EE (ed): Advances in Molecular and Cell Biology. Amsterdam, Elsevier, 2004, p 115.
106. Schaefer BM, Caracciolo V, Frishman WH, et al: Gender, ethnicity, and genes in cardiovascular disease. Part 2: Implications for pharmacotherapy. Heart Dis 5:202, 2003.
107. Sudhir K, Komesaroff PA: Clinic review 110. Cardiovascular actions of estrogens in men. J Clin Endocrinol Metab 84:3411, 1999.
108. Turner ME, Jenkins C, Milsted A, et al: Sex chromosomes. In Bittar EE (ed): Advances in Molecular and Cell Biology. Amsterdam, Elsevier, 2004, p 1.
109. Shearman AM: Hormone receptor polymorphisms. In Bittar EE (ed): Advances in Molecular and Cell Biology. Amsterdam, Elsevier, 2004, p 59.
110. Kunnas TA, Laippala P, Penttila A, et al: Association of polymorphism of human [alpha] oestrogen receptor gene with coronary artery disease in men: A necropsy study. Br Med J 321:273, 2000.
111. Shearman AM, Cupples LA, Demissie S, et al: Association between estrogen receptor alpha gene variation and cardiovascular disease. JAMA 290:2263, 2003.
112. Siest G, Ferrari L, Accaoui MJ, et al: Pharmacogenomics of drugs affecting the cardiovascular system. Clin Chem Lab Med 41:590, 2003.
113. Williams JA, Hurst SI, Bauman J, et al: Reaction phenotyping in drug discovery: Moving forward with confidence? Curr Drug Metab 4:527, 2003.

chapter 6

Atherosclerosis

Peter Libby

The view of atherosclerosis has evolved markedly in recent years. Previously regarded as a segmental disease, we now appreciate increasingly its diffuse nature. The traditional clinical focus on atherosclerosis has emphasized coronary artery disease. The attention of physicians, in general, and cardiovascular specialists, in particular, has now expanded to embrace other arterial beds, including the peripheral and cerebrovascular arterial beds.

Formerly considered an inevitable and relentlessly progressive degenerative process, we now recognize that, quite to the contrary, atherogenesis progresses at varied paces. Increasing clinical and experimental evidence indicates that atheromatous plaques can evolve in vastly different fashions. Atheromata display a much more dynamic nature than previously thought possible, both from a structural and biologic point of view. Plaques not only progress but also may regress and alter their qualitative characteristics in ways that may influence their clinical behavior.

Concepts of the pathobiology of atherosclerosis have likewise undergone perpetual revision. During much of the 20th century, most considered atherosclerosis a cholesterol storage disease. The recognition of the key role of interactions of vascular cells; blood cells including leukocytes and platelets; and lipoproteins challenged this older model in the latter decades of the 20th century.[1] Current thinking further broadens this schema, incorporating an appreciation of the global metabolic status of individuals, extending far beyond the traditional risk factors, as triggers to the atherogenic process.

This chapter will delineate the concepts of the widespread and diffuse distributions of atherosclerosis and its clinical manifestations, and also describe progress in understanding its fundamental biology.

RISK FACTORS FOR ATHEROSCLEROSIS: TRADITIONAL, EMERGING, AND THOSE ON THE RISE

Traditional Risk Factors for Atherosclerosis

Cholesterol

Since the dawn of the 20th century, experimental data have repeatedly shown a link between plasma cholesterol levels and formation of atheromata.[2] Pioneering work performed in Russia in the early 20th century showed that consumption by rabbits of a cholesterol-rich diet caused formation of arterial lesions that shared features with human atheromata. By mid-century, the application of the ultracentrifuge to the analysis of plasma proteins led to the recognition that various classes of lipoproteins transported cholesterol and other lipids through the aqueous medium of the blood. Multiple epidemiologic studies verified a link between one cholesterol-rich lipoprotein particle in particular, low-density lipoprotein (LDL), and risk for coronary heart disease. The characterization of familial hypercholesterolemia as a genetic disease provided further evidence that linked LDL cholesterol levels with coronary heart disease.[3] Heterozygotes for this condition had markedly elevated risk for atherosclerotic disease. Individuals homozygous for familial hypercholesterolemia commonly develop coronary heart disease within the first decade of life.

The elucidation of the LDL-receptor pathway and the proof that mutations in the LDL receptor cause familial hypercholesterolemia provided proof positive of LDL's role in atherogenesis; however, the *cholesterol hypothesis* of atherogenesis still encountered skepticism.[4,5] Many critics—some lay people and some respected professionals—questioned aspects of the cholesterol theory of atherogenesis.[6] Critics pointed out that dietary cholesterol levels did not always correlate with cholesterolemia.[7] The lack of proof that either dietary or drug intervention could modify outcomes dogged proponents of the cholesterol hypothesis of atherogenesis.

Ultimately, controlled clinical trials that lowered LDL by interventions including partial intestinal bypass, bile acid–binding resins, and the statin class of drugs showed reductions in coronary events and vindicated the cholesterol hypothesis.[8] In appropriately powered trials conducted with sufficiently potent agents, lipid-lowering also reduced overall mortality. However, the very success of these interventions suggested that there must be more to atherogenesis than cholesterol because a majority of events still occurred despite increasingly aggressive control of LDL cholesterol levels. Of course, aspects of the lipoprotein profile other than LDL can influence atherogenesis (see later). However, as atherosclerotic events commonly occurred in individuals with average levels of the major lipoprotein classes, it remains clear that a full understanding of atherogenesis requires consideration of factors other than blood lipids.

Systemic Arterial Hypertension

The relationship between arterial blood pressure and mortality emerged early from actuarial studies. Insurance underwriters had a major financial stake in mortality prediction. A simple measurement of blood pressure with a cuff sphygmomanometer powerfully predicted longevity. Data emerging from the Framingham Study and other observational cohorts verified a relationship between systemic arterial pressure and coronary heart disease events.[9] Concordant observations from experimental animals and epidemiologic studies bolstered the link between hypertension and atherosclerosis.

As in the case of high cholesterol, clinical evidence that pharmacologic reduction in blood pressure could reduce coronary heart disease events proved fairly elusive. Early intervention studies readily showed decreases in stroke and congestive heart failure endpoints following administration of antihypertensive drugs.[10] Studies that indicated clear-cut reductions in coronary heart disease events with antihypertensive treatment have accumulated much more recently.[11] Another study testing the efficacy in cardiovascular event reduction of equally effective blood pressure lowering by a calcium channel blocker and an angiotensin-converting enzyme inhibitor includes an intracoronary ultrasound substudy that may shed light on the mechanism of the relationship between hypertension and atherosclerosis.[12]

Mechanistically, antihypertensive drug therapy likely benefits atherosclerosis and its complications by hypotensive and other actions. For example, the recent Losartan Intervention for Endpoint (LIFE) Reduction in Hypertension Study showed a striking incremental benefit of the angiotensin receptor blocker that indicated modulatory effects of angiotensin II on outcomes independent of blood pressure, despite equal degrees of blood pressure control with a β-blocker or an angiotensin receptor blocker.[13] Yet, another large randomized clinical trial, the Antihypertensive and Lipid-Lowering Treatment to Prevent Heart Attack Trial (ALL-HAT), showed little advantage to an angiotensin receptor blocker over either a calcium channel antagonist or a β–adrenergic blocking agent.[14]

Clinical observations provide strong additional support for the concept that hypertension itself can promote atherogenesis. Atherosclerosis of the pulmonary arteries seldom occurs in individuals with normal pulmonary artery pressures. Even in relatively young patients with pulmonary hypertension, pulmonary arterial atheromata occur quite commonly. This "experiment of nature" supports the direct proatherogenic effect of hypertension in humans.

Cigarette Smoking

Tobacco abuse and cigarette smoking, in particular, accentuate the risk of cardiovascular events. In the context of noncoronary arterial disease, tobacco smoking appears particularly important (see Chapter 15). Some have speculated that the rapid restoration of baseline rates of cardiovascular events after smoking cessation indicates that tobacco use alters the risk of thrombosis rather than accentuating atherogenesis per se.[15] Classic studies in nonhuman primates have shown little effect of 2 to 3 years of cigarette smoke inhalation on experimental atherosclerosis in the presence of moderate hyperlipidemia.[16,17]

Tobacco smoke, both first- and second-hand, impairs endothelial vasodilator functions—an index of arterial health.[18,19] Cigarette smoking seems to contribute particularly to abdominal aortic aneurysm formation. The mechanistic link between cigarette smoking and arterial aneurysm formation may resemble that invoked in the pathogenesis of smoking-related emphysema. Studies in genetically altered mice that inhale tobacco smoke have delineated a role for elastolytic enzymes such as matrix metalloproteinase (MMP)-12 in the destruction of lung extracellular matrix.[20] Smoke-induced inflammation appears to release tumor necrosis factor-α (TNF-α) from macrophages that can elevate the activity of elastolytic enzymes and promote pulmonary emphysema. A similar mechanism might well promote the destruction of elastic laminae in the tunica media of the abdominal aorta characteristic of aneurysm formation.

Age

Multiple observational studies have identified age as a potent risk factor for atherosclerotic events. Indeed, in the current cardiovascular risk algorithm based on the Framingham Study, age contributes substantially to risk calculation.[21] Owing to the demographics of the US population, we should witness a marked expansion in the elderly population, particularly women, in coming years. Although age-adjusted rates of cardiovascular disease may appear stable or even declining in men, the actual burden of disease in the elderly will increase because of their sheer number. In view of the expanding elderly population, evidence that supports the mutability of atherosclerosis assumes even greater importance (see below).

Gender

Male gender also contributes to heightened cardiovascular risk in numerous observational studies. The mechanisms for this increased burden of disease may reflect male-related pro-atherogenic factors and/or lack of protection conferred by female gender. As cardiovascular risk increases post-menopause in women, many previously attributed the vascular protection enjoyed by pre-menopausal women to estrogen. However, estrogen therapy in women (in the recent large-scale clinical trials) and in men (in the older Coronary Drug Project study) seems to confer hazard rather than benefit in the circumstances studied.[22,23] Thus estrogen, certainly in combination with progesterone, does not provide a panacea for protection against cardiovascular events.[24] The decrease in high-density lipoprotein (HDL) levels in blood following menopause might explain part of the apparent protection from the cardiovascular risk of the pre-menopausal state.

High Density Lipoprotein (HDL)

The Framingham risk algorithm recognizes lower strata of HDL, below 40 mg/dl in both women and men, as a risk factor.[25] Numerous concordant population studies have pointed to the importance of HDL as an atheroprotective lipoprotein fraction. Indeed, low HDL appears more common than does high LDL in patients who come to cardiac catheterization and display angiographically significant coronary artery disease.[26]

Numerous animal studies have established a protective effect of HDL or its major apolipoprotein (apo) AI. The mechanisms by which HDL may protect against atherosclerosis include promotion of reverse lipid transport.[27] Furthermore, nascent HDL particles can take up cholesterol from macrophages and other cells in a process that depends on the ATP binding cassette transporter 1 (ABCA1). In addition, HDL can have antiinflammatory effects. One mechanism of HDL's arterial protective effect may relate to its ability to bind and carry certain enzymes that can catabolize and inactivate oxidized phospholipids deemed mediators of inflammation during atherogenesis.[28] These antioxidant enzymes include paraoxonase-1 and platelet-activating factor acetylhydrolase, also known as lipoprotein-associated phospholipase A_2 ($LpPLA_2$).

Emerging Risk Factors for Atherosclerosis

Homocysteine

Homocysteine, a product of amino acid metabolism, may contribute to atherothrombosis.[29] Individuals with genetic defects that lead to elevated homocysteine levels (e.g., homocystinuria, commonly due to deficiency in cystathionine β–synthase) have a thrombotic diathesis. In vitro, treatment with homocysteine and related compounds can alter aspects of vascular cell function related to atherogenesis. Reliable clinical tests for hyperhomocystinemia exist. Although clearly associated with elevated thrombotic risk in patients with homocystinuria, elevated levels of homocysteine in unselected populations only weakly predict cardiovascular risk[30-32] (Fig. 6-1). The Homocysteine Lowering Trialists Collaboration has called for large-scale randomized trials of dietary supplementation with folic acid in high-risk populations to evaluate whether lowering blood homocysteine levels reduces the risk of vascular disease.[33] The scientific answer to this question may emerge from the SEARCH trial.[34] The enrichment of cereals and flour

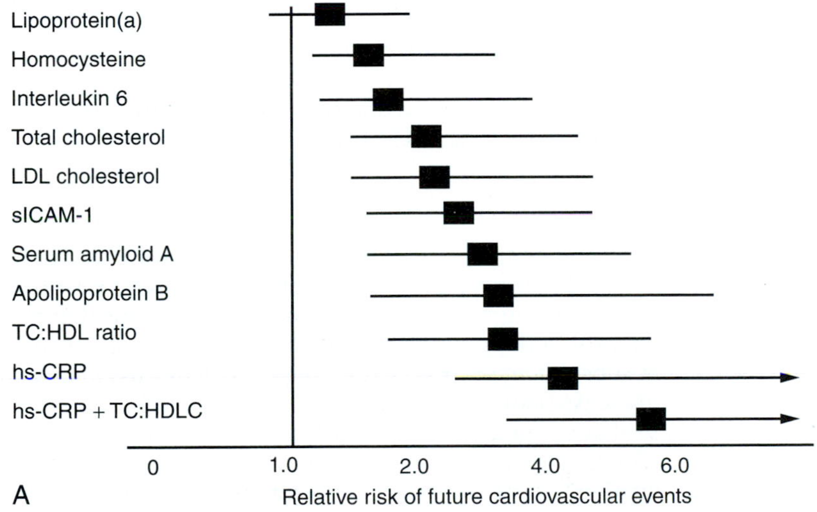

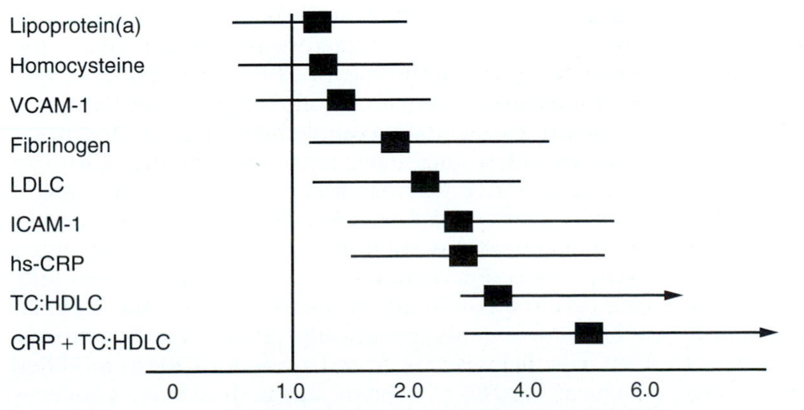

FIGURE 6-1. Predictive power of some established and emerging risk markers for coronary and peripheral atherosclerosis. Relative risk for overall cardiovascular events **(A)** and incidence of peripheral arterial disease **(B)** from the Women's Health Study and the Physicians' Health Study, respectively. The whisker plots show the point estimates and confidence intervals for various emerging and established risk factors for atherosclerotic complications. The rank, order, and magnitude of risk of peripheral arterial disease in the Women's Health Study and of cardiovascular events in the Physicians' Health Study due to these established and emerging risk factors resembles that reported earlier (*not shown*). hs-CRP, C-reactive protein measured by the high sensitivity assay; LDLC, low density lipoprotein cholesterol; sICAM-1, soluble intercellular adhesion molecule-1; TC:HDL ratio, total cholesterol: high density lipoprotein ratio; TC:HDLC, total cholesterol:high density lipoprotein cholesterol; VCAM-1, soluble vascular cell adhesion molecule. (Reproduced with permission from Ridker PM: Clinical application of C-reactive protein for cardiovascular disease detection and prevention. Circulation 107:363, 2003; Ridker PM, Stampfer MJ, Rifai N: Novel risk factors for systemic atherosclerosis: A comparison of C-reactive protein, fibrinogen, homocysteine, lipoprotein(a), and standard cholesterol screening as predictors of peripheral arterial disease. JAMA 285:2481, 2001.)

with folate in the United States is shifting dietary intake and will presumably cause a secular shift in blood homocysteine levels in the American population.

Lipoprotein(a)

Lipoprotein(a) Lp(a) (commonly pronounced "L P little A"), consists of a low-density lipoprotein particle with apolipoprotein a (apo a)—covalently attached to the apo B, the major apolipoprotein of LDL particles.[35] Apolipoprotein a should not be confused with apolipoprotein A, the family that includes apolipoprotein AI, the principal apolipoprotein of HDL. Lp(a) has considerable heterogeneity, determined genetically, and related to the number of repeats of a structural motif known as a "kringle" in the apo a moiety of the special lipoprotein particle. The structural resemblance of apo a to plasminogen suggested that Lp(a) may inhibit fibrinolysis. The heterogeneity of Lp(a) has frustrated attempts to develop a standardized assay.[36] Moreover, Lp(a) levels in the general population have high skew. Most individuals lie in the lower range of distribution with a few "outliers" in the higher levels of Lp(a). Black Americans have a higher frequency of elevated Lp(a). Those with Lp(a) levels substantially above normal do appear at increased cardiovascular risk.[37] However, as in the case of homocysteine, Lp(a) in large populations only weakly predicts future cardiovascular disease (see Fig. 6-1).

Fibrinogen

Fibrinogen, the substrate of thrombin, provides the major meshwork of arterial thrombi. Levels of fibrinogen increase in inflammatory states as part of the acute-phase response. A consistent body of observational evidence has established a link between elevated levels of fibrinogen and cardiovascular risk.[30,38,39] Standardization of assays for fibrinogen has proved difficult. Moreover, diurnal variation in plasma fibrinogen levels weakens its potential as a biomarker of cardiovascular risk, despite its obvious biological plausibility as a major participant in thrombosis. Fibrin deposition in plaques, first hypothesized by von Rokitansky in the mid-19th century, provides evidence of fibrinogen's involvement in atherogenesis.[40,41]

Infection

The possibility that infectious agents or responses to infection may contribute to atherogenesis or precipitate atherosclerotic events has periodically captured the fancy of students of atherosclerosis. Many infectious agents might plausibly contribute to aspects of atherogenesis by direct cytopathic effect or by virtue of mediators they release or elicit as part of a host defense. The hemodynamic stresses of acute infection, as well as accentuated thrombotic risk or impaired fibrinolysis due to acute-phase reactants, such as fibrinogen or plasminogen activator inhibitor-1 (PAI-1), might well transiently heighten the risk for thrombotic complications of atherosclerosis.[42] Seroepidemiologic studies have suggested links between exposure to both viral and bacterial pathogens and various measures of atherosclerosis or risk of atherosclerotic events.[43-45] However, prospective studies properly controlled for confounding factors have shown weak, if any, correlation of antibody titers against various microbial or viral pathogens and cardiovascular events.[45-47] More recent formulations of the "infectious theory" of atherosclerosis have invoked the concept of "pathogen burden," suggesting that experience with more than one microorganism may potentiate atherosclerosis.[48]

The recognition that some 40% of human atherosclerotic plaques disclose evidence for the presence of *Chlamydia pneumoniae* has focused considerable interest on this particular pathogen in the context of atherogenesis. After publication of some promising pilot trials, several large-scale and adequately powered clinical trials began. The Weekly Intervention with Zithromax against Atherosclerosis and Related Disorders (WIZARD) Trial tested the hypothesis that weekly azithromycin for a period of 12 weeks would reduce recurrent cardiovascular events in survivors of myocardial infarction. WIZARD was the first adequately powered randomized trial to test such a hypothesis. This study did not show a decrease in the composite cardiovascular event endpoints prespecified by the investigators.[49] Other recent large scale trials have also shown no benefit of longer-term azithromycin or gatifloxacin administration on recurrent coronary events.[50,50a,50b] Thus, although there is considerable and intriguing evidence that infectious agents or their products may potentiate atherosclerosis or precipitate events in at least some cases, no data yet substantiate antibiotic therapy as a treatment for atherosclerosis.[51]

Inflammation and Atherosclerosis

The recognition that inflammation provides a unifying theme for many of the pathophysiologic alterations that occur during atherogenesis has garnered considerable interest and increasing acceptance over the last decade. A subsequent section of this chapter will discuss in detail the links between inflammatory processes and risk factors and atherogenesis and complications of atherosclerosis. The emergence of C-reactive protein (CRP) as a validated marker of prospective cardiovascular risk in several categories of individuals has spawned countless studies proposing other inflammatory markers as potential predictors of atherosclerotic risk.[52-54] Although some markers of inflammation, such as fibrinogen and PAI-1, have clear-cut roles as mediators as well as markers, the evidence regarding the role of CRP as an effector as well as an indicator of inflammation remains unsettled.

Known to facilitate complement fixation for many years, recent studies have examined whether CRP can alter behavior or vascular wall cells in a way that might directly promote atherosclerosis or its complications. The concentrations used in many in vitro studies often exceed those encountered in plasma at levels that indicate elevated risk of atherosclerotic events. Some experiments in rodents genetically altered to overexpress CRP have likewise suggested a role for CRP in modified vascular function.[55] Once again, however, concerns regarding the relevance of the levels of CRP expression achieved in these gain-of-function experiments require careful consideration in interpreting their applicability to human subjects.

Genetic Predisposition

The example of familial hypercholesterolemia recounted above provides an irrefutable illustration of the link between gene mutation and atherosclerosis. The accelerated development of molecular genetic technology and the increasing ease of identifying and cataloging genetic polymorphisms have facilitated the search for genetic variants that predispose toward atherosclerosis or its complications. Monogenic conditions, such as familial hypercholesterolemia, do not appear to explain the majority of the burden or risk of atherosclerotic disease. The quest for genetic polymorphisms that predispose toward atherosclerosis has yielded many potential candidates. Some of recent interest include the MEF-2A transcription factor in families with a predisposition toward premature atherosclerosis.[56] Other recent studies identified variants in 5-lipoxygenase or its activating protein or in lymphotoxin-α that may influence atherogenesis or risk of myocardial infarction.[57-60]

The acceptance of various associations between single nucleotide polymorphisms (SNPs) or haplotypes with cardiovascular risk requires validation on independent populations with substantial numbers of events. Thus far, few polymorphisms have met this test for reliability. In the future, genetic markers of atherosclerotic risk should nonetheless prove increasingly important in risk stratification, selection of therapies, and understanding pathophysiology.

Risk Factors on the Rise

We are witnessing a transition in the pattern of atherosclerotic risk factors in the United States. Unfortunately, it appears as if the rest of the world will soon follow suit in this shifting spectrum of atherosclerotic risk. Certain traditional atherosclerotic risk factors are on the wane. For example, at least in the United States, rates of smoking are declining, particularly in men. In addition, dissemination of effective antihypertensive therapies has provided a means to reduce the degree or prevalence of this traditional atherosclerotic risk factor. Although many patients do not achieve the currently established targets for blood pressure, effective therapies for this risk factor have become much more widely implemented in recent decades.[61-63]

We have made striking progress in combating high levels of LDL, a major traditional risk factor for atherosclerosis, as discussed earlier. In particular, the introduction of the statins and accumulating evidence of their effectiveness as preventive therapies, combined with their relative ease of use and tolerability, should foster a secular trend toward lower LDL levels in the higher-risk segments of our population.

Although we justly derive considerable satisfaction from these pharmacologic inroads into the traditional profile of cardiovascular risk, we are losing ground rapidly in other respects.[64] The astounding increase in obesity in the U.S. population in merely the last decade represents a change in body habitus of substantial proportion in what amounts to an instant on an evolutionary timescale.[65,66] Short of major disasters or famines, this kind of rapid shift in body habitus may have no precedent in the evolution of our species. From the perspective of cardiovascular risk, the metabolic alterations that accompany this increased girth of our population should sound an alarm. Current data point to a significant increase in the prevalence of the metabolic syndrome.[64]

TABLE 6-1 CRITERIA FOR THE METABOLIC SYNDROME*

Risk Factor	Defining Level
Abdominal obesity† (waist circumference‡)	
Men	>102 cm (>40 in)
Women	>88 cm (>35 in)
Triglycerides	≥150 mg/dL
HDL-C	
Men	<40 mg/dL
Women	<50 mg/dL
Blood pressure	≥130/≥85 mm Hg
Fasting glucose	≥110 mg/dL

*Diagnosis is established when ≥3 of these risk factors are present.
†Abdominal obesity is more highly correlated with metabolic risk factors than is increased body mass index (BMI).
‡Some men develop metabolic risk factors when circumference is only marginally increased.
HDL-C, high density lipoprotein-cholesterol.
From the Expert Panel on Detection, Evaluation, and Treatment of High Blood Cholesterol in Adults. JAMA 285:2486, 2001.

The National Cholesterol Education Project Adult Treatment Panel III (ATPIII) arbitrarily defined five components of the metabolic syndrome (Table 6-1).[21] Individuals with any three components have the metabolic syndrome by ATPIII criteria. Note that LDL, the traditional focus of guidelines and therapies, does not figure among the metabolic syndrome criteria. Instead, lower ranges of HDL and higher levels of triglycerides characterize the metabolic syndrome. Thus, we may witness a shift in lipid risk factor burden from primarily LDL to the dyslipidemia of the metabolic syndrome and diabetes, characterized by lower HDL and higher triglycerides. The very success of the statin category of drugs in reducing LDL cholesterol will likely contribute to the increased importance of the dyslipidemia of the metabolic syndrome in the future.

Although individuals with the metabolic syndrome commonly have dyslipidemia, their levels of LDL cholesterol may be average or even below average. This finding may provide false reassurance to physicians and patients alike. Although the LDL cholesterol level in such patients may not show particular elevation, the quality of the lipoprotein particles may prove particularly atherogenic. LDL particles in those with high levels of triglycerides and low levels of HDL tend to be small and dense. Such small, dense LDL particles appear to bind to proteoglycans in the arterial intima with more avidity. Their retention in the intima may facilitate their oxidative modification.[67] Thus, small, dense LDL particles may have particularly atherogenic properties.

Hyperglycemia

An additional criterion for the metabolic syndrome, hyperglycemia, may also independently contribute to the pathogenesis of atherosclerosis. In the presence of higher levels of glucose, the nonenzymatic glycation and other types of oxidative posttranslational modification of various macromolecules increases. Hemoglobin A1c, a glycated form of this oxygen-carrying pigment, reflects this biochemical process. The accumulation of glycated macromolecules ultimately leads to the formation of complex condensates known as advanced glycation end products, or AGEs.[68,69] Considerable evidence supports a role for advanced glycation end products as triggers for the inflammatory responses implicated in atherogenesis. A cell surface receptor for AGEs known as RAGE appears to transduce proinflammatory signals when occupied by AGE-modified ligands (Fig. 6-2). RAGE stimulation reportedly increases the production of reactive oxygen species and leads to activation of a master transcription factor, nuclear factor-kappa B (NF-κB).[70] NF-κB in turn stimulates the transcription of a cassette of proinflammatory genes including cytokines, chemokines, leukocyte adhesion molecules, and other proinflammatory mediators implicated in atherogenesis (see later). This and other mechanisms link hyperglycemia and insulin resistance to aspects of host defenses considered essential for the atherogenic process.

Interactions of Risk Factors with Cells in the Arterial Wall and Leukocytes During Atherogenesis

We increasingly understand atherosclerosis as a process that involves cellular interactions with risk factors such as high levels of LDL. This contemporary view contrasts with the previous notions that the arterial wall passively accumulated cholesterol. This cross-talk among cells of varying types during atherogenesis involves more than just the intrinsic cells of the arterial wall, the endothelium, and vascular smooth muscle cells (see Chapters 1 and 2). Indeed, the mononuclear phagocyte probably also contributes importantly to atherogenesis. The normal endothelium resists prolonged contact with leukocytes, including blood monocytes, the precursors of the tissue macrophages that accumulate in atheromata. A mechanism involving the expression of particular leukocyte adhesion molecules on the endothelial surface likely mediates the recruitment of blood monocytes to sites of formation of the earliest atherosclerotic lesions.

Adhesion molecules considered important in this process include members of the selectin superfamily, such as P-selectin. Leukocytes passing through the arterial circulation can bind to patches of endothelial cells expressing P-selectin, which mediates a rolling or saltatory slowing of the leukocytes.[71] The more permanent adhesion of the tethered white cell depends on the expression of another category of leukocyte adhesion molecule expressed on the endothelial surface at sites prone to lesion formation. Such adhesion molecules, members of the IgG superfamily, include vascular cell adhesion molecule-1 (VCAM-1).[72] Both P-selectin and VCAM-1, among other adhesion molecules, show increased expression in regions of human atherosclerotic plaques and on the macrovascular endothelium overlying nascent atherosclerotic plaques in experimental animals. While other leukocyte adhesion molecules doubtless participate in this capture of blood leukocytes, considerable evidence from genetically altered mice supports the essential involvement of P-selectin and VCAM-1 in lesion formation.[72,73]

Once firmly bound to the endothelial surface, white blood cells must receive chemoattractant stimuli to penetrate into the intima. Many such signals exist. Among them, monocyte chemoattractant protein-1 (MCP-1) may play a particularly important role. Again, experiments in genetically altered mice support the involvement of MCP-1 in the formation of experimental atherosclerotic lesions.[74] Other chemokines, such as the cell surface–associated molecule fractalkine, may also contribute to this process.[75-78]

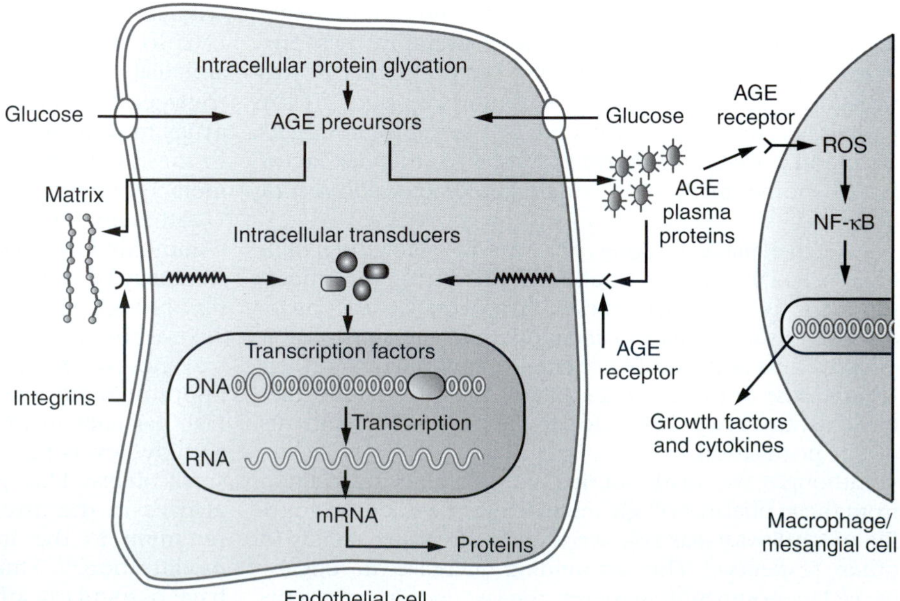

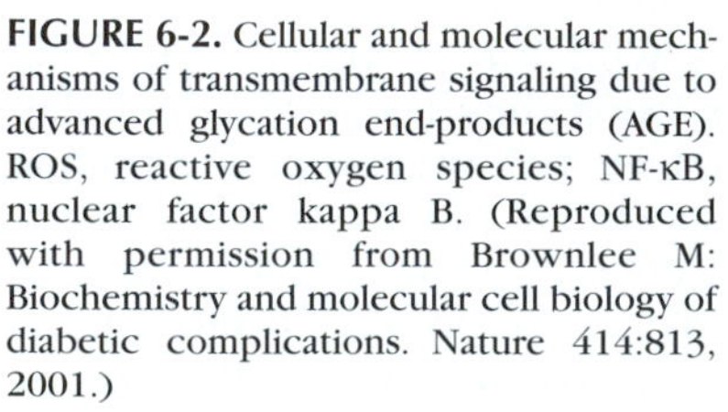

FIGURE 6-2. Cellular and molecular mechanisms of transmembrane signaling due to advanced glycation end-products (AGE). ROS, reactive oxygen species; NF-κB, nuclear factor kappa B. (Reproduced with permission from Brownlee M: Biochemistry and molecular cell biology of diabetic complications. Nature 414:813, 2001.)

In addition to mononuclear phagocytes, T lymphocytes accumulate in human atherosclerotic plaques, where they may play important regulatory roles. Adhesion molecules such as intracellular adhesion molecule-1 (ICAM-1), overexpressed by endothelial cells overlying atheromata, may participate in the adhesion of T lymphocytes along with VCAM-1. In addition, a trio of chemokines induced by the T cell activator, interferon gamma, may promote the chemoattraction of adherent T cells into the arterial intima.[79] Mast cells, long recognized as a part of the leukocyte population in the arterial adventitia, also localize within the intimal lesions of atherosclerosis. Although vastly outnumbered by macrophages, some believe that mast cells subserve specific functions that contribute to lesion formation or complication.[80] The chemokine exotaxin may participate in the recruitment of mast cells to the arterial intima.[81]

Once present in the arterial intima, these various classes of leukocytes undergo diverse activation reactions that may potentiate atherogenesis. For example, monocytes mature into macrophages in the atherosclerotic plaque, where they overexpress a series of scavenger receptors that can capture modified lipoproteins that accumulate in the atherosclerotic intima.[82-84] Because their levels do not decrease as cells accumulate cholesterol, these scavenger receptors permit the formation of foam cells, a hallmark of the atheromatous plaque. Macrophages within the atherosclerotic intima proliferate and become a rich source of mediators that may contribute to the progression of atherosclerosis including reactive oxygen species and proinflammatory cytokines.

One of the key signals for macrophage activation, macrophage-colony stimulating factor (M-CSF), can enhance scavenger receptor expression and promote replication of macrophages and their production of proinflammatory cytokines. Experiments in mutant mice have shown an important role for M-CSF in formation of atheromata.[85-87]

The T cells in the atherosclerotic plaque also display markers of chronic activation. Gamma interferon, a strong activating stimulus for T cells, localizes in plaques. Indicators of the action of gamma interferon, such as induction of the class II major histocompatibility antigen molecules, provide evidence for the biologic activity of gamma interferon in atherosclerotic plaques.[88] Recent work has shown that interleukin-18, expressed in atheromata, may participate in gamma interferon production within the plaque and thus amplify the adaptive immune response that appears to operate in lesions.[89]

Once recruited to the intima, the white blood cells can perpetuate and amplify the ongoing inflammatory response that led to their recruitment. The function of the "professional phagocytes" adds to the proinflammatory mediators elaborated by the intrinsic vascular wall cells and perpetuates and amplifies the local inflammatory response.

Atherosclerosis Progression

The recruitment of blood leukocytes and their activation in the arterial intima sets the stage for the progression of atherosclerosis. The proinflammatory mediators produced by these various cell types lead to the elaboration of factors that can stimulate the migration of smooth muscle cells from the tunica media into the intima. The normal human tunica intima contains resident smooth muscle cells. Growth factors produced locally by activated leukocytes provide a paracrine stimulus to smooth muscle cell proliferation. Activated smooth muscle cells also appear capable of producing growth factors that can stimulate their own proliferation or that of their neighbors, an autocrine pathway of proliferation.[90]

Other mediators present in atheromatous plaques, such as transforming growth factor beta (TGF-β), can augment the production of macromolecules of the extracellular matrix, including interstitial collagen. Thus "maturing" atherosclerotic lesions assume fibrous as well as fatty characteristics. Ultimately, the established atherosclerotic plaque develops a central lipid core encapsulated in fibrous extracellular matrix. In particular, the fibrous cap, the layer of connective tissue overlying the lipid core and separating it from the lumen of the artery, forms during the phase of lesion progression.

Another characteristic of the advancing atherosclerotic plaque, calcification, also involves tightly regulated biological functions. The expression of certain calcium-binding proteins within the plaque may sequester calcium hydroxyapatite. Such deposits, far from fixed, can undergo resorption as well as deposition. Reminiscent of bone metabolism, activated macrophages within the plaque appear to function as osteoclasts. Indeed, mice deficient in M-CSF, the macrophage activator, show increased accumulation of calcified deposits.[87,91] This observation supports the dynamic nature of the calcium accretion in the plaque.

Thus, during the phase of progression of atherosclerotic plaques, migration and proliferation of smooth muscle cells, accumulation of extracellular matrix, and calcification lead to the transition from the fatty streak, dominated by the lipid-laden macrophages known as foam cells, to the fibrocalcific plaque that can produce arterial stenoses and other complications of the disease. Although this phase of lesion progression in humans may begin in youth, it often continues for many decades. Notably, atherosclerotic plaques often produce no symptoms during this generally prolonged phase of lesion evolution. Although traditionally viewed as a disease of middle and later life, the seeds of atherosclerosis are sown much earlier. This recognition highlights the importance of early and aggressive reduction of risk factors, best accomplished by lifestyle modification rather than pharmacological intervention during the formative phase of the disease process.

THE DIVERSITY OF ATHEROSCLEROSIS

Heterogeneity of Atherosclerosis Lesions

Although most practitioners and laymen have focused in the past on atherosclerosis of the coronary arteries, we now recognize increasingly that atherosclerosis reaches beyond the coronary bed. Atherosclerosis lies at the root of many strokes. Although peripheral arterial disease jeopardizes limb more than life, the limitation of exercise capacity and the considerable burden of nonhealing ulcers and other complications of peripheral arterial disease render this manifestation of atherosclerosis important from both a medical and economic point of view (see Chapters 15 and 16). In addition, atherosclerotic involvement of the renal arteries contributes to end-stage renal disease and refractory hypertension in many instances (see Chapter 21).

From a pathophysiologic perspective, atherosclerosis in different distributions of the arterial tree has more in common than not. Although the fundamental cellular and molecular events that underlie atherosclerosis in various arterial trees seem similar, certain complications appear distinct. For example, ectasia and eventual aneurysm formation affect the atherosclerotic abdominal aorta more commonly than do stenosis and thrombosis leading to total aortic occlusion. In addition, the aorta, and particularly the proximal portions of its trunk, appear especially important as a source for atheroemboli that may cause cerebral or renal infarction.[92] Atherosclerosis of the extracranial vessels that perfuse the brain often develop stenosis. However, ulceration of carotid plaques with embolization of atheromatous material commonly causes transient ischemic attacks or monocular blindness.[93]

Some of the regional variations in the expressions of atherosclerosis may depend on embryologic factors. Endothelial cells in different regions of the arterial tree can display considerable heterogeneity, as determined by a variety of markers. Developmental biologists have long recognized that smooth muscle cells found in various segments of the arterial tree may have distinct embryologic origins. For example, smooth muscle cells in the ascending aorta and other arteries of the upper body derive from neural crest cells rather than mesenchyme.[94] Thus, smooth muscle cells can arise even from different germ layers in the lower body and neurectoderm in certain upper body arteries. The developmental biology of arteriogenesis and the determination of smooth muscle and endothelial cell lineages constitute a frontier of contemporary vascular biology research. For example, recent work suggests that both endothelial cells and smooth muscle cells may derive from bone marrow postnatally in injured, diseased, or transplanted arteries.[95-97] This recognition has not only intrinsic scientific interest but also may have therapeutic implications for regenerative medicine.

Atherosclerosis: A Focal or Diffuse Disease?

We classically understand atherosclerosis as a segmental process. Much of our traditional diagnostic armamentarium and treatment modalities aim to identify stenoses and restore flow by revascularization.

However, we recognize increasingly the diffuse nature of atherosclerosis. Classic comparison of histopathological examination with angiograms showed that the arteriogram vastly underestimates the involvement of coronary arteries by atherosclerosis.[98] More recently, the application of intravascular ultrasound has renewed our appreciation of the diffuse nature of coronary atherosclerosis.[99] Arterial stenoses often cause ischemia and bring the patient to the attention of clinicians. Various noninvasive modalities can disclose ischemia. Contrast angiography readily localizes the focal stenoses that most often cause demand ischemia. Yet, cross-sectional images obtained by intravascular ultrasound reveal that segments of arteries that appear absolutely normal by angiogram may nonetheless harbor a substantial burden of atherosclerotic disease.

The process of arterial remodeling during atherogenesis explains this apparent paradox. During much of its life history, an atherosclerotic plaque grows in an outward, or abluminal, direction. Thus, the plaque can grow silently without producing stenosis. Morphometric studies in nonhuman primates by Clarkson and colleagues first called attention to this compensatory enlargement of arteries that preserves the lumen during atherogenesis.[100] Oft-cited studies by Glagov and colleagues established the relevance of this process to human coronary atherosclerosis.[101] We now recognize that encroachment on the lumen occurs relatively late in the life history of an atheromatous plaque.

Well-performed and systematic histopathologic studies have shown that atherosclerotic disease begins early in life. In the Pathobiological Determinants of Atherosclerosis in Youth (PDAY) study, the aortas and coronary arteries of Americans aged 34 years or under who died noncardiac deaths revealed consistent involvement of the dorsal surface of the abdominal aorta by both fatty and raised arterial plaque. The coronary arteries, including the proximal portion of the left anterior descending coronary artery, also disclosed involvement even in this young population.[102] The Bogalusa Heart Study also showed a correlation between risk factors during life and the degree of atherosclerotic involvement at autopsy.[103] These systematic observations agree with reports of a substantial burden of coronary arterial atherosclerosis in young American male casualties during the Korean and Vietnam wars.[104] Indeed, maternal hypercholesterolemia associates with fatty streak formation in fetuses.[105,106]

These various data indicate that atherosclerosis is far more diffuse than we believed only a few years ago. The process begins much earlier in life than generally acknowledged. Indeed, intravascular ultrasound studies have shown one in six American teenagers has significant atherosclerotic involvement of the coronary arteries.[107] These findings have considerable importance for understanding the pathophysiology of the clinical manifestations of atherosclerosis. They also have important implications for the management of this disease (see later).

Shear Stress and Atheroprotection: Why Atherosclerosis Begins Where It Does

The foregoing section emphasizes the diffuse nature of atherosclerosis in adults. However, both in humans and experimental animals, atherosclerosis begins in certain stereotyped locales. The predilection of atherosclerosis for branch points and flow dividers appears quite consistent across species.

Why do these sites have a predisposition to early atherogenesis? Decades of sophisticated biomechanical analysis have established that atheromata tend to form at sites of disturbed blood flow, particularly areas of low shear stress.[108] Endothelial cells can somehow sense shear stress. For example, in areas of laminar shear stress in vivo and in monolayers of cultured cells in vitro, endothelial cells align their long axes parallel to the direction of flow. At branch points and dividers in the arterial tree, the well-ordered cobblestone array of the endothelial monolayer changes: cells show more polygonal and irregular shapes. Areas of low shear stress show heightened endothelial cell turnover, increased permeability, and prolonged retention of lipoprotein particles in the subendothelial regions of the intima. Such data, accumulated over many decades, began to provide answers to the question, "What goes awry at sites of lesion predilection?"

More recent data have inspired a different and complementary hypothesis to explain the focality of atherosclerosis initiation. Using the techniques of modern molecular biology, transcriptional profiling provides a "snapshot" of the expression of a large number of genes in a single experiment. The pattern of genes expressed by endothelial cells subjected to controlled physiologic levels of laminar shear stress in vitro differs strikingly from that of resting endothelial cells in vitro. A number of genes differentially expressed by endothelial cells experiencing laminar shear stress appear to have "atheroprotective" functions. Pioneering work performed by Topper working with Gimbrone identified putative atheroprotective genes as selectively augmented by laminar shear flow.[109] These findings suggested that regions of undisturbed, laminar shear stress enjoy tonic endogenous antioxidant, vasodilatory, and anti-inflammatory properties conferred by the function of these putative "atheroprotective" genes. For example, superoxide dismutase can catabolize the highly reactive superoxide anion (O_2^-). Cyclooxygenase-2 can give rise to the vasodilatory and anti-aggregatory arachidonic acid metabolite prostacyclin. The endothelial isoform of nitric oxide synthase (eNOS) produces the endogenous vasodilator, antithrombotic, and anti-inflammatory mediator nitric oxide (·NO).[109] Nitric oxide also exerts anti-inflammatory actions by combating leukocyte adhesion to the activated endothelial cell.[110]

At regions of disturbed flow, for example near branch points and flow dividers, the expression of these endogenous atheroprotective genes should decline. Indeed, elegant studies by Collins and Cybulsky indicate that areas predisposed to lesion formation show activation of NF-κB, the master regulator of inflammatory gene expression.[111] Because nitric oxide can antagonize the activation of NF-κB, the absence of laminar flow in these regions may well explain, at least in part, the tendency of nascent atheromata to form at such sites.

Thus, atherosclerosis is both a focal and diffuse disease. It begins focally for reasons we understand in increasing detail. The stenoses that cause flow-limiting lesions tend to localize in similar regions. Much of our diagnostic and therapeutic activity in contemporary cardiology and vascular medicine has focused on these stenoses. However, we appreciate increasingly the diffuse distribution of atherosclerosis and the systemic nature of the risk factors that promote its development.

The Pathophysiology of the Thrombotic Complications of Atherosclerosis

As noted, flow-limiting stenoses have driven much of the diagnostic and therapeutic activity in clinical atherosclerosis for many decades. Patients with flow-limiting lesions often experience symptoms due to ischemia: angina pectoris in the coronary circulation and intermittent claudication in peripheral arterial disease. We can readily diagnose ischemia by various noninvasive modalities. We can localize stenoses by angiographic techniques, both invasive and noninvasive. The percutaneous and surgical approaches that relieve ischemia caused by focal stenoses have proved effective in relieving ischemia as well.

However, we now recognize that in many cases, acute thrombosis does not occur on the most tightly narrowed segments of an artery. The best illustration of this counterintuitive observation arises from analyses of fatal coronary thromboses. Various lines of clinical evidence suggest that a minority of fatal coronary thrombi occur where stenoses exceed 60%. Thus, many occlusive thrombi complicate lesions that neither limit flow nor meet traditional angiographic criteria for "significance." Fewer data exist regarding the substrates for thrombosis in noncoronary arteries; however, in peripheral and carotid arteries, inflammation, tightly linked to mechanisms of thrombosis, characterizes atherosclerotic lesions. Intraplaque hemorrhage appears quite common in carotid plaques that cause cerebral ischemic disease as well.[112]

Although most fatal myocardial infarctions occur at sites of noncritical stenosis, it does not follow that high-grade stenoses cause fewer heart attacks than less obstructive lesions. Indeed, on a "per lesion basis," the tighter stenoses are more likely to give rise to acute myocardial infarction.[113] Because the noncritically stenotic lesions outnumber the "tight" stenoses, the total risk attributable to the less stenotic lesions exceeds the risk due to the less numerous lesions that cause higher-grade stenoses.

A common confusion surrounds the distinction between lesion size and degree of stenosis. Based on our traditional angiographic view of atherosclerosis, many assume that lesions that cause high-grade stenoses are larger than those that cause less obstruction. This fallacy fails to consider the importance of outward remodeling or compensatory enlargement. The outward growth of most atherosclerotic plaques before they begin to encroach on the lumen protects the lumen from obstruction and conceals the growing lesion from visualization by angiography until the latter stages of its evolution. Thus, low-grade stenoses do *not* equate with smaller plaques. Indeed, larger and eccentrically remodeled plaques may cause acute coronary syndromes more frequently than smaller plaques that do not exhibit compensatory enlargement and/or produce greater degrees of stenosis.[113,114]

Concordant evidence from several avenues of investigation suggests that a physical disruption of the atherosclerotic plaque, rather than a critical degree of stenosis, can commonly precipitate arterial thromboses. Four mechanisms of plaque disruption may cause thrombosis or rapid plaque expansion (Fig. 6-3). A through-and-through fracture of the plaque's fibrous cap causes most

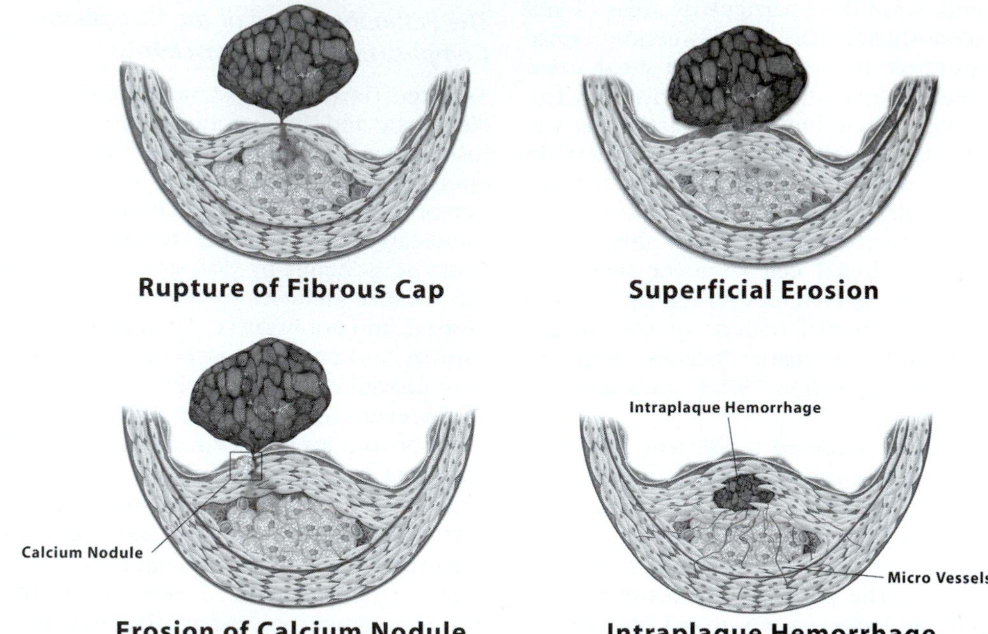

FIGURE 6-3. Mechanisms of plaque disruption. Rupture of the fibrous cap (*upper left*) causes two thirds to three quarters of fatal coronary thrombosis. Superficial erosion (*upper right*) occurs in one-fifth to one quarter of all cases of fatal coronary thrombosis. Certain populations, such as diabetic individuals and women, appear more susceptible to superficial erosion as a mechanism of plaque disruption and thrombosis. Erosion of a calcium nodule may also cause plaque disruption and thrombosis (*lower left*). In addition, the friable microvessels in the base of the atherosclerotic plaque may rupture and cause intraplaque hemorrhage (*lower right*). The consequent local generation of thrombin may stimulate smooth muscle proliferation, migration, and collagen synthesis, promoting fibrosis and plaque expansion on a subacute basis. Severe intraplaque hemorrhage can cause sudden lesion expansion by a mass effect acutely as well. (Reproduced with permission from Libby P, Theroux P: Pathophysiology of coronary artery disease. Circulation 111:3481-3488, 2005).

fatal coronary thromboses (see Fig. 6-3). Our group hypothesized some time ago a model of the pathophysiology of this common mechanism of atherosclerotic plaque disruption that focused on the metabolism of interstitial collagen.[115] This extracellular matrix macromolecule accounts for much of the biomechanical strength of the plaque's fibrous cap. Further hypothesizing that inflammation regulates the metabolism of interstitial forms of collagen and might regulate the stability of an atherosclerotic plaque (Fig. 6-4), we found that certain proinflammatory cytokines expressed in the atherosclerotic plaque can inhibit the ability of the smooth muscle cell to synthesize new collagen required to repair and maintain the integrity of the plaque's fibrous cap. Notably, gamma interferon can inhibit interstitial collagen gene expression in human vascular smooth muscle cells.[116]

The interstitial collagen triple helix resists breakdown by most proteases. We described the overexpression of proteolytic enzymes specialized in the catabolism of collagen in the atherosclerotic plaque, and further demonstrated that inflammatory mediators found in the atheroma can enhance the expression of these collagenolytic enzymes, members of the matrix metalloproteinase (MMP) family.[117,118] Cells in human atheromata overexpress all three members of the human interstitial collagenase family (MMP-1, -13, and -8).[119-122] Our group has furnished evidence that collagen breakdown actually occurs in situ in human atherosclerotic plaques.[121] These findings indicate that the interstitial collagenase MMPs exist in their active rather than their precursor zymogen forms.[123] Furthermore, the demonstration of collagenolysis in situ indicates that these collagenases overwhelm their endogenous inhibitors including the tissue inhibitors of MMPs (TIMPs). Our group also ascribed a hitherto unknown function to tissue factor pathway inhibitor-2 (TFPI-2) as a potent collagenase inhibitor. Although we find little regulation of TIMPs in atherosclerotic lesions,

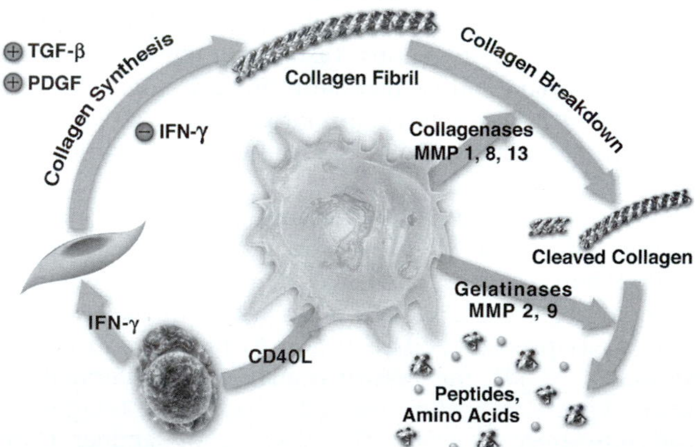

FIGURE 6-4. The relationship between inflammation and collagen metabolism in the atherosclerotic plaque. The T lymphocyte can elaborate interferon gamma (IFN-γ) that reduces the ability of the smooth muscle cell to synthesize new collagen. The T cell also can stimulate the macrophage through CD40 ligation to elaborate the interstitial collagenases MMP-1, -8, and -13—which can make the initial cleavage in the collagen fibril. The elaboration of gelatinases such as MMP-2 and -9 can contribute to the further cleavage of collagen fragments to peptides and amino acids. Transforming growth factor-beta (TGF-β) and platelet-derived growth factor (PDGF) from autocrine or paracrine sources, including degranulating platelets, can promote collagen synthesis by smooth muscle cells.

MMP = matrix metalloproteinases, CD40L = CD40 ligand.

TFPI-2, abundant in normal arteries, shows decreased levels in atherosclerotic lesions.[124] Thus, a preponderance of proteases over their inhibitors prevails in the atherosclerotic plaque. Colocalization of proteases with inflammatory cells and regulation of their expression by products of inflammatory cells strongly implicate disordered collagen metabolism as a key mechanism for atherosclerotic plaque destabilization. Recent experiments in genetically altered mice have demonstrated formally the importance of collagen catabolism in the regulation of the steady-state level of this extracellular matrix macromolecule in experimental atheromata.[125]

Superficial erosion of the endothelial monolayer constitutes an important cause of a minority of coronary thromboses (see Fig. 6-3). Women, diabetic individuals, hypertriglyceridemics, and the elderly appear to have a higher frequency of superficial erosion as a cause of fatal thrombosis than do younger, male hypercholesterolemic individuals.[126,127] Various molecular and cellular mechanisms may underlie superficial erosion. Excessive proteolysis of extracellular matrix macromolecules that make up the subendothelial basement membrane may predispose toward endothelial desquamation and superficial erosion.[128] Apoptosis, or programmed death, of endothelial cells may also promote superficial erosion. Various proinflammatory stimuli can sensitize endothelial cells to apoptosis.[129] In addition, hypochlorous acid, a product of myeloperoxidase, an enzyme found in leukocytes in atherosclerotic plaques, can provoke endothelial cell apoptosis.[130] Local generation of tissue factor from dying endothelial cells may also contribute to thrombosis at sites of superficial erosion.[130]

Atherosclerotic plaques often harbor rich plexuses of microvessels.[131] The neovascularization of plaques provides an additional portal for trafficking of leukocytes that may promote the inflammatory process. Neovessels in the plaque, like those in the diabetic retina, may be friable and fragile. Intraplaque hemorrhage due to disruption of microvessels may cause sudden plaque expansion (see Fig. 6-3). Local generation of thrombin and other mediators associated with coagulation in situ may promote lesion growth. For example, platelet-derived growth factor (PDGF) and transforming growth factor-beta (TGF-β), as well as PF-4, released by platelets at sites of microvascular hemorrhage and intramural thrombosis may hasten local fibrosis.[116] Thrombin can stimulate smooth muscle cell migration, division, and collagen synthesis.[132] Thus, microvascular disruption, while not provoking an occlusive thrombus, may promote lesion evolution nonetheless.

Erosion through the intima of a calcified nodule represents another less common form of atherosclerotic plaque disruption associated with thrombosis (see Fig. 6-3). The active metabolism of calcium hydroxyapatite with its accretion and removal, as described above, can contribute to calcium accumulation in regions of atherosclerotic plaques.[91] The tendency of atheromata to accumulate calcium has given rise to clinical testing. Increasing evidence supports the contention that the amount of coronary artery calcification correlates with the burden of atherosclerotic disease.[133] Moreover, emerging data suggest a correlation between calcium score and risk of future cardiovascular events. However, we await the results of larger and longer studies on unselected populations to assess whether or not calcium scoring can provide prognostic information beyond that available from established risk algorithms or other biomarkers currently under study. The notion that arterial calcification bears a relationship to atherosclerosis complication holds considerable sway. Yet, current biologic understanding and preliminary clinical evidence suggest that coronary lesions most likely to cause thrombosis contain less calcium than lesions that cause flow-limiting stenoses and ischemia.[134] Thus, the calcified lesions may actually have less propensity to disrupt and provoke coronary thrombosis than those with little calcium.

The Mutability of the Atherosclerotic Plaque

The classic concept of atherosclerosis assumed a steady, relentless, and continuous progression of the disease. However, serial angiographic studies suggest that stenoses evolve in a discontinuous fashion with periods of relative quiescence punctuated by spurts in growth.[135,136] Our current understanding of plaque pathobiology suggests a plausible mechanism to explain this angiographically discontinuous evolution of arterial stenoses. Careful study of the coronary arteries of individuals who succumb to noncardiac death, and of coronary arteries perfusion-fixed in the operating room from hearts of transplantation recipients with ischemic cardiomyopathy, as well as observations on cholesterol-fed nonhuman primates, all indicate that areas of plaque disruption or superficial erosion with nonocclusive mural thrombus formation occur frequently.[137-140] The picture that arises from an amalgamation of these human and experimental observations indicates that most plaque disruptions with thrombosis in situ do not proceed to a total occlusion and, indeed, usually pass unnoticed by the patient or physician (Fig. 6-5). For various reasons, plaque disruptions with mural thrombosis may not proceed to a disastrous total thrombosis in all events. In many patients, the endogenous fibrinolytic mechanisms or antithrombotic effects of dietary or pharmacologic intervention may prevent thrombi from propagating. Larger arteries such as the aorta have sufficient flow to prevent mural thrombi from progressing to total occlusion in most instances. Indeed, although inspection of the aortas of many patients with atherosclerosis discloses many ulcerated lesions with mural thrombi, aortic occlusion due to thrombosis fortunately occurs relatively rarely (Fig. 6-6).

The failure of most mural thrombi to progress to total occlusion does not imply that such events have a benign course. Although subclinical at the time that they occur, the mural thrombi elicit a local "wound healing" response that tends to promote plaque progression. Indeed, one of the types of "crisis" in the history of a plaque that can lead to its sudden evolution, as disclosed by serial angiographic studies, likely reflects such a scenario (see Fig. 6-5). A localized plaque disruption with mural thrombus can engender a healing response induced by platelet products released at short range, such as TGF-β, a potent stimulus to collagen gene expression by smooth muscle cells. PDGF, also released during platelet aggregation, stimulates

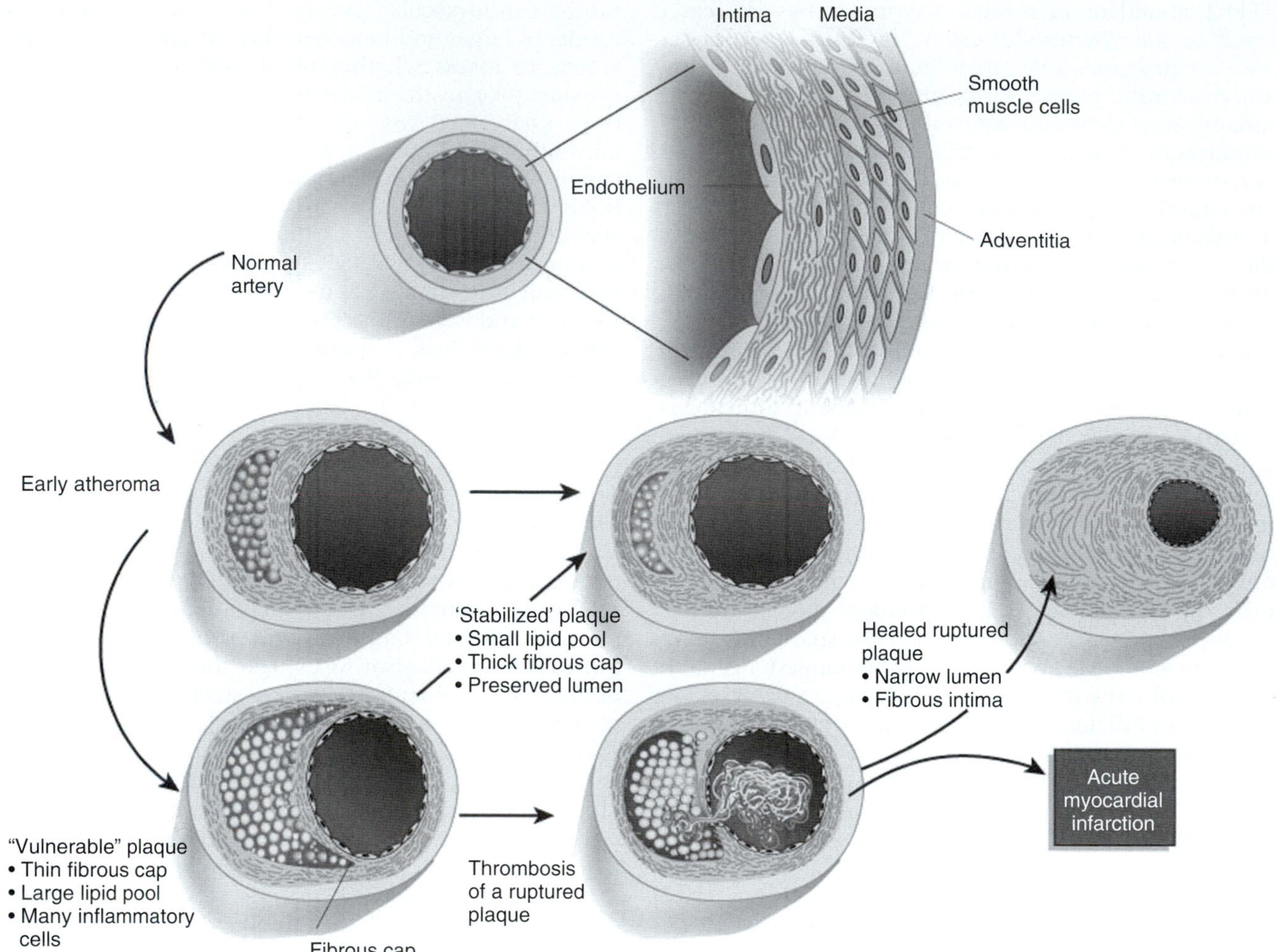

FIGURE 6-5. (See also Color Plate 6-5.) Schematic of the life history of an atheroma. The normal human coronary artery has a typical trilaminar structure. The endothelial cells in contact with the blood in the arterial lumen rest on a basement membrane. The intimal layer in adult humans generally contains a small amount of smooth muscle cells scattered within the intimal extracellular matrix. The internal elastic lamina forms the barrier between the tunica intima and the underlying tunica media. The media consists of multiple layers of smooth muscle cells, much more tightly packed than in the diffusely thickened intima, and embedded in a matrix rich in elastin as well as collagen. In early atherogenesis, recruitment of inflammatory cells and the accumulation of lipids leads to formation of a lipid-rich core, as the artery enlarges in an outward, abluminal direction to accommodate the expansion of the intima. If inflammatory conditions prevail and risk factors such as dyslipidemia persist, the lipid core can grow, and proteinases secreted by the activated leukocytes can degrade extracellular matrix, whereas proinflammatory cytokines such as interferon-gamma can limit the synthesis of new collagen. These changes can thin the fibrous cap and render it friable and susceptible to rupture.

When the plaque ruptures, blood coming in contact with the tissue factor in the plaque coagulates; platelets activated by thrombin generated from the coagulation cascade, as well as by contact with collagen in the intimal compartment, instigate thrombus formation. If the thrombus occludes the vessel persistently, an acute myocardial infarction can result (the dusky blue area in the anterior wall of the left ventricle, (*lower right*). The thrombus may eventually resorb due to endogenous or therapeutic thrombolysis. However, a wound-healing response triggered by thrombin generated during blood coagulation can stimulate smooth muscle proliferation. Platelet-derived growth factor (PDGF) released from activated platelets stimulates smooth muscle cell migration.

Transforming growth factor-beta (TFG-β), also released from activated platelets, stimulates interstitial collagen production. This increased migration, proliferation, and extracellular matrix synthesis by smooth muscle cells thickens the fibrous cap and causes further expansion of the intima, often now in an inward direction constricting the lumen. Such stenotic lesions produced by the luminal encroachment of the fibrosed plaque may restrict flow, particularly under situations of increased cardiac demand, leading to ischemia, commonly provoking symptoms such as *angina pectoris*. Such advanced stenotic plaques, being more fibrous, may prove less susceptible to rupture and renewed thrombosis. Lipid lowering can reduce lipid content and calm the intimal inflammatory response, yielding a more stable plaque with a thick fibrous cap and a preserved lumen (*center*). (Reproduced with permission from Libby P: Inflammation in atherosclerosis. Nature 420:868, 2002.)

smooth muscle migration. Thrombin locally generated at sites of thrombosis can stimulate smooth muscle cell proliferation, migration, and collagen gene expression. All of these molecular and cellular mechanisms conspire to promote a round of smooth muscle cell migration, proliferation, and local collagen synthesis. Quite plausibly, this scenario leads to evolution from a lipid-rich plaque with abundant inflammatory cells to a more fibrous lesion, rich in connective tissue, often with a paucity of inflammatory cells due to their death or departure, accretion of calcium deposits, and a relative lack of lipid accumulation. Careful study of atheromata obtained at autopsy does show signs of healed plaque disruption in some fibrous lesions (Fig. 6-7).[141]

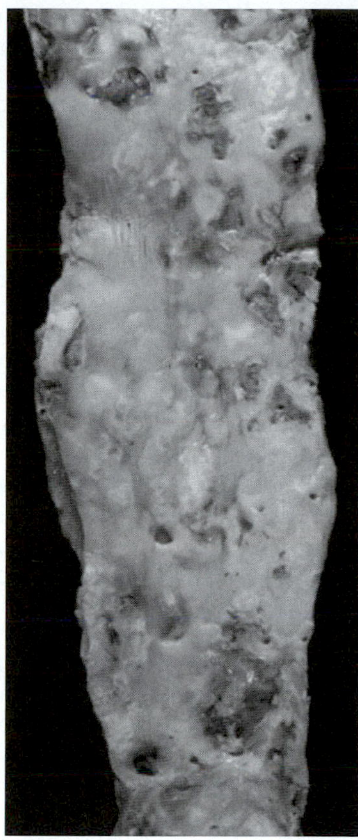

FIGURE 6-6. (See also Color Plate 6-6.) Widespread atheromatous involvement of the abdominal aorta in a patient with atherosclerosis. Note the variety of atheromata in different stages of evolution within a few centimeters of one another. There are ulcerated plaques, raised lesions, and fatty streaks, among other types of lesions demonstrated in this example.

The biologic scenario described above depicts a life history of the atherosclerotic plaque more dynamic than heretofore recognized (see Fig. 6-5). The heterogeneity of human atherosclerotic plaques, a concept now gaining considerable currency, highlights the importance of the qualitative characteristics of a lesion, not just its size. Whereas previous concepts emphasized the structure of atherosclerotic plaques, contemporary thinking accords a greater contribution to the biologic characteristics of the plaque as well.

"Stable" vs. "Vulnerable" Plaques

This recognition of the heterogeneity of atherosclerotic plaques has fostered the adoption of a dichotomous view of atheromata: "stable" versus "vulnerable" plaques.[138] The notion of the *vulnerable plaque* has engendered considerable interest by pathologists and practitioners alike. Current cardiologic parlance uses the term *vulnerable plaque* as shorthand for a particular type of lesion characterized by a thin fibrous cap, large lipid core, and surfeit of inflammatory cells. Use of this term and its opposite, the so-called *stable* plaque, extends findings largely obtained at postmortem examination of intact human beings. Although the dichotomization of plaques into *vulnerable* and *stable* provides a useful shorthand, we should exercise care in extrapolating morphologic findings uncritically to foretell clinical complications.

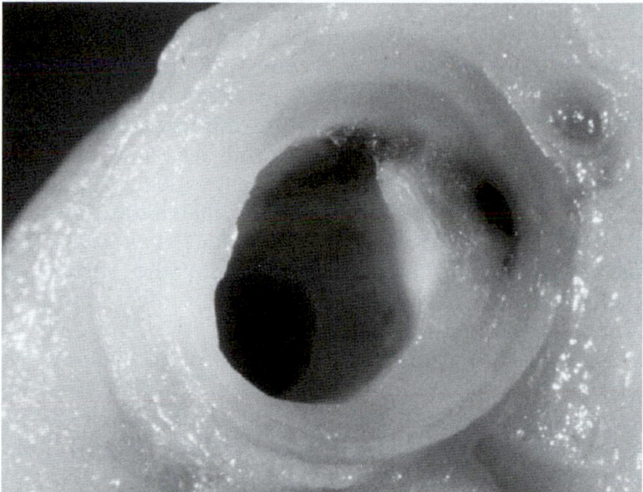

A

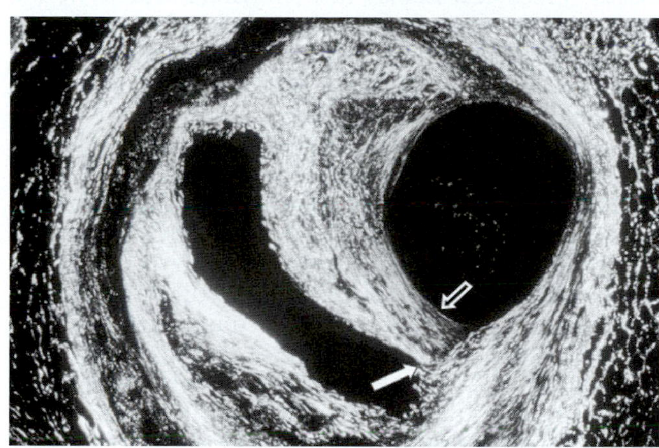

B

FIGURE 6-7. (See also Color Plate 6-7.) Hemorrhage, thrombosis, and plaque healing as a mechanism of atheroma progression. **A,** Photograph of a coronary artery with a plaque rupture that has led to an intraplaque hematoma without an occlusive thrombus. As explained in the text, thrombin and platelet products such as platelet-derived growth factor (PDGF) and transforming growth factor-beta (TGF-β) elaborated locally at the site of microthrombosis and hematoma formation can stimulate fibrosis. **B,** This Sirius-red-stained preparation of a cross-section of a coronary artery shows an area of plaque rupture (*solid arrow*) that healed to cause further accretion of a layer of collagen (*open arrow*) and luminal encroachment. This example illustrates the "archaeology" of the atherosclerotic plaque: distant plaque rupture followed by healing and fibrosis with progression of the lesion to stenosis. Note that the arterial lumen at the time of the original plaque rupture would not have shown a critical narrowing. (These figures were kindly provided by the late Prof. Michael J. Davies.)

This pigeon-holing of plaques has engendered considerable effort to develop methods for identifying so-called vulnerable or high risk lesions. However, such a simple dichotomous view of atherosclerosis oversimplifies a disease of staggering complexity. For example, considerable evidence suggests that a given arterial tree has not one but many vulnerable plaques. Angioscopic and intravascular ultrasonographic study of coronary arteries, as well as interpretation of angiographic observations, supports the multiplicity of disrupted plaques in patients with acute coronary syndromes.[142-144,144a] Inflammation may link "instability" of coronary and carotid plaques in the same individuals.[145] As previously mentioned, the aorta in atherosclerotic individuals often shows multiple ulcerated lesions, often within millimeters of fatty streaks, raised fibrous lesions, and resorbing, healing thrombi (see Fig. 6-5). Thus, the quest to identify a single vulnerable plaque probably underestimates the complexity of the clinical challenge. Our broader view of the risk of atherosclerotic complications seeks the vulnerable patient and targets intervention more widely than to a single so-called vulnerable plaque.

How could one approach such a "vulnerable patient"? Here are grounds for considerable optimism. Atherosclerosis, both experimental and human, exhibits a mutability not imagined until recently. Indeed, lipid lowering and other manipulations can alter features of plaques paramount to the clinical expression of the disease. Preclinical studies have shown that lipid lowering by diet or by treatment with statins can alter features of plaques associated with vulnerability in humans.[146-148] Likewise, treatment with angiotensin-converting enzyme (ACE) inhibitors can confer characteristics of stability on experimentally produced plaques in rabbits.[149] A number of studies in atherosclerosis-prone mice have demonstrated that interruption of inflammatory signaling pathways or manipulation of TGF-β, the anti-inflammatory and pro-fibrotic cytokine, can alter features of plaques associated with their propensity to rupture and provoke thrombosis.[150,151] In addition to structural changes relating to the collagen content of plaques that may determine their biomechanical integrity, interventions such as lipid lowering can reduce the expression of tissue factor, hence lowering the thrombogenic potential of the atherosclerotic plaque.[152]

Clinical studies have begun to illustrate the potential mutability of atherosclerosis, abundantly demonstrated in animals by the experiments described above. Infusion of apolipoprotein A-1 Milano can cause modest reductions in the volume of atherosclerotic plaques as monitored by intravascular ultrasound.[153] Aggressive lipid- lowering therapy with a potent statin can likewise arrest the accumulation of atherosclerotic plaque as determined by serial ultrasonographic study.[154] Careful histological correlations with magnetic resonance imaging likewise disclose evidence for the mutability of atherosclerotic plaques in intact human beings.[155] These preclinical and clinical observations together provide grounds for considerable optimism regarding our ability to manipulate the character of atherosclerotic plaques in ways that can benefit patient outcomes. The disease appears much more mutable than many had dared hope in years gone by.

ATHEROSCLEROSIS: A SYSTEMIC DISEASE

Our traditional medical focus on atherosclerosis as a segmental disease caused by cholesterol accumulation has undergone an accelerated revision. We increasingly understand the global nature of factors that encompass the entire metabolic state of the patient, not just the serum cholesterol level. As the spectrum of risk factors in our population shifts, our attention must likewise broaden to encompass not just hypercholesterolemia but the dyslipidemia associated with the metabolic syndrome and diabetes. As elevated LDL cholesterol and smoking recede as risk factors in our society, we must expand our traditional thinking about atherogenesis to acknowledge the increasing contribution of obesity and insulin resistance.

We also recognize increasingly the importance of atherosclerosis beyond the coronary arteries. Our purview should now embrace the entire arterial tree with all of its beds. We must strive to fill the knowledge gaps about regional differences in human atherosclerosis as well as differences in the biology and clinical manifestations of atherosclerosis associated with the shifting pattern of risk factors.

Our comprehension of the pathophysiology of atherosclerosis has undergone a revolution in recent decades. There is no reason to believe that emerging data and deeper understanding of this process will not continue to change our concepts of this disease in the future. We should take immense satisfaction in the therapeutic inroads furnished by contemporary pharmacologic tools. The reduction in coronary heart disease and cerebrovascular events accruing from such treatments as the statins and ACE inhibitors has changed medicine irrevocably and provides striking benefits to patients. The therapeutic advances that have emerged from the application of progress in basic science and have proved effective in randomized clinical trials furnish cardiovascular medicine with an enviable and unparalleled database for the practice of evidence-based medicine.

Yet, much remains undone. Despite the previously mentioned victory of clinical science, the majority of cardiovascular events still occur despite optimal therapy that addresses multiple facets of our current understanding of the pathophysiology of this disease.[155a] Our challenge for the future is clear. We must strive to turn the tide on the alarming trends toward increased cardiovascular risk due to obesity and physical inactivity. We must not relent in our quest to advance the scientific understanding of atherogenesis and the translation to innovative therapies to address the residual and ever-growing burden of disease.

Many of the current landmark studies in the cardiovascular arena have focused on death and acute coronary syndromes as "major adverse coronary events." These endpoints offer relative ease of study, adjudication, and quantification. However, we must not lose sight of the enormous impediment to quality of life due to intermittent claudication caused by peripheral arterial disease, and loss of ability to communicate and live independently due to cerebrovascular disease. In addition to the human costs of these manifestations of noncoronary atherosclerosis, our society shoulders a substantial economic burden due to the ravages of peripheral arterial and cerebrovascular disease. We must pursue these issues with the same fervor we have traditionally accorded to coronary artery disease. This goal will become even more important as elder segments of our population continue to increase in numbers due to changing demographics. The powerful tools available to investigators today provide grounds for optimism. Further inroads against the residual morbidity and mortality from atherosclerosis will emerge from future application of basic science to alter the biology of this disease, regarded not so long ago as an inevitable companion of the aging process.

REFERENCES

1. Ross R: The pathogenesis of atherosclerosis: A perspective for the 1990s. Nature 362:801, 1993.
2. Libby P, Aikawa M, Schonbeck U: Cholesterol and atherosclerosis. Biochim Biophys Acta 1529:299, 2000.
3. Brown MS, Goldstein JL: A receptor-mediated pathway for cholesterol homeostasis. Science 232:232, 1986.
4. Steinberg D: Thematic review series: The pathogenesis of atherosclerosis. An interpretive history of the cholesterol controversy: Part I. J Lipid Res 45:1583, 2004.
5. Steinberg D: Thematic review series: The pathogenesis of atherosclerosis. An interpretive history of the cholesterol controversy, Part II: The early evidence linking hypercholesterolemia to coronary disease in humans. J Lipid Res 46(2):179, 2004.
6. Oliver MF: Might treatment of hypercholesterolaemia increase non-cardiac mortality? Lancet 337:1529, 1991.
7. Moore TJ: The cholesterol myth. The Atlantic Monthly 264:37, 1989.
8. Genest J, Libby P, Gotto M Jr: Lipoprotein disorders and cardiovascular disease. In Zipes DP, Libby P, Bonow R, et al (eds): Heart Disease: A Textbook of Cardiovascular Medicine. 7th ed. Philadelphia, Elsevier; 2005, p 1013.
9. Levy D, Merz CN, Cody RJ, et al: Hypertension detection, treatment and control: Acall to action for cardiovascular specialists. J Am Coll Cardiol 34:1360, 1999.
10. Gifford RW Jr: Review of the long-term controlled trials of usefulness of therapy for systemic hypertension. Am J Cardiol 63:8B, 1989.
11. Turnbull F: Effects of different blood-pressure-lowering regimens on major cardiovascular events: Results of prospectively-designed overviews of randomised trials. Lancet 362:1527, 2003.
12. Nissen SE, Tuzcu EM, Libby P, et al: Effect of antihypertensive agents on cardiovascular events in patients with coronary disease and normal blood pressure: The CAMELOT study: A randomized controlled trial. JAMA 292:2217, 2004.
13. Dahlof B, Devereux RB, Kjeldsen SE, et al: Cardiovascular morbidity and mortality in the Losartan Intervention for Endpoint Reduction in Hypertension study (LIFE): A randomised trial against atenolol. Lancet 359:995, 2002.
14. Julius S, Kjeldsen SE, Weber M, et al: Outcomes in hypertensive patients at high cardiovascular risk treated with regimens based on valsartan or amlodipine: The VALUE randomised trial. Lancet 363:2022, 2004.
15. Fuster V, Gotto AM, Libby P, et al: 27th Bethesda Conference: Matching the intensity of risk factor management with the hazard for coronary disease events. Task Force 1. Pathogenesis of coronary disease: The biologic role of risk factors. J Am Coll Cardiol. 27:964, 1996.
16. McGill HC Jr: The cardiovascular pathology of smoking. Am Heart J 115:250, 1988.
17. McGill HC Jr: Smoking and the pathogenesis of atherosclerosis. Adv Exp Med Biol 273:9, 1990.
18. Celermajer DS, Sorensen KE, Georgakopoulos D, et al: Cigarette smoking is associated with dose-related and potentially reversible impairment of endothelium-dependent dilation in healthy young adults. Circulation 88:2149, 1993.
19. Deanfield J: Passive smoking and early arterial damage. Eur Heart J 17:645, 1996.
20. Churg A, Wang RD, Tai H, et al: Macrophage metalloelastase mediates acute cigarette smoke-induced inflammation via tumor necrosis factor-alpha release. Am J Respir Crit Care Med 167:1083, 2003.
21. Executive summary of the third report of the national cholesterol education program (NCEP) expert panel on detection, evaluation, and treatment of high blood cholesterol in adults (Adult Treatment Panel III). JAMA 285:2486, 2001.
22. Wenger NK: You've come a long way, baby: Cardiovascular health and disease in women: Problems and prospects. Circulation 109:558, 2004.
23. Stamler J: The coronary drug project—findings with regard to estrogen, dextrothyroxine, clofibrate and niacin. Adv Exp Med Biol 82:52, 1977.
24. Mosca L, Appel LJ, Benjamin EJ, et al: Evidence-based guidelines for cardiovascular disease prevention in women. Circulation 109:672, 2004.
25. Third report of the national cholesterol education program (NCEP) expert panel on detection, evaluation, and treatment of high blood cholesterol in adults (Adult Treatment Panel III) final report. Circulation 106:3143, 2002.
26. Genest J Jr, Cohn J: Plasma triglyceride-rich lipoprotein and high density lipoprotein disorders associated with atherosclerosis. J Invest Med 46:351, 1998.
27. Tall AR, Jiang X, Luo Y, et al: 1999 George Lyman Duff Memorial Lecture: Lipid transfer proteins, HDL metabolism, and atherogenesis. Arterioscler Thromb Vasc Biol 20:1185, 2000.
28. Navab M, Anantharamaiah GM, Reddy ST, et al: The oxidation hypothesis of atherogenesis: The role of oxidized phospholipids and HDL. J Lipid Res 45:993, 2004.
29. Handy DE, Loscalzo J: Homocysteine and atherothrombosis: Diagnosis and treatment. Curr Atheroscler Rep 5:276, 2003.
30. Ridker PM, Stampfer MJ, Rifai N: Novel risk factors for systemic atherosclerosis: A comparison of C-reactive protein, fibrinogen, homocysteine, lipoprotein(a), and standard cholesterol screening as predictors of peripheral arterial disease. JAMA 285:2481, 2001.
31. Homocysteine Studies Collaboration: Homocysteine and risk of ischemic heart disease and stroke: A meta-analysis. JAMA 288:2015, 2002.
32. Wilson PW: Homocysteine and coronary heart disease: How great is the hazard? JAMA 288:2042, 2002.
33. Homocysteine Lowering Trialists' Collaboration: Lowering blood homocysteine with folic acid based supplements: Meta-analysis of randomised trials. BMJ 316:894, 1998.
34. Clarke R, Collins R: Can dietary supplements with folic acid or vitamin B6 reduce cardiovascular risk? Design of clinical trials to test the homocysteine hypothesis of vascular disease. J Cardiovasc Risk 5:249, 1998.
35. Scanu AM, Nakajima K, Edelstein C: Apolipoprotein(a): Structure and biology. Front Biosci 6:D546, 2001.
36. Scanu AM: Lp(a) lipoprotein—coping with heterogeneity. N Engl J Med 349:2089, 2003.
37. Stein JH, Rosenson RS: Lipoprotein Lp(a) excess and coronary heart disease. Arch Intern Med 157:1170, 1997.
38. Koenig W: Fibrinogen and coronary risk. Curr Cardiol Rep 1:112, 1999.
39. Montalescot G, Collet JP, Choussat R, et al: Fibrinogen as a risk factor for coronary heart disease. Eur Heart J 19 (Suppl H):H11, 1998.
40. Rokitansky K: The organs of circulation. In Swaine WE, Moore CH, Sieveking E, Day Ge (transl.): A Manual of Pathological Anatomy. Philadelphia, Blanchard and Lea; 1855, vol. IV, p.201.
41. Bini A, Wu D, Schnuer J, et al: Characterization of stromelysin 1 (MMP-3), matrilysin (MMP-7), and membrane type 1 matrix metalloproteinase (MT1-MMP) derived fibrin(ogen) fragments D-dimer and D-like monomer: NH2-terminal sequences of late-stage digest fragments. Biochemistry 38:13928, 1999.
42. Libby P, Egan D, Skarlatos S: Roles of infectious agents in atherosclerosis and restenosis: An assessment of the evidence and need for future research. Circulation 96:4095, 1997.
43. Danesh J, Collins R, Peto R: Chronic infections and coronary heart disease: Is there a link? Lancet 350:430, 1997.
44. Danesh J: Coronary heart disease, *Helicobacter pylori*, dental disease, *Chlamydia pneumoniae*, and cytomegalovirus: Meta-analyses of prospective studies. Am Heart J 138:S434, 1999.
45. Danesh J, Whincup P, Lewington S, et al: *Chlamydia pneumoniae* IgA titres and coronary heart disease; prospective study, and meta-analysis. Eur Heart J 23:371, 2002.
46. Ridker PM: Inflammation, infection, and cardiovascular risk: How good is the clinical evidence? Circulation 97:1671, 1998.
47. Ridker PM: Are associations between infection and coronary disease causal or due to confounding? Am J Med 106:376, 1999.
48. Zhu J, Nieto FJ, Horne BD, et al: Prospective study of pathogen burden and risk of myocardial infarction or death. Circulation 103:45, 2001.
49. O'Connor CM, Dunne MW, Pfeffer MA, et al: Azithromycin for the secondary prevention of coronary heart disease events: The WIZARD study: A randomized controlled trial. JAMA 290:1459, 2003.
50. Gelfand EV, Cannon CP: Antibiotics for secondary prevention of coronary artery disease: An ACES hypothesis but we need to PROVE IT. Am Heart J 147:202, 2004.

50a. Grayston JT, Kronmal RA, Jackson LA, et al: Azithromycin for the secondary prevention of coronary events. N Engl J Med 352:1637, 2005.
50b. Cannon CP, Braunwaid E, McCabe CH, et al: Antibiotic treatment of *Chlamydia pneumoniae* after acute coronary syndrome. N Engl J Med 352:1646, 2005.
51. Kalayoglu MV, Libby P, Byrne GI: *Chlamydia pneumoniae* as an emerging risk factor in cardiovascular disease. JAMA 288:2724, 2002.
52. Libby P, Ridker PM: Inflammation and atherosclerosis: Role of C-reactive protein in risk assessment. Am J Med 116 (Suppl) 6A:9S, 2004.
53. Ridker PM: High-sensitivity C-reactive protein, inflammation, and cardiovascular risk: From concept to clinical practice to clinical benefit. Am Heart J 148:S19, 2004.
54. Willerson JT, Ridker PM: Inflammation as a cardiovascular risk factor. Circulation 109:II2, 2004.
55. Danenberg HD, Szalai AJ, Swaminathan RV, et al: Increased thrombosis after arterial injury in human C-reactive protein-transgenic mice. Circulation 108:512, 2003.
56. Wang L, Fan C, Topol SE, et al: Mutation of MEF2A in an inherited disorder with features of coronary artery disease. Science 302:1578, 2003.
57. Dwyer JH, Allayee H, Dwyer KM, et al: Arachidonate 5-lipoxygenase promoter genotype, dietary arachidonic acid, and atherosclerosis. N Engl J Med 350:29, 2004.
58. Helgadottir A, Manolescu A, Thorleifsson G, et al: The gene encoding 5-lipoxygenase activating protein confers risk of myocardial infarction and stroke. Nat Genet 36:233, 2004.
59. Ozaki K, Ohnishi Y, Iida A, et al: Functional SNPs in the lymphotoxin-alpha gene that are associated with susceptibility to myocardial infarction. Nat Genet 32:650, 2002.
60. Ozaki K, Inoue K, Sato H, et al: Functional variation in LGALS2 confers risk of myocardial infarction and regulates lymphotoxin-alpha secretion in vitro. Nature 429:72, 2004.
61. Chobanian AV: Control of hypertension—an important national priority. N Engl J Med 345:534, 2001.
62. Chobanian AV, Bakris GL, Black HR, et al: The Seventh Report of the Joint National Committee on Prevention, Detection, Evaluation, and Treatment of High Blood Pressure: The JNC 7 report. JAMA 289:2560, 2003.
63. Lenfant C, Chobanian AV, Jones DW, et al: Seventh report of the Joint National Committee on the Prevention, Detection, Evaluation, and Treatment of High Blood Pressure (JNC 7): resetting the hypertension sails. Hypertension 41:1178, 2003.
64. Ford ES, Giles WH, Dietz WH: Prevalence of the metabolic syndrome among US adults: Findings from the third National Health and Nutrition Examination Survey. JAMA 287:356, 2002.
65. Mokdad AH, Bowman BA, Ford ES, et al: The continuing epidemics of obesity and diabetes in the United States. JAMA 286:1195, 2001.
66. Mokdad AH, Ford ES, Bowman BA, et al: Prevalence of obesity, diabetes, and obesity-related health risk factors, 2001. JAMA 289:76, 2003.
67. Williams KJ, Tabas I: The response-to-retention hypothesis of atherogenesis reinforced. Curr Opin Lipidol 9:471, 1998.
68. Brownlee M: Biochemistry and molecular cell biology of diabetic complications. Nature 414:813, 2001.
69. Naka Y, Bucciarelli LG, Wendt T, et al: RAGE axis: Animal models and novel insights into the vascular complications of diabetes. Arterioscler Thromb Vasc Biol 24:1342, 2004.
70. Thurberg B, Collins T: The nuclear factor-kappa B/inhibitor of kappa B autoregulatory system and atherosclerosis. Curr Opin Lipidol 9:387, 1998.
71. Burger PC, Wagner DD: Platelet P-selectin facilitates atherosclerotic lesion development. Blood 101:2661, 2003.
72. Cybulsky MI, Iiyama K, Li H, et al: A major role for VCAM-1, but not ICAM-1, in early atherosclerosis. J Clin Invest 107:1255, 2001.
73. Dong ZM, Brown AA, Wagner DD: Prominent role of P-selectin in the development of advanced atherosclerosis in ApoE-deficient mice. Circulation 101:2290, 2000.
74. Gu L, Okada Y, Clinton S, et al: Absence of monocyte chemoattractant protein-1 reduces atherosclerosis in low-density lipoprotein-deficient mice. Mol Cell 2:275, 1998.
75. Peters W, Charo IF: Involvement of chemokine receptor 2 and its ligand, monocyte chemoattractant protein-1, in the development of atherosclerosis: Lessons from knockout mice. Curr Opin Lipidol 12:175, 2001.
76. Lesnik P, Haskell CA, Charo IF: Decreased atherosclerosis in CX3CR1-/- mice reveals a role for fractalkine in atherogenesis. J Clin Invest 111:333, 2003.
77. Boisvert WA, Curtiss LK, Terkeltaub RA: Interleukin-8 and its receptor CXCR2 in atherosclerosis. Immunol Res 21:129, 2000.
78. Cybulsky MI, Hegele RA: The fractalkine receptor CX3CR1 is a key mediator of atherogenesis. J Clin Invest 111:1118, 2003.
79. Mach F, Sauty A, Iarossi AS, et al: Differential expression of three T lymphocyte-activating CXC chemokines by human atheroma-associated cells. J Clin Invest 104:1041, 1999.
80. Kovanen PT: Role of mast cells in atherosclerosis. Chem Immunol 62:132, 1995.
81. Haley KJ, Lilly CM, Yang JH, et al: Overexpression of eotaxin and the CCR3 receptor in human atherosclerosis: Using genomic technology to identify a potential novel pathway of vascular inflammation. Circulation 102:2185, 2000.
82. Platt N, Haworth R, Darley L, et al: The many roles of the class A macrophage scavenger receptor. Int Rev Cytol 212:1, 2002.
83. Febbraio M, Hajjar DP, Silverstein RL: CD36: A class B scavenger receptor involved in angiogenesis, atherosclerosis, inflammation, and lipid metabolism. J Clin Invest 108:785, 2001.
84. Nicholson AC, Han J, Febbraio M, et al: Role of CD36, the macrophage class B scavenger receptor, in atherosclerosis. Ann N Y Acad Sci 947:224, 2001.
85. Smith JD, Trogan E, Ginsberg M, et al: Decreased atherosclerosis in mice deficient in both macrophage colony-stimulating factor (op) and apolipoprotein E. Proc Natl Acad Sci U S A 92:8264, 1995.
86. Qiao JH, Tripathi J, Mishra NK, et al: Role of macrophage colony-stimulating factor in atherosclerosis: Studies of osteopetrotic mice. Am J Pathol 150:1687, 1997.
87. Rajavashisth T, Qiao JH, Tripathi S, et al: Heterozygous osteopetrotic (op) mutation reduces atherosclerosis in LDL receptor-deficient mice. J Clin Invest 101:2702, 1998.
88. Hansson GK, Libby P, Schonbeck U, et al: Innate and adaptive immunity in the pathogenesis of atherosclerosis. Circ Res 91:281, 2002.
89. Gerdes N, Sukhova GK, Libby P, et al: Expression of interleukin (IL)-18 and functional IL-18 receptor on human vascular endothelial cells, smooth muscle cells, and macrophages: Implications for atherogenesis. J Exp Med 195:245, 2002.
90. Geng YJ, Libby P: Progression of atheroma: A struggle between death and procreation. Arterioscler Thromb Vasc Biol 22:1370, 2002.
91. Doherty TM, Asotra K, Fitzpatrick LA, et al: Calcification in atherosclerosis: Bone biology and chronic inflammation at the arterial crossroads. Proc Natl Acad Sci U S A 100:11201, 2003.
92. Macleod MR, Amarenco P, Davis SM, et al: Atheroma of the aortic arch: An important and poorly recognised factor in the aetiology of stroke. Lancet Neurol 3:408, 2004.
93. Park AE, McCarthy WJ, Pearce WH, et al: Carotid plaque morphology correlates with presenting symptomatology. J Vasc Surg 27:872, 1998.
94. Bergwerff M, Verberne ME, DeRuiter MC, et al: Neural crest cell contribution to the developing circulatory system: Implications for vascular morphology? Circ Res 82:221, 1998.
95. Hill JM, Zalos G, Halcox JP, et al: Circulating endothelial progenitor cells, vascular function, and cardiovascular risk. N Engl J Med 348:593, 2003.
96. Shimizu K, Sugiyama S, Aikawa M, et al: Host bone-marrow cells are a source of donor intimal smooth-muscle-like cells in murine aortic transplant arteriopathy. Nat Med 7:738, 2001.
97. Saiura A, Sata M, Hirata Y, et al: Circulating smooth muscle progenitor cells contribute to atherosclerosis. Nat Med 7:382, 2001.
98. Arnett EN, Isner JM, Redwood DR, et al: Coronary artery narrowing in coronary heart disease: Comparison of cineangiographic and necropsy findings. Ann Intern Med 91:350, 1979.
99. Ziada KM, Kapadia SR, Tuzcu EM, et al: The current status of intravascular ultrasound imaging. Curr Probl Cardiol 24:541, 1999.
100. Clarkson TB, Prichard RW, Morgan TM, et al: Remodeling of coronary arteries in human and nonhuman primates. JAMA 271:289, 1994.
101. Glagov S, Weisenberg E, Zarins C, et al: Compensatory enlargement of human atherosclerotic coronary arteries. N Engl J Med 316:371, 1987.
102. Strong JP, Malcom GT, McMahan CA, et al: Prevalence and extent of atherosclerosis in adolescents and young adults: Implications for prevention from the Pathobiological Determinants of Atherosclerosis in Youth Study. JAMA 281:727, 1999.

103. Li S, Chen W, Srinivasan SR, et al: Childhood cardiovascular risk factors and carotid vascular changes in adulthood: The Bogalusa Heart Study. JAMA 290:2271, 2003.
104. Virmani R, Robinowitz M, Geer JC, et al: Coronary artery atherosclerosis revisited in Korean War combat casualties. Arch Pathol Lab Med 111:972, 1987.
105. Napoli C, D'Armiento FP, Mancini FP, et al: Fatty streak formation occurs in human fetal aortas and is greatly enhanced by maternal hypercholesterolemia. Intimal accumulation of low density lipoprotein and its oxidation precede monocyte recruitment into early atherosclerotic lesions. J Clin Invest 100:2680, 1997.
106. Napoli C, Glass CK, Witztum JL, et al: Influence of maternal hypercholesterolaemia during pregnancy on progression of early atherosclerotic lesions in childhood: Fate of Early Lesions in Children (FELIC) study. Lancet 354:1234, 1999.
107. Tuzcu EM, Kapadia SR, Tutar E, et al: High prevalence of coronary atherosclerosis in asymptomatic teenagers and young adults: Evidence from intravascular ultrasound. Circulation 103:2705, 2001.
108. Davies PF, Polacek DC, Shi C, et al: The convergence of haemodynamics, genomics, and endothelial structure in studies of the focal origin of atherosclerosis. Biorheology 39:299, 2002.
109. Gimbrone MA Jr, Topper JN, Nagel T, et al: Endothelial dysfunction, hemodynamic forces, and atherogenesis. Ann N Y Acad Sci 902:230, 2000.
110. De Caterina R, Libby P, Peng HB, et al: Nitric oxide decreases cytokine-induced endothelial activation. Nitric oxide selectively reduces endothelial expression of adhesion molecules and proinflammatory cytokines. J Clin Invest 96:60, 1995.
111. Collins T, Cybulsky MI: NF-kappa B: Pivotal mediator or innocent bystander in atherogenesis? J Clin Invest 107:255, 2001.
112. Montauban van Swijndregt AD, Elbers HR, Moll FL, et al: Cerebral ischemic disease and morphometric analyses of carotid plaques. Ann Vasc Surg 13:468, 1999.
113. Falk E, Shah P, Fuster V: Coronary plaque disruption. Circulation 92:657, 1995.
114. Bezerra HG, Higuchi ML, Gutierrez PS, et al: Atheromas that cause fatal thrombosis are usually large and frequently accompanied by vessel enlargement. Cardiovasc Pathol 10:189, 2001.
115. Libby P: The molecular bases of the acute coronary syndromes. Circulation 91:2844, 1995.
116. Amento EP, Ehsani N, Palmer H, et al: Cytokines and growth factors positively and negatively regulate interstitial collagen gene expression in human vascular smooth muscle cells. Arterioscler Thromb Vasc Biol 11:1223, 1991.
117. Galis Z, Muszynski M, Sukhova G, et al: Cytokine-stimulated human vascular smooth muscle cells synthesize a complement of enzymes required for extracellular matrix digestion. Circ Res 75:181, 1994.
118. Mach F, Schoenbeck U, Bonnefoy J-Y, et al: Activation of monocyte/macrophage functions related to acute atheroma complication by ligation of CD40. Induction of collagenase, stromelysin, and tissue factor. Circulation 96:396, 1997.
119. Galis Z, Sukhova G, Lark M, et al: Increased expression of matrix metalloproteinases and matrix degrading activity in vulnerable regions of human atherosclerotic plaques. J Clin Invest 94:2493, 1994.
120. Nikkari ST, O'Brien KD, Ferguson M, et al: Interstitial collagenase (MMP-1) expression in human carotid atherosclerosis. Circulation 92:1393, 1995.
121. Sukhova GK, Schonbeck U, Rabkin E, et al: Evidence for increased collagenolysis by interstitial collagenases-1 and -3 in vulnerable human atheromatous plaques. Circulation 99:2503, 1999.
122. Herman MP, Sukhova GK, Libby P, et al: Expression of neutrophil collagenase (matrix metalloproteinase-8) in human atheroma: A novel collagenolytic pathway suggested by transcriptional profiling. Circulation 104:1899, 2001.
123. Libby P, Lee RT: Matrix matters. Circulation 102:1874, 2000.
124. Herman MP, Sukhova GK, Kisiel W, et al: Tissue factor pathway inhibitor-2 is a novel inhibitor of matrix metalloproteinases with implications for atherosclerosis. J Clin Invest 107:1117, 2001.
125. Fukumoto Y, Deguchi JO, Libby P, et al: Genetically determined resistance to collagenase action augments interstitial collagen accumulation in atherosclerotic plaques. Circulation 110:1953, 2004.
126. Farb A, Burke A, Tang A, et al: Coronary plaque erosion without rupture into a lipid core. A frequent cause of coronary thrombosis in sudden coronary death. Circulation 93:1354, 1996.
127. Virmani R, Burke AP, Farb A, et al: Pathology of the unstable plaque. Prog Cardiovasc Dis 44:349, 2002.
128. Rajavashisth TB, Liao JK, Galis ZS, et al: Inflammatory cytokines and oxidized low density lipoproteins increase endothelial cell expression of membrane type 1-matrix metalloproteinase. J Biol Chem 274:11924, 1999.
129. Slowik MR, Min W, Ardito T, et al: Evidence that tumor necrosis factor triggers apoptosis in human endothelial cells by interleukin-1-converting enzyme-like protease-dependent and -independent pathways. Lab Invest 77:257, 1997.
130. Sugiyama S, Kugiyama K, Aikawa M, et al: Hypochlorous acid, a macrophage product, induces endothelial apoptosis and tissue factor expression: Involvement of myeloperoxidase-mediated oxidant in plaque erosion and thrombogenesis. Arterioscler Thromb Vasc Biol 24:1309, 2004.
131. Barger A, Beeuwkes IR, Lainey L, et al: Hypothesis: Vasa vasorum and neovascularization of human coronary arteries. N Engl J Med 310:175, 1984.
132. Coughlin SR: Sol Sherry lecture in thrombosis: How thrombin 'talks' to cells: Molecular mechanisms and roles in vivo. Arterioscler Thromb Vasc Biol 18:514, 1998.
133. Greenland P, LaBree L, Azen SP, et al: Coronary artery calcium score combined with Framingham score for risk prediction in asymptomatic individuals. JAMA 291:210, 2004.
134. Beckman JA, Ganz J, Creager MA, et al: Relationship of clinical presentation and calcification of culprit coronary artery stenoses. Arterioscler Thromb Vasc Biol 21:1618, 2001.
135. Bruschke AV, Kramer J Jr, Bal ET, et al: The dynamics of progression of coronary atherosclerosis studied in 168 medically treated patients who underwent coronary arteriography three times. Am Heart J 117:296, 1989.
136. Yokoya K, Takatsu H, Suzuki T, et al: Process of progression of coronary artery lesions from mild or moderate stenosis to moderate or severe stenosis: A study based on four serial coronary arteriograms per year. Circulation 100:903, 1999.
137. Davies MJ, Woolf N, Rowles PM, et al: Morphology of the endothelium over atherosclerotic plaques in human coronary arteries. Br Heart J 60:459, 1988.
138. Davies MJ: Stability and instability: The two faces of coronary atherosclerosis. The Paul Dudley White Lecture, 1995. Circulation 94:2013, 1996.
139. Faggiotto A, Ross R, Harker L: Studies of hypercholesterolemia in the nonhuman primate. I. Changes that lead to fatty streak formation. Arteriosclerosis 4:323, 1984.
140. Faggiotto A, Ross R: Studies of hypercholesterolemia in the nonhuman primate. II. Fatty streak conversion to fibrous plaque. Arteriosclerosis 4:341, 1984.
141. Burke AP, Kolodgie FD, Farb A, et al: Healed plaque ruptures and sudden coronary death: Evidence that subclinical rupture has a role in plaque progression. Circulation 103:934, 2001.
142. Goldstein JA, Demetriou D, Grines CL, et al: Multiple complex coronary plaques in patients with acute myocardial infarction. N Engl J Med 343:915, 2000.
143. Asakura M, Ueda Y, Yamaguchi O, et al: Extensive development of vulnerable plaques as a pan-coronary process in patients with myocardial infarction: An angioscopic study. J Am Coll Cardiol 37:1284, 2001.
144. Rioufol G, Finet G, Ginon I, et al: Multiple atherosclerotic plaque rupture in acute coronary syndrome: A three-vessel intravascular ultrasound study. Circulation 106:804, 2002.
144a. Libby P: Act local, act global: Inflammation and the multiplicity of "vulnerable" coronary plaques. J Am Coll Cardiol 45:1600, 2005.
145. Lombardo A, Biasucci LM, Lanza GA, et al: Inflammation as a possible link between coronary and carotid plaque instability. Circulation 109:3158, 2004.
146. Libby P, Aikawa M: Stabilization of atherosclerotic plaques: New mechanisms and clinical targets. Nat Med 8:1257, 2002.
147. Aikawa M, Rabkin E, Okada Y, et al: Lipid lowering by diet reduces matrix metalloproteinase activity and increases collagen content of rabbit atheroma: A potential mechanism of lesion stabilization. Circulation 97:2433, 1998.
148. Bustos C, Hernandez-Presa MA, Ortego M, et al: HMG-CoA reductase inhibition by atorvastatin reduces neointimal inflammation in a rabbit model of atherosclerosis. J Am Coll Cardiol 32:2057, 1998.

149. Hernandez-Presa MA, Bustos C, Ortego M, et al: ACE inhibitor quinapril reduces the arterial expression of NF-kappa B-dependent proinflammatory factors but not of collagen I in a rabbit model of atherosclerosis. Am J Pathol 153:1825, 1998.
150. Lutgens E, Gijbels M, Smook M, et al: Transforming growth factor-beta mediates balance between inflammation and fibrosis during plaque progression. Arterioscler Thromb Vasc Biol 22:975, 2002.
151. Hansson GK, Robertson AK: TGF-beta in atherosclerosis. Arterioscler Thromb Vasc Biol 24:e137, 2004.
152. Aikawa M, Voglic SJ, Sugiyama S, et al: Dietary lipid lowering reduces tissue factor expression in rabbit atheroma. Circulation 100:1215, 1999.
153. Nissen SE, Tsunoda T, Tuzcu EM, et al: Effect of recombinant ApoA-I Milano on coronary atherosclerosis in patients with acute coronary syndromes: A randomized controlled trial. JAMA 290:2292, 2003.
154. Nissen SE, Tuzcu EM, Schoenhagen P, et al: Effect of intensive compared with moderate lipid-lowering therapy on progression of coronary atherosclerosis: A randomized controlled trial. JAMA 291:1071, 2004.
155. Zhao XQ, Yuan C, Hatsukami TS, et al: Effects of prolonged intensive lipid-lowering therapy on the characteristics of carotid atherosclerotic plaques in vivo by MRI: A case-control study. Arterioscler Thromb Vasc Biol 21:1623, 2001.
155a. Libby P: The forgotten majority: Unfinished business in cardiovascular risk reduction. J Am Coll Cardiol 2005 [In press].

chapter 7

Pathophysiology of Vasculitis

Peter Libby

The pathophysiologic mechanisms that underlie vasculitis include elements of virtually all effector limbs of host defenses, including innate and adaptive immunities. Various classification schemes separate the vasculitides into primary and secondary families, and categorize them by the size of the afflicted vessel. Whereas Chapter 41 provides a detailed classification of the vasculitides, this chapter focuses on the primary vasculitides and, for pedagogic purposes, considers the pathophysiologic mechanisms of vasculitis in two broad categories (1) mechanisms that underlie small vessel vasculitis; and (2) mechanisms involved in medium- and large-sized arteritides. Although this categorization represents an oversimplification, it provides an organizational framework for discussing elements of humoral immunity, involved chiefly in primary small vessel vasculitides, and cellular immunity—likely the central mechanism underlying vasculitides of medium- and large-sized arteries.

PATHOPHYSIOLOGY OF SMALL VESSEL VASCULITIS

The Chapel Hill Consensus Conference included conditions such as Wegener's granulomatosis, Churg-Strauss syndrome, microscopic polyangiitis, Henoch-Schönlein purpura, essential cryoglobulinemic vasculitis, and cutaneous leukocytoclastic angiitis—among the small vessel vasculitides.[1] Many, but not all, cases of small vessel vasculitis occur in conjunction with elevated levels of antineutrophil cytoplasmic antibodies (ANCA).[2,3] In particular, Wegener's granulomatosis, Churg-Strauss syndrome, and microscopic polyangiitis associate strongly with ANCA. Importantly, many of the ANCA-positive small vessel vasculitides involve the kidney.[4]

The principal antigens recognized by ANCA are the neutrophil enzymes myeloperoxidase (MPO) and proteinase-3 (Table 7-1); some ANCA may recognize human neutrophil elastase as well. The antigens recognized by ANCA usually localize within the polymorphonuclear leukocyte (PMN). When primed by such stimuli as tumor necrosis factor-α (TNF-α) or when undergoing apoptosis, PMNs can release these antigens or express them on the cell surface. When released in soluble form, proteinases such as proteinase-3 and neutrophil elastase readily bind to widely distributed and abundant antiproteinases that may mask their recognition by ANCA. Circulating ANCA can also complex with these antigens. Such complexes, however, form preferentially when the proteinase antigens remain associated with the neutrophil cell surface. Proteinase-3 expressed on the endothelial cell surface may also serve as a stimulus to ANCA production and a recognition target for ANCA (Fig. 7-1).

Individuals who express primarily MPO-directed versus proteinase-3–directed ANCA may have distinct clinical courses.[5] The possible clinical dichotomy between these patient categories may relate to the functions of the target antigens. For example, binding to ANCA may protect MPO from clearance and inactivation by ceruloplasmin, increasing the ability of this enzyme to produce the highly oxidant species hypochlorous acid (HOCl). HOCl has many properties that may contribute to the pathophysiology of vasculitis, including the stimulation of endothelial apoptosis.[6]

Not all patients with small vessel vasculitis have ANCA-positive serology, thus indicating that some small vessel vasculitides may not involve mechanisms other than this humoral response. However, low titer antibodies may explain the negative serology in some cases. Additionally, "atypical" ANCA directed against antigens other than MPO or proteinase-3 may participate in the pathogenesis of vasculitis.[2]

Owing to the inconstent association of ANCA with small vessel vasculitides and their presence in some patients with nonvasculitic illnesses, a pathogenic role for ANCA has remained uncertain; however, recent studies in mutant mice have demonstrated unequivocally that ANCA can prove pathogenic under experimental conditions. In a landmark study, Xiao and colleagues immunized mice lacking endogenous myeloperoxidase due to targeted gene inactivation with exogenous mouse myeloperoxidase.[7] Transfer of splenocytes from these

TABLE 7-1 PATHOPHYSIOLOGIC MECHANISMS OF VASCULITIS

	Small-Vessel Vasculitides	Medium to Large Vessel Vasculitides
Effectors	Antibody/complement	T cells, dendritic cells
Histologic features	Necrotic lesions	Fibroproliferative lesions • Concentric • Granulomatous • Elastin fragmentation
Candidate antigen(s)	Antigens recognized by ANCAs • Myeloperoxidase • Proteinase-3	Unknown
Effector elastase(s)	Neutrophil elastase	• Matrix metalloproteinases-9 and -12 • Cathepsins K and S

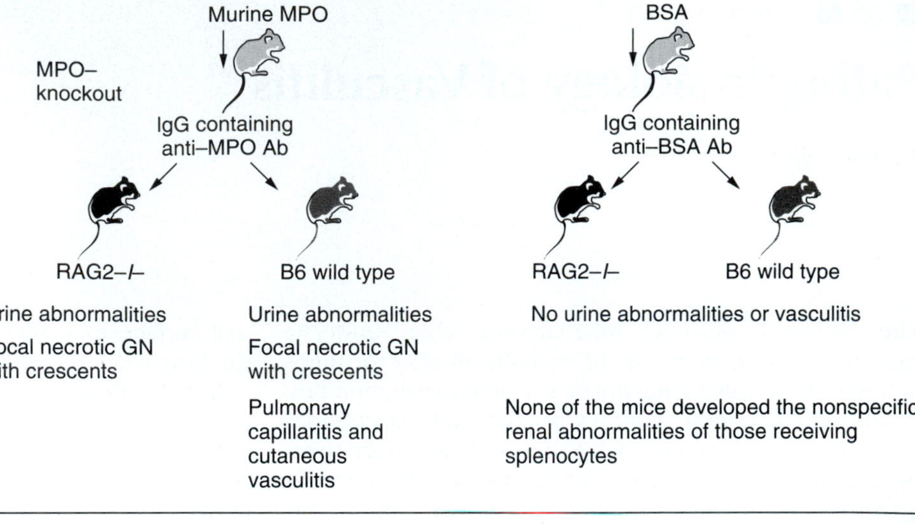

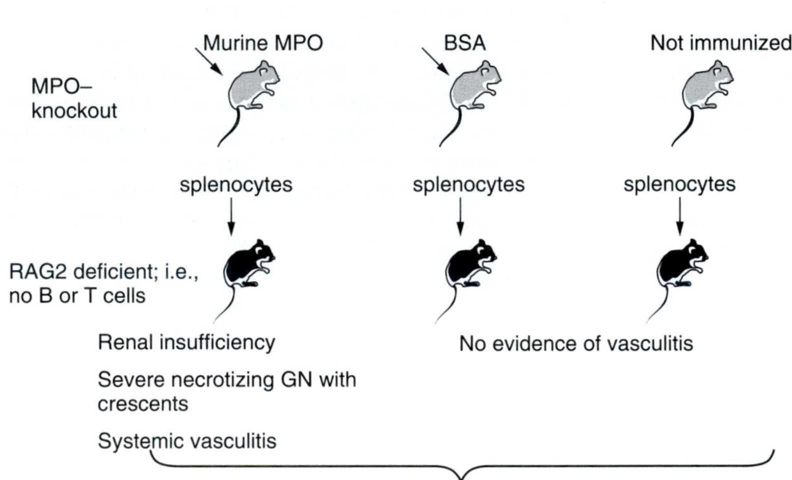

FIGURE 7-1. MPO-ANCA mice are pathogenic. (Data from Xiao H, Herringa P, Hu P, et al: Antineutrophil cytoplasmic autoantibodies specific for myeloperoxidase cause glomerulonephritis and vasculitis in mice. J Clin Invest 110:955, 2002. Reproduced with permission from Day CJ, Hewins P, Savage CO: New directions in the pathogenesis of ANCA-associated vasculitis. Clin Exp Rheumatol 21:S35, 2003.)

MPO-immunized mice into immunodeficient mice caused severe necrotizing crescentic glomerulonephritis. In some cases, a systemic necrotizing and granulomatous vasculitis affected lung capillaries as well as the renal microvasculature (see Fig. 7-1). Purified anti-MPO immunoglobulin G (IgG) isolated from the MPO-immunized mice caused renal, pulmonary, and cutaneous small vessel vasculitis. The antibody transfer experiments showed involvement somewhat less severe than adoptive transfer of splenocytes, indicating that aspects of cellular, as well as humoral, immunity may contribute to, or potentiate, the primarily humoral pathogenesis of small vessel vasculitis associated with MPO-ANCA.[7] ANCA may provoke vasculitis in several ways, and it may increase the activation and adherence of neutrophils to endothelial cells.[8] Exposure of neutrophils, "primed" by exposure to TNF-α, to MPO-ANCA can cause a respiratory burst that produces reactive oxygen species, such as superoxide anion and hydrogen peroxide—proinflammatory mediators that can injure endothelial cells and activate smooth muscle cells.[9] ANCA binding to neutrophils can activate a number of intracellular signaling pathways and heighten the sensitivity of PMN to classic stimulants such as formyl peptides.[2,10]

The ANCA-positive vasculitides have a solid experimental and clinical evidence base that supports a pathogenic role for ANCA in the development of vasculitis. These findings illustrate the importance of humoral immunity in the pathogenesis of this category of vasculitides; however, it is important to recognize that the cellular immune response may regulate aspects of the primarily humoral immune pathogenesis of the small vessel vasculitides. For example, the balance between the Th1 (γ-interferon predominant) helper T cell responses versus Th2 slanted reactions (IL-4 predominant) may modulate the expression of small vessel vasculitides; a Th1 response may associate with the localized variant of Wegener's granulomatosis than with the generalized form.[11]

Some of the secondary vasculitides provide clear-cut examples of the involvement of antibodies in vasculitis. In particular, the cryoglobulinemic vasculitis associated with hepatitis C virus infection frequently involves a polyclonal elevation of IgG and IgM antibodies, perhaps in response to polyclonal activation of B cells. In some cases, the mixed cryoglobulins in patients with chronic hepatitis C virus infection may contain ANCA, illustrating the overlap between primary and secondary vasculitides.[12]

These antibodies may lead to classic immune complex disease.[13,14] The mechanism of vascular damage in immune complex disease involves complement activation. IgM- or IgG-containing antigen-antibody complexes (immune complexes) can bind to complement factor 1 (C1), lead to assembly of C3 convertase, and yield activation of C3, C4, and C5. Ultimately, assembly of the membrane attack complex (MAC, composed of oligomers of C9 and other terminal complement components) can damage endothelial cells by forming pores in their plasma membrane (Fig. 7-2). Circulating immune complexes (IC) can be trapped in subendothelial basement membrane at sites where interendothelial separation has occurred. These trapped IC will then activate complement and can engage neutrophils and monocytes via their FcRs. Anaphylatoxins (fragments of C3a, C4a, and C5a) generated during activation of the classical complement pathway can recruit granulocytes and monocytes and activate mast cells at sites of immune complex deposition in vessels. These leukocytes can amplify local inflammation and aggravate and perpetuate the vasculitic response. Given the ubiquity of viral infections and antigen-specific antibody responses, circulation of viral antigen-antibody complexes probably occur frequently. The relative rarity of symptomatic or sustained vasculitis in common viral infections probably relates to the tight control of the complement system, which, like many protease cascades, is subject to intricate regulation by endogenous inhibitors.

The Churg-Strauss syndrome, which characteristically occurs in individuals with asthma, comprises a special case of small vessel vasculitis. Tissue accumulation of eosinophils and peripheral blood eosinophilia characterize this disease. This particular eosinophil-driven form of small vessel vasculitis appears to result from prolonged survival of eosinophils due to an excess of soluble CD95, which antagonizes apoptosis usually mediated by engagement of CD95 on the eosinophil surface, a mechanism that usually holds the eosinophil population tonically in check. Indeed, patients with the Churg-Strauss syndrome have elevated levels of soluble CD95, and CD95 ligation appears important in regulating eosinophil apoptosis.[15,16]

PATHOGENESIS OF THE MEDIUM- AND LARGE-SIZED ARTERIAL VASCULITIDES

The pathologic hallmark of the medium- and large-sized artery vasculitides, fibroproliferation with or without granuloma formation, implicates the active cellular immune response. The stimuli that drive the arteritis in Takayasu's and Kawasaki's diseases and in polyarteritis nodosa remain unknown. Recent work has advanced considerably the elucidation of the pathogenesis of giant cell arteritis, and more detailed consideration of the current state of knowledge of the pathogenesis of this

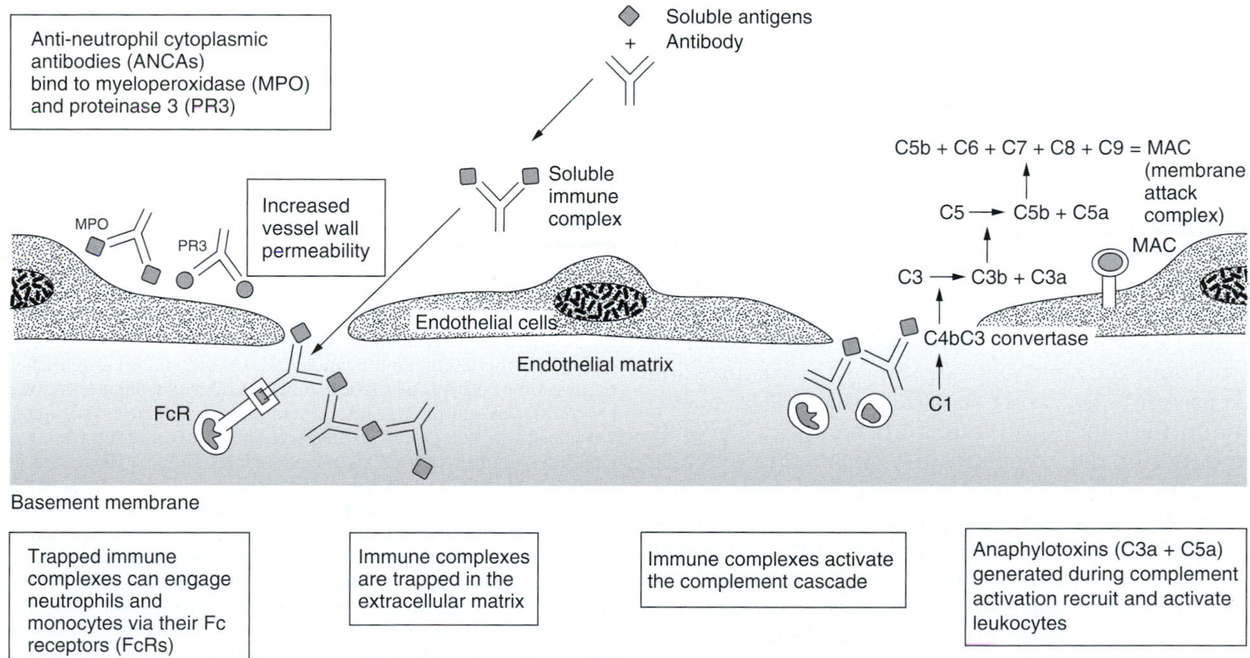

FIGURE 7-2. Some mechanisms of small vessel vasculitides. In the resting PMN, antigens such as myeloperoxidase (MPO) or proteinase-3 (PR3) remain localized within cells and hidden from the immune system. On priming or activation, cells can release or exteriorize MPO or PR3, displaying these antigens on their cell membrane (as depicted on the left-most endothelial cell). In addition, apoptotic bodies elaborated by dying PMN can furnish externally disposed MPO and PR3 to the immune system (*not shown*). Binding of antibodies known as ANCAs (antineutrophil cytoplasmic antibodies) can activate PMN, enhancing their adhesion to endothelial cells (middle endothelial cell). The activated PMN can undergo an oxidative burst, producing high levels of reactive oxygen species such as superoxide anion or hypochlorous acid. These reactive oxygen species can injure endothelial cells. The release of neutrophil elastase can digest the basement membrane, leading to the classic picture of a necrotizing vasculitis affecting the small vessels of the glomerulus, the lung, or the skin. The formation of immune complexes can activate cells directly by binding to Fc receptors, and also unleash complement. The activation of the complement cascade can injure endothelial cells directly by ultimately triggering assembly of the pore-forming membrane-attack complex (MAC). Activation of the complement pathway can also generate anaphylotoxins that can further recruit and activate leukocytes. Similar mechanisms are involved in the secondary vasculitides, such as those associated with endocarditis and serum sickness, and in systemic lupus erythematosus and rheumatoid arthritis.

disease will provide a framework for understanding the cell types and effector mechanisms involved in large-vessel vasculitides in general. Weyand and colleagues have provided strong experimental evidence for the critical involvement of CD4-positive T lymphocytes in the pathogenesis of giant cell arteritis. These ingenious experiments involve grafting human temporal artery specimens from patients with giant cell arteritis into immunodeficient mice. Ablation of the human T lymphocytes by administering anti-T cell antibodies to these mice halts the inflammatory process in the xenografted human arterial specimen.[17]

The initiating stimulus for medium and large vessel arteritis remains uncertain. The predisposition of certain populations, particularly those of Northern European extraction, suggests a genetic component. Some have hypothesized that infectious processes trigger medium and large artery vasculitides; however, the recovery of organisms such as *Chlamydia pneumoniae* or *Mycoplasma pneumoniae* from lesions has not proved reproducible. Some experimental results support the presence of antigens that can stimulate T cells in extracts of the lesions of giant cell arteritis or Takayasu's arteritis. Such extracts contain constituents that can activate T cell lines isolated from the lesions.[18] The biochemical nature of these putative antigens remains undefined.

The inflammatory process that initiates mid- and large-sized artery vasculitis may originate in the adventitia. The normal arterial adventitia contains resting dendritic cells. When activated, the dendritic cell functions importantly as an antigen-presenting cell (Fig. 7-3). Dendritic cells patrol their environment, engulfing and presenting antigens to T helper cells that typically bear the CD4 marker. The unactivated dendritic cell usually inhibits T cell stimulation, a process known as *tolerization*; however, the activated dendritic cell can trigger the cellular immune response. The normal arterial tunica media appears "immunoprivileged" (i.e., it usually does not support afferent signaling to the cellular immune system). This immunoprivilege may result from the local expression of the characteristic Th1 cytokine γ-interferon.[19]

In arteries affected by giant cell arteritis, dendritic cells become activated as disclosed by their expression of the markers CD86 and CD83. Dendritic cells can accumulate in the media and intima of the artery. The activated dendritic cell expresses the chemokine receptor CCR-7 that can bind a trio of chemokine ligands, CCL-18, -19, and -21. These chemoattractant cytokines, overexpressed in the inflamed artery wall, can attract dendritic cells into the nascent vasculitic lesion. The recruited and activated dendritic cells can now effectively present antigen to T lymphocytes and stimulate the afferent limb of cellular immunity.

When activated, T cells can secrete cytokines such as γ-interferon and express CD40 ligand on their surface. These effectors of the activated T lymphocyte act as strong stimuli for macrophage activation. The activated macrophages can then form granulomas. The accumulating macrophages can fuse into multinucleated giant cells, one of the histologic hallmarks of granuloma formation. T cell-driven macrophage activation classically instigates the delayed-type hypersensitivity response

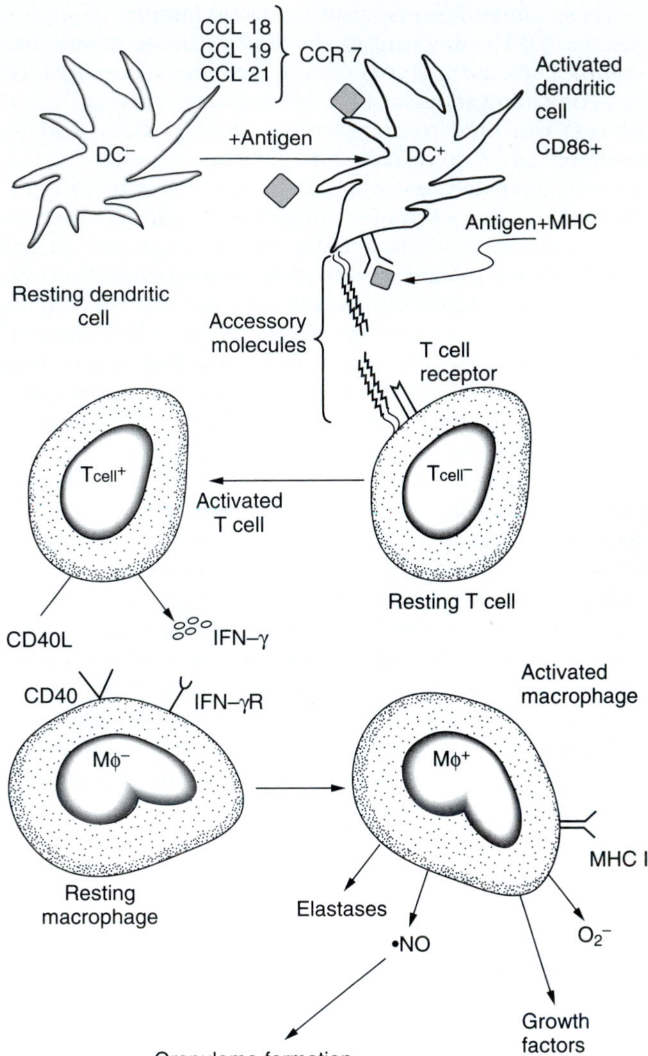

FIGURE 7-3. Some mechanisms of small vessel vasculitides. The resting dendritic cell (DC−) can actually exert an inhibitory influence on T cells. DC− localized in the adventitia may provide a check on T cell activation in the normal arterial wall. When appropriately stimulated, the activated dendritic cell (DC+) expresses markers such as CD86. The expression of chemokine receptor-7 (CCR-7) allows recruitment of DC+ by the chemokine ligands CCL-18, -19, and -21. High levels of expression of class II histocompatibility antigens facilitate the presentation of foreign peptides to T lymphocytes. When activated, the CD4-positive T cell (T cell +) augments production of interferon γ and expresses high levels of CD40 ligand on its surface. These and other stimuli can activate the resting macrophage (MΦ−) by engagement of cognate receptors on its surface. The stimulated macrophage (MΦ+) can secrete multiple mediators of the fibroproliferative response involved in the intimal expansion characteristic of large- and medium-cell arteritides, including growth factors and cytokines, and reactive oxygen species, such as superoxide anion (O_2^-) or reactive nitrogen species such as nitric oxide (•NO). The activated macrophage also augments expression of class II major histocompatibility antigens (MHC) that enhance the cell type's antigen-presenting function. Elastolytic and other proteinases secreted by the activated macrophage can contribute to arterial remodeling in inflamed vessels. Coalescence of activated macrophages creates the multinucleated giant cell characteristic of the granulomas that form in these arteritides. These mechanisms participate in the pathogenesis of giant cell arteritis and other medium- and large-vessel arteritides.

(DTH) characteristic of granulomatous disease. For example, the cutaneous reaction to injected purified protein derivative from tubercle bacilli elicits a T cell-driven macrophage response believed to replicate the initial steps in formation of granulomas (e.g., those characteristic of infection with the tubercle bacillus).

The activated macrophage can release multiple mediators that participate in the fibroproliferative process that characterizes medium and large artery vasculitis. Production of mediators such as transforming growth factor-β can stimulate collagen synthesis as well as that of other constituents of the extracellular matrix.[20] This fibrogenic response contributes to the expansion of intimal volume characteristic of these arteritides. Mitogenic and chemoattractant factors released from activated macrophages can also stimulate smooth muscle migration and proliferation. For example, activated macrophages can produce platelet-derived growth factor, fibroblast growth factor family members, and other stimulators of smooth muscle multiplication and directed migration.[21] The activated macrophage also produces reactive oxygen species and lipid hydroperoxides that can injure endothelial cells and further amplify arterial injury.

The elastic laminae in medium- and large-sized arteries affected by giant cell arteritis typically do not show severe dissolution; however, fragmentation of the internal elastic lamina can occur. Elastolysis mediated by elastolytic enzymes of the matrix metalloproteinase family (e.g., MMP-9 and MMP-12) or elastolytic cathepsins secreted by macrophages stimulated by CD40 ligand or other proinflammatory cytokines contribute to elastic fiber fragmentation. This elastolysis can promote the migration of smooth muscle cells and remodeling characteristic of intima expansion. In some cases, arterial ectasia or aneurysm formation occurs in advanced giant cell arteritis or frequently as a chronic complication of Kawasaki's disease. In this case, the elastin destruction and digestion of other extracellular matrix macromolecules likely pave the way for arterial expansion. Compared with the small vessel vasculitides, medium- and large-sized arteritides do not involve extensive necrosis. A concentric fibroproliferative expansion of the intima with or without granuloma formation rather than cell death predominates (see Table 7-1).

The detailed comparative pathogenesis of giant cell arteritis and Takayasu's arteritis is incomplete. HLA-DRB1*04 and DRB1*01 appear associated with susceptibility to giant cell arteritis and polymyalgia rheumatica[22]; however, Takayasu's arteritis appears related to HLA-B52 and -B39.[23] Many of the T cells found in Takayasu lesions bear γ, δ markers rather than markers of α, β T lymphocytes. Because heat shock proteins are elevated in Takayasu's arteritis lesions and can interact with γ, δ T cells, heat shock proteins, such as HSP-65, constitute a candidate antigen in this disease.

SUMMARY OF PATHOGENIC MECHANISMS IN THE VASCULITIDES

This chapter has dichotomized the pathophysiologic mechanisms of vasculitis, those that affect primarily small vessels and those that characteristically involve medium- and large-sized arteries (see Table 7-1). Although exceptions and overlap clearly exist, the small vessel vasculitides appear more driven by antibodies and activated PMNs than the cells of the adaptive immune response, such as T cells and dendritic cells involved in the initiation of medium- and large-sized arteritis. Activated PMNs appear to serve as the major effector in the small vessel vasculitides. In contrast, the macrophage, recruited in response to dendritic cell–T lymphocyte control, likely accounts for much of the tissue response characteristic of the medium- and large-vessel arteritides. The antigens that drive small vessel vasculitides include myeloperoxidase and proteinase-3, the common stimuli for ANCA development. The antigenic drivers of medium- and large-sized arteritides remain unknown.

Necrosis, the histologic hallmark of small vessel vasculitides, occurs in all lesions whether they affect the glomerular capillaries, the pulmonary microvasculature, or small vessels in the skin. In contrast, rapid formation of concentric intimal lesions characterized by accumulations of extracellular matrix and smooth muscle cells occurs during the formation of the medium- and large-sized arteritides. The histologic hallmark of these arteritides, the granuloma, usually does not involve necrosis or widespread elastolysis; rather, the formation of giant cells derived from macrophages characterizes these lesions of medium- and large-sized arteritis. The pathogenesis of both types of vasculitis appears to involve oxidative stress as typified by production of reactive oxygen species, including superoxide anion and myeloperoxidase-derived HOCl. Elastolysis in the small vessel vasculitides, however, probably involves neutrophil elastase rather than the metalloelastases or cysteinyl elastases characteristically elaborated by mononuclear phagocytes stimulated by Th1 cytokines.

Future goals of investigation in this field include delineation of the antigens involved in instigating the medium- and large-sized arteritides. We should aim to achieve a greater understanding of the differences between giant cell arteritis and polymyalgia rheumatica (that in some ways resembles a forme fruste of giant cell arteritis), and Takayasu's arteritis. Immunogenetic components may well participate in these distinct manifestations of arteritis.

Northern Europeans display the greatest susceptibility to giant cell arteritis, whereas Asian and Hispanic populations seem most at risk for Takayasu's arteritis. As we understand better the specific triggers for the inflammatory processes involved in these various forms of vasculitis, we should strive to target therapies more precisely and develop finer diagnostic tools. Ultimately, deeper insight into pathogenesis may permit us to prevent and treat effectively these often serious and debilitating diseases of the vasculature.

Acknowledgments

I thank Drs. Andrew Lichtman, Richard N. Mitchell, and Rene Packard for their critical reading of this manuscript and Karen E. Williams for her editorial expertise.

REFERENCES

1. Jennette JC, Falk RJ, Andrassy K, et al: Nomenclature of systemic vasculitides: Proposal of an international consensus conference. Arthritis Rheum 37:187, 1994.
2. Day CJ, Hewins P, Savage CO: New developments in the pathogenesis of ANCA-associated vasculitis. Clin Exp Rheumatol 21:S35, 2003.
3. Kallenberg CGM, Cohen Tervaert JW: Autoantibodies in vasculitis. In Hoffman GS, Weyand CM (eds): Inflammatory Diseases of Blood Vessels. New York, Marcel Dekker, 2002, p 37.
4. Rutgers A, Heeringa P, Tervaert JW: The role of myeloperoxidase in the pathogenesis of systemic vasculitis. Clin Exp Rheumatol 21:S55, 2003.
5. Franssen CF, Stegeman CA, Kallenberg CG, et al: Antiproteinase 3- and antimyeloperoxidase-associated vasculitis. Kidney Int 57:2195, 2000.
6. Sugiyama S, Kugiyama K, Aikawa M, et al: Hypochlorous acid, a macrophage product, induces endothelial apoptosis and tissue factor expression: Involvement of myeloperoxidase-mediated oxidant in plaque erosion and thrombogenesis. Arterioscler Thromb Vasc Biol 24:1309, 2004.
7. Xiao H, Heeringa P, Hu P, et al: Antineutrophil cytoplasmic autoantibodies specific for myeloperoxidase cause glomerulonephritis and vasculitis in mice. J Clin Invest 110:955, 2002.
8. Radford DJ, Luu NT, Hewins P, et al: Antineutrophil cytoplasmic antibodies stabilize adhesion and promote migration of flowing neutrophils on endothelial cells. Arthritis Rheum 44:2851, 2001.
9. Hewins P, Savage C: Anti-neutrophil cytoplasm antibody associated vasculitis. Int J Biochem Cell Biol 35:277, 2003.
10. Hattar K, Sibelius U, Bickenbach A, et al: Subthreshold concentrations of anti-proteinase 3 antibodies (c-ANCA) specifically prime human neutrophils for fMLP-induced leukotriene synthesis and chemotaxis. J Leukoc Biol 69:89, 2001.
11. Mueller A, Holl-Ulrich K, Feller AC, et al: Immune phenomena in localized and generalized Wegener's granulomatosis. Clin Exp Rheumatol 21:S49, 2003.
12. Lamprecht P, Gutzeit O, Csernok E, et al: Prevalence of ANCA in mixed cryoglobulinemia and chronic hepatitis C virus infection. Clin Exp Rheumatol 21:S89, 2003.
13. Misiani R: Virus-associated vasculitides: Pathogenesis. In Hoffman GS, Weyand CM (eds): Inflammatory Diseases of Blood Vessels. New York, Marcel Dekker, 2002, p 553.
14. Vassilopoulos D, Calabrese LH: Virus-associated vasculitides: Clinical aspects. In Hoffman GS, Weyand CM (eds): Inflammatory Diseases of Blood Vessels. New York, Marcel Dekker, 2002, p 565.
15. Muschen M, Warskulat U, Perniok A, et al: Involvement of soluble CD95 in Churg-Strauss syndrome. Am J Pathol 155:915, 1999.
16. Hellmich B, Ehlers S, Csernok E, et al: Update on the pathogenesis of Churg-Strauss syndrome. Clin Exp Rheumatol 21:S69, 2003.
17. Brack A, Geisler A, Martinez-Taboada VM, et al: Giant cell vasculitis is a T cell-dependent disease. Mol Med 3:530, 1997.
18. Martinez-Taboada V, Hunder NN, Hunder GG, et al: Recognition of tissue residing antigen by T cells in vasculitic lesions of giant cell arteritis. J Mol Med 74:695, 1996.
19. Dal Canto AJ, Swanson PE, O'Guin AK, et al: IFN-gamma action in the media of the great elastic arteries: A novel immunoprivileged site. J Clin Invest 107:R15, 2001.
20. Amento EP, Ehsani N, Palmer H, et al: Cytokines and growth factors positively and negatively regulate interstitial collagen gene expression in human vascular smooth muscle cells. Arterioscler Thromb Vasc Biol 11:1223, 1991.
21. Raines E, Rosenfeld M, Libby P: The role of macrophages. In Fuster V, Topol EJ, Nabel EG, (eds): Atherothrombosis and Coronary Artery Disease, 2nd ed. Philadelphia, Lippincott Williams & Wilkins, 2004, p 505.
22. Haworth S, Ridgeway J, Stewart I, et al: Polymyalgia rheumatica is associated with both HLA-DRB1*0401 and DRB1*0404. Br J Rheumatol 35:632, 1996.
23. Seko Y: Takayasu's arteritis: Pathogenesis. In Hoffman GS, Weyand CM (eds): Inflammatory Diseases of Blood Vessels. New York, Marcel Dekker, 2002, p 443.

chapter 8

Thrombosis

Jane E. Freedman
Joseph Loscalzo

Thrombosis of either the venous or arterial circulation is a major cause of morbidity and mortality. Under normal circumstances, the hemostatic process is a delicate balance of pro- and antithrombotic factors in the vasculature. Advances in understanding the mechanisms of thrombosis, as well as the development of new techniques for studying its regulation, have led to a clearer understanding of thrombotic disease as well as the availability of new classes of antithrombotic drugs.

Initially, characterization of arachidonic acid metabolism in platelets furthered an understanding of the therapeutic usefulness of cyclooxygenase inhibitors in vascular disease, most notably, aspirin. The discovery and characterization of platelet receptors, such as the adenosine diphosphate (ADP) receptor and glycoprotein IIb/IIIa, have been associated with the development of novel classes of antiplatelet drugs, such as thienopyridine derivatives and glycoprotein IIb/IIIa receptor antagonists, respectively. Further knowledge of receptor pathways and their inhibitors as well as developing concepts in the interaction of thrombosis and inflammation will continue to advance our understanding of thrombosis.

Multiple mechanisms contribute to the development of thrombosis, most notably the coagulation and fibrinolytic cascades, platelet activation, and the condition of the vessel wall. Further descriptions of the normal pathways regulating hemostasis and the coagulation cascade can be found in Chapter 4, and more complete discussions of venous thrombosis and hypercoagulability are found in Chapters 53 and 54.

Platelets, Thrombosis, and Vascular Disease

Thrombus formation within a vessel is the precipitating event in multiple vascular disease processes, including myocardial infarction, thrombotic cerebrovascular events, and venous thrombosis; however, the pathophysiological processes regulating these diseases are distinct. In venous thrombosis, primary hypercoagulable states reflecting defects of the proteins of coagulation and fibrinolysis or secondary hypercoagulable states involving abnormalities of blood vessels and blood flow lead to thrombosis (see Chapters 53 and 54). Distinct from venous thrombosis and thromboembolism, arterial thrombosis is highly dependent on the vessel wall and platelet. In the setting of coronary stenoses, rupture of atheromatous plaque in relatively mildly stenosed vessels and subsequent thrombus formation is believed to underlie the majority of acute coronary syndromes.[1] Both superficial intimal injury caused by endothelial denudation and deep intimal injury caused by plaque rupture expose collagen and von Willebrand factor to platelets (Fig. 8-1).[1] Platelets then adhere directly to collagen or indirectly via the binding of von Willebrand

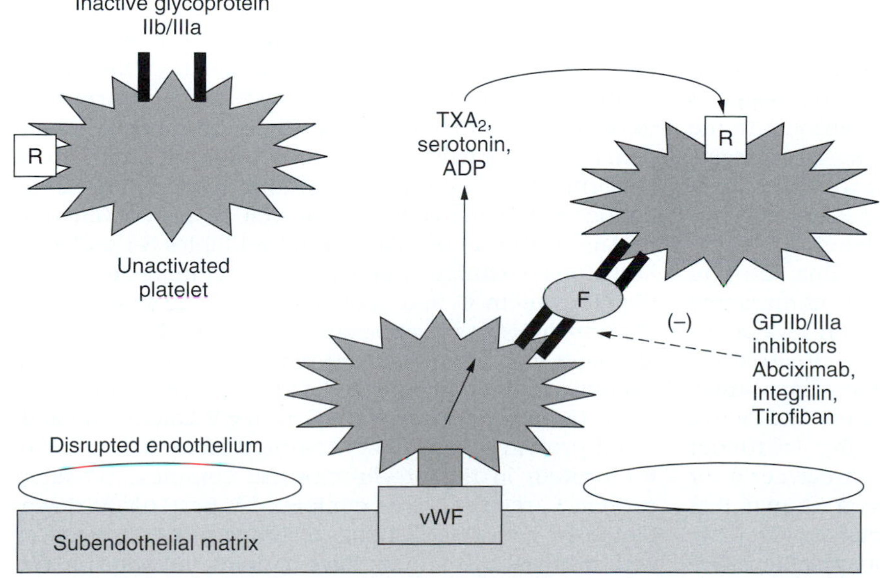

FIGURE 8-1. Damage or vascular injury exposes subendothelial von Willebrand factor (vWF) to the circulating blood. Platelets adhere to the site of injury when GPIb/V/IX expressed on the platelet surface binds to the subendothelial vWF. This event triggers the synthesis and release of thromboxane A_2 (TXA_2), serotonin, and adenosine diphosphate (ADP), which induces local activation of platelets by activating specific receptors (R). These events cause a conformational change in glycoprotein (GP IIb/IIIa) enabling the high affinity binding of fibrinogen (F). As local platelet activation and recruitment occur, fibrinogen bivalently bonds to activated platelet GPIIb/IIIa receptors resulting in thrombus formation (homotypic aggregates).

factor to glycoprotein Ib/IX to matrix. Local platelet activation (by tissue factor-mediated thrombin generation or by collagen) stimulates further thrombus formation and additional platelet recruitment by supporting cell-surface thrombin formation and releasing ADP, serotonin, and thromboxane A_2.[2] Thrombus forms as platelets aggregate via the binding of bivalent fibrinogen to glycoprotein IIb/IIIa. In support of these mechanisms, increased platelet-derived thromboxane A_2 and prostaglandin metabolites have been detected in patients with acute coronary syndromes.[3] These pathways regulating thrombosis will be described in further detail subsequently.

Activation and recruitment of platelets are tightly regulated. Adhesion of platelets to the endothelium and platelet activation are prevented by several mechanisms, including endothelial cell production of prostacyclin, nitric oxide (NO), and ecto-AD(T)Pase.[4,5] ATP induces aggregation in whole blood via conversion of ATP to ADP by ecto-ATPases on leukocytes. Agents that prevent adenosine removal may inhibit this process, and reduced aggregation at high concentrations of ATP (>100 μmol/L) may be a consequence of inhibition by ATP of ADP action at ADP receptors.[6] Prostacyclin, released by the vessel wall, inhibits platelet function via cAMP and its effects are also mediated by high-affinity prostanoid receptors found on the platelet.[7]

In addition, NO inhibits platelet activation,[8,9] prevents thrombosis,[10] and inhibits the normal activation-dependent increase in the expression of platelet surface glycoproteins, including P-selectin and the integrin glycoprotein IIb-IIIa complex.[11] Nitric oxide inhibits platelet function by stimulating soluble guanylyl cyclase to produce cyclic GMP (cGMP). This action results in the stimulation of cGMP-dependent protein kinase leading to a reduction in fibrinogen binding to glycoprotein IIb/IIIa and modulation of phospholipase A_2- and C-mediated responses.[12] In addition, NO attenuates the oxidation of arachidonate[13] and inhibits the agonist-dependent increase in platelet cytosolic free calcium in cGMP-dependent[14] and cGMP-independent manners.[15]

Activated platelets from patients with acute coronary syndromes produce significantly less NO as compared with patients with stable coronary artery disease.[16] This decrease in NO production is significant even after controlling for cardiovascular risk factors and the extent of atherosclerotic disease. This observation suggests that impaired platelet-derived NO may contribute to the development of acute coronary syndromes by influencing platelet function or recruitment and consequent thrombus formation. Supportive of these observations is a study showing that platelets from patients with acute myocardial infarction and unstable angina, despite aspirin treatment, are still partially activated as measured by platelet surface expression of P-selectin and active glycoprotein IIb/IIIa.[17] For both patients with atrial fibrillation and with unstable angina or acute myocardial infarction, surface expression of P-selectin and active glycoprotein GPIIb/IIIa was reduced by treatment with nitric oxide donors, including nitroglycerin or S-nitrosoglutathione. It has recently been shown that atrial fibrillation is associated with a marked decrease in endocardial NOS expression and bioavailable NO.[18] This study suggests that organized atrial contraction is needed to maintain normal endocardial expression of NOS and to inhibit the associated thromboembolism.[18]

Thrombosis has also been attributed to NO deficiency in noncardiac clinical thrombotic disorders. In patients with recurrent forms of thrombotic microangiopathy, including hemolytic uremic syndrome and thrombotic thrombocytopenic purpura, there is evidence that endothelial damage is a crucial feature in the development of microvascular thrombosis. Patients with these disease states have elevated plasma concentrations of NO metabolites, and serum from these patients enhances NO release when incubated with cultured endothelial cells. Importantly, superoxide production and lipid peroxidation are also enhanced,[19] suggesting that the interaction of these reactive oxygen species with NO reduces its bioactivity by increasing its oxidative state, potentially leading to enhanced thrombus formation.

VENOUS THROMBOSIS

The hemostatic process in the vasculature is also tightly controlled by prothrombotic mechanisms of coagulation activation (see also Chapter 4). After vascular injury, the hemostatic pathway is activated with the initiation of the coagulation cascade primarily owing to exposure of tissue factor. This leads to the formation of thrombin and the subsequent conversion of fibrinogen to fibrin monomer. This process occurs simultaneously as platelets adhere to the exposed extracellular matrix and contribute to the platelet-fibrin thrombus. This prothrombotic process is also regulated by the endogenous anticoagulants, antithrombin III, tissue factor pathway inhibitor, and activated protein C (APC) and its cofactor protein S. During coagulation, the fibrinolytic system is activated by plasminogen activators, that lead to the production of plasmin and contribute to the degradation of the fibrin clot.[20]

Genetic Abnormalities Associated with Venous Thrombosis

Thrombosis, particularly in the venous system, is regulated by abnormalities of the vasculature, the blood components, or rheology (Virchow's triad). Contributing to the risk factors that predispose to thrombosis include genetic abnormalities of blood components. These abnormalities include loss-of-function mutations of endogenous anticoagulants as well as gain-of-function mutations of procoagulant proteins (Tables 8-1 and 8-2). Mutations of natural anticoagulants, including antithrombin III, protein C, and protein S, were the first genetic abnormalities to be associated with thrombophilia and, although rare, are associated with an increased risk for venous thromboembolism.[20] Other polymorphisms in the protein C pathway include factor V Leiden and activated protein C resistance. Activated factor V is a cofactor protein in the prothrombinase complex. Activated protein C regulates this complex by proteolytic degradation of factor Va. Patients resistant to the activity of activated protein C may have a point mutation in the

TABLE 8-1 GENETIC POLYMORPHISMS AND THROMBOSIS

Polymorphism
Protein C Anticoagulant Pathway
Factor V Leiden: 1691G→A (Arg506Gln)
Thrombomodulin 1481C→T (Ala455Val)
Procoagulant Proteins
Fibrinogen-multiple polymorphisms
Prothrombin 20210G→A
Factor VII-multiple polymorphisms
Fibrinolytic Proteins
Plasminogen activator inhibitor (PAI-1)—multiple polymorphisms
Tissue plasminogen activator (t-PA)—multiple polymorphisms
Plasminogen deficiency—multiple polymorphisms
Dysfibrinogenemia—multiple polymorphisms
Homocysteine
Cystathionine β-synthase 833T→C
5,10-methylene tetrahydrofolate reductase (MTHFR) 677C→T
Platelet Receptors
GPIIIa Leu33Pro
GPIb variable number of tandem repeats (VNTR)
Thrombin receptor PAR-1-5061→D

From Kottke-Marchant K: Genetic polymorphisms associated with venous and arterial thrombosis: An overview. Arch Pathol Lab Med 126:295, 2002.

factor V gene located on chromosome 1 called *factor V Leiden*.[21] This mutation is relatively common in the white population (2% to 15%) but is infrequent in blacks and Asians. Thrombin plays a central role in hemostasis and a mutation associated with increased prothrombin levels is associated with the prothrombin 20210G→A mutation.[20] This mutation is found in fewer than 2% of the normal population but has been detected in up to 20% of individuals with venous thrombosis.[22] Other polymorphisms associated with altered risk of venous thromboembolism include fibrinogen mutations and factor VII polymorphisms. Polymorphisms of methylene tetrahydrofolate reductase as well as hyperhomocystinemia have been shown to be independent risk factors for venous thrombosis and arterial vascular disease.[20]

TABLE 8-2 PREVALENCE OF GENETIC ABNORMALITIES ASSOCIATED WITH VENOUS THROMBOEMBOLISM

Genetic Abnormality	General Population (%)	Patients with Venous Thrombosis (%)
Protein C deficiency	0.14-0.5	3.2
Protein S deficiency	—	2.2
Antithrombin (AT) deficiency	0.02-0.17	1.1
Activated protein C (APC) resistance	3.6-6.0	21
Prothrombin G20210A	1.7-3.0	6.2

From Anderson FA, Jr, Spencer FA: Risk factors for venous thromboembolism. Circulation. 107:I9, 2003.

Also known to promote (venous and arterial) thrombosis are antiphospholipid antibodies, a family of autoantibodies that recognize combinations of phospholipids (including cardiolipin) or phospholipid-binding proteins (including β_2-glycoprotein I). It has been hypothesized that the presence of these antibodies causes endothelial cells to express adhesion molecules and cytokines, express tissue factor, reduce expression of surface-bound plasminogen and plasminogen activators, and induce oxidant injury to the vascular endothelium.[23] Criteria for diagnosis of the antiphospholipid syndrome include vascular thrombotic events with the presence of anticardiolipin antibodies or lupus anticoagulant antibodies.

ARTERIAL THROMBOSIS

General Mechanisms and their Pharmacologic Regulation

On platelet stimulation, arachidonic acid is liberated from membrane phospholipids by phospholipase A_2 and C (Fig. 8-2). The catalytic activities of prostaglandin (PG) H-synthase sequentially metabolize arachidonic acid to generate PGG_2 and, subsequently, PGH_2. PGH-synthase possesses two catalytic sites. The first, a bis-oxygenase (cyclooxygenase), is responsible for the formation of PGG_2 and a hydroperoxidase function then catalyzes a net two-electron reduction in the 15-hydroperoxyl group of PGG_2 to produce PGH_2.[24] Aspirin induces the irreversible loss of the enzyme's cyclooxygenase activity by selectively acetylating the hydroxyl group of a single serine residue at position 529 (Ser^{529}) without altering the enzyme's hydroperoxidase activity. Other specific synthases then modify PGH_2 to generate the prostaglandins D_2, E_2, $F_{2\alpha}$, and I_2, as well as thomboxane (TX) A_2, which mediate distinct cellular functions—including regulation of platelet activation and aggregation.[25]

Platelets synthesize and release TXA_2 on stimulation with the agonists collagen, thrombin, or ADP.[26,27] The TXA_2 released by platelets then binds to platelet thromboxane receptors.[26,27] Engagement of the platelet TXA_2 receptor activates phospholipase C and liberates intracellular calcium. The increase in intracellular calcium amplifies platelet aggregation and results in the synthesis and release of additional TXA_2 and ADP from activated platelets. Both TXA_2 and ADP participate in a positive feedback loop that leads to irreversible aggregation.

In both normal subjects and in patients with atherosclerotic vascular disease, aspirin produces a dose-dependent inhibition of platelet cyclooxygenase activity after the administration of a single oral dose. The inhibitory effect of aspirin occurs in as quickly as 5 minutes after administration as a result of the acetylation of platelet cyclooxygenase. Because of aspirin's irreversible inhibition of cyclooxygenase and the inability of platelets to synthesize new protein, aspirin's effect is maintained for the life span of the platelet (7 to 10 days). Cyclooxygenase activity returns only as new platelets are formed and released into the circulation.

Aspirin reduces acute coronary and cerebrovascular events[28,29] such as unstable angina, myocardial infarction,

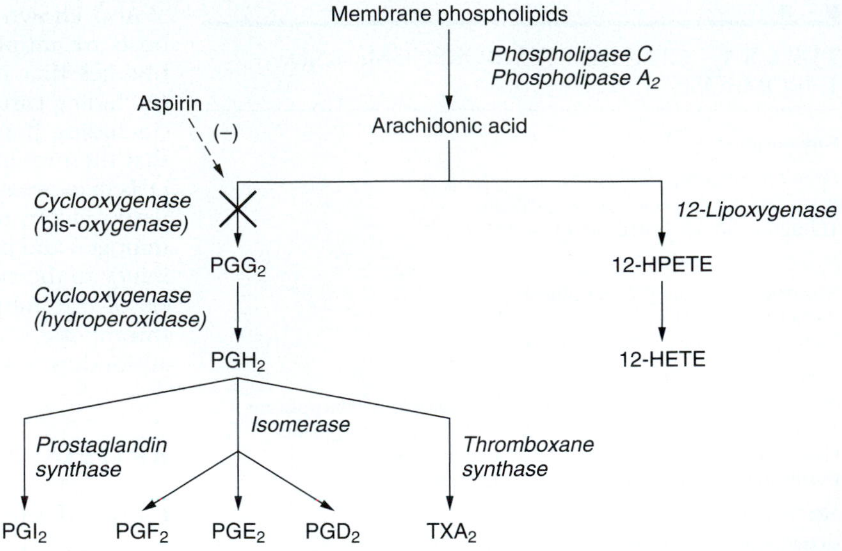

FIGURE 8-2. Metabolism of arachidonic acid in platelets. Arachidonic acid is metabolized through two catalytic pathways mediated by cyclooxygenase and lipoxygenase generating thomboxane A_2 (TXA_2) and 12-hydroxyeicosatetraenoic (12-HETE), respectively.

sudden cardiac death, and stroke. The inhibitory effects of aspirin are pronounced when using relatively weak platelet agonists but are less so pronounced against stronger agonists, such as thrombin, that can induce platelet activation in the absence of TXA_2. Importantly, the majority of platelet responses remain unaffected by aspirin treatment. Aspirin does not inhibit shear stress-induced platelet activation and platelet adhesion. Aspirin may also have a relatively high incidence of resistance and has been associated with a greater than threefold increase in the risk of major adverse effects in patients found to be resistant by platelet function studies.[30,31]

In platelets, arachidonic acid is also metabolized by lipoxygenase (see Fig. 8-2).[32] 12-Lipoxygenase metabolizes arachidonic acid to 12-hydroperoxyeicosatetraenoic acid (HPETE). HPETE is then reduced to 12(S)-hydroxyeicosatetraenoic (12[S]-HETE), which may also play a role in the regulation of platelet aggregation.[33] In vitro, 12-HETE potentiates platelet aggregation[33] and a specific inhibitor of 12-HETE in platelets, OPC-29030, has been shown to inhibit agonist-induced platelet aggregation and 12-HETE production.[34] OPC-29030 also inhibits activation of the glycoprotein IIb/IIIa receptor in vitro—suggesting that platelet-derived 12-HETE plays a role in mediating platelet aggregation.

Although many of aspirin's pharmacologic actions are related to its ability to inhibit prostaglandin and thromboxane biosynthesis and mediate thrombosis, aspirin also has endothelial-specific effects that can subsequently modulate platelet function. Incubation of aspirin with endothelial cells leads to the formation of a class of eicosanoids formed by acetylated prostaglandin H synthase (PGHS-2) and 5-lipoxygenase interactions that are potent inhibitors of leukotriene B_4-mediated adhesion of neutrophils to endothelial cells.[35]

Erythrocytes and endothelial cells secrete ADP that contributes to hemostasis, thrombus formation, and vascular occlusion by stimulating platelet aggregation. The ADP secreted from the dense granules of stimulated platelets potentiates platelet aggregation.[32,36,37] In the platelet, ADP induces a rapid influx of external calcium, mobilizes calcium from intracellular stores, and inhibits the inhibition of adenylyl cyclase.

Transduction of ADP-induced signaling events involves the binding of ADP to purinergic receptors on the platelet surface. Current evidence suggests the presence of three distinct ADP receptors, classified as $P2X_1$, $P2Y_1$, and P_{2T} ($P2T_{AC}$ and $P2T_{ADP}$) (Fig. 8-3).[36-40] The $P2X_1$ receptor, a ligand-gated ion channel, mediates rapid, transient calcium influx and does not appear to play a role in platelet aggregation.[41] ADP stimulation of the $P2Y_1$ G_q-coupled receptor activates phospholipase C, thereby causing internal calcium mobilization.[40,41] Activation of the $P2Y_1$ receptor is believed to be responsible for mediating ADP-induced platelet shape change[41] in addition to ADP-induced platelet aggregation. Additional evidence to support the role of the $P2Y_1$ receptor in platelet aggregation comes from studies of platelets from $P2Y_1$-null mice that fail to aggregate in response to ADP.[42,43]

The activation of both the P_{T2} and $P2Y_1$ receptors are essential for ADP-induced platelet aggregation.[41,44] Recent evidence indicates that activation of the platelet $P2Y_1$ receptor mediates the initial rapid response to ADP determining the maximal rate of ADP-induced platelet aggregation.[44] The degree of sustained platelet aggregation, however, is believed to be due to ADP-activation of the P_{2T} receptor.[44] Selective antagonism of the P_{2T} receptor with AR-C69931MX indicates that the P_{2T} receptor plays a role in sustaining and amplifying ADP-induced aggregation.[45]

Two thienopyridine derivatives, ticlopidine and clopidogrel, are clinically used inhibitors of ADP-induced platelet aggregation. Both drugs are mechanistically and structurally similar; however, owing to a lower incidence of severe neutropenia and other adverse effects associated with ticlopidine, clopidogrel is primarily used in clinical settings.[46] The antiplatelet effect of clopidogrel is due to irreversible inhibition of ADP binding to platelet purinergic receptors.[47,48] Metabolism of clopidogrel by the hepatic cytochrome P450-1A enzyme system to an

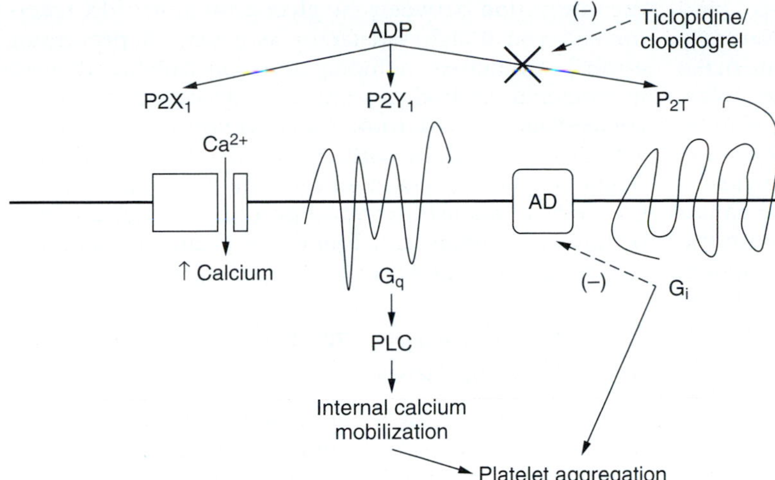

FIGURE 8-3. The platelet membrane contains three distinct ADP P_2 receptor subtypes classified as $P2X_1$, $P2Y_1$, and P_{2T}. ADP induces platelet aggregation via activation of both the $P2Y_1$ and P_{2T} receptors. Activation of the P_{2T} receptor leads to the inhibition of adenylyl cyclase (AD) mediating a fall in the levels of cyclic AMP. Activation of the P_{2T} receptor sustains ADP-induced aggregation; thienopyridines inhibit this purine-mediated process. The G protein, Gq, initiates platelet shape change by mobilizing calcium (Ca^{2+}). The G protein, G_i, is coupled to the ADP receptor and mediates adenylyl cyclase inhibition, which is essential for full aggregation. PLC; phospholipase C.

active metabolite[47,48] is essential for its in vivo antiplatelet effects.[47,48] This metabolite of clopidogrel displays the same in vivo effects as seen in vitro, such as inhibition of adenylyl cyclase and inhibition of ADP-induced aggregation.[47,48] A daily dose of clopidogrel (75 mg) is more effective than aspirin in reducing risk for ischemic events in patients with acute myocardial infarction, recent ischemic stroke, or peripheral arterial disease.[46]

Although platelets lack a nucleus, they possess many of the signaling pathways found in nucleated cells. The activation of platelets results in a rapid series of a variety of signal transduction events including tyrosine kinase activation, serine/threonine kinase activation, and lipid kinase activities. In unstimulated platelets, the major platelet integrin glycoprotein IIb/IIIa is maintained in an inactive conformation and functions as a low-affinity adhesion receptor for fibrinogen.[49] After stimulation, the interaction between fibrinogen and glycoprotein IIb/IIIa forms intracellular bridges between platelets leading to platelet aggregation (see Fig. 8-1). A conformational change in the extracellular domain of glycoprotein IIb/IIIa enables the high affinity binding of soluble plasma fibrinogen as a result of a complex network of inside-out signaling events.[50] This primary, reversible phase of platelet aggregation is precipitated by a series of extremely rapid and complex signaling pathways that are currently incompletely characterized.[51]

The glycoprotein IIb/IIIa receptor serves as a bidirectional conduit with glycoprotein IIb/IIIa-mediated signaling (outside-in signaling) occurring immediately after the binding of fibrinogen and initiating intracellular signaling that further stabilizes the aggregate. The initial phase of outside-in signaling contributes to further activate the integrin glycoprotein IIb/IIIa via integrin clustering and the formation of a complex network of signaling and structural cytoskeletal proteins. Calcium mobilization, tyrosine phosphorylation, activation of phosphoinositide metabolism, and cytoskeletal reorganization result from the activation of glycoprotein IIb/IIIa. This series of events transforms platelet aggregation from a reversible to an irreversible process.

Although aspirin and clopidogrel are effective antiplatelet agents, they are relatively weak antiaggregatory drugs. Drugs that specifically target the glycoprotein IIb/IIIa receptor and prevent the binding of fibrinogen have been developed to inhibit this final common pathway for platelet aggregation.[52] Antagonism of the glycoprotein IIb/IIIa receptor inhibits platelet aggregation irrespective of the platelet activator (see Fig. 8-1).

Murine monoclonal antibodies were the first antagonists of the glycoprotein IIb/IIIa receptor to be developed.[53] Platelet aggregation is completely inhibited by blockade of 80% of the surface glycoprotein IIb/IIIa receptors.[54] A high affinity antibody inhibits platelet function by engaging glycoprotein IIb/IIIa, thereby preventing the binding of fibrinogen to activated platelets. It has also been shown to bind to the vitronectin ($\alpha_v\beta_3$) receptor that is present on platelets.[55] Therefore, as an antagonist of not only the glycoprotein IIb/IIIa, but also the vitronectin receptor, the c7E3 antibody, abciximab, may provide additional clinical benefits by inhibiting vitronectin-mediated thrombin generation. The c7E3 antibody also possesses a slow, yet appreciable, dissociation rate from platelets.[56]

Multiple clinical trials have shown inhibition of glycoprotein IIb/IIIa to be a highly effective antithrombotic strategy.[57] The first phase III trial, the Evaluation of c7E3 in Preventing Ischemic Complications (EPIC), administered a 0.25 mg/kg bolus of c7E3 Fab followed by a 12-hour infusion of 10 μg/min to patients undergoing angioplasty or directed atherectomy.[57] Administration of c7E3 led to a 35% reduction in the incidence of acute ischemic events and a 26% reduction in recurrent ischemic events was noted at 6 months. In a subsequent study, the Evaluation of PTCA to Improve Long-Term Outcome by c7E3 Glycoprotein IIb/IIIa Receptor Blockade (EPILOG), the incidence of death was reduced at 30 days (68%) and at 6 months (46%) in patients who received c7E3.[58]

Several ligands of integrins, including fibrinogen and von Willebrand factor, possess one of the two amino acid sequences 95 to 97 (Arg-Gly-Asp or RGD) and 572 to 575

(Arg-Gly-Asp-Ser or RGDS) that enable them to bind to the activated glycoprotein IIb/IIIa receptor. Naturally occurring RGD-containing peptides isolated from snake venoms that compete with fibrinogen for the glycoprotein IIb/IIIa receptor binding site inhibit platelet aggregation.[59] These low molecular weight, cysteine-rich polypeptides, collectively known as disintegrins, block the crucial interaction between the RGD amino acid sequence of the ligand and the binding site on the glycoprotein IIb/IIIa receptor that is essential for inducing the conformational change of the receptor. These RGD-containing peptides, however, lack specificity for the glycoprotein IIb/IIIa receptor and can inhibit the binding of many other RGD-dependent integrins to their receptors.

Although the therapeutic usefulness of the naturally occurring disintegrins is limited because of transient thrombocytopenia and immunogenicity, the RGD and Lys-Gly-Asp (KGD) motifs became the template for the development of other glycoprotein IIb/IIIa receptor antagonists. The synthetic cyclic KGD peptide, integrilin, was one of the earliest glycoprotein IIb/IIIa antagonist peptides developed. Nonpeptide antagonists that are designed to mimic the charge and conformation of the RGD sequence have also been developed. These include lamifiban, xemilofiban, and tirofiban. These nonpeptide mimetics are unique in that they have the potential for oral administration that initially was believed to be useful for long-term antiplatelet therapy; however, several oral glycoprotein IIb/IIIa inhibitors have been evaluated and their use has not been associated with clinical benefit.[60-63] The oral glycoprotein IIb/IIIa inhibitors have a steep dose-response curve that requires constant dose titration and monitoring. The lack of a surrogate marker for efficacy, platelet activity, and safety further complicates the use of oral administration of glycoprotein IIb/IIIa inhibitors for prolonged periods of time.

The glycoprotein Ib/V/IX adhesive receptor, which is expressed on both platelets and endothelial cells, plays an important role in both platelet adhesion and activation. Damage to the blood vessel wall exposes subendothelial von Willebrand factor and collagen to the circulating blood. When such vascular injury occurs in the microcirculation and stenosed arteries, the glycoprotein Ib/V/IX receptor expressed on the platelet surface binds to the exposed von Willebrand factor causing platelets to adhere to the subendothelium at the site of injury even under rapid flow conditions. In addition to anchoring the platelet to the injured vessel wall, glycoprotein Ib/V/IX is able to transduce signals that lead to platelet activation. Von Willebrand factor-bound glycoprotein Ib/V/IX induces a conformational change in the glycoprotein IIb/IIIa receptor (outside-in signaling) transforming it from an inactive low affinity state to an active state that binds von Willebrand factor or fibrinogen with high affinity. The glycoprotein Ib/V/IX receptor is unique in that it is responsible for the initial adhesion of the platelet to the subendothelial matrix.

Given the important role the glycoprotein Ib/V/IX receptor plays in platelet adhesion and aggregation, it has become an attractive target for the development of antiplatelet drugs. Drugs have been developed that target the interaction between the glycoprotein Ib/V/IX receptor and von Willebrand factor as a way of preventing arterial thrombosis, including anti–von Willebrand factor monoclonal antibodies[64] and the glycoprotein Ib/V/IX antagonists isolated from snake venoms.[65,66] Recently, a study examined the antithrombotic efficacy of the Fab fragments of the novel murine monoclonal antibody, 6B4, raised against the glycoprotein Ib/V/IX receptor of human platelets and found significant inhibition of thrombus generation.[67]

Genetic Polymorphisms and Arterial Thrombosis

Genetic alteration of blood components may lead to enhanced thrombosis. Through the recognition of familial tendencies in thrombosis, genetic abnormalities in the coagulation system have been found. As previously discussed, those initially described were mutations that led to a loss of function of endogenous anticoagulants, including antithrombin III, protein C, or protein S (see Tables 8-1 and 8-2).[20] Other mutations have been associated with enhanced thrombotic function such as factor V Leiden or increased coagulation factors (prothrombin G20210A). Alteration of the fibrinolytic cascade have also been linked with alteration in thrombosis; however, numerous mutations may result in dysfunction of these proteins, which has made genetic testing difficult. In addition, many studies of polymorphisms have been association studies that are prone to error and have had inconsistent outcomes. Although the vast number of polymorphisms studied have been factors in the coagulation cascade (see Tables 8-1 and 8-2),[20] numerous other associations have been reported. This has included abnormalities in homocysteine metabolism and platelet surface glycoproteins (see Table 8-1). Functional effects of many of these polymorphisms have not been ascertained. Although most of these abnormalities have been associated with venous thrombosis, a recent large, population-based study suggested that heritable factors play a major role in determining platelet aggregation as compared with environmental covariates.[68] The study also reported that the platelet glycoprotein *IIIa Pl^{A2}* and fibrinogen *Hind III* polymorphisms contributed <1% to the overall variance. This study concluded "that data are sparse regarding the genetic epidemiology of abnormal platelet aggregability," and future studies are needed to identify key genetic variants regulating platelet function.[68]

Recently, the role of eNOS polymorphisms in thrombosis has been examined. Several polymorphic variants of the eNOS gene have been described, and the most extensively characterized variant is the 894-G/T polymorphism in exon 7 of the gene resulting in a glutamate or aspartate at position 298. The 894T allele is associated with higher plasma levels of nitrogen oxides in healthy individuals.[69] Epidemiologic studies have shown an increased risk of hypertension, myocardial infarction, and stroke in patients homozygous for the Glu298Asp variant.[70,71,72] Another eNOS polymorphism, designated ecNOS4a, has been identified on intron 4 and has been associated with premature coronary artery disease, and also with a history of myocardial infarction.[73]

Polymorphisms in the promoter region and exon 7 have been associated with lower levels of platelet-derived NO.[74]

Other genetic abnormalities that may regulate thrombosis are polymorphisms of glutathione peroxidase. Glutathione peroxidase is a selenium-containing enzyme, and selenium deficiency has been reported in patients with acute myocardial infarction and coronary atherothrombotic disease.[75] Glutathione peroxidase potentiates the inhibition of platelet function by NO by decreasing LOOH concentrations.[76] Impairment of this process can lead to a clinical thrombotic disorder as shown in two brothers with thrombotic strokes in childhood.[77] A similar deficiency has been reported in five other families who experienced childhood strokes.[78]

THE INTERACTION OF THROMBOSIS AND INFLAMMATION

Accumulating information suggests that inflammation plays an important role during the acute thrombotic phase of unstable coronary syndromes. Recent data demonstrate that patients with acute coronary syndromes have not only increased interactions between platelets (homotypic aggregates), but also increased interactions between platelets and leukocytes (heterotypic aggregates) detectable in circulating blood. These aggregates form when platelets are activated and undergo degranulation, after which they adhere to circulating leukocytes. Platelets bind via P-selectin (CD62P) expressed on the surface of activated platelets to the leukocyte receptor, P-selectin glycoprotein ligand-1 (PSGL-1).[24] This association leads to increased expression of CD11b/CD18 (Mac-1) on leukocytes,[79] which itself supports interactions with platelets, perhaps via bivalent fibrinogen linking this integrin with its platelet surface counterpart, glycoprotein IIb/IIIa.[80,81]

The binding of platelets and monocytes in acute coronary syndromes highlights the interaction between inflammation and thrombosis in cardiovascular disease. Plaque rupture promotes activation of the inflammatory response, and increased expression of tissue factor initiates extrinsic coagulation. The expression of tissue factor on both endothelial cells and monocytes is partially regulated by proinflammatory cytokines including tumor necrosis factor and IL-1.[82] In addition to initiating coagulation, tissue factor interacts with P-selectin, accelerating fibrin formation and deposition.[82] Platelet surface P-selectin also induces the expression of tissue factor on monocytes[83] and enhances monocyte cytokine expression,[84] as well as promotes CD11b/CD18 expression.[79] This prothrombotic process is regulated by production of endothelium-derived NO that reduces endotoxin- and cytokine-induced expression of tissue factor.[85]

In addition to platelet-monocyte aggregates, measurement of the immunomodulator, soluble CD40 ligand (CD40L or CD154), also reflects the interface between thrombosis and inflammation. The CD40 ligand is a trimeric, transmembrane protein of the tumor necrosis factor family and, with its receptor CD40, is an important contributor to the inflammatory processes leading to atherosclerosis and thrombosis.[86] Many immunologic and vascular cells have been found to express CD40 and/or CD40 ligand, and both have been clearly shown to be present in human atheroma.[87] In platelets, CD40 ligand is rapidly translocated to the surface after stimulation and is upregulated in fresh thrombus.[86] The surface-expressed CD40 ligand is then cleaved from the platelet over a period of minutes to hours, subsequently generating a soluble fragment (soluble CD40 ligand).[88] Although also shed from stimulated lymphocytes, it is estimated that greater than 95% of the circulating CD40 ligand is derived from platelets.[88] Soluble CD40 ligand has been shown to be associated with increased cardiovascular risk in apparently healthy women.[87] Soluble CD40 ligand can identify patients at high risk of acute coronary syndromes,[89] and this increased risk associated with elevated soluble CD40 ligand levels is reduced by abciximab treatment. These observations suggest that soluble CD40 ligand can be used to identify patients with enhanced thrombotic risk.

Although the presence of soluble CD40 ligand as well as heterotypic aggregates reflects platelet activation during a cardiac event, it is not known if these immunomodulators themselves play a role in the acute thrombotic process. On endothelial cells or monocytes, the engagement of CD40 with CD40 ligand leads to the synthesis of adhesion molecules, chemokines, and tissue factor, and causes the activation of matrix metalloproteinases that are known to contribute to atherothrombotic pathophysiology. Soluble CD40 ligand has a lysine-arginine-glutamic acid (KGD) motif that allows for its binding to platelet glycoprotein IIb/IIIa. It is possible that such binding is blocked in the setting of glycoprotein IIb/IIIa inhibitors, potentially altering the clot-stabilizing properties of soluble CD40 ligand.[88]

EVALUATION OF THROMBOSIS AND THROMBOTIC PROPENSITY

Laboratory evaluation for hypercoagulability differs depending on whether the thrombotic event is venous or arterial in origin. Evaluation of venous thromboembolism includes examination of protein C, protein S, and antithrombin deficiency. Other tests may include factor V Leiden, activated protein C resistance, antiphospholipid antibodies, and homocysteine levels. Further workup for venous thrombotic events is discussed in Chapters 53 and 54.

Arterial thrombosis including myocardial infarction, unstable angina, or peripheral arterial disease, normally occurs in the setting of atherosclerosis. Importantly, elevated cholesterol level is an established risk factor for arterial thrombosis in the setting of atherosclerosis. Studies have shown that decreasing low-density lipoprotein cholesterol reduces thrombotic risk.[90] Antiphospholipid antibodies, including lupus anticoagulant and anticardiolipin antibodies, have been associated with an increased risk of venous and arterial thromboses. Prospective studies have shown that these antibodies are associated with an enhanced risk of myocardial infarction.[90] Homocysteine, in addition to being a risk factor for venous thrombosis, has been associated with enhanced arterial thrombotic risk.[90,91] Although not all of the prospective studies in general populations have found an association between homocysteine and risk of death or myocardial infarction, most of the studies in the atherosclerotic patient populations have shown enhanced risk. Clearly, studies showing that lowering homocysteine reduces cardiovascular disease will be of great interest.

REFERENCES

1. Davies MJ,Thomas AC: Thrombosis and acute coronary-artery lesions in sudden cardiac ischemic death. N Engl J Med 310:1137, 1984.
2. Santos MT, Valles J, Marcus AJ, et al: Enhancement of platelet reactivity and modulation of eicosanoid production by intact erythrocytes: A new approach to platelet activation and recruitment. J Clin Invest 87:571, 1991.
3. Fitzgerald DJ, Roy L, Catella F, et al: Platelet activation in unstable coronary disease. N Engl J Med 315:983, 1986.
4. de Graaf JC, Banga JD, Moncada S, et al: Nitric oxide functions as an inhibitor of platelet adhesion under flow conditions. Circulation 85:2284, 1992.
5. Radomski MW, Palmer MJ, Moncada S: The role of nitric oxide and cGMP in platelet adhesion to vascular endothelium. Biochem Biophys Res Commun 148:1482, 1987.
6. Stafford NP, Pink AE, White AE, et al: Mechanisms involved in adenosine triphosphate-induced platelet aggregation in whole blood. Arterioscler Thromb Vasc Biol 23:1928, 2003.
7. Kahn NN, Bauman WA, Sinha AK: Loss of high-affinity prostacyclin receptors in platelets and the lack of prostaglandin-induced inhibition of platelet-stimulated thrombin generation in subjects with spinal cord injury. Proc Natl Acad Sci U S A 93:245, 1996.
8. Stamler J, Mendelsohn ME, Amarante P, et al: *N*-acetylcysteine potentiates platelet inhibition by endothelium-derived relaxing factor. Circ Res 65:789, 1989.
9. Cooke JP, Stamler J, Andon N, et al: Flow stimulates endothelial cells to release a nitrovasodilator that is potentiated by reduced thiol. Am J Physiol 259:H804, 1990.
10. Shultz PJ, Raij L: Endogenously synthesized nitric oxide prevents endotoxin-induced glomerular thrombosis. J Clin Invest 90:1718, 1992.
11. Michelson AD, Benoit SE, Furman MI, et al: Effects of nitric oxide/endothelium-derived relaxing factor on platelet surface glycoproteins. Am J Physiol 270:H1640, 1996.
12. Radomski M, Moncada S: Regulation of vascular homeostasis by nitric oxide. Thromb Haemost 70:36, 1993.
13. Wirthumer-Hocke C, Silberbauer K, Sinzinger H: Effect on nitroglycerin and other organic nitrates on the in vitro biosynthesis of arachidonic acid-metabolites in washed human platelets. Prostaglandins Leuko Med 15:317, 1984.
14. Negrescu E, Sazonova L, Baldenkov G, et al: Relationship between the inhibition of receptor-induced increase in cytosolic free calcium concentration and the vasodilator effects of nitrates in patients with congestive heart failure. Int J Cardiol 26:175, 1990.
15. Trepakova ES, Cohen RA, Bolotina VM: Nitric oxide inhibits capacitative cation influx in human platelets by promoting sarcoplasmic/endoplasmic reticulum Ca^{2+}-ATPase-dependent refilling of Ca^{2+} stores. Circ Res 84:201, 1999.
16. Freedman JE, Ting B, Hankin B, et al: Impaired platelet production of nitric oxide in patients with unstable angina. Circulation 98:1481, 1998.
17. Langford E, Wainwright R, Martin J: Platelet activation in acute myocardial infarction and angina is inhibited by nitric oxide donors. Arterioscler Thromb Vasc Biol 16:51, 1996.
18. Cai H, Li Z, Goette A, Mera F, et al: Downregulation of endocardial nitric oxide synthase expression and nitric oxide production in atrial fibrillation: Potential mechanisms for atrial thrombosis and stroke. Circulation 106:2854, 2002.
19. Noris M, Ruggenenti P, Todeschini M, et al: Increased nitric oxide formation in recurrent thrombotic microangiopathies: A possible mediator of microvasclar injury. Am J Kidney Dis 27:790, 1996.
20. Kottke-Marchant K: Genetic polymorphisms associated with venous and arterial thrombosis: An overview. Arch Pathol Lab Med 126:295, 2002.
21. Bertina RM, Koeleman BP, Koster T, et al: Mutation in blood coagulation factor V associated with resistance to activated protein C. Nature 369:64, 1994.
22. Rosendaal FR, Doggen CJ, Zivelin A, et al: Geographic distribution of the 20210 G to A prothrombin variant. Thromb Haemost 79:706, 1998.
23. Levine JS, Branch DW, Rauch J: The antiphospholipid syndrome. N Engl J Med 346:752, 2002.
24. Rinder HM, Bonan JL, Rinder CS, et al: Dynamics of leukocyte-platelet adhesion in whole blood. Blood 78:1730, 1991.
25. Park JW, Ma M, Ruedi JM, et al: The cytosolic components of the respiratory burst oxidase exist as a M(r) approximately 240,000 complex that acquires a membrane-binding site during activation of the oxidase in a cell-free system. J Biol Chem 267:17327, 1992.
26. Smith WL: Prostanoid biosynthesis and mechanisms of action. Am J Physiol 263:F181, 1992.
27. Smith WL, DeWitt DL, Shimokawa T, et al: Molecular basis for the inhibition of prostanoid biosynthesis by nonsteroidal anti-inflammatory agents. Stroke 21:IV24, 1990.
28. Hirsh J, Dalen JE, Fuster V, et al: Aspirin and other platelet-active drugs: The relationship among dose, effectiveness, and side effects. Chest 108:247S, 1995.
29. Randomized trial of intravenous heparin versus recombinant hirudin for acute coronary syndromes. The Global Use of Strategies to Open Occluded Coronary Arteries (GUSTO) IIa Investigators. Circulation 90:1631, 1994.
30. Eikelboom JW, Hankey GJ: Aspirin resistance: A new independent predictor of vascular events? J Am Coll Cardiol 41:966, 2003.
31. FitzGerald GA: Parsing an enigma: The pharmacodynamics of aspirin resistance. Lancet 361:542, 2003.
32. Clutton P, Folts JD, Freedman JE: Pharmacological control of platelet function. Pharmacol Res 44:255, 2001.
33. Sekiya F, Takagi J, Usui T, et al: 12S-hydroxyeicosatetraenoic acid plays a central role in the regulation of platelet activation. Biochem Biophys Res Commun 179:345, 1991.
34. Katoh A, Ikeda H, Murohara T, et al: Platelet-derived 12-hydroxyeicosatetraenoic acid plays an important role in mediating canine coronary thrombosis by regulating platelet glycoprotein IIb/IIIa activation. Circulation 98:2891, 1998.
35. Claria J, Serhan CN: Aspirin triggers previously undescribed bioactive eicosanoids by human endothelial cell-leukocyte interactions. Proc Natl Acad Sci U S A 92:9475, 1995.
36. Cattaneo M, Lombardi R, Zighetti ML, et al: Deficiency of (33P)2MeS-ADP binding sites on platelets with secretion defect, normal granule stores and normal thromboxane A2 production: Evidence that ADP potentiates platelet secretion independently of the formation of large platelet aggregates and thromboxane A2 production. Thromb Haemost 77:986, 1997.
37. Gachet C, Cattaneo M, Ohlmann P, et al: Purinoceptors on blood platelets: Further pharmacological and clinical evidence to suggest the presence of two ADP receptors. Br J Haematol 91:434, 1995.
38. Daniel JL, Dangelmaier C, Jin J, et al: Role of intracellular signaling events in ADP-induced platelet aggregation. Thromb Haemost 82:1322, 1999.
39. Daniel JL, Dangelmaier C, Jin J, et al: Molecular basis for ADP-induced platelet activation. I. Evidence for three distinct ADP receptors on human platelets. J Biol Chem 273:2024, 1998.
40. Fagura MS, Dainty IA, McKay GD, et al: P2Y1-receptors in human platelets which are pharmacologically distinct from P2Y(ADP)-receptors. Br J Pharmacol 124:157, 1998.
41. Jin J, Kunapuli SP: Coactivation of two different G protein-coupled receptors is essential for ADP-induced platelet aggregation. Proc Natl Acad Sci U S A 95:8070, 1998.
42. Leon C, Hechler B, Freund M, et al: Defective platelet aggregation and increased resistance to thrombosis in purinergic P2Y(1) receptor-null mice. J Clin Invest 104:1731, 1999.
43. Leon C, Vial C, Gachet C, et al: The P2Y1 receptor is normal in a patient presenting a severe deficiency of ADP-induced platelet aggregation. Thromb Haemost 81:775, 1999.
44. Jarvis GE, Humphries RG, Robertson MJ, et al: ADP can induce aggregation of human platelets via both P2Y(1) and P(2T) receptors. Br J Pharmacol 129:275, 2000.

45. Storey RF, Sanderson HM, White AE, et al: The central role of the P(2T) receptor in amplification of human platelet activation, aggregation, secretion and procoagulant activity. Br J Haematol 110:925, 2000.
46. A randomised, blinded, trial of clopidogrel versus aspirin in patients at risk of ischaemic events (CAPRIE). CAPRIE Steering Committee. Lancet 348:1329, 1996.
47. Savi P, Pereillo JM, Uzabiaga MF, et al: Identification and biological activity of the active metabolite of clopidogrel. Thromb Haemost 84:891, 2000.
48. Savi P, Combalbert J, Gaich C, et al: The antiaggregating activity of clopidogrel is due to a metabolic activation by the hepatic cytochrome P450-1A. Thromb Haemost 72:313, 1994.
49. Savage B, Ruggeri ZM: Selective recognition of adhesive sites in surface-bound fibrinogen by glycoprotein IIb-IIIa on nonactivated platelets. J Biol Chem 266:11227, 1991.
50. Naik UP, Patel PM, Parise LV: Identification of a novel calcium-binding protein that interacts with the integrin alpha IIb cytoplasmic domain. J Biol Chem 272:4651, 1997.
51. Clemetson KJ: Platelet activation: Signal transduction via membrane receptors. Thromb Haemost 74:111, 1995.
52. Lefkovits J, Plow EF, Topol EJ: Platelet glycoprotein IIb/IIIa receptors in cardiovascular medicine. N Engl J Med 332:1553, 1995.
53. Coller BS, Scudder LE: Inhibition of dog platelet function by in vivo infusion of F(ab′)2 fragments of a monoclonal antibody to the platelet glycoprotein IIb/IIIa receptor. Blood. 66:1456, 1985.
54. Coller BS, Scudder LE, Beer J, et al: Monoclonal antibodies to platelet glycoprotein IIb/IIIa as antithrombotic agents. Ann N Y Acad Sci.614:193, 1991.
55. Coller BS, Seligsohn U, West SM, et al: Platelet fibrinogen and vitronectin in Glanzmann thrombasthenia: Evidence consistent with specific roles for glycoprotein IIb/IIIA and alpha v beta 3 integrins in platelet protein trafficking. Blood 78:2603, 1991.
56. Coller BS, Folts JD, Scudder LE, et al: Antithrombotic effect of a monoclonal antibody to the platelet glycoprotein IIb/IIIa receptor in an experimental animal model. Blood 68:783, 1986.
57. Use of a monoclonal antibody directed against the platelet glycoprotein IIb/IIIa receptor in high-risk coronary angioplasty. The EPIC Investigation. N Engl J Med 330:956, 1994.
58. Platelet glycoprotein IIb/IIIa receptor blockade and low-dose heparin during percutaneous coronary revascularization. The EPILOG Investigators. N Engl J Med 336:1689, 1997.
59. Dennis MS, Henzel WJ, Pitti RM, et al: Platelet glycoprotein IIb-IIIa protein antagonists from snake venoms: Evidence for a family of platelet-aggregation inhibitors. Proc Natl Acad Sci U S A 87:2471, 1990.
60. O'Neill WW, Serruys P, Knudtson M, et al: Long-term treatment with a platelet glycoprotein-receptor antagonist after percutaneous coronary revascularization. EXCITE Trial Investigators. Evaluation of Oral Xemilofiban in Controlling Thrombotic Events. N Engl J Med 342:1316, 2000.
61. Cannon CP, McCabe CH, Wilcox RG, et al: Oral glycoprotein IIb/IIIa inhibition with orbofiban in patients with unstable coronary syndromes (OPUS-TIMI 16) trial. Circulation 102:149, 2000.
62. Curtin R, Fitzgerald DJ: A cold start for oral glycoprotein IIb/IIIa antagonists. Eur Heart J 21:1992, 2000.
63. Chew DP, Bhatt DL, Sapp S, et al: Increased mortality with oral platelet glycoprotein IIb/IIIa antagonists: A meta-analysis of phase III multicenter randomized trials. Circulation. 103:201, 2001.
64. Yamamoto H, Vreys I, Stassen JM, et al: Antagonism of vWF inhibits both injury induced arterial and venous thrombosis in the hamster. Thromb Haemost 79:202, 1998.
65. Chang MC, Lin HK, Peng HC, et al: Antithrombotic effect of crotalin: A platelet membrane glycoprotein Ib antagonist from venom of Crotalus atrox. Blood 91:1582, 1998.
66. Yeh CH, Chang MC, Peng HC, et al: Pharmacological characterization and antithrombotic effect of agkistin: A platelet glycoprotein Ib antagonist. Br J Pharmacol 132:843, 2001.
67. Cauwenberghs N, Meiring M, Vauterin S, et al: Antithrombotic effect of platelet glycoprotein Ib-blocking monoclonal antibody Fab fragments in nonhuman primates. Arterioscler Thromb Vasc Biol 20:1347, 2000.
68. O'Donnell CJ, Larson MG, Feng D, et al: Genetic and environmental contributions to platelet aggregation: The Framingham heart study. Circulation 103:3051, 2001.
69. Lacolley P, Gautier S, Poirier O, et al: Nitric oxide synthase gene polymorphisms, blood pressure and aortic stiffness in normotensive and hypertensive subjects. J Hypertens 16:31, 1998.
70. Shimasaki Y, Yasue H, Yoshimura M, et al: Association of the missense Glu298Asp variant of the endothelial nitric oxide synthase gene with myocardial infarction. J Am Coll Cardiol 31:1506, 1998.
71. Elbaz A, Poirier O, Moulin T, et al: Association between the Glu298Asp polymorphism in the endothelial constitutive nitric oxide synthase gene and brain infarction. The GENIC Investigators. Stroke 31:1634, 2000.
72. Hingorani AD, Liang CF, Fatibene J, et al: A common variant of the endothelial nitric oxide synthase (Glu298→Asp) is a major risk factor for coronary artery disease in the UK. Circulation 100:1515, 1999.
73. Wang XL, Sim AS, Badenhop RF, et al: A smoking-dependent risk of coronary artery disease associated with a polymorphism of the endothelial nitric oxide synthase gene. Nat Med 2:41, 1996.
74. Tanus-Santos JE, Desai M, Deak LR, et al: Effects of endothelial nitric oxide synthase gene polymorphisms on platelet function, nitric oxide release, and interactions with estradiol. Pharmacogenetics 12:407, 2002.
75. Keaney J, Stamler J, Folts J, et al: NO forms a stable adduct with serum albumin that has potent antiplatelet properties in vivo. Clin Res 40:194A, 1992.
76. Freedman JE, Frei B, Welch GN, et al: Glutathione peroxidase potentiates the inhibition of platelet function by S-nitrosothiols. J Clin Invest. 96:394, 1995.
77. Freedman JE, Loscalzo J, Benoit SE, et al: Decreased platelet inhibition by nitric oxide in two brothers with a history of arterial thrombosis. J Clin Invest. 97:979, 1996.
78. Inbal A, Kenet G, Freedman J, et al: Impaired NO-mediated inhibition of platelet aggregation and P-selectin expression by plasma from patients with childhood stroke. Thromb Haemost. Supplement:304, PS-1245, 1997.
79. Neumann FJ, Zohlnhofer D, Fakhoury L, et al: Effect of glycoprotein IIb/IIIa receptor blockade on platelet-leukocyte interaction and surface expression of the leukocyte integrin Mac-1 in acute myocardial infarction. J Am Coll Cardiol 34:1420, 1999.
80. Gawaz MP, Loftus JC, Bajt ML, et al: Ligand bridging mediates integrin alpha IIb beta 3 (platelet GPIIB- IIIA) dependent homotypic and heterotypic cell-cell interactions. J Clin Invest 88:1128, 1991.
81. Simon DI, Ezratty AM, Francis SA, et al: Fibrin(ogen) is internalized and degraded by activated human monocytoid cells via Mac-1 (CD11b/CD18): A nonplasmin fibrinolytic pathway. Blood 82:2414, 1993.
82. Shebuski RJ, Kilgore KS: Role of inflammatory mediators in thrombogenesis. J Pharmacol Exp Ther 300:729, 2002.
83. Celi A, Pellegrini G, Lorenzet R, et al: P-selectin induces the expression of tissue factor on monocytes. Proc Natl Acad Sci U S A 91:8767, 1991.
84. Neumann FJ, Marx N, Gawaz M, et al: Induction of cytokine expression in leukocytes by binding of thrombin-stimulated platelets. Circulation 95:2387, 1997.
85. Yang Y, Loscalzo J: Regulation of tissue factor expression in human microvascular endothelial cells by nitric oxide. Circulation 101:2144, 2000.
86. Henn V, Slupsky JR, Grafe M, et al: CD40 ligand on activated platelets triggers an inflammatory reaction of endothelial cells. Nature 391:591, 1998.
87. Schonbeck U, Varo N, Libby P, et al: Soluble CD40L and cardiovascular risk in women. Circulation 104:2266, 2001.
88. Andre P, Prasad KS, Denis CV, et al: CD40L stabilizes arterial thrombi by a beta3 integrin-dependent mechanism. Nat Med 8:247, 2002.
89. Freedman JE: CD40 ligand-assessing risk instead of damage? N Engl J Med. 348:1163, 2003.
90. Van Cott EM, Laposata M, Prins MH: Laboratory evaluation of hypercoagulability with venous or arterial thrombosis. Arch Pathol Lab Med 126:1281, 2002.
91. Anderson FA, Jr, Spencer FA: Risk factors for venous thromboembolism. Circulation. 107:I9, 2003.

chapter 9

The History and Physical Examination

Joshua A. Beckman
Mark A. Creager

The ubiquitous nature of arteries, veins, and lymphatic vessels allows for any region of the body to develop vascular disease. This chapter describes the vascular medical history and physical examination, which are the core components of the evaluation of patients with vascular diseases. Application of these methods and the tailored use of special examination maneuvers facilitates the diagnosis of vascular disease, especially when used in conjunction with vascular tests described elsewhere in this section. This chapter will review the cardinal complaints of patients with vascular disease, and then the physical findings associated with common arterial, venous, and lymphatic diseases. More specific features of the vascular history and examination are discussed in the relevant chapters of each vascular disease.

VASCULAR HISTORY

The medical history is the foundation of the physician-patient interaction, guiding the physical examination, testing, and treatment decisions. A comprehensive medical history can identify the diagnosis the vast majority of the time, whereas an inadequate one can result in excess testing and inappropriate therapy.

Arterial Disease

Symptoms of arterial disease typically arise as a result of either arterial stenoses or occlusions, although aneurysms also may cause symptoms. The important historical features of arterial disease in select regional circulations are reviewed subsequently.

Peripheral Arterial Disease

Peripheral arterial disease (PAD) is one of the most common clinical manifestations of atherosclerosis, in addition to carotid and coronary artery disease. Approximately 50% of patients with PAD have symptoms, described below as typical or atypical, and the remainder are asymptomatic. The importance of making the diagnosis of PAD, even in the absence of symptoms, derives from the prognostic information implicit with its diagnosis (see Chapter 14). Notably, patients with PAD often have coexisting coronary and cerebrovascular atherosclerosis, and are sixfold more likely than patients without PAD to die of cardiovascular disease.[1]

Therefore, the history of patients with PAD should seek to determine whether the patient has known risk factors for atherosclerosis, and also to determine whether or not there are other clinical manifestations of atherosclerosis. History should elicit information regarding dyslipidemia, diabetes mellitus, hypertension, family history of premature atherosclerosis, or cigarette smoking. Historical evidence of coronary artery disease, including prior myocardial infarction, symptoms of angina, or prior coronary revascularization procedures and history of stroke or symptoms of cerebrovascular ischemia, including hemiparesis, hemiparesthesia, aphasia, or amaurosis fugax, should be sought and documented.

Intermittent Claudication

A cardinal symptom of PAD is intermittent claudication (see Chapter 17). Claudication occurs when limb skeletal muscle ischemia is produced with effort, as increased muscle energy requirements are not served by sufficient augmentation in blood supply. Symptoms develop *intermittently* with activity, because the blood flow limitation imposed by peripheral arterial stenosis typically does not compromise muscular function at rest. Claudication is variably described as aching, heaviness, burning, fatigue, cramping, and/or tightness in the affected limb. The symptoms occur with reproducible amounts of exercise; e.g., one block of walking, one flight of stairs, or 5 minutes on a bicycle. The discomfort may develop in any muscular portion of the leg including the buttocks, hip, thigh, calf, or foot. The areas of the limb to develop discomfort are related to the arterial segments with stenoses. Iliac artery disease typically produces hip or buttock claudication, whereas femoral artery disease causes thigh or calf claudication. Arm claudication is unusual, but may occur in patients with innominate, subclavian, axillary, or brachial artery stenosis. Cessation of activity relieves the exercising muscle's demand-supply mismatch and enables restoration of oxidative metabolism. Therefore, patients typically report that discontinuation of activity relieves the discomfort after several minutes. Atypical symptoms of PAD, however, also occur and these include reduction of leg discomfort despite continued effort, gait disturbance, and slower walking speed.[2] Patients with intermittent claudication often slow their walking speed by one third to moderate muscle use and prolong walking distance. Thus, when a physician discusses walking impairment, patients may report no change in distance walked before symptoms occur, despite a progressive decline in functional ability.[3]

Several questionnaires for PAD have been devised and validated. These provide a standard to accompany the interview when querying patients about symptoms of PAD. The Rose questionnaire was the initial PAD-related questionnaire, but limited diagnostic sensitivity limits its usefulness.[4,5] The San Diego questionnaire is a modified version of the Rose questionnaire and a more reliable instrument to assess intermittent claudication (see Chapter 14).[6] The disease-specific Walking Impairment questionnaire has been validated and can be used to assess walking difficulty in patients with PAD. It has four subscales: severity of pain with walking, distance, speed, and stair climbing.[7]

Critical Limb Ischemia

Critical limb ischemia (CLI) occurs when limb blood flow is inadequate to meet the metabolic demands of the tissues at rest.[8] This may cause persistent pain, especially in the acral portions of the leg: the toes, ball of the foot, or heel. Additional foot symptoms include sensitivity to cold, joint stiffness, and hypesthesia. As a consequence of the effects of gravity on perfusion pressure, patients may observe worsening of pain with leg elevation, or even when the feet are in bed, and reduction in pain with limb dependency; e.g., when the feet hang over the bed onto the floor. CLI may cause tissue breakdown (ulceration) or gangrene.

Acute Limb Ischemia

Acute limb ischemia occurs most often as a result of embolism or in situ thrombosis (see Chapter 46).[9] Other causes include arterial dissection or trauma. The presentation of acute arterial occlusion ranges from the asymptomatic loss of a pulse, to worsened claudication, to the sudden onset of severe pain at rest. Symptoms may develop suddenly over several hours, or over several days. Acute ischemic symptoms are more likely to occur when no or few collateral vessels are present, rather than when there is a well-developed collateral network. Acute arterial occlusion may cause symptoms in any portion of the leg distal to the obstruction. The five 'Ps': pain, pallor, poikilothermia, paresthesias, and paralysis, characterize the historical features and findings of patients with acute limb ischemia. The severity of symptoms does not discriminate among etiologies.

Atheroembolism

Atheroembolism is the embolization of atherosclerotic debris that compromises distal arteries (see Chapter 47). Atheroemboli vary in composition, from the larger fibroplatelet particles that occlude small arteries to cholesterol emboli, nanometers in size, which occlude arterioles. Causes of atheroemboli include catheterization and cardiovascular surgery, but approximately one half of the events occur without a known precipitant.[10]

Symptoms reflect the occlusion of the small, distal vessels in the limb, and patients will commonly present with calf, foot, or toe pain, and areas of violaceous discoloration or cyanosis in the toes (blue toe syndrome). The symptoms develop hours to days after the event; ulcerations may develop and are slow to resolve. Symptoms may be unilateral or bilateral, depending on the origin of emboli proximal to or beyond the aortic bifurcation. If atheroemboli arise proximal to the renal arteries, renal insufficiency is a potential sequela.

Other Peripheral Arterial Diseases

Uncommon diseases of the peripheral arteries should be considered in patients with claudication or evidence of ischemia, but whose age falls below that typically affected by atherosclerosis or in those with atypical symptoms. These diseases include Takayasu's arteritis (see Chapter 42) and giant cell arteritis (see Chapter 43); thromboangiitis obliterans (see Chapter 44); and vascular compression syndromes—such as those affecting the thoracic outlet, iliac artery, and popliteal artery (see Chapter 64).

Takayasu's arteritis is a vasculitis that generally occurs between the ages of 20 and 40 years. Women are more likely to develop the disease than are men. Constitutional and vascular symptoms occur. These include fevers, weight loss, fatigue, arthralgias, and myalgias—and may be present months to years without overt evidence of vascular disease. Approximately 50% of patients complain of muscle or joint pains, and headache has been reported in up to 40% of patients. More than 50% of the patients will have a diminished pulse or claudication of an upper extremity. Approximately 30% of patients will report neck pain and have a tender carotid artery; i.e., carotodynia. Lightheadedness is also common, and it may be secondary to vertebral arterial involvement.

Patients with *giant cell arteritis* (GCA) are typically more than the age of 50 years. GCA predominantly affects the branches of the thoracic aorta and the intracranial arteries. Approximately 50% of the patients have constitutional symptoms related to inflammation. Fifty percent of patients have coexisting polymyalgia rheumatica. The most common complaint is headache, which typically affects the occipital or temporal region, and occurs in more than 60% of the patients with GCA. In patients with headache, scalp tenderness may occur. Partial or complete visual loss develops in 20% of patients, and approximately 50% of patients with visual loss report amaurosis fugax. Patients may present with upper limb claudication; 40% of patients report jaw claudication. Tongue claudication and swallowing difficulties are less common.

Thromboangiitis obliterans (TAO) (Buerger's disease) is a small to medium vessel vasculitis that affects the distal vessels of the arms or legs, and usually occurs before 40 years of age in persons who smoke cigarettes.[11] It affects men more than it affects women. The classic triad of TAO is claudication, Raynaud's phenomenon, and superficial thrombophlebitis. Claudication of the hands or feet may progress to ulceration of the fingers or toes.[11]

Neurovascular Compression Syndromes

Claudication in the upper extremities raises the possibility of thoracic outlet syndrome (see Chapter 64).[12] Compression of the axillary or subclavian artery by a cervical rib, abnormal insertion of the scalene anticus muscle, or apposition of the clavicle and first rib may result in arterial compression during head turning, arm use above or behind the head, or arm extension, and cause weakness, burning, aching, or fatigue in the arms. Examples include wall-painting, hair washing, and housecleaning.

Popliteal artery entrapment should be considered in a young person with leg claudication.[13] Anatomic variants of the popliteal artery may result in its compression by the gastrocnemius muscle during exercise and can cause symptoms of claudication.

Vasospastic Diseases

Raynaud's phenomenon is the most common vasospastic disorder (see Chapter 48).[14] The digits become pale or cyanotic during local or environmental cold exposure. The fingers are most commonly affected, but the toes develop symptoms in 40% of patients. Less commonly involved areas include the tongue, nose, and ear lobes. Patients may report paresthesias or pain in the digits if ischemia persists. With rewarming and the release of vasospasm, digital rubor may develop as a result of reactive hyperemia. A pulsating or flushed feeling may accompany the hyperemic phase. All color phases are not required for diagnosis. Indeed, with an appropriate history, the diagnosis can be made with only one color change.

There are two categories of Raynaud's phenomenon, primary and secondary. Differentiating between the two forms is important because of the information it provides about cause and prognosis. Primary Raynaud's disease is benign, typically affects the fingers (and toes) symmetrically, and recovery is predictable with rewarming. Seventy to 80% of patients with Raynaud's disease are women. In patients with secondary Raynaud's phenomenon, pallor may occur in only one or several digits. In severe cases, cyanosis is unremitting and tissue loss may occur. Raynaud's phenomenon that has its onset after age 45 years should prompt an investigation for an underlying cause. The history should include questions to elicit evidence of disease or conditions that cause secondary Raynaud's phenomenon, including connective tissue disorders, arterial occlusive disease, trauma (vibration, hypothenar hand injury), neurovascular compression syndromes, blood dyscrasias, and drug use.

Acrocyanosis is a vascular disorder characterized by a bluish discoloration of the hands and feet that is exacerbated by cold exposure (see Chapter 49). Unlike Raynaud's phenomenon, the discoloration is not confined to the digits and pallor does not occur. Warming, however, can ameliorate the cyanosis and restore normal skin color. Acrocyanosis typically occurs in persons aged 20 to 45 years and women are affected more often than men.

Pernio is a vascular inflammatory disorder in which skin lesions and swelling occur in fingers and toes, particularly in cold, moist climates (see Chapter 51). Other exposed portions of the body may be affected. The typical lesions described by the patient are pruritic and painful blisters or superficial ulcers.

Cerebrovascular Diseases

The complex regional pain syndromes, reflex sympathetic dystrophy (RSD), and causalgia are associated with limb symptoms, often following a relatively minor injury (see Chapter 52). Hand or foot pain is a frequent complaint. This may be associated with hyperpathia, hyperesthesias, coolness, cyanosis, hyperhidrosis, and swelling. The symptoms typically are out of proportion to the severity of the initial injury. Patients may observe brittle nails that develop ridges and report muscle, skin, and subcutaneous tissue wasting, and limited joint mobility in the affected limb.

Renal Artery Stenosis

There are no symptoms elicited by history that are specific to renal artery stenosis. Unlike other end organs, symptoms of chronic renal ischemia are not localized to the kidney, but reflect the systemic pathophysiologic alterations that result from activation of the renin angiotensin system and disturbances of salt and water balance. Historical clues that raise suspicion of renal artery stenosis include the onset of hypertension before age 30 years or after age 55 years; malignant hypertension; hypertension refractory to three concurrently prescribed antihypertensive medications; azotemia subsequent to administration of an angiotensin-converting enzyme inhibitor or angiotensin receptor blocker; unexplained azotemia; recurrent congestive heart failure; and episodic pulmonary edema (see Chapter 22). Renal artery stenosis should be considered in patients with these clinical clues, particularly if they have evidence of atherosclerosis in other regional circulations—such as coronary artery disease, peripheral arterial disease, or aortic disease.

Mesenteric Artery Disease

Most patients with atherosclerosis of the celiac, superior mesenteric, or inferior mesenteric arteries are asymptomatic unless two, or all three, of these arteries are occluded. Symptoms of chronic mesenteric ischemia include postprandial epigastric or midabdominal pain, that may radiate to the back (see Chapter 26). The onset of abdominal discomfort is 15 to 30 minutes after eating and the symptoms may persist for several hours. Patients tend to avoid food to prevent these symptoms and weight loss ensues.

Carotid Artery Disease

The majority of patients with significant stenoses of the common or internal carotid arteries are asymptomatic. Symptoms, when they occur, may be temporary (minutes to hours) indicating a transient ischemic attack (TIA) or fixed, indicating a stroke. The symptoms of carotid artery disease (see Chapter 30) reflect those of the neural territory supplied by its principal intracranial branch, the middle cerebral artery, and includes contralateral hemiparesis, hemiparesthesia, and aphasia. Ipsilateral amaurosis fugax or blindness may also occur because the ophthalmic artery is supplied by the internal carotid artery. The prevalence of carotid artery disease is increased in patients with coronary artery disease or peripheral artery disease, both of which increase the risk of stroke by two- to fourfold.

The Venous and Lymphatic Systems

A history soliciting evidence of venous and lymphatic diseases is required when patients complain of leg pain or swelling, or express concerns regarding leg ulcers, varicose veins, or localized inflammation on a limb. In patients presenting with leg edema, the history should seek to determine whether the swelling is secondary to venous or lymphatic diseases, trauma, arthritis, or whether it is associated with a systemic condition—such as congestive heart failure, cirrhosis, nephrotic syndrome, renal insufficiency, or endocrinopathy (hypothyroidism or Cushing's syndrome).

Deep Vein Thrombosis (DVT)

Patients with thrombosis of a deep vein (see Chapter 53) of a limb may present with swelling or discomfort, or no symptoms at all. Symptoms are usually, albeit not always, unilateral. Historical queries should seek potential causes of DVT when it is suspected. Information regarding recent trauma, surgery, hospitalization, prolonged period of immobility, cancer, thrombophilia, or family history of venous thrombosis should be acquired. An uncommon cause of left leg DVT is May-Thurner syndrome in which the left iliac vein is compressed by the right iliac artery. In patients with arm symptoms, questions should seek evidence of indwelling catheters or cancer, because these are the most common causes of upper extremity DVT. In addition, a history of repetitive arm motion should be sought when considering the possibility of Paget-Schroetter syndrome, in which compression of the axillo-subclavian vein by muscular, tendinous, or bony components of the thoracic outlet may cause thrombosis. Thrombosis or extrinsic compression of the superior vena cava may cause symptoms of superior vena cava syndrome, which include headache, face and neck fullness and flushing, and bilateral arm swelling.

Superficial Thrombophlebitis

Thrombosis of a superficial vein is a local phenomenon that manifests with pain and tenderness over the affected vein. Predisposing factors sought by history include intravenous catheters, varicose veins, and malignancy. It is important to consider the possibility of malignancy, especially pancreatic, lung, and ovarian cancers in patients with recurrent or migratory superficial thrombophlebitis (i.e., Trousseau's syndrome). Uncommon disorders associated with superficial thrombophlebitis include thromboangiitis obliterans and Behçet's syndrome.

Chronic Venous Insufficiency

Venous insufficiency (see Chapter 56) should be considered in patients who present with chronic unilateral or bilateral leg swelling. Causes of venous insufficiency include deep venous obstruction and deep venous valvular incompetence. Approximately 30% of patients with DVT will ultimately develop chronic venous insufficiency.[15,16] Valvular incompetence may be a consequence of recanalized venous thrombus or a primary valvular abnormality. Queries should address the duration of leg swelling, knowledge of prior DVT, presence of focal hyperpigmentation, pain, pruritus, or ulcers. Symptoms may include a heavy, dull, or "bursting" sensation of the edematous leg. Patients may report that discomfort in the affected leg increases with dependency and improves with leg elevation. Some individuals with severe leg swelling note that calf discomfort worsens with walking, a symptom termed *venous claudication*.

Varicose Veins

Most patients with varicose veins (see Chapter 55) do not have specific symptoms, but present to a physician's office with cosmetic concerns. Symptoms of varicose veins include leg discomfort or aching, particularly with prolonged standing. These symptoms are most likely to occur along long segments of the greater and lesser saphenous veins and their tributaries. Burning or pruritus may develop, particularly if complicated by accompanying skin ulceration.

Lymphedema

Lymphedema should be considered in patients who present with limb swelling (see Chapter 60). Lymphedema may affect the arms or legs. It is usually unilateral, although it can be bilateral. Lymphedema should be suspected if limb swelling occurs early in life, particularly during childhood or adolescence. Congenital lymphedema typically appears at birth or shortly thereafter. Lymphedema praecox often manifests around puberty, but can occur any time before age 35. Lymphedema tarda generally occurs after age 35. Lymphedema is also associated with genetic disorders such as Turner's and Noonan's syndromes. It is important to elicit a history of conditions that may predispose a patient to lymphedema, including recurrent skin infection, lymphangitis, filariasis, trauma, malignancy of the lymphatic system, and radiation or surgical resection of lymph nodes and lymphatic vessels as adjunctive therapy for cancer.

Lymphangitis

Patients with lymphangitis may report an erythematous patch or linear streak that affects the limb and tends to propagate proximally over time. The erythematous area may be painful and tender. These patients usually present with systemic signs of infection, including fever and shaking chills. History might determine whether lesions induced by trauma or infection may have served as portals of entry.

VASCULAR EXAMINATION

As in any comprehensive physical examination, vital signs, including blood pressure, heart rate, and respiratory rate, should be assessed and recorded. The blood pressure should be measured in both arms, and preferably in the supine, seated, and upright positions. The overall appearance of the patient should be noted.

The vascular examination includes inspection, palpation, and auscultation of vascular structures in many areas of the body. A systematic approach ensures a complete evaluation. Thus, the examination described in this chapter will cover principal anatomic regions that are particularly relevant to the peripheral vasculature. The heart, lungs, and neurologic and musculoskeletal systems should be examined, but details of these examinations are beyond the scope of this chapter.

Limbs

The limbs should be inspected carefully, assessing their appearance, symmetry, color, and evidence of edema or muscle wasting.

Pulse Examination

The pulse examination of the arms and legs is a critical part of the vascular examination. Asymmetry, decreased intensity, or absence of pulses provides clinical evidence of PAD and indicate the location of stenotic lesions. Some examiners describe pulses as absent, diminished, or normal, or use a numeric scale, e.g., from 0 (absent) to 2+ (normal). Bounding pulses may be evidence of aortic valve insufficiency, and dilated, expansive pulses may be a sign of ectasia or aneurysm.

The pulses of the arms, including the brachial, radial, and ulnar pulses should be palpated using two or three fingertips. The brachial pulse is superficial and in the medial third of the antecubital fossa. The radial pulse, also superficial, can be found over the stylus of the radius near the base of the thumb (Fig. 9-1). The ulnar pulse is palpated on the volar aspect of the wrist, over the head of the ulnar bone. Wrist support by the examiner improves pulse detection by decreasing overlying muscle tension.

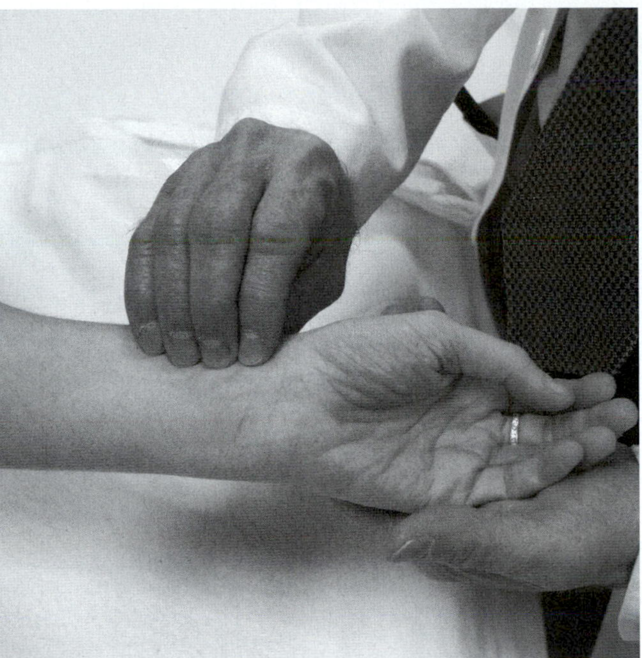

FIGURE 9-1. Palpation of the radial pulse. The examiner, using three or four fingers, lightly palpates the superficial radial pulse over the stylus of the radius near the base of the thumb.

The pulse examination of the leg, including the femoral, popliteal, posterior tibial, and dorsalis pedis pulses, should be undertaken with the subject in the supine position. The femoral pulse is located deep, below the inguinal ligament, approximately midway between the symphysis pubis and the iliac spine. Obesity may obscure local landmarks. Lateral rotation of the leg, pannus retraction and two hands may be required for adequate palpation. On occasion, the increase in flow velocity may create a thrill in the common or superficial femoral artery that is appreciated by palpation of the femoral pulse or a bruit that can be heard with auscultation. Palpation of the popliteal pulse can be difficult. The leg should be straight, yet relaxed to decrease overlying muscle stiffness. The popliteal pulse should be palpated with three fingers from each hand while the thumbs are applying moderate opposing force to the top of the knee (Fig. 9-2). The popliteal pulse typically can be found at the junction of the medial and lateral thirds of the fossa. In contrast to superficial pulses such as the radial or dorsalis pedis pulse, the popliteal pulse is diffuse and deep. Widened popliteal pulses may be indicative of a popliteal artery aneurysm. The posterior tibial pulse can be found slightly below and behind the medial malleolus. Counter pressure with the thumb and passive dorsiflexion of the foot may increase the

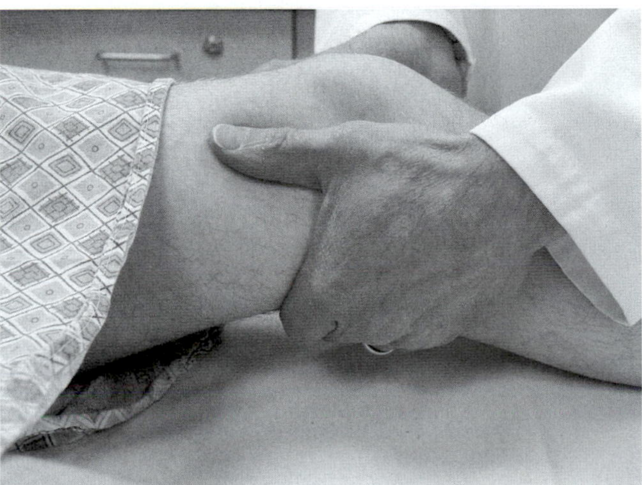

FIGURE 9-2. Palpation of the popliteal pulse. The popliteal pulse requires moderate pressure for its appreciation. The examiner uses both thumbs for moderate opposing force while placing digits two, three, and four in the lateral third of the popliteal fossa. The patient's leg should be relaxed while the examiner induces a mild flexion. The pulse is not typically appreciated immediately, requiring a few seconds for its recognition. Rapid pulse appreciation may indicate the presence of an aneurysm.

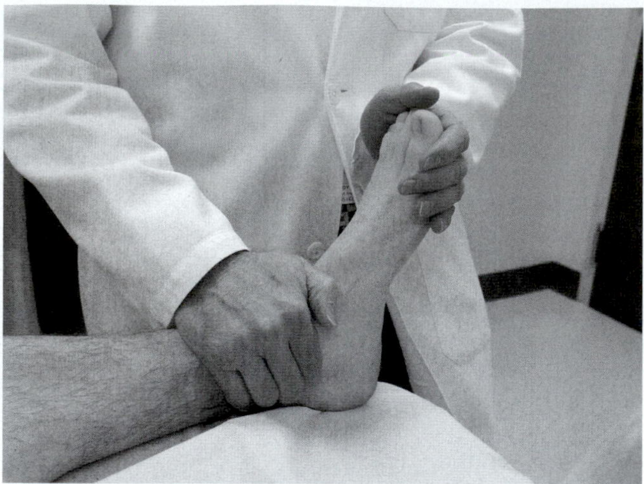

FIGURE 9-3. Palpation of the posterior tibial pulse. The posterior tibial pulse resides slightly below and behind the medial malleolus. It should be approached from the lateral aspect, with the digits applied to the lower curvature of the malleolus. Passive dorsiflexion of the foot may enhance appreciation of the pulse.

likelihood of palpation (Fig. 9-3). The posterior tibial pulse should be present. Its absence is diagnostic for PAD. In contrast, the dorsalis pedis pulse, which can be appreciated just lateral to the extensor tendon on the dorsum of the foot, normally may be absent in 5% to 10% of the population.

The Allen Test

The radial and ulnar arteries supply blood flow to the hand. Within the hand, these arteries form the superficial and deep palmar arches, enabling blood supply to the digits from either vessel. A congenitally incomplete arch has been found in 5% to 10% of the population. Disease states associated with interruption of the palmar arch include connective-tissue diseases such as the CREST variant of scleroderma, vasculitides (e.g., thromboangiitis obliterans), and thromboemboli. The Allen test can differentiate between a complete and an incomplete palmar arch. The examiner occludes both the radial and ulnar pulses (Fig. 9-4). The patient then opens and closes the fist several times, creating palmar pallor. On release of one pulse, normal skin color should return within seconds. The other artery is then tested and observed similarly. Persistent pallor is indicative of an incomplete palmar arch or an occluded artery distal to the remaining pulse occluded by the examiner.

Nearly three quarters of all patients with thromboangiitis obliterans will have a positive Allen test. Approximately 50% of all patients with Buerger's disease will report Raynaud's phenomenon. Digital ischemia in these patients is more likely to progress and cause persistent cyanosis and lead to digital ulcers. Patients with thromboangiitis obliterans also may develop migratory superficial thrombophlebitis, which appears as painful, tender red nodules.

Thoracic Outlet Maneuvers

Thoracic outlet syndrome results from compression of the neurovascular bundle as it leaves the thoracic cavity. Each component of the bundle may be affected, including the brachial plexus, subclavian/axillary artery, and subclavian/axillary vein.

Thoracic outlet maneuvers seek to elicit positional interruption of arterial flow. During the examination, the physician holds the radial pulse in one hand and maneuvers the arm with the other. The subclavian artery is auscultated in the supraclavicular fossa. An abnormal thoracic outlet maneuver is characterized by the development of a subclavian bruit followed by the loss of the radial pulse. Several thoracic outlet maneuvers have been

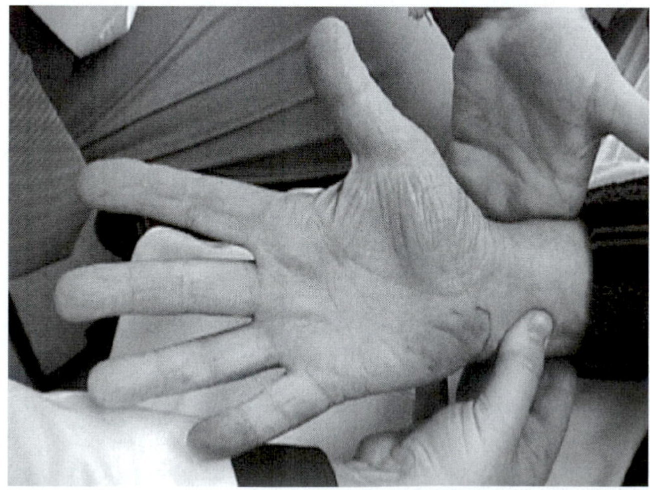

A

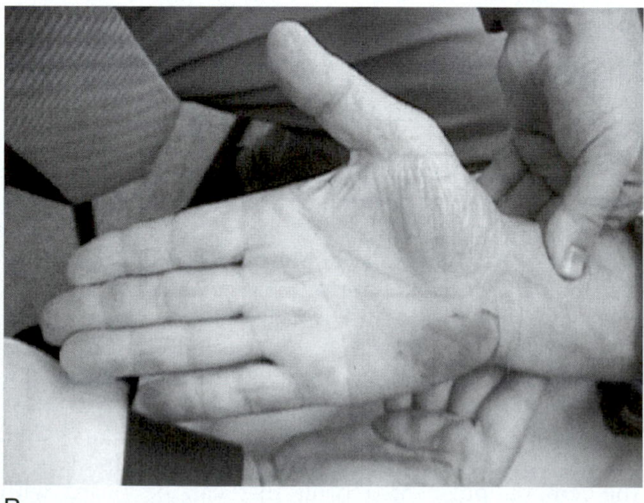

B

FIGURE 9-4. The Allen test. The Allen test determines the presence or absence of a complete palmar arch. Both radial and ulnar pulses are occluded while the patient opens and closes the hand to create palmar pallor. Once pallor is evident, the examiner releases one pulse. In this example, the patient presented with persistent fifth digit and hypothenar cyanosis. **A,** The release of the radial artery pulse results in the expected hyperemia and palmar erythema. **B,** In contrast, release of the ulnar artery pulse does not result in palmar erythema, indicating a proximal occlusion in the ulnar segment of the palmar arch. This test is considered a positive Allen test.

described and each may be relevant to compression at different sites in the thoracic outlet. Each side is examined in sequence. The Adson maneuver assesses the segment of the subclavian artery in the scalene triangle. The patient rotates his or her head toward the symptomatic side and extends the neck, (i.e., looking up and over the shoulder) and simultaneously performs an exaggerated inspiration. The costoclavicular maneuvers assess the segment of the subclavian artery coursing between the clavicle and first rib. The patient thrusts the shoulders back and inferiorly. The hyperabduction maneuver evaluates the subclavian artery as it courses near the insertion of the pectoralis major muscle. The patient is seated and the head is looking forward. The arm is abducted 180° to a position along the side of the head. The abduction of the arm to 90° may be combined with external rotation in the evaluation of symptoms suggestive of thoracic outlet syndrome (Fig. 9-5). This maneuver is often used to assess subclavian venous or arterial compression during ultrasonography or angiography. When used in patients who have a clinical suspicion for thoracic outlet syndrome, the sensitivity and specificity for these provocative tests are 72% and 53%, respectively.[17] Routine application of these maneuvers is not warranted, however, because up to 50% of the population may have a positive finding. Indeed, in one study of 64 randomly selected subjects, the application of these maneuvers in a nonspecific manner overdiagnosed the syndrome more than threefold.[18]

Limb Ischemia

Skin color and temperature can provide information about the severity of limb arterial perfusion. The feet, hands, fingers, and toes should be examined for temperature, skin color, and nails for evidence of fragility and pitting. Limb temperature can best be appreciated using the back of the examiner's hand, and enables detection of the temperature changes of adjacent segments on the ipsilateral limb and comparison with the contralateral limb. The presence of foot pallor while the leg is horizontal is indicative of poor perfusion and may be a sign of ischemia. Foot pallor may be precipitated in patients with PAD who do not have critical limb ischemia by elevating the patient's leg to 60° for 1 minute. Also, repetitive dorsiflexion and plantar flexion of the foot may precipitate pallor on the sole of the foot when PAD is present. To qualitatively assess collateral blood flow, the leg then is lowered as the patient moves to the seated position, to elicit rubor, indicative of reactive hyperemia, and determine pedal vein refill time. The time to development of dependent rubor is indicative of the severity of PAD. Severe PAD and poor collateral blood flow may prolong reactive hyperemia by more than 30 seconds; normally, pedal venous refill occurs in less than 15 seconds. Moderate PAD subserved by collateral vessels is suspected if venous refill is 30 to 45 seconds, whereas severe disease with poor collateral development likely is present when venous filling time is longer than 1 minute.

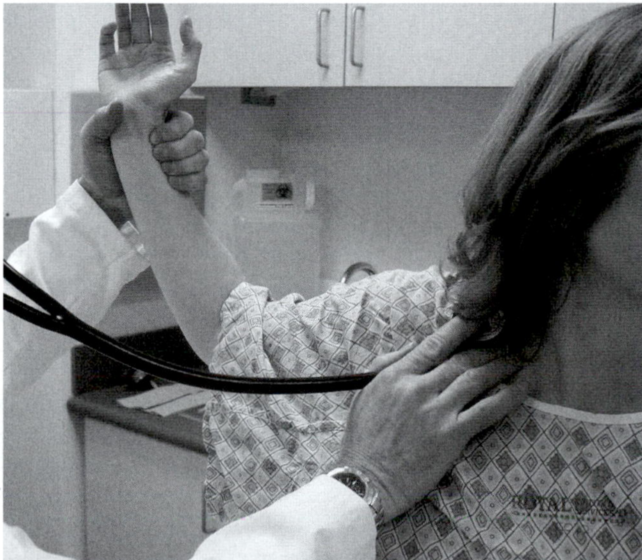

FIGURE 9-5. The hyperabduction maneuver. In the evaluation of the thoracic outlet syndrome, the hyperabduction maneuver is used to evaluate the subclavian artery as it courses near the insertion of the pectoralis major muscle. The patient initially sits looking forward while the arm is abducted 90°. During the maneuver, the radial pulse should be palpated while the subclavian artery is auscultated. The loss of the pulse or the development of a subclavian artery bruit is a positive study. External rotation of the head may be used as well, as demonstrated in the figure.

Ulcers

Ischemia arising from arterial occlusive disease or emboli may cause the formation of ischemic ulcers (see Chapter 62). The ulcers tend to be small, annular, pale, and desiccated (Fig. 9-6). They are usually located in distal areas of the limbs, such as the toes, heel, or fingertips. Ischemic ulcers vary in size, but may be as small as 3 mm in diameter. Arterial ischemic ulcers are tender. Neurotrophic ulcers, which develop in patients with diabetes, typically occur at sites of trauma, such as areas of callus formation, bony prominences, or parts of the foot exposed to mild chronic trauma caused by

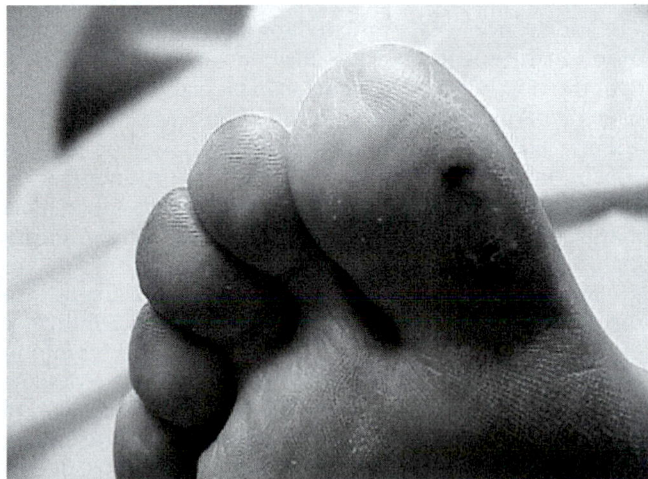

FIGURE 9-6. Digital ulceration. This patient complained of a persistent feeling of cold and pain in her toes. She reported areas of blue nodules that were painful. On examination, a discrete ulcer was noted in the area of greatest pain. The patient was diagnosed with pernio.

ill-fitting shoes. Ischemic ulcers also develop in diabetic patients with PAD and may have features of neuropathic ulcers. Without proper treatment, ulceration may progress to tissue necrosis and gangrene. Gangrene can be characterized as an area of dead tissue that blackens, mummifies, and sloughs.

Digital Vasospasm

It is unusual for patients with Raynaud's phenomenon to present to the physician's office during an attack in which the fingers are blanched. Moreover, it is difficult to precipitate digital ischemia in these patients, even with local cold exposure, such as placing the hands in ice water. Digital ischemia may be apparent in patients with fixed obstructive lesions of the digital arteries. Persistent digital ischemia may occur in patients with connective tissue disorders—such as scleroderma or systemic lupus erythematosus, atheroemboli, thromboangiitis obliterans, or atherosclerosis. The fingers and toes are cool and appear cyanotic or pale. Fissures, pits, ulcerations, or necrosis or gangrene may be evident on the ischemic digits (see Fig. 9-6).

Livedo Reticularis

Livedo reticularis can be described as a lace-like or net-like pattern in the skin (Fig. 9-7). The "laces" may vary in color from red to blue and surround a central area of clearing. Cold exposure exacerbates the changes in hue. Both primary and secondary forms may occur and may be complicated by ulceration. The primary benign form is more common in women. The secondary forms are usually associated with vasculitis, atheroemboli, hyperviscosity syndromes, endocrine abnormalities, and infections. In the secondary forms of livedo reticularis, the lesions may be more diffuse and ominous. Purpuric lesions and cutaneous nodules that progress to ulceration in response to cold may develop.

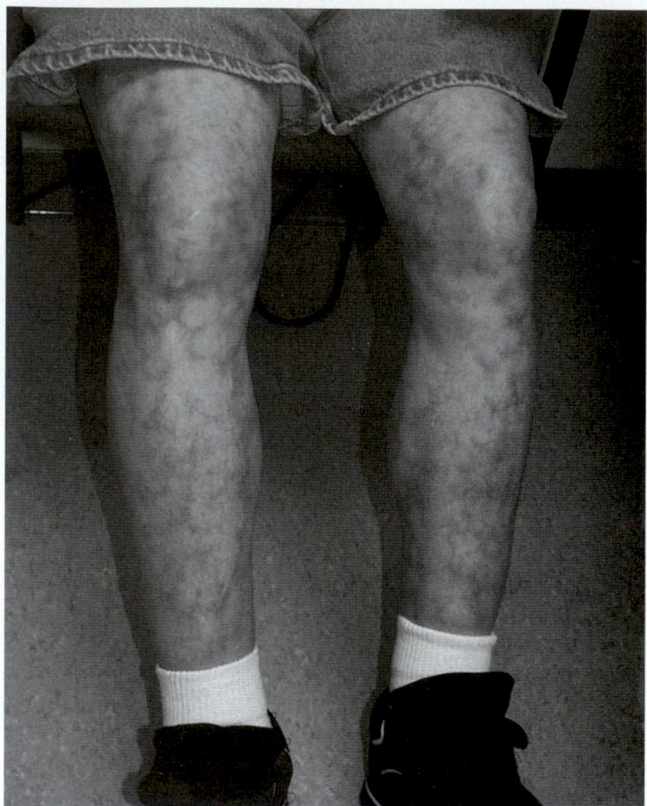

FIGURE 9-7. (See also Color Plate 9-7.) Livedo reticularis. This patient was referred to a vascular specialist for livedo reticularis. Note the lace-like pattern of superficial skin vessels surrounding a clear area. This patient reported these findings were chronic and without symptoms. Secondary causes were excluded and a diagnosis of idiopathic livedo reticularis was made.

Edema

The limbs should be evaluated for edema. The most common location is in the legs, adjacent to the malleoli and over the tibia. With deep digital palpation, the development of a divot or finger impression is indicative of pitting edema. Edema can be graded in each leg or arm as absent, mild, moderate, or severe or on a numeric scale of 4, with 0 being the absence of edema. Unilateral edema may be evidence of deep vein thrombosis, chronic venous insufficiency, or lymphedema.

The most common physical findings of deep vein thrombosis include unilateral leg swelling, warmth, and erythema. The affected vein may be tender. A common femoral vein cord is detected by palpating along its course just below the inguinal ligament vein, and a superficial femoral vein cord would be appreciated along the anteromedial aspect of the thigh. In the absence of obvious edema, a subtle clue includes the unilateral absence of contours of the thigh, calf, or ankle. Muscular groups subtended by the thrombosed vein may be edematous as a result of poor venous drainage conferring a boggy feeling to the affected calf or thigh muscles. The inflammation associated with a thrombosis may make the leg feel warm.

Homans's sign is nonspecific and misses the diagnosis as commonly as it makes it. In John Homans' essay on lower extremity venous thrombosis, he states, "The clinical signs of a deep thrombosis of the muscles of the calf are entirely lacking when the individual lies or even reclines in bed. It is possible there may be a little discomfort upon forced dorsiflexion of the foot (tightening of the posterior muscles) but it is not yet clear whether or not this is a sign upon which to depend."[19]

The presence of thrombus just below the skin makes the diagnosis of superficial thrombophlebitis relatively easy. The patient may present with local venous engorgement, a palpable cord, warmth, erythema, or tenderness.

Chronic Venous Insufficiency

With chronic venous insufficiency, the physical examination may demonstrate fibrosis, tenderness, excoriation, and skin induration from hyperkeratosis, cellulitis, and ulceration (Fig. 9-8). Chronic venous edema may impart hemosiderin deposition in the skin, and confer a brawny appearance, typically in the pretibial calf. The severity of chronic venous disease may be classified using the CEAP

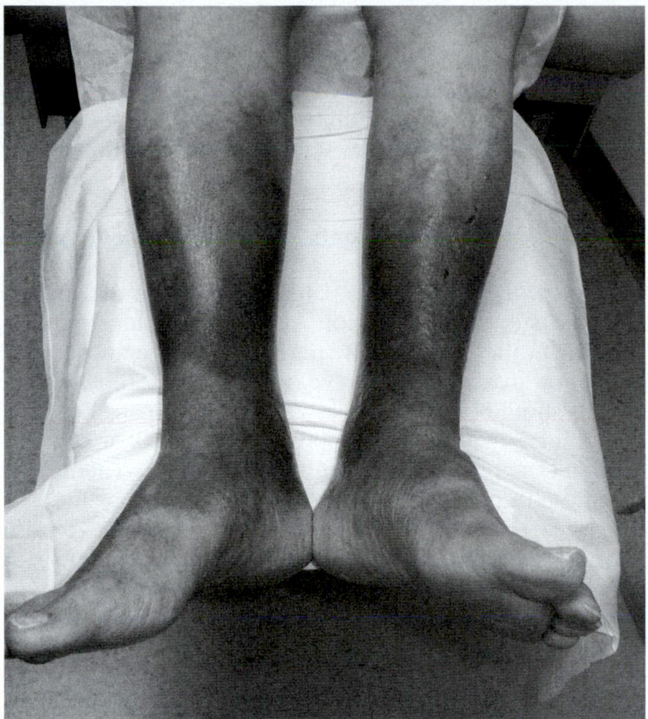

FIGURE 9-8. (See also Color Plate 9-8.) The skin changes of chronic venous insufficiency. Chronic venous insufficiency and edema result in the deposition of hemosiderin causing the darkening and toughening of the skin giving the calf a brawny appearance. Note the small, superficial venous ulcers mid-calf above the shin.

(*C*linical signs, *E*tiology, *A*natomy, *P*athophysiology) classification (Table 9-1).[20]

Venous ulcers, in contrast to the circumscribed, pallid arterial ulcers, are large with irregular borders, erythematous, and moist giving the skin a shiny appearance. They are usually located near the medial or lateral malleolus. Venous ulcers may be painless, but many are associated with pain.[21-23]

Varicose Veins

Varicose veins are dilated, serpentine, superficial veins. If they cluster, they may feel and appear like a bunch of grapes. Varicose veins should be inspected and palpated. Areas of erythema, tenderness, or induration may identify superficial thrombophlebitis. Varicose veins are most prominent with leg dependence (e.g., with standing). Once filled, the veins may be balloted and a fluid wave may be detected. Venous telangiectasias, also known as ***spider veins***, are commonly mistaken for varicose veins (Fig. 9-9). The spider veins are small, cutaneous veins typically in a caput medusa pattern.

Superficial venous varicosities may be primary or result from deep venous thrombosis or insufficiency. An examiner can distinguish between superficial venous insufficiency and deep venous insufficiency at the bedside using the Brodie-Trendelenberg test. With the patient lying supine, the leg is elevated to 45° and a tourniquet applied after the veins have drained. The patient then stands. The veins below the tourniquet should fill slowly. If venous refill distal to the site of tourniquet application occurs in less than 30 seconds, this is evidence of an incompetent deep and perforator system. Slower refills suggest a competent deep and perforator system. The varicose veins are examined on tourniquet release.

TABLE 9-1 CEAP* CLINICAL CLASSIFICATION

Class	Clinical Signs
0	No visible or palpable signs of venous disease
1	Telangiectasis or reticular veins
2	Varicose veins
3	Edema
4	Skin changes ascribed to venous disease (e.g., pigmentation, venous eczema, lipodermatosclerosis)
5	Skin changes as defined above with healed ulceration
6	Skin changes as defined above with active ulceration

*Clinical signs, *E*tiology, *A*natomy, *P*athophysiology.

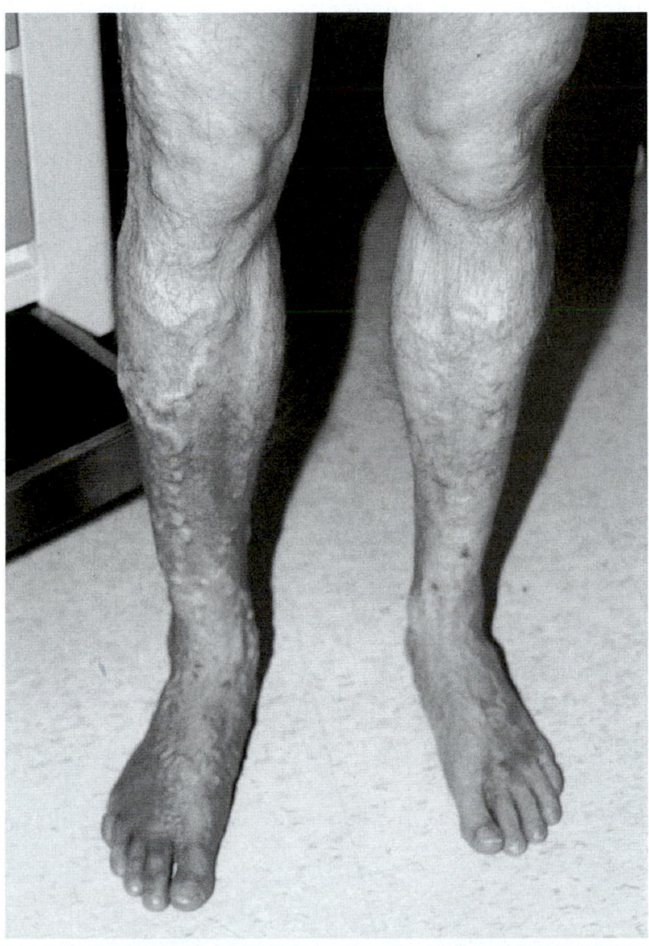

FIGURE 9-9. Varicose veins. This patient required many right heart catheterizations to follow his congenital heart disease. As a result, he developed an inferior vena caval occlusion and a marked increase in his lower extremity venous pressures. He developed severe, bilateral varicose veins. Note the extensive varicosities extend into both feet. The patient suffered several venous hemorrhages at the union of his first and second right digits prior to therapy with compression stockings and leg elevation.

Superficial venous insufficiency will be confirmed with rapid retrograde superficial venous filling.

The Perthes test can differentiate between deep venous insufficiency and a deep venous obstruction as a cause of varicose veins. Have the patient stand and, when the superficial veins are engorged, apply a tourniquet around the mid-thigh. Have the patient walk for 5 minutes. If the varicose veins collapse below the level of the tourniquet, the perforator veins are competent and the deep veins are patent. If the superficial veins remain engorged, either the superficial and/or communicating veins are incompetent. If the varicose veins increase in prominence and walking causes leg pain, the deep veins are occluded.

Lymphedema

During the initial stages of lymphedema, the leg swelling will be similar to venous insufficiency, soft and pitting. Extension of the edema into the foot to the origin of the toes, may help to differentiate lymphedema from venous edema (Fig. 9-10). In addition, the inability to pinch skin on the toes, the Stemmer sign, may also differentiate early lymphedema from venous edema. Subsequently, the limb becomes wood-like as the progressive deposition of protein-rich fluid causes induration and fibrosis of the affected tissues. Lymphedema increases the production of subcutaneous and adipose tissue, thickening the skin. When the leg feels wooden, the edema is no longer pitting, the limb is enlarged, and the skin may appear verrucous at the toes. Palpation for lymphadenopathy should be performed when considering secondary causes of lymphedema.

Lymphangitis

Lymphangitis can usually be visualized as a red streak that extends proximally from an inciting lesion. If left untreated, the entire limb may become edematous, erythematous, and warm without evidence of venous congestion or impairment of arterial flow. Commonly, the regional lymph nodes are indurated.

Neck Examination

The neck is inspected for any areas of swelling or asymmetry. The jugular venous pressure is assessed to investigate the possibility of a volume overloaded state or congestive heart failure. Patients typically are placed at 45° and the height of jugular venous pressure is estimated. If necessary, the angle of head elevation should be adjusted to see the top of the jugular venous column.

The carotid arteries are palpated between the trachea and the sternocleidomastoid muscles. In older patients especially, the carotid body may be sensitive and carotid palpation may induce bradycardia and hypotension. The pulses should be symmetric with a rapid upstroke. Pulse asymmetry may indicate a proximal carotid or brachiocephalic stenosis. Parvus and tardus pulses (decreased amplitude and a delayed, slow upstroke) may indicate aortic valve stenosis or proximal occlusive disease. Stenosis of the carotid bifurcation or internal carotid artery usually does not affect carotid pulse contour or amplitude. Occasionally, a severe stenosis will create a thrill that can be appreciated by palpation.

The carotid pulses are auscultated to elicit evidence of bruits. Bruits are caused by blood flow turbulence as a result of arterial stenosis, extrinsic compression, aneurysmal dilation, or arteriovenous connection. The bell of the stethoscope is recommended to appreciate the low frequency bruits and to eliminate any adventitious sounds heard through the diaphragm. The entire cervical portion of each carotid artery should be auscultated, including the segment near the angle of the jaw where the carotid bifurcation is often located (Fig. 9-11). Auscultation of the subclavian arteries for bruits is performed in the supraclavicular fossa and between the lateral aspect of the clavicle and pectoralis muscle. Although the proximal location of a bruit defines the area of turbulent flow, a bruit may be appreciated for an additional several centimeters. The sensitivity and specificity of a carotid bruit for the presence of stenosis ranges from 50% to 79% and 61% to 91%.[24] The pitch of bruits increases with worsening severity.

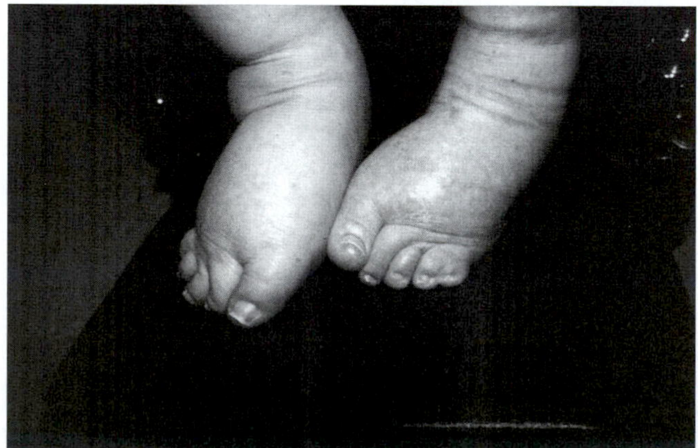

FIGURE 9-10. Lymphedema. Extension of the edema into the foot to the level of the toe is a useful physical sign to differentiate between venous edema and lymphedema. The swelling of the foot ending abruptly at the toes is called the "squared toe" sign.

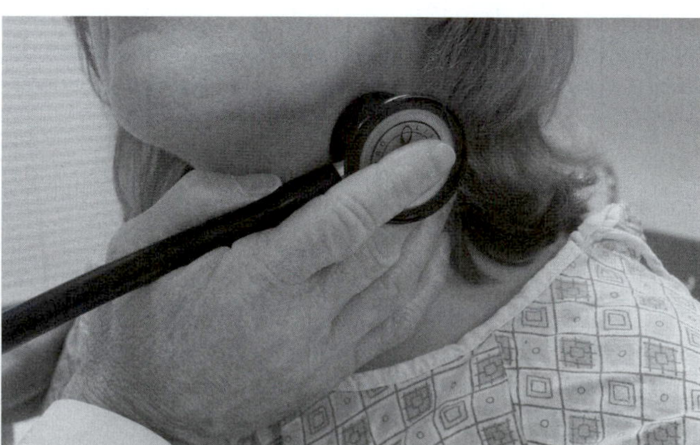

FIGURE 9-11. Auscultation of the carotid artery. To appreciate low-tone bruits, the examiner should use the bell of the stethoscope and apply mild to moderate pressure. The entire length of the artery should be examined, with particular attention paid to the region just below the jaw—at the approximation of the carotid artery bifurcation.

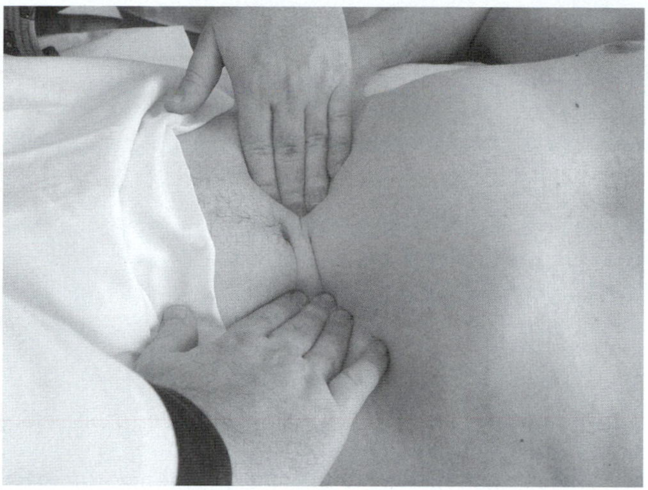

FIGURE 9-12. Abdominal palpation for aneurysm. The examiner, using progressively increasing force, palpates until the aorta can be defined between both sets of fingers. The examiner should appreciate lateral pulsation with every heart beat. Aneurysm sizing is performed by estimating the distance between the closest fingers of each hand.

Continuation of the bruit into diastole is another marker of severity and implies an advanced stenosis. Paradoxically, severe stenosis causing subtotal arterial occlusion may not evoke an audible bruit.

Abdominal Vascular Examination

The vascular examination of the abdomen is performed as the patient lies supine on the examining table with legs outstretched. From this position the abdominal wall should be relaxed and not rigid. Prior to palpation, the abdomen should be inspected. Engorged superficial veins in the abdomen have the possibility of inferior vena cava obstruction. After the inspection, all four quadrants are auscultated with the stethoscope. The presence of bruits is indicative of aortic or branch vessel occlusive disease. Bruits may arise as a result of mesenteric, renal, or aortic disease. Following auscultation, the abdomen is palpated for masses and to detect an aortic aneurysm. Deepest palpation can generally be obtained by gradually increasing pressure in the midline using both hands (Fig. 9-12). In asthenic patients, the aorta can be palpated. In subjects with a waist size greater than 40 inches, the likelihood of palpating an aneurysm is quite limited.

The presence of an aneurysm can be determined when there is a distinct and expansive pulsatile configuration to the aorta. An aneurysm should be sized by determining the lateral borders with both hands, and the space estimated with a measuring tape. Tenderness during the abdominal vascular examination is unusual and may suggest aneurysmal expansion, an inflammatory aneurysm, or a contained rupture. Non-aortic pathologies, including appendicitis, cholecystitis, diverticulitis, and peritonitis, are more common causes of tenderness.

REFERENCES

1. Criqui MH, Langer RD, Fronek A, et al: Mortality over a period of 10 years in patients with peripheral arterial disease. N Engl J Med 326:381, 1992.
2. McDermott MM, Greenland P, Liu K, et al: Leg symptoms in peripheral arterial disease: Associated clinical characteristics and functional impairment. JAMA 286:1599, 2001.
3. McDermott MM, Liu K, Greenland P, et al: Functional decline in peripheral arterial disease: Associations with the ankle brachial index and leg symptoms. JAMA 292:453, 2004.
4. Rose G: The diagnosis of ischemic heart pain and intermittent claudication in field surveys. Bull World Health Organ 27:645, 1962.
5. Coyne KS, Margolis MK, Gilchrist KA, et al: Evaluating effects of method of administration on Walking Impairment Questionnaire. J Vasc Surg 38:296, 2003.
6. Criqui MH, Denenberg JO, Bird CE, et al: The correlation between symptoms and non-invasive test results in patients referred for peripheral arterial disease testing. Vasc Med 1:65, 1996.
7. Regensteiner JG, Gardner A, Hiatt WR: Exercise testing and exercise rehabilitation for patients with peripheral arterial disease: Status in 1997. Vasc Med 2:147, 1997.
8. Rajagopalan S, Grossman PM: Management of chronic critical limb ischemia. Cardiol Clin 20:535, 2002.
9. Strandness DE, Jr: Acute arterial occlusion. Heart Dis Stroke 2:322, 1993.
10. Fukumoto Y, Tsutsui H, Tsuchihashi M, et al: The incidence and risk factors of cholesterol embolization syndrome, a complication of cardiac catheterization: A prospective study. J Am Coll Cardiol 42:211, 2003.
11. Olin JW. Thromboangiitis obliterans (Buerger's disease). N Engl J Med 343:864, 2000.
12. Mackinnon SE, Novak CB: Thoracic outlet syndrome. Curr Prob Surg 39:1070, 2002.
13. Lambert AW, Wilkins DC: Popliteal artery entrapment syndrome. Br J Surg 86:1365, 1999.
14. Wigley FM: Clinical practice: Raynaud's phenomenon. N Engl J Med 347:1001, 2002.
15. Prandoni P, Lensing AW, Cogo A, et al: The long-term clinical course of acute deep venous thrombosis. Ann Intern Med 125:1, 1996.
16. Heldal M, Seem E, Sandset PM, et al: Deep vein thrombosis: A 7-year follow-up study. J Intern Med 234:71, 1993.
17. Gillard J, Perez-Cousin M, Hachulla E, et al: Diagnosing thoracic outlet syndrome: Contribution of provocative tests, ultrasonography, electrophysiology, and helical computed tomography in 48 patients. Joint Bone Spine 68:416, 2001.
18. Warrens AN, Heaton JM: Thoracic outlet compression syndrome: The lack of reliability of its clinical assessment. Ann R Coll Surg Engl 69:203, 1987.
19. Homans J: Venous thrombosis in the lower limbs: Its relation to pulmonary embolism. Am J Surg 38:316, 1937.
20. Beebe HG, Bergan JJ, Bergqvist D, et al: Classification and grading of chronic venous disease in the lower limbs: A consensus statement. Int Angiol 14:197, 1995.
21. Phillips T, Stanton B, Provan A, et al: A study of the impact of leg ulcers on quality of life: Financial, social, and psychologic implications. J Am Acad Dermatol 31:49, 1994.
22. de Araujo T, Valencia I, Federman DG, et al: Managing the patient with venous ulcers. Ann Intern Med 138:326, 2003.
23. Nemeth KA, Harrison MB, Graham ID, et al: Pain in pure and mixed aetiology venous leg ulcers: A three-phase point prevalence study. J Wound Care 12:336, 2003.
24. Magyar MT, Nam EM, Csiba L, et al: Carotid artery auscultation—anachronism or useful screening procedure? Neurol Res 24:705, 2002.

chapter 10

Vascular Laboratory Testing

Marie Gerhard-Herman
Joshua A. Beckman
Mark A. Creager

Vascular laboratory technology offers many cost-effective applications in the practice of vascular medicine.[1] Vascular testing includes both physiologic testing and duplex ultrasonography. Physiologic testing includes segmental pressure measurements, pulse volume recordings, continuous wave Doppler, and plethysmography. These tests employ sphygmomanometric cuffs, Doppler instruments, and plethysmographic recording devices. Duplex ultrasonography combines gray scale and Doppler imaging with spectral and color Doppler, and is used for the majority of vascular laboratory tests. An ultrasound machine should be equipped with vascular software and two transducers/probes, 5- to 12-MHz transducers for the neck and extremities and 2.25- to 3.5-MHz transducers for the abdomen.

LIMB PRESSURE MEASUREMENT AND PULSE VOLUME RECORDINGS

Limb segmental systolic blood pressure measurements and pulse volume recordings are used to confirm a clinical diagnosis of peripheral arterial disease (PAD) and further define the level and extent of the obstruction. Segmental pressures are typically measured in conjunction with segmental limb plethysmography (pulse volume recordings). These techniques are used predominantly in the lower extremities, but are also applicable to the arms. Both procedures are performed using sphygmomanometric cuffs that are appropriately sized to the diameter of the limb segment under study. The patient rests in the supine position for at least 10 minutes prior to measuring limb pressures. Commercially available machines with automatic cuff inflation are able to digitally store the pressures and waveforms. A continuous-wave (CW) Doppler instrument with a 4- to 8-MHz transducer frequency is used to detect the arterial flow signal. The cuff is quickly inflated to a suprasystolic pressure, and then slowly deflated until a flow signal occurs. The cuff pressure at which the flow signal is detected is the systolic pressure in the arterial segment beneath the cuff. For example, if the cuff is on the high thigh and the sensor is over the posterior tibial artery at the ankle, the measured pressure is reflective of the proximal superficial and deep femoral arteries beneath the cuff, as well as any collateral arteries, and not the posterior tibial artery. The Doppler flow signal from a vessel at the ankle is typically used for all limb measurements. It is more accurate, although less convenient, to place the Doppler transducer probe close to the cuff being inflated.

Sphygmomanometric cuffs are positioned on each arm above the antecubital fossa, on the upper portion of each thigh (high thigh), on the lower portions of the thighs above the patella (low thigh), on the calves below the tibial tubercle, and on the ankles above the malleoli. Typically, foot pressures are measured by insonating the posterior tibial and anterior tibial arteries at the ankle level. Both arm pressures at the brachial artery are determined. A difference of greater than 20 mm Hg between the arm pressures indicates the presence of stenosis on the side of the lower pressure. Pressure measurements are made at the high thigh, low thigh, calf and ankle levels with a tibial signal selected as the flow indicator. The lower extremity pressure evaluation should begin at the ankle level and proceed proximally. Patients who are found to have a normal pressure measurement at rest may require a treadmill exercise test to detect PAD. If disease distal to the ankle is suspected, pedal or digital artery obstruction can be evaluated with cuffs sized appropriately for the toes.

Segmental Doppler Pressure Interpretation

Segmental limb pressures are compared with the highest arm pressure. The ankle pressures are used to calculate the ankle-brachial indices (ABI) for each extremity. This is accomplished by dividing each of the ankle pressures by the higher of the brachial artery pressures.[2] A normal ABI is between 1.0 and 1.3. Studies that evaluated the ABI in healthy subjects and patients with PAD confirmed by arteriography found that an ABI of less than or equal to 0.97 was diagnostic of PAD with 99% specificity and 94% sensitivity.[3,4] In the general population, an ABI cutoff of 0.97 might be less specific for severe disease, prompting many laboratories to use an ABI of less than or equal to 0.90 as a discriminant value to diagnose PAD. Pressures are compared between levels. A 20 mm Hg or greater reduction in pressures from one level to the next is considered significant and indicates stenosis between those two levels. In healthy subjects, the high thigh pressure determined by cuff typically exceeds the brachial artery pressure by approximately 30 mm Hg. A thigh/brachial index of 1.1 or greater is interpreted as normal, and an index of less than 0.9 indicates stenosis proximal to the thigh (Fig. 10-1). When the high thigh pressures are low compared with the arm pressure, the site of obstruction

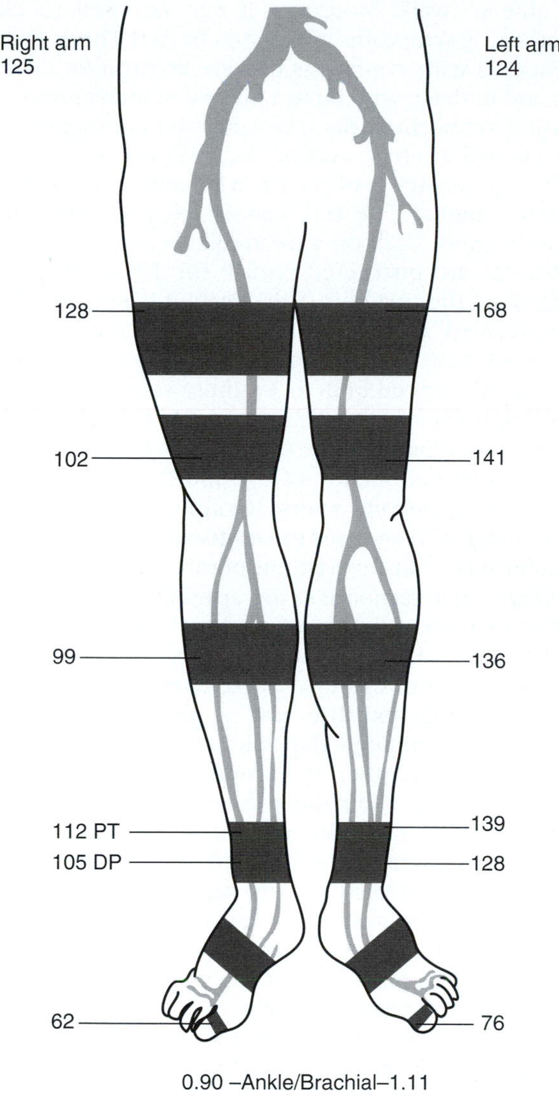

FIGURE 10-1. Segmental pressure measurements. The right high thigh pressure is less than the brachial pressure, suggesting possible right iliofemoral artery stenosis. An additional pressure gradient is noted in the right thigh. The ankle brachial index is abnormal at the right leg. In the left leg, the ankle brachial index is normal; therefore, there is no evidence of arterial disease in the left leg at rest.

could be in the aorta or in the ipsilateral iliac artery, common femoral artery, or proximal superficial femoral artery (see Fig. 10-1). If only one high thigh pressure is less than the brachial pressure, then an ipsilateral iliofemoral artery stenosis is inferred.

In the presence of severe vascular calcification, systolic pressures cannot be determined because the vessels are noncompressible. An index of 1.3 or greater suggests vascular calcification artifact and makes interpretation of the pressure measurement unreliable. The presence or absence of a significant pressure gradient cannot be determined in the presence of vascular calcification artifact. In this setting the toe brachial index (TBI) is a useful measurement. The TBI is the ratio of the systolic pressure in the toe to the brachial artery systolic pressure. To perform the procedure, a cuff is placed on a toe. Typically, the great toe is used. The pulse waveform is obtained by photoplethysmography. The cuff is inflated to suprasystolic pressure and then deflated. Systolic pressure is determined as the pressure at which the waveform reappears. A normal value for TBI is 0.60 ± 0.17.

Pulse Volume Recording Interpretation

The same cuffs used to measure segmental pressures may be attached to a plethysmographic instrument and used to record the change in volume of a limb segment with each pulse, and the pulse volume. The pulse volume waveform evaluation allows assessment of arterial flow in regions of calcified vessels because the test does not rely on cuff occlusion of the calcified artery. Each cuff is inflated in sequence to a predetermined reference pressure, up to 65 mm Hg. The change in volume in the limb segment causes a corresponding change in pressure in the cuff throughout the cardiac cycle. Interpretation of the pulse volume recording (PVR) requires calibration of the amount of air in the cuff.

A pulse volume waveform is recorded for each limb segment. PVR analysis is based on evaluation of waveform shape, signal, and amplitude (Fig. 10-2). The configuration of the normal pulse volume waveform resembles the arterial pressure waveform, and is composed of a sharp systolic upstroke followed by a downstroke that contains a prominent dicrotic notch. A hemodynamically significant stenosis manifests as a change in the PVR contour toward a tardus parvus waveform. The slope and amplitude are less when there is more severe disease. Severity of PAD can be defined by the slope of the upstroke and the amplitude of the pulse volume (see Fig. 10-2).

Pulse waveforms can also be obtained using photoplethysmography, recording reflected infrared light. In photoplethysmography, the signal is proportional to the quantity of red blood cells in the cutaneous circulation; it does not measure volume changes. Waveform shape is assessed in a similar fashion in pulse volume and photoplethysmography recordings.

TRANSCUTANEOUS OXIMETRY

By exploiting the variations in color absorbance of oxygenated and deoxygenated hemoglobin, transcutaneous oximetry can determine the state of blood oxygenation. Oximeters use two light frequencies, red at 600 to 750 nm and infrared at 800 to 1050 nm, to differentiate oxygenated and deoxygenated hemoglobin. Deoxygenated blood absorbs more red light, whereas oxygenated blood absorbs more infrared light. Oximeters typically employ both an emitter and receiver. Red and infrared light is emitted and passes through a relatively translucent structure, such as the finger or earlobe. A photodetector determines the ratio of red and infrared light received to derive blood oxygenation. When measured continuously, oxygenation peaks with each heartbeat as fresh, oxygenated blood arrives in the zone of measurement. The normal values for oxygen tension are from 50 to 75 mm Hg. One probe is placed on the chest as a control to ensure that the oxygen tension is from 50 to 75 mm Hg.

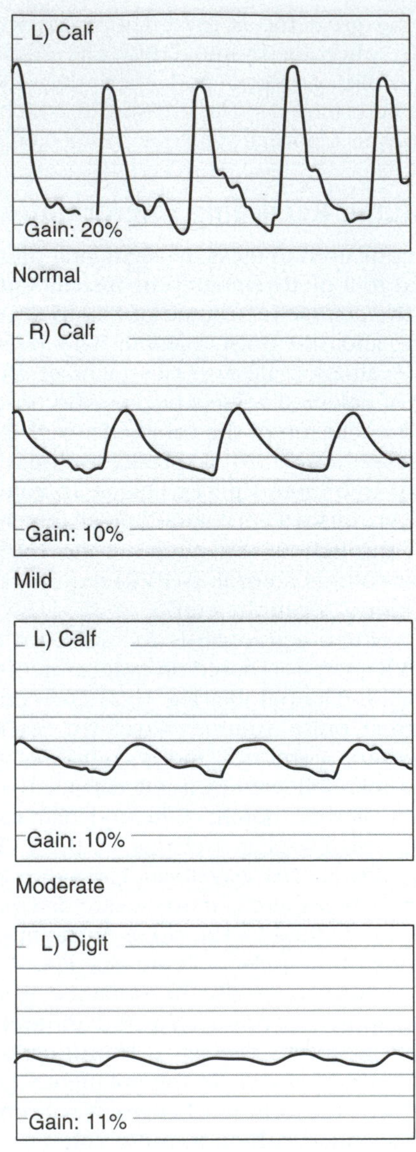

FIGURE 10-2. Pulse volume recording. The normal waveform has a sharp upstroke, dicrotic notch, and a period of diastasis. The mildly abnormal waveform has a delay in the upstroke and no dicrotic notch. The moderately abnormal waveform has a delay in upstroke, flat systolic peak, and diminished amplitude. The severely abnormal waveform has a flat systolic peak and very diminished amplitude.

A second probe is placed on the limb in the area of interest. Measurements are obtained from the probe, which is sequentially positioned from proximal to distal segments of the limb. The normal limb TcO_2 should approximate that of the chest. Transcutaneous oximetry is most often used to determine the level of amputation. A value of >20 mm Hg can predict healing at the site with 80% accuracy.[5] This measurement is not affected by arterial calcification.

Exercise Testing for Peripheral Artery Disease

Exercise testing is an adjunctive physiologic test to evaluate PAD. It is useful to assess functional capacity and determine the distance patients with claudication are able to walk. Moreover, it can be used to clarify whether leg symptoms are related to PAD. This is relevant in patients with symptoms that are atypical for claudication and in those who have a history of intermittent claudication, yet normal ABIs at rest. Relative contraindications to treadmill exercise testing for PAD include: rest pain in the leg, shortness of breath with minimal exertion, or unstable angina. The test cannot be performed if the patient cannot walk on a treadmill.

Patients are instructed to fast for 12 hours prior to walking on the treadmill. The constant load treadmill test is performed at a speed of 2 miles per hour and an incline of 12%. Graded exercise protocols increase the grade and/or speed in 2- to 3-minute stages. The Gardner protocol is the most commonly used graded protocol to evaluate walking exercise capacity.[6] It begins at a speed of 2 mph and an incline of 0% and the grade increases by 2% progressively every 2 minutes, allowing for a wider range of responses to be measured. It is often used to determine clinical trial endpoints, such as change in walking time in response to therapy. Other graded exercise protocols, such as the Bruce protocol, are not commonly used because the rapid rate of speed and incline limits the assessment of exercise capacity in claudicants.

The treadmill exercise test is terminated when the patient cannot continue due to leg claudication, chest pain, or is limited by other symptoms such as shortness of breath or fatigue. The patient then immediately lies down on the stretcher. The ankle pressures are obtained starting with the symptomatic leg, followed by the highest brachial pressure. The pressures are repeated approximately every 1 to 2 minutes until they return to baseline. Data recorded from the exercise test should include ankle pressures, length of time the patient was able to walk, time required for the pressures to return to baseline, nature and location of the patient's symptoms, and reason for discontinuing test. A decrease in ABI of more than 20% immediately following exercise is diagnostic for PAD. The time before ankle pressure returns to normal is increased in more severe disease (e.g., from 1 minute in mild disease to 10 minutes in more severe disease).

PHYSICAL PRINCIPLES OF ULTRASONOGRAPHY

Ultrasound Image Creation

An ultrasound transducer, or probe, emits sound waves in discrete bundles or pulses into the tissue of interest. On encountering a tissue, a portion of the waves is reflected back to the transducer. The fraction of returning waves depends on the density and size of the tissue examined. The depth of tissue is determined by the time required for pulse emission and return. Thus, by integrating the number of returning pulses and the time required for return, a B-mode, or gray-scale image may be created. The time for wave reflection decreases with higher ultrasound probe frequencies. Transducer probes with higher frequencies image superficial tissues better than probes with lower frequencies, but lose depth imaging because of attenuation of the returning emitted pulses.

Improvements in technology have permitted a widening of the band width of vascular transducers, facilitating the analysis of harmonics of the fundamental frequency. A harmonic represents a whole number multiple of the emitted frequency. Because the tissue compresses and expands in response to the application of ultrasound, the fundamental wave may become distorted, impairing image quality. The distortion, however, also creates harmonics of the original frequency that can be detected by the transducer. By detecting only the fundamental frequency and its harmonics, artifact, such as speckle and reverberation, may be reduced to create a clearer image.

Detection of Blood Flow

Normal blood flow is laminar in a straight segment of an artery. If thought of as a telescopic series of flow rings, blood moves forward most rapidly in the middle ring and velocity decreases in the outer rings as blood comes closer to the vessel wall. The cardiac cycle, defined by its pulsatile nature of flow, causes a continual variation in blood flow velocity, highest with systole and lowest with diastole. The concentric or laminar flow of blood may be disturbed at a normal branching point or with abnormal vessel contours, such as those caused by atherosclerotic plaque. Disturbed, or turbulent flow causes a much greater loss of pressure than does laminar flow.

Determination of flow velocity is a mainstay of vascular ultrasonography. Abnormalities in the vessel wall cause changes in flow velocity and permit the detection and assessment of stenotic regions within the vessel. Flow in a normal vessel is proportional to the difference of pressure between the proximal and distal end of the vessel. The prime determinant or limitation of flow is the radius of the vessel because volume of blood flow is determined by the fourth power of the radius. For example, a 50% reduction in vessel radius causes a greater than 90% reduction in blood flow. Thus, blood flow represents an example of Poiseuille's law, which determines flow of a viscous fluid through a tube. Specifically,

$$Q = \frac{\pi \times \Delta P \times r^4}{8\eta L}$$

where Q = the volume of flow, ΔP = pressure at inflow point − pressure at outflow, r = radius, η = viscosity, and L = tube length. Because blood viscosity, blood vessel length, and pressure remain relatively stable, the most important determinant of blood flow is vessel lumen size.

Vascular ultrasonography can depict flow velocity by taking advantage of Doppler shift frequencies. The frequency will shift, either positively or negatively, depending on the direction of blood flow. The variables, which determine the size of the shift, include the speed of sound, the speed of the moving object, and the angle between the transmitted beam and the moving object. Christoph Doppler described this relationship using the following equation:

$$F_d = (2\ F_t \bullet V \bullet \cos\theta) \div c$$

where F_d is the Doppler frequency shift; F_t is the Doppler frequency transmitted from the probe; V is the velocity of flow; cos is the cosine, θ is the angle between the beam and direction of the moving object, and c is the velocity of sound.

Artifact

Although a highly reliable imaging modality, ultrasound does suffer from occasional image artifact. Dense objects, such as vessel wall calcium deposits permit few sound waves to penetrate, diminishing imaging of deeper tissues. Tissue imaging enhancement may be noted when below echo-free or liquid-filled zones. Tissue interfaces may generate multiple sound-wave reflections causing "additions" to the tissue. Refraction of the sound pulse may cause improper placement of a structure of an image and shadowing at the edge of a large structure. Highly reflective surfaces may create mirror images because the reflecting tissue alters the timing of the returning sound wave. The mirror image should be equidistant from the reflecting surface or tissue.

Gray Scale (B Mode) Imaging

Ultrasound images are generated using a pulse echo system. The position of the tissue interface is determined by the time between pulse generation and returning echo. Each returning echo is displayed as a gray dot on a video screen using a brightness mode (B mode), in which the brightness of the dot depends on the strength of the reflected wave. A 2-D image is created by sequentially transmitting waves in multiple directions within a single plane and combining the reflected echoes into a single display. The image can be refreshed rapidly, permitting real-time display of the gray-scale image. The surface of interest should be perpendicular to the ultrasound beam to obtain the brightest echo with B-mode imaging. This is readily achieved in vascular imaging because the neck, extremity, and visceral vessels generally lie parallel to the surface of the transducer. Higher frequency probes are used to image vessels close to the surface and lower frequency probes are used to image deeper vessels. Details of the vessel wall can be seen more clearly with the use of harmonics. The wide band width of transducers allows analysis of returning harmonics (whole number multiples) of the fundamental frequency.

Spectral Doppler Waveform Analysis

Velocity recordings are obtained with an angle of 60 degrees between the Doppler insonation beam and the flow. In ultrasound practice, the optimal angle of measurement between the beam and blood flow is 60 degrees. Although maximal shift is detected at 0 degrees, this angle cannot be reliably obtained in vascular imaging because the vessels are parallel to the surface of the body. Insonation angles below and above 60 degrees influence the measurement, such that small reductions in the insonation angle may alter velocity by 10%, whereas small increases in insonation angle may change flow velocity by 25% (Fig. 10-3). Thus, the sample volume cursor is placed parallel to the inner wall, and a Doppler[7,8] angle from 30 to 60 degrees between the wall and the insonation

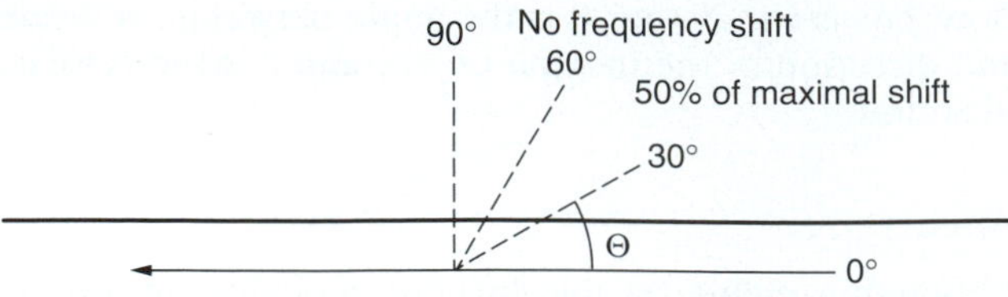

FIGURE 10-3. The Doppler angle is the angle between the insonation beam and the sample cursor aligned with flow. The *dashed lines* represent different insonation beams. The *solid arrow* represents the direction of flow and the position of the Doppler sample cursor. The velocity is determined using the Doppler equation, with the cosine (cos) in the denominator. The cos 0 degrees = 1, cos 30 degrees = 0.86, cos 60 degrees = 0.5, and cos 90 degrees = 0. c, velocity of sound; Fd, Doppler frequency shift; Ft, transmitted Doppler frequency; V, velocity.

beam (or flow jet) is used. A normal peripheral artery Doppler waveform consists of a narrow, sharply defined tracing. This indicates that all blood cells are moving at an equivalent speed at any time in the cardiac cycle.[9] Waveforms are also characterized as high resistance due to limited flow during diastole (e.g., normal peripheral arterial Doppler velocity waveform), or low resistance with continuous flow during diastole as when downstream resistance arterioles are widely dilated or there is contiguity with low-resistance circuits (e.g., normal internal carotid artery velocity waveform) (Fig. 10-4).[10] The normal high resistance waveform is typically triphasic. The first component is caused by initial high-velocity forward flow during ventricular systole. A range of normal peak systolic velocity (PSV) measurements have been defined[11] for each arterial segment as described later in this chapter.

The second phase of the waveform consists of early diastolic flow reversal, as the left ventricular pressure falls below the aortic pressure prior to aortic valve closure. The final or third component is a small amount of forward flow when there is elastic recoil of vessel walls. Flow is typically not uniform or laminar at bifurcations and sites of stenosis; at these sites flow becomes turbulent. For these locations, the spectral Doppler waveform reflects the fact that blood cells move with varying velocities. Instead of a narrow, well-defined tracing (see Fig. 10-4), spectral broadening becomes evident

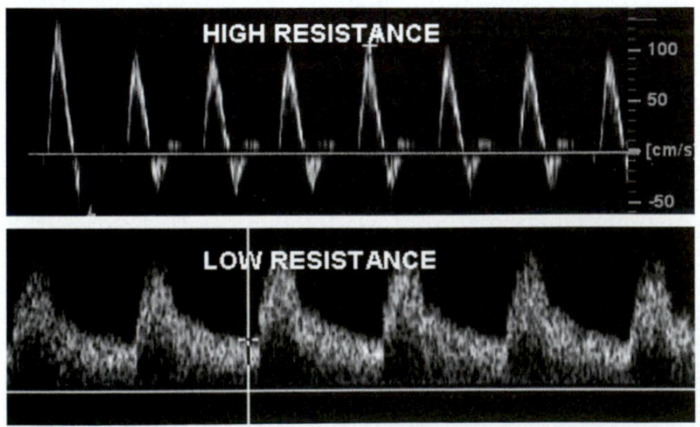

FIGURE 10-4. High and low resistance waveforms. These two waveforms are distinguished by the absence (high resistance) and a presence (low resistance) of flow during diastole.

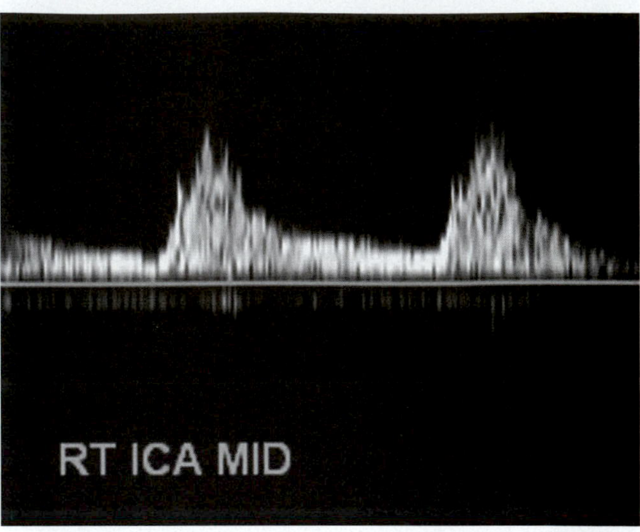

FIGURE 10-5. Post-stenotic waveform. The waveform has a delay in upstroke, diminished amplitude, and marked turbulence.

(Fig. 10-5), with partial or complete filling-in of the area under the spectral waveform. This third, or late, diastolic component is usually absent in atherosclerotic vessels that have lost compliance or elasticity.

Color Doppler

Color Doppler is the phase or frequency shift information that is contained in the returning echoes and processed in real time to form a velocity map over the entire imaging field. Doppler frequency-shift data are available for every point imaged. This information is then superimposed on the gray-scale image to provide a composite real-time display of both anatomy and flow. When motion is detected, it is assigned a color, typically red or blue, determined by whether the frequency shift is toward or away from the probe. Color assignment is arbitrary and can be altered by the user, but most choose to assign the color red to arteries and blue to veins. With increasing Doppler frequency shifts, the hue and intensity of the color display change, with a progressive desaturation of the color and a shift toward white at the highest detectable velocities. The pulse repetition frequency (velocity) scale determines the degree of color saturation and filling of the vessel lumen. The pulse repetition frequency (radio frequency pulses per second from the probe) is adjusted so that in a normal vessel, laminar flow appears as a homogeneous color. The color appearance changes throughout the cardiac cycle. Increasing flow velocity and turbulence in the region of a stenosis results in the production of a high-velocity jet and an abrupt change in the color-flow pattern (Fig. 10-6). Color aliasing occurs at the site of stenosis when the flow velocity exceeds the Nyquist limit (i.e., when the Doppler frequency shift exceeds one half the pulse repetition frequency). Aliasing causes the color display to appear as if there is an abrupt reversal in the direction of the flow (wraparound). This suggests a high velocity flow jet, requiring confirmation by pulsed-wave Doppler analysis. Color persistence is a continuous flow

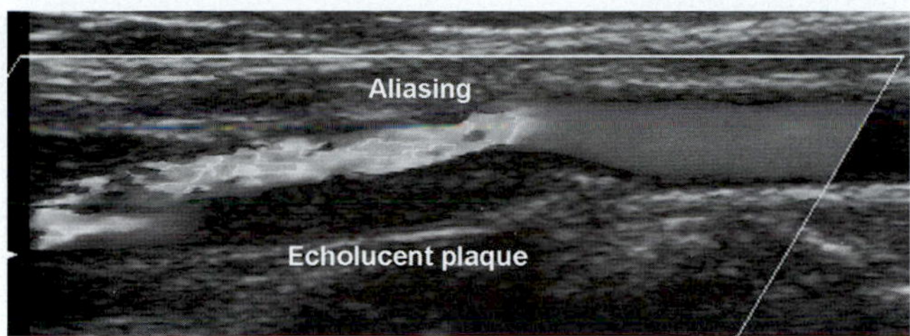

FIGURE 10-6. (See also Color Plate 10-6.) Aliasing at the site of arterial stenosis. There is an abrupt change as the velocity exceeds the Nyquist limits. An echolucent (dark) plaque is evident at the site of stenosis.

signal that is the color of the forward direction only, in contrast to the alternating color in normal arteries.[12] There is loss of early diastolic flow reversal. Color persistence corresponds to the monophasic spectral Doppler waveform and is indicative of severe stenosis. Post-stenotic regions display mosaic patterns indicating turbulent flow (see Fig. 10-6). A color bruit in the surrounding soft tissue also indicates flow disturbance. This color artifact is associated with turbulence and occurs with flow disturbances associated with high-velocity jets. The color bruit is particularly useful in locating postcatheterization arteriovenous fistulae.

Assessment of Arterial Stenosis

Characteristic duplex ultrasound features of a stenosis include elevated systolic velocity, elevated end-diastolic velocity, color aliasing, color bruit, spectral broadening of the Doppler waveform, post-stenotic flow, and post-stenotic turbulence. An auditory "thump" occurs in the presence of total arterial occlusion. Doppler velocity measurements are the main tools used to evaluate stenosis severity. When flow rate is constant, a decrease in vessel cross-sectional area is balanced by an increase in velocity.[13] As blood flow turbulence increases, spectral broadening of the Doppler waveform becomes a clear indicator of turbulent flow seen in the post-stenotic region. The post-stenotic waveform is dampened with a delayed upstroke (see Fig. 10-3).[14] If no post-stenotic turbulence can be identified, inappropriate angle alignment or a tortuous vessel should be suspected. Power (or amplitude) Doppler is a complementary imaging technique that displays the total strength or amplitude of the returning Doppler signal.[15] In comparison with conventional color flow imaging, color-flow sensitivity is increased by a factor of 3 to 5 times with power Doppler. This enhanced dynamic range can depict very slow flow in the area of a subtotal occlusion that may not be detected by conventional color-flow Doppler. Contrast agents can also help to differentiate between occlusion and high-grade stenosis in carotid and renal arteries, and especially in cases where multiple renal arteries are present.[16]

CAROTID DUPLEX ULTRASOUND

The standard carotid duplex examination includes assessment of the carotid arteries, as well as the vertebral, subclavian, and brachiocephalic arteries. Indications for this test include a bruit, transient ischemic attack, amaurosis fugax, stroke, and surveillance after revascularization.[17] The examination begins with a gray-scale survey of the extracranial carotid arteries in transverse and longitudinal views. The operator images the region from the clavicle to the angle of the jaw, in both the anterolateral and posterolateral views.[18] The common carotid artery (CCA) is typically medial to the internal jugular vein, and the bifurcation is often located near the cricoid cartilage. The internal carotid artery (ICA) is usually posterolateral, with an origin diameter greater than that of the anteromedially located external carotid artery (ECA).

Carotid artery stenosis can be focal, and flow patterns can normalize within a short distance. Therefore, the pulse-wave sample volume should be methodically advanced along the length of the vessel; color Doppler may be used for guidance in delineating areas of abnormal flow requiring change in the position of the sample volume (Fig. 10-7). Representative velocity measurements should be recorded from the proximal, mid- and distal CCA. The CCA spectral waveform is a combination of the ECA and ICA waveforms, with greater diastolic flow than the ECA, but less than that of the ICA. Atherosclerosis, when present, is usually most evident at the ICA origin, whereas fibromuscular dysplasia may be more evident distally. Using spectral Doppler, the sample volume is advanced throughout the entire ICA. At a minimum, peak-systolic velocity (PSV) and end-diastolic velocity (EDV) from the proximal-, mid-, and distal-ICA segments should be recorded. The vertebral artery is then located posterior to the carotid artery. The vertebral artery and vein

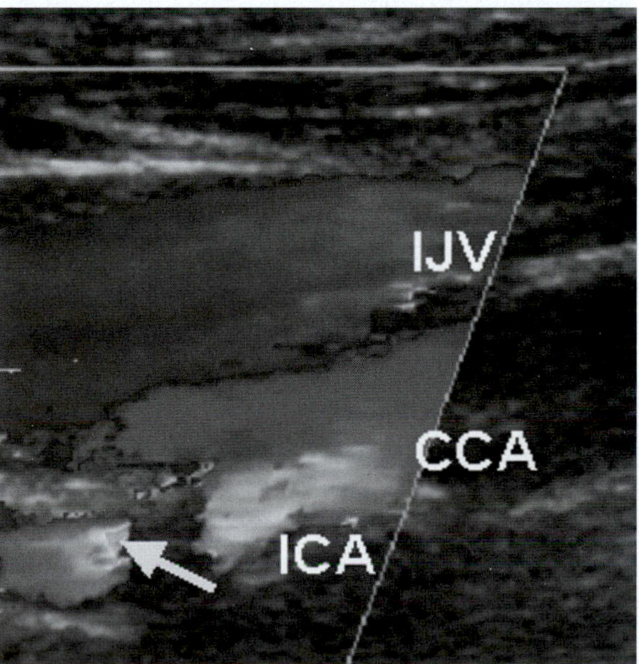

FIGURE 10-7. (See also Color Plate 10-7.) Carotid bifurcation. A calcified lesion obscures the color Doppler signal in the proximal internal carotid artery (ICA). The presence of aliasing distal to the calcification artifact (*arrow*) is helpful in identifying possible stenosis with the pulsed-wave Doppler sample volume. The transducer should be rocked side to-side in this situation in an attempt to see the flow in the region of calcification. CCA, common carotid artery; IJV, internal jugular vein.

lie between the spinous processes. The vertebral artery is followed as far cephalad as possible, sampling the spectral Doppler in the accessible portions of the vertebral artery.

Distinguishing the internal and external carotid artery (ECA) is critical to the examination (Fig. 10-8). The ECA is usually smaller, more anteromedial, and has less diastolic flow than the ICA. The external carotid artery will also have branches in the cervical region, whereas the internal carotid artery will not. A direct comparison of the waveforms from the two vessels is critical. A velocity waveform obtained from the proximal vessel or the site of maximal velocity should be obtained while intermittently tapping on the preauricular branch of the temporal artery. The intermittent tapping is reflected clearly in the diastolic portion of the ECA waveform, but not in the ICA waveform (Fig. 10-9).

The interpretation of the spectral waveforms is based on parameters such as peak systolic velocity, end-diastolic velocity, shape, and the extent of spectral broadening (Fig. 10-10).[19] There are a number of criteria that have been proposed, each having their own strengths and weaknesses (Table 10-1).[19] Peak systolic velocity criteria for ICA stenosis have identified a cut point of 230 cm/sec as the threshold for detecting greater than 70% stenosis, and 125 cm/sec as the cut point for identifying greater than 50% stenosis. Criteria that include end-diastolic velocity use a cut point of greater than 140 cm/sec to identify greater than 80% stenosis. The ratio of the peak ICA systolic velocity to the mid-CCA velocity may be particularly useful in determining the presence or stenosis in the hemodynamic setting of low cardiac output or critical aortic stenosis. At a minimum, the velocity criteria must distinguish less than 50% stenosis, 50% to 69% stenosis, and greater than 70% stenosis. Selection of criteria for use in an individual laboratory requires review of the published parameters and selection

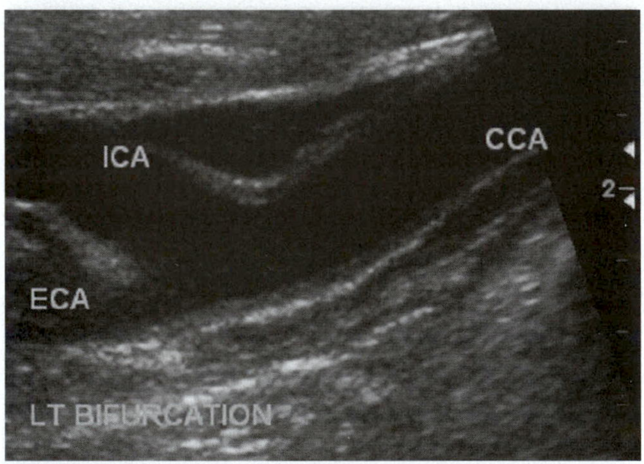

A

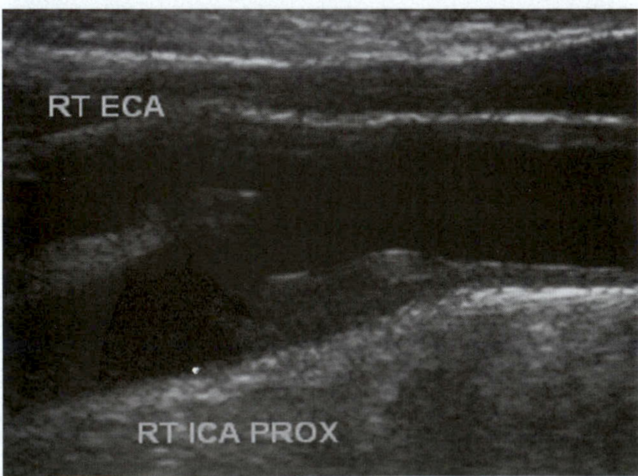

B

FIGURE 10-8. Carotid bifurcation. In both **A** and **B**, the ICA diameter is greater than that of the ECA. The position alone is not adequate to distinguish ECA from ICA. ECA, external carotid artery; ICA, internal carotid artery.

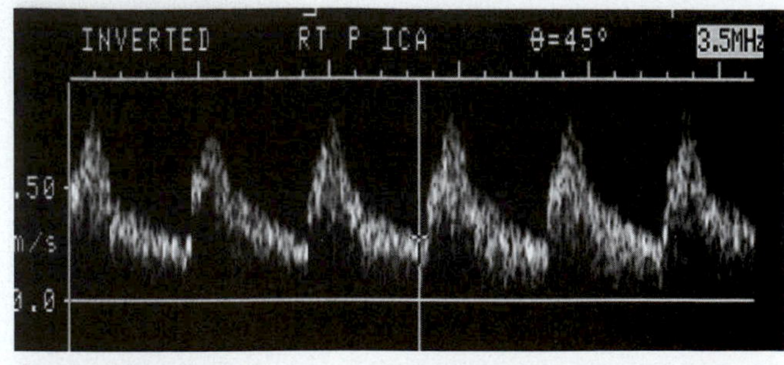

A

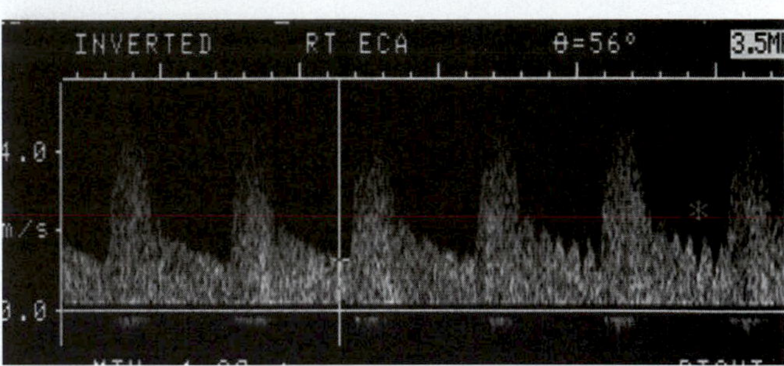

B

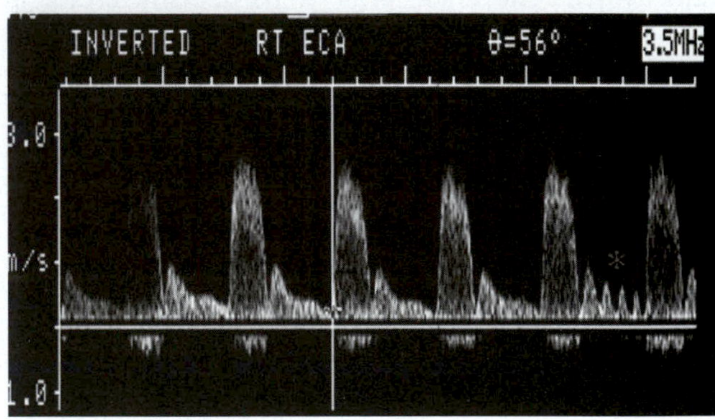

C

FIGURE 10-9. Spectral waveforms of the internal and external carotid arteries during intermittent tapping of the ipsilateral temporal artery. **A,** has no clear "tapping" pattern and is therefore likely ICA. **B,** has high-peak-systolic velocity (PSV) of 400 cm/sec. Tapping (*asterisk*) clearly identified in the diastolic component of the waveform identifies the artery as the ECA and indicates that the high PSV represents ECA stenosis. **C,** The typical ECA waveform is high resistance with low-peak systolic velocity and obvious tapping pattern of the temporal artery during diastole. ECA, external carotid artery; ICA, internal carotid artery.

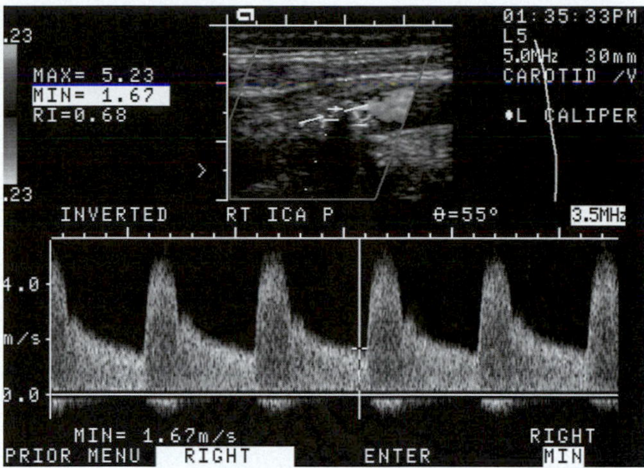

FIGURE 10-10. (See also Color Plate 10-10.) Internal carotid artery stenosis. The pulsed-wave sample volume is placed at the site of aliasing. The peak-systolic velocity is elevated to 523 cm/sec. The end-diastolic velocity is elevated to 167 cm/sec. There is marked spectral broadening. The waveform resembles that in Fig. 10-9C, except that the "temporal tap" is not reflected in the diastolic portion of the waveform.

of those that are appropriate to the laboratory practice. Individual vascular laboratories must validate the results of their own criteria for stenosis against a suitable standard, such as arteriography.

Waveform analysis depends on evaluation of acceleration, diastolic flow, direction of flow, and comparison to the contralateral vessel. If the internal carotid artery is totally occluded, there will be absent or severely diminished diastolic flow in the ipsilateral CCA (Fig. 10-11). A delay in the upstroke suggests more proximal stenosis. For example, severe stenosis of the brachiocephalic artery will result in dampened right CCA waveforms. A step-up in systolic velocity in the cervical portion of the CCA indicates stenosis, with doubling indicating at least 50% stenosis and tripling indicating at least 75% stenosis.

TABLE 10-1 CRITERIA FOR INTERNAL CAROTID ARTERY STENOSIS

Diameter Reduction	PSV	ICA PSV/CCA PSV	EDV
0	<100	no spectral broadening	<40
1-29	<100	<2	<40
30-49	101-124	<2	<40
50-59	>125	>2 and <3.2	<40
60-69	>230	3.2-4.0	40-110
70-79	>230	>4.0	110-140
80-95	>230	>4.0	>140
96-99			string flow
100			no flow

This table summarizes multiple criteria—including peak-systolic velocity alone, peak-systolic and end-diastolic velocities, and ICA/CCA ratio. CCA, common carotid artery; EDV, end-diastolic volume; ICA, internal carotid artery; PSV, peak-systolic velocity.

From Grant EG, Benson CB, Moneta GL, et al: Carotid artery stenosis: Gray-scale and Doppler US diagnosis—Society of Radiologists in Ultrasound Consensus Conference. Radiology 229:340, 2003.

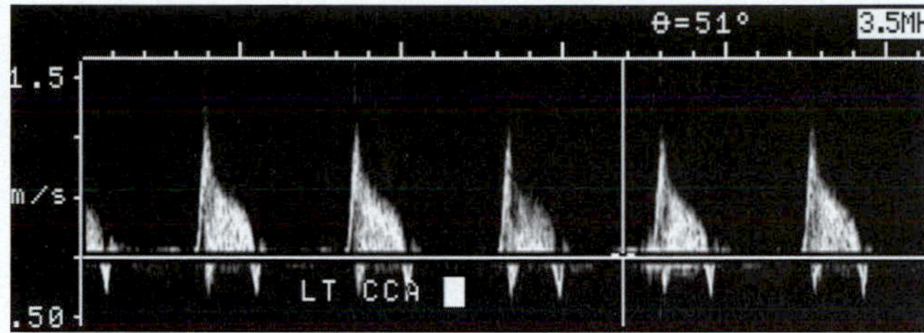

FIGURE 10-11. Absent diastolic flow in the CCA suggesting the presence of total occlusion of the ipsilateral ICA. CCA, common carotid artery; ICA, internal carotid artery.

Waveform evaluation is particularly valuable in the vertebral artery because the segments within the bone cannot be directly evaluated with ultrasound. Specific velocity criteria have not been developed for vertebral artery stenosis. Velocities greater than 125 cm/sec and dampened waveforms are two indicators of vertebral artery stenosis. Absent flow in the vertebral artery is confirmed when flow is detected in the vertebral vein, but not in the vertebral artery. Retrograde flow in the vertebral artery is referred to as subclavian steal (i.e., the subclavian circulation is stealing from the cerebral circulation). Reverse flow is confirmed by comparing the direction of vertebral artery flow with that of the carotid artery (Fig.10-12). Reverse flow typically will have a diminished diastolic component because flow is into the high resistance bed of the subclavian artery (Fig. 10-13). If flow is cephalad, but the diastolic component is markedly diminished or reversed, subclavian steal can be elicited by reexamining flow after arm exercise or following deflation of a blood pressure cuff that had been inflated to suprasystolic pressures on the ipsilateral arm. These maneuvers will increase demand in the subclavian bed, and vertebral flow will completely reverse in the setting of subclavian stenosis proximal to the vertebral origin. The vast majority of these patients with subclavian stenosis are asymptomatic.

The subclavian artery is evaluated as close to the origin as possible. The probe is placed longitudinally above

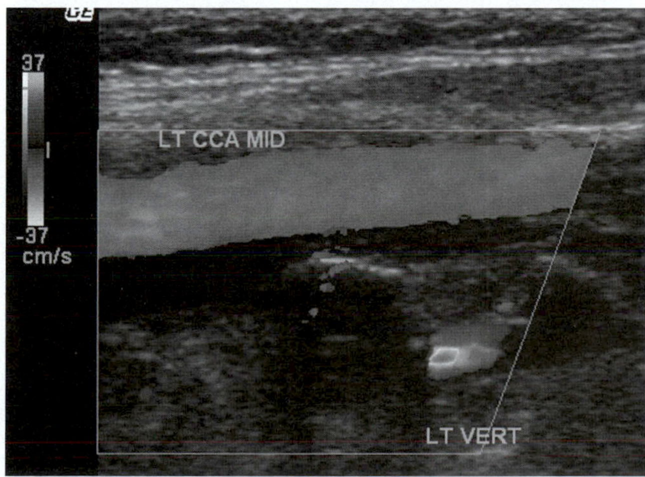

FIGURE 10-12. (See also Color Plate 10-12.) Color Doppler of the CCA and vertebral arteries demonstrating antegrade carotid flow and retrograde vertebral flow. CCA, common carotid artery.

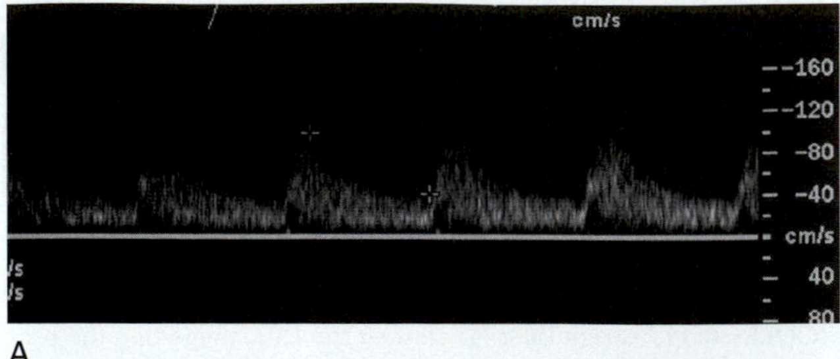

A

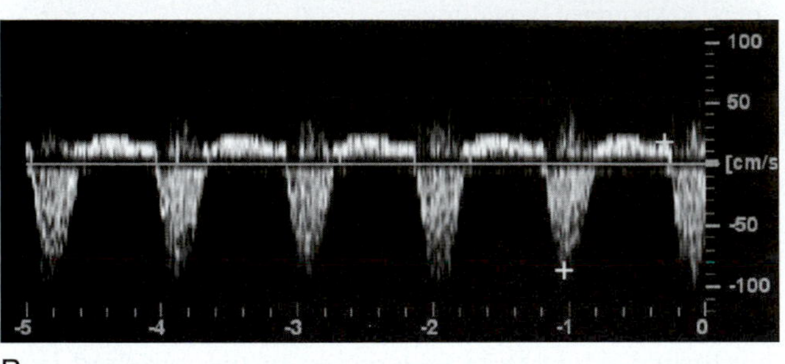

B

FIGURE 10-13. Spectral waveform of normal, antegrade vertebral flow (**A**) with low resistance waveform and (**B**) reversed, retrograde vertebral flow with high resistance waveform.

the clavicle and angled to obtain a scanning plane below the clavicle. Color Doppler surveillance is used to detect nonlaminar flow. The Doppler spectrum is obtained throughout the vessel. A doubling of the peak systolic velocity is consistent with ≥50% stenosis.

Plaque and Arterial Wall Characterization

Gray-scale imaging is used to evaluate carotid plaque and arterial wall characteristics. Atherosclerotic plaque is evident on ultrasound examination as material that thickens the intima and protrudes into the arterial lumen. Plaque surface and echo characteristics can be determined and described. Ulceration refers to an excavation within the plaque containing flow. Echolucent plaque is characterized as plaque that is less echogenic than the surrounding muscle, and is often first detected by the presence of abnormal color flow (Fig. 10-14). The volume of plaque is appreciated best in the transverse view (Fig. 10-15) and with 3-D reconstruction.

Another potential technique to characterize plaque content and activity is contrast-enhanced ultrasound to detect ulceration and inflammation (Fig. 10-16A). Activated leukocytes attached to the inflamed vessel wall may bind the shells of lipid microbubbles, which are detectable by ultrasound. Contrast also can be used to define the plaque-lumen interface in the presence of echolucent plaque. The plaque thickness can be severely overestimated or underestimated in the longitudinal image, and is best evaluated in transverse images. Ultrasound can also evaluate findings such as wall edema or dissection in the carotid wall (see Fig. 10-16B). Dissection can originate in the ICA or extend from the arch into the CCA. A flap separates the true and false lumen. The flap may be apparent on gray-scale imaging, but generally requires color or contrast for elucidation.

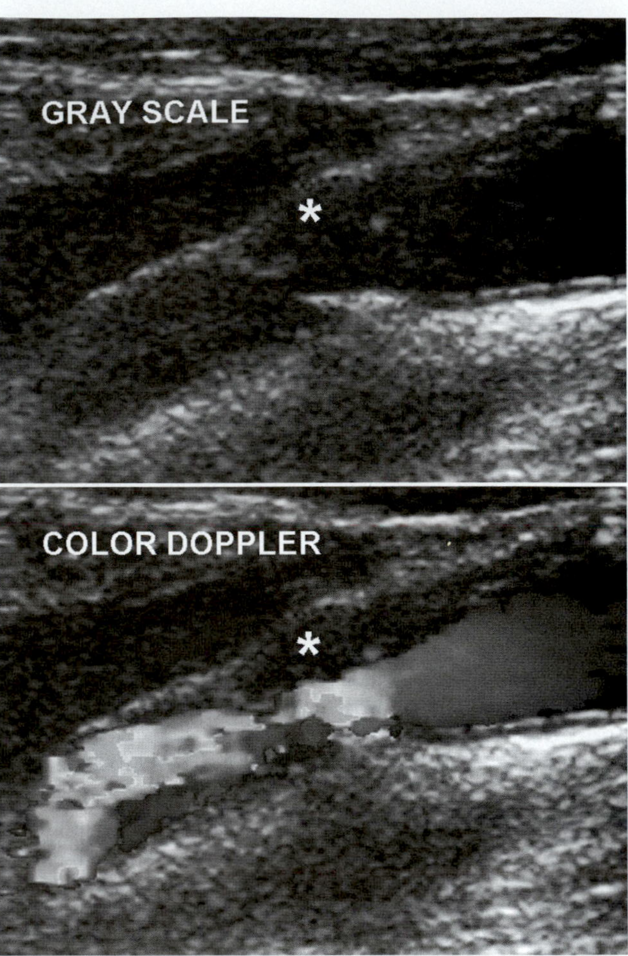

FIGURE 10-14. (See also Color Plate 10-14.) Echolucent plaque is indicated (*asterisk*) in the gray-scale and Doppler image of this internal carotid artery.

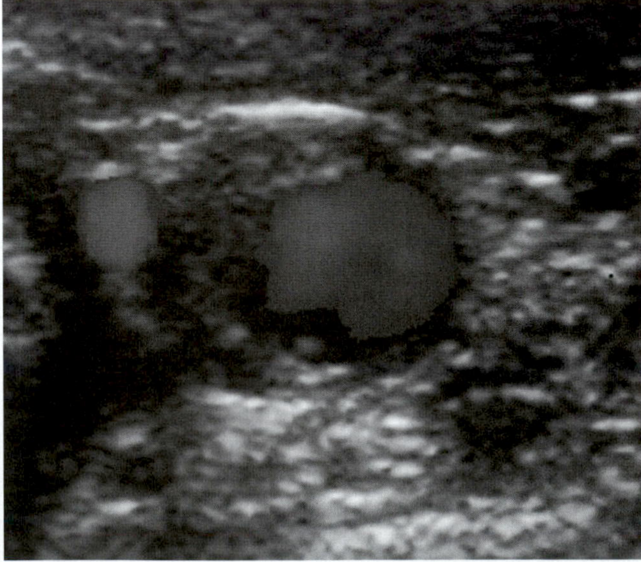

FIGURE 10-15. (See also Color Plate 10-15.) Transverse view of the internal carotid artery origin with atherosclerotic plaque of mixed echogenicity evident in the left half of the vessel.

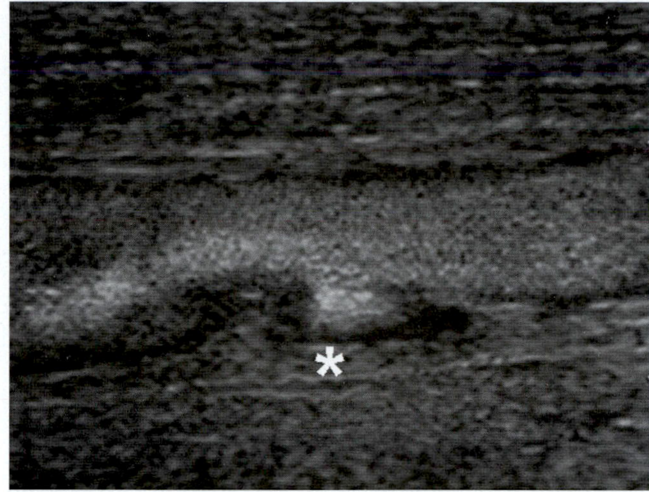

A

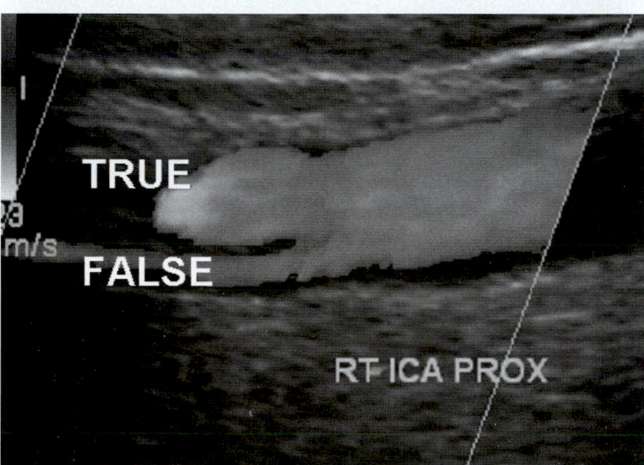

B

FIGURE 10-16. (See also Color Plate 10-16.) Arterial wall characteristics. **A,** Ulceration of atherosclerotic plaque in the common carotid artery. Contrast is evident within an echolucent plaque (*asterisk*). **B,** Dissection of the internal carotid artery (ICA) with flow evident in both the true and false lumina.

A flutter is occasionally identified in the down-slope of the waveform on the affected side. Evaluation should identify the proximal and distal extents of dissection, and the flow velocities in the true lumen.

Carotid Intimal Medial Thickness

Carotid ultrasonography has traditionally been used to evaluate the presence of obstructive atherosclerosis in the setting of symptomatic cerebrovascular disease or asymptomatic carotid bruit. More recently, carotid ultrasonography has been performed in epidemiologic studies to detect nonobstructive plaque and intimal-medial thickness (IMT).[20] IMT refers to the distance from the intima lumen interface to the media adventitia border (Fig. 10-17). Protocols have measured ICA, CCA, ICA plus CCA and carotid bulb IMT. The measurement yield and reproducibility appear to be greatest for the far wall CCA IMT measurement. The measurement is most commonly made from longitudinal images with the assistance of semi-automated edge detection software. There

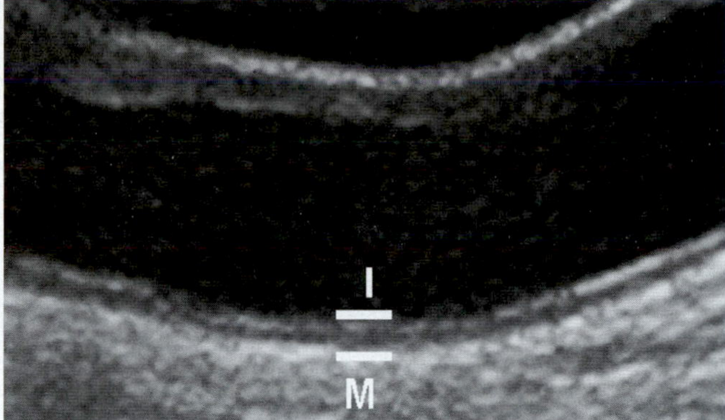

FIGURE 10-17. Internal medial thickness (IMT). The distance between the intima lumen border (I) and the media adventitia border (M).

is variability in this measurement from systole to diastole, and by age and gender. A single threshold value for abnormal IMT has not been determined. Ideally, threshold values derived from large population-based studies should be used in the evaluation of IMT. Both findings correlate with cardiovascular morbidity and mortality.[20] Indeed, the presence of carotid plaque resulting in 50% stenosis is included in the Adult Treatment Panel III guidelines as a coronary heart disease equivalent.

ABDOMINAL AORTA EVALUATION

Abdominal ultrasound is used to diagnose and follow abdominal aortic aneurysms. An ultrasound machine with a low-frequency transducer (e.g., 2.5 MHz) is used to determine the aneurysm size, shape, location (infrarenal or suprarenal) and distance from other arterial segments. The patient is required to fast prior to the study because bowel gas will obscure imaging. Aortic ultrasound scanning begins with the patient supine and the transducer placed in a subxiphoid position. The aorta is located slightly left of midline. The abdominal aorta from the diaphragm to the bifurcation is evaluated using three sonographic views: the sagittal plane (A-P diameter), transverse plane (A-P diameter and transverse diameters) and coronal plane (longitudinal and transverse diameters). Diameter is measured from outer wall to outer wall. If overlying bowel gas obstructs the aorta from view, patients are instructed to lie in the decubitus position and the aorta is visualized via the coronal plane through either flank.[21] As the transducer is moved caudally, the celiac trunk will be evident branching into the common hepatic and splenic arteries (Fig. 10-18). The superior mesenteric artery originates approximately 1 cm distal to the celiac trunk (Fig. 10-19). Next, the right renal artery may be seen emerging from the aorta and traveling under the inferior vena cava. The left renal vein then crosses over the aorta, and the left renal artery will be seen posterior to the vein. The inferior mesenteric artery is the final branch arising from the aorta before it bifurcates into the iliac vessels. Spectral Doppler evaluation of the celiac and mesenteric vessels will demonstrate low-resistance waveforms following a meal and high resistance waveforms in the normal, fasting patient

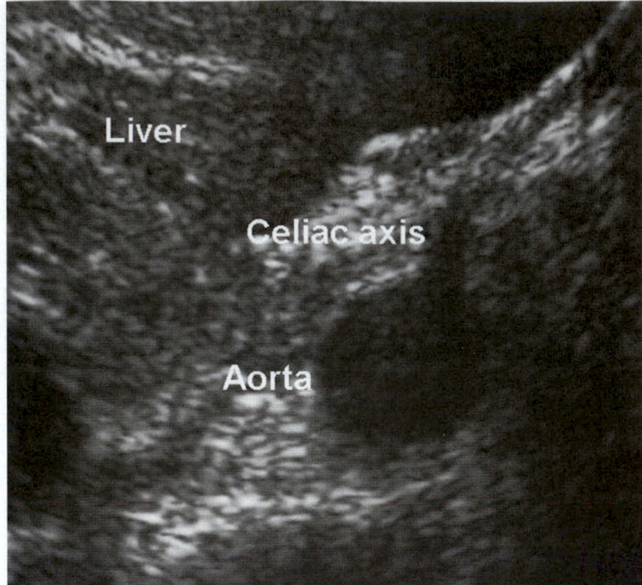

FIGURE 10-18. Celiac trunk originating from the abdominal aorta.

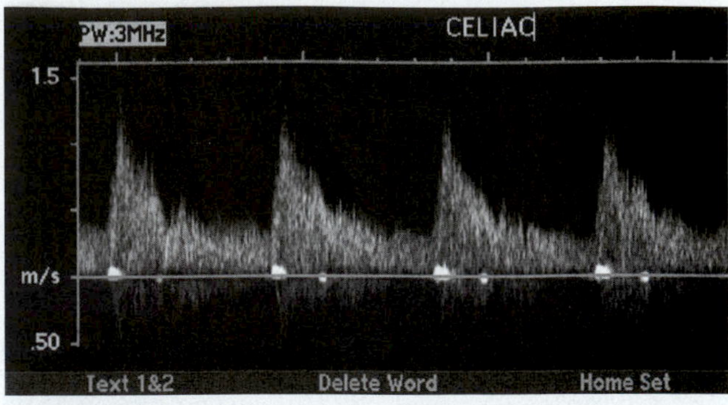

A

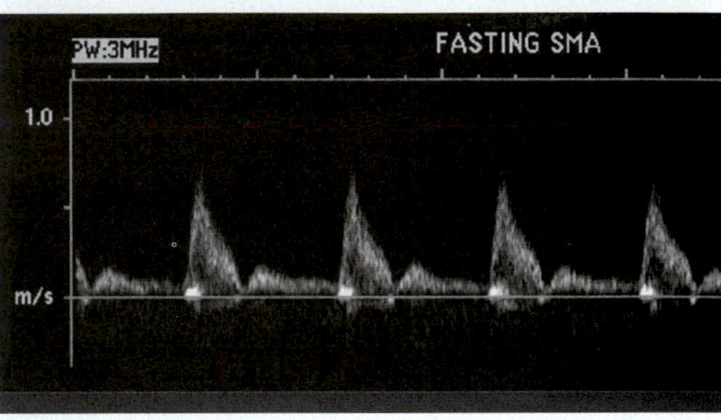

B

FIGURE 10-20. A, Postprandial spectral waveform in the celiac trunk. **B,** Fasting spectral waveform in the superior mesenteric artery (SMA).

(Fig. 10-20). In contrast, evaluation of the normal renal arteries demonstrates low-resistance waveforms.

An abdominal aortic aneurysm is defined as an aortic diameter of at least 1.5 times the adjacent normal segment, or a distal aorta diameter of greater than 3.0 cm (Fig.10-21). Normal abdominal aortic diameters range from 1.4 to 3.0 cm.[22] The shape of the abdominal aortic aneurysm is described as saccular, fusiform, or cylindrical. The majority of abdominal aortic aneurysms are fusiform in shape, located below the renal arteries, and involve one or both of the iliac arteries. Atherosclerotic plaque, mural thrombus, and dissection can be detected in the wall of the aneurysm.[23-25]

Ultrasound evaluation is also performed after endograft repair of abdominal aortic aneurysm. Flow within the graft is evaluated with longitudinal and transverse imaging. Endoleak is diagnosed when there is flow outside the graft, but within the aneurysm. Dissection, pseudoaneurysm and thrombus within the graft are other potential complications[26] that can be detected using ultrasound evaluation.

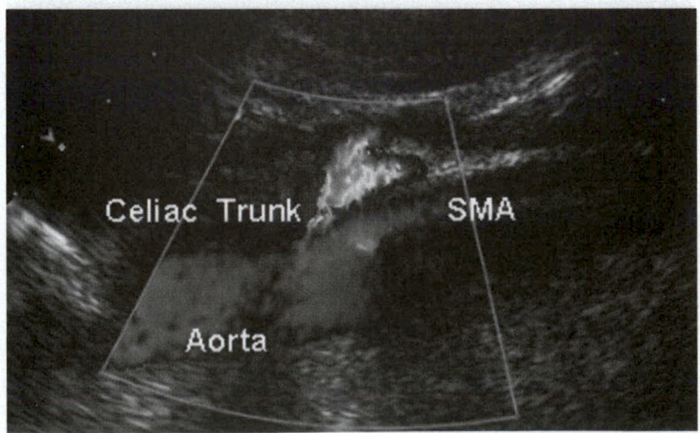

FIGURE 10-19. (See also Color Plate 10-19.) Proximity of the origin of the celiac trunk (bifurcating into hepatic and splenic arteries) and the origin of the superior mesenteric artery (SMA).

RENAL ARTERY DUPLEX ULTRASONOGRAPHY

Atherosclerotic renal artery stenosis is recognized as a cause of hypertension, and may contribute to decline

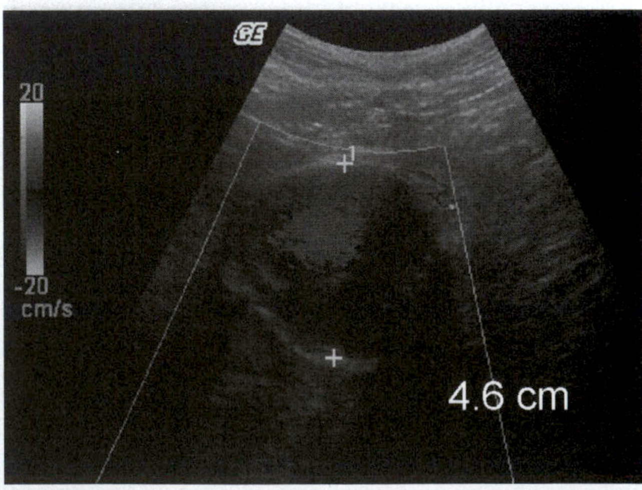

FIGURE 10-21. (See also Color Plate 10-21.) Transverse image of the abdominal aorta with a diameter of 4.6 cm indicating aneurysm. The dropout of acoustic echoes in the right lower corner of this image is due to bowel gas.

in renal function (see Chapter 22). Duplex ultrasound of the renal arteries includes spectral Doppler evaluations of the aorta, the renal arteries and renal parenchyma, and B-mode determination of kidney size. Abdominal obesity and bowel gas are barriers to adequate renal artery duplex examination (see Fig. 10-21).

A longitudinal view of the aorta is obtained with the patient in the supine position. The origins of the celiac artery and superior mesenteric artery (SMA) are seen on the anterior aspect of the aorta cephalad to the renal arteries. The peak systolic velocity in the aorta is then recorded using a 60-degree Doppler angle. The probe is turned transverse to localize the renal arteries. The Doppler cursor is "walked" from the aorta into the ostium of the renal artery. The right renal artery is generally seen most easily. It is followed from the origin to the hilum of the kidney. The left lateral decubitus position can also be used for examination of the right renal artery. The left renal artery is best evaluated in the right lateral decubitus position using a posterolateral transducer position. Ideally, the renal arteries are evaluated from two views to ensure that stenosis is not missed. Kidney length is measured with the patient in the decubitus position.

Color and spectral Doppler are obtained throughout the course of each renal artery. A low velocity range and a low wall filter setting are used in the spectral Doppler evaluations of the segmental renal arteries and the hilar flow. The renal artery normally has a low resistance waveform. A ≥60% renal artery stenosis is characterized by a renal-to-aortic peak systolic velocity ratio of >3.5, combined with a peak systolic velocity within the stenosis of >180 cm/sec. Elevated end-diastolic velocity ≥150 cm/sec suggests ≥80% stenosis (Fig. 10-22).[27,28] Low systolic flow, post-stenotic turbulence, and a color mosaic appearance indicate subtotal occlusion of the renal artery (Fig. 10-23). Low parenchymal Doppler velocities support the diagnosis of an occluded renal artery in those cases where no flow can be detected in the renal artery. In addition, the ipsilateral kidney is often small, <9 cm in length. The overall sensitivity of duplex ultrasonography for renal artery stenosis is 98% and specificity is 98% compared with arteriography.[27]

Measurement of the resistive index is used to evaluate renal parenchymal disease. Spectral Doppler waveforms are obtained from at least three regions of each kidney. The resistive index (RI) is calculated using the formula, $RI = [1-(V_{min} \div V_{max})] \times 100$, where V_{min} denotes end diastolic velocity and V_{max} denotes peak systolic velocity. In severe renal artery stenosis, where there is significant renal parenchymal disease, the end-diastolic velocity is

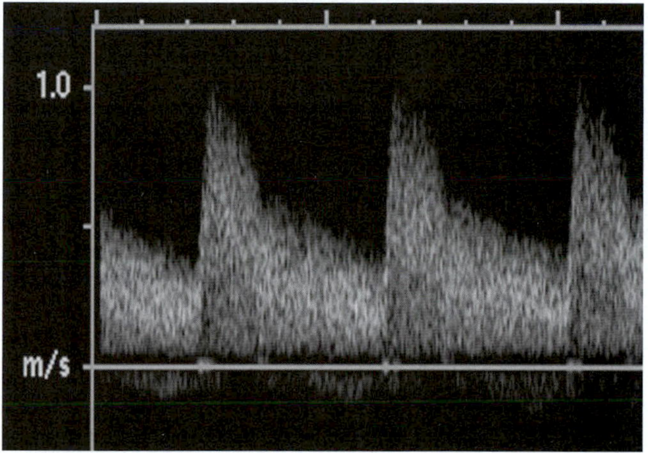

A

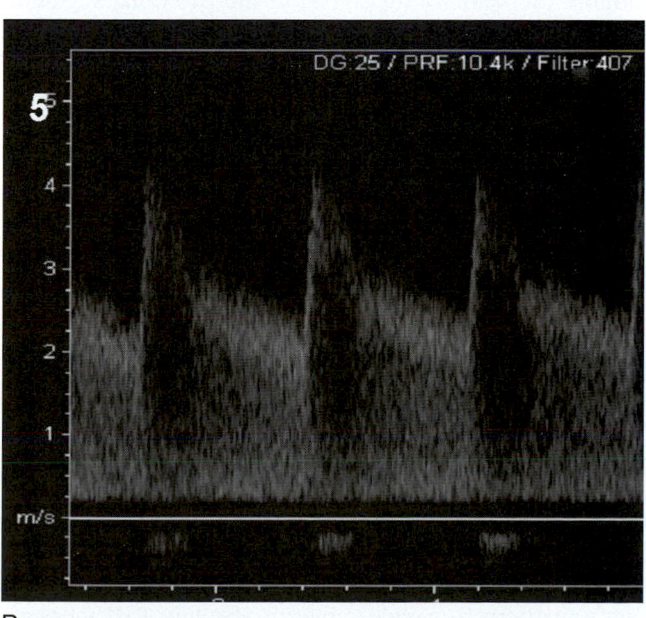

B

FIGURE 10-22. **A,** Normal renal artery peak systolic velocity <100 cm/ sec and low resistance waveform. **B,** Elevated systolic (>500 cm/ sec) and diastolic (>200 cm/sec) velocities consistent with renal artery stenosis.

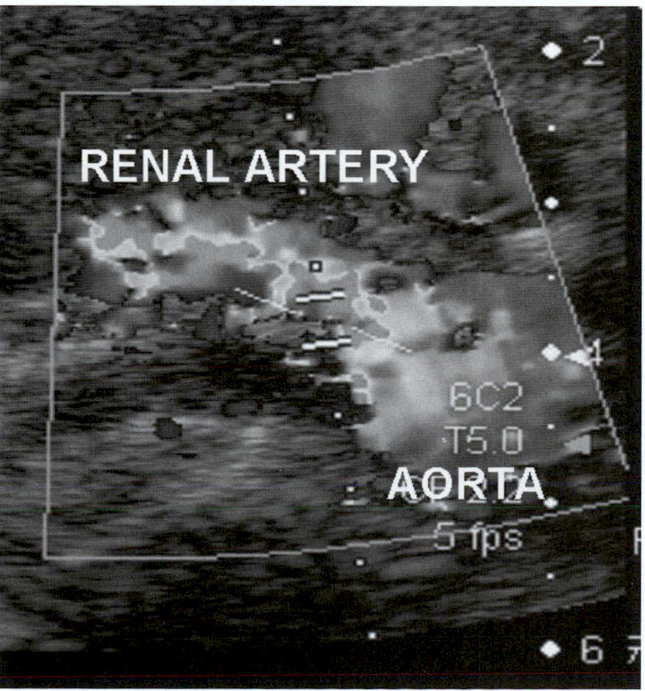

FIGURE 10-23. (See also Color Plate 10-23.) Transverse Doppler image of the origin of the right renal artery. Turbulent flow is evident in the renal artery origin, suggesting the presence of atherosclerotic plaque and the possibility of stenosis.

often low. A resistive index >0.70 suggests significant parenchymal renal disease[29,30] and may have implications regarding the outcome of therapy.

PERIPHERAL ARTERIAL ULTRASONOGRAPHY

Ultrasound of the lower extremities is used in the diagnosis of PAD in the setting of claudication, limb pain, or ulcers.[11] It is also indicated following lower extremity revascularization and in planning therapy for known PAD. The goal of the examination is to elucidate the location and severity of limb arterial stenoses.[31] The study is tailored to individual requirements and can be limited to a given arterial segment, extended to evaluate both lower extremities in their entirety, or to evaluate the upper extremity.

Color Doppler is used initially to detect normal or abnormal flow states throughout the arterial segments or bypass grafts being evaluated.[32] Laminar flow is visible in the absence of disease (Fig. 10-24), whereas turbulence and aliasing are present at the sites of disease. When an abnormal flow pattern is detected by color Doppler, pulsed (spectral) Doppler sampling is used to characterize the degree of stenosis. The pulse Doppler signal is then acquired through the arterial segments. Peak systolic velocity (PSV) determination and waveform analyses are the primary parameters used to quantify and localize disease. Peak systolic velocity measurements are obtained at the level of the lesion, and from vascular segments proximal and distal to the lesion. Aneurysmal dilation is another etiology for abnormal color flow. The velocities will decrease as the diameter doubles at the site of the aneurysm. The superficial femoral and popliteal arteries are both sites of aneurysm (Fig. 10-25).

Peripheral arterial stenosis is categorized by pulsed-wave Doppler examination as percentage reduction of luminal diameter that is mild (0% to 19%), moderate (20% to 49%), or severe (50% and greater).[11] With mild stenosis, there is some spectral broadening and a slight increase in PSV. With moderate stenosis, there is increased spectral broadening and a rise in PSV that is less than double that of the proximally sampled segment. Pulsed Doppler interrogation at the level of a severe stenosis reveals marked spectral broadening and a monophasic waveform. The waveform loses its normal diastolic reverse flow component and flow is forward throughout the cardiac cycle. Also, the PSV is more than double the velocity measured in the proximal segment. An occlusion is present when flow is absent within an arterial segment. If there are no collateral vessels, high-resistance waveforms are present in the artery proximal to the occlusion. Antegrade diastolic flow is present in the proximal artery if there are collateral vessels. The reconstituted distal artery will have the characteristic post-stenotic, tardus et parvus waveform.[33] This Doppler waveform is particularly important to recognize because it signifies a proximal high-grade lesion.

Duplex ultrasound examination is accurate for diagnosing PAD.[34] The comparison of duplex ultrasound evaluation with arteriography to detect significant stenoses in patients with symptomatic aortoiliac and femoropopliteal disease reveals a high sensitivity (82%) and specificity (92%) for identifying significant stenoses.[31] Using both color and pulsed-wave Doppler increases the sensitivity (87% to 88%) and specificity (95% to 99%).[35] Ratios of PSV between the stenosis and the proximal artery are preferred over the absolute PSV measurements for the classification of peripheral arterial stenosis because there is a wide range of absolute PSV measurements obtained in normal and abnormal patients.[36] There is a stronger correlation between PSV ratio and degree of stenosis than between absolute PSV and degree of stenosis. PSV ratios of 2 and 7 correspond to stenoses ≥50% and

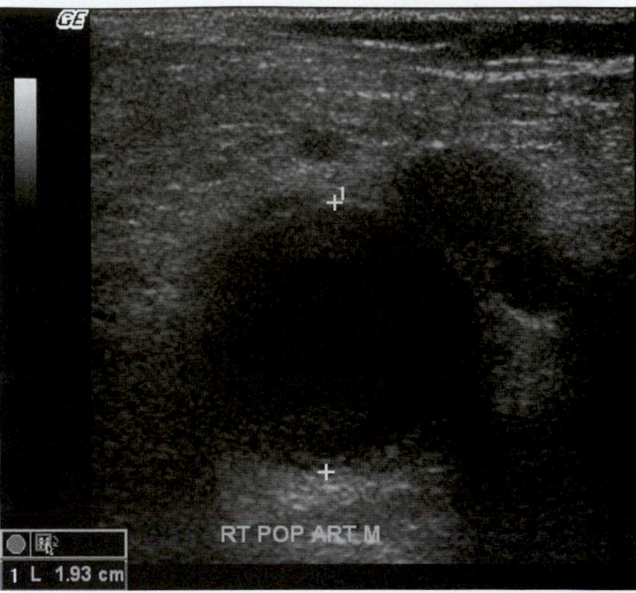

FIGURE 10-25. Gray-scale image of popliteal artery aneurysm. Aneurysm is defined by a 1.5× or greater increase in arterial diameter compared with the proximal segment. Thrombus develops in these aneurysms and can result in occlusion or distal embolization.

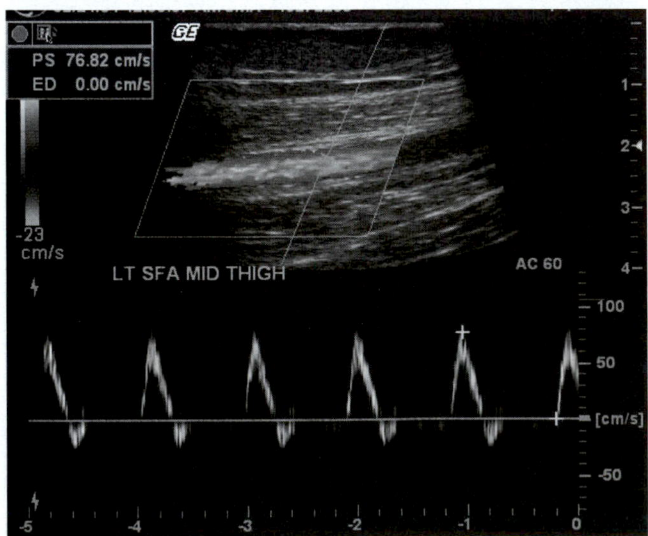

FIGURE 10-24. (See also Color Plate 10-24.) Duplex ultrasound of a superficial femoral artery (SFA) stent. Laminar flow is evident in the Doppler image. The peak systolic velocity of 76 cm/sec is within normal limits.

≥90%, respectively. There are conflicting data regarding the precision of the duplex ultrasound examination in the determination of stenosis severity when serial stenoses are present.[37,38]

Extremity Arterial Ultrasound Following Revascularization

Ultrasound evaluation following endovascular procedures is performed to detect recurrence of stenoses at sites of intervention. The concept is similar to that for graft surveillance (i.e., early detection of lesions assists in identifying the need for reintervention to maintain arterial patency).[39] Duplex ultrasonography is performed following the intervention prior to discharge; 1, 3, and 6 months postintervention; then yearly. The color Doppler and pulsed-wave Doppler evaluations focus on the vessel proximal to the site of intervention, at the site of intervention, and distal to the site of intervention. Waveform analysis is used to categorize stenosis in a manner similar to that used in native vessels.[40] A doubling of peak systolic velocity is consistent with hemodynamically significant stenosis (Fig. 10-26).[41,42] Increases in velocity measurements and change in waveform shape from triphasic to monophasic on serial examinations suggest developing stenosis, and warrant close interval follow-up and consideration for revision.

Graft surveillance is extremely useful in efforts to preserve the patency of peripheral arterial bypass grafts. Graft failure in the first month is usually caused by technical factors. Between 1 month and 2 years postoperatively, it is often due to intimal hyperplasia. Graft failure after 2 years is likely the result of progression of atherosclerotic disease. The 5-year primary patency rate for an infrainguinal vein bypass graft ranges from 60% to 85%.[43] Surgical revision of these stenoses identified with ultrasound surveillance improves the 5-year patency rate to 82% to 93%.[44,45] By contrast, segmental pressure measurements have not proved useful to predict bypass graft thrombosis. To detect graft abnormalities before frank graft failure, standard graft surveillance protocols recommend duplex ultrasound evaluation at 1, 3, and 6 months during the first postoperative year, and 12 months thereafter. The location and type of graft are identified before performing the ultrasound examination. Scanning techniques in the supine patient are similar to native arterial examinations. Color Doppler is used initially to scan the entire graft. The color pulse repetition frequency is adjusted so focal stenoses or arteriovenous fistulae appear as regions of aliasing, persistence, or bruit color flash artifact. Based on color Doppler findings, pulsed Doppler interrogation is used to determine the PSV. Sampling is done routinely at the proximal native artery, proximal anastomosis, throughout the graft, distal anastomosis, distal native vessel, and throughout sites of flow disturbance. These measurements are used also for serial comparison during subsequent examinations.

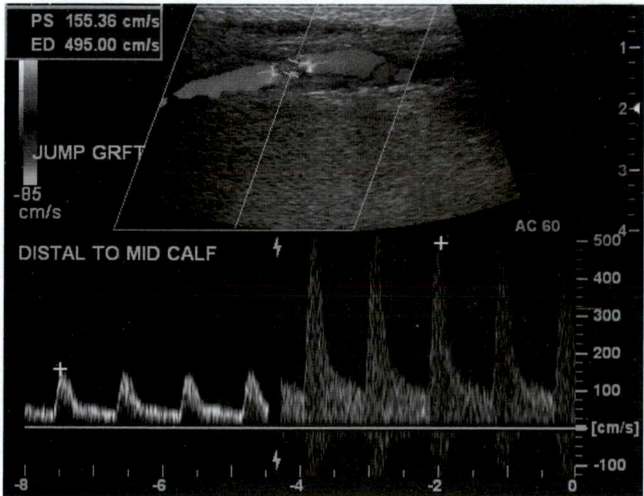

FIGURE 10-26. (See also Color Plate 10-26.) Duplex ultrasound of peripheral bypass graft. The proximal velocity is 155 cm/sec and increases to 495 cm/sec at the site of stenosis. Aliasing of the Doppler is also evident at the site of stenosis.

Pulsed Doppler is used to determine PSV ratios within the graft similar to its use in the native arterial examination. A segment distal (rather than proximal) to the lesion may be chosen for the ratio when there is a diameter mismatch in the graft or there are tandem lesions proximal to the flow disturbance. Doubling of the velocity ratio indicates a significant graft stenosis (greater than 50% diameter reduction) with a sensitivity of 95% and specificity of 100%.[41,42] Vein graft lesions have been classified using PSV (1) a minimal stenosis (<20%) has PSV ratio up to 1.4 with a PSV of less than 125 cm/sec; (2) a moderate stenosis (20% to 50%) has a PSV ratio of 1.5 to 2.4 with a PSV up to 180 cm/sec; (3) a severe stenosis (50% to 75%) has a PSV ratio of 2.5 to 4 with a PSV of more than 180 cm/sec; and (4) a high-grade stenosis (>75%) has a PSV ratio greater than 4 with a PSV greater than 300 cm/sec.[46] Intervention is recommended for lesions categorized as severe or high grade. Detection of low-flow velocities within the graft with pulsed Doppler suggests either proximal or distal stenosis. Low velocity flow can also be caused by large graft diameter or poor arterial inflow. Nonetheless, velocities within a functioning graft that are less than 45 cm/sec indicate that subsequent graft failure is likely to occur.[44] Other worrisome findings are a significant decrease or increase in PSV on serial examination.

PSEUDOANEURYSM

A pseudoaneurysm is a contained arterial rupture. A hole through all layers of the arterial wall results in extravasation of blood which is then enclosed by the surrounding soft tissues.[47] Any patient who has undergone an arterial puncture for arteriography and experiences sudden pain at the access site, or is found to have pulsatile mass or a bruit on auscultation over the access site, should be evaluated for the presence of pseudoaneurysm.

Ultrasound evaluation is performed in the region of the puncture. Spectral waveforms are obtained in the native artery proximal and distal to the site of puncture, and in the femoral vein proximal and distal to the site of puncture. Color Doppler evaluation should focus on detecting an extravascular collection of flowing blood,

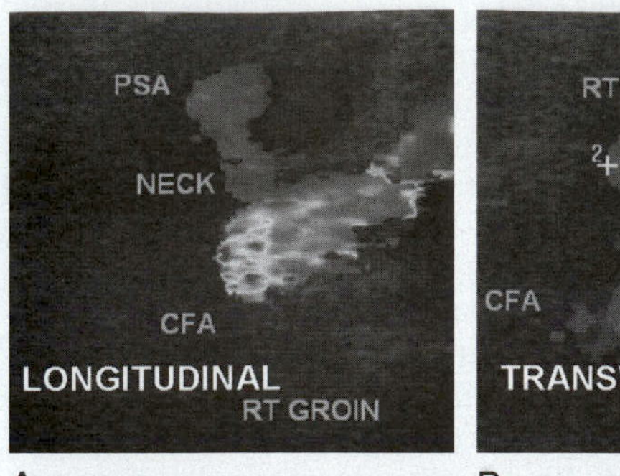

A

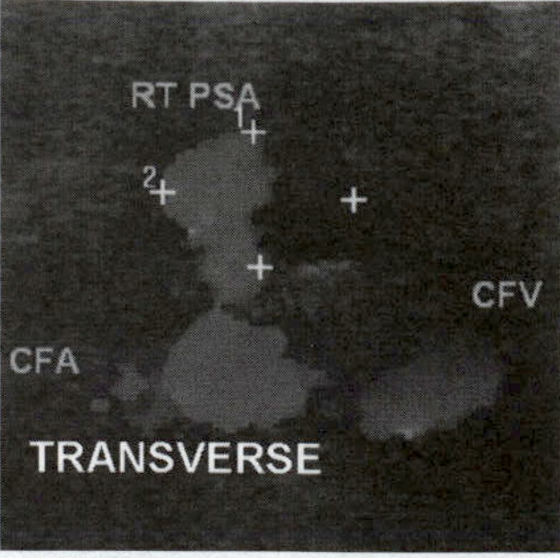

B

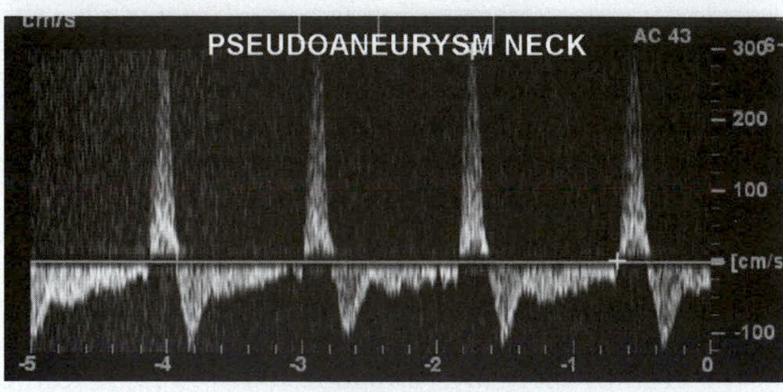

C

FIGURE 10-27. (See also Color Plate 10-27.) Doppler evaluations of a pseudoaneurysm (PSA). The "yin-yang" appearance of the PSA cavity is evident in the longitudinal (**A**) and transverse (**B**) images. Whereas the artery lengthens in the longitudinal image, the contained rupture sac of the PSA retains its saccular shape. Pulsed Doppler placed in the neck of the pseudoaneurysm demonstrates the pathognomonic "to-and-fro" pattern of bidirectional flow into and out of the contained rupture (**C**).

most commonly anterior to the native artery (Fig. 10-27).[48] Posterior extravasation is less common. The neck is the connection between the native artery and the pseudoaneurysm sac. The neck is identified by a "to and fro" pattern of the Doppler waveform that is pathognomonic for pseudoaneurysm (see Fig. 10-27).[49] This waveform results from systolic flow out of the native artery into the contained rupture, and diastolic flow back into the native artery. In addition to the to and fro signal in the neck, the segment of native artery proximal to the origin of the pseudoaneurysm may have a lower resistance waveform when compared with that found in the artery distal to the pseudoaneurysm.

There are several options for treatment of pseudoaneurysms including observation,[50] surgical repair,[51,52] manual compression,[47] ultrasound-guided compression,[53] or thrombin injection.[54] Ultrasound-guided compression is performed with visualization of the pseudoaneurysm neck while compressing until flow is absent in the neck. Pressure is applied for 20 minutes, and may need to be maintained for much longer before thrombosis of the pseudoaneurysm sac is achieved.[55-57] Reported success rate of compression varies from 60% to 80%. Ultrasound-guided thrombin injection is best suited for those pseudoaneurysms with a long, narrow neck. Thrombin injection is contraindicated in those with allergy to bovine thrombin, and in those with overlying skin infections, in the presence of ipsilateral arteriovenous fistula, and in those with active limb ischemia. The injection is performed under sterile conditions, using a syringe equipped with a three-way stopcock. The needle is placed into the sac while drawing back gently on the syringe. The tip of the needle is seen in the cavity and blood return is noted. The stopcock is then switched to a position open to the thrombin, and 0.1 to 0.2 ml of thrombin are injected. The duplex ultrasound examination should include final pictures documenting thrombosis of the pseudoaneurysm, and a patent artery of origin. Complications of thrombin injection include limb ischemia if thrombin enters the native artery and causes a thrombus to form, and anaphylaxis.

ARTERIOVENOUS FISTULAE

Arteriovenous fistulae occur secondary to trauma, including catheterization or are created intentionally for dialysis.[58] The duplex ultrasound findings include turbulent and pulsatile venous flow.[59] The turbulence may result in a color "bruit" adjacent to the vein, caused by vibration of the surrounding soft tissue.[60] Arterial flow proximal to the fistula will have a low resistance pattern, rather than the typical high resistance peripheral waveform (Fig. 10-28). The arterial flow distal to the fistula will have a high resistance waveform. The venous flow pattern at the connection will resemble an arterial waveform. The actual arteriovenous connection may be too small to be seen in postcatheterization arteriovenous fistulae.

Evaluation of dialysis fistulae uses specific criteria for the Doppler spectra obtained from arterial inflow and venous outflow.[61] Peak systolic velocity is recorded throughout the native system and the graft. The arterial limb should demonstrate high velocities and continuous forward flow with a low-resistance waveform.[62] The venous limb is expected to have slightly lower velocities. The normal peak systolic velocity at the anastomosis is

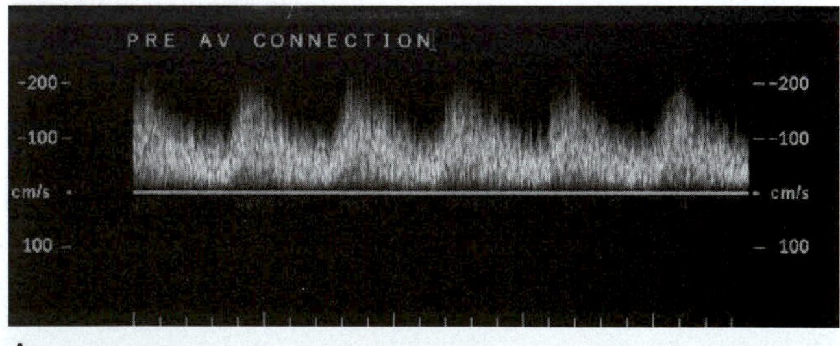

A

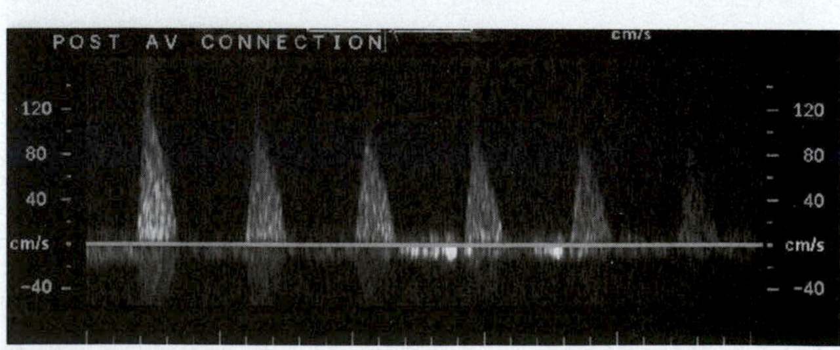

B

FIGURE 10-28. Spectral Doppler evaluation of a peripheral artery proximal before (**A**) and distal (**B**) to an arteriovenous connection. The low resistance pattern in **A** occurs because the artery is flowing into the high-capacitance venous bed.

300 cm/sec. The normal outflow vein has a peak systolic velocity greater than 180 cm/sec and appears distended. Peak systolic velocity less than 150 cm/sec indicates a fistula in jeopardy of failure. The fistula may result in arterial steal from the distal circulation. If this is suspected, the direction of distal flow should be evaluated before and after compression of the arteriovenous fistula.

VENOUS DUPLEX ULTRASOUND

Duplex examination of the extremity veins enables accurate noninvasive evaluation for deep vein thrombosis (DVT). Normal veins have thin walls and an echo-free lumen. The vein lumen can be obliterated (compressed) with a small amount of extrinsic pressure (Fig. 10-29). The walls do not coapt, however, when the lumen contains thrombus, even when enough pressure is applied to distort the shape of an adjacent artery. Vein compressibility is best tested in an image plane transverse to the vein axis. Veins are characterized by anatomical location as deep or superficial, and as proximal or distal. The major veins of the thigh and arm are larger in diameter than the corresponding arteries. Extremity veins have valves, which permit only cephalad flow, and these increase in number from proximal to distal. Valve sinuses are widened areas of the lumen that accommodate the valve cusps.

Doppler evaluation of flow in normal veins has four important characteristics (1) respirophasic variation; (2) augmentation with distal compression; (3) unidirectional flow toward the heart; (4) and abrogation of flow in the lower extremities by the Valsalva maneuver. Complete analysis of venous spectral waveforms requires comparison of the waveforms from both right and left limbs. The presence of a flattened, unvarying waveform (loss of respirophasic variation in flow) on one side compared with the other suggests the presence of more proximal obstruction of venous return proximal to the site of the Doppler interrogation.

Neck and Upper Extremity Venous Duplex Ultrasound

Neck and upper extremity duplex evaluation includes assessments of the internal jugular, subclavian, axillary, brachial, cephalic, and basilic veins. The innominate veins and the superior vena cava cannot be evaluated with duplex ultrasound because of their location within the bony thorax. The examination begins with evaluation of the internal jugular (Fig. 10-30) and subclavian veins. The subclavian vein can be imaged from a supraclavicular or subclavicular approach. The arm is extended in a comfortable position for the evaluation of the axillary vein, paired brachial veins, basilic vein (medial), and cephalic vein (lateral). The examination includes color and spectral Doppler evaluation of flow in all of these veins. Loss of respirophasic variation in the waveform in the subclavian or axillary veins suggests the presence of more proximal venous obstruction (due to thrombosis or extrinsic compression) (Fig. 10-31). The subclavian vein cannot be compressed where it lies directly below the clavicle, and venous thrombosis is suspected when flow is absent or echogenic material is seen within the lumen.

Loss of compressibility is the pathognomonic feature of venous thrombosis. As the thrombus progresses from acute to chronic, there is increased echogenicity of the thrombus and decreased diameter of the vein. Over time, collateral veins may develop and recanalization may occur in the thrombosed vessel. In the upper arm, both superficial and deep venous systems have a significant role in venous drainage. The majority of upper extremity deep vein thromboses are secondary to indwelling venous catheters, pacemaker leads or hypercoagulability. Primary upper extremity deep vein thrombosis is a rare disorder that is idiopathic, attributed to effort thrombosis (Paget-Schrotter syndrome), or related to thoracic outlet

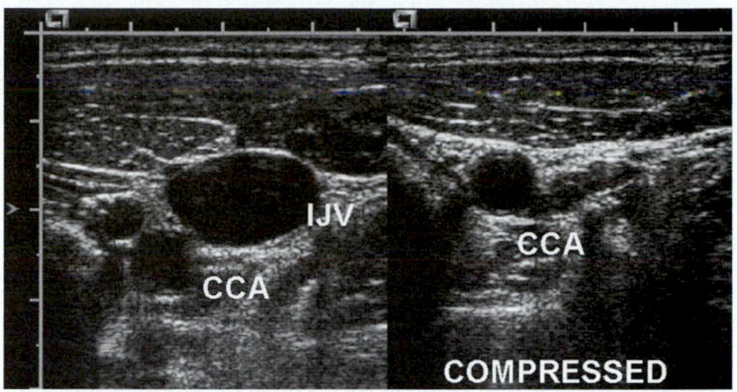

FIGURE 10-30. Transverse gray-scale imaging of the internal jugular vein and common carotid artery without compression (*left*) and with gentle compression (*right*) obliterating the lumen of the vein. CCA, common carotid artery; IJV, internal jugular vein.

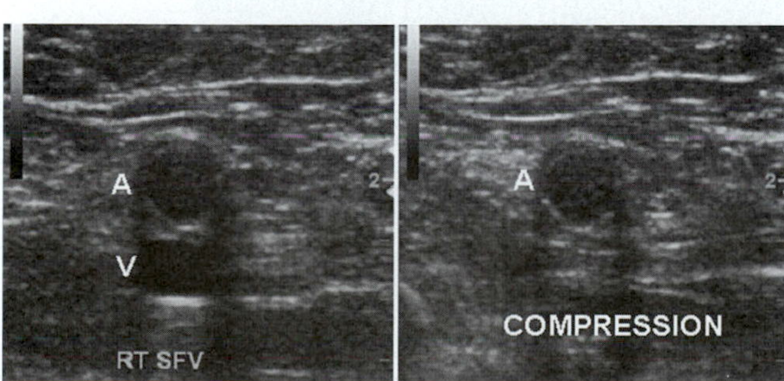

FIGURE 10-29. Transverse gray-scale imaging of the superficial femoral artery (A) and vein (V) (*left*). With gentle compression (*right*) the artery is unchanged and the vein is obliterated.

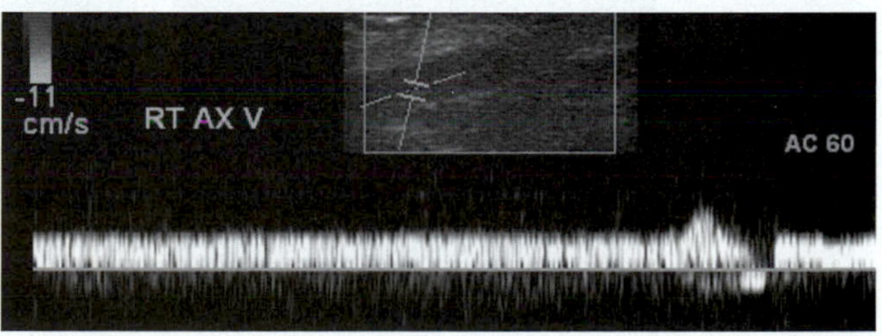

FIGURE 10-31. Spectral Doppler evaluation of the axillary vein demonstrating loss of phasic variation in flow with respiration. This finding suggests more proximal venous obstruction. The increase in flow on the right results from compression of the forearm (augmenting venous return).

obstruction.[63] An unusual etiology of noncompressible veins is intravascular tumor. This is suspected when the echogenic material within the lumen appears to extend through the vessel wall and may contain arterial flow signals.

Lower Extremity Venous Duplex Ultrasound

The venous ultrasound examination to evaluate the presence or absence of leg DVT begins at the inguinal ligament with identification of the common femoral vein and extends to the calf.[64] The proximal deep veins evaluated include the common femoral, superficial femoral, and popliteal veins. The deep calf veins include posterior tibial, peroneal, gastrocnemius (sural), and soleal veins. Special attention is given to the saphenofemoral and saphenopopliteal junctions because thrombus in the superficial veins of these regions deserve more aggressive treatment than thrombus limited to other parts of the superficial venous system. The examination includes color and spectral Doppler evaluation of flow in all these veins (Fig. 10-32). Loss of respirophasic variation in the waveform of the common femoral vein suggests the presence of obstruction proximal to the site of Doppler interrogation which is preventing venous return. Augmentation of flow with calf compression is not prevented by proximal venous obstruction. Proximal obstruction may be caused by extrinsic compression or venous thrombosis.

B-mode transverse images are used to determine compressibility along the entire course of the veins examined. Normally, the vein walls fully coapt with gentle pressure. Lack of compressibility, which occurs because of a thrombosis in the vein, is the most reliable finding for determining venous thrombosis.[65] With acute thrombosis, there is low echogenicity of the intraluminal thrombus and the vein is dilated. As the thrombus ages, it becomes more echogenic and less central within the lumen. The vein diameter decreases as the thrombus retracts. Recanalization occurs and flow can be detected by pulsed or color Doppler. The thrombus often appears eccentric and adjacent to the vein wall. When image quality is poor because of significant soft tissue edema, it is not possible to exclude the presence of small, nonocclusive thrombi. Sensitivity for the detection of common femoral vein thrombosis is 91%, and for both the superficial femoral and popliteal veins is 94%.[66]

Duplex ultrasound is accurate for the diagnosis of deep calf vein thrombosis in symptomatic patients, as long as the calf veins can be seen clearly (Fig. 10-33).[67] Sensitivity of compression ultrasound for deep calf vein thrombosis is 94% and specificity is 100% when compared with angiography.[68] The small calf veins cannot be visualized well in all patients. However, the specificity and positive-predictive value are high even when those individuals with poor calf vein images are included in the evaluation.[68] Thus, the diagnosis of DVT is made when calf veins are seen and cannot be compressed.

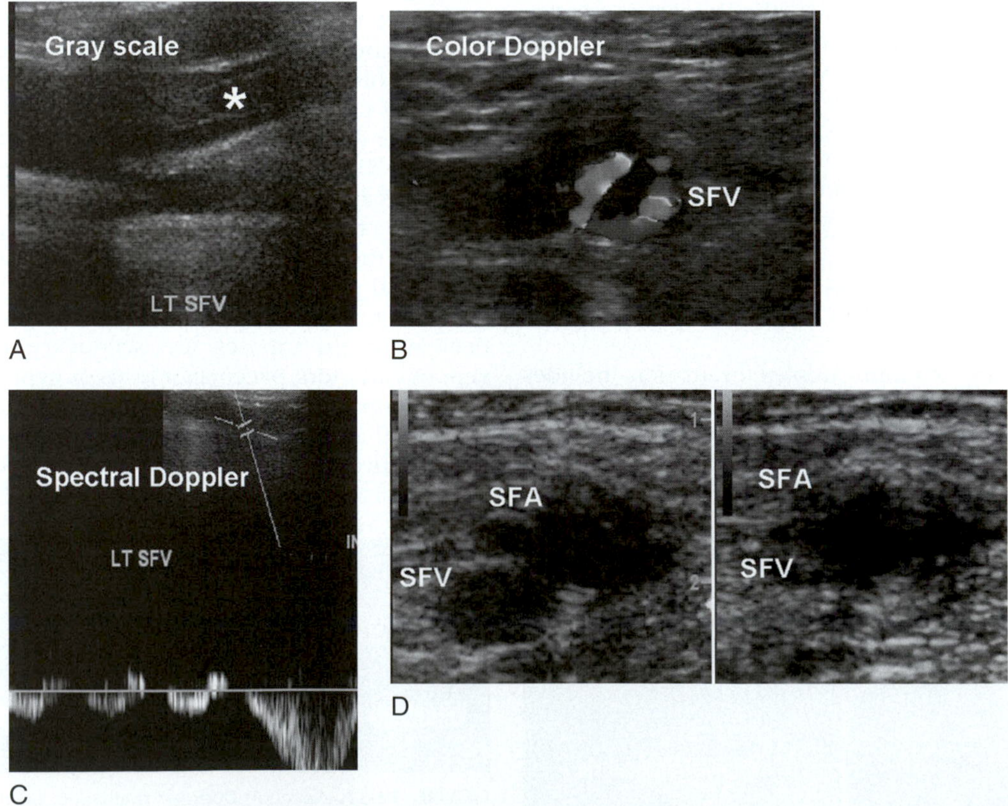

FIGURE 10-32. (See also Color Plate 10-32.) Ultrasound evaluation of the femoral vein thrombosis. **A,** Gray imaging with echogenic material (*asterisk*) seen within the lumen of the superficial femoral vein (SFV). **B,** Doppler in the superficial femoral vein shows a flow void within the lumen. **C,** Spectral Doppler demonstrates diminished flow with respirophasic variation. **D,** Superficial femoral artery (SFA) and vein without (*left*) and with (*right*) compression; the vein is only partially obliterated due to thrombus.

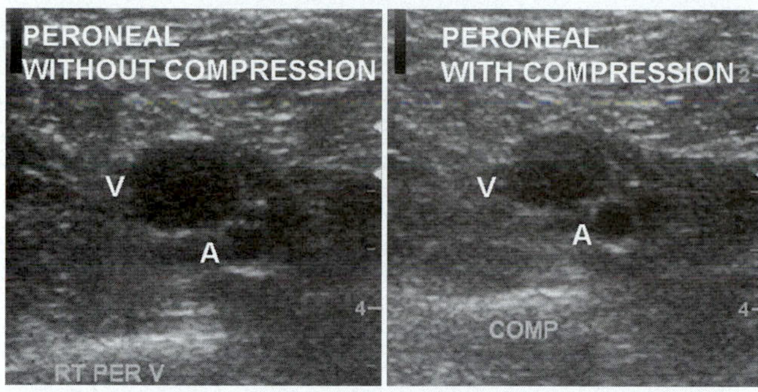

FIGURE 10-33. Transverse gray-scale imaging of the peroneal veins of the calf. The vein appears dilated in the noncompression image on the *left*. The vein lumen is not obliterated by gentle compression indicating the presence of calf-vein thrombosis. A, artery; V, vein.

Lower extremity venous ultrasound testing is often ordered when a patient is undergoing evaluation for pulmonary embolism. This test will provide information about the presence or absence of venous thrombosis, but will not determine whether or not someone has had a pulmonary embolism. At least 30% of the individuals with pulmonary embolism do not have lower extremity venous thrombosis.[69,70]

Duplex Ultrasound Evaluation of Venous Insufficiency

The use of duplex ultrasound has been extended to detect reflux or obstruction and determine the anatomical extent of venous disease in patients with chronic venous insufficiency.[71] This development has been facilitated by the use of color Doppler imaging to provide instant determination of the direction of blood flow. A 4- to 7-MHz linear array transducer is used. The saphenofemoral junction is examined first with the patient standing and then in the supine, reverse Trendelenburg position. Compressibility is determined in transverse views of the veins. A longitudinal view of the saphenofemoral junction is then obtained.

One of two maneuvers can be used to elicit reflux. The first is the Valsalva maneuver. Intra-abdominal pressure increases as the patient bears down, and venous outflow from the legs decreases. The venous return from the legs increases with release of the maneuver.[72] The second is thigh cuff inflation and deflation. Venous return is stopped with inflation of a cuff to arterial diastolic pressure. There is a transient increase in venous return that accompanies cuff deflation. Color flow is evaluated before and after one of these two maneuvers to elicit reflux.[73] Baseline antegrade flow is displayed by blue color Doppler. Red color after the maneuver indicates retrograde flow. Reflux is present if red color persists for >0.5 seconds after either maneuver. Spectral Doppler can also be used to evaluate reflux. The Doppler cursor is placed midstream with an angle of 60 degrees with respect to the wall. Reverse flow >0.5 seconds in duration is consistent with reflux. Ideally, the remainder of the examination is performed with the patient standing with the weight on the leg that is not being examined.

The extent of reflux can be determined by repeating this assessment throughout the deep and superficial veins of the leg. For evaluation of the lesser saphenous and popliteal veins, the patient sits on the edge of the examination table with his/her foot resting on a stool. The probe is placed over the popliteal fossa. The gastrocnemius veins can be seen between the popliteal (which is deep) and lesser saphenous (which is superficial) vein. Compressibility and reflux following a Valsalva maneuver are determined in these veins. The posterior tibial and peroneal veins are assessed for reflux using the posteromedial and anterolateral views.

Perforating veins are vessels connecting superficial and deep veins. Incompetent perforating veins are identified by sliding the transducer up and down dilated superficial varicose veins. Color Doppler is then used while distal compression of the superficial vein is performed. The presence of different colors during compression and release indicates that the direction of venous flow changes with compression and relief. This finding is diagnostic of reflux in the perforator veins.

PLETHYSMOGRAPHIC EVALUATION OF VENOUS REFLUX

Duplex ultrasound identifies reflux in individual veins, and plethysmographic methods evaluate the volume of venous reflux in the limb.[74] Air plethysmography is a simple screening test that has the potential to provide a complete analysis of venous hemodynamics. The chamber is filled with air to 6 mm Hg and connected to a pressure transducer and recorder.[75] Changes in the volume of the leg as a result of emptying or filling veins produce changes in the pressure of the air chamber. Recordings are made with the patient supine, and the leg elevated at a 45-degree angle. The patient then stands with the leg flexed slightly and bearing weight on the nonstudy leg. Venous filling time and venous volume are determined. The time until the volume plateaus after the raised limb is dropped is the venous filling time. Venous volumes of 80 to 150 ml are normal. The venous filling index (VFI) correlates best with the clinical severity of reflux.

$$\text{VFI} = .90\ (\text{venous volume}) \div .9\ (\text{venous filling time})$$

Values <2 ml/sec indicate the absence of significant reflux, whereas values >10 ml/sec indicate high risks of edema, skin changes, and ulceration.

Post-exercise plethysmography can be used to evaluate the ejecting capacity of the calf muscle pump. Venous volume is measured at rest, and again post-exercise. The rest volume minus the post-exercise volume equals the ejected volume. The ejection fraction, is the ejected volume/rest volume × 100. Calf ejection fractions <40% indicate patients most likely to benefit from deep vein reconstruction.[76]

VASCULAR LABORATORY ACCREDITATION

Laboratory accreditation is obtained through organizations such as the Intersocietal Commission for the

Accreditation of Vascular Laboratories (www.icavl.org) and the American College of Radiology (www.acr.org). The accreditation process reviews the educational credentials of the interpreting physicians and sonographers, as well as laboratory procedures. It provides excellent standards for setting up examination protocols and quality assurance programs.

REFERENCES

1. Boyajian RA, Otis SM: Integration and added value of the modern noninvasive vascular laboratory in vascular diseases management. J Neuroimaging 12:148, 2002.
2. Pascarelli EF, Bertrand CA: Comparison of blood pressures in the arms and legs. N Engl J Med 270:693, 1964.
3. Ouriel K, Zarins CK: Doppler ankle pressure: An evaluation of three methods of expression. Arch Surg 117:1297, 1982.
4. Carter SA: Clinical measurement of systolic pressures in limbs with arterial occlusive disease. JAMA 207:1869, 1969.
5. Wutschert R, Bounameaux H: Determination of amputation level in ischemic limbs. Reappraisal of the measurement of TcPo2. Diabetes Care 20:1315, 1997.
6. Gardner AW, Skinner JS, Cantwell BW, et al: Progressive vs. single-stage treadmill tests for evaluation of claudication. Med Sci Sports Exerc 23:402, 1991.
7. Philips D, Beach K, Primozich J: Should results of ultrasound Doppler criteria be reported in units of frequency or velocity? Ultrasound Med Biol 15:205, 1989.
8. Logason K, Barlin T, Jonsson M, et al: The importance of Doppler angle of insonation on differentiation between 50-69% and 70-99% carotid artery stenosis. Eur J Endovasc Surg 21:311, 2001.
9. Strandness DE, Jr., Schultz RD, Sumner DS, et al: Ultrasonic flow detection. A useful technic in the evaluation of peripheral vascular disease. Am J Surg 113:311, 1967.
10. Rohren EM, Kliewer MA, Carroll BA, et al: A spectrum of Doppler waveforms in the carotid and vertebral arteries. AJR Am J Roentgenol 181:1695, 2003.
11. Jager K: Non-invasive mapping of lower limb arterial lesions. Ultrasound Med Biol 11:515, 1985.
12. Pellerito J: Color persistence: Indicator of hemodynamically significant peripheral arterial stenosis. Radiology 181:89, 1991.
13. Needham TN: Review of pressure and flow in the arterial system. J Vasc Tech 26:27, 2002.
14. Kotval PS: Doppler waveform parvus and tardus. A sign of proximal flow obstruction. J Ultrasound Med 8:435, 1989.
15. Rubin J: Power Doppler US: A potentially useful alternative to mean frequency-based color Doppler US. Radiology 190:853, 1994.
16. Langholz J, Schlief R, Schurmann R, et al: Contrast enhancement in leg vessels. Clin Radiol 51 Suppl 1:31, 1996.
17. Medicare services of Missouri draft policy for non-invasive vascular studies.
18. Langlois Y, Roederer G, Strandness DJ: Ultrasonic evaluation of carotid bifurcation. Echocardiography 4:141, 1987.
19. Grant EG, Benson CB, Moneta GL, et al: Carotid artery stenosis: Gray-scale and Doppler US diagnosis—Society of Radiologists in Ultrasound Consensus Conference. Radiology 229:340, 2003.
20. O'Leary DH, Polak JF, Kronmal RA, et al: Carotid-artery intima and media thickness as a risk factor for myocardial infarction and stroke in older adults. Cardiovascular Health Study Collaborative Research Group. N Engl J Med 340:14, 1999.
21. Steiner E, Rubens D, Weiss SL, et al: Sonographic examination of the abdominal aorta through the left flank: A prospective study. J Ultrasound Med 5:499, 1986.
22. Yucel EK, Fillmore DJ, Knox TA, et al: Sonographic measurement of abdominal aortic diameter: Interobserver variability. J Ultrasound Med 10:681, 1991.
23. Harter LP, Gross BH, Callen PW, et al: Ultrasonic evaluation of abdominal aortic thrombus. J Ultrasound Med 1:315, 1982.
24. Clayton MJ, Walsh JW, Brewer WH: Contained rupture of abdominal aortic aneurysms: Sonographic and CT diagnosis. AJR Am J Roentgenol 138:154, 1982.
25. King PS, Cooperberg PL, Madigan SM: The anechoic crescent in abdominal aortic aneurysms: Not a sign of dissection. AJR Am J Roentgenol 146:345, 1986.
26. Blum U, Voshage G, Lammer J, et al: Endoluminal stent-grafts for infrarenal abdominal aortic aneurysms. N Engl J Med 336:13, 1997.
27. Olin JW, Piedmonte MR, Young JR, et al: The utility of duplex ultrasound scanning of the renal arteries for diagnosing significant renal artery stenosis. Ann Intern Med 122:833, 1995.
28. Hoffmann U, Edwards JM, Carter S, et al: Role of duplex scanning for the detection of atherosclerotic renal artery disease. Kidney Int 39:1232, 1991.
29. Malatino LS, Polizzi G, Garozzo M, et al: Diagnosis of renovascular disease by extra- and intrarenal Doppler parameters. Angiology 49:707, 1998.
30. Radermacher J, Chavan A, Bleck J, et al: Use of Doppler ultrasonography to predict the outcome of therapy for renal-artery stenosis. N Engl J Med 344:410, 2001.
31. Kohler T: Duplex scanning for diagnosis of aortoiliac and femoropopliteal disease: A prospective study. Circulation 76:1074, 1987.
32. Hatsukami TS, Primozich J, Zierler RE, et al: Color Doppler characteristics in normal lower extremity arteries. Ultrasound Med Biol 18:167, 1992.
33. Bude R: Pulsus tardus: Its cause and potential limitations in detection of arterial stenosis. Radiology 190:779, 1994.
34. Leng GC, Whyman MR, Donnan PT, et al: Accuracy and reproducibility of duplex ultrasonography in grading femoropopliteal stenoses. J Vasc Surg 17:510, 1993.
35. Cossman D: Comparison of dye arteriography to arterial mapping with color-flow duplex imaging in the lower extremities. J Vasc Surg 10:522, 1989.
36. Ranke C, Creutzig A, Alexander K: Duplex scanning of the peripheral arteries: Correlation of the peak velocity ratio with angiographic diameter reduction. Ultrasound Med Biol 18:433, 1992.
37. Allard L, Cloutier G, Durand LG, et al: Limitations of ultrasonic duplex scanning for diagnosing lower limb arterial stenoses in the presence of adjacent segment disease. J Vasc Surg 19:650, 1994.
38. Moneta GL, Yeager RA, Taylor LM, Jr., et al: Hemodynamic assessment of combined aortoiliac/femoropopliteal occlusive disease and selection of single or multilevel revascularization. Semin Vasc Surg 7:3, 1994.
39. Kinney EV, Bandyk DF, Mewissen MW, et al: Monitoring functional patency of percutaneous transluminal angioplasty. Arch Surg 126: 743, 1991.
40. Ahn S: Reporting standards for lower extremity arterial endovascular procedures. J Vasc Surg 17:1103, 1993.
41. Polak J: Early detection of saphenous vein arterial bypass graft stenosis by color assisted duplex sonography: A prospective study. Am J Roentgenol 154:857, 1990.
42. Polak J: Determinations of the extent of lower extremity peripheral arterial disease with color-assisted duplex sonography: Comparison with angiography. Am J Roentgenol 155:1085, 1990.
43. Mills J, Bandyk D: Surgical management of femoropopliteal occlusive disease. In Breda S (ed): Vascular Diseases: Surgical and Interventional Therapy. New York, Churchill Livingstone, 1994, p. 493.
44. Donaldson M, Mannick J, Whittemore A: Causes of primary graft failure after in situ saphenous vein bypass grafting. J Vasc Surg 15:113, 1992.
45. Bergamini T: Experience with in situ saphenous vein bypasses during 1981 to 1989. Determinant factors of long-term patency. J Vasc Surg 13:137, 1991.
46. Bandyk D: Nature and management of duplex abnormalities encountered during infrainguinal vein bypass grafting. J Vasc Surg 24:430, 1996.
47. Kronzon I: Diagnosis and treatment of iatrogenic femoral artery pseudoaneurysm: A review. J Am Soc Echocardiogr 10:236, 1997.
48. Lacy JH, Box JM, Connors D, et al: Pseudoaneurysm: Diagnosis with color Doppler ultrasound. J Cardiovasc Surg 31:727, 1990.
49. Abu-Yousef MM, Wiese JA, Shamma AR: The "to-and-fro" sign: Duplex Doppler evidence of femoral artery pseudoaneurysm. AJR Am J Roentgenol 150:632, 1988.
50. Toursarkissian B, Allen BT, Petrinec D, et al: Spontaneous closure of selected iatrogenic pseudoaneurysms and arteriovenous fistulae. J Vasc Surg 25:803, 1997.
51. Kent K, McArle C, Kennedy B, et al: A prospective study of the clinical outcome of femoral pseudoaneurysms and arteriovenous fistulas induced by arterial puncture. J Vasc Surg 17:125, 1993.

52. Rivers SP, Lee ES, Lyon RT, et al: Successful conservative management of iatrogenic femoral arterial trauma. Ann Vasc Surg 6:45, 1992.
53. Cox GS, Young JR, Gray BR, et al: Ultrasound-guided compression repair of postcatheterization pseudoaneurysms: Results of treatment in one hundred cases. J Vasc Surg 19:683, 1994.
54. Kang SS, Labropoulos N, Mansour MA, et al: Expanded indications for ultrasound-guided thrombin injection of pseudoaneurysms. J Vasc Surg 31:289, 2000.
55. Mohler ER III, Mitchell ME, Carpenter JP, et al: Therapeutic thrombin injection of pseudoaneurysms: A multicenter experience. Vasc Med 6:241, 2001.
56. La Perna L, Olin JW, Goines D, et al: Ultrasound-guided thrombin injection for the treatment of postcatheterization pseudoaneurysms. Circulation 102:2391, 2000.
57. Taylor BS, Rhee RY, Muluk S, et al: Thrombin injection versus compression of femoral artery pseudoaneurysms. J Vasc Surg 30:1052, 1999.
58. Roubidoux MA, Hertzberg BS, Carroll BA, et al: Color flow and image-directed Doppler ultrasound evaluation of iatrogenic arteriovenous fistulas in the groin. J Clin Ultrasound 18:463, 1990.
59. Rose SC: Noninvasive vascular laboratory for evaluation of peripheral arterial occlusive disease. Part III—Clinical applications: Nonatherosclerotic lower extremity arterial conditions and upper extremity arterial disease. J Vasc Interv Radiol 12:11, 2001.
60. Pinheiro L, Jain S, Nanda NC, et al: Diagnosis of arteriovenous fistula between common iliac artery and vein by color Doppler flow imaging. Am Heart J 122:592, 1991.
61. Polkinghorne KR, McMahon LP, Becker GJ: Pharmacokinetic studies of dalteparin (Fragmin), enoxaparin (Clexane), and danaparoid sodium (Orgaran) in stable chronic hemodialysis patients. Am J Kidney Dis 40:990, 2002.
62. Barnes RW: Noninvasive assessment of arteriovenous fistula. Angiology 29:691, 1978.
63. Joffe HV, Goldhaber SZ: Upper-extremity deep vein thrombosis. Circulation 106:1874, 2002.
64. Lensing AW, Prandoni P, Brandjes D, et al: Detection of deep-vein thrombosis by real-time B-mode ultrasonography. N Engl J Med 320:342, 1989.
65. Raghavendra BN, Horii SC, Hilton S, et al: Deep venous thrombosis: Detection by probe compression of veins. J Ultrasound Med 5:89, 1986.
66. Vogel P, Laing FC, Jeffrey RB, Jr., et al: Deep venous thrombosis of the lower extremity: US evaluation. Radiology 163:747, 1987.
67. Polak JF, Culter SS, O'Leary DH: Deep veins of the calf: Assessment with color Doppler flow imaging. Radiology 171:481, 1989.
68. Dauzat MM, Laroche JP, Charras C, et al: Real-time B-mode ultrasonography for better specificity in the noninvasive diagnosis of deep venous thrombosis. J Ultrasound Med 5:625, 1986.
69. Lohr JM, James KV, Deshmukh RM, et al: Allastair B. Karmody Award. Calf vein thrombi are not a benign finding. Am J Surg 170:86, 1995.
70. Hull RD, Hirsh J, Carter CJ, et al: Pulmonary angiography, ventilation lung scanning, and venography for clinically suspected pulmonary embolism with abnormal perfusion lung scan. Ann Intern Med 98:891, 1983.
71. Kalodiki E, Nicolaides AN: Out of a recent CVI consensus: Some features of a basic statement. Int Angiol 21:2, 2002.
72. Szendro G, Nicolaides AN, Zukowski AJ, et al: Duplex scanning in the assessment of deep venous incompetence. J Vasc Surg 4:237, 1986.
73. van Bemmelen PS, Bedford G, Beach K, et al: Quantitative segmental evaluation of venous valvular reflux with duplex ultrasound scanning. J Vasc Surg 10:425, 1989.
74. Welch HJ, Faliakou EC, McLaughlin RL, et al: Comparison of descending phlebography with quantitative photoplethysmography, air plethysmography, and duplex quantitative valve closure time in assessing deep venous reflux. J Vasc Surg 16:913, 1992.
75. Miyazaki K, Nishibe T, Kudo F, et al: Hemodynamic changes in stripping operation or saphenofemoral ligation of the greater saphenous vein for primary varicose veins. Ann Vasc Surg, 2004.
76. Christopoulos D, Nicolaides AN, Cook A, et al: Pathogenesis of venous ulceration in relation to the calf muscle pump function. Surgery 106:829, 1989.

chapter 11

Magnetic Resonance Imaging

Piotr Sobieszczyk
Martin J. Lipton
E. Kent Yucel

The relatively high incidence of morbidity and the expense associated with traditional x-ray angiography have spurred development of noninvasive methods for safe and accurate imaging of the vascular system. Nephrotoxic contrast agents and ionizing radiation have hindered contrast CT angiography. Duplex ultrasound is operator- and patient body habitus-dependent and limited in many anatomical regions by bowel gas, tissue depth, and bone. Magnetic resonance angiography (MRA), although not without its own limitations, has gained widespread acceptance as the modality of choice for many vascular imaging applications. The rapid growth of this imaging modality is the function of continuing improvements in image acquisition strategies. Contrast-enhanced MRA (CE-MRA) is capable of providing images with high spatial resolution and fewer artifacts during acquisition times that are much shorter than traditional noncontrast MR methods. MR angiography refers to the processing of MRI slices into projectional angiograms, that can be rotated in 3-D.

THE PHYSICS OF MRA

Magnetic resonance imaging uses the inherent magnetic properties of human tissue and the ability of contrast agents to alter them. MR imaging depends on the detection of magnetic moment created by single protons in the omnipresent hydrogen atoms. Because any moving electrical charge produces a magnetic field, spinning protons produce small magnetic fields and can be thought of as little magnets or "spins." When a patient is placed in the bore of a large magnet (i.e., MR scanner) hydrogen protons align with the externally applied, static magnetic field (B_0) to create a net magnetization vector. On a quantum level, most protons will distribute randomly either with or against the scanner's B_0, canceling each other out. However, a slight excess of spins aligns with the field causing net magnetization of the tissue. The time needed for this alignment to take place is described by the longitudinal relaxation time, T1, and is one of the MR features that varies between tissues and can be used as a basis of MR contrast.

Spinning protons wobble or "precess" about the axis of B_0. The frequency of the wobble is proportional to the strength of B_0. If a radio frequency (RF) pulse is applied at the resonance frequency of the wobble, protons can absorb energy and jump to a higher energy state. This RF pulse deflects the protons, and thus the net magnetization vector, away from the major axis of the applied magnetic field. The net magnetization vector tips from longitudinal to the transverse plane (transverse magnetization). The protons are "flipped" by the RF pulse and the net magnetization vector is deflected by a "flip angle." The stronger the RF applied, the greater the angle of deflection for the magnetization. Common flip angles for spin echo are 90° and 180°; for gradient echo MRI, flip angles typically range between 10° and 70°. After the RF pulse tips the spins out of alignment with the main magnetic field, new protons begin to align with the main magnetic field at a rate determined by the T1 relaxation time.

Energy is given off as the spins go from the high to low energy states. The absorbed RF energy is retransmitted at the resonance frequency and can be detected with RF antennas or coils placed around the patient. These signals make up the MR images. The process of excitation of protons with externally applied RF field is repeated at short intervals to form images. This MR parameter is referred to as the time of repetition or TR. For conventional anatomic MR imaging, TR is typically 0.5 to 2 seconds, whereas in MRA, TR ranges from 30 msec to less than 5 msec.

When the spins are tipped to the transverse plane, they are all precessing in phase. The speed of wobbling depends on the strength of the magnetic field that the proton experiences. Some protons spin faster whereas others spin slower, and they quickly get out of phase relative to each other. As this process of dephasing takes place, the MR signal fades away and decays. This loss of phase is termed T2 relaxation time or transverse relaxation. T2, like T1, is unique for every type of tissue and provides an additional basis for contrast on MR images.

In addition to the intrinsic T2 of tissue, inhomogenicity of B_0 results in rapid loss of transverse magnetization. The relaxation time that reflects the sum of these random defects with tissue T2 is called T2*. In order to obtain an MRI signal, these spins must be brought back in phase, producing a signal, or echo. The time at which it happens is referred to as echo time (TE). In spin echo imaging technique, the echo is obtained by using a refocusing 180° RF pulse. As soon as the spins are back in phase, they start to go out of phase again. Another 180° RF pulse can be applied to generate a second echo and so on. Signal loss at longer echo times reflects tissue T2. In gradient echo imaging, the echo is obtained by gradient reversal rather than a radiofrequency pulse. Because this includes effects from tissue homogenicity, TE-dependent signal loss reflects T2*. Recently, gradient echo sequences (balanced gradient echo, steady-state free precession [SSFP]) have been developed which are insensitive to magnet field inhomogeneities and reflective of actual tissue T2.

Longitudinal and transverse magnetizations occur simultaneously but are two different processes that reflect properties of various tissues in the body. Because T1 is a measure of signal recovery, tissues with short T1 are bright, whereas tissues with long T1 are dark. Fat has a very short T1. Because T2 is a measure of signal loss, tissues with short T2 are dark and those with long T2 are bright. Simple fluids, such as cerebrospinal fluid and urine, have the longest T2. To differentiate between the tissues based on these relaxation times, MR images can be designed to be T1-weighted, T2-weighted, or proton-density weighted. If there is little intrinsic difference in contrast between structures, exogenous contrast agents can be used to improve sensitivity and specificity of MR.

To form an actual MR image, the signals obtained from tissues must be localized in space. Additional external, time-varying magnetic fields are applied to spatially encode the MR signal and form cross-sectional images. Here gradients are required to fully define the location of the MR signal in space. In 2-D MRI, these are slice-selection, frequency-encoding, and phase-encoding gradients. In 3-D MRI, the slice-selection gradient is replaced by second phase-encoding gradient.

The echoes are digitized and stored in a data acquisition matrix called k-space. This is composed of two axes in 2-D MRI (frequency and phase-encoding) and three axes in 3-D MRI (frequency and two phase-encoding). The number of lines in each direction of the matrix determines the resolution of the image. Fourier transformation is used to convert the k-space data into a familiar image by breaking a signal into a sum of sine waves with various frequencies, phases, and amplitudes. An important feature of k-space is that tissue contrast is determined by the center of k-space (central phase encoding lines), whereas the periphery of the k-space encodes the image detail. The order in which k-space lines are collected can be varied and strongly influences tissue contrast. For example, in contrast-enhanced MRA, the central, contrast-defining portion of k-space may be acquired early in the scan (centric acquisition) during peak intra-arterial contrast concentration to maximize arterial contrast. In addition to simple, line-by-line k-space acquisition schemes, more complex schemes have been described, such as spiral k-space imaging, which starts acquiring data in the center of the k-space and then moves out to the periphery in a spiral trajectory.

Slice-selective gradients applied along the z-axis will form axial images; those along the y-axis will yield coronal images, and the x-axis gradients will provide sagittal images. An oblique slice can be selected by a combination of two or more gradients. The ability to image in arbitrary planes is a feature of MRI that differentiates it from CT.

MR Angiography Techniques

MR angiography relies on selective imaging of moving blood in multiple, thin cross-sectional slices. A series of contiguous slices may then be assembled to encompass the anatomic volume of interest. Signals from the blood vessels are maximized, whereas signals from the stationary tissues are suppressed. This allows the use of computer reconstruction algorithms to reformat images from a volume of tissue into images similar to those provided by conventional x-ray angiography (Table 11-1).

Two basic MRA imaging modalities depict blood as either black or white. The most traditional "black blood"

TABLE 11-1 TYPES OF MRA SEQUENCES

Name of Sequence	Description	2D or 3D	Gating Useful	Flow Quantification Possible	Applications
Time of flight	Bright vessels produced by inflow of blood with full magnetization into a slice or volume where the magnetization has been reduced by radiofrequency saturation	Both	Occasionally	No	Intracranial, carotid, pedal
Phase contrast	Bright vessels produced by the application of flow encoding radiofrequency pulses that produce a phase image where intensity is proportional to velocity	Both	Occasionally	Yes	None in current practice
Dynamic contrast-enhanced	Bright vessels produced by the rapid infusion of gadolinium contrast with timing of the scan to arterial and/or venous transit; mask subtraction may be used	3D	No	No	Carotid, chest, abdomen, extremity runoff
Post-contrast	Bright vessels produced by equilibrium enhancement of gadolinium contrast with fat saturation	Both	No	No	Veins, aorta
Black blood	Dark vessels produced by the use of an inversion prepulse to null the signal of blood based on its T1 recovery time	2D	Necessary	No	Plaque imaging

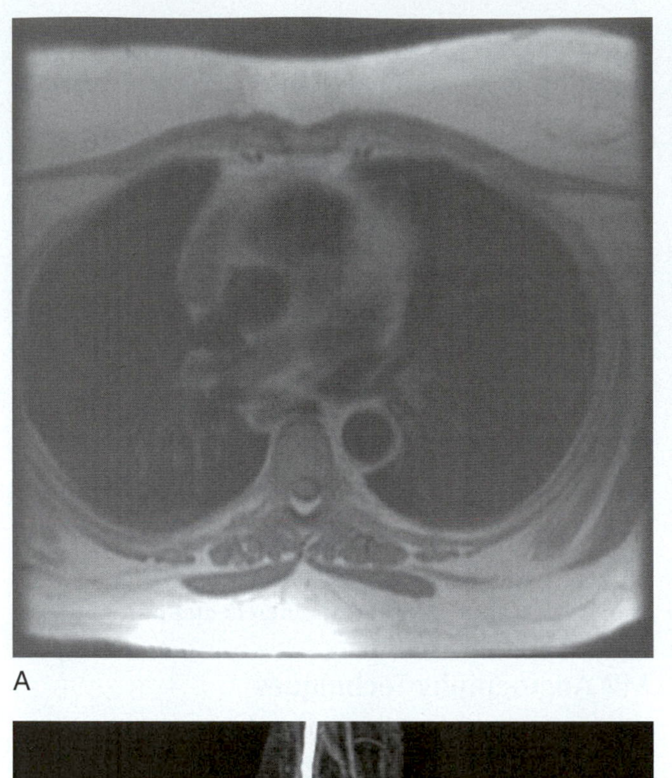
A

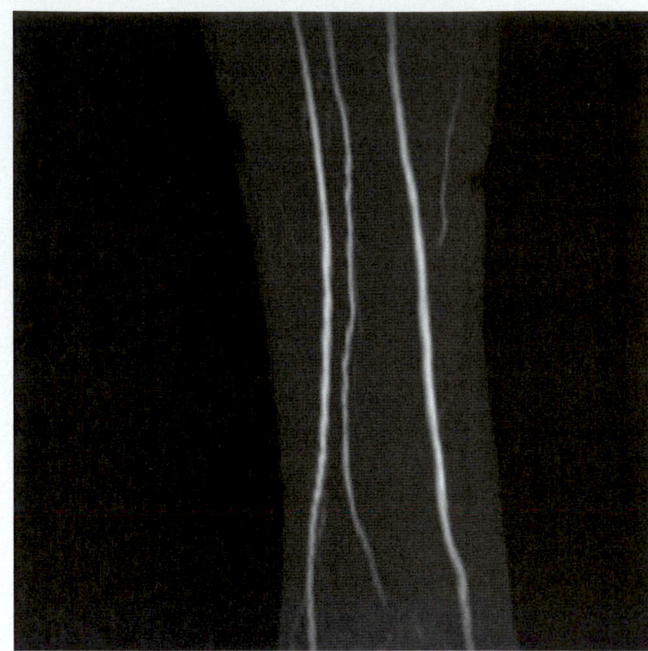
B

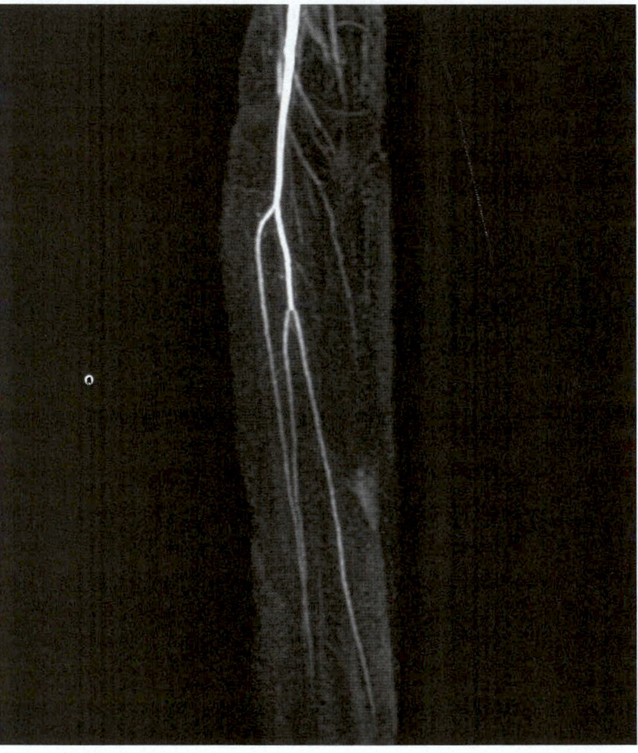
C

FIGURE 11-1. "Black blood" and "bright blood" imaging techniques. **A,** shows a cross-sectional T1-weighted image of the ascending and descending aorta. The lumen appears black. **B,** shows a time of flight (TOF) image of the tibial arteries. The vessel lumen appears bright. **C,** shows a gadolinium-enhanced image of the popliteal artery and its trifurcation into tibial arteries.

technique uses standard spin echo (SE) sequences (Fig. 11-1A). The excitation RF pulse is applied at 90° and is followed by a refocusing pulse at 180°. If the imaging slice cuts across a vessel, then, depending on the flow velocity and time interval between the pulses, the blood volume originally excited by the first pulse may not "see" the second pulse. This results in a black-appearing signal void in the vessel lumen. Selecting thin sections or long echo times can further emphasize this flow void. This technique allows detailed examination of the arterial wall morphology. Fast spin echo sequences, where a long train of echoes is obtained by use of repeated 180° pulses, produce images more rapidly. A new generation of black blood sequences is the double inversion-recovery fast spin echo approach. This uses two consecutive inversion pulses, the first to null or blacken the blood everywhere in the coil and the second to restore magnetization in the slice being imaged. Between these pulses and image production, blood within the slice is replaced by nulled blood from outside. This produces more reliable black blood than conventional approaches, making this sequence ideal for examining wall thickness, dissection flaps, and the presence of mural thrombus or inflammation.[1] This provides a clear advantage over traditional x-ray angiography.

"Bright blood" MRA techniques use gradient echo (GRE) sequences and are generally divided into those measuring signal amplitude (time of flight, TOF) and those based on phase effects (phase contrast, PC). In each GRE sequence, a single RF pulse is applied in short time intervals, eliminating signal loss due to flow void. The stationary protons occupying a given tissue slice do not have sufficient time to relax to their equilibrium state.

TOF-MRA techniques depend on the inflow of unsaturated protons in blood from outside the field of view (FOV) into the stationary tissue within a section that is already saturated by its exposure to repeated RF pulses. These "saturated" protons are unable to contribute signal to the image. The signals in the stationary tissues of gradient echo images used in MRA are, therefore, typically low. The "unsaturated" protons in blood flowing into the imaging plane have not experienced the RF pulses and yield maximum signal: the unsaturated blood appears bright compared with the background tissue (see Fig. 11-1B). The time required for the blood to flow through an image slice and the effect that has on blood's signal is known as TOF. Saturation of signals can occur in vessels with slow-moving blood due to repeated RF excitation in the acquisition plane. This can create artifacts in vessels with stenotic lesions or reduced blood flow.

TOF techniques can be obtained in 2-D or 3-D. The 2-D TOF uses multiple sequentially acquired overlapping thin slices to form an image. It can be obtained during the breath-hold to minimize motion artifact. However, spatial misregistration can occur as patients cannot hold their breath at the same level each time and typically only one to two slices are acquired per breath-hold. 2-D TOF has good sensitivity for identifying vessels with slow flow because blood must move only 3 to 5 mm to refresh a slice. 3-D TOF consists of gradient echo acquisition of a volume into which blood is flowing. The advantage of this technique is higher signal-to-noise ratio and improved resolution. The thick volumes of tissue imaged require rapid flow to fully refresh signals within the arteries. It is thus flow dependent and fails in areas of low flow. It is superior in vessels with rapid, steady flow without respiratory motion. Additional saturation pulses can be applied to eliminate signal from veins. Segmented gradient echo sequence with cardiac triggering can be used to eliminate arterial pulsation artifacts.

A successful TOF image requires the section thickness to be thin enough to allow for sufficient inflow between RF pulse repetitions, but thick enough to ensure adequate signal-to-noise ratio (SNR) and anatomic coverage. Section thickness of 3 to 4 mm is used for large vessels and section thickness of 1 to 2 mm is used for smaller vessels. Spatial presaturation pulses are applied above or below the imaged slice or volume to eliminate unwanted signal from arteries or veins, depending on which part of the vascular tree is being imaged. Optimal TR for TOF is 20 to 50 milliseconds. Short TR keeps background tissues saturated, but it must be long enough to allow for satisfactory inflow of unsaturated blood between successive repetitions. The best flip angle is usually 30° to 60°. With phasic flow in the extremities, systolic flow signal may be increased (because of greater transverse magnetization created) and the distal flow may be decreased creating view-to-view intensity changes and phase artifacts from pulsatile variations. This pulsation artifact is greatest at higher flip angles. Cardiac gating can be used to minimize these artifacts at the expense of increased imaging time.

While TOF uses differences in the signal amplitude to differentiate between stationary and flowing spins, phase contrast technique (PC) observes the phase shifts of signals. Moving spins experience different phase shifts in the presence of the applied magnetic fields used in MRA. The strength and orientation of the applied magnetic field are varied to encode different phase shifts for flowing protons relative to stationary protons. The faster the spins are moving, the greater is their phase shift, and protons of flowing blood may be discriminated from stationary protons. The phase shifts result in a contrast between moving and stationary tissues and form the basis for phase contrast imaging. Pairs of images are acquired that have different sensitivities to flow and are then subtracted to cancel background signal, leaving only the signal from flowing blood. Phase shift is proportional to the velocity, allowing flow quantification with this modality. PC acquisitions may be acquired in 2-D or 3-D. Phase-contrast, although used rarely in angiography today, offers a reliable way to quantify the amount and direction of flow. PC requires long imaging times: two data sets in each direction are acquired by using flow-encoding gradients of opposite polarity and up to three measurements in the orthogonal planes are needed to image flow in all directions.

The visualization of the arterial system with these techniques (PC and TOF) is adequate[2] but has limitations. The acquisition times can be long and prevent imaging within the time span of a single breath-hold. This increases the chance of movement artifacts. Some of the limitations are caused by flow-related artifacts such as in plane saturation and phase dispersion. Flow-based imaging also has limits in areas of slow flow such as aneurysms. Overgrading of stenotic lesions is most commonly a manifestation of signal loss in the areas of complex flow. Undergrading is a matter of inadequate spatial resolution. Complex, turbulent flow pattern in areas of stenoses can create signal loss and mimic a critical lesion. This is due to "intravoxel dephasing." An accelerated flow across a stenosis consists of a wide distribution of velocities and, thus, a large distribution of proton phases. In the smallest volume element, "voxel" of the image, this distribution of phases can result in cancellation rather than coherent addition of signals and accounts for the presence of signal voids at the site of stenosis. A short echo time TE minimizes flow-phase dispersion artifacts. Phase dispersion is further decreased when voxel size is minimized using thin sections. Small voxels and short TE are most easily obtained with 3-D TOF methods, but the biggest drawback of the thick volumes used with 3-D techniques is that slow or recirculating flow can become saturated. The MOTSA (multiple overlapping thin-slab acquisitions) technique of sequential 3-D TOF gives better flow enhancement than single slab 3-D TOF techniques and less dephasing than 2-D techniques. Its drawback is the need for substantial overlap of adjacent slabs, which increases the acquisition time.

The introduction of CE-MRA has revolutionized MR angiography.[3,4] This technique overcomes many of the limitations of traditional "bright blood" modalities: respiratory motion artifacts, poor SNR, flow and saturation-related artifacts (see Fig. 11-1C). Gadolinium increases the signal intensity of blood on contrast enhanced 3-D T1-weighted (spoiled) gradient echo images. Blood contrast is not flow dependent. It is determined by the concentration of contrast agent within the arterial system while imaging data are being collected. Reliable images can be acquired irrespective of whether flow is laminar, turbulent, or stagnant. This technique acquires large-volume data sets in coronal or sagittal orientation within a single breath-hold during the first pass of the contrast material. The contrast agent, gadolinium, is a heavy metal but becomes inert when bound to a chelator. Intravenous administration of gadolinium-DTPA results in a marked reduction of the T1 or longitudinal relaxation time of blood and, therefore, reduces the effects of spin saturation—so problematic in the 3-D TOF sequences. Moreover, the very short TE reduces spin dephasing and allows accurate evaluation of vascular stenoses.

Multiple refinements have resulted in a technique that is much faster than TOF-MRA. The development of high-performance gradient systems with ultra-short repetition TR and TE has shortened the acquisition time in CE-MRA to allow imaging within a single breath-hold and to minimize motion artifacts. Administration of agents shortening T1 allows selective visualization of contrast-containing structures and better visualization of circuitous collaterals. Digital subtraction, spoiling, and fat saturation techniques suppress background signal and enhance the signal from the contrast agent in the vessels. The subtracted data sets can be post-processed to provide 3-D projectional images. The CE-MRA still provides a luminogram, and conventional or fast SE images are needed for a complete study so that the true lumen diameter and presence of thrombus can be established.

Optimal images are generated when gadolinium concentration is highest in the vessel of interest. To make blood bright compared with background tissues, the gadolinium bolus must be administered in a way that ensures the majority of the contrast to be present in the arterial tree. This requires exact timing of the arrival of the gadolinium bolus. Acquisition prior to contrast arrival creates a "ringing" artifact, whereas late acquisition creates venous and tissue enhancement contaminating the arterial signal. This is especially problematic in MRA of the extremities, where the images are obtained in multiple segments. Contrast transit time can be affected by low cardiac output, valvular regurgitation, large abdominal aneurysms, and flow-limiting stenoses. Proper timing can be achieved by an empiric estimation of transit time or a test bolus in the anatomic field of interest. Alternatively, with automated triggering, a pulse sequence can be designed to sense the arrival of contrast and automatically trigger image acquisition. MR fluoroscopy allows the user to visualize the arrival of the contrast bolus directly on the image and manually trigger the start of the scan. Larger doses of contrast are needed for the longer acquisition times used in areas that require higher spatial resolution, such as the lower extremities.

Imaging during the arterial phase of gadolinium infusion takes advantage of higher arterial SNR and eliminates overlapping venous enhancement. This is a brief moment in time, but several methods allow slower MR acquisition to capture that moment. Phase reordering (mapping k-space) technique acquires central k-space data (i.e., the low spatial frequency data) when contrast concentration in arteries is high, but relatively lower in veins. This allows a relatively long MR acquisition to achieve the image contrast associated with the shorter arterial phase of the contrast bolus. It is critical to time contrast bolus for maximum arterial gadolinium concentration during acquisition of central k-space data.

Contrast-enhanced MRA is limited by venous and soft tissue enhancement. It not only passes into venous structures, dependent on the arteriovenous transit time of the tissue, but also rapidly leaks out of the vascular compartment creating significant tissue enhancement. New "blood pool" agents, which are currently undergoing clinical trials, are retained within blood vessels and selectively enhance the blood pool on T1-weighted MR images. These use either gadolinium compounds that bind to albumin or are large enough to stay within the vascular space or ultra-small iron particle. Another agent, gadobenate, has higher T1 relaxivity because of its capacity for weak and transient interaction with serum albumin and may be expected to provide greater vascular signal intensity enhancement and, hence, greater diagnostic efficacy at doses comparable with those used for the current gadolinium agents. It is approved for imaging use in Europe but is under clinical investigation in the United States. It provides a higher and longer-lasting vascular signal enhancement in the abdominal aorta compared with gadolinium, which does not interact with proteins.[5]

Metal objects, such as surgical clips, can lead to artifacts in MRA. The increasing use of stents in the arterial tree has important implications for MRA. Cavagna and colleagues evaluated CE-MRA imaging of seven stent types in aortic, iliac, and popliteal positions.[6] Only a few of the commonly used stents permitted visualization of the lumen. Stents containing ferromagnetic metals create significant susceptibility artifacts. This results in significant signal loss and precludes proper visualization of the stent lumen even with gadolinium-enhanced MRA. Some nitinol, tantalum, or polytetrafluoroethylene based devices, on the other hand, have been shown to have decreased artifact on CE-MRA.

Post-Processing Techniques

The superiority of MRA rests in its ability to display vessels in a projective format similar to standard x-ray angiography. Post-processing techniques of 2-D or 3-D gradient echo data produce images in any desired plane and improve evaluation of overlapping vessels (Table 11-2).

TABLE 11-2 TYPES OF POST-PROCESSING TECHNIQUES

Technique	Description
Multiplanar reformatting (MPR)	Production of cross-sectional images in planes different from the acquisition plane
Maximum intensity pixel (MIP) projection	Production of full- or partial-volume projection images along any desired axis from a stack of image slices
Volume rendering	Manipulation of MRI slices to produce full volumetric images; structures segmented for viewing by the application of intensity thresholds and removal of unwanted structures

The origins of the left common carotid artery and the left subclavian artery, for example, overlap in frontal projection, whereas the origins of the right subclavian artery and the right common carotid artery overlap in the oblique views. Similarly, the origins of the renal arteries are best seen in the frontal or slightly oblique views, whereas the celiac and superior mesenteric arteries are best seen on lateral projections. X-ray angiography requires multiple injections to assess the origins of these vessels, whereas MRA post-processing techniques allow rotation of the image to the desired viewing angle.

The maximum intensity projection (MIP) is the most common reconstruction technique (Fig. 11-2A). In the first step, multiple thin MRA slices are obtained and arranged sequentially to cover the anatomic volume of interest. The maximum intensity projection algorithm then selects the brightest pixel in a projection at any arbitrary angle chosen by the operator to create a projection image. By reduction of pixel size and suppression of the signal of stationary tissue, the quality of MIP can be substantially improved. The reduction of pixel size is accomplished by use of large acquisition matrix along a smaller field of view. The technique fails in areas of poor flow contrast, such as margins of blood vessels and small vessels with reduced flow, which may be obscured by overlap with brighter stationary tissue. The lower intensity features of blood vessels may be lost and the apparent vessel lumen may be falsely narrowed, overestimating a stenosis or limiting visualization of small vessels. MIP images can also imitate stenoses at the site of surgical clips. It is thus imperative to always review the source images.

Multiplanar reformats (MPR) are frequently used as a rapid problem-solving tool. They are tomograms produced in a plane different from that of the acquisition. They are best suited to 3-D acquisitions where resolution is comparable in all directions and especially useful for contrast-enhanced MRA where the acquisition plane is chosen to maximize scanning efficiency rather than optimal vessel display.

Shaded-surface display (SSD) generates a binary image when contiguous voxels above a preset threshold are modeled as a single structure with depth relationships depicted by shading from an imaginary light source, giving a 3-D appearance (see Fig. 11-2B and C). This requires extensive editing to produce images of high quality. An incorrect setting of a threshold may imply or remove lesions, but the advantage of this technique lies in its excellent anatomic detail. The volume rendering post-processing technique provides high-quality 3-D images. It is a two-step process consisting of classification and rendering. The classification step determines tissue types and assigns brightness levels and colors to each voxel, creating a voxel intensity histogram. Rendering stage involves image projection to form a simulated 3-D image. Relative voxel attenuation is then conveyed using gray scale in the final image. These techniques require the use of advanced image-processing workstations and can take substantial operator time. For these reasons, because of its lower dependence on operator skill, and because of the high vessel-background contrast available with MRA, MIP and MPR are usually the post-processing methods of choice for MRA images. SSD and volume rendering are reserved for special situations where their display capabilities outweigh the effort required to produce them.

CLINICAL APPLICATIONS

Extracranial Carotid Arteries

The most common pathologic processes affecting the extracranial carotid arteries are atherosclerosis, inflammatory diseases of the arterial wall, and dissection (see Chapter 29). Of these, atherosclerosis is by far the most common and affects primarily the carotid bifurcation. 2-D and 3-D TOF methods as well as CE-MRA have been used in imaging the carotid arteries (Fig. 11-3). 2-D TOF excels in identifying areas of slow flow and distinguishes near from complete arterial occlusion. 3-D TOF, on the other hand, has much better resolution but fails in areas of slow flow. Turbulent flow in the carotid bifurcation, where most of the lesions occur, can cause artifacts in TOF and overestimate lesion severity. CE-MRA has mostly replaced the noncontrast techniques. The transcranial blood flow is remarkable for the rapid arteriovenous transit time. For this reason, venous superimposition can severely limit CE-MRA in this vascular bed. A number of techniques have been developed within CE-MRA to solve this problem. The dynamic or time-resolved variant of CE-MRA accelerates image acquisition and reduces the venous signal contamination. Unfortunately, poor spatial resolution of this technique limits its clinical use. Nevertheless, in some studies this technique reached a sensitivity of 98% and specificity of 86% for stenoses greater than 70%.[7] CE-MRA with linear k-space ordering and fluoroscopic triggering, as well as CE-MRA with elliptical centric k-space ordering have recently become the techniques of choice in carotid MRA. When these techniques are used, CE-MRA achieves a sensitivity of 100% and specificities of 84% to 100% for stenoses and 70% to 99% for vascular occlusion. The low specificity of CE-MRA is due to stenosis overestimation by MRA.[8] In a community setting, CE-MRA achieved sensitivity of 92% and specificity of 62%, misclassifying lesions by overcalling

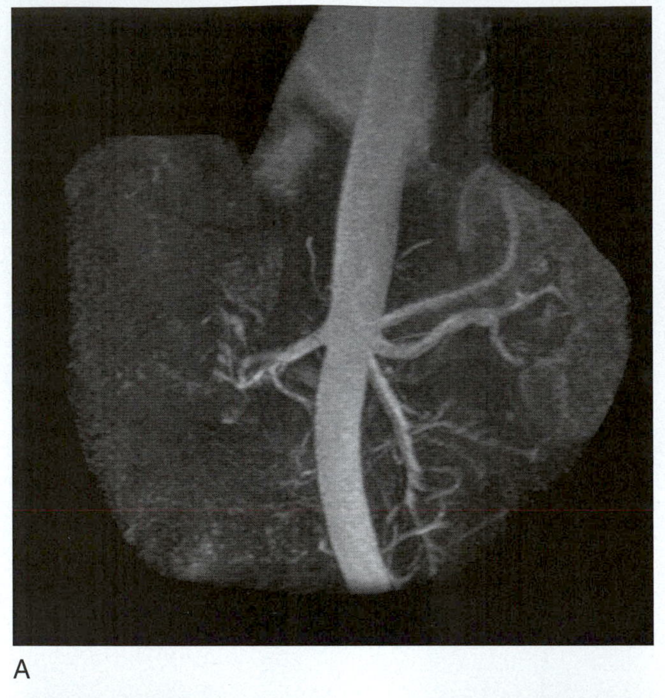
A

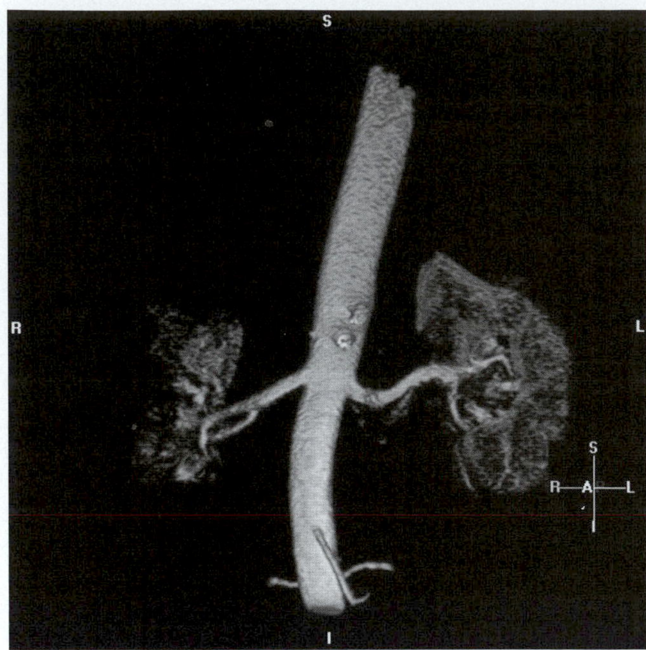

B

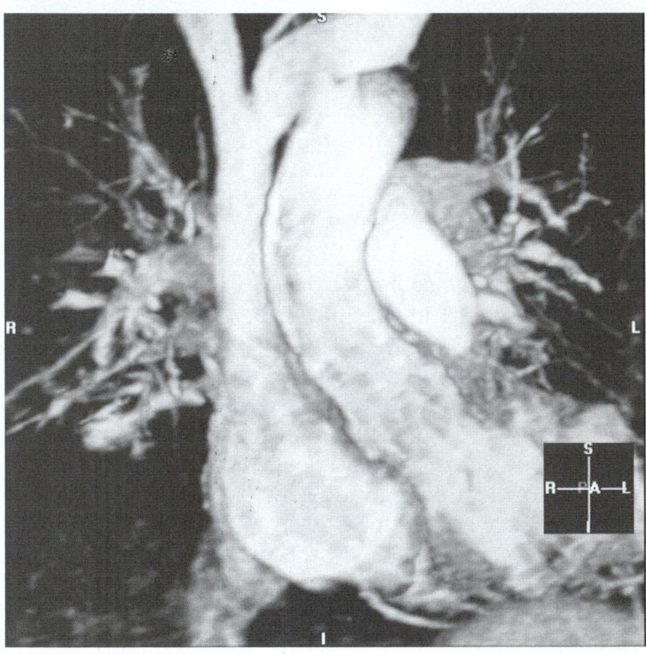

C

FIGURE 11-2. Post-processing techniques. **A,** shows a maximum intensity projection (MIP) reconstruction of the abdominal aorta. **B,** shows a surface-shaded post-processing of the same vessel. **C,** shows a shaded surface reconstruction of the heart.

the severity of stenosis in 24% of studies.[9] An overall assessment of MRA accuracy in carotid artery evaluation is made difficult by the ever-changing technology and heterogeneity of study methods and patient characteristics. Nevertheless, a recent meta-analysis evaluated 26 studies using contrast and noncontrast techniques and confirmed a high sensitivity and specificity for detecting 70% to 99% stenosis.[10] Source images must be reviewed carefully to avoid overestimation of the lesion severity in an area of turbulent flow. The best tool for initial investigation of carotid artery stenosis is still duplex ultrasound—but in cases with positive or unclear findings, CE-MRA is an excellent adjunctive test.

Thoracic Aorta and its Branches

The ever-increasing speed of 3-D CE-MRA allows imaging of the thoracic aorta to be performed within a single breath-hold. ECG gating permits synchronization of data acquisition with the cardiac cycle. These advances have

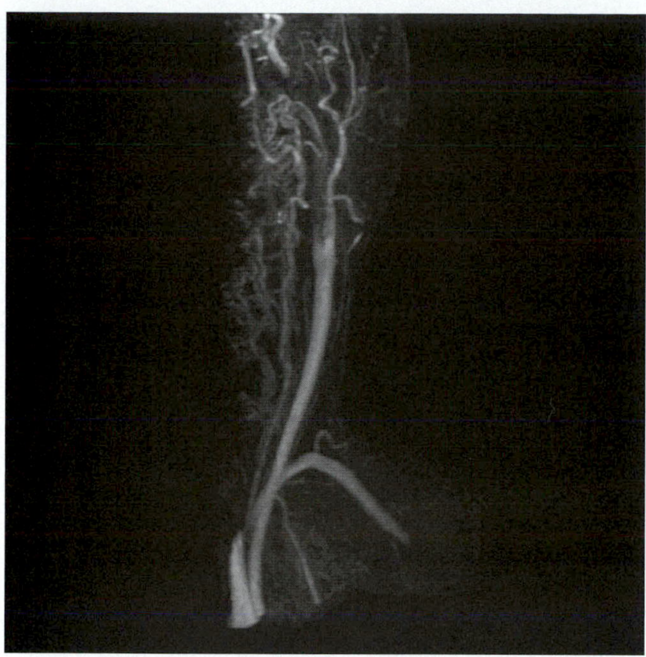

FIGURE 11-3. Carotid artery disease. The left internal carotid artery dissection resulted in a thrombotic occlusion of the proximal vessel. The internal carotid artery reconstitutes more distally.

eliminated motion artifacts and propelled MRA as the imaging modality of choice for evaluation of the thoracic aorta in a stable patient.

Aortic Dissection

Among the four imaging modalities used in the diagnosis of aortic dissection (see Chapter 34), MRA has the highest sensitivity and specificity in diagnosing types A and B aortic dissections. Similarly, it is 100% sensitive for detection of intramural hematoma.[11] MRA offers information beyond the mere diagnosis of dissection. Multiplanar reconstructions identify the location and extent of the intimal tear and its relationship to the branch vessels. Cine images of the proximal aorta can identify aortic regurgitation complicating type A dissection. Cross-sectional delayed phase images allow identification of aortic wall pathology such as intramural hematoma or ulceration. On T1-weighted spin-echo sequences, the intramural hematoma can be seen as a concentric thickening of the wall with increased intramural signal intensity. Inflammatory changes can be seen as arterial wall enhancement. Magnetic resonance imaging is superior to conventional CT in differentiating acute intramural hematoma from atherosclerotic plaque and chronic intraluminal thrombus.[12] It is also well suited for evaluation of penetrating atherosclerotic ulcers, defined as ulcerated atherosclerotic lesions penetrating the elastic lamina and forming a hematoma within the media of the aortic wall. This condition is distinct from the classic aortic dissection and aortic rupture. Although life-threatening complications such as aortic rupture are rare, patients with penetrating atherosclerotic ulcers must be closely followed, particularly during the first month after diagnosis. Signs of expanding intramural hematoma or impending rupture, as well as inability to control pain and blood pressure changes, should prompt surgical treatment.[12]

Comprehensive aortic magnetic resonance examinations of the thoracic aorta currently include multiple nonenhanced and contrast-enhanced sequences, that hinder prompt evaluation of unstable, acutely ill patients. Recent reports suggest the noncontrast MRA techniques can determine the presence or absence of aortic dissection with 100% accuracy in less than 4 minutes.[13] The constraints of time and local expertise, however, make CT a more appropriate technique in initial evaluation of an unstable patient. MRA, however, plays an important role in the long-term follow-up of patients with surgically or medically managed disease of the thoracic aorta.[14]

Thoracic Aortic Aneurysm

Imaging of any arterial aneurysm requires consideration of the slow flow through the lesion. Long contrast travel time has to be anticipated to allow filling of the entire aorta. MRA can demonstrate the location and size of an aneurysm, presence of a mural thrombus, and its relationship to the branch vessels (Fig. 11-4). The 3-D CE-MRA provides a luminogram and, just like conventional angiograms, can underestimate the size of an aneurysm. Cross-sectional spin-echo images are thus crucial in evaluating aneurysmal size. The accuracy of CE-MRA in the diagnosis of thoracic aortic aneurysm has been well established.[15,16]

Arch Vessel Disease

Occlusive disease of the great vessels is usually a consequence of atherosclerosis. Vasculitis, fibromuscular dysplasia, and radiation arteriopathy also can lead to branch vessel stenoses with symptoms of upper extremity claudications, subclavian steal, or cerebrovascular ischemia. The ability to rotate MIP projections in 3-D allows precise evaluation of the branch vessel origin, free of confounding effects of the overlying vessels (Fig. 11-5). CE-MRA is a well-established tool for rapid and accurate definition of brachiocephalic and subclavian artery occlusive disease.[17] CE-MRA has a potential pitfall in that susceptibility effects associated with high concentrations of contrast in the subclavian vein after ipsilateral arm injection can decrease subclavian artery signal. This may be misinterpreted as subclavian artery disease. For this reason, right arm injection is generally preferred, unless clinical concern is focused on the right subclavian artery.

Congenital Abnormalities

Developmental abnormalities of the arch and aortic coarctation are depicted well on MRA (see Chapter 65). Aortic coarctation, the most common congenital abnormality, appears as a discrete narrowing of the aorta distal to the left subclavian artery. MRA has been validated against x-ray angiography and is especially helpful in assessing anatomy of a tortuous aorta and numerous collaterals accompanying the coarctation.[18] A complete 3-D view of the coarctation allows rotation around the

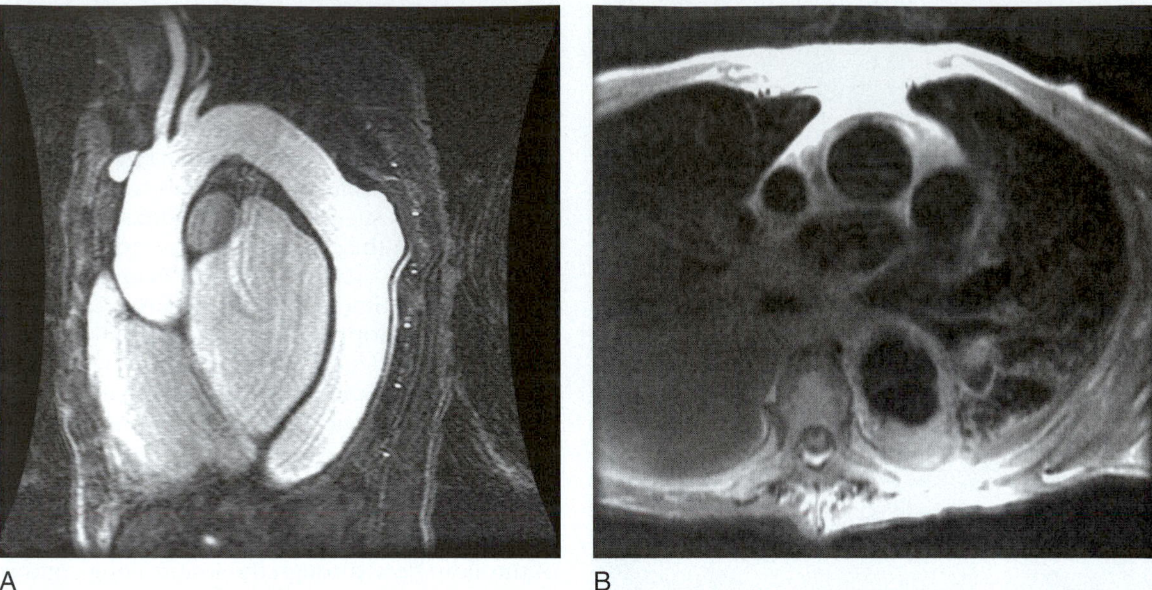

FIGURE 11-4. Thoracic aortic aneurysm. **A,** shows gadolinium-enhanced image of a descending aortic aneurysm. **B,** a T1-weighted cross-sectional image shows eccentric thrombus lining the arterial wall of the descending aorta.

lesion and visualization of the relationship with the adjacent structures. Collateral flow assessment with MR velocity mapping can accurately evaluate the hemodynamic importance of a coarctation.[19] Cine MR imaging also permits diagnosis of a bicuspid valve and possible aortic stenosis, frequently associated with coarctation. Such additional information is crucial for planning therapy. MRA also provides a noninvasive modality for regular follow-up of patients with previous intervention for coarctation, to screen for re-coarctation or aneurysm formation.[20]

MRA also can distinguish between coarctation and pseudocoarctation. Pseudocoarctation is a rare, asymptomatic anomaly in the descending thoracic aorta and is characterized by an elongated, redundant thoracic aorta with buckling distal to the origin of the left subclavian artery. It is of no hemodynamic importance and there is no pressure gradient across the buckled segment. It has been regarded as a benign condition although several reports demonstrate that complications may occur.[21] Therefore, close follow-up of patients with pseudocoarctation is indicated.

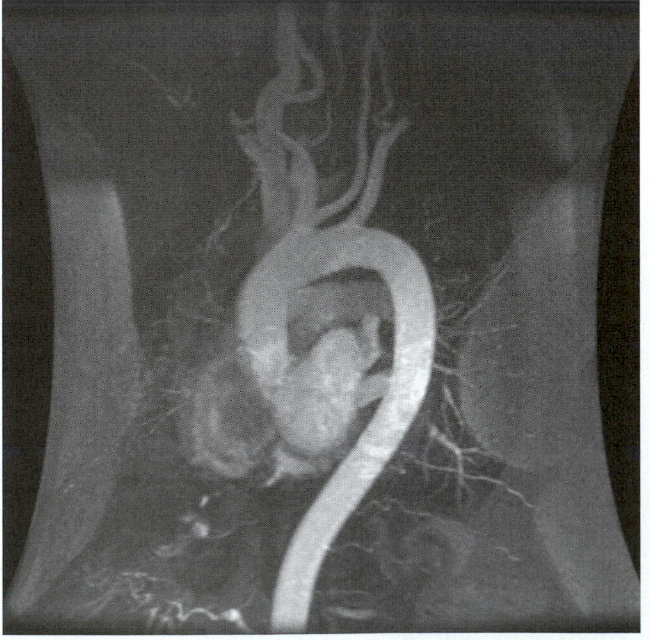

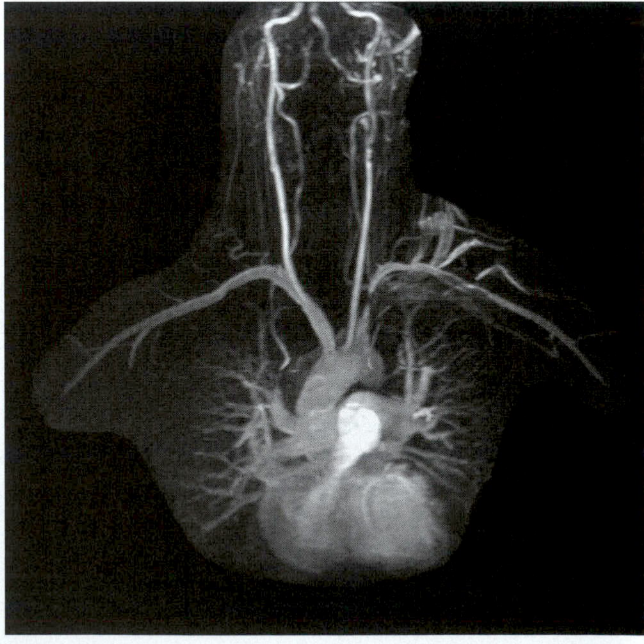

FIGURE 11-5. A, shows a gadolinium-enhanced image of the aortic arch and the great vessels. **B,** shows a maximum intensity projection (MIP) reconstruction of the aortic arch and stenosis of the proximal left subclavian artery in a patient with atherosclerosis.

Thoracic Outlet Syndrome

Thoracic outlet syndrome results from the compression of the neurovascular bundle as it leaves the thoracic inlet (see Chapter 64). The neurovascular bundle is composed of the subclavian artery, the subclavian vein, and the brachial plexus. The symptoms of thoracic outlet or inlet syndrome are most often caused by compression of the nerves of the brachial plexus, which is involved in up to 98% of cases. The remainder may be due to vascular compression. MRI and MRA accurately demonstrate the anatomy of the brachial plexus, as well as any arterial or venous compression or occlusion.[22] Imaging during abduction and adduction of the arm can confirm the clinical diagnosis of vascular compression. The relationship of the vascular structures to the first rib and subclavius muscle can be defined for treatment purposes.[23]

Pulmonary Vessels

The increasing use of radiofrequency ablation for treatment of atrial fibrillation has enlisted MRA for preprocedural definition of pulmonary vein anatomy and post-procedural surveillance of stenotic complications.[24] MRA allows accurate assessments of the number, location, and size of the pulmonary veins—information crucial for planning electrophysiologic procedures (Fig. 11-6).

Diagnosis of pulmonary embolus using MRA is attractive in theory, but has not been widely accepted. It is not readily available in the emergency setting and requires breath-holding longer than that with CTA. It is very accurate for large, proximal thrombi but so far has lacked the resolution for small, distal thrombi.[25,26] It is not the optimal tool in an unstable patient unless contrast allergy or renal failure precludes the use of CT. Other pulmonary arterial lesions, such as aneurysms and stenotic lesions, are well suited for MRA imaging.

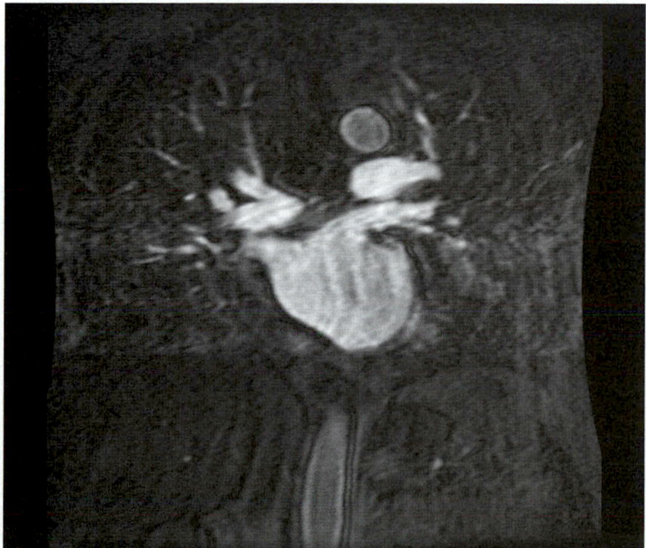

FIGURE 11-6. Left atrium. Coronal slice of the left atrium showing the size and location of the superior pulmonary veins.

Peripheral Arterial Disease of the Lower and Upper Extremities

Peripheral arterial disease (PAD) is most commonly due to atherosclerosis (see Chapters 14 and 17). Patients referred for MRA typically have claudication or nonhealing vascular ulcers. Claudication implies arterial flow reserve reduction and inability to augment flow to meet the increased metabolic demand of exercise. Severe flow impairment at rest results in ulceration of the digits and limb-threatening ischemia. Other conditions altering arterial flow to the legs include peripheral arterial aneurysms, popliteal artery entrapment, cystic adventitial disease, Buerger's disease, giant cell and Takayasu's arteritis and, rarely, fibromuscular dysplasia.

Arterial imaging of patients with PAD is challenging because it requires evaluation of the arterial tree from the aortic bifurcation to the level of the ankle and foot. The entire tree must be imaged because most patients have multiple lesions. Surgical as well as percutaneous interventions depend on the identification of all occlusive lesions—as well as evaluation of inflow and outflow vessels. Surgical planning requires identification of potential proximal and distal anastomotic sites.

Traditional 2-D TOF peripheral arterial MRA imaging has been successful in detecting stenoses greater than 50% with 85% to 92% sensitivity and 81% to 88% specificity.[27,28] It is also effective for the smaller infrapopliteal vessels. However, excessive scan time, often greater than 2 hours has limited the applicability of this technique in the peripheral vascular tree. Additional pitfalls of TOF include flow artifacts caused by pulsatile nature of the flow, although ECG gating has been used to improve image quality. Spatial presaturation pulses can be placed below the slice being imaged to minimize the venous signal, but this may also eliminate flow signal in collateral and reconstituted vessels.

The fundamental challenge in peripheral CE-MRA has been balancing the accurate imaging of the entire length of the vascular tree with the imaging capabilities of the system. The FOV available in MR is limited to 450 to 500 mm and requires image acquisition from pelvis to the foot to be done in three or four overlapping stages. Generally, the timing of the bolus is optimized for the first station (abdomen and pelvis) and then imaging is performed as rapidly as possible to try to keep up with the flow of the contrast material down the distal arteries. Image quality in the first station (Fig. 11-7) is excellent but often suboptimal in the third as gadolinium enters the venous system with resulting venous contamination of the image. This is especially true in patients with short arteriovenous transit time, often the case in severely ischemic limbs, where precise definition of the tibial arteries is especially important. On average, contrast reaches the common femoral artery in 24 seconds, with only an additional 5 and 7 seconds needed to reach the popliteal artery and the ankle, respectively.[29] The mean time window of arterial enhancement (i.e., time to venous enhancement) is 49 seconds in the pelvis, 45 seconds in the thigh, and 35 seconds in the calf. The travel time to the femoral arteries correlates with the presence of aortic aneurysm, increasing age, male gender, history of myocardial

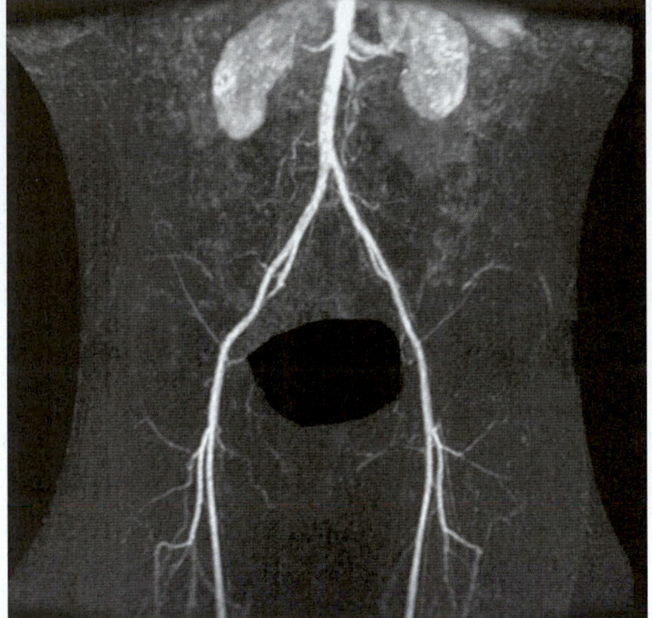

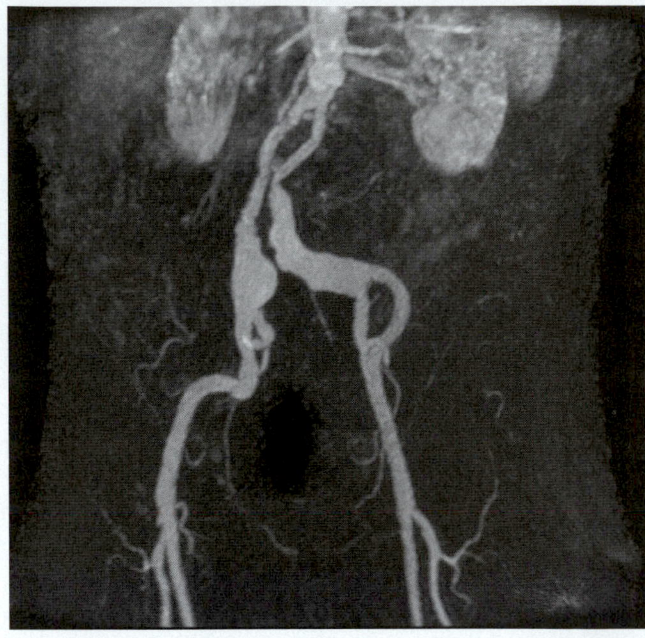

FIGURE 11-7. A, shows normal aortic bifurcation and pelvic vessels. **B,** shows atherosclerotic changes of the aortic bifurcation and common iliac artery aneurysms.

infarction, and diabetes. The motion of the MR table and imaging time currently available are not fast enough to keep up with gadolinium flow in an average patient. To achieve optimum results with bolus chase, the current imaging times of 20 to 30 seconds per station should be accelerated to 5 to 6 seconds per station, including table movement. This problem is compounded by the higher resolution (and consequent longer scan times) required for the tibial arteries.

A hybrid technique has been successfully used to overcome these limitations. A stationary contrast-enhanced scan is obtained of the tibial arteries in the calf, followed by a bolus-chase MRA for the iliac and femoral stations. A supplementary 2-D-TOF scan may be used to image the foot. For bolus-chase MRA, 40 ml of gadolinium is typically administered at a slow rate of 0.3 to 1.0 ml/sec. The rate of infusion should be adjusted so that the length of the contrast bolus duration matches roughly the time required to acquire the critical k-space data for the overlapping stations. Published results with the CE-MRA bolus-chase method are reasonably good. It reliably and accurately depicts peripheral arterial stenosis more than 50% with sensitivity of 81% to 95% and specificity of 91% to 98% (Fig. 11-8).[30-33] It has been evaluated for use in postoperative graft surveillance with 100% sensitivity and specificity reported for evaluable segments.[34] Recently, time-resolved imaging technique has been shown to be effective in infrapopliteal imaging. Morasch and coworkers used a stepping-table technique with multilevel contrast timing and segmented contrast infusion to image the lower extremity arterial tree. This combination of dual-time imaging and dual-injection techniques achieved an overall sensitivity of 99% and specificity of 97% when compared with x-ray angiography and surgical findings. Diagnostic quality in the calf and foot vessels was superior to conventional CE-MRA bolus-chase method.[35] All bolus-chase techniques require a multistation localizer and matching pre-contrast coronal 3-D acquisition at each location to ensure proper anatomic coverage. These images also serve as a mask for image subtraction, which can significantly improve arterial contrast at these relatively low injection rates.

CE-MRA can be used for imaging of pedal arteries (Fig. 11-9). A recent study of 37 patients with critical leg ischemia compared conventional x-ray angiography, 3-D CE-MRA and duplex ultrasound to identify pedal artery best suitable for bypass targets. The 30-day patency was used as a primary validation measure. CE-MRA was shown to be equivalent to x-ray angiography, although venous contamination and bolus timing were occasional problems.[36] Konkus and associates modified the standard three-station CE-MRA to obtain a four-station study including the feet.[37] Biphasic contrast infusion allowed prolonged, preferential arterial enhancement and accurate imaging of the pedal arteries.

MRA has also been used in the evaluation of popliteal artery entrapment syndrome and cystic adventitial disease. Popliteal artery entrapment is an uncommon congenital syndrome of anomalous relationship between the popliteal artery and surrounding muscular structures. It can be a source of ischemic symptoms in the lower extremity in young adults. MRI defines the anatomic relationships and MRA allows accurate evaluation of vascular compromise during provocative plantar flexion and at rest.[38,39] Cystic adventitial disease accounts for 1 in 1200 cases of calf claudication. A mucin-containing cyst in the popliteal artery wall compromises arterial flow and causes claudication. Water signal makes the cyst appear hyperintense on T2-weighted images and the MRA reveals popliteal artery stenosis.[38,40]

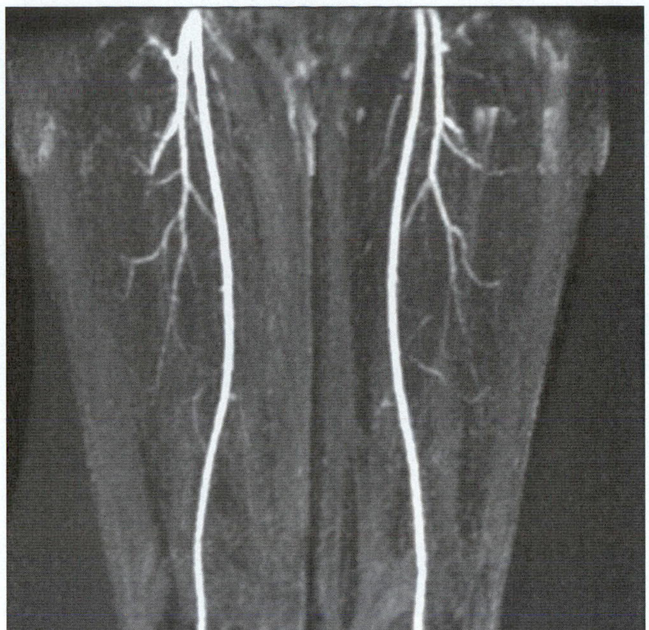

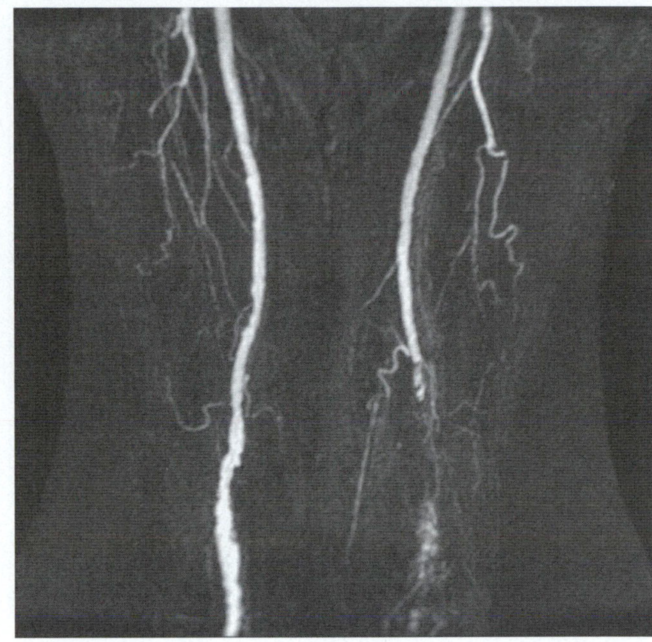

FIGURE 11-8. A, shows normal anatomy of bilateral superficial femoral arteries. **B,** shows occluded left superficial femoral artery and ectatic, aneurysmal right popliteal artery segment.

Vascular syndromes of the upper extremities often stem from the disease of the subclavian artery such as subclavian artery stenosis and aneurysm or thoracic outlet obstruction. Small vessel vasculitis and trauma can require imaging of the forearm and hand (Fig. 11-10). Spatial resolution of MRA in arteries of the hand has been inferior to conventional angiography but can provide some information.[41] The acquisition window is restricted to the few seconds between full enhancement of the arteries and beginning of venous contamination. Blood pressure cuff inflation proximally to the imaged area can extend imaging time and permit a fourfold increase in resolution. This allows visualization of the palmar, metacarpal, and digital arteries.[42]

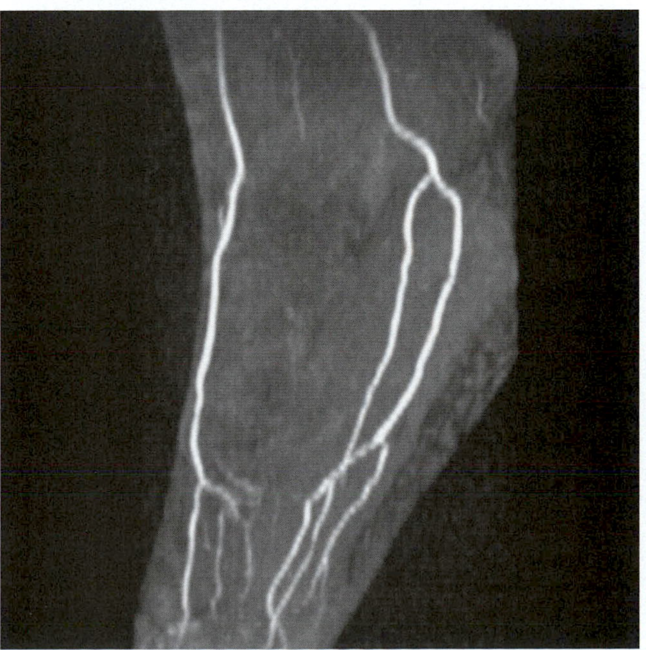

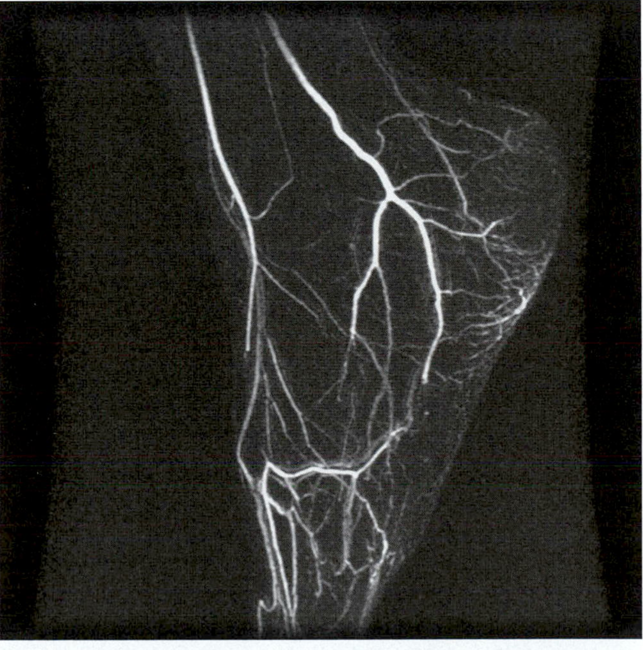

FIGURE 11-9. A, shows a time of flight (TOF) image of normal pedal arteries. **B,** is a CE-MRA maximum intensity projection (MIP) reconstruction of pedal arteries in a patient with cryoglobulinemia and small vessel vasculitis. Arteries of the pedal arch are occluded. Moderate venous enhancement is present.

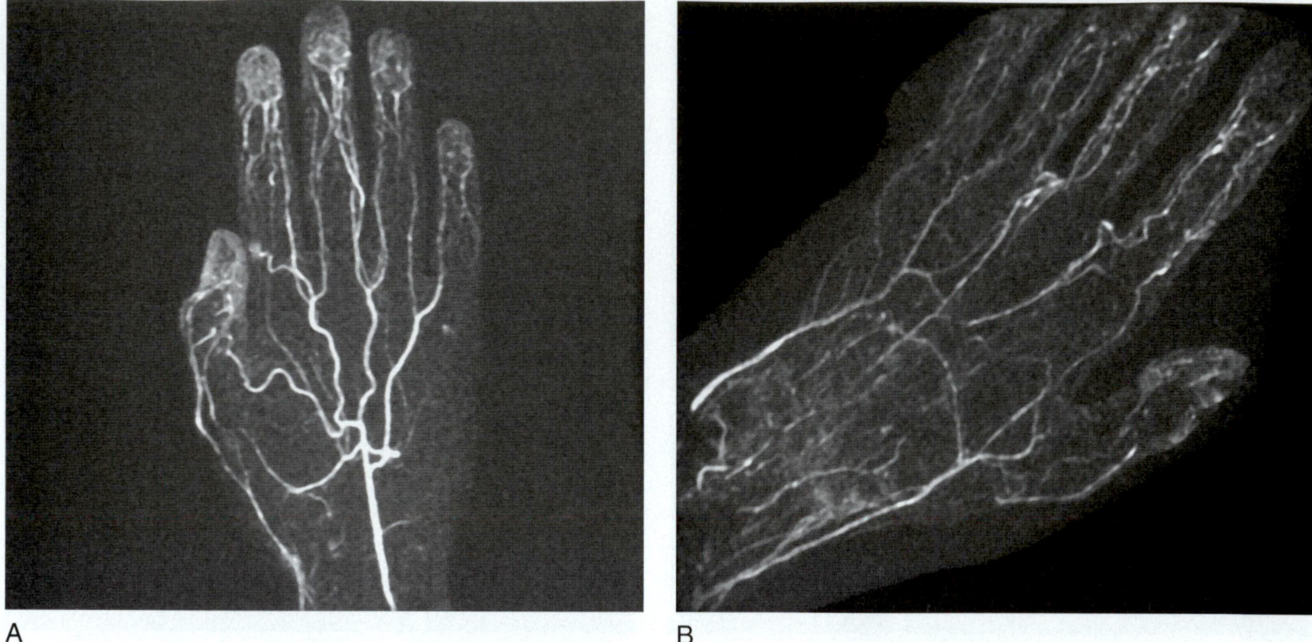

FIGURE 11-10. CE-MRA of the hand. **A,** shows a dominant ulnar supply to the hand in a patient with absent radial artery. **B,** shows the left hand of a patient with radiation-induced arteriopathy. The ulnar and radial arteries are patent. The common palmar and proper palmar arteries are small in caliber and diffusely irregular in their contour.

A reliable estimate of the overall sensitivity and specificity of MRA in evaluation of peripheral arterial occlusive disease is difficult. A review of the diagnostic performance of TOF- and CE-MRA suggests that 2-D TOF-MRA has sensitivity of 64% to 100% and specificity of 68% to 96%, whereas CE-MRA achieves 92% to 100% sensitivity and 91% to 99% specificity.[43]

MRA is an ever-evolving modality.[44,45] The innovations in peripheral MRA focus on achieving higher resolution to better visualize smaller distal vessels and decreasing scanning time to image distal arterial segments before venous enhancement. Development of an affordable, dedicated vascular coil, currently a research tool, will improve signal and spatial resolution. New acquisition techniques and higher field strength scanners continue to improve speed and image resolution. Parallel imaging techniques, such as simultaneous acquisition of spatial harmonics and sensitivity encoding (SENSE) can reduce the imaging time by a factor of two to three, increase spatial resolution, and decrease venous contamination.[46] The technique of segmental volume acquisition ("shoot and scoot") segments the 3-D such that only the central portions of the k-space (low spatial frequency data) are acquired during the initial pass that takes place during the arterial phase of the contrast bolus. The remaining k-space data are acquired later during the second pass that occurs during the delayed phase. Segmental volume acquisition provides high spatial resolution data sets and enables more efficient data acquisition because the time-critical portions of k-space (the center of k-space) are preferentially acquired during the arterial phase of the bolus. Another innovation is the time-resolved 3-D TRICKS digital subtraction MRA. Time-resolved acquisitions, such as 3-D TRICKS, reduce the time needed to acquire a standard 3-D data set from 20 seconds to a frame rate of 2 seconds per 3-D volume. TRICKS combines the repeated sampling of the critical central k-space views with temporal interpolation of the less frequently sampled periphery of k-space to produce a series of time-resolved 3-D images. This technique obviates the need for timing tests and a separate acquisition of precontrast images for mask mode subtraction. Swan and colleagues evaluated three-station, time-resolved TRICKS 3-D CE-MRA of the peripheral vessels in 69 patients with symptomatic PAD and compared its diagnostic accuracy with conventional angiography.[47] The sensitivity of MRA for occlusion was 89% and the specificity was 97%. In evaluating stenosis greater than 50%, it was 87% sensitive and 90% specific. This technique, completed in less than 30 minutes, proved to be a robust, easy to use, and accurate method of imaging PAD.

MRA of the Abdominal Vessels

The vascular anatomy of the abdomen lends itself well to CE-MRA imaging. The celiac trunk arises from the anterior aspect of the aorta at a level of T12 and L1. It divides into left gastric, splenic, and hepatic arteries. This pattern is seen in 65% to 75% of individuals. The superior mesenteric artery (SMA) arises from the anterior surface of the aorta at about L1. The inferior mesenteric artery (IMA), the smallest of the mesenteric arteries, arises from the anterior or left anterolateral aspect of the aorta at the level of L3. The renal arteries arise from the abdominal aorta at the superior margin of L2—immediately caudal to the origin of the SMA. About 32% of individuals have multiple unilateral, renal arteries, whereas 12% have bilateral supranumerary arteries. An independent superior renal pole artery is observed in up to 7% and inferior pole artery in about 5% of persons tested.

CE-MRA produces high contrast between vessels and surrounding organs and is superior to conventional x ray-angiography in its ability to provide a panoramic view of the abdominal arteries and veins during a single bolus of contrast (Fig. 11-11). The most common indications for abdominal MRA are evaluation of renal artery stenosis (RAS), assessment of abdominal aortic aneurysm, evaluation of aortic dissection, or occlusion and diagnosis of suspected mesenteric stenosis. Abdominal aorta and its branches can be reliably imaged within a single breath-hold. This is best performed in the coronal or oblique coronal 3-D prescription. Origins of the ventrally originating branches, such as SMA and IMA may be best seen on a sagittal acquisition. Because MRA is a lumenogram, each study should include spin-echo axial images to allow exact measurement of the aortic diameter and evaluation of the aortic wall, as well as any potential intra-abdominal pathology. Prior to contrast injection, an unenhanced breath-hold, 3-D MRA should be performed to ensure that the 3-D volume is appropriately placed and includes the vascular territory of interest and to serve as a mask for subtraction. The study should include at least two post-contrast acquisitions (arterial and delayed phase). This does not significantly prolong the study and can provide valuable information, especially about venous structures. This is especially crucial if the blood flow is slow, as is the case in large abdominal aneurysms or aortic dissections with slow flow in the false lumen. The initial arterial phase MRA may be completed before the arrival of sufficient contrast concentration in the slow-flow aortic segment being imaged. When used in renal artery imaging, this approach adds information about renal parenchymal enhancement. Doses of 20 to 30 ml of gadolinium, administered at 2 ml/second, are usually sufficient for imaging of the abdominal aorta on gadolinium-enhanced 3-D MRA. The larger dose is recommended for patients with known large abdominal aneurysms, aortic dissection, or aortic occlusion because this ensures sufficiently high arterial gadolinium concentration for adequate visualization of all segments. Newer MRA techniques, such as TRICKS and multicoil imaging (such as SENSE), can provide faster acquisition times, making even temporally-resolved imaging possible, without compromising spatial resolution.

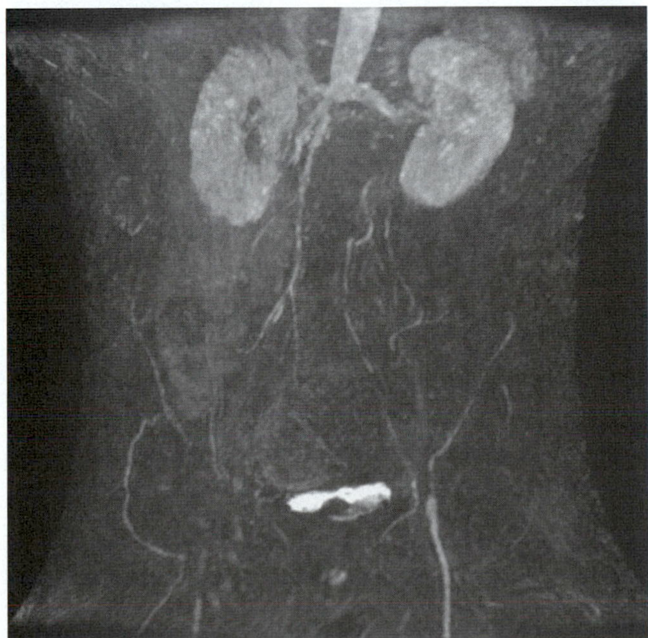

FIGURE 11-11. Occluded infrarenal aorta in a patient with Leriche's syndrome.

Renal Artery Imaging

MRA has become the modality of choice for the diagnosis of RAS (Fig. 11-12). It is especially attractive because it does not employ nephrotoxic agents. Both TOF and PC techniques have been used for evaluation of RAS. Long imaging time, limited accuracy in grading the stenoses, and lack of detection of supranumerary arteries have prevented widespread use of these techniques. CE-MRA, with its independence from flow effects, has revolutionized renal artery imaging. The 3-D, dynamic spoiled-gradient echo sequence is repeated three times for pre-contrast, arterial phase, and delayed venous phase images. The 3-D data is post-processed with the construction of MIP and MPR images. Post-stenotic dilation and delayed renal parenchymal enhancement are additional signs of significant stenosis.

The critical issue in renal artery imaging is spatial resolution, especially for the distal renal artery. There is persistent craniocaudal motion of the distal renal artery even during fast, breath-hold CE-MRA.[48] The observed, average net renal displacement during breath-hold CEMRA can be greater than the typically used voxel size and further compromises image accuracy in distal renal arteries. The recent use of SENSE techniques to decrease acquisition time may improve distal renal artery image quality.

The diagnosis of stenosis can be challenging in fibromuscular dysplasia because the changes of alternating webs and dilations may be subtle on MRA and occur in the distal arterial segments, limiting the usefulness of MRA for this diagnosis.

The aorta does not move significantly with respiration, and the linear breath-hold drift for the kidney tapers to near zero at the renal artery ostium. This allows optimal imaging of atherosclerotic lesions that occur in the proximal segment of renal arteries. MRA is highly reliable for diagnosis of atherosclerotic RAS. A recent meta-analysis reviewed 25 studies from 1985 to 2001, which, in a blinded fashion, compared conventional x-ray angiography with MRA.[49] A total of 998 patients underwent renal artery MRA: 499 patients with noncontrast techniques and 499 patients with gadolinium enhanced 3-D MRA. The sensitivity and specificity of noncontrast MRA for detecting stenoses greater than 50% were 94% and 85%, respectively, whereas CE-MRA reached 97% and 93% sensitivity and specificity. This analysis reflected technology available up to 1999. MRA is firmly established as a preferred modality for evaluation of renovascular

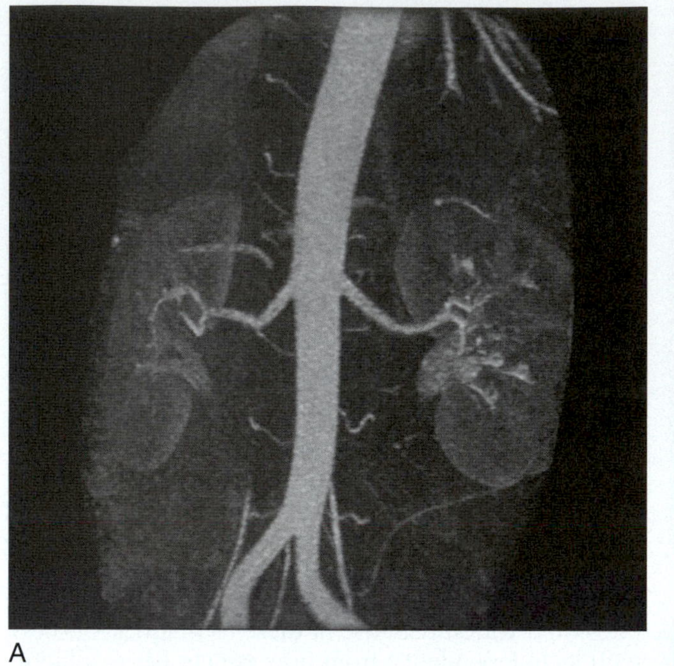
A

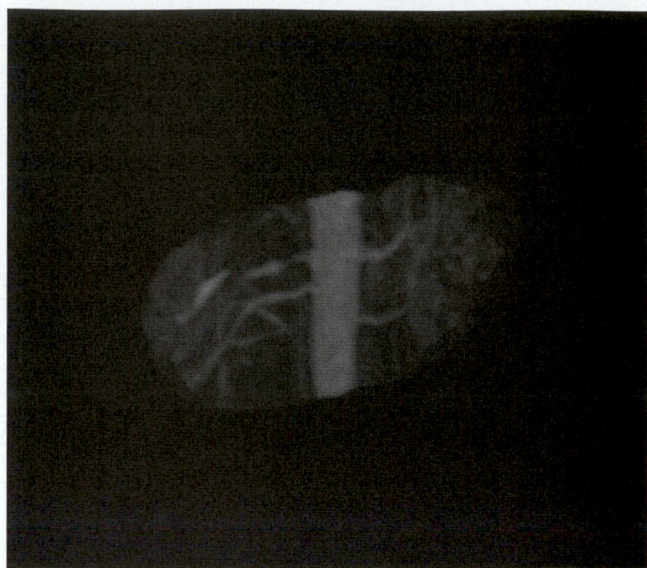
B

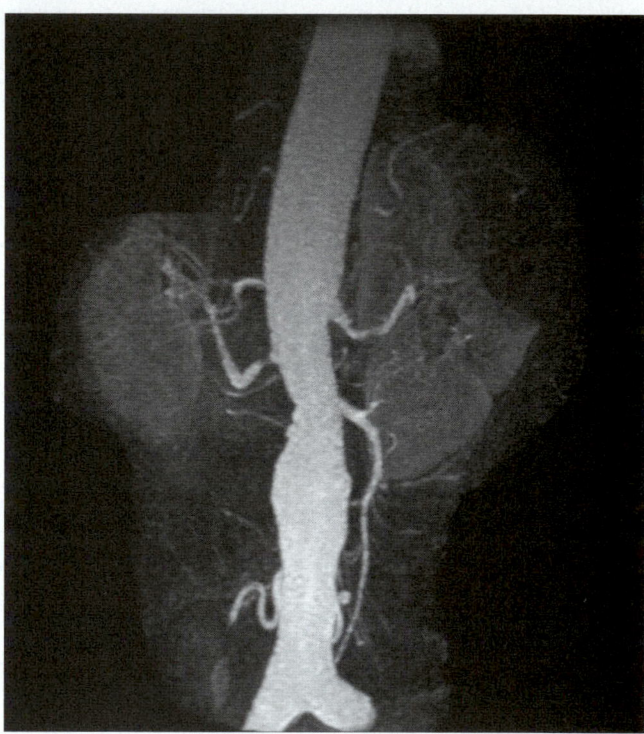
C

FIGURE 11-12. Renal artery disease. **A,** shows normal-appearing renal arteries. **B,** shows right renal artery stenosis. **C,** shows bilateral accessory renal arteries and occlusive disease of the right renal artery.

hypertension,[50] especially in the age group in whom atherosclerotic disease predominates.

Abdominal Aorta Imaging

Abdominal aortic aneurysm is typically fusiform and is due to atherosclerosis and degeneration of the arterial wall (see Chapter 37). A saccular aneurysm should raise the possibility of an infectious mycotic aneurysm. An aneurysm is often defined as enlargement of arterial diameter of 50% or more from its normal caliber, usually 3 cm or greater for the abdominal aorta. The size of the aneurysm is best measured on spin-echo images. Proper evaluation should also assess the proximal and distal extent of the aneurysm and its relationship to the visceral branch vessels. Gadolinium-enhanced 3-D MRA fulfills these requirements (Fig. 11-13). It can identify the main and supranumerary renal arteries and the mesenteric

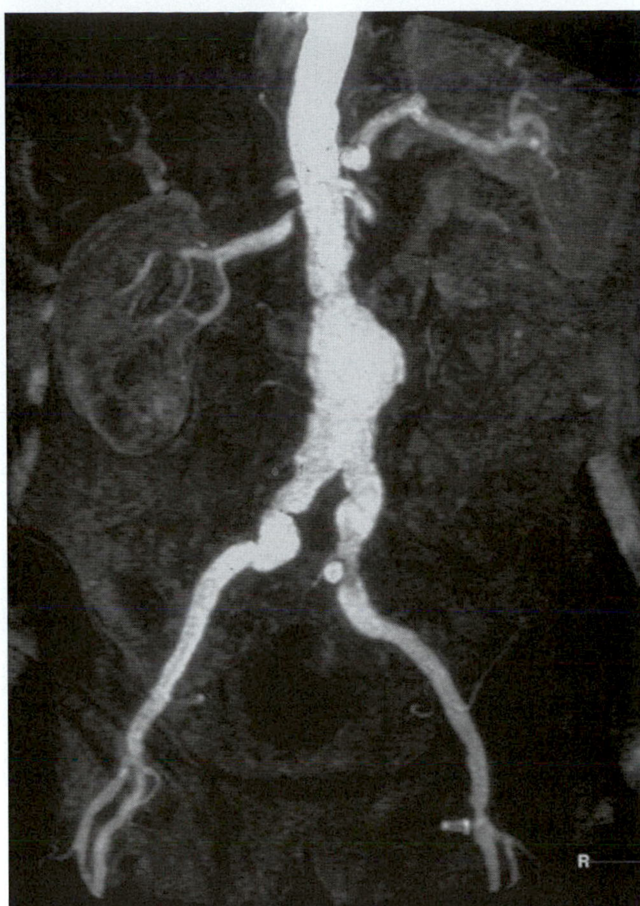

FIGURE 11-13. Abdominal aortic aneurysm.

vessels and define their relationship to the aneurysm. MRA is very accurate in the diagnosis and characterization of abdominal aneurysms.[51]

Aortic stent grafts have emerged as a treatment option for management of aortic aneurysms. CT has been generally favored as the modality of choice for pre-procedural staging and post-stenting endoleak surveillance. MRA can reliably provide all the pre-procedural data[52] except for the amount of calcification. It has been hindered by stent artifacts, which limit post-procedural follow-up studies. A growing use of nitinol and PTFE devices, which yield minimal artifact on CE-MRA, may overcome this limitation. Cejna and colleagues evaluated the accuracy of 3-D CE-MRA in follow-ups of patients with endoluminally treated aortic aneurysm and compared it with CTA. In patients with nitinol stent grafts, MRA was at least as sensitive as CTA.[53] MRA is safe for nonferromagnetic stents and does not induce heating and stent deflection.[54,55]

Abdominal Aortic Dissection

Evaluation of aortic dissection in the abdomen involves detection of the exit site, extension of the tear, and involvement of the visceral branches (see Chapter 34). The celiac trunk and SMA are rarely compromised because, in most cases, they arise from the true lumen. Often, the intimal flap extends into the visceral artery, separating the vessel into two channels. One of them is supplied by the true and the other by the false lumen. Thrombosis of the false lumen or compression of the true lumen in the celiac trunk can lead to hepatic or splenic infarcts. Obstruction of the mesenteric artery can lead to mesenteric ischemia. Asymmetric renal enhancement can be due to renal artery obstruction. Arteries supplied exclusively by the false lumen are rarely compromised.

The distal extension of the dissection often spirals and may be difficult to image with traditional modalities. 3-D MRA reliably depicts the true and false channels of a spiraling aortic dissection (Fig. 11-14). MPR post-processing of 3-D data sets enable the selective viewing of individual aortic branch vessels and identification of their blood supply as coming from the true or false lumen. Delayed-phase imaging is recommended because slow flow in the false lumen may not adequately fill with contrast during the initial acquisition. In a study of 90 patients with aortic dissection extending to the abdomen, 3-D CE-MRA, when compared with x-ray angiography and intraoperative findings, correctly diagnosed all cases.[16]

Mesenteric Arteries

Most patients will not develop symptoms of chronic mesenteric ischemia unless two of the three mesenteric arteries are occluded (see Chapter 25). CE-MRA is accurate for evaluating the origins of mesenteric and celiac vessels where the majority of stenoses develop. Holland and coworkers reported 100% sensitivity and specificity of CE-MRA in detecting celiac, superior mesenteric, and internal mesenteric artery lesions.[56] Similar observation was made in a study of 125 patients with mesenteric ischemia using dual phase CE-MRA.[57] More recent technology using 3-D fat-suppressed CE-MRA can correctly assess abnormalities in 75% of first order branching, 60% of second order branching, and 50% of third order branching of the SMA.[58] Delayed acquisitions can be diagnostically helpful in demonstrating delayed enhancement of bowel.

MRA is currently not ideal for evaluation of acute mesenteric ischemia. It is not able to demonstrate nonocclusive low flow states or embolization of smaller, distal branch vessels. MRA is a reasonable tool for evaluations of chronic mesenteric occlusion, mesenteric artery aneurysm formation, and vasculitis affecting the mesenteric arteries.

Portal System

Another advantage of CE-MRA relies on its ability to provide simultaneous views of the inferior vena cava, hepatic veins, and the portal veins. The advent of fast CE-MRA makes it possible to obtain images in arterial, portal, and systemic venous phases. 3-D MRA is used extensively prior to liver transplantation to define portal vascular anatomy and exclude the presence of thrombosis.[59,60]

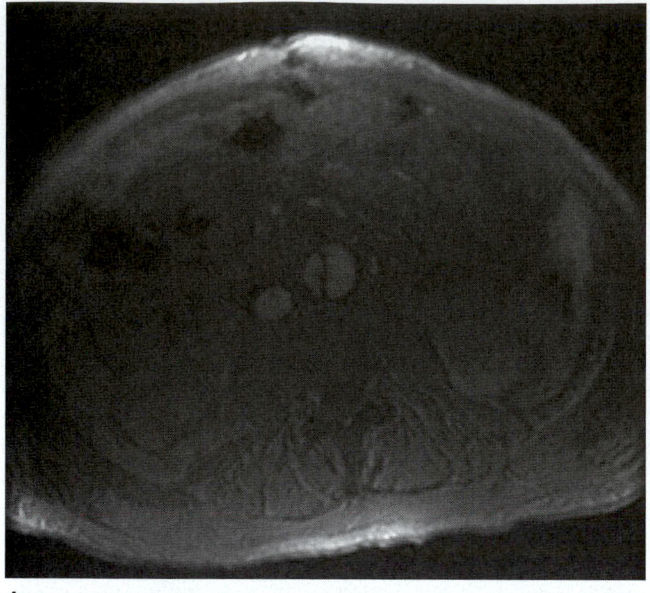

A

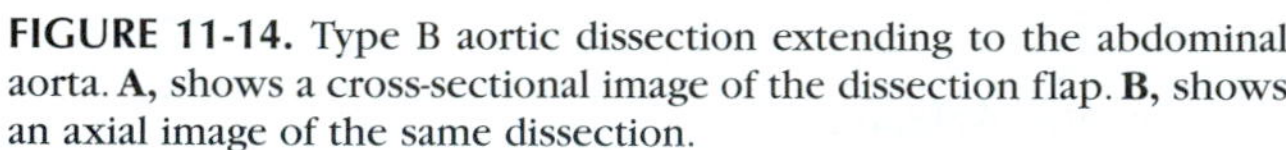

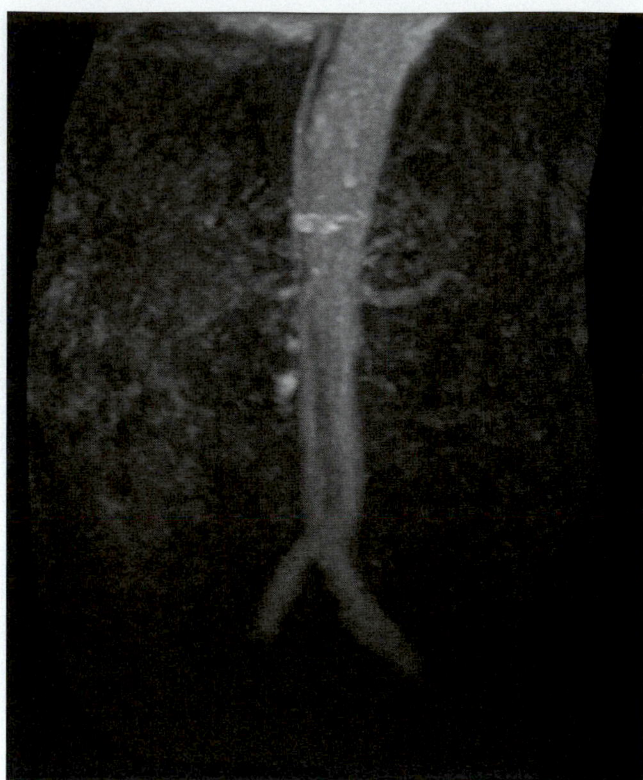

B

FIGURE 11-14. Type B aortic dissection extending to the abdominal aorta. **A,** shows a cross-sectional image of the dissection flap. **B,** shows an axial image of the same dissection.

Inflammatory Diseases of the Arterial Wall

MRA has become an important modality for diagnosing and serial follow-ups of patients with suspected large vessel vasculitis. MRA provides the advantages of axial, sagittal, and coronal imaging with good spatial resolution. The normal aortic wall is barely perceptible on conventional MR imaging. Vascular wall edema and thickening are features of vasculitis that are present early in disease before lumen changes are angiographically apparent. Vessel wall morphology is well seen on spin-echo, cross-sectional images. Post-contrast imaging can demonstrate mural enhancement. Other wall abnormalities seen in vasculitis include ulceration, dissection, stenosis, occlusion, and aneurysmal enlargement.

Takayasu's Arteritis

Takayasu's arteritis (TA) is an inflammatory disease of the aorta and it branches (see Chapter 42). It typically affects young women. Diagnosis is difficult to establish in the early stages because of nonspecific symptoms and lack of reliable serologic markers. Signs and symptoms of arterial stenoses, occlusion, or aneurysm constitute late, irreversible manifestations of this disease. Conventional angiographic methods do not provide information on vessel wall morphology and cannot provide corroborative diagnostic information until significant large vessel anatomical changes have occurred. Helical contrast CT is hindered by high density of contrast in the lumen, which causes artifacts in the adjacent vessel wall. CTA is suboptimal for imaging of mural changes, especially early changes in pulmonary arteries.[61] Traditional cross-sectional and contrast MR techniques, on the other hand, are well suited for evaluation of the mural changes in the arterial vessels that signal early disease.

Typical CE-MRA findings suggestive of TA include stenoses of the aorta and its major branches (Fig. 11-15A and B). Left subclavian artery is the most commonly involved vessel, followed by renal and carotid arteries.[62] In as many as 50% of patients, MRA may demonstrate pulmonary arterial system abnormalities with occlusion of peripheral pulmonary vessels.[63] Aneurysmal enlargement of the aorta can be seen on MRA in 9.5% of patients. Sensitivity and specificity of CE-MRA are both estimated to be 100%.[63]

The inflammatory markers are unreliable in following disease activity. Persistent erythrocyte sedimentation rate (ESR) elevation can be seen during clinical remission in 56% of cases, whereas surgical biopsy specimens in patients with clinically inactive disease show active inflammation in 44% of cases.[62] This has focused interest on using MRA to identify early changes of vasculitis and to assess disease activity. This can be achieved by evaluating wall morphology and wall enhancement. The normal aortic wall is almost imperceptibly thin on MR imaging. Traditional, cross-sectional T1-weighted noncontrast sequencies show circumferential, diffuse, 3- to 10-mm thickening of the arterial wall before development of stenoses (see Fig. 11-15C).[61] T2 signal is sensitive to

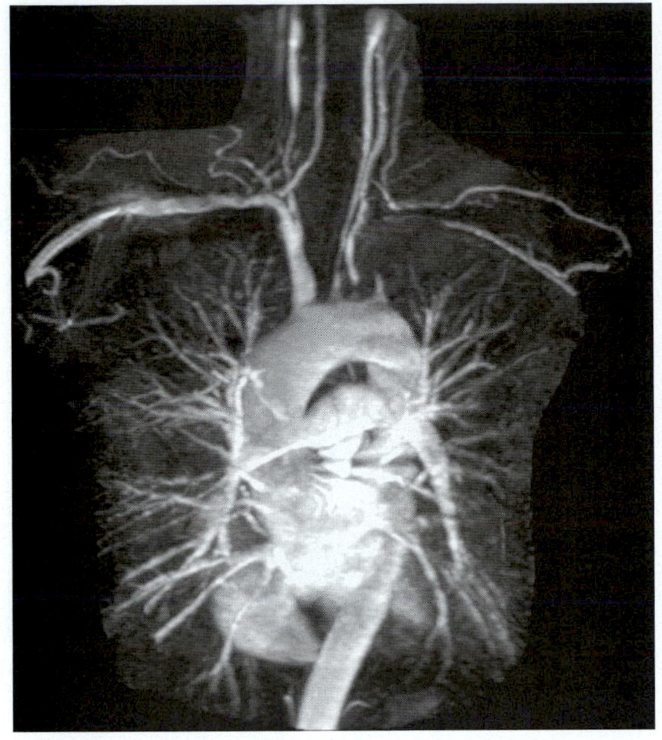

A

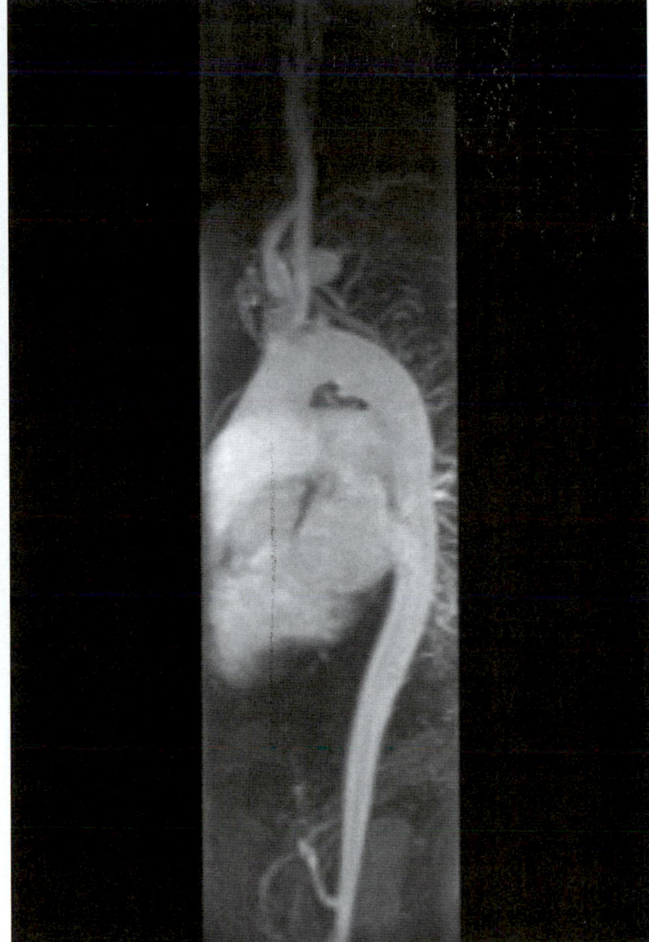

B

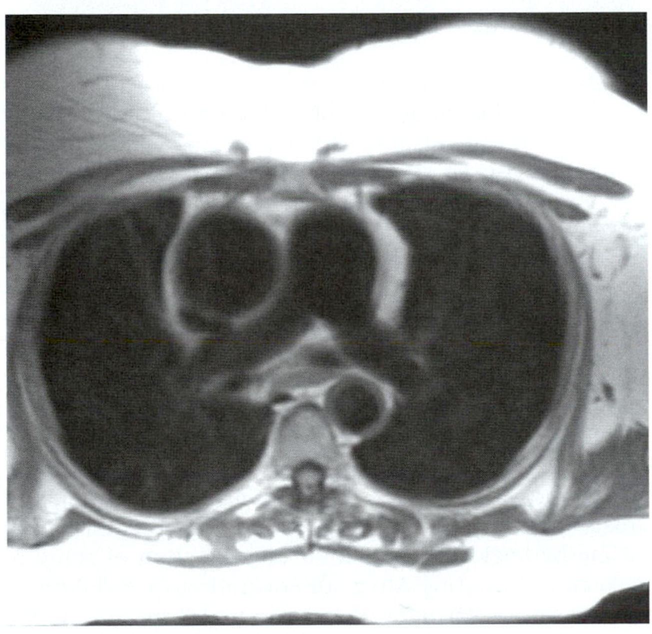

C

FIGURE 11-15. Takayasu's arteritis. **A,** shows the aortic arch and great vessels in a woman with Takayasu's arteritis. Note occluded left subclavian artery and stenoses of the left vertebral and bilateral carotid arteries. **B,** shows smooth, diffuse tapering of the descending aorta in a patient with Takayasu's arteritis. **C,** shows a T1-weighted cross-sectional image of the ascending and descending aorta in a patient with Takayasu's arteritis. There is circumferential thickening of the descending aortic wall suggestive of active inflammation.

water content and mural edema appears as bright T2 signal. Short inversion time inversion recovery (STIR) technique is a pulse sequence that may be slightly more sensitive to edema than conventional T2, particularly when employed with the black blood imaging technique. Such "edema weighted" MRA sequences have been reported to demonstrate acute inflammatory changes of arteritis in these areas.[64] The inherent MR signal changes related to alterations in distribution of water in the edematous, inflamed tissue make the wall of active disease appear bright. The initial excitement about this technique has been dampened by subsequent studies that showed that MR-identified wall edema can be present in 94%, 81%, and 56% of studies obtained during periods of unequivocal active disease, uncertain activity, and apparent clinical remission, respectively.[65] Moreover, ESR and CRP did not correlate with clinical assessment or MR evidence of vascular edema. The presence of edema did not correlate with the occurrence of new anatomic changes found on subsequent studies. All these studies suffer from lack of histopathologic correlation. Edema-weighted MR cannot be reliably used as the only modality to assess disease activity. It is possible that edema may remain during tissue remodeling after inflammation is resolved.

CE-MRA has been evaluated in determination of disease activity.[66] Mural enhancement on post-contrast T1-weighted images reflects increased vascularity and excessive leakage of contrast from the vasa vasorum. Late post-contrast phase imaging may demonstrate persistent wall enhancement. This probably indicates a more acute stage of disease. The degree of aortic wall enhancement can be assessed by measuring signal intensity and comparing it with that of the myocardium. Strong enhancement of the arterial wall on CE-MRA, where signal intensity of the thickened aortic wall is higher than that of the myocardium, suggests active inflammation. These findings were concordant with clinical findings of disease activity, ESR, and CRP levels—and they improved with therapy.[66] The sensitivity of CE-MRA T1-weighted imaging in the detection of active inflammation appears to be superior to T2-weighted techniques but also remains unproved in the absence of histopathologic correlation. The previously noted pitfall of CE-MRA in the subclavian artery after ipsilateral arm injection should be recalled when evaluating the subclavian artery. Current evaluation of vessel wall edema and inflammation should include T2-weighted, pre- and post-contrast T1-weighted spin-echo sequences and 3D-MR angiography with contrast. Axial, coronal, sagittal and, when appropriate, oblique views should be obtained.

Giant Cell Arteritis

Giant cell arteritis (GCA) is a large vessel inflammatory disease affecting primarily older patients (see Chapter 43). MRA is useful in diagnosing thoracic aortic aneurysm associated with this disease. Involvement of large peripheral arteries, such as subclavian arteries, is also reliably diagnosed by MRA (Fig. 11-16). However, data regarding MRA evaluation of giant cell arteritis come primarily from case reports. Standard 2-D TOF-MRA has been shown to identify superficial temporal artery narrowing in a case of documented giant cell arteritis.[67] MRA also has been shown to be helpful for diagnosis and follow-up of giant cell arteritis.[68,69] Anders used parasagittal fat-saturated T1-weighted SE images to visualize proximal portions of the frontal and parietal branches of temporal superficial arteries in GCA,[70] but biopsy remains the standard.

MR Venography

Techniques used in MR venography (MRV) differ from those employed in MRA because of the differences in flow and disease patterns. Noncontrast MRV, such as TOF and PC, and contrast-enhanced CE MRV can be used in imaging the venous system. 2-D TOF has the advantage of being able to cover a large area and detect slow flow. It is thus ideal for venous imaging. Its disadvantages are decreased resolution and saturation of in-plane flow. 3-D TOF is not practical for venous imaging. The PC technique is challenged by long scan duration, sensitivity to flow dephasing, and image degradation from extravascular motion. For these reasons its applicability to MRV is quite limited.

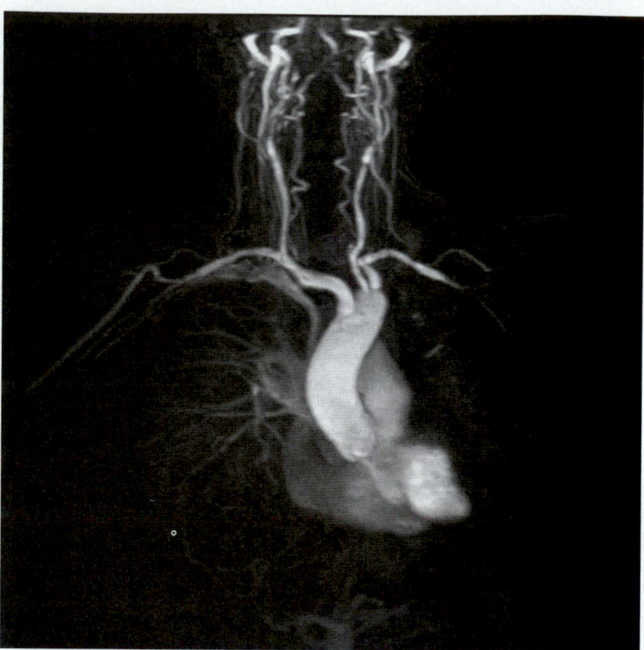

FIGURE 11-16. Giant cell arteritis. Elderly woman with giant cell arteritis developed bilateral arm claudication. Both subclavian arteries have smooth, tapered stenoses in the mid- to distal segments.

3-D CE-MRV can be performed with the indirect method of injecting nondiluted contrast at a distant venous site and imaging the vein of interest during the venous phase of contrast enhancement. Considerable dilution occurs as the contrast reaches the target area, so contrast is less than for CE-MRA. A direct technique, analogous to a conventional venogram, involves administration of diluted contrast (usually 1:20 dilution) in a peripheral vein distal to the target area and imaging of the draining venous system. This technique provides excellent contrast-to-noise ratio but limits images to the veins draining at the site of injection.

MRI can detect the T1 signal of the thrombus itself. There is a predictable reduction in the T1 of the clot, which provides a high-signal intensity on T1-weighted images. This T1 reduction depends on the formation of methemoglobin and allows identification of acute to subacute thrombus. After administration of gadolinium, inflammatory changes that take place in the setting of acute DVT lead to stranding on spin-echo or post-contrast imaging in the perivascular tissues. A pattern of peripheral, mural enhancement is seen around an acutely thrombosed vein in CE-MRV, appearing as a "bull's-eye" sign (Fig. 11-17). This pattern disappears with time as thrombus organizes and inflammation resolves. These changes help to differentiate acute from chronic thrombosis.

Deep Vein Thrombosis

Venous imaging by ultrasonography and conventional venography has several limitations. Ultrasound is operator dependent and suffers from the inability to image the

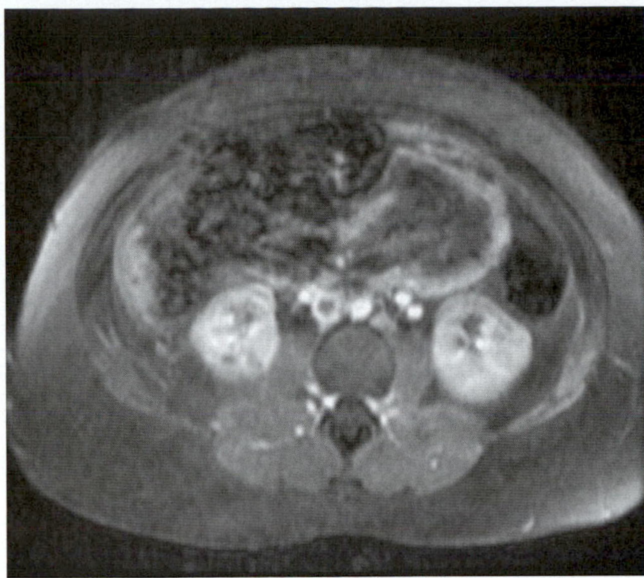

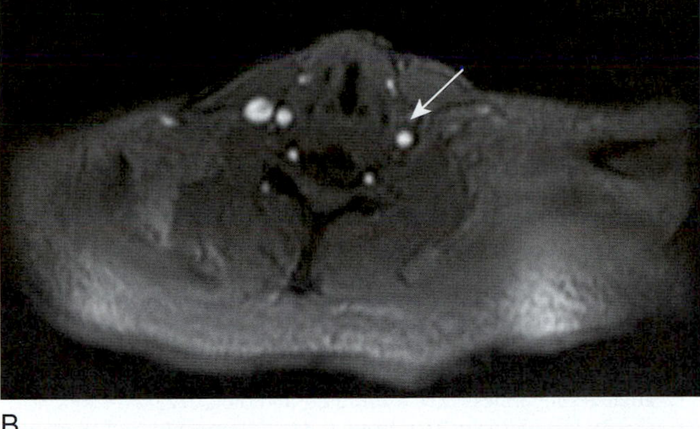

FIGURE 11-17. MR venography in deep vein thrombosis. **A,** shows acute thrombosis of the inferior vena cava with the classic "bulls-eye" appearance. **B,** shows chronic occlusive thrombosis of the left internal jugular vein (*arrow*).

central venous system. Venography is invasive and uses iodinated contrast and radiation. CT venograms also require nephrotoxic contrast and suffer from low venous contrast enhancement. 2-D TOF has been the modality of choice, but CE-MRA is used more and more frequently. Many studies have established accuracy of 2-D TOF in diagnosing deep vein thrombosis (DVT) (see Chapter 53).[71,72] This modality can achieve 100% sensitivity and 96% specificity for detection of a DVT in the large proximal deep venous system extending from the popliteal veins to the inferior vena cava (IVC). 3-D CE-MRA is also accurate in the superficial and perforating veins with slow flow and retrograde flow.[73]

MRV is useful in evaluating renal vein thrombosis. This condition affects about 0.5% of population and is difficult to diagnose. The most concerning cause is renal cell carcinoma. This malignancy extends into the renal vein in 20% of cases, into the IVC in 10% of patients, and reaches the right atrium in 2% of cases.[74] MRV has been validated for evaluating the extent of renal vein thrombosis[75] and provides additional anatomic information crucial for surgical planning. MRV using spin-echo and gradient-echo techniques has a sensitivity of 100%.[76] Retrospective analysis by Narumi and colleagues[77] showed 100% sensitivity and 98% specificity for detection and characterization of venous involvement by tumor. CE-MRA is especially useful because it can show enhancement of tumor thrombus. Gadolinium enhancement can differentiate between bland and tumor thrombus with 89% sensitivity and 96% specificity.[75] Ovarian vein thrombosis is especially difficult to evaluate with ultrasound techniques. 2-D TOF proved superior to CT and duplex ultrasound with sensitivity and specificity of 100%.[78]

Central veins are well visualized by CE-MRA. Spontaneous occlusion of SVC is very rare and most commonly it is a consequence of neoplastic compression, compression by arterial aneurysm, or goiter. Catheter-related thrombosis is becoming more frequent. MRV can be very helpful in planning central venous catheter placement in patients with chronic venous occlusion from repeated catheter placement. The IVC and iliac veins can be occluded from compression by lymph nodes and organomegaly as well as DVT. MRV is useful for identifying the extent and cause of venous occlusion in the pelvis and abdomen.

Congenital Venous Anomalies

Congenital absence of suprarenal IVC can occur in 0.5% of the general population and in some cases culminates in massive lower extremity thrombosis.[79] MRV can delineate the congenital anomalies and assess their patency.

REFERENCES

1. Toussaint JF, LaMuraglia GM, Southern JF, et al: Magnetic resonance images lipid, fibrous, calcified, hemorrhagic, and thrombotic components of human atherosclerosis in vivo. Circulation 94:932, 1996.
2. Yucel EK, Anderson CM, Edelman RR, et al: AHA scientific statement. Magnetic resonance angiography: Update on applications for extracranial arteries. Circulation 100:2284, 1999.
3. Prince MR, Yucel EK, Kaufman JA, et al: Dynamic gadolinium-enhanced three-dimensional abdominal MR arteriography. J Magn Reson Imaging 3:877, 1993.
4. Prince MR: Gadolinium-enhanced MR aortography. Radiology 191:155, 1994.
5. Kroencke TJ, Wasser MN, Pattynama PM, et al: Gadobenate dimeglumine-enhanced MR angiography of the abdominal aorta and renal arteries. AJR Am J Roentgenol 179:1573, 2002.
6. Cavagna E, Berletti R, Schiavon F: In vivo evaluation of intravascular stents at three-dimensional MR angiography. Eur Radiol 11:2531, 2001.
7. Lenhart M, Framme N, Volk M, et al: Time-resolved contrast-enhanced magnetic resonance angiography of the carotid arteries: Diagnostic accuracy and inter-observer variability compared with selective catheter angiography. Invest Radiol 37:535, 2002.
8. Wutke R, Lang W, Fellner C, et al: High-resolution, contrast-enhanced magnetic resonance angiography with elliptical centric k-space ordering of supra-aortic arteries compared with selective x-ray angiography. Stroke 33:1522, 2002.

9. Johnston DC, Eastwood JD, Nguyen T, et al: Contrast-enhanced magnetic resonance angiography of carotid arteries: Utility in routine clinical practice. Stroke 33:2834, 2002.
10. Westwood ME, Kelly S, Berry E, et al: Use of magnetic resonance angiography to select candidates with recently symptomatic carotid stenosis for surgery: Systematic review. BMJ 324:198, 2002.
11. Moore AG, Eagle KA, Bruckman D, et al: Choice of computed tomography, transesophageal echocardiography, magnetic resonance imaging, and aortography in acute aortic dissection: International Registry of Acute Aortic Dissection (IRAD). Am J Cardiol 89:1235, 2002.
12. Hayashi H, Matsuoka Y, Sakamoto I, et al: Penetrating atherosclerotic ulcer of the aorta: Imaging features and disease concept. Radiographics 20:995, 2000.
13. Pereles FS, McCarthy RM, Baskaran V, et al: Thoracic aortic dissection and aneurysm: Evaluation with nonenhanced true FISP MR angiography in less than 4 minutes. Radiology 223:270, 2002.
14. Cesare ED, Giordano AV, Cerone G, et al: Comparative evaluation of TEE, conventional MRI and contrast-enhanced 3D breath-hold MRA in the post-operative follow-up of dissecting aneurysms. Int J Card Imaging 16:135, 2000.
15. Hartnell GG, Finn JP, Zenni M, et al: MR imaging of the thoracic aorta: Comparison of spin-echo, angiographic, and breath-hold techniques. Radiology 191:697, 1994.
16. Prince MR, Narasimham DL, Jacoby WT, et al: Three-dimensional gadolinium-enhanced MR angiography of the thoracic aorta. AJR Am J Roentgenol 166:1387, 1996.
17. Cosottini M, Zampa V, Petruzzi P, et al: Contrast-enhanced three-dimensional MR angiography in the assessment of subclavian artery diseases. Eur Radiol 10:1737, 2000.
18. Godart F, Labrot G, Devos P, et al: Coarctation of the aorta: Comparison of aortic dimensions between conventional MR imaging, 3D MR angiography, and conventional angiography. Eur Radiol 12:2034, 2002.
19. Holmqvist C, Stahlberg F, Hanseus K, et al: Collateral flow in coarctation of the aorta with magnetic resonance velocity mapping: Correlation to morphological imaging of collateral vessels. J Magn Reson Imaging 15:39, 2002.
20. Bogaert J, Kuzo R, Dymarkowski S, et al: Follow-up of patients with previous treatment for coarctation of the thoracic aorta: Comparison between contrast-enhanced MR angiography and fast spin-echo MR imaging. Eur Radiol 10:1847, 2000.
21. Taneja K, Kawlra S, Sharma S, et al: Pseudocoarctation of the aorta: Complementary findings on plain film radiography, CT, DSA, and MRA. Cardiovasc Intervent Radiol 21:439, 1998.
22. Panegyres PK, Moore N, Gibson R, et al: Thoracic outlet syndromes and magnetic resonance imaging. Brain 116 (Pt 4):823, 1993.
23. Esposito MD, Arrington JA, Blackshear MN, et al: Thoracic outlet syndrome in a throwing athlete diagnosed with MRI and MRA. J Magn Reson Imaging 7:598, 1997.
24. Kato R, Lickfett L, Meininger G, et al: Pulmonary vein anatomy in patients undergoing catheter ablation of atrial fibrillation: Lessons learned by use of magnetic resonance imaging. Circulation 107:2004, 2003.
25. Gupta A, Frazer CK, Ferguson JM, et al: Acute pulmonary embolism: Diagnosis with MR angiography. Radiology 210:353, 1999.
26. Yucel EK: Pulmonary MR angiography: Is it ready now? Radiology 210:301, 1999.
27. Baum RA, Rutter CM, Sunshine JH, et al: Multicenter trial to evaluate vascular magnetic resonance angiography of the lower extremity. American College of Radiology Rapid Technology Assessment Group. JAMA 274:875, 1995.
28. Yucel EK, Kaufman JA, Geller SC, et al: Atherosclerotic occlusive disease of the lower extremity: Prospective evaluation with two-dimensional time-of-flight MR angiography. Radiology 187:637, 1993.
29. Prince MR, Chabra SG, Watts R, et al: Contrast material travel times in patients undergoing peripheral MR angiography. Radiology 224:55, 2002.
30. Khilnani NM, Winchester PA, Prince MR, et al: Peripheral vascular disease: Combined 3D bolus chase and dynamic 2D MR angiography compared with x-ray angiography for treatment planning. Radiology 224:63, 2002.
31. Ho KY, Leiner T, de Haan MW, et al: Peripheral vascular tree stenoses: Evaluation with moving-bed infusion-tracking MR angiography. Radiology 206:683, 1998.
32. Meaney JF, Ridgway JP, Chakraverty S, et al: Stepping-table gadolinium-enhanced digital subtraction MR angiography of the aorta and lower extremity arteries: Preliminary experience. Radiology 211:59, 1999.
33. Ruehm SG, Hany TF, Pfammatter T, et al: Pelvic and lower extremity arterial imaging: Diagnostic performance of three-dimensional contrast-enhanced MR angiography. AJR Am J Roentgenol 174:1127, 2000.
34. Bertschinger K, Cassina PC, Debatin JF, et al: Surveillance of peripheral arterial bypass grafts with three-dimensional MR angiography: Comparison with digital subtraction angiography. AJR Am J Roentgenol 176:215, 2001.
35. Morasch MD, Collins J, Pereles FS, et al: Lower extremity stepping-table magnetic resonance angiography with multilevel contrast timing and segmented contrast infusion. J Vasc Surg 37:62, 2003.
36. Hofmann WJ, Forstner R, Kofler B, et al: Pedal artery imaging—A comparison of selective digital subtraction angiography, contrast enhanced magnetic resonance angiography and duplex ultrasound. Eur J Vasc Endovasc Surg 24:287, 2002.
37. Konkus CJ, Czum JM, Jacobacci JT: Contrast-enhanced MR angiography of the aorta and lower extremities with routine inclusion of the feet. AJR Am J Roentgenol 179:115, 2002.
38. Elias DA, White LM, Rubenstein JD, et al: Clinical evaluation and MR imaging features of popliteal artery entrapment and cystic adventitial disease. AJR Am J Roentgenol 180:627, 2003.
39. Atilla S, Akpek ET, Yucel C, et al: MR imaging and MR angiography in popliteal artery entrapment syndrome. Eur Radiol 8:1025, 1998.
40. Crolla RM, Steyling JF, Hennipman A, et al: A case of cystic adventitial disease of the popliteal artery demonstrated by magnetic resonance imaging. J Vasc Surg 18:1052, 1993.
41. Krause U, Pabst T, Kenn W, et al: High resolution contrast enhanced MR-angiography of the hand arteries: Preliminary experiences. Vasa 31:179, 2002.
42. Wentz KU, Frohlich JM, von Weymarn C, et al: High-resolution magnetic resonance angiography of hands with timed arterial compression (tac-MRA). Lancet 361:49, 2003.
43. Nelemans PJ, Leiner T, de Vet HC, et al: Peripheral arterial disease: Meta-analysis of the diagnostic performance of MR angiography. Radiology 217:105, 2000.
44. Hood MN, Ho VB, Foo TK, et al: High-resolution gadolinium-enhanced 3D MRA of the infrapopliteal arteries. Lessons for improving bolus-chase peripheral MRA. J Magn Reson Imaging 20:543, 2002.
45. Carroll TJ, Grist TM: Technical developments in MR angiography. Radiol Clin North Am 40:921, 2002.
46. Maki JH, Wilson GJ, Eubank WB, et al: Utilizing SENSE to achieve lower station sub-millimeter isotropic resolution and minimal venous enhancement in peripheral MR angiography. J Magn Reson Imaging 15:484, 2002.
47. Swan JS, Carroll TJ, Kennell TW, et al: Time-resolved three-dimensional contrast-enhanced MR angiography of the peripheral vessels. Radiology 225:43, 2002.
48. Vasbinder GB, Maki JH, Nijenhuis RJ, et al: Motion of the distal renal artery during three-dimensional contrast-enhanced breath-hold MRA. J Magn Reson Imaging 16:685, 2002.
49. Tan KT, van Beek EJ, Brown PW, et al: Magnetic resonance angiography for the diagnosis of renal artery stenosis: A meta-analysis. Clin Radiol 57:617, 2002.
50. Vasbinder GB, Nelemans PJ, Kessels AG, et al: Diagnostic tests for renal artery stenosis in patients suspected of having renovascular hypertension: A meta-analysis. Ann Intern Med 135:401, 2001.
51. Prince MR, Narasimham DL, Stanley JC, et al: Gadolinium-enhanced magnetic resonance angiography of abdominal aortic aneurysms. J Vasc Surg 21:656, 1995.
52. Lutz AM, Willmann JK, Pfammatter T, et al: Evaluation of aortoiliac aneurysm before endovascular repair: Comparison of contrast-enhanced magnetic resonance angiography with multidetector row computed tomographic angiography with an automated analysis software tool. J Vasc Surg 37:619, 2003.
53. Cejna M, Loewe C, Schoder M, et al: MR angiography vs CT angiography in the follow-up of nitinol stent grafts in endoluminally treated aortic aneurysms. Eur Radiol 12:2443, 2002.
54. Shellock FG, Shellock VJ: Metallic stents: Evaluation of MR imaging safety. AJR Am J Roentgenol 173:543, 1999.
55. Engellau L, Olsrud J, Brockstedt S, et al: MR evaluation ex vivo and in vivo of a covered stent-graft for abdominal aortic aneurysms:

Ferromagnetism, heating, artifacts, and velocity mapping. J Magn Reson Imaging 12:112, 2000.
56. Holland GA, Dougherty L, Carpenter JP, et al: Breath-hold ultrafast three-dimensional gadolinium-enhanced MR angiography of the aorta and the renal and other visceral abdominal arteries. AJR Am J Roentgenol 166:971, 1996.
57. Gaa J, Laub G, Edelman RR, et al: [First clinical results of ultrafast, contrast-enhanced 2-phase 3D-angiography of the abdomen.] Rofo 169:135, 1998.
58. Shirkhoda A, Konez O, Shetty AN, et al: Mesenteric circulation: Three-dimensional MR angiography with a gadolinium-enhanced multiecho gradient-echo technique. Radiology 202:257, 1997.
59. Vosshenrich R, Fischer U: Contrast-enhanced MR angiography of abdominal vessels: Is there still a role for angiography? Eur Radiol 12:218, 2002.
60. Laissy JP, Trillaud H, Douek P: MR angiography: Noninvasive vascular imaging of the abdomen. Abdom Imaging 27:488, 2002.
61. Tanigawa K, Eguchi K, Kitamura Y, et al: Magnetic resonance imaging detection of aortic and pulmonary artery wall thickening in the acute stage of Takayasu arteritis. Improvement of clinical and radiologic findings after steroid therapy. Arthritis Rheum 35:476, 1992.
62. Kerr GS, Hallahan CW, Giordano J, et al: Takayasu arteritis. Ann Intern Med 120:919, 1994.
63. Yamada I, Nakagawa T, Himeno Y, et al: Takayasu arteritis: Diagnosis with breath-hold contrast-enhanced three-dimensional MR angiography. J Magn Reson Imaging 11:481, 2000.
64. Flamm SD, White RD, Hoffman GS: The clinical application of 'edema-weighted' magnetic resonance imaging in the assessment of Takayasu's arteritis. Int J Cardiol 66 Suppl 1:S151, 1998.
65. Tso E, Flamm SD, White RD, et al: Takayasu arteritis: Utility and limitations of magnetic resonance imaging in diagnosis and treatment. Arthritis Rheum 46:1634, 2002.
66. Choe YH, Han BK, Koh EM, et al: Takayasu's arteritis: Assessment of disease activity with contrast-enhanced MR imaging. AJR Am J Roentgenol 175:505, 2000.
67. Mitomo T, Funyu T, Takahashi Y, et al: Giant cell arteritis and magnetic resonance angiography. Arthritis Rheum 41:1702, 1998.
68. Harada S, Mitsunobu F, Kodama F, et al: Giant cell arteritis associated with rheumatoid arthritis monitored by magnetic resonance angiography. Intern Med 38:675, 1999.
69. Roberts WN, DeMeo JH, Breitbach SA: Well-imaged large vessel vasculitis attributed to anticardiolipin antibody. Arthritis Rheum 37:1254, 1994.
70. Anders HJ, Sigl T, Sander A, et al: Gadolinium contrast magnetic resonance imaging of the temporal artery in giant cell arteritis. J Rheumatol 26:2287, 1999.
71. Spritzer CE, Arata MA, Freed KS: Isolated pelvic deep venous thrombosis: Relative frequency as detected with MR imaging. Radiology 219:521, 2001.
72. Carpenter JP, Holland GA, Baum RA, et al: Magnetic resonance venography for the detection of deep venous thrombosis: Comparison with contrast venography and duplex Doppler ultrasonography. J Vasc Surg 18:734, 1993.
73. Ruehm SG, Zimny K, Debatin JF: Direct contrast-enhanced 3D MR venography. Eur Radiol 11:102, 2001.
74. Nguyen BD, Westra WH, Zerhouni EA: Renal cell carcinoma and tumor thrombus neovascularity: MR demonstration with pathologic correlation. Abdom Imaging 21:269, 1996.
75. Laissy JP, Menegazzo D, Debray MP, et al: Renal carcinoma: Diagnosis of venous invasion with Gd-enhanced MR venography. Eur Radiol 10:1138, 2000.
76. Kallman DA, King BF, Hattery RR, et al: Renal vein and inferior vena cava tumor thrombus in renal cell carcinoma: CT, US, MRI and venacavography. J Comput Assist Tomogr 16:240, 1992.
77. Narumi Y, Hricak H, Presti JC, Jr, et al: MR imaging evaluation of renal cell carcinoma. Abdom Imaging 22:216, 1997.
78. Kubik-Huch RA, Hebisch G, Huch R, et al: Role of duplex color Doppler ultrasound, computed tomography, and MR angiography in the diagnosis of septic puerperal ovarian vein thrombosis. Abdom Imaging 24:85, 1999.
79. Minniti S, Visentini S, Procacci C: Congenital anomalies of the venae cavae: Embryological origin, imaging features and report of three new variants. Eur Radiol 12:2040, 2002.

chapter 12

CT Angiography

U. Joseph Schoepf
Martin J. Lipton
Thomas G. Flohr

Computed transmission tomography (CT) was introduced in the early 1970s and has revolutionized not only diagnostic radiology but the practice of medicine in general. It was the first technology to marry a computer to a medical imaging machine, the first to display x-ray images in cross-section, and the first modality to herald a new era of digital imaging. The scout view, which is now part of every CT scan, is a digital computerized radiograph and is fundamental for accurate scan level localization. CT, therefore, led the way for the development of digital subtraction angiography (DSA), magnetic resonance imaging (MRI), positron emission tomography (PET) and digital echocardiography. Indeed, many of the same principles and methods used in these later modalities were based on CT technology.

The remarkably high contrast resolution (density range) of CT allows intravenous iodinated contrast agents to provide sufficient vascular enhancement to compete favorably with conventional intra-arterial angiography. Several fundamental issues determine clinical usefulness for specific diagnostic applications. These include spatial, temporal, and contrast resolution, field of view, x-ray scan speed, and geometry, as well as how well protocols match scan acquisition to optimal vascular contrast enhancement in structures of interest.

Computed tomography angiography (CTA) has now become a reality. Initially, conventional whole body single-slice CT was too slow to be competitive with invasive catheter angiography. Nevertheless, feasibility was established for almost every area by single-slice studies. Furthermore, electron beam CT (EBCT) demonstrated the great potential of CT for cardiovascular diagnosis. However, it required several generations of CT scanner development over two decades before multislice CT (MSCT) made CTA part of the clinical routine. Multislice CT has become almost ubiquitously available. In fact, most scanner manufacturers have discontinued production of traditional single-slice CT scanners; since the introduction of the first 4-slice systems in the late nineties, manufacturers have leapfrogged each other with the introduction of ever-faster scanners with additional detector rows and more sophisticated image acquisition techniques.

This chapter discusses the basic principles of MSCT and explains how this technology is progressively replacing more invasive diagnostic vascular imaging for virtually every organ system, both in the arterial and venous circulation. Modern MSCT scanners can acquire hundreds of CT scans within seconds, resulting in vast data observer sets for analysis. Image interpretation has, therefore, evolved with routine post-processing methods for image display, analysis, and quantitation. These methods will be discussed as well as the strengths and weaknesses of CTA, including radiation dose concerns.

EVOLUTION OF SPIRAL CT: FROM SINGLE-SLICE TO MULTISLICE CT

The introduction of spiral CT in the early nineties[1-3] constituted a fundamental evolutionary step in the development and ongoing refinement of CT-imaging techniques. For the first time, volume data could be acquired without misregistration of anatomical detail. Volume data became the very basis for CT angiography. The ability to acquire volume data also paved the way for the development of 3-D image processing techniques such as multiplanar reformations (MPR), maximum intensity projections (MIP), surface-shaded displays (SSP), and volume rendering techniques (VRT), which have become a vital component of medical imaging today.

Ideally, volume data is of high spatial resolution and isotropic in nature, i.e., each image data element ("voxel") is of equal dimensions in all three spatial axes, as a basis for image display in arbitrarily oriented imaging planes. For most clinical scenarios, however, single-slice spiral CT with one-second gantry rotation time is unable to fulfill these prerequisites. To avoid motion artifacts and to optimally use the contrast bolus, CT angiography needs to be completed within a certain time frame of a patient breath-hold (25- to 30-seconds). If a large scan range, such as the entire aorta (≈60 cm), has to be covered within a single breath-hold, a thick collimation of 5 to 8 mm must be used. This results in a considerable mismatch between longitudinal (z-) resolution along the patient axis, which is determined by the collimated slice width, and the in-plane resolution of ordinarily 0.5 to 0.7 mm. Thus, with single-slice spiral CT the ideal of isotropic resolution can be achieved only for very limited scan ranges.[4]

Strategies to achieve more substantial volume coverage with improved longitudinal resolution include the simultaneous acquisition of more than one slice at a time and a reduction of the gantry rotation time. Apart from a dedicated 2-slice system for cardiac applications introduced in 1984, the first step toward multislice acquisition in general radiology was a 2-slice CT scanner introduced in 1993. In 1998, eventually, all major CT manufacturers introduced MSCT systems, which provided considerable improvement of scan speed and longitudinal resolution and better use of the available x-ray power.[5-7] These systems typically offered simultaneous acquisition of four slices at a rotation time of 0.5 second.

Simultaneous acquisition of *M* slices results in an *M*-fold increase in speed if all other parameters, such as slice thickness, are unchanged. This increased performance of MSCT compared to single-slice CT allowed for the optimization of CT angiography. The examination time for standard protocols could be significantly reduced. This proved to be of immediate clinical benefit for the quick and comprehensive assessment of trauma victims and of critically ill or noncooperative patients. Alternatively, the scan range that could be covered within a certain scan time was extended by a factor of *M*. This is relevant to CT angiography with extended coverage, for example of the lower extremity runoff. The most important clinical benefit, however, proved to be the ability to scan a given anatomical volume within a given scan time with substantially reduced slice width, at *M* times with increased longitudinal resolution. This way, for many clinical applications, the goal of isotropic resolution was within reach. Examinations of the entire thorax or abdomen could now routinely be performed with 1 mm or 1.25 mm collimated slice width. Despite these promising advances, clinical challenges and limitations remained for 4-slice CT systems. True isotropic resolution for routine applications had not yet been achieved because the longitudinal resolution of about 1 mm does not fully match the in-plane resolution of about 0.5 to 0.7 mm in a routine scan of the chest or abdomen. For large volumes, such as CT angiography of the lower extremity runoff, thicker (i.e., 2.5 mm) collimated slice width had to be used to complete the scan within a reasonable time frame. Scan times were often too long to allow for image acquisition during pure arterial phase. For a CTA of the circle of Willis, for instance, a scan range of about 100 mm must be covered. With 4-slice CT, at 1-mm slice width and 0.5-second gantry rotation time, this volume can be covered in about 9-second scan time, not fast enough to avoid venous overlay—assuming a cerebral circulation time of less than 5 seconds.

As a next step, the introduction of an 8-slice CT system in 2000 enabled shorter scan times, but did not yet provide improved longitudinal resolution (thinnest collimation 8 × 1.25 mm). The latter was achieved with the introduction of 16-slice and 64-slice CT,[8] which made it possible to routinely acquire substantial anatomical volumes with isotropic sub-millimeter spatial resolution and scan times of less than 10 seconds for 300 mm coverage. Although in-plane spatial resolution is not substantially improved, the two major advantages of fast MSCT acquisition are true isotropic through-plane resolution and short acquisition time that enables high-quality examinations in severely debilitated and severely dyspneic patients.

Traditional CT applications have been enhanced and strengthened by the remarkable, yet incremental, improvement in scanner performance by the addition of more detector rows. Conventional MSCT also dramatically expanded into areas previously considered beyond the scope of conventional CT scanners, such as cardiac imaging—with the addition of ECG gating capability. With a gantry rotation time of 0.5 second and dedicated image reconstruction approaches, the temporal resolution for the acquisition of a transaxial image was improved to 250 msec and less, which proved to be sufficient for motion-free imaging of the heart in the mid- to end-diastolic phase at slow to moderate heart rates (i.e., up to 65 beats/min).[9-11] With 4 simultaneously acquired slices, coverage of the entire heart volume with thin slices (i.e., 4 × 1 mm or 4 × 1.25 mm collimation) within a single breath-hold became feasible. The increased longitudinal resolution, combined with improved contrast resolution of modern CT systems, enabled noninvasive visualization of the coronary arteries. The initial clinical studies demonstrated MSCT's potential to not only detect but, to some degree, also characterize noncalcified and calcified plaques in the coronary arteries based on their CT attenuation.[12,13] The limitations of 4- and 8-slice CT systems, however, so far have prevented the successful integration of CT coronary angiography into routine clinical algorithms: Stents or heavily calcified arteries constitute a diagnostic dilemma, mainly because of partial volume artifacts as a consequence of insufficient longitudinal resolution. For patients with higher heart rates, careful selection of separate reconstruction intervals for different coronary arteries has been mandatory. The breath-hold time of about 40 seconds required to cover the entire heart volume (~12 cm) with 4-slice CT is almost impossible to comply with for patients with manifest heart disease. The ongoing technical refinement of MSCT, however, holds promise of gradually overcoming some of these limitations. The most important steps toward this goal are gantry rotation times faster than 0.5 second; for improved temporal resolution and robustness of use, 16-slice or 64-slice sub-millimeter acquisition for increased longitudinal resolution and shorter breath-hold times; and novel, sophisticated approaches for image acquisition and reconstruction.

MULTISLICE CT IMAGE ACQUISITION

Spiral Acquisition

For clinical purposes different slice widths must be available to adjust the optimum scan speed, longitudinal resolution, and image noise for each application. With a single-slice CT detector, different slice widths are obtained by prepatient collimation ("bundling") of the x-ray beam (Fig. 12-1). A very elementary model of an *M*-slice CT detector consists of *M* detector rows: only for $M = 2$, however, different slice widths can be realized by prepatient collimation. For *M* greater than 2, this simple design principle encounters its limitations and has to be replaced by more flexible concepts requiring more than *M* detector rows to simultaneously acquire *M* slices. Different manufacturers of MSCT scanners introduced different detector designs. To be able to select different slice-widths, all scanners electronically combine several detector rows into a smaller number of slices according to the selected beam width.

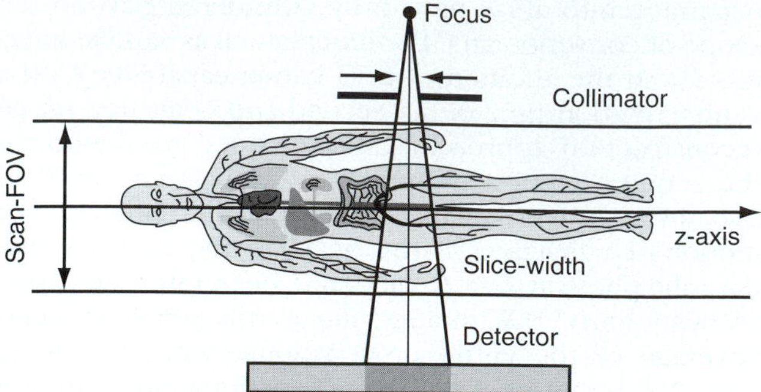

FIGURE 12-1. Illustration of prepatient collimation of the x-ray beam to obtain different collimated slice widths with a single-slice CT detector.

For established 4-slice CT systems, two detector types are commonly used. The fixed array detector consists of detector elements with equal sizes in the longitudinal direction. A representative example for this scanner type, the GE Lightspeed scanner, has 16 detector rows, each of them defining 1.25 mm slice width.[6,7,14] The total coverage in the longitudinal direction is 20 mm; because of geometric magnification the actual detector is about twice as wide. By combination of the signals of the individual detector rows, the following slice widths are realized: 4 × 1.25 mm, 4 × 2.5 mm, 4 × 3.75 mm, and 4 × 5 mm (Fig. 12-2A). The same detector design is used for the 8-slice version of this system, providing 8 × 1.25 mm and 8 × 2.5 mm slice width.

A different approach uses an adaptive array detector design, which comprises detector rows with different sizes in the longitudinal direction.[5] Scanners of this type, the Philips Mx8000 4-slice scanner and the Siemens SOMATOM Sensation 4 scanner, have 8 detector rows. Their widths in the longitudinal direction range from 1 mm to 5 mm and allow for the following slice widths: 2 × 0.5 mm, 4 × 1 mm, 4 × 2.5 mm, 4 × 5 mm, 2 × 8 mm, and 2 × 10 mm (see Fig. 12-2B).

The selection of the slice width determines the intrinsic longitudinal resolution of a scan. In a "step and shoot" axial mode, any multiple of the slice width of one detector slice can be obtained by adding the detector signals during image reconstruction. In a spiral mode, the effective slice width is adjusted independently in the spiral interpolation process during image reconstruction. Hence, from the same data set both narrow slices for high-resolution detail or for 3-D post-processing and wide slices for better contrast resolution or quick review and filming may be derived.

All recently introduced 16-slice CT systems have adaptive array detectors. A representative example of this scanner type, the Siemens SOMATOM Sensation 16 scanner, uses 24 detector rows.[8,15] The 16 central rows define 0.75-mm slice width, the 4 outer rows on both sides define 1.5-mm slice width (see Fig. 12-2C). The total coverage in the longitudinal direction is 24 mm. By appropriate combination of the signals of the individual detector rows, either 12 or 16 slices with 0.75-mm or 1.5-mm slice width can be acquired simultaneously. The GE Lightspeed 16 scanner uses a similar design, which provides 16 slices with either 0.625-mm or 1.25-mm slice width. The total coverage in the longitudinal direction is 20 mm. Yet another design, which is implemented in the Toshiba Aquilion scanner, allows the use of 16 slices with either 0.5-mm, 1-mm, or 2-mm slice width and a total z-coverage of 32 mm.

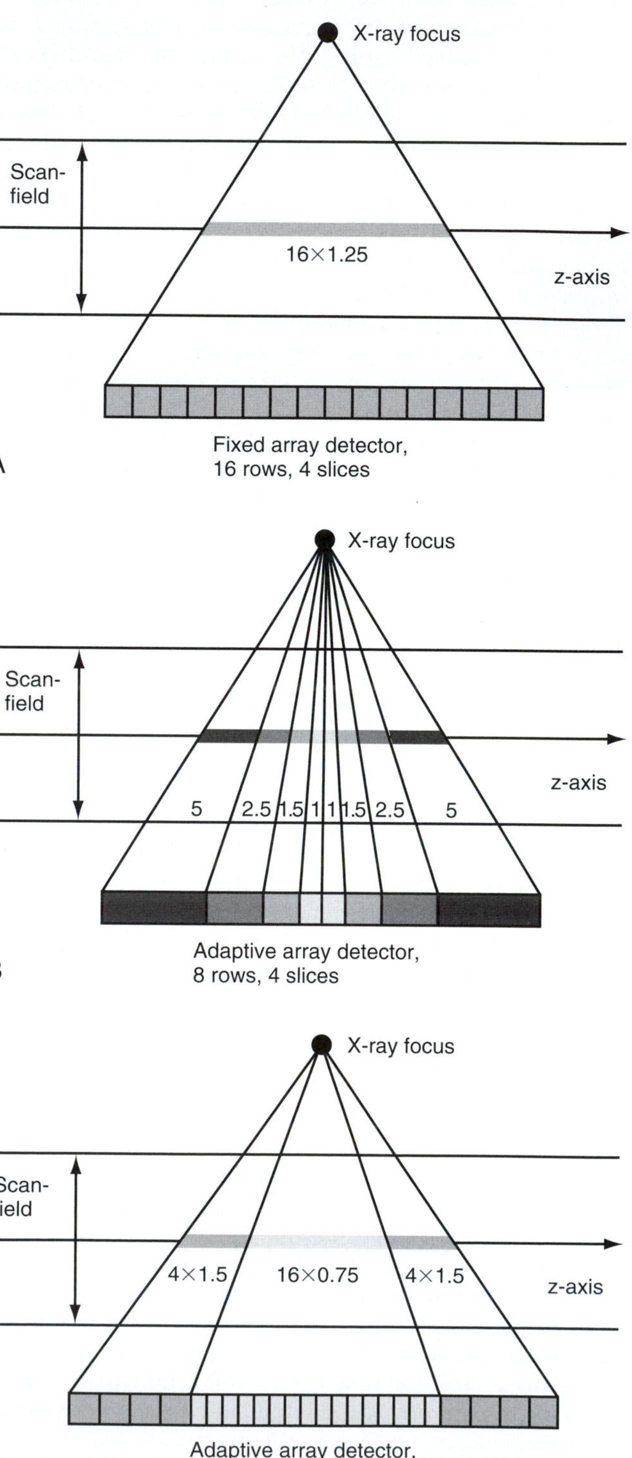

FIGURE 12-2. Examples of fixed array detectors and adaptive array detectors used in commercially available 4-slice and 16-slice CT systems.

ECG-Synchronized Scan and Image Reconstruction Techniques

One of the most exciting new applications of MSCT is the ability to image the heart and cardiovascular anatomy without motion artifacts. In 1984, electron-beam CT was introduced as the first system to enable ECG-synchronized CT scan acquisition of cardiac anatomy.[16] With presently available electron-beam CT scanners, the routine protocol for evaluation of cardiac anatomy and of the coronary arteries ordinarily comprises 3-mm slice width, a temporal resolution of 100 msec and prospective ECG triggering (see later) for sequential acquisition of transaxial images consistently at the same phase of the cardiac cycle, typically during diastole.[17]

Coronary arteries are small and complex 3-D structures. The diameter of coronary vessels tapers from typically 5 mm in the left main coronary artery to 1 mm luminal diameter in the distal left anterior descending coronary artery.[18] For adequate visualization of the small, tortuous, and complex anatomy of the coronary artery tree and of subtle pathology along the vessel course, an isotropic (i.e., equal voxel dimensions in x-, y- and z-axes) or near isotropic in-plane and through-plane spatial resolution of less than 1 mm is necessary. With the protocols that are ordinarily used for high resolution imaging of the coronary arteries, current MSCT scanner systems provide an in-plane resolution of 0.5 mm and an effective through-plane (z)-resolution of 0.6 to 0.8 mm,[15] which is approaching the requirements for successful noninvasive imaging of the coronary arteries.[19] To differentiate a 10% to 20% coronary artery stenosis, however, CT systems will need to provide an isotropic spatial resolution of at least 0.3 mm.[15]

Motion artifacts that are caused by cardiac pulsation can be minimized in high resolution CT studies of the heart via scanning or reconstructing scan projection data at a time point with the least cardiac motion, ordinarily in the diastolic phase of the heart cycle. For most practical purposes, a heart-rate independent temporal resolution of 100 msec or less allows for elimination of most cardiac motion, if images are acquired (prospective triggering) or reconstructed (retrospective gating) during diastole. The heart phases can be determined from a simultaneously recorded ECG signal. Two different ECG synchronization techniques are most commonly employed for cardiac CT scanning, prospective ECG triggering and retrospective ECG gating.

ECG-Synchronized CT Scan Acquisition: Prospective Triggering

Prospective ECG triggering has long been used in conjunction with electron-beam CT and single-slice spiral CT.[17,20-22] A trigger signal is derived from the patient's ECG—based on a prospective estimation of the present RR-interval—and the scan is started at a defined time point after a detected R-wave, usually during diastole. With MSCT, several sections are simultaneously acquired during one scan acquisition with a cycle time that ordinarily allows image acquisition at every other heart beat.[23] Generally this strategy results in shorter breath-hold times compared with single-slice CT techniques, and respiratory artifacts are less likely to occur. To improve temporal resolution, scan data are acquired only during a partial scanner rotation (~ 2/3 of a rotation with 240 to 260° projection data) that covers the minimum amount of data required for image reconstruction. Conventional partial scan reconstruction based on fan beam projection data results in a temporal resolution that equals the acquisition time of the partial scan. Optimized temporal resolution can be achieved with parallel-beam-based "half-scan" reconstruction algorithms that provide a temporal resolution of one half the rotation time in a center area of the scan field of view (e.g., 250 msec for 500 msec rotation time and 210 msec for 420 msec rotation time). This way prospective ECG triggering is the most dose-efficient way of ECG-synchronized scanning because only the very minimum of scan data needed for image reconstruction is acquired.[24] However, usually only quite thick slices (3 mm with electron-beam CT, 2.5 to 3 mm with 4- to 8-slice CT, 1.5 mm with 16-slice CT) is being used for prospectively ECG-triggered acquisition. Thus, resulting data sets are less suitable for 3-D reconstruction of small cardiac anatomy. Also, prospectively ECG-triggered technique greatly depends on a regular heart rate of the patient and is bound to result in misregistration in the presence of arrhythmia.

ECG-Synchronized CT Scan Acquisition: Retrospective Gating

An alternative approach for ECG-synchronized CT scan acquisition is retrospective ECG gating (Fig. 12-3).

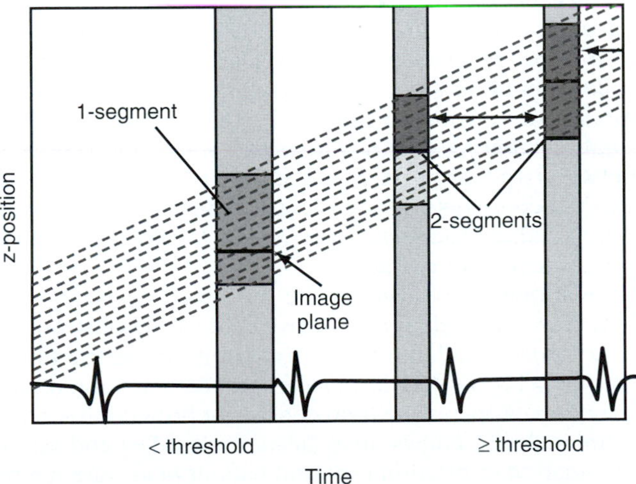

FIGURE 12-3. Schematic illustration of an adaptive segmented image reconstruction approach for ECG-gated multidetector-row CT scanning. Dashed lines indicate the z-positions of the detector slices, which continuously and linearly change position relative to the patient with constant spiral feed. The ECG signal is simultaneously recorded during scan acquisition and is displayed at the bottom of the diagram. At heart rates below a certain predefined threshold, one segment of consecutive multislice spiral data is used for image reconstruction. At higher heart rates, two (or more) subsegments from adjacent heart cycles contribute to the partial scan data segment. In each cardiac cycle, a stack of images is reconstructed at different z-positions covering a small subvolume of the heart, which is indicated as a box. The combination of subvolumes from all heart cycles during the scan provides a continuous 3-D data set of the entire heart.

This strategy generally enables greater flexibility for phase-consistent image reconstruction when examining patients with changing heart rates during scan acquisition. Retrospective ECG gating requires multislice spiral scanning with slow table motion and simultaneous recording of the ECG trace that is used for retrospective linkage of scan data with particular phases of the cardiac cycle.[8,25] Retrospectively ECG-gated CT scan acquisition of the heart requires a highly overlapping spiral scan with a spiral table speed adapted to the heart rate to ensure complete phase-consistent coverage of the heart with overlapping image slices. Most multislice CT scanners provide scan protocols with fixed overlapping spiral pitch between 0.25 and 0.375 that result in gapless volume coverage for heart rates above ~40 beats/min. The spiral pitch is defined as the table feed per rotation divided by the collimation width of all detector slices. Reconstruction of image stacks at the exact phase of the heart cycle enables continuous and phase-consistent coverage of the entire heart and adjacent anatomy in the selected scan range (see Fig. 12-3). Ordinarily a stack of images is reconstructed at every heart beat, enabling faster scan coverage as compared with prospectively ECG-triggered multislice CT scanning. Continuous spiral acquisition enables reconstruction of overlapping image slices and, thus, a longitudinal spatial resolution of about 20% below the slice width can be achieved (e.g., 2.5-mm for 3.0-mm slices, 1.0-mm for 1.25-mm slices, 0.8-mm for 1.0-mm slices, and 0.6-mm for 0.75-mm slices).[15,26] For these reasons, retrospectively ECG-gated scan acquisition is the preferred method for contrast-enhanced high spatial resolution imaging of small cardiac structures, especially of the coronary arteries. For image reconstruction at every heart beat, fan beam data of a partial rotation (usually 240° to 260°) is used that results in a temporal resolution equivalent to one half of the rotation time in a centered region of interest (250-msec for 500-msec rotation time and 210-msec for 420-msec rotation time).[15,25,26] A multislice spiral interpolation between the projections of adjacent detector rows is used to compensate for table movement and to provide a well-defined slice-sensitivity profile for images without spiral movement artifacts.

Temporal resolution can be improved by using scan data from more than one heart cycle for reconstruction of a single axial image ("segmented reconstruction") (see Fig. 12-3).[26-29] The partial scan data set for reconstruction of one image then consists of projection sectors from multiple consecutive heart cycles. Depending on the relation of rotation time and patient heart rate, a temporal resolution between rotation-time/2 and rotation-time/2M is present (M equals the number of projection sectors and the number of used heart cycles). Despite theoretically better temporal resolution, segmented reconstruction algorithms do not regularly provide superior image quality[29] because the algorithms are very sensitive to changing heart rates.

Usually diastole is chosen for image reconstruction of cardiac and coronary morphology as the phase of the cardiac cycle with the least motion; however, due to the highly overlapping scan acquisition, image data can be reconstructed for each x-, y- and z-position within the scanned volume over the entire course of the cardiac cycle. This allows for retrospective selection of reconstruction points that provide best relative image quality in an individual patient and for anatomy with special motion patterns.[30,31] To improve phase consistency in the presence of arrhythmia, individual image stacks can be discarded or their reconstruction interval arbitrarily shifted within the cardiac cycle, so that ideally reconstruction always coincides with the same interval during diastole at each level of the cardiac volume.[25] In addition to the structural information that is derived from image reconstruction during diastole, additional reconstructions of the same scan data set in different phases of the cardiac cycle can be used as a byproduct of retrospectively ECG-gated scan acquisitions for analysis of basic cardiac function parameters—such as end-diastolic volume, end-systolic volume; and ejection fraction.[32-34]

Radiation Dose and Dose Efficiency

Radiation exposure of the patient by computed tomography and the resulting potential radiation hazard has recently gained considerable attention both in the public and in the scientific literature.[35,36] The typical effective patient dose of selected CT protocols is 1 to 2 mSv for a head examination, 5 to 7 mSv for a chest CT, and 8 to 11 mSv for CT of the abdomen and pelvis.[37,38] This radiation exposure must be appreciated in the context of the average annual background radiation, which is 3.6 mSv in the United States. Despite its undoubted clinical benefits, multislice scanning is often considered to require increased patient dose compared with single-slice CT. Indeed, a certain increase in radiation dose is unavoidable owing to the underlying physical principles.

In the x-ray tube of a CT scanner a small area on the anode plate, the focal spot, emits x-ray beams that penetrate the patient and are registered by the detector. A collimator between x-ray tube and patient, the prepatient collimator, is used to shape the beam and to establish the dose profile. In general, the collimated dose profile is a trapezoid in the longitudinal direction. In the umbral region, that is the plateau region of the trapezoid, x-rays emitted from the entire area of the focal spot illuminate the detector. In the penumbra regions, only a part of the focal spot illuminates the detector, while the prepatient collimator blocks off other parts. With single-slice CT, the entire trapezoidal dose profile can contribute to the detector signal and the collimated slice width is determined as the full width at half maximum (FWHM) of this trapezoid. The relative dose use of a single-slice CT system can, therefore, be close to 100%. With MSCT, in most cases only the plateau region of the dose profile is used to ensure equal signal level for all detector elements. The penumbra region is then discarded, either by a postpatient collimator or by the intrinsic self-collimation of the multislice detector, and represents "wasted" dose. The relative contribution of the penumbra region increases with decreasing slice width, and it decreases with increasing number of simultaneously acquired images. This is demonstrated in Figure 12-4, which compares the "minimum width" dose profiles

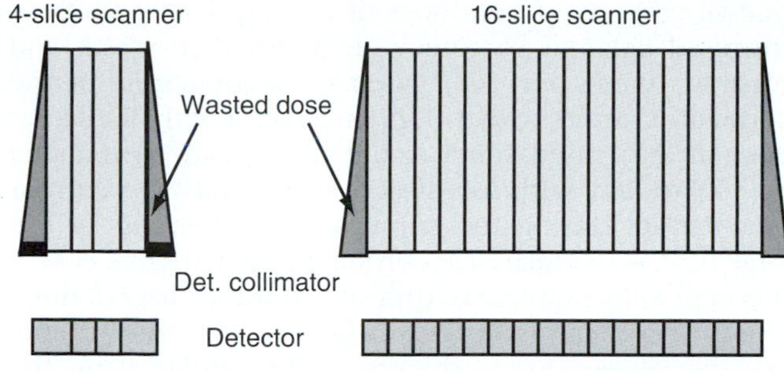

FIGURE 12-4. Dose profiles for a 4-slice CT system and a 16-slice CT system with identical collimated width of one detector slice. The relative contribution of the penumbra region, which represents wasted dose, decreases with increasing number of simultaneously acquired slices. Det, detector.

for a 4-slice CT system and a corresponding 16-slice CT system with equal width of one detector slice. Correspondingly, the relative dose utilization at 4 × 1 mm with 4-slice CT is 70% or less, depending on the scanner type. With 16-slice CT systems and sub-millimeter slices, dose utilization can be improved up to 84%, again depending on scanner type. Some MSCT systems offer special implementations of even more dose-efficient modes that use a portion of the penumbral region. Thus, unlike the transition from single-slice CT to 4-slice CT systems, a further increase in radiation exposure with the more widespread availability of 16-slice CT systems is not expected.

A clinically appropriate measure for dose is the weighted computerized tomographic dose index $CTDI_w$, which uses the absorbed dose in a Lucite phantom as an approximation of the dose delivered to a cross-section of the patient's anatomy. $CTDI_w$ is measured using a 16 cm Lucite phantom for head and a 32 cm Lucite phantom for body and determined as one third of the CTDI value in the phantom center plus two thirds of the CTDI value at the periphery (see Appendix).

Concepts for Radiation Dose Reduction

The most important factor for reducing radiation exposure is the adaptation of the radiation dose to patient size and weight.[39-41]

As a general rule, the dose necessary to maintain constant image noise has to be doubled if the patient diameter is increased by 4 cm. Correspondingly, for patients 4 cm smaller than average, one half the standard dose is sufficient for maintaining adequate image quality. Dose reduction can be achieved by mAs reduction and lower kV settings.

Another means to reduce radiation exposure is to adapt the x-ray tube voltage to the intended application. In contrast-enhanced studies, such as CT angiography, the contrast-to-noise ratio for fixed patient dose increases with decreasing x-ray tube voltage. As a consequence, to obtain the desired contrast-to-noise ratio, patient dose can be reduced by choosing lower kV settings. The potential for dose saving is more significant for smaller patient diameter. Ideally, 80 kV should be used for CT angiography in order to reduce patient dose. Clinical studies have confirmed these findings and demonstrated a potential for dose reduction of about 50% when using 80 kV instead of 120 kV for performing CT angiography. In reality, however, the maximum x-ray tube current available at 80 kV is generally not sufficient to scan bigger patients, which limits the routine application of this approach. Therefore, use of 100 kV appears as a suitable compromise and the method of choice for performing CT angiography. Figure 12-5 shows CT pulmonary angiography in a patient with pulmonary embolism, acquired on a 16-slice scanner at 100 kV and 120 mAs. The effective patient radiation dose for this scan was 2.3 mSv, 25% less than for the standard 120 kV protocol. 100 kV has been

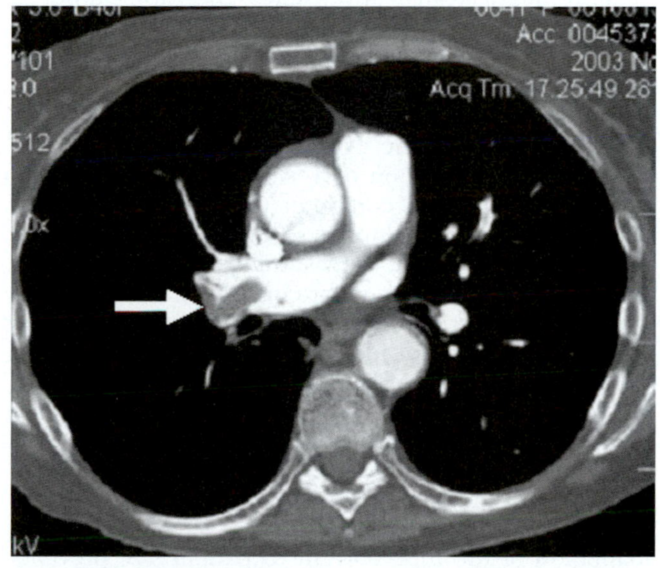

A

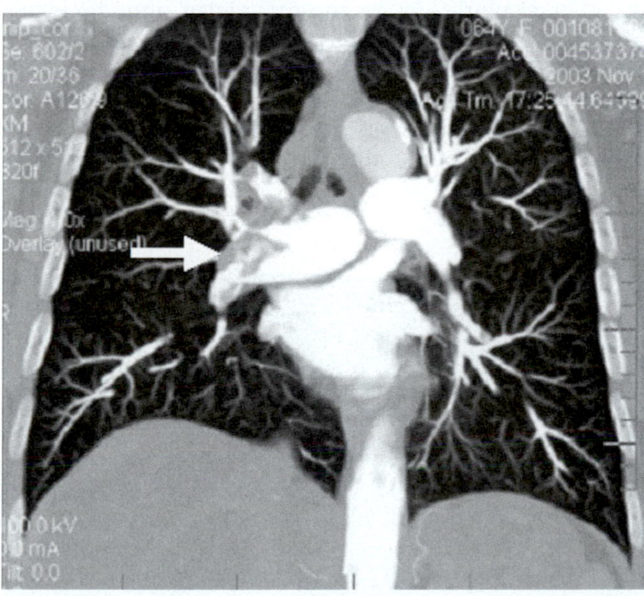

B

FIGURE 12-5. Thorax examination of a patient with pulmonary embolism (*arrow*) acquired on a 16-slice scanner at 100 kV and 120 mAs. Effective patient dose for this scan was 2.3 mSv, 25% less than for the standard 120 kV protocol. Axial section **(A)** and coronal maximum intensity projection **(B)**.

recommended as the standard mode for thoracic and abdominal CT angiography, and dose savings of 30% without loss of diagnostic information have been reported.

An approach which finds increased implementation in clinical practice is anatomic tube current modulation. With this technique the tube output is adapted to the patient geometry during each rotation of the scanner to compensate for strongly varying x-ray attenuation in asymmetric body regions such as the shoulders and pelvis. The variation of the tube output is either predefined by an analysis of the localizer scan (topogram, scout view) or determined online by evaluating the signal of a single detector row. With use of this technique and depending on the body region, the radiation dose can be reduced by 15% to 35% without degrading image quality. In more sophisticated approaches, the tube output is modified according to the patient geometry not only during each rotation, but also in the longitudinal direction to maintain adequate dose when moving to different body regions, as for instance, when moving from thorax to abdomen (automatic exposure control). In a typical scenario, the attenuation of a "standard-sized" patient is stored in the control computer for each body region. This attenuation corresponds to the mAs setting of the standard protocol. If the actual attenuation of the patient deviates from the "standard" attenuation, the tube output is adapted correspondingly. Figure 12-6 shows the variation of the mAs output for a CT scan of the chest and abdomen of a 6-year-old child. Although the standard protocol with 165 mAs was used—which would have resulted in a significantly higher radiation dose than necessary in a standard mode of operation—the average mAs value throughout the scan was adjusted to 38 mAs by means of automatic exposure control. Automatic adaptation of the tube current to patient size prevents both over- and under-irradiation, considerably simplifies the clinical workflow for the technician, and eliminates the need for look-up tables of patient weight and size for adjusting the mAs settings.

Radiation dose for ECG-synchronized scanning for cardiac applications has been a topic of considerable controversy.[37,38] Recent studies based on 4-slice CT systems find an effective patient dose of roughly 1 mSv for ECG-triggered calcium scoring with 3-mm slice width and roughly 10-mSv for ECG gated CT angiography of the coronary arteries with 1/1.25-mm slice width. Radiation dose in ECG-gated spiral examinations can be reduced by 30% to 50% with use of ECG-controlled tube current modulation. During the spiral scan, the output of the x-ray tube is modulated according to the patient's ECG.[42] It is kept at its nominal output only during a user-defined phase of the cardiac cycle, in general the mid- to end-diastolic phase. During the rest of the cardiac cycle, the tube output is typically reduced to 20% of its nominal value, although not switched off entirely to allow for image reconstruction throughout the entire cardiac cycle. Thus, even though the signal-to-noise ratio is decreased at certain phases of the cardiac cycle, the low-dose images are still sufficient for evaluation of functional parameters, such as ejection fraction, should this information be desired.

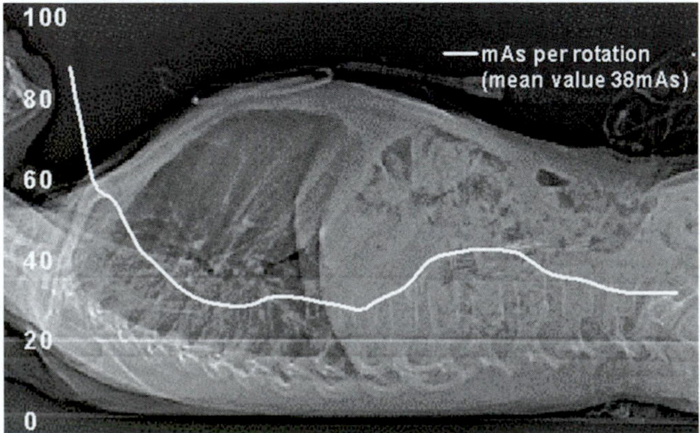

FIGURE 12-6. Automatic exposure control: Variation of the mAs-value for a chest-abdomen scan of a 6-year-old child. Although the standard protocol with 165 mAs was used, the average mAs value throughout the scan was adjusted to 38 mAs with use of automatic exposure control.

VASCULAR APPLICATIONS: MULTISLICE CT ANGIOGRAPHY FROM HEAD TO TOE

Vascular applications benefit from multislice technology in several ways, including shorter scan time, extended scan range, and improved longitudinal resolution.

Most protocols benefit from a combination of these advantages. The near isotropic spatial resolution in routine examinations enables 3-D rendering of diagnostic quality. The widespread availability of MSCT technology has already begun to change the traditional perception of CT imaging. In CT, distinction is traditionally made between longitudinal and in-plane resolution. This distinction is based mainly on historical reasons. Before the introduction of spiral CT, longitudinal resolution was determined by slice width only, while the reconstruction algorithm determined in-plane resolution. With spiral CT, slice width is no longer the only factor determining transverse resolution, but the spiral interpolation function also comes into play. MSCT now allows for reconstruction of arbitrary slice widths from a given slice width by using z-filter techniques, as long as the desired slice width is not smaller than the collimation. The potential to trade off z-axis resolution with image noise for the very same data set is the most important benefit of z-filter reconstruction. In many applications, data acquisition with narrow slices is recommended independent of the slice width desired for primary viewing. The distinction between longitudinal and in-plane resolution will gradually become a historical curiosity, and the traditional axial slice will lose its clinical importance. In its place interactive viewing and manipulation of isotropic volume images will become commonplace, with only the key slices or views in arbitrary directions recorded and stored.

The introduction of spiral scanning with 16 submillimeter slices constituted a breakthrough on the way toward true isotropic resolution for routine clinical applications. Improved longitudinal resolution is combined with considerably reduced scan times, facilitating examination of uncooperative patients and reducing the amount of contrast material needed.

Neurologic Applications—Supra-Aortic Vessels

CT angiography of intracranial and cervical vessels exemplifies the improvements that have been observed since the advent of multislice CT. The advantage of the noninvasive assessment of intracranial arteries has long been recognized.[43-45] Accurate imaging information is mandatory, especially for preoperative evaluation prior to surgical clipping or endovascular treatment in patients with ruptured or nonruptured (Fig. 12-7) intracranial aneurysms. CT angiography allows accurate delineation of the aneurysm neck, shape, orientation, its relationship to the feeding vessel, and important adjacent bone structures (see Fig. 12-7).[46] Recent studies show that the sensitivity of CTA for the detection of very small cerebral aneurysms is higher than that of DSA with equal specificity and high interoperator reliability,[46] making this technique the method of choice for the prospective, noninvasive evaluation of patients with suspected cerebral aneurysmal disease. Visualization of calcium (Fig. 12-8) for the characterization of atherosclerotic lesions is a significant advantage of CT over competing imaging modalities.

Conventional CT techniques for visualization of the intracranial vasculature require large amounts of contrast material and relatively long scan times to obtain high-quality images.

CTA of the intracranial or cervical vessels thus strikingly benefits from the quick and detailed scanning technology of multislice CT. Isotropic volume data sets generated by multislice CT provide the necessary spatial resolution for intuitive visualization of often small-sized and tortuous vessels. Using these kinds of data, high quality 2-D and 3-D renderings of minute vascular anatomy can be produced, employing techniques, such as multiplanar reconstruction (MPR), maximum intensity projections (MIP), surface shaded display (SSD) or volume rendering (VRT). With multislice CT, the ever-accelerating scan speed now allows acquisition of extensive volumes (Fig. 12-9) with sub-millimeter resolution from the aortic arch to the circle of Willis during pure arterial phase, without venous enhancement that would get in the way of 3-D post-processing techniques. CT angiography of the carotid arteries and the circle of Willis with 16 × 0.75 mm slice width, 0.5-second rotation time and a pitch of 1.5 requires only 9 seconds for a scan range of about 300 mm (table feed 36 mm/second). Optimal anatomic detail can be achieved by using 0.5-mm slices, which enables isotropic scanning of the fine arteries of the circle of Willis. Evaluation of the supra-aortic vessels with 16-slice CT is particularly useful in emergency situations because CT allows for a quick diagnosis with optimized patient access. For patients with suspicion of ischemic stroke, both the status of the vessels supplying the brain and the location of the intracranial occlusion can be assessed in the same examination. Brain perfusion CT can be performed using the same modality with the goal of differentiating irreversibly damaged brain tissue from reversibly impaired tissue at risk. The combined use of nonenhanced CT, perfusion CT, and CT angiography may rapidly provide comprehensive information regarding the extent of ischemic damage in acute stroke patients.

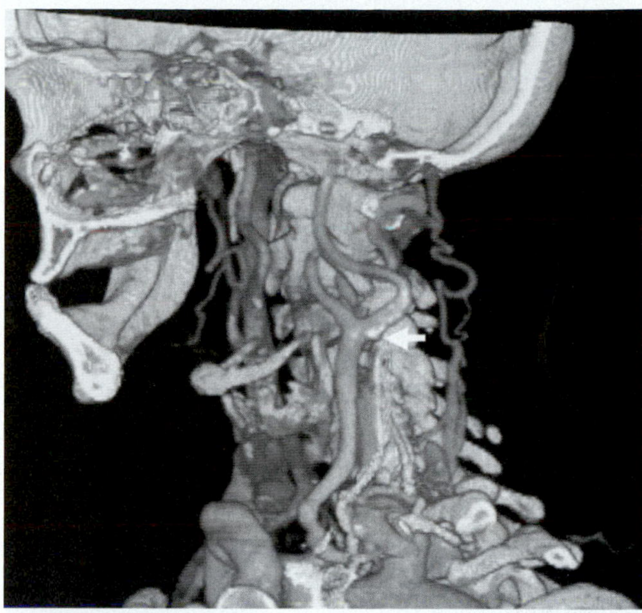

FIGURE 12-8. (See also Color Plate 12-8.) Multislice CT angiography of the carotid arteries with a 4-slice CT scanner. Nonstenotic calcified plaques in the left internal carotid artery near the bifurcation. Characterization of atherosclerotic lesions by means of visualization of calcium (*arrow*) is a significant advantage of CT over competing imaging modalities. The speed of multislice CT allows scanning of the entire length of the carotids with 1-mm spatial resolution along the z-axis without significant venous enhancement that would get in the way of 3-D post-processing. Colored volume rendering technique.

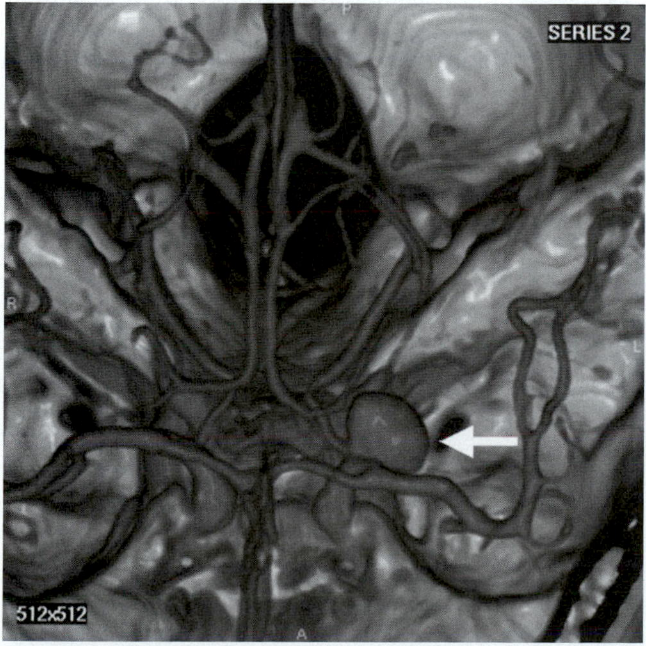

FIGURE 12-7. (See also Color Plate 12-7.) Aneurysm (*arrow*) of the left internal carotid artery seen craniofrontally with a 4-slice CT scanner. Colored volume rendering technique. The shape and location of the aneurysm and the spatial relationship with its feeding vessel is intuitively visualized.

CT Angiography for Pulmonary Embolism

In many institutions, spiral CT is becoming the first line imaging test for the assessment of patients with suspected acute pulmonary embolism in daily clinical practice (see Chapter 54). Both mediastinal and

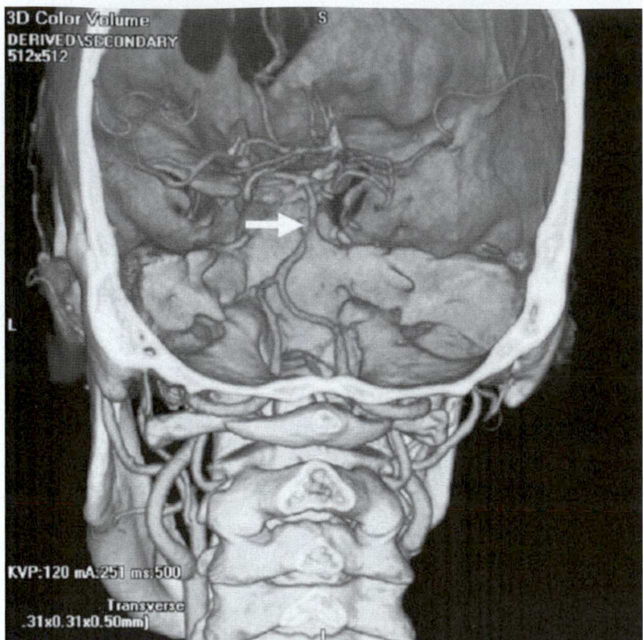

FIGURE 12-9. (See also Color Plate 12-9.) Stenosis of the basilar artery (*arrow*) is shown with a 16-slice CT scanner. Colored volume rendering technique.

parenchymal structures are evaluated, and thrombus is directly visualized (Fig. 12-10). Many patients with an initial suspicion of pulmonary embolism receive other diagnoses as a result of spiral CT,[47] some of which are potentially life-threatening diseases, such as aortic dissection, pneumonia, lung cancer, and pneumothorax.[48] With spiral CT, a specific etiology for patients' symptoms and important additional diagnoses can be established in many cases.[49] The interobserver agreement for spiral CT is better than that for nuclear scintigraphy for pulmonary embolism.[48,50] Spiral CT also appears to be the most cost-effective test in the diagnostic algorithm of pulmonary embolism.[51]

The main impediment for spiral CT has been limitations of this modality for the accurate detection of small peripheral emboli.[52-54] Early studies comparing conventional single-slice spiral CT to selective pulmonary angiography demonstrated the high accuracy of spiral CT for the detection of PE from the main pulmonary artery to the segmental arterial level,[52,55,56] but suggested that subsegmental pulmonary emboli may be overlooked by spiral CT scanning. With older generations of conventional single-slice spiral CT scanners, false negative rates of up to 30% were reported.[52-54]

Although the accuracy of conventional single-slice spiral CT for the detection of isolated peripheral emboli may be limited, encouraging data are accumulating on the high negative predictive value of a normal spiral CT study.[57-61] According to these retrospective[57-59] and prospective[60,61] studies, patient outcome is not adversely affected if anticoagulation is withheld based on a negative spiral CT study. The negative predictive value of a normal spiral CT study is high, compares very favorably with catheter pulmonary angiography, and approaches 98%, regardless if underlying lung disease is present.[58] The frequency of a subsequent clinical diagnosis of pulmonary embolism or deep venous thrombosis after a negative spiral CT pulmonary angiogram is low and is lower than that after a negative or low-probability V-Q scan.[57] Thus even single-slice spiral CT appears to be a reliable imaging tool for excluding clinically relevant pulmonary embolism; it appears that anticoagulation can be safely withheld when the spiral CT scan is normal and of good diagnostic quality.[57,59-61]

Remaining concerns regarding the accuracy of spiral CT for pulmonary embolism detection have been overcome by the introduction of multislice CT. To cover substantial parts of the human anatomy with ever-finer spatial resolution has obvious advantages for imaging pulmonary embolism. Shorter breath-hold times benefit patients with underlying lung disease and reduce the percentage of nondiagnostic CT scans.[62] High-resolution multidetector-row spiral CT data can be transformed easily for 2-D and 3-D visualization. This may, in some instances, improve pulmonary embolism diagnosis but

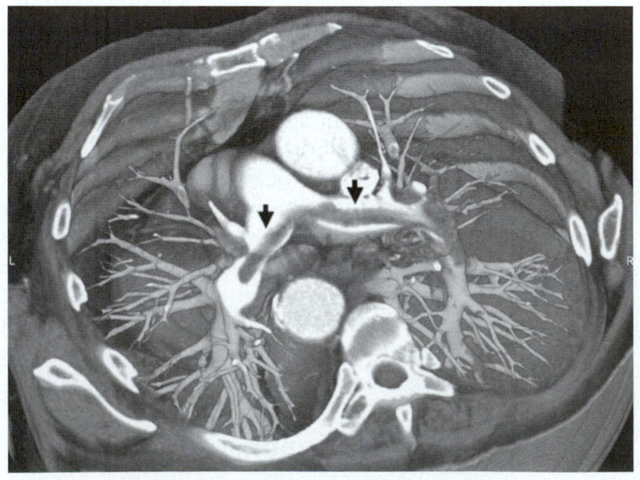
A

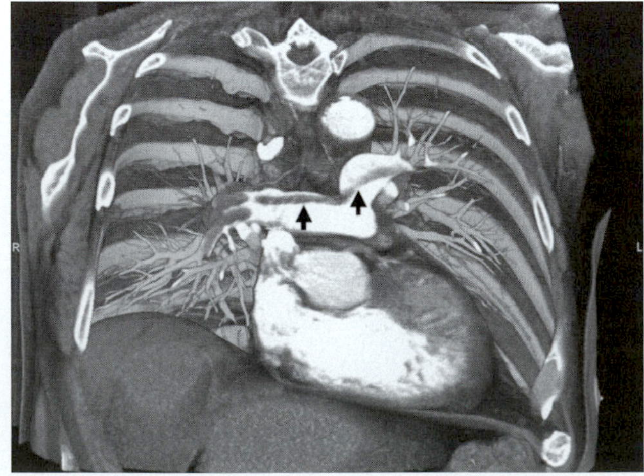
B

FIGURE 12-10. Contrast-enhanced 16-slice CT examination showing a "saddle embolus" (*arrows*) extending into both central pulmonary arteries in a 72-year-old man. Volume-rendered display seen from a dorsocranial **(A)** and oblique coronal **(B)** perspectives.

is generally of greater importance for conveying information on localization and extent of embolic disease in a more intuitive display format (see Fig. 12-10). Probably the most important advantage of multidetector-row spiral CT is improved diagnosis of small peripheral emboli (Fig. 12-11). The degree of accuracy that could be achieved for the visualization of subsegmental pulmonary arteries and for the detection of emboli in these vessels with previously available modalities (single-slice, dual-slice, and electron-beam CT) was found to range between 61% and 79%.[52,63-65] The high spatial resolution (i.e., 0.6 × 0.6 × 0.6 mm in x-, y- and z-extension) of MSCT data sets now allows evaluation of pulmonary vessels down to sixth order branches and significantly increases the detection rate of segmental and subsegmental pulmonary emboli.[10,66,67] This improved detection rate is likely due to the accurate analysis of progressively smaller vessels by use of thinner sections. The interobserver correlation for confident diagnosis of subsegmental emboli with high-resolution multidetector-row spiral CT exceeds the reproducibility of selective pulmonary angiography.[10,68,69] The true accuracy of multidetector-row spiral CT for the detection of small peripheral emboli in patients with suspected pulmonary embolism will be difficult to determine. As a direct result of high-resolution imaging capabilities, small peripheral clots that may have gone unnoticed in the past are now frequently seen, often in patients with minor symptoms. It appears highly unlikely that pulmonary angiography will be performed on a patient merely to prove the presence of a small (2 to 3 mm) isolated embolus. Thus, the lack of a clinically available standard for the diagnosis of pulmonary embolism suggests that the medical community should replace theoretical and academic discussions on the relative value of different imaging modalities with more realistic approaches toward pulmonary embolism diagnosis based on patient outcome.

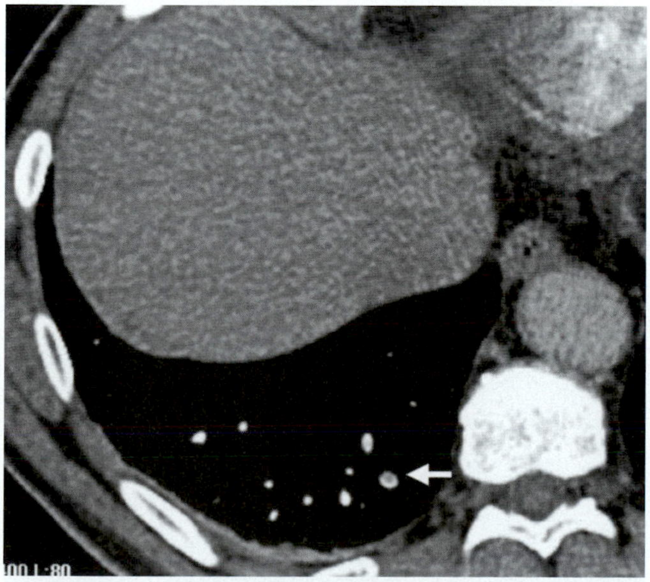

FIGURE 12-11. A 16-slice CT study showing isolated peripheral pulmonary embolus (*arrow*) in the right lower lobe of a 72-year-old man with acute right-sided pleuritic chest pain. Total scan time: 10 seconds. Emboli in subsegmental and smaller pulmonary arteries were previously considered a limitation of CT. These perceived limitations should be overcome with the advent of 16-slice CT.

MSCT Coronary Angiography

The greatest challenge for noninvasive imaging is the reliable assessment of the coronary arteries, because of their small size, tortuous 3-D anatomy, and fast continuous motion. Owing to the overwhelming importance of coronary artery disease in Western societies, accurate noninvasive evaluation of coronary arteries is a coveted goal. No noninvasive modality has achieved this as yet. However, MSCT coronary angiography currently appears to best fulfill the requirements for noninvasive morphologic assessment of the coronary arteries, based on its combination of unprecedented acquisition speed, spatial resolution, and robustness of use.

Contrast-enhanced CT angiography has been recognized as the preferred diagnostic strategy for the evaluation of coronary artery anomalies (Fig. 12-12) because the information that can be obtained from volumetric imaging on the origin and anatomic course of aberrant vessels by far surpasses conventional angiography. MRI is limited in determining the distal coronary course.[70] Therefore, CT is the preferred modality for evaluating small collaterals, fistulas, and vessels originating outside the normal sinuses.[71]

Noninvasive imaging for determining patency or occlusion of bypass grafts (Fig. 12-13) had moved into the scope of CT at very early stages of this technology.[72-74] Patency of venous and arterial bypass grafts could be determined with greater than 90% sensitivity and specificity using contrast-enhanced single-slice spiral CT.[75,76] The challenge for noninvasive bypass graft imaging, which has not been resolved, is less a simple differentiation between patent versus occluded grafts, but a more clinically relevant complex functional assessment of bypass flow,[77,78] accurate detection of graft lesions, and reliable visualization of (distal) anastomoses. Data on the accuracy of CT for the detection and grading of hemodynamically significant graft stenosis are still sparse. In a somewhat larger patient population investigated with 4-slice CT, an overall sensitivity and specificity for bypass occlusion of 97% and 98%, respectively, was reported. After exclusion of 38% of grafts which could not be evaluated, sensitivity for detection of high-grade graft stenosis was 75% with 92% specificity.[79]

The accuracy of CT coronary angiography for noninvasive detection of coronary artery stenosis is an area of active research. Depending on study design and the number of patients or arteries excluded from analysis, most published series using electron-beam CT or 4-slice multidetector-row CT technology found the sensitivity of noninvasive CT angiography for the detection of hemodynamically significant coronary artery stenosis within proximal coronary arteries (Fig. 12-14) to range between 80% and 90%.[10,80-82] According to literature, the accuracy of CT surpasses the accuracy of MRI for the detection of coronary artery stenosis.[83-85] The advent of faster CT scanner generations with added detector elements increases the number of assessable coronary arteries[86] and improves the overall accuracy of noninvasive CT coronary angiography for stenosis detection.[86,87] Initial clinical experience with 0.37-second gantry rotation

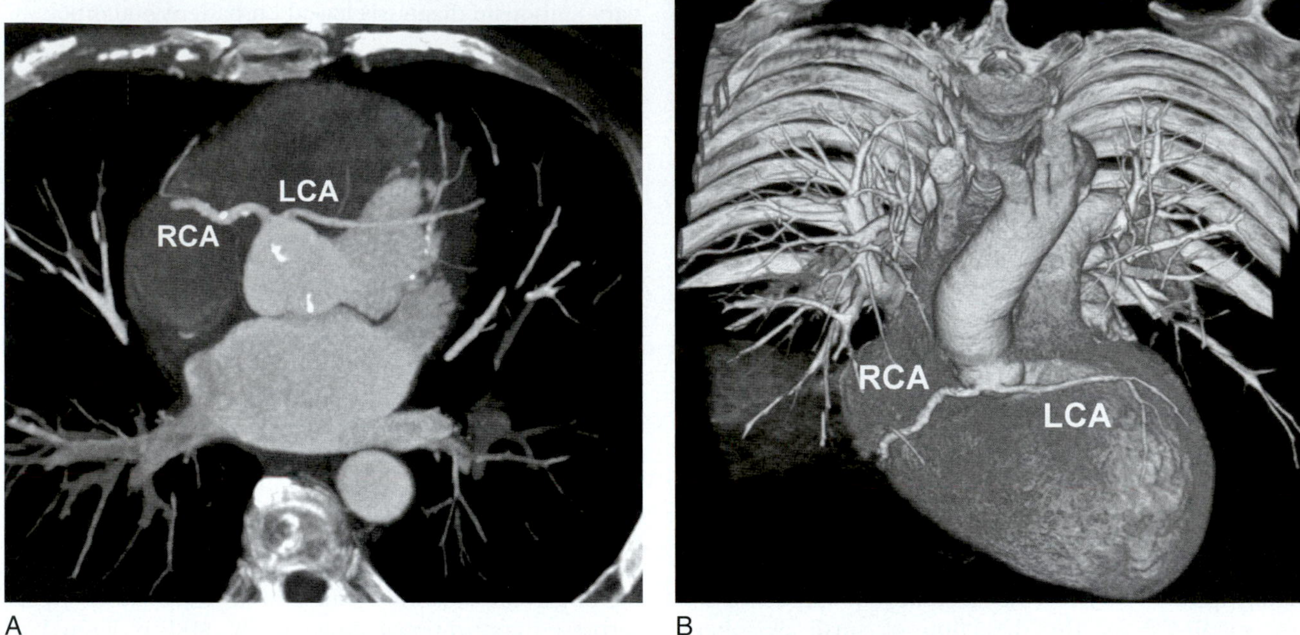

FIGURE 12-12. (See also Color Plate 12-12.) A 42-year-old man with anomalous origin and course of the left coronary artery (LCA). Retrospectively ECG-gated 16-slice CT coronary angiography displayed as axial maximum intensity projection **(A)** and colored volume rendering **(B)**. The vessel originates medial to the origin of the right coronary artery (RCA) and crosses the median line before giving off branches supplying the left side of the myocardium.

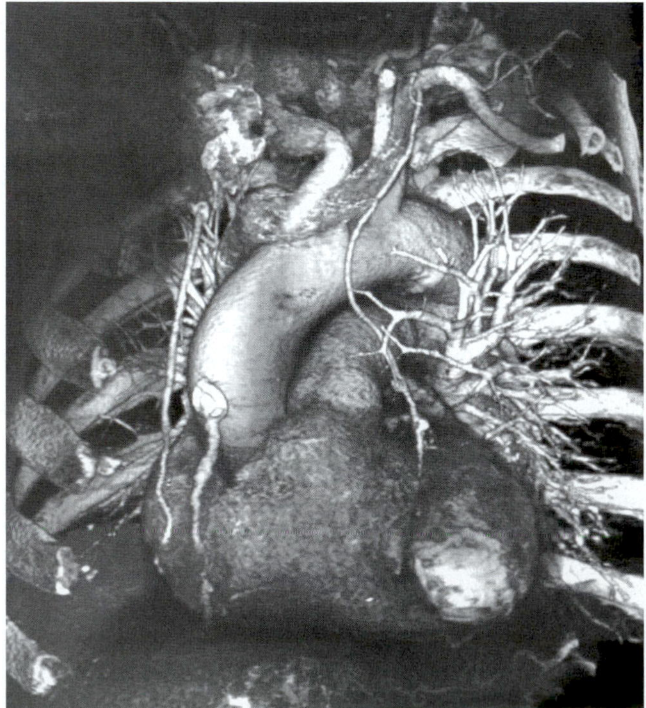

FIGURE 12-13. (See also Color Plate 12-13.) Patient with left internal mammary artery (LIMA) bypass graft to the left anterior descending (LAD) coronary artery and saphenous bypass graft to the right coronary artery. Note calcified aneurysm in the apex of the left ventricle as sequelae of ischemic heart disease. Colored 3-D volume-rendered display enables visualization of native and graft vessels in their relationship to surrounding thoracic anatomy.

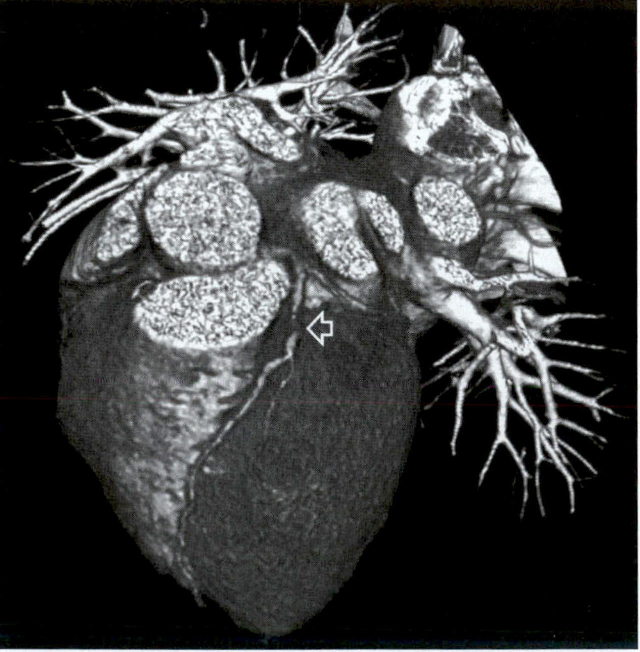

FIGURE 12-14. High-grade stenosis (*arrow*) of the proximal left anterior descending coronary artery. Colored volume-rendered display of a contrast-enhanced 4-slice multidetector-row CT coronary angiogram.

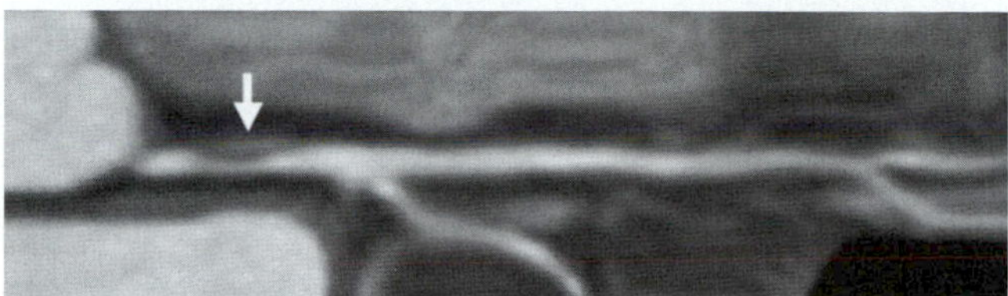

FIGURE 12-15. Hemodynamically significant stenosis (*arrow*) in the proximal left anterior descending coronary artery caused by a noncalcified, soft-tissue density lesion. Intuitive visualization of the entire course of the artery is achieved by displaying a curved multiplanar reformat along an automatically generated centerline of the vessel.

indicates improved image quality because of reduced cardiac motion and increased clinical robustness at higher heart rates, thereby potentially reducing the number of patients requiring heart rate control.

The majority of published studies found an encouragingly high negative predictive value of a negative CT coronary angiogram (97% with 16-slice multidetector-row CT).[10,11,81,82,86-88] This high negative predictive value suggests a potentially important role of noninvasive CT coronary angiography for reliably ruling out significant coronary artery disease in the large population of patients with equivocal clinical presentation and findings, who currently undergo a costly invasive work-up for excluding the remote possibility of stenotic coronary artery disease.

An inherent advantage of CT for imaging of the coronary arteries is the cross-sectional nature of this technology. Conventional catheter angiography, widely accepted as the standard for the detection of coronary artery disease owing to its unsurpassed spatial resolution, displays only the vessel lumen and the degree of luminal narrowing in a cast-like manner, but fails to visualize the coronary artery wall.[89] In contrast, the ability of contrast-enhanced CT to delineate calcified and noncalcified lesions (Fig. 12-15) within the coronary artery wall that may or may not cause luminal stenosis has been demonstrated.[12,13,90-94]

The potential of contrast-enhanced CT to noninvasively assess atherosclerotic plaque within the vessel wall[12,13,90-95] has sparked considerable scientific interest and may provide more valuable insight in the intricate pathogenesis of coronary atherosclerosis.

Imaging of the Aorta and Its Thoracic and Abdominal Branches

In aortic imaging, the high-speed large volume covering capabilities of multislice CT has dramatically improved diagnosis and patient comfort. 16-slice CT angiography of the chest and abdomen with submillimeter slices can be completed in a single breath-hold of about 17 seconds for a scan range of 600 mm (Fig. 12-16). When true isotropic

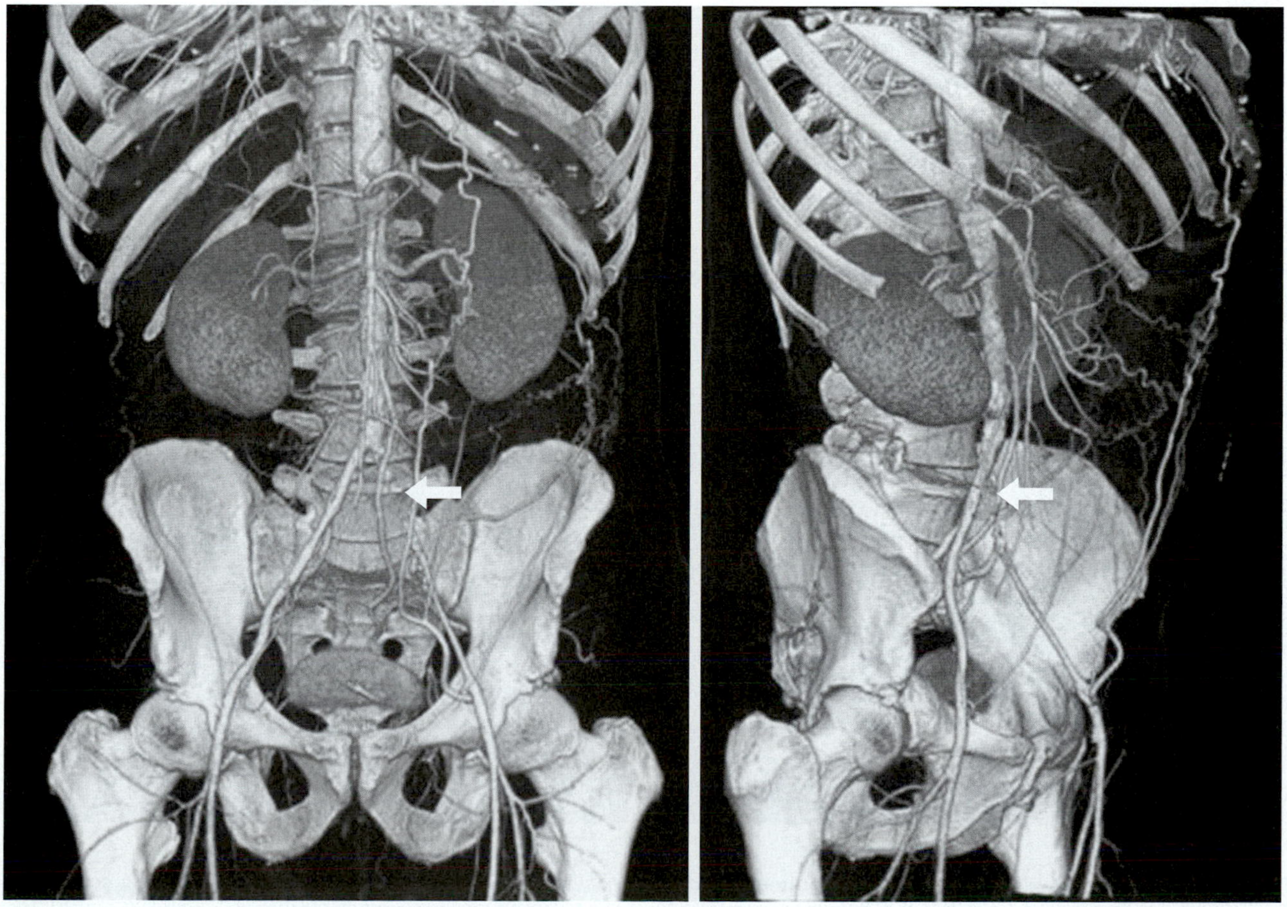

A B

FIGURE 12-16. (See also Color Plate 12-16.) Case study illustrating the clinical performance of 16-slice CT: patient with occlusion (*arrow*) of the left common iliac artery, scanned with 16 × 0.75 mm collimation. Frontal **(A)** and oblique **(B)** views.

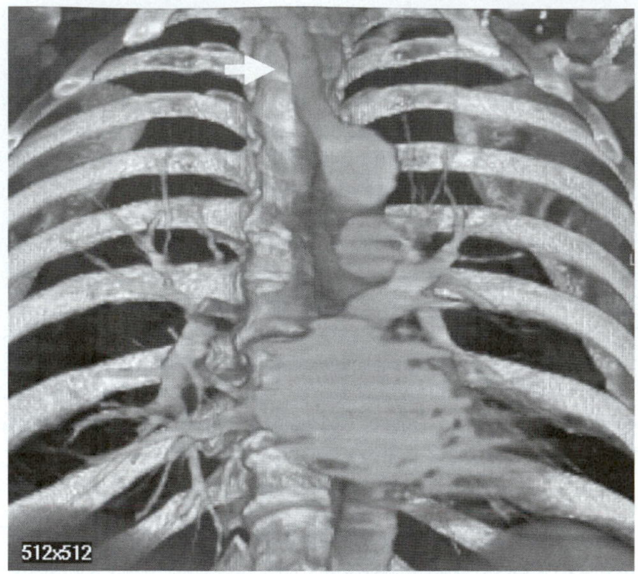

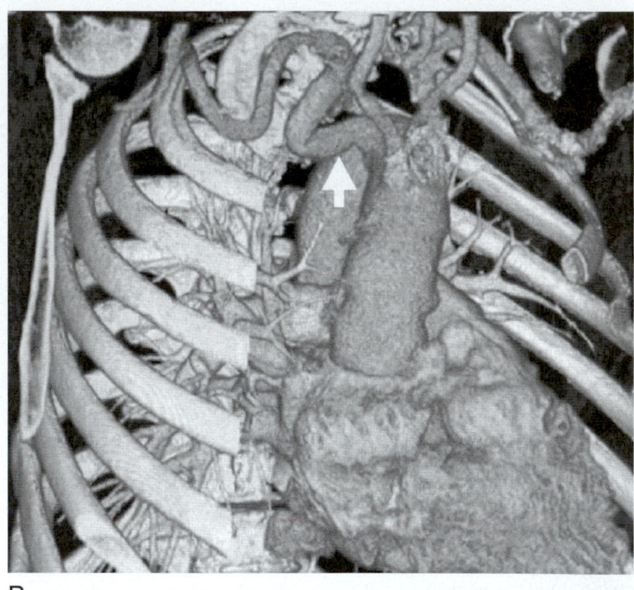

FIGURE 12-17. (See also Color Plate 12-17.) Two patients with aberrant right subclavian arteries (*arrow*). **A,** A 4-slice MSCT study with 4 × 1 mm collimation and 29-second total scan time and **B,** 16-slice CT acquisition with 16 × 0.75 mm collimation and 7-second total scan time. Note substantially improved spatial resolution and image quality with high-resolution 16-slice CT, despite significantly shorter scan time.

resolution is not required, the use of 16 × 1.25 mm/16 × 1.5 mm slices enables even shorter examination times or extended scan ranges. Whole-body CT angiography with 1500 mm scan range, 16 × 1.5 mm slice width, 0.5-second rotation time and pitch 1.25 (table feed 30 mm/sec) can be completed in only 26 seconds. The high scan speed has substantially reduced contrast medium requirements.

CT angiography can evaluate congenital (Fig. 12-17) and acquired aortic disease.[96,97] It is valuable for surgical planning (Fig. 12-18) and for following patients after cardiovascular interventions. Fast high-resolution image acquisition with multislice CT becomes particularly important for the initial diagnosis and follow-up of acute aortic injury, notably aortic transection or dissection (see Chapter 34).[98] If pathology of the aortic root is suspected, prospective or retrospective ECG synchronization[25] of the scan acquisition significantly reduces cardiac pulsation artifacts. With 4-slice CT systems, the scan time necessary to cover the entire thoracic aorta with thin slices and

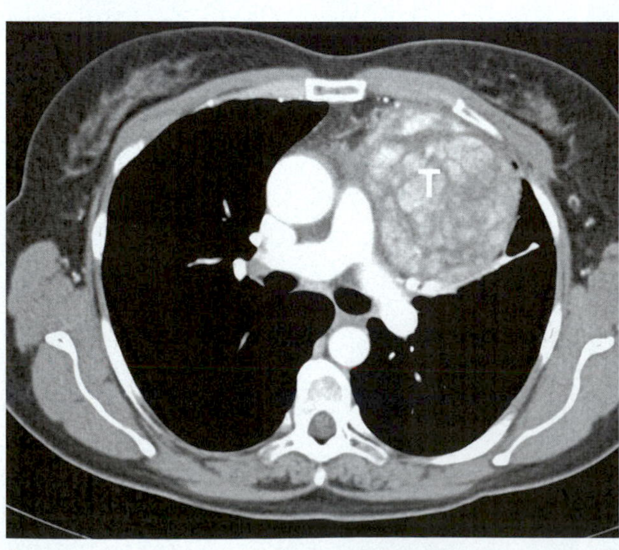

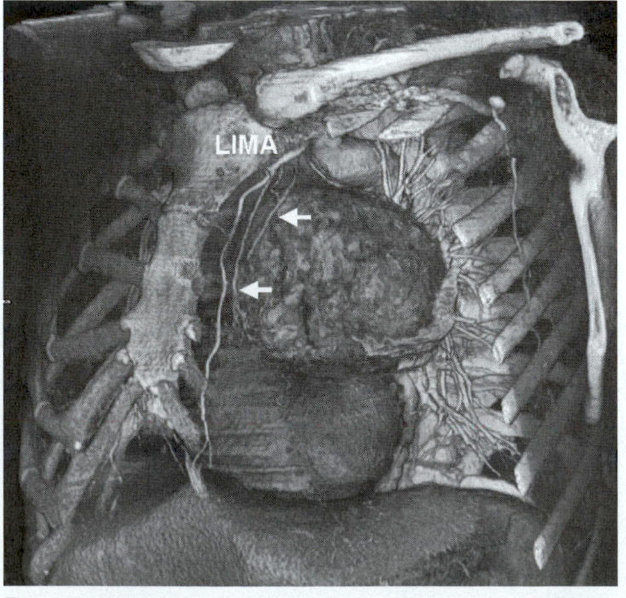

FIGURE 12-18. (See also Color Plate 12-18.) Invasive thymoma. **A,** Contrast-enhanced axial image shows an intensely enhancing nodular mediastinal tumor (T) with adjacent atelectasis. **B,** Color enhanced 3-D volume-rendered image effectively shows enlarged left internal mammary artery (LIMA) and tumor neovasculature (*arrows*). Preoperative information on the vascular supply of the tumor was invaluable in surgical planning. The extent of the vessels was not demonstrated on the axial images.

high through-plane resolution exceeds the breath-hold capabilities of most patients, if retrospective ECG gating is to be used. Thus, with 4-slice CT, retrospectively ECG-gated acquisitions require use of thicker slices to cover the entire course of the thoracic aorta, which suppresses cardiac motion artifacts but sacrifices through-plane resolution for intuitive 3-D visualization. With the advent of current generation multislice CT systems, such trade-offs no longer exist. MSCT now allows retrospectively ECG-gated high-resolution acquisition of the entire aorta (Fig. 12-19), which effectively eliminates cardiac motion as a source of potential diagnostic pitfalls and preserves the near isotropic nature of multislice CT data sets.

In the abdomen traditional and common indications for performing noninvasive CT angiography[99] include detection and postoperative surveillance of aneurysmal

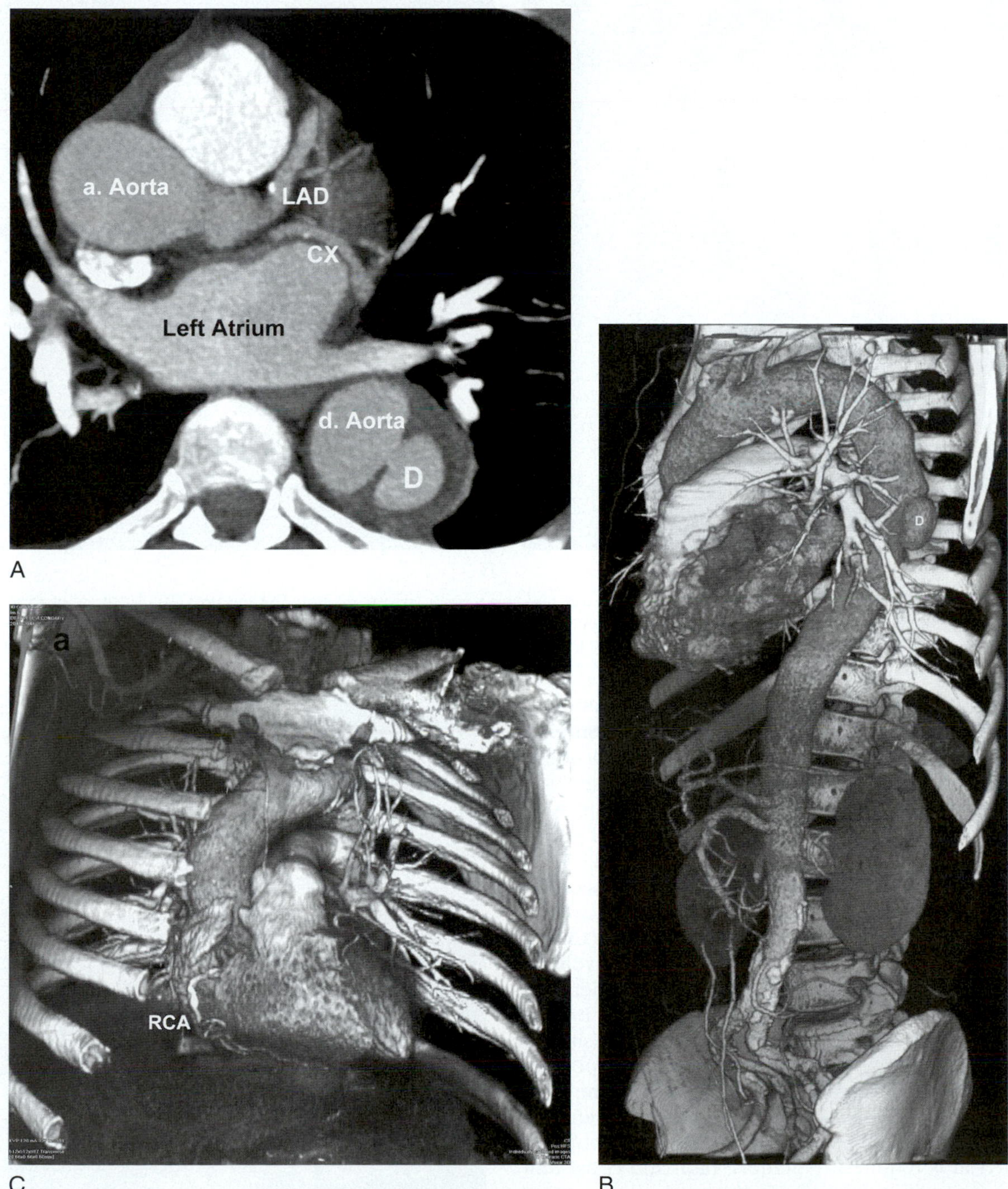

FIGURE 12-19. Contrast-enhanced 16-slice CT of the thoracic and abdominal aorta with retrospective ECG gating. **A,** Axial maximum intensity projection at the level of the left atrium shows type B dissection (D) in the descending aorta and circumscribed atherosclerotic calcified nodules in the wall of the left anterior descending (LAD) and left circumflex (CX) coronary arteries. The entire data set is displayed as 3-D volume rendering **(B)** seen from a left oblique anterior perspective. Enlarged views of the thoracic vasculature **(C)** enable evaluation of the distal posterior descending branch of the right coronary artery (RCA), thus enabling a comprehensive assessment of multiple systemic manifestations of atherosclerotic disease by a single contrast-enhanced ECG-gated 16-slice CT angiography study.

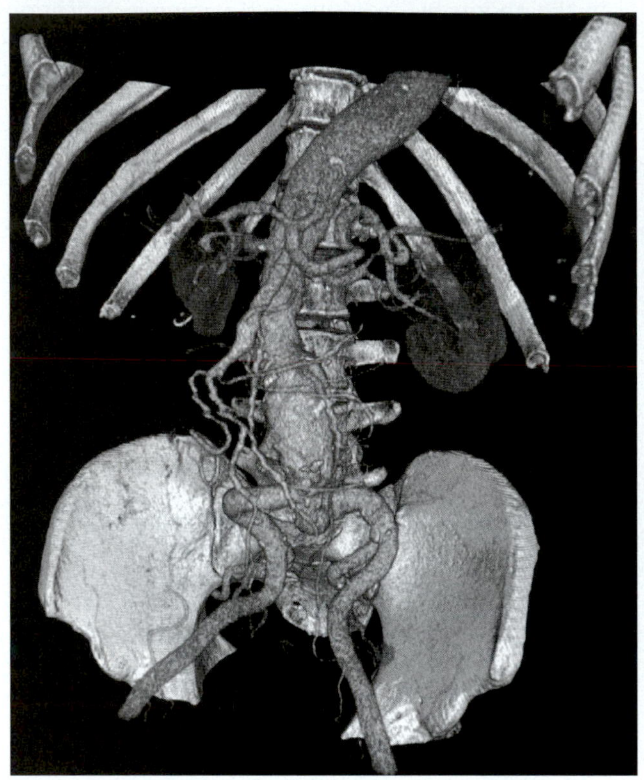

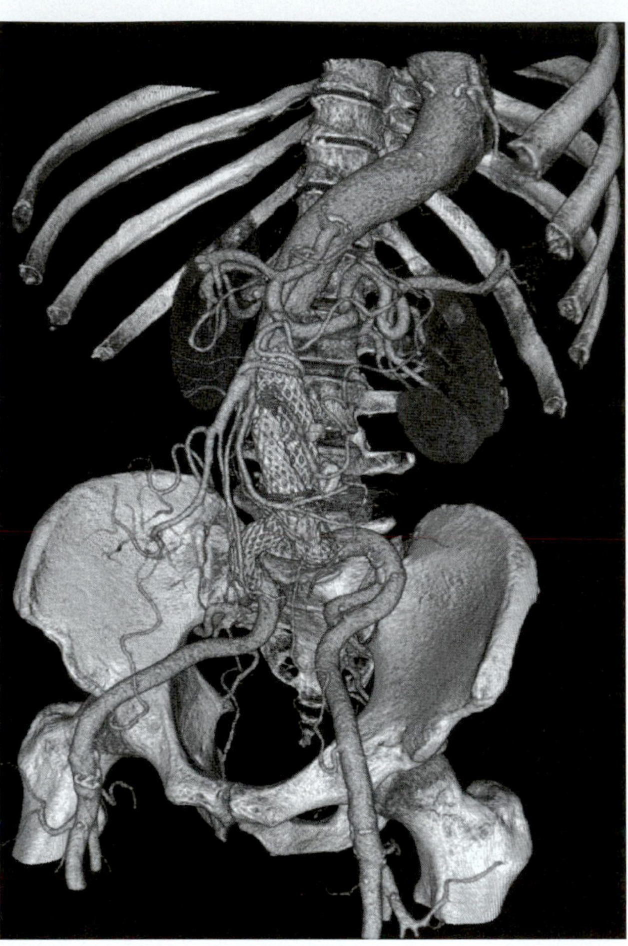

A B

FIGURE 12-20. (See also Color Plate 12-20.) A 62-year-old man with abdominal aortic aneurysm before **(A)** and after **(B)** placement of an aortic stent. The patient underwent contrast-enhanced CT for preinterventional evaluation of the abdominal aorta and the aneurysm and for therapeutic planning **(A)**. After successful placement of the stent, the CT scan demonstrates effective exclusion of the aneurysm and restitution of the aortic lumen **(B)**.

disease (Fig. 12-20),[100-102] tumor staging for evaluation of vascular invasion (e.g., in pancreatic cancer[100] and surgical planning prior to resection of tumors). Other indications are a clinical suspicion of ischemic bowel disease,[103,104] renal artery stenosis[105,106] (Fig. 12-21) in patients with hypertension of unresolved origin, or evaluation of potential renal donors prior to related organ donation.[107] The typical coverage for investigation of the branches of the abdominal aorta should cover the volume from the origin of the celiac trunk to the aortic bifurcation. With conventional single-slice CT the scan time to cover this volume with thin slices exceeds the ability of most patients to hold their breath, thus impairing image quality by breathing artifacts. Thin slices, however, are a prerequisite for the reliable evaluation of smaller-sized arteries, especially of those with a course oblique to the scan plane (i.e., renal arteries, see Fig. 12-21) that are difficult to analyze with thicker slices. Also, a relatively large quantity of contrast material is required to achieve high and consistent arterial opacification throughout the scan.

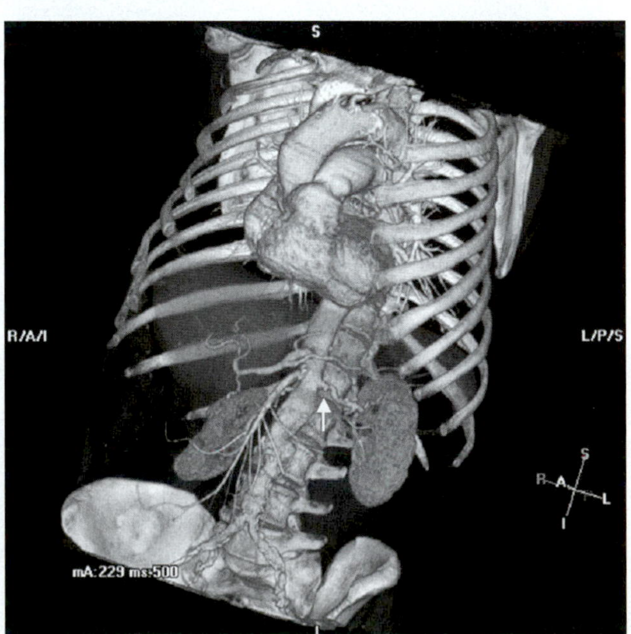

FIGURE 12-21. A 16-slice CT angiogram of the thoracic and abdominal vessels. Despite extensive volume coverage, stenosis of the left renal artery (*arrow*) with atherosclerotic wall changes is clearly visualized, based on a full-body CT angiogram.

Extremity Runoff Studies

One of the most striking examples of new applications made possible by multislice CT is noninvasive imaging

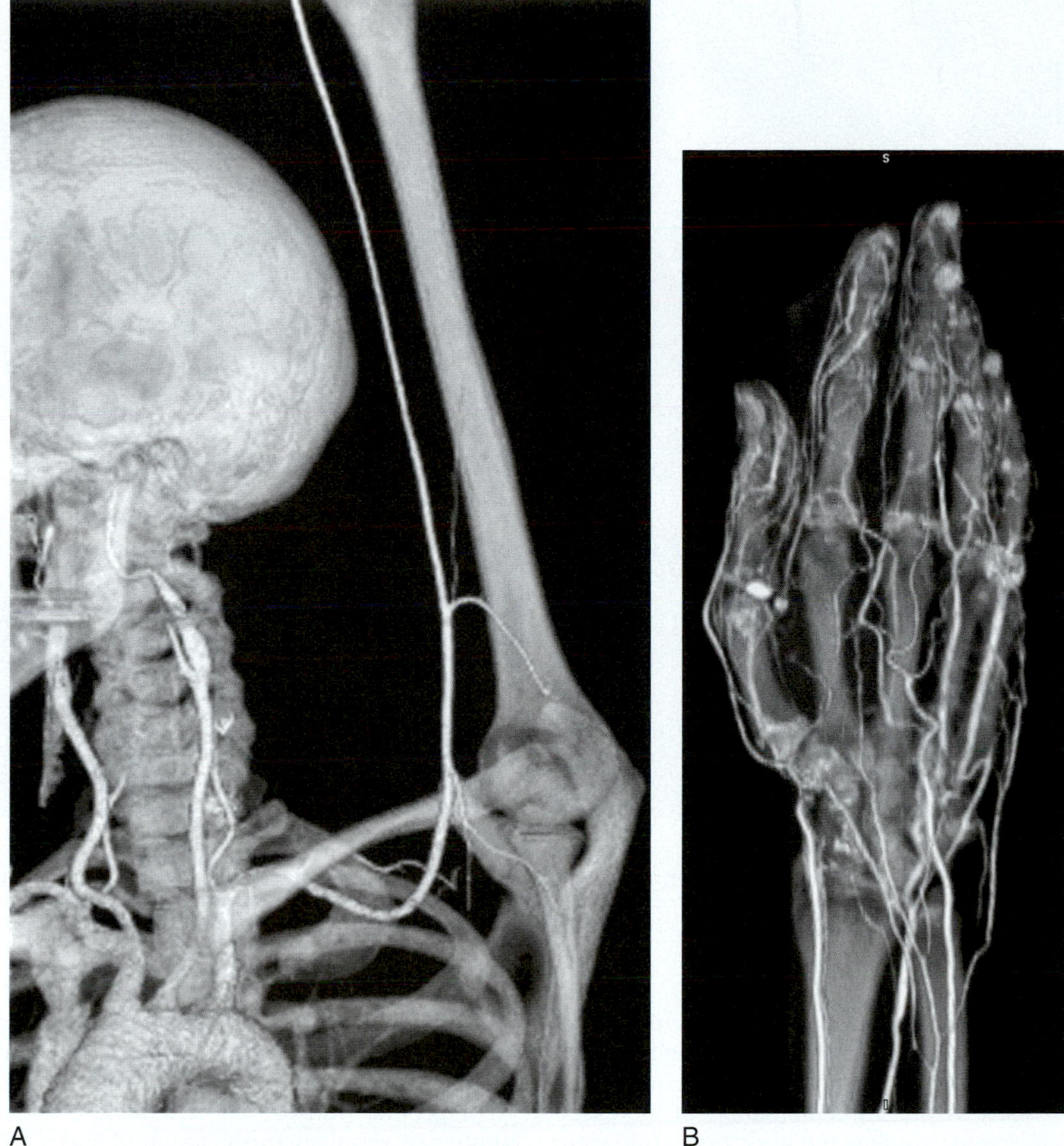

FIGURE 12-22. A 16-slice CT angiogram of the right upper extremity in a 39-year-old woman with Takayasu's arteritis. 3-D volume-rendered display of the proximal **(A)** and distal **(B)** arm vessels is of sufficient spatial resolution and diagnostic quality to obviate the need for invasive catheter angiography.

of the entire upper (Fig. 12-22) and, more importantly, of the lower (Figs. 12-23 and 12-24) extremities[108,109] with sufficiently high spatial resolution to perform peripheral arteriography (see Figs. 12-22B and 12-24B) (see Chapter 17). Before the introduction of multislice CT, only limited coverage of peripheral extremity vessels was feasible.[110] Traditionally, invasive angiography has been used as a first line modality for the evaluation of lower extremity arteries. However, if no therapeutic intervention is planned (e.g., removal of thrombi, dilation, or stenting) a noninvasive modality may be preferable over invasive angiography as the initial diagnostic test. For surgical planning, visualization of popliteal vessels (see Fig. 12-24) is of paramount importance for determining the site for insertion of a surgical bypass graft. To this end, magnetic resonance angiography for noninvasive imaging of the lower extremity runoff is increasingly gaining ground at many institutions and is continuously being refined for this particular application. While multislice CT generally may not be the initial choice of a noninvasive modality for evaluation of lower extremity arteries because of the use of ionizing radiation and demanding post-processing requirements, there are instances when CT may be employed as a suitable and robust first line test. Examples include patients with contraindications for undergoing MR angiography or cases where superior spatial resolution of multislice CT compared to MR facilitates noninvasive visualization of small-sized vessels in the calves for surgical planning.

CT ANGIOGRAPHY: FUTURE PERSPECTIVES

Multislice CT has become widely available and provides truly isotropic submillimeter imaging for virtually any application. This technology sets today's benchmark in

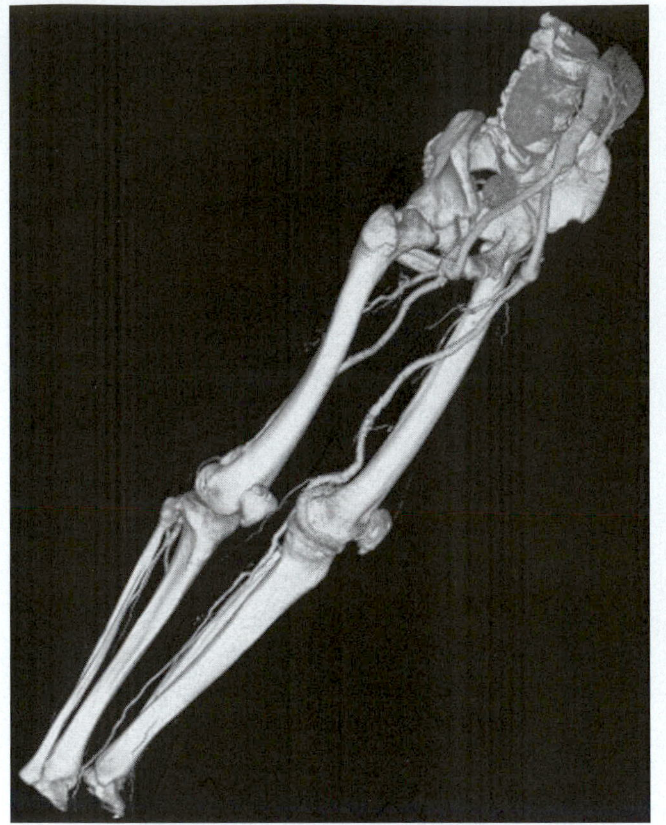

A

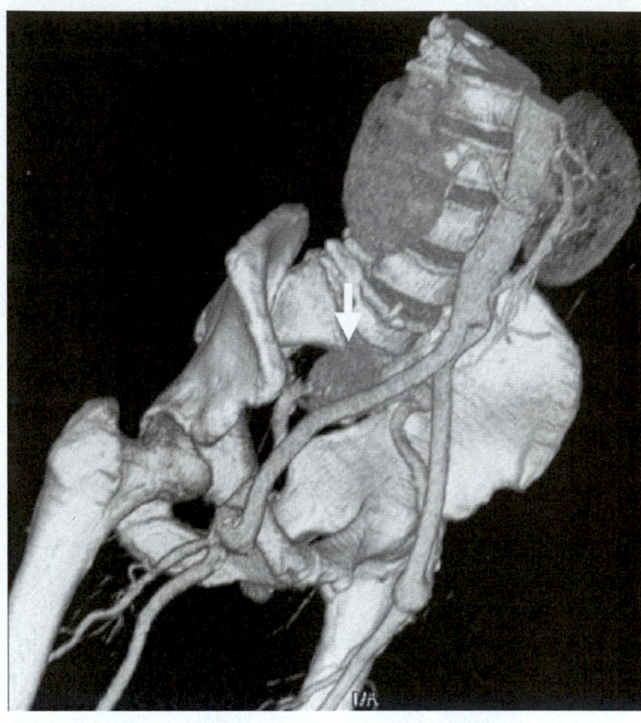

B

FIGURE 12-23. A 4-slice CT angiogram of lower-extremity runoff in a patient with an aneurysm (shown by *arrow* in **B**) of the right internal iliac artery. A range from the renal arteries to the ankles is covered with 4 × 2.5 mm slice width. Total scan time: 40 seconds. Colored volume-rendered display of the entire scan range **(A)**, and detailed visualization of the abdominal and pelvic arteries **(B)**.

spatial resolution for noninvasive cardiovascular imaging. As motion artifacts in patients with higher heart rates remain the most important challenge for multislice CTA, we will witness the implementation of increased gantry rotation speed, which is the most preferable strategy for providing robust clinical performance. Obviously, significant development efforts are needed to account for the substantial increase in mechanical forces (~17G for 0.42-second rotation time; >33G for 0.3-second rotation time) and increased data transmission rates. Rotation times of less than 0.2 second (mechanical forces >75G), required to provide a temporal resolution of less than 100 msec appear to be beyond today's mechanical limits. An alternative to further increased rotation speed is to reconsider a scanner concept with multiple tubes and multiple detectors that has already been described in the early times of CT.[111,112]

Because of its ease of use and its widespread availability, general purpose CT continues to evolve into the most widely used diagnostic modality for routine examinations. CT provides morphologic information only; in combination with other modalities; however, functional and metabolic information can also be obtained. Therefore, combined systems for obtaining comprehensive structural and functional diagnoses will gain increasing importance in the near future. The combination of state-of-the-art MSCT with PET scanners, for instance, opens a wide spectrum of applications—ranging from oncological staging to comprehensive neurologic and cardiac examinations. The clinical potential of these scanners is currently being evaluated.

For general purpose CT, a moderate increase of the number of simultaneously acquired slices will occur in the near future. A new generation of CT systems with 32, 40, and 64 simultaneously acquired slices is currently being introduced. However, in contrast to the transition from single-slice to 4-slice and 16-slice CT, clinical performance will improve only incrementally with a further increase of the number of simultaneously acquired slices. The achievable clinical benefit will have to be carefully considered in the light of the necessary technical efforts and cost. Clinical progress can more likely be expected from further improved spatial resolution rather than from an increase in the volume coverage speed. In clinical reality, the latter only rarely is a limiting factor since the introduction of 16-slice CT. Until all relevant examinations can be performed in a comfortable breathhold of not more than 10 seconds, a further increase of the slice number will not provide significant clinical benefit.

At this point, a qualitative enhancement of CT may again bring substantial clinical progress (e.g., by the introduction of area detectors large enough to cover entire organs, such as the heart, the kidneys, or the brain, in one axial scan [~120 mm scan range]). With these systems, dynamic volume scanning would become feasible,

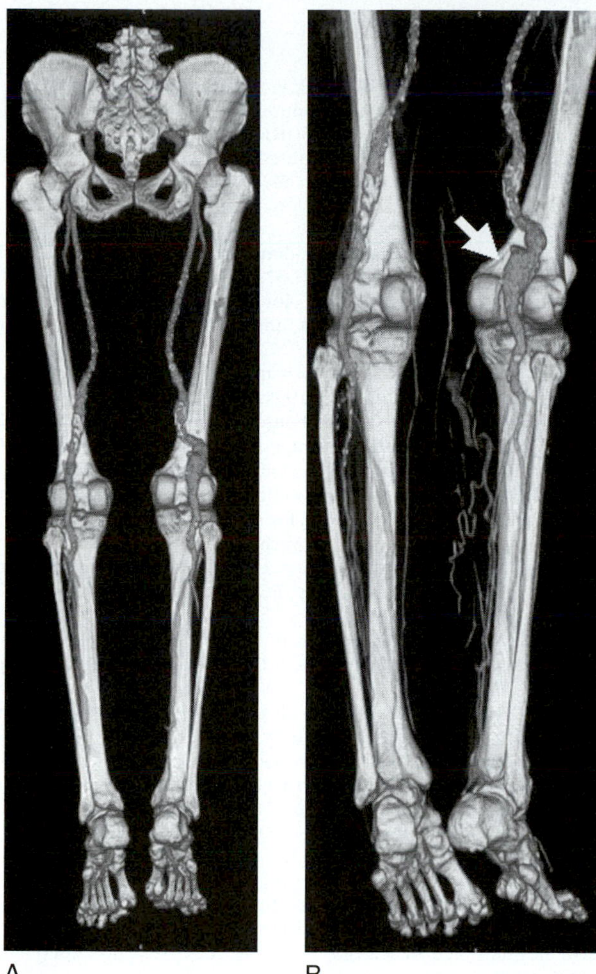

FIGURE 12-24. A 16-slice CT angiogram of lower-extremity runoff in a patient with aneurysmal dilation (shown by *arrow* in **B**) of the popliteal arteries. A range from the renal arteries to the toes is covered with 16 × 1.5 mm slice width. Total scan time: 22 seconds. Colored volume-rendered display of the entire scan range **(A)**, and detailed visualization of the distal runoff **(B)**.

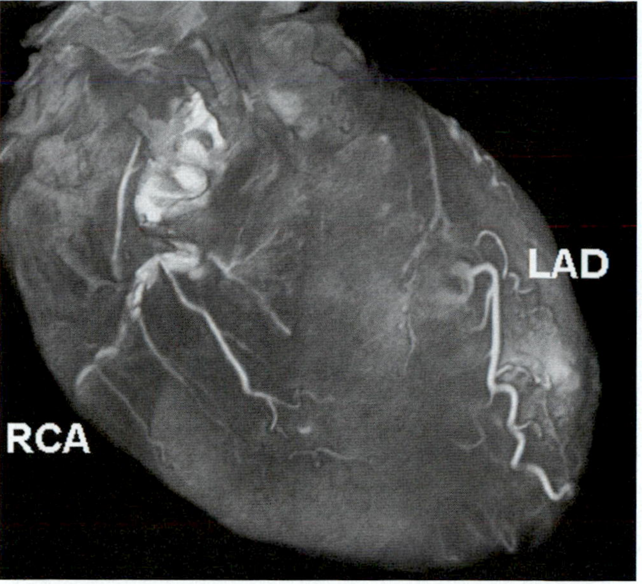

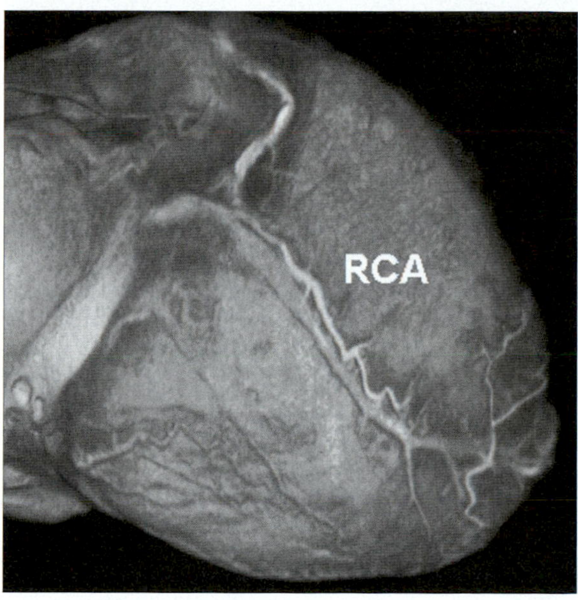

FIGURE 12-25. (See also Color Plate 12-25.) Flat panel CT volume acquisition of a stationary human cadaveric heart specimen. Display in colored volume rendering technique seen from anterior **(A)** and inferior **(B)** projections. Coronary arteries filled with iodinated contrast media. Isotropic in-plane and through-plane resolution of 0.25 mm enables visualization of small caliber marginal branches of the partially calcified right (RCA) and left anterior descending (LAD) coronary arteries.

opening a whole spectrum of new applications, such as functional or volume perfusion studies. Area detector technology is currently under development, but no commercially available system fulfills the requirements of medical CT with regard to contrast resolution and fast data read-out. Prototype systems use CSI-ASI flat panel detector technology, originally used for conventional catheter angiography, which is limited in low contrast resolution and scan speed. Because of the intrinsic slow signal decay of flat panel detectors, rotation times of at least 20 seconds are needed to acquire a sufficient number of projections (≥600). These detectors cover a 25 × 25 × 18 cm^3 scan field of view with an isotropic spatial resolution of 0.25 mm^3. Thus, spatial resolution of such systems is excellent. Excessive dose requirements, however, preclude the examination of larger objects. Initial experimental results are limited to small, high-contrast objects, such as contrast-filled vessel specimens (Fig. 12-25). The combination of area detectors that provide sufficient image quality with fast gantry rotation speeds will be a promising technical concept for medical CT systems. The vast spectrum of potential applications may bring about another quantum leap in the evolution of medical CT imaging; however, such systems will probably not be available in the near future.

APPENDIX: RADIATION DOSE IN SINGLE-SLICE AND MULTISLICE SPIRAL CT

Both for single-slice CT and multislice CT, the pitch p is given by

$$p = \text{tablefeed per rotation/total width of the collimated beam,} \quad (1)$$

according to IEC specifications.[34] For $p < 1$ data acquisition occurs with overlap in the z-direction, for $p > 1$ data acquisition occurs with gaps.

A clinically appropriate measure for the dose is the weighted computerized tomographic dose index $CTDI_w$,[34] which is determined from the $CTDI_{100}$ measurements in a 16-cm Lucite phantom for head and in a 32-cm Lucite phantom for body according to the following equation[33]:

$$CTDI_w = 1/3\ CTDI_{100}\,(\text{center}) + 2/3\ CTDI_{100}\,(\text{periphery}) \quad (2)$$

$CTDI_w$, given in mGy, is always measured in an axial scan mode. It depends on scanner geometry and beam prefiltration as well as on x-ray tube voltage, tube current mA and gantry rotation time t_{rot}. The product of mA and t_{rot} is the mAs value of the scan. To obtain a parameter characteristic for the scanner used, it is helpful to eliminate the mAs dependence and to introduce a normalized $(CTDI_w)_n$ given in mGy/mAs:

$$CTDI_w = mA \times t_{rot} \times (CTDI_w)_n = mAs \times (CTDI_w)_n \quad (3)$$

$CTDI_w$ is a measure for the dose in a single axial scan. To represent the dose in a spiral scan, it is essential to account for gaps or overlaps between the radiation dose profiles from consecutive rotations of the x-ray source.[33] For this purpose $CTDI_{vol}$, the volume $CTDI_w$, has been introduced:

$$CTDI_{vol} = 1/p \times CTDI_w = mAs \times 1/p \times (CTDI_w)_n \quad (4)$$

The factor $1/p$ accounts for the increasing dose accumulation with decreasing spiral pitch due to the increasing spiral overlap. In principle, equation 4 holds for single-slice CT as well as for multislice CT. In single-slice CT, a higher pitch is often used to reduce patient dose, at the expense of a wider SSP and loss of transverse resolution. The image noise, however, is independent of the pitch. In multislice CT, the situation is more complex. Most multislice CT scanners use z filtering approaches, such as the Adaptive Axial Interpolation, for image reconstruction. With z filtering the image noise decreases with decreasing pitch if the tube current mA is left unchanged, due to the increasing transverse sampling density (overlapping spiral sampling). To maintain constant image noise, different mA settings depending on the spiral pitch have to be chosen. Some manufacturers semi-automatically adjust the mA settings if the pitch of a spiral scan is changed. Some others adapt the tube current (mA) to the pitch as an automatic procedure.[4,17,26,47] The user selects a certain image noise level and, hence, a certain image quality by choosing an "effective" mAs value $(mAs)_{eff}$, which is simply the product of tube current and irradiation time of each slice:

$$(mAs)_{eff} = mA \times t_{rot} \times 1/p = mAs \times 1/p \quad (5)$$

To keep $(mAs)_{eff}$ constant, the tube current mA is increased directly proportional to p. Using the effective mAs concept and inserting equation 5 into equation 4, the dose of a multislice spiral scan is simply given by

$$CTDI_{vol} = (mAs)_{eff} \times (CTDI_w)_n \quad (6)$$

The spiral dose with this concept is, therefore, constant and equal to the dose of a sequential scan with the same mAs.

REFERENCES

1. Kalender W, Seissler W, Klotz E, et al: Spiral volumetric CT with single-breath-hold technique, continuous transport, and continuous scanner rotation. Radiology 176:181, 1990.
2. Crawford CR, King KF: Computed tomography scanning with simultaneous patient translation. Med Phys 17:967, 1990.
3. Kalender WA: Technical foundations of spiral CT. Seminars in ultrasound, CT & MR 15:81, 1994.
4. Kalender WA: Thin-section three-dimensional spiral CT: Is isotropic imaging possible? Radiology 197:578, 1995.
5. Klingenbeck-Regn K, Schaller S, Flohr T, et al: Subsecond multi-slice computed tomography: Basics and applications. Eur J Radiol 31:110, 1999.
6. McCollough CH, Zink FE: Performance evaluation of a multi-slice CT system. Med Phys 26:2223, 1999.
7. Hu H, He HD, Foley WD, et al: Four multidetector-row helical CT: Image quality and volume coverage speed. Radiology 215:55, 2000.
8. Flohr T, Bruder H, Stierstorfer K, et al: New technical developments in multislice CT, part 2: Sub-millimeter 16-slice scanning and increased gantry rotation speed for cardiac imaging. Rofo Fortschr Geb Rontgenstr Neuen Bildgeb Verfahr 174:1022, 2002.
9. Achenbach S, Ulzheimer S, Baum U, et al: Noninvasive coronary angiography by retrospectively ECG-gated multislice spiral CT. Circulation 102:2823, 2000.
10. Becker C, Knez A, Leber A, et al: Detection of coronary artery stenoses with multislice helical CT. J Comput Assist Tomogr 26:750, 2002.
11. Knez A, Becker C, Leber A, et al: Usefulness of multislice spiral computed tomography angiography for determination of coronary artery stenoses. Am J Cardiol 88:1191, 2001.
12. Schroeder S, Kopp AF, Baumbach A, et al: Noninvasive detection and evaluation of atherosclerotic coronary plaques with multislice computed tomography. J Am Coll Cardiol 37:1430, 2001.
13. Schroeder S, Kopp AF, Baumbach A, et al: Non-invasive characterisation of coronary lesion morphology by multi-slice computed tomography: A promising new technology for risk stratification of patients with coronary artery disease. Heart 85:576, 2001.
14. Hu H: Multi-slice helical CT: Scan and reconstruction. Med Phys 26:5, 1999.
15. Flohr T, Schoepf U, Kuettner A, et al: Advances in cardiac imaging with 16-section CT systems. Acad Radiol 10:386, 2003.
16. Lipton M, Higgins C, Farmer D, et al: Cardiac imaging with a high-speed Cine-CT Scanner: Preliminary results. Radiology 152:579, 1984.
17. McCollough C, Morin R: The technical design and performance of ultrafast computed tomography. Radiol Clin North Am 32:521, 1994.
18. Funabashi N, Kobayashi Y, Perlroth M, et al: Coronary artery: Quantitative evaluation of normal diameter determined with electron-beam CT compared with cine coronary angiography: Initial experience. Radiology 226:263, 2003.
19. NIH: Research, development and evaluation of minimally invasive systems for detection and quantification of atherosclerotic lesions in coronary arteries in humans. In NHLBI R (Ed): NIH. Washington, DC, NIH, US Dept. HHS, 1982, p 83.
20. Schoepf UJ, Becker CR, Bruening RD, et al: Electrocardiographically gated thin-section CT of the lung. Radiology 212:649, 1999.
21. Becker CR, Jakobs TF, Aydemir S, et al: Helical and single-slice conventional CT versus electron beam CT for the quantification of coronary artery calcification. AJR Am J Roentgenol 174:543, 1999.
22. Becker CR, Knez A, Jakobs TF, et al: Detection and quantification of coronary artery calcification with electron-beam and conventional CT. Eur Radiol 9:620, 1999.
23. Ohnesorge B, Becker C, Flohr T, et al: Multislice CT in Cardiac Imaging: Technical Principles, Clinical Application and Future Developments. Berlin, Heidelberg, London, New York, Springer, p 140.
24. Schoepf UJ, Becker CR, Obuchowski NA, et al: Multi-slice computed tomography as a screening tool for colon cancer, lung cancer and coronary artery disease. Eur Radiol 11:1975, 2001.
25. Ohnesorge B, Flohr T, Becker C, et al: Cardiac imaging by means of electrocardiographically gated multisection spiral CT: Initial experience. Radiology 217:564, 2000.

26. Flohr T, Ohnesorge B: Heart rate adaptive optimization of spatial and temporal resolution for electrocardiogram-gated multislice spiral CT of the heart. J Comput Assist Tomogr 25:907, 2001.
27. Kachelriess M, Ulzheimer S, Kalender WA. ECG-correlated imaging of the heart with subsecond multislice spiral CT. IEEE Trans Med Imaging 19:888, 2000.
28. Wicky S, Rosol M, Hamberg L, et al: Evaluation of retrospective multisector and half scan ECG-gated multidetector cardiac CT protocols with moving phantoms. J Comput Assist Tomogr 26:768, 2002.
29. Halliburton S, Stillman A, Flohr T, et al: Do segmented reconstruction algorithms for cardiac multi-slice computed tomography improve image quality? Herz 28:20, 2003.
30. Hong C, Becker CR, Huber A, et al: ECG-gated reconstructed multidetector row CT coronary angiography: Effect of varying trigger delay on image quality. Radiology 220:712, 2001.
31. Kopp AF, Schroeder S, Kuettner A, et al: Coronary arteries: Retrospectively ECG-gated multi-detector row CT angiography with selective optimization of the image reconstruction window. Radiology 221:683, 2001.
32. Juergens K, Grude M, Fallenberg E, et al: Using ECG-gated multidetector CT to evaluate global left ventricular function in patients with coronary artery disease. AJR Am J Roentgenol 179:1545, 2002.
33. Mahnken A, Spuntrup E, Wildberger J, et al: Quantification of cardiac function with multislice spiral CT using retrospective EKG-gating: Comparison with MRI. Rofo Fortschr Geb Rontgenstr Neuen Bildgeb Verfahr 175:83, 2003.
34. Saito K, Saito M, Komatu S, et al: Real-time four-dimensional imaging of the heart with multi-detector row CT. Radiographics 23:8e, 2003.
35. Nickoloff EL, Alderson PO: Radiation exposure to patients from CT: Reality, public perception, and policy. AJR Am J Roentgenol 177: 285, 2001.
36. Brenner D, Elliston C, Hall E, et al: Estimated risks of radiation-induced fatal cancer from pediatric CT. AJR Am J Roentgenol 176: 289, 2001.
37. McCollough C: Patient dose in cardiac computed tomography. Herz 28:1, 2003.
38. Morin R, Gerber T, McCollough C: Radiation dose in computed tomography of the heart. Circulation 107:917, 2003.
39. Donelly L, Emry K, Brody A: Minimizing radiation dose for pediatric body applications of single-detector helical CT: Strategies at a large children's hospital. AJR Am J Roentgenol 176:303, 2001.
40. Frush DP, Soden B, Frush KS, et al: Improved pediatric multidetector body CT using a size-based color-coded format. AJR Am J Roentgenol 178:721, 2002.
41. Wildberger JE, Mahnken AH, Schmitz-Rode T, et al: Individually adapted examination protocols for reduction of radiation exposure in chest CT. Invest Radiol 36:604, 2001.
42. Jakobs T, Becker C, Ohnesorge B, et al: Multislice helical CT of the heart with retrospective ECG gating: Reduction of radiation exposure by ECG-controlled tube current modulation. Eur J Radiol 12:1081, 2002.
43. Katz DA, Marks MP, Napel SA, et al: Circle of Willis: Evaluation with spiral CT angiography, MR angiography, and conventional angiography. Radiology 195:445, 1995.
44. Preda L, Gaetani P, Rodriguez Y, et al: Spiral CT angiography and surgical correlations in the evaluation of intracranial aneurysms. Eur Radiol 8:739, 1998.
45. Korogi Y, Takahashi M, Katada K, et al: Intracranial aneurysms: Detection with three-dimensional CT angiography with volume rendering—comparison with conventional angiographic and surgical findings. Radiology 211:497, 1999.
46. Villablanca JP, Jahan R, Hooshi P, et al: Detection and characterization of very small cerebral aneurysms by using 2D and 3D helical CT angiography. AJNR: Am J Neuroradiol 23:1187, 2002.
47. Hull R, Raskob GE, Ginsberg JS, et al: A noninvasive strategy for the treatment of patients with suspected pulmonary embolism. Arch Intern Med 154:289, 1994.
48. van Rossum AB, Pattynama PM, Mallens WM, et al: Can helical CT replace scintigraphy in the diagnostic process in suspected pulmonary embolism? A retrolective-prolective cohort study focusing on total diagnostic yield. Eur Radiol 8:90, 1998.
49. Garg K, Welsh CH, Feyerabend AJ, et al: Pulmonary embolism: Diagnosis with spiral CT and ventilation-perfusion scanning—correlation with pulmonary angiographic results or clinical outcome. Radiology 208:201, 1998.
50. Blachere H, Latrabe V, Montaudon M, et al: Pulmonary embolism revealed on helical CT angiography: Comparison with ventilation-perfusion radionuclide lung scanning. AJR Am J Roentgenol 174: 1041, 2000.
51. van Erkel AR, van Rossum AB, Bloem JL, et al: Spiral CT angiography for suspected pulmonary embolism: A cost-effectiveness analysis. Radiology 201:29, 1996.
52. Goodman LR, Curtin JJ, Mewissen MW, et al: Detection of pulmonary embolism in patients with unresolved clinical and scintigraphic diagnosis: Helical CT versus angiography. AJR Am J Roentgenol 164:1369, 1995.
53. Drucker EA, Rivitz SM, Shepard JA, et al: Acute pulmonary embolism: Assessment of helical CT for diagnosis. Radiology 209:235, 1998.
54. Perrier A, Howarth N, Didier D, et al: Performance of helical computed tomography in unselected outpatients with suspected pulmonary embolism. Ann Intern Med 135:88, 2001.
55. Cauvain O, Remy-Jardin M, Remy J, et al: [Spiral CT angiography in the diagnosis of central pulmonary embolism: Comparison with pulmonary angiography and scintigraphy]. Rev Mal Respir 13:141, 1996.
56. Teigen CL, Maus TP, Sheedy PF II, et al: Pulmonary embolism: Diagnosis with contrast-enhanced electron beam CT and comparison with pulmonary angiography. Radiology 194:313, 1995.
57. Goodman LR, Lipchik RJ, Kuzo RS, et al: Subsequent pulmonary embolism: Risk after a negative helical CT pulmonary angiogram—prospective comparison with scintigraphy. Radiology 215:535, 2000.
58. Remy-Jardin M, Tillie-Leblond I, Szapiro D, et al: CT angiography of pulmonary embolism in patients with underlying respiratory disease: Impact of multislice CT on image quality and negative predictive value. Eur Radiol 12:1971, 2002.
59. Swensen SJ, Sheedy PF II, Ryu JH, et al: Outcomes after withholding anticoagulation from patients with suspected acute pulmonary embolism and negative computed tomographic findings: A cohort study. Mayo Clin Proc 77:130, 2002.
60. Musset D, Parent F, Meyer G, et al: Diagnostic strategy for patients with suspected pulmonary embolism: A prospective multicentre outcome study. Lancet 360:1914, 2002.
61. van Strijen MJ, de Monye W, Schiereck J, et al: Single-detector helical computed tomography as the primary diagnostic test in suspected pulmonary embolism: A multicenter clinical management study of 510 patients. Ann Intern Med 138:307, 2003.
62. Ghaye B, Remy J, Remy-Jardin M: Non-traumatic thoracic emergencies: CT diagnosis of acute pulmonary embolism: The first 10 years. Eur Radiol 12:1886, 2002.
63. Mayo JR, Remy-Jardin M, Muller NL, et al: Pulmonary embolism: Prospective comparison of spiral CT with ventilation-perfusion scintigraphy. Radiology 205:447, 1997.
64. Qanadli SD, Hajjam ME, Mesurolle B, et al: Pulmonary embolism detection: Prospective evaluation of dual-section helical CT versus selective pulmonary arteriography in 157 patients. Radiology 217: 447, 2000.
65. Becker CR, Knez A, Leber A, et al: [Initial experiences with multislice detector spiral CT in diagnosis of arteriosclerosis of coronary vessels]. Radiologe 40:118, 2000.
66. Ghaye B, Szapiro D, Mastora I, et al: Peripheral pulmonary arteries: How far in the lung does multi-detector row spiral CT allow analysis? Radiology 219:629, 2001.
67. Patel S, Kazerooni EA, Cascade PN: Pulmonary embolism: Optimization of small pulmonary artery visualization at multidetector row CT. Radiology 227:455, 2003.
68. Diffin D, Leyendecker JR, Johnson SP, et al: Effect of anatomic distribution of pulmonary emboli on interobserver agreement in the interpretation of pulmonary angiography. AJR Am J Roentgenol 171:1085, 1998.
69. O'Malley PG, Feuerstein IM, Taylor AJ: Impact of electron beam tomography, with or without case management, on motivation, behavioral change, and cardiovascular risk profile: A randomized controlled trial. JAMA 289:2215, 2003.
70. Angelini P, Velasco JA, Flamm S: Coronary Anomalies: Incidence, Pathophysiology, and Clinical Relevance. Circulation 105:2449, 2002.
71. Mesurolle B, Qanadli S, Merad M, et al: Anomalous origin of the left coronary artery arising from the pulmonary trunk: Report of an adult case with long-term follow-up after surgery. Eur Radiol 9: 1570, 1999.

72. Brundage B, Lipton M, Herfkens R, et al: Detection of patent coronary bypass grafts by computed tomography. A preliminary report. Circulation 61:826, 1980.
73. Daniel W, Dohring W, Stender H, et al: Value and limitations of computed tomography in assessing aortocoronary bypass graft patency. Circulation 67:983, 1983.
74. Godwin J, Califf R, Korobkin M, et al: Clinical value of coronary bypass graft evaluation with CT. AJR Am J Roentgenol 140:649, 1983.
75. Tello R, Costello P, Ecker C, et al: Spiral CT evaluation of coronary artery bypass graft patency. J Comput Assist Tomogr 17:253, 1993.
76. Engelmann M, von Smekal A, Knez A, et al: Accuracy of spiral computed tomography for identifying arterial and venous coronary graft patency. Am J Cardiol 80:569, 1997.
77. Lu B, Dai RP, Jing BL, et al: Evaluation of coronary artery bypass graft patency using three-dimensional reconstruction and flow study on electron beam tomography. J Comput Assist Tomogr 24:663, 2000.
78. Tello R, Hartnell G, Costello P, et al: Coronary artery bypass graft flow: Qualitative evaluation with cine single-detector row CT and comparison with findings at angiography. Radiology 224:913, 2002.
79. Ropers D, Ulzheimer S, Wenkel E, et al: Investigation of aorto-coronary artery bypass grafts by multislice spiral computed tomography with electrocardiographic-gated image reconstruction. Am J Cardiol 88:792, 2001.
80. Achenbach S, Moshage W, Ropers D, et al: Value of electron-beam computed tomography for the noninvasive detection of high-grade coronary-artery stenoses and occlusions. N Engl J Med 339:1964, 1998.
81. Nieman K, Oudkerk M, Rensing BJ, et al: Coronary angiography with multi-slice computed tomography. Lancet 357:599, 2001.
82. Achenbach S, Giesler T, Ropers D, et al: Detection of coronary artery stenoses by contrast-enhanced, retrospectively electrocardiographically-gated, multislice spiral computed tomography. Circulation 103:2535, 2001.
83. Regenfus M, Ropers D, Achenbach S, et al: Noninvasive detection of coronary artery stenosis using contrast-enhanced three-dimensional breath-hold magnetic resonance coronary angiography. J Am Coll Cardiol 36:44, 2000.
84. Kim W, Danias P, Stuber M, et al: Coronary magnetic resonance angiography for the detection of coronary stenoses. N Engl J Med 345:1863, 2001.
85. Bogaert J, Kuzo R, Dymarkowski S, et al: Coronary artery imaging with real-time navigator three-dimensional turbo-field-echo MR coronary angiography: Initial experience. Radiology 226:707, 2003.
86. Nieman K, Cademartiri F, Lemos PA, et al: Reliable noninvasive coronary angiography with fast submillimeter multislice spiral computed tomography. Circulation 106:2051, 2002.
87. Ropers D, Baum U, Pohle K, et al: Detection of coronary artery stenoses with thin-slice multi-detector row spiral computed tomography and multiplanar reconstruction. Circulation 107:664, 2003.
88. Kopp AF, Schroeder S, Kuettner A, et al: Non-invasive coronary angiography with high resolution multidetector-row computed tomography. Results in 102 patients. Eur Heart J 23:1714, 2002.
89. Topol E, Nissen S: Our preoccupation with coronary luminology: The dissociation between clinical and angiographic findings in ischemic heart disease. Circulation 92:2333, 1995.
90. Becker CR, Knez A, Ohnesorge B, et al: Imaging of noncalcified coronary plaques using helical CT with retrospective ECG gating. AJR Am J Roentgenol 175:423, 2000.
91. Kopp AF, Schroeder S, Baumbach A, et al: Non-invasive characterisation of coronary lesion morphology and composition by multislice CT: First results in comparison with intracoronary ultrasound. Eur Radiol 11:1607, 2001.
92. Kopp A, Kuttner A, Heuschmid M, et al: Multidetector-row CT cardiac imaging with 4 and 16 slices for coronary CTA and imaging of atherosclerotic plaques. Eur Radiol 12:S17, 2002.
93. Leber A, Knez A, White C, et al: Composition of coronary atherosclerotic plaques in patients with acute myocardial infarction and stable angina pectoris determined by contrast-enhanced multislice computed tomography. Am J Cardiol 91:714, 2002.
94. Becker C, Nikolaou K, Muders M, et al: Ex vivo coronary atherosclerotic plaque characterization with multi-detector-row CT. Eur Radiol 12:12, 2003.
95. Fayad Z, Fuster V, Nikolaou K, et al: Computed tomography and magnetic resonance imaging for noninvasive. Circulation 106: 2026, 2002.
96. Costello P, Ecker CP, Tello R, et al: Assessment of the thoracic aorta by spiral CT. AJR Am J Roentgenol 158:1127, 1992.
97. Rubin G: Helical CT angiography of the thoracic aorta. J Thorac Imaging 12:128, 1997.
98. Raptopoulos V, Sheiman RG, Phillips DA, et al: Traumatic aortic tear: Screening with chest CT. Radiology 182:667, 1992.
99. Rubin GD, Dake MD, Semba CP: Current status of three-dimensional spiral CT scanning for imaging the vasculature. Radiol Clin North Am 33:51, 1995.
100. Raptopoulos V, Steer ML, Sheiman RG, et al: The use of helical CT and CT angiography to predict vascular involvement from pancreatic cancer: Correlation with findings at surgery. AJR Am J Roentgenol 168:971, 1997.
101. Armerding MD, Rubin GD, Beaulieu CF, et al: Aortic aneurysmal disease: Assessment of stent-graft treatment—CT versus conventional angiography. Radiology 215:138, 2000.
102. Tillich M, Hill BB, Paik DS, et al: Prediction of aortoiliac stent-graft length: Comparison of measurement methods. Radiology 220: 475, 2001.
103. Johnson PT, Heath DG, Kuszyk BS, et al: CT angiography with volume rendering: Advantages and applications in splanchnic vascular imaging. Radiology 200:564, 1996.
104. Laghi A, Iannaccone R, Catalano C, et al: Multislice spiral computed tomography angiography of mesenteric arteries. Lancet 358:638, 2001.
105. Galanski M, Prokop M, Chavan A, et al: Renal arterial stenoses: Spiral CT angiography. Radiology 189:185, 1993.
106. Wittenberg G, Kenn W, Tschammler A, et al: Spiral CT angiography of renal arteries: Comparison with angiography. Eur Radiol 9:546, 1999.
107. Hofmann LV, Smith PA, Kuszyk BS, et al: Three-dimensional helical CT angiography in renal transplant recipients: A new problem-solving tool. AJR Am J Roentgenol 173:1085, 1999.
108. Rubin GD, Shiau MC, Leung AN, et al: Aorta and iliac arteries: Single versus multiple detector-row helical CT angiography. Radiology 215:670, 2000.
109. Rubin GD, Schmidt AJ, Logan LJ, et al: Multi-detector row CT angiography of lower extremity arterial inflow and runoff: Initial experience. Radiology 221:146, 2001.
110. Raptopoulos V, Rosen MP, Kent KC, et al: Sequential helical CT angiography of aortoiliac disease. AJR Am J Roentgenol 166:1347, 1996.
111. Robb R, Ritman E: High speed synchronous volume computed tomography of the heart. Radiology 133:655, 1979.
112. Ritman EL, Kinsey JH, Robb RA, et al: Three-dimensional imaging of heart, lungs, and circulation. Science 210:273, 1980.

■ ■ ■ chapter 13

Peripheral Arterial Angiography

Christopher J. White

Invasive contrast angiography is the standard method for diagnosing peripheral arterial disease (PAD) and against which all other methods are compared for accuracy. Angiography provides the "road map" on which therapeutic decisions are based. Knowledge of the vascular anatomy and its normal variations is a core element in the skill set required to safely perform peripheral vascular angiography and intervention.

Imaging Equipment

There are multiple excellent radiographic equipment vendors, and many different room layout schemes that are suitable for performing peripheral vascular angiography. However, if both cardiac and noncardiac types of peripheral vascular angiography are to be performed in the same room, then the equipment options become much more limited.

One angiographic suite that is designed to perform both coronary and peripheral vascular angiography is a "dual-plane" system (Fig. 13-1). Dual-plane encompasses a layout with two independent C-arm image intensifiers, operated by a single x-ray generator and one computer. Dual-plane is not a biplane system, which is the simultaneous operation of an anteroposterior (AP) and lateral (LAT) image acquisition system. In a dual-plane system, the cardiac C-arm is a three mode, 9-inch image intensifier, and the noncardiac C-arm should be as large as possible, usually a 15-inch or 16-inch image intensifier. For peripheral vascular imaging, particularly bilateral lower extremity runoff angiography, an image intensifier smaller than 15 inches may not be able to include both legs in the same field. The noncardiac C-arm must be capable of head-to-toe digital imaging.

The ability to angulate the image intensifier is necessary to resolve bifurcation lesions and to optimally image aorto-ostial branch lesions. Of the many imaging options available, the most often used include digital subtraction angiography, roadmapping, and a stepping table for lower extremity (digital subtraction) runoff angiography.

Radiographic Contrast

Ionic low-osmolar or nonionic radiographic contrast is required for contrast angiography in the peripheral vessels to avoid patient discomfort. Low-osmolar contrast agents

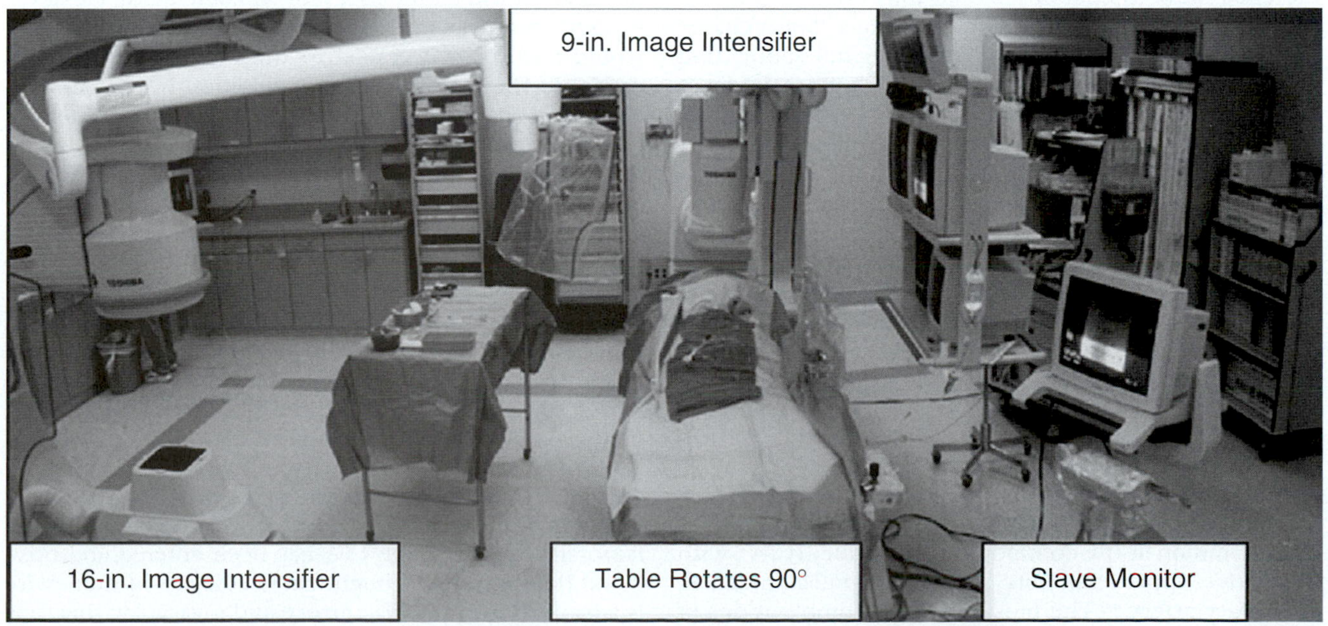

FIGURE 13-1. Dual-plane catheterization laboratory. Note two C-arm image intensifiers (9- and 16-inch) with the catheterization table able to rotate 90°.

produce fewer side effects—such as nausea, vomiting, and local pain—leading to better patient tolerability.[1] In addition, low-osmolar agents deliver a lesser osmotic load and, thereby, a lower intravascular volume, which may be important in patients with impaired left ventricular and renal function. Digital subtraction angiography is often preferred because nonvascular structures are removed and less contrast is required.

Alternatives to iodine-based radiographic contrast include carbon dioxide (CO_2) and gadolinium (gadopentetate dimeglumine).[2,3] It is recommended that CO_2 not be used for angiograms above the diaphragm, to minimize the risk of distal embolization and stroke.[4-6] Gadolinium, traditionally used with magnetic resonance imaging, is relatively nontoxic at a recommended dose not exceeding 0.4 mmol/Kg.[7]

Imaging Technique

Many of the technical aspects of diagnostic cardiac imaging also apply to the performance of angiography of the aorta and the peripheral vasculature. The basic principle of vascular angiography is to not only visualize the target lesion, but to demonstrate the inflow and outflow vascular segments. The inflow anatomy constitutes the vascular segment preceding the target lesion and the outflow constitutes the vascular segment immediately distal to the target vessel and includes the runoff bed. For example, the inflow segment for the common iliac artery is the infrarenal aorta and the outflow segment is the external iliac and femoral vessels. The runoff bed would be the tibioperoneal vessels to the foot.

It is important for patients' safety, when performing selective arterial imaging, that a "coronary" manifold with pressure measurement is used to monitor the hemodynamic status of the patient and to ensure that damping of the catheter has not occurred prior to injecting contrast. The use of pressure monitoring during selective angiography can prevent a myriad of complications—including the creation of dissections and air injection.

Angiography may be performed using a "bolus chase" cineangiographic method or with a digital subtraction stepping mode. The bolus chase technique involves injecting a bolus of contrast at the inflow of the territory, then "panning" or manually moving the image intensifier to follow the bolus of contrast through the target lesion and into the run-off segment. In digital subtraction stepping mode, the patient lies motionless on the angiographic table. A "mask" of the segments to be imaged is taken, and then contrast is injected. The table moves in steps to image the contrast filled vessels from which the mask is then subtracted, leaving only the contrast-filled vascular structures.

OBTAINING VASCULAR ACCESS

Vascular access for noncardiac diagnostic angiography is most common at the common femoral artery (CFA), with alternative upper extremity sites at the radial, brachial, or axillary artery.[8,9] The most common complications of angiographic procedures involve vascular access sites.

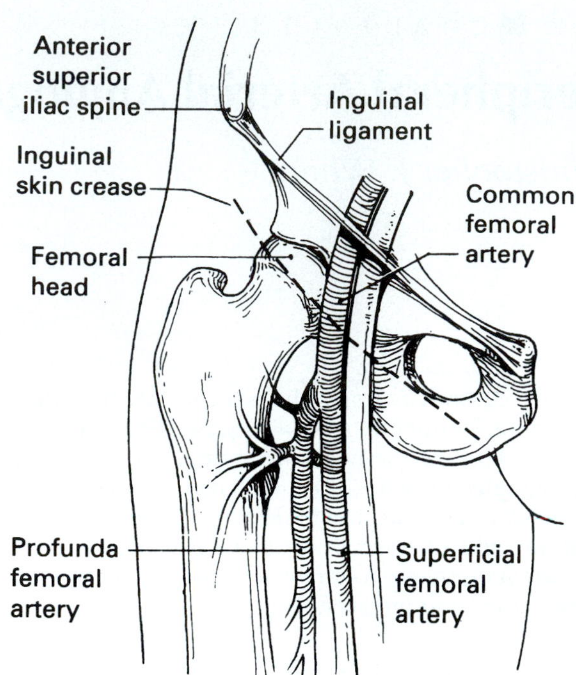

FIGURE 13-2. Schematic of common femoral artery anatomic landmarks.

A thorough understanding of the relationship of the CFA to anatomic landmarks is necessary to ensure safe CFA puncture (Fig. 13-2). The femoral artery and vein lie below the inguinal ligament, which is a band of dense fibrous tissue connecting the anterior superior iliac spine to the pubic tubercle. The inguinal skin crease, which is variable in location, is shown as a dotted line. The inguinal skin crease is located caudal to the bifurcation of the CFA in three fourths of all limbs.[10]

The most important landmark for femoral access is the head of the femur. In a morphologic study using CT images, there was not a single case in which a puncture would have passed cranial to the inguinal ligament or caudal to the femoral artery bifurcation if the CFA was entered at the level of the center of the femoral head.[11] Caudal to the femoral head, the CFA is encased in the femoral sheath and bifurcates to the superficial femoral artery (SFA) medially and the deep femoral artery (DFA) laterally. With these anatomic observations in mind, the importance of osseous support and entry of the needle into the CFA at the center of the femoral head is obvious.

Anatomic landmarks are initially identified by palpation of the anterior superior iliac spine and the pubic tubercle to locate the inguinal ligament, and the position of the femoral head is confirmed fluoroscopically. Depending on the amount of subcutaneous fat, a skin incision should be made 1 to 2 cm caudal to the level of the center of the femoral head. The needle is directed in an oblique direction while palpating the CFA over the center of the femoral head. Once the CFA has been entered and brisk blood flow returns through the needle, a soft guidewire is advanced into the iliac artery and a vascular sheath is inserted to secure vascular access.

Complications of CFA puncture are most commonly related to arterial entry either too high or too low. When the puncture is too high, a retroperitoneal hemorrhage may occur.[12-14] The presence of loose connective tissue in the retroperitoneal space can lead to large hematomas. The lack of osseous support and the presence of a tense inguinal ligament at the arterial puncture site make manual compression difficult. Low punctures may be complicated by formation of arteriovenous fistulas, false aneurysms, and hematomas.[15-17]

ABDOMINAL AORTOGRAPHY AND LOWER EXTREMITY RUNOFF

For abdominal aortography, vascular access with a 4 to 6 Fr catheter is obtained in the CFA, although brachial or radial access may also be used. The angiographic catheter (e.g., pigtail, tennis racquet, omni flush) is positioned in the abdominal aorta so that the tip of the catheter reaches the level of the last rib. A power injector is used to deliver 20 to 30 ml of contrast at 15 ml/sec for digital subtraction (Fig. 13-3). Either biplane angiography or two separate angiograms may be obtained, if needed, with single plane systems.

Three visceral (mesenteric) arterial branches, the celiac trunk, the superior mesenteric artery (SMA), and the inferior mesenteric artery (IMA) arise from the anterior surface of the abdominal aorta (Fig. 13-4). The renal arteries originate from the lateral aspect of the abdominal aorta at the level of L-1 to L-2. The AP projection allows visualization of the aorta, renal arteries, and iliac artery bifurcation, whereas the LAT view demonstrates the origin of the celiac trunk and mesenteric arteries. Commonly, in the AP view, the proximal portion of the SMA obscures

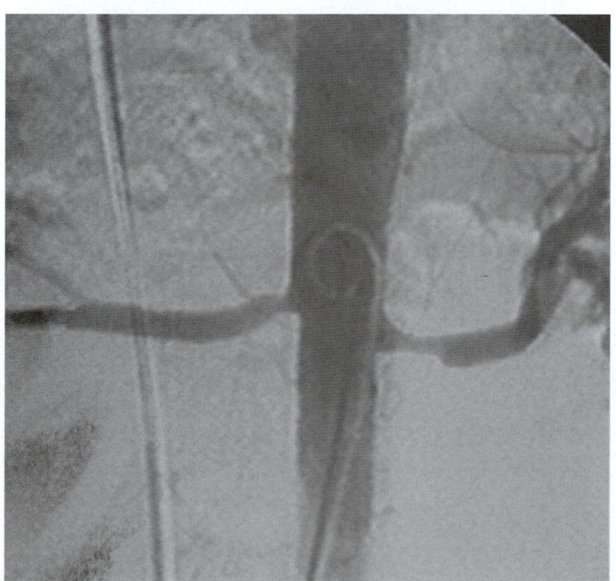

FIGURE 13-3. Femoral access: Pigtail catheter contrast injection of 20 ml/sec for 30 ml (5° LAO) using a DSA technique. Note the bilateral renal artery stenosis. DSA, digital subtraction angiography; LAO, left anterior oblique.

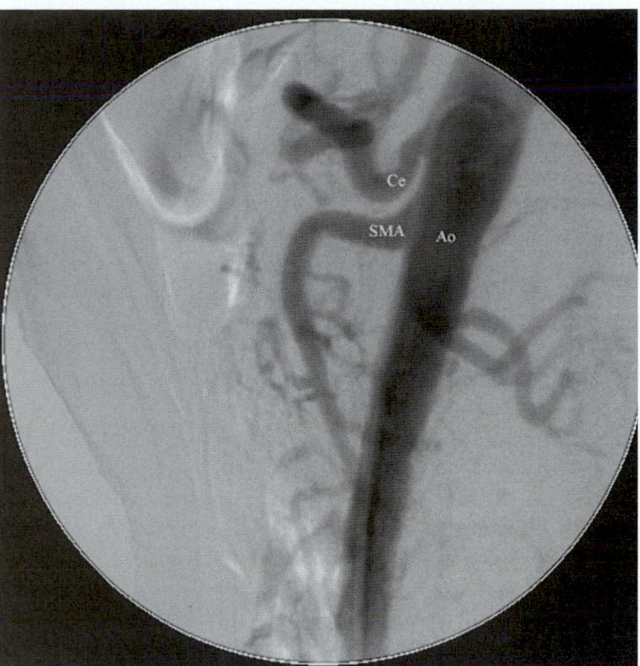

FIGURE 13-4. Femoral access: Lateral aortogram. Aorta (Ao) with celiac trunk (Ce) and superior mesenteric artery (SMA) arising from the anterior surface of the aorta.

the origin of the right renal artery. When this occurs, selective angiography of the renal artery may be required to visualize the origin of this vessel.

Generally, a nonselective abdominal aortogram is obtained before selective renal angiography using a large format (9- to 16-inch) image intensifier with digital subtraction imaging. The nonselective aortogram demonstrates the level at which the renal arteries arise, the presence of any accessory renal arteries and their location, the severity and location of aortoiliac pathology, and the presence of significant renal artery stenosis. To optimize viewing of the renal arteries, the angiographic catheter should be placed below the origin of the SMA, and the image intensifier should be positioned such that the superior, inferior, and lateral borders of both kidneys are visualized. The ostia of the renal arteries are often better seen with slight rotation of the image intensifier, usually left anterior oblique (LAO).

Selective Renal Angiography

Selective renal angiography is indicated to identify suspected renovascular disease. Selective renal artery engagement allows the measurement of pressure gradients, particularly if ostial lesions are suspected. When measuring pressure gradients across lesions, it is important that the smallest catheter possible is used (i.e., ≤ 4 Fr), so as to not create an artificial gradient. The 0.014-inch pressure wire (RADI) is the optimal method of pressure gradient measurement. Usually selective renal angiography is performed with 4- to 6-Fr diagnostic catheters (Fig. 13-5) and a 9-inch image intensifier. Selective renal angiography is performed using hand

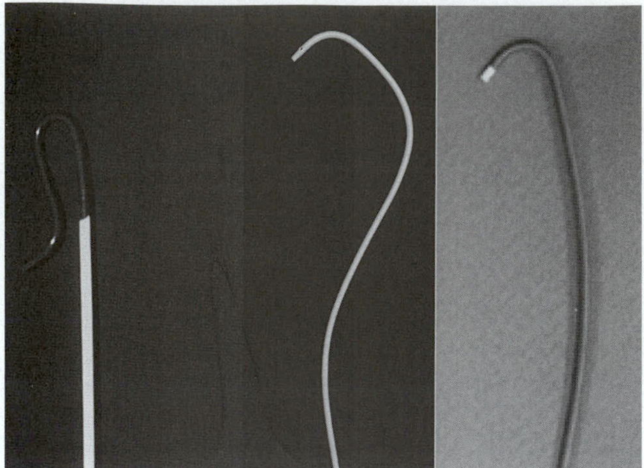

FIGURE 13-5. Selective renal angiographic catheters. *Left*: Sos; *Middle*: Cobra; *Right*: internal mammary artery (IMA) catheter.

injections with shallow oblique angulations to optimize visualization of the renal ostia (Figs. 13-6 and 13-7). Caudal or cranial angulation (15° to 20°) may occasionally be necessary for better visualization of some ostial lesions. An optimal image will reveal the ostial portion of the renal artery and the distal branches at the cortex of the kidney.

Selective Mesenteric Angiography

As is the case for the renal arteries, nonselective aortography (AP and LAT) generally precedes selective angiography. Once the origin of the mesenteric vessels have been identified, selective angiography may be carried out in the lateral and oblique views using 4- to 6-Fr catheters

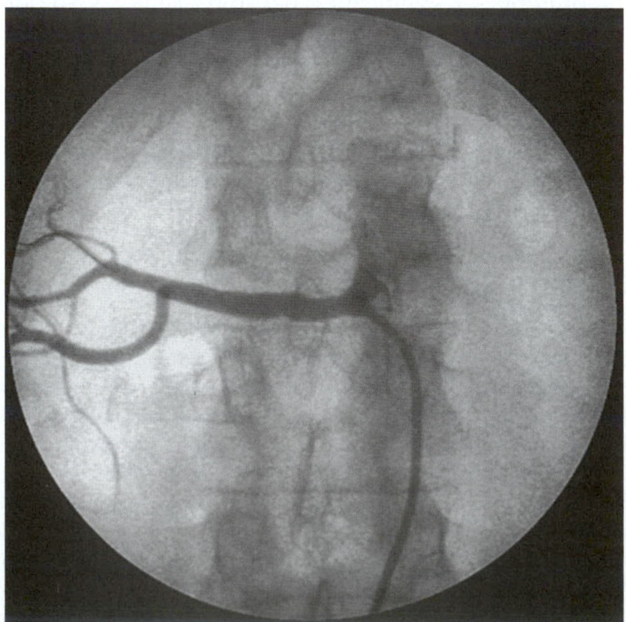

FIGURE 13-6. Femoral access: Internal mammary artery (IMA) catheter selectively engaged in right renal artery.

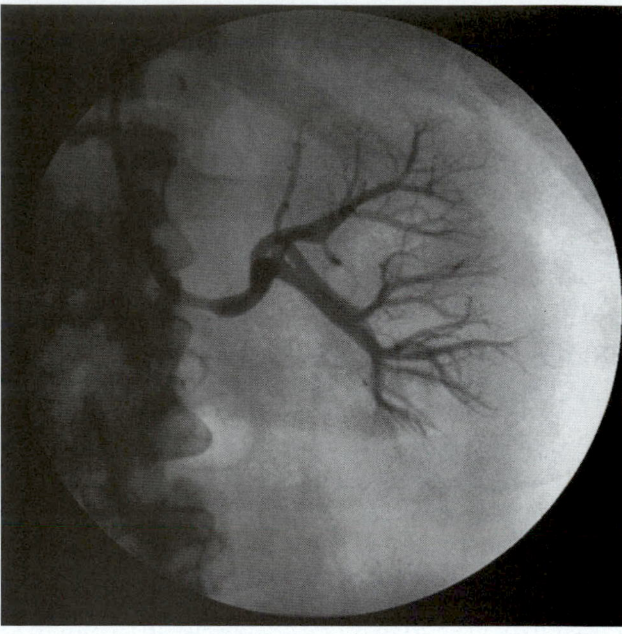

FIGURE 13-7. Upper extremity access: Selective left renal artery engagement with a multipurpose catheter.

(Fig. 13-8). The celiac trunk, SMA, and IMA arteries arise from the anterior surface of the aorta. There commonly are collaterals between the mesenteric vessels, and it is uncommon for stenosis or occlusion of a single branch to cause clinical symptoms.

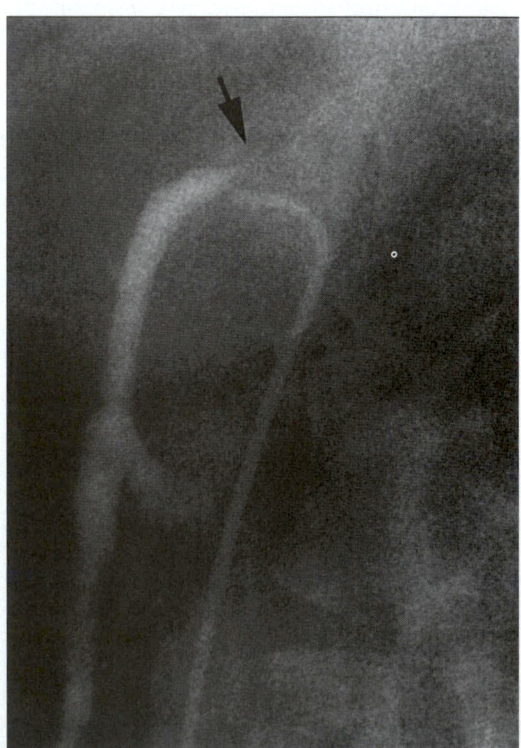

FIGURE 13-8. Selective superior mesenteric angiography in the lateral (LAT) projection with an internal mammary artery (IMA) catheter. Note the ostial stenosis (*arrow*).

The mesenteric arteries often arise at an inferior (caudal) angle from the abdominal aorta, for which a shepherd's crook catheter is helpful, from a femoral access, for selective engagement. Alternatively, upper extremity vascular access allows the mesenteric arteries to be engaged with a multipurpose-shaped catheter. Analogous to the renal arteries, selective engagement of the mesenteric arteries also allows measurement of the pressure gradient. Selective angiographic images in multiple views are obtained with hand injections of contrast.

Aortoiliac and Lower Extremity Angiography

The abdominal aorta bifurcates into the common iliac arteries (CIA), which bifurcate into the internal (IIA) and external (EIA) iliac arteries (Fig. 13-9). The internal iliac artery is often referred to as the *hypogastric* artery because this vessel commonly provides collateral circulation to the viscera. The external iliac artery emerges from the pelvis just posterior to the inguinal ligament. At the level of the inguinal ligament, two small branches originate from the EIA: the inferior epigastric artery, which follows a medial direction, and the deep iliac circumflex artery, which takes a lateral and superior direction.

On crossing the inguinal ligament, the EIA becomes the common femoral artery (CFA), which lies over the femoral head. When it reaches the lower third of the femoral head, the CFA divides into the superficial femoral artery (SFA) and profunda femoris or deep femoral artery (DFA). The DFA runs posterolaterally along the femur. The SFA continues down the anteromedial thigh, and in its distal portion dives deeper to enter Hunter's (adductor) canal and emerges as the popliteal artery (Fig. 13-10).

The popliteal artery, below the knee bifurcates into the anterior tibial (AT) artery and the tibioperoneal trunk (TPT). The AT artery runs laterally and anterior to the tibia toward the foot, and continues onto the foot as the dorsalis pedis (DP) artery. The TPT bifurcates into the posterior tibial (PT) and peroneal arteries (Fig. 13-11). The PT courses posterior and medially in the calf, whereas the peroneal artery runs near the fibula between the AT and PT arteries. On the dorsum of the foot, the DP artery has lateral and medial tarsal branches. After the PT artery passes behind the medial malleus, it divides into medial and lateral plantar arteries. The lateral plantar and distal DP arteries join to form the plantar arch.

Vascular access, for diagnostic aortic angiography with lower extremity runoff imaging, is obtained in the CFA, preferentially in the least symptomatic extremity, although upper extremity access may also be used. A 4- to 6-Fr pigtail catheter is positioned above the aortic bifurcation. The preferred technique is to use digital subtraction angiography (DSA) with a stepping table and a large

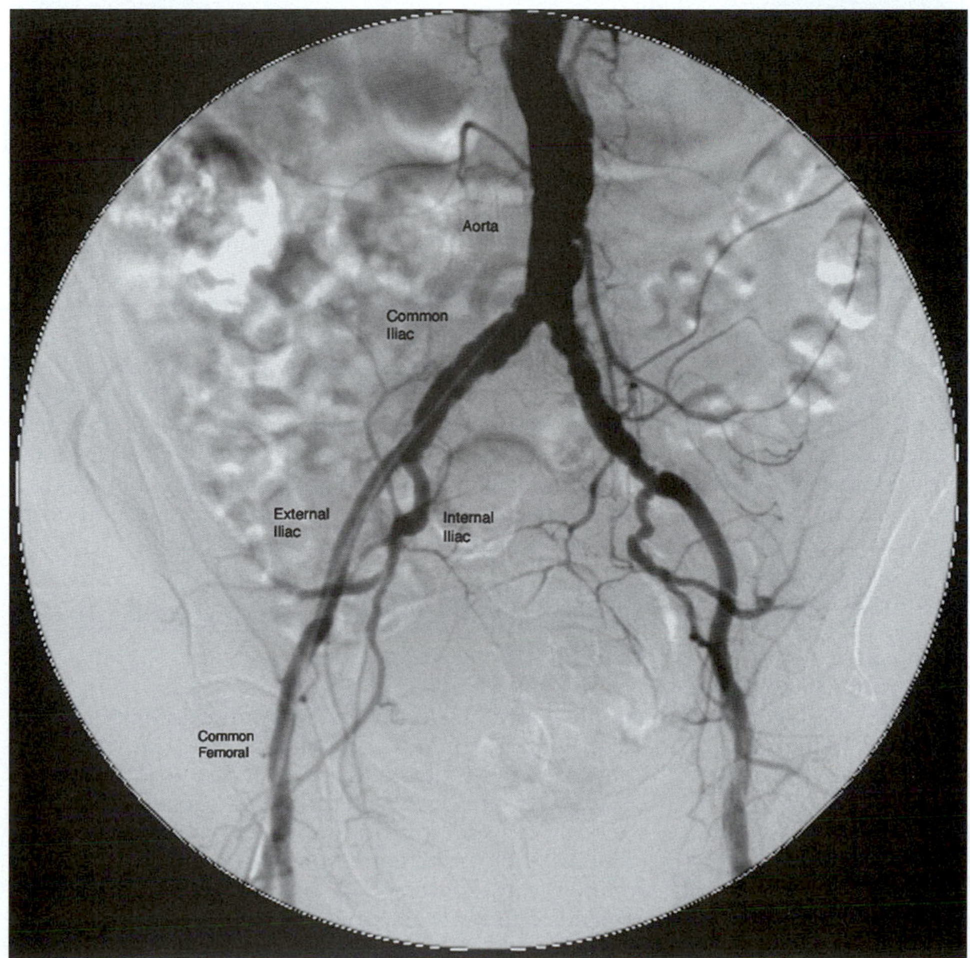

FIGURE 13-9. Aortoiliac angiography. Pigtail catheter contrast injection of 20 ml/sec for a total of 30 ml.

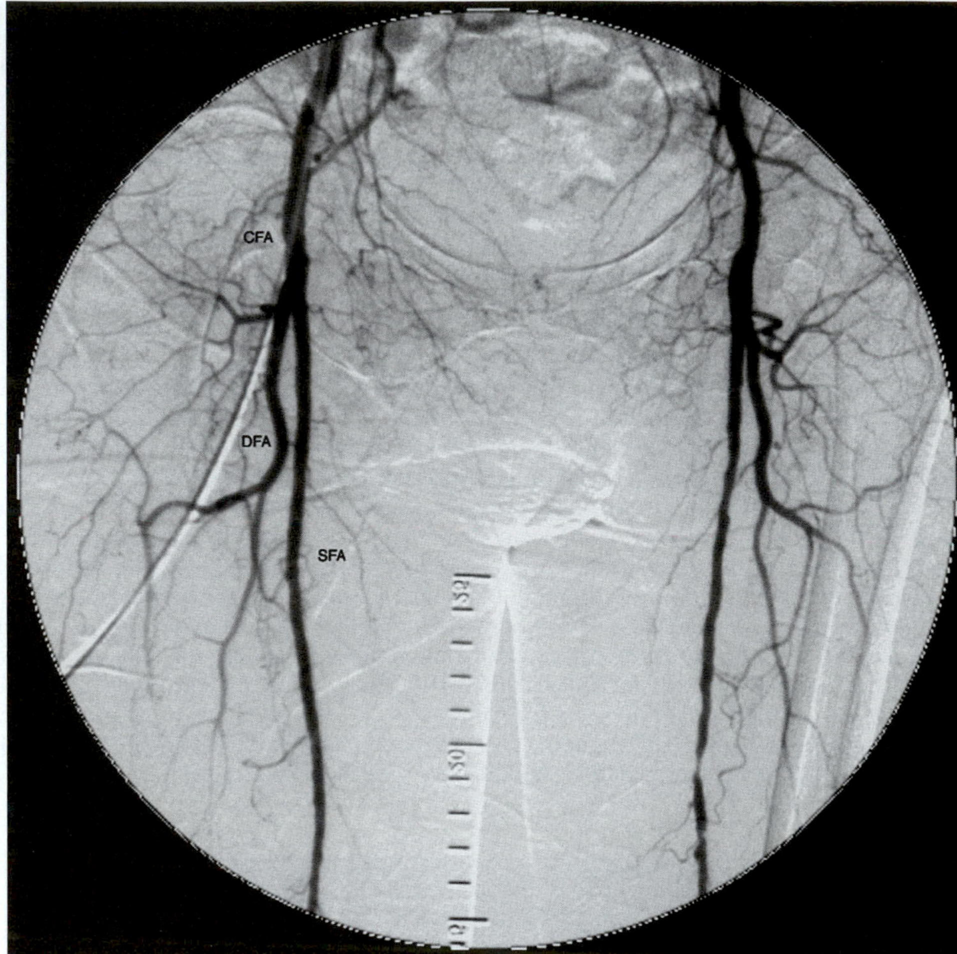

FIGURE 13-10. Common femoral arteries (CFA) branching into the deep femoral artery (DFA) and superficial femoral artery (SFA).

(15- or 16-inch) format image intensifier so that both legs are imaged together. A single bolus of nonionic contrast is injected from the catheter at the aortic bifurcation at 8 to 12 ml/sec for a total of 70 to 120 ml and sequential images are obtained from the aorta to the feet.

Selective angiograms performed in angulated views of a particular artery or arterial segments are useful when anatomic clarification is needed. One option is to place a diagnostic catheter at different levels in the iliac, femoral, or popliteal artery for a more detailed examination of a particular arterial segment. If access has been obtained in the CFA and the arterial segment in question is located in the contralateral extremity, a diagnostic internal mammary catheter (or a shepherd's crook catheter) is positioned at the level of the aortic bifurcation with the tip of the catheter selectively engaged in the contralateral common iliac artery (Fig. 13-12). An angled glidewire (Terumo, BSC, Watertown, MA) is advanced to the common femoral artery and the diagnostic catheter is advanced over the glidewire to the area of interest.

There are several angiographic views that are important to mention because they help to clarify anatomical detail. In the AP view there is often overlapping of the origin of the external and internal iliac arteries, and ostial stenoses in either or both vessels may be missed. The contralateral oblique view (20°) with 20° of caudal angulation is very useful to separate these vessels (Fig. 13-13).

Overlap at the origin of the superficial (SFA) and deep femoral (DFA) arteries commonly occurs in the AP projection and can be improved with a 20° to 30° lateral oblique view.[18] Another common source of artifact may occur when the tibial arteries overlie the relatively radiodense bony periosteum of the tibia or fibula. In that case, slight angulation will move the artery in question off of the bony density to allow better visualization.

AORTIC ARCH AND BRACHIOCEPHALIC VESSELS

The aortic arch includes portions of the ascending, transverse, and descending aorta (Fig. 13-14). The transverse portion of the thoracic aorta gives rise to the brachiocephalic trunk proximally, the left common carotid artery in the mid-portion, and the left subclavian artery in its distal portion. In 10% to 20% of the cases, the left common carotid artery may originate from the brachiocephalic trunk, an anatomical variation known as a

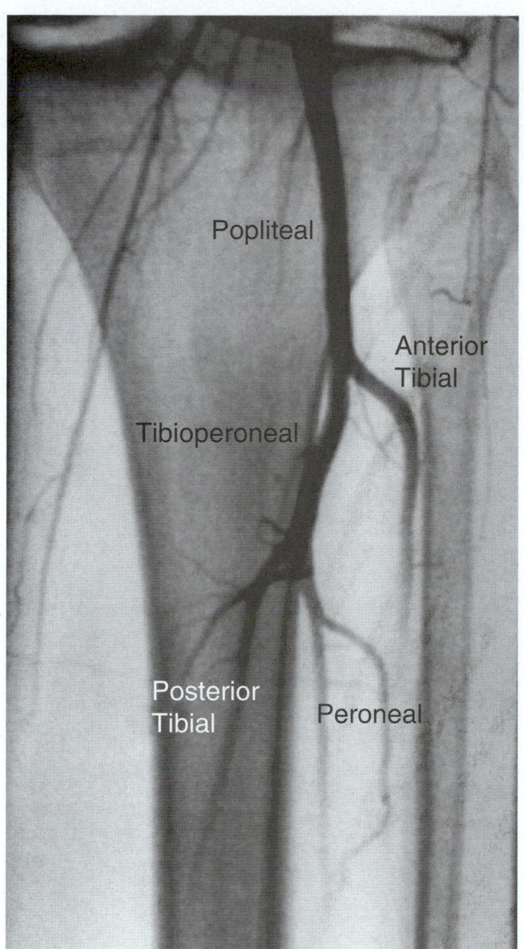

FIGURE 13-11. Left popliteal artery bifurcates into the anterior tibial (lateral), and the tibioperoneal trunk, which then divides into the posterior tibial (medial) and peroneal arteries.

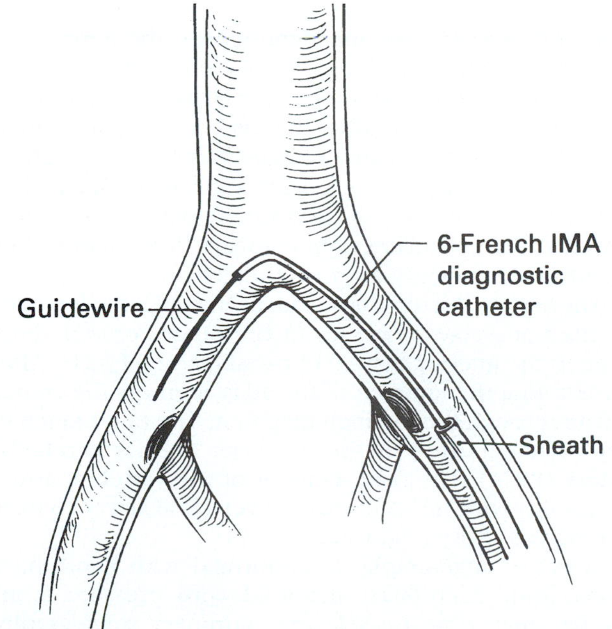

FIGURE 13-12. Drawing illustrating contralateral iliac access for selective angiography.

bovine arch (Fig. 13-15).[19] Other less common variations include the left vertebral artery—originating directly from the aortic arch, between the left common carotid artery and the left subclavian artery, and the right subclavian artery—originating from the aortic arch distal to the origin of the left subclavian artery.

Thoracic aortography is commonly performed for the diagnosis of pathologic entities such as stenoses of the origin of the great vessels, aneurysms, aortic dissection, coarctation of the aorta, patent ductus arteriosus, vascular rings, as well as for the evaluation of vascular injuries such as blunt or penetrating chest trauma.[20] Vascular access is most often obtained at the common femoral artery, although the brachial or radial approaches are also useful. A pigtail catheter is advanced into the ascending aorta and positioned proximal to the brachiocephalic trunk. Using a power injector, radiographic contrast material is injected at 15 to 20 ml/sec for a total of 40 ml to 60 ml. The LAO projection (30° to 60°) separates the ascending from the descending aorta and allows good visualization of the origin of the great vessels (see Fig. 13-14).

The brachiocephalic trunk, left common carotid, and subclavian arteries originate in the transverse thoracic aorta. The brachiocephalic trunk or innominate artery divides into the right common carotid artery and the right subclavian artery. The common carotid arteries run lateral to the vertebral bodies and bifurcate into the external and the internal carotid arteries at about the level of the fourth cervical vertebra (Fig. 13-16). In its extracranial portion, the internal carotid artery has no branches. On entering the skull, the internal carotid artery makes a sharp turn at the carotid siphon, and thereafter, divides into the anterior (ACA) and middle (MCA) cerebral arteries, which with the anterior communicating artery form the anterior portion of the circle of Willis (Fig. 13-17).

CAROTID ANGIOGRAPHY

Selective carotid angiography is usually performed after obtaining an aortic arch aortogram in the LAO view, which allows the operator to visualize the origin of the brachiocephalic trunk and left common carotid artery. Using that same LAO angle, the brachiocephalic trunk is engaged with either angled or Shepherd's crook catheters (Fig. 13-18).

Once the origin of the common carotid artery has been engaged, the catheter is advanced into the common carotid artery over an atraumatic 0.035-inch guidewire. Care must be taken to clear the catheters and manifold of air and debris before injecting into the carotid artery. Carotid angiograms are obtained in the anteroposterior, oblique, and lateral views.

Because of the dense bony structure of the skull, it is necessary to use digital subtraction techniques to obtain diagnostic images of the intracranial vascular anatomy. A 12-inch or larger image intensifier is ideal for intracranial angiography, but image intensifiers from 9 to 16 inches are acceptable. It is important to emphasize the importance of using DSA for the intracranial portion of the internal carotid artery and its branches in the anteroposterior

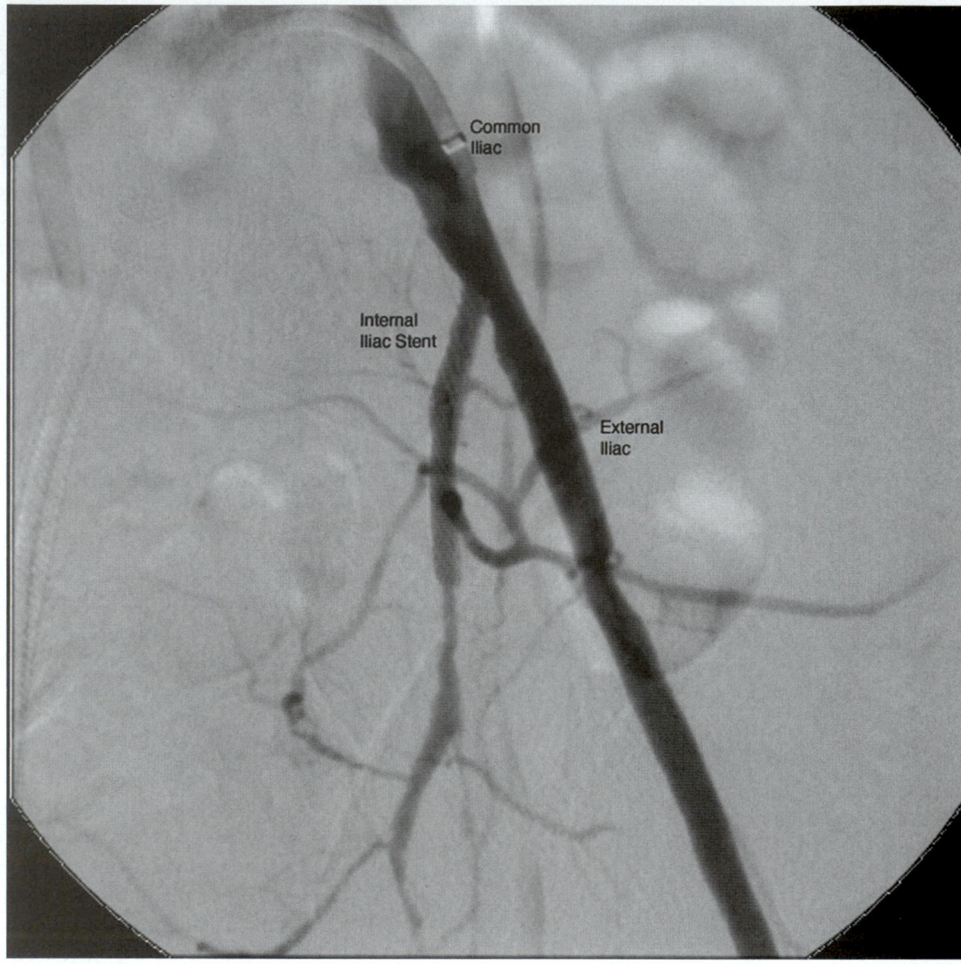

FIGURE 13-13. Selective left common iliac angiography (20° LAO and 20° caudal view) demonstrating the origin of the internal iliac artery (ostial stent present) and the external iliac artery. LAO, left anterior oblique.

and lateral views. This enables an assessment of the circle of Willis and demonstrates the presence of any collateral circulation.

SUBCLAVIAN ANGIOGRAPHY

Important branches of the subclavian artery include the vertebral (superior) and internal mammary (inferior) arteries (Fig. 13-19). The vertebral artery, the first branch and usually the largest branch of the subclavian artery, arises from the superior and posterior surface of the subclavian. The right or left subclavian arteries are selectively engaged with a 4- to 6-Fr angiographic catheter. The AP view usually discloses the area of stenosis often located in the proximal subclavian artery (the left subclavian artery is affected three to four times as frequently as the right subclavian artery.)[21] In patients with a tortuous proximal left subclavian artery, a steep RAO view with caudal angulation may help to show a proximal stenosis. If the proximal portion of the right subclavian artery is suspected as having a lesion, the AP view may not show the stenosis because of overlap with the origin of the right common carotid artery. A steep RAO caudal view (40° to 60° RAO and 15° to 20° caudal), will usually separate the ostium of these two vessels (Fig. 13-20).

VERTEBRAL ANGIOGRAPHY

The vertebral arteries are identified on the aortic arch aortogram. Often a nonselective injection of contrast in the subclavian artery near the origin of the vertebral artery is performed to view ostial lesions.[22] Cranial angulation (30° to 40°), with shallow oblique views (RAO or LAO), may be necessary to view the origin (see Fig. 13-19). Selective angiography is performed with a 4- to 6-Fr angled catheter (Judkins right coronary, Berenstein, Cobra, or internal mammary artery catheter).

The vertebral artery runs cranially through the foramina of the transverse processes of the other cervical vertebrae to the inferior surface of the skull (Fig. 13-21). After penetrating the foramen of the atlas, it enters the cranial cavity through the foramen magnum. The first branch of the vertebral artery is the posterior inferior cerebellar artery (PICA). The final segment of the vertebral artery then joins with the contralateral vertebral artery to form the basilar artery (Fig. 13-22).

Selective angiography is performed with hand injections, using a coronary manifold with pressure monitoring, analogous to selective coronary angiography. Anteroposterior and lateral views of the extracranial and intracranial course of the vertebral and basilar arteries should be performed with a DSA technique. Similar to

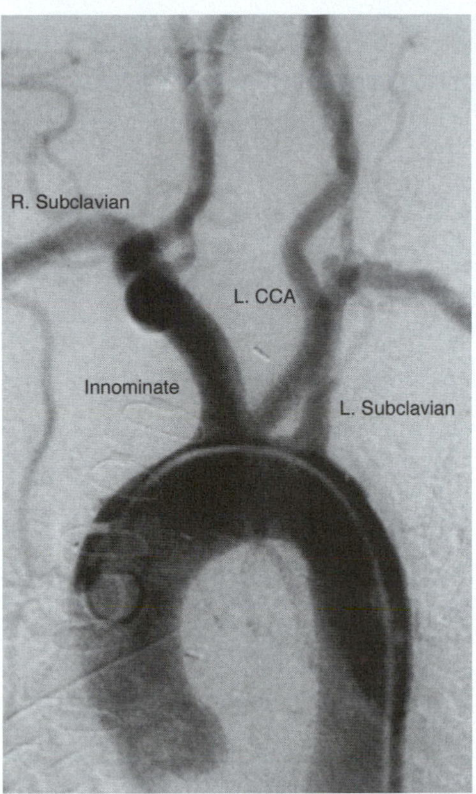

FIGURE 13-14. Aortic arch and brachiocephalic vessels. Digital subtraction angiogram injection of 15 ml per second of contrast material for 3 seconds with image obtained at 30° LAO. CCA, common carotid artery; LAO, left anterior oblique.

views of the anterior cerebral circulation, it is important to image the posterior circulation that contributes to the circle of Willis.

COMPLICATIONS OF PERIPHERAL VASCULAR ANGIOGRAPHY

Complications of peripheral vascular angiography, as with cardiac catheterization, may lead to significant morbidity or even mortality.[8,9,23] Complications may be thought of in three categories: (1) access site related; (2) systemic; or (3) catheter induced.[24] The best strategy to minimize these complications is to anticipate and avoid them.

Access Site Related

Vascular-access-related complications include hematoma formation, retroperitoneal hemorrhage, pseudoaneurysm formation, arteriovenous fistula creation, and infection. Access site bleeding is the most frequent complication following femoral arterial access. The management of access site bleeding depends on the severity and hemodynamic consequences of bleeding. In general, access site bleeding may be controlled by manual or mechanical compression and reversal of anticoagulation. If bleeding continues despite these steps, more aggressive therapies—including percutaneous intervention or surgical therapy—may be considered.[25]

The signs and symptoms of retroperitoneal bleeding include hypotension, abdominal distention or fullness, and pain.[26,27] The diagnosis of retroperitoneal bleeding may be confirmed by computed tomography (CT) or abdominal/ pelvic ultrasound. If retroperitoneal bleeding is suspected, anticoagulation should be reversed and discontinued. Volume resuscitation with crystalloid solutions and/or blood products should be administered if volume depletion is clinically evident. Alternatively, if bleeding causes hemodynamic embarrassment, emergency angiography from the contralateral femoral access site may be performed to find the bleeding site. Once the bleeding site has been identified, tamponade of bleeding with balloon occlusion will stabilize the patient. If prolonged balloon inflation is not effective in stopping the blood loss, consideration may be given to placing a covered stent (Wallgraft, BSC, Watertown, MA) to seal the leak. Open surgical repair may also be considered.[25,28]

A pseudoaneurysm occurs when a hematoma continues to communicate with the arterial lumen. Low arterial access (superficial femoral artery or profunda femoris artery entry) has been associated with pseudoaneurysm formation.[29] Other risk factors include female sex, age greater than 70 years, diabetes mellitus, and obesity.

Patients with pseudoaneurysms often present with pain at the access site several days following the intervention. On physical examination, a pulsatile hematoma may be present with a systolic bruit. Management of a femoral pseudoaneurysm is dependent on its size, severity of symptoms, and need for continued anticoagulation. A small pseudoaneurysm (≤2 cm) may be observed and often will resolve spontaneously. Larger pseudoaneurysms may be treated with ultrasound-guided compression, percutaneous thrombin injection, endovascular coil insertion, or with covered stents. Surgical repair of pseudoaneurysms is usually reserved for the failure of less invasive approaches.[25,28,30]

An arteriovenous fistula (AVF) complicates vascular access when the needle punctures the femoral artery and the overlying vein, creating a fistulous communication when the sheath is removed. The risk of creating an AVF is increased by either a high or low femoral puncture, multiple puncture attempts, or prolonged clotting times. Fistulae may not be clinically evident for several days following the procedure. Clinically, an AVF is characterized by a continuous to-and-fro murmur over the access site. In some cases, there may be a swollen and tender extremity due to venous dilation, and in severe circumstances arterial insufficiency (steal syndrome) may occur. The diagnosis of a suspected AVF may be confirmed by color flow Doppler ultrasound.

Most AVFs following femoral access are small, not hemodynamically significant, and close spontaneously. Symptomatic AVFs require closure to prevent increased shunting and distal swelling and tenderness.[30] Surgical repair, the traditional therapy for closure of catheterization-related AVFs, when necessary, has been displaced by percutaneous methods. Once again, surgical correction is reserved for those patients who fail a less invasive approach.

Vascular access closure devices are designed to facilitate hemostasis and to reduce the time to ambulation and to decrease hospital length of stay. All of the currently

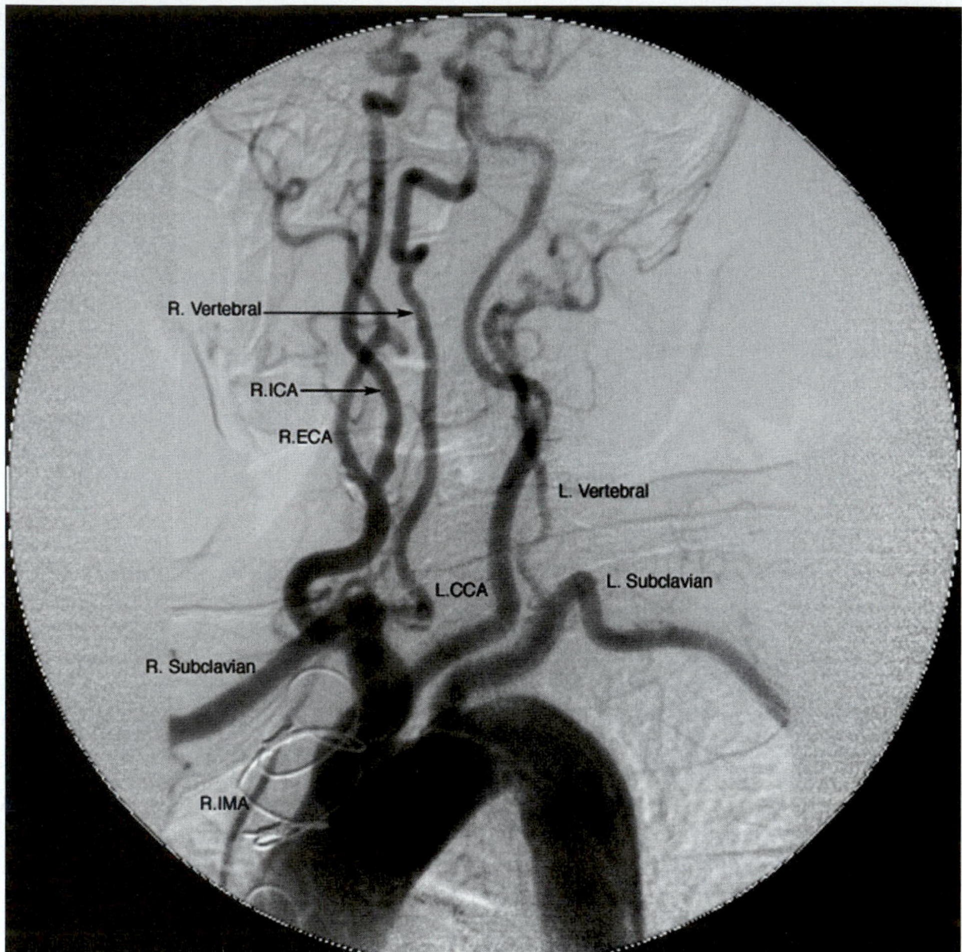

FIGURE 13-15. Bovine aortic arch angiogram injection of 15 ml of contrast per second for 3 seconds (total 45 ml contrast) at 45° LAO. LAO, left anterior oblique; L.CCA, left common carotid artery; R.ECA, right external carotid artery; R.ICA, right internal carotid artery; R.IMA, right internal mammary artery.

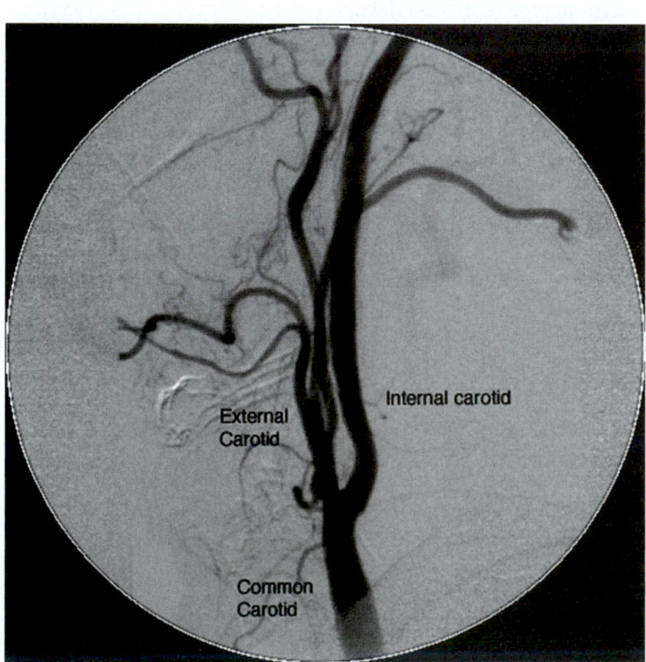

FIGURE 13-16. Common carotid bifurcation. External carotid artery is marked by the presence of branch vessels.

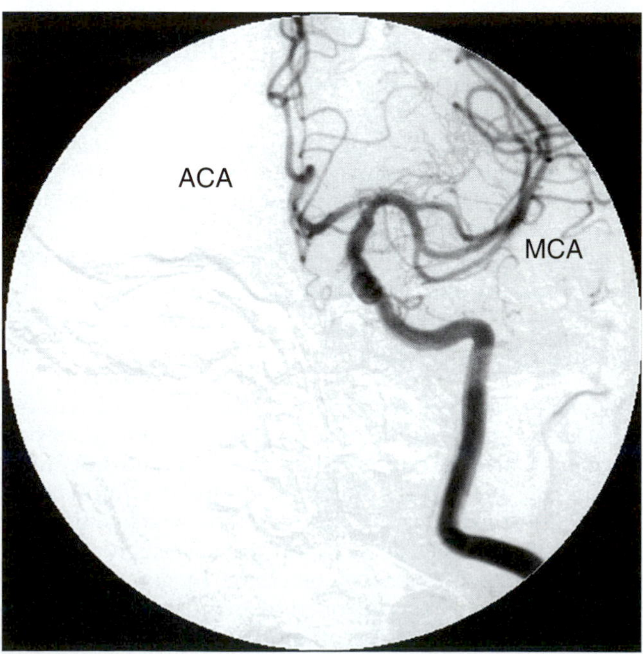

FIGURE 13-17. Intracranial carotid arteries (AP view). The internal carotid artery branches into the middle cerebral artery (MCA) and anterior cerebral artery (ACA). AP, anteroposterior.

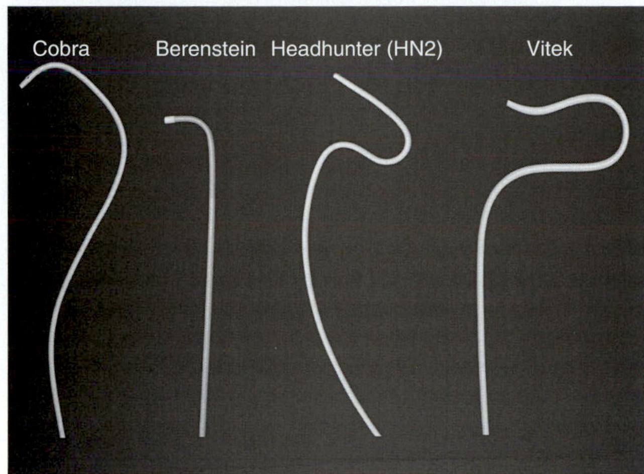

FIGURE 13-18. Commonly used brachiocephalic and carotid angiographic catheters.

FDA-approved devices in the United States have shown favorable results. However, these devices are prone to specific complications and have not been demonstrated to reduce access site complications.[31]

Systemic Complications

Systemic complications relate to allergic and anaphylactoid reactions, as well as nephrotoxicity caused by iodinated contrast agents. Allergic or anaphylactoid reactions occur in fewer than 3% of cases, and fewer than 1% require hospitalization.[32]

Nonoliguric creatinine elevation peaking within 1 to 2 days and returning to baseline by 7 days is the usual clinical scenario of contrast nephrotoxicity. Patients at risk for contrast-induced nephropathy are those with baseline chronic renal insufficiency, diabetes mellitus, multiple myeloma, and those who are receiving other nephrotoxic drugs, such as aminoglycosides. All patients in general, but those at risk to develop contrast-induced nephropathy in particular, should be well hydrated before and after the procedure, and the amount of contrast volume must be minimized. A recently published randomized trial has suggested that in patients with renal insufficiency, the use of Iodopaque (iso-osmolar, nonionic) is less nephrotoxic than Omnipaque (low-osmolar, nonionic) contrast.[33] *N*-Acetylcysteine (Mucomyst) has been shown to protect against contrast nephropathy in a randomized controlled trial in patients with renal insufficiency.[34]

Diuretics do not protect against contrast-induced nephrotoxicity.[35] Hydration with half-normal saline for 12 hours before and after the procedure provides better protection against creatinine rise than does the

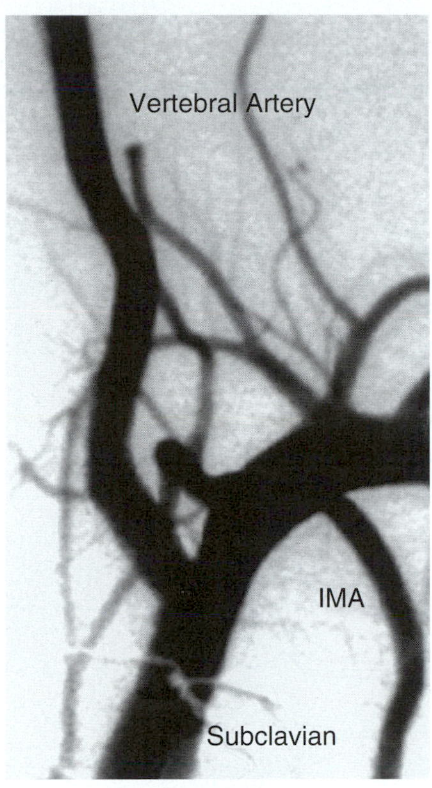

FIGURE 13-19. Left subclavian angiogram showing the vertebral artery arising superiorly and the internal mammary artery (IMA) arising inferiorly.

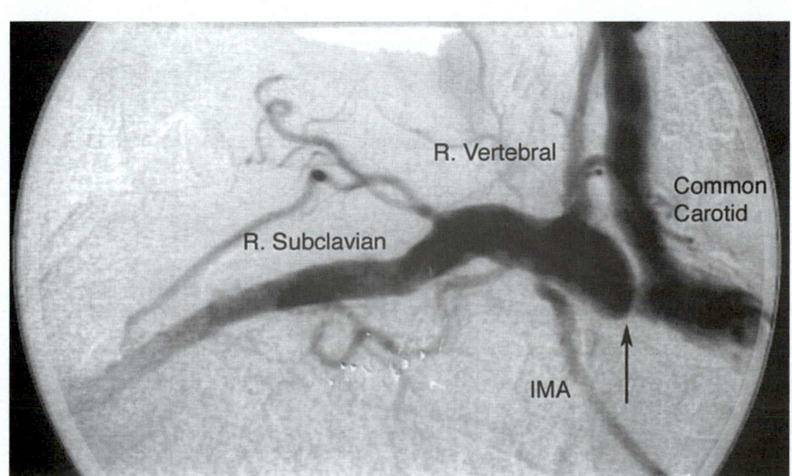

FIGURE 13-20. Proximal right subclavian stenosis (*arrow*), seen best at 40° RAO and 20° of caudal angulation. IMA, interior mammary artery; RAO, right anterior oblique.

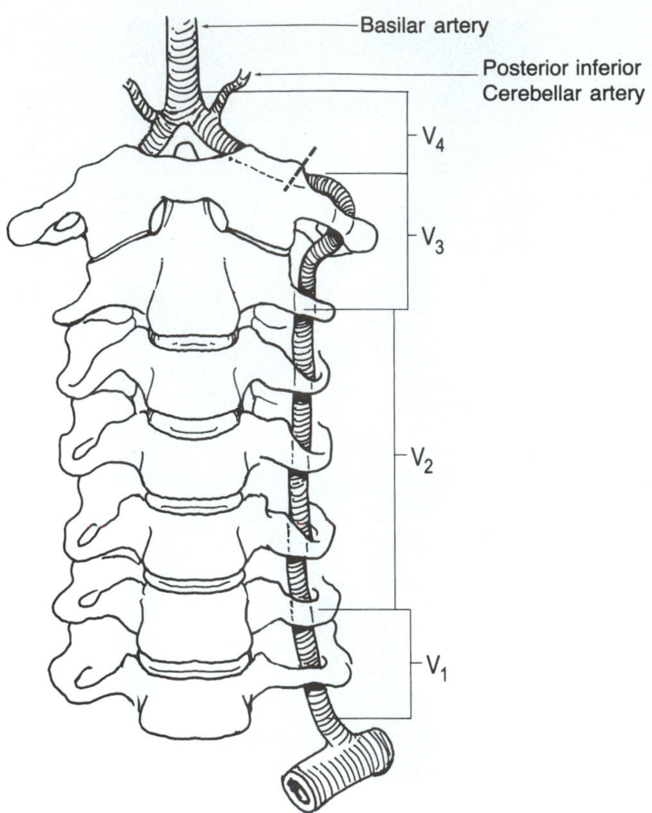

FIGURE 13-21. Drawing of the vertebral artery, divided into four anatomic segments, coursing through the cervical spine foramina.

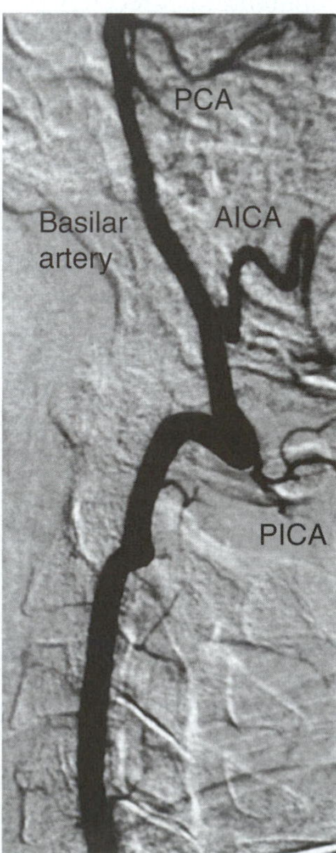

FIGURE 13-22. Proximal vertebral artery segment visualized with subclavian angiography. AICA, anterior inferior cerebellar artery; PCA, posterior cerebral artery; PICA, posterior inferior cerebellar artery.

combination of hydration and diuretics.[36] Two prospective trials have demonstrated that mannitol does not reduce contrast nephropathy.[37,38]

Catheter Related Complications

When the aorta or brachiocephalic vessels are manipulated during a thoracic aortogram, stroke is a rare but potentially devastating complication.[8,39,40] In general, asymptomatic patients have a lower risk, whereas patients who undergo angiography in the setting of transient ischemic events have a slightly higher complication rate. Patients who develop a neurologic complication should have an immediate neurologic assessment, and an emergency CT scan should be obtained. In the presence of intracerebral hemorrhage, anticoagulants and antiplatelet agents should be reversed. If an embolic stroke has occurred, one option is to perform catheter-directed thrombolysis and/or angioplasty.

Atheroembolism is another cause of renal insufficiency following angiography. Unlike contrast-induced nephropathy, renal dysfunction after atheroembolization usually develops slowly (weeks to months) and some of these patients progress to renal failure. The diagnosis is confirmed by tissue examination (biopsy) and treatment is supportive. Systemic manifestations of atheroembolism include livedo reticularis, abdominal or foot pain, and purple toes associated with systemic eosinophilia (blue toe syndrome).[41]

REFERENCES

1. Krouwels M, Overbach E, Guit G: Iohexol versus ioxaglate in lower extremity angiography: A comparative randomized double-blind study in 80 patients. Eur J Radiol 22:133, 1996.
2. Spinosa D, Angle J, Hagspiel K, et al: Feasibility of gadodiamide compared with dilute iodinated contrast material for imaging of the abdominal aorta and renal arteries. J Vasc Interv Radiol 11:733, 2000.
3. Diaz L, Pabon I, Garcia J, et al: Assessment of CO_2 arteriography in arterial occlusive disease of the lower extremities. J Vasc Interv Radiol 11:163, 2000.
4. Hawkins IF: Carbon dioxide digital subtraction arteriography. Am J Roentgenol 139:19, 1982.
5. Kerns S, Hawkins I: Carbon dioxide digital subtraction angiography: Expanding applications and technical evolution. Am J Radiol 164:735, 1995.
6. Caridi J, Hawkins I: CO_2 digital subtraction angiography: Potential complications and their prevention. J Vasc Interv Radiol 8:383, 1997.
7. Kaufman J, Geller S, Waltman A: Renal insufficiency: Gadopentetate dimeglumine as a radiographic contrast agent during peripheral vascular interventional procedures. Radiology 198:383, 1996.
8. Armstrong P, Han D, Baxter J, et al: Complication rates of percutaneous brachial artery access in peripheral vascular angiography. Ann Vasc Surg 17:107, 2003.
9. McIvor J, Rhymer J: 245 Transaxillary arteriograms in arteriopathic patients: Success rate and complications. Clin Radiol 45:390, 1992.
10. Greenfield A: Femoral, popliteal and tibial arteries: Percutaneous transluminal angioplasty. Am J Roentgenol 135:927, 1980.
11. Lechner G, Jantsch H, Waneck R, et al: The relationship between the common femoral artery, the inguinal crease, and the inguinal ligament; a guide to accurate angiographic puncture. Cardiovasc Intervent Radiol 11:165, 1988.
12. Dotter CT, Judkins MP: Transluminal treatment of arteriosclerotic obstruction: Description of a new technic and a preliminary report of its application. Circulation 30:654, 1964.

13. Spijkerboer A, Scholten F, Mali W, et al: Antegrade puncture of the femoral artery: Morphologic study. Radiology 176:57, 1990.
14. Bouhoutsos J, Morris T: Femoral artery complications after diagnostic procedures. Br Med J 3:396, 1973.
15. Hessel S, Adams D, Abrams H: Complications of angiography. Radiology 138:273, 1981.
16. Altin R, Flicker S, Naidech H: Pseudoaneurysm and arteriovenous fistula after femoral artery catheterization: Association with low femoral punctures. Am J Roentgenol 152:629, 1989.
17. Rapoport S, Sniderman K, Morse S, et al: Pseudoaneurysm: A complication of faulty technique in femoral arterial puncture. Radiology 154:529, 1985.
18. Beales J, Adcock F, Frawley J, et al: The radiological assessment of disease of the profunda femoris artery. Br J Radiol 44:854, 1971.
19. Kadir S: Regional anatomy of the thoracic aorta. In Kadir S (ed): Atlas of Normal and Variant Angiographic Anatomy. Philadelphia, WB Saunders, 1991, p 19.
20. Schainfield R, Jaff M: Angiography of the aorta and peripheral arteries. In Baim D, Grossman W (eds): Grossman's Cardiac Catheterization, Angiography and Intervention. Philadelphia, Lippincott Williams & Wilkins, 2000, p 293.
21. Zelenock GB, Cronenwett JL, Graham LM, et al: Brachiocephalic arterial occlusions and stenoses. Manifestations and management of complex lesions. Arch Surg 120:370, 1985.
22. Courtheoux P, Tournade A, Theron J, et al: Transcutaneous angioplasty of vertebral artery atheromatous ostial stricture. Neuroradiology 27:259, 1985.
23. AbuRahma A, Robinson P, Boland J, et al: Complications of arteriography in a recent series of 707 cases: Factors affecting outcome. Ann Vasc Surg 7:122, 1993.
24. Singh H, Cardella J, Cole P, et al: Quality improvement guidelines for diagnostic arteriography. J Vasc Interv Radiol 13:1, 2002.
25. Samal AK, White CJ: Percutaneous management of access site complications. Catheter Cardiovasc Interv 57:12, 2002.
26. Sreeram S, Lumsden A, Miller J, et al: Retroperitoneal hematoma following femoral arterial catheterization: A serious and often fatal complication. Am J Surg 59:94, 1993.
27. Kent K, Moscucci M, Mansour K, et al: Retroperitoneal hematoma after cardiac catheterization: Prevalence, risk factors, and optimal management. J Vasc Surg 20:905, 1994.
28. Kazmers A, Meeker C, Nofz K, et al: Nonoperative therapy for post-catheterization femoral artery pseudoaneurysms. Am J Surg 63:199, 1997.
29. Kim D, Orron D, Skillman J, et al: Role of superficial femoral artery puncture in the development of pseudoaneurysm and arteriovenous fistula complicating percutaneous transfemoral cardiac catheterization. Cath Cardiovasc Diagn 25:91, 1992.
30. Waigand J, Uhlich F, Gross C, et al: Percutaneous treatment of pseudoaneurysms and arteriovenous fistulas after invasive vascular procedures. Cathet Cardiovasc Intervent 47:157, 1999.
31. Toursarkissian B, Mejia A, Smilanich R, et al: Changing patterns of access site complications with the use of percutaneous closure devices. Vasc Surg 35:203, 2001.
32. Bettmann MA, Heeren T, Greenfield A, et al: Adverse events with radiographic contrast agents: Results of the SCVIR Contrast Agent Registry. Radiology 203:611, 1997.
33. Aspelin P, Aubry P, Fransson S, et al: Nephrotoxic effects in high-risk patients undergoing angiography. N Eng J Med 348:491, 2003.
34. Chow W, Chan T, Lo S, et al: Acetylcysteine for prevention of acute deterioration of renal function following elective coronary angiography and intervention: A randomized controlled trial. JAMA 289:553, 2003.
35. Weinstein J, Heyman S, Brevis M: Potential deleterious effects of furosemide in radiocontrast nephropathy. Nephron 62:413, 1992.
36. Solomon R, Werner C, Mann D, et al: Effects of saline, mannitol and furosemide on acute decreases in renal function induced by radiocontrast agents. N Eng J Med 331:1416, 1994.
37. Stevens M, McCullough P, Tobin K, et al: A prospective randomized trial of prevention measures in patients at high risk for contrast nephropathy. J Am Coll Cardiol 33:403, 1999.
38. Rudnick M, Goldfarb S, Wexler L, et al: Nephrotoxicity of ionic and nonionic contrast media in 1196 patients: A randomized trial. Kidney Int 47:254, 1995.
39. Willinsky R, Taylor S, Terbrugge K, et al: Neurologic complications of cerebral angiography: Prospective analysis of 2,899 procedures and review of the literature. Radiology 227:522, 2003.
40. Fayed A, White C, Ramee S, et al: Carotid and cerebral angiography performed by cardiologists: Cerebrovascular complications. Cathet Cardiovasc Intervent 55:277, 2002.
41. Rosman H, Davis T, Reddy D, et al: Cholesterol embolization: Clinical findings and implications. J Am Coll Cardiol 15:1296, 1990.

chapter 14

The Epidemiology of Peripheral Arterial Disease

Michael H. Criqui
John Ninomiya

Peripheral arterial disease (PAD) is generally defined as partial or complete obstruction of one or more peripheral arteries caused by atherosclerosis. Although the term PAD is sometimes inclusive of all peripheral arteries, in this chapter PAD refers to atherosclerotic occlusive disease of the lower extremities. PAD is associated with many of the same risk factors as atherosclerotic cardiovascular and cerebrovascular diseases, and is very common among the elderly. PAD that exhibits typical symptomatology, usually in the form of leg pain brought about by walking, has been conservatively estimated to reduce quality of life in at least 2 million Americans, and in some cases leads to a need for surgical revascularization or amputation.[1] Many millions more have measurable asymptomatic disease, or disease with atypical symptoms. Both symptomatic and asymptomatic PAD have been shown to be associated with a sharply elevated risk of mortality due to coronary and cerebrovascular disease.

SYMPTOMS AND MEASURES OF PAD IN EPIDEMIOLOGY

It was recognized as long ago as the 18th century that an insufficient blood supply to the legs could cause pain and dysfunction in the same way that deficient coronary circulation could lead to angina. This type of pain is known as intermittent claudication and is characterized as leg pain or discomfort that is associated with walking and relieved by rest. Intermittent claudication is generally indicative of exercise-induced ischemic pain caused by PAD.

Early studies of PAD focused primarily on claudication as the chief symptomatic manifestation of PAD. A number of patient questionnaires have been developed to uniformly identify claudication and to distinguish it from other types of leg pain. The first of these was the Rose questionnaire, also referred to as the World Health Organization questionnaire.[2] The San Diego Claudication Questionnaire is a modification of the Rose questionnaire that additionally captures information on the laterality of symptoms.[3] The interviewer-administered form of the San Diego Claudication Questionnaire appears in Table 14-1.

Ankle-Brachial Index

Although intermittent claudication is an important manifestation of PAD, it is not pathognomonic. Atherosclerosis may have been developing for many years before claudication begins, and the extent to which it occurs is influenced by factors other than disease per se, such as the patient's level of activity.[4] Furthermore, the definitional distinctions used to separate claudication from other leg pain make claudication more specific to arterial disease, but less sensitive to other types of pain that may in some cases be related to arterial disease. Spinal stenosis can cause leg pain during exercise that is similar to claudication. For these reasons, another method of diagnosing PAD was needed.

Low blood pressure at the ankle was proposed as a test for PAD as early as 1950[5] and led to the development of a simple measure called the ankle-brachial index (ABI). The ABI is the ratio of the systolic blood pressure at the ankle to that in the arm. An abnormally low value of ABI is indicative of atherosclerosis of the lower extremities. The ABI has been shown to have good receiver operating curve characteristics as a test for PAD. Although there is no definitive cut point above which disease is always absent and below which disease is always present, an ABI of less than or equal to 0.9 is commonly used in both clinical practice and epidemiologic research to diagnose PAD. The ABI is also sometimes referred to as the ankle-brachial pressure index (ABPI)[6] and the ankle-arm index (AAI).[7]

As a test for ABI-based PAD, claudication has been shown to have very high specificity but very low sensitivity. For example, in the Rotterdam Study, 99.4% of subjects with ABI equal to or greater than 0.9 did not have claudication; but only 6.3% of subjects with ABI of less than 0.9 had claudication.[8] In a study of elderly women in the United States, the percentages were 93.3% and 18.3%, respectively.[4] Based on this, PAD based on ABI criteria is much more common than claudication in the general population, and large numbers of patients without claudication can be shown to have asymptomatic PAD based on ABI.

To validate the ABI and the huge burden of previously unrecognized asymptomatic disease that it implied, early studies compared the ABI-based diagnosis with

TABLE 14-1 SAN DIEGO CLAUDICATION QUESTIONNAIRE*

		Right	Left
1. Do you get pain or discomfort in either leg or either buttock on walking?	No...........	1	1
(If no, stop)	Yes..........	2	2
2. Does this pain ever begin when you are standing still or sitting?	No...........	1	1
	Yes..........	2	2
3. In what part of the leg or buttock do you feel it?			
a. Pain includes calf/calves	No...........	1	1
	Yes..........	2	2
b. Pain includes thigh/thighs	No...........	1	1
	Yes..........	2	2
c. Pain includes buttock/buttocks	No...........	1	1
	Yes..........	2	2
4. Do you get it when you walk uphill or hurry?	No...........	1	1
	Yes..........	2	2
	Never walks uphill/hurries....	3	3
5. Do you get it when you walk at an ordinary pace on level ground?	No...........	1	1
	Yes..........	2	2
6. Does the pain ever disappear while you are walking?	No...........	1	1
	Yes..........	2	2
7. What do you do if you get it when you are walking?	Stop or slow down.............	1	1
	Continue on.................	2	2
8. What happens to it if you stand still?	Lessened or relieved..........	1	1
(if unchanged, stop)	Unchanged......	2	2
9. How soon?	10 minutes or less...........	1	1
	More than 10 minutes.......	2	2

*Interviewer administered version.
1. **No Pain**—1 = 1
2. **Pain at rest**—1 = 2 and 2 = 2
3. **Non-calf**—1 = 2 and 2 = 1 and 3a = 1 and 3b = 2 or 3c = 2
4. **Non-Rose calf**—1 = 2 and 2 = 1 and 3a = 2, and not Rose
5. **Rose**—1 = 2 and 2 = 1 and 3a = 2 and 4 = 2 or 3 (and if 4 = 3, then 5 = 2), and 6 = 1 and 7 = 1 and 8 = 1 and 9 = 1

angiography, which was considered the "gold standard" for the visualization of atherosclerosis in the legs. Two such studies are often cited, in which the sensitivity and specificity of the ABI were shown to be in the 97% to 100% range.[9,10] However, because angiography presents some risk to patients, it was not ethical to perform angiography on patients who were not suspected to have PAD. Therefore, these studies involved comparisons of patients with angiographically confirmed PAD with young, healthy patients assumed not to have PAD. The sensitivities and specificities calculated are therefore based on the ability of the ABI to discriminate between extremes of disease and wellness. If measured among patients seen in routine clinical practice or the population in general, the specificity of the ABI remains in the 97%+ range, but the sensitivity is somewhat less, in part due to some PAD patients with stiff peripheral arteries and false-negative ABIs.[11,12]

The ABI has been demonstrated to have strong associations with cardiovascular disease (CVD) risk factors and disease outcomes. In the Cardiovascular Health Study cohort, a dose-response relationship was demonstrated between ABI and cardiovascular disease risk factors, as well as both clinical and subclinical cardiovascular disease.[13] In a study in Edinburgh, asymptomatic patients with an ABI of less than 0.9 were shown to have a higher risk of developing claudication and higher mortality.[14] In a clinical study, patients with an ABI of less than 0.9 who did not have exertional leg pain were shown to have poorer lower extremity functioning, even after adjustment for traditional risk factors and comorbidities.[15] The ABI correlates with the ability to exercise as measured on an accelerometer[16] and an ABI of less than 0.6 is related to the development of walking impairment.[17] Thus, even aside from its association with claudication, the ABI is related to the types of functional outcomes, risk factors, and associated diseases that one would expect of a measure of PAD. The ABI has also been shown to have high intra- and inter-rater reliability.[18]

In practice, the ABI is measured using a blood pressure cuff, a standard sphygmomanometer, and Doppler instrument to detect pulses. The pressure measurements are made with the patient at rest in a supine position for 5 minutes prior to measurement. The ankle pressure is measured in both legs at the dorsalis pedis and posterior tibial arteries. The higher pressure measurement in each ankle has traditionally been used as the numerator of the ABI for that ankle. Using the lower or average pressure can substantially change estimates of PAD prevalence; one study reported 47% prevalence based on the higher pressure versus 59% based on the lower.[16] Results of two recent studies support the use of the average of dorsalis pedis and posterior tibial pressures as the ankle pressure for each leg, based on superior reproducibility in repeated tests and closer statistical association with leg function.[16,19] However, the relative predictive value of the higher versus the average (or perhaps the lower) of the two ankle pressures for CVD risk factors or clinical events has not yet been evaluated. Practice also differs as to the brachial pressure used as the denominator of the ABI; the same brachial pressure is usually used for both the left and right ABIs in the same patient, but that pressure may be the right arm, the average of both arms, or the highest of both arms. A recent study supports the use of the average of the left and right arms, based on superior reproducibility,[19] but another study shows a strong correlation between PAD and subclavian stenosis, suggesting the highest arm pressure should be used in the ABI calculation.[20] Based on the numerators and denominators described, separate ABIs are calculated for the left and right legs of each subject. In epidemiologic analyses, the unit of analysis is either the leg, with appropriate statistical adjustments for intrasubject correlation; or the subject, with disease status classified based on the "worst" limb; i.e., the limb with the lowest ABI.

The ABI has several limitations as a measure of PAD. Occlusive disease distal to the ankle is not detected by the ABI; other measures, such as pressure ratios using pressures measured in the toe, are required for detecting such distal disease. The ABI is also sensitive to the height of the patient, with taller patients having slightly higher ABIs; it is unlikely these differences are related to real differences in PAD.[21,22] Similarly, it has been noted in several studies that the ABI of the left leg tends to be slightly lower on average than the ABI of the right leg.[21,22]

Arterial calcification (medial calcinosis) can make the arteries of the ankle incompressible, and lead to artificially high values of the ABI. This is particularly common in patients with diabetes.[23,24] Values of the ABI above 1.5 are often excluded in epidemiologic analyses, and should be viewed with suspicion clinically.[4,13,25-27] In two large population-based studies in the United States, the proportion of patients with such elevated values was around one half of 1%.[13,27] Some investigators use the more conservative cut point of 1.3. New evidence suggests 1.4 may be a good compromise.[28]

INCIDENCE AND PREVALENCE OF PAD

Although uncommon among younger people, the prevalence of PAD rises sharply with age to include a substantial proportion of the elderly population. Figure 14-1 shows some ABI-based estimates of PAD prevalence by age from six large studies.[8,11,13,29-31] In four of the studies, the standard ABI of less than 0.9 criterion was used; in the Limburg Study, PAD was diagnosed based on two ABI measurements of less than 0.95,[30] whereas in the Rancho Bernardo Study, a combination of a conservative ABI cut point of 0.8 and other noninvasive tests was used.[11] Although the estimates vary, prevalence appears to be well under 5% before age 50, around 10% by age 65,

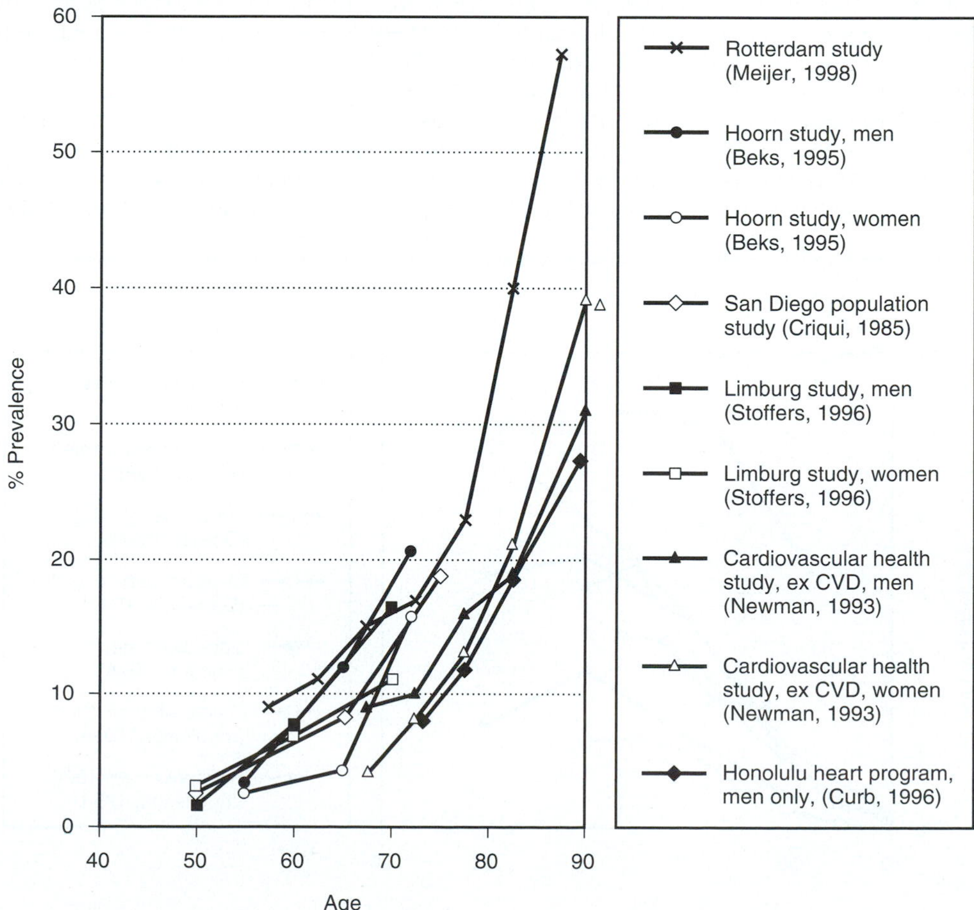

FIGURE 14-1. PAD prevalence: Estimates based on ankle-brachial index from six large studies.

and in excess of 25% in patients 80 years of age or older. All studies show this stronger-than-linear relationship of prevalence to age, although there is some variability in the age at which prevalence begins to increase most dramatically.

Estimates of PAD incidence are reported somewhat less frequently in the literature, with more data based on claudication incidence than on ABI. With respect to claudication, data from the Framingham Study show claudication in men rising from less than 0.4 per 1000 per year in men aged 35 to 45 years to more than 6 per 1000 per year in men aged 65 years and older.[32] Incidence among women ranged from 40% to 60% lower by age, although estimates in men and women were similar by age 65 to 74. In a group of Israeli men, the incidence of claudication ranged from 6.3 per 1000 per year at ages 40 to 49 to 10.5 per 1000 at age 60 and greater.[1] In a study of 4570 men from Quebec, claudication incidence rose from 0.7 per 1000 per year at ages 35 to 44, to 3 per 1000 per year at ages 45 to 54, 7 per 1000 per year at ages 55 to 63, and 9 per 1000 at age 65 and greater.[33] In the Speedwell Study, which followed English men aged 45 to 63 years for 10 years, claudication incidence per 1000 per year ranged from 3.1 in the youngest to 4.9 in oldest age group based on age at baseline examination.[34] A higher incidence of 15.5 per 1000 per year was reported among men and women aged 55 to 74 in the Edinburgh Artery Study; however, this study did not apply strict Rose criteria for probable claudication.[35]

In the Reykjavik Study, Ingolfsson and colleagues used Poisson regression techniques to conclude that intermittent claudication rates among Icelandic men dropped significantly between 1968 and 1986; among 50-year-old men, their estimate of the rate of claudication dropped from 1.7 per 1000 per year in 1970 to 0.6 per 1000 per year in 1984, whereas in 70-year olds, the rate of claudication dropped from 6.0 to 2.0.[36] The authors attributed this to decreased smoking and cholesterol levels. The design and duration of this study were uniquely suited to the estimation of long-term trends in disease incidence; comparable studies for other populations are not available. The potential for trends of this magnitude should be considered in reviewing the results of other studies. Figure 14-2 shows incidence rates by age for various studies identifying PAD based on claudication.[1,32-34,36]

There are very few ABI-based studies of PAD incidence, given the time and resources required to periodically retest study subjects for incident disease. In the Limburg PAOD Study, incidence rates for PAD were based on two ABI measurements of less than 0.95. Among men, annual incidence was 1.7 per 1000 at ages 40 to 54; 1.5 per 1000 at ages 55 to 64; and 17.8 per 1000 at ages 65 and greater. Annual incidence in women was higher: 5.9, 9.1, and 22.9 per 1000, respectively, for the same age groups.[37]

Sex differences in the incidence and prevalence of PAD are less clear than those in other cardiovascular disease. Claudication incidence and prevalence have usually been found to be higher in men than in women. For example, in the Framingham Study, annual claudication incidence for all ages combined was 7.1 per 1000 in men versus 3.6 per 1000 in women, for a male to female ratio of 1.97.[32] In the Framingham Offspring Study, claudication prevalence was 1.9% in men versus 0.8% in women (ratio = 2.38), whereas in the Rotterdam Study it was 2.2% in men versus 1.2% in women (ratio = 1.83).[8,27] However, the Edinburgh Artery Study and the Limburg PAOD Study found relatively low male to female ratios of claudication prevalence of 1.11 and 1.2, respectively.[21,30]

The case for an excess of disease among males is even weaker for PAD diagnosed based on ABI. This is true even in those studies finding a clear male excess with respect to claudication. For example, in the Framingham Offspring Study mentioned earlier, PAD based on ABI

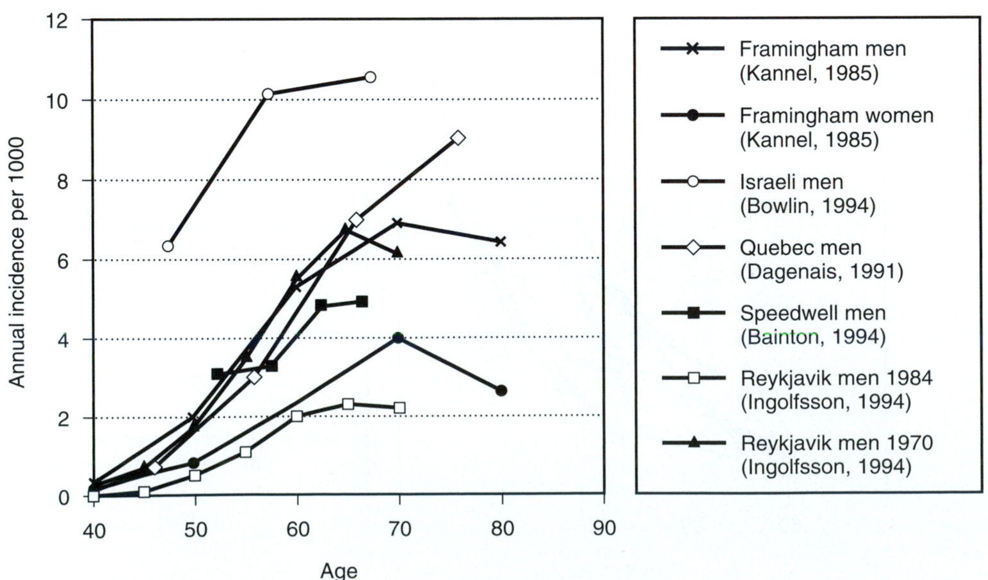

FIGURE 14-2. PAD incidence: Estimates based on claudication from five large studies.

was found in 3.9% of men and 3.3% of women, for a ratio of 1.18.[27] In the Rotterdam Study, ABI-based PAD was actually lower in men than in women, with prevalences of 16.9% and 20.5% for a ratio of 0.82.[8] The Limburg PAOD Study, which reported a low male to female ratio for claudication, reported a similarly low ratio of 1.1 for ABI-based PAD.[30] A population-based study from Southern Italy found prevalences of PAD based on ABI of less than 0.9 to be very similar in men and women, with male to female ratios by age of .89 to .99.[38] In the Cardiovascular Health Study, ABI of less than 0.9 was somewhat more prevalent in men (13.8%) than in women (11.4%) (ratio = 1.21), but the association of disease with sex was not significant after adjustment for age and CVD status.[13] In the Atherosclerosis Risk in Communities (ARIC) Study, PAD prevalence based on ABI was actually lower in men than in women among both African-Americans (3.3% vs. 4.0%) and whites (2.3% vs. 3.3%).[39]

The greater male excess observed for symptomatic versus ABI-diagnosed disease may be related to severity of disease. A prevalence study in Southern California found that the excess of disease among males increased with the severity of PAD.[11] In a recent presentation of data by the MESA (Multi-Ethnic Study of Atherosclerosis) researchers, in a multi-ethnic population of more than 6000 persons, PAD prevalence (ABI of less than or equal to 0.9) was similar in men and women (roughly 4% in both sexes), but borderline values of ABI (>0.9 and <1.0) were much higher in women (11% vs. 5%).[40]

PAD RISK FACTORS

The section that follows reviews the existing evidence for the association of various possible risk factors with PAD. It begins with a discussion of traditional risk factors long implicated in atherosclerotic processes underlying coronary heart and cerebrovascular disease; and then moves on to a discussion of emerging or "novel" risk factors. Where applicable, information on interaction between risk factors and the impact of risk factors on the natural history of disease are also provided.

The study of PAD epidemiology raises a number of methodological issues that should be kept in mind while reviewing the literature. As discussed earlier, the definition of disease has evolved over time, with earlier studies focusing more on claudication, as measured using Rose and other criteria, and later studies using the ABI, with a value of less than or equal to 0.9—now widely used to define disease. These different potential definitions are noted throughout.

Methodologically, the strongest epidemiologic evidence for a causal relationship between disease and putative risk factors comes of studies of incident disease. Such studies usually involve the measurement of risk factors at a baseline examination, with subsequent tracking of incident disease among the subjects. Acute events such as myocardial infarction and stroke lend themselves to such study, because the date of onset of disease is generally documented in the records of health care providers and recalled by subjects. Conversely, the onset of PAD as defined by ABI is often asymptomatic, and in any case is unlikely to be documented other than through periodic reexamination of all the subjects, which involves substantial time and expense. For that reason, many studies of PAD risk factors are based on cross-sectional associations; i.e., the association between current disease status and current risk factor measurements. Although such studies are potentially informative, the reported associations cannot conclusively prove causation because it is not known if the risk factor preceded the disease or vice versa. Caution should, therefore, be exercised in reviewing the results of such cross-sectional studies, particularly where reverse causation is plausible. For example, low physical activity might cause claudication, but claudication might just as plausibly cause low physical activity.

It is necessary to adjust for multiple potential risk factors in a single statistical model to accurately estimate the unique contribution of any single risk factor, because the potential risk factors for PAD are themselves interrelated in various ways. The estimates presented subsequently are based on such multiple adjustment for all traditional PAD risk factors, except as noted. Null findings may indicate the lack of a real association, but may also be based on insufficient sample size. Most of the null findings discussed below are based on failure of the risk factor of interest to remain statistically significant in stepwise regression models, which vary as to their algorithms for variable selection.

The following discussion of risk factors focuses on the results from four large epidemiologic studies, which are referred to as index studies (Table 14-2). These studies each had over 3000 subjects drawn from the general population, and included both men and women. These studies are similar enough in their selection and manner of measuring risk factors, and in their statistical analyses, to allow reasonable comparisons for most of the common risk factors. Although the discussion draws on data from many other studies (see Table 14-2 for a partial list), data are presented from these four studies across all the conventional cardiovascular disease risk factors to provide some consistency and comparability for the reader, and as a check against potential biases that might be introduced by selecting all the studies to present for each risk factor in a more ad hoc fashion.

Smoking

Smoking is one of the strongest risk factors for PAD in virtually all studies. Studies vary as to their measurement of smoking, often combining a categorical assessment of smoking status (current, past, or never) with some measure of current or historical volume of smoking; these multiple approaches to measurement make comparisons difficult. However, even with some type of additional adjustment for volume of smoking, current smoking versus nonsmoking has been shown to at least double the odds of PAD in most studies, with some estimates as high as a four times greater risk among smokers than others. Among the index studies, current smoking (vs. never or former/never) resulted in 2.0 to 2.7 times higher odds of PAD in the three studies using such categorization; however, in two of these studies, the

TABLE 14-2 POPULATION-BASED STUDIES OF PAD

Study Name	First Author, Year[1]	No. of Subjects	Country	Population Characteristics	Study Design	PAD Endpoint
Index Studies						
Framingham Study	Murabito, 1997	5209	United States		Cross-sectional	IC
Framingham Offspring Study	Murabito, 2002	3313	United States		Longitudinal	ABI < .9
Cardiovascular Health Study	Newman, 1993	5084	United States	Ages 65+	Cross-sectional	ABI < .9
Rotterdam Study	Meijer, 2000	6450	Netherlands		Cross-sectional	ABI < .9 (<.7 also studied)
Other Large Studies						
Honolulu Heart Program	Curb, 1996	3450	United States	Japanese-American men	Cross-sectional and Longitudinal	ABI < .9
Edinburgh Artery Study	Fowkes, 1992	1592	Scotland		Cross-sectional	ABI and reactive hyperemia
Limburg PAOD Study	Hooi, 2001	2327	Netherlands		Longitudinal	ABI < .95, 2×
Israeli Ischemic Heart Disease Project	Bowlin, 1994	10059	Israel	Middle-aged men	Longitudinal	IC
Reykjavik Study	Ingolfsson, 1994	9141	Iceland	Men only	Longitudinal	IC
Quebec Cardiovascular Study	Dagenais, 1991	4570	Canada	Men only	Longitudinal	IC
Physicians' Health Study	Ridker, 2001	14916	United States	Male physicians	Nested Case-Control	IC or PAD surgery

[1]Where multiple papers were published, this refers to the paper most frequently referenced herein.

models also included pack-years of smoking as a significant variable. The fourth index study included only current packs/day, showing a doubling of the odds of PAD for each pack per day smoked (Table 14-3). All of the large, population-based studies that were reviewed found a significant, independent association between PAD and smoking.

Cessation of smoking among patients with claudication has been shown to improve various functional and physiological measures related to PAD, as well as reducing mortality.[41-43] However, because symptomatic PAD patients have long been advised to quit smoking, it is possible that observational comparisons of patients who quit smoking with those who do not are confounded by other differences in compliance with medical advice between the two groups. Randomized trials of this question would raise ethical issues. However, substantial bias is unlikely given the large effect size for cigarette smoking.

Aside from the large increase in risk associated with it, smoking is the traditional risk factor for which the best case can be made for a more important role in PAD than in other atherosclerotic diseases. In a comparison of risk factors conducted in the same large cohort, Fowkes and colleagues found smoking to be associated with a significantly higher relative risk for PAD compared with other cardiovascular diseases; smoking was the only traditional cardiovascular disease risk factor for which the odds ratio differed significantly between PAD and other cardiovascular diseases.[44]

Diabetes

Diabetes is strongly associated with an elevated risk of PAD, although the evidence for an independent role in multivariable analysis is not entirely consistent. Three of the four index studies found diabetes, dichotomized

TABLE 14-3 SMOKING AS A PAD RISK FACTOR

Study	Variable	Odds Ratio	95% CI Low	95% CI High
Framingham Study	Current packs/day	1.96	1.69	2.25
Framingham Offspring Study	Current smoker (vs. former or never)	2.00	1.10	3.40
	Pack-years of smoking	1.03	1.02	1.03
Cardiovascular Health Study	Current smoker (vs. former or never)	2.55	1.76	3.68
	Pack-years of smoking	1.01	1.01	1.02
Rotterdam Study	Current smoker (vs. never)	2.69	1.67	4.33
	Former smoker (vs. never)	1.15	0.75	1.78

based on different criteria, to be associated with PAD after multivariable adjustment, with odds ratios ranging from 1.89 to 4.05;[7,13,45] the Framingham Offspring Study found such an association on an age- and sex-adjusted basis, but not in multivariable models.[27]

Among other large, population-based studies, multivariable logistic regression models have often shown a relationship with diabetes as a categorical variable[1,29,31,37] or various blood sugar measures as linear variables.[34] Other null findings for diabetes or blood sugar measures were seen in the Edinburgh Artery Study[44] and the Reykjavik Study.[36]

More severe and/or longstanding diabetes appears to be more strongly related to PAD. In the Hoorn Study, it was shown that known diabetes was associated with PAD in multivariable analysis, whereas newly diagnosed diabetes was only of borderline significance and impaired glucose tolerance was not associated with PAD.[29] In that study, after excluding known diabetics, none of the common glycemic indices that were tested were significantly associated with PAD based on ABI, although significant associations were observed when the PAD criteria were broadened to include patients with additional criteria. Studies conducted in patients with diabetes have shown that duration of diabetes and use of insulin are associated with PAD.[46-48]

Outcomes of PAD in diabetic patients have been shown to be worse. In one study, diabetic patients with PAD were five times more likely to have an amputation than other patients with PAD; they also had more than three times the odds of mortality.[49] There is also some evidence to support a somewhat different anatomic distribution of disease, with more disease in arteries distal to the knee in diabetic versus nondiabetic persons.[49,50]

Lipids

As is the case in cardiovascular disease epidemiology, the challenge of defining the roles of the various lipid fractions in PAD lies in identifying the strongest independent risk factors from among multiple correlated measures. Results from the index studies appear in Table 14-4.

Total cholesterol was the first lipid measure to be examined as a potential risk factor for PAD and has been the most widely studied. Total cholesterol was examined as a potential risk factor in all four of the index studies, and was significantly associated with PAD in multivariable analysis in three; in the remaining study, total cholesterol was significant in univariate analysis, but dropped out of multivariable models in which other lipid measures were considered.[27] Similarly, in other studies, total cholesterol has usually been found to be associated with PAD[1,31,36,44] with occasional null findings in multivariable analyses in which other lipid measures are considered.[34,51] One of the few null findings for total cholesterol as the sole lipid measure was an analysis of the Quebec Cardiovascular Study cohort.[33]

High-density lipoprotein cholesterol (HDL-C) has been shown to be protective against PAD in most studies where it was evaluated, usually in models that also considered total cholesterol. HDL-C was included among the potential risk factors in three of the four index studies, and was significantly associated with PAD in multivariable analysis in all three. In two studies both HDL-C and total cholesterol were significant in multivariable analysis, whereas in one study HDL-C (but not total cholesterol) was significant. Other studies have also shown a protective effect of HDL-C.[31,51]

Two measures that combine total and HDL cholesterol into a single number have been proposed. Bowlin and colleagues found that non-HDL cholesterol (total cholesterol minus HDL cholesterol) was significantly associated with incident claudication in a large cohort of Israeli men; neither total cholesterol nor HDL cholesterol were significantly associated with disease in models that included non-HDL cholesterol.[1] In a comparison of incident cases of claudication with healthy controls in the Physician's Health Study, Ridker and colleagues found that the ratio of total to HDL cholesterol was the lipid measure most strongly associated with disease, with patients in the highest quartile having 3.9 times the claudication risk of patients in the lowest quartile; screening for other lipid fractions was judged to have little clinical usefulness beyond measurement of this ratio.[52]

TABLE 14-4 LIPID MEASURES AS PAD RISK FACTORS

Study	Variable	Odds Ratio	95% CI Low	95% CI High
Framingham Study[1]	Total cholesterol (10 mg/dL)	1.05	1.02	1.07
Framingham Offspring Study[2]	HDL cholesterol (5 mg/dL)	0.90	0.80	1.00
Cardiovascular Health Study[3]	Total cholesterol (10 mg/dL)	1.10	1.06	1.14
	HDL cholesterol (5 mg/dL)	0.95	0.90	1.00
Rotterdam Study[4]	Total cholesterol (10 mg/dL)	1.05	1.01	1.08
	HDL cholesterol (5 mg/dL)	0.93	0.87	1.00

[1]Only total cholesterol was tested.
[2]Hypercholesterolemia (>= 240 mg/dL or medication) and triglycerides dropped out of stepwise logistic regression model.
[3]Triglycerides dropped out of stepwise logistic regression model.
[4]Triglycerides not tested.

The evidence for high triglycerides as an independent risk factor for PAD is fragmentary. Early case-control studies showed a very consistent relationship between triglycerides and PAD, suggesting a uniquely strong relationship with PAD; however, large, population-based cohort studies employing multivariable modeling later called this into question.[44,53] Among the index studies, only two included triglycerides among the potential risk factors evaluated. In both cases, triglycerides were significant in univariate analysis, but dropped out of multivariable models based on stepwise logistic regression.[13,27] Similarly, in the Edinburgh Artery Study cohort and in a large study of geriatric patients in the United States, triglycerides were not significantly associated with PAD after adjustment for other lipid meaures.[44,51] However, other studies have shown triglycerides to be significantly and independently associated with PAD in multivariable analysis.[34,46,54] There is also some evidence suggesting that elevated triglycerides may have a special role in disease progression or more severe PAD.[44,55]

In summary, although total cholesterol, HDL-C, and triglycerides all appear to be associated with PAD on a univariate basis, in multivariable analysis triglycerides frequently drop out as an independent risk factor. Although it has been the most extensively studied, it is not clear that total cholesterol is the strongest independent risk factor for PAD; in one comparison of PAD patients with healthy controls, it was found that mean total cholesterol did not differ significantly, whereas triglycerides, very low-density lipoprotein (VLDL) cholesterol, low-density lipoprotein (LDL) cholesterol, high-density lipoprotein (HDL) cholesterol, and the total-to-HDL cholesterol ratio all did.[56] Total and HDL cholesterol seem to provide distinct information, although these may lend themselves to summarization in a single ratio or difference. Because many early studies considered only total cholesterol, the full resolution of the question of which lipid measures are the most strongly and independently related to PAD awaits the completion of additional large-scale studies that assess all of the relevant lipid risk factors. Irrespective of results from multivariable analysis, simple descriptive statistics and clinical observation both suggest that PAD patients are frequently diabetic or insulin resistant, with the typical dyslipidemia of insulin resistance (i.e., low HDL and high triglycerides).

Hypertension and Blood Pressure

The association of hypertension with PAD has been demonstrated in most studies in which blood pressure was studied. All four of the index studies reported a significant association between hypertension as a categorical variable and PAD. The lowest reported odds ratio was 1.32 as reported in the Rotterdam Study; this is somewhat understated relative to the others, as it was based on a model that included both a categorical hypertension variable and an adjustment for systolic blood pressure level, which was also significant.[7] Other than this, odds ratios for hypertension ranged from 1.50 to 2.20.

Most other large, population-based studies have also found a significant, independent association of hypertension or systolic blood pressures with PAD.[33,34,37,44] Where both systolic and diastolic pressures were considered, systolic pressure was usually found to be associated with PAD, whereas diastolic pressure was not significantly associated[7,13,57] or had a nonlinear relationship with PAD.[31]

Two large studies found no relationship of blood pressure with PAD. In the Israeli Ischemic Heart Disease Project cohort, neither systolic nor diastolic blood pressure was associated with claudication,[1] whereas in the Reykjavik Study systolic and diastolic blood pressures were significantly associated with claudication in cross-sectional but not longitudinal models.[36] It is interesting to note that both of these studies appear to have used blood pressure as a linear term in their models; most other recent large studies have used a categorization of subjects into normotensive and hypertensive groups, based on systolic and diastolic pressures as well as hypertension medication use. Both of the null findings also come from studies in which claudication was the outcome of interest. It has been speculated that elevated central perfusion pressure as indicated by (axial) blood pressure will sometimes delay the onset of claudication by increasing blood pressure in the lower extremities, which—if true—would obscure the relationship of hypertension with underlying disease processes.[58] However, randomized trials of blood pressure lowering in PAD patients do not report worsened claudication.

Although the relative risks associated with hypertension are modest in some studies, its high prevalence, particularly among older patients, make it a significant contributor to the total burden of PAD in the population. For example, in one large study from the Netherlands, the odds ratio for hypertension was 1.32, but its attributable risk (a measure of the proportion of PAD in the population attributable to hypertension) was 17.0%, which was second only to current smoking in this group.[7] In the Framingham Study, 30% of the risk of claudication in the population was attributable to blood pressure in excess of 160/100.[45]

Obesity

To date, the preponderance of evidence fails to support a consistent, independent positive association between obesity and PAD. In one of the few large studies with a positive finding, Bowlin and colleagues estimated an odds ratio of 1.24 (95% CI = 1.05 to 1.46) for incident claudication related to a 5.0 kg/m^2 difference in body mass index (BMI) in a study of 10,059 Israeli men.[1]

Two of the index studies and a number of other large, population-based studies have failed to find a significant association between obesity and PAD or claudication after multivariable adjustment.[7,27,36,37,51] There have also been many studies, including the other two index studies, in which higher relative weight or BMI was actually shown to be protective against PAD. In the Framingham Study, claudication was significantly inversely related to relative weight in men in multivariable analysis, and appeared to have a "U-shaped" nonlinear relationship with relative weight in women.[32] In an analysis from the Edinburgh Artery Study, BMI was significantly associated with less disease in preliminary multivariable analysis, although BMI was excluded from the paper's final multivariable model because it "suggested a counterintuitive effect".[44] The Cardiovascular Health Study found higher BMI to be significantly protective against PAD after multivariable adjustment in a large sample of Medicare beneficiaries.[13] BMI was significantly protective against PAD (defined based on a combination of ABI, Doppler flow curves, and history of surgery) in the Hoorn Study.[29] Similarly, the odds of PAD among subjects in the highest quintile of BMI compared with the lowest quintile were found to be significantly reduced in a cross-sectional analysis of elderly Japanese American men.[31] Subjects with higher BMI were again shown to be at significantly lower risk of PAD in a study of Taiwanese subjects with diabetes.[59]

Obesity has been implicated in the etiology of other risk factors for PAD, such as hypertension, type II diabetes, and dyslipidemia. In epidemiology, adjusting for factors that are on the causal pathway between a risk factor and disease is known to attenuate the observed strength of that risk factor. Therefore, estimates of risks related to obesity in multivariable models are estimates of the risk of obesity that artificially ignore most of the mechanisms by which obesity might reasonably cause PAD. In a few cases, unadjusted models or models adjusted only for age and sex show a significant association with PAD, even though obesity was nonsignificant or protective after multivariable adjustment.[27,44,51] However, in other studies, obesity was found to be either protective or nonsignificant even in unadjusted models, or models adjusted only for age and sex.[7,13,31,32,34] Thus, the failure to find more cases of positive association between PAD and obesity is not simply an artifact of adjusting for factors on the causal pathway in multivariable modeling, but seems to suggest a real lack of consistent evidence that such a relationship exists at all.

Unaccounted for in the multivariable analyses just cited is possible residual confounding by cigarette smoking, which is strongly associated with both PAD and lower BMI. In addition, chronic illness in older persons, where PAD is most common, may lead to weight loss, allowing for a spurious inverse correlation between obesity and PAD.

As in coronary heart disease epidemiology, there is some evidence to suggest that central adiposity, rather than obesity per se, may be more closely related to an increased risk of PAD. Vogt and colleagues found that, after adjustment for BMI, higher waist/hip ratio (WHR) was associated with significantly higher risk of PAD.[4] In a group of patients with diabetes, it was shown that WHR, but not BMI or body fat percentage, was associated with PAD.[46]

Alcohol Consumption

Evidence for a protective effect of light-to-moderate alcohol consumption, as seen in coronary heart disease, is less consistent for PAD. Two of the four index studies considered alcohol intake; neither showed alcohol to be significantly associated with PAD in either age- and sex-adjusted or multivariable models.[7,27] However, in a later analysis of data from one of these studies, a significant protective effect was found in women but not in men.[60] Conversely, a protective effect of alcohol was seen in men but not women in the Edinburgh Artery Study, but this association disappeared after adjustment for social class.[61] In Native Americans, a protective effect of alcohol was seen in multivariable analysis,[62] but in elderly Japanese American men, alcohol intake was found to increase rather than decrease the risk of incident PAD.[31] Data from the Physician's Health Study suggest that a protective effect related to moderate alcohol consumption may exist.[63] In that study, there was no univariate association between alcohol and claudication incidence, but adjustment for cigarette smoking "unmasked" a significant protective association, reflecting the positive correlation of alcohol consumption with smoking, a strong risk factor for PAD. Based on this, it seems possible that incomplete adjustment for smoking in other studies might allow residual confounding that would obscure any protective effect of alcohol, despite multivariable adjustment.[60]

Race and Ethnicity

Data on the association of race with PAD are limited, because many of the large studies of PAD have been conducted in non-Hispanic white groups. A recent review of ethnicity and PAD concluded that there are at present "no large population-based studies assessing the prevalence of PAD in non-caucasians".[64]

Several studies suggest a higher risk of PAD among blacks. The Cardiovascular Health Study, a study of 5084 Medicare beneficiaries in the United States, found that non-white (mostly black) race was associated with an odds ratio of 2.12 for PAD after adjustment for traditional risk factors.[13] A study of 933 women, aged 65 years and older, found a higher percentage of black subjects among the PAD (36.3%) versus non-PAD (24.8%) groups.[15] In the Atherosclerosis Risk in Communities Study, Zheng and colleagues found that PAD prevalence was higher in African-Americans versus whites in both men (3.3% vs. 2.3%) and women (4.0% vs. 3.3%).[39] The San Diego Population Study recently reported an unadjusted relative risk of 3.4 for blacks vs. non-Hispanic whites, which was reduced to 2.6 after adjustment for hypertension and diabetes.[12] Additional analyses also showed no evidence of a greater sensitivity of blacks to traditional CVD risk factors. It remains to be seen whether other risk factors, such as markers of inflammation, account for the remaining difference, or whether black race confers additional risk independent of all known risk factors. Interestingly, hospital-based studies suggest that the anatomic distribution of disease may differ in blacks, with a higher percentage of distal disease in black subjects, even after adjustment for diabetes and other cardiovascular risk factors.[64]

Data on other races and ethnic groups are even more fragmentary. One study showed, compared with non-Hispanic whites, a slightly lower prevalence of PAD in Hispanics and Asians after multivariable adjustment, although neither result achieved statistical significance.[12] In another study, Asians were reported to have lower PAD prevalence than comparable non-Hispanic white subjects.[31] A study of Native Americans suggested PAD prevalence comparable with that in non-Hispanic whites.[62]

Homocysteine

The association of homocysteine with PAD has been examined in a number of studies, with conflicting results. A 1995 meta-analysis of early case-control studies conducted in the late 1980s and early 1990s suggested an odds ratio of 6.8 for a 5 μmol/L difference in fasting homocysteine (tHcy).[65] To put this in perspective, the differences between the 25th and 75th percentiles of tHcy among controls in the Physician's Health Study and a study of women in the Netherlands were between 3.5 and 4.0 μmol/L.[52,66] The 5 μmol/L difference noted above is, therefore, not unreasonable as the difference between low and high tHcy levels in the population. In that light, an odds ratio of 6.8 might make homocysteine the single most powerful risk factor for PAD. Interestingly, the odds ratio for PAD in the meta-analysis was strikingly higher than the odds ratios for coronary artery disease and cerebrovascular disease, which were below 2 in the same study.

However, more recent studies have produced much lower and frequently nonsignificant estimates of the PAD risk associated with homocysteine. In a large European case-control study, Graham and colleagues estimated an odds ratio of 1.7 for subjects in the top quintile of homocysteine for their control group versus all other subjects—a result of only borderline statistical significance.[67] One population-based study from the Netherlands found a 1.44 odds ratio for a 5 μmol/L difference in fasting tHcy, based on an extreme definition of PAD involving surgery or an ABI of less than 0.5.[68] However, an analysis of a subset of the Rotterdam Study cohort found no significant relationship between tHcy and PAD, based either on the conventional 0.9 ABI cut-off or on a 0.7 ABI cut-off for severe disease.[7] Similarly, a nested case-control study using the Physician's Health Study cohort failed to find any association between quartiles of fasting tHcy and claudication.[52] A recent case-control study of young women in the Netherlands also failed to find any significant association between fasting homocysteine and symptomatic PAD.[66] Among patients with PAD, disease progression based on ABI was not significantly different in patients with the highest and lowest 20% of homocysteine levels.[69]

At this point, although it is still possible that homocysteine may be an independent risk factor for PAD, it appears that the early results summarized in the 1995 meta-analysis may have overstated the importance of homocysteine. This may be related to the quality of the studies included in the meta-analysis, which included primarily small case-control studies.[65]

C-Reactive Protein and Fibrinogen

C-reactive protein and fibrinogen are two inflammatory markers that have been shown to be associated with PAD in a number of studies. In an analysis from the Physician's Health Study, each was found to be significantly associated with PAD in multivariable models, with odds ratios for the upper versus lower population quartiles of 2.2 for fibrinogen and 2.8 for C-reactive protein.[52] However, adding both variables to risk prediction models did not improve the accuracy of prediction, because they are significantly intercorrelated. C-reactive protein was not studied in any of the index studies; however, fibrinogen was included in three of the four studies, and was significantly associated with PAD in multivariable analysis in two of them.[7,27] Other studies have also reported significant and independent associations of PAD with C-reactive protein[66] and fibrinogen.[31]

OTHER RISK FACTORS

A variety of other potential risk factors for PAD have been examined. In several studies, various measures of oral health have been shown to be independently associated with PAD, possibly based on common inflammatory pathways.[70] A study in young women found that self-reported history of various types of infectious diseases, such as chicken pox, shingles, mumps, pneumonia, chronic bronchitis, or peptic ulcer, was independently and significantly related to PAD.[66] Another study found that a history of arthritis was associated with PAD as diagnosed by ABI.[4]

Psychosocial factors were found to be associated with PAD in one large cohort in Scotland,[71] whereas in a large study of Israeli men, anxiety, job-related stress, and manner of coping with job-related conflicts were all significantly related to incident claudication even after adjustment for traditional risk factors.[1] Among patients with PAD, depressive symptoms were found to be associated with poorer lower extremity functioning.[72]

Genetic factors appear to have a role in PAD, but data are limited. In a study of fraternal and identical twins, Carmelli and colleagues estimated that 48% of the variability in ABI could be explained by additive genetic effects.[73] It has also been shown that familial hypercholesterolemia, a genetic disorder, is related to a higher prevalence of PAD.[74]

Other possible risk factors for which some supporting data exist include antiphospholipid antibodies,[75,76] hypothyroidism,[77] and sedentary lifestyle.[78] Possible protective effects have been reported for antioxidants[79] and hormone replacement therapy.[80] However, the Women's Health Initiative randomized clinical trial of combined estrogen/progestin therapy showed no effect on incidence of PAD.[81]

INTERACTION AND RISK FACTOR COMPARISONS

Some research has been conducted into potential variations in the significance and strength of the various risk factors as they are estimated in different subgroups and for different PAD-related outcomes.

Differences in the relative strength and significance of risk factors in men and women have been examined in several studies. Many of these studies have concluded that risk factors do not differ substantially in men and women. In the Rotterdam Study, separate models for men and women were compared and failed to reveal differences in risk factors for PAD.[7] In the large Framingham and Framingham Offspring cohorts, testing for statistical interactions between sex and risk factors failed to provide any evidence of such interactions.[27,45] One study of Medicare beneficiaries in the United States (ages 65 and older) found similar risk factor associations with ABI in men and in women, the exceptions being total and LDL cholesterol levels, which were related to ABI in women but not in men.[13]

Meijer and colleagues looked at whether severe PAD, diagnosed based on ABI of less than 0.7, had different risk factors than ABI diagnosed based on the traditional cut-point of 0.9.[7] In their analysis, the direction and magnitude of odds ratios were similar for most risk factors under the two criteria. The point estimates suggested that age and current smoking were greater risk factors for conventionally-defined PAD, whereas diabetes was more important for severe PAD; however, the 95% confidence intervals overlapped in all cases.

Many of the risk factors that have been studied for their relationship to PAD were originally identified as risk factors for ischemic heart disease. In the most formal comparison of the relative significance and strength of risk factors for PAD versus ischemic heart disease, the same risk factors were analyzed for their association with the two diseases in the Edinburgh Artery Study cohort.[44] In that study, only the association with smoking was significantly different for PAD versus ischemic heart disease, with a higher association with PAD. Especially strong or consistent relationships to PAD that were suggested for triglycerides and homocysteine were generally not borne out in later studies, as described earlier. In general, with the exception of smoking and possibly more severe diabetes, most risk factors do not seem to differ greatly in their associations with PAD and ischemic heart disease.

PROGRESSION OF PAD

Little is known about the early natural history of PAD, particularly the progression from asymptomatic to early symptomatic disease. The average annual change in ABI has been estimated as −0.01 and −0.02 in various groups.[82,83] However, these figures may be somewhat misleading, because an average change in ABI masks a variety of changes of different directions and magnitudes.

A more meaningful approach may be to look at the percentage of the population achieving some categorically defined measure of change. Nicoloff and colleagues found that in 5 years, 37% of patients experienced a significant (≥0.15) worsening of ABI, whereas 22% of patients experienced clinical progression of PAD based on a change in symptoms or a need for surgical intervention.[84] Among 415 English smokers with PAD referred for a surgical opinion, about one half experienced a significant (≥0.14) drop in ABI over the following 48 months.[55] In a group of German PAD patients, PAD was reported to progress in 18.6% of patients during an average follow-up of 64 months, based on a variety of criteria including change in ABI.[85] Bird and colleagues defined a ranked series of six categories of PAD defined based on ABI and other tests; in a study of patients referred to a vascular laboratory, 30.2% of limbs progressed to a more serious category of PAD over an average follow-up time of 4.6 years, but 22.8% of limbs regressed to a less severe category during the same period.[82]

In a study based on angiography, 9.1% of patients annually were found to have evidence of progression of PAD.[86] In a study using development of rest pain or gangrene as the criteria for PAD progression, PAD progressed in 2.5% of patients annually.[87] In the latter study, it was noted that PAD progressed at a rate approximately three times greater in the first year following diagnosis than in subsequent years.[87] Because many studies of PAD progression have used subjects whose recruitment is linked to the referral for diagnostic testing, estimates of progression from such studies may be appropriate only for newly diagnosed populations, particularly if follow-up time is short.

Data on risk factors associated with progression of PAD are relatively sparse. One report showed age, diabetes, classic claudication, previous intervention, and PAD in the contralateral leg to be independently predictive of PAD progression.[82] One study of English smokers with PAD identified hypertriglyceridemia as the most important independent risk factor for progression of PAD and onset of critical ischemia.[55] Hemorheologic factors have been shown to be associated with an increased risk of need for vascular intervention.[88] Patients with premature PAD (onset of symptoms at or before age 45) appear to have more rapid progression of disease and generally poorer outcomes.[89-93]

CO-PREVALENCE OF PAD AND OTHER ATHEROSCLEROTIC DISEASE

Given the common risk factors for PAD and other cardiovascular and cerebrovascular diseases, it is not surprising that cross-sectionally, people with PAD are more likely to have these other disorders, and vice versa. Among 5084 Medicare beneficiaries in the Cardiovascular Health Study, the prevalence of history of myocardial infarction was 2.5 times as high in subjects with PAD (based on ABI < 0.9) versus those without; for angina, congestive heart failure, stroke, and TIA, the prevalences were 1.9, 3.3, 3.1, and 2.3 times as high, respectively.[13] Conversely, the prevalence of PAD was 2.1 times as high in patients with a history of myocardial infarction versus those without; the corresponding ratios for angina, congestive heart failure, stroke and TIA were 1.7, 2.6, 2.4, and 2.1, respectively.[13] Other studies have found similar cross-sectional correlations.[39,94,95] Subjects with PAD have also been shown to have an elevated prevalence of carotid artery stenosis[96,97] and a modest but significant correlation between the severities of the two diseases has been demonstrated.[98]

PAD AS A PREDICTOR OF MORTALITY AND MORBIDITY

Going beyond the cross-sectional associations discussed earlier, it has been shown that PAD is prospectively related to morbidity or mortality from other types of atherosclerotic disease, even after adjustment for known common risk factors. Although PAD seems unlikely to directly cause these other diseases, the presence of PAD may serve as a marker for underlying atherosclerotic processes or susceptibilities affecting other vascular beds. These prospective relationships are clinically important, to the extent that the PAD has prognostic value independent of other known risk factors.

Attempts to elucidate this association epidemiologically began with studies of patients having symptomatic PAD in the form of intermittent claudication. Elevated mortality rates among subjects with claudication were reported in the 1970s and 1980s in the Framingham cohort, although this excess risk was markedly attenuated when subjects with baseline cerebrovascular and coronary heart disease were excluded.[32,99,100] Similarly, a 1982 Finnish study failed to find an association between claudication and total or cardiovascular mortality in men after adjustment for cardiovascular risk factors and baseline cardiovascular disease.[101] Other studies demonstrated increased mortality risk among claudicants, but did not fully adjust for the conventional cardiovascular risk factors.[33,87,102] However, in the largest and most methodologically rigorous study of its kind, data from the 18,403 men in the Whitehall cohort were used to show that after adjusting for cardiovascular risk factors, claudication was a significant predictor of cardiovascular disease mortality, even after excluding subjects with baseline disease.[103]

The development of the ankle-brachial index (ABI) and other noninvasive measures of peripheral arterial disease permitted further investigation of the association of PAD and cardiovascular disease. In 1985, it was first demonstrated that a combination of noninvasive measures, including ABI, were prospectively related to all-cause mortality, even after adjustment for cardiovascular risk factors and exclusion of subjects with baseline cardiovascular disease.[104] Relative risks in this study were in the range of 4 to 5; a later reanalysis of the same cohort with additional mortality follow-up demonstrated elevated relative risks for cardiovascular disease and coronary heart disease in particular, with no significant increase in noncardiovascular death.[105]

In the 1990s, a number of other prospective studies confirmed that ABI was related to cardiovascular disease, based on either mortality or combined mortality and morbidity. This was found to be true in a variety of populations: vascular laboratory patients,[25,106] elderly patients with hypertension,[107] elderly women,[108] an employment-based cohort from Belgium,[109] the Edinburgh Artery Study cohort from Scotland,[14] and the Cardiovascular Health Study cohort.[26] Most of these studies controlled for various known cardiovascular disease risk factors and the presence of cardiovascular disease at baseline. The relative risks reported ranged from roughly 2 to 5. Many of these studies also found PAD to be significantly associated with incident coronary heart disease in particular, although the very large Cardiovascular Health Study failed to find such associations for either total myocardial infarction or angina.[26]

The data regarding the association of PAD with cerebrovascular disease are less conclusive. A 1991 study showed a strong association between multiple noninvasive measures of PAD and cerebrovascular disease morbidity and mortality, with risk ratios of 3.3 for men and 9.0 for women after multivariable adjustment.[110] Data from the Edinburgh Artery Study also showed such an association based on ABI, although after multivariable adjustment, the association persisted for nonfatal but not fatal stroke.[14] However, data from the Cardiovascular Health Study failed to show a relationship between low ABI and incident stroke.[26] Another large study, the Atherosclerosis Risk in Communities (ARIC) Study, showed a significant association between ABI as a continuous variable and ischemic stroke after multivariable adjustment, but failed to show such association when ABI was categorized based on a 0.80 cut-point.[111]

Table 14-5 provides a summary of studies of the association of PAD with various mortality and morbidity outcomes. The table is limited to studies using a noninvasive measure of PAD (usually ABI at various cut-points) and logistic or proportional hazards regression models, with multivariable adjustment for conventional cardiovascular risk factors; results are shown with multivariable adjustment, and after exclusion of subjects with baseline cardiovascular disease where such exclusion was attempted.

SUMMARY AND CONCLUSION

PAD is the atherosclerotic obstruction of the arteries of the lower extremities. The most common symptom of PAD is intermittent claudication, which is pain in the legs associated with walking that is relieved by rest. However, noninvasive measures such as the ankle-brachial index show that asymptomatic PAD is several times more common in the population than intermittent claudication. PAD prevalence is sharply age-related, rising to more than 10% among patients in their 60s and 70s. Prevalence appears to be higher among men versus women for moderate-to-severe disease. The major risk factors for PAD are similar to those for cardiovascular and cerebrovascular disease, with some differences in the relative importance of factors. Smoking is a particularly strong risk factor for PAD. PAD is cross-sectionally associated with cardiovascular and cerebrovascular disease. After adjustment for known cardiovascular disease risk factors, PAD is associated with an increased risk of cardiovascular and cerebrovascular disease, morbidity, and mortality.

With the general aging of the population, it seems likely that PAD will be increasingly common in the future. The diagnosis and treatment of PAD in its asymptomatic stage may prove highly beneficial, particularly with respect to interventions aimed at ameliorating risk factors common to atherosclerotic disease of the several vascular beds.

TABLE 14-5 PAD AS A PREDICTOR OF CORONARY HEART AND CEREBROVASCULAR DISEASE MORBIDITY AND MORTALITY

Study	PAD Measurement	Hazard Ratio	95% CI Lower	95% CI Upper	Model Specifications
Total Mortality					
Criqui, 1992	Large-vessel PAD (multiple criteria)	3.10	1.80	5.30	Adjusted for conventional risk factors; excludes subjects with baseline angina, MI, stroke
Newman, 1993	ABI < 0.9	3.40	1.60	7.10	Adjusted for conventional risk factors; excludes subjects with baseline cardiovascular disease
Vogt, 1993	ABI < 0.9	3.10	1.50	6.70	Adjusted for conventional risk factors; excludes subjects with baseline cardiovascular disease
Kornitzer, 1995	ABI < 0.9	2.07	0.90	4.77	Adjusted for conventional risk factors other than blood pressure; excludes baseline coronary heart disease
Jager, 1999	ABI < 0.9	1.50	0.79	2.84	Adjusted for conventional risk factors
Newman, 1999	ABI < 0.9	1.62	1.24	2.12	Adjusted for conventional risk factors; excludes subjects with baseline cardiovascular disease
Hooi, 2002	ABI < 0.7 (vs. > 0.95)	2.10	1.60	2.80	Adjusted for conventional risk factors
Cardiovascular Disease Mortality					
Criqui, 1992	Large-vessel PAD (multiple criteria)	6.30	2.60	15.00	Adjusted for conventional risk factors; excludes subjects with baseline angina, MI, stroke
Vogt, 1993	ABI < 0.9	4.50	1.50	6.70	Adjusted for conventional risk factors; excludes subjects with baseline cardiovascular disease
Kornitzer, 1995	ABI < 0.9	3.29	1.02	10.57	Adjusted for conventional risk factors other than blood pressure: excludes baseline coronary heart disease
Jager, 1999	ABI < 0.9	2.36	0.92	6.09	Adjusted for conventional risk factors
Newman, 1999	ABI < 0.9	2.03	1.22	3.37	Adjusted for conventional risk factors; excludes subjects with baseline cardiovascular disease
Hooi, 2002	ABI < 0.7 (vs. > 0.95)	2.30	1.70	3.10	Adjusted for conventional risk factors
Coronary Heart Disease Mortality					
Criqui, 1992	Large-vessel PAD (multiple criteria)	6.30	2.60	15.00	Adjusted for conventional risk factors; excludes subjects with baseline cardiovascular disease
Kornitzer, 1995	ABI < 0.9	3.63	1.11	11.84	Adjusted for conventional risk factors other than blood pressure excludes baseline coronary heart disease
Cardiovascular Morbidity					
Newman, 1993	ABI < 0.9	2.10	1.10	4.10	Adjusted for conventional risk factors
Hooi, 2002	ABI < 0.7 (vs. > 0.95)	1.70	1.30	2.40	Adjusted for conventional risk factors
Myocardial Infarction					
Newman, 1999	ABI < 0.9	1.40	0.90	2.17	Adjusted for conventional risk factors; excludes subjects with baseline cardiovascular disease
Stroke					
Newman, 1999	ABI < 0.9	1.12	0.74	1.70	Adjusted for conventional risk factors; excludes subjects with baseline cardiovascular disease

REFERENCES

1. Bowlin SJ, Medalie JH, Flocke SA, et al: Epidemiology of intermittent claudication in middle-aged men. Am J Epidemiol 140:418, 1994.
2. Rose GA: The diagnosis of ischaemic heart pain and intermittent claudication in field surveys. Bull WHO 27:645, 1962.
3. Criqui MH, Denenberg JO, Bird CE, et al: The correlation between symptoms and non-invasive test results in patients referred for peripheral arterial disease testing. Vasc Med 1:65, 1996.
4. Vogt MT, Cauley JA, Kuller LH, et al: Prevalence and correlates of lower extremity arterial disease in elderly women. Am J Epidemiol 137:559, 1993.
5. Winsor T: Influence of arterial disease on the systolic blood pressure gradients of the extremity. Am J Med Sci 220:117, 1950.
6. Hooi JD, Stoffers HE, Kester AD, et al: Peripheral arterial occlusive disease: Prognostic value of signs, symptoms, and the ankle-brachial pressure index. Med Decis Making 22: 99, 2002.
7. Meijer WT, Grobbee DE, Hunink MG, et al: Determinants of peripheral arterial disease in the elderly: The Rotterdam study. Arch Intern Med 160:2934, 2000.
8. Meijer WT, Hoes AW, Rutgers D, et al: Peripheral arterial disease in the elderly: The Rotterdam Study. Arterioscler Thromb Vasc Biol 18:185, 1998.
9. Yao ST, Hobbs JT, Irvine WT: Ankle systolic pressure measurements in arterial disease affecting the lower extremities. Br J Surg 56: 676, 1969.
10. Ouriel K, McDonnell AE, Metz CE, et al: Critical evaluation of stress testing in the diagnosis of peripheral vascular disease. Surgery 91:686, 1982.

11. Criqui MH, Fronek A, Barrett-Connor E, et al: The prevalence of peripheral arterial disease in a defined population. Circulation 71:510, 1985.
12. Criqui MH, Vargas V, Ho E, et al: Ethnicity and peripheral arterial disease: The San Diego Population Study. Presented at the Asia-Pacific Scientific Forum—The Genomics Revolution: Bench to Bedside to Community and the 42nd Annual Conference on Cardiovascular Disease Epidemiology and Prevention, Honolulu, HI, April 26, 2002. Circulation 105:e113, 2002.
13. Newman AB, Siscovick DS, Manolio TA, et al: Ankle-arm index as a marker of atherosclerosis in the Cardiovascular Health Study. Cardiovascular Heart Study (CHS) Collaborative Research Group. Circulation 88:837, 1993.
14. Leng GC, Fowkes FG, Lee AJ, et al: Use of ankle brachial pressure index to predict cardiovascular events and death: A cohort study. BMJ 313:1440, 1996.
15. McDermott MM, Fried L, Simonsick E, et al: Asymptomatic peripheral arterial disease is independently associated with impaired lower extremity functioning: The women's health and aging study. Circulation 101:1007, 2000.
16. McDermott MM, Criqui MH, Liu K, et al: Lower ankle/brachial index, as calculated by averaging the dorsalis pedis and posterior tibial arterial pressures, and association with leg functioning in peripheral arterial disease. J Vasc Surg 32:1164, 2000.
17. McDermott MM, Ferrucci L, Simonsick EM, et al: The ankle brachial index and change in lower extremity functioning over time: The Women's Health and Aging Study. J Am Geriatr Soc 50:238, 2002.
18. de Graaff JC, Ubbink DT, Legemate DA, et al: Interobserver and intraobserver reproducibility of peripheral blood and oxygen pressure measurements in the assessment of lower extremity arterial disease. J Vasc Surg 33:1033, 2001.
19. Aboyans V, Lacroix P, Lebourdon A, et al: The intra- and interobserver variability of ankle-arm blood pressure index according to its mode of calculation. J Clin Epidemiol 56:215, 2003.
20. Shadman R, Criqui MH, Bundens WP, et al: Subclavian stenosis: Prevalence, risk factors, and association with other cardiovascular diseases. Presented at the American Federation for Medical Research Western Regional Meeting, Carmel, CA, January 29-February 1, 2003. J Investig Med 2003;51.
21. Fowkes FG, Housley E, Cawood EH, et al: Edinburgh Artery Study: Prevalence of asymptomatic and symptomatic peripheral arterial disease in the general population. Int J Epidemiol 20:384, 1991.
22. Hiatt WR, Hoag S, Hamman RF: Effect of diagnostic criteria on the prevalence of peripheral arterial disease: The San Luis Valley Diabetes Study. Circulation 91:1472, 1995.
23. Kreines K, Johnson E, Albrink M, et al: The course of peripheral vascular disease in non-insulin-dependent diabetes. Diabetes Care 8:235, 1985.
24. Orchard TJ, Strandness DE, Jr: Assessment of peripheral vascular disease in diabetes. Report and recommendations of an international workshop sponsored by the American Heart Association and the American Diabetes Association, 18-20 September 1992, New Orleans, Louisiana. Diabetes Care 16:1199, 1993.
25. McKenna M, Wolfson S, Kuller L: The ratio of ankle and arm arterial pressure as an independent predictor of mortality. Atherosclerosis 87:119, 1991.
26. Newman AB, Shemanski L, Manolio TA, et al: Ankle-arm index as a predictor of cardiovascular disease and mortality in the Cardiovascular Health Study. The Cardiovascular Health Study Group. Arterioscler Thromb Vasc Biol 19:538, 1999.
27. Murabito JM, Evans JC, Nieto K, et al: Prevalence and clinical correlates of peripheral arterial disease in the Framingham Offspring Study. Am Heart J 143:961, 2002.
28. Wang JC, Criqui MH, Denenberg JO, et al: Variations in leg pain in peripheral arterial disease. Presented at the American Federation for Medical Research Western Regional Meeting, Carmel, CA, January 29-February 1, 2003. J Investig Med 2003;51.
29. Beks PJ, Mackaay AJ, de Neeling JN, et al: Peripheral arterial disease in relation to glycaemic level in an elderly Caucasian population: The Hoorn study. Diabetologia 38:86, 1995.
30. Stoffers HE, Rinkens PE, Kester AD, et al: The prevalence of asymptomatic and unrecognized peripheral arterial occlusive disease. Int J Epidemiol 25:282, 1996.
31. Curb JD, Masaki K, Rodriguez BL, et al: Peripheral artery disease and cardiovascular risk factors in the elderly. The Honolulu Heart Program. Arterioscler Thromb Vasc Biol 16:1495, 1996.
32. Kannel WB, McGee DL: Update on some epidemiologic features of intermittent claudication: The Framingham Study. J Am Geriatr Soc 33:13, 1985.
33. Dagenais GR, Maurice S, Robitaille NM, et al: Intermittent claudication in Quebec men from 1974-1986: The Quebec Cardiovascular Study. Clin Invest Med 14:93, 1991.
34. Bainton D, Sweetnam P, Baker I, et al: Peripheral vascular disease: Consequence for survival and association with risk factors in the Speedwell prospective heart disease study. Br Heart J 72:128, 1994.
35. Leng GC, Lee AJ, Fowkes FG, et al: Incidence, natural history and cardiovascular events in symptomatic and asymptomatic peripheral arterial disease in the general population. Int J Epidemiol 25:1172, 1996.
36. Ingolfsson IO, Sigurdsson G, Sigvaldason H, et al: A marked decline in the prevalence and incidence of intermittent claudication in Icelandic men 1968-1986: A strong relationship to smoking and serum cholesterol—the Reykjavik Study. J Clin Epidemiol 47:1237, 1994.
37. Hooi JD, Kester AD, Stoffers HE, et al: Incidence of and risk factors for asymptomatic peripheral arterial occlusive disease: A longitudinal study. Am J Epidemiol 153:666, 2001.
38. Gallotta G, Iazzetta N, Milan G, et al: Prevalence of peripheral arterial disease in an elderly rural population of southern Italy. Gerontology 43:289, 1997.
39. Zheng ZJ, Sharrett AR, Chambless LE, et al: Associations of ankle-brachial index with clinical coronary heart disease, stroke and preclinical carotid and popliteal atherosclerosis: The Atherosclerosis Risk in Communities (ARIC) Study. Atherosclerosis 131:115, 1997.
40. McDermott MM, Liu K, Criqui MH: The ankle-brachial index and subclinical atherosclerosis: The Multi-Ethnic Study of Atherosclerosis. Presented at the 43rd Annual Conference on Cardiovascular Disease Epidemiology and Prevention, Miami, FL, March 6, 2003. Circulation 107:e7001, 2003.
41. Faulkner KW, House AK, Castleden WM: The effect of cessation of smoking on the accumulative survival rates of patients with symptomatic peripheral vascular disease. Med J Aust 1: 217, 1983.
42. Quick CR, Cotton LT: The measured effect of stopping smoking on intermittent claudication. Br J Surg 69 Suppl: S24, 1982.
43. Jonason T, Bergstrom R: Cessation of smoking in patients with intermittent claudication: Effects on the risk of peripheral vascular complications, myocardial infarction and mortality. Acta Med Scand 221:253, 1987.
44. Fowkes FG, Housley E, Riemersma RA, et al: Smoking, lipids, glucose intolerance, and blood pressure as risk factors for peripheral atherosclerosis compared with ischemic heart disease in the Edinburgh Artery Study. Am J Epidemiol 135:331, 1992.
45. Murabito JM, D'Agostino RB, Silbershatz H, et al: Intermittent claudication: A risk profile from The Framingham Heart Study. Circulation 96:44, 1997.
46. Katsilambros NL, Tsapogas PC, Arvanitis MP, et al: Risk factors for lower extremity arterial disease in non-insulin-dependent diabetic persons. Diabet Med 13:243, 1996.
47. Tseng CH: Prevalence and risk factors of peripheral arterial obstructive disease in Taiwanese type 2 diabetic patients. Angiology 54:331, 2003.
48. Kallio M, Forsblom C, Groop PH, et al: Development of new peripheral arterial occlusive disease in patients with type 2 diabetes during a mean follow-up of 11 years. Diabetes Care 26:1241, 2003.
49. Jude EB, Oyibo SO, Chalmers N, et al: Peripheral arterial disease in diabetic and nondiabetic patients: A comparison of severity and outcome. Diabetes Care 24:1433, 2001.
50. Haltmayer M, Mueller T, Horvath W, et al: Impact of atherosclerotic risk factors on the anatomical distribution of peripheral arterial disease. Int Angiol 20:200, 2001.
51. Ness J, Aronow WS, Ahn C: Risk factors for symptomatic peripheral arterial disease in older persons in an academic hospital-based geriatrics practice. J Am Geriatr Soc 48:312, 2000.
52. Ridker PM, Stampfer MJ, Rifai N: Novel risk factors for systemic atherosclerosis: A comparison of C-reactive protein, fibrinogen, homocysteine, lipoprotein(a), and standard cholesterol screening as predictors of peripheral arterial disease. JAMA 285:2481, 2001.
53. Fowkes FG: Epidemiology of atherosclerotic arterial disease in the lower limbs. Eur J Vasc Surg 2:2831, 1988.
54. Cheng SW, Ting AC, Wong J: Fasting total plasma homocysteine and atherosclerotic peripheral vascular disease. Ann Vasc Surg 11:217, 1997.

55. Smith I, Franks PJ, Greenhalgh RM, et al: The influence of smoking cessation and hypertriglyceridaemia on the progression of peripheral arterial disease and the onset of critical ischaemia. Eur J Vasc Endovasc Surg 11:402, 1996.
56. Mowat BF, Skinner ER, Wilson HM, et al: Alterations in plasma lipids, lipoproteins and high density lipoprotein subfractions in peripheral arterial disease. Atherosclerosis 131:161, 1997.
57. Criqui MH, Deneberg JO, Langer RD, et al: Peripheral arterial disease and hypertension. In Izzo JL, Black HR (eds): Hypertension Primer. Dallas, American Heart Association, 2003, p 250.
58. Dormandy J, Heeck L, Vig S: Predictors of early disease in the lower limbs. Semin Vasc Surg 12:109, 1999.
59. Tseng CH: Prevalence and risk factors of peripheral arterial obstructive disease in Taiwanese type 2 diabetic patients. Angiology 54:331, 2003.
60. Vliegenthart R, Geleijnse JM, Hofman A, et al: Alcohol consumption and risk of peripheral arterial disease: The Rotterdam Study. Am J Epidemiol 155: 332, 2002.
61. Jepson RG, Fowkes FG, Donnan PT, et al: Alcohol intake as a risk factor for peripheral arterial disease in the general population in the Edinburgh Artery Study. Eur J Epidemiol 11:9, 1995.
62. Fabsitz RR, Sidawy AN, Go O, et al: Prevalence of peripheral arterial disease and associated risk factors in American Indians: The Strong Heart Study. Am J Epidemiol 149:330, 1999.
63. Camargo CA, Jr, Stampfer MJ, Glynn RJ, et al: Prospective study of moderate alcohol consumption and risk of peripheral arterial disease in U.S. male physicians. Circulation 95:577, 1997.
64. Hobbs SD, Wilmink AB, Bradbury AW: Ethnicity and peripheral arterial disease. Eur J Vasc Endovasc Surg 25:505, 2003.
65. Boushey CJ, Beresford SA, Omenn GS, et al: A quantitative assessment of plasma homocysteine as a risk factor for vascular disease. Probable benefits of increasing folic acid intakes. JAMA 274:1049, 1995.
66. Bloemenkamp DG, van den Bosch MA, Mali WP, et al: Novel risk factors for peripheral arterial disease in young women. Am J Med 113:462, 2002.
67. Graham IM, Daly LE, Refsum HM, et al: Plasma homocysteine as a risk factor for vascular disease. The European Concerted Action Project. JAMA 277:1775, 1997.
68. Hoogeveen EK, Kostense PJ, Beks PJ, et al: Hyperhomocysteinemia is associated with an increased risk of cardiovascular disease, especially in non-insulin-dependent diabetes mellitus: A population-based study. Arterioscler Thromb Vasc Biol 18:133, 1998.
69. Taylor LM, Jr, Moneta GL, Sexton GJ, et al: Prospective blinded study of the relationship between plasma homocysteine and progression of symptomatic peripheral arterial disease. J Vasc Surg 29:8, 1999.
70. Hung HC, Willett W, Merchant A, et al: Oral health and peripheral arterial disease. Circulation 107:1152, 2003.
71. Whiteman MC, Deary IJ, Fowkes FG: Personality and social predictors of atherosclerotic progression: Edinburgh Artery Study. Psychosom Med 62:703, 2000.
72. McDermott MM, Greenland P, Guralnik JM, et al: Depressive symptoms and lower extremity functioning in men and women with peripheral arterial disease. J Gen Intern Med 18:461, 2003.
73. Carmelli D, Fabsitz RR, Swan GE, et al: Contribution of genetic and environmental influences to ankle-brachial blood pressure index in the NHLBI Twin Study. National Heart, Lung, and Blood Institute. Am J Epidemiol 151:452, 2000.
74. Kroon AA, Ajubi N, van Asten WN, et al: The prevalence of peripheral vascular disease in familial hypercholesterolaemia. J Intern Med 238:451, 1995.
75. Taylor LM, Jr, Chitwood RW, Dalman RL, et al: Antiphospholipid antibodies in vascular surgery patients: A cross-sectional study. Ann Surg 220:544, 1994.
76. Lam EY, Taylor LM, Jr, Landry GJ, et al: Relationship between antiphospholipid antibodies and progression of lower extremity arterial occlusive disease after lower extremity bypass operations. J Vasc Surg 33:976, 2001.
77. Mya MM, Aronow WS: Increased prevalence of peripheral arterial disease in older men and women with subclinical hypothyroidism. J Gerontol A Biol Sci Med Sci 58:68, 2003.
78. Asgeirsdottir LP, Agnarsson U, Jonsson GS: Lower extremity blood flow in healthy men: Effect of smoking, cholesterol, and physical activity—a Doppler study. Angiology 52:437, 2001.
79. Klipstein-Grobusch K, den Breeijen JH, Grobbee DE, et al: Dietary antioxidants and peripheral arterial disease: The Rotterdam Study. Am J Epidemiol 154:145, 2001.
80. Westendorp IC, in't Veld BA, Grobbee DE, et al: Hormone replacement therapy and peripheral arterial disease: The Rotterdam Study. Arch Intern Med 160:2498, 2000.
81. Hsia J, Criqui MH, Rodabough R, et al: Estrogen plus progestin and the risk of peripheral arterial disease: The Women's Health Initiative. Circulation 109:620, 2004.
82. Bird CE, Criqui MH, Fronek A, et al: Quantitative and qualitative progression of peripheral arterial disease by non-invasive testing. Vasc Med 4:15, 1999.
83. Fowkes FG, Lowe GD, Housley E, et al: Cross-linked fibrin degradation products, progression of peripheral arterial disease, and risk of coronary heart disease. Lancet 342: 84, 1993.
84. Nicoloff AD, Taylor LM, Jr, Sexton GJ, et al: Relationship between site of initial symptoms and subsequent progression of disease in a prospective study of atherosclerosis progression in patients receiving long-term treatment for symptomatic peripheral arterial disease. J Vasc Surg 35:38, 2002.
85. Taute BM, Glaser C, Taute R, et al: Progression of atherosclerosis in patients with peripheral arterial disease as a function of angiotensin-converting enzyme gene insertion/deletion polymorphism. Angiology 53:375, 2002.
86. Walsh DB, Gilbertson JJ, Zwolak RM, et al: The natural history of superficial femoral artery stenoses. J Vasc Surg 14:299, 1991.
87. Jelnes R, Gaardsting O, Hougaard Jensen K, et al: Fate in intermittent claudication: Outcome and risk factors. Br Med J (Clin Res Ed) 293:1137, 1986.
88. Smith FB, Lowe GD, Lee AJ, et al: Smoking, hemorheologic factors, and progression of peripheral arterial disease in patients with claudication. J Vasc Surg 28:129, 1998.
89. McCready RA, Vincent AE, Schwartz RW, et al: Atherosclerosis in the young: A virulent disease. Surgery 96:863, 1984.
90. Pairolero PC, Joyce JW, Skinner CR, et al: Lower limb ischemia in young adults: Prognostic implications. J Vasc Surg 1:459, 1984.
91. Hallett JW, Jr, Greenwood LH, Robison JG: Lower extremity arterial disease in young adults: A systematic approach to early diagnosis. Ann Surg 202:647, 1985.
92. Valentine RJ, MacGillivray DC, DeNobile JW, et al: Intermittent claudication caused by atherosclerosis in patients aged forty years and younger. Surgery 107:560, 1990.
93. Levy PJ, Hornung CA, Haynes JL, et al: Lower extremity ischemia in adults younger than forty years of age: A community-wide survey of premature atherosclerotic arterial disease. J Vasc Surg 19:873, 1994.
94. Criqui MH, Denenberg JO, Langer RD, et al: The epidemiology of peripheral arterial disease: Importance of identifying the population at risk. Vasc Med 2:221, 1997.
95. Ness J, Aronow WS: Prevalence of coexistence of coronary artery disease, ischemic stroke, and peripheral arterial disease in older persons, mean age 80 years, in an academic hospital-based geriatrics practice. J Am Geriatr Soc 47:1255, 1999.
96. Alexandrova NA, Gibson WC, Norris JW, et al: Carotid artery stenosis in peripheral vascular disease. J Vasc Surg 23:645, 1996.
97. Pilcher JM, Danaher J, Khaw KT: The prevalence of asymptomatic carotid artery disease in patients with peripheral vascular disease. Clin Radiol 55:56, 2000.
98. Long TH, Criqui MH, Vasilevskis EE, et al: The correlation between the severity of peripheral arterial disease and carotid occlusive disease. Vasc Med 4:135, 1999.
99. Kannel WB, Skinner JJ, Jr, Schwartz MJ, et al: Intermittent claudication: Incidence in the Framingham Study. Circulation 41:875, 1970.
100. Kannel WB, Shurtleff D: The natural history of arteriosclerosis obliterans. Cardiovasc Clin 3:37, 1971.
101. Reunanen A, Takkunen H, Aromaa A: Prevalence of intermittent claudication and its effect on mortality. Acta Med Scand 211:249, 1982.
102. Kallero KS: Mortality and morbidity in patients with intermittent claudication as defined by venous occlusion plethysmography: A ten-year follow-up study. J Chronic Dis 34:455, 1981.
103. Smith GD, Shipley MJ, Rose G: Intermittent claudication, heart disease risk factors, and mortality: The Whitehall Study. Circulation 82:1925, 1990.
104. Criqui MH, Coughlin SS, Fronek A: Noninvasively diagnosed peripheral arterial disease as a predictor of mortality: Results from a prospective study. Circulation 72:768, 1985.

105. Criqui MH, Langer RD, Fronek A, et al: Mortality over a period of 10 years in patients with peripheral arterial disease. N Engl J Med 326:381, 1992.
106. McDermott MM, Feinglass J, Slavensky R, et al: The ankle-brachial index as a predictor of survival in patients with peripheral vascular disease. J Gen Intern Med 9:445, 1994.
107. Newman AB, Sutton-Tyrrell K, Vogt MT, et al: Morbidity and mortality in hypertensive adults with a low ankle/arm blood pressure index. JAMA 270:487, 1993.
108. Vogt MT, Cauley JA, Newman AB, et al: Decreased ankle/arm blood pressure index and mortality in elderly women. JAMA 270:465, 1993.
109. Kornitzer M, Dramaix M, Sobolski J, et al: Ankle/arm pressure index in asymptomatic middle-aged males: An independent predictor of ten-year coronary heart disease mortality. Angiology 46:211, 1995.
110. Criqui MH, Langer RD, Fronek A, et al: Coronary disease and stroke in patients with large-vessel peripheral arterial disease. Drugs 42 Suppl 5:16, 1991.
111. Tsai AW, Folsom AR, Rosamond WD, et al: Ankle-brachial index and 7-year ischemic stroke incidence: The ARIC study. Stroke 32:1721, 2001.

■ ■ ■ chapter 15

Pathophysiology of Intermittent Claudication

William R. Hiatt
Eric P. Brass

Peripheral arterial disease (PAD) is a systemic disorder that commonly coexists with coronary and carotid disease, placing the patient at high risk of cardiovascular events including myocardial infarction and ischemic stroke.[1,2] The pathophysiology of atherothrombosis has been previously described (see Chapter 6).[3,4] The focus of this chapter is on the pathophysiology of claudication, the major symptom of PAD.

PAD of the lower extremity is often associated with the classic symptom of intermittent claudication, which is an exercise-induced discomfort in the calf that is associated with reversible muscle ischemia. Claudication is derived from the Latin word *claudicato*, meaning to limp, which is typical of the gait pattern of the patient who experiences claudication when walking. Claudication is characterized by a cramping and aching in the affected muscle. The discomfort develops only during exercise, steadily increases during the walking activity to a point where the patient has to stop, and then is quickly relieved by rest without change of position. Patients with claudication have severe limitations in exercise performance and walking ability. When compared with healthy individuals of the same age, patients with claudication have a 50% to 60% reduction in peak treadmill performance, reflecting a disability similar to that of patients with severe congestive heart failure.[5,6] This laboratory-defined functional impairment is manifested as a marked decrease in ambulatory activity and the physical dimension of several quality-of-life instruments.[7]

Although classic claudication defined by a questionnaire may occur in less than one half of the patients with PAD, all patients with PAD have reductions in ambulatory activity and daily functional capacity.[8,9] Even "asymptomatic" patients with PAD have a marked reduction in quality of life.[10] Thus the major goals of treatment are to prevent the progression of systemic atherosclerosis leading to fatal and nonfatal ischemic events, and to relieve the symptoms of claudication and enhance quality of life. Understanding the pathophysiologic mechanisms that underlie the development and progression of atherosclerosis and ischemic symptoms is critical in the overall management of the patient with PAD and the development of potential new therapies. Table 15-1 summarizes the major pathophysiologic mechanisms contributing to intermittent claudication that are reviewed in this chapter.

HEMODYNAMICS AND INTERMITTENT CLAUDICATION

Role of Muscle Blood Flow During Exercise

At rest and during submaximal and maximal exercise, muscle oxygen consumption is a function of oxygen delivery (pulmonary oxygen uptake, oxygen content of

TABLE 15-1 ABNORMALITIES OBSERVED IN PERIPHERAL ARTERIAL DISEASE

Changes in PAD	Possible Consequences
Hemodynamic	
Arterial stenosis/occlusion	Pressure drop across stenosis Inability to increase flow relative to demand
Collateral formation	Partial compensation for arterial stenosis
Increased blood viscosity	Reduced flow
Endothelial dysfunction	Altered arteriolar regulation of flow
Muscle capillary proliferation	Increased oxygen diffusion capacity
Oxidant Stress	
Free radical generation	Endothelial and muscle injury
White cell activation	Contributes to oxidant injury
Mitochondrial DNA deletions	Reflection of mitochondrial oxidant stress/injury
Structural	
Distal axonal denervation	Muscle weakness
Reinnervation	Partial compensation
Type II fiber loss	Decreased muscle mass/strength
Metabolic	
Increased oxidative enzymes	Partial compensation for flow and metabolic abnormalities
Short chain acylcarnitine	Reflects altered oxidative metabolism Muscle accumulation related to performance
Decreased activity of complexes I and III of electron transport chain	Reduced potential for generation of ATP; increased production of reactive oxygen species, and altered metabolic intermediate accumulation

hemoglobin, and cardiac output driving muscle blood flow) and oxygen extraction by mitochondria. In healthy humans, maximal muscle oxygen consumption is determined primarily by maximal oxygen delivery rather than mitochondrial metabolic rate.[11,12] Muscle mitochondrial oxidative capacity remains tightly coupled with maximal exercise capacity and increases with exercise training.[13] At the onset of submaximal exercise, skeletal muscle rapidly extracts oxygen from hemoglobin, producing deoxyhemoglobin.[14] The kinetics of the changes in tissue oxygen uptake are tightly coupled to pulmonary oxygen consumption to maintain a balance between oxygen delivery and oxygen utilization. In PAD, arterial occlusions limit the increase in blood flow during exercise. Resting blood flow is impaired only in the more severe manifestation of PAD—critical leg ischemia. The determinants of blood flow and oxygen delivery are described subsequently.

Determinants of Large Vessel Flow

At any given systemic blood pressure, the major determinant of flow velocity in a normal regional circulation is the peripheral resistance of the vascular bed that is supplied by the major conduit vessels. This basic relationship can be expressed as

$$\text{flow} = \text{pressure} \div \text{resistance}$$

In healthy subjects, exercise is a major stimulus for vasodilation with a decrease in peripheral resistance, which when combined with an increase in systemic pressure results in a large increase in arterial flow. Normal arteries have the capacity to support large volumetric increases in blood flow without a significant drop in pressure across the large and medium conduit vessels (Fig. 15-1). In contrast, the arterial occlusive disease process in PAD places fixed resistance elements into the circulation, and thus initiates the multiple pathophysiologic processes that manifest clinically as claudication in patients with PAD (see Fig. 15-1). The major factors that determine the pressure drop across a stenosis with arterial disease include blood flow and the resistance induced in the circulation by the stenosis which is defined by the length and internal radius of the stenosis, and blood viscosity. These parameters have been classically described by the Poiseuille equation defining the relationships between resistance, pressure, and flow

$$\text{Pressure drop across stenosis} = \text{flow}\left[8L\eta\right] \div \pi r^4$$

Where L = length of stenosis, r = internal radius, and η= viscosity.

This equation makes clear that the radius or cross-sectional area of the stenosis is the dominant factor in determining the drop in pressure and flow across a

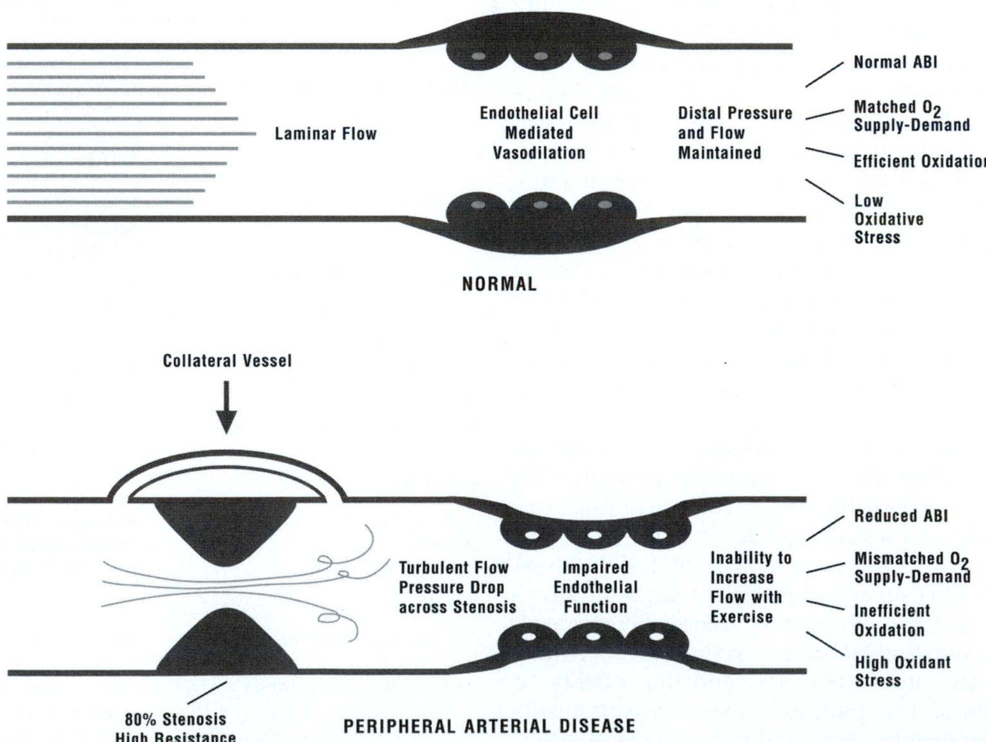

FIGURE 15-1. Normal arterial function. In healthy arteries (*top*) flow is laminar and endothelial function is normal. Therefore, blood flow and oxygen delivery match muscle metabolic demand at rest and exercise. Muscle metabolism is efficient, resulting in low oxidative stress. In contrast, in peripheral arterial disease (*bottom*) the arterial stenosis results in turbulent flow. The loss of kinetic energy results in a pressure drop across the stenosis. Collateral vessels are of high resistance and only partially compensate for the arterial stenosis. In addition, endothelial function is impaired resulting in further loss of vascular function. These changes limit the blood flow response to exercise, resulting in a mismatch of oxygen delivery to muscle metabolic demand. Changes in skeletal muscle metabolism further compromise the efficient generation of high energy phosphates. Oxidant stress—the result of inefficient oxidation—further impairs endothelial function and muscle metabolism.

stenosis because a 50% reduction in the cross-sectional diameter of the vessel results in a 16-fold increase in resistance of the stenosis. In addition, dissipation of energy occurs as blood flow traverses a stenosis that is, in part, determined by the morphology of the stenosis and blood viscosity.[15] The resultant pressure drop is easily quantified and diagnosed clinically with use of the ankle-brachial index (ABI), which defines the ratio of blood pressures in the ankle and the arm.[16] Whereas the ABI is approximately 1.10 in healthy subjects, it is below 0.90 in patients with PAD.[17]

In PAD, a common angiographic finding is multilevel disease. For example, a patient with mild claudication may have only an iliac artery stenosis, but a patient with moderately severe claudication could have occlusive disease in the iliac and femoral or popliteal circulations. Patients with critical leg ischemia almost always have disease affecting multiple arterial segments such as the iliac, femoral, and tibial vessels. Based on the Poiseuille's equation, increases in length of an individual stenosis will not have a major impact on blood flow and pressure drop. Nevertheless, the hemodynamic effect of two equivalent lesions in series is double that of a single lesion.[18] Thus, several individual noncritical stenoses may become hemodynamically significant when combined in series in the same limb.[18,19] Similarly, the systemic nature of the atherosclerosis means that these patients develop multiple localized arterial lesions, increasing the number of muscle beds affected, and limiting alternate conduits for blood flow.

The hemodynamic significance of an arterial stenosis is not only a function of the percent stenosis, but also linear flow velocity across the lesion.[20,21] For example, resting blood flow velocity in the femoral artery may be as low as 10 to 20 cm/second, corresponding to a downstream calf blood flow of 1 to 2 ml/100 ml/minute.[22] When a large vessel stenosis is imposed into the system at this resting flow velocity, any loss of kinetic energy across the stenosis does not initially perturb distal flow because of a compensatory decrease in peripheral resistance. This would, in fact, result in an increase in linear flow velocity at the point of maximal stenosis to maintain a constant volumetric flow to the tissue. Once the stenosis becomes greater than 90% occlusive, changes in peripheral resistance can no longer compensate and then distal flow rapidly decreases to zero with increasing degrees of stenosis from 90% to 100%. In this example, the critical arterial stenosis needed to reduce distal blood flow is 90%. With exercise in the normal extremity, flow velocity may increase to 150 cm/second resulting in a calf flow of 15 ml/100 ml/minute.[22] At these higher flow velocities, an arterial stenosis of only 50% could be hemodynamically significant, where laminar flow is lost and there is an apparent increase in resistance across the stenosis due to turbulent flow. These changes result in a relative decrease in distal flow delivery at a stenosis greater than 50%, whereas the same lesion would not decrease distal flow or pressure at rest. These hemodynamic parameters have clinical significance. For example, in a patient with a single iliac stenosis of 50%, the calf blood flow, pulse examination, and ankle-brachial index may be normal at rest. However, when flow velocity increases with exercise, the same iliac lesion becomes hemodynamically significant, resulting in a loss of pedal pulses due to the decrease in ankle pressure distal to the stenosis. The decrease in the ankle pressure with exercise reflects the fact that the exercise-induced demand for increase in flow is limited by the arterial stenosis and therefore cannot match the fall in peripheral resistance, so pressure must decrease. With exercise, the increase in flow velocity crossing the critical arterial stenosis further worsens the hemodynamic changes.

Blood Flow Response to Exercise in Intermittent Claudication

At rest, patients with claudication have no ischemic leg symptoms. This is because blood flow and leg oxygen consumption tend to be normal and well matched.[23-25] Importantly, at the onset of leg exercise, patients with PAD demonstrate a normal initial rise in leg blood flow and leg oxygen consumption.[23-26] With a graded increase in exercise intensity, there is an initial linear increase in flow. As exercise intensity increases, blood flow reaches a plateau that is limited by the arterial obstructions. The severity of the arterial disease (defined by the ABI) is correlated to the maximal increase in flow.[27] Following the cessation of exercise, the hyperemic phase (increased flow over resting levels) is prolonged in PAD relative to healthy controls. Despite the plateau in oxygen delivery during exercise, further increases in oxidative work output are supported by increased muscle oxygen extraction.[28] Nonoxidative ATP production also contributes to the muscle energy requirements.[29] Importantly, muscle ischemia is not simply related to the lack of increase in blood flow, but rather to the resultant mismatch between the demands for bioenergetics and the flow supply (see Fig. 15-1).

Although arterial flow limitations are of critical importance in the pathophysiology of claudication, the hemodynamic status of the limb is poorly correlated with exercise performance. Most studies have shown that resting ankle blood pressure (or ABI) and exercise blood flow do not predict treadmill walking time,[25,26,30] whereas other studies have shown a weak positive correlation.[31-33] This lack of consistent relationship between ABI and claudication-limited exercise capacity is surprising—especially given the relationship between ABI and exercise-induced peak blood flow. Thus, factors distal to the arterial obstruction likely contribute to the functional limitations in PAD.

Endothelial Regulation of Flow

Blood flow to skeletal muscle is also determined by endothelial and microcirculatory factors (see Fig. 15-1). Nitric oxide is central to the physiologic regulation of arteriolar tone and to a lesser degree contributes to the regulation of the hyperemic response to exercise. However, nitric oxide and prostaglandins are major determinates of the increase in blood flow and its optimal distribution during exercise in normal subjects.[34,35,36] Patients with atherosclerosis have a systemic abnormality in endothelial function that is associated with impaired vasodilation and enhanced platelet aggregation.[37,38] The primary mediator of endothelial injury is felt to be oxidant stress from the generation of superoxide anion.[39,40]

Consistent with the above, abnormalities in endothelium-dependent vasodilation have been observed in PAD.[41] Thus, altered oxygen delivery to exercising skeletal muscle in PAD is related not only to the large vessel occlusive process, but also to endothelial dysfunction, which is not just localized to the ischemic limb, but is systemic in nature.

Rheology and Hemodynamics in Peripheral Arterial Disease

Blood flow in large arteries is, in part, a function of viscosity, as described by the Poiseuille's equation (see earlier). Systemic abnormalities in blood rheology and blood viscosity have been described in PAD. For example, patients with PAD have increased blood concentrations of fibrinogen, von Willebrand factor, and plasminogen activator inhibitor—as well as fibrin turnover.[42-44] These changes may also affect blood flow characteristics in the microcirculation, but none of these factors has been directly correlated with claudication-limited exercise performance.

CHANGES IN MUSCLE STRUCTURE AND FUNCTION IN PERIPHERAL ARTERIAL DISEASE

In healthy humans, exercise requires a coordinated recruitment of appropriate muscle fiber types to meet the demands of specific exercise conditions. With low intensity, repetitive contractions, there is a recruitment of type I oxidative, slow twitch fibers that have high mitochondrial content. Depending on the exercise intensity, the fuel sources are a balance of fat and carbohydrate oxidation. In contrast, rapid, forceful muscle contractions require the recruitment of type II, glycolytic, fast twitch fibers. These fibers have fewer mitochondria than type I fibers, and have easy fatigability. Type II fibers have two subtypes: IIa fibers demonstrate intermediate oxidative and contractile properties and type IIb fibers have the greatest capacity for force generation.

Patients with PAD develop several histologic abnormalities in their skeletal muscle. Muscle biopsy studies have shown a decrease in type II, fast twitch fiber area that is associated with muscle weakness.[45] These observations have been extended to patients with critical leg ischemia where decreases in skeletal muscle myosin isoforms for types IIa and IIb fibers were observed.[46]

Skeletal muscle from patients with claudication also demonstrates extensive denervation using histologic criteria. The denervation injury has been confirmed by electrophysiologic testing, and these abnormalities are progressive over time.[47] These changes in skeletal muscle fiber type and neurologic function are correlated with a decrease in muscle strength.

Several gait abnormalities have also been described in claudication.[48] The findings are primarily of a slowed walking speed due to decreased step length and cadence. Gait stability is also favored over walking speed. Whether these gait abnormalities are related to the muscle denervation and weakness are unknown. These observations may explain, in part, why the reduced exercise performance in a patient with claudication cannot be entirely explained by alterations in limb blood flow and pressure.

In addition to changes in muscle fibers, muscle capillarity is increased in skeletal muscle from patients with PAD.[49] If the capillary architecture is normal, this suggests that distal diffusion is not limiting for oxygen delivery in PAD. The increased capillarity may be in compensation for the reduction in large vessel blood flow, and these changes in peripheral diffusion (higher conductance) may have functional relevance.[50]

OXIDATIVE INJURY IN PERIPHERAL ARTERIAL DISEASE

Animal models have shown that both ischemia, and ischemia-reperfusion, are associated with oxidative stress due to the production of free radicals.[51,52] Patients with claudication do not deliver sufficient oxygen to exercising muscle and have a prolonged hyperemic phase with recovery from exercise.[53] Muscle ischemia during exercise and reperfusion after claudication-limited exercise are associated with an increase in oxidant stress.[54,55] For example, blood levels of malondialdehyde (a marker of free radical generation) are elevated at rest in PAD, and increase further with exercise.[54,56] These patients also have systemic evidence of neutrophil and platelet activation, and endothelial injury.[57-61] The oxidative stress observed in PAD may be part of a broad spectrum of inflammatory responses to systemic atherosclerosis and enhanced by exercise in PAD.[62]

The production of oxygen-free radicals may be a unifying mechanism of skeletal muscle injury in PAD (Fig. 15-2). Repeated episodes of ischemia during exercise, and reperfusion during recovery, may promote oxidant injury to endothelial cells, muscle mitochondria, muscle fibers, and distal motor axons. Oxidative injury to these tissues may, in turn, promote the chronic changes in muscle structure and metabolism leading to loss of function in PAD that cannot be explained simply by a reduction in blood flow and oxygen delivery.

Mitochondria are the major source of free radicals within the cell and, therefore, mitochondrial DNA is an important marker of oxidant injury.[63-65] Muscle mitochondrial oxidative damage in patients with PAD is readily demonstrated as the accumulation of somatic mutations in mitochondrial DNA. For example, patients with PAD have an increased frequency of a mitochondrial DNA 4977 bp deletion mutation.[66] This is a common finding in other tissues under conditions of oxidative stress. More importantly, muscle mitochondria from patients with PAD have specific defects in key steps of the electron transport chain (see Fig. 15-2). These steps have been previously identified as targets of oxidative injury in myocardial perfusion-reperfusion models.[67] Mitochondrial oxidative injury may represent a positive feedback system, as electron transport chain impairment increases mitochondrial free radical production, which

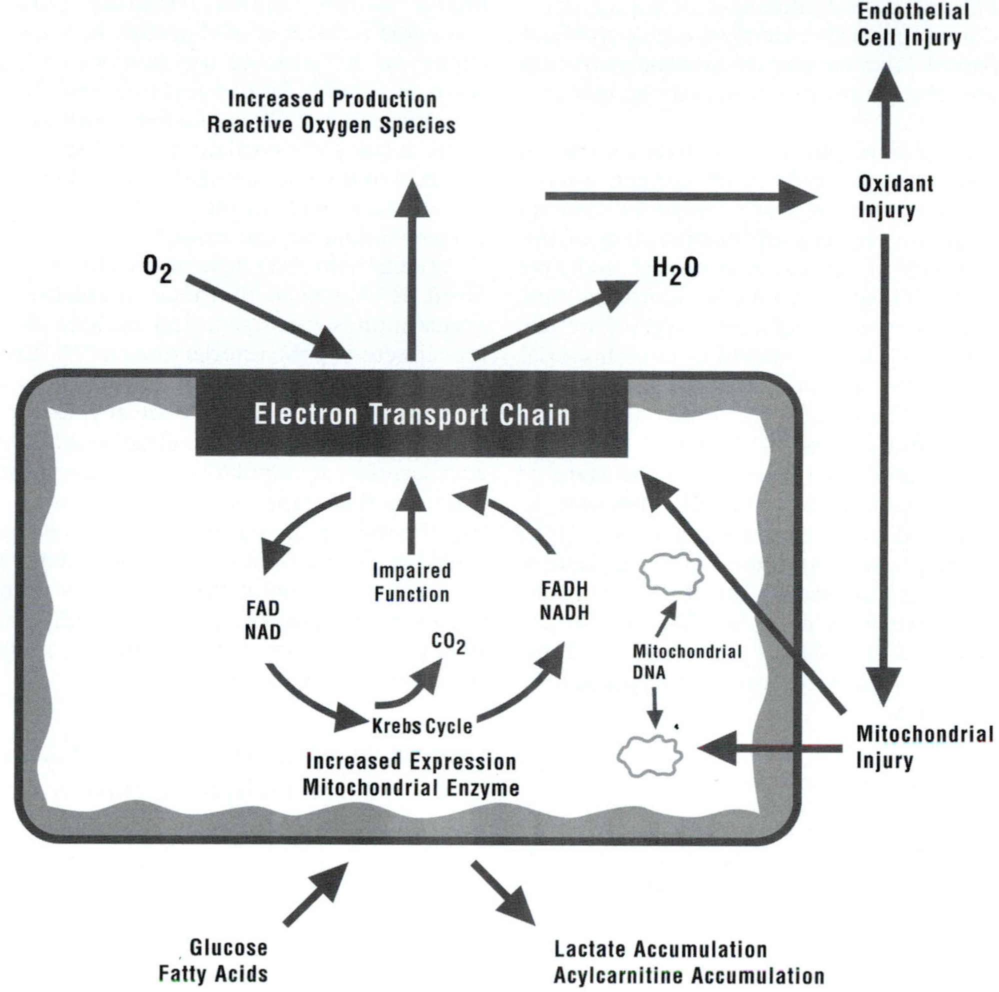

FIGURE 15-2. Alterations in muscle metabolism in peripheral arterial disease. Oxidant stress results in endothelial and mitochondrial injuries that cause mitochondrial DNA deletions and impairment of electron transport chain function. The sequelae are an increase in expression of mitochondrial enzymes and accumulation of lactate and acylcarnitines.

results in more electron transport dysfunction.[68] Such mechanisms may eventually result in cell loss due to apoptosis.[69,70]

Strategies to reduce or modulate the oxidant stress may be important to prevent not only atherosclerotic disease progression, but also to protect skeletal muscle from oxidant injury. Supplementation with the antioxidant vitamin C has been shown to improve endothelial function in patients with diabetes.[71] However, long-term administration of vitamins C and E did not improve endothelial function in patients with cardiovascular disease.[72] In animals, ischemia-reperfusion injury of skeletal muscle (defined as microvascular vasoconstriction and plugging and inhibition of nitric oxide production) could be prevented by a combination of antioxidant vitamins and L-arginine.[73] Important challenges remain concerning the development of antioxidant therapy. A relevant antioxidant should target specific subcellular locations (for example mitochondria) and must not be capable of propagating oxidative injury. Thus, it remains unclear how oxidant stress can be optimally modulated in PAD, or if antioxidants will favorably alter the pathophysiology of claudication.

SKELETAL MUSCLE METABOLISM AND CLAUDICATION

When patients with PAD exercise, skeletal muscle blood flow is insufficient to meet metabolic demand as described. This limitation in the blood flow response to exercise has metabolic consequences. In persons with PAD, muscle oxygen saturation and phosphocreatine levels are normal at rest, but at the onset of exercise, oxygen saturation decreases to very low levels and phosphocreatine is used preferentially compared with control subjects at equivalent exercise work loads.[53] The hemodynamic limitations are also correlated with a slowed resynthesis of phosphocreatine during the recovery phase from exercise. These metabolic changes would be expected simply from a reduced oxygen supply from the arterial disease.

Patients with PAD also have changes in oxidative metabolism that appear intrinsic to the skeletal muscle. A potential site of impairment of oxidative metabolism in PAD is the electron transport chain, which is vulnerable to free radical injury.[74] Skeletal muscle from legs affected by PAD had a reduced activity of mitochondrial NADH dehydrogenase of complex I and ubiquinol-cytochrome c oxidoreductase (complex III).[75] These observations suggest that electron transport chain activity is impaired due to the ischemia-reperfusion injury in PAD, and may contribute to metabolic dysfunction in PAD.

Altered mitochondrial respiration may have functional consequences. For example, pulmonary oxygen uptake kinetics are slowed at the onset of exercise in patients with PAD.[5] The kinetic changes are independent of the hemodynamic severity of the vascular disease and may thus relate to the muscle metabolic abnormalities. Consistent with the slowed ventilatory oxygen kinetics, patients with PAD have altered control of mitochondrial respiration. A number of investigators have used ^{31}P-MRS to evaluate the control of respiration in the muscle of control subjects and patients with PAD.[76] Using the muscle ADP concentration as a marker of the state of mitochondrial respiration, mitochondrial function in PAD was characterized by an increased level of ADP to maintain cellular respiration. An altered ADP-respiratory control relationship is unusual in human chronic diseases, but is characteristic of inherited disorders of the electron transport chain.[76] Given these observations, PAD muscle energetics cannot entirely be explained by the reduced blood flow.

Mitochondrial Expression

Muscle mitochondrial content and mitochondrial enzyme activities reflect the functional state of the individual. Skeletal muscle mitochondrial oxidative enzyme activities increase with exercise training and decrease with prolonged bed rest or inactivity.[77,78] In healthy subjects, muscle mitochondrial content is positively correlated with peak oxygen uptake, indicating the importance of muscle oxidative capacity in determining the exercise performance of the individual.[79] In PAD, the marked limitation in walking activity and resultant sedentary behavior, would be expected to result in a decrease in muscle mitochondrial enzyme content and activity (detraining). In contrast, several studies have shown an increased mitochondrial content in muscle of patients with PAD.[80-82] This increased mitochondrial expression appears to be a direct consequence of, and is proportionate to, the severity of the occlusive disease as assessed by leg hemodynamics.[80] Thus, alterations in skeletal muscle mitochondria in PAD appear to reflect the severity of the underlying occlusive disease process. An increased mitochondrial content might improve oxygen extraction under ischemic conditions, or could reflect a compensatory mechanism for any intrinsic abnormality in mitochondrial oxidative capacity. Interestingly, increased mitochondrial expression is also associated with inherited disorders of mitochondrial electron transport, suggesting a mechanistic and functional link with the acquired disorder in PAD discussed earlier.[83]

Accumulation of Metabolic Intermediates

During normal metabolic conditions, fuel substrates such as fatty acids, protein, and carbohydrates are converted to acyl-CoA intermediates for oxidative metabolism in the Krebs cycle. These coenzyme A-coupled intermediates are linked to the cellular carnitine pool through the reversible transfer of acyl groups between carnitine and coenzyme A.[84] One of the functions of carnitine is to serve as a buffer for the acyl-CoA pool by the formation of acylcarnitines. Thus, during conditions of metabolic stress, incomplete oxidation or utilization of an acyl-CoA will lead to their accumulation. Transfer of the acyl group to carnitine will result in the accumulation of the corresponding acylcarnitine.[85]

Patients with PAD have alterations in carnitine metabolism, as evidenced by the accumulation of short-chain acylcarnitines in plasma and skeletal muscle from the legs affected by the arterial disease.[6,86] This accumulation of acylcarnitines implies that acyl-CoA is not being efficiently oxidized, given that the acyl-CoA pool is in equilibrium with the acylcarnitine pool. Importantly, the acylcarnitine accumulation may have functional significance in that patients with the greatest accumulation had the most reduced treadmill exercise performance.[86] Thus, the degree of metabolic abnormality (as defined by acylcarnitine accumulation) is a better predictor of treadmill exercise performance than the ABI, emphasizing the importance of altered skeletal muscle metabolism in the pathophysiology of claudication.

Impact of Metabolic Agents, Carnitine, and Pyruvate Dehydrogenase Modifiers

Ranolazine, dichloroacetate, glucose-insulin-potassium solutions, L-carnitine, and propionyl-L-carnitine alter ischemic muscle metabolism by shifting the balance of fuels oxidized from fatty acids toward glucose.[87] This metabolic shift is associated with an improvement in the ratio of adenosine triphosphate (ATP) production to oxygen used, which is advantageous when oxygen is limiting. A recent study demonstrated that ranolazine improved exercise performance in patients with angina, in many respects a cardiac equivalent to claudication, without any changes in systemic hemodynamics.[88] Orally administered L-carnitine and propionyl-L-carnitine may have metabolic benefits by providing an additional source of carnitine to buffer the cellular acyl CoA pool. In this way, carnitine may enhance glucose oxidation under ischemic conditions.[89] Propionyl-CoA generated from propionyl-L-carnitine may also improve oxidative metabolism through its anaplerotic actions in priming the Krebs cycle secondary to succinyl-CoA production. Propionyl-L-carnitine has been shown to improve treadmill performance and quality of life in patients with claudication.[90,91]

The observed effects of these metabolic modifiers in PAD provide clinical evidence that alterations in muscle metabolism have functional importance, and they contribute to the pathophysiology of claudication. Treatment with metabolic agents that do not alter systemic or local hemodynamics, can improve the clinical and functional status of the patient.

MECHANISM OF BENEFIT OF EXERCISE TRAINING

Exercise training is an important treatment for claudication.[92] A rigorous, supervised program of treadmill-based walking exercise can induce a training response characterized by large improvements in treadmill exercise performance, peak oxygen consumption, and quality of life. The benefits and mechanisms of improvement have been reviewed.[92] Possible mechanisms underlying the training response in PAD include improvements in endothelial vasodilator function, skeletal muscle metabolism, blood viscosity, and a reduction in systemic inflammation.[92] Exercise training may also improve leg blood flow and oxygen delivery, but the observed changes are inconsistent and not generally correlated with the training response. In addition to hemodynamic and metabolic mechanisms, improvements in the biomechanics of walking also contribute to increased walking ability by decreasing the oxygen requirements to sustain a given level of constant load exercise.[93] The clinical response also appears to be specific to the type of exercise used in the training program. A training regimen based on treadmill walking produces greater functional improvements when compared with strength training.[93]

Exercise training can be related to the metabolic alterations in PAD detailed earlier. Physical training is an important modifier of mitochondrial expression and can thus change the intracellular environment resulting from the demands of exercise. Improved metabolic function may be a final common mechanism for the diverse responses induced by training. Consistent with this concept, training of PAD subjects is associated with decreases in plasma and muscle acylcarnitine contents that are related to the magnitude of exercise improvement derived from the training.[82] A metabolic component to the training benefit also is consistent with the greater impact of aerobic training as compared with strength training.[93]

Thus, progressive walking exercise addresses many aspects of the nonhemodynamic components of the pathophysiology of claudication. That the benefit of exercise training is as effective in improving exercise performance as a successful revascularization, provides further evidence that the components of the pathophysiology of claudication that are not directly related to large vessel hemodynamics contribute significantly to the functional limitations in these patients.[94]

CONCLUSIONS

Patients with PAD and claudication have a profound limitation in their exercise performance. The large vessel obstructions impair the delivery of oxygenated blood to skeletal muscle during exercise resulting in a supply-demand mismatch. Arterial hemodynamics and large vessel blood flow, however, do not fully account for the exercise limitations observed in patients with claudication. Changes in the microcirculation, and skeletal muscle structure and metabolic function significantly contribute to the disease pathophysiology. Understanding these multiple components of exercise limitation provides insight into treatment approaches that address the spectrum of abnormalities seen in patients with claudication.

REFERENCES

1. Ness J, Aronow WS: Prevalence of coexistence of coronary artery disease, ischemic stroke, and peripheral arterial disease in older persons, mean age 80 years, in an academic hospital-based geriatrics practice. J Am Geriatr Soc 47:1255, 1999.
2. Hertzer NR, Beven EG, Young JR, et al: Coronary artery disease in peripheral vascular patients: A classification of 1000 coronary angiograms and results of surgical management. Ann Surg 199:223, 1984.
3. Libby P: Vascular biology of atherosclerosis: Overview and state of the art. Am J Cardiol 91:3A, 2003.
4. Geng YJ, Libby P: Progression of atheroma: A struggle between death and procreation. Arterioscler Thromb Vasc Biol 22:1370, 2002.
5. Bauer TA, Regensteiner JG, Brass EP, Hiatt WR: Oxygen uptake kinetics during exercise are slowed in patients with peripheral arterial disease. J Appl Physiol 87:809, 1999.
6. Hiatt WR, Nawaz D, Brass EP: Carnitine metabolism during exercise in patients with peripheral vascular disease. J Appl Physiol 62:2383, 1987.
7. McDermott MM, Greenland P, Liu K, et al: Leg symptoms in peripheral arterial disease: Associated clinical characteristics and functional impairment. JAMA 286:1599, 2001.
8. Criqui MH, Fronek A, Klauber MR, et al: The sensitivity, specificity, and predictive value of traditional clinical evaluation of peripheral arterial disease: Results from noninvasive testing in a defined population. Circulation 71:516, 1985.
9. McDermott MM, Mehta S, Liu K, et al: Leg symptoms, the ankle-brachial index, and walking ability in patients with peripheral arterial disease. J Gen Intern Med 14:173, 1999.
10. Vogt MT, Cauley JA, Kuller LH, Nevitt MC: Functional status and mobility among elderly women with lower extremity arterial disease: The study of osteoporotic fractures. J Am Geriatr Soc 42:923, 1994.
11. Richardson RS, Grassi B, Gavin TP, et al: Evidence of O_2 supply-dependent VO_2 max in the exercise-trained human quadriceps. J Appl Physiol 86:1048, 1999.
12. Richardson RS, Leigh JS, Wagner PD, Noyszewski EA: Cellular PO_2 as a determinant of maximal mitochondrial O(2) consumption in trained human skeletal muscle. J Appl Physiol 87:325, 1999.
13. Rasmussen UF, Rasmussen HN, Krustrup P, et al: Aerobic metabolism of human quadriceps muscle: In vivo data parallel measurements on isolated mitochondria. Am J Physiol Endocrinol Metab 280:E301, 2001.
14. Grassi B, Pogliaghi S, Rampichini S, et al: Muscle oxygenation and pulmonary gas exchange kinetics during cycling exercise on-transitions in humans. J Appl Physiol 95:149-158, 2003.
15. Young DF, Tsai FY: Flow characteristics in models of arterial stenoses. II. Unsteady flow. J Biomech 6:547, 1973.
16. Carter SA: Clinical measurement of systolic pressures in limbs with arterial occlusive disease. JAMA 207:1869, 1969.
17. Hiatt WR, Hoag S, Hamman RF: Effect of diagnostic criteria on the prevalence of peripheral arterial disease: The San Luis Valley diabetes study. Circulation 91:1472, 1995.
18. Flanigan DP, Tullis JP, Streeter VL, et al: Multiple subcritical arterial stenoses: Effect on poststenotic pressure and flow. Ann Surg 186:663, 1977.
19. Karayannacos PE, Talukder N, Nerem RM, et al: The role of multiple noncritical arterial stenoses in the pathogenesis of ischemia. J Thorac Cardiovasc Surg 73:458, 1977.
20. Young DF, Cholvin NR, Kirkeeide RL, Roth AC: Hemodynamics of arterial stenoses at elevated flow rates. Circ Res 41:99, 1977.
21. Demer L, Gould KL, Kirkeeide R: Assessing stenosis severity: Coronary flow reserve, collateral function, quantitative coronary arteriography, positron imaging, and digital subtraction angiography: A review and analysis. Prog Cardiovasc Dis 30:307, 1988.
22. Lewis P, Psaila JV, Morgan RH, et al: Common femoral artery volume flow in peripheral vascular disease. Br J Surg 77:183, 1990.
23. Pentecost BL: The effect of exercise on the external iliac vein blood flow and local oxygen consumption in normal subjects, and in those with occlusive arterial disease. Clin Sci 27:437, 2003.
24. Hlavova J, Linhart J, Prerovsky I, et al: Leg blood flow at rest, during and after exercise in normal subjects and in patients with femoral artery occlusion. Clin Sci 29:555, 1965.

25. Hillestad LK: The peripheral blood flow in intermittent claudication IV: The significance of the claudication distance. Acta Med Scand 173:467, 2003.
26. Folse R: Alterations in femoral blood flow and resistance during rhythmic exercise and sustained muscular contractions in patients with arteriosclerosis. Surg Gynecol Obstet 121:767, 1965.
27. Sumner DS, Strandness DE, Jr: The relationship between calf blood flow and ankle blood pressure in patients with intermittent claudication. Surgery 65:763, 1969.
28. Maass U, Alexander K: Effect of treadmill exercise on blood gases and acid-base balance in patients with intermittent claudication. Z Kardiol 72:537, 1983.
29. Hansen JE, Sue DY, Oren A, Wasserman K: Relation of oxygen uptake to work rate in normal men and men with circulatory disorders. Am J Cardiol 59:669, 1987.
30. Pernow B, Zetterquist S: Metabolic evaluation of the leg blood flow in claudicating patients with arterial obstructions at different levels. Scand J Clin Lab Invest 21:277, 1968.
31. Sorlie D, Myhre K: Lower leg blood flow in intermittent claudication. Scand J Clin Lab Invest 38:171-179, 1978.
32. Gardner AW, Ricci MA, Case TD, Pilcher DB: Practical equations to predict claudication pain distances from a graded treadmill test. Vasc Med 1:91-96, 1996.
33. Gardner AW, Skinner JS, Cantwell BW, Smith LK: Prediction of claudication pain from clinical measurements obtained at rest. Med Sci Sports Exerc 24:163-170, 1992.
34. Gordon MB, Jain R, Beckman JA, Creager MA: The contribution of nitric oxide to exercise hyperemia in the human forearm. Vasc Med 7:163-168, 2002.
35. Kinlay S, Creager MA, Fukumoto M, et al: Endothelium-derived nitric oxide regulates arterial elasticity in human arteries in vivo. Hypertension 38:1049, 2001.
36. Boushel R, Langberg H, Gemmer C, et al: Combined inhibition of nitric oxide and prostaglandins reduces human skeletal muscle blood flow during exercise. J Physiol 543:691, 2002.
37. Anderson TJ, Gerhard MD, Meredith IT, et al: Systemic nature of endothelial dysfunction in atherosclerosis. Am J Cardiol 75: 71B-74B, 1995.
38. Lieberman EH, Gerhard MD, Uehata A, et al: Flow-induced vasodilation of the human brachial artery is impaired in patients <40 years of age with coronary artery disease. Am J Cardiol 78:1210, 1996.
39. Ohara Y, Peterson TE, Harrison DG: Hypercholesterolemia increases endothelial superoxide anion production. J Clin Invest 91:2546, 1993.
40. Tsao PS, Buitrago R, Chang H, et al: Effects of diabetes on monocyte-endothelial interactions and endothelial superoxide production in fructose-induced insulin-resistant and hypertensive rats. Circulation 92:A2666, 1995.
41. Liao JK, Bettmann MA, Sandor T, et al: Differential impairment of vasodilator responsiveness of peripheral resistance and conduit vessels in humans with atherosclerosis. Circ Res 68:1027, 1991.
42. Ernst EEW, Matrai A: Intermittent claudication, exercise, and blood rheology. Circulation 76:1110-1114, 1987.
43. Woodburn KR, Lowe GD, Rumley A, et al: Relation of haemostatic, fibrinolytic, and rheological variables to the angiographic extent of peripheral arterial occlusive disease. Int Angiol 14:346, 1995.
44. Ernst EE, Matrai A: Intermittent claudication, exercise, and blood rheology. Circulation 76:1110, 1987.
45. Regensteiner JG, Wolfel EE, Brass EP, et al: Chronic changes in skeletal muscle histology and function in peripheral arterial disease. Circulation 87:413, 1993.
46. Steinacker JM, Opitz-Gress A, Baur S, et al: Expression of myosin heavy chain isoforms in skeletal muscle of patients with peripheral arterial occlusive disease. J Vasc Surg 31:443, 2000.
47. England JD, Ferguson MA, Hiatt WR, Regensteiner JG: Progression of neuropathy in peripheral arterial disease. Muscle Nerve 18:380, 1995.
48. Scherer SA, Bainbridge JS, Hiatt WR, Regensteiner JG: Gait characteristics of patients with claudication. Arch Phys Med Rehabil 79:529, 1998.
49. McGuigan MR, Bronks R, Newton RU, et al: Muscle fiber characteristics in patients with peripheral arterial disease. Med Sci Sports Exerc 33:2016, 2001.
50. Sala E, Noyszewski EA, Campistol JM, et al: Impaired muscle oxygen transfer in patients with chronic renal failure. Am J Physiol Regul Integr Comp Physiol 280:R1240, 2001.
51. Karmazyn M: Ischemic and reperfusion injury in the heart: Cellular mechanisms and pharmacologic interventions. Can J Physiol Pharmacol 69:719, 1991.
52. Turrens JF, Beconi M, Barilla J, et al: Mitochondrial generation of oxygen radicals during reoxygenation of ischemic tissues. Free Radic Res Commun 2:681, 1991.
53. Kemp GJ, Roberts N, Bimson WE, et al: Mitochondrial function and oxygen supply in normal and in chronically ischemic muscle: A combined 31P magnetic resonance spectroscopy and near infrared spectroscopy study in vivo. J Vasc Surg 34:1103, 2001.
54. Hickman P, Harrison DK, Hill A, et al: Exercise in patients with intermittent claudication results in the generation of oxygen derived free radicals and endothelial damage. Adv Exp Med Biol 361:565, 1994.
55. Ciuffetti G, Mercuri M, Mannarino E, et al: Free radical production in peripheral vascular disease: A risk for critical ischaemia? Int Angiol 10:81, 1991.
56. Belch JJ, Mackay IR, Hill A, et al: Oxidative stress is present in atherosclerotic peripheral arterial disease and further increased by diabetes mellitus. Int Angiol 14:385, 1995.
57. Edwards AT, Blann AD, Suarez-Mendez VJ, et al: Systemic responses in patients with intermittent claudication after treadmill exercise. Br J Surg 81:1738, 1994.
58. Edwards AT, Blann AD, Suarez-Mendez VJ, et al: Systemic responses in patients with intermittent claudication after treadmill exercise. Br J Surg 81:1738, 1994.
59. Kirkpatrick UJ, Mossa M, Blann AD, McCollum CN: Repeated exercise induces release of soluble P-selectin in patients with intermittent claudication. Thromb Haemost 78:1338, 1997.
60. Blann AD, Farrell A, Picton A, McCollum CN: Relationship between endothelial cell markers and arterial stenosis in peripheral and carotid artery disease. Thromb Res 97:209, 2000.
61. Edwards AT, Blann AD, Suarez-Mendez VJ, et al: Systemic responses in patients with intermittent claudication after treadmill exercise. Br J Surg 81:1738, 1994.
62. Signorelli SS, Mazzarino MC, Di Pino L, et al: High circulating levels of cytokines (IL-6 and TNF alpha), adhesion molecules (VCAM-1 and ICAM-1) and selectins in patients with peripheral arterial disease at rest and after a treadmill test. Vasc Med 8:15, 2003.
63. Wallace DC: Diseases of the mitochondrial DNA. Annu Rev Biochem 61:1175, 1992.
64. Tritsehler H-J, Meduri R: Mitochondrial DNA alterations as a source of human disorders. Neurology 43:280, 1993.
65. Melov S, Shoffner JM, Kaufman A, Wallace DC: Marked increase in the number and variety of mitochondrial DNA rearrangements in aging human skeletal muscle. Nucleic Acids Res 23:4122, 1995.
66. Bhat HK, Hiatt WR, Hoppel CL, Brass EP: Skeletal muscle mitochondrial DNA injury in patients with unilateral peripheral arterial disease. Circulation 99:807, 1999.
67. Rouslin W, Ranganathan S: Impaired function of mitochondrial electron transfer complex I in canine myocardial ischemia: Loss of flavin mononucleotide. J Mol Cell Cardiol 15:537-542, 1983.
68. Shigenaga MK, Hagen TM, Ames BN: Oxidative damage and mitochondrial decay in aging. Proc Natl Acad Sci U S A 91:10771, 1994.
69. Kumar D, Jugdutt BI: Apoptosis and oxidants in the heart. J Lab Clin Med 142:288, 2003.
70. Sastre J, Pallardo FV, Vina J: The role of mitochondrial oxidative stress in aging. Free Radic Biol Med 35:1, 2003.
71. Ting HH, Timimi FK, Boles KS, et al: Vitamin C improves endothelium-dependent vasodilation in patients with non-insulin-dependent diabetes mellitus. J Clin Invest 97:22, 1996.
72. Kinlay S, Behrendt D, Fang JC, et al: Long-term effect of combined vitamins E and C on coronary and peripheral endothelial function. J Am Coll Cardiol 43:629, 2004.
73. Nanobashvili J, Neumayer C, Fuegl A, et al: Combined L-arginine and antioxidative vitamin treatment mollifies ischemia-reperfusion injury of skeletal muscle. J Vasc Surg 39:868, 2004.
74. Rouslin W: Mitochondrial complexes I, II, III, IV, and V in myocardial ischemia and autolysis. Am J Physiol 244:H743, 1983.
75. Brass EP, Hiatt WR, Gardner AW, Hoppel CL: Decreased NADH dehydrogenase and ubiquinol-cytochrome c oxidoreductase in peripheral arterial disease. Am J Physiol 280:H603, 2001.
76. Kemp GJ, Taylor DJ, Thompson CH, et al: Quantitative analysis by 31P magnetic resonance spectroscopy of abnormal mitochondrial oxidation in skeletal muscle during recovery from exercise. NMR Biomed 6:302, 1993.

77. Holloszy JO, Coyle EF: Adaptations of skeletal muscle to endurance exercise and their metabolic consequences. J Appl Physiol 56:831, 1984.
78. Wibom R, Hultman E, Johansson M, et al: Adaptation of mitochondrial ATP production in human skeletal muscle to endurance training and detraining. J Appl Physiol 73:2004, 1992.
79. Wang H, Hiatt WR, Barstow TJ, Brass EP: Relationships between muscle mitochondrial DNA content, mitochondrial enzyme activity and oxidative capacity in man: Alterations with disease. Eur J Appl Physiol 80:22, 1999.
80. Jansson E, Johansson J, Sylven C, Kaijser L: Calf muscle adaptation in intermittent claudication: Side-differences in muscle metabolic characteristics in patients with unilateral arterial disease. Clin Physiol 8:17, 1988.
81. Lundgren F, Dahllof AG, Schersten T, Bylund-Fellenius AC: Muscle enzyme adaptation in patients with peripheral arterial insufficiency: Spontaneous adaptation, effect of different treatments and consequences on walking performance. Clin Sci 77:485, 1989.
82. Hiatt WR, Regensteiner JG, Wolfel EE, et al: Effect of exercise training on skeletal muscle histology and metabolism in peripheral arterial disease. J Appl Physiol 81:780, 1996.
83. Haller RG, Lewis SF, Estabrook RW, et al: Exercise intolerance, lactic acidosis, and abnormal cardiopulmonary regulation in exercise associated with adult skeletal muscle cytochrome c oxidase deficiency. J Clin Invest 84:155, 1989.
84. Bieber LL: Carnitine. Ann Rev Biochem 57:261, 1988.
85. Brass EP, Hoppel CL: Relationship between acid-soluble carnitine and coenzyme A pools in vivo. Biochem J 190:495, 1980.
86. Hiatt WR, Wolfel EE, Regensteiner JG, Brass EP: Skeletal muscle carnitine metabolism in patients with unilateral peripheral arterial disease. J Appl Physiol 73:346, 1992.
87. Schofield RS, Hill JA: Role of metabolically active drugs in the management of ischemic heart disease. Am J Cardiovasc Drugs 1:23, 2001.
88. Chaitman BR, Pepine CJ, Parker JO, et al: Effects of ranolazine with atenolol, amlodipine, or diltiazem on exercise tolerance and angina frequency in patients with severe chronic angina: A randomized controlled trial. JAMA 291:309, 2004.
89. Broderick TL, Quinney HA, Lopaschuk GD: Carnitine stimulation of glucose oxidation in the fatty acid perfused isolated working rat heart. J Biol Chem 267:3758, 1992.
90. Brevetti G, Perna S, Sabba C, et al: Propionyl-L-carnitine in intermittent claudication: Double-blind, placebo-controlled, dose titration, multicenter study. J Am Coll Cardiol 26:1411-1416, 1995.
91. Hiatt WR, Regensteiner JG, Creager MA, et al: Propionyl-L-carnitine improves exercise performance and functional status in patients with claudication. Am J Med 110:616l, 2001.
92. Stewart KJ, Hiatt WR, Regensteiner JG, Hirsch AT: Exercise training for claudication. N Engl J Med 347:1941, 2002.
93. Hiatt WR, Wolfel EE, Meier RH, Regensteiner JG: Superiority of treadmill walking exercise vs. strength training for patients with peripheral arterial disease: Implications for the mechanism of the training response. Circulation 90:1866, 1994.
94. Lundgren F, Dahllof A, Lundholm K, et al: Intermittent claudication—surgical reconstruction or physical training? A prospective randomized trial of treatment efficiency. Ann Surg 209:346, 1989.

chapter 16

Pathophysiology of Critical Limb Ischemia

Dean Patterson
Jill J. F. Belch

Ischemia of a degree that endangers the limb, or part of it, is known as critical limb ischemia (CLI). CLI occurs when the essential supply of nutrients falls below the cut-off level that will sustain tissue viability. *Chronic CLI,* therefore, refers to patients with "chronic ischemic rest pain, ulcers, or gangrene attributable to objectively proven arterial occlusive disease."[1] The incidence of CLI is 400 to 1000/million per year and one new patient will develop CLI for every 100 patients with peripheral arterial disease (PAD).[1] Hemodynamic measures of PAD associated with CLI include an ankle systolic pressure less than 50 mm Hg in nondiabetic persons or toe systolic pressures less than 30 mm Hg in diabetic persons. Although acute limb ischemia may be due to large vessel thromboembolism, most cases of CLI are the result of the progressive process of atherosclerosis. CLI sometimes can be caused by thromboangiitis obliterans (Buerger's disease) and other vasculitides.

The overall prognosis of patients with CLI is poor. Approximately 12% to 18% of CLI subjects are dead within 6 to 12 months of diagnosis and one third have lost their limb.[2] Thus, only 50% of the patients with CLI will be alive with two limbs 6 to 12 months after diagnosis. Mobility postamputation depends on the level of amputation, but is often limited, with only 22% of patients with an above-knee amputation walking again and 30% being bed bound.[3] This may be due to the diffuse nature of atherothrombosis,[4] such that mobility is limited by angina or stroke, or to the inability of this usually elderly population to acquire the level of fitness required to support the use of an artificial limb.

It is important that the pathophysiology of CLI be understood in order to develop effective treatments and prevent amputation. Many of the risk factors that contribute to CLI are similar to those of intermittent claudication (see Chapter 14). These and additional pathophysiologic processes within the macro- and microcirculations will be reviewed.

SYSTEMIC RISK FACTORS

Chronic CLI is the end result of peripheral atherosclerotic arterial occlusive disease, which is associated with increasing age, hypertension, hypercholesterolemia, cigarette smoking, diabetes, and hyperhomocysteinemia (see Chapter 14).[5,6] These risk factors, alone and in combination, contribute to the progression of symptomatic PAD from intermittent claudication to CLI.

Age

Age is a continuous variable affecting limb outcome. Major amputations are more common in the elderly. In a population with a mean age of 70 years, each year of age increases the risk of having an amputation by 2%, and the risk of not recovering from CLI by about 1%.[7] In a 3-year prospective study in Sweden, 45% of the amputees were at least 80 years old.[8] In a Danish study, the incidence of amputation rose from 0.0003% in persons aged 40 years to 0.23% in persons 80 years old.[9]

Smoking

Cigarette smoking increases both the risk of developing PAD and its progression. The risks associated with smoking apply to all ages and increase with the number of cigarettes smoked.[10] Major amputation is more common among patients with intermittent claudication who are heavy smokers[11] and who continue to smoke[12] than among nonsmokers. The amputation rate is between 11% and 23% in those who continued to smoke, compared with less than 10% in those who were smoking abstinent.[13] There is greater graft failure rate in subjects who smoke.[14] In patients with CLI who have undergone revascularization, graft patency rates are improved and amputation rates are reduced by smoking cessation.

Diabetes

Diabetes is a particularly important risk factor because it is frequently associated with severe PAD and neuropathy.[15] Diabetes adversely modifies the course of PAD and is the commonest cause of nontraumatic amputation, accounting for 45% to 70% of these.[16] Atherosclerosis develops at a younger age in patients with diabetes and progresses rapidly. Moreover, atherosclerosis affects more distal vessels in patients with diabetes; the deep femoral, popliteal, and tibial arteries are frequently affected. Furthermore, the presence of diabetes is associated with poor results following endovascular intervention because distal lesions are less amenable to revascularization.[17] Patients with diabetes and symptomatic PAD have been shown to have greater arterial stiffness than those without symptoms.[18]

Atherosclerosis in distal arteries in combination with diabetic neuropathy contributes to the higher rates of limb loss in diabetic patients with PAD who develop CLI.[19] Thus, these patients have a 10-fold increased rate of amputation compared to patients without diabetes,[20,21] and they tend to have amputations at an earlier age.[22] One study reported the progression of CLI to gangrene to be 40% in diabetic patients compared with 9% in nondiabetic patients.[23] Patients with diabetes who smoke or who have high homocysteine levels have additive risk.[24,25] Patients with diabetes are less likely than nondiabetic patients to recover from CLI.[7]

Lipids and Hypertension

There generally are no specific studies to link dyslipidemia and hypertension to the pathophysiology of CLI. One study reported that decreases in the prevalence of hypertension, over a 9-year period, were associated with reduced rates of lower limb arterial reconstruction and amputation.[26] The role of low-density lipoprotein (LDL) in the pathophysiology of atherosclerosis has been extensively studied in areas other than PAD.[27] There is some evidence that LDL predicts the presence of PAD,[28] but it is not known whether it predicts CLI. Similarly, it is not known whether lipid-lowering therapy prevents CLI or affects limb viability in patients with CLI.

Inflammation and Procoagulant Markers

Inflammation and endogenous procoagulants may be causally related to CLI. High sensitivity C-reactive protein (CRP), a marker of inflammation, may have a direct role in mediating plaque formation, rupture, and thrombosis.[29] CRP increases expression of intercellular and vascular adhesion molecules (ICAM, VCAM), monocyte chemoattractant protein (MCP-1), angiotensin type 1(AT_1) receptor, endothelin, vascular smooth muscle, reactive oxygen species, and endothelial cell apoptosis.[30,31] Also, CRP decreases the activity of endothelial nitric oxide synthase and attenuates angiogenesis.[32] Von Willebrand factor (vWF) may be an index of endothelial damage/dysfunction.[33] Elevated levels of vWF occur in both coronary and peripheral atherosclerotic disease[34] and predict adverse outcome.[35] Tissue factor is a procoagulant that normally is expressed only at extravascular sites and in the adventitial layer of blood vessels. However, raised plasma tissue factor levels, possibly arising from the endothelium and/or monocytes, have been reported in patients with PAD and ischemic heart disease.[36] Elevated levels of tissue factor may be related to endothelial damage and detachment.[37,38] Endothelial detachment exposes the underlying matrix, which, in the presence of increased tissue factor in the circulating blood, leads to hypercoagulability.

Fibrinogen plays a key role in the coagulation cascade and platelet aggregation, and also is a major determinant of plasma viscosity. Each of these properties is important in the pathogenesis of CLI. Fibrinogen is associated with vascular disorders and is linked to endothelial damage.[39] Increasing levels of fibrinogen are associated with a fall in ankle brachial index[40] and the clinical progression to CLI.[41] Fibrinogen, as the precursor of fibrin, may affect the balance between clot formation and dissolution in CLI. Raised plasma levels of D-dimer, an index of intravascular thrombus formation and fibrin turnover, also occur in PAD and may have prognostic relevance in terms of progression to CLI.[42] D-dimer predicts poor results following intravascular interventions.[17]

Hyperhomocysteinemia is associated with atherosclerosis.[43] There is a high incidence of hyperhomocysteinemia in PAD patients with rest pain,[44] notably in younger women.[45,46] Homocysteine adversely affects the endothelium, platelet function, and blood clotting, but at an average level substantially greater than in most PAD patients. Homocysteine levels do not predict outcome in patients with CLI who undergo revascularization procedures.[17]

Elevated levels of isoeicosanoids, potent mediators of numerous homeostatic biologic functions and inflammation, occur in patients with hypercholesterolemia,[47] and in those with unstable angina.[48] Levels are raised in the atherosclerotic plaques of those patients who progress to revascularization procedures.[49] One of these eicosanoids, thromboxane, contributes to platelet activation and vascular smooth muscle contraction[50] and proliferation, and its blockade by aspirin has been demonstrated to reduce the number of ischemic events in subjects with angina.[51,52] The vascular response to thromboxane is increased in the presence of advanced atherosclerosis,[53] a prominent feature of CLI.

Viscosity

Plasma viscosity is increased in CLI and remains raised even after revascularization.[39,54] Plasma viscosity is associated with worsening symptoms of PAD,[55] and may be correlated with its progression to CLI.[56] When coupled with the changes in the blood cell characteristics, these changes result in a further reduction in microcirculatory blood flow.

MACROVASCULAR MECHANISMS

Obstructive vascular disease underpins the pathophysiology of both intermittent claudication and CLI (Fig. 16-1). Blood flow to the limb is increasingly limited by the number and severity of occlusive lesions. Patients with sequential lesions affecting proximal and distal limb arteries are more likely to develop CLI than those with isolated stenosis. Progression of the disease from intermittent claudication to chronic CLI is modulated by collateral vessel development and other compensatory mechanisms. As atherosclerosis progresses, compensatory enlargement of preexisting collateral blood vessels can occur, thus delaying the clinical presentation of CLI. This is usually enough to prevent CLI in patients with occlusive lesions at a single level. Patients with lesions at two or more levels (e.g., aortoiliac and femoral artery occlusive disease) may have CLI, despite seemingly adequate collateral vessels as a result of additive reductions in perfusion pressure imposed by multiple occlusive lesions. Distal obstructions are predictive of a higher amputation rate and likelihood of persistent CLI.[7]

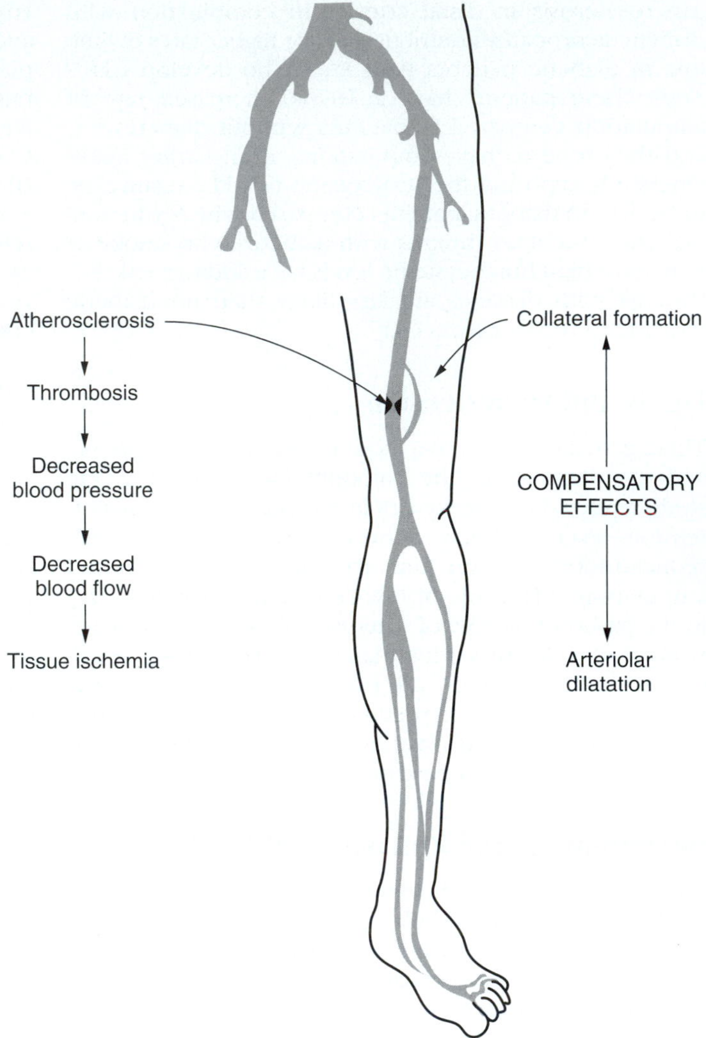

FIGURE 16-1. The macrocirculation in critical limb ischemia. Atherosclerotic plaques, and related thrombotic occlusions, decrease perfusion pressure and blood flow in the limb. If the impaired blood flow is unable to accommodate the metabolic requirements of the tissue—particularly the skin of the foot—pain, ulceration, necrosis and gangrene may ensue. Compensatory mechanisms that modulate the reduction in perfusion pressure and flow include collateral blood vessel development and local autoregulatory phenomena that induce vasodilation in resistance vessels.

In CLI, disease tends to be diffuse with complex atherosclerotic plaque composed of fibrous lesions and calcification. Rupture of unstable plaques, characterized by thin fibrous caps, rich lipid cores that rupture with consequent occlusion of the lumen by a thrombus, occurs in acute coronary syndromes. It is likely, but not proved, that this process occurs in some cases of CLI.[57]

MICROVASCULAR MECHANISMS

The microcirculation contributes to the maintenance of skin integrity. Multiple factors may disturb microcirculatory physiology in CLI, including low intravascular pressure, interstitial and endothelial edema, arteriolar vasospasm, abnormal vasomotion, microthromboses, platelet aggregates, rigid adhesive leukocytes, and blood cell/platelet aggregates (Fig. 16-2).

The microvascular environment in CLI is characterized by reduced capillary density, reduced media-to-lumen ratio in subcutaneous small arteries, and vessel wall thinning (due to remodeling).[58] There is an abnormal contractile response and impaired arteriolar dilation. The responses

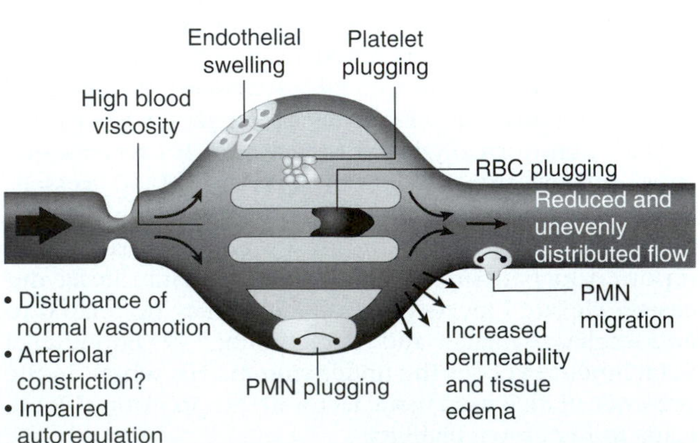

FIGURE 16-2. Microcirculatory mechanisms in critical limb ischemia. Mechanisms that may contribute to impaired microcirculatory blood flow in critical limb ischemia include abnormal vasomotion, endothelial swelling, interstitial edema, microthromboses, red blood cell and leukocyte plugging, and platelet aggregates. PMN, polymorphonuclear; RBC, red blood cells. (From Brevetti G, Corrado S, Marone VD: Microcirculation and tissue metabolism in peripheral arterial disease. Clin Hemorheol Microcirc 21:245, 1999.)

to both endothelium-dependent and endothelium-independent vasodilators specific for guanylate cyclase-mediated responses are altered in CLI.[59] The normal vasoconstrictor response on rising from the supine to the sitting position is diminished in patients with mild arterial disease[60] and is either absent or there is a paradoxic rise in skin perfusion in CLI.[61] This explains, in part, why a patient with CLI is more comfortable with the limb in the dependent position. Dependency, however, favors capillary hypertension and filtration of fluid in excess. The resultant edema, commonly seen in patients with CLI, compresses nutritive capillaries and increases the oxygen diffusion distance, further contributing to the ischemic process. Also, there is a severely altered pattern of skin blood flow assessed by laser Doppler fluxmetry, with reduced prevalence of slow waves and increased prevalence of fast waves, in patients with CLI.[62] Capillary-to-skin transit times are increased in CLI and there is inadequate nutrient delivery.[63] Accumulation and activation of inflammatory cells lead to progressive tissue damage and increased capillary permeability and edema.

In CLI, the endothelium may become swollen and more permeable; cellular junctions are weakened, and intercellular spaces enlarge. Turbulent shear forces acting on these weakened areas lead to endothelial detachment and circulating endothelial cells. The presence of excessive numbers of circulating endothelial cells has been demonstrated in various vascular disease states including CLI.[64,65] Endothelial dysfunction is characterized by decreased nitric oxide bioactivity and increased release of the potent vasoconstrictor, endothelin. Endothelin receptors are over-expressed in the skeletal muscles of CLI patients.[66] Endothelin levels predict death at 3 years in patients with CLI undergoing amputation.[67] Elevated levels of fibroblast growth factor, but not of vascular endothelial growth factor (VEGF) occur in CLI.[68] Dysfunctional endothelium also contributes to a procoagulant state characterized by decreased secretion of tissue plasminogen activator, increased secretion of plasminogen activator inhibitor-1 (PAI-1), activation and increased reactivity of platelets, local production of tissue factor, and exposure of collagen.[69] Elevated von Willebrand factor levels are indicative of endothelial damage.[33] Although current data on this is limited to date, the numbers of circulating endothelial cells seems to be related to serum von Willebrand factor and tissue factor levels.[64]

Thus, once lesions have developed, endothelial dysfunction may exacerbate the development of CLI, by abnormally reducing vascular perfusion, producing factors that decrease plaque stability, and augmenting the thrombotic response to plaque rupture described earlier.[70,71] Inflammation and thrombosis ensues, leading to progressive tissue damage and increased capillary permeability and edema.[63]

The Role of Blood Cells in Critical Limb Ischemia

One prominent feature of CLI is the formation of cellular plugs and microthrombi (see Fig. 16-2). Thrombosis plays a key role in the progression of disease in PAD to CLI.[57] The platelet count and platelet activation are increased in CLI.[39,72] Activated platelets interact with endothelial receptors releasing the potent vasoconstrictor, thromboxane, further promoting vasoconstriction and platelet activation.

Leukocytes play an important role in ischemic disease via the formation of microemboli and induction of oxidative damage.[73] The white cell count predicts patients with CLI who will require future amputation.[74] Leukocyte adhesion is increased in CLI. This may be due to increased endothelial expression of the adhesion molecules, VCAM-1 and E-selectin.[39] These adherent cells further decrease lumen diameter. Activated neutrophils[75] then adhere to other leukocytes and blood cells, which further narrow the vessel lumen, and through release of mediators, increase vessel wall damage. Activated leukocytes found in many vascular diseases are abnormally rigid, potentially exacerbating microvascular occlusion in CLI.[76] In experimental animals with hind limb ischemia, neutrophils activate matrix metalloproteinases, MMP-2 and MMP-9.[77]

The flexibility and deformability of red blood cells are reduced in CLI and may obstruct flow through capillaries.[78,79] Also, red blood cells release ATP when exposed to hypoxic conditions.[80] Activation of P2 receptors on the endothelium may induce vasodilation via release of nitric oxide and prostaglandins.[81,82]

Conclusion

CLI is a state characterized by severe impairment of blood flow to the limb, whereby the metabolic requirements of the tissue are not met. Multiple occlusive lesions of the limb arteries coupled with functional and structural changes in the microcirculation are responsible for inadequate tissue perfusion and the formation of skin ulcers and necrosis. Age, smoking, and diabetes are major risk factors for CLI. Inflammatory mediators and endogenous procoagulants contribute to the development and progression of CLI. Blood components, such as red cells, white cells, and platelets, aggregate and perturb blood flow in the microcirculation. Revascularization procedures are the mainstay of treatment for CLI. Further understanding of the pathophysiologic disturbances that occur in CLI may lead to additional strategies to preserve limb viability and improve symptoms.

REFERENCES

1. Management of peripheral arterial disease (PAD). TransAtlantic Inter-Society Consensus (TASC). Eur J Vasc Endovasc Surg 19 Suppl A:Si, 2000.
2. Criqui MH, Langer RD, Fronek A, et al: Mortality over a period of 10 years in patients with peripheral arterial disease. N Engl J Med 326:381, 1992.
3. Second European Consensus Document on chronic critical leg ischemia. Circulation 84:IV1, 1991.
4. Aronow WS, Ahn C: Prevalence of coexistence of coronary artery disease, peripheral arterial disease, and atherothrombotic brain infarction in men and women ≥62 years of age. Am J Cardiol 74:64, 1994.
5. Tegos TJ, Kalodiki E, Sabetai MM, et al: The genesis of atherosclerosis and risk factors: A review. Angiology 52:89, 2001.
6. Libby P. Vascular biology of atherosclerosis: Overview and state of the art. Am J Cardiol 91:3A, 2003.

7. Bertele V, Roncaglioni C: Predictors of clinical outcome in critical leg ischaemia. Critical Ischaemia 11:93, 2001.
8. Liedberg E, Persson BM: Age, diabetes and smoking in lower limb amputation for arterial occlusive disease. Acta Orthop Scand 54:383, 1983.
9. Eickhoff JH, Hansen HJ, Lorentzen JE: The effect of arterial reconstruction on lower limb amputation rate. An epidemiological survey based on reports from Danish hospitals. Acta Chir Scand Suppl 502:181, 1980.
10. Cronenwett JL, Warner KG, Zelenock GB, et al: Intermittent claudication. Current results of nonoperative management. Arch Surg 119:430, 1984.
11. McGrath MA, Graham AR, Hill DA, et al: The natural history of chronic leg ischemia. World J Surg 7:314, 1983.
12. Jonason T, Ringqvist I: Factors of prognostic importance for subsequent rest pain in patients with intermittent claudication. Acta Med Scand 218:27, 1985.
13. Hirsch AT, Treat-Jacobson D, Lando HA, et al: The role of tobacco cessation, antiplatelet and lipid-lowering therapies in the treatment of peripheral arterial disease. Vasc Med 2:243, 1997.
14. Wiseman S, Powell J, Greenhalgh R, et al: The influence of smoking and plasma factors on prosthetic graft patency. Eur J Vasc Surg 4:57, 1990.
15. Carrington AL, Abbott CA, Griffiths J, et al: Peripheral vascular and nerve function associated with lower limb amputation in people with and without diabetes. Clin Sci (Lond) 101:261, 2001.
16. Diabetes-related amputations of lower extremities in the Medicare population—Minnesota, 1993-1995. MMWR Morb Mortal Wkly Rep 47:649, 1998.
17. Laxdal E, Eide GE, Wirsching J, et al: Homocysteine levels, haemostatic risk factors and patency rates after endovascular treatment of the above-knee femoro-popliteal artery. Eur J Vasc Endovasc Surg 28:410, 2004.
18. Taniwaki H, Shoji T, Emoto M, et al: Femoral artery wall thickness and stiffness in evaluation of peripheral vascular disease in type 2 diabetes mellitus. Atherosclerosis 158:207, 2001.
19. Beckman JA, Creager MA, Libby P: Diabetes and atherosclerosis: Epidemiology, pathophysiology, and management. JAMA 287:2570, 2002.
20. Wrobel JS, Mayfield JA, Reiber GE: Geographic variation of lower-extremity major amputation in individuals with and without diabetes in the Medicare population. Diabetes Care 24:860, 2001.
21. Da Silva A, Widmer LK, Ziegler HW, et al: The Basle longitudinal study: Report on the relation of initial glucose level to baseline ECG abnormalities, peripheral artery disease, and subsequent mortality. J Chronic Dis 32:797, 1979.
22. Hierton T, James U: Lower extremity amputation in Uppsala county 1947-1969. Incidence and prosthetic rehabilitation. Acta Orthop Scand 44:573, 1973.
23. Kannel WB: Risk factors for atherosclerotic cardiovascular outcomes in different arterial territories. J Cardiovasc Risk 1:333, 1994.
24. Ciccarone E, Di Castelnuovo A, Assanelli D, et al: Homocysteine levels are associated with the severity of peripheral arterial disease in Type 2 diabetic patients. J Thromb Haemost 1:2540, 2003.
25. Pell JP, Fowkes FGR: Risk factors for critical limb ischaemia. Epidemiol Update 2:19, 1997.
26. Feinglass J, Brown JL, LoSasso A, et al: Rates of lower-extremity amputation and arterial reconstruction in the United States, 1979 to 1996. Am J Public Health 89:1222, 1999.
27. Cote MC, Ligeti R, Cutler BS, et al: Management of hyperlipidemia in patients with vascular disease. J Vasc Nurs 21:63, 2003.
28. Drexel H, Steurer J, Muntwyler J, et al: Predictors of the presence and extent of peripheral arterial occlusive disease. Circulation 94:II199, 1996.
29. Verma S, Buchanan MR, Anderson TJ: Endothelial function testing as a biomarker of vascular disease. Circulation 108:2054, 2003.
30. Libby P, Ridker PM, Maseri A: Inflammation and atherosclerosis. Circulation 105:1135, 2002.
31. Blake GJ, Ridker PM: Novel clinical markers of vascular wall inflammation. Circ Res 89:763, 2001.
32. Verma S, Wang CH, Li SH, et al: A self-fulfilling prophecy: C-reactive protein attenuates nitric oxide production and inhibits angiogenesis. Circulation 106:913, 2002.
33. Boneu B, Abbal M, Plante J, et al: Letter: Factor-VIII complex and endothelial damage. Lancet 1:1430, 1975.
34. Blann AD, Seigneur M, Steiner M, et al: Circulating endothelial cell markers in peripheral vascular disease: Relationship to the location and extent of atherosclerotic disease. Eur J Clin Invest 27:916, 1997.
35. Thompson SG, Kienast J, Pyke SD, et al: Hemostatic factors and the risk of myocardial infarction or sudden death in patients with angina pectoris. European Concerted Action on Thrombosis and Disabilities Angina Pectoris Study Group. N Engl J Med 332:635, 1995.
36. Falciani M, Gori AM, Fedi S, et al: Elevated tissue factor and tissue factor pathway inhibitor circulating levels in ischaemic heart disease patients. Thromb Haemost 79:495, 1998.
37. Makin AJ, Blann AD, Chung NA, et al: Assessment of endothelial damage in atherosclerotic vascular disease by quantification of circulating endothelial cells. Relationship with von Willebrand factor and tissue factor. Eur Heart J 25:371, 2004.
38. Yang Y, Loscalzo J: Regulation of tissue factor expression in human microvascular endothelial cells by nitric oxide. Circulation 101:2144, 2000.
39. Woodburn KR, Rumley A, Lowe GD, et al: Fibrinogen and markers of fibrinolysis and endothelial damage following resolution of critical limb ischaemia. Eur J Vasc Endovasc Surg 10:272, 1995.
40. Philipp CS, Cisar LA, Kim HC, et al: Association of hemostatic factors with peripheral vascular disease. Am Heart J 134:978, 1997.
41. Koksch M, Zeiger F, Wittig K, et al: Haemostatic derangement in advanced peripheral occlusive arterial disease. Int Angiol 18:256, 1999.
42. Lassila R, Peltonen S, Lepantalo M, et al: Severity of peripheral atherosclerosis is associated with fibrinogen and degradation of cross-linked fibrin. Arterioscler Thromb 13:1738, 1993.
43. Kuller LH, Evans RW: Homocysteine, vitamins, and cardiovascular disease. Circulation 98:196, 1998.
44. Spark JI, Laws P, Fitridge R: The incidence of hyperhomocysteinaemia in vascular patients. Eur J Vasc Endovasc Surg 26:558, 2003.
45. van den Berg M, Stehouwer CD, Bierdrager E, et al: Plasma homocysteine and severity of atherosclerosis in young patients with lower-limb atherosclerotic disease. Arterioscler Thromb Vasc Biol 16:165, 1996.
46. van den Bosch MA, Bloemenkamp DG, Mali WP, et al: Hyperhomocysteinemia and risk for peripheral arterial occlusive disease in young women. J Vasc Surg 38:772, 2003.
47. Reilly MP, Pratico D, Delanty N, et al: Increased formation of distinct F2-isoprostanes in hypercholesterolemia. Circulation 98:2822, 1998.
48. Cipollone F, Ciabattoni G, Patrignani P, et al: Oxidant stress and aspirin-insensitive thromboxane biosynthesis in severe unstable angina. Circulation 102:1007, 2000.
49. Mallat Z, Nakamura T, Ohan J, et al: The relationship of hydroxyeicosatetraenoic acids and F2-isoprostanes to plaque instability in human carotid atherosclerosis. J Clin Invest 103:421, 1999.
50. Yamada T, Fujino T, Yuhki K, et al: Thromboxane A2 regulates vascular tone via its inhibitory effect on the expression of inducible nitric oxide synthase. Circulation 108:2381, 2003.
51. Sachinidis A, Flesch M, Ko Y, et al: Thromboxane A2 and vascular smooth muscle cell proliferation. Hypertension 26:771, 1995.
52. Ikonomidis I, Andreotti F, Nihoyannopoulos P: Reduction of daily life ischaemia by aspirin in patients with angina: Underlying link between thromboxane A2 and macrophage colony-stimulating factor. Heart 90:389, 2004.
53. Lopez JA, Armstrong ML, Piegors DJ, et al: Effect of early and advanced atherosclerosis on vascular responses to serotonin, thromboxane A2, and ADP. Circulation 79:698, 1989.
54. Parsson H, Holmberg A, Siegbahn A, et al: Activation of coagulation and fibrinolytic systems in patients with CLI is not normalized after surgical revascularisation. Eur J Vasc Endovasc Surg 27:186, 2004.
55. Smith FB, Lowe GD, Lee AJ, et al: Smoking, hemorheologic factors, and progression of peripheral arterial disease in patients with claudication. J Vasc Surg 28:129, 1998.
56. Poredos P, Zizek B: Plasma viscosity increase with progression of peripheral arterial atherosclerotic disease. Angiology 47:253, 1996.
57. Makin A, Silverman SH, Lip GY: Peripheral vascular disease and Virchow's triad for thrombogenesis. QJM 95:199, 2002.
58. Jacobs MJ, Ubbink DT, Kitslaar PJ, et al: Assessment of the microcirculation provides additional information in critical limb ischaemia. Eur J Vasc Surg 6:135, 1992.
59. Hillier C, Sayers RD, Watt PA, et al: Altered small artery morphology and reactivity in critical limb ischaemia. Clin Sci (Lond) 96:155, 1999.

60. Eickhoff JH, Engell HC: Changes after arterial reconstruction in the forefoot local vasoconstrictor response to increased venous transmural pressure. Eur J Clin Invest 12:313, 1982.
61. Ubbink DT, Jacobs MJ, Tangelder GJ, et al: Posturally induced microvascular constriction in patients with different stages of leg ischaemia: Effect of local skin heating. Clin Sci (Lond) 81:43, 1991.
62. Rossi M, Carpi A: Skin microcirculation in peripheral arterial obliterative disease. Biomed Pharmacother 58:427, 2004.
63. Anvar MD, Khiabani HZ, Kroese AJ, et al: Alterations in capillary permeability in the lower limb of patients with chronic critical limb ischaemia and oedema. Vasa 29:106, 2000.
64. Makin AJ, Blann AD, Chung NAY, et al: Assessment of endothelial damage in atherosclerotic vascular disease by quantification of circulating endothelial cells: Relationship with von Willebrand factor and tissue factor. Eur Heart J 25:371, 2004.
65. Dignat-George F, Sampol J: Circulating endothelial cells in vascular disorders: New insights into an old concept. Eur J Haematol 65:215, 2000.
66. Tsui JC, Baker DM, Biecker E, et al: Evidence for the involvement of endothelin-1 but not urotensin-II in chronic lower limb ischaemia in man. Eur J Vasc Endovasc Surg 25:443, 2003.
67. Newton DJ, Khan F, McLaren M, et al: Endothelin-1 levels predict 3-year survival in patients who have amputation for critical leg ischaemia. Br J Surg 92:1377, 2005.
68. Palmer-Kazen U, Wariaro D, Luo F, et al: Vascular endothelial cell growth factor and fibroblast growth factor 2 expression in patients with critical limb ischemia. J Vasc Surg 39:621, 2004.
69. Behrendt D, Ganz P: Endothelial function. From vascular biology to clinical applications. Am J Cardiol 90:40L, 2002.
70. Radomski MW, Palmer RM, Moncada S: The role of nitric oxide and cGMP in platelet adhesion to vascular endothelium. Biochem Biophys Res Commun 148:1482, 1987.
71. Diodati JG, Dakak N, Gilligan DM, et al: Effect of atherosclerosis on endothelium-dependent inhibition of platelet activation in humans. Circulation 98:17, 1998.
72. Cassar K, Bachoo P, Ford I, et al: Platelet activation is increased in peripheral arterial disease. J Vasc Surg 38:99, 2003.
73. Ernst E, Hammerschmidt DE, Bagge U, et al: Leukocytes and the risk of ischemic diseases. JAMA 257:2318, 1987.
74. Belch JJ, Sohngen M, Robb R, et al: Neutrophil count and amputation in critical limb ischaemia. Int Angiol 18:140, 1999.
75. Ciuffetti G, Lombardini R, Pasqualini L, et al: Leucocyte-endothelial interactions in chronic critical limb ischaemia. Ann Ital Med Int 11:170, 1996.
76. Belch JJ: The relationship between white blood cells and arterial disease. Curr Opin Lipidol 5:440, 1994.
77. Plitas G, Gagne PJ, Muhs BE, et al: Experimental hindlimb ischemia increases neutrophil-mediated matrix metalloproteinase activity: A potential mechanism for lung injury after limb ischemia. J Am Coll Surg 196:761, 2003.
78. Ambrus JL, Ambrus CM, Taheri SA, et al: Red cell flexibility and platelet aggregation in patients with chronic obstructive vascular disease (COAD) and study of therapeutic approaches. Angiology 35:418, 1984.
79. Cella G, De Haas H, Kakkar VV, et al: Blood viscosity and red cell deformability in peripheral vascular disease. Haematologica 64:611, 1979.
80. Ellsworth ML, Forrester T, Ellis CG, et al: The erythrocyte as a regulator of vascular tone. Am J Physiol 269:H2155, 1995.
81. Wang L, Olivecrona G, Gotberg M, et al: ADP acting on P2Y13 receptors is a negative feedback pathway for ATP release from human red blood cells. Circ Res 96:189, 2005.
82. Gonzalez-Alonso J, Olsen DB, Saltin B: Erythrocyte and the regulation of human skeletal muscle blood flow and oxygen delivery: Role of circulating ATP. Circ Res 91:1046, 2002.

chapter 17

Peripheral Arterial Disease: Clinical Evaluation

Joshua A. Beckman
Mark A. Creager

The least often recognized of the commonly occurring manifestations of atherosclerosis is peripheral arterial disease (PAD). Epidemiological studies suggest that between 8 and 12 million people in the United States have PAD.[1,2] Among 2174 participants aged 40 years and older from the 1999 to 2000 National Health and Nutrition Examination Survey (NHANES), the prevalence of PAD was 4.3%.[2] Put differently, for every four patients in the United States with coronary artery disease, there are three with PAD. Despite its relative frequency, predictable patient population, and prognostic implications for life and limb, many cardiovascular physicians do not undertake the clinical evaluation of PAD. This chapter will focus on the history, physical examination, and diagnostic tests important to the management of limb atherosclerosis.

HISTORY

The diagnosis of PAD begins with clinical suspicion in the typical patient population. This includes avid questioning and seeking to elicit historical evidence of limb and systemic atherosclerosis. Clinical suspicion should be heightened in older persons, in those with coronary or cerebral atherosclerosis, and in patients with atherosclerotic risk factors such as diabetes or tobacco use. PAD is uncommon before the age of 40 years. In a free-living, southern California population, the prevalence of PAD increased from 2.5% among subjects aged 40 to 59 years to 18.8% in subjects aged 70 to 79 years.[3] In the Rotterdam study, the frequency of PAD increased from 9% in patients aged 55 to 59 years to 57% in patients aged 85 to 89 years.[4] Increased rates of PAD have been demonstrated in patients with coronary artery disease, diabetes, and renal failure.[5-7] In an older, hypertensive population participating in the Systolic Hypertension in the Elderly Program (SHEP), the prevalence of PAD was 25% in white men, 38% in black men, 23% in white women, and 41% in black women.[8] In the PAD Awareness, Risk, and Treatment: New Resources for Survival (PARTNERS) program, a study of 6979 patients in 350 primary care practices across the United States, ankle brachial index (ABI) screening was performed in subjects older than age 70, or older than age 50 if they were smokers or had diabetes.[9] In this primary care population, 29% of those screened with an ABI met the criteria for PAD.

Despite the relative frequency of disease, the diagnosis of PAD is not often considered because the majority of patients with PAD are asymptomatic. Indeed, in the Edinburgh Artery Study (a cross-sectional survey of 1592 men and women aged 55 to 74 years), the prevalence of PAD was 21.5%, but only 4.5% of the subjects had symptoms.[10] Similarly, in the PARTNERS program, only 11% of the PAD patients had classic symptoms.[9] Similar data have been reported in other large cross-sectional studies.[11,12] Even in high-risk subgroups with a higher population frequency of PAD, the diagnosis may be missed because PAD is often asymptomatic. The decision to look for PAD in the outpatient should be predicated on the pretest probability of finding it. The application of the PARTNERS criteria, for example, demonstrated the importance of risk factors in enriching the population with PAD to make ABI screening worthwhile. Thus, the presence of risk factors for atherosclerosis should lower the threshold for routine screening.

Cigarette smoking may be the most potent of the classic risk factors to promote the development of PAD (Table 17-1). Large epidemiologic studies have demonstrated an increase in the risk of both asymptomatic and symptomatic PAD, ranging between 1.7- and 5.6-fold compared with nonsmokers.[4,13-18] In the Rotterdam study, male smokers had a 1.7-fold increased risk and female smokers had a 1.2-fold increased risk of PAD.[4] Similarly, in the Edinburgh Artery Study, the risk of PAD in smokers was increased by 5.6-fold.[18] Data from the Framingham study demonstrate a dose-response relationship between smoking and the risk of the symptomatic

TABLE 17-1 EFFECT OF CIGARETTE SMOKING AND DIABETES ON DEVELOPING PERIPHERAL ARTERIAL DISEASE AND INTERMITTENT CLAUDICATION

Author	*N*	Age	Population	Relative Risk
Peripheral Arterial Disease				
Meijer	7715	>55	Current smokers	M 1.7/F 1.2
Fowkes	1592	55-74	Current smokers	5.6
Newman	5084	>64	Diabetes	3.8
Beks	5209	50-74	Diabetes on meds	3.0
Intermittent Claudication				
Kannel	5209	55-64	1-20 Cigarettes	M 1.5/F 1.2
			≥20 Cigarettes	M 3.9/F 1.8
Smith	18,385	40-64	Current smokers	3.3
Bowlin	8343	40-65	Diabetes	1.9
Kannel	5209	55-84	Subjects with	M 3.5/F 8.6

F, female; M, male.

form of PAD, intermittent claudication.[19] Men who smoked 1 to 20 cigarettes per day faced a 50% increase in risk, whereas those who smoked more than 20 cigarettes per day suffered a 3.9-fold increase in risk compared with nonsmokers. Smoking not only causes the premature development of PAD,[9] it exacerbates its development in the elderly. In a prospective study of men and women whose mean age was 80 years, smoking increased Charcot foot.[25]

Diabetes mellitus increases the risk of PAD two- to fourfold in large epidemiologic studies (see Table 17-1).[20-22] Patients with diabetes are more likely to have absent pedal pulses and femoral artery bruits.[23] In the Cardiovascular Health Study, whose participants were aged 65 years or older, a history of diabetes increased the risk of developing PAD by nearly fourfold.[21] Similarly, in the Hoorn study, a stepwise increase in PAD frequency could be demonstrated with worsening diabetes. Subjects with normal glucose tolerance tests had a 7% prevalence of PAD, whereas patients with diabetes on multiple hypoglycemic medications had a 20.9% prevalence.[22] Like smoking, diabetes hastens the progression of PAD, increasing the frequency of symptom development. In the Framingham cohort, the presence of glycosuria increased the risk of intermittent claudication by 3.5-fold in men and 8.6-fold in women.[19] Diabetes in any form increases the risk of claudication by approximately 2.5-fold.[24] Diabetes reduces lower extremity functioning beyond PAD because of diabetes-inherent problems, such as neuropathy and Charcot foot.[25]

Symptoms of Peripheral Arterial Disease

The most commonly ascribed symptom that develops as a result of PAD is intermittent claudication (IC). The word, "claudication," derives from the Latin *claudicatio*, which was used to describe the limp gait of a lame horse. As defined in the Rose questionnaire,[26] claudication is the development of an ischemic muscular pain on exertion. The pain can be characterized as aching, burning, heaviness, feeling leaden, tightness, or cramping. The pain should originate in a muscular bed, such as the calf, thigh, hip, or buttock, and not localize to a joint. The area of the worst blood flow limitation usually subtends the site of muscular discomfort. For example, patients who develop hip or buttock discomfort with walking most likely have distal aorta or iliac artery occlusive disease, whereas patients with calf claudication likely have superficial femoral or popliteal arterial stenoses or occlusions. Reduction of muscular work on activity cessation rebalances available blood supply with muscle demand and quickly resolves the pain. Both time or activity to pain onset and time to pain resolution should be consistent and predictable. The distance walked to the onset of leg discomfort is called the "initial claudication distance," and the maximal distance that the patient can walk without stopping because of leg discomfort is called the "absolute claudication distance." Several classification schemes are used to categorize the severity of claudication, including the Fontaine[27] (Table 17-2) and Rutherford classifications (Table 17-3).[27] When the interview is complete, the physician should have insight into the nature of discomfort, how long it has been present, the typical duration of exercise required to cause the discomfort, and the amount of rest necessary to relieve the symptoms.

TABLE 17-2 FONTAINE CLASSIFICATION

Stage	Description
I	Asymptomatic, ABI < 0.9
II	Intermittent claudication
III	Daily rest pain
IV	Focal tissue necrosis

ABI, ankle brachial index.

Classic symptoms of claudication do not represent all patients with PAD, including those with functional limitations. The application of questionnaires for claudication, such as the World Health Organization/Rose questionnaire or the Walking Impairment Questionnaire,[26,28] may underestimate PAD prevalence by 50%.[3,4,10,11,29-34] Recent data from McDermott and colleagues indicate that complaints other than claudication are common.[35] They evaluated functional tolerance across a range of symptoms in a cross-sectional analysis of patients with and without PAD.[36] In this study, PAD patients demonstrated several types of leg discomfort, including leg pain at rest and with walking, pain with walking alone requiring cessation of activity, and pain that the patients could "walk through." This variety of presentations would be missed with questioning only for classic symptoms. Moreover, the type of discomfort predicted function. Patients with pain at rest and with walking had worse functional capacity than those whose pain occurred with walking and stopped with walking cessation, and those who were able to "walk through" the pain. The quality of leg pain, whether it is atypical or classic, does not predict the severity of reduction in limb perfusion pressure as measured by the ABI.[37]

The presence of intermittent claudication has important prognostic implications regarding functional capacity and mortality. Three quarters of patients with intermittent claudication will have stable symptoms over the next 10 years; approximately 25% will progress to more disabling claudication or critical limb ischemia requiring revascularization or culminating in amputation.[27] The level of impairment is roughly equivalent to New York

TABLE 17-3 RUTHERFORD CLASSIFICATION

Grade	Category	Description
0	0	Asymptomatic
I	1	Mild claudication
I	2	Moderate claudication
I	3	Severe claudication
II	4	Ischemic rest pain
III	5	Minor tissue loss
IV	6	Major tissue loss

Heart Association Class III congestive heart failure or chronic obstructive pulmonary disease.[38] Moreover, they will suffer a mortality more than twice that of the general population, approximately 30% at 5 years.[39]

Differential Diagnosis of Claudication

Once exercise-related exertion has been established, several alternate vascular and nonvascular diagnoses should be considered (Table 17-4). Vascular disorders include popliteal artery entrapment (see Chapter 64), compartment syndrome, fibromuscular dysplasia, venous insufficiency (see Chapter 56), and vasculitis (see Chapters 41 through 44). Popliteal artery entrapment typically occurs in very active persons or athletes. Because of an abnormal origin of the medial (or, less commonly, lateral) head of the gastrocnemius muscle, the popliteal artery may be compressed with walking and yield symptoms of claudication. Endofibrosis of the external iliac artery, a relatively rare occurrence in highly trained cyclists and other endurance athletes, may cause claudication. Fibromuscular dysplasia (FMD) is a noninflammatory arterial occlusive disease that most commonly affects the renal and carotid arteries, but may involve other arterial beds (see Chapter 65).[40] Any of the arteries in the lower extremities may be affected, but the iliac arteries are the most common. The fibroplasias may involve the intima, media, or adventitial layer of the artery. The most common variety is medial fibroplasia. It can be diagnosed from the "string of beads" appearance on angiography and by its predilection for the nonbranching points of vessels. The etiology of fibromuscular dysplasia remains unknown.

Increased calf muscle size with exercise may inhibit venous outflow, cause exertional compartment syndrome—in which tissue pressure is increased and microvascularity flow is impeded—and bring about complaints of calf pain or tightness with exertion. The symptoms improve with leg elevation after exercise cessation. Venous claudication may occur as a result of iliofemoral thrombosis with poor collateral vein formation.[41] When venous outflow is impaired, the increase in arterial inflow with exercise increases venous pressure markedly and causes a severe tightness or bursting sensation in the limb. Patients may report improvement in symptoms with leg elevation following exercise cessation. These patients frequently have leg edema. Vasculitides, such as Takayasu's arteritis, giant cell arteritis, and thromboangiitis obliterans, are infrequent causes of claudication.

Nonvascular causes of exertional leg pain include lumbar radiculopathy, hip and knee arthritis, and myositis. Perhaps the most common nonvascular diagnosis is lumbar radiculopathy causing nerve-based pain.[42,43] Patients may complain of leg pain or paresthesias as a result of compression of the lumbar nerve roots from disc herniation or degenerative osteophytes. The paresthesias or pain tends to affect the posterior aspect of the leg and occurs with specific positions, such as standing, or develops at the beginning of ambulation. These symptoms may improve with continued walking or when leaning forward because pressure on the nerve roots is reduced.

Osteoarthritis of the hip or knee may cause pain associated with walking. The pain may be confused with IC because it typically occurs with exercise. The discomfort, however, is usually referable to a joint, such as the hip or knee. It can be distinguished from claudication in that the level of activity required to precipitate symptoms varies and does not resolve rapidly with activity cessation.

Critical Limb Ischemia

Critical limb ischemia (CLI) is the most debilitating manifestation of PAD (Fig. 17-1). The TransAtlantic Inter-Society Consensus (TASC) Working Group estimates that the incidence of CLI is between 300 and 1000 persons per million per year.[27] In a northern Italian population, the incidence of CLI in the population older than 45 years is 450 per million persons per year, and the incidence of amputation is 112 per million persons per year.[44] In Finland, the incidence of amputation is 216 per million people per year, whereas the corresponding incidence of arterial

TABLE 17-4 NONATHEROSCLEROTIC CAUSES OF EXERTIONAL LEG PAIN

Nonatherosclerotic Arterial Disease
Atheroembolism
Vasculitis
Extravascular compression
Popliteal artery entrapment
Adventitial cysts
Fibromuscular dysplasia
Endofibrosis of the internal iliac artery
Venous Claudication
Compartment Syndrome
Lumbar Radiculopathy
Spinal Stenosis
Hip/Knee Arthritis
Myositis

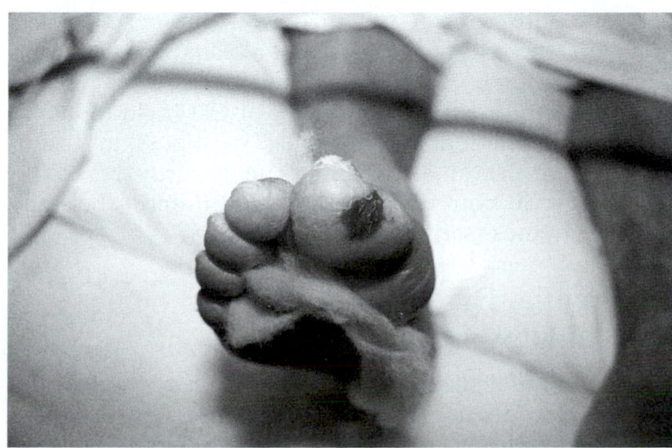

FIGURE 17-1. A nonhealing first-digit ulcer with overlying eschar.

reconstructions is 203 per million inhabitants per year.[45] Across the globe, the frequency of amputation varies from 28 per million people per year in Madrid to 439 amputations per million people per year among Navajo Americans.[46] These numbers should be interpreted cautiously because the incidence of amputation, even in the United States, varies eightfold depending mainly on the presence or absence of a vascular surgeon.[47]

Diabetes and smoking increase the risk of developing CLI. Diabetes is the cause of most nontraumatic lower extremity amputations in the United States.[48] Diabetes increases the risk of amputation nearly fourfold, even with similar levels of blood flow limitation as in nondiabetic patients.[49] For diabetic persons aged 65 to 74 years, the relative risk of amputation is nearly 24-fold that of patients without diabetes.[55] In a population of 2990 diabetic patients in a primary care setting, the 4-year incidence of amputations was 2.2%, and it was 10% in patients with foot sores or ulcers.[50] Cigarette smoking also increases the risk that PAD will progress to CLI. In a study of 343 consecutive patients with IC, 16% of those who continued to smoke developed CLI—compared with none in those who were able to stop smoking.[51] In 190 patients undergoing lower extremity revascularization followed for 3 years, those who smoked more than 15 cigarettes per day had a 10-fold higher risk (21%) of amputation compared with those who smoked fewer than 15 cigarettes per day (2%).[52] In fact, patients who do not smoke or do not have diabetes represent less than 20% of all patients requiring amputation.[53]

CLI occurs as a consequence of tissue ischemia at rest and it manifests as foot pain, nonhealing ulcers, or tissue gangrene. The pain is often severe and unremitting, and localized to the acral portion of the foot or toes, notably at the site of ulceration or gangrene. Blood flow limitation is so severe that the gravitational effects of leg position may affect symptoms. Patients commonly report that leg elevation worsens pain. This is typically worse at night when the patient is in bed and the leg, now at heart level, no longer benefits from the dependent position. Placing the foot on the floor beside the bed is a common action used by patients to reduce pain. The inability to use the leg and chronically placing the leg in a dependent position may cause peripheral edema, a finding that is occasionally mistaken for venous disease in these patients. With severe ischemia, any skin perturbation, including the use of bedclothes or blankets, may cause pain; in ischemic neuropathy, this causes a lancinating pain in the foot. Other symptoms of CLI include hypesthesia, cold intolerance, muscular weakness, and joint stiffness of the affected limb. The severity of CLI is categorized in both the Fontaine and Rutherford classification schemes (see Tables 17-2 and 17-3).

Differential Diagnosis of Critical Limb Ischemia

The differential diagnosis of CLI includes vascular and nonvascular diseases (Table 17-5). Atheroembolism or blue toe syndrome occurs when components of large-vessel atherosclerotic plaque embolize to distal vessels (Fig. 17-2) (see Chapter 47). The embolized material is composed of fibroplatelet debris and cholesterol crystals. A common cause of atheroembolism is iatrogenic disturbance of the vessel, whether from catheterization or surgery.[54,55] Several features may help in differentiating atheroembolism from traditional critical limb ischemia. The patients typically have pulses palpable down into the feet because the emboli require a patent pathway to the distal portions of the extremities. Other clinical clues include new renal insufficiency and blood eosinophilia. On examination, the patient will have areas of cyanosis or violaceous discoloration of the toes or portions of the feet and areas of livedo reticularis.

Acute limb ischemia may occur from thrombosis in situ or from thromboemboli of large fibro-platelet accumulations that originate in the heart or large arteries, and occlude conduit arteries (see Chapter 46).[56] These patients have an accelerated course and may present with the five "p's" of acute ischemia: pain, pallor, poikilothermia, paresthesia, and paralysis. Other causes of limb ischemia include vasospasm, thromboangiitis obliterans, other vasculitides, and connective tissue disorders (see Chapters 41, 44, and 48). Other causes of ulcers include neuropathy, venous disease, and trauma (see Chapter 62). Nonvascular causes of foot pain include neuropathy, arthritides such as gout, fasciitis, and trauma (see Table 17-4).

TABLE 17-5 DIFFERENTIAL DIAGNOSIS OF CRITICAL LIMB ISCHEMIA

Ischemia
Atherosclerosis
Atheroemboli
Acute arterial occlusion
In situ thrombosis
Emboli
Vasculitis
Thromboangiitis obliterans
Scleroderma
Systemic lupus erythematosus
MCTD
Cryoglobulinemia
Vasospasm
Raynaud's phenomenon
Acrocyanosis
Ulcers
Neuropathy
Venous insufficiency
Trauma
Pain
Neuropathy
Arthritis
Gout
Rheumatoid arthritis
Fasciitis
Trauma

MCTD, mixed connective tissue disease.

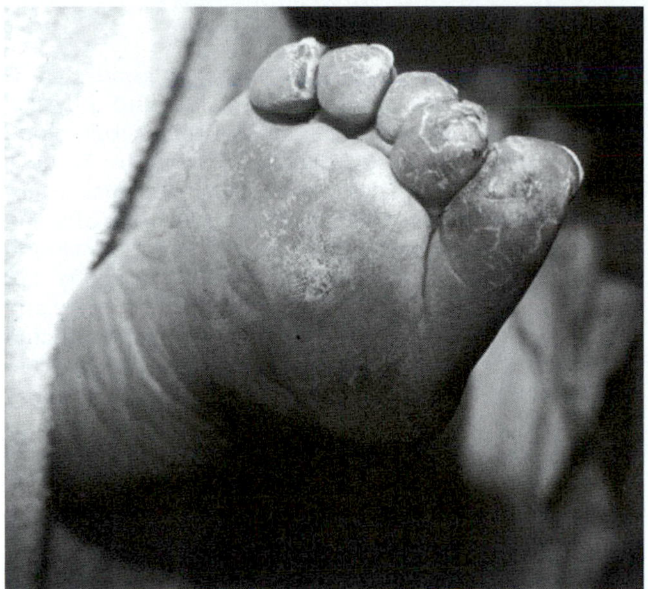

FIGURE 17-2. Atheroembolism after catheterization. Note the areas of cyanosis and surrounding livedo reticularis. This patient had a palpable dorsalis pedis pulse.

Physical Examination

A comprehensive physical examination that includes the general appearance of the patient, integument, heart, lungs, abdomen, and limbs should be performed during the initial patient encounter to elucidate evidence of systemic disease and provide insight into cause and manifestation of the patient's vascular disease. The entire vascular system should be examined. Blood pressure is measured in each arm. A blood pressure difference of 10 mm Hg or more may be indicative of innominate, subclavian, axillary, or brachial artery stenosis. The carotid, brachial, radial, ulnar, femoral, popliteal, dorsalis pedis, and posterior tibial pulses should be palpated in every patient (Fig. 17-3). Several pulse-descriptive schemes have been promulgated. One is to grade the pulses as 0 (absent), 1 (diminished), and 2 (normal). A very prominent or forceful pulse may occur in patients with aortic regurgitation or high cardiac output states. The absence of any pulse in the lower extremity, except in the dorsalis pedis, is suggestive of PAD. The dorsalis pedis pulse is not palpable in 2% to 12% of healthy patients.[57-59] The absence of a peripheral pulse may indicate a significant stenosis between the present and absent pulse. Occasionally, pulses may be palpable below the level of a significant stenosis. This most commonly occurs in the setting of iliac artery disease when there may be sufficient collateral vessels to maintain perfusion to distal arteries. The abdominal aorta should also be palpitated if permitted by body habitus to elicit evidence of aortic aneurysm. A widened pulse in the abdomen or over a peripheral artery (e.g., the popliteal artery) may be indicative of an aneurysm. Once palpated, the abdomen and several peripheral vessels also should be auscultated. Palpation of an expansile or pulsatile periumbilical mass is indicative of an abdominal aortic aneurysm. Proper auscultation of normal vessels with a stethoscope should reveal no sound. Bruits should be sought over the carotid and subclavian arteries, in the abdomen, in the lower back, and over the femoral arteries. The presence of a bruit, indicative of turbulent blood flow, typically occurs as a result of arterial stenosis, but may indicate extrinsic compression or arteriovenous malformation. Vessels with no flow, resulting from complete occlusion, do not convey bruits.

A skin examination should be performed looking for alterations in temperature, edema, signs of active or healed lesions, or the signs of chronic ischemia—including thin shiny skin, thickened yellow nails, and loss of hair. Foot or toe cyanosis or pallor may be a forerunner of ulceration. Inspection of the skin may reveal trophic signs of chronic ischemia, including sympathetic denervation (impaired hair growth or impaired sweating) and sensorimotor neuropathy (lack of vibratory sense). CLI may cause muscle and subcutaneous tissue atrophy, hair loss, petechiae, and thin or encrusted skin. In CLI, the toes and foot are cool and pallor may be present when the foot is in the neutral (or horizontal) position. Changes in skin appearance with elevation and dependency may provide a gauge for PAD severity. The leg should be elevated to 45° to 60° for 1 minute. If pallor develops quickly (within 10 to 15 seconds), severe PAD is likely.

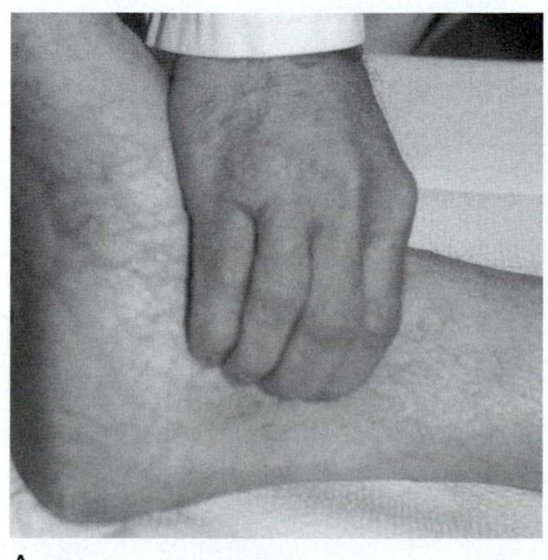

A

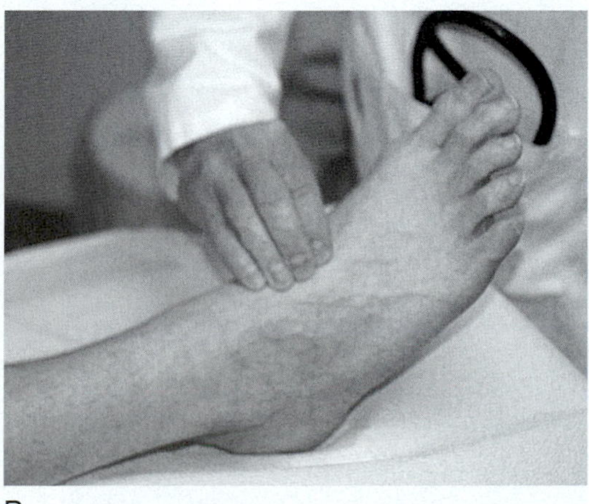

B

FIGURE 17-3. Palpation of the pedal pulses. **A,** Palpation of the posterior tibial (PT) pulse. The examiner should place his/her fingers in the curve below the malleolus with light pressure and reposition as needed. The application of passive foot dorsiflexion occasionally makes PT palpation easier. **B,** The dorsalis pedis pulse is typically appreciated within one cm of the dorsum, most prominent near the navicular bone.

After 1 minute, the patient sits up and the leg is placed in a dependent position. The time to pedal vein refill should be recorded. Ischemic-induced arteriolar and venular dilation may lead to the development of a violaceous appearance of the foot with dependency, called "dependent rubor" (Fig. 17-4). Normal refill occurs rapidly, typically within 10 to 15 seconds. Prolongation of venous filling or the development of numbness beyond 1 minute suggests severe PAD.

Arterial fissures most commonly develop in the heel, toes, in the web space between the toes, or in segments subjected to pressure (the ball of the foot). Arterial ulcers are circumscribed, tender, and prone to infection. The base of the ulcer is usually pale. The ulcers, in contrast to venous ulcers, are dry; however, the devitalized tissue is prone to infection, which may generate a purulent exudate. The ulcer may be covered by an eschar. In CLI, gangrene most commonly occurs in the digits, but may occur on the ball of the foot or heel. In the absence of infection, gangrene tends to be dry and the skin is mummified.

Two classification schemes are used to categorize the clinical assessment of patients with peripheral arterial disease: the Fontaine Stage Classification of PAD and the Rutherford Categorical Classification of PAD. In the system described by Fontaine, the severity of PAD is classified into 1 of 4 stages—ranging from asymptomatic in stage 1; IC in stage 2; daily rest pain in stage 3; and focal tissue necrosis in stage 4 (see Table 17-2). The Rutherford system employs seven categories, dividing the severity of claudication into three categories (mild, moderate, and severe) and critical limb ischemia into three categories (rest pain, minor tissue loss, and major tissue loss) (see Table 17-3).

Office-Based Ankle Brachial Index

Measurement of the ABI is a simple method that is employed to corroborate the historical and physical findings of PAD. The ABI is the ratio of the systolic blood pressure at the ankle and brachial artery. The latter is an estimate of central aortic pressure. Brachial artery systolic blood pressure is measured in both arms and ankles using a handheld 5 or 10 MHz Doppler ultrasound device and sphygmomanometric cuff. The cuffs are placed on each arm above the antecubital fossa and above each ankle. The cuffs are sequentially inflated above systolic pressure and then are slowly depressurized. The Doppler probe, placed over the brachial artery and the dorsalis pedis and posterior tibial arteries, monitors the pressure (Fig. 17-5). As the cuff is slowly deflated, the reappearance of a Doppler signal indicates the systolic pressure at the level of the cuff. Brachial artery pressures must be measured in both arms because atherosclerosis may occur in subclavian and axillary arteries. Therefore, the higher of the two brachial systolic blood pressures is used for reference in the ABI calculation. Hence, the ABI is the systolic pressure at each ankle divided by the higher pressure of the two brachial artery pressures; thus, an ABI may be generated for each leg. When assessing foot perfusion, the ABI uses the highest of the pedal pressures in each leg.[60] Both pedal pressures (dorsalis pedis and posterior tibial artery) are considered when seeking evidence of atherosclerosis. Some have suggested that ankle pressure used to calculate ABI should be an average of the two pedal pressures.[61]

The normal systolic pressure at the ankle should be at least the same as in the arm, thus yielding an ABI of

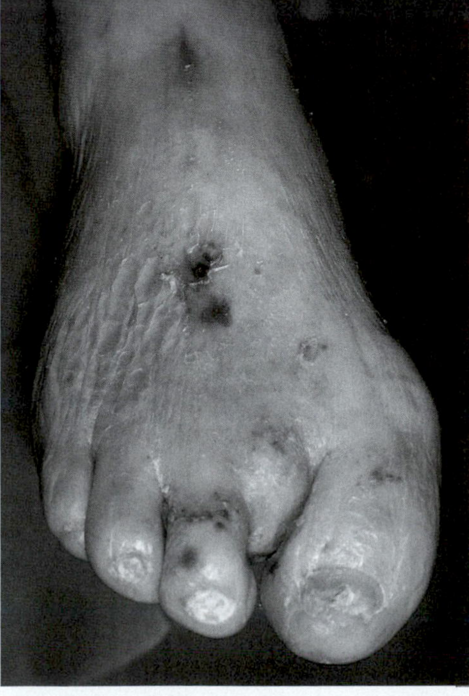
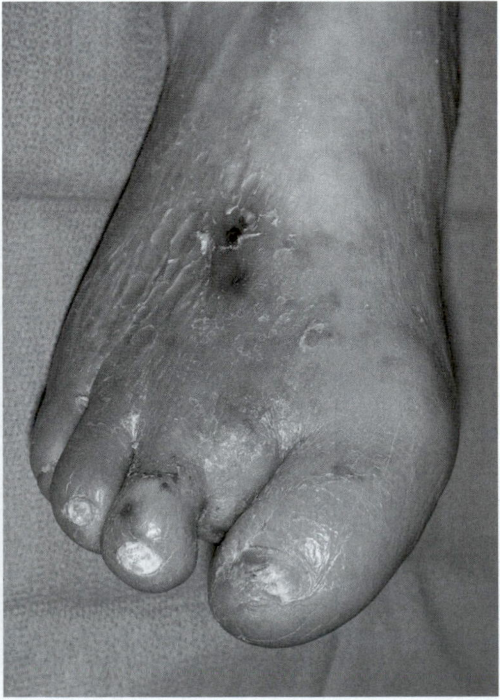

FIGURE 17-4. Dependent rubor. This patient with severe PAD (note the previously amputated second digit) develops a ruborous appearance of the forefoot with dependent positioning as a result of arteriolar and venular dilation.

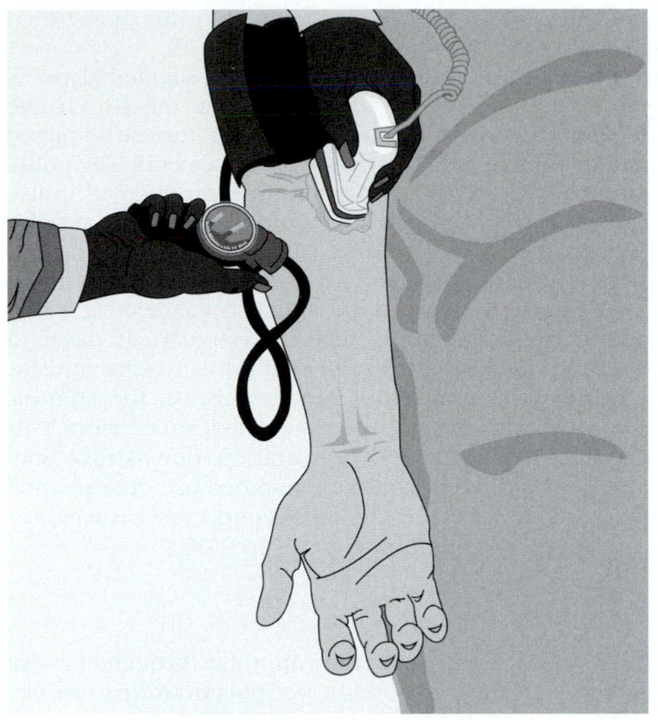

A

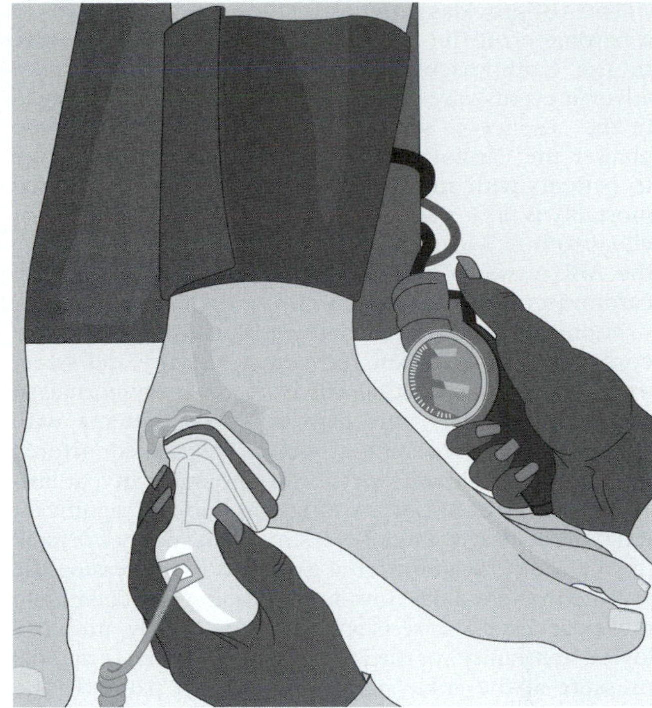

B

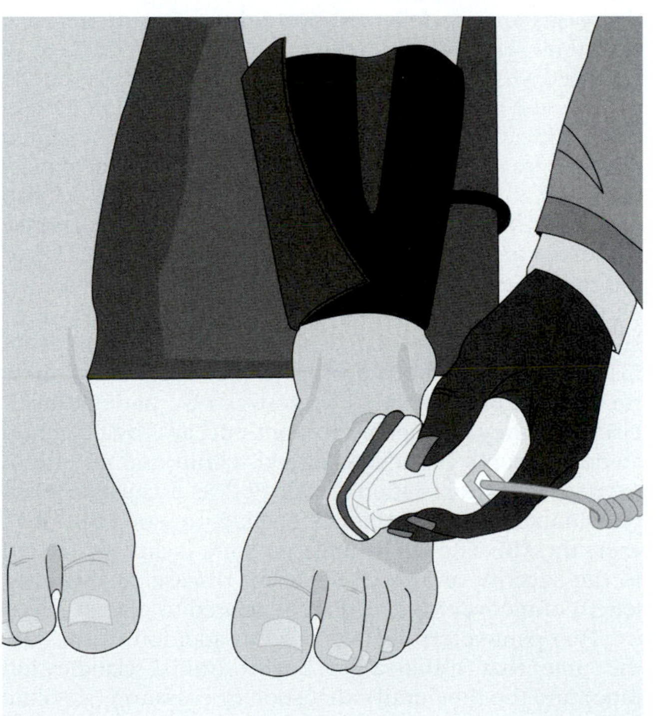

C

FIGURE 17-5. Measurement of the ankle brachial index (ABI). Brachial artery systolic blood pressure is determined in both arms and both ankles using a handheld 5 or 10 MHz Doppler ultrasound and sphygmomanometric cuff. Because atherosclerosis may occur in subclavian and axillary arteries, brachial artery pressures must be measured in both arms **(A)**. The higher of the two brachial systolic blood pressures is used as the reference pressure in the ABI calculation. In each ankle, the pressure should be measured at the dorsalis pedis **(B)** and posterior tibial pulse **(C)**. Hence, the ABI is the quotient of the highest systolic pressure at each ankle divided by the highest pressure of the two brachial artery pressures.

1.0 or greater. As a result of reflected arterial pressure waves, healthy persons tend to have an ABI ranging from 1.0 to 1.3. Recognizing an intrinsic (up to 10%) variability of blood pressure when measured sequentially, as ankle pressures are not measured simultaneously, an abnormal ABI consistent with the diagnosis of PAD is categorized as less than or equal to 0.9. The ABI is a reliable determinant of PAD, with a sensitivity ranging from 79% to 95% and specificity of 96% to 100%.[62,63] An ABI of less than or equal to 0.4 is extremely abnormal and is typically present in patients with CLI. Arterial calcification may introduce a false elevation in ABI, typically 1.3 or greater, as a result of noncompressible vessels at the ankle. Arterial calcification occurs more commonly in patients with diabetes or end-stage renal disease, and in the elderly.[7,64]

The ABI provides prognostic information because it is a barometer of the burden of systemic atherosclerosis. In the Cardiovascular Health Study, the incidence of adverse events rose as the ABI dropped below 1.0, even in the absence of symptoms.[21] The lower the ABI, the greater the cardiovascular morbidity and mortality.[65,66] In patients with an ABI less than or equal to 0.7, 5-year mortality is 30% and in patients with an ABI less than or equal to 0.4, 5-year mortality is 50%.[67] Thus, measuring the ABI provides both an assessment of PAD and of cardiovascular risk.

There are limitations to the ABI measurement. The correlation between ABI, functional capacity, and symptoms is weak. The resting ABI is occasionally normal in patients with PAD; this may occur in patients with aortoiliac stenoses and a well-collateralized arterial system that maintains perfusion pressure. In patients with a normal ABI but a strong suspicion of significant PAD, office-based exercise testing may be performed. Exercise accentuates arterial gradients by increasing the turbulence across the flow-limiting lesion and decreasing muscular arteriolar resistance to significantly attenuate lower extremity perfusion pressure. In fact, arterial pressure at the ankle may reach zero in patients who develop claudication, recovering more than 10 minutes after exercise cessation. In the office, stair climbing or active pedal plantar flexion[68] may be used to elicit symptoms and document a decrease in ankle pressure (and ABI) to confirm the diagnosis of IC.

Noninvasive Laboratory Testing for Peripheral Arterial Disease

For patients in whom revascularization is considered, such as those with CLI or disabling claudication, the location and severity of disease should be evaluated by additional noninvasive testing. There are two general formats of noninvasive testing to discern the location and severity of PAD: physiologic testing and anatomic imaging.

Physiologic Testing

Physiologic or functional testing most commonly occurs in a noninvasive vascular laboratory (see Chapter 10). Measurement of limb segmental systolic pressures employs methods similar to the measurement of the ABI (Fig. 17-6). Sphygmomanometric cuffs are placed on the proximal thigh, distal thigh, calf, and ankle. The cuffs are inflated sequentially to suprasystolic pressure and then deflated to determine systolic pressure at each site. A Doppler probe is placed on the posterior tibial or dorsalis pedis artery. Arterial stenosis or occlusion will decrease the perfusion pressure. Arterial pressure gradients of more than 20 mm Hg between thigh cuffs and 10 mm Hg between cuffs below the knee indicate the presence of a stenosis. The test has an 86% predictive accuracy.[69] As with the ABI, the most common source of error for the test is vascular calcification. In the setting of vascular calcification, a toe brachial index may be obtained. Pressures in the toe may be measured with strain gauge photoplethysmography.[70,71] Pressure is measured in the toes and a ratio of toe pressure to brachial artery pressure is generated; a value of less than or equal to 0.7 is consistent with PAD.[72,73]

Pulse volume recordings (PVRs) or segmental pneumatic plethysmography determines the relative change in limb volume with each pulse and can be obtained along with segmental pressure measurements. The pulse-volume waveform represents the product of pulse pressure and vascular wall compliance. In a healthy subject, the pulse-volume waveform is similar to a normal arterial pressure waveform and includes rapid upstroke, dicrotic notch, and downstroke (see Fig. 17-6). The waveform changes when it is recorded distal to a significant stenosis as perfusion pressure falls. Initially, there is a loss of the dicrotic notch. As the stenosis worsens, waveform upstroke (anacrotic slope) is delayed, the amplitude is less, and the downstroke (catacrotic slope) is slower. The combined use of segmental pressure measurements and PVRs improves the accuracy of identifying significant stenosis to 95%.[69]

Treadmill Testing

As described earlier, eliciting symptoms through exercise may permit the diagnosis of peripheral arterial disease, despite a normal or near-normal ABI. When a vessel has a significant stenosis, increasing flow through the lesion decreases energy delivered beyond the area of stenosis. Treadmill exercise increases blood flow through a stenosed vessel and can increase the sensitivity of the ABI. In the vascular laboratory, a diagnosis of IC and a quantification of exercise tolerance may be obtained through treadmill exercise testing. Many protocols exist to test walking ability, but each falls into one of two types: constant or graded exercise. In constant exercise protocols (e.g., Carter protocol), a specific speed (1.5 to 2.0 miles per hour) and treadmill grade (0% to 12%) is chosen, whereas in the graded exercise protocols (e.g., Hiatt or Gardner protocol), speed and/or treadmill grade may increase.[74] In both protocols, the brachial and ankle pressures are determined pretest at rest, patients exercise until they are unable to continue, and brachial and ankle pressures are redetermined within one minute of exercise cessation. Patients with PAD as a cause of exercise limitation will have a fall in ankle pressure, thus lowering the ABI. The fall in ankle pressure is directly related to the severity of arterial occlusive disease. Analogously, length of recovery is also directly related to disease severity. Two parameters are recorded in addition to the ABI, the time that claudication begins (initial claudication time), and the time until exhaustion or cessation (absolute claudication time). Variability of walking distance is greater in the constant exercise protocols than the graded protocols, making the latter more commonly used.

Anatomic Imaging of the Peripheral Circulation

Defining arterial anatomy is not typically necessary to make the diagnosis of PAD, but is required for patients who will be undergoing revascularization. Following is a discussion of the major methods used to image peripheral arteries.

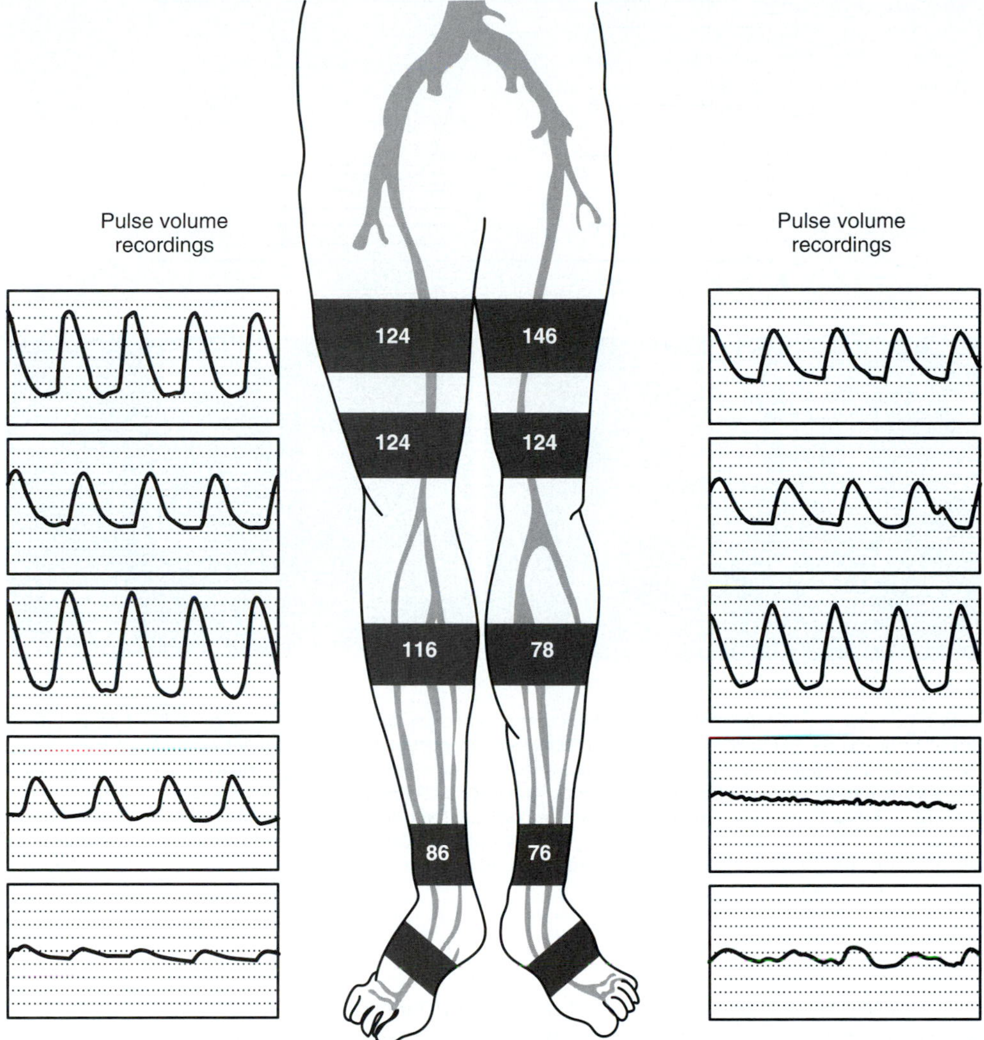

FIGURE 17-6. Segmental pressure measurements. Sequential Doppler pressures are measured by placing sphygmomanometric cuffs on the proximal thigh, distal thigh, calf, and ankle. The cuffs are inflated above systolic pressure and then slowly depressurized. Simultaneously, a Doppler probe, placed over the dorsalis pedis or posterior tibial artery, monitors the pressure. As the cuff is slowly deflated, the reappearance of a Doppler signal indicates the systolic pressure at the level of the cuff which permits blood flow. Arterial stenosis or occlusion will decrease the perfusion pressure. Arterial pressure gradients between cuffs indicate the presence of a stenosis. In this example, arterial pressures (mm Hg) are noted in the location of each sphygmomanometric cuff. The patient has evidence of a systolic gradient between both upper thigh cuffs, suggestive of right iliac and/or common femoral arterial occlusive disease, and a gradient between the right calf and ankle, suggestive of arterial occlusive disease in the infrapopliteal arteries. The diminished pressure in the left calf suggests a significant gradient between the lower thigh cuff and calf cuff, indicative of distal superficial femoral artery and/or popliteal artery occlusive disease.

Duplex Ultrasonography

Duplex ultrasonography of the lower extremities is performed in most vascular laboratories (see Chapter 10). The combination of B-mode ultrasound, color Doppler imaging, and pulsed-Doppler velocity analysis can accurately identify the location and severity of atherosclerotic lesions in the legs. Normally, flow through each arterial segment should be laminar, with a uniform, homogeneous color appearance. Blood flow becomes turbulent and velocity increases at sites of sclerosis, creating areas of color discordance. Pulsed-Doppler measurements in the area of stenosis demonstrate increased flow velocity and spectral broadening.

Applying the concepts of Poiseuille's law regarding the movement of incompressible viscous fluids through a tube, the ratio of peak systolic velocity in the area of a stenosis is compared with the normal area of artery proximal to the stenosis. A ratio greater than or equal to 2 is consistent with stenosis greater than or equal to 50% (Fig. 17-7).[75-77] In a meta-analysis of 14 studies performed over 10 years, the sensitivity and specificity of color-guided Doppler analysis was 93% and 95%, respectively.[78] Duplex ultrasonography is less accurate at the site of calcified plaque because of the acoustic shadowing caused by the dense calcium.[79] Serial stenoses are more difficult to diagnose because ultrasound diagnosis relies on comparing peak arterial velocities between adjacent segments, and there are altered hemodynamics between sequential stenoses.[79] Single-center studies have found that ultrasound may be used alone in planning both percutaneous and surgical peripheral revascularization.[60,80-82]

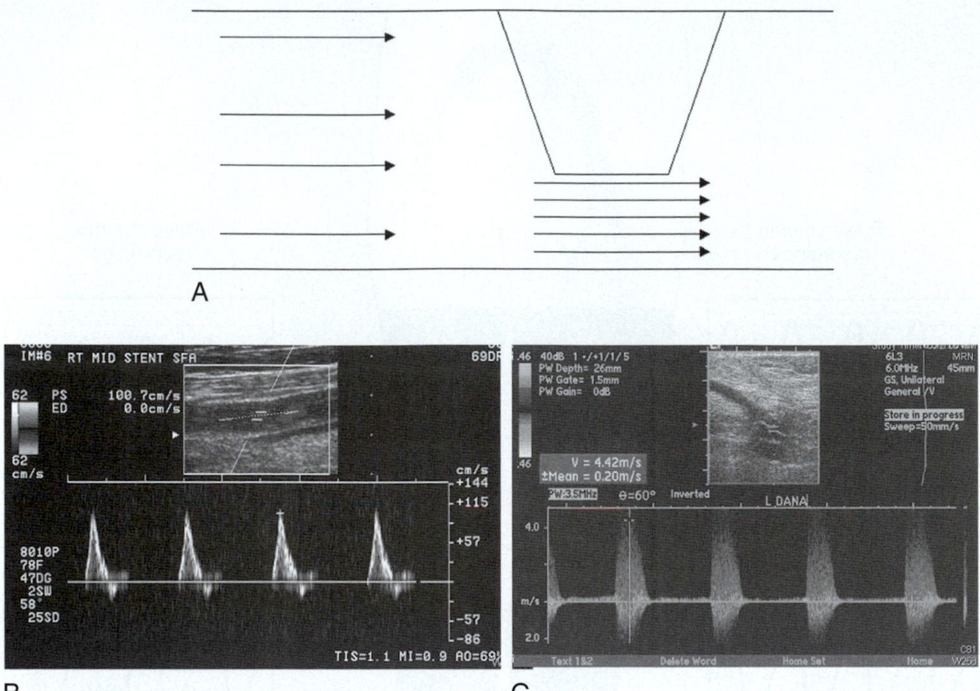

FIGURE 17-7. **A,** Poiseuille's law defines the movement of a incompressible viscous fluid through a tube. Fluid entry into the tube must equal its exit; thus, the ratio of peak-systolic velocity in the area of a stenosis is proportional to the segment of normal vessel proximal to the stenosis. When the ratio is greater than 2, a stenosis of more than 50% is diagnosed. The sensitivity and specificity of a duplex ultrasound evaluation in the determination of stenoses equal to or greater than 50% range from 90% to 95%. Normal arterial flow velocity is approximately 100 cm per second. **B,** A Doppler ultrasound is passed through a recently placed superficial femoral artery stent, demonstrating a normal flow velocity. This is indicative of a patent stent without evidence of restenosis. **C,** A Doppler ultrasound is passed through the distal anastomosis of a femoral-popliteal bypass graft, demonstrating a flow velocity of 4.4 meters/second. This is consistent with a greater than 75% stenosis. The velocity in the proximal normal segment is 1.3 meters/second (*not shown*).

Duplex ultrasonography is also used in the postoperative surveillance of arterial bypass grafts. A program of routine ultrasound surveillance is more likely to diagnose significant bypass graft stenoses than is history, physical examination, or ABI.[83-85] Clinical trials have evaluated the efficacy of ultrasound surveillance as a strategy to identify graft stenosis and prompt repair before graft occlusion occurs.[86] One study randomized 156 patients to serial ultrasonography or ABI. Patients were referred for angiography, and then corrective revascularization if greater than or equal to 50% stenosis was identified by ultrasound, or if the ABI decreased by 0.15 compared with the postoperative baseline.[87] Assisted primary cumulative vein graft patency in the ultrasound group was 78% compared with 53% in the ABI group after 3 years. In other randomized studies, however, no benefit was found for ultrasound compared with ABI 1 year after surgery.[88,89] The data for surveillance for synthetic bypass grafts[87,90-92] and after angioplasty[93,94] are less robust than for vein grafts.

Magnetic Resonance Angiography

Magnetic resonance angiography (MRA) is an accurate imaging modality to diagnose PAD, visualize peripheral arteries, and determine the location of stenoses (see Chapter 11). Several techniques have been developed to image the arterial tree, including black blood, phase contrast, time of flight, and contrast-enhanced MRA.[95] The application of two magnetic pulses to suppress the signal in the vessel lumen yields a dark appearance of flowing blood, with the vessel wall remaining white. The selective removal of blood from the image causes the lumen to appear black, and the technique is therefore called *black blood*.[95] When the phase shift of moving electron spins in flowing blood is compared with the surrounding stable tissue, blood volume and velocity can be measured to permit assessment of blood flow.[95] The application of electrocardiographic gating, while interrogating the flow-related enhancement of spins into a partially saturated area, provides a time of flight (TOF) angiogram.[96,97] In a multicenter study, the diagnostic accuracy of TOF MRA was comparable in patients with PAD to that in contrast angiography.[98] Limitations of a flow-based TOF MRA include lengthy acquisition types, turbulence, nonlinear vascular structures, and retrograde flow.[99,103,104] Most MRAs are performed using contrast, most commonly, gadolinium.[95] Contrast-enhanced magnetic resonance angiography provides a high-resolution angiogram.

Contrast-enhanced TOF MRA is useful as a noninvasive imaging test to define lower extremity vascular anatomy. In a meta-analysis comparing contrast-enhanced MRA with TOF MRA, the contrast-enhanced study had a much greater diagnostic accuracy.[99] The use of contrast has improved scan quality and efficiency, and enhanced

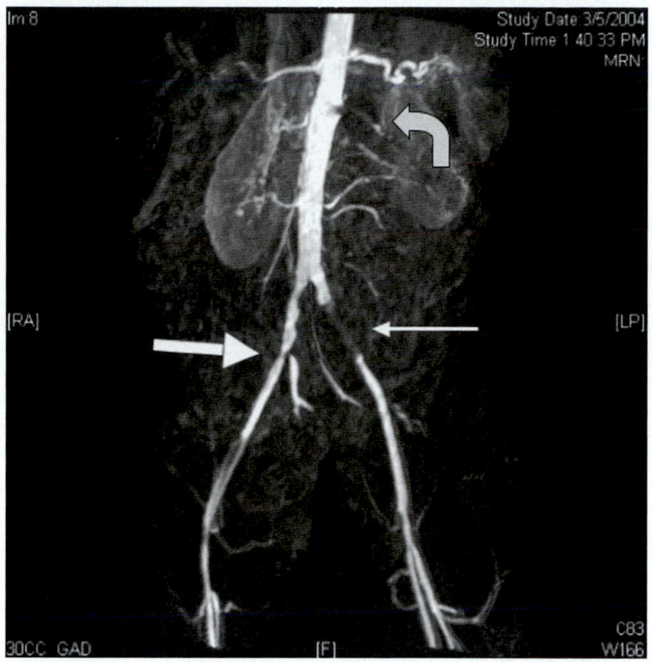

FIGURE 17-8. A gadolinium-enhanced MRA. This MRA was performed in a patient with Takayasu's arteritis. Several findings are notable. The patient has an occluded left renal artery, and the right internal iliac artery has a severe stenosis (*thick arrow*). At the *thin arrow* is an area of dropout as a result of image interference by a previously placed stent. The *curved arrow* indicates an occluded left upper renal artery.

vessel visualization and identification, especially in distal vessels (Fig. 17-8).[100,101] MRA can identify the presence of stenoses and reveal distal vessels suitable for bypass not demonstrated by contrast angiography.[102-104] In one study, time-resolved MRA had a sensitivity of 96% and specificity of 97% for stenoses greater than 50%, 97.8% sensitivity and 99.2% specificity for occlusions in PAD patients.[105] One potential limitation is a tendency for MRA to overestimate lesion severity.[106] Similar benefits and limitations exist in the imaging of bypass grafts. MRA has a sensitivity as high as 91% for the identification of arterial bypass graft stenoses,[107] but overestimates lesion severity in up to 30% of stenoses.[108,109] A sound strategy may involve the use of MRA initially because of the noninvasive nature of the test and its superior identification of bypass vessels, reserving digital subtraction angiography for cases requiring greater definition.[110] Technologic advancement is rapid in MRA, improving detection and identification of arterial occlusive disease. As imaging protocols and techniques, such as three-dimensional MRA imaging, gain acceptance and are made commonly available, MRA may ultimately be used as a stand-alone evaluation prior to revascularization.[111-113]

Computed Tomographic Angiography

Computed tomographic (CT) angiography has recently undergone rapid improvements in technology and imaging, allowing its entry into peripheral vascular imaging (see Chapter 12). Much of this advance results from the development of multidetector-row CT scanners and improved resolution of arteries. Single-detector devices are limited in their ability to resolve stenotic lesions because of thick image slices (5 mm).[114,115] With four-detector systems, image slice thickness is 3 mm. Eight-detector systems improve resolution to 1.25 mm, whereas the machines with 16 detectors can resolve down to 1 mm.[116] The availability of higher resolution to scanners is particularly relevant for smaller and more distal arteries.

In studies using four or more detector CT scanners, CT angiography achieved an 87% to 100% sensitivity and 88% to 100% specificity for the detection of occlusions, and 73% to 93% sensitivity and 94% to 100% specificity for the detection of stenoses greater than 75% in the femoral and popliteal arteries.[117] As scanner number increases, newer CT scanners should have even greater accuracy.

CT angiography is commonly presented using a maximal intensity projection (MIP) or with a volume rendering technique (VRT) (Fig. 17-9). The MIP algorithm displays only the pixel with the highest intensity along a ray perpendicular to the plane of projection. This algorithm creates a 2-D projectional image similar in appearance to MRA or contrast angiography. Volume rendering applies

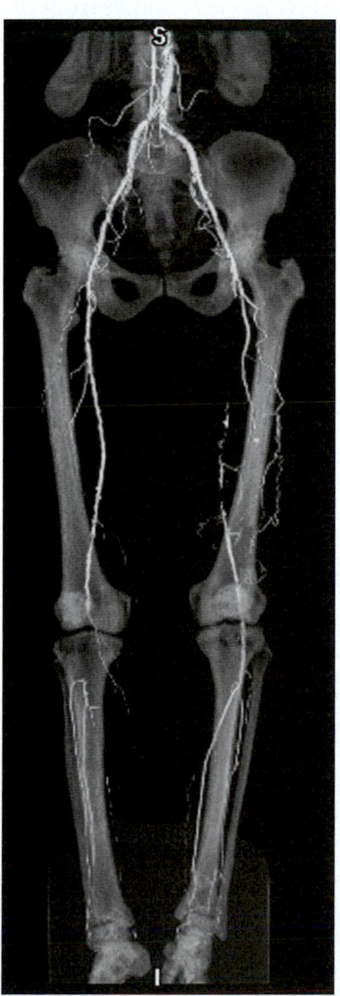

FIGURE 17-9. Volume-rendered CT angiogram of the lower extremities. Note the superficial femoral artery occlusion and collateral formation depicted by this study. (Image provided courtesy of Dr. Joseph Schoepf.)

shades of gray to pixels of varying density.[118] Fourier transfer functions allow modification of the relative contribution of various pixel values. Volume rendering considers pixels that are only partially filled with contrast material. Arterial calcification limits imaging with both CT techniques. Optimal techniques used for post-processing are being developed.[116] As resolution improves, CT angiography may become a regular instrument in the diagnostic armamentarium because of its rapid study time (typically less than 1 minute) or because of the 75% reduction in ionizing radiation compared with angiography.

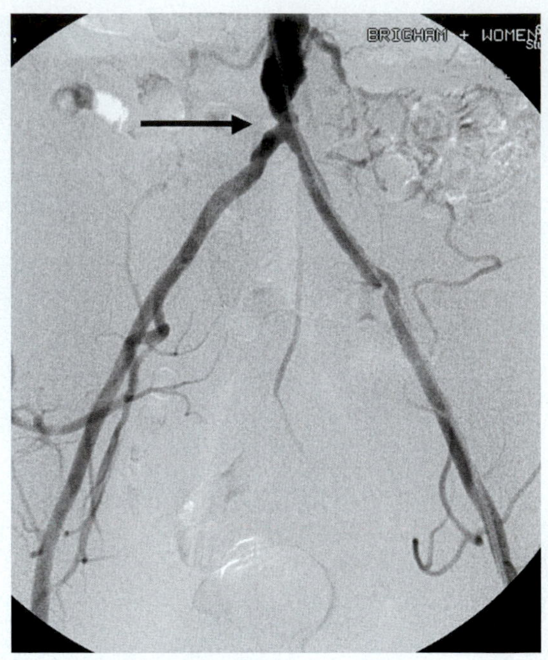

FIGURE 17-10. Contrast abdominal angiogram demonstrating a significant aortic stenosis just proximal to the bifurcation into the iliac arteries (*arrow*).

Contrast Angiography

Contrast angiography is the most venerable and widely available method for imaging arterial anatomy (see Chapter 13). Angiography commonly serves as the standard for determining the sensitivity and specificity of newer techniques and is an excellent method to clarify arterial anatomic queries (Fig. 17-10).[110] Technical improvements in equipment, including smaller catheters, image resolution, and digital subtraction, have enhanced the capability of angiography. Digital subtraction eliminates bony and soft-tissue shadows from the angiographic

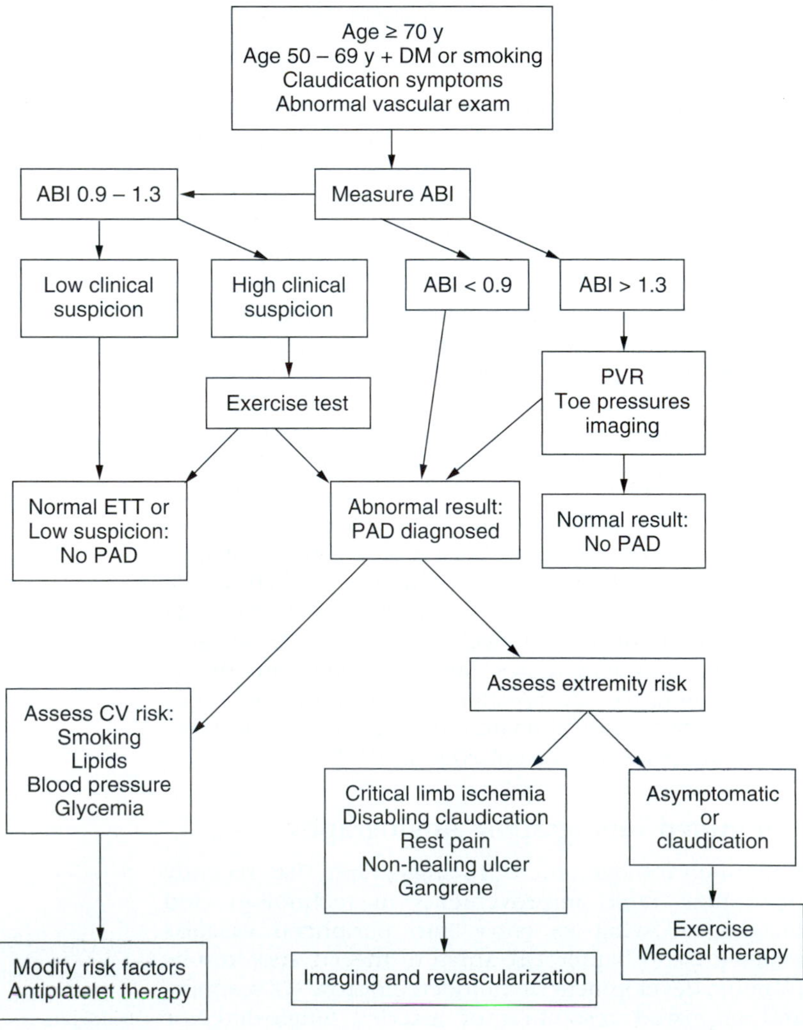

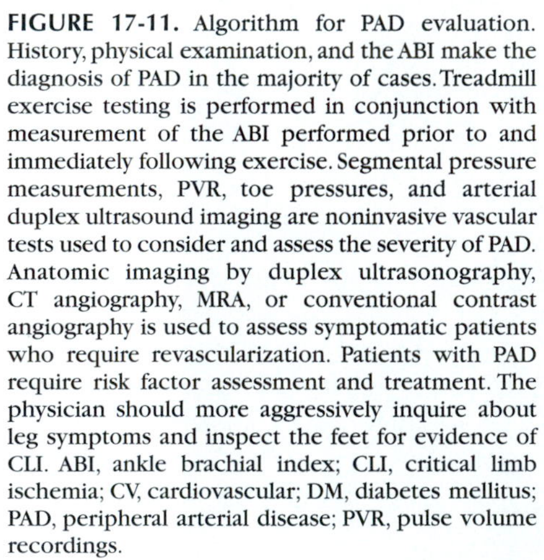

FIGURE 17-11. Algorithm for PAD evaluation. History, physical examination, and the ABI make the diagnosis of PAD in the majority of cases. Treadmill exercise testing is performed in conjunction with measurement of the ABI performed prior to and immediately following exercise. Segmental pressure measurements, PVR, toe pressures, and arterial duplex ultrasound imaging are noninvasive vascular tests used to consider and assess the severity of PAD. Anatomic imaging by duplex ultrasonography, CT angiography, MRA, or conventional contrast angiography is used to assess symptomatic patients who require revascularization. Patients with PAD require risk factor assessment and treatment. The physician should more aggressively inquire about leg symptoms and inspect the feet for evidence of CLI. ABI, ankle brachial index; CLI, critical limb ischemia; CV, cardiovascular; DM, diabetes mellitus; PAD, peripheral arterial disease; PVR, pulse volume recordings.

image, enhancing angiographic detail. Despite the wide acceptance of angiography as a reliable method for defining arterial anatomy, its invasive nature, requirement for contrast, nephrotoxicity, risk of atheroembolism, and risk of pseudoaneurysms or arteriovenous fistula continue to foster the development of alternative angiographic methods.

Summary

An algorithm for the evaluation of the patient with PAD is depicted in Figure 17-11. The diagnosis and evaluation of PAD is required in patients predisposed to develop PAD because of age or the presence of atherosclerotic risk factors and in patients whose history or examination are suggestive of PAD. An office evaluation should include measurement of ABI. An exercise test with measurement of the ABI after exercise is appropriate if the resting ABI is normal, yet clinical suspicion remains high. Patients with noncompressible ankle vessels should be referred to a vascular laboratory for additional testing, including segmental pressure measurements, pulse-volume recordings, and/or duplex ultrasonography. Symptomatic patients, particularly those with CLI who are being treated for revascularization, should undergo anatomic imaging with CT, MRA, or conventional carotid angiography.

REFERENCES

1. Belch JJ, Topol EJ, Agnelli G, et al: Critical issues in peripheral arterial disease detection and management: A call to action. Arch Intern Med 163:884, 2003.
2. Selvin E, Erlinger TP: Prevalence of and risk factors for peripheral arterial disease in the United States: Results from the National Health and Nutrition Examination Survey, 1999-2000. Circulation 110:738, 2004.
3. Criqui MH, Coughlin SS, Fronek A: Noninvasively diagnosed peripheral arterial disease as a predictor of mortality: Results from a prospective study. Circulation 72:768, 1985.
4. Meijer WT, Hoes AW, Rutgers D, et al: Peripheral arterial disease in the elderly: The Rotterdam Study. Arterioscler Thromb Vasc Biol 18:185, 1998.
5. Ciccone M, Di Noia D, Di Michele L, et al: The incidence of asymptomatic extracoronary atherosclerosis in patients with coronary atherosclerosis. Int Angiol 12:25, 1993.
6. Elhadd TA, Jung RT, Newton RW, et al: Incidence of asymptomatic peripheral arterial occlusive disease in diabetic patients attending a hospital clinic. Adv Exp Med Biol 428:45, 1997.
7. Leskinen Y, Salenius JP, Lehtimaki T, et al: The prevalence of peripheral arterial disease and medial arterial calcification in patients with chronic renal failure: Requirements for diagnostics. Am J Kidney Dis 40:472, 2002.
8. Newman AB, Sutton-Tyrrell K, Kuller LH: Lower-extremity arterial disease in older hypertensive adults. Arterioscler Thromb 13:555, 1993.
9. Hirsch AT, Criqui MH, Treat-Jacobson D, et al: Peripheral arterial disease detection, awareness, and treatment in primary care. JAMA 286:1317, 2001.
10. Fowkes FG, Housley E, Cawood EH, et al: Edinburgh Artery Study: Prevalence of asymptomatic and symptomatic peripheral arterial disease in the general population. Int J Epidemiol 20:384, 1991.
11. Stoffers HE, Rinkens PE, Kester AD, et al: The prevalence of asymptomatic and unrecognized peripheral arterial occlusive disease. Int J Epidemiol 25:282, 1996.
12. Hooi JD, Kester AD, Stoffers HE, et al: Incidence of and risk factors for asymptomatic peripheral arterial occlusive disease: A longitudinal study. Am J Epidemiol 153:666, 2001.
13. Bowlin SJ, Medalie JH, Flocke SA, et al: Epidemiology of intermittent claudication in middle-aged men. Am J Epidemiol 140:418, 1994.
14. Bainton D, Sweetnam P, Baker I, et al: Peripheral vascular disease: Consequence for survival and association with risk factors in the Speedwell prospective heart disease study. Br Heart J 72:128, 1994.
15. Smith GD, Shipley MJ, Rose G: Intermittent claudication, heart disease risk factors, and mortality. The Whitehall Study. Circulation 82:1925, 1990.
16. Ingolfsson IO, Sigurdsson G, Sigvaldason H, et al: A marked decline in the prevalence and incidence of intermittent claudication in Icelandic men 1968-1986: A strong relationship to smoking and serum cholesterol—the Reykjavik Study. J Clin Epidemiol 47:1237, 1994.
17. Ness J, Aronow WS, Ahn C: Risk factors for symptomatic peripheral arterial disease in older persons in an academic hospital-based geriatrics practice. J Am Geriatr Soc 48:312, 2000.
18. Fowkes FG, Housley E, Riemersma RA, et al: Smoking, lipids, glucose intolerance, and blood pressure as risk factors for peripheral atherosclerosis compared with ischemic heart disease in the Edinburgh Artery Study. Am J Epidemiol 135:331, 1992.
19. Kannel WB, Shurtleff D: The Framingham Study. Cigarettes and the development of intermittent claudication. Geriatrics 28:61, 1973.
20. Hiatt WR, Hoag S, Hamman RF: Effect of diagnostic criteria on the prevalence of peripheral arterial disease. The San Luis Valley Diabetes Study. Circulation 91:1472, 1995.
21. Newman AB, Siscovick DS, Manolio TA, et al: Ankle-arm index as a marker of atherosclerosis in the Cardiovascular Health Study. Cardiovascular Heart Study (CHS) Collaborative Research Group. Circulation 88:837, 1993.
22. Beks PJ, Mackaay AJ, de Neeling JN, et al: Peripheral arterial disease in relation to glycaemic level in an elderly Caucasian population: The Hoorn study. Diabetologia 38:86, 1995.
23. Abbott RD, Brand FN, Kannel WB: Epidemiology of some peripheral arterial findings in diabetic men and women: Experiences from the Framingham Study. Am J Med 88:376, 1990.
24. Murabito JM, D'Agostino RB, Silbershatz H, et al: Intermittent claudication. A risk profile from The Framingham Heart Study. Circulation 96:44, 1997.
25. Dolan NC, Liu K, Criqui MH, et al: Peripheral artery disease, diabetes, and reduced lower extremity functioning. Diabetes Care 25:113, 2002.
26. Rose GA: The diagnosis of ischaemic heart pain and intermittent claudication infield surveys. Bulletin of the World Health Organization 27:645, 1962.
27. Dormandy JA, Rutherford RB: Management of peripheral arterial disease (PAD). TASC Working Group. TransAtlantic Inter-Society Consensus (TASC). J Vasc Surg 31:S1, 2000.
28. Regensteiner JG, Steiner JF, Panzer RJ, et al: Evaluation of walking impairment by questionnaire in patients with peripheral arterial disease. J Vasc Med Biol 2:142, 1990.
29. Schroll M, Munck O: Estimation of peripheral arteriosclerotic disease by ankle blood pressure measurements in a population study of 60-year-old men and women. J Chronic Dis 34:261, 1981.
30. Postiglione A, Cicerano U, Gallotta G, et al: Prevalence of peripheral arterial disease and related risk factors in elderly institutionalized subjects. Gerontology 38:330, 1992.
31. Binaghi F, Fronteddu PF, Cannas F, et al: Prevalence of peripheral arterial occlusive disease and associated risk factors in a sample of southern Sardinian population. Int Angiol 13:233, 1994.
32. Bo M, Zanocchi M, Gallo R, et al: Prevalence and risk factors of peripheral arterial disease among older patients living in nursing homes [letter]. J Am Geriatr Soc 44:738, 1996.
33. Curb JD, Masaki K, Rodriguez BL, et al: Peripheral artery disease and cardiovascular risk factors in the elderly. The Honolulu Heart Program. Arterioscler Thromb Vasc Biol 16:1495, 1996.
34. Newman AB, Shemanski L, Manolio TA, et al: Ankle-arm index as a predictor of cardiovascular disease and mortality in the Cardiovascular Health Study. The Cardiovascular Health Study Group. Arterioscler Thromb Vasc Biol 19:538, 1999.
35. McDermott MM, Mehta S, Greenland P: Exertional leg symptoms other than intermittent claudication are common in peripheral arterial disease. Arch Intern Med 159:387, 1999.
36. McDermott MM, Greenland P, Liu K, et al: Leg symptoms in peripheral arterial disease: Associated clinical characteristics and functional impairment. JAMA 286:1599, 2001.
37. McDermott MM, Mehta S, Liu K, et al: Leg symptoms, the ankle-brachial index, and walking ability in patients with peripheral arterial disease. J Gen Intern Med 14:173, 1999.

38. Ware JE, Jr: The status of health assessment 1994. Annu Rev Public Health 16:327, 1995.
39. Jelnes R, Gaardsting O, Hougaard Jensen K, et al: Fate in intermittent claudication: Outcome and risk factors. Br Med J (Clin Res Ed) 293: 1137, 1986.
40. Slovut DP, Olin JW: Fibromuscular dysplasia. N Engl J Med 350: 1862, 2004.
41. Delis KT, Bountouroglou D, Mansfield AO. Venous claudication in iliofemoral thrombosis: Long-term effects on venous hemodynamics, clinical status, and quality of life. Ann Surg 239:118, 2004.
42. Lipetz JS: Pathophysiology of inflammatory, degenerative, and compressive radiculopathies. Phys Med Rehabil Clin N Am 13:439, 2002.
43. Goldstein B: Anatomic issues related to cervical and lumbosacral radiculopathy. Phys Med Rehabil Clin N Am 13:423, 2002.
44. Catalano M: Epidemiology of critical limb ischaemia: North Italian data. Eur J Med 2:11, 1993.
45. Luther M, Kantonen I, Lepantalo M, et al: Arterial intervention and reduction in amputation for chronic critical leg ischaemia. Br J Surg 87:454, 2000.
46. Group TG: Epidemiology of lower extremity amputation in centres in Europe, North America and East Asia: The global lower extremity amputation study group. Br J Surg 87:328, 2000.
47. Wrobel JS, Mayfield JA, Reiber GE: Geographic variation of lower-extremity major amputation in individuals with and without diabetes in the Medicare population. Diabetes Care 24:860, 2001.
48. Diabetes-related amputations of lower extremities in the Medicare population—Minnesota, 1993-1995. MMWR Morb Mortal Wkly Rep 47:649, 1998.
49. Jude EB, Oyibo SO, Chalmers N, et al: Peripheral arterial disease in diabetic and nondiabetic patients: A comparison of severity and outcome. Diabetes Care 24:1433, 2001.
50. Moss SE, Klein R, Klein BE: The prevalence and incidence of lower extremity amputation in a diabetic population. Arch Intern Med 152:610, 1992.
51. Jonason T, Bergstrom R: Cessation of smoking in patients with intermittent claudication: Effects on the risk of peripheral vascular complications, myocardial infarction and mortality. Acta Med Scand 221:253, 1987.
52. Lassila R, Lepantalo M. Cigarette smoking and the outcome after lower limb arterial surgery. Acta Chir Scand 154:635, 1988.
53. Liedberg E, Persson BM: Age, diabetes and smoking in lower limb amputation for arterial occlusive disease. Acta Orthop Scand 54:383, 1983.
54. Bayne SR, Donovan DL, Henthorne WA: A rare complication in elective repair of an abdominal aortic aneurysm: Multiple transmural colonic infarcts secondary to atheroemboli. Ann Vasc Surg 8:290, 1994.
55. Fukumoto Y, Tsutsui H, Tsuchihashi M, et al: The incidence and risk factors of cholesterol embolization syndrome, a complication of cardiac catheterization: A prospective study. J Am Coll Cardiol 42:211, 2003.
56. Dormandy J, Heeck L, Vig S: Acute limb ischemia. Semin Vasc Surg 12:148, 1999.
57. Silverman JJ: The incidence of palpable dorsalis pedis and posterior tibial pulsations in soldiers: An analysis of over 1,000 infantry soldiers. Am Heart J 32:82, 1946.
58. Sun YQ, Zhu DL: Absent dorsalis pedis and posterior tibial pulsations in normal young Chinese. A survey of 1,728 young people. Chin Med J (Engl) 96:643, 1983.
59. Robertson GS, Ristic CD, Bullen BR: The incidence of congenitally absent foot pulses. Ann R Coll Surg Engl 72:99, 1990.
60. Ascher E, Mazzariol F, Hingorani A, et al: The use of duplex ultrasound arterial mapping as an alternative to conventional arteriography for primary and secondary infrapopliteal bypasses. Am J Surg 178:162, 1999.
61. McDermott MM, Criqui MH, Liu K, et al: Lower ankle/brachial index, as calculated by averaging the dorsalis pedis and posterior tibial arterial pressures, and association with leg functioning in peripheral arterial disease. J Vasc Surg 32:1164, 2000.
62. Lijmer JG, Hunink MG, van den Dungen JJ, et al: ROC analysis of noninvasive tests for peripheral arterial disease. Ultrasound Med Biol 22:391, 1996.
63. Fowkes FG: The measurement of atherosclerotic peripheral arterial disease in epidemiological surveys. Int J Epidemiol 17:248, 1988.
64. Ishimura E, Okuno S, Kitatani K, et al: Different risk factors for peripheral vascular calcification between diabetic and nondiabetic haemodialysis patients—importance of glycaemic control. Diabetologia 45:1446, 2002.
65. Vogt MT, McKenna M, Anderson SJ, et al: The relationship between ankle-arm index and mortality in older men and women. J Am Geriatr Soc 41:523, 1993.
66. Sikkink CJ, van Asten WN, van't Hof MA, et al: Decreased ankle/brachial indices in relation to morbidity and mortality in patients with peripheral arterial disease. Vasc Med 2:169, 1997.
67. McKenna M, Wolfson S, Kuller L: The ratio of ankle and arm arterial pressure as an independent predictor of mortality. Atherosclerosis 87:119, 1991.
68. McPhail IR, Spittell PC, Weston SA, et al: Intermittent claudication: An objective office-based assessment. J Am Coll Cardiol 37:1381, 2001.
69. Rutherford RB, Lowenstein DH, Klein MF: Combining segmental systolic pressures and plethysmography to diagnose arterial occlusive disease of the legs. Am J Surg 138:211, 1979.
70. Bone GE, Pomajzl MJ: Toe blood pressure by photoplethysmography: An index of healing in forefoot amputation. Surgery 89:569, 1981.
71. Ramsey DE, Manke DA, Sumner DS. Toe blood pressure: A valuable adjunct to ankle pressure measurement for assessing peripheral arterial disease. J Cardiovasc Surg (Torino) 24:43, 1983.
72. Carter SA, Tate RB: Value of toe pulse waves in addition to systolic pressures in the assessment of the severity of peripheral arterial disease and critical limb ischemia. J Vasc Surg 24:258, 1996.
73. Brooks B, Dean R, Patel S, et al: TBI or not TBI: That is the question. Is it better to measure toe pressure than ankle pressure in diabetic patients? Diabet Med 18:528, 2001.
74. Hiatt WR, Hirsch AT, Regensteiner JG, et al: Clinical Trials for Claudication: Assessment of exercise performance, functional status, and clinical end points. Circulation 92:614, 1995.
75. Moneta GL, Yeager RA, Lee RW, et al: Noninvasive localization of arterial occlusive disease: A comparison of segmental Doppler pressures and arterial duplex mapping. J Vasc Surg 17:578, 1993.
76. Pinto F, Lencioni R, Napoli V, et al: Peripheral ischemic occlusive arterial disease: Comparison of color Doppler sonography and angiography. J Ultrasound Med 15:697, 1996.
77. Ranke C, Creutzig A, Alexander K. Duplex scanning of the peripheral arteries: Correlation of the peak velocity ratio with angiographic diameter reduction. Ultrasound Med Biol 18:433, 1992.
78. de Vries SO, Hunink MG, Polak JF: Summary receiver operating characteristic curves as a technique for meta-analysis of the diagnostic performance of duplex ultrasonography in peripheral arterial disease. Acad Radiol 3:361, 1996.
79. Allard L, Cloutier G, Durand LG, et al: Limitations of ultrasonic duplex scanning for diagnosing lower limb arterial stenoses in the presence of adjacent segment disease. J Vasc Surg 19:650, 1994.
80. van der Heijden FH, Legemate DA, van Leeuwen MS, et al: Value of Duplex scanning in the selection of patients for percutaneous transluminal angioplasty. Eur J Vasc Surg 7:71, 1993.
81. Ligush J, Jr, Reavis SW, Preisser JS, et al: Duplex ultrasound scanning defines operative strategies for patients with limb-threatening ischemia. J Vasc Surg 28:482, 1998.
82. Proia RR, Walsh DB, Nelson PR, et al: Early results of infragenicular revascularization based solely on duplex arteriography. J Vasc Surg 33:1165, 2001.
83. Mills JL, Harris EJ, Taylor LM, Jr, et al: The importance of routine surveillance of distal bypass grafts with duplex scanning: A study of 379 reversed vein grafts. J Vasc Surg 12:379, 1990.
84. Laborde AL, Synn AY, Worsey MJ, et al: A prospective comparison of ankle/brachial indices and color duplex imaging in surveillance of the in situ saphenous vein bypass. J Cardiovasc Surg (Torino) 33:420, 1992.
85. Taylor PR, Tyrrell MR, Crofton M, et al: Colour flow imaging in the detection of femoro-distal graft and native artery stenosis: Improved criteria. Eur J Vasc Surg 6:232, 1992.
86. Westerband A, Mills JL, Kistler S, et al: Prospective validation of threshold criteria for intervention in infrainguinal vein grafts undergoing duplex surveillance. Ann Vasc Surg 11:44, 1997.
87. Lundell A, Lindblad B, Bergqvist D, et al: Femoropopliteal-crural graft patency is improved by an intensive surveillance program: A prospective randomized study. J Vasc Surg 21:26, 1995.

88. Ihlberg L, Luther M, Tierala E, et al: The utility of duplex scanning in infrainguinal vein graft surveillance: Results from a randomised controlled study. Eur J Vasc Endovasc Surg 16:19, 1998.
89. Ihlberg L, Luther M, Alback A, et al: Does a completely accomplished duplex-based surveillance prevent vein-graft failure? Eur J Vasc Endovasc Surg 18:395, 1999.
90. Lalak NJ, Hanel KC, Hunt J, et al: Duplex scan surveillance of infrainguinal prosthetic bypass grafts. J Vasc Surg 20:637, 1994.
91. Dunlop P, Sayers RD, Naylor AR, et al: The effect of a surveillance programme on the patency of synthetic infrainguinal bypass grafts. Eur J Vasc Endovasc Surg 11:441, 1996.
92. Calligaro KD, Musser DJ, Chen AY, et al: Duplex ultrasonography to diagnose failing arterial prosthetic grafts. Surgery 120:455, 1996.
93. Sacks D, Robinson ML, Summers TA, et al: The value of duplex sonography after peripheral artery angioplasty in predicting subacute restenosis. AJR Am J Roentgenol 162:179, 1994.
94. Spijkerboer AM, Nass PC, de Valois JC, et al: Iliac artery stenoses after percutaneous transluminal angioplasty: Follow-up with duplex ultrasonography. J Vasc Surg 23:691, 1996.
95. Tatli S, Lipton MJ, Davison BD, et al: From the RSNA refresher courses: MR imaging of aortic and peripheral vascular disease. Radiographics 23 Spec No:S59, 2003.
96. Steffens JC, Link J, Schwarzenberg H, et al: Lower extremity occlusive disease: Diagnostic imaging with a combination of cardiac-gated 2D phase-contrast and cardiac-gated 2D time-of-flight MRA. J Comput Assist Tomogr 23:7, 1999.
97. Quinn SF, Sheley RC, Semonsen KG, et al: Aortic and lower-extremity arterial disease: Evaluation with MR angiography versus conventional angiography. Radiology 206:693, 1998.
98. Baum RA, Rutter CM, Sunshine JH, et al: Multicenter trial to evaluate vascular magnetic resonance angiography of the lower extremity. American College of Radiology Rapid Technology Assessment Group. JAMA 274:875, 1995.
99. Nelemans PJ, Leiner T, de Vet HC, et al: Peripheral arterial disease: Meta-analysis of the diagnostic performance of MR angiography. Radiology 217:105, 2000.
100. Rofsky NM, Adelman MA: MR angiography in the evaluation of atherosclerotic peripheral vascular disease. Radiology 214:325, 2000.
101. Sharafuddin MJ, Stolpen AH, Sun S, et al: High-resolution multiphase contrast-enhanced three-dimensional MR angiography compared with two-dimensional time-of-flight MR angiography for the identification of pedal vessels. J Vasc Interv Radiol 13:695, 2002.
102. Dorweiler B, Neufang A, Kreitner KF, et al: Magnetic resonance angiography unmasks reliable target vessels for pedal bypass grafting in patients with diabetes mellitus. J Vasc Surg 35:766, 2002.
103. Owen RS, Carpenter JP, Baum RA, et al: Magnetic resonance imaging of angiographically occult runoff vessels in peripheral arterial occlusive disease. N Engl J Med 326:1577, 1992.
104. Kreitner KF, Kalden P, Neufang A, et al: Diabetes and peripheral arterial occlusive disease: Prospective comparison of contrast-enhanced three-dimensional MR angiography with conventional digital subtraction angiography. AJR Am J Roentgenol 174:171, 2000.
105. Krause UJ, Pabst T, Kenn W, et al: Time-resolved contrast-enhanced magnetic resonance angiography of the lower extremity. Angiology 55:119, 2004.
106. Winterer JT, Schaefer O, Uhrmeister P, et al: Contrast enhanced MR angiography in the assessment of relevant stenoses in occlusive disease of the pelvic and lower limb arteries: Diagnostic value of a two-step examination protocol in comparison to conventional DSA. Eur J Radiol 41:153, 2002.
107. Bendib K, Berthezene Y, Croisille P, et al: Assessment of complicated arterial bypass grafts: Value of contrast-enhanced subtraction magnetic resonance angiography. J Vasc Surg 26:1036, 1997.
108. Dorenbeck U, Seitz J, Volk M, et al: Evaluation of arterial bypass grafts of the pelvic and lower extremities with gadolinium-enhanced magnetic resonance angiography: Comparison with digital subtraction angiography. Invest Radiol 37:60, 2002.
109. Loewe C, Cejna M, Schoder M, et al: Contrast material-enhanced, moving-table MR angiography versus digital subtraction angiography for surveillance of peripheral arterial bypass grafts. J Vasc Interv Radiol 14:1129, 2003.
110. Brillet PY, Vayssairat M, Tassart M, et al: Gadolinium-enhanced MR angiography as first-line preoperative imaging in high-risk patients with lower limb ischemia. J Vasc Interv Radiol 14:1139, 2003.
111. Cronberg CN, Sjoberg S, Albrechtsson U, et al: Peripheral arterial disease: Contrast-enhanced 3D MR angiography of the lower leg and foot compared with conventional angiography. Acta Radiol 44:59, 2003.
112. Steffens JC, Schafer FK, Oberscheid B, et al: Bolus-chasing contrast-enhanced 3D MRA of the lower extremity: Comparison with intraarterial DSA. Acta Radiol 44:185, 2003.
113. Bezooijen R, van den Bosch HC, Tielbeek AV, et al: Peripheral arterial disease: Sensitivity-encoded multiposition MR angiography compared with intraarterial angiography and conventional multiposition MR angiography. Radiology 231:263, 2004.
114. Rieker O, Duber C, Schmiedt W, et al: Prospective comparison of CT angiography of the legs with intraarterial digital subtraction angiography. AJR Am J Roentgenol 166:269, 1996.
115. Tins B, Oxtoby J, Patel S: Comparison of CT angiography with conventional arterial angiography in aortoiliac occlusive disease. Br J Radiol 74:219, 2001.
116. Becker CR, Wintersperger B, Jakobs TF: Multi-detector-row CT angiography of peripheral arteries. Semin Ultrasound CT MR 24:268, 2003.
117. Martin ML, Tay KH, Flak B, et al: Multidetector CT angiography of the aortoiliac system and lower extremities: A prospective comparison with digital subtraction angiography. AJR Am J Roentgenol 180:1085, 2003.
118. Lawler LP, Fishman EK: Multi-detector row CT of thoracic disease with emphasis on 3D volume rendering and CT angiography. Radiographics 21:1257, 2001.

chapter 18

Medical Treatment of Peripheral Arterial Disease

Heather L. Gornik
Mark A. Creager

The treatment of patients with peripheral arterial disease (PAD) must take into consideration two principal themes (1) the risk of adverse cardiovascular events that are related to systemic atherosclerosis, including myocardial infarction and death; and (2) limb-related symptoms and prognosis, including functional capacity, quality of life, and limb viability. The risk of myocardial infarction, stroke, or death related to cardiovascular disease is increased three- to six-fold in patients with PAD (see Chapter 14). Functional limitations imposed by PAD, including symptoms of limb claudication, impaired walking ability, and critical limb ischemia, adversely affect quality of life and restrict patients' ability to participate in many basic vocational and recreational activities. This chapter, therefore, is divided into two major sections. The first section reviews the evidence to support aggressive risk factor modification and antiplatelet therapy for patients with PAD to reduce adverse cardiovascular events. The second section reviews the physical and medical therapies used to treat patients with intermittent claudication and critical limb ischemia. Catheter-based revascularization for PAD is reviewed in Chapter 19, and surgical revascularization for PAD is reviewed in Chapter 20.

RISK FACTOR MODIFICATION AND ANTIPLATELET THERAPY

Smoking Cessation

Tobacco smoking is strongly associated with the development and progression of PAD, with the risk of PAD among smokers as high as three-fold to that of nonsmokers (see Chapter 14).[1-4] Smoking cessation, therefore, is a critical component of risk factor modification for patients with PAD. Epidemiologic studies have established that smoking cessation improves both cardiovascular and limb-related outcomes among patients with PAD. Given the established hazards of cigarette smoking, it would be unethical to conduct a randomized clinical trial of smoking cessation.

Smoking cessation has salutary effects on claudication symptoms, exercise physiology, and limb-related outcomes in patients with symptomatic PAD. Patients with intermittent claudication who quit smoking have longer pain-free walking times and maximal walking times when compared with patients who continue to smoke.[5] In a prospective study of patients with intermittent claudication followed with serial noninvasive vascular testing over a period of 10 months, patients who quit smoking had significant improvements in maximal treadmill walking distance and post-exercise ankle pressure, whereas ongoing smokers had no changes in these parameters.[6] Smoking cessation is also associated with improved clinical outcomes in patients with PAD. In a Swedish study, patients with intermittent claudication who were active smokers or who had quit within 6 months were followed prospectively for the development of limb-related and cardiovascular outcomes.[7] At 7 years of follow-up, ongoing tobacco smoking was associated with the development of critical limb ischemia and was also an independent predictor of the need for surgical revascularization. Indeed, only patients who continued to smoke developed rest pain during the follow-up period. Ongoing smoking was also associated with the development of myocardial infarction and a trend toward decreased overall survival at 10 years of follow-up.

Continued cigarette smoking is associated with adverse outcome among patients with PAD referred for vascular surgery. In a prospective study of patients referred for femoropopliteal arterial bypass grafting, ongoing tobacco use was associated with a significant reduction in the one-year cumulative patency rate of both venous and prosthetic lower extremity bypass grafts.[8] In an Australian study of patients who underwent lumbar sympathectomy or lower extremity bypass grafting for symptomatic PAD, patients who quit smoking following surgery had dramatically improved 5-year survival rates when compared with patients who continued to smoke (Fig. 18-1).[9] The majority of the deaths that occurred in the postoperative patients were due to a major vascular event, whereas the remaining deaths were due to other smoking-related illnesses, namely COPD and lung cancer. The degree of ongoing tobacco use following revascularization may also be predictive of adverse events. In a registry study of patients who underwent their first arterial revascularization procedure, patients categorized as heavy smokers (>15 cigarettes per day) had significantly reduced overall survival when compared with moderate smokers (<15 cigarettes per day).[10] In addition, there was a 10-fold higher amputation rate among heavy smokers when compared with moderate smokers at 3 years' follow-up.

Despite the multiple benefits of smoking cessation in patients with PAD, it is an extremely difficult goal to

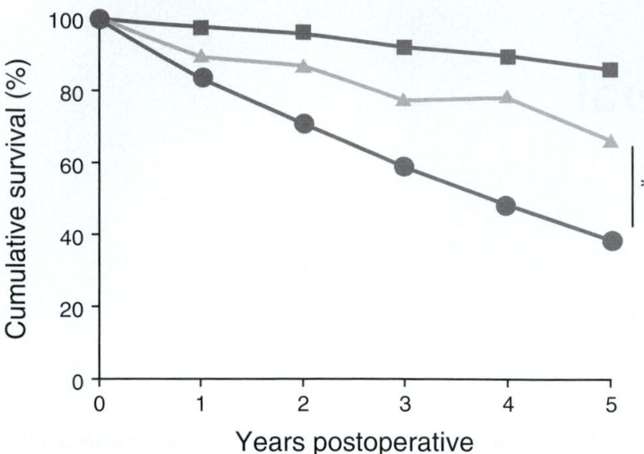

FIGURE 18-1. Smoking cessation is associated with improved cumulative survival after lower extremity revascularization surgery or lumbar sympathectomy. Patients who continue to smoke are compared with patients who quit smoking and historical age-matched controls from the Australian census. ■, Australian census; ▲, ceased smokers; ●, continuing smokers; *$P < .01$. (Reproduced with permission from Faulkner, KW, House AK, Castleden WM: The effect of cessation of smoking on the accumulative survival rates of patients with symptomatic peripheral vascular disease. Med J Aust 1[5]:217, 1983.)

accomplish and initial success rates are low. The efficacy of physician advice in achieving smoking cessation is less than 5%.[11] The success rate is at least 10-fold higher when smoking cessation advice and encouragement are given to patients at risk for myocardial infarction or patients who have survived a myocardial infarction. Smoking cessation programs may be more successful when coupled with nicotine replacement therapy. Most recently, the antidepressant bupropion has been demonstrated to improve tobacco abstinence rates at 12 months relative to placebo when used alone or in combination with the nicotine patch.[12] The efficacy of achieving smoking cessation among patients with PAD has not been studied. Novel approaches to smoking cessation is an area in grave need of research.

Recommendations

Smoking cessation advice, as well as encouragement of cessation efforts, should be key components of the office visit. For patients motivated to quit smoking, nicotine replacement therapy and/or bupropion should be prescribed. These efforts may be incorporated into a formal smoking cessation program, which includes longitudinal counseling on an individual basis or in a small group.

Lipid-Lowering Therapy

Dyslipidemia is well established as a risk factor for the development of atherosclerotic vascular disease, including coronary artery disease (CAD) and cerebrovascular disease (CVD). In addition, epidemiologic studies have established dyslipidemia, specifically total and low-density lipoprotein (LDL) cholesterol, as a risk factor for the development of atherosclerosis in the peripheral circulation (see Chapter 14).[1,13,14] There is a less established association between low levels of high density lipoprotein (HDL) cholesterol and the development of claudication.[1,15,16] The association, if any, between elevated triglycerides and PAD is controversial.[15,16] Due to the association of dyslipidemia and vascular disease, lipid-lowering therapy has been extensively investigated as a clinical strategy to prevent myocardial ischemia, stroke, and death in patients with systemic atherosclerosis. Many of these studies have specifically addressed the use of lipid-lowering therapy in patients with PAD.

Angiographic Trials

The Cholesterol Lowing Atherosclerosis Study (CLAS) investigated the effect of cholesterol-lowering therapy with colestipol hydrochloride and niacin on the angiographic progression of peripheral atherosclerosis in men with CAD.[17] After 2 years of treatment, there was a significant regression in femoral atherosclerotic plaque burden among patients randomized to colestipol and niacin, particularly in proximal lesions and high-grade stenoses. In contrast, the Probucol Quantitative Regression Swedish Trial (PQRST) found no effect of intensive lipid-lowering therapy with probucol plus cholestyramine, compared with placebo plus cholestyramine, on femoral artery atherosclerosis among hyperlipidemic patients with femoral atherosclerosis.[18] Patients were followed over a 3-year period. Patients randomized to cholestyramine plus placebo had a slight but significant improvement in two angiographic measures of atherosclerotic burden, plaque roughness, and arterial lumen volume. The 24% decline in HDL cholesterol among patients treated with probucol compared with the placebo group may have contributed to the negative findings of the study.

Clinical Outcome Trials

Given convincing epidemiologic evidence that established dyslipidemia as a risk factor for the development of atherosclerosis and subsequent cardiovascular events, multiple randomized clinical trials have investigated the use of lipid lowering agents for the prevention of death and other major cardiovascular events in high-risk patients. Many of these studies predate the availability of the highly effective HMG CoA reductase inhibitors ("statin" drugs) that have now become accepted as first-line therapy for dyslipidemia. Statins decrease cholesterol synthesis via potent inhibition of the hepatic enzyme HMG CoA reductase.[19]

In one of the early intervention trials with prolonged clinical follow-up, the Program on the Surgical Control of the Hyperlipidemias (POSCH) investigators studied the use of a partial ileal bypass to lower cholesterol and prevent cardiovascular events among survivors of myocardial infarction.[20] This surgical procedure bypasses the distal portion of the small intestine, the site of dietary cholesterol absorption, with the creation of an ileocecostomy. Patients were followed for a mean of 9.7 years. There was a 35% reduction in the composite endpoint of death due to CAD or confirmed nonfatal myocardial infarction among patients randomized to surgery. Randomization to partial ileal bypass surgery was associated with a significant reduction in the incidence of symptomatic PAD and in the incidence of asymptomatic PAD, as defined as an ABI of less than 0.95. Serial angiography demonstrated a significant decrease in the progression of coronary atherosclerosis and a trend toward decreased development of peripheral atherosclerosis among patients randomized to surgery. Despite the findings of the POSCH study, the invasive nature of the ileal bypass procedure, and its potential for severe adverse events (i.e., bowel obstruction, chronic diarrhea, nephrolithiasis, and gallstones) did not translate to widespread clinical application of the technique. The POSCH study, however, served as the springboard for modern randomized clinical trials of lipid-lowering pharmacotherapy for patients with atherosclerotic vascular disease.

The development of highly effective and safe agents, particularly the HMG CoA reductase inhibitors, as well as the fibrates and novel compounds, has allowed for the widespread application of lipid lowering therapy to patients with hyperlipidemia and atherosclerotic vascular disease. During the past decade, multiple large, randomized clinical trials have established the role of lipid-lowering pharmacotherapy, primarily with statins, in the secondary prevention of cardiovascular events among patients with CAD (Table 18-1).[21-24] Although these studies were not designed to specifically investigate the long-term benefit of lipid-lowering therapy in patients with PAD, the findings are of great relevance in these patients as most patients with PAD have either symptomatic or asymptomatic coronary atherosclerosis.[25,26] Recently, the Heart Protection Study broadened the indication for cholesterol-lowering therapy to include patients with atherosclerosis in any major vascular territory.[27]

The Scandinavian Simvastatin Survival Study (4S) was the first major clinical trial to demonstrate the survival benefit of aggressive lipid-lowering therapy with statins in hypercholesterolemic patients with CAD (see Table 18-1).[22] In secondary analyses, the 4S investigators examined the effect of simvastatin on the development of symptoms and signs of atherosclerotic vascular disease, including claudication and the appearance of a vascular bruit during semi-annual physical examinations of the study participants.[28] There was no significant difference in the detection of new or worsening femoral bruits, although this endpoint was likely limited by interobserver variability and the limited sensitivity of the physical examination. During a semi-annual query for adverse events, 2.3% of patients randomized to simvastatin, compared with 3.6% of patients randomized to placebo, reported new or progressive intermittent claudication. This finding has been confirmed in subsequent studies of the use of HMG-CoA reductase inhibitors for the treatment of symptomatic claudication, as discussed later in this chapter.[29,30]

The Cholesterol and Recurrent Events (CARE) and the Long-Term Intervention with Pravastatin in Ischaemic Disease (LIPID) trials expanded the potential for the use of statins in patients with CAD to include those with moderate cholesterol levels.[23] Although neither of these studies included prespecified PAD endpoints, both studies demonstrated a significant reduction in the relative risk of stroke among patients randomized to statin therapy (see Table 18-1).

The Heart Protection Study extended the use of statins to the secondary prevention of cardiovascular events in patients with atherosclerosis in any major vascular bed and to the primary prevention of cardiovascular events in high-risk patients, particularly diabetics.[27,31] Eligible patients included those with documented CAD, cerebrovascular disease, or PAD, or patients without documented atherosclerotic vascular disease believed to be at high-risk of a major vascular event due to diabetes or multiple cardiac risk factors. Patients enrolled in the study of the basis of PAD had intermittent claudication, had undergone lower extremity revascularization, or had objective evidence of "leg artery stenosis." Patients were randomized to simvastatin or placebo, as well as antioxidant vitamins or placebo, in a 2×2 factorial design. The majority of patients randomized in the study had a history of CAD (65%). Of these, 30% of patients had PAD. Patients were followed for a mean of 5 years. There was a 13% reduction in the relative risk of all-cause mortality among patients randomized to simvastatin, due largely to a 17% reduction in the risk of vascular death. Among patients randomized to simvastatin, there was a striking 38% relative reduction in the incidence of first nonfatal myocardial infarction. Overall, there was a 24% reduction in the first occurrence of any major vascular event among patients randomized to simvastatin. This benefit was evident in patients enrolled by all criteria, including those without CAD, but with atherosclerosis in other vascular beds. Patients enrolled on the basis of PAD alone, with no documented CAD, had a 19% reduction in incidence of first major vascular event if randomized to simvastatin. Although limb-related outcomes were not studied in detail, there was a significant 15% reduction in the incidence of noncoronary revascularization procedures (i.e., carotid endarterectomy, percutaneous intervention, or peripheral revascularization) among patients randomized to simvastatin. On the basis of the Heart Protection Study, as well as other recent trials of lipid-lowering for the secondary prevention of cardiovascular events, the National Cholesterol Education Program (NCEP) has recently established an LDL goal of less than 100 mg/dL as the therapeutic target in patients at risk for the development of cardiovascular events, and an LDL goal of <70 mg/dL as a more aggressive option for those patients at highest risk of a recurrent event.[32,33]

Non-LDL cholesterol, particularly low HDL cholesterol, has been identified as an independent risk factor for the development of CAD.[34,35] Pharmacologic agents that raise HDL cholesterol, such as fibric acid derivatives and niacin, have not been as widely studied as agents that lower total and LDL cholesterol (i.e., the statins) for the secondary prevention of cardiovascular events in patients with atherosclerotic vascular disease. The Veterans Affairs High-Density Lipoprotein Cholesterol Intervention Trial (VA-HIT) investigators randomized men with documented CAD and low HDL cholesterol to gemfibrozil or placebo (see Table 18-1).[21] After a median 5.1 years of follow-up, there was a 22% reduction in the primary composite endpoint of death from CAD or nonfatal myocardial infarction in patients randomized to gemfibrozil. The incidence of peripheral vascular surgery, the only PAD endpoint studied, was not significantly

TABLE 18-1 SIGNIFICANT FINDINGS OF MAJOR RANDOMIZED CLINICAL TRIALS OF CHOLESTEROL-LOWERING THERAPY IN ATHEROSCLEROTIC VASCULAR DISEASE

Study	Drug (daily dose)	Patient Population	Number Randomized	Baseline Cholesterol	Follow-Up	Primary Endpoint	Vascular Endpoints
Scandinavian Simvastatin Survival Study (4S)[22,28]	Simvastatin (20-40 mg)	Angina pectoris or history of MI (>6 months) Total cholesterol 213-309 mg/dL	4444	Total: 261 mg/dL LDL: 188 mg/dL	5.4 years	30% ⇓ total mortality	30% ⇓ cerebrovascular event 48% ⇓ carotid bruit 38% ⇓ intermittent claudication
Cholesterol and Recurrent Events Trial (CARE)[23]	Pravastatin (40 mg)	Recent MI (within 3-20 months) Total cholesterol < 240 mg/dL	4159	Total: 209 mg/dL LDL: 139 mg/dL	5.0 years	24% ⇓ fatal coronary artery disease or nonfatal MI	31% ⇓ stroke
Long-Term Intervention with Pravastatin in Ischaemic Disease Study (LIPID)[24]	Pravastatin (40 mg)	Acute MI or hospitalization for unstable angina (within 3-36 months) Total cholesterol 155-271 mg/dL	9014	Total: 218 mg/dL LDL: 150 mg/dL	6.1 years	24% ⇓ death from coronary artery disease	19% ⇓ stroke
MRC/BHF Heart Protection Study [27,31]	Simvastatin (40 mg)	Atherosclerotic vascular disease (CAD, CVD, PAD) patients at high risk for cardiovascular event (DM) Total cholesterol >135 mg/dL	20,536	Total: 5.9 mmol/liter (228 mg/dL) LDL: 3.4 mmol/L (131 mg/dL)	5.0 years	13% ⇓ all cause mortality 17% ⇓ vascular death	25% ⇓ stroke 15% ⇓ noncoronary revascularization
Veterans Affairs High-Density Lipoprotein Cholesterol Intervention Study (VA-HIT)[21]	Gemfibrozil (600 mg)	Documented CAD HDL < 40 mg/dL LDL < 140 mg/dL TGs < 300 mg/dL	2531	Total: 175 mg/dL LDL: 112 mg/dL HDL: 32 mg/dL	5.1 years	22% ⇓ fatal coronary artery disease or nonfatal MI (composite endpoint)	25% ⇓ confirmed stroke (-NS-, $P = .10$) 59% ⇓ TIA 65% ⇓ Carotid endarterectomy

CAD, coronary artery disease; CVD, cerebrovascular disease; DM, diabetes mellitus; HDL, high-density lipoprotein; LDL, low-density lipoprotein; MI, myocardial infarction; PAD, peripheral arterial disease; TGs, triglycerides; TIA, transient ischemic attack.

different within the treatment groups. Although early evidence suggests that pharmacologic therapies targeting non-LDL cholesterol may have a role in the primary or secondary prevention of cardiovascular events in patients with CAD, the role of such therapies in the management of patients with PAD is entirely uncertain.

Recommendations

On the basis of multiple, large randomized clinical trials, all patients with PAD should be treated with an HMG CoA reductase inhibitor to a target LDL cholesterol of less than 100 mg/dL.[36] Statins should be prescribed for all patients with PAD regardless of whether or not they have documented CAD. Owing to the findings of the Heart Protection Study, patients with PAD and normal cholesterol levels should also be treated with statin therapy.[33] There is no specific clinical evidence to support the treatment of low HDL cholesterol with fibrates in patients with PAD, although it is a reasonable extrapolation of clinical trials for patients with concomitant CAD. To date, no large clinical trial has investigated the role of combination therapy (i.e., statin plus fibrate or statin plus ezetimibe) in patients with atherosclerotic vascular disease, although combination therapy should be considered for a patient with atherosclerotic vascular disease and persistent dyslipidemia (i.e., LDL cholesterol >100 mg/dL) despite high doses of statins.[33]

Treatment of Hypertension

Control of hypertension is critical for the prevention of stroke, myocardial infarction, and congestive heart failure. Blood pressure control can be achieved with a number of pharmacologic agents, either individually or in combination, and large, randomized clinical trials have demonstrated the benefits of pharmacotherapy on clinical outcomes, including death.[37,38] Although patients with hypertension and PAD are at an increased risk of serious vascular events, few studies have specifically addressed the benefit of blood pressure lowering in this population.

Effect of Blood Pressure Lowering on Claudication

Traditional clinical teachings and conventional medical wisdom have alleged that intensive blood pressure lowering, particularly with β-adrenergic blockers, may worsen symptoms in patients with claudication and PAD.[39-41] This is a particularly important issue because patients with PAD often have compelling indications for β-adrenergic blockers. Several small clinical trials have directly investigated this clinical issue. Roberts and colleagues randomized 20 patients with PAD and hypertension to one of three β blockers (pindolol, atenolol, and labetalol) or the ACE inhibitor captopril for each of four 1-month treatment intervals in a crossover study.[42] There was a significant reduction in pain-free and maximal-walking distance documented during the labetalol and pindolol arms and a trend toward reduced walking distances with atenolol. Patients had no significant decline in treadmill exercise capacity during treatment with captopril. Solomon and colleagues studied the effect of atenolol and the calcium channel blocker nifedipine given alone and in combination in patients with intermittent claudication.[43] There was no significant effect of atenolol or nifedipine, when given alone, on pain-free walking distance or total walking distance. The combination of atenolol and nifedipine resulted in small (9%) but statistically significant reduction in total walking distance. Despite these findings, there was no effect of the combination of atenolol and nifedipine on subjective assessment of leg fatigue. In a meta-analysis of small randomized controlled clinical trials of the use of β blockers in patients with PAD and intermittent claudication, there was no significant effect on pain-free or maximal walking distance among patients treated with β blockers.[44] The Solomon study was not included in the analysis. Of the 11 studies included in the analysis, only the study by Roberts and coworkers demonstrated an adverse effect of β blockers.

The safety of blood pressure-lowering therapy, specifically with β-adrenergic blockers, in patients with PAD and claudication is of great importance. A substantial percentage of patients with PAD have concomitant CAD. In these patients, specifically those with myocardial infarction, treatment with a β-adrenergic blocker has been demonstrated to be a lifesaving therapy in large, multicenter randomized clinical trials.[45,46]

β-Adrenergic blockers are also crucial for the management of symptomatic angina pectoris in patients with CAD. In addition, β-adrenergic blockers are a key component of the perioperative management of patients with PAD and claudication undergoing lower extremity revascularization surgery.[47,48]

More recently, Overlack and colleagues investigated the effect of blood pressure-lowering therapy on the severity of select comorbid illnesses in patients with essential hypertension.[49] Patients with hypertension and one of many comorbidities, including PAD, dyslipidemia, diabetes mellitus, CAD, renal insufficiency with proteinuria, COPD, and arthritis, were randomized to treatment with the ACE inhibitor, perindopril, or placebo. Patients were followed for a total of 6 weeks for the development of adverse events related to their comorbid conditions. A subgroup of patients had significant symptomatic PAD, rigorously defined as a pain-free walking distance of 80 to 200 meters (Fontaine IIb), and an imaging study that demonstrated evidence of iliac or femoral arterial occlusive disease. Patients with ankle pressures of less than 70 mm Hg were excluded. Among the patients with PAD, there was no difference in the pain-free or maximal walking distance between the perindopril and placebo groups, although walking distance increased modestly in both groups above baseline. None of the PAD patients reported worsening claudication. Demonstration of the safety of ACE inhibitors in the majority of patients with claudication is very important, particularly given the findings of recent trials that have established the importance of this class of agents in the prevention of cardiovascular events.[50]

Clinical Outcome Trials

Two major clinical trials have investigated the potential benefits of blood pressure-lowering therapy in the prevention of cardiovascular events in patients with PAD. The Appropriate Blood Pressure Control in Diabetes (ABCD) trial studied the effect of intensive blood pressure control compared with moderate blood pressure control on the occurrence of cardiovascular events and renal insufficiency in diabetic patients.[51,52] Normotensive (diastolic blood pressure 80 to 90 mm Hg) and hypertensive (diastolic blood pressure greater than 90 mm Hg) diabetic patients were enrolled. The hypertensive patients were randomized to receive either enalapril or nisoldipine as first-line therapy. The normotensive patients were randomized to intensive blood pressure treatment (with further randomization to one of the two study drugs) to achieve a reduction in diastolic pressure of 10 mm Hg, or standard therapy, in which case they received placebo. Patients were followed for a mean of 5 years. In a substudy of the diabetic patients in the normotensive cohort, the effect of intensive blood pressure treatment among patients with PAD was investigated.[51] Among the 220 normotensive patients randomized to intensive blood pressure treatment, there was a 65% reduction in the relative risk of myocardial infarction, stroke, or cardiovascular death. There was a strong inverse relationship between baseline ABI and the risk of a cardiovascular event. Intensive blood pressure control negated this relationship and normalized the odds of a cardiovascular event toward that of patients with a normal ABI (Fig. 18-2). The benefit of intensive blood pressure control was evident even in patients with a severely decreased ABI, a subset of patients that had been excluded from prior studies.[49] There were too few patients with PAD to analyze data for enalapril and nisoldipine separately. The findings of the ABCD trial emphasize the importance of intensive blood pressure control in diabetic patients with PAD.

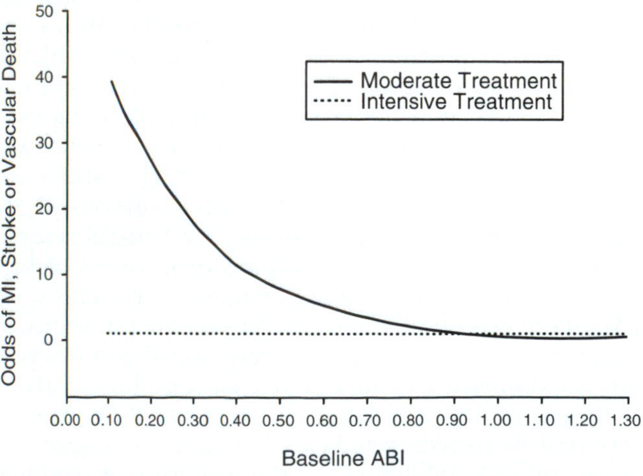

FIGURE 18-2. Intensive blood pressure with enalapril or nisoldipine decreases the odds of a major vascular event among diabetic patients with peripheral arterial disease. Results from the Appropriate Blood Pressure Control in Diabetics (ABCD) Trial. The inverse correlation of ankle-brachial index and odds of a major vascular event are not present among patients randomized to the intensive blood pressure control group. ABI, ankle-brachial index. (Reproduced with permission from Mehler PS, Coll JR, Estacio R, et al: Intensive blood pressure control reduces the risk of cardiovascular events in patients with peripheral arterial disease and type 2 diabetes. Circulation 107[5]:753, 2003.)

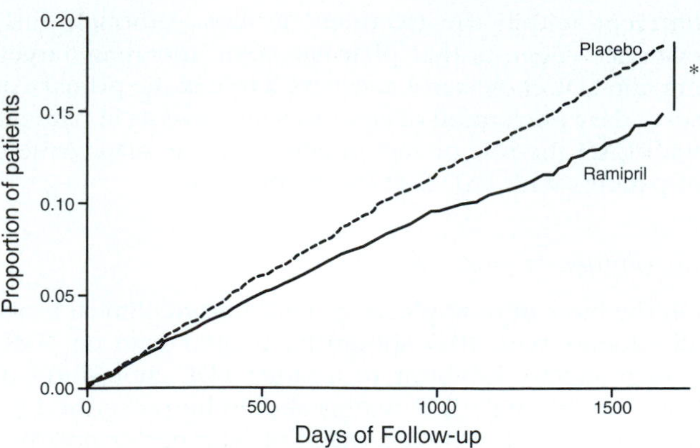

FIGURE 18-3. Ramipril reduces the incidence of myocardial infarction, stroke, or cardiovascular death among high-risk patients with atherosclerotic vascular disease or diabetes mellitus. *$P < .001$. (Reproduced with permission from Yusuf S, Sleight P, Pogue J, et al: Effects of an angiotensin-converting-enzyme inhibitor, ramipril, on cardiovascular events in high-risk patients. The Heart Outcomes Prevention Evaluation Study Investigators. N Engl J Med 342[3]:145, 2000.)

The Heart Outcomes Prevention Evaluation (HOPE) investigators tested the efficacy of the ACE inhibitor ramipril for the primary and secondary prevention of cardiovascular events in high-risk patients.[50] Patients were enrolled on the basis of established atherosclerotic vascular disease (CAD, prior stroke, or PAD) or diabetes mellitus with additional cardiac risk factors. Forty-four percent of patients randomized had evidence of PAD, as manifested by a history of claudication with an abnormal ankle-brachial index (ABI) of less than 0.8, limb revascularization procedure, amputation, or angiographic evidence of arterial stenosis.[53] Patients were randomized to receive ramipril or placebo, as well as vitamin E supplements or placebo in a 2×2 factorial design. At a mean of 5 years of follow-up, there was a 22% reduction in the primary composite endpoint of myocardial infarction, stroke, or cardiovascular death among patients randomized to ramipril (Fig. 18-3). In subgroup analysis, the benefit of ramipril was present regardless of baseline blood pressure. The benefit of ramipril on the composite endpoint was present among the subgroup of patients with PAD. The benefit of ramipril was likely due to cardiovascular benefits other than its blood pressure-lowering properties because the mean decrease in blood pressure among patients randomized to active therapy was very small. The findings of the HOPE trial indicate that patients with PAD should be treated with an ACE inhibitor—regardless of baseline blood pressure or the presence or absence of diabetes.

Recommendations

Blood pressure control is an important component of cardiovascular risk reduction among patients with PAD, and all patients with PAD should undergo blood pressure assessment routinely. Any class of antihypertensive agents, including β blockers, can be safely prescribed for blood pressure lowering, although ACE inhibitors should be considered as the first line agent. Caution should be exercised when managing the patient with critical limb ischemia because aggressive blood pressure lowering may be detrimental in this small subset of patients. Even normotensive patients with PAD may benefit from ACE-inhibitor therapy. Aggressive blood pressure control is particularly important for diabetic patients with PAD.

Control of Diabetes Mellitus

Multiple epidemiologic studies have established a strong association between diabetes mellitus and PAD (see Chapter 14).[1,4,13,54] The relative risk of PAD is 2 to 4 times that of nondiabetic patients. The presence of diabetes is associated with adverse limb-related outcomes among patients with documented PAD, including the need for amputation.[55,56] In addition, diabetes is associated with a markedly increased risk of a major cardiovascular event, including myocardial ischemia, stroke, and death. During recent decades, there have been new therapeutic options for achieving glycemic control in diabetic patients, particularly the insulin sensitizing agents metformin and the thiazolidinediones ("glitazones"). Sulfonylureas and insulin remain mainstays of therapy in certain subsets of diabetic patients. Whereas clinical trials have established the vital importance of rigorous glycemic control for the prevention of microvascular complications in diabetic patients, the benefits of glycemic control for the prevention of major cardiovascular events has not been definitively established.

Clinical Outcome Trials

The Diabetes Control and Complications Trial (DCCT) Research Group investigated whether intensive glycemic control could improve clinical outcomes in diabetic patients.[57] Young patients (ages 13 to 39 years) with type 1 diabetes mellitus, with and without retinopathy, were randomized to one of two glycemic control strategies: intensive therapy, with an insulin pump or frequent injections to maintain blood sugar as close to normal as possible, or conventional therapy with once or twice daily insulin injections. The development or progression of retinopathy was the primary endpoint of the study, and the low cardiovascular risk profile of the study population reflected this goal. PAD endpoints included the development of claudication, persistent loss of a pedal pulse, and need for a revascularization procedure or limb amputation. Patients were followed for a mean of 6.5 years. Among patients randomized to intensive glycemic control, there were significant reductions in the development and progression of retinopathy and proteinuria and the development of sensorimotor neuropathy when compared with patients treated with conventional glycemic control. Owing to the young average age of the patient population, there were few deaths or major macrovascular events in either treatment group. Nonetheless, randomization to intensive glycemic control was associated with a nonsignificant 42% reduction in peripheral vascular and coronary events (Fig. 18-4).[58] Perhaps more importantly, however, randomization to intensive glycemic control was protective against the development of elevated total and LDL cholesterol—risk factors for the future development of cardiovascular events in this young patient population.

The United Kingdom Prospective Diabetes Study 33 (UKPDS 33) was designed to complement the findings of

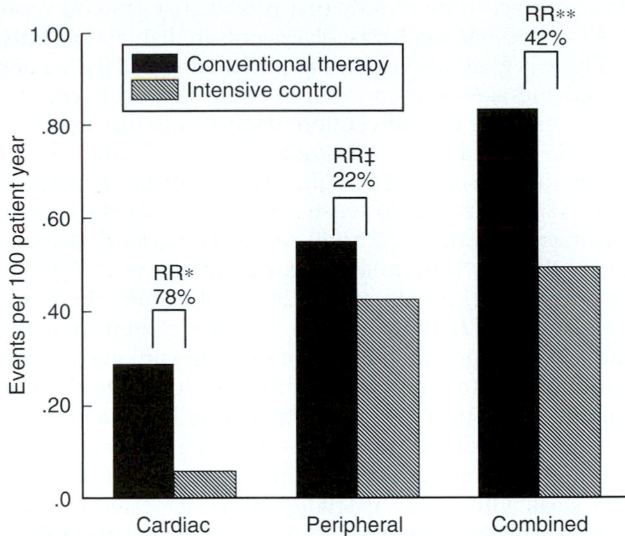

FIGURE 18-4. Effect of intensive glycemic control on the incidence of macrovascular events among type 1 diabetic patients in the DCCT trial. Cardiac events are defined as myocardial infarction, revascularization for coronary artery disease, development of angina with abnormal noninvasive testing or coronary angiogram, or cardiac or sudden death. Peripheral arterial disease events are defined as amputation, need for revascularization procedure, or claudication with confirmatory testing. The combined endpoint includes cardiac and peripheral arterial disease events. *P = .07; ‡, NS; **,0.08. (Adapted with permission from the Effect of Intensive Diabetes Management on Macrovascular Events and Risk Factors in the Diabetes Control and Complications Trial. Am J Cardiol 75[14]:894,1995.)

the DCCT by investigating the effect of intensive glycemic control (with sulfonylureas or insulin) on the incidence of macrovascular events in type 2 diabetic patients. An earlier study of glycemic control strategies in type 2 diabetic persons found no cardiovascular benefit of intensive therapy with insulin and an excess of cardiovascular deaths among patients treated with the sulfonylurea, tolbutamide.[59] This early finding generated concern regarding the safety and potential cardiovascular toxicity of sulfonylureas with prolonged use in diabetic patients. In UKPDS 33, patients were randomized to intensive therapy with insulin or one of three sulfonylureas or to conventional treatment with a prescribed diabetic diet, and were followed for a median of 10 years.[60] Although there were no differences in the treatment groups with regard to total mortality, cardiac mortality, or diabetes-related mortality, there was a 16% reduction in the relative risk of myocardial infarction in the group randomized to intensive therapy. There was also a 39% reduction in the relative risk of amputation in the intensive therapy group, which did not achieve statistical significance. There were too few deaths attributable to PAD to allow for comparison. Consistent with the findings of the DCCT, there was a highly significant 25% reduction in the relative risk of microvascular complications among patients randomized to intensive glycemic control, including the need for retinal surgery. Although the UKPDS 33 study reaffirmed the importance of glycemic control in the prevention of microvascular complications in diabetic patients, the findings with regard to macrovascular endpoints were underwhelming, and there has yet to be a study that proves that glycemic control can prevent cardiovascular events in diabetic patients.

There is great interest in the potential use of the insulin sensitizing agents, metformin and the thiazolidinediones (glitazones) for the prevention of cardiovascular events in diabetic patients. In a substudy of UKPDS (UKPDS 34), newly diagnosed, overweight type 2 diabetic patients were randomized to intensive therapy with the insulin sensitizing agent metformin or a prescribed diabetic diet.[61] Patients were followed for a median of 10.7 years. In contrast to the sulfonylurea arm of the study, there was a significant 42% reduction in diabetes-related mortality and a 36% reduction in all-cause mortality among patients randomized to metformin therapy compared with patients randomized to diet. There was no difference in the incidence of PAD endpoints between the two groups, although the total number of clinical events related to PAD was small. Other recent studies have suggested that the insulin sensitizing agents (i.e., metformin and the thiazolidinediones) may improve the cardiovascular risk profile among diabetic patients.[62,63] The Veterans Affairs Diabetes Trial will investigate the effect of intensive glycemic control with insulin-sensitizing agents on cardiovascular endpoints in high-risk type 2 diabetic patients.[64]

Recommendations

The American Diabetes Association has published guidelines for the medical care of diabetic patients with and without PAD.[65,66] To prevent microvascular complications, all diabetic patients should be treated aggressively with insulin or oral agents, alone or in combination, with a goal hemoglobin A1c of less than 7%. The optimal choice of glucose-lowering agent has not been well established, although metformin should be considered as a first-line agent for overweight diabetic patients. Periodic foot examination by health care providers and patient education regarding preventive foot care are also critical for diabetic patients, particularly given the prevalence of peripheral neuropathy. The American Diabetic Association recommends ankle-brachial index measurement for all diabetic persons above the age of 50 years and for diabetic persons younger than 50 years who have additional PAD risk factors, such as tobacco use.

Treatment of Hyperhomocysteinemia

Hyperhomocysteinemia is a disorder associated with derangements of the metabolic pathway involved in the metabolism of the essential amino acid methionine.[67] Hyperhomocysteinemia occurs as the result of an inherited defect of one of the enzymes involved in transsulfuration or remethylation of homocysteine, or can occur as a result of malnutrition and deficiency of key cofactors for these enzymatic reactions (i.e., folic acid and vitamins B_6 and B_{12}). Hyperhomocysteinemia is also associated with end-stage renal disease, although the mechanism by which this occurs is not well established.[67] Inherited homocystinuria, the most striking form of hyperhomocysteinemia, is due to homozygous deficiency of the enzyme cystathionine β-synthase, a critical enzyme of the transsulfuration pathway of homocysteine. Homocystinuria is associated with mental retardation, ectopia lentis, and premature coronary and peripheral atherosclerosis. Among heterozygotes for cystathionine β-synthase deficiency, homocysteine levels are significantly lower (on the order of 20 to 40 μmol/L vs. up to 400 μmol/L for homozygotes), although there is also a predisposition to premature atherosclerosis.[67,68] Multiple epidemiologic studies have established an association between an elevated plasma homocysteine level and development and progression of CAD and cerebrovascular disease.[67,69] Extensive epidemiologic evidence has also established hyperhomocysteine as an independent risk factor for asymptomatic PAD and the clinical progression of symptomatic PAD.[70-73] In addition to premature atherosclerosis, elevated levels of homocysteine are associated with a hypercoagulable state characterized by a tendency toward venous and arterial thrombosis.[67,74]

As elevated plasma homocysteine levels are associated with low levels of the enzymatic cofactors folic acid, vitamin B_6, and vitamin B_{12}, vitamin supplementation is an obvious therapeutic consideration for the treatment of hyperhomocysteinemia. A number of clinical trials have investigated the effect of vitamin supplementation on plasma homocysteine concentrations. A meta-analysis by the Homocysteine Lowering Trialists' Collaboration reported on 1114 patients enrolled in 12 randomized controlled trials of vitamin supplementation.[75] Median pretreatment blood homocysteine concentration was 11.8 μmol/L. The meta-analysis reported that the greatest reduction in plasma homocysteine levels with vitamin supplementation occurred among the patients with the highest pretreatment homocysteine concentrations (>18.5 μmol/L) and lowest plasma folate concentrations. Folic acid supplementation reduced plasma homocysteine concentrations by an average of 25% with no incremental improvement in homocysteine levels with doses above 0.5 mg, even in patients with the highest baseline homocysteine levels. The addition of vitamin B_{12} supplementation (mean 0.5 mg daily) to folic acid produced a small incremental (7%) decline in homocysteine levels, whereas the addition of vitamin B_6 (mean 16.5 mg daily) to folic acid supplementation had no additive homocysteine-lowering effect.

Although the effectiveness of supplementation with folic acid and vitamin B_{12} in lowering plasma homocysteine levels has been established, no large, randomized clinical trials have determined the clinical benefit of vitamin therapy on the prevention of cardiovascular endpoints in patients with hyperhomocysteinemia. One small trial of healthy siblings of patients with hyperhomocysteinemia and premature atherosclerotic vascular disease (PAD, CAD, or CVD before the age of 56 years) randomized siblings to combination vitamin therapy with 5 mg folic acid and 250 mg vitamin B_6 or placebo.[76] Siblings with and without evidence of hyperhomocysteinemia were enrolled. Subjects continued therapy for a period of 2 years and were followed for the development of CAD (abnormal stress test), PAD (abnormal ABI or lower extremity arterial duplex scan), and cerebrovascular disease (abnormal carotid artery duplex scan). Among patients randomized to vitamins, fasting plasma homocysteine levels fell from 14.7 to 7.4 μmol/L (a nearly 50% decline); there was an 18% decline in the placebo group. There was no significant difference in the development of PAD or asymptomatic cerebrovascular disease among the two groups. Among the patients randomized to aggressive vitamin therapy, there was a decrease in the incidence of an abnormal stress test. Large clinical trials that investigate the effectiveness of homocysteine-lowering therapy for the prevention of cardiovascular events and limb-related outcomes in patients with PAD are in progress.[77]

Recommendations

Although no randomized trials have established the efficacy of homocysteine-lowering therapy for the prevention of cardiovascular events in patients with PAD, treatment is inexpensive and safe. A fasting plasma homocysteine level may be measured in all patients with PAD, and should be determined in patients with PAD that has developed at a young age or is unexpected given the absence of traditional risk factors. Among patients with PAD who have fasting plasma homocysteine levels greater than 14 μmol/L, it is reasonable to prescribe folic acid (0.5 to 5 mg daily) and vitamin B_{12} supplementation (0.2-1 mg daily). Treatment with folic acid alone may exacerbate the neurologic manifestations of vitamin B_{12} deficiency. Vitamin B_6 is not effective in lowering homocysteine levels, and should not be routinely prescribed. The optimal target for homocysteine levels in patients receiving vitamin supplementation has not been established.

Antiplatelet Therapy

The pivotal role of antiplatelet agents, particularly aspirin, in the secondary prevention of death and myocardial infarction in patients with CAD has been established by large randomized clinical trials.[78,79] The role of antiplatelet therapy in the management of patients with PAD continues to evolve, with important evidence gleaned from subset analyses of large clinical trials directed primarily at the prevention of cardiovascular events in patients with and without CAD.

Although epidemiologic studies suggested a role for aspirin in the primary prevention of cardiovascular events, one clinical trial found no significant benefit and an excess of adverse events among healthy British male physicians randomized to high-dose aspirin therapy (500 mg daily).[80] The Physicians' Health Study sought to investigate the benefit of low-dose aspirin therapy in the primary prevention of cardiovascular mortality.[81] Healthy male physicians were randomized to aspirin (325 mg orally every other day) or placebo and beta-carotene supplements or placebo in a 2 × 2 factorial design and followed for a mean of 5.0 years. There was no benefit of aspirin therapy in terms of the primary endpoint—cardiovascular death; however, there was a striking 44% reduction in the relative risk of myocardial infarction among physicians randomized to aspirin therapy. The benefit of aspirin therapy in the prevention of myocardial infarction was observed only in physicians who were 50 years of age or older. There was a nonsignificant trend toward an excess of stroke among patients randomized to aspirin therapy, a finding that was due largely to an excess of hemorrhagic stroke among the aspirin group.

In a subsequent substudy, the effect of low-dose aspirin on the incidence of PAD endpoints was investigated.[81,82] Among physicians randomized to low-dose aspirin therapy, there was a 46% reduction in the incidence of lower extremity revascularization surgery. The benefit of low-dose aspirin therapy in the prevention of lower extremity revascularization was greatest among physicians who had reported intermittent claudication at the time of enrollment in the study. Despite the impressive effect on revascularization, low-dose aspirin therapy had no effect on self-report of new claudication. The benefit of aspirin may be greatest in the prevention of thrombosis at the site of existing high-grade atherosclerotic plaques, rather than in the delay of progression of atherosclerosis and the development of new stenoses.

Recently, the Antithrombotic Trialists' Collaboration updated the 1994 meta-analysis of the evidence supporting the use of antiplatelet agents in the management of high-risk patients with atherosclerotic vascular disease.[78] The initial meta-analysis determined that antiplatelet therapy, primarily aspirin at a moderate dose of 75 to 325 mg daily, significantly reduced the odds of a major vascular event among high-risk patients with atherosclerosis by 27%.[79] Also, antiplatelet therapy was effective for the prevention of both coronary and peripheral artery bypass graft occlusion, with a reduction in the relative risk of graft occlusion of approximately one third.[84]

In the updated analysis, a total of 287 randomized trials, with more than 200,000 patients, were included.[83] Studies of antiplatelet agents versus control and studies involving direct comparisons of different antiplatelet agents were included. Confirming the original findings, there was a 22% reduction in the odds of a serious vascular event (vascular death, nonfatal myocardial infarction, or nonfatal stroke) among high-risk patients treated with antiplatelet agents. The benefit appeared to be greatest among studies that enrolled patients on the basis of high-risk criteria—such as prior or acute myocardial infarction, PAD, or atrial fibrillation. Among the 42 studies that enrolled 9214 high-risk patients on the basis of PAD, there was a 23% reduction in the odds of a major vascular event among patients randomized to antiplatelet therapy. The benefit of antiplatelet therapy was consistent across all PAD enrollment criteria, including intermittent claudication and surgical lower extremity revascularization. Of note, 2304 patients in this category were enrolled in a study that randomized PAD patients to treatment with a nonaspirin antiplatelet agent, picotamide, or placebo.[85] Picotamide is a dual antiplatelet agent that inhibits thromboxane A_2 synthase and antagonizes the thromboxane A_2 receptor of platelets.

The Antithrombotic Trialists' Collaboration studied a number of antiplatelet regimens, alone and in combination, in the prevention of vascular events among high-risk patients. Among seven trials with direct comparison of aspirin at different doses, there was no benefit of high-dose (500 to 1000 mg daily) versus medium-dose (75 to

325 mg) aspirin on the odds of a major vascular event. Three trials, involving approximately 3500 patients, compared low-dose aspirin (less than 75 mg daily) with standard doses of more than 75 mg daily. There was a trend toward greater reduction in the odds of a major vascular event among patients treated with more than 75 mg of aspirin daily, although this comparison did not achieve statistical significance. In the analysis of head-to-head trials of antiplatelet agents versus aspirin, there was no class of agents that significantly reduced the odds of a vascular event to a greater extent than aspirin, with the exception of the thienopyridines—clopidogrel and ticlopidine. There was also a nonsignificant trend toward a minor benefit of combination therapy with aspirin plus dipyridamole versus aspirin alone in the prevention of major vascular events.

Large multicenter randomized clinical trials have investigated the use of the antiplatelet agent clopidogrel in the secondary prevention of cardiovascular events. Clopidogrel is a thienopyridine derivative that inhibits platelet aggregation by antagonism of the adenosine diphosphate receptor.[19] Clopidogrel is less likely to cause serious adverse hematologic side effects, particularly neutropenia and thrombotic thrombocytopenic purpura, than its analog, ticlopidine. Pooled analysis of early clinical trials suggested a trend toward a marginal benefit of ticlopidine over aspirin in the prevention of myocardial infarction, stroke, or vascular death.[79] The Clopidogrel versus Aspirin in Patients at Risk of Ischaemic Events (CAPRIE) study built on this finding and investigated the benefit of clopidogrel versus aspirin in the secondary prevention of cardiovascular events.[86] Patients with recent myocardial infarction (within 35 days), ischemic stroke (within 6 months), or symptomatic PAD were randomized to clopidogrel (75 mg daily) or aspirin (325 mg daily). Patients enrolled on the basis of PAD had intermittent claudication and an abnormal ABI (ABI < 0.85) or had undergone leg amputation or revascularization. A total of 19,185 randomized patients were followed for the development of the primary composite endpoint of first occurrence of ischemic stroke, myocardial infarction, or vascular death. After a mean 1.9 years of follow-up, there was an 8.7% relative-risk reduction in the annual event rate of the primary endpoint among patients randomized to clopidogrel. The benefit of clopidogrel over aspirin was greatest among the subgroup of patients enrolled on the basis of symptomatic PAD, with a relative-risk reduction of the composite endpoint of 23.8% (Fig. 18-5). There was no increase in minor or major bleeding episodes associated with clopidogrel, although there was an increased incidence of gastrointestinal hemorrhage among patients randomized to aspirin.

Dual antiplatelet therapy, namely the combination of aspirin and clopidogrel, for the secondary prevention of cardiovascular events has been studied among patients with acute coronary syndromes, a subset of patients at very high risk for the development of a recurrent major vascular event. The Clopidogrel in Unstable Angina to Prevent Recurrent Events (CURE) investigators randomized 12,562 patients with active unstable angina pectoris or non-ST segment elevation myocardial infarction to receive aspirin (75 to 325 mg) and either clopidogrel (300 mg bolus followed by 75 mg daily) or placebo for a mean duration of 9 months.[87] There was a 20% relative risk reduction in the primary endpoint of cardiovascular death, nonfatal myocardial infarction, or stroke among patients randomized to clopidogrel plus aspirin. Although the CURE trial did not specifically enroll patients on the basis of PAD, the findings further suggest the potential benefit for combination therapy with aspirin and a thienopyridine for the secondary prevention of vascular events in patients with atherosclerosis. The CHARISMA study, which will further address the role of combination antiplatelet therapy for the prevention of cardiovascular events in high-risk patients, is ongoing.[88] This study, which has randomized more than 15,000 patients, will investigate the benefit of combination antiplatelet therapy in a subset of patients with PAD.

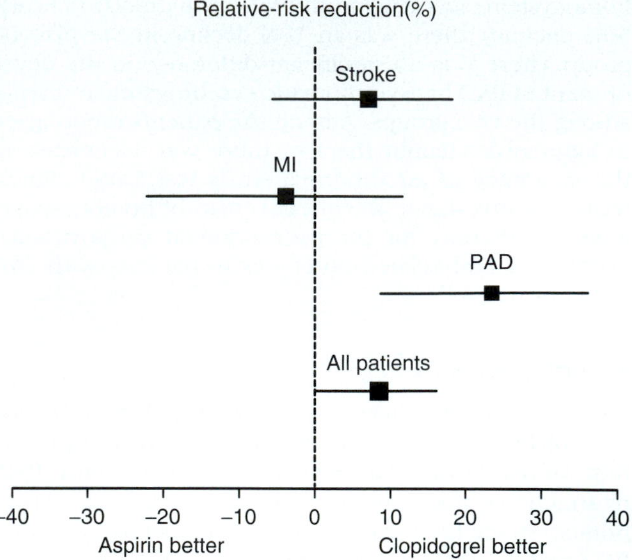

FIGURE 18-5. Clopidogrel decreases the risk of the composite endpoint of stroke, myocardial infarction, or vascular death relative to aspirin among high-risk patients with atherosclerotic vascular disease. Relative risk reduction for each subgroup of patients is displayed with 95% confidence intervals. The benefit of clopidogrel is particularly pronounced among the subset of patients with peripheral arterial disease. MI, myocardial infarction; PAD, peripheral arterial disease. (Reproduced with permission from the CAPRIE Steering Committee: A randomised, blinded, trial of clopidogrel versus aspirin in patients at risk of ischaemic events (CAPRIE). Lancet 348[9038]:1329, 1996.)

Recommendations

In light of the 20% to 25% reduction in serious vascular events attributable to antiplatelet therapy among patients with atherosclerotic vascular disease, all patients with PAD, regardless of concomitant CAD or CVD, should receive antiplatelet therapy. Aspirin should be prescribed at a dose of 75 to 325 mg daily. Aspirin therapy is particularly important among patients undergoing surgical or percutaneous revascularization procedures and should be continued perioperatively—or initiated as soon as possible postoperatively—if it had not been prescribed previously. Clopidogrel is a therapeutic alternative among patients intolerant of aspirin (e.g., gastrointestinal distress, allergy, or bronchospasm), and can also be considered as the initial choice for patients with PAD.[89] With the exception of patients with acute coronary syndrome or those undergoing percutaneous coronary or peripheral interventions, there is currently insufficient evidence to support dual antiplatelet therapy with aspirin and clopidogrel for the secondary prevention of cardiovascular events. The results of ongoing clinical trials will clarify the role of dual antiplatelet therapy for secondary prevention among high-risk patients with atherosclerotic vascular disease.

Anticoagulant Therapy

Few clinical trials have specifically addressed the role of anticoagulant therapy, typically with the vitamin K antagonist, warfarin, in the management of patients with PAD. In contrast, many clinical trials have investigated the use of anticoagulant therapy for the secondary prevention of cardiovascular events in patients with CAD. Anand and Yusuf recently updated a meta-analysis of all randomized trials of oral anticoagulant therapy for CAD published through 1999, involving more than 20,000 patients.[90,91] Separate analyses were performed for each intensity of oral anticoagulation therapy (low-intensity—[International Normalized Ratio] INR < 2.0; moderate-intensity INR 2.0 to 3.0; high-intensity INR > 2.8) and for concomitant antiplatelet therapy with aspirin. The primary endpoint was the composite of cardiovascular death, myocardial infarction, or stroke. The incidence of major bleeding was analyzed for each dosing regimen. Low-intensity oral anticoagulation was of no benefit when used in combination with aspirin among patients with CAD. In contrast, the combination of moderate-to-high intensity oral anticoagulation plus aspirin was associated with a statistically significant 12% reduction in the occurrence of the composite endpoint when compared with aspirin alone. Moderate-to-high intensity oral anticoagulation, without aspirin, was associated with a 21% reduction in the incidence of the primary endpoint—when compared with aspirin. The incidence of major bleeding among patients randomized to moderate-to-high intensity oral anticoagulation was twice that of those randomized to aspirin monotherapy, although the addition of aspirin to moderate-to-high intensity oral anticoagulation did not further increase the rate of hemorrhage. High-intensity oral anticoagulation was associated with a 43% reduction in the odds of the primary endpoint relative to control. Unfortunately, the benefit came at a high cost with a markedly increased incidence of major bleeding episodes (4.6% oral anticoagulation vs. 0.7% control). No data were available for the comparison of high-intensity anticoagulation to aspirin.

With the exception of the management of acute limb ischemia (see Chapter 46), there is no established role for anticoagulant therapy in the routine management of patients with PAD. A recent review of three small clinical trials found that anticoagulant therapy had no benefit on walking capacity, limb-related outcomes, or cardiovascular outcomes among patients with intermittent claudication.[92] As a result of the lack of compelling efficacy data, the American College of Chest Physicians Conference on Antithrombotic and Thrombolytic Therapy has recently issued a recommendation opposing the routine use of oral anticoagulant therapy in patients with intermittent claudication.[93] The one potential exception to this recommendation is the use of oral anticoagulant therapy in patients with PAD following lower extremity revascularization. The Dutch Bypass Oral Anticoagulants or Aspirin investigators randomized patients following infrainguinal bypass grafting to high-intensity warfarin therapy (target INR 3.0 to 4.5) or aspirin (80 mg daily) within 5 days of surgery.[94] Patients were followed for development of the primary endpoint of graft occlusion, as well as for cardiovascular events. After a mean of 21 months' follow-up, there was no significant overall difference in the rate of graft occlusion between the oral anticoagulation and aspirin groups. Subset analyses, however, demonstrated a significant reduction (31%) in the rate of graft occlusion among patients with venous conduit bypass grafts randomized to oral anticoagulation compared with aspirin. In contrast, among patients with nonvenous grafts (i.e., prosthetic conduit), aspirin reduced the incidence of graft occlusion more effectively than oral anticoagulation. This finding was somewhat counterintuitive. Oral anticoagulation halved the incidence of ischemic stroke, but was associated with a more than threefold increase in the incidence of hemorrhagic stroke. Overall, oral anticoagulation was associated with a nearly twofold increase in the incidence of a major bleeding episode (4.7% anticoagulation vs. 2.5% aspirin).

Recommendations

Anticoagulation is not routinely recommended for patients with PAD. Compliance with antiplatelet therapy (i.e., aspirin or clopidogrel) should be the primary goal for all patients, particularly as antiplatelet therapy (as discussed earlier) has been demonstrated to reduce the incidence of cardiovascular events and prevent death in these patients. Anticoagulation therapy may be indicated following an episode of acute limb ischemia treated with thrombolytic therapy or may be warranted due to the presence of concomitant risk factors for thromboembolism, such as atrial fibrillation or the presence of a mechanical heart valve. In these cases, it should generally be combined with low-dose aspirin. Aspirin remains the treatment of choice to prevent bypass graft failure following surgical lower extremity arterial revascularization, although high-intensity oral anticoagulation with warfarin is an alternative regimen for patients with venous grafts. The potential benefit of anticoagulant therapy over aspirin must be balanced against the high cost of therapy and the significant risk of major hemorrhage associated with its use.

TREATMENT OF INTERMITTENT CLAUDICATION AND CRITICAL LIMB ISCHEMIA

Physical and pharmacologic therapies should be considered in the treatment plan of patients with symptomatic PAD. These include supersized exercise rehabilitation and foot care. Drugs available for the treatment of intermittent claudication include cilostazol and pentoxifylline. Investigative pharmacotherapies include prostaglandins, metabolic agents, angiogenic growth factors, and statins. The evidence supporting and reflecting the efficacy of drug therapy for intermittent claudication and critical limb ischemia is reviewed subsequently. Endovascular and surgical reconstructions for the treatment of disabling claudication are reviewed in Chapters 19 and 20.

Exercise Training

Supervised exercise training programs improve walking duration, speed, and walking distance in patients with intermittent claudication. Two separate meta-analyses have supported the efficacy of supervised exercise training. One meta-analysis of 21 randomized and nonrandomized trials found that pain-free walking distance and maximal walking distance increased by 180% and 120%, respectively.[95] Another meta-analysis that included 10 randomized trials found that supervised exercise training improved maximal walking distance by 150%.[96] Strength or resistance training is not as effective as treadmill training in improving walking distances in patients with claudication.[97] Unsupervised exercise training programs are not as effective as supervised programs.[98,99] Comparative studies have found that home-based unsupervised exercise training programs result in negligible improvement, whereas supervised exercise training increased maximal walking time approximately 80% to 140% after 3 months.[98,99]

Several mechanisms have been proposed to explain the improvement in walking distance that results from exercise training. These include collateral blood vessel development; enhancement in endothelium-dependent, nitric oxide-mediated, vasodilation of the microcirculation; improved hemorrheology; increased oxidative capacity of calf skeletal muscle; and better walking biomechanics.[100] Exercise training has been found to improve collateral blood flow in animal models of hind limb ischemia.[101,102] Exercise-induced angiogenesis has been attributed to upregulation of angiogenic growth factors such as vascular endothelial growth factors (VEGF).[103,104] Increased expression and activity of endothelial nitric oxide synthase (eNOS), and production of nitric oxide (NO) may contribute to angiogenesis.[102,104-106] In humans, several studies have found that exercise training improves maximal calf blood flow following exercise and due to reactive hyperemia following an ischemic stimulus.[107,108] There was no effect of exercise training on resting calf blood flow in these studies. Exercise training enhances endothelium-dependent vasodilation in peripheral conduit arteries and thereby may contribute to improved blood flow and walking time in claudicants.[109,110] Improvement in skeletal muscle metabolic function, and specifically oxidative capacity, occurs with exercise training and may be relevant to the improvement in walking capacity experienced by patients with intermittent claudication.[111,112] Also, exercise training may improve walking distance by altering biomechanics and adapting patterns of walking that are more efficient, engaging skeletal muscle less affected by ischemia, and improving gate stability.[113]

Recommendations

A program of supervised exercise training is recommended as an initial treatment modality for patients with intermittent claudication.[89] Exercise programs should use a treadmill or a track and take place in sessions of 45 to 60 minutes at least 3 times per week for a minimum of 12 weeks. Prior to beginning exercise rehabilitation, patients should undergo a comprehensive cardiovascular risk assessment that includes a history, physical examination, and ascertainment of all relevant atherosclerotic risk factors. An electrocardiogram monitored exercise tolerance test (ETT), tailored to the patient's symptoms and ability, should be performed to assess the development of any exercise-induced cardiac symptoms, heart rate and blood pressure responses, ST segment depression, and arrhythmias. It also may serve as a baseline evaluation of the time to the onset of claudication and the maximal walking time that is tolerated on the treadmill by the patient. During the training session, patients should be encouraged to walk until symptoms of moderate severity develop. Following a rest period and resolution of symptoms, walking should resume until symptoms recur. This cycle should be repeated as many times as needed during the 45- to 60-minute period.

Foot Care

Careful attention to foot care is indicated to reduce the likelihood of skin breakdown and infection, and is particularly important in diabetic persons with vascular disease and in patients with critical limb ischemia. Treatment of ulcers is discussed in Chapter 62. Patients' feet should be kept clean. Moisturizing lotion should be applied to prevent drying and fissuring. Well-fitted shoes should be worn to reduce the likelihood of pressure-induced necrosis, and stockings made of natural, absorbent fibers are recommended. The patient is advised to inspect the skin of the feet frequently so that minor abrasions can be tended to promptly. Elastic support stockings generally should be avoided because they may restrict cutaneous blood flow.

In patients with ischemia at rest, conservative measures include placing the affected limb in a dependent position below heart level to increase perfusion pressure and oxygen tension in ischemic tissues. In cases where edema, which may impair healing, is present, the limb should be kept horizontal instead. Sheepskin should be placed beneath the heels of the feet because pressure against bed sheets accounts for the frequent occurrence of skin breakdown at those sites. A footboard should be used to cradle the blankets over the feet in a fashion that minimizes frictional trauma. Wisps of cotton inserted between the toes for separation help protect the digits from intertriginous friction and moisture. Unless infection with purulence is present, dryness is preferred to soaks, except in a limited fashion, to permit intermittent cleansing. Gentle warmth is recommended to minimize vasoconstriction, but excessive heat should be avoided. Fungal onycholysis should be treated with appropriate antimicrobial preparations to reduce the likelihood of cutaneous breakdown leading to bacterial superinfection.

In general, caution must be exercised in the use of topical medications because of the possibility of local inflammatory reactions. Open sores should be kept clean, and cultures should be obtained, but antibiotic medications are not always effective, in part because of impaired delivery to ischemic tissue. Plain roentgenographic examinations of underlying bone may be helpful in assessing the possibility of osteomyelitis, for which antibiotic therapy generally is given. Passive physical therapy may proceed to progressive weight bearing and ambulation but must be accompanied by careful attention to foot care, the use of absorbent, natural-fiber (preferably cotton) socks, and soft, nonconstrictive, properly fitted shoes.

Vasodilator Drugs

Vasodilator drugs have undergone extensive investigation for the treatment of patients with claudication and critical limb ischemia. It is tempting to assume that treatment with a medication that reduces arteriolar resistance would be effective for patients with PAD as nitrates and calcium channel blockers are for patients with angina. In general, however, vasodilator drug therapy has been disappointing for relief of intermittent claudication. The differences in the pathophysiology of limb and myocardial ischemia may promote insight into the disparate efficiency of vasodilator drugs. Vasodilator therapy may decrease myocardial oxygen demand, but is not likely to affect skeletal muscle oxygen demand. Therefore, to be effective, vasodilators would have to improve the blood supply to exercising muscle. When an obstructive arterial lesion produces critical stenosis, distal perfusion pressure is reduced. Intramuscular arterioles normally dilate in response to the metabolic demands of limb exercise, but flow augmentation is blunted in patients with proximal stenotic disease. Also, distal pressure falls during exercise, leading to accumulation of the ischemic metabolites believed to mediate the symptom of claudication. These substances potentiate local vasodilation, and perfusion pressure falls, no longer balancing the extravascular compressive force exerted by exercising muscle within the tissue compartment. The distal vasculature virtually collapses under these circumstances, and this mechanism may not be mitigated by vasodilator therapy. Indeed, vasodilator drugs, including β-adrenergic agonists (isoproterenol, nylidrin), α-adrenergic antagonists (reserpine, guanethidine, tolazoline), calcium channel blockers, nitrates, and others (isoxsuprine, cyclandelate) have been evaluated in clinical trials. None increases blood flow in exercising skeletal muscle subtended by significant arterial obstructive lesions, nor do any of these improve symptoms of intermittent claudication or objective measures of exercise capacity. Nonetheless, one drug with vasodilator properties, cilostazol, has been reported to improve walking distance in patients with claudication.

Cilostazol

Cilostazol was approved by the United States Food and Drug Administration in 1999 for use in patients with intermittent claudication. As a phosphodiesterase III inhibitor, cilostazol increases cyclic adenosine monophosphate (cAMP), causes vasodilation, and inhibits platelet aggregation.[114-117] The precise mechanism of action whereby cilostazol may improve symptoms of claudication, however, is not known.

A meta-analysis of six placebo-controlled, randomized trials, comprising 1751 patients with claudication, found that cilostazol (50 to 100 mg twice daily) significantly improved pain-free and maximal walking distance compared with placebo[118] (Fig. 18-6). Of the trials that used a graded treadmill protocol, cilostazol improved maximal walking distance by 40%, compared with 20% in those randomized to placebo. In trials that used a constant load treadmill protocol, cilostazol improved maximal walking distance by 76% compared with 20% in those treated with placebo. In addition, quality of life questionnaires indicated that cilostazol improved patients' perception of walking distance, walking speed, and overall function. The efficacy of cilostazol in patients with critical limb ischemia has not been evaluated.

The side effects of cilostazol include headache in approximately 25%, palpitations in approximately 15%, and diarrhea or abnormal stool in 15% to 20%.[119] The U.S. Food and Drug Administration has advised that cilostazol not be administered to patients with congestive heart failure. The reason for this advisory is that other phosphodiesterase III inhibitors, such as milrinone or vesnarinone, when studied in patients with congestive heart failure were associated with increased mortality.[120,121] Cilostazol per se has not been associated with increased

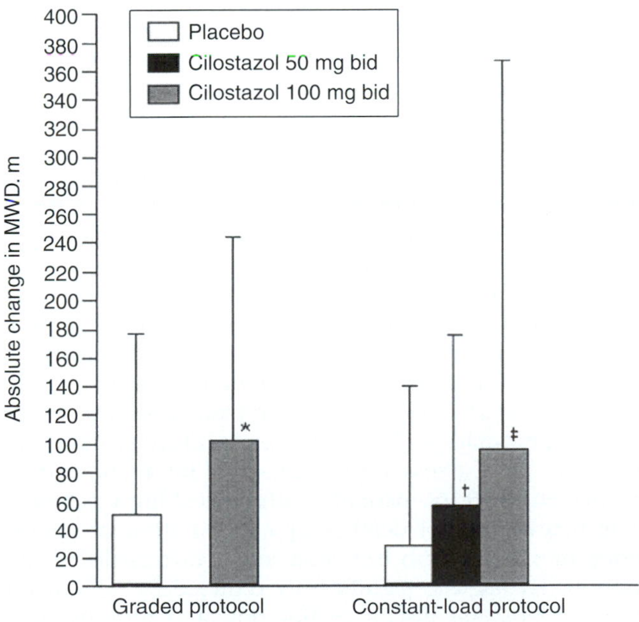

FIGURE 18-6. Cilostazol improves maximal walking distance in patients with claudication. Meta-analysis of six randomized, controlled trials. Mean improvement ± standard deviation is shown. Graded protocols did not include a 50 mg group. **P* <.0001 vs. placebo; †*P* < .0011 vs. placebo; ‡*P* < .0001 vs. placebo. BID, twice daily; m, meters; mg, milligrams; MWD, maximal walking distance. (Reproduced with permission from Regensteiner JG, Ware JE, Jr, McCarthy, et al: Effect of cilostazol on treadmill walking, community-based walking ability, and health-related quality of life in patients with intermittent claudication due to peripheral arterial disease: Meta-analysis of six randomized controlled trials. J Am Geriatr Soc 50[12]:1939, 2002.)

mortality rates, but has not been studied in a heart failure population. Cilostazol is primarily metabolized in the liver by the CYP3A4 isoenzyme. Prescription of the low dose (50 mg twice a day) of cilostazol is recommended for patients who concurrently take medications that are known to inhibit CYP3A4, including diltiazem, fluconazole, erythromycin, and other macrolide antibiotics.

Recommendations

Cilostazol is an effective therapy to improve walking distance in patients with intermittent claudication.[89] Physicians should be aware of the side effect profile and are advised not to administer this medication to patients with congestive heart failure.

Prostaglandins

Vasodilator prostaglandins have undergone somewhat extensive investigation for the treatment of patients with intermittent claudication or critical limb ischemia. This class of drugs includes prostaglandin E_1 (PGE_1), prostacyclin, and its analogs beraprost and iloprost. The efficacy of vasodilator prostaglandins, administered intra-arterially or intravenously, has been assessed in patients with intermittent claudication and in patients with critical limb ischemia. Intravenous administration of PGE_1 for 4 to 8 weeks to patients with intermittent claudication increased pain-free and maximal walking distance in one study.[122-125] In contrast, intravenous prostacyclin or its analog taprostene, was found not to improve walking distance in a systematic review of clinical trials of prostanoids for the treatment of claudication.[125] Two placebo-controlled trials of oral beraprost administered for 6 months had conflicting results, one showing improvement and one showing no change in pain-free or maximal walking distance.[126,127] In one placebo-controlled trial, iloprost administered for 6 months was no more effective than placebo in improving pain-free or maximal walking distance (Creager, personal communication).

Short-term (i.e., 3 to 4 days) intra-arterial or intravenous administration of PGE_1, iloprost, or ciprostene is not effective in ameliorating critical limb ischemia[128] but, when administered parenterally for longer periods of time (7 to 28 days), may reduce pain, ulcer size, or the risk of amputation.[128] The Ischemia Cronica degli Arti Inferiori study assessed the efficacy of intravenous PGE_1 or placebo in 1560 patients with critical limb ischemia. The relative risk of death, major amputation or persistence of critical limb ischemia, acute myocardial infarction, or stroke was significantly reduced by 13% at the time of hospital discharge but not at 6 months. After 6 months of treatment, there was no difference between groups in death or amputation, but there was a greater chance in resolution of critical limb ischemia in those survivors who did not have amputation.[129] Two randomized, placebo-controlled studies assessed the effect of oral iloprost on critical limb ischemia.[130] There was no apparent benefit of iloprost in terms of reducing the risk of the primary endpoint of amputation or death, but a modest benefit in terms of resolution of ulcers and rest pain in those who survived without amputation. Side effects of prostaglandins include flushing, headache, and gastrointestinal distress.

Recommendations

The use of oral or intravenous vasodilator prostaglandins, such as beraprost and iloprost, is not recommended to improve walking distance in patients with intermittent claudication.[89] In addition, these drugs are not effective therapy to reduce the risk of amputation or death in patients with critical limb ischemia. Parenteral administration of PGE_1 or iloprost for 7 to 28 days may improve ulcer healing or reduce pain in patients with critical limb ischemia, but such efficacy would be limited to a small percentage of patients.[89]

Calcium Channel Blockers

The efficacy of calcium channel blockers in patients with intermittent claudication has been evaluated in several small clinical trials. Nifedipine failed to improve exercise tolerance as assessed by pedal ergometry in a randomized, placebo-controlled trial.[131] In another placebo-controlled trial comparing nifedipine with atenolol, alone or in combination, nifedipine did not improve pain-free or absolute walking distance.[43] In one placebo-controlled, dose-ranging, crossover trial, verapamil improved pain-free walking distance by 29% and maximal walking distance by 49%.[132] There have been no subsequent trials with verapamil reported to confirm these findings.

Hemorrheologic Agents

Pentoxifylline

Pentoxifylline is a methylxanthine derivative that was approved by the U.S. Food and Drug Administration for treatment of patients with intermittent claudication in 1984. It is purported to decrease blood and plasma viscosity, improve red and white blood cell deformability, inhibit neutrophil adhesion and activation, and decrease plasma fibrinogen, although not all studies have confirmed these findings.[133-135] One meta-analysis of 11 trials comprising 612 patients found that pentoxifylline (600 to 1200 mg daily) improved pain-free walking distance by 29 meters, and maximal claudication distance by 48 meters.[136] Another meta-analysis of six randomized, double-blinded, placebo-controlled trials found that pentoxifylline improved pain-free walking distance by 21 meters and maximal claudication distance by 44 meters.[137] The meta-analyses did not include a large, randomized, placebo-controlled trial of 698 patients with intermittent claudication, of whom 232 received pentoxifylline, 227 received cilostazol, and 239 received placebo.[119] In this trial, there was no difference in pain-free walking distance or maximal walking distance between the pentoxifylline and the placebo-treated group after 24 weeks of treatment. Pain-free and maximal walking distance increased in the cilostazol group compared with both placebo and pentoxifylline.

The efficacy of pentoxifylline to improve critical limb ischemia has been studied in two placebo-controlled trials. In one study, patients with critical limb ischemia were randomized to treatment with intravenous pentoxifylline, 600 mg twice daily, or placebo for up to 21 days. The severity of rest pain was significantly reduced in the patients treated with pentoxifylline compared with those treated with placebo.[138] Yet, in another placebo-controlled trial, pentoxifylline, 600 mg intravenously, was administered to patients with critical limb ischemia. There was no significant difference in pain relief between the placebo and pentoxifylline treatment groups.[139] It is not known whether pentoxifylline facilitates ulcer healing or reduces the risk of amputation in patients with critical limb ischemia. Side effects of pentoxifylline include dyspepsia, nausea, and vomiting, eructation, flatus, bloating, and dizziness. Side effects requiring discontinuation of the drug occur in up to 9.6% of patients.

Recommendations

The clinical efficacy of pentoxifylline for intermittent claudication is not well established. Improvement in claudication distance is very modest, at best, and falls within a range that may not be clinically recognized by the patient. Pentoxifylline is not useful in the treatment of critical limb ischemia.

Metabolic Agents

Symptoms of intermittent claudication may be related, in part, to abnormalities in skeletal muscle metabolism (see Chapter 15). Therefore, drugs that favorably affect oxidative metabolism may confer benefit by enhancing skeletal muscle function even without improving blood supply. L-Carnitine and its derivative propionyl-L-carnitine, enhance glucose oxidation and oxidative metabolism via the Krebs cycle by providing a source of carnitine.[140] Three placebo-controlled trials have assessed the efficacy of propionyl-L-carnitine in patients with intermittent claudication.[141-143] In these studies, propionyl-L-carnitine, administered as a 1 g dose orally, twice each day, improved maximal walking distance by 54% to 73%, whereas those randomized to placebo increased maximal walking distance 25% to 46% (Fig. 18-7). Propionyl-L-carnitine improved physical function, walking speed and distance as assessed by quality-of-life questionnaires.[143,144] Propionyl-L-carnitine was not associated with any significant adverse side effect. Propionyl-L-carnitine, has potential merit for the treatment of intermittent claudication, but should be considered investigational at this time.

Ranolazine is a piperazine derivative that inhibits fatty acid oxidation, activates pyruvate dehydrogenase, and shifts metabolism toward carbohydrate oxidation, thereby increasing efficiency of oxygen utilization.[145] Ranolazine improves exercise capacity and decreases angina frequency in patients with coronary artery disease, but the drug has not been investigated in patients with PAD.[146,147]

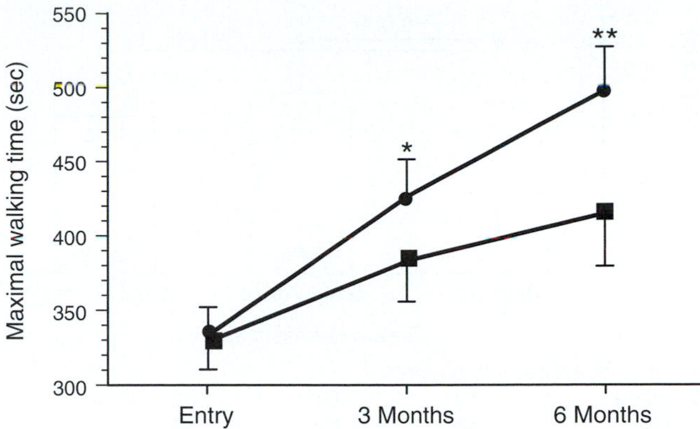

FIGURE 18-7. Propionyl-L-carnitine improves maximal walking time in patients with claudication. Maximal walking times for 155 patients with disabling claudication randomized to active therapy or placebo are presented at baseline, at 3 months, and at 6 months following randomization. **P* < .001; ***P* < .001; ■ placebo; ● propionyl-L-carnitine 2 grams daily. Sec, seconds. (Adapted from text with permission from Hiatt WR, Regensteiner JG, Creager MA, et al: Propionyl-L-carnitine improves exercise performance and functional status in patients with claudication. Am J Med 110[8]:616).

Angiogenic Growth Factors

Angiogenic growth factors are undergoing investigation for the treatment of PAD. This class of drugs includes vascular endothelial growth factor (VEGF), fibroblast growth factor (FGF), and hypoxia-inducible factor-1 (HIF-1). Angiogenic growth factors have the potential to promote collateral blood vessel formation and thereby increase blood flow to the ischemic limbs of patients with PAD. They may be administered as recombinant proteins or by gene transfer using plasmid DNA or an adenoviral vector that encodes the angiogenic growth factor.[148] VEGF, bFGF, and HIF-1α increase collateral blood vessels and improve blood flow in animal models of hindlimb ischemia.[149-152]

Vascular Endothelial Growth Factor

Several, nonrandomized, open-label studies found that intra-arterial gene transfer therapy of $pHVEGF_{165}$ increased collateral blood vessels, as assessed by magnetic resonance imaging or digital subtracted angiography in patients with PAD.[153,154] $pHVEGF_{165}$ administration improved blood flow and increased the ABI in some of the patients that participated in these trials.[154] A randomized, placebo-controlled trial of intramuscular $VEGF_{121}$ was conducted in patients with unilateral intermittent claudication. VEGF was administered as 10 intramuscular injections to the affected leg in total doses of 4×10^9 or 4×10^{10} particle units. There was no significant improvement in pain-free or maximal walking distance after 12 or 26 weeks.[155]

Fibroblast Growth Factor

A nonrandomized study of patients with critical limb ischemia observed that intramuscular injection of plasmid DNA encoding FGF-1 reduced pain and ulcer size

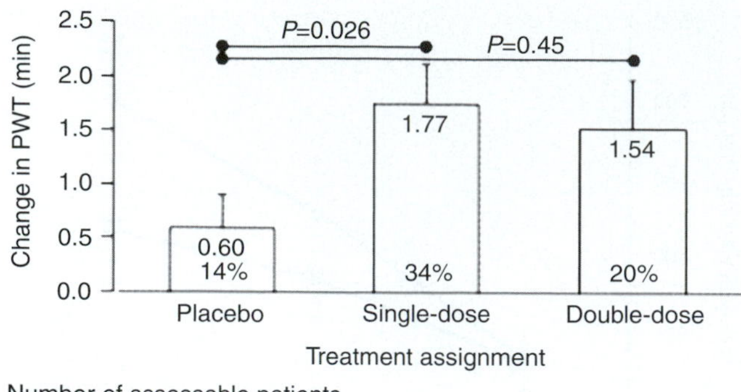

Number of assessable patients			
Baseline	63	66	61
Day 90	58	62	54

FIGURE 18-8. A single intra-arterial dose of recombinant fibroblast growth factor-2 improves maximal walking time in patients with intermittent claudication. Results of the TRAFFIC study. Percent change is relative to log-transformed baseline. There is no additional benefit of a second dose of rFGF-2. PWT, maximal (peak) walking time; rFGF-2, recombinant fibroblast growth factor-2. (Reproduced with permission from Lederman RJ, Mendelsohn FO, Anderson RD, et al: Therapeutic angiogenesis with recombinant fibroblast growth factor-2 for intermittent claudication (the TRAFFIC study): A randomised trial. Lancet 359:2053, 2002.)

and increased the ABI.[156] Recombinant FGF-2, administered directly into the femoral artery, was studied in a placebo-controlled study (Fig. 18-8).[157] Patients were randomized to receive FGF-2, 30 μg/kg, on one occasion only, or on two occasions 30 days apart, or placebo. One-time administration of FGF-2 increased peak walking time at 90 days by 34% compared with 14% for placebo. Yet, there was no significant improvement in peak walking time compared with placebo when FGF-2 was administered on two occasions.

Other Growth Factors

Del-1 (developmentally regulated endothelial locus 1) is an extracellular matrix protein that stimulates angiogenesis.[158] Administration of a plasmid expressing Del-1 via intramuscular injections to patients with claudication did not improve maximal walking distance when compared with placebo.[159]

Hypoxia inducible factor-1 (HIF-1α) is an inducible transcriptional regulatory factor. In conditions of low oxygen tension, HIF-1α binds to hypoxia-responsive elements in the promoter/enhancer region of target genes inducing those encoding VEGF-A, platelet derived growth factor (PDGF), angiotensin-1, and inducible nitric oxide synthase (iNOS).[160-162] Clinical trials are in progress to determine the effect of intramuscular injection of an adenovirus encoding HIF-1α in patients with critical limb ischemia and claudication.

Stem Cell Therapy

Infusion of endothelial progenitor cells to mice in an experiment model of hindlimb ischemia has been shown to improve blood flow and capillary density in the ischemic hindlimb and reduce the rate of limb loss.[163] Bone marrow-mononuclear cells include endothelial progenitor cells. Intramuscular injection of autologous

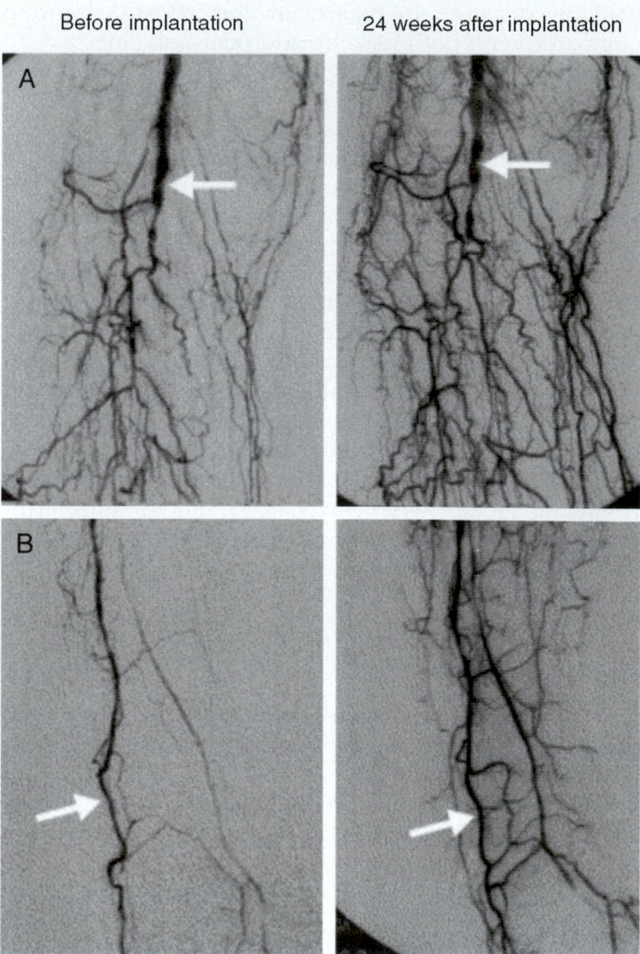

FIGURE 18-9. Angiographic demonstration of lower extremity collateral formation in a patient with critical limb ischemia treated with mononuclear stem cells. **A,** demonstrates angiogenesis in the knee and upper tibial region before and 24 days after stem-cell infusion. **B,** demonstrates angiogenesis in the lower leg and ankle. Arrows denote reference points in each vascular segment before and after stem cell infusion. (Reproduced with permission from Tateishi-Yuyama E, Matsubara H, Murohara T, et al: Therapeutic angiogenesis for patients with limb ischaemia by autologous transplantation of bone-marrow cells: A pilot study and a randomised controlled trial. Lancet 360:427, 2002.)

bone marrow-derived mononuclear cells improve collateral blood vessel formation in animal models of myocardial and hindlimb ischemia.[164,165] As a result of these preclinical studies, the effect of autologous implantation of bone marrow-derived mononuclear cells was studied in patients with PAD manifested as limb ischemia.[166] Injection of bone marrow-mononuclear cells compared with peripheral blood mononuclear cells reduced rest pain and improved pain-free walking time. The improvement was sustained for 24 weeks. Angiographic evidence of collateral blood vessel formation was present in many of the patients who received bone marrow-derived mononuclear cells (Fig. 18-9).

Statins

As discussed earlier in this chapter, lipid-lowering therapy with statins reduces the risk of adverse cardiovascular events in patients with atherosclerosis including those with PAD. As discussed earlier, post-hoc analysis of the Scandinavian Simvastatin Survival Study found that simvastatin reduced the risk of new or worsening claudication.[28] Several prospective studies have found that statin therapy improved symptoms of claudication in patients with intermittent claudication. One placebo-controlled trial found that atorvastatin, 80 mg per day, for 12 months improved pain-free walking time by 63% compared with 38% in the placebo group (Fig. 18-10).[29] In other studies, 6 and 12 months of treatment with simvastatin, 40 mg per day, improved pain-free and maximal walking distance.[30,167]

There are several potential mechanisms whereby statin therapy may improve symptoms of claudication. These include reduction in plaque size, improvement in vasomotor regulation of blood flow, particularly in the microcirculation, and promotion of angiogenesis. It is not likely that reduction of plaque size accounts for the improvement in symptoms. This is because angiographic studies have shown that treatment with statins induces only very mild changes in vascular lumen size, and these are unlikely to affect blood flow through a stenotic artery.[168] In the studies that have examined the effect of statins on patients with claudication, there have been no, or only very minor, changes in the ABI.[29,167] Endothelial function, particularly in the peripheral resistance vessels, is impaired in patients with atherosclerosis including those with PAD.[169] Statin therapy has been shown to improve endothelial function in patients with coronary artery disease.[170,171] Therefore, statin therapy may improve blood flow to the microcirculation and thereby ameliorate symptoms of claudication. Animal studies have found that hypercholesterolemia inhibits angiogenesis.[172] This inhibition may be reduced when cholesterol concentration is lowered by statin therapy, enabling collateral formation to occur. In addition, statins have been shown to increase circulating endothelial progenitor cells, independent of cholesterol reduction, and thereby may have a proangiogenic effect.[173]

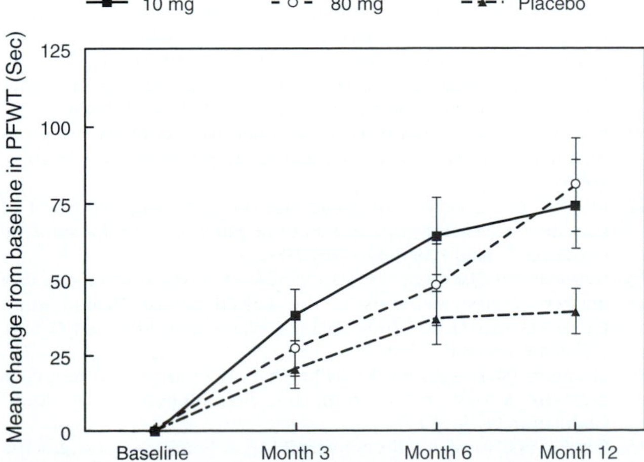

FIGURE 18-10. Atorvastatin improves pain-free walking time in patients with intermittent claudication. * $P = .025$ for 80-mg dose at 12 months. PFWT, pain-free walking time. (Reproduced with permission from Mohler ER, III, Hiatt WR, Creager MA: Cholesterol reduction with atorvastatin improves walking distance in patients with peripheral arterial disease. Circulation 108:1481, 2003.)

Nutriceuticals and Alternative Therapies

Dietary supplements with nutrients, herbs, and vitamins such as L-arginine, ginkgo biloba, and vitamin E, as well as ethylenediaminetetraacetic acid (EDTA), have been studied as complementary therapeutic strategies to improve functional capacity in patients with intermittent claudication. The available evidence supporting and refuting these holistic therapies is reviewed below because vascular specialists are frequently queried by their patients about these remedies.

L-Arginine

Endothelium-derived nitric oxide (NO) is synthesized from its precursor, L-arginine, by endothelial nitric oxide synthase (eNOS) (see Chapter 5). Endothelium-dependent vasodilation, mediated by NO, contributes to the physiologic regulation of blood flow at rest and during exercise.[174-176] NO activates guanylyl cyclase on subjacent vascular smooth muscle and increases cyclic guanosine monophosphate (cGMP) and thereby causes vasodilation. Endothelium-dependent vasodilation is abnormal in conduit and resistance vessels in patients with PAD.[169]

In one study, L-arginine, administered intravenously at a dose of 8 g twice each day, for 3 weeks, improved pain-free walking distance by 230% and maximal walking distance by 155%.[123] Another study examined the effect of a food bar containing L-arginine (3.3 g), as well as B complex and antioxidant vitamins, on walking distance in patients with intermittent claudication.[177] Pain-free and maximal walking distance improved by 66% and 23%, respectively, following 2 weeks of therapy in patients eating two bars per day. A larger placebo-controlled trial assessing the affect of this L-arginine-enriched food bar had been completed several years ago, but the results have not been reported (Creager, personal communication). In light of the limited studies with L-arginine in patients with intermittent claudication, it is premature to make any recommendations regarding its efficacy.

Vitamin E

Vitamin E (α-tocopherol) is a lipid-soluble antioxidant that has undergone evaluation in patients with intermittent claudication. It inhibits the oxidation of polyunsaturated fatty acid. Vitamin E may improve erythrocyte deformability and improve blood flow through the microcirculation because polyunsaturated fatty acids are incorporated into the erythrocyte membrane. A Cochrane database systematic review evaluated five placebo-controlled trials of vitamin E in patients with intermittent claudication.[178] The trials, conducted between 1953 and 1975, were small and measured different outcomes, precluding any conclusions regarding the efficacy of vitamin E for intermittent claudication. Both the Heart Protection Study (HPS) and the Heart Outcomes Prevention Evaluation (HOPE) study failed to demonstrate any efficacy of vitamin E on adverse cardiovascular events in patients with atherosclerosis including those with PAD.[27,50] Therefore, vitamin E is not recommended as therapy for patients with PAD, including those with intermittent claudication.

Ginkgo Biloba

Ginkgo biloba is an herb whose major constituents include flavonoids and terpene lactones, such as ginkgolides and bilobalide. Ginkgo may have antioxidant, antiplatelet, and hemorrheologic actions.[179] It is one of the top-selling herbal medicinal products in the United States.

A meta-analysis of eight randomized, placebo-controlled trials found that in recipients of ginkgo, the pain-free claudication distance was 34 meters more than in patients receiving placebo.[180] In the largest trial, 24 weeks of ginkgo treatment improved pain-free and maximal walking distance by 45 and 61 meters, respectively; whereas placebo improved these by 21 and 25 meters, respectively.[181] Doses employed in clinical trials range from 120 to 320 mg per day. The most common dosage is 40 mg 3 times daily. The potential adverse effects of ginkgo include gastrointestinal symptoms, headache, nausea, vomiting, bleeding, or allergic skin reactions.[179] *Ginkgo biloba* is also associated with adverse interactions with many common prescription medications. *Ginkgo biloba* has been associated with cerebral hemorrhage in case reports.[182] *Ginkgo biloba* may be considered as an alternative therapy for treatment of claudication, but its efficacy is probably of marginal clinical importance.

Disodium Ethylenediaminetetraacetic Acid (EDTA)

EDTA combines with polyvalent cations, including calcium ions, to form a soluble nonionic complex that can be excreted. It requires intravenous administration and is usually administered 2 or more times per week. The rationale for using EDTA in patients with atherosclerosis, including those with PAD, is to leech calcium out of atherosclerotic plaque, induce plaque regression, and reduce the severity of stenosis. Also, EDTA may decrease metal ion-dependent formation of reactive oxygen species and metal ion-dependent lipid peroxidation.[183] There is limited biologic evidence to support its efficacy in atherosclerosis.[184] The Program to Assess Alternative Treatment Strategies to Achieve Health (PATCH) assessed the effect of EDTA on endothelium-dependent vasodilation in patients with coronary artery disease. Up to 33 treatments of intravenous EDTA over a 6-month period caused no changes in peripheral endothelial function.[185] One clinical trial found no effect of EDTA on the severity of atherosclerosis in patients with PAD.[186] Two systematic reviews evaluated four placebo controlled trials that assessed the efficacy of EDTA in patients with intermittent claudication.[187,188] These reviews found no evidence that EDTA improves pain-free or maximal walking distance in patients with intermittent claudication. Potential serious adverse effects of EDTA include hypocalcemia, renal insufficiency, and proteinuria. Additional side effects include gastrointestinal and musculoskeletal symptoms, hypertension, tachycardia, and fever. Based on lack of efficacy, and safety concerns, EDTA should not be used to treat patients with intermittent claudication.

Conclusion

Patients with PAD are at increased risk for adverse cardiovascular events, such as myocardial infarction, stroke, and death. Risk factor modification and antiplatelet therapy are critical components of the management of all patients with PAD. Supervised exercise rehabilitation and the phosphodiesterase inhibitor, cilostazol, improve walking distance in patients with claudication. Unfortunately, the pharmacologic armamentarium for the treatment of claudication is limited. Promising new therapies for claudication, particularly angiogenic growth factors and stem cells, are undergoing extensive clinical investigation. The success of these initiatives will define the future role of medical therapy for PAD and intermittent claudication.

REFERENCES

1. Bowlin SJ, Medalie JH, Flocke SA, et al: Epidemiology of intermittent claudication in middle-aged men. Am J Epidemiol 140:418, 1994.
2. Smith GD, Shipley MJ, Rose G: Intermittent claudication, heart disease risk factors, and mortality: The Whitehall Study. Circulation 82:1925, 1990.
3. Kannel WB, Shurtleff D: The Framingham Study: Cigarettes and the development of intermittent claudication. Geriatrics 28:61, 1973.
4. Meijer WT, Hoes AW, Rutgers D, et al: Peripheral arterial disease in the elderly: The Rotterdam Study. Arterioscler Thromb Vasc Biol 18:185, 1998.
5. Gardner AW: The effect of cigarette smoking on exercise capacity in patients with intermittent claudication. Vasc Med 1:181, 1996.
6. Quick CR, Cotton LT: The measured effect of stopping smoking on intermittent claudication. Br J Surg 69 Suppl:S24, 1982.
7. Jonason T, Bergstrom R: Cessation of smoking in patients with intermittent claudication: Effects on the risk of peripheral vascular complications, myocardial infarction and mortality. Acta Med Scand 221:253, 1987.
8. Powell JT, Greenhalgh RM: Changing the smoking habit and its influence on the management of vascular disease. Acta Chir Scand Suppl 555:99, 1990.
9. Faulkner KW, House AK, Castleden WM: The effect of cessation of smoking on the accumulative survival rates of patients with symptomatic peripheral vascular disease. Med J Aust 1:217, 1983.
10. Lassila R, Lepantalo M: Cigarette smoking and the outcome after lower limb arterial surgery. Acta Chir Scand 154:635, 1988.
11. Law M, Tang JL: An analysis of the effectiveness of interventions intended to help people stop smoking. Arch Intern Med 155:1933, 1995.
12. Jorenby DE, Leischow SJ, Nides MA, et al: A controlled trial of sustained-release bupropion, a nicotine patch, or both for smoking cessation. N Engl J Med 340:685, 1999.
13. Newman AB, Siscovick DS, Manolio TA, et al: Ankle-arm index as a marker of atherosclerosis in the Cardiovascular Health Study. Cardiovascular Heart Study (CHS) Collaborative Research Group. Circulation 88:837, 1993.
14. Murabito JM, D'Agostino RB, Silbershatz H, et al: Intermittent claudication: A risk profile from the Framingham Heart Study. Circulation 96:44, 1997.
15. Fowkes FG, Housley E, Riemersma RA, et al: Smoking, lipids, glucose intolerance, and blood pressure as risk factors for peripheral atherosclerosis compared with ischemic heart disease in the Edinburgh Artery Study. Am J Epidemiol 135:331, 1992.
16. Mowat BF, Skinner ER, Wilson HM, et al: Alterations in plasma lipids, lipoproteins, and high density lipoprotein subfractions in peripheral arterial disease. Atherosclerosis 131:161, 1997.

17. Blankenhorn DH, Azen SP, Crawford DW, et al: Effects of colestipol-niacin therapy on human femoral atherosclerosis. Circulation 83:438, 1991.
18. Walldius G, Erikson U, Olsson AG, et al: The effect of probucol on femoral atherosclerosis: The Probucol Quantitative Regression Swedish Trial (PQRST). Am J Cardiol 74:875, 1994.
19. Opie L, Gersh BJ: Drugs for the Heart. 2001, Philadelphia, WB Saunders.
20. Buchwald H, Varco RL, Matts JP, et al: Effect of partial ileal bypass surgery on mortality and morbidity from coronary heart disease in patients with hypercholesterolemia: Report of the Program on the Surgical Control of the Hyperlipidemias (POSCH). N Engl J Med 323:946, 1990.
21. Rubins HB, Robins SJ, Collins D, et al: Gemfibrozil for the secondary prevention of coronary heart disease in men with low levels of high-density lipoprotein cholesterol. Veterans Affairs High-Density Lipoprotein Cholesterol Intervention Trial Study Group. N Engl J Med 341:410, 1999.
22. Scandinavian Simvastatin Survival Study Group: Randomised trial of cholesterol lowering in 4444 patients with coronary heart disease: The Scandinavian Simvastatin Survival Study (4S). Lancet 344:1383, 1994.
23. Sacks FM, Pfeffer MA, Moye LA, et al: The effect of pravastatin on coronary events after myocardial infarction in patients with average cholesterol levels: Cholesterol and Recurrent Events Trial investigators. N Engl J Med 335:1001, 1996.
24. Prevention of cardiovascular events and death with pravastatin in patients with coronary heart disease and a broad range of initial cholesterol levels: The Long-Term Intervention with Pravastatin in Ischaemic Disease (LIPID) Study Group. N Engl J Med 339:1349, 1998.
25. Hirsch AT, Criqui MH, Treat-Jacobson D, et al: Peripheral arterial disease detection, awareness, and treatment in primary care. JAMA 286:1317, 2001.
26. Zheng ZJ, Sharrett AR, Chambless LE, et al: Associations of ankle-brachial index with clinical coronary heart disease, stroke, and preclinical carotid and popliteal atherosclerosis: The Atherosclerosis Risk in Communities (ARIC) Study. Atherosclerosis 131:115, 1997.
27. MRC/BHF Heart Protection Study of cholesterol lowering with simvastatin in 20,536 high-risk individuals: A randomised placebo-controlled trial. Lancet 360:7, 2002.
28. Pedersen TR, Kjekshus J, Pyorala K, et al: Effect of simvastatin on ischemic signs and symptoms in the Scandinavian simvastatin survival study (4S). Am J Cardiol 81:333, 1998.
29. Mohler ER, III, Hiatt WR, Creager MA: Cholesterol reduction with atorvastatin improves walking distance in patients with peripheral arterial disease. Circulation 108:1481, 2003.
30. Aronow WS, Nayak D, Woodworth S, et al: Effect of simvastatin versus placebo on treadmill exercise time until the onset of intermittent claudication in older patients with peripheral arterial disease at six months and at one year after treatment. Am J Cardiol 92:711, 2003.
31. MRC/BHF Heart Protection Study of cholesterol-lowering therapy and of antioxidant vitamin supplementation in a wide range of patients at increased risk of coronary heart disease death: Early safety and efficacy experience. Eur Heart J 20:725, 1999.
32. Cannon CP, Braunwald E, McCabe CH, et al: Intensive versus moderate lipid lowering with statins after acute coronary syndromes. N Engl J Med 350:1495, 2004.
33. Grundy SM, Cleeman JI, Merz CN, et al: Implications of recent clinical trials for the National Cholesterol Education Program Adult Treatment Panel III guidelines. Circulation 110:227, 2004.
34. Gordon DJ, Rifkind BM: High-density lipoprotein: The clinical implications of recent studies. N Engl J Med 321:1311, 1989.
35. Goldbourt U, Yaari S, Medalie JH: Isolated low HDL cholesterol as a risk factor for coronary heart disease mortality: A 21-year follow-up of 8000 men. Arterioscler Thromb Vasc Biol 17:107, 1997.
36. Executive Summary of the Third Report of the National Cholesterol Education Program (NCEP) Expert Panel on Detection, Evaluation, and Treatment of High Blood Cholesterol in Adults (Adult Treatment Panel III). JAMA 285:2486, 2001.
37. Psaty BM, Lumley T, Furberg CD, et al: Health outcomes associated with various antihypertensive therapies used as first-line agents: A network meta-analysis. JAMA 289:2534, 2003.
38. Major outcomes in high-risk hypertensive patients randomized to angiotensin-converting enzyme inhibitor or calcium channel blocker vs. diuretic: The Antihypertensive and Lipid-Lowering Treatment to Prevent Heart Attack Trial (ALLTHAT). JAMA 288:2981, 2002.
39. Lip GY, Makin AJ: Treatment of hypertension in peripheral arterial disease. Cochrane Database Syst Rev: CD003075, 2003.
40. Frishman WH: Beta-adrenergic receptor blockers: Adverse effects and drug interactions. Hypertension 11:II21, 1988.
41. Rodger JC, Sheldon CD, Lerski RA, et al: Intermittent claudication complicating beta-blockade. Br Med J 1:1125, 1976.
42. Roberts DH, Tsao Y, McLoughlin GA, et al: Placebo-controlled comparison of captopril, atenolol, labetalol, and pindolol in hypertension complicated by intermittent claudication. Lancet 2:650, 1987.
43. Solomon SA, Ramsay LE, Yeo WW, et al: Beta blockade and intermittent claudication: Placebo controlled trial of atenolol and nifedipine and their combination. Br Med J 303:1100, 1991.
44. Radack K, Deck C: Beta-adrenergic blocker therapy does not worsen intermittent claudication in subjects with peripheral arterial disease: A meta-analysis of randomized controlled trials. Arch Intern Med 151:1769, 1991.
45. Norwegian Multicentre Study Group: Timolol-induced reduction in mortality and reinfarction in patients surviving acute myocardial infarction. N Engl J Med 304:801, 1981.
46. A randomized trial of propranolol in patients with acute myocardial infarction. I. Mortality results. JAMA 247:1707, 1982.
47. Poldermans D, Boersma E, Bax JJ, et al: The effect of bisoprolol on perioperative mortality and myocardial infarction in high-risk patients undergoing vascular surgery: Dutch Echocardiographic Cardiac Risk Evaluation Applying Stress Echocardiography Study Group. N Engl J Med 341:1789, 1999.
48. Mangano DT, Layug EL, Wallace A, et al: Effect of atenolol on mortality and cardiovascular morbidity after noncardiac surgery. Multicenter Study of Perioperative Ischemia Research Group [published erratum appears in N Engl J Med 1997 Apr 3;336(14):1039]. N Engl J Med 335:1713, 1996.
49. Overlack A, Adamczak M, Bachmann W, et al: ACE-inhibition with perindopril in essential hypertensive patients with concomitant diseases: The Perindopril Therapeutic Safety Collaborative Research Group. Am J Med 97:126, 1994.
50. Yusuf S, Sleight P, Pogue J, et al: Effects of an angiotensin-converting-enzyme inhibitor, ramipril, on cardiovascular events in high-risk patients: The Heart Outcomes Prevention Evaluation Study Investigators [published erratum appears in N Engl J Med 2000 Mar 9;342(10):748]. N Engl J Med 342:145, 2000.
51. Mehler PS, Coll JR, Estacio R, et al: Intensive blood pressure control reduces the risk of cardiovascular events in patients with peripheral arterial disease and type 2 diabetes. Circulation 107:753, 2003.
52. Estacio RO, Jeffers BW, Hiatt WR, et al: The effect of nisoldipine as compared with enalapril on cardiovascular outcomes in patients with non-insulin-dependent diabetes and hypertension. N Engl J Med 338:645, 1998.
53. The HOPE (Heart Outcomes Prevention Evaluation) Study: The design of a large, simple randomized trial of an angiotensin-converting enzyme inhibitor (ramipril) and vitamin E in patients at high risk of cardiovascular events. Can J Cardiol 12:127, 1996.
54. Adler AI, Stevens RJ, Neil A, et al: UKPDS 59: Hyperglycemia and other potentially modifiable risk factors for peripheral vascular disease in type 2 diabetes. Diabetes Care 25:894, 2002.
55. Bowers BL, Valentine RJ, Myers SI, et al: The natural history of patients with claudication with toe pressures of 40 mm Hg or less. J Vasc Surg 18:506, 1993.
56. Jude EB, Oyibo SO, Chalmers N, et al: Peripheral arterial disease in diabetic and nondiabetic patients: A comparison of severity and outcome. Diabetes Care 24:1433, 2001.
57. The Diabetes Control and Complications Trial Research Group: The effect of intensive treatment of diabetes on the development and progression of long-term complications in insulin-dependent diabetes mellitus. N Engl J Med 329:977, 1993.
58. Effect of intensive diabetes management on macrovascular events and risk factors in the Diabetes Control and Complications Trial. Am J Cardiol 75:894, 1995.
59. Knatterud GL, Klimt CR, Levin ME, et al: Effects of hypoglycemic agents on vascular complications in patients with adult-onset diabetes. VII. Mortality and selected nonfatal events with insulin treatment. JAMA 240:37, 1978.

60. UK Prospective Diabetes Study Group: Intensive blood glucose control with sulphonylureas or insulin compared with conventional treatment and risk of complications in patients with type 2 diabetes (UKPDS 33). Lancet 352:837,1998.
61. UK Prospective Diabetes Study (UKPDS) Group: Effect of intensive blood-glucose control with metformin on complications in overweight patients with type 2 diabetes (UKPDS 34). Lancet 352:854, 1998.
62. Abbasi F, Chu JW, McLaughlin T, et al: Effect of metformin treatment on multiple cardiovascular disease risk factors in patients with type 2 diabetes mellitus. Metabolism 53:159, 2004.
63. Gilling L, Suwattee P, DeSouza C, et al: Effects of the thiazolidinediones on cardiovascular risk factors. Am J Cardiovasc Drugs 2:149, 2002.
64. Abraira C, Duckworth W, McCarren M, et al: Design of the cooperative study on glycemic control and complications in diabetes mellitus type 2: Veterans Affairs Diabetes Trial. J Diabetes Complications 17:314, 2003.
65. American Diabetes Association: Standards of medical care for patients with diabetes mellitus. Diabetes Care 26 Suppl 1:S33, 2003.
66. American Diabetes Association: Peripheral arterial disease in people with diabetes. Diabetes Care 26:3333, 2003.
67. Welch GN, Loscalzo J: Homocysteine and atherothrombosis. N Engl J Med 338:1042, 1998.
68. Boers GH, Smals AG, Trijbels FJ, et al: Heterozygosity for homocystinuria in premature peripheral and cerebral occlusive arterial disease [see comments]. N Engl J Med 313:709, 1985.
69. Stampfer MJ, Malinow MR, Willett WC, et al: A prospective study of plasma homocyst(e)ine and risk of myocardial infarction in U.S. physicians. JAMA 268:877, 1992.
70. Taylor LM, Jr, DeFrang RD, Harris EJ, Jr, et al: The association of elevated plasma homocyst(e)ine with progression of symptomatic peripheral arterial disease. J Vasc Surg 13:128, 1991.
71. Darius H, Pittrow D, Haberl R, et al: Are elevated homocysteine plasma levels related to peripheral arterial disease? Results from a cross-sectional study of 6880 primary care patients. Eur J Clin Invest 33:751, 2003.
72. Malinow MR, Kang SS, Taylor LM, et al: Prevalence of hyperhomocyst(e)inemia in patients with peripheral arterial occlusive disease. Circulation 79:1180, 1989.
73. van den Bosch MA, Bloemenkamp DG, Mali WP, et al: Hyperhomocysteinemia and risk for peripheral arterial occlusive disease in young women. J Vasc Surg 38:772, 2003.
74. den Heijer M, Koster T, Blom HJ, et al: Hyperhomocysteinemia as a risk factor for deep-vein thrombosis. N Engl J Med 334:759, 1996.
75. Homocysteine Lowering Trialists' Collaboration. Lowering blood homocysteine with folic acid based supplements: Meta-analysis of randomised trials. Br Med J 316:894, 1998.
76. Vermeulen EG, Stehouwer CD, Twisk JW, et al: Effect of homocysteine-lowering treatment with folic acid plus vitamin B_6 on progression of subclinical atherosclerosis: A randomised, placebo-controlled trial. Lancet 355:517, 2000.
77. Clarke R: Homocysteine-lowering trials for prevention of heart disease and stroke. Semin Vasc Med 5:215, 2005.
78. Antithrombotic Trialists Collaboration: Collaborative meta-analysis of randomised trials of antiplatelet therapy for prevention of death, myocardial infarction, and stroke in high risk patients.[erratum appears in Br Med J 2002 Jan 19;324(7330):141]. Br Med J 324:71, 2002.
79. Antiplatelet Trialists' Collaboration: Collaborative overview of randomised trials of antiplatelet therapy—I: Prevention of death, myocardial infarction, and stroke by prolonged antiplatelet therapy in various categories of patients. [published erratum appears in Br Med J 1994 Jun 11;308(6943):1540]. Br Med J 308:81, 1994.
80. Peto R, Gray R, Collins R, et al: Randomised trial of prophylactic daily aspirin in British male doctors. Br Med J (Clin Res Ed) 296:313, 1988.
81. Steering Committee of the Physicians' Health Study Research Group: Final report on the aspirin component of the ongoing Physicians' Health Study. N Engl J Med 321:129, 1989.
82. Goldhaber SZ, Manson JE, Stampfer MJ, et al: Low-dose aspirin and subsequent peripheral arterial surgery in the Physicians' Health Study. Lancet 340:143, 1992.
83. Collaborative meta-analysis of randomised trials of antiplatelet therapy for prevention of death, myocardial infarction, and stroke in high risk patients. Br Med J 324:71, 2002.
84. Antiplatelet Trialists' Collaboration: Collaborative overview of randomised trials of antiplatelet therapy—II: Maintenance of vascular graft or arterial patency by antiplatelet therapy. Br Med J 308:159, 1994.
85. Balsano F, Violi F: Effect of picotamide on the clinical progression of peripheral vascular disease: A double-blind placebo-controlled study. The ADEP Group. Circulation 87:1563, 1993.
86. CAPRIE Steering Committee: A randomised, blinded, trial of clopidogrel versus aspirin in patients at risk of ischaemic events (CAPRIE). Lancet 348:1329, 1996.
87. Yusuf S, Zhao F, Mehta SR, et al: Effects of clopidogrel in addition to aspirin in patients with acute coronary syndromes without ST-segment elevation. N Engl J Med 345:494, 2001.
88. Bhatt DL, Topol EJ: Clopidogrel added to aspirin versus aspirin alone in secondary prevention and high-risk primary prevention: Rationale and design of the Clopidogrel for High Atherothrombotic Risk and Ischemic Stabilization, Management, and Avoidance (CHARISMA) trial. Am Heart J 148:263, 2004.
89. ACC/AHA Guidelines for the Management of Peripheral Arterial Disease. http://www.acc.org/clinical/guidelines/pad/summary.pdf
90. Anand SS, Yusuf S: Oral anticoagulants in patients with coronary artery disease. J Am Coll Cardiol 41:S62, 2003.
91. Anand SS, Yusuf S: Oral anticoagulant therapy in patients with coronary artery disease: A meta-analysis [published erratum appears in JAMA 2000 Jul 5;284(1):45]. JAMA 282:2058, 1999.
92. Cosmi B, Conti E, Coccheri S: Anticoagulants (heparin, low molecular weight heparin and oral anticoagulants) for intermittent claudication. Cochrane Database Syst Rev:CD001999, 2001.
93. Clagett GP, Sobel M, Jackson MR, et al: Antithrombotic therapy in peripheral arterial occlusive disease: The Seventh ACCP Conference on Antithrombotic and Thrombolytic Therapy. Chest 126:609S, 2004.
94. Efficacy of oral anticoagulants compared with aspirin after infrainguinal bypass surgery. The Dutch Bypass Oral Anticoagulants or Aspirin Study: A randomised trial. Lancet 355:346, 2000.
95. Gardner AW, Poehlman ET: Exercise rehabilitation programs for the treatment of claudication pain: A meta-analysis. JAMA 274:975, 1995.
96. Leng GC, Fowler B, Ernst E: Exercise for intermittent claudication. Cochrane Database Syst Rev: CD000990, 2004.
97. Regensteiner JG, Steiner JF, Hiatt WR: Exercise training improves functional status in patients with peripheral arterial disease. J Vasc Surg 23:104, 1996.
98. Regensteiner JG, Meyer TJ, Krupski WC, et al: Hospital vs. home-based exercise rehabilitation for patients with peripheral arterial occlusive disease. Angiology 48:291, 1997.
99. Degischer S, Labs KH, Hochstrasser J, et al: Physical training for intermittent claudication: A comparison of structured rehabilitation versus home-based training. Vasc Med 7:109, 2002.
100. Stewart KJ, Hiatt WR, Regensteiner JG, et al: Exercise training for claudication. N Engl J Med 347:1941, 2002.
101. Mathien GM, Terjung RL: Muscle blood flow in trained rats with peripheral arterial insufficiency. Am J Physiol 258:H759, 1990.
102. Lloyd PG, Yang HT, Terjung RL: Arteriogenesis and angiogenesis in rat ischemic hindlimb: Role of nitric oxide. Am J Physiol Heart Circ Physiol 281:H2528, 2001.
103. Prior BM, Yang HT, Terjung RL: What makes vessels grow with exercise training? J Appl Physiol 97:1119, 2004.
104. Laufs U, Werner N, Link A, et al: Physical training increases endothelial progenitor cells, inhibits neointima formation, and enhances angiogenesis. Circulation 109:220, 2004.
105. Buckwalter JB, Curtis VC, Valic Z, et al: Endogenous vascular remodeling in ischemic skeletal muscle: A role for nitric oxide. J Appl Physiol 94:935, 2003.
106. Niebauer J, Maxwell AJ, Lin PS, et al: Impaired aerobic capacity in hypercholesterolemic mice: Partial reversal by exercise training. Am J Physiol 276:H1346, 1999.
107. Hiatt WR, Regensteiner JG, Hargarten ME, et al: Benefit of exercise conditioning for patients with peripheral arterial disease. Circulation 81:602, 1990.
108. Gardner AW, Katzel LI, Sorkin JD, et al: Exercise rehabilitation improves functional outcomes and peripheral circulation in

patients with intermittent claudication: A randomized controlled trial. J Am Geriatr Soc 49:755, 2001.
109. Brendle DC, Joseph LJ, Corretti MC, et al: Effects of exercise rehabilitation on endothelial reactivity in older patients with peripheral arterial disease. Am J Cardiol 87:324, 2001.
110. Gokce N, Vita JA, Bader DS, et al: Effect of exercise on upper and lower extremity endothelial function in patients with coronary artery disease. Am J Cardiol 90:124, 2002.
111. Hiatt WR, Regensteiner JG, Wolfel EE, et al: Effect of exercise training on skeletal muscle histology and metabolism in peripheral arterial disease. J Appl Physiol 81:780, 1996.
112. Brass EP: Skeletal muscle metabolism as a target for drug therapy in peripheral arterial disease. Vasc Med 1:55, 1996.
113. Gardner AW, Forrester L, Smith GV: Altered gait profile in subjects with peripheral arterial disease. Vasc Med 6:31, 2001.
114. Igawa T, Tani T, Chijiwa T, et al: Potentiation of anti-platelet aggregating activity of cilostazol with vascular endothelial cells. Thromb Res 57:617, 1990.
115. Woo SK, Kang WK, Kwon KI: Pharmacokinetic and pharmacodynamic modeling of the antiplatelet and cardiovascular effects of cilostazol in healthy humans. Clin Pharmacol Ther 71:246, 2002.
116. Tanaka T, Ishikawa T, Hagiwara M, et al: Effects of cilostazol: A selective cAMP phosphodiesterase inhibitor on the contraction of vascular smooth muscle. Pharmacology 36:313, 1988.
117. Oida K, Ebata K, Kanehara H, et al: Effect of cilostazol on impaired vasodilatory response of the brachial artery to ischemia in smokers. J Atheroscler Thromb 10:93, 2003.
118. Regensteiner JG, Ware JE, Jr, McCarthy WJ, et al: Effect of cilostazol on treadmill walking, community-based walking ability, and health-related quality of life in patients with intermittent claudication due to peripheral arterial disease: Meta-analysis of six randomized controlled trials. J Am Geriatr Soc 50:1939, 2002.
119. Dawson DL, Cutler BS, Hiatt WR, et al: A comparison of cilostazol and pentoxifylline for treating intermittent claudication. Am J Med 109:523, 2000.
120. Packer M, Carver JR, Rodeheffer RJ, et al: Effect of oral milrinone on mortality in severe chronic heart failure: The PROMISE Study Research Group. N Engl J Med 325:1468, 1991.
121. Cohn JN, Goldstein SO, Greenberg BH, et al: A dose-dependent increase in mortality with vesnarinone among patients with severe heart failure. Vesnarinone Trial Investigators. N Engl J Med 339:1810, 1998.
122. Diehm C, Balzer K, Bisler H, et al: Efficacy of a new prostaglandin E1 regimen in outpatients with severe intermittent claudication: Results of a multicenter placebo-controlled double-blind trial. J Vasc Surg 25:537, 1997.
123. Boger RH, Bode-Boger SM, Thiele W, et al: Restoring vascular nitric oxide formation by L-arginine improves the symptoms of intermittent claudication in patients with peripheral arterial occlusive disease. J Am Coll Cardiol 32:1336, 1998.
124. Mangiafico RA, Messina R, Attina T, et al: Impact of a 4-week treatment with prostaglandin E1 on health-related quality of life of patients with intermittent claudication. Angiology 51:441, 2000.
125. Reiter M, Bucek RA, Stumpflen A, et al: Prostanoids for intermittent claudication. Cochrane Database Syst Rev: CD000986, 2004.
126. Lievre M, Morand S, Besse B, et al: Oral Beraprost sodium, a prostaglandin I(2) analogue, for intermittent claudication: A double-blind, randomized, multicenter controlled trial. Beraprost et Claudication Intermittente (BERCI) Research Group. Circulation 102:426, 2000.
127. Mohler ER, III, Hiatt WR, Olin JW, et al: Treatment of intermittent claudication with Beraprost sodium, an orally active prostaglandin I2 analogue: A double-blinded, randomized, controlled trial. J Am Coll Cardiol 41:1679, 2003.
128. Second European Consensus Document on chronic critical leg ischemia. Circulation 84:IV1, 1991.
129. The ICAI Study Group: Prostanoids for chronic critical leg ischemia: A randomized, controlled, open-label trial with prostaglandin E1. Ischemia Cronica degli Arti Inferiori. Ann Intern Med 130:412, 1999.
130. The Oral Iloprost in Severe Leg Ischaemia Study Group: Two randomised and placebo-controlled studies of an oral prostacyclin analogue (Iloprost) in severe leg ischaemia. Eur J Vasc Endovasc Surg 20:358, 2000.
131. Lewis P, Psaila JV, Davies WT, et al: Nifedipine in patients with peripheral vascular disease. Eur J Vasc Surg 3:159, 1989.
132. Bagger JP, Helligsoe P, Randsbaek F, et al: Effect of verapamil in intermittent claudication A randomized, double- blind, placebo-controlled, cross-over study after individual dose- response assessment. Circulation 95:411, 1997.
133. Rao KM, Simel DL, Cohen HJ, et al: Effects of pentoxifylline administration on blood viscosity and leukocyte cytoskeletal function in patients with intermittent claudication. J Lab Clin Med 115:738, 1990.
134. Schratzberger P, Dunzendorfer S, Reinisch N, et al: Mediator-dependent effects of pentoxifylline on endothelium for transmigration of neutrophils. Immunopharmacology 41:65, 1999.
135. Dawson DL, Zheng Q, Worthy SA, et al: Failure of pentoxifylline or cilostazol to improve blood and plasma viscosity, fibrinogen, and erythrocyte deformability in claudication. Angiology 53:509, 2002.
136. Hood SC, Moher D, Barber GG: Management of intermittent claudication with pentoxifylline: Meta-analysis of randomized controlled trials. CMAJ 155:1053, 1996.
137. Girolami B, Bernardi E, Prins MH, et al: Treatment of intermittent claudication with physical training, smoking cessation, pentoxifylline, or nafronyl: A meta-analysis. Arch Intern Med 159:337, 1999.
138. The European Study Group: Intravenous pentoxifylline for the treatment of chronic critical limb ischaemia. Eur J Vasc Endovasc Surg 9:426, 1995.
139. Norwegian Pentoxifylline Multicenter Trial Group: Efficacy and clinical tolerance of parenteral pentoxifylline in the treatment of critical lower limb ischemia: A placebo controlled multicenter study. Int Angiol 15:75, 1996.
140. Broderick TL, Quinney HA, Lopaschuk GD: Carnitine stimulation of glucose oxidation in the fatty acid perfused isolated working rat heart. J Biol Chem 267:3758, 1992.
141. Brevetti G, Perna S, Sabba C, et al: Propionyl-L-carnitine in intermittent claudication: Double-blind, placebo-controlled, dose titration, multicenter study. J Am Coll Cardiol 26:1411, 1995.
142. Brevetti G, Diehm C, Lambert D: European multicenter study on propionyl-L-carnitine in intermittent claudication. J Am Coll Cardiol 34:1618, 1999.
143. Hiatt WR, Regensteiner JG, Creager MA, et al: Propionyl-L-carnitine improves exercise performance and functional status in patients with claudication. Am J Med 110:616, 2001.
144. Brevetti G, Perna S, Sabba C, et al: Effect of propionyl-L-carnitine on quality of life in intermittent claudication. Am J Cardiol 79:777, 1997.
145. Stanley WC: Myocardial energy metabolism during ischemia and the mechanisms of metabolic therapies. J Cardiovasc Pharmacol Ther 9 Suppl 1:S31, 2004.
146. Chaitman BR, Pepine CJ, Parker JO, et al: Effects of ranolazine with atenolol, amlodipine, or diltiazem on exercise tolerance and angina frequency in patients with severe chronic angina: A randomized controlled trial. JAMA 291:309, 2004.
147. Chaitman BR, Skettino SL, Parker JO, et al: Anti-ischemic effects and long-term survival during ranolazine monotherapy in patients with chronic severe angina. J Am Coll Cardiol 43:1375, 2004.
148. Isner JM, Asahara T: Angiogenesis and vasculogenesis as therapeutic strategies for postnatal neovascularization. J Clin Invest 103:1231, 1999.
149. Tsurumi Y, Takeshita S, Chen D, et al: Direct intramuscular gene transfer of naked DNA encoding vascular endothelial growth factor augments collateral development and tissue perfusion. Circulation 94:3281, 1996.
150. Yang HT, Deschenes MR, Ogilvie RW, et al: Basic fibroblast growth factor increases collateral blood flow in rats with femoral arterial ligation. Circ Res 79:62, 1996.
151. Takeshita S, Zheng LP, Brogi E, et al: Therapeutic angiogenesis: A single intraarterial bolus of vascular endothelial growth factor augments revascularization in a rabbit ischemic hind limb model. J Clin Invest 93:662, 1994.
152. Vincent KA, Shyu KG, Luo Y, et al: Angiogenesis is induced in a rabbit model of hindlimb ischemia by naked DNA encoding an HIF-1alpha/VP16 hybrid transcription factor. Circulation 102:2255, 2000.

153. Baumgartner I, Pieczek A, Manor O, et al: Constitutive expression of phVEGF165 after intramuscular gene transfer promotes collateral vessel development in patients with critical limb ischemia. Circulation 97:1114, 1998.
154. Isner JM, Baumgartner I, Rauh G, et al: Treatment of thromboangiitis obliterans (Buerger's disease) by intramuscular gene transfer of vascular endothelial growth factor: Preliminary clinical results. J Vasc Surg 28:964, 1998.
155. Rajagopalan S, Mohler ER, III, Lederman RJ, et al: Regional angiogenesis with vascular endothelial growth factor in peripheral arterial disease: A phase II randomized, double-blind, controlled study of adenoviral delivery of vascular endothelial growth factor 121 in patients with disabling intermittent claudication. Circulation 108:1933, 2003.
156. Comerota AJ, Throm RC, Miller KA, et al: Naked plasmid DNA encoding fibroblast growth factor type 1 for the treatment of end-stage unreconstructible lower extremity ischemia: Preliminary results of a phase I trial. J Vasc Surg 35:930, 2002.
157. Lederman RJ, Mendelsohn FO, Anderson RD, et al: Therapeutic angiogenesis with recombinant fibroblast growth factor-2 for intermittent claudication (the TRAFFIC study): A randomised trial. Lancet 359:2053, 2002.
158. Ho HK, Jang JJ, Kaji S, et al: Developmental endothelial locus-1 (Del-1), a novel angiogenic protein: Its role in ischemia. Circulation 109:1314, 2004.
159. A phase II multicenter, randomized, double-blind, placebo-controlled trial of plasmid Del-1 (developmentally regulated endothelial locus 1) in subjects with intermittent claudication secondary to peripheral arterial disease: DELTA1-PAD. Circulation 110: III-521, 2004.
160. Wenger RH, Gassmann M: Oxygen(es) and the hypoxia-inducible factor-1. Biol Chem 378:609, 1997.
161. Guillemin K, Krasnow MA: The hypoxic response: Huffing and HIFing. Cell 89:9, 1997.
162. Wang GL, Jiang BH, Rue EA, et al: Hypoxia-inducible factor 1 is a basic-helix-loop-helix-PAS heterodimer regulated by cellular O_2 tension. Proc Natl Acad Sci U S A 92:5510, 1995.
163. Kalka C, Masuda H, Takahashi T, et al: Transplantation of ex vivo expanded endothelial progenitor cells for therapeutic neovascularization. Proc Natl Acad Sci U S A 97:3422, 2000.
164. Shintani S, Murohara T, Ikeda H, et al: Augmentation of postnatal neovascularization with autologous bone marrow transplantation. Circulation 103:897, 2001.
165. Kamihata H, Matsubara H, Nishiue T, et al: Implantation of bone marrow mononuclear cells into ischemic myocardium enhances collateral perfusion and regional function via side supply of angioblasts, angiogenic ligands, and cytokines. Circulation 104:1046, 2001.
166. Tateishi-Yuyama E, Matsubara H, Murohara T, et al: Therapeutic angiogenesis for patients with limb ischaemia by autologous transplantation of bone-marrow cells: A pilot study and a randomised controlled trial. Lancet 360:427, 2002.
167. Mondillo S, Ballo P, Barbati R, et al: Effects of simvastatin on walking performance and symptoms of intermittent claudication in hypercholesterolemic patients with peripheral vascular disease. Am J Med 114:359, 2003.
168. Brown BG, Zhao XQ, Sacco DE, et al: Lipid lowering and plaque regression: New insights into prevention of plaque disruption and clinical events in coronary disease. Circulation 87:1781, 1993.
169. Liao JK, Bettman MA, Sandor T, et al: Differential impairment of vasodilator responiveness of peripheral resistance and conduit vessels in humans with atherosclerosis. Circ Res 68:1027, 1991.
170. Treasure CB, Klein JL, Weintraub WS, et al: Beneficial effects of cholesterol-lowering therapy on the coronary endothelium in patients with coronary artery disease. N Engl J Med 332:481, 1995.
171. Anderson TJ, Meredith IT, Yeung AC, et al: The effect of cholesterol-lowering and antioxidant therapy on endothelium-dependent coronary vasomotion. N Engl J Med 332:488, 1995.
172. Van Belle E, Rivard A, Chen D, et al: Hypercholesterolemia attenuates angiogenesis but does not preclude augmentation by angiogenic cytokines. Circulation 96:2667, 1997.
173. Vasa M, Fichtlscherer S, Adler K, et al: Increase in circulating endothelial progenitor cells by statin therapy in patients with stable coronary artery disease. Circulation 103:2885, 2001.
174. Gordon MB, Jain R, Beckman JA, et al: The contribution of nitric oxide to exercise hyperemia in the human forearm. Vasc Med 7:163, 2002.
175. Duffy SJ, New G, Tran BT, et al: Relative contribution of vasodilator prostanoids and NO to metabolic vasodilation in the human forearm. Am J Physiol 276:H663, 1999.
176. Maxwell AJ, Schauble E, Bernstein D, et al: Limb blood flow during exercise is dependent on nitric oxide. Circulation 98:369, 1998.
177. Maxwell AJ, Anderson BE, Cooke JP: Nutritional therapy for peripheral arterial disease: A double-blind, placebo-controlled, randomized trial of HeartBar. Vasc Med 5:11, 2000.
178. Kleijnen J, Mackerras D: Vitamin E for intermittent claudication. Cochrane Database Syst Rev:CD000987, 2000.
179. Ernst E: The risk-benefit profile of commonly used herbal therapies: Ginkgo, St. John's Wort, Ginseng, Echinacea, Saw Palmetto, and Kava. Ann Intern Med 136:42, 2002.
180. Pittler MH, Ernst E: Ginkgo biloba extract for the treatment of intermittent claudication: A meta-analysis of randomized trials. Am J Med 108:276, 2000.
181. Peters H, Kieser M, Holscher U: Demonstration of the efficacy of ginkgo biloba special extract EGb 761 on intermittent claudication: A placebo-controlled, double-blind multicenter trial. Vasa 27:106, 1998.
182. De Smet PA: Herbal remedies. N Engl J Med 347:2046, 2002.
183. Lamas GA, Ackermann A: Clinical evaluation of chelation therapy: Is there any wheat amidst the chaff? Am Heart J 140:4, 2000.
184. Evans DA, Tariq M, Sujata B, et al: The effects of magnesium sulphate and EDTA in the hypercholesterolaemic rabbit. Diabetes Obes Metab 3:417, 2001.
185. Anderson TJ, Hubacek J, Wyse DG, et al: Effect of chelation therapy on endothelial function in patients with coronary artery disease: PATCH substudy. J Am Coll Cardiol 41:420, 2003.
186. Sloth-Nielsen J, Guldager B, Mouritzen C, et al: Arteriographic findings in EDTA chelation therapy on peripheral arteriosclerosis. Am J Surg 162:122, 1991.
187. Ernst E: Chelation therapy for peripheral arterial occlusive disease: A systematic review. Circulation 96:1031, 1997.
188. Villarruz MV, Dans A, Tan F: Chelation therapy for atherosclerotic cardiovascular disease. Cochrane Database Syst Rev:CD002785, 2002.

chapter 19

Catheter-Based Intervention

Christopher J. White

The concept of nonsurgical revascularization of the lower extremities was initiated by Charles Dotter[1] and further advanced by Andreas Gruntzig with the development of balloon catheters that could safely dilate vascular stenoses.[2] Peripheral vascular intervention is a safe and effective means of restoring blood flow in select patients with lower extremity ischemia.[3]

Multiple specialties have contributed to the advancement of the field of peripheral vascular intervention over the past several decades. Experienced interventional cardiologists have successfully brought coronary skills and techniques to the peripheral vasculature.[4] No specialty program (cardiology, radiology, or surgery) offered training that satisfied the entire skill set needed to perform peripheral vascular intervention (Table 19-1). The recognition of this unmet need for a trained cadre of clinicians to care for patients with peripheral arterial disease prompted the development of a cardiology fellowship training program core curriculum document (COCATS-11) by the American College of Cardiology.[5]

PATIENT AND LESION SELECTION CRITERIA

Indications

Anatomic and Functional Criteria

Patient selection for nonsurgical revascularization depends on both anatomical and functional criteria. Anatomic criteria include the ability to gain vascular access, a reasonable likelihood of crossing the lesion with a guidewire, and the expectation that a catheter can be advanced to the lesion. A favorable procedural result is more likely for a stenosis than for a total occlusion, for aortoiliac than for femoral-popliteal disease, and in patients with claudication rather than limb salvage situations.[6,7]

The availability of endovascular stents (balloon expandable and self-expanding) has significantly extended the anatomical subset of patients that may be considered candidates for percutaneous revascularization, particularly for long lesions and occlusions. The rate-limiting step for nonsurgical revascularization of the aortoiliac vessels is the ability to pass a guidewire across the lesion. Regardless of the balloon dilation result, the option of stent placement offers a reliable and reproducible method to recanalize these vessels.

Patients with access site complications following invasive vascular or coronary procedures are often candidates for percutaneous intervention.[8] In patients with hypotension and a high suspicion of bleeding after femoral artery access, diagnostic angiography from the contralateral femoral artery will often confirm the bleeding site and provide an opportunity to obtain hemostasis with balloon tamponade.

Asymptomatic patients with anatomically suitable lesions may be considered candidates for intervention to facilitate vascular access, such as for intra-aortic counterpulsation balloon placement or for coronary intervention. Symptomatic patients with suitable anatomic lesions should have failed medical therapy for life-style limiting claudication or demonstrate critical limb ischemia to be considered candidates for revascularization therapy. When considering a patient with limb-threatening ischemia (gangrene, nonhealing ulcer, or rest pain) for percutaneous intervention, it is likely that multilevel disease will be manifest and that simply improving "inflow" without addressing the more distal flow-limiting lesions may fail to solve the problem.

TABLE 19-1 REQUIRED SKILL ELEMENTS FOR OPTIMAL PERIPHERAL VASCULAR INTERVENTION

Skill Element	
Cognitive	The fund of knowledge for vascular disease, including the natural history, pathophysiology, diagnostic methods, and treatment alternatives
Technical	Includes competence in both diagnostic angiography and interventional techniques, such as the use and selection of balloons, guidewires, stents, and emboli protection devices
Clinical	The ability to manage inpatients, interpret laboratory tests, admitting privileges, obtain informed consent, and assessment of risk-to-benefit ratio

Contraindications

Anatomic relative contraindications to intervention include lesions likely to generate atheroemboli and lesions that are undilatable due to calcification. Clinical relative contraindications would include instances in which the risks of the procedure would outweigh the potential benefits.

TECHNICAL AND PROCEDURAL CONSIDERATIONS

Preprocedure

General Measures

Prior to performing peripheral vascular intervention, the patient should have a general medical evaluation with specific attention directed to the status of the cardiovascular system. Atherosclerosis is a systemic disease and appropriate risk factor modification, screening tests for cardiovascular diseases, and optimization of medical therapy should be performed.

Prior to performing lower extremity intervention, it is necessary to objectively determine the functional status of the patient. This can be done with a complete history, physical examination, and noninvasive testing. If the patient is ambulatory, a rest and exercise assessment of the ankle-brachial index (ABI) with pulse volume recordings should be performed to assess the baseline functional status. The use of other noninvasive assessments such as vascular ultrasound, or alternative imaging modalities—such as MRA or CTA—may be used at the discretion of the physician.

When planning a lower extremity intervention, it is necessary that the anatomy and status of the inflow and outflow vessels be determined. This is usually done with invasive diagnostic angiography, but in select patients, ultrasound imaging, MRA, or CTA may be adequate.

Premedication

The only premedication requirement for peripheral vascular intervention is aspirin therapy (81 mg to 325 mg daily). The use of other antiplatelet agents, (clopidogrel or ticlopidine) is optional because there is no evidence that their use improves procedural success or decreases complications, as has been shown for coronary artery intervention.

Procedure

Anticoagulation

There is no standard for anticoagulation therapy, except to state that intravenous heparin, in a dose range of 2500 to 5000 IU, is commonly used. In general, the activated clotting time (ACT) is kept between 250 and 300 seconds during the procedure. At the end of the case, anticoagulation may be reversed with protamine sulfate. At the present time, there is no evidence that the use of glycoprotein IIb/IIIa platelet-receptor antagonists, low-molecular-weight heparins, or antithrombins improve procedural efficacy or safety for peripheral vascular intervention.

Vascular Access

The first step to ensure a successful procedure is to plan the appropriate vascular access. The majority of peripheral vascular interventions can be performed from several access sites (i.e., brachial, common femoral, or popliteal artery). However, some cases require a specific access to achieve a successful result. Consequently, familiarity with a variety of vascular access sites and techniques is one of the most important components of the basic skill set for peripheral vascular intervention. The ability to gain both retrograde and antegrade common femoral access is a required skill for the interventionalist. An infrapopliteal target lesion may be best approached with antegrade femoral access, whereas a proximal superficial femoral artery lesion may require a retrograde femoral access and a contralateral approach. Occasionally, bilateral retrograde femoral artery access is desirable, for example, when treating common iliac bifurcation lesions. Specific guidelines and techniques for obtaining vascular access are addressed in Chapter 13.

Equipment Choices

Guidewire

A major technical decision point for the operator is to decide whether to use an 0.014-inch, 0.018-inch, or 0.035-inch guidewire-based system for intervention. Trade-offs include lower profiles, smaller sheath sizes, and increased flexibility for the smallest coronary systems, balanced against increased support and pushability for the larger profile 0.035-inch systems. It is recommended that the interventional laboratory be stocked with at least two of the three lines of equipment to allow for flexibility in the approach to patients with different requirements. In general, the lowest profile system with the smallest vascular access sheath possible that will accommodate the necessary angioplasty equipment should be used.

The use of "glidewires" should be carefully restricted to instances when their unique properties are necessary because these wires are more difficult to control than conventional guidewires and are prone to vascular perforation. Their lack of a "transition point" makes them ideal for negotiating abrupt angles—such as gaining contralateral femoral access. Their lubricated coating makes them attractive tools for crossing occlusions. Ideally, once they have achieved the desired result, it is wise to exchange for a safer and more controllable wire.

Balloon Catheters

A wide variety of monorail and over-the-wire balloon catheters are available that are suitable for dilating lower extremity lesions. They come in a variety of diameters with balloon lengths up to 10 cm. Both semi-compliant and non-compliant materials are available for use. A pressure manometer is recommended to monitor balloon inflation pressure. Although no optimal inflation pressure or duration has been determined, it is generally recommended that the balloon be inflated with adequate pressure to ensure full expansion of the lesion. Neither the rate of balloon inflation nor the duration of balloon inflation have been shown to impact either safety or efficacy of the procedure.

Stents

Stents are either balloon expandable or self-expanding. Balloon expandable stents are intended for use within the axial skeleton to protect them from external compression. This generally limits their use to the iliac arteries; however coronary balloon expandable stents are occasionally used to salvage failed angioplasty in below-knee vessels. Balloon expandable stents may be deployed with more precision than self-expanding stents, although there is some shortening associated with their expansion. Self-expanding stents resist compression and are elastic. Their flexible nature allows them to be delivered in longer lengths and they will fit themselves to a tapering artery. Self-expanding stents may be made of nitinol or a stainless steel alloy. At this time, there is no evidence that either material is associated with any safety or efficacy advantage.[9] Recently, experimental studies with drug-eluting stents have been reported, and it is hoped that further development of these "antiproliferative" stents will have a favorable impact on restenosis in difficult-to-treat arteries.[10]

Adjunctive Devices

Other adjunctive devices, such as laser catheters, atherectomy catheters (rotational and directional), brachytherapy catheters, cryotherapy balloons, and cutting balloons have been developed, tested, and aggressively marketed. At this time, with the possible exception of the brachytherapy catheters, there is no evidence that these devices bring any added value, efficacy, or safety to percutaneous lower extremity revascularization.

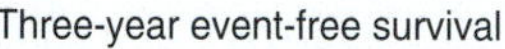

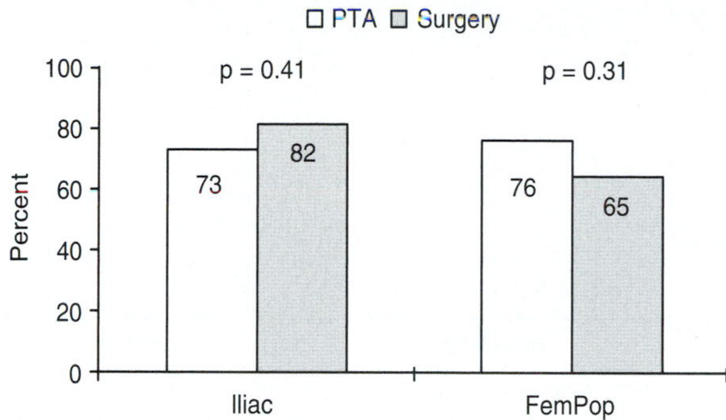

FIGURE 19-1. Randomized trial of percutaneous transluminal angioplasty (PTA) versus surgery. (From Wilson SE, Wolf GL, Cross AP: Percutaneous transluminal angioplasty versus operation for peripheral arteriosclerosis: Report of a prospective randomized trial in a selected group of patients. J Vasc Surg 9:1, 1989.)

CLINICAL OUTCOMES

Aortoiliac Vessels

Balloon Angioplasty

Ideal patient and lesion subsets for balloon angioplasty have been proposed (Table 19-2).[11] The procedural success rate for balloon angioplasty of these "optimal" lesions is expected to be greater than 90% with a 5-year patency rate of successfully dilated lesions of between 54% to 78%.[12-14] The procedural success rate and long-term patency rates are lower for occlusions, which have a 78% to 98% procedural success and 48% to 85% patency at 3 years.[15,16]

These results compare favorably with surgical results in patients following aortoiliac and aortofemoral bypass revascularizations which have a 74% to 95% 5-year patency.[6] In one reported surgical series of 105 consecutive patients undergoing aortofemoral bypass (58% for symptomatic claudication), the operative mortality rate was 5.7%; the early graft failure rate was 5.7%; and the 2-year patency was 92.8%.[17] A randomized comparison of PTA with surgery for 157 iliac lesions, reported no difference in the 3-year cumulative event-free rate for study-related deaths, amputations, and revascularization failure between surgery (81.8%) and PTA (73.1%) (Fig. 19-1).[18] In a second randomized controlled trial of surgery versus angioplasty in 102 patients with severe claudication and limb-threatening ischemia, there was no difference at 1 year for the hemodynamic effect of revascularization by either angioplasty or surgery (Fig. 19-2).[19] Therefore, the current recommendations, based on these clinical trials, is to prefer percutaneous therapy before surgical therapy if a patient is a candidate for either procedure.

Stent Placement

The use of endovascular stents has improved the results of balloon angioplasty of these vessels (Figs. 19-3 and 19-4).[20-22] There has been debate about whether stent architecture or composition (i.e., nitinol versus stainless steel) has any effect on restenosis rates. The recently completed CRISP trial failed to show any difference in outcomes between nitinol (Smart, Cordis, Miami Lakes, FL) and stainless steel (Wallstent, Boston Scientific Corp., Watertown, MA) iliac artery stents at 1 year (Fig. 19-5).[9]

TABLE 19-2 ILIAC BALLOON ANGIOPLASTY ANATOMIC LESION CRITERIA*

Type A	Type B	Type C	Type D
Single < 3 cm stenosis	Single stenosis 3-10 cm in length, not involving CFA	Bilateral 5-10 cm stenosis not involving CFA	Diffuse, multiple unilateral stenoses
CIA or EIA	Two stenoses <5 cm in length not involving the CFA	Unilateral EIA occlusion, without CFA involvement	Unilateral occlusions of both CIA and EIA
Unilateral or bilateral	Unilateral CIA occlusion	Unilateral EIA stenosis involving CFA	Bilateral EIA occlusion
		Bilateral CIA occlusion	Diffuse disease involving the aorta and both iliac arteries
			Iliac stenoses in patients with an abdominal aortic aneurysm

*Lesions are stratified from those most commonly treated with balloons (type A) to those more commonly treated with surgery (type D). CIA, common iliac artery; EIA, external iliac artery. From Dormandy JA, Rutherford RB: Management of peripheral arterial disease (PAD). TASC Working Group. TransAtlantic Inter-Society Consensus (TASC). J Vasc Surg 31:S1, 2000.

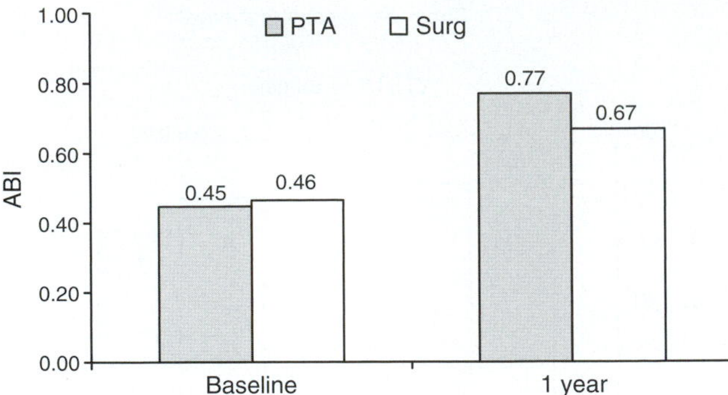

FIGURE 19-2. Comparison of percutaneous transluminal angioplasty (PTA) versus surgery. ABI, ankle-brachial index. (From Holm J, Arfvidsson B, Jivegard L, et al: Chronic lower limb ischaemia. A prospective randomised controlled study comparing the 1-year results of vascular surgery and percutaneous transluminal angioplasty (PTA). Eur J Vasc Surg 5:517, 1991.)

The result of primary iliac stent placement (without regard to the predilation balloon result) of balloon expandable stents has been reported in a multicenter trial in 486 patients followed for up to 4 years (mean 13.3 ± 11 months).[23] Using a life-table analysis, clinical benefit was present in 91% of the patients at 1 year, 84% at 2 years, and 69% at 43 months of follow-up. The angiographic patency rate of the iliac stents was 92%. Complications occurred in 10% and were predominantly related to the arterial access site.

Stent placement following a suboptimal angioplasty result (provisional stent placement) has been reported in 184 iliac lesions after failed or suboptimal balloon angioplasty outcomes.[24] A 91% procedural success rate and a 6-month patency rate of 99% was achieved for iliac lesions. Long-term follow-up demonstrated a 4-year primary patency rate of 86% and a secondary patency rate of 95% for iliac arteries. Excellent results for provisional stent placement with self-expanding stents have been reported in patients following failed or suboptimal angioplasty in iliac lesions.[25] Vorwerk and colleagues demonstrated excellent outcomes for provisional iliac stent placement in aortoiliac lesions. They reported primary patency at 1 year of 95%, 2 years of 88%, and 4 years of 82% in 118 treated lesions.[26]

A Dutch trial compared the use of primary with provisional iliac stent placement in a randomized trial. Pressure gradients across the lesions after primary stent placement (5.8 ± 4.7 mm Hg) were significantly lower than after balloon angioplasty alone (8.9 ± 6.8 mm Hg), but not after provisional stenting (5.9 ± 3.6 mm Hg) in the PTA group.[27] The procedural success rate, defined as a postprocedural gradient of less than 10 mm Hg, revealed no difference between the two treatment strategies, (primary stenting = 81% versus PTA plus provisional stenting = 89%). By employing a provisional stenting strategy, stent placement was avoided in 63% of the lesions, and still achieved an equivalent hemodynamic result compared with primary stenting. Long-term follow-up will be necessary to evaluate and confirm the efficacy of this approach.

A recent observational study compared the nonrandomized results of iliac stenting with surgery in patients with TASC types B and C lesions.[28] The authors found no difference for limb salvage and patient survival at 5 years, but vessel patency was reduced in limbs with poor runoff with stents compared with surgery.

Current clinical practice is primary stent placement and this is supported by a meta-analysis that involved more than 2000 patients.[29] Procedural success was higher in the primary stent group and there was a 43% reduction in long-term (4-year) failures for aortoiliac stent placement compared with balloon angioplasty alone. A European randomized trial of primary iliac (Palmaz) stent placement versus balloon angioplasty also favored primary stent placement by demonstrating a 4-year patency of

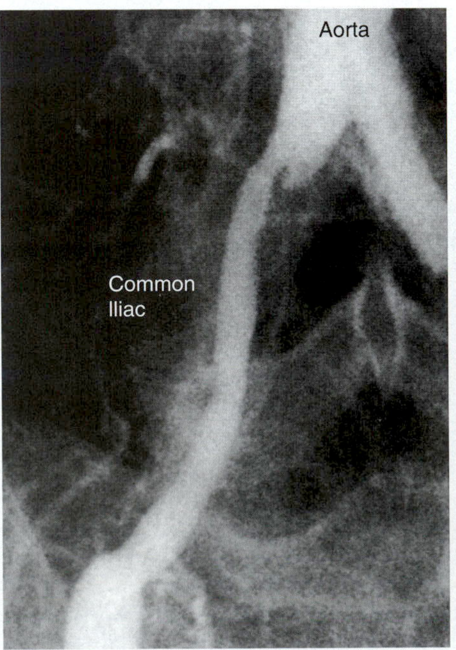

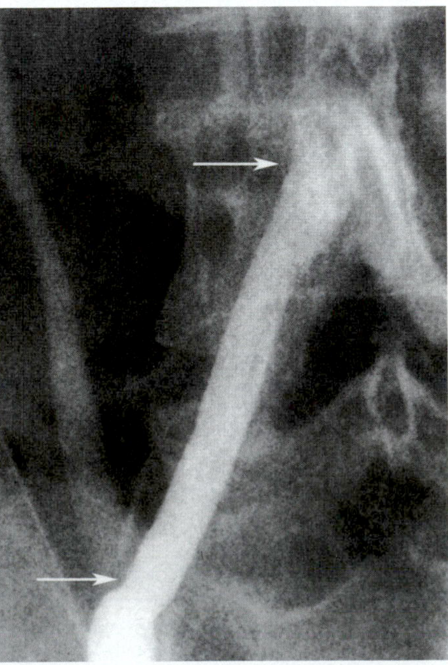

FIGURE 19-3. *Left*: Baseline image of a right common iliac lesion after balloon angioplasty. *Right*: Angiogram following stent placement.

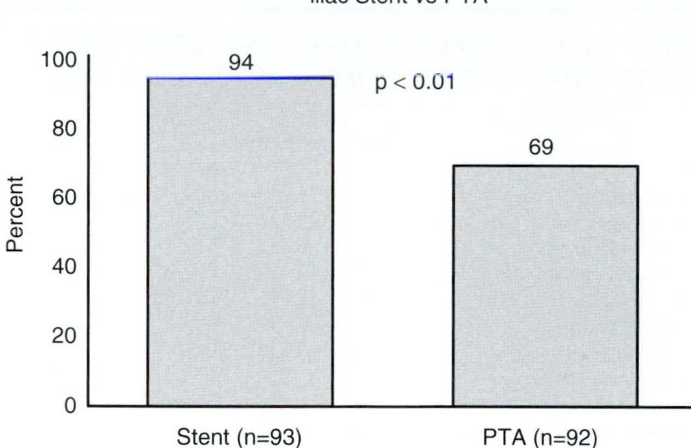

FIGURE 19-4. Randomized trial of iliac stents versus angioplasty. PTA, percutaneous transluminal angioplasty. (From Richter GM, Roeren T, Noeldge G, et al: [Initial long-term results of a randomized 5-year study: Iliac stent implantation versus PTA]. Vasa Suppl 35:192, 1992.)

94% for the stent group versus a 69% patency for the balloon angioplasty group (see Fig. 19-4).[30]

Iliac stent placement may also be used as an adjunctive procedure to lower extremity surgical bypass operations. In select patients, a combined approach using angioplasty and surgery can be a safe and effective method of revascularization. Peterkin and coworkers reported the results of combined iliac intervention and infrainguinal bypass in 46 patients with a 93% 5-year limb salvage rate and a 72% 5-year angioplasty patency rate.[31] In another report, 70 consecutive patients with and without "in-flow" iliac artery lesions were treated with angioplasty or stenting before femoral-femoral bypass. After a 7-year follow-up, those with iliac angioplasty or stent placement did as well as those without iliac artery disease.[32]

These results suggest that percutaneous intervention can provide adequate long-term in-flow and allow femoral-femoral bypass as an alternative to aortobifemoral bypass in patients at increased risk for a major operation. The approach for symptomatic patients with multilevel atherosclerosis of the lower extremity is to plan a strategy that will relieve the patient's symptoms with the lowest morbidity. This includes involvement by both the vascular surgeon and the interventional cardiologist, and a combined approach is used when indicated.

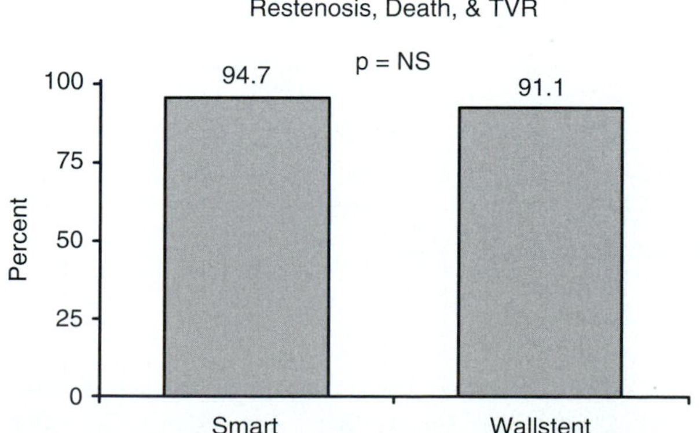

FIGURE 19-5. Bar graph showing the 1-year results of the CRISP trial. TVR, target vessel revascularization. (From Ponec D: Cordis Randomized Iliac Stent Project (CRISP). Presented at the Annual Society of Interventional Radiology, 2003. (Accessed at http://www.jnj.com/news/jnj_news/20030331_124524.htm).

Femoral-Popliteal Vessels

Balloon Angioplasty

Percutaneous angioplasty has a primary success rate between 70% and 97% for femoropopliteal atherosclerotic lesions, with the success rate being higher for stenoses than for total occlusions.[33,34] Reported patency rates for successfully dilated femoral-popliteal lesions range between 50% and 70% at 3 to 5 years.[35]

A European study reported the results of a randomized trial comparing femoral balloon angioplasty with medical therapy for patients with single-leg claudication.[36] At the 6-month follow-up assessment the balloon angioplasty group could walk further before the onset of symptoms, and had a significantly higher ABI. The most important benefit for the PTA group, however, was improved vessel patency. Only 3.6% of patients in the PTA group had developed an occlusion compared with 41.2% in the medically treated group ($P < .001$) (Table 19-3). At the 2-year follow-up, the walking and ABI benefit for PTA were no longer apparent; however the PTA group had fewer occluded arteries and a lesser degree of stenosis in the patent arteries.[37]

Two additional trials comparing PTA with medical therapy for patients with claudication and lower extremity peripheral arterial disease have been reported. Perkins and colleagues reported late follow-up in 37 patients randomized to PTA or medical therapy for unilateral, stable claudication.[38] They found that the PTA group had statistically better ABI, but those patients in the exercise program had greater improvements in walking distance and symptom improvement. Another prospective matched cohort study of 526 patients with intermittent claudication undergoing surgery, intervention, or medical therapy reported significant advantages for the revascularization groups compared with conservative medical therapy.[39] Patients with surgery and angioplasty had significantly better functional improvement than medical management patients, that included physical functioning, bodily pain, and walking distance. Importantly, patients with the highest ABI had the most improvement suggesting that the degree of revascularization correlated with a successful outcome.

TABLE 19-3 MEDICAL THERAPY VERSUS PTA FOR FEMORAL LESIONS AT 6 MONTHS' FOLLOW-UP

6-Month Follow-Up Result	PTA	MED	*P* Value
Walk ≥ 1 km	68%	39%	<.05
Onset of symptoms on treadmill	667	172	<.05
Ankle-brachial index	0.88	0.74	<.01
Occluded artery	3.6%	41.2%	<.001

MED, medical therapy; PTA, percutaneous transluminal angioplasty. From Whyman MR, Fowkes FG, Kerracher EM, et al: Randomised controlled trial of percutaneous transluminal angioplasty for intermittent claudication. Eur J Vasc Endovasc Surg 12:167, 1996.

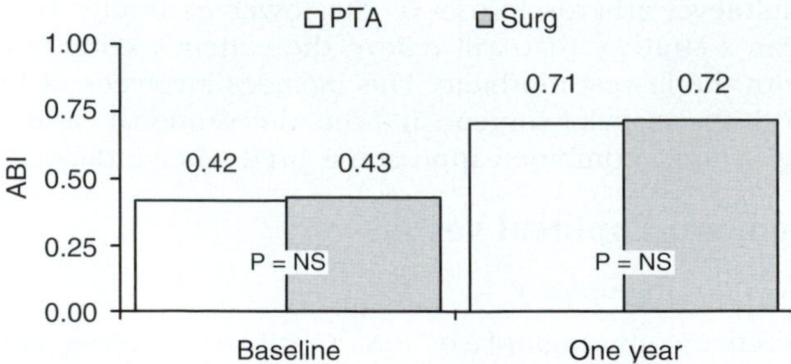

FIGURE 19-6. Randomized trial of percutaneous transluminal angioplasty (PTA) versus surgery. ABI, ankle-brachial index. (From Holm J, Arfvidsson B, Jivegard L, et al: Chronic lower limb ischaemia. A prospective randomised controlled study comparing the 1-year results of vascular surgery and percutaneous transluminal angioplasty [PTA]. Eur J Vasc Surg 5:517, 1991).

Two randomized trials of patients with femoral-popliteal lesions showed equivalent hemodynamic improvement and patency for PTA compared with surgical bypass.[18,19] There were no significant differences between the two groups at late follow-up for study related deaths, amputations, and late interventions (see Fig. 19-1; Fig. 19-6). The authors concluded that in lesions that are amenable to either angioplasty or surgery, PTA should be chosen first for its lower morbidity and cost and equivalent long-term results.

The long-term patency of femoral-popliteal angioplasty depends on clinical as well as anatomic variables.[13,40,41] Clinical factors that negatively affect the long-term patency of PTA include female sex, diabetes, and the presence of rest pain or threatened limb loss. Technical factors that correlate with long-term failure of angioplasty include longer lesion length, multiple versus single lesions, lesion eccentricity, and a poor angiographic appearance post-angioplasty.

The status of the distal runoff bed impacts the long-term success of PTA in the femoral-popliteal vessels. In one study of 370 patients undergoing angioplasty for lower limb ischemia, patients with less than one vessel runoff had a 3-year patency of only 25%, compared with 78% in patients with a two- or three-vessel runoff.[13] Minar and colleagues analyzed restenosis at 2 years in 207 patients following successful femoropopliteal angioplasty and used a multivariate analysis to assess variables affecting restenosis (Table 19-4).[42]

Stent Placement

Self-expanding stents are preferred in this location because of the risk of stent compression from external trauma. Early nonrandomized clinical series suggested that superficial femoral artery (SFA) stent placement could be accomplished with a very high primary success rate, and that the restenosis rates were the lowest in the larger diameter arteries, shorter lesions, and with fewer stents placed.[24,25]

A meta-analysis compared SFA stent placement with balloon angioplasty over the period between 1993 to 2000.[43] A total of 923 balloon dilations and 473 stent placements were compared. In contrast to results of SFA

TABLE 19-4 VARIABLES AFFECTING RESTENOSIS FOLLOWING FEMOROPOPLITEAL ANGIOPLASTY

	Two-Year Patency (%)	*P* Value
Claudication	64	.06
Limb threat	50	
2-3 vessel runoff	68	.02
0-1 vessel runoff	49	
Stenosis (single)	74	.06
Stenosis (multiple)	63	
Occlusion (<10 cm)	59	.06
Occlusion (10 cm)	47	
Diabetes (+)	68	.05
Diabetes (−)	54	
Male	68	.06
Female	56	

From Minar E, Ahmadi A, Koppensteiner R, et al: Comparison of effects of high-dose and low-dose aspirin on restenosis after femoropopliteal percutaneous transluminal angioplasty. Circulation 91:2167, 1995.

balloon angioplasty, long-term vessel patency after stent placement was minimally affected by the clinical indication or the lesion morphology (Fig. 19-7). However, compared with SFA balloon angioplasty, stent placement did yield better results in patients with occlusions and critical limb ischemia.

The U.S. Food and Drug Administration approved the IntraCoil stent (Sulzer, Minneapolis, MN) in 2001 for the primary treatment of symptomatic atherosclerotic disease in the femoral-popliteal arteries (Fig. 19-8). This was based on data from 266 patients entered into a pivotal U.S. randomized trial. Patients were included in the trial if they had (1) symptomatic leg ischemia and they were candidates for balloon angioplasty; (2) stenoses 15-cm long or occlusions 12-cm long; and (3) target lesion proximal to the tibial artery bifurcation. At 9 months there was no difference in target lesion revascularization (TLR) between the stent group (14.3%) and the balloon group (16.1%, P = NS); however there was an advantage for the stent in the longer lesion lengths (Figs. 19-9 and 19-10).

The current evidence-based recommendation regarding femoral-popliteal artery stents is to use them in a

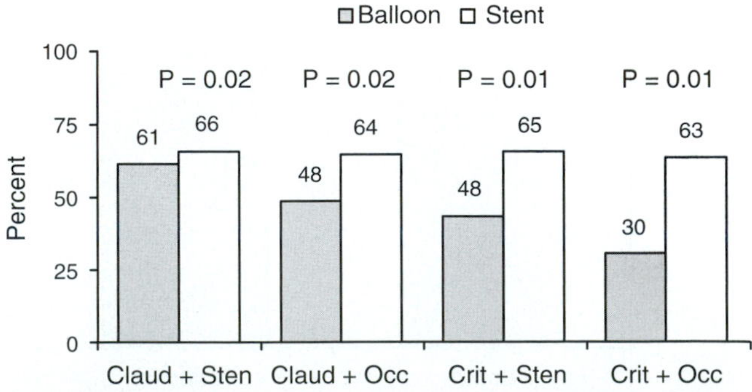

FIGURE 19-7. Meta-analysis of superficial femoral artery percutaneous transluminal angioplasty (PTA) versus stent. ABI, ankle-brachial index. (From Muradin GS, Bosch JL, Stijnen T, et al: Balloon dilation and stent implantation for treatment of femoropopliteal arterial disease: Meta-analysis. Radiology 221:137, 2001.)

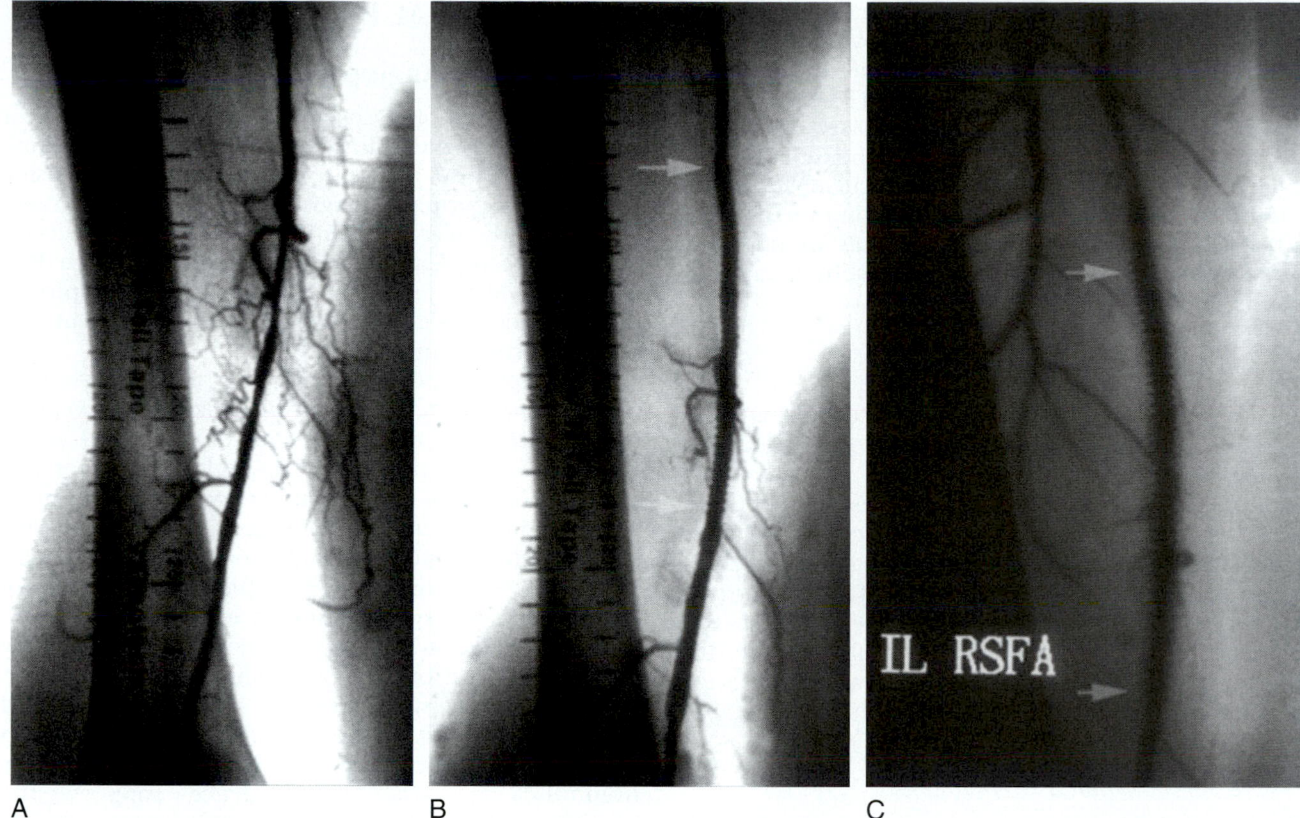

FIGURE 19-8. **A,** Baseline angiogram of distal superficial femoral artery (SFA) stenosis. **B,** Post-stent (VascuCoil) placement. Stent is at *arrow*. **C,** Six-month follow-up with patent SFA stent segment. IL RSFA, right superficial femoral artery.

"provisional" strategy. That is, stents should be reserved, in general, for salvage of a failed balloon angioplasty result in femoral-popliteal arteries. An exception to this may favor stent placement in patients with longer lesions, occlusions, and those with limb-threatening ischemia where there is evidence of superior stent performance compared with balloon angioplasty.[43]

Drug-Eluting Stents

Most recently, data on a small number ($n=36$) of patients randomized to either a bare metal self-expanding stent or a drug-eluting (sirolimus) self-expanding stent (Smart, Cordis, Miami Lakes, FL) have been reported.[10] At 6 months, the restenosis rate was 0% in the sirolimus group and 23.5% in the uncoated stent group ($P=.10$). There were no occlusions in the sirolimus group, whereas one patient in the uncoated stent group had an occlusion. These trials are currently being expanded and larger numbers of patients are being tested.

Brachytherapy Trials

Late patency is lower for angioplasty and stent placement for femoral popliteal lesions due to the proliferative intimal response after intervention. In an attempt to

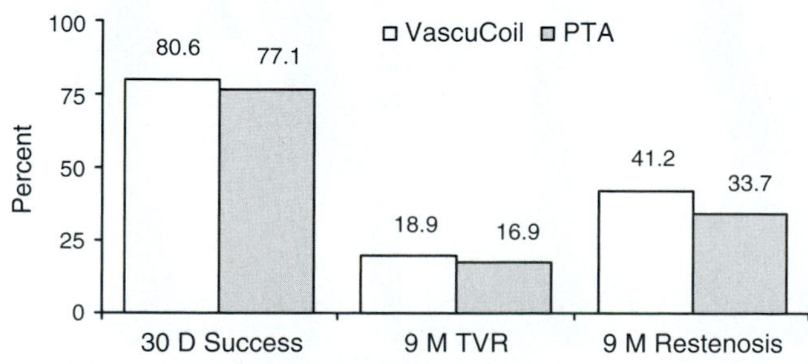

FIGURE 19-9. VascuCoil pivotal FDA approval data. (*P is* not significant for all.) 30 D success, 30-day success; 9 M TVR, 9-month target vessel revascularization; 9 M Restenosis, 9-month restenosis; PTA, percutaneous transluminal angioplasty.

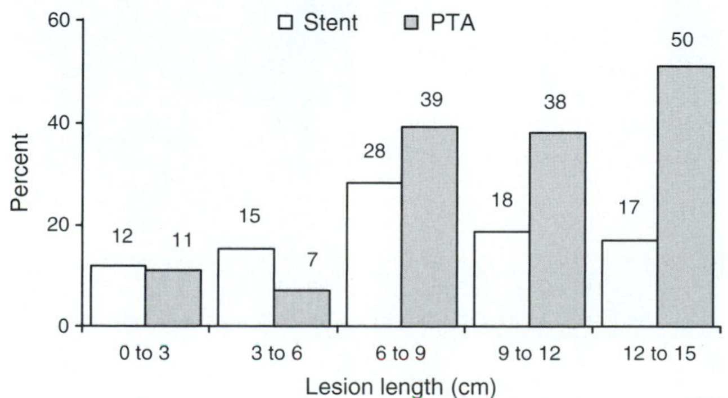

FIGURE 19-10. VascuCoil pivotal FDA approval data for restenosis stratified by lesion length. PTA, percutaneous transluminal angioplasty.

reduce the intimal hyperplasia after intervention, the use of radiation, in the form of brachytherapy, has been investigated. A randomized trial comparing brachytherapy (^{192}Ir, 12 Gy) and balloon angioplasty (PTA + BT) with percutaneous transluminal angioplasty (PTA) in 113 patients has demonstrated a benefit for the brachytherapy group. The overall recurrence rate at 6 months was 28.3% in the PTA + BT group versus 53.7% in the PTA group ($P < .05$). Current trials are underway to investigate the usefulness of brachytherapy for in-stent restenosis.[44,45]

Laser-Assisted Angioplasty

There has been the expectation that by "debulking" atherosclerotic plaque, the primary patency of the SFA could be improved. The PELA (Peripheral Excimer Laser Angioplasty) trial randomized 251 patients to either PTA or laser-assisted PTA in patients with claudication and a total SFA occlusion.[46] There was no difference in clinical events or patency rates at 1 year of follow-up. There is currently no convincing evidence that laser-assisted angioplasty adds any benefit to conventional therapy.[47,48] The one area that the laser may be of help is in crossing total occlusions that are not crossable with a guidewire (Fig. 19-11).

Cutting Balloon Angioplasty

The cutting balloon is approved in the coronary circulation for "undilatable" lesions.[49] There is no good evidence base to extend the indications for this device at this time. Certainly, there is no evidence to suggest benefit for placing undersized coronary cutting balloons in large peripheral arteries, or in large peripheral stents with in-stent restenosis.

INFRAPOPLITEAL INTERVENTION

Tibioperoneal Angioplasty

Below-knee angioplasty has been generally reserved for cases of threatened limb loss due to critical limb ischemia because of the technical difficulty in using conventional peripheral angioplasty equipment in these vessels and the fear of potential limb loss, should a complication occur. Early published experience with PTA demonstrated the feasibility of a percutaneous approach documenting procedural success rates greater than 80% for tibioperoneal angioplasty.[50]

The adoption and use of coronary angioplasty equipment improved the results of below-knee intervention (Fig. 19-12). In 111 patients with tibioperoneal angioplasty for claudication (47%), tissue loss (27%), or rest pain (26%), Dorros and coworkers reported a primary success rate of 90% for all lesions, including a 99% success rate for stenoses and a 65% success rate for occlusions.[51,52] At the time of hospital discharge 95% of the patients were symptomatically improved.

Two more recent trials have demonstrated the efficacy and attractiveness of an initial percutaneous approach to select patients with critical limb ischemia and infrapopliteal vascular disease.[52,53] The limb salvage rate in these patients treated with PTA after 2 to 5 years ranges from 85% to 91%. This evidence supports the contention that angioplasty of the tibioperoneal vessels should not necessarily be reserved for limb salvage situations; however, caution is still advised in patient selection because the surgical options are limited if angioplasty fails.

Optimal treatment of infrapopliteal disease requires appropriate patient and lesion selection for treatment. Focal stenoses have the best outcomes, with fewer than

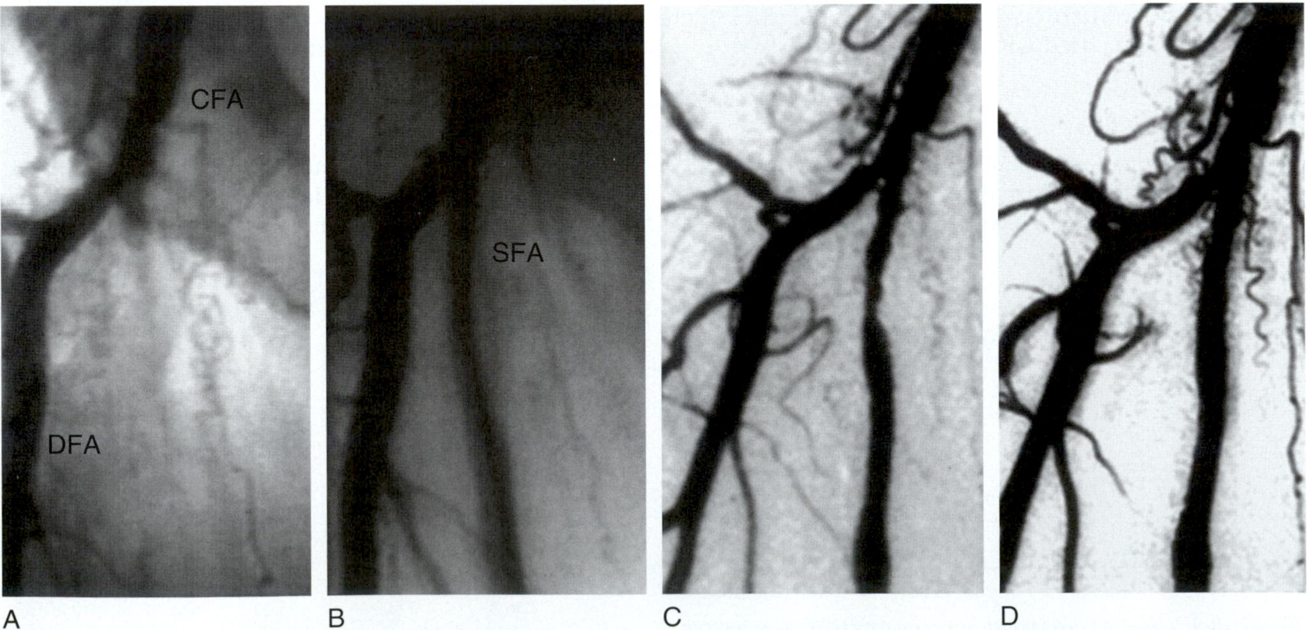

FIGURE 19-11. A, Baseline angiogram showing patent deep femoral artery (DFA) and occluded superficial femoral artery (SFA). **B,** Angiogram immediately following laser-assisted angioplasty (PELA). **C,** Angiogram at 6-month follow-up with restenosis of proximal SFA. **D,** Post-balloon result of restenosis at 6 months. CFA, common femoral artery.

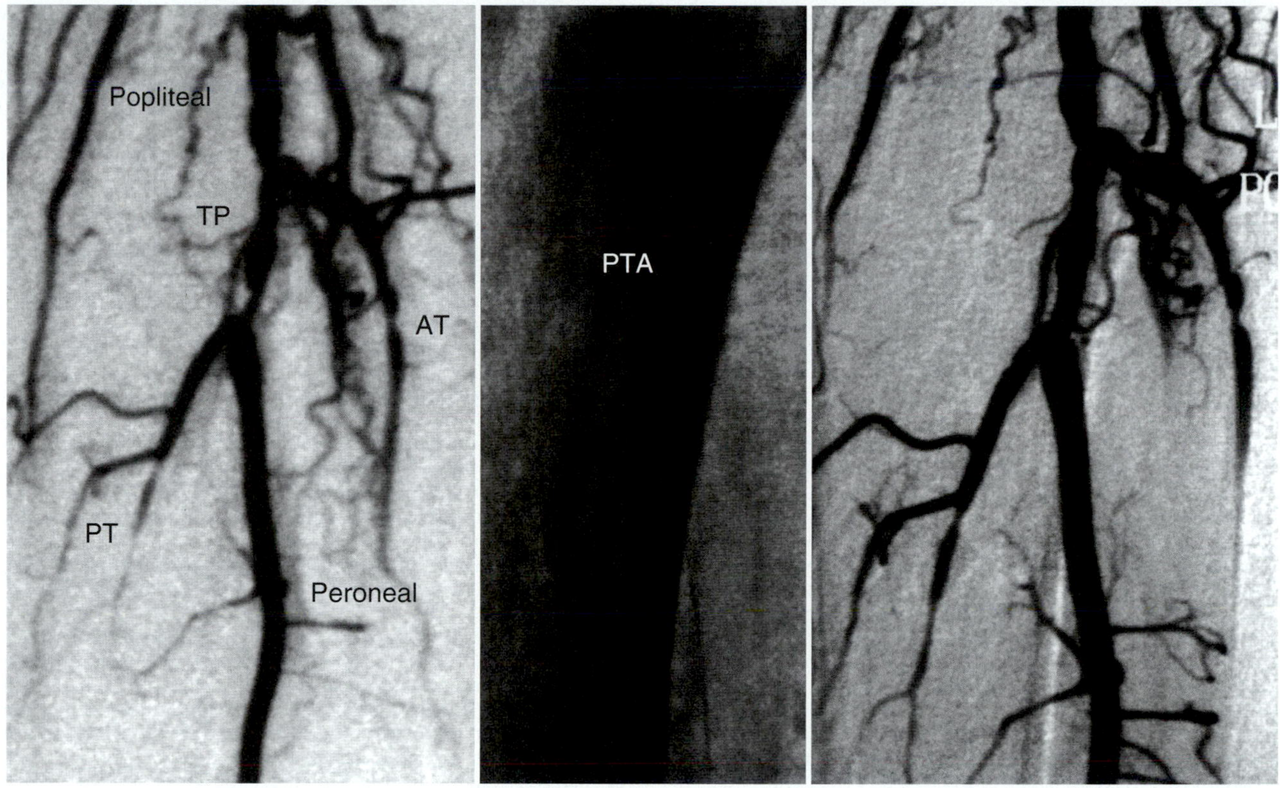

FIGURE 19-12. *Left*: Baseline angiogram of severe stenosis of tibioperoneal (TP) artery. *Middle*: Balloon angioplasty. *Right*: Final angiogram. AT, anterior tibial artery; PT, posterior tibial artery; PTA, percutaneous transluminal angioplasty.

five separate lesions associated with a higher success rate. The goal of therapy is measured by relief of rest pain, healing of ulcers, and avoiding amputation, not necessarily by long-term vessel patency. When trying to heal ischemic ulcers, the basic principle is that it takes more oxygenated blood flow to heal a wound than to maintain tissue integrity. Recent clinical trials suggest that percutaneous therapy can result in long-term limb salvage in more than 80% of patients and should be considered the current standard of treatment in patients with limb-threatening ischemia who are candidates for endovascular intervention.[53]

Conclusion

Percutaneous revascularization therapy is rapidly replacing surgical therapies as the initial treatment of choice for lower extremity vascular diseases. Of the new devices, stents appear to have improved the outcomes for iliac lesions, but their role in infrainguinal revascularization should be limited to bail-out use, after failed or failing angioplasty. Adjunctive devices such as atherectomy, laser, brachytherapy, and cutting balloons have a very limited role in the treatment of lower extremity ischemic lesions and should only be used after failure of balloon angioplasty. The emergence of drug-eluting stents, with their anti-restenotic properties, are eagerly awaited. If drug eluting stents prove to be as effective in preserving late-patency as they have in coronary arteries, this would establish the primacy of percutaneous therapy for lower extremity revascularization.

REFERENCES

1. Dotter CT, Judkins MP: Transluminal treatment of arteriosclerotic obstruction: Description of a new technic and a preliminary report of its application. Circulation 30:654, 1964.
2. Gruntzig A, Hopff H: [Percutaneous recanalization after chronic arterial occlusion with a new dilator-catheter (modification of the Dotter technique) (author's transl)]. Dtsch Med Wochenschr 99:2502, 1974.
3. Isner JM, Rosenfield K: Redefining the treatment of peripheral artery disease: Role of percutaneous revascularization. Circulation 88:1534, 1993.
4. White CJ, Ramee SR, Collins TJ, et al: Initial results of peripheral vascular angioplasty performed by experienced interventional cardiologists. Am J Cardiol 69:1249, 1992.
5. Beller GA, Bonow RO, Fuster V, et al: ACC Revised Recommendations for Training in Adult Cardiovascular Medicine Core Cardiology Training II (COCATS 2) (Revision of the 1995 COCATS Training Statement), 2002.
6. Johnston KW: Balloon angioplasty: Predictive factors for long-term success. Semin Vasc Surg 3:117, 1989.
7. Wilson SE, Sheppard B: Results of percutaneous transluminal angioplasty for peripheral vascular occlusive disease. Ann Vasc Surg 4:94, 1990.
8. Samal AK, White CJ: Percutaneous management of access site complications. Catheter Cardiovasc Interv 57:12, 2002.
9. Ponec D: Cordis Randomized Iliac Stent Project (CRISP). Presented at the Annual Society of Interventional Radiology, 2003. (Accessed at http://www.jnj.com/news/jnj_news/20030331_124524.htm).
10. Duda SH, Pusich B, Richter G, et al: Sirolimus-eluting stents for the treatment of obstructive superficial femoral artery disease: Six-month results. Circulation 106:1505, 2002.
11. Dormandy JA, Rutherford RB: Management of peripheral arterial disease (PAD). TASC Working Group. TransAtlantic Inter-Society Consensus (TASC). J Vasc Surg 31:S1, 2000.
12. Johnston KW: Iliac arteries: Reanalysis of results of balloon angioplasty. Radiology 186:207, 1993.

13. Jeans WD, Armstrong S, Cole SE, et al: Fate of patients undergoing transluminal angioplasty for lower-limb ischemia. Radiology 177:559, 1990.
14. Tegtmeyer CJ, Hartwell GD, Selby JB, et al: Results and complications of angioplasty in aortoiliac disease. Circulation 83:I53, 1991.
15. Casarella WJ: Noncoronary angioplasty. Curr Probl Cardiol 11:141, 1986.
16. Gallino A, Mahler F, Probst P, et al: Percutaneous transluminal angioplasty of the arteries of the lower limbs: A 5-year follow-up. Circulation 70:619, 1984.
17. Ameli FM, Stein M, Provan JL, et al: Predictors of surgical outcome in patients undergoing aortobifemoral bypass reconstruction. J Cardiovasc Surg (Torino) 31:333, 1990.
18. Wilson SE, Wolf GL, Cross AP: Percutaneous transluminal angioplasty versus operation for peripheral arteriosclerosis: Report of a prospective randomized trial in a selected group of patients. J Vasc Surg 9:1, 1989.
19. Holm J, Arfvidsson B, Jivegard L, et al: Chronic lower limb ischaemia: A prospective randomised controlled study comparing the 1-year results of vascular surgery and percutaneous transluminal angioplasty (PTA). Eur J Vasc Surg 5:517, 1991.
20. Sullivan TM, Childs MB, Bacharach JM, et al: Percutaneous transluminal angioplasty and primary stenting of the iliac arteries in 288 patients. J Vasc Surg 25:829, 1997.
21. Laborde JC, Palmaz JC, Rivera FJ, et al: Influence of anatomic distribution of atherosclerosis on the outcome of revascularization with iliac stent placement. J Vasc Interv Radiol 6:513, 1995.
22. Palmaz JC, Garcia OJ, Schatz RA, et al: Placement of balloon-expandable intraluminal stents in iliac arteries: First 171 procedures. Radiology 174:969, 1990.
23. Palmaz JC, Laborde JC, Rivera FJ, et al: Stenting of the iliac arteries with the Palmaz stent: Experience from a multicenter trial. Cardiovasc Intervent Radiol 15:291, 1992.
24. Henry M, Amor M, Ethevenot G, et al: Palmaz stent placement in iliac and femoropopliteal arteries: Primary and secondary patency in 310 patients with 2-4-year follow-up. Radiology 197:167, 1995.
25. Zollikofer CL, Antonucci F, Pfyffer M, et al: Arterial stent placement with use of the Wallstent: Midterm results of clinical experience. Radiology 179:449, 1991.
26. Vorwerk D, Gunther RW, Schurmann K, et al: Aortic and iliac stenoses: Follow-up results of stent placement after insufficient balloon angioplasty in 118 cases. Radiology 198:45, 1996.
27. Tetteroo E, Haaring C, van der Graaf Y, et al: Intraarterial pressure gradients after randomized angioplasty or stenting of iliac artery lesions. Dutch Iliac Stent Trial Study Group. Cardiovasc Intervent Radiol 19:411, 1996.
28. Timaran CH, Prault TL, Stevens SL, et al: Iliac artery stenting versus surgical reconstruction for TASC (TransAtlantic Inter-Society Consensus) type B and type C iliac lesions. J Vasc Surg 38:272, 2003.
29. Bosch JL, Hunink MG: Meta-analysis of the results of percutaneous transluminal angioplasty and stent placement for aortoiliac occlusive disease. Radiology 204:87, 1997.
30. Richter GM, Roeren T, Noeldge G, et al: [Initial long-term results of a randomized 5-year study: Iliac stent implantation versus PTA]. Vasa Suppl 35:192, 1992.
31. Peterkin GA, Belkin M, Cantelmo NL, et al: Combined transluminal angioplasty and infrainguinal reconstruction in multilevel atherosclerotic disease. Am J Surg 160:277, 1990.
32. Perler BA, Williams GM: Does donor iliac artery percutaneous transluminal angioplasty or stent placement influence the results of femorofemoral bypass? Analysis of 70 consecutive cases with long-term follow-up. J Vasc Surg 24:363, 1996.
33. Capek P, McLean GK, Berkowitz HD: Femoropopliteal angioplasty: Factors influencing long-term success. Circulation 83:I70, 1991.
34. Morgenstern BR, Getrajdman GI, Laffey KJ, et al: Total occlusions of the femoropopliteal artery: High technical success rate of conventional balloon angioplasty. Radiology 172:937, 1989.
35. Casarella WJ: Percutaneous transluminal angioplasty below the knee: New techniques, excellent results. Radiology 169:271, 1988.
36. Whyman MR, Fowkes FG, Kerracher EM, et al: Randomised controlled trial of percutaneous transluminal angioplasty for intermittent claudication. Eur J Vasc Endovasc Surg 12:167, 1996.
37. Whyman MR, Fowkes FG, Kerracher EM, et al: Is intermittent claudication improved by percutaneous transluminal angioplasty? A randomized controlled trial. J Vasc Surg 26:551, 1997.
38. Perkins JM, Collin J, Creasy TS, et al: Exercise training versus angioplasty for stable claudication: Long and medium term results of a prospective, randomised trial. Eur J Vasc Endovasc Surg 11:409, 1996.
39. Feinglass J, McCarthy WJ, Slavenksy R, et al: Functional status and walking ability after lower extremity bypass grafting or angioplasty for intermittent claudication: Results from a prospective outcomes study. J Vasc Surg 31:93, 2000.
40. Stokes KR, Strunk HM, Campbell DR, et al: Five-year results of iliac and femoropopliteal angioplasty in diabetic patients. Radiology 174:977, 1990.
41. Hewes RC, White RI Jr, Murray RR, et al: Long-term results of superficial femoral artery angioplasty. AJR Am J Roentgenol 146:1025, 1986.
42. Minar E, Ahmadi A, Koppensteiner R, et al: Comparison of effects of high-dose and low-dose aspirin on restenosis after femoropopliteal percutaneous transluminal angioplasty. Circulation 91:2167, 1995.
43. Muradin GS, Bosch JL, Stijnen T, et al: Balloon dilation and stent implantation for treatment of femoropopliteal arterial disease: Meta-analysis. Radiology 221:137, 2001.
44. Minar E, Pokrajac B, Maca T, et al: Endovascular brachytherapy for prophylaxis of restenosis after femoropopliteal angioplasty: Results of a prospective randomized study. Circulation 102:2694, 2000.
45. Waksman R, Laird JR, Jurkovitz CT, et al: Intravascular radiation therapy after balloon angioplasty of narrowed femoropopliteal arteries to prevent restenosis: Results of the PARIS feasibility clinical trial. J Vasc Interv Radiol 12:915, 2001.
46. Laird JR: Peripheral Excimer Laser Angioplasty (PELA) Trial Results: Presented at the late breaking clinical trials. TCT Annual Meeting, September 2002; www.tctmd.com.
47. Scheinert D, Laird JR Jr, Schroder M, et al: Excimer laser-assisted recanalization of long, chronic superficial femoral artery occlusions. J Endovasc Ther 8:156, 2001.
48. Steinkamp HJ, Rademaker J, Wissgott C, et al: Percutaneous transluminal laser angioplasty versus balloon dilation for treatment of popliteal artery occlusions. J Endovasc Ther 9:882, 2002.
49. Engelke C, Sandhu C, Morgan RA, et al: Using 6-mm cutting balloon angioplasty in patients with resistant peripheral artery stenosis: Preliminary results. AJR Am J Roentgenol 179:619, 2002.
50. Matsi PJ, Manninen HI, Suhonen MT, et al: Chronic critical lower-limb ischemia: Prospective trial of angioplasty with 1-36 months' follow-up. Radiology 188:381, 1993.
51. Dorros G, Lewin RF, Jamnadas P, et al: Below-the-knee angioplasty: Tibioperoneal vessels, the acute outcome. Cathet Cardiovasc Diagn 19:170, 1990.
52. Dorros G, Jaff MR, Dorros AM, et al: Tibioperoneal (outflow lesion) angioplasty can be used as primary treatment in 235 patients with critical limb ischemia: Five-year follow-up. Circulation 104:2057, 2001.
53. Soder HK, Manninen HI, Jaakkola P, et al: Prospective trial of infrapopliteal artery balloon angioplasty for critical limb ischemia: Angiographic and clinical results. J Vasc Interv Radiol 11:1021, 2000.

■ ■ ■ chapter 20

Reconstructive Surgery

Matthew T. Menard
Michael Belkin

The clinical manifestations and complications of atherosclerosis are the most common therapeutic challenge encountered by vascular surgeons. The tendency for lesions to develop at specific anatomic sites and follow recognizable patterns of progression was appreciated as long ago as the late 1700s by the extraordinary British anatomist and surgeon, John Hunter. Considered one of the forefathers of vascular surgery, his dissections of atherosclerotic aortic bifurcations remain on view at the Hunterian museum in London and presage the disease process that Leriche would give name to 150 years later.[1]

The modern era of surgical reconstruction for complex atherosclerotic occlusive disease began in earnest in 1947, when the Portuguese surgeon J. Cid dos Santos successfully endarterectomized a heavily diseased common femoral artery.[2] Four years later, Wylie and coworkers in San Francisco extended this new technique to the aortoiliac level.[3] At the same time, and building on the pioneering work of Alexis Carrel,[4] Kunlin[5] would report the first long segment vein bypass in the lower extremity. It would be another 10 years before synthetic grafts were being regularly used for aortic bypass grafting and the first efforts to extend vein grafting to the tibial level were described by McCaughan.[6] Tremendous advances in the understanding of atherosclerosis biology and the ability to treat arterial occlusive disease percutaneously have dramatically affected the treatment algorithms for arterial insufficiency in recent years. This chapter will review the current role for the surgical management of aortoiliac and infrainguinal arterial occlusive disease.

AORTOILIAC OCCLUSIVE DISEASE

Chronic obliterative atherosclerosis of the distal aorta and iliac arteries commonly manifests as symptomatic arterial insufficiency of the lower extremities. Disease in this location is seen often in combination with occlusive disease of the femoropopliteal arteries, producing a range of symptoms from mild claudication to more severe levels of tissue loss and critical ischemia. Patients with hemodynamic impairment limited to the aortoiliac system may have intermittent claudication of the calf muscles alone or involvement of the thigh, hip, and/or buttocks. If the disease distribution also targets the hypogastric vessels, patients may additionally suffer from difficulty in achieving and maintaining an erection resulting from inadequate perfusion of the internal pudendal arteries. The equivalent impact of impaired pelvic perfusion in women remains poorly understood but has more recently attracted investigative attention.[7] A well-characterized constellation of symptoms and signs known as the Leriche syndrome associated with aortoiliac occlusive disease in the male includes thigh, hip, or buttock claudication, atrophy of the leg muscles, impotence, and reduced femoral pulses.[8]

Although atherosclerotic disease limited to the aortoiliac region commonly gives rise to claudication of varying degrees, it is rarely associated with lower extremity ischemic rest pain or ischemic tissue loss. This is largely the result of adequate collateralization around the point of obstruction via lumbar, sacral, and circumflex iliac vessels that serves to reconstitute the infrainguinal system with enough well-perfused arterial blood to ensure sufficient resting tissue perfusion (Fig. 20-1). A well-recognized exception to this general observation arises in the situation of embolic disease. The so-called *blue toe syndrome* represents a situation where atherosclerotic debris breaks free from an aortic or iliac plaque and embolizes to the distal vessels.[9,10] Wire manipulation during coronary or peripheral angiographic procedures and cross-clamping across a calcific aortic plaque during cardiac surgery are common sources of such emboli. The terminal target of the microembolic particles, be they cholesterol crystals, calcified plaque, thrombus, or platelet aggregates, is typically the small vessels of the toes.

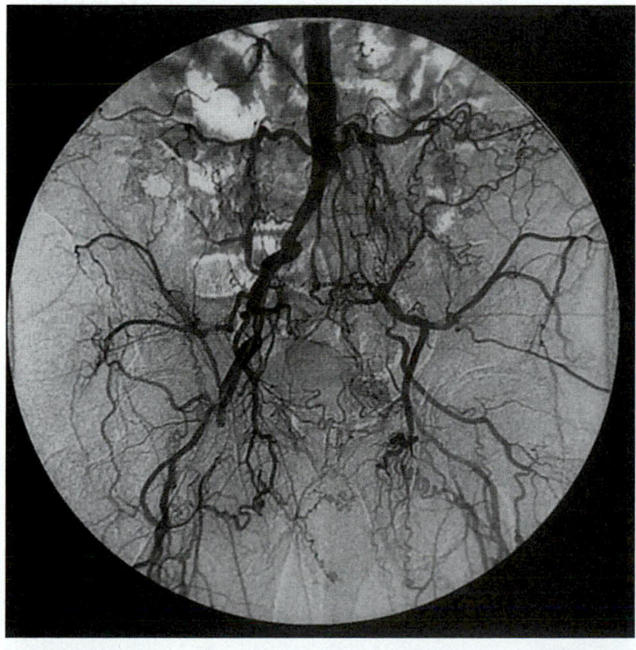

FIGURE 20-1. Aortoiliac occlusive disease results in a variable degree of collateralization. Here the left hypogastric artery is reconstituted via prominent distal lumbar collaterals and the right hypogastric artery. Hypogastric collaterals are in turn perfusing the femoral cirmcumflex vessels.

If aortoiliac occlusive disease is found in combination with femoropopliteal occlusive disease, ischemic rest pain or even more severe perfusion impairment leading to ischemic tissue loss or gangrene is not uncommon.[11] Such progressive disease, affecting multiple levels of the peripheral vasculature tree, is most frequently encountered in the elderly. Approximately, one third of patients operated on for symptomatic aortoiliac occlusive disease have orificial profunda femoris occlusive disease and more than 40% have superficial femoral artery occlusions. Aortoiliac disease typically begins at the distal aorta and common iliac artery origins, and slowly progresses proximally and distally over time.[12] This progression is quite variable, but may ultimately extend to the level of the renal arteries or result in total aortic occlusion.

A particularly virulent form of atherosclerotic arterial disease is often found in young women smokers.[13] Radiographic imaging in this subset of patients typically reveals atretic, narrowed vasculature with diffusely calcific atherosclerotic changes. Frequently, a focal stenosis is found posteriorly near the aortic bifurcation. This particular distribution of disease and the characteristic patient profile have been referred to as the small aorta syndrome (Fig. 20-2).[14] Such patients invariably have an extensive smoking history, with or without other typical factors for atherosclerosis. Given the diminutive size of the aorta and iliac vessels, the durability of endovascular intervention is generally inferior in these patients, particularly in the face of continued cigarette use.

The diagnosis of aortoiliac occlusive disease is generally made based on patient symptomatology, physical examination, and noninvasive tests such as segmental pressure measurements and pulse volume recordings (see Chapter 17). Following the diagnosis of aortoiliac disease and the decision to pursue intervention, further imaging is warranted. In many centers, magnetic resonance angiography (MRA) has supplanted contrast angiography as the initial imaging study of choice. Advances have solved many of the technical limitations of earlier studies, and reliable roadmaps to guide operative planning are now reproducibly obtainable (see Chapter 11). Should a lesion amenable to percutaneous therapy be identified, angiography is then pursued. In cases in which a good quality roadmap is obtained with MRA and the clinical situation or anatomic pattern is unfavorable to a percutaneous approach, surgery can, in most instances, be planned directly from the MRA, obviating the need for traditional subtraction angiography.[15]

In the minority of cases necessitating digital subtraction angiography for preoperative planning, a retrograde femoral approach is typically used, whereas the transbrachial approach serves as a useful alternative in patients with particularly challenging anatomy.[16] Additional lateral and oblique views of the abdominal aorta are advised if concomitant mesenteric or renal occlusive disease is present and multiple projections of the iliac and femoral bifurcations are essential in clarifying the extent of disease in these regions (see Chapter 13). Finally, full runoff views of the lower extremities are needed to assess the presence or absence of femoropopliteal or crural disease. In ambiguous cases, pull back pressure measurements, both before and after the administration of a systemic vasodilator, such as papaverine or nitroglycerine, or the application of a tourniquet to induce reactive hyperemia, can be useful in documenting the hemodynamic significance of a particular stenotic zone.[17] The use of gadolinium[18] or carbon dioxide[19] as contrast agents in patients with compromised renal function can minimize or eliminate the nephrotoxic effects associated with standard iodinated contrast medium.

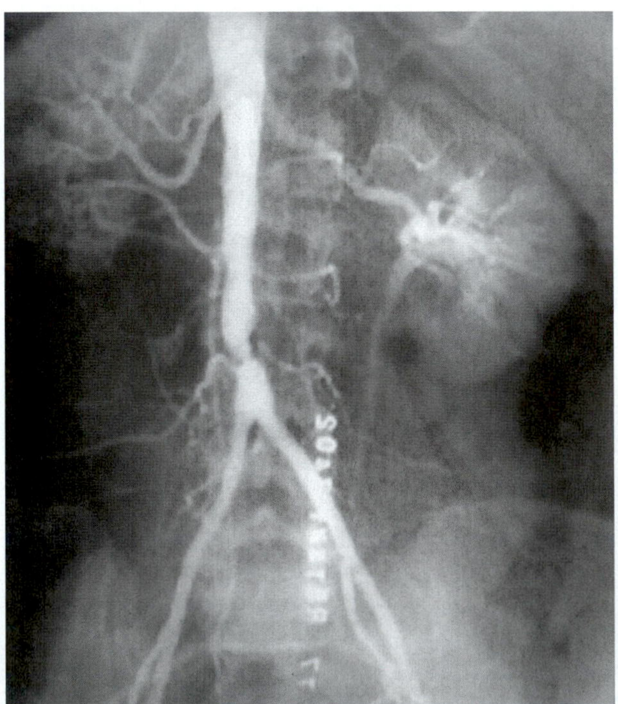

FIGURE 20-2. Aortoiliac occlusive disease may consist of a short segment stenosis localized to the distal aorta, a lesion particularly common in young female smokers. Such a lesion may be amenable to endarterectomy.

Management

Risk factor modification remains a cornerstone of the management of aortoiliac occlusive disease (see Chapter 18). Smoking cessation, blood pressure control, and aggressive efforts at cholesterol lowering should be addressed with every patient with atherosclerotic disease. Strong evidence exists supporting the benefit of a structured walking program[20] in increasing the walking distance of patients with claudication. The benefit of walking outside of a structured regimen with close follow-up is more debatable.[21] Medical management with pentoxifylline or, more recently, cilostazol, has benefit in a subset of patients and is a reasonable first line approach to improve claudication symptoms.[22]

There has been a considerable change in the management approach to claudication in recent years. Anyone suffering from disabling claudication, rest pain, or ischemia-related tissue loss continues to warrant serious consideration for arteriography and either percutaneous or surgical intervention. Previously, however, such aggressive treatment would have been considered inappropriate for claudication that was not clearly disabling.

As percutaneous treatment has become increasingly safer and more effective, however, and its application spread to increasingly more arterial beds, the indications for transluminal angioplasty have correspondingly increased (see Chapter 19). Such a sea-change in the overall management approach to aortoiliac disease has had a dramatic impact on the numbers of patients now proceeding to open surgery. Just as the escalating use of renal angioplasty and stenting for renal occlusive disease has led to a considerable drop in open surgical renal artery reconstructions, the rising popularity and success of aortic and iliac balloon angioplasty and stenting as first line therapy has noticeably reduced the volume of aortoiliac reconstructive procedures performed in this country.

When medical therapy or percutaneous treatment has proven to be inadequate or is technically inadvisable, open surgical revascularization remains indicated for those patients with aortoiliac disease and disabling claudication, ischemic rest pain and ischemic ulceration or gangrene. Patients with nighttime foot rest pain or tissue loss usually have multisegment disease and the decision whether to perform both supra- and infrainguinal revascularization procedures or to perform only an inflow procedure is guided by the severity of the ischemia.[11,23-25] In general, patients presenting with significant tissue loss or gangrene are much more likely to require simultaneous or staged inflow and outflow procedures.

The numerous surgical options available to the trained vascular surgeon allow tailoring of the approach to the particular overall and anatomic situation of each patient. Historically, the reconstructive options for aortoiliac occlusive disease include aortoiliac endarterectomy, aortobifemoral bypass, and so-called *extra-anatomic revascularization* in the form of iliofemoral, femorofemoral, or axillofemoral grafting.

Endarterectomy

Aortic endarterectomy was commonly performed in the early era of aortoiliac reconstruction.[26,27] Although it is particularly suited to localized disease limited to the distal aorta or promixal iliac arteries, it has proven to be less reliable for disease involving the entire infrarenal aorta and extending into the external iliac arteries.[28,29] The obvious benefit of endarterectomy is the elimination of the need for a prosthetic graft, removing the possibility of the myriad late graft-related complications. The long-term patency of limited endarterectomy is excellent and on par with bypass procedures.[30] However, the number of patients suitable for this reconstructive approach is small and continues to diminish in the era of endoluminal reconstruction. Experience with endarterectomy during one's training or early surgical career is another important factor influencing the choice of therapy offered because significant technical expertise is required and many surgeons in the current era have limited familiarity with this approach.

Aortobifemoral Bypass

Aortobifemoral bypass remains the mainstay of operative treatment for aortoiliac occlusive disease. During the last 20 years, the procedure has supplanted both aortic endarterectomy and aortoiliac bypass procedures. In the latter case, this change was largely driven by the recognition of subsequent graft failure due to progression of native iliac arterial disease.[28,31] Early experience with aortobifemoral grafting in the 1970s was associated with a 5% to 8% 30-day operative mortality rate.[29,30,32,33] Over the recent decades, mortality rates of 1% have been reported, on par with those of elective abdominal aortic aneurysm repair.[34,35]

Typically one half of patients proceeding to surgery for aortoiliac occlusive disease will have significant coronary artery disease; even more will have hypertension and almost 80% will be current or earlier cigarette smokers.[34] The reduced mortality and morbidity seen in recent years are, in large part, due to advances in the management of concomitant coronary disease. Specifically, the importance and benefit of better preoperative identification of patients in need of initial coronary revascularization, awareness of the benefit of waiting an interval period following coronary stenting before proceeding with major noncoronary vascular surgery, improved perioperative pharmacologic management of patients with impaired myocardium, and more focused efforts to tailor operative and postoperative fluid administration to the individual patient's myocardial reserve are all well-recognized.[36,37] General advances in postoperative intensive care unit management, including pulmonary care, infection control, and blood product utilization, have further contributed to the progress seen.

Current early patency rates for aortobifemoral bypass grafting are excellent, approaching 100% in many reporting institutions. Five-year patency rates are greater than 80%[30,32-34,38] whereas 10 year rates are near 75%.[30] There are multiple reasons for the improved patency. The current graft material used by most surgeons for aortoiliac reconstruction is a knitted Dacron prosthesis, which has enhanced hemostatic properties and tends to have a more stable pseudointima than earlier-used woven grafts.[39,40] More attention is paid to avoiding graft redundancy and to ensuring a good size match between the graft and the recipient vessels. Grafts are more routinely extended beyond the iliac level to the femoral vessels, which not only improves exposure and makes for a technically easier distal anastomosis but is also associated with less graft thrombosis from unanticipated progression of atherosclerotic disease in the external iliac vessels.[31] With meticulous skin preparation, close attention to draping, careful surgical technique, and judicious use of a short course of intravenous antibiotic therapy, the feared higher rate of graft infection from placing the distal dissection at the groins has not materialized.[41] An exception to this general practice is recommended in certain circumstances, however. For example, patients with hostile groin creases from prior surgery or radiation therapy or obese, diabetic patients with an intertriginous rash at the inguinal crease will all likely be better served by performing the distal anastomosis at the external iliac level if their anatomy for such is suitable.

The increased awareness of the critical role played by the deep femoral artery in preserving long-term patency of aortobifemoral grafts[30,33,42,43] has also undoubtedly contributed to the better results seen. This awareness parallels a better overall appreciation for the importance of establishing adequate outflow at the femoral level in achieving higher early and late graft patency rates and sustained symptom relief. The true impact of concomitant superficial femoral artery disease is unclear from the literature. Some reports have indicated similar patency rates between those patients with and without superficial femoral artery occlusion,[23,24] whereas others have suggested late patency rates are reduced in this setting.[41,44] What has definitely been shown is the benefit of a profundaplasty in the presence of significant superficial and profunda femoral occlusive disease.[45,46] Some authors have even recommended that a profundaplasty should be carried out in every case of superficial artery occlusion, even in the absence of orificial profunda disease, arguing that a "functional" obstruction on the order of 50% stenosis is present in these patients.[47] Although this position has not been universally adopted, it is now common practice to extend the hood of the distal anastomosis over the origin of the profunda femoral artery to enhance the graft outflow, especially in situations in which the superficial femoral artery is occluded or severely diseased. In the presence of significant common femoral or profunda femoral origin plaque, an extensive endarterectomy and/or profundaplasty is indicated (Fig. 20-3). In these circumstances, it is preferable to close the endarterectomized recipient bed with a vein, bovine pericardial or Dacron patch, onto which the distal anastomosis can then be attached, rather than creating a long femoris patch with the graft limb.[42]

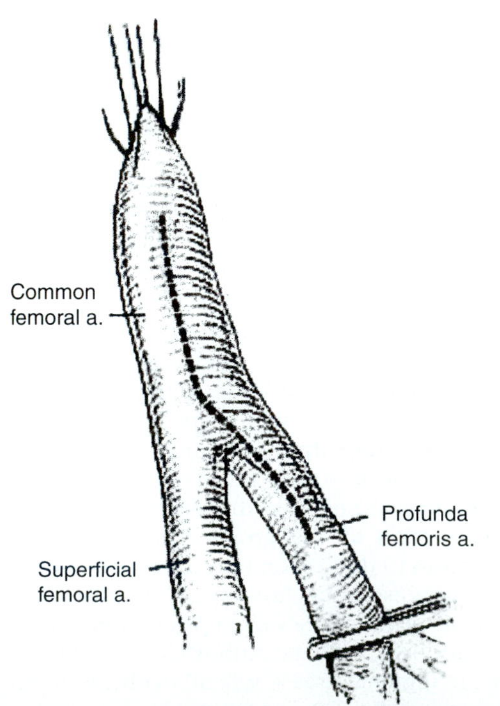

FIGURE 20-3. In the setting of superficial femoral artery and orificial profunda femoral artery disease, extending the common femoral arteriotomy into the origin of the profunda and performing a profundaplasty prior to completing the distal anastomosis of the aortobifemoral bypass will improve outflow and maximize graft patency.

There are several technical considerations related to aortobifemoral bypass grafting that are the subject of considerable and passionate debate. The first involves the manner of the proximal anastomotic creation. Advocates of an end-to-end configuration claim that it facilitates a more comprehensive thromboendarterectomy of the proximal stump and allows for a direct, more in-line flow pattern, with less turbulence and more favorable flow characteristics.[48] The obviation of competitive flow through the excluded iliac vessels with this approach is likely more of theoretical rather than real benefit. Certainly, with concomitant aneurysmal disease or complete aortic occlusion extending up to the level of the renal arteries, end-to-end grafting is indicated. Creation of an end-to-side anastomosis can at times be technically challenging in a heavily diseased aorta partially occluded by a side-biting clamp. A lower rate of proximal suture line pseudoaneurysms and better long-term patency rates have been found in some series.[49] Stapling or oversewing of the distal aorta with the end-to-end technique minimizes the immediate risk of clamp-induced emboli to the lower extremities following release of the distal clamp. Finally, those in favor of this approach claim the ability to more effectively close the retroperitoneum, particularly after resection of a short segment of the infrarenal aorta, results in lower rates of late graft infection and aortoenteric fistulae, although there is no direct evidence to support this assertion.

There are certain circumstances when an end-to-side proximal anastomotic configuration is advantageous. The most common indication involves those patients with occluded external iliac arteries, in whom interruption of forward aortic flow may result in loss of perfusion to an important hypogastric or inferior mesenteric artery and consequent significant pelvic ischemia. Colon ischemia (1% to 2%),[50] or even more rarely, paraplegia secondary to cauda equina syndrome (<1%),[51] are additional complications that can be avoided by an end-to-side configuration. Although advocated by some,[52] routine preservation of a patent IMA is not universally practiced.

Operative Management

The operative procedure is performed under general endotracheal anesthesia, with an epidural catheter placed for postoperative pain control. The patient is sterilely prepped and draped from the mid-chest to the mid-thighs. The femoral vessels are first exposed through bilateral longitudinal, oblique incisions, thereby reducing the time in which the abdomen is open and the viscera exposed. The extent of exposure of the femoral vessels necessary is dictated by the severity of disease and the level of reconstruction planned for the common femoral artery and its bifurcation. Next, the inferior aspect of the retroperoneal tunnel through which the graft will course to reach the femoral region is begun with digital manipulation posterior to the inguinal ligament and tracking along the anterior aspect of the external iliac artery. Antibiotic soaked sponges are then placed in the groin wounds and attention is turned to the aortic dissection.

The proximal reconstruction is performed via a midline laparotomy. In general, the aortic dissection is limited to the region between the renal arteries and the inferior mesenteric artery. This allows avoidance of extensive dissection anterior to the aortic bifurcation, where the autonomic nerve plexus regulating erection and ejaculation in men sweeps over the aorta. An intriguing recent survey indicated no significant differences in the rate of sexual dysfunction with open compared with endovascular repair of abdominal aortic aneurysms, suggesting the effects of aortic dissection in this area are perhaps less important than typically believed.[53]

In situations where significant aortic calcification extends up to the level of the renal arteries, it may be necessary to continue the aortic dissection to the suprarenal or even the supraceliac level to allow for safe proximal clamp placement. Alternatively, proximal control may be obtained by intraluminal balloon deployment. If end-to-side repair is planned, circumferential dissection of the aortic segment to be clamped is recommended, as gaining control of any lumbar or accessory renal vessels encountered prior to performing the aortotomy helps to avoid troublesome backbleeding. The superior aspect of the graft limb tunnels are then completed, taking care to maintain a course anterior to the common iliac vessels but posterior to the ureters. Between 5000 and 7000 units of heparin are then administered, with additional heparin given throughout the procedure to maintain the activated clotting time near the target range of 250 to 300 seconds. After allowing sufficient time for the heparin to circulate, atraumatic vascular clamps are placed above the inferior mesenteric artery and just below the renal arteries. The distal clamp is applied first to avoid any distal embolization of plaque dislodged with placement of the proximal clamp. If an end-to-end anastomosis is planned, the aorta is transected 1 to 2 cm below the proximal clamp and a short segment of the distal aortic cuff is excised (Fig. 20-4A). This results both in better exposure of the aortic neck and a more precise proximal reconstruction and also allows the graft to lie flat against the vertebral column rather than anteriorly oriented, facilitating later retroperitoneal coverage. If necessary, a thromboendarterectomy of the infrarenal neck is carried out at this point (see Fig. 20-4B). The anastomosis is performed with a running suture of no. 3-0 polypropylene (see Fig. 20-4C). The distal aorta is then oversewn with two layers of a running monofilament suture or stapled with a surgical stapler. If an end-to-side anastomosis is performed, an anterior longitudinal arteriotomy is carried out after placement of proximal and distal transaortic clamps. If necessary, an endarterectomy is performed and the anastomosis carried out after the graft is beveled appropriately (see Fig. 20-4D). If there is minimal plaque present, the distal anastomosis is performed to the common femoral artery and individual dissection of the superficial femoral and profunda femoral arteries is not necessary.

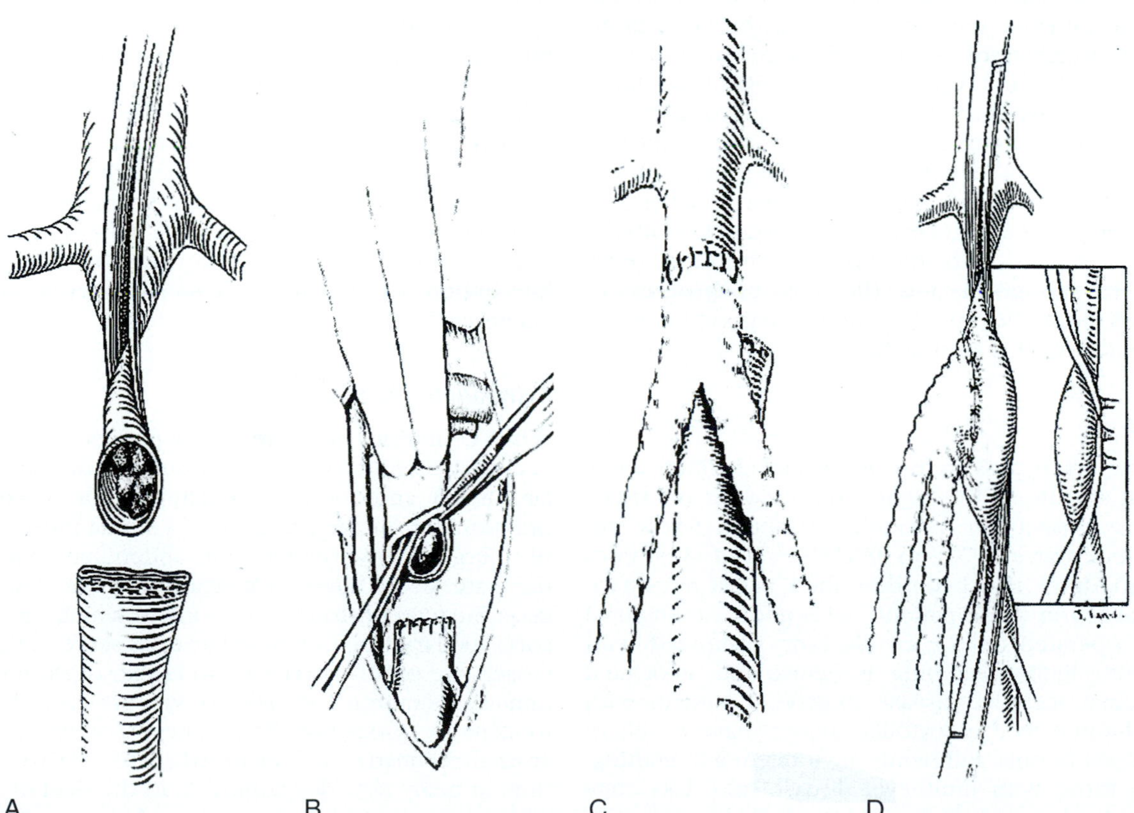

FIGURE 20-4. The end-to-end proximal anastomosis for aortofemoral reconstruction is initiated with the infrarenal aorta cross-clamp placed in an anterior/posterior direction as close to the origin of the renal arteries as possible. The aorta is transected 1 to 2 cm below the proximal clamp. A short segment of distal aortic cuff is excised and the aorta is stapled or over-sewn just proximal to the origin of the inferior mesenteric artery (**A**). If necessary, a thromboendarterectomy of the aortic cuff is carried out (**B**). The end-to-end configuration allows the graft to lie flat against the vertebral column and results in less turbulent flow (**C**). An end-to-side configuration is required to preserve antegrade pelvic perfusion in situations where retrograde flow would be compromised due to heavily diseased or occluded external iliac arteries (**D**).

Another point of some debate concerns the optimal management of patients with multilevel occlusive disease. The question frequently arises as to whether or under what circumstances a concomitant or staged outflow procedure should be performed. It is generally believed that up to 80% of patients with both inflow and outflow disease will be substantially improved following aortofemoral bypass grafting.[11,23] Other reports, however, have suggested that between as many as one quarter to one third of such patients will not have significant symptomatic relief with an inflow procedure alone.[24] Although no single parameter exists to reliably guide the surgeon to know in which circumstances a combined procedure is optimal, the severity of distal ischemia is probably the most important factor to be considered. The overall medical condition of the patients and their ability to tolerate a prolonged operative procedure is also clearly important. Finally, the status of the profunda femoral artery must be taken into consideration. In the presence of superficial femoral artery occlusion, a profunda that is atretic or extensively diseased may well be unable to provide sufficient collateral runoff to the foot.

If, on the one hand, the bypass procedure is undertaken for claudication alone or mild rest pain, restoring adequate inflow may provide sufficient and relatively durable symptomatic relief. If, on the other hand, significant tissue loss is present, a combined inflow and outflow procedure is likely warranted if limb salvage is to be achieved. If several operating teams are used, performing both procedures at the same time can be done in an acceptably timely fashion and has been found to be safe. Indeed, several recent reports found no significant differences in operative mortality or perioperative morbidity in patients undergoing concurrent inflow and outflow procedures compared with those having major inflow reconstruction alone.[54,55] Although staged revascularization may be preferable in certain circumstances, both the risk of wound and graft infection resulting from redissection in the groin and the risk of progressive tissue loss during the initial recuperative period must be considered with this approach.

Results

Aortobifemoral bypass grafting is associated with patency rates that are among the highest reported for any major arterial reconstruction. As indicated above, 5-year primary patency rates of 70% to 88%[30,32,33] and 10-year rates of 66% to 78%[30] have been described. Better rates have been realized in those patients with good infrainguinal outflow operated on for claudication compared with those with limb-threatening ischemia and associated infrainguinal occlusive disease. In general, patients with disease limited to the aortoiliac region have excellent relief of symptoms following aortobifemoral grafting, whereas those with multilevel disease have less complete levels of symptom diminution. Perioperative mortality rates average 4%, whereas 5-year survival rates between 70% and 75% have been reported.[32,56,57] This latter rate is notably less than the 5-year survival rate of age-matched control population but on par with that typically seen for claudicants in general.

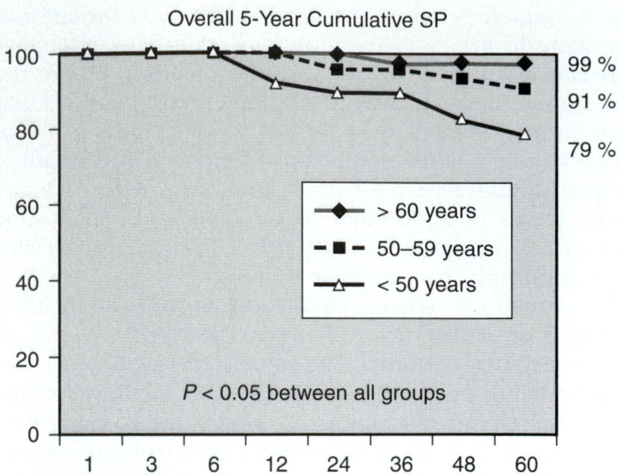

FIGURE 20-5. Overall 5-year cumulative secondary patency rates in a recent cohort of patients undergoing aortobifemoral bypass grafting, indicating an inverse relationship between age and graft patency.[34]

Although the early and late mortality rates are similar across different age groups, the 5-year primary and secondary patency rates are significantly increased with each increase in age group.[34] Reed and colleagues reported that primary patency rates were 66%, 87%, and 96% and secondary patency rates were 79%, 91%, and 98% (Fig. 20-5), respectively, for those younger than 50 years of age, those 50 to 59 years of age, and those older than 60 years of age.[34] It seems prudent, based on these findings, to apply caution in the application of aortobifemoral bypass grafting for younger patients with virulent aortoiliac disease. The potential impact of graft failure and need for subsequent complex interventions should be considered, especially given the longer life expectancy of younger patients. Full utilization of all medical and endovascular options appears to be the best first line option for younger patients with severe aortoiliac occlusive disease.

Extra-anatomic Bypass

When comorbid disease renders a patient with aortoiliac occlusive disease particularly unsuitable for major vascular surgery and aortic cross-clamping, or when sepsis, prior surgery, or the presence of a stoma presents a hostile surgical environment for abdominal exploration, there are several alternatives available to the vascular surgeon. Such reconstructive options, in which the thoracic aorta, axillary, iliac or femoral arteries serve as the donor vessels, are generally referred to as extra-anatomic to distinguish them from the in-line flow represented by an aortobifemoral procedure. The concept of extra-anatomic arterial reconstruction emerged in the 1950s during a time of many new developments in the field of vascular surgery. Freeman and Leeds provided one of the first descriptions in 1952 in their report of the use of the superficial femoral artery as the conduit for a crossover femorofemoral bypass graft.[58] These approaches are also called on in desperate situations represented by infection of a previously placed aortic graft.

Axillobifemoral Bypass

Axillobifemoral bypass grafting was introduced by Blaisdell[59] in the early 1960s and has since enjoyed increasing popularity as an alternative to aortobifemoral bypass. This is largely due to the reliability of the axillary artery as a donor vessel and the minimal morbidity incurred, making it a particularly appealing option for patients with significant operative risk from comorbid disease. It is also appropriate in patients with significant aortoiliac occlusive disease of the distal aorta and the iliac arteries in the setting of intra-abdominal sepsis, a history of multiple prior abdominal operations, intra-abdominal adhesions, or prior pelvic irradiation. Of note, LoGerfo and colleagues[60] have shown that axillobifemoral grafting has improved long-term patency compared with axillounifemoral grafting, presumably owing to the increased flow afforded by the second outflow limb.

Although usually performed under general anesthesia, it is possible to carry out the procedure using a combination of local anesthesia and intravenous conscious sedation. In the event that one arm has a higher blood pressure or a stronger pulse, that side should be selected as the donor site. If both sides are equal, the right axillary artery is chosen because evidence suggests there is a lower risk of arterial occlusive disease developing in the right subclavian artery compared with the left.

The axillary artery is exposed through a short infraclavicular incision parallel to the clavicle in the deltopectoral groove. The pectoralis major muscle is then bluntly separated between the clavicular and sternal heads and the pectoralis minor muscle is identified and typically divided, enhancing exposure and allowing more space for the graft as it courses from the axilla to the subcutaneous space. The axillary artery medial to the pectoralis minor is then isolated because the proximal anastomosis is optimally placed as close to the chest as possible to minimize the risk of kinking or graft avulsion during rotational shoulder movement. Avoiding more lateral dissection further reduces the risk of injuring the medial and lateral cords of the brachial plexus as they emerge anteriorly to form the median nerve. A tunnel is created between the axillary and femoral arteries in the subcutaneous space, tracking deep to the pectoralis major muscle and inferiorly along the mid-axillary line before coursing medial to the anterior superior iliac spine; this latter orientation is important to avoid kinking of the conduit in the sitting position. Long, rigid tunneling devices with a removable central obturator are specifically designed for this step and have helped to lower the incidence of graft infection by obviating the need for counterincisions.

The common femoral arteries are then dissected through standard bilateral short groin incisions and a second subcutaneous tunnel is fashioned between them in an extrafascial, suprapubic plane. A Dacron or polytetrafluoroethylene graft, typically 8 mm in diameter, is then drawn through the tunnel. Although there is no convincing evidence that one graft material is superior to the other, several reports support the common practice of using an externally reinforced graft.[61,62] Newer grafts are available that are prefigured in an axillobifemoral configuration, thereby reducing from four to three the number of anastomoses needed. As in aortobifemoral bypass grafting, unrestricted outflow should be ensured by carrying the hood of the femoral grafts down over the profunda orifice and performing an endarterectomy or profundaplasty when necessary. If a prefigured graft is unavailable, the origin of the cross-femoral graft can be tailored to the body habitus of the patient. In most cases, the graft is taken off the distal hood of the descending axillofemoral graft. In particularly obese individuals, however, it may be preferable to move the takeoff more proximally to prevent kinking at the level of the inguinal ligament. Orienting the takeoff of the crossover graft at an acute angle to give an "S-shaped" final configuration has been associated with higher patency rates in some studies.[63]

Many of the complications following axillofemoral grafting are directly related to the graft and are potentially avoidable. Disruption of the proximal anastomosis can be minimized by proper orientation of the proximal hood and ensuring that the descending limb of the graft is free from undue tension.[64] Kinking and subsequent thrombosis of the graft can be reduced by strict attention to tunnel position and use of a reinforced conduit. Given the minimal physiologic insult, most patients undergoing axillofemoral grafting are ambulatory and able to tolerate a regular diet on the first postoperative day.

The reported long-term patency rates of axillofemoral grafts have varied significantly, ranging from as low as 29% to as high as 85%.[61,65-67] Favorable results were reported by Passman and colleagues,[68] who achieved 5-year patency rates of 74% and a long-term limb salvage rate of 89% and who are vocal advocates of a wider use for this approach. In general, axillobifemoral grafting should be reserved for high-risk patients with significant tissue loss in danger of limb loss, and not be used for the treatment of claudication.

Femorofemoral Bypass

Femorofemoral bypass grafts are ideally suited to those patients with preserved flow in both the aorta and one iliac branch, but occlusion or severe stenosis of the contralateral iliac not amenable to percutaneous treatment (Figs. 20-6 and 20-7A and B). Although possible to perform under local anesthesia in high-risk patients, it is best carried out under regional or general anesthesia. On occasion, it has been performed in an intensive care unit setting in the particular instance of a leg rendered acutely ischemic by the placement of an intra-aortic balloon pump. The technical details are identical to those of the crossover component of the axillobifemoral grafting discussed earlier. The suprapubic tunnel is created in a gentle C-curve just superficial to the deep fascia and can in most instances be completed by blunt finger dissection approaching from both groin incisions. Although some surgeons advocate placement of the tunnel beneath the rectus sheath, this is a minority view. Again, if warranted by the presence of significant concomitant femoral disease, an endarterectomy or profundaplasty is indicated prior to completion of the proximal or distal anastomosis.

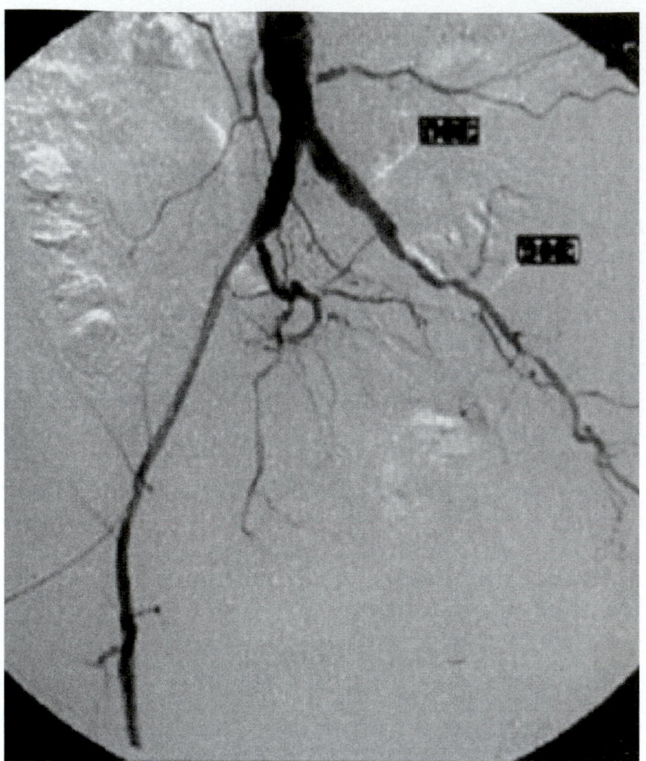

FIGURE 20-6. An oblique view digital subtraction angiogram indicating a long segment total occlusion of the left external iliac artery. Extra-anatomic left-to-right femorofemoral or iliofemoral bypass grafting would be appropriate options for this anatomic disease distribution (see also Fig. 20-7).

Graft failure due to progression of inflow disease following femorofemoral grafting is less problematic than one might predict. Some investigators have argued that the increased flow through the donor iliac artery following the restoration of bilateral outflow, in essence shifting the aortic bifurcation to a more distal point, serves to impede the further development of atherosclerotic disease. Animal studies correlating blood flow and shear stress with intimal hyperplasia lend support to this explanation.[69] Maini and Mannick reported a 5-year cumulative patency rate of 80%.[70] This is similar to other reports in the literature[71-73] and compares favorably with the 85% rate seen with conventional aortobifemoral bypass grafting.[34]

With its high patency rates and the low associated morbidity, cross-femoral grafting is an excellent option in patients with favorable anatomy. Given the risk of late graft failure from progression of inflow disease and the potential need to reintervene on previously dissected femoral beds should a later aortobifemoral graft be needed; however, it has traditionally been advised to proceed directly to aortobifemoral grafting in good-risk patients with any evidence of atherosclerotic disease in the aorta or patent iliac vessels. In the current era, aortic or iliac angioplasty and/or stenting in combination with cross-femoral grafting is a viable alternative in this setting, particularly for those patients at increased operative risk.

Iliofemoral Bypass

Iliofemoral grafting is another alternative to aortobifemoral grafting for a select group of patients with

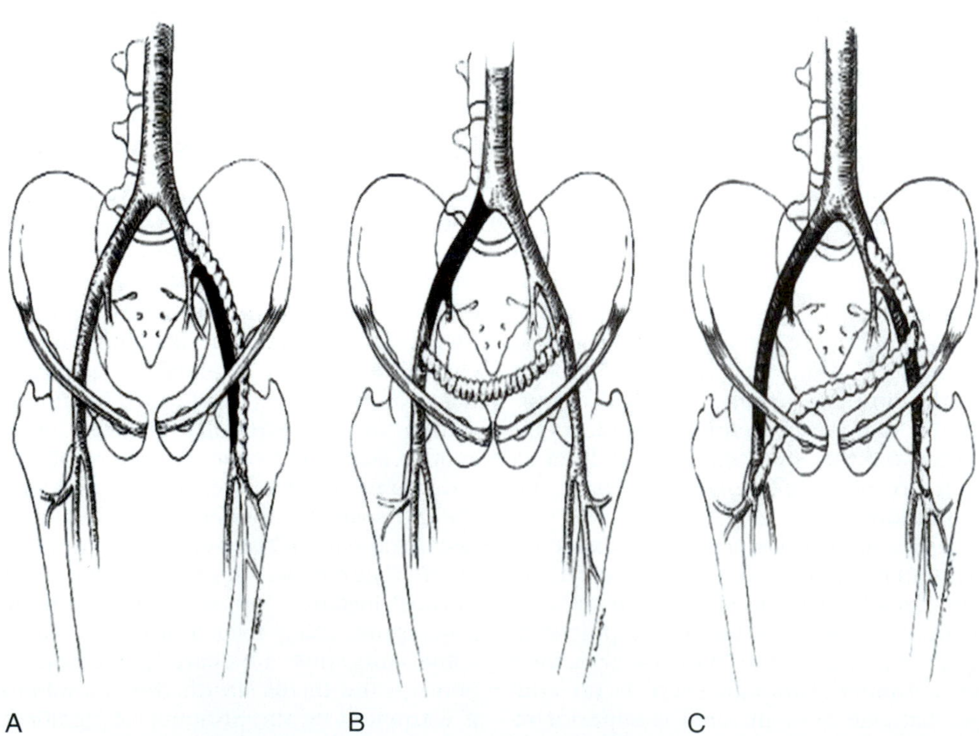

FIGURE 20-7. A patent common or external iliac artery may be used as a donor vessel for the (**A**) iliofemoral, (**B**) ilioiliac, or (**C**) ilio-bifemoral bypass grafts depicted. The lesions depicted in **A** and **B** would also be appropriate for femorofemoral grafts, whereas the lesion in **C** would be appropriate for aortobifemoral or axillobifemoral grafting.

hemodynamically significant disease limited to the external iliac artery (see Fig. 20-6). Currently, most patients with this anatomic pattern of disease would typically undergo an attempt at percutaneous recanalization of a tightly stenotic or long segment external iliac occlusion. Indeed, as the success rates with such efforts increase, the number of iliofemoral bypass grafts performed has continued to fall. However, if the percutaneous approach is unsuccessful, an iliofemoral bypass remains an excellent surgical option as it can be performed with minimal morbidity and cardiopulmonary insult and avoids the long descending limb necessitated by an axillofemoral graft (see Fig. 20-7). As the grafts are situated within the pelvis, they are also better protected from kinking, infection, and thrombosis than from either axillofemoral or femorofemoral grafts. Less disturbance of inguinal lymph nodes and lymphatic channels typically occurs with the more limited dissection necessary. Either the ipsilateral common iliac or proximal external iliac artery can serve as the donor site, and if need be, a bifurcated graft can be used and taken to both femoral vessels. Alternatively, bilateral iliofemoral grafts or an ilio-iliac graft can be fashioned as appropriate. Iliac exposure can be achieved through an oblique suprainguinal "transplant" incision and development of the retroperitoneal plane, which affords excellent proximal exposure even in the obese patient. Care must be taken in isolating the donor vessel and tunneling the graft to avoid injury to the ureter coursing over the iliac bifurcation. If a crossover graft is used, it can be tunneled retroperitoneally in the iliac fossa or across the properitoneum deep to the rectus sheath.

In early experience with iliac origin grafts reported by Couch and colleagues, there were no operative deaths and a 77% 4-year patency rate.[74] Nearly one half of these patients were operated on for limb salvage in the face of critical ischemia. In those patients undergoing revascularization with bilateral iliofemoral grafts, the 4-year patency rates were 92%, whereas an 85% patency rate was seen if both the superficial and deep femoral vessels were patent.[74] Other reported series of iliofemoral bypass grafting have indicated similar patency rates.[72,75]

Thoracic Aorto-to-Femoral Artery Bypass

As early as 1961, Blaisdell and colleagues reported on a novel extra-anatomic bypass from the descending thoracic aorta to the femoral artery, followed by a femorofemoral bypass.[76] Although carried out in the setting of sepsis after a ruptured aneurysm repair and not for occlusive disease, it provided a new alternative when the infrarenal aorta was inaccessible or inappropriate as a donor vessel. The procedure is performed through a thoracotomy incision, typically entering the chest through the eighth or ninth interspace. A muscle-sparing technique in which the lattisimus dorsi muscle is not divided aids in postoperative pain management. The distal descending thoracic aorta is circumferentially dissected enough to allow for clamp control, with care taken to avoid injury to the adjacently positioned esophagus. A tunnel is fashioned by separating the diaphragm from the posterior chest wall over a distance of two finger-breadths. In 1994, Criado and Keagy[77] reviewed the literature and summarized 193 reconstructions taken off the descending thoracic aorta. Not unexpectedly, the majority were performed for thrombosis or infection of a previously placed aortic graft, although some primary procedures undertaken in the setting of a "hostile" abdomen were included. Cumulative 5-year primary and secondary patency rates of 73% and 83%, respectively, were obtained and the operative mortality rate was 6%.[77]

Laparoscopic Revascularization

There is an increasing interest in applying laparoscopic techniques to the treatment of aortic occlusive disease, reflected in a small, but growing, body of literature of individual case series.[78,79] Some surgeons have favored a more limited approach using hand-assisted techniques and smaller incisions,[80] whereas others have championed the use of complete laparoscopic or robot-assisted revascularization.[78,81] The purported benefits of shorter hospital stays, less perioperative pain and postoperative complications are balanced against longer operative times and the lack of long-term data to support the durability of this alternative approach. It remains at present an extremely technically challenging procedure with a significant learning curve. As the technology advances and improvement is seen with anastomotic devices and instrumentation, the role of aortofemoral bypass will likely expand and become more defined.

INFRAINGUINAL ARTERIAL OCCLUSIVE DISEASE

Infrainguinal arterial occlusive disease is the most prevalent manifestation of chronic arterial occlusive disease encountered and treated by the vascular surgeon. Isolated disease of the superficial femoral artery typically manifests as calf-muscle claudication, whereas patients with multilevel disease involving the superficial femoral, popliteal and tibial arteries generally have rest pain or ischemic tissue loss. The ischemia ulcerations usually begin as small, dry ulcers of the toes or heel area, and progress to frankly gangrenous changes of the forefoot or heel with greater degrees of arterial insufficiency. Several identifiable patterns of disease are recognized, with smokers typically having disease limited to the superficial femoral artery and corresponding symptoms of claudication. Diabetes most often targets the popliteal and tibial vessels, and patients may present with frank tissue necrosis with no history of claudication.

Infrainguinal reconstruction for the treatment of peripheral vascular occlusive disease has been increasingly successful for both long-term palliation of intermittent claudication and for the salvage of limbs threatened by critical ischemia. Although there are certainly times when primary amputation represents the safest and most advisable solution in the face of irreversible ischemia, particularly in cases where extensive infection or tissue necrosis is present, an attempt at reconstruction is almost always indicated when a limb is threatened by severe ischemia. Improvements in perioperative management and surgical technique have allowed progressively more distal reconstructions to be successfully completed in an older, sicker, and challenging patient population. In general, high rates of relief for claudication and up to an 80% to 90% limb salvage rate may be anticipated for patients with critical ischemia at institutions devoted to peripheral bypass surgery.

The two major indications for surgical intervention of infrainguinal arterial occlusive disease are claudication and limb-threatening critical ischemia. Claudication is a relative indication, given the natural history of the disease; of patients with claudication, only 1% per year will ultimately progress to limb loss.[82,83] As such, it remains a subjective assessment on the parts of both patient and surgeon as to the relative degree of disability a given level of claudication pain represents.

Role of Percutaneous Transluminal Angioplasty

Of relevance in this regard is the significant shift in the indications for percutaneous intervention for infrainguinal occlusive disease witnessed in recent years. As the associated risks of balloon angioplasty and stenting have fallen and the relative success rates have risen, the threshold for offering endovascular treatment to claudicants has considerably decreased. Patients once considered appropriate only for risk-factor modification, exercise therapy, and medical treatment are now increasingly being offered percutaneous revascularization as a secondary or even primary treatment option (see Chapter 19).

Similarly, occlusive disease of the tibial vessels, once thought to be the exclusive domain of operative bypass, is increasingly being treated percutaneously. The impact of these trends on the natural history of the disease, and to what extent the expanding reach of percutaneous therapy will affect subsequent operative management in a given patient, remains to be seen. Certainly, as the enthusiasm for less-invasive options has spread to include the infrapopliteal level, the relative roles of surgical and percutaneous intervention are further being redefined. Newer generation atherectomy devices, cold balloon angioplasty and flexible stents designed to withstand the unique torsional forces of the leg or with drug-eluting capability may significantly improve the patency and durability rates currently seen.[84,85] Until the efficacy of infrainguinal percutaneous intervention is better defined, however, surgical revascularization remains the standard for any patient with critical limb ischemia. For patients with favorable anatomy and significant operative risk, and for the treatment of claudication in general, percutaneous therapy has assumed a more primary role.

Both duplex ultrasonography and MRA are increasingly used as first line modalities in the assessment of patients with infrainguinal occlusive disease (see Chapters 10, 11, and 17). Although a growing literature supports the use of duplex scanning as a stand-alone preoperative mapping modality,[86] this requires a highly dedicated vascular laboratory and, to date, has not gained wide acceptance. MRA is particularly useful as a noninvasive screening test to determine the suitability for percutaneous therapy. Although in some instances, operative planning may be based solely on MRA scanning if high-quality time of flight and gadolinium-enhanced images are obtained,[87,88] in many cases surgeons are reluctant to proceed to surgery without the confirmation afforded by standard contrast angiography. This is particularly true if the distal target is at the tibial or pedal level, where MRA technology remains more limited.

Operative Management

Infrainguinal bypass can be performed under general anesthesia, or in the appropriate patient, regional spinal or epidural anesthesia. The multiple sites of dissection and the harvesting of saphenous vein or an alternative vein conduit make these procedures particularly suited to a two-team approach. The time saved, particularly in cases involving potentially more tedious arm vein or lesser saphenous vein harvesting, has direct benefit in minimizing the total anesthetic load and physiologic insult to the patient. Typically, the site proposed for the distal anastomosis is explored first to ascertain whether the preoperative imaging was accurate in predicting the suitability of the target vessel. On occasion, the operation is begun with an on-table angiogram to clarify the anatomy if preoperative imaging was deferred or ambiguous.

The above-knee popliteal vessel is easily exposed through a medial thigh incision, with subsequent posterolateral retraction of the sartorius muscle. The popliteal artery, with its accompanying vein and nerve, is found just posterior to the femur. The vessel is palpated to determine the presence of atherosclerotic plaque, which will guide the extent of dissection and the optimal bypass target site. The below-knee popliteal artery is also exposed through a medial incision in the proximal calf (Fig. 20-8). If the saphenous vein is to be harvested, the incision is made directly over the vein to minimize the creation of devascularized skin flaps. With the exposed vein carefully protected, the incision is carried through the deep muscular fascia and the medial head of the gastrocnemius is reflected posterolaterally to expose the below-knee popliteal fossa. The distal popliteal artery is then dissected free from the adjacent tibial nerve posteriorly and popliteal vein medially. If the distal target is the tibioperoneal trunk, the dissection is continued along the anteromedial surface of the distal popliteal artery after dividing the origin of the soleus muscle from the tibia (Fig. 20-9). In instances in which the below-knee popliteal artery has previously been exposed or where sepsis is involved, a lateral approach with excision of a segment of proximal fibula is a useful alternative approach to the below-knee popliteal artery.

Although exposure of the proximal posterior and peroneal vessels can be gained by extending the tibioperoneal trunk dissection distally, more distal exposure of these vessels is best gained through targeted medial incisions. The posterior tibial artery is found more medially on the reflected soleus muscle, whereas the peroneal artery is deeper and more lateral. The posterior tibial artery at the level of the ankle is a relatively easier target given the proximity of the vessel to the skin surface. The initial incision is made just posterior to the medial malleolus, and the artery is exposed by division of the

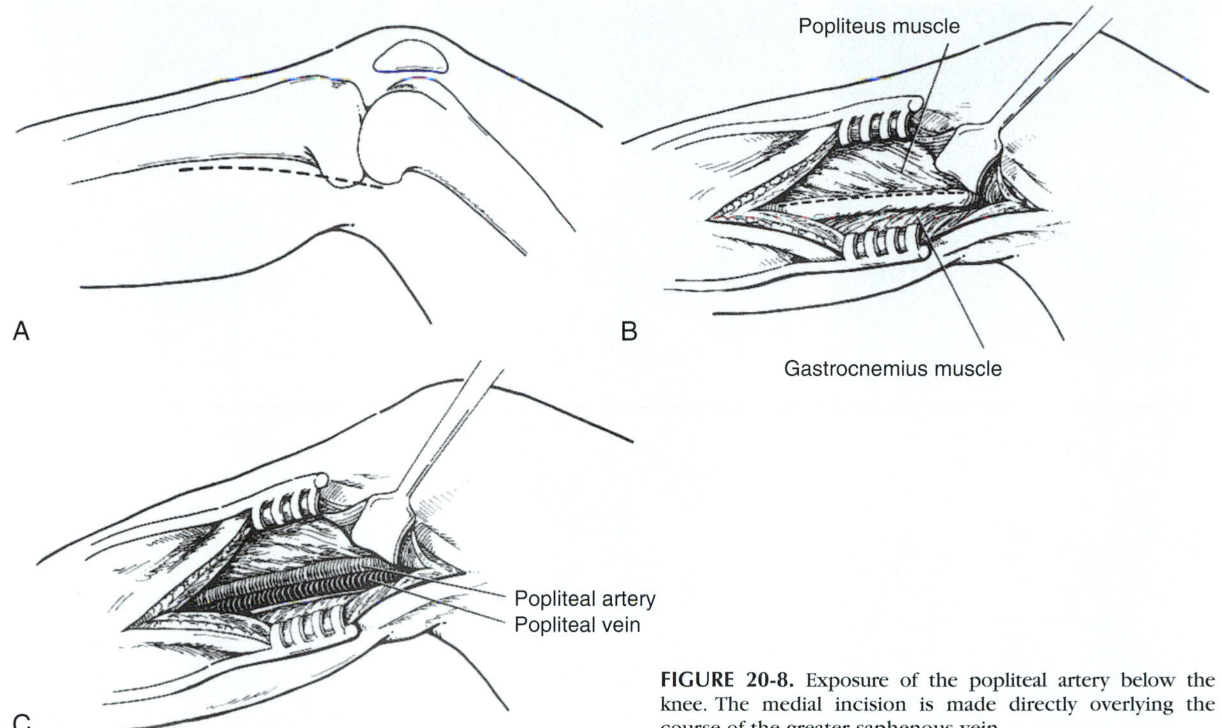

FIGURE 20-8. Exposure of the popliteal artery below the knee. The medial incision is made directly overlying the course of the greater saphenous vein.

overlying retinaculum. Further distal dissection allows access to the bifurcation and medial and lateral plantar branches.[89] The anterior tibial artery is typically approached from the anterolateral aspect of the calf (see Fig. 20-9) and is found deep within the anterior compartment with the adjacent deep peroneal nerve and anterior tibial veins. The dorsalis pedis artery is easily exposed through an axial incision on the dorsum of the foot just lateral to the extensor hallucis longus tendon (see Fig. 20-9).

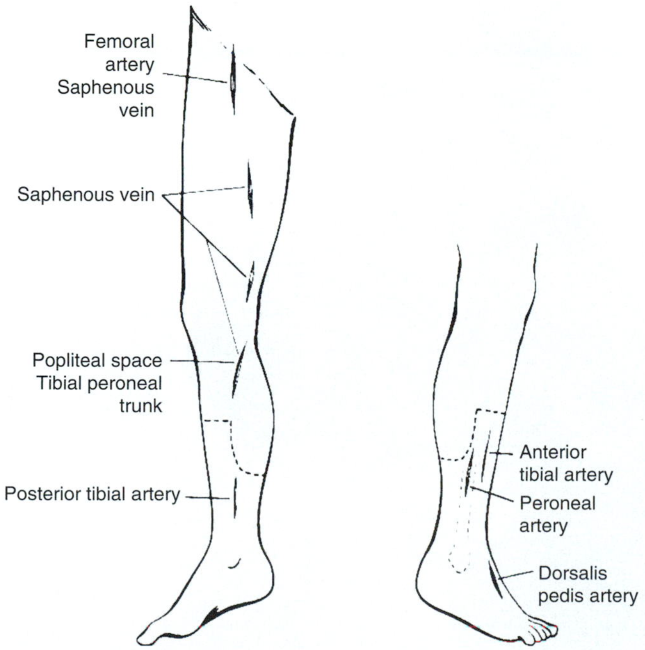

Following exposure of the distal anastomotic target vessel, the site of the proximal anastomosis is dissected. For patients with superficial femoral artery disease, this will most commonly be at the level of the common femoral artery. The artery is mobilized as described above, from the level of the inguinal ligament to its terminal bifurcation. The distal extent of this dissection is dictated by the presence of concomitant femoral plaque. Lymphatic tissue overlying the femoral vessels is best ligated and divided to prevent the postoperative development of lymph fistulas or lymphoceles. If an extensive endarterectomy or profundaplasty is required, the proximal profunda femoral artery is dissected along its proximal length accordingly.

If all or part of the superficial femoral artery is spared of significant atherosclerotic involvement, the proximal anastomosis can be moved distally as dictated by the particular anatomic pattern of disease, and a so-called "distal origin graft" can be fashioned (Fig. 20-10).[90] This situation is particularly applicable to the diabetic population, where infrapopliteal disease is the rule and sparing of the superficial femoral and popliteal arteries is not uncommon. It is also used in situations where conduit is sparse, and a moderately diseased proximal vessel is accepted as an inflow source for a more distal origin bypass graft in the interests of performing a fully autologous vein graft rather than using prosthetic material. An increasingly popular approach when only limited conduit is available is to combine, either concurrently in the operating room or as a staged preoperative procedure,

Femoral artery
Saphenous vein
Saphenous vein
Popliteal space
Tibial peroneal trunk
Posterior tibial artery
Anterior tibial artery
Peroneal artery
Dorsalis pedis artery

FIGURE 20-9. Placement of incisions for femoropopliteal and femorotibial bypass and for greater saphenous vein harvest. These should avoid the incision lines for a below-knee amputation.

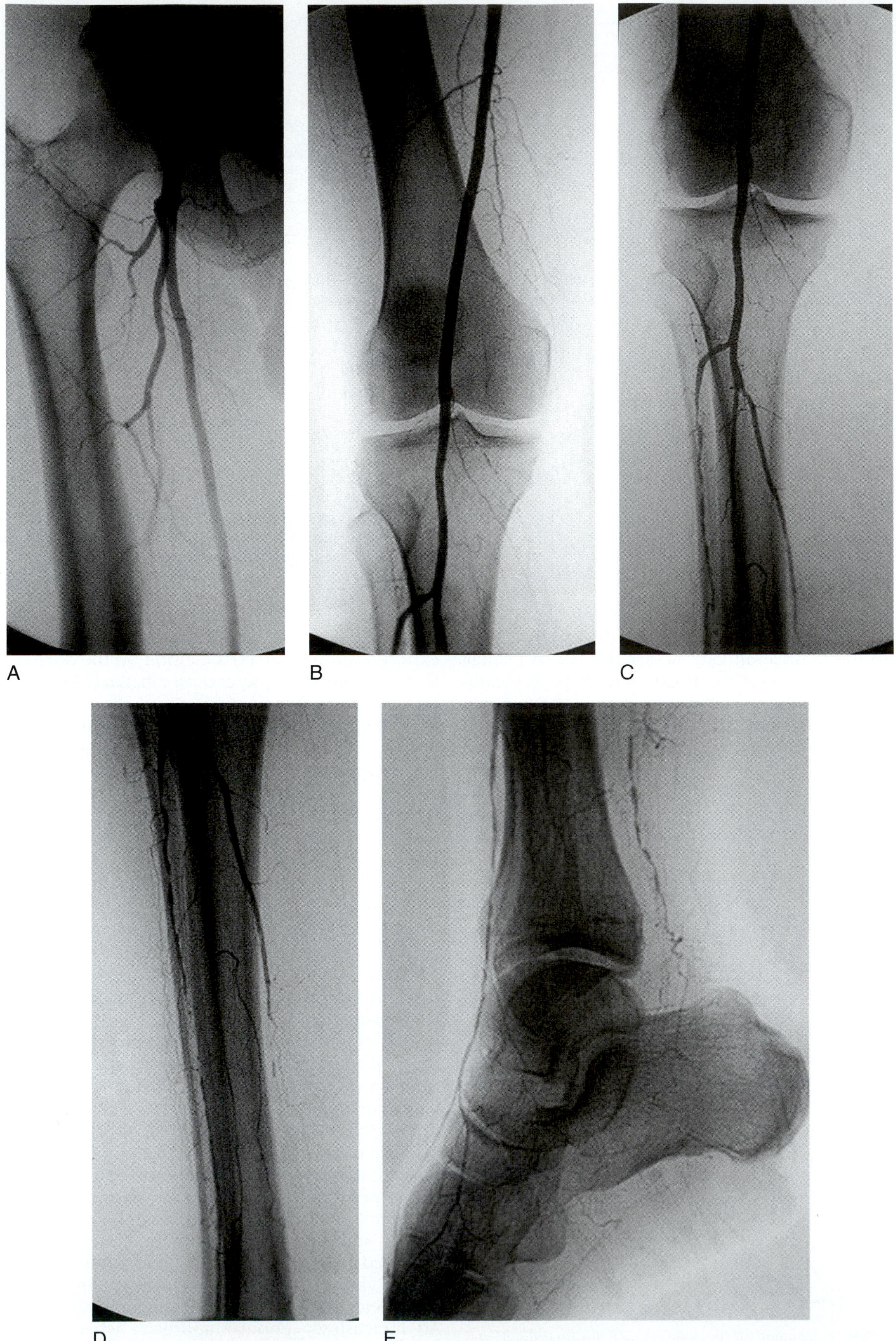

FIGURE 20-10. **A-E**, Arteriogram indicating preservation of the superficial femoral artery and popliteal arteries with mid-calf occlusions of all three infrageniculate vessels. This anatomic pattern of disease is amenable to "distal origin" vein grafting from the below-knee popliteal or proximal posterior tibial artery to the dorsalis pedis artery.

catheter-based treatment of the superficial femoral or popliteal artery inflow with more distal bypass.[90]

Autogenous Vein Bypass

In general, infrainguinal bypass surgery is best performed with autogenous vein conduit, preferably the ipsilateral greater saphenous vein, if available.[91] This is particularly true for grafts extending below the knee, where prosthetic conduits of Dacron or PTFE have significantly poorer patency rates. The first report of a femoropopliteal bypass graft using autogenous greater saphenous vein in a reversed orientation was by Kunlin in 1951.[5] Given the orientation of the vein valves, the vein is reversed such that the distal end of the vein is sewn to the proximal inflow artery and the larger proximal end of the vein is sewn to the distal outflow artery. The vein is harvested through a long incision overlying the course of the vein or by more tedious but less invasive sequential skip incisions with intervening cutaneous skin bridges (see Fig. 20-9). All side branches are ligated and, after harvest, the vein is cannulated and gently dilated with a solution containing heparin and papaverine to assess its suitability. Veins with chronic fibrosis or that fail to dilate to a diameter of 3 mm or greater will likely have poor long-term function.

For prosthetic grafts, a tunnel is usually fashioned through the subsartorial plane between the groin incision and the above-knee popliteal space in the interests of protecting the graft from subsequent infection. For vein conduits, it remains the surgeon's preference as to whether the graft is tunneled deeply or in a superficial location in the subcutaneous space. The more superficial configuration greatly facilitates ongoing clinical examination and ultrasonographic surveillance as well as later surgical revision, but it carries a risk of graft exposure—should there be wound-healing problems. Occlusion from trauma to grafts placed superficially has been of theoretical but not practical concern.

The order of anastomoses is surgeon dependent, with strong feelings expressed in each camp. Before occluding the target vessel, the patient is systemically anticoagulated with 5,000 to 10,000 units of heparin. The artery is then clamped proximally and distally and incised, the vein spatulated, and a beveled anastomosis is carried out. Typically a 5-0 monofilament suture of Prolene is used for the femoral anastomosis, a 6-0 suture is used at the popliteal level, and a very fine 7-0 suture is used at the tibial or pedal level. If the target tibial vessel is deep within the calf and visibility is challenging, a technique of "parachuting" the heel of the distal anastomosis is often employed. After completing the first anastomosis, the graft is carefully marked to ensure against mechanical twisting or kinking of the graft during the tunneling process. One of the benefits of performing the proximal anastomosis first is that following release of the clamps, adequacy of flow through the graft can be assessed.

Occasionally, such extensive calcification of the target vessel is encountered that the risk of a significant injury from clamping, even with the minimally traumatic clamps in use today, is prohibitively high. In such cases, proximal inflow and distal artery backbleeding can be controlled by occlusion balloons placed intraluminally. For distal anastomoses at the knee or more distal level, another alternative technique is the use of a proximally placed sterile pneumatic tourniquet. This is particularly advantageous when sewing to diminutive distal tibial or pedal targets, where the impact of a crush injury or plaque dislodgment on graft function could be considerable. Removing the need for clamps by using the tourniquet has two more advantages. First, it improves the operative visibility. Second, and more importantly, given that less longitudinal and circumferential dissection is needed, the degrees of vessel spasm and venous bleeding that frequently accompany vessel exposure at this level are kept to a minimum.

Flow through the graft and the outflow arteries is assessed following completion of the bypass with a continuous-wave Doppler. Ideally, a contrast angiogram is also performed after directly cannulating the proximal graft (Fig. 20-11); this allows for immediate repair of any technical defects, for example intraluminal thrombus, twisting or kinking of the graft, or retained valve cusps, that are identified (Fig. 20-12).[92] Intraoperative completion duplex ultrasonography is a sensitive screen for hemodynamically significant abnormalities within the graft.[93,94]

Current reports of the 5-year results of reversed saphenous vein graft using modern techniques have been excellent, with primary and secondary patency rates of 75% and 80%, respectively, and limb salvage rates of 90%.[95,96]

In-Situ Grafting

There has been ongoing enthusiasm in some circles for in-situ vein bypass grafting, whereby except for its proximal and distal extent, the greater saphenous vein is left undisturbed in its native bed. This technique was first described in 1962[97] but was later popularized by Leather and Karmody in the late 1970s.[98] Recent reports of in-situ saphenous vein grafting have indicated 5-year graft patency rates approaching 80% and limb salvage rates of 84% to 90%.[96,99-101]

The approach minimizes trauma to the vein during excision and handling and in theory enhances preservation of the vasovasorum and endothelium. It further lowers the considerable risk of wound healing complications seen with traditional vein harvesting and facilitates the creation of more technically precise anastomoses because the proximal and distal vein diameters are more closely matched to those of the inflow and outflow target vessels (Fig. 20-13). The extent of the proximal vein mobilization is dictated by the location of the saphenofemoral junction relative to the proposed site of the proximal anastomosis. It may at times be necessary to perform an endarterectomy of the superficial femoral artery if the length of proximal vein is insufficient. Lysis of the valve cusps is obligatory given the nonreversed configuration, and is facilitated by newer, less traumatic valvulotomes that function safely through the blinded segments of undissected graft. Critics of this technique argue that the advantages listed have not translated into improved graft function or patency. They further argue that the time required and dissection involved in finding and ligating substantial side branches—which can develop into

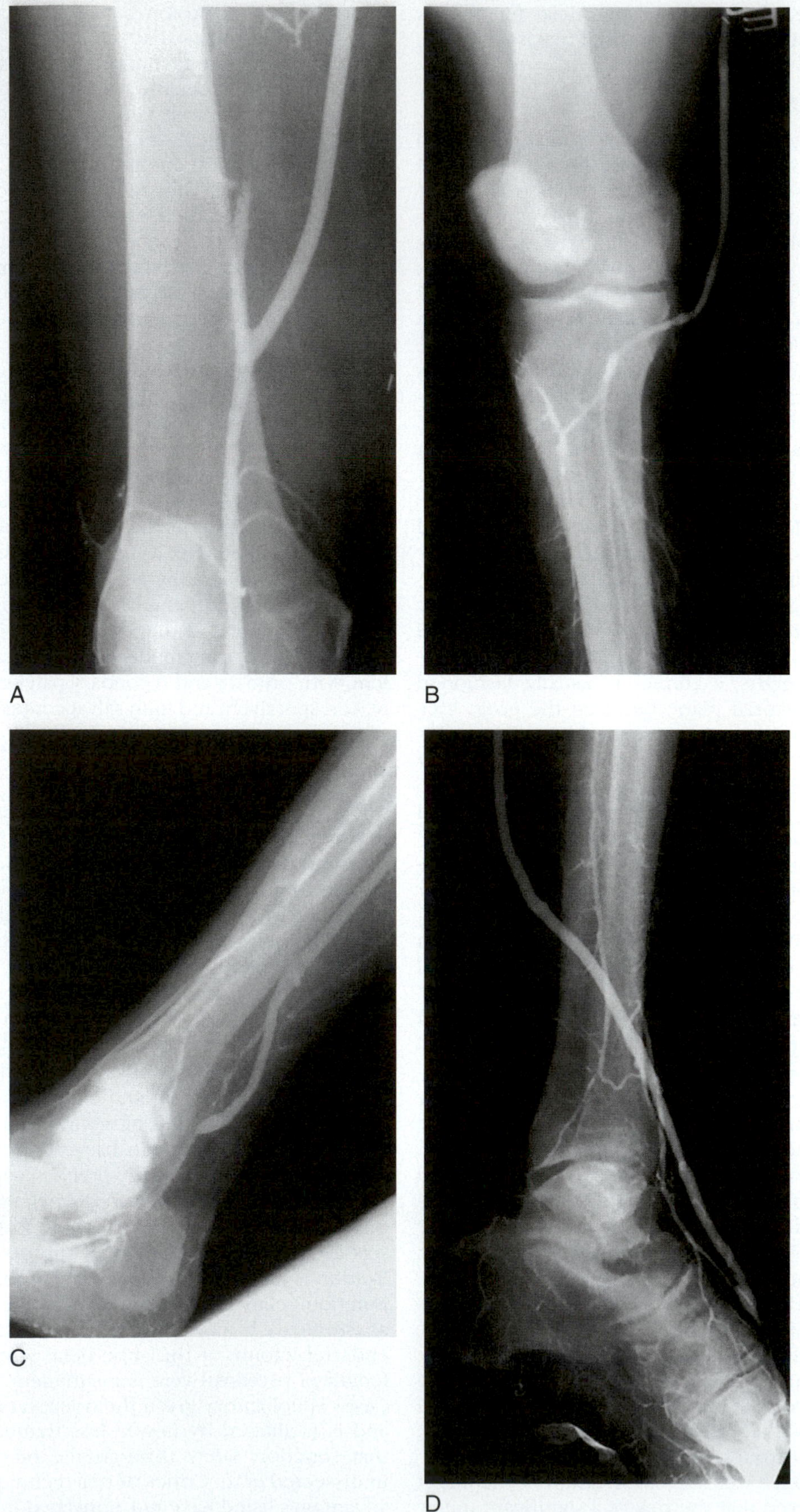

FIGURE 20-11. Intraoperative completion arteriograms of distal anastomoses to the above-knee popliteal (**A**), below-knee popliteal (**B**), distal posterior tibial (**C**), and dorsalis pedis (**D**) arteries.

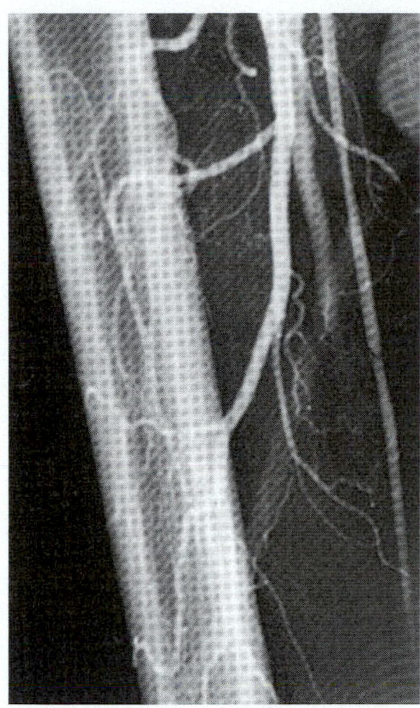

FIGURE 20-12. Intraoperative completion arteriogram of an in-situ femoropopliteal vein graft indicating a retained valve—visualized as a filling defect in the graft, and a persistent arteriovenous fistula.

physiologically important arteriovenous fistulae that "steal" distal flow—obviates the stated benefits of this approach. Newer techniques using angioscopy and endoluminal coiling[102] of larger side branches may help to minimize these concerns.

Angioscopic-assisted valve lysis has been employed for more than a decade, but has not gained widespread favor. Although there is a significant learning curve with this technology, and operative times—at least initially—are significantly prolonged, advocates cite fewer wound complications, shorter hospital stays, and decreased recuperative periods as potential benefits. Proponents of routine angioscopy for direct visualization of valve lysis stress its particular utility in demonstrating such unsuspected endoluminal venous pathology as phlebitic strictures, webs, and fibrotic valve cusps.[103] This adjunct may be particularly useful in cases in which arm vein is used, when endoluminal pathology is more frequently encountered and is presumably partly responsible for suboptimal results.[104]

Nonreversed Saphenous Vein Grafts

Recognizing the many practical advantages inherent to the in-situ technique, Belkin and colleagues and others have modified the approach to infrainguinal bypass grafting with venous conduit to incorporate several of the same principles.[105] In particular, if the harvested vein is tapered to any significant extent, it is used in a nonreversed fashion. By optimizing the size matching between the artery and vein at both the proximal and distal anastomosis sites as discussed earlier, one can often use smaller veins than would be suitable for reversed vein grafting. The nonreversed configuration also allows preservation of the saphenous vein hood, which extends the available conduit length and is especially beneficial when the femoral artery is thick walled and diseased.

The vein is harvested and dilated in a similar fashion to reversed vein grafts and the cusps of the proximal valve of the greater saphenous vein are excised under direct vision with fine Potts scissors. There are currently two main types of valvulotomes available. The modified Mills valvulotome is a short, metal, hockey stick-shaped cutter that can be introduced through the distal end of the vein or through the side branches. After the proximal anastomosis is performed, and with the perfused conduit on gentle stretch, the valves are carefully lysed in a sequential fashion by pulling the valvulotome inferiorly. An alternative, recently designed self-centering valvulotome allows lysis of all valves in a single pass and is believed by some to be less traumatic. Once acceptable pulsatile flow is ensured, the distal anastomosis is performed in the standard fashion.

It is important to note that similar patency rates have consistently been demonstrated regardless of which technique is applied,[100,101] and so surgeon preference and comfort level are acceptable reasons for choosing one method over another.

Prosthetic Bypass

It is recommended that infrainguinal bypass surgery be performed with saphenous vein or an autologous substitute whenever feasible, given the clearly demonstrated enhanced patency rates.[91,106] Some institutions more frequently rely on prosthetic grafts. When the distal target is the above-knee popliteal artery and the tibial outflow is relatively well preserved, this is an acceptable approach because patency rates in this situation approach those of vein grafts.[107] A variety of surgical adjunctive procedures, from patching the distal anastomotic target vessel to the creation of a distal arteriovenous fistula or various autogenous vein cuffs interposed between the distal prosthetic and the target artery, have all been attempted as a means of improving the patency rates of grafts extending below the knee.[108] More recently, flared grafts designed to minimize turbulence and shear stress between the prosthetic and native vessel have gained some popularity. Polyester (Dacron) and PTFE grafts are the two main types of prosthetics available and, as in other anatomic positions, available data show generally equal results with either choice. The entire procedure is carried out through two small proximal and distal incisions between which the graft is tunneled anatomically. The selection of a 6- or 8-mm graft is dictated by the size of the native vessels.

Reoperative Bypass Surgery

As the patient population treated by vascular surgeons has increased in age, and more and more challenging cases are accepted for primary treatment, there has been a corresponding increase in the incidence of reoperative bypass surgery performed for infrainguinal arterial occlusive disease. Such reoperative procedures are particularly challenging, both because of the scarring present at the inflow and ouflow target sites and because there is typically a lack of ipsilateral greater saphenous vein. Whenever possible, the first problem is addressed by choosing anastomotic sites just above or below the previous touchdown

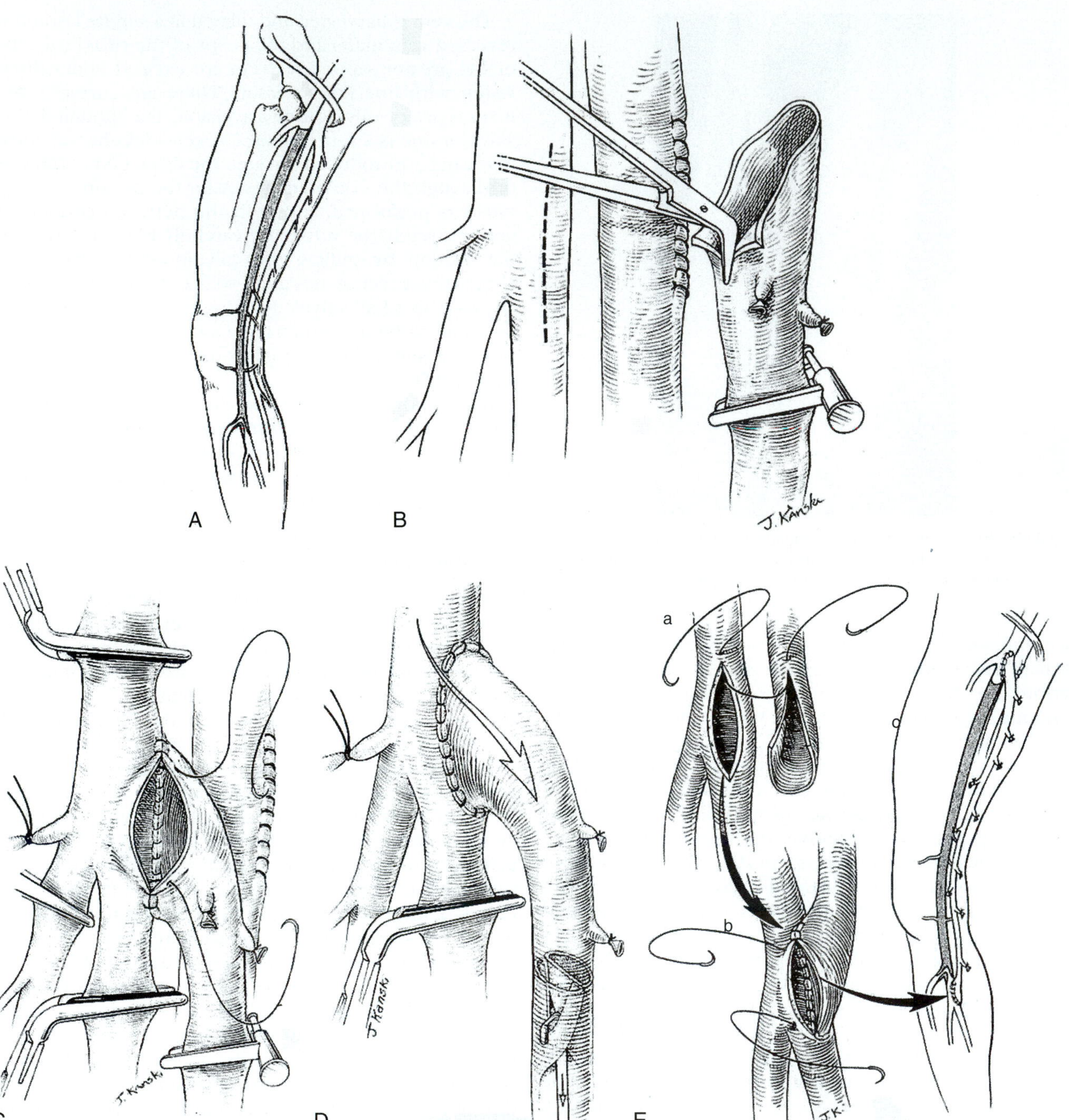

FIGURE 20-13. In the in-situ method of infrainguinal reconstruction, the saphenous vein is left undisturbed in its native bed except at the proximal and distal anastomotic sites—in this case, the common femoral artery and the tibioperoneal trunk, respectively (**A**). The saphenofemoral junction is transected in the groin, the venotomy in the femoral vein is over-sewn, and the proximal end of the saphenous vein spatulated in preparation for anastomosis (**B**). After the first venous valve is excised under direct vision, the graft is anastomosed end-to-side to the femoral artery (**C**). Flow is then restored through the vein graft and the valvulotome passed from the distal end to lyse the residual valves (**D**) before the distal anastomosis is performed (**E**).

points, thereby avoiding dissection through often densely scarred tissue planes. When ipsilateral greater saphenous vein is absent due to prior infrainguinal or coronary artery bypass surgery or prior saphenous vein stripping, there are a number of alternative conduit sites available. Chew and colleagues studied the consequence of using the contralateral greater saphenous vein in these situations and found it to be the optimal conduit; despite the presumably high incidence of contralateral lower extremity as well as coronary occlusive disease in this population, the short- and long-term impacts were found to be minimal.[109]

In the absence of any greater saphenous vein, preoperative venous duplex ultrasonography is employed to evaluate the cephalic and basilic veins of the arms and the lesser saphenous veins of the legs in an effort to

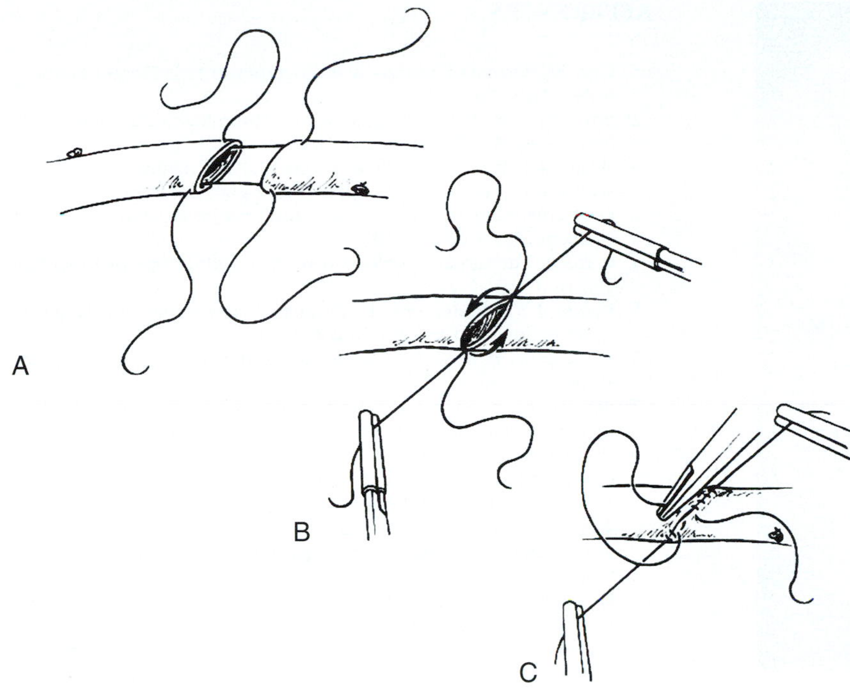

FIGURE 20-14. Creation of a composite graft from two or more segments of arm vein or lesser saphenous vein is sometimes necessary to obtain the desired length of fully autogenous conduit for infrainguinal bypass. A widely spatulated venovenostomy is optimal.

determine the best conduit available. Often the veins distal to the antecubital crease are scarred and of small caliber, but their more proximal counterparts are often of excellent size and quality. The use of arm veins, in general, can be extremely technically challenging and for that reason it has not been universally adopted. The dissection of the basilic vein can be particularly tedious because it has multiple side branches and lies adjacent to several important nerves. Because arm veins are often relatively short, a venovenostomy is often required to create composite grafts long enough to complete the arterial reconstruction (Fig. 20-14). This is performed with generous spatulation of each vein hood to create a widely patent vein-to-vein anastomosis. Given their thin-walled nature, arm vein grafts are also quite prone to twisting and kinking, and special care must to taken during the tunneling process to avoid these problems. The more proximal arm veins can be relatively large, and it is often advantageous to use one or more of the segments in a nonreversed fashion to better match the graft to the inflow vessel size.

Not surprisingly, the results of reoperative infrainguinal bypass surgery do not match those of primary reconstruction. With autogenous vein, 5-year patency rates of 60% and limb salvage rates of 70% to 80% have been reported.[109,110] Coumadin is often used postoperatively in patients with compromised outflow or in whom the conduit was of marginal quality and has been associated with improved long-term patency.[111]

Post Reconstruction Management

Many of the patients undergoing surgical reconstruction for arterial insufficiency will require one or more adjunctive operative procedures of their foot. Small, uninfected ulcerations of the toe or foot often can be safely managed conservatively. However, larger, gangrenous lesions of the toe, forefoot, or heel usually require débridement of all necrotic tissue at the completion of the revascularization procedure. If the ischemia is particularly severe or infection is present, toe or transmetatarsal amputation may be necessary to achieve a margin of healthy tissue. This is particularly important in patients with diabetes or end-stage renal disease, in whom persistent infection or necrosis can result in limb loss, despite the presence of a well-revascularized extremity. The wounds are usually left open and treated with saline wet-to-dry dressings or newer, vacuum sponge dressings. Serial débridements on the ward or in the operating room are often necessary for the larger wounds, which can then be surgically closed after an interval healing period or allowed to slowly close via secondary intention.

Unless otherwise contraindicated, all patients are maintained indefinitely on an antiplatelet regimen with either aspirin or clopidogrel following surgical bypass. As stated earlier, in cases in which a graft is at increased risk of failure, such as in the redo setting or when compromised outflow or a marginal conduit was accepted, the antiplatelet agent may be supplemented with coumadin.[111] Aggressive risk factor modification in the form of smoking cessation, lipid reduction, exercise, blood pressure management, and diabetic blood sugar control is of further paramount importance in minimizing the risk of disease progression or recurrence.[112] More immediately, aggressive rehabilitation maximizes the chances of and shortens the time to a return to full function after extensive reconstructive surgery.

Graft Failure and Surveillance

Postoperative graft failures are typically classified according to the time interval from surgery as early, intermediate,

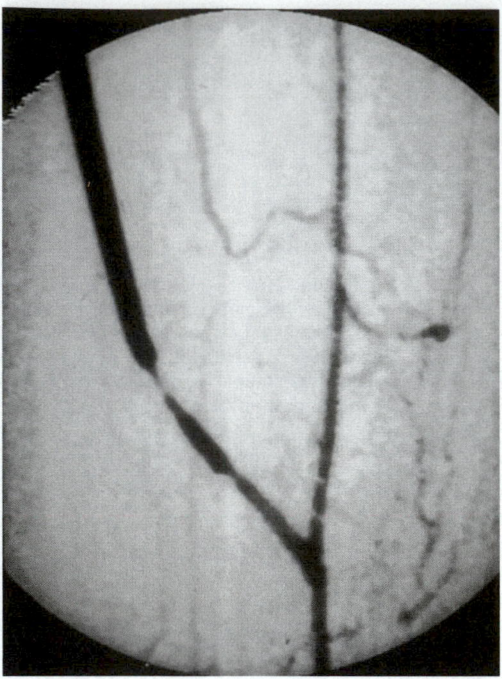

FIGURE 20-15. Arteriogram demonstrating severe stenosis of distal graft from intimal hyperplasia, likely at prior valve site.

or late. Graft thrombosis occurring within 30 days, so-called early graft failures, are generally believed to be due to technical or judgment errors by the surgeon. Included in this list would be such technical errors as twists, kinks, incompletely lysed valves, or anastomotic defects, as well as judgment errors in using a poor-quality vein or targeting an outflow vessel with inadequate runoff to support the graft. Intermediate graft failures include those between 30 days and 2 years and are generally attributed to the proliferation of intimal hyperplasia at the anastomoses or prior valve sites within the graft (Fig. 20-15). Randomized trials are currently underway to determine the impact of genetic modulation of vein grafts on the development of intimal hyperplasia, and hold some promise in reducing or minimizing this significant cause of vein graft failure.[113] Late graft failures occurring beyond 2 years are typically due to progression of atherosclerotic occlusive disease within the inflow or outflow arteries.

Given the known incidence of graft failure and the potentially dire consequence in terms of limb salvage or preservation of limb function in a patient with limited options for secondary or tertiary bypass, the ability to maintain graft patency through early identification and prompt correction of graft stenoses is of paramount importance.[114] Serial postoperative surveillance scanning with a duplex ultrasound has proved an excellent means of accurately identifying hemodynamically significant stenoses within the vein graft that threaten the graft patency.[115] Subsequent confirmation by angiography and prophylactic treatment by percutaneous cutting balloon angioplasty, surgical patch angioplasty, or interposition grafting of significant lesions minimizes the risk of graft thrombosis and ensures optimal long-term graft patency.

REFERENCES

1. Gray EA: Portrait of a surgeon: A biography of John Hunter. London, Robert Hale, 1952.
2. dos Santos JC: Sur la desobstion des thromboses arterielles anciennes. Mem Acad Chir 73:409, 1947.
3. Wylie EJ, Kerr E, Davies O: Experimental and clinical experiences with the use of fascia lata applied as a graft about major arteries after thromboendarterectomy and aneurysmorrhaphy. Surg Gynecol Obstet 93:257, 1951.
4. Carrel A: The surgery of blood vessels, etc. John Hopkins Hosp Bull 190:18, 1907.
5. Kunlin J: Le traitement de l'ischemie arteritique par la greffe veineuse longue. Rev Chir 70:206, 1951.
6. McCaughan JJ, Jr: Surgical exposure of the distal popliteal artery. Surgery 44:536, 1958.
7. Berman JR, Berman LA, Goldstein I: Female sexual dysfunction: Incidence, pathophysiology, evaluation and treatment options. Urology 54:385, 1999.
8. Leriche R, Morel A: The syndrome of thrombotic obliteration of the aortic bifurcation. Ann Surg 127:193, 1948.
9. Wingo JP, Nix ML, Greenfield LJ, Barnes RW: The blue toe syndrome: Hemodynamic and therapeutic correlates of outcome. J Vasc Surg 3:475, 1986.
10. Karmody AM, Powers SR, Monaco VJ, et al: "Blue toe" syndrome. Arch Surg 111:1263, 1976.
11. Brewster DC, Perler BA, Robison JG, et al: Aortofemoral graft for multilevel occlusive disease: Predictors of success and need for distal bypass. Arch Surg 117:1593, 1982.
12. Imparata AM, Kim G, Davidson T, et al: Intermittent claudication: Its natural course. Surgery 78:795, 1975
13. Cronenwett JL, Davis JT, Gooch JB, et al: Aortoiliac occlusive disease in women. Surgery 88:775, 1980.
14. Caes F, Cham B, Van den Brande P, et al: Small artery syndrome in women. Surg Gynecol Obstret 161:165, 1985.
15. Carpenter JP, Owen RS, Holland GA, et al: Magnetic resonance angiography of the aorta, iliac and femoral arteries. Surgery 116:17, 1994.
16. Seldinger SE: Catheter replacement of needle in percutaneous arteriography: New technique. Acta Radiol 39:368, 1953.
17. Udoff EJ, Barth KH, Harrington DP, et al: Hemodynamic significance of iliac artery stenosis: Pressure measurements during angiography. Radiology 132:289, 1979.
18. Spinosa DJ, Kaufmann JA, Hartwell GD: Gadolinium chelates in angiography and interventional radiology: A useful alternative to iodinated contrast media for angiography. Radiology 223:326, 2002.
19. Back MR, Caridi JG, Hawkins IF, et al: Angiography with carbon dioxide (CO_2). Surg Clin North Am 78: 575, 1998.
20. Nehler MR, Hiatt WR: Exercise therapy for claudication. Ann Vasc Surg 13:109, 1999.
21. Regensteiner JG, Meyer TJ, Krupski WC: Hospital versus home-based exercise rehabilitation for patients with peripheral arterial occlusive disease. Angiology 48:291, 1997.
22. Dawson DL, Cutler BS, Hiatt WR, et al: A comparison of cilostazol and pentoxifylline for treating intermittent claudication. Am J Med 109:523, 2000.
23. Martinez BD, Hertzer NR, Beven EG: Influence of distal arterial occlusive disease on prognosis following aortobifemoral bypass. Surgery 88:795, 1980.
24. Hill DA, McGrath MA, Lord RSA, et al: The effect of superficial femoral artery occlusion on the outcome of aortofemoral bypass for intermittent claudication. Surgery 87:133, 1980.
25. Harris PL, Cave-Bigley DJ, McSweeney L: Aortofemoral bypass and the role of concomitant femorodistal reconstruction. Br J Surg 72:317, 1985.
26. Darling RC, Linton RR: Aortoiliofemoral endarterectomy for atherosclerotic occlusive disease. Surgery 110:1458, 1975.
27. Barker WF, Cannon JA: An evaluation of endarterectomy. Arch Surg 66:488, 1953.
28. Crawford ES, Manning LG, Kelly TF: "Redo" surgery after operations for aneurysm and occlusion of the abdominal aorta. Surgery 81:41, 1977.
29. Perdue GD, Long WD, Smith RB III: Perspective concerning aortofemoral arterial reconstruction. Ann Surg 173:940, 1971.
30. Brewster DC, Darling RC: Optimal methods of aortoiliac reconstruction. Surgery 84:739, 1978.

31. Baird RJ, Feldman P, Miles JT, et al: Subsequent downstream repair after aorta-iliac and aorta-femoral bypass operations. Surgery 82:785, 1977.
32. Crawford ES, Bombcrger RA, Glaeser DH, et al: Aortoiliac occlusive disease: Factors influencing survival and function following reconstructive operation over a twenty-five year period. Surgery 90:1055, 1981.
33. Malone JM, Moore WS, Goldstone J: The natural history of bilateral aortofemoral bypass grafts for ischemia of the lower extremities. Arch Surg 110:1300, 1975.
34. Reed AB, Conte MS, Donaldson MC, et al: The impact of patient age and aortic size on the results of aortobifemoral bypass grafting. J Vasc Surg 37:1219, 2003.
35. Menard MT, Chew DK, Chan RK, et al: Outcome in patients at high risk after open surgical repair of abdominal aortic aneurysm. J Vasc Surg 37:285, 2003.
36. Whittemore AD, Clowes AW, Hechtman HB, et al: Aortic aneurysm repair: Reduced operative mortality associated with maintenance of optimal cardiac performance. Ann Surg 173:940, 1971.
37. Kaluza GL, Joseph J, Lee JR, et al: Catastrophic outcomes of noncardiac surgery soon after coronary stenting. J Am Coll Cardiol 35:1288, 2000.
38. Mozersky DJ, Summer DS, Strandness DE: Long-term results of reconstructive aortoiliac surgery. Am J Surg 123:503, 1972.
39. Cooley DA, Wukasch DC, Bennett JG, et al: Double velour knitted Dacron grafts for aortoiliac vascular replacements. Paper presented at Vascular Graft Symposium, National Institutes of Health, Bethesda, Md, November 5, 1976.
40. Yates SG, Barros D'Sa AA, Berger K, et al: The preclotting of porous arterial prosthesis. Ann Surg 188:611, 1978.
41. Nevelsteen A, Wouters L, Suy R: Aorto-femoral Dacron reconstruction for aortoiliac occlusive disease: A 25 year survey. Eur J Vasc Surg 5:179, 1991.
42. Malone JM, Goldstone J, Moore WS: Autogenous profundaplasty: The key to long-term patency in secondary repair of aortofemoral graft occlusion. Ann Surg 188:817, 1978.
43. Morris GC, Jr, Edwards W, Cooley DA, et al: Surgical importance of profunda femoris artery. Arch Surg 82:32, 1961.
44. Rutherford RB, Jones DN, Martin MS, et al: Serial hemodynamic assessment of aortobifemoral bypass. J Vasc Surg 4:428, 1986.
45. Bernhard VM, Ray LI, Militello JP: The role of angioplasty in the profunda femoris artery in revascularization of the ischemic limb. Surg Gynecol Obstet 142:840, 1976.
46. Malone JM, Goldstone J, Moore WS: Autogenous profundaplasty: The key to long-term success and need for distal bypass. Arch Surg 117:1593, 1982.
47. Berguer R, Higgins RF, Cotton LT: Geometry, blood flow, and reconstruction of the deep femoral artery. Am J Surg 130:68, 1975.
48. Juleff RS, Brown OW, McKain MM, et al: The influence of competitive flow on graft patency. J Cardiovasc Surg 33:415, 1992.
49. Pierce GE, Turrentine M, Stringfield S, et al: Evaluation of end-to-side vs. end-to-end proximal anastomosis in aortobifemoral bypass. Arch Surg 117:1580, 1982.
50. Brewster DC, Franklin DP, Cambria RP, et al: Intestinal ischemia complicating abdominal aortic surgery. Surgery 109:447, 1991.
51. Gloviczki P, Cross SA, Stanson AW, et al: Ischemic injury to the spinal cord or lumbosacral plexus after aorto-iliac reconstruction. Am J Surg 162:131, 1991.
52. Seegar JM, Coe DA, Kaelin LD, et al: Routine reimplantation of patent inferior mesenteric arteries limits colon infarction after aortic reconstructions. J Vasc Surg 15:635, 1992.
53. Prinssen M, Buskens E, Blankensteijn JD: Sexual dysfunction after conventional or endovascular AAA repair: Results of a randomized trial. Paper presented at 17th International Congress of Endovascular Interventions, Phoenix, February 12, 2004.
54. Nypaver TJ, Ellenby MI, Mendoza O, et al: A comparison of operative approaches and parameters of success in multilevel arterial occlusive disease. J Am Coll Surg 179:449, 1994.
55. Dalman RL, Taylor LM, Jr, Moneta GL, et al: Simultaneous operative repair of multilevel lower extremity occlusive disease. J Vasc Surg 13:211, 1991.
56. Malone JM, Moore WS, Goldstone J: Life expectancy following aortofemoral arterial grafting. Surgery 81:551, 1977.
57. Szilagyi DE, Hageman JH, Smith RF, et al: A thirty-year survey of the reconstructive surgical treatment of aortoiliac occlusive disease. J Vasc Surg 3:421, 1986.
58. Freeman NE, Leeds FH: Operations on large arteries. Calif Med 77:229, 1952.
59. Blaisdell FW, Hall AD: Axillary-femoral artery bypass for lower extremity ischemia. Surgery 54:563, 1963.
60. LoGerfo FW, Johnson WC, Carson JD, et al: A comparison of the late patency rates of axillo-bilateral femoral and axillo-unilateral femoral grafts. Surgery 81:33, 1977.
61. Harris EJ, Taylor LM, McConnell DB, et al: Clinical results of axillobifemoral bypass using externally supported polytetrafluoroethylene. J Vasc Surg 12:416, 1990.
62. El-Massry S, Saad E, Sauvage LR, et al: Axillofemoral bypass using externally-supported, knitted Dacron grafts: A follow-up through twelve years. J Vasc Surg 17:107, 1993.
63. Broome A, Christenson JT, Ekloff B, et al: Axillofemoral bypass reconstructions in sixty-one patients with leg ischemia. Surgery 88:673, 1980.
64. Taylor LM, Park TC, Edwards JM, et al: Acute disruption of polytetrafluoroethylene grafts adjacent to axillary anastomoses: A complication of axillofemoral grafting. J Vasc Surg 20:520, 1994.
65. Donaldson MC, Louras JC, Buckman CA: Axillofemoral bypass: A tool with a limited role. J Vasc Surg 3:757, 1986.
66. Ascer E, Veith FJ, Gupta SK, et al: Comparison of axillounifemoral and axillobifemoral bypass operations. Surgery 97:169, 1985.
67. Rutherford RB, Patt A, Pearce WH: Extra-anatomic bypass: A closer look. J Vasc Surg 6:437, 1987.
68. Passman MA, Taylor LM, Moneta GL, et al: Comparison of axillofemoral and aortofemoral bypass for aortoiliac occlusive disease. J Vasc Surg 23:263, 1996.
69. Berguer R, Higgins RJ, Reddy DJ: Intimal hyperplasia: An experimental study. Arch Surg 115:332, 1980.
70. Maini BS, Mannick JA: Effect of arterial reconstruction on limb salvage. Arch Surg 113:1297, 1978.
71. Plecha FR, Plecha FM: Femorofemoral bypass grafts: Ten years experience. J Vasc Surg 1:555, 1984.
72. Harrington ME, Harrington EB, Haimov M, et al: Iliofemoral versus femorofemoral bypass: The case for an individualized approach. J Vasc Surg 16:841, 1992.
73. Schneider JR, Besso SR, Walsh DB, et al: Femorofemoral versus aortobifemoral bypass: Outcome and hemodynamic results. J Vasc Surg 19:43, 1994.
74. Couch NP, Clowes AW, Whittemore AD, et al: The iliac-origin graft arterial graft: A useful alternative for iliac occlusive disease. Surgery 97:183, 1985.
75. Kalman PG, Hosang M, Johnston KW, et al: Unilateral iliac disease: The role of iliofemoral bypass. J Vasc Surg 6:139, 1987.
76. Blaisdell FW, DeMattei GA, Gauder PG: Extraperitoneal thoracic aorta to femoral bypass grafts as replacement for an infected aortic bifurcation prosthesis. Am J Surg 102:583, 1961.
77. Criado E, Keagy BA: Use of the descending thoracic aorta as an inflow source in aortoiliac reconstruction: Indications and long-term results. Ann Vasc Surg 8:38, 1994.
78. Dion YM, Gracia CR: A new technique for laparoscopic aortobifemoral grafting in occlusive aortoiliac disease. J Vasc Surg 26:685, 1997.
79. Ahn SS, Hiyama DT, Rudkin GH, et al: Laparoscopic aortobifemoral bypass. J Vasc Surg 26:128, 1997.
80. Kelly JJ, Kercher KW, Gallagher KA, et al: Hand-assisted laparoscopic aortobifemoral bypass versus open bypass for occlusive disease. J Laparoendosc Adv Surg Tech A12:339, 2002.
81. Wisselink W, Cuesta MA, Gracia C, et al: Robot-assisted laparoscopic aortobifemoral bypass for aortoiliac occlusive disease: A report of two cases. J Vasc Surg 36:1079, 2002.
82. McAllister FF: The fate of patients with intermittent claudication managed non-operatively. Am J Surg 132:593, 1976.
83. Walsh DB, Gilbertson JJ, Zwolak RM, et al: The natural history of superficial femoral artery stenoses. J Vasc Surg 14:299, 1991.
84. Faries PF, Morrisey NJ, Teodorescu V, et al: Recent advances in peripheral angioplasty and stenting. Angiology 53:617, 2002.
85. Duda SH, Poerner TC, Wiesenger B, et al: Drug-eluting stents: Potential applications for peripheral arterial occlusive disease. J Vasc Interv Radiol 14:291, 2003.
86. Grassbaugh JA, Nelson PR, Rzucidlo EM, et al: Blinded comparison of preoperative duplex ultrasound scanning and contrast arteriography for planning revascularization at the level of the tibia. J Vasc Surg 37:1186, 2003.

87. Baum RA, Rutter CM, Sunshine JH, et al: Multicenter trial to evaluate vascular magnetic resonance angiography of the lower extremity. JAMA 274:875, 1995.
88. Koelemay MJ, Lijmer JG, Stoker J, et al: Magnetic resonance angiography for the evaluation of lower extremity arterial disease: A meta-analysis. JAMA 285:1338, 2001.
89. Ascher E, Veith FJ, Gupta SK: Bypasses to plantar arteries and other tibial branches: An extended approach to limb salvage. J Vasc Surg 8:434, 1988.
90. Reed AB, Conte MS, Belkin M, et al: Usefulness of autogenous bypass grafts originating distal to the groin. J Vasc Surg. 35:48, 2002.
91. Vieth FJ, Gupta SK, Ascer E, et al: Six-year prospective multicenter randomized comparison of autologous saphenous vein and expanded polytetrafluoroethylene graft in infrainguinal arterial reconstruction. J Vasc Surg 3:104, 1986.
92. Baxter BT, Rizzo RJ, Flinn WR, et al: A comparative study of intraoperative angioscopy and completion arteriography following femorodistal bypass. Arch Surg 125:997, 1990.
93. Gilbertson JJ, Walsh DB, Zwolak RM, et al: A blinded comparison of angiography, angioscopy, and duplex scanning in the intraoperative evaluation of in situ saphenous vein bypass grafts. J Vasc Surg 15:121, 1992.
94. Bandyk D, Johnson B, Gupta A, et al: Nature and management of duplex abnormalities encountered during infrainguinal vein bypass grafting. J Vasc Surg 24:430, 1996.
95. Taylor LM, Edwards JM, Porter JM: Present status of reversed vein bypass grafting: Five-year results of a modern series. J Vasc Surg 11:193, 1990.
96. Fogle MA, Whittemore AD, Couch NP, et al: A comparison of in situ and reversed saphenous vein grafts for infrainguinal reconstruction. J Vasc Surg 5:46, 1987.
97. Hall KV: The great saphenous vein used "in situ" as an arterial shunt after extirpation of vein valves. Surgery 51:492, 1962.
98. Leather RP, Powers SR, Karmody AM: A reappraisal of the in situ saphenous vein arterial bypass: Its use in limb salvage. Surgery 86:453, 1979.
99. Donaldson MC, Mannick JA, Whittemore AD: Femoral-distal bypass with in situ greater saphenous vein: Long-term results using Mills valvulotome. Ann Surg 213:457, 1991.
100. Moody AP, Edwards PR, Harris PL: In situ versus reversed femoropoplitial vein grafts: Long-term follow-up of a prospective, randomized trial. Br J Surg 79:750, 1992.
101. Wengerter KR, Veith FJ, Gupta SK, et al: Prospective randomized multicenter comparison of in situ and reversed vein infrapopliteal bypasses. J Vasc Surg 13:189, 1991.
102. Rosenthal D, Dickson C, Rodriquez F, et al: Infrainguinal endovascular in situ saphenous vein bypass: Ongoing results. J Vasc Surg 20:389, 1994.
103. Panetta Tf, Marin ML, Veith FJ, et al: Unsuspected pre-existing saphenous vein pathology: An unrecognized cause of vein bypass failure. J Vasc Surg 15:102, 1992.
104. Marcaccio EJ, Miller A, Tannenbaum GA, et al: Angioscopically directed interventions improve arm vein bypass grafts. J Vasc Surg 17:994, 1993.
105. Belkin M, Knox J, Donaldson MC, et al: Infrainguinal arterial reconstruction with nonreversed greater saphenous vein. J Vasc Surg 24:957, 1996.
106. Whittemore AD, Kent KC, Donaldson MC, et al: What is the proper role of polytetrafluoroethylene grafts in infrainguinal reconstruction? J Vasc Surg 10:299, 1989.
107. Quinones-Baldrich WJ, Prego AA, Ucelay-Gomez R, et al: Long-term results of infrainguinal revascularization with polytetrafluoroethylene: A ten-year experience. J Vasc Surg 16:209, 1992.
108. Miller JH, Foreman RK, Ferguson L, et al: Interposition vein cuff for anastomosis of prosthesis to small artery. Aust NZ J Surg 54:283, 1984.
109. Chew DK, Owens CD, Belkin M, et al: Bypass in the absence of ipsilateral greater saphenous vein: Safe superiority of the contralateral greater saphenous vein. J Vasc Surg 35:1085, 2002.
110. Belkin M, Conte MS, Donaldson MC, et al: Preferred strategies for secondary infrainguinal bypass: Lessons learned from 300 consecutive reoperations. J Vasc Surg 21:282, 1995.
111. Sarac TP, Huber TS, Back MR, et al: Warfarin improves the outcome of infrainguinal vein bypass grafting at high risk for failure. J Vasc Surg 28:446, 1998.
112. Creager MA: Medical management of peripheral arterial disease. Cardiol Rev. 9:238, 2001.
113. Mann MJ, Whittemore AD, Donaldson MC, et al: Ex-vivo gene therapy of human vascular bypass grafts with E2F: The PREVENT single-centre, randomized, controlled trial. Lancet 354:1493, 1999.
114. Veith FJ, Weiser RK, Gupta SK, et al: Diagnosis and management of failing lower extremity arterial reconstructions prior to graft occlusion. J Cardiovasc Surg 25:381, 1984.
115. Bandyk DF, Schmitt DD, Seabrook GR, et al: Monitoring functional patency of in situ saphenous vein bypasses: The impact of a surveillance protocol and elective revision. J Vasc Surg 9:286, 1989.

chapter 21

Renal Artery Disease: Pathophysiology

Stephen C. Textor
Lilach O. Lerman

Vascular disease affecting the renal arteries presents complex challenges to clinicians. Partly as a result of recent advances in vascular imaging, more patients than ever before are being identified with some degree of atherosclerotic or fibromuscular renovascular disease. Many of these lesions are of minor hemodynamic importance at the time of detection. Some reach a degree at which perfusion pressures and intrarenal hemodynamics are altered, leading to changes in blood pressure regulation and renal function. These can produce a variety of recognizable clinical syndromes[1] as illustrated in Figure 21-1, which range from modest changes in systemic arterial pressure to impaired volume control associated with congestive cardiac failure to threatened viability of the kidney, sometimes designated *ischemic nephropathy*. Understanding the pathways by which renovascular disease affects cardiovascular and renal disease is important for diagnosis and for defining optimal management using tools to block the renin-angiotensin system and to restore the circulation. This chapter will focus on the pathophysiologic events underlying these syndromes.

Most renovascular lesions are the result of atherosclerosis. With the aging of the U.S. and other Western populations and reduced mortality from stroke and coronary disease, the prevalence of vascular disease in other vascular beds reaching clinically "critical" levels appears to be increasing.[1a] Understanding the variety of clinical manifestations of these lesions, the potential for disease progression, and the benefits and limitations of vascular repair are essential for vascular medicine specialists. This chapter will examine the pathophysiology of renovascular lesions regarding blood pressure control, ischemic nephropathy, and clinical syndromes—such as "flash" pulmonary edema. Specific issues regarding diagnostic evaluation and management will be addressed elsewhere.

A wide range of lesions can affect the renal blood supply, some of which are summarized in Table 21-1. Historically, recognition of renovascular disease resulted from searching for underlying causes of hypertension. This followed the seminal observations of Goldblatt more than 60 years ago[2] that renal artery constriction produced a rise in arterial pressure in the dog. These studies were among the first to establish a primary role of the kidney in overall blood pressure regulation. Renovascular hypertension produced by a "clipped" renal artery remains among the most widely studied experimental forms of angiotensin-dependent hypertension.[3]

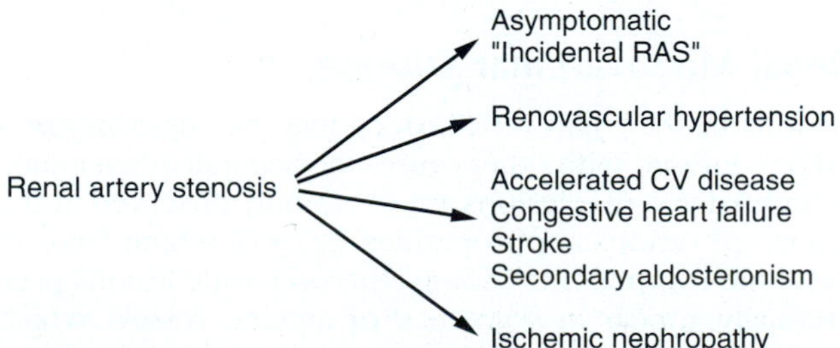

FIGURE 21-1. Renal artery stenosis produces a broad range of manifestations, ranging from "incidental" disease with no hemodynamic effect to deteriorating kidney function and accelerating cardiovascular morbidity. (Modified from Textor SC: Managing renal arterial disease and hypertension. Curr Opin Cardiol 18:260, 2003, with permission.)

TABLE 21-1 VASCULAR LESIONS THAT PRODUCE RENAL HYPOPERFUSION AND RENOVASCULAR HYPERTENSION SYNDROME

Unilateral Disease (analogous to one-clip, two-kidney hypertension)
Unilateral atherosclerotic renal artery stenosis
Unilateral fibromuscular dysplasia (FMD)
Medial fibroplasia
Perimedial fibroplasia
Intimal fibroplasia
Medial hyperplasia
Renal artery aneurysm
Arterial embolus
Arteriovenous fistula (congenital/traumatic)
Segmental arterial occlusion (posttraumatic)
Extrinsic compression of renal artery (e.g., pheochromocytoma)
Renal compression (e.g., metastatic tumor)
Bilateral Disease or Solitary Functioning Kidney (analogous to one-clip, one-kidney model)
Stenosis to a solitary functioning kidney
Bilateral renal arterial stenosis
Aortic coarctation
Systemic vasculitis (e.g., Takayasu's arteritis, polyarteritis)
Atheroembolic disease
Vascular occlusion due to endovascular aortic stent graft

EPIDEMIOLOGY OF RENAL ARTERIAL DISEASE

Fibromuscular disease may be identified in 1% to 3% of normal kidney donors subjected to angiography before donor nephrectomy.[4] Of those patients developing clinical hypertension and referred for revascularization, more than 85% are female with a predilection for disease in the right renal artery.[5] The location of these lesions is most commonly in the mid-portion and distal segments of the renal artery, distal to the ostium. A variety of fibromuscular lesions have been described, but the most common is medial fibroplasia.[6] Occasionally, such lesions may be found in the carotid and other vascular beds, but most commonly they are limited to the renal arteries. Most do not progress to impair renal function, although some lead to arterial dissection and/or thrombosis with ultimate loss of the kidney. Among recent interventional series, the prevalence of fibromuscular lesions has fallen to 16%.[7]

Atherosclerosis is the most common cause of renal arterial disease. Its presence and severity are related to age and the presence of other atherosclerotic diseases in the descending aorta and lower extremities. One population-based series indicates that among 834 subjects older than 65 years, significant renal artery stenosis (defined as a Doppler peak systolic velocity above 1.8 m/s) can be identified in 6.8% of the general population, regardless of race.[8] Recent series of carotid, coronary, and peripheral angiography indicate that the prevalence of renovascular disease corresponds to overall atherosclerotic burden. Incidental renal arterial occlusive disease (>50% stenosis) has been reported in 19% to 24% of patients with coronary disease, and in 35% to 50% of those with iliac artery and more distal peripheral arterial occlusive disease.[9] As expected, risk factors predicting the presence of renal artery stenosis include smoking, hyperlipidemia, hypertension, and diabetes. A corollary observation is that renovascular hypertension resulting from these lesions is now most commonly superimposed gradually on preexisting "essential" hypertension. Hence, the blood pressure response and cure rates after successful restoration of blood flow to the kidney are limited by preexisting conditions.

PATHOPHYSIOLOGIC CONSEQUENCES OF RENOVASCULAR DISEASE

Under basal conditions, renal blood flow is among the highest of all organs. This feature reflects the kidney's filtration function with less than 10% of delivered oxygen being sufficient to maintain renal metabolic needs. Importantly, a fall in renal blood flow is accompanied by decreased oxygen consumption, partly due to reduced metabolic demands of filtration and tubular solute reabsorption. Reduced renal blood flow can be sustained without a measurable change in total kidney oxygen consumption (as assessed by renal vein oxygen tension) or stimulation of erythropoietin release.[10] These observations argue against a direct lack of oxygen as a primary trigger for either hypertension or renal tissue injury, and cast doubt on the use of the term *ischemic* nephropathy. Alternative terms proposed included *azotemic renovascular disease* or *hypoperfusion injury*.[11] Nonetheless, vascular stenosis leading to diminished renal perfusion eventually does lead to renal tissue injury and interstitial fibrosis.

Subcritical Levels of Stenosis

The majority of renal arterial lesions that compromise renal function are caused by gradually developing atherosclerosis of the renal vascular bed. As noted earlier, between 19% and 24% of patients undergoing cardiac catheterization have "incidental" renal lesions producing more than a 50% cross-sectional stenosis[12] for whom the presence of renal artery stenosis is a strong independent predictor of mortality. Moreover, nonobstructive renal artery stenosis (20% to 50% decrease in renal arterial luminal diameter) can be found in an additional 28% of patients undergoing cardiac catheterization[12] and 48% of patients undergoing aortography for peripheral vascular disease.[13] Although lesions producing less than a 50% reduction in arterial luminal diameter are not considered hemodynamically significant, the relationships between resting pressure gradients and angiographic degree of stenosis are curvilinear and only approximate. In some individuals, there can be an abrupt fall in post-stenotic pressures beyond a subcritical range (Fig. 21-2).[14] In some patients with controlled blood pressures, arterial pressure gradients can be observed beyond even mild stenoses[15]; at 50% stenosis severity, the mean pressure gradient may exceed 20 mm Hg.[14] A trans-lesion pressure gradient leading to a decrease in renal perfusion pressure, especially when superimposed on intrarenal disease, may contribute to adverse renal outcomes. Kidneys with a baseline renal artery disease classified as moderate (less than 60% stenosis) have an 11.7% 2-year cumulative incidence of renal atrophy (defined radiologically as a loss of kidney size)[16] and a 28% cumulative incidence of renal artery disease progression, although progression to total renal artery occlusion is uncommon.[17] Increased severity of renal artery stenosis in patients undergoing cardiac catheterization has an adverse effect on survival, with the 4-year adjusted survival rate for patients with a 50% stenosis decreasing to 70% as compared with 89% in patients without renal artery stenosis.[18] Therefore, relatively minor stenosis in the renal artery might have some long-term functional implications, especially in the presence of additional risk factors or coexisting renal disease.

Renal Microvascular Disease

Lesions in the main renal artery may be superimposed on or confused with other causes for ischemic renal injury. Intrarenal vascular lesions are commonly observed in the course of various nephropathies, many of which have an ischemic component.[19] Some atherosclerotic lesions preferentially appear in segmental or arcuate vessels, which are beyond sites amenable to vascular repair with current technologies. Risk factors such as diabetes, hypertension, atherosclerosis, and aging elicit vasoconstriction or structural changes leading to intrarenal small vessel disease and ischemic injury similar to those observed in large vessel disease. The loss of microvessels and

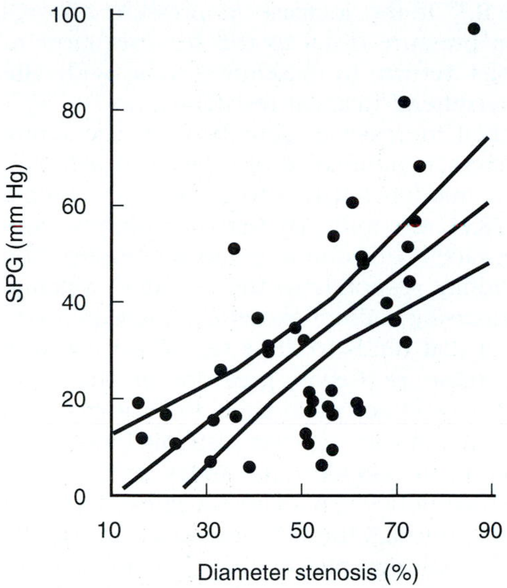

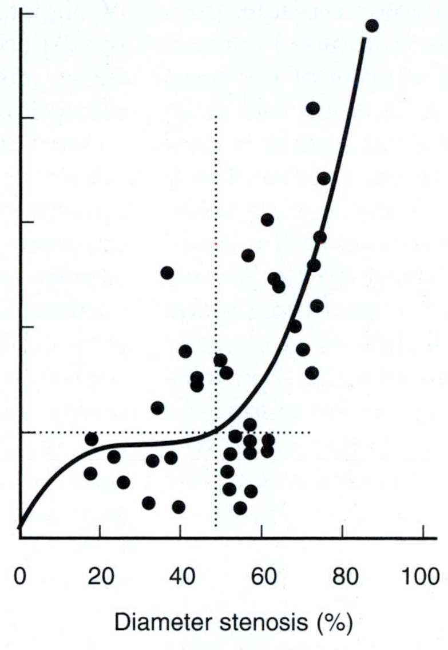

FIGURE 21-2. Relationship between radiologically evident vessel stenosis and measured pressure gradient in atherosclerotic renal artery disease. These data indicate that minor stenosis has minimal hemodynamic effect, but that more severe stenosis is associated with a precipitous rise in pressure gradients across the lesion. SPG, systolic pressure gradient. (From Gross CM, Kramer J, Weingartner O, et al: Determination of renal arterial stenosis severity: Comparison of pressure gradient and vessel diameter. Radiology 220:751, 2001, with permission.)

impaired capillary repair correlate with the development of glomerular and tubulointerstitial scarring[20] and may lead to end-stage renal failure. Renal microvascular disease distal to a stenosis in the renal artery may perpetuate and exacerbate renal parenchymal injury and may blunt renal recovery. The presence of small microvessel injury is difficult to verify but may account for changes in diastolic blood flow, such as those producing changes in renal resistance index. Elevations of renal resistance index are strong predictors of poor outcome in many renal diseases, including renovascular disease.[21]

Critical Renal Artery Stenosis

High-grade vascular stenosis eventually leads to a decrease in renal perfusion pressure. "Critical" stenosis is identified when it produces a fall in renal blood flow and glomerular filtration rate. During experimental renal artery occlusion, the kidney sustains autoregulation of blood flow through a range of perfusion pressures from 200 mm Hg to approximately 80 mm Hg. The mechanisms of autoregulation include myogenic responses to changes in wall tension, release of vasoactive substances, and the tubulo-glomerular feedback. The latter responds to decreased renal perfusion pressure and salt delivery by decreasing vascular resistance distal to the obstruction. In addition, the kidney activates multiple pathways that elevate systemic blood pressure during a fall in renal perfusion pressure, an effect which tends to restore renal perfusion and sustain renal blood flow at the expense of arterial hypertension (Fig. 21-3). Consequently, as long as systemic arterial pressure is allowed to rise, a fall in renal blood flow does not occur until renal arterial diameter is reduced by 65% to 75%. The critical level of acute renal artery stenosis leading to a decrease in renal blood flow in dogs is approximately two thirds luminal obstruction.[22]

When the reduction of renal perfusion pressure develops gradually, additional mechanisms are recruited that protect the kidney from the functional and morphologic consequences observed after acute ischemic injury.[23,24] These include development of collateral vessels and redistribution of intrarenal blood flow from the cortex to the medulla. Renal cortical blood flow autoregulates more efficiently than that of the outer medulla, which is continuously at the verge of anoxia. During chronic reduction of renal blood flow, medullary perfusion is relatively maintained by adaptive mechanisms at the expense of cortical blood flow. When post-stenotic renal artery pressures eventually fall, either due to progressive vascular occlusion or to reduction of systemic blood pressures by drug therapy, renal volume decreases.

In clinical terms, renal *atrophy* is defined as a loss of renal length by at least one centimeter, and a difference in size between the two kidneys is suggestive of unilateral renal artery stenosis (or a higher grade of stenosis in one

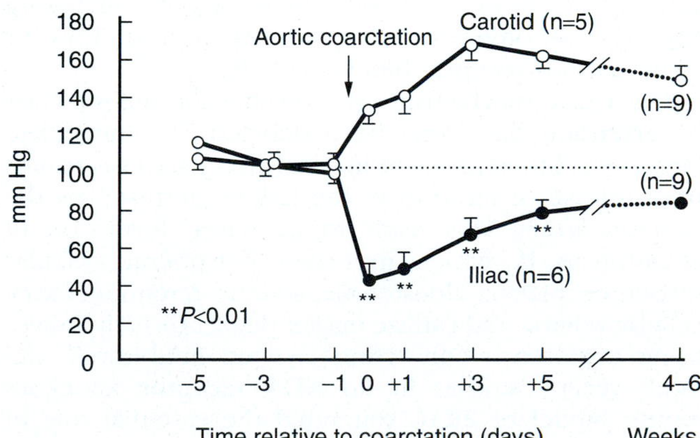

FIGURE 21-3. Development of arterial hypertension after placement of a renal artery clip lesion in a conscious rat aortic coarctation model. Post-stenotic pressures (iliac artery) rise to near baseline levels at the expense of systemic arterial pressures (carotid). Despite a significant pressure gradient, renal perfusion is maintained. Reduction of systemic pressures, however, lowers renal perfusion and activates pressor systems, including the renin-angiotensin system (see text). (Reproduced with permission from Textor SC, Smith-Powell L: Post-stenotic arterial pressure, renal haemodynamics and sodium excretion during graded pressure reduction in conscious rats with one- and two-kidney coarctation hypertension. J Hypertens 6:311, 1988.)

of the kidneys). A decrease in renal volume results from a decrease in filling pressure, filtrate, and blood content of the kidney, as well as structural atrophy of the renal tubules due to apoptosis and necrosis. Apoptosis is an active, preprogrammed form of cell death, which is intricately regulated and distinct from cellular necrosis. These changes may be reversible because tubular cells show vigorous potential for regeneration. However, if a blood flow deficit persists, permanent damage to the kidney may occur. As mentioned earlier, decreased renal blood flow is often accompanied by a decline in glomerular filtration rate (GFR) and inhibition of tubular epithelial transport, which limit renal oxygen consumption and maintain oxygen saturation. Hence, the kidney is not conventionally considered to suffer ischemia until an extreme decrease in renal blood flow develops.

Renovascular Hypertension

Goldblatt and colleagues were the first to show in 1934 that obstruction of the renal artery is followed by an increase in systemic blood pressure.[2] The characteristics of renovascular hypertension depend to a large extent on the status of the kidneys. Unilateral renal artery stenosis may be present with an intact contralateral renal artery (the experimental form is termed *two-kidney, one-clip*, or 2K1C). This model is characterized by counter-regulatory processes in the contralateral kidney leading to sodium excretion in response to elevated arterial pressure ("pressure natriuresis") (Fig. 21-4 A and B). Alternatively, renal artery stenosis may affect a solitary kidney (*one-kidney, one-clip*, or 1K1C) (Fig. 21-5 A and B). Bilateral renal artery stenosis and 1K1C lead to more severe renovascular hypertension, although bilateral renal artery stenosis may behave similarly to 2K1C if one kidney is significantly less ischemic than the other. Patients with this constellation of findings have higher mortality, are more prone to circulatory congestion, and are more likely to experience deterioration of kidney function during administration of antihypertensive agents, including angiotensin-converting enzyme (ACE) inhibitors or angiotensin II receptor blockers (ARBs).

The exact mechanisms responsible for renovascular hypertension have long been debated. The immediate increase in blood pressure in renal artery stenosis results from release of renin from the kidney perfused by the stenotic artery. This leads to increased formation of angiotensin II, which increases peripheral vascular resistance, plasma aldosterone, sodium retention, extracellular volume, and cardiac output (Fig. 21-6). Early studies using angiotensin-converting enzyme inhibitors[25] and more recent studies in an ATIA receptor knockout mouse model of 2K1C reiterated the essential role of angiotensin II in mediating Goldblatt hypertension during its initial phase.[26] Blockade of angiotensin action in experimental models prevents the initial series of events and delays the development of renovascular hypertension indefinitely. Activation of the sympathetic nervous system also plays an important role in the pathogenesis of renovascular hypertension,[27] primarily via the renal afferent nerves. Both the peripheral and central components of the autonomic system are also under the influence of angiotensin II.[27] If the increase in pressure restores renal perfusion pressure distal to the stenosis, most of these alterations return to baseline levels, with the exception of peripheral vascular resistance.

After the initial increase in activity from the renin-angiotensin system, maintenance of renovascular hypertension in 1K1C models appears to depend on volume expansion. In 2K1C, the interplay between plasma-renin activity and extracellular volume is more complex. The contralateral kidney responds to the elevated systemic pressure by increasing sodium excretion (pressure natriuresis), an effect that tends to drive the blood pressure down and decrease perfusion pressure of the post-stenotic kidney. This effect again leads to an increase in renin release, which in turn elevates systemic blood pressure, and so on. In high-grade renal artery stenosis, this cycle of events may induce extracellular volume depletion and renal failure. Although these features are consistently demonstrated in experimental models, human renovascular hypertension frequently has elements of both 1K and 2K pathophysiology, particularly when the function of the contralateral kidney is compromised.

It is important to recognize that activation of the systemic renin-angiotensin system is temporary in renovascular hypertension. After a period of time, circulating levels of plasma-renin activity and angiotensin fall, despite sustained elevation of peripheral vascular resistance. This may be the result both of a slow-response to angiotensin II through which low levels of angiotensin have pressor actions and of recruitment of additional mechanisms of vasoconstriction. The latter include activation of vasoconstrictor lipoxygenase products, oxidative stress, and endothelin. Additional rise in pressure results from an imbalance between vasoconstrictors and vasodilators, such as that derived from decreased bioavailability of nitric oxide. An important role is ascribed to dissociation among systemic blood pressure levels, extra-cellular volume, and inappropriate levels of angiotensin II.[28] The complexity of these relationships partly explains the failure of measuring any single pathway to predict blood pressure responses to renal revascularization.[29]

Accelerated Hypertension and Pulmonary Edema

Series of patients referred for renal revascularization in the last decade have included older patients with more widespread atherosclerotic disease than ever before.[9,30] This reflects improved medical care leading to better blood pressure control and reduced mortality from coronary and cerebrovascular diseases. Patient demographics commonly include more women than men and a high prevalence of coronary disease, heart failure, and cerebrovascular disease. In some cases, suspicion arises regarding renal artery stenosis because of rapid acceleration of these processes, particularly the rapid rise in arterial pressure in a previously stable patient. When untreated, a cycle of malignant phase hypertension and hyponatremia (attributed to the dipsogenic action of angiotensin II) may ensue. In other cases, symptoms include recent progression of hypertension followed by neurological symptoms of an acute stroke.

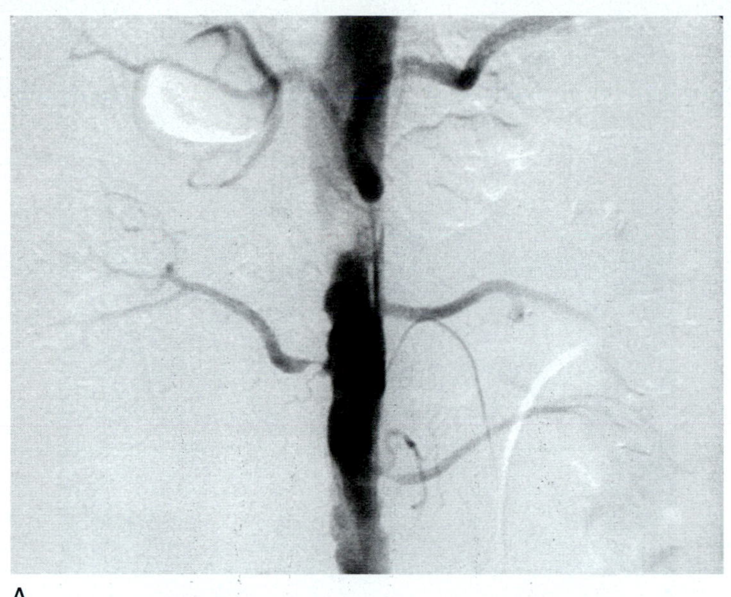

A

Unilateral Renal Artery Stenosis

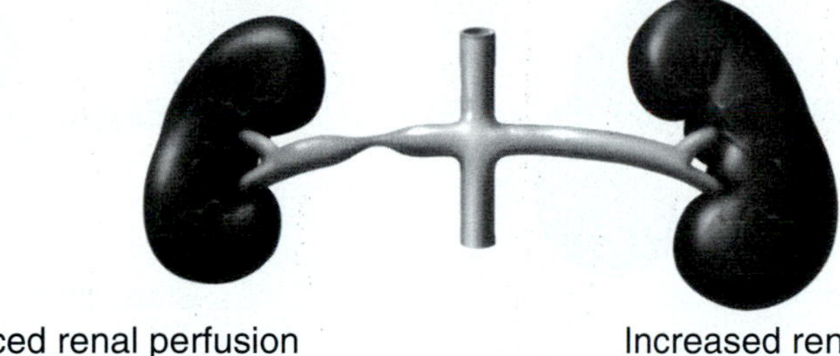

Reduced renal perfusion → ↑ Renin-angiotensin system (RAS), ↑ Renin, ↑ Angiotensin II, ↑ Aldosterone → Angiotensin II-dependent hypertension

Increased renal perfusion → Supressed RAS; Increased Na^+ excretion (pressure natriuresis)

Effect of blockade of RAS

Reduced arterial pressure

Enhanced lateralization of diagnostic tests

Glomerular filtration rate (GFR) in stenotic kidney may fall

Diagnostic tests

Plasma renin activity elevated

Laterlized features (e.g., renin levels in renal veins, captopril-enhanced renography)

B

FIGURE 21-4. A, Angiogram of unilateral renal arterial stenosis with well-preserved vascular supply to the contralateral kidney. **B,** Schematic illustrating the pathophysiology of unilateral renovascular hypertension (two-kidney, one-clip). The stenotic kidney responds to reduced perfusion with activation of the renin-angiotensin system producing widespread effects, including a rise in arterial pressure. Elevated pressures, however, subject the nonstenotic kidney to "pressure natriuresis" leading to asymmetric sodium excretion, a fall in blood pressure, and continued stimuli to the stenotic kidney. Such asymmetry is the basis for diagnostic testing, such as captopril renography and renal vein renin measurements.

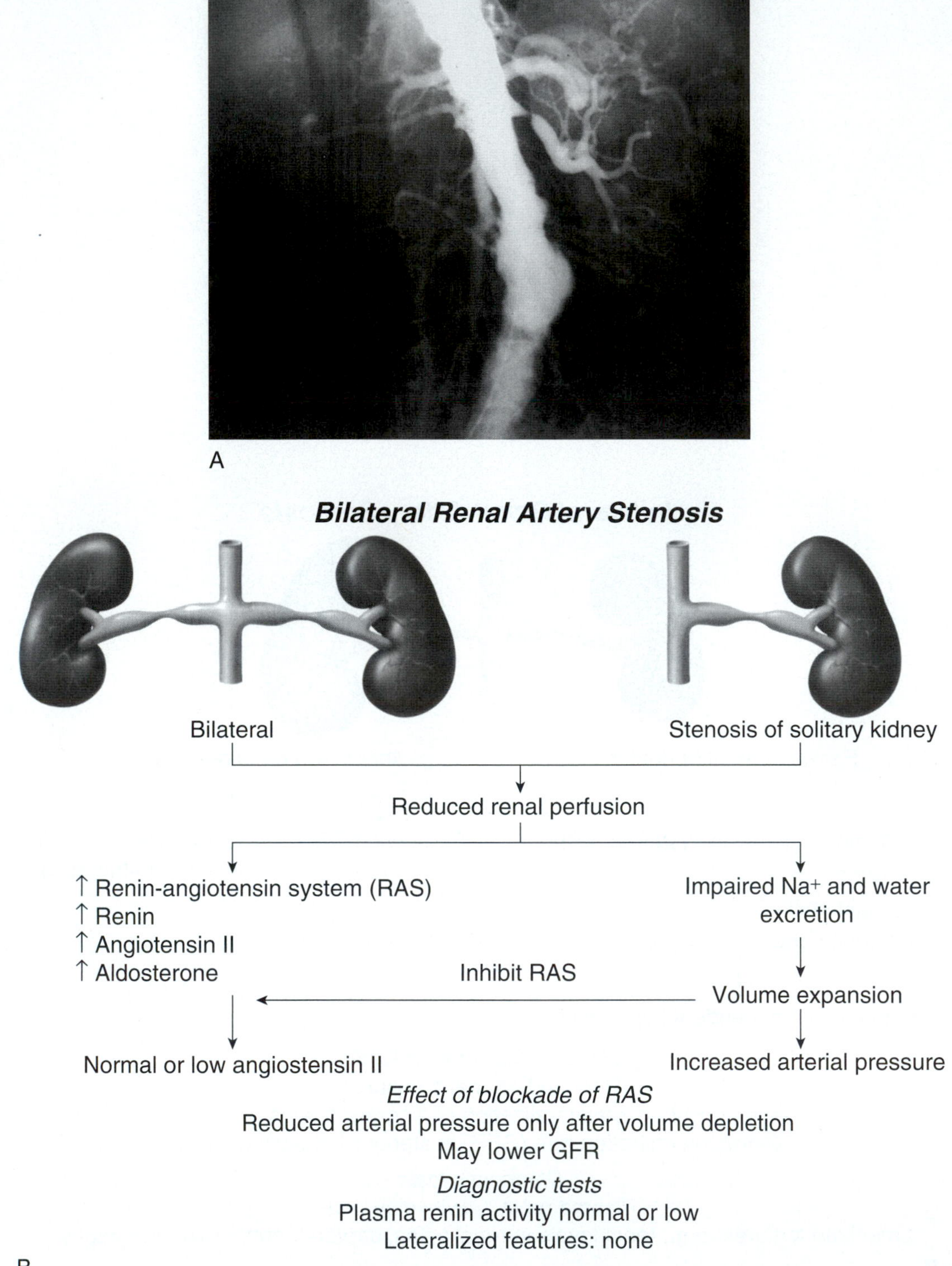

FIGURE 21-5. **A,** Angiogram illustrating renal artery stenosis affecting the entire renal mass—in this case a solitary functioning kidney. The contralateral kidney is occluded. **B,** Schematic illustrating the pathophysiology of renovascular hypertension in which stenosis affects the entire renal mass. In the absence of a normal contralateral kidney, sodium retention occurs and hypertension is heavily dependent on volume mechanisms.

Some patients develop cycles of worsening congestive heart failure out of proportion to left ventricular dysfunction, sometimes designated "flash" pulmonary edema.[31] Many of these patients have bilateral disease or stenosis to a solitary functioning kidney. When volume expands, renal function may improve slightly at the price of hypertension and circulatory congestion. Sudden pulmonary edema may partly reflect diastolic dysfunction precipitated by a rapid rise in afterload,[32] in addition to impaired sodium excretion as a result of renal

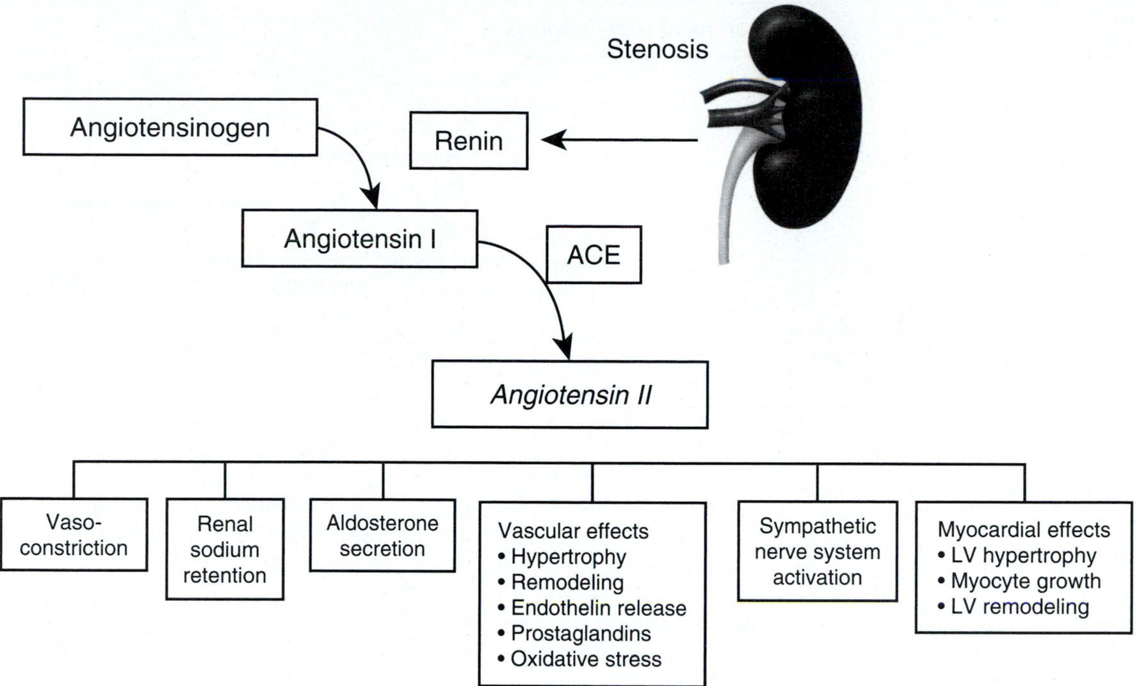

FIGURE 21-6. Actions of angiotensin II in the generation of renovascular hypertension. In addition to direct effects on vascular tone and sodium homeostasis, angiotensin II modulates and induces vasoconstriction by several independent mechanisms, including oxidative stress. Induction of "slow pressor" responses are associated with reduction of circulating levels of plasma-renin activity and loss of demonstrable pressure dependence on angiotensin II (see text). LV, left ventricular.

hypoperfusion. During volume depletion, serum creatinine commonly rises with evidence of prerenal azotemia. This condition warrants recognition, because several series indicate that cycles of symptomatic exacerbation and hospitalization can be improved with successful renal revascularization.[33-35]

Renal Hypoperfusion Injury: Ischemic Nephropathy

The precise mechanisms responsible for irreversible renal scarring in ischemic nephropathy in the absence of true ischemia have not been fully elucidated. They are likely related to interaction among several systems activated in the kidney, the most prominent among which is the renin-angiotensin system.

Renal Vasoactive Hormonal Systems: Angiotensin II

Renal hypoperfusion is accompanied by activation of the renin-angiotensin system, a mechanism normally designed to regulate volume homeostasis and maintain GFR during a transient decrease in renal perfusion pressure. Angiotensin II maintains glomerular capillary pressure and GFR by way of its predominant vasoconstrictor effect on the efferent arteriole. The importance of angiotensin II for preserving GFR is most evident under conditions of reduced preglomerular arterial pressures, particularly under conditions of volume depletion.[36] This feature underlies the fall in GFR sometimes observed following administration of angiotensin-converting enzyme inhibitors to patients with renal artery stenosis, particularly when the entire renal mass is affected.

The range of angiotensin II effects in the kidney includes induction of cell hypertrophy and hyperplasia, and stimulation of hormone synthesis and ion transport. Its renal actions are mediated primarily through ATI receptors expressed on endothelial, epithelial, and vascular cells. Chronic activation of ATI receptors in renal ischemic injury[37] may elicit local inflammatory and fibrogenic responses. Angiotensin II has been implicated in the stimulation of vascular smooth muscle and mesangial cell growth, platelet aggregation, generation of superoxide, activation of adhesion molecules and macrophages, infiltration of inflammatory cells, increased expression of extracellular matrix (ECM) proteins, and induction of proto-oncogenes.

The intrarenal effects of angiotensin II during renal ischemia are modulated by interactions with other humoral systems (Fig. 21-7). Vasodilator prostaglandins attenuate vasoconstriction caused by angiotensin II and may limit ischemia caused by elevated levels of this hormone.[38] Nitric oxide negates many actions of angiotensin II, modulates the effects of angiotensin II on the afferent arteriole and the proximal tubule, and downregulates ACE and AT1 gene expression.[39] By contrast, endothelin-1 regulates renal angiotensin-converting enzyme expression, mediates some of the vascular effects of angiotensin II and amplifies its pressor effects, and activates a similar signal transduction pathway for growth- and differentiation-related genes. Thromboxane A_2, a vasoconstrictor metabolite of arachidonic acid, is also released within the kidney by angiotensin II and

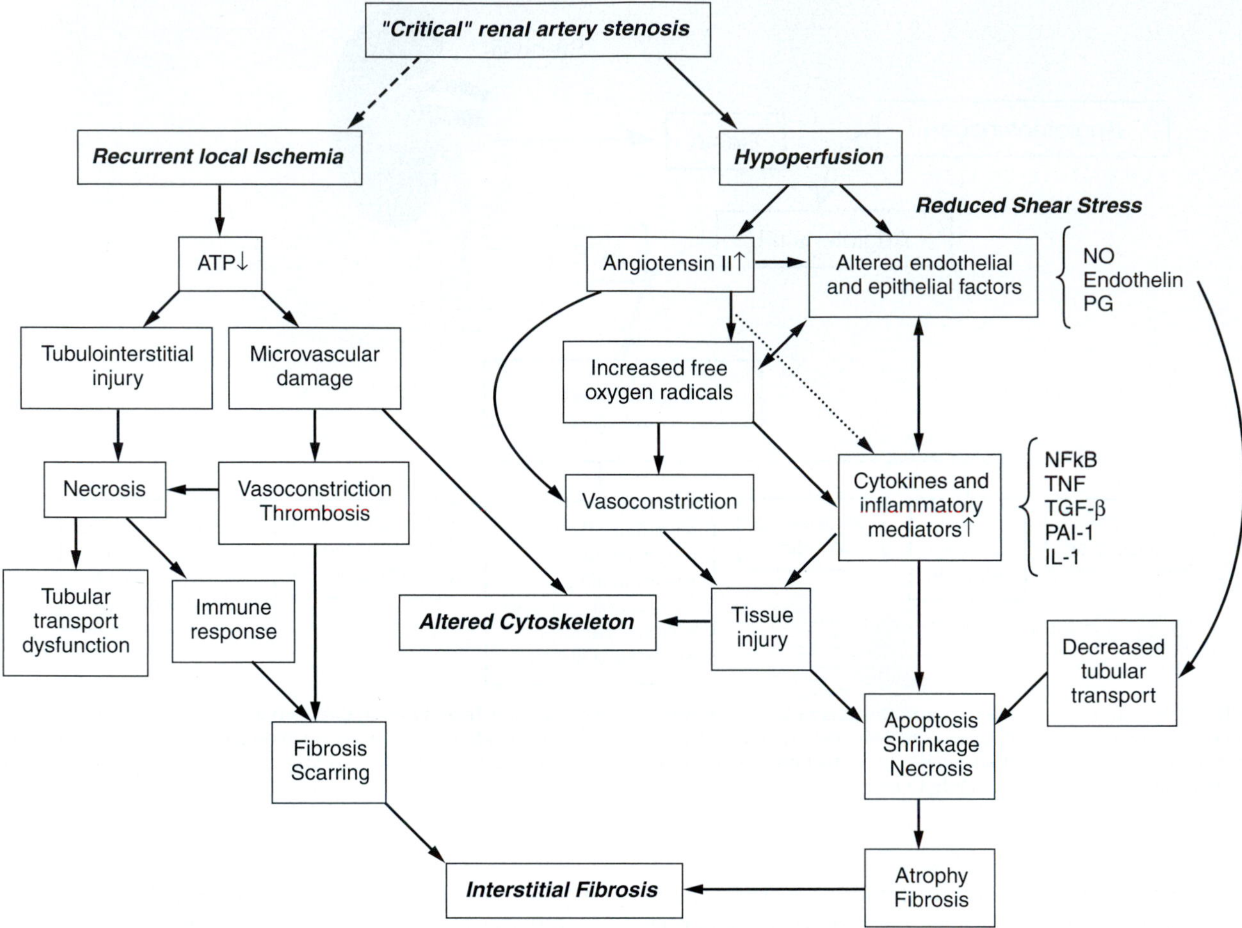

FIGURE 21-7. Proposed pathways by which renal hypoperfusion activates fibrogenic mechanisms within the kidney and ultimately produce irreversible parenchymal injury and interstitial fibrosis. Both intermittent local ischemia (*shown on the left*) and vasoconstrictor-mediated cytokine-mediated pathways (*right*) participate in this process. ATP, adenosine triphosphate; IL-1, interleukin-1; NFkB, nuclear factor κB ; PAI, plasminogen activator inhibitor; TGF-β, transforming growth factor-β; TNF, tumor necrosis factor. (From Lerman L, Textor SC: Pathophysiology of ischemic nephropathy. Urol Clin North Am 28:793, 2001.)

mediates much of the pressor and renal hemodynamic responses to angiotensin II.[40] Thus, angiotensin II is involved in renal adaptive response to ischemia, but long-term activation of the renin-angiotensin system and its interaction with other humoral systems can lead to progressive destruction of renal tissue.

Nitric Oxide in the Kidney

Nitric oxide is synthesized from L-arginine within the kidney by a family of nitric oxide synthases, and plays a crucial role in the regulation of renal hemodynamics and excretory function. The differential expression, localization, and regulation of three isoforms of nitric oxide synthase (NOS) expressed in the kidney, namely neuronal (nNOS), inducible (iNOS), and endothelial (eNOS) isoforms, contribute to diverse intrarenal actions.[41] Consequently, nitric oxide reduces renal vascular tone, increases sodium excretion by inhibiting solute transport in the proximal tubule and collecting duct, and nitric oxide released from the macula densa participates in tubulo-glomerular feedback by modulating vascular tone of the afferent arteriole. In addition, it has antithrombotic actions, inhibits growth-related responses to injury, and modulates the aforementioned renal actions of angiotensin II. Nitric oxide further buffers many processes implicated in the pathogenesis of tissue injury in renovascular disease, including growth of vascular smooth muscle cells, mesangial cell hypertrophy and hyperplasia, and synthesis of ECM. Regulation of renal blood flow, however, becomes less dependent on eNOS-derived nitric oxide and more dependent on prostaglandins as renal artery stenosis progresses[42] because of a decrease in renal perfusion pressure and vascular shear stress distal to the stenosis, which are the primary stimuli to eNOS.

The role of nitric oxide in renal tissue ischemia is complex. The iNOS isoform is upregulated during renal ischemia,[43] and generates nitric oxide fluxes that can be cytotoxic to renal epithelial cells and contributes to tubular injury, both by decreasing the activity of the eNOS isoform and by formation of the oxidant peroxynitrite.

Endothelins

The *endothelin* peptides comprise a family of peptides produced and released from endothelial cells that have potent and long-lasting vasoconstrictor effects on the renal microcirculation and modify tubular function. Endothelin release can be stimulated by angiotensin II, thrombin, transforming growth factor (TGF)-β, and other cytokines (e.g., tumor necrosis factor-α, interleukin-1-β). Tissue levels of endothelin-1 are increased in the post-stenotic kidney,[44] and, in fact, in most forms of renal failure, and may persist for days after resolution of the initial injury. Chronic blockade of the endothelin A receptor directly inhibits cellular growth and gene expression, and in ischemic acute renal failure provides long-term functional and morphologic benefits greater than those observed during simultaneous blockade of both the A and B receptors,[45] likely because of the role of the latter in eliminating salt.

Prostaglandins

Prostaglandins are cyclooxygenase-dependent derivatives of arachidonic acid that have important roles in maintaining renal blood flow and glomerular filtration. Biosynthesis of vasodilator prostaglandins, like prostacyclin and prostaglandin E_2, protects the kidney against the effects of prolonged ischemia or extreme environmental changes and prevents hypoxic tissue injury. In renal artery stenosis, they selectively prevent preglomerular constriction, and thus limit a fall in GFR in the kidney perfused by a stenotic artery,[46] potentially through regulatory interactions with nitric oxide. Conversely, thromboxane A_2 is an endothelium-derived vasoconstrictor prostaglandin that is upregulated in kidneys with renovascular disease.[47] It is released within the kidney by reactive oxygen species or angiotensin II, modulates some of the deleterious effects of angiotensin II and endothelin-1, and contributes to the progression of kidney disease.[48] Blockade of thromboxane A_2 receptors improves urine volume, glomerular filtration rate, and renal plasma flow in ischemic kidneys, and exerts a variety of beneficial effects that reduce the severity of ischemic damage.

Oxidative Stress

A growing body of evidence implicates increased generation of reactive radical species in the mechanisms of renal injury in renovascular disease.[49,50] Angiotensin II is a potent stimulus for superoxide production via the membrane NADH/NADPH oxidase system, and xanthine oxidase is also an important source of oxygen-free radicals during renal ischemia. Increased oxidative stress can promote the formation of a variety of vasoactive mediators, including endothelin-1, leukotrienes, and prostaglandin F_2 α-isoprostanes—endogenous products of lipid peroxidation. In addition, a chemical reaction between superoxide anion and nitric oxide not only decreases the bioavailability of nitric oxide but also leads to the production of toxic species (e.g., peroxynitrite [$ONOO^-$]). In mesangial cells, superoxide promotes hypertrophy and ECM production, by both interaction with nitric oxide and by acting as an intracellular signal for growth-related responses, such as activation of mitogen-activated protein kinase.[51] Reactive oxygen species are implicated in the pathogenesis of ischemic renal injury by causing lipid peroxidation of cell and organelle membranes and disrupting the structural integrity and capacity for cell transport and energy production, especially in the proximal tubule. Activation of growth factors and cytokines, such as nuclear factor κB,[52] may also play an important role in the mechanism of action of angiotensin II and reactive oxygen species. Studies in humans confirm that oxidative stress contributes to the impairment in endothelium-dependent vasodilation observed in patients with renovascular hypertension, which can be reversed with successful renal revascularization.[53]

The fibrogenic factors TGF-β, tissue inhibitor of metalloproteinases (TIMP)-1, and plasminogen activator inhibitor (PAI)-1, which are upregulated in post-stenotic kidneys,[52] are important mediators of ECM synthesis that characterizes progression of renal tissue injury. Early induction of TGF-β via the ATI receptor plays a major role in tissue fibrosis[54] by increasing type IV collagen deposition, and may play a role in the interstitial scarring observed in chronic renal injury characterized by increased activity of intrarenal angiotensin II.[55] TGF-β interacts with endothelin and several growth factors and cytokines in promoting progressive interstitial fibrosis,[56] but also participates in post-ischemic renal healing.

Tubular Cells

Acute ischemic renal failure is characterized by a rapid decline in adenosine triphosphate (ATP) that leads to secondary cascades of cellular injury, including increases in intracellular calcium, activation of phospholipases, and generation of oxygen radicals, which cause significant surface membrane damage.[57] The susceptible proximal tubule cells are primarily responsible for the pathophysiological and clinical aspects of ischemic acute renal failure. Of central importance are disruption and dissociation of the actin cytoskeleton and associated surface membrane structures that occur rapidly and are dependent on the severity and duration of ischemic injury.[58] These alterations may be secondary to activation and relocation of the actin-associated protein actin depolymerizing factor/cofilin and β-1 integrin to the apical membrane. ATP depletion also induces necrotic cell death[59] by inducing opening of a plasma membrane "death channel," which is normally kept closed in ischemic tissue by tissue glycine and decreased pH. The epithelial brush border may disappear, in association with apical membrane blebbing, interruption of cell-to-cell junctions, and subsequently epithelial desquamation. Detachment of tubule cells and microvilli contributes to backleak of glomerular filtrate and formation of intraluminal aggregations of exfoliated cells, proteins, and glycoproteins—such as fibronectin—resulting in tubular obstruction. The functional ramifications of these changes are substantial in terms of tubular reabsorption, function of the intercellular tight junction, impaired cell-substrate adhesion, and integral membrane protein function.

Tubulointerstitial Injury

In patients with atherosclerotic renal artery stenosis, the severity of pathologic tissue damage is an important determinant and predictor of renal functional outcome.[60]

The earliest and most prominent pathologic feature in renal ischemia is tubulointerstitial injury, which is considered to be the best prognostic factor in all nephropathies, and may subsequently contribute to the development of hypertension. The early phase of tubulointerstitial injury involves cellular activation, migration of mononuclear cells into the interstitium, leukocyte-endothelial interactions, and release of inflammatory products by myofibroblasts/activated-fibroblasts. An altered antigenic profile of the tubular epithelium may initiate a cell-mediated immune response, and be accompanied by interstitial inflammatory infiltrates composed of B lymphocytes, T-helper lymphocytes, and macrophages.[61] Although the tubular lesions are initially reversible, tubulointerstitial injury may lead to irreversible fibrosis. A plethora of fibrogenic factors have been implicated in the development of renal fibrosis following ischemic injury, such as TGF-β1, PAI-1, TIMP-1, α_1(IV) collagen, fibronectin-EIIIA (FN-EIIIA), tissue transglutaminase,[62] and others, which may increase synthesis of ECM. Recent evidence suggests that in the context of atherosclerosis, matrix degradation is also impaired—so the overall matrix turnover balance favors fibrosis.

Glomerulosclerosis

In human atherosclerotic renal artery stenosis, glomerulosclerosis is a relatively late sequela and is exacerbated by long duration, preexisting renal injury, and comorbid clinical conditions. In experimental models of chronic moderate renal artery stenosis, glomerular lesions are initially minimal. Ischemia may elicit global or focal segmental glomerulosclerosis, manifested as segmental collapse or sclerosis, with or without reactive podocyte hypertrophy and proliferation. Initiation of glomerular cell apoptosis, thickening of the basement membrane, and expansion of the mesangial ECM involve progression of glomerulosclerosis.[63] The presence of glomeruli that are not connected to normal tubule segments correlates with the concomitant decrease in GFR.

RENAL ARTERIAL DISEASE AND MORTALITY: THE ROLE OF DISEASE PROGRESSION

Follow-up studies of patients with incidentally identified renal arterial disease[18] indicate that renal artery stenosis independently predicts subsequent mortality. Rarely is this risk due to progressive renal disease alone, but more commonly to associated cardiovascular events. Mortality is remarkably similar in those treated with medical management or renal revascularization,[64-66] although few randomized trials address this issue directly. Death is most commonly related to cardiovascular events and only infrequently is progressive renal failure the primary cause of death.[64,66] Some authors suggest that atherosclerotic disease affecting the kidney is a general marker of the degree of "atherosclerotic burden." Others argue that renovascular disease exacerbates these conditions and accelerates cardiovascular mortality directly.[67] Available data do not support a direct role for renal revascularization to improve overall survival, although observational series indicate that patients experiencing an improvement in GFR after successful revascularization do, in fact, have reduced cardiovascular mortality over several years of follow-up.[68]

Survival is reduced for patients with bilateral renal arterial disease or stenosis to a solitary functioning kidney. Prospective studies using Doppler ultrasound indicate that atherosclerotic lesions can progress in severity over periods of 3 to 5 years.[17] The risks of progression are related to initial severity of the stenotic lesion and systolic blood pressure levels. It must be emphasized that clinical manifestations of renal arterial disease within an individual patient may change over time. It is important that clinicians identify these transitions to consider interventions timed to when they are most likely to be effective.[69]

Specific decisions regarding management of patients with renovascular disease depend heavily on recognizing the clinical syndromes that develop as a result of these lesions. As with many other forms of peripheral vascular disease, the opportunity to benefit patients is greatest in those with overt clinical manifestations of the disease. Understanding the pathophysiology underlying the clinical syndromes identified here will assist the clinician in choosing patients most likely to benefit from intervention.

REFERENCES

1. Textor SC: Managing renal arterial disease and hypertension. Curr Opin Cardiol 18:260, 2003.

1a. Schneider E, Guralnik J: The aging of America: Impact on health care costs. JAMA 263:2335, 1990.

2. Goldblatt H, Lynch J, Hanzal RE, et al: Studies on experimental hypertension I: The production of persistent elevation of systolic blood pressure by means of renal ischemia. J Exp Med 59:347, 1934.

3. Martinez-Maldonado M: Pathophysiology of renovascular hypertension. Hypertension 17:707, 1991.

4. Cragg AH, Smith TP, Thompson BH, et al: Incidental fibromuscular dysplasia in potential renal donors: Long-term clinical follow-up. Radiology 172:145, 1989.

5. Maxwell MH, Bleifer KH, Franklin SS, et al: Cooperative Study of Renovascular Hypertension: Demographic analysis of the study. JAMA 220:1195, 1972.

6. Harrison EG, McCormack LJ: Pathologic classification of renal arterial disease in renovascular hypertension. Mayo Clin Proc 46:161, 1971.

7. Krijnen P, van Jaarsveld BC, Steyerberg EW, et al: A clinical prediction rule for renal artery stenosis. Ann Int Med 129:705, 1998.

8. Hansen KJ, Edwards MS, Craven TE, et al: Prevalence of renovascular disease in the elderly: A population based study. J Vasc Surg 36:443, 2002.

9. Conlon PJ, O'Riordan E, Kalra PA: Epidemiology and clinical manifestations of athersclerotic renal artery stenosis. Am J Kidney Dis 35:573, 2000.

10. Wiecek A, Kokot F, Kuczera M, et al: Plasma erythropoietin concentration in renal venous blood of patients with unilateral renovascular hypertension. Nephrol Dial Transplant 7:221, 1992.

11. Textor SC, Wilcox CS: Renal artery stenosis: A common, treatable cause of renal failure? Annu Rev Med 52:421, 2001.

12. Rihal CS, Textor SC, Breen JF, et al: Incidental renal artery stenosis among a prospective cohort of hypertensive patients undergoing coronary angiography. Mayo Clin Proc 77:309, 2002.

13. Iglesias JI, Hamburger RJ, Feldman L, et al: The natural history of incidental renal artery stenosis in patients with aortoiliac vascular disease. Am J Med 109:642, 2000.

14. Gross CM, Kramer J, Weingartner O, et al: Determination of renal arterial stenosis severity: Comparison of pressure gradient and vessel diameter. Radiology 220:751, 2001.
15. Sigmund G, Hettinger M, Block T, et al: Evaluation of renal artery stenosis: Comparison of angiography and invasive blood pressure measurement and doppler ultrasound. ROFO FortschrGebRontgenstrNeuen Bildgeb Verfahr 172:615, 2000.
16. Caps MT, Zierler RE, Polissar NL, et al: Risk of atrophy in kidneys with atherosclerotic renal artery stenosis. Kidney Int 53:735, 1998.
17. Caps MT, Perissinotto C, Zierler RE, et al: Prospective study of atherosclerotic disease progression in the renal artery. Circulation 98:2866, 1998.
18. Conlon PJ, Little MA, Pieper K, et al: Severity of renal vascular disease predicts mortality in patients undergoing coronary angiography. Kidney Int 60:1490, 2001.
19. Meyrier A, Hill GW, Simon P: Ischemic renal diseases: New insights into old entities. Kidney Int 54:2, 1998.
20. Kang DH, Kanellis J, Hugo C, et al: Role of the microvascular endothelium in progressive renal disease. J Am Soc Nephrol 13:806, 2002.
21. Radermacher J, Chavan A, Bleck J, et al: Use of Doppler ultrasonography to predict the outcome of therapy for renal-artery stenosis. N Engl J Med 344:410, 2001.
22. Pemsel HK, Thermann M: The haemodynamic effects of renal artery stenosis. ROFO FortschrGebRontgenstrNukearmed 129:189, 1978.
23. Textor SC, Smith-Powell L: Post-stenotic arterial pressure, renal haemodynamics and sodium excretion during graded pressure reduction in conscious rats with one- and two-kidney coarctation hypertension. J Hypertens 6:311, 1988.
24. Lerman L, Textor SC: Pathophysiology of ischemic nephropathy. Urol Clin North Am 28:793, 2001.
25. DeForrest JM, Knappenberger RC, Antonaccio MJ, et al: Angiotensin II is a necessary component for the development of hypertension in the two-kidney, one clip rat. Am J Cardiol 49:1515, 1982.
26. Cervenka L, Horacek V, Vaneckova I, et al: Essential role of AT1-A receptor in the development of 1K1C hypertension. Hypertension 40:735, 2002.
27. Fink GD: Long-term sympatho-excitatory effect of angiotensin II: A mechanism of spontaneous and renovascular hypertension. Clin Exp Pharmacol Physiol 24:91, 1997.
28. Reckelhoff JF, Romero, JC: Role of oxidative stress in angiotensin-induced hypertension. Am J Physiol 284:R893, 2003.
29. Safian RD, Textor SC: Medical progress: Renal artery stenosis. N Engl J Med 344:431, 2001.
30. Textor SC, McKusick M: Renovascular hypertension and ischemic nephropathy: Angioplasty and stenting. In Brady HR, Wilcox CS (eds): Therapy in Nephrology and Hypertension. London, WB Saunders, 2003, p 599.
31. Messina LM, Zelenock GB, Yao KA, et al: Renal revascularization for recurrent pulmonary edema in patients with poorly controlled hypertension and renal insufficiency: A distinct subgroup of patients with arteriosclerotic renal artery occlusive disease. J Vasc Surg 15:73, 1992.
32. Gandhi SK, Powers JC, Nomeir AM, et al: The pathogenesis of acute pulmonary edema associated with hypertension. N Engl J Med 344:17, 2001.
33. Missouris CG, Belli AM, MacGregor G: "Apparent" heart failure: A syndrome caused by renal artery stenoses. Heart 83:152, 2000.
34. Pickering TG, Herman L, Devereux RB, et al: Recurrent pulmonary oedema in hypertension due to bilateral renal artery stenosis: Treatment by angioplasty or surgical revascularisation. Lancet 2:551, 1988.
35. Gray BH, Olin JW, Childs MB, et al: Clinical benefit of renal artery angioplaty with stenting for the control of recurrent and refractory congestive heart failure. Vasc Med 7:275, 2002.
36. Hall JE: Renal function in one-kidney, one-clip hypertension and low renin essential hypertension. Am J Hyper 4:523s, 1991.
37. Kontogiannis J, Burns KD: Role of AT1 angiotensin II receptors in renal ischemic injury. Am J Physiol 274:F79, 1998.
38. Stebbins CL, Symons JD, Hageman KS, et al: Endogenous prostaglandins limit angiotensin-II induced regional vasoconstriction in conscious rats. J Cardiovasc Pharmacol 42:10, 2003.
39. Ichiki T, Usui M, Kato M, et al: Downregulation of angiotensin II type 1 receptor gene transcription by nitric oxide. Hypertension 31:342, 1998.
40. Wilcox CS, Welch WJ: Angiotensin II and thromboxane in the regulation of blood pressure and renal function. Kidney Int 38:S81, 1990.
41. Kone BC, Baylis C: Biosynthesis and homeostatic roles of nitric oxide in the normal kidney. Am J Physiol 272:F561, 1997.
42. Tokuyama H, Hayashi K, Matsuda H, et al: Stenosis-dependent role of nitric oxide and prostaglandins in chronic renal ischemia. Am J Physiol 282:F859, 2002.
43. Chade AR, Rodriguez-Porcel M, Grande JP, et al: Distinct renal injury in early atherosclerosis and renovascular disease. Circulation 106:1165, 2002.
44. Firth JD, Ratcliffe PJ: Organ distribution of the three rat endothelin messenger RNAs and the effects of ischemia on renal gene expression. J Clin Invest 90:1023, 1992.
45. Forbes JM, Hewitson TD, Becker GJ, et al: Simultaneous blockade of endothelin A and B receptors in ischemic acute renal failure is detrimental to long-term kidney function. Kidney Int 59:1333, 2001.
46. Milot A, Lambert R, Lebel M, et al: Prostaglandins and renal function in hypertensive patients with unilateral renal artery stenosis and patients with essential hypertension. J Hypertens 14:765, 1996.
47. Anderson CB, Tannenbaum JS, Sicard GA, et al: Renal thromboxane synthesis in excised kidney distal to renovascular lesions. JAMA 251:3118, 1984.
48. Salvati P, Ferti C, Ferrario RG, et al: Role of enhanced glomerular synthesis of thromboxane A2 in progressive kidney disease. Kidney Int. 38:447, 1990.
49. Schocken DD, Arrieta MI, Leaverton PE, et al: Prevalence and mortality rate of congestive heart failure in the United States. J Am Coll Cardiol 20:301, 1992.
50. Lerman LO, Nath KA, Rodriguez-Porcel M, et al: Increased oxidative stress in experimental renovascular hypertension. Hypertension 37:541, 2001.
51. Jaimes EA, Galceran JM, Raij L: Angiotensin II induces superoxide anion production by mesangial cells. Kidney Int 54:775, 1998.
52. Chade AR, Rodriguez-Porcel M, Grande JP, et al: Mechanisms of renal structural alterations in combined hypercholesterolemia and renal artery stenosis. Aterioscler Vasc Thromb Biol 23:1295, 2003.
53. Higashi Y, Sasaki S, Nakagawa K, et al: Endothelial function and oxidative stress in renovascular hypertension. N Engl J Med 346:1954, 2002.
54. Tomita H, Egashira K, Ohara Y, et al: Early induction of transforming growth factor-beta via angiotensin II type 1 receptors contributes to cardiac fibrosis induced by long-term blockade of nitric oxide synthesis in rats. Hypertension 32:273, 1998.
55. Wolf G, Mueller E, Stahl RA, et al: Angiotensin II-induced hypertrophy of cultured murine proximal tubular cells is mediated by endogenous transforming growth factor-beta. J Clin Invest 92:1366, 1993.
56. Eddy AA: Molecular insights into renal interstitial fibrosis. J Am Soc Nephrol 7:2495, 1996.
57. Kellerman PS: Cellular and metabolic consequences of chronic ischemia on kidney function. Semin Nephrol 16:33, 1996.
58. Sutton TA, Molitoris BA: Mechanisms of cellular injury in ischemic acute renal failure. Semin Nephrol 18:490, 1998.
59. Bonventre JV, Weinberg JM: Recent advances in the pathophysiology of ischemic acute renal failure. J Am Soc Nephrol 14:199, 2003.
60. Wright JR, Duggal A, Thomas R, et al: Clinicopathological correlation in biopsy-proven atherosclerotic nephropathy: Implications for renal functional outcome in atherosclerotic renovascular disease. Nephrol Dial Transplant 16:765, 2001.
61. Truong LD, Farhood A, Tasby J, et al: Experimental chronic renal ischemia: Morphologic and immunologic studies. Kidney Int 41:1676, 1992.
62. Johnson TS, El-Koriaie AF, Skill NJ, et al: Tissue transglutaminase and the progression of human renal scarring. J Am Soc Nephrol 14:2052, 2003.
63. Makino H, Sugiyama H, Kashihara N: Apoptosis and extracellular matrix-cell interactions in kidney disease. Kidney Int 77 (supplement):S67, 2000.
64. Chabova V, Schirger A, Stanson AW, et al: Outcomes of atherosclerotic renal artery stenosis managed without revascularization. Mayo Clin Proc 75:437, 2000.
65. Dorros G, Jaff M, Mathiak L, et al: Multicenter Palmaz stent renal artery stenosis revascularization registry report: Four-year follow-up of 1,058 successful patients. Catheter Cardiovasc Interv 55:182, 2002.

66. Uzzo RG, Novick AC, Goormastic M, et al: Medical versus surgical management of atherosclerotic renal artery stenosis. Transplantation Proc 34:723, 2002.
67. Rimmer JM, Plante DA, Madias NE: Therapeutic decision making in renal vascular hypertension. In Novick AC, Scoble J, Hamilton G, (eds): Renal Vascular Disease. London, WB Saunders, 1996, p 245.
68. Kennedy DJ, Colyer WR, Brewster PS, et al: Renal insufficiency as a predictor of adverse events and mortality after renal artery stent placement. Am J Kidney Dis 14:926, 2003.
69. Textor SC: Progressive hypertension in a patient with "incidental" renal artery stenosis. Hypertension 40:595, 2002.

chapter 22

Renal Artery Stenosis: Clinical Evaluation

Jonathan E.E. Fisher
Jeffrey W. Olin

More than 60 million Americans have primary (essential) hypertension. Renovascular disease and renal parenchymal disease are the most common secondary causes of hypertension after obesity, excess alcohol ingestion, drug abuse, and oral contraceptive use are excluded.

The presence of anatomic renal artery stenosis (RAS) does not necessarily establish that the hypertension or renal failure is caused by the RAS. Incidentally discovered renal artery stenosis is quite common, whereas renovascular hypertension occurs only in 1% to 5% of all patients with hypertension.[1,2] Approximately 90% of all renovascular disease is caused by atherosclerosis.[3] Fibromuscular dysplasia (FMD) is the second most common cause of RAS. Patients with atherosclerotic RAS are typically older than the age of 55 and have the usual risk factors for atherosclerosis, whereas FMD is most common in young women. The predominant clinical manifestation of FMD is hypertension, whereas atherosclerotic RAS may manifest with hypertension, renal failure (ischemic nephropathy), and/or recurrent episodes of CHF and "flash" pulmonary edema.[4] Although atherosclerotic RAS most often occurs at the ostium or the proximal portion of the renal artery, FMD usually occurs in the mid- to distal renal artery and its primary branches (Fig. 22-1).

The effects of atherosclerosis on the coronary and carotid arteries are well recognized; however, involvement of the renal arteries is frequently overlooked. In addition to the sequelae of RAS (hypertension, renal failure), patients with atherosclerotic RAS succumb prematurely from myocardial infarction and stroke.[5-7] Thus, early diagnosis and treatment are of vital importance to avoid the consequences of RAS. When considering the diagnosis of renal artery stenosis, it is useful to think in terms of the circumstances in which renal artery stenosis is likely to occur (Table 22-1).

Hypertension

Individuals who develop hypertension between the ages of 30 and 55 usually have primary (essential) hypertension. If the initial diagnosis of hypertension is made before the age of 30, it is usually due to FMD if other known secondary causes (obesity, oral contraceptive use, drug abuse, or parenchymal renal disease) have been excluded. Because atherosclerosis occurs in older individuals, it is usually the cause of RAS after the age of 55. Although renal artery stenosis can be associated with both systolic and diastolic hypertension, the diagnosis of renal artery stenosis should be seriously considered in individuals who present with new-onset diastolic hypertension after the age of 55—primarily because diastolic blood pressure usually declines after age 55 in normal individuals. It is not uncommon for patients to have primary hypertension for many years, and as they age, develop atherosclerotic RAS. This cohort of patients may have had well-controlled blood pressure that suddenly becomes more difficult to control. It should also be recognized that patients may have anatomically significant renal artery stenosis and no hypertension at all. Dustan and colleagues reviewed 149 aortograms and found that approximately one half of patients with greater than 50% RAS did *not* have hypertension.[8] Therefore, the mere presence of RAS and hypertension does not necessarily mean that one condition is causing the other. Accelerated or malignant hypertension has also been associated with a very high prevalence of RAS. Davis and colleagues demonstrated that renovascular hypertension was present in 32% of 76 white patients and 11% of 29 black patients studied with grade III or IV hypertensive retinopathy.[9] Resistant hypertension is defined as failure to normalize blood pressure to less than 140/90 mm Hg following an optimal medical regimen consisting of at least three drugs with different mechanisms of action, including a diuretic.[10] The diagnosis of renovascular disease should be strongly considered in patients with true drug-resistant hypertension.

Renal Abnormalities

Gifford and colleagues found that 71% of patients (53 of 75 patients) with an atrophic kidney had severe stenosis or complete occlusion of the renal artery supplying the small kidney.[11] Three studies have shown that if there is a discrepancy in the size between the two kidneys or if one kidney is atrophic, the contralateral renal artery (normal-sized kidney) is severely stenotic approximately 60% of the time.[1,11,12] Therefore, the presence of an atrophic kidney or a discrepancy in size between the two kidneys demands a thorough investigation for the presence of renovascular disease.

There are numerous reports suggesting that patients who develop azotemia while receiving ACE inhibitors have bilateral RAS, RAS to a solitary functioning kidney, or decompensated CHF in the sodium-depleted state.[13-17]

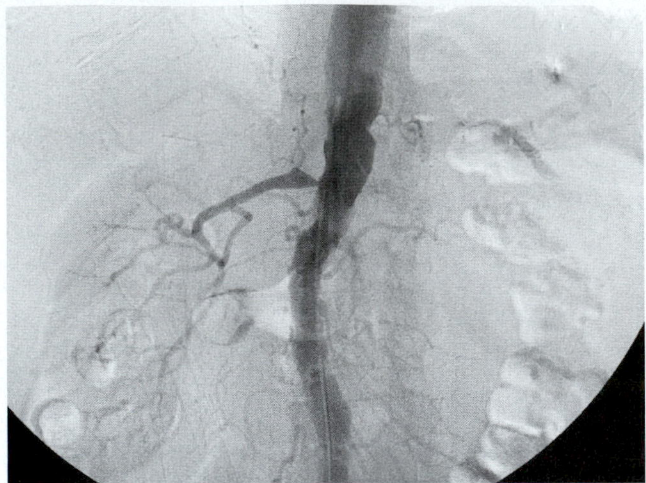

A

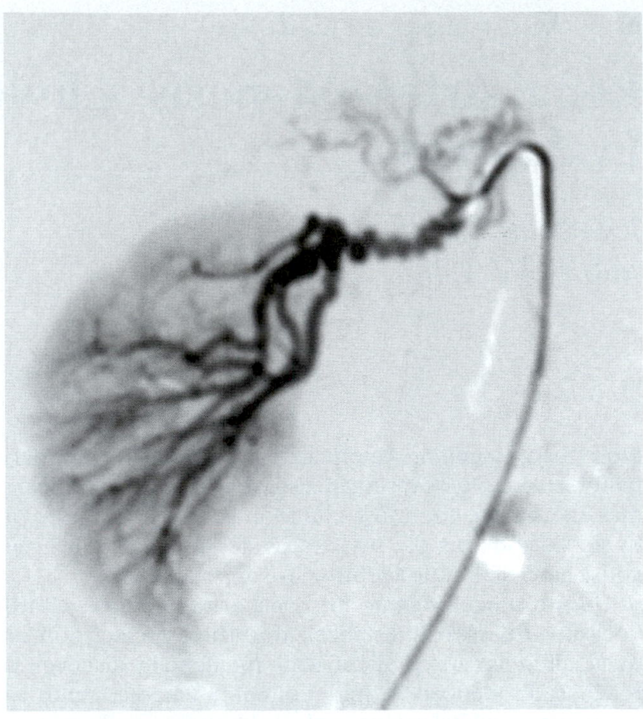

B

FIGURE 22-1. **A,** Digital subtraction angiogram showing the typical features of atherosclerotic renal artery stenosis. Note that the right renal artery has a severe stenosis at the origin. The left renal artery is occluded and a nephrogram is not visualized. **B,** Digital subtraction angiogram demonstrating medial fibroplasia located in the mid- to distal part of the right renal artery. Note the "beading" with the beads larger than the normal caliber of the artery, which is typical of medial fibroplasia. (From Slovut D, Olin JW: Fibromuscular dysplasia. N Engl J Med 350:1862, 2004.)

These clinical scenarios are absolute indications for investigation because they usually reflect the presence of severe RAS to the entire functioning renal mass, thus placing the patient in jeopardy of renal failure. The mechanisms of acute and chronic renal failure in patients with renal artery stenosis are discussed in detail in Chapter 21.

There are no prospective studies evaluating how often atherosclerotic renovascular disease leads to end-stage renal disease (ESRD). Scoble and colleagues found that atherosclerotic renovascular disease was the cause of ESRD in 14% of patients starting dialysis therapy.[18,19] In a retrospective review over a 20-year period in 683 patients, 83 (12%) patients had documented RAS as a cause of ESRD. Because arteriography was performed only in patients with suspected RAS, it is entirely possible that the true incidence of RAS as a cause of ESRD was underestimated. Renal artery stenosis must be excluded in every patient starting dialysis if a clear-cut etiology for the ESRD is not known because the mortality in this patient population is extremely high. In the series by Malloux and associates, the median survival in patients with ESRD secondary to RAS was 25 months, whereas the 2-, 5-, and 10-year survival rates were 56%, 18%, and 5%, respectively.[6,7]

Effects of Renal Artery Stenosis on the Heart

Recurrent CHF and "flash" pulmonary edema not related to ischemic heart disease can result from bilateral RAS (or unilateral RAS to a single functioning kidney). In a renal artery stent series, 39 patients (19% of all patients undergoing renal artery stent implantation from 1991 to 1997) had recurrent episodes of CHF or "flash" pulmonary edema as the primary indication for renal artery stenting.[20] Nineteen of 39 patients had moderate-to-severe left ventricular systolic function. Although not completely understood, the mechanism of CHF may be related in part to the inability to use ACE inhibitors or angiotensin receptor blockers (ARBs), to the direct adverse effects of

TABLE 22-1 CLINICAL CLUES SUGGESTING RENAL ARTERY STENOSIS

Hypertension
Hypertension onset age less than 30 or more than 55 years
Malignant or accelerated hypertension
Resistant hypertension (BP > 140/90 despite appropriate three-drug regimen including a diuretic)
Loss of blood pressure control in a previously well-controlled patient
Renal Abnormalities
Acute renal failure precipitated by an angiotensin-converting enzyme inhibitor or angiotensin receptor blocking agent
Unexplained azotemia
Patient receiving renal replacement therapy (dialysis) without a definite known cause of the end-stage renal disease
Atrophic or small kidney
Cardiac Disease
Recurrent congestive heart failure or "flash" pulmonary edema
Angina disproportionate to coronary anatomy
Presence of Atherosclerosis in Other Vascular Beds
Peripheral arterial disease
Aortoiliac occlusive disease
Aortic aneurysm
Multivessel coronary artery disease

angiotensin II on myocardial function, or to the inability to control volume adequately. If coronary ischemia has been excluded as a cause of CHF, renal revascularization (surgical or percutaneous stenting) is a very effective method of treatment in these individuals.[20-22]

One retrospective study demonstrated improvement in anginal symptoms in patients undergoing renal artery stent implantation. The mechanism of such improvement is not clearly delineated, but 88% of these patients had improved blood pressure control after stenting. This effect may account, at least in part, for decreased anginal symptoms.[23]

Presence of Atherosclerosis in Other Vascular Beds

Several series have examined the prevalence of renovascular disease in patients who have atherosclerotic disease elsewhere. To determine the prevalence of atherosclerotic RAS, Olin and colleagues studied 395 consecutive patients who had undergone arteriography as part of an evaluation for either an abdominal aortic aneurysm, aortoiliac occlusive disease, or peripheral arterial disease (Table 22-2).[1] These patients did not have the usual clinical clues to suggest RAS. High-grade bilateral renal artery disease was present in approximately 13% of patients. In addition, 76 patients had an aortogram performed for suspected renal artery stenosis and RAS was present in 70% of these subjects. Other studies have shown that 22% to 59% of patients with peripheral arterial disease have significant RAS.[24]

It has also been established that RAS is common in patients with coronary artery disease. Of 7758 patients undergoing cardiac catheterization during a 78-month period, 3987 underwent aortography at the time of catheterization to screen for RAS.[25] One hundred ninety-one (4.8%) had greater than 75% RAS and 0.8% had severe bilateral disease. In a Mayo Clinic series, renal arteries were studied at the time of cardiac catheterization in patients with hypertension.[26] Ninety percent of the renal arteries were adequately visualized and no complications occurred from the aortogram. Renal artery stenosis greater than 50% was present in 19.2%, RAS greater than 70% in 7%, and bilateral RAS was present in 3.7% of patients. The likelihood of significant RAS is markedly increased in patients with more than two coronary artery lesions.[27] A prospective study of the long-term natural histories of patients undergoing cardiac catheterization and renal angiography is needed to determine whether diagnosing RAS in this setting improves patient outcome measures. Renal artery disease is also associated with atherosclerotic disease in the carotid arteries. Louie and associates demonstrated that 46% of patients with greater than 60% RAS also had greater than 50% carotid stenosis.[28] All of these studies support the fact that atherosclerotic RAS is a manifestation of systemic atherosclerosis and reinforce the concept of treating the entire patient, not just the circulatory bed involved at a given point in time.

The presence of RAS, even before the development of ESRD, portends a poor prognosis. Patient survival decreases as the severity of RAS increases, with 2-year survival rates of 96% in patients with unilateral RAS, 74% in patients with bilateral RAS, and 47% in patients with stenosis or occlusion to a solitary functioning kidney.[29] Dorros and associates demonstrated that as the serum creatinine increases, the survival decreases in patients with atherosclerotic RAS.[30] The 3-year probability of survival was 92 ± 4% for patients with a serum creatinine less than 1.4 mg/dL, 74 ± 8% for patients with a serum creatinine of 1.5 to 1.9 mg/dL, and 51 ± 8% for patients with a serum creatinine greater than 2.0 mg/dL.

Long-term survival was investigated at Duke University in a cohort of 1235 patients who underwent abdominal aortography at the time of cardiac catheterization. The 4-year survival rate of subjects without RAS was 88% versus 57% for those with RAS (Fig. 22-2).[29]

Physical Examination

The physical examination is generally not helpful in the diagnosis of RAS. Evidence of coronary, cerebral, or peripheral arterial disease is associated with a higher likelihood of renal artery disease because of the systemic nature of atherosclerosis. A systolic abdominal bruit is common and nonspecific; however, the presence of a systolic/diastolic bruit especially over the epigastrium may point to underlying renal artery disease.[31] The presence of a diastolic component to the bruit indicates that the degree of narrowing of the artery is severe because there is continued flow during diastole.[32] A systolic/diastolic bruit more often occurs in patients with fibromuscular disease (53%) than in patients who have atherosclerotic disease (12.5%). The presence of a bruit is helpful for

TABLE 22-2 PREVALENCE OF ATHEROSCLEROTIC RENAL ARTERY STENOSIS

≥ 50% Stenosis	Abdominal Aortic Aneurysm (n = 109)	Aortoiliac Occlusive Disease (n = 21)	Peripheral Arterial Disease (n = 189)	Renal Artery Stenosis (n = 76)
All patients	41 (38%)	7 (33%)	74 (39%)	53 (70%)*
Diabetic patients	6 (50%)	1 (33%)	34 (50%)**	10 (71%)
Nondiabetic patients	35 (36%)	6 (33%)	40 (33%)	43 (69%)*

*P < .001
**P < .02
From Olin JW, Melia M, Young JR, et al: Prevalence of atherosclerotic renal artery stenosis in patients with atherosclerosis elsewhere. Am J Med 88:46N, 1990.

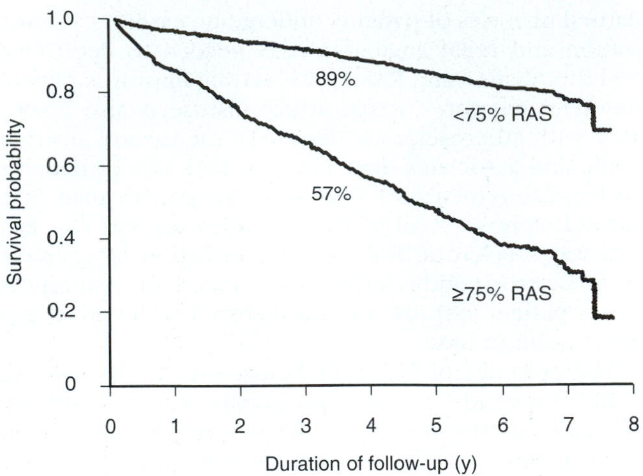

FIGURE 22-2. Four-year survival rates in 1235 patients undergoing abdominal aortography at the time of cardiac catheterization based on the presence or absence of renal artery stenosis (RAS). In those patients with less than 75% stenosis, the 4-year survival rate was 89%; in patients with greater than 75% stenosis, the 4-year survival rate was only 57%. (From Conlon P, O'Riordan E, Kalra P: New insights into the epidemiologic and clinical manifestations of atherosclerotic renovascular disease. Am J Kidney Dis 35:573, 2000.)

diagnosis, but the absence does not exclude the diagnosis of either atherosclerotic renovascular disease or FMD.

DIAGNOSIS OF RENOVASCULAR DISEASE

In the past, indirect methods of assessing the renal arteries were commonly used to diagnose RAS. Intravenous urography is obsolete as a screening tool due to its poor sensitivity and specificity.[33] Plasma renin activity (PRA) as a stand-alone screening test is not reliable for diagnosing or excluding renal artery disease. Elevated PRA may manifest in approximately 15% of patients with essential hypertension. In addition, patients with bilateral disease or disease to a solitary functioning kidney may have normal or low PRA due to extracellular volume expansion, the position of the patient during the test, or medication use. The test is less accurate in azotemic patients and in African-American patients.[34] The captopril test (plasma renin measurement before and after administration of captopril) is not an ideal screening test and is rarely used. Renal vein renin measurement is not a useful test to screen for RAS; in addition, it has little value in determining who will benefit from revascularization. This test is rarely used to make clinical decisions, except under unusual circumstances.

Imaging modalities have become the first line tests for the diagnosis of RAS. Imaging has become so sophisticated and accurate that it is seldom necessary to perform catheter-based angiography for the *diagnosis* of renal artery disease. The ideal imaging procedure should[35]

1. identify the main renal arteries as well as accessory vessels;
2. localize the site of stenosis or disease;
3. determine the type of disease present (e.g., atherosclerosis or FMD);
4. provide evidence for the hemodynamic significance of the lesion;
5. determine the likelihood of a favorable response to revascularization;
6. identify associated pathology (i.e., abdominal aortic aneurysm, renal mass, etc.) that may have an impact on the treatment of the renal artery disease; and
7. detect restenosis after percutaneous or surgical revascularization.

None of the available imaging modalities fulfills all of these criteria. The three most commonly used techniques for renal artery imaging are duplex ultrasound, computed tomographic angiography (CTA), and magnetic resonance angiography (MRA). Which of the imaging modalities is used as the first line test depends on local expertise, availability in a given institution, and cost (Fig. 22-3). Other factors that may play a role in determining the optimal screening test are patient body habitus, renal function, and patient claustrophobia.

Duplex Ultrasonography

Duplex ultrasonography (see Chapter 10) is the least expensive of the imaging modalities and provides information about the degree and location of stenosis, kidney size, and other associated disease processes such as obstruction, renal mass, or abdominal aortic aneurysm. It may also help predict which patients can expect an improvement in blood pressure control or renal function after renal artery revascularization.[36] Duplex ultrasound can be performed without altering the antihypertensive regimen and does not require potentially nephrotoxic contrast.

Duplex ultrasonography combines B-mode ultrasound and Doppler examination. Improvements in ultrasound hardware, software, and transducer technology are responsible for improved visualization of the arteries and more precise Doppler interrogation of the entire artery. Renal artery ultrasound should be performed from both anterior and oblique (or posterior [flank]) approaches (Figs. 22-4 and 22-5). In the longitudinal view, the peak systolic flow velocity in the aorta is recorded at the level of the renal arteries. The aortic velocity and the highest renal artery peak systolic velocity (PSV) are used to calculate the renal aortic ratio (RAR).[37,38]

The renal arteries are best visualized in a transverse (short axis) view. Using the B-mode image and a 60-degree angle of insonance, the arteries are interrogated with pulse-wave Doppler. The Doppler should be swept through the artery from its origin to the renal hilum, which will allow the examiner to survey the artery for velocity shifts along the entire course of the renal artery. Velocities should be recorded at the origin, proximal, mid-, and distal arterial segments. From an oblique approach, the renal artery can be visualized at the renal hilum and followed to the aorta. By studying the patient from an anterior and an oblique approach, Doppler velocity measurements are obtained in two views ensuring that a focal stenosis is not missed and that the angle of insonation is correct. Because medial fibroplasia most often occurs in the mid- to distal renal artery, the oblique

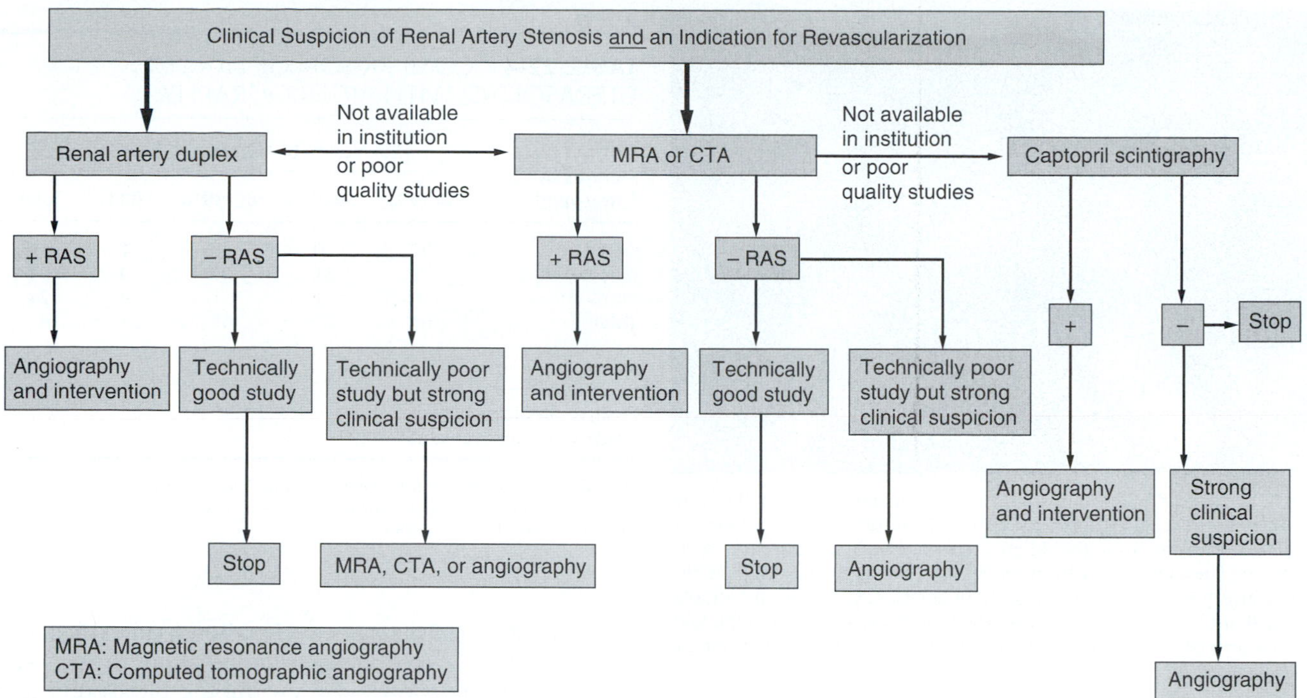

FIGURE 22-3. Algorithm for the diagnosis of renal artery stenosis. (From Carman TL, Olin JW: Diagnosis of renal artery stenosis: What is the optimal diagnostic test? Curr Interv Cardiol Rep 2:111, 2000.)

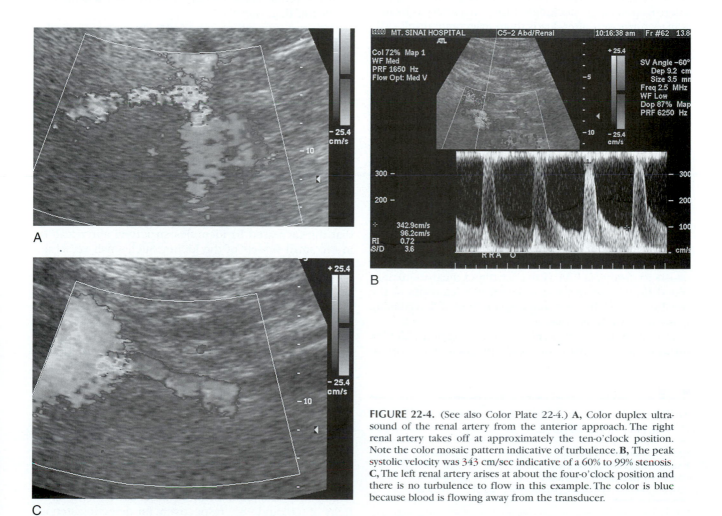

FIGURE 22-4. (See also Color Plate 22-4.) **A,** Color duplex ultrasound of the renal artery from the anterior approach. The right renal artery takes off at approximately the ten-o'clock position. Note the color mosaic pattern indicative of turbulence. **B,** The peak systolic velocity was 343 cm/sec indicative of a 60% to 99% stenosis. **C,** The left renal artery arises at about the four-o'clock position and there is no turbulence to flow in this example. The color is blue because blood is flowing away from the transducer.

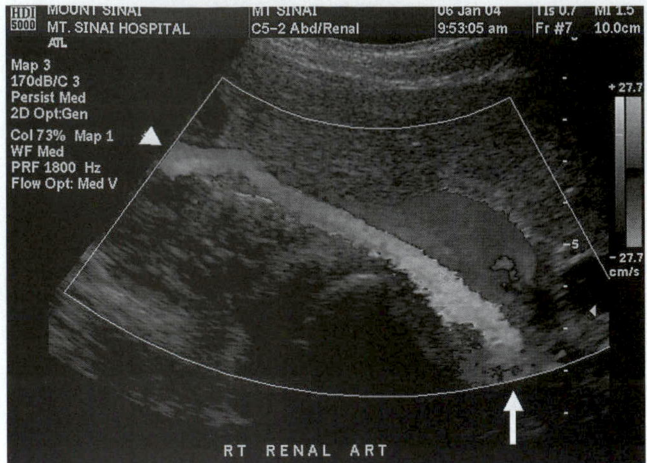

FIGURE 22-5. Duplex ultrasound of the renal artery from the right oblique approach. This approach allows the ultrasonographer to image the renal artery from the kidney (*arrowhead*) back to the aorta (*arrow*). Therefore, one can measure the velocity at the origin of the renal artery from another approach. In addition, fibromuscular dysplasia will not be overlooked because the lesions usually occur in the mid- to distal renal artery. This normal renal artery has uniform flow and no turbulence.

approach is particularly good for detecting this type of stenosis. It is important to note that segmental Doppler interrogation (spot-checking) of the renal artery velocities is inadequate and often leads to an inaccurate result.[37-39]

The RAR, the ratio of the PSV in the renal arteries to the PSV in the aorta, is used to classify the degree of stenosis (Table 22-3). A three-category classification scheme is commonly used: 0% to 59% stenosis, 60% to 99% stenosis, and occlusion. When the aortic velocity is less than 40 cm/second or greater than 100 cm/second, the RAR is not an accurate representation of the degree of stenosis. In these instances, if the PSV is greater than 200 cm/second and turbulence is present on color flow, the stenosis would be classified as 60% to 99%. When there is a discrepancy in kidney size of 1.5 cm or greater, the ultrasonographer should search very carefully for the presence of RAS or an occluded renal artery.

The acceleration time (AT), acceleration index (AI), and resistive index (RI) have been used by some investigators to *diagnose* RAS. However, direct measurement of blood flow velocities in the visualized segments of the renal arteries is the most accurate method of determining if significant RAS is present.

Overall, when compared with angiography, duplex ultrasound has sensitivities and specificities of 84% to 98% and 62% to 99%, respectively, when used to diagnose RAS.[38,40,41-44] In a prospective blinded study, there was a very good correlation between duplex ultrasound and angiography (Table 22-4). In addition, it was determined that if the end diastolic velocity was greater than 150 cm/second, then the degree of stenosis was likely to be greater than 80%.[37]

There are two other important advantages of duplex ultrasonography. One study demonstrated that duplex ultrasonography can accurately identify patients likely to have a favorable clinical outcome after surgical or catheter-based renal revascularization.[36] One hundred thirty-eight patients with greater than 50% RAS underwent renal artery angioplasty or surgery for blood pressure control or preservation of renal function. A renal RI of 80 or greater identified patients in whom angioplasty or surgery was not associated with improved blood pressure, renal function, or kidney survival. Ninety-seven percent of patients with an increased renal RI demonstrated no improvement in blood pressure and 80% had no improvement in renal function. The authors suggested that the increased RI identifies structural abnormalities in the small vessels of the kidney. Such small vessel disease is typical of long-standing hypertension associated with nephrosclerosis or glomerulosclerosis.[45] The RI is easy to measure, and is calculated by the formula {[1-(end-diastolic velocity/PSV)] × 100} (Fig. 22-6). Using a 0° angle, the PSV and end diastolic velocity are measured in the parenchyma of the kidney. If this study is confirmed, it could be a major step forward in predicting which patients will improve after renal revascularization.

The second major advantage of duplex ultrasonography is its ability to detect restenosis after percutaneous therapy or surgical bypass (Fig. 22-7).[46-48] Unlike MRA (which may be affected by artifact or scatter produced by the stent), ultrasound transmission through the stent is not a problem. CTA has not been adequately studied in this respect. Hudspeth and colleagues compared angiography with duplex ultrasound for follow-up of RAS after angioplasty and demonstrated a sensitivity and specificity of 69% and 98%, respectively, for detecting stenosis

TABLE 22-3 DUPLEX CRITERIA FOR DIAGNOSIS OF RENAL ARTERY STENOSIS

RAR < 3.5 and PSV < 200 cm/s	0-59%
RAR ≥ 3.5 and PSV > 200 cm/s	60-99%
RAR > 3.5 and EDV ≥ 150 cm/s	80-99%
Absent flow, low amplitude parenchymal signal	Occluded

EDV, end diastolic velocity; PSV, peak systolic velocity; RAR, renal to aortic ratio.

TABLE 22-4 COMPARISON OF DUPLEX ULTRASOUND WITH ARTERIOGRAPHY

Stenosis by Ultrasound	STENOSIS BY ARTERIOGRAPHY 0-59%	60-79%	80-99%	100%	Total
0-59%	62	0	1	1	64
60-99%	1	31	67	0	99
100%	0	1	1	22	24
Total	63	32	69	23	187

Sensitivity	0.98
Specificity	0.98
Positive predictive value	0.99
Negative predictive value	0.97

From Olin JW, Piedmonte MR, Young JR, et al: The utility of duplex ultrasound scanning of the renal arteries for diagnosing significant renal artery stenosis. Ann Intern Med 122:833, 1995.

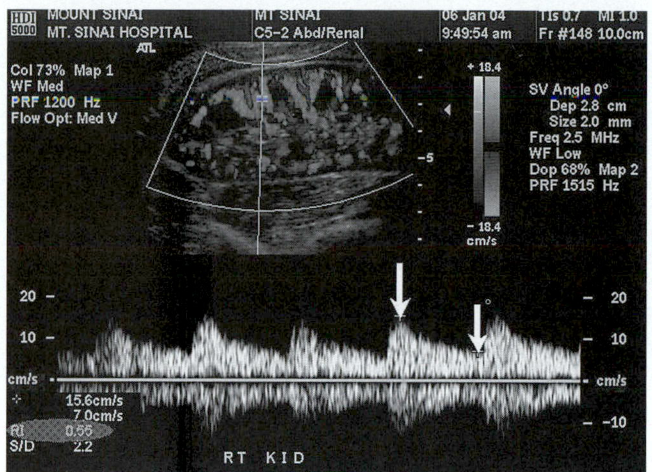

FIGURE 22-6. Measurement of the RI {[1-(end-diastolic velocity/PSV)] × 100}. The parenchyma of the kidney is visualized. Note the blood flow within the kidney. The Doppler angle is zero degrees to optimize the Doppler waveform. The color velocity scale is set low to optimize color flow. By measuring the PSV (*left arrow*) and end diastolic velocity (*right arrow*), the ultrasound machine calculates RI. This is shown in the gray area at the bottom left portion of this image (RI = 0.55 × 100 = 55). PSV, peak systolic velocity; RI, resistive index.

greater than 60%.[47] In a more contemporary series, Bakker and coworkers showed that duplex ultrasound was an excellent technique to detect restenosis after stent implantation (see Fig. 22-7). In 33 consecutive patients using threshold values of 226 cm/sec for PSV and 2.7 for renal to aortic ratio, sensitivities and specificities were 100% and 90%, and 100% and 84%, respectively.[48] All patients who have undergone percutaneous intervention should be placed in a surveillance program in an attempt to identify restenosis and treat it before the artery occludes. Following PTA and stent implantation, a renal artery duplex should be obtained at 6 months, 12 months, and yearly thereafter.[4]

There are several limitations of duplex ultrasound. It is technically demanding and requires a steep learning curve, and it is particularly challenging in the obese individual. The sensitivity of identifying accessory renal arteries is only approximately 67%.[40] In addition, in approximately 5% of patients there is too much bowel gas to allow for an adequate study and thus the patient must return to be studied at a later date.

Magnetic Resonance Angiography

Magnetic resonance angiography (see Chapter 11) of the renal arteries can be performed rapidly with excellent image quality. The two advantages of MRA are that there is no nephrotoxicity from the contrast agents and the images are obtained without the use of ionizing radiation. MRA allows direct visualization of the aorta and renal arteries as well as assessment of renal size. Absolute blood flow rate and glomerular filtration rate (GFR) can be determined.[49] There is recent evidence that functional renal perfusion can be assessed by MRA.[50,51]

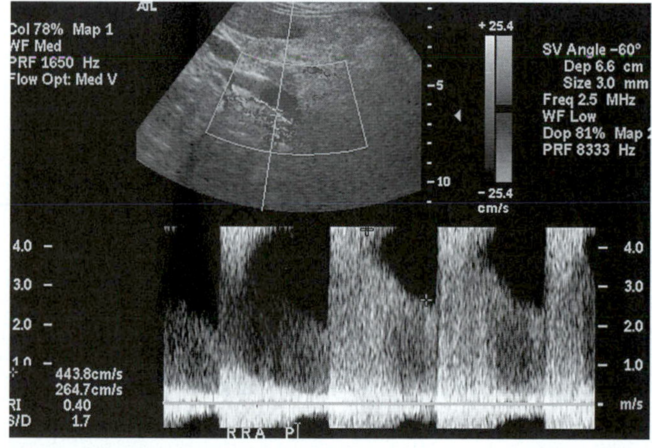

A

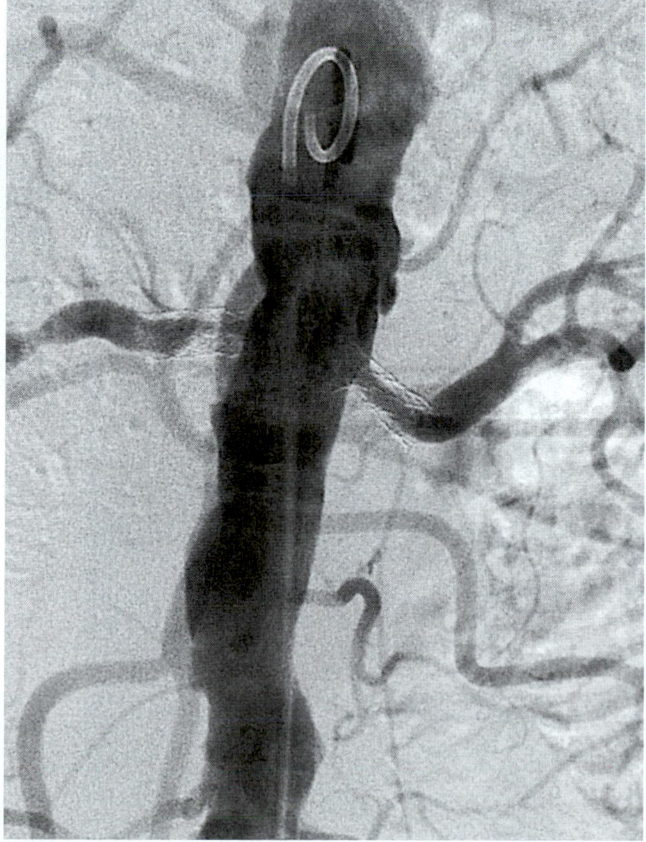

B

FIGURE 22-7. **A,** Duplex ultrasound demonstrating severe stenosis on the first surveillance ultrasound 6 months after bilateral renal artery stent implantation. There is turbulence on the image. The PSV in the right renal artery is 444 cm/sec and the end diastolic velocity is 265 cm/sec with a renal-to-aortic ratio of 7.4. This is consistent with an 80% to 99% stenosis. **B,** Digital subtraction angiogram of the same patient demonstrating severe bilateral in-stent restenosis, right more severe than left. PSV, peak systolic velocity.

Contrast-enhanced 3-D MRA has become the standard because of the ability to produce 3-D angiographic images with excellent image quality and improved speed of acquisition.[39,50,52,53] Contrast-enhanced 3-D MRA uses an injected gadolinium-based contrast medium followed by rapid 3-D MRI. Gadolinium chelate is not nephrotoxic and may be used in patients with renal insufficiency, CHF, or a contrast allergy. Blood appears bright, and stationary tissues have a dark appearance. The use of gadolinium shortens image acquisition time to 20 to 40 seconds, significantly limiting artifact due to patient movement and respiration.[54] Because signal intensity with gadolinium is concentration-dependent and not flow-based, visualization of small vessels is better than with other MRI techniques and low-flow related artifacts are diminished.[55] Contrast-enhanced MRA is performed using fast 3-D spoiled gradient echo recalled pulse sequences. These pulse sequences are available primarily at higher magnetic field strengths (1.0 or 1.5 Tesla). Because hundreds of images are acquired, 3-D image processing is subsequently performed to project vessels in views of high diagnostic interest.

Advanced MR methods use techniques such as partial k-space sampling, rectangular field of view, and real-time fluoroscopic imaging to further improve image quality. Additional slices can be acquired in the slice select direction by interpolating between adjacent acquired slices to improve the smoothness of the reconstructed 3-D images.[56]

TABLE 22-5 ACCURACY OF 3-D GADOLINIUM MR ANGIOGRAPHY FOR RENAL ARTERY STENOSIS

Author	Year	Patients	Sensitivity (%)	Specificity (%)
Snidow[65]	1996	47	100	89
Hany[63]	1997	39	93	98
De Cobelli[61]	1997	55	100	97
Rieumont[64]	1997	30	100	71
Bakker[57]	1998	54	97	92
Schoenberg[58]	1999	50	94	100
Hahn[59]	1999	22	91	79
Fain[62]	2001	25	97	92

Abdominal MRA is being used increasingly to evaluate the abdominal aorta and its branches, particularly the renal arteries. MRA has a sensitivity of 91% to 100% and a specificity of 71% to 100% for detecting RAS (Table 22-5, Fig. 22-8).[57-65] MRA, however, is not useful for monitoring

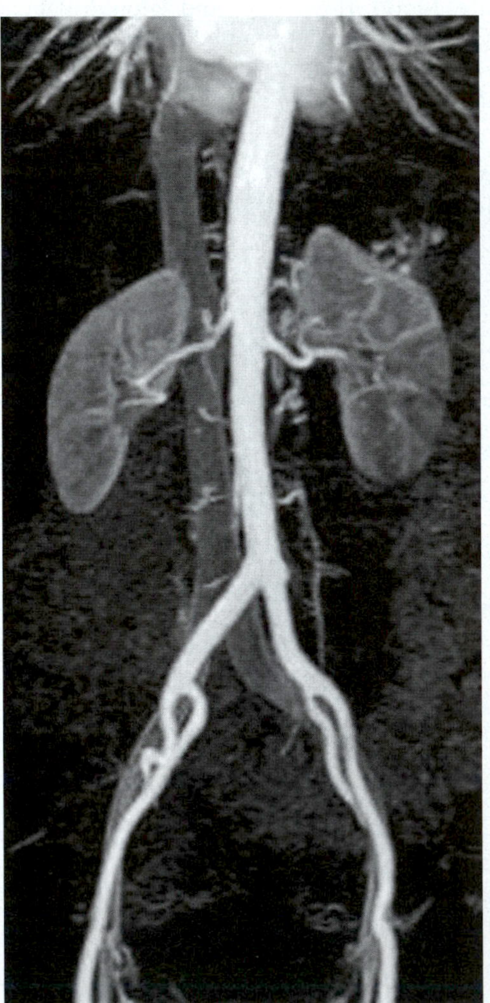

A

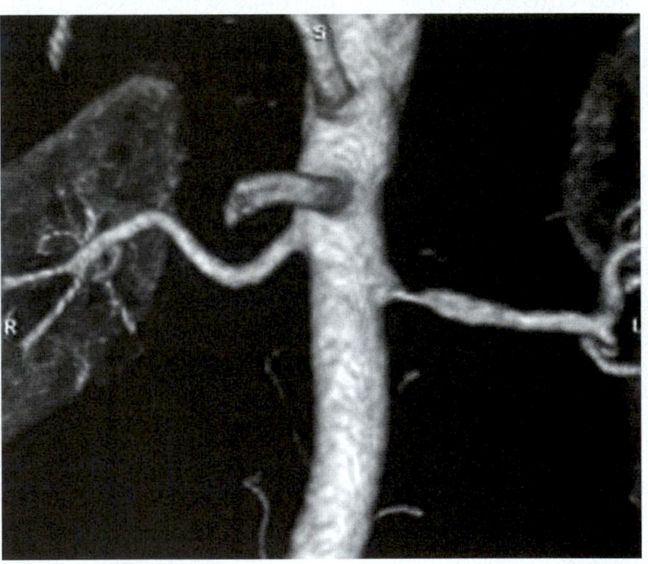

B

FIGURE 22-8. A, 3-D Gadolinium-enhanced magnetic resonance angiogram demonstrating normal renal arteries bilaterally. There is an excellent view of the aorta from the diaphragm to the inguinal ligament. By imaging a large field-of-view one can be certain not to miss an accessory renal artery. The kidneys are also well seen with this technology. The inferior vena cava can be seen in the background. **B,** Severe atherosclerotic renal artery stenosis of the left renal artery. The right renal artery was normal.

patients after renal artery angioplasty and stenting because of artifact produced by the stent. In the near future, MRI-compatible stents should be available.[66]

As with CTA, the patient must be able to breath-hold and remain motionless during image acquisition. Moreover, MRA may not be possible for patients with claustrophobia and those with metal clips, pacemakers, or other metallic devices. For these reasons, MRA is most useful in patients after an inconclusive preliminary work-up for RAS or in those with a high clinical suspicion for renovascular hypertension or with contraindications to other imaging modalities.

Kidneys, adrenal glands, and surrounding soft tissues are evaluated by T1- and T2-weighted image acquisition. Time-of-flight (high velocity jet within stenosis appears black due to signal loss), phase contrast (gadolinium injection allows phase-shift difference detection and rendering of renal arterial blood flow), and maximal intensity projection are the most widely applied MRA imaging techniques. After 20 minutes of source image acquisition, an additional 30 to 45 minutes of reformatting are required. As with CTA, software allows for both 2- and 3-D reconstruction, which increases the diagnostic yield. Proper equipment, software, and technical expertise are critical for optimal renal MRA and account for significant variability of study quality between institutions.

MRA is limited by its high cost and by artifacts (respiration, peristalsis, vessel tortuosity, accessory arteries). It also has a tendency to overestimate stenosis severity and may miss accessory renal arteries if the field-of-view is too narrow.

Computed Tomographic Angiography

Computed tomographic angiography (see Chapter 12) is a vascular imaging technique that can be performed rapidly and safely for the assessment of renal artery disease as well as other vascular applications. Multidetector-row CTA provides excellent image quality with higher resolution than could be obtained previously with single detector-row technology. Current multidetector-row scanners acquire up to 64 simultaneous interweaving helices. The advantages of CTA over catheter-based angiography are:[67-71]

- volumetric acquisition demonstrating better visualization of the anatomy from multiple angles and in multiple planes after a single acquisition;
- improved visualization of soft tissues and other adjacent anatomic structures;
- less invasive and thus fewer complications; and
- lower cost.

CTA has several advantages over MRA, such as higher spatial resolution, absence of flow-related phenomena that may distort MRA images, and capability to visualize calcification and metallic implants such as endovascular stents or stent grafts. The disadvantages of CTA compared with MRA are exposure to ionizing radiation as well as the need for potentially nephrotoxic iodinated contrast. Its potential nephrotoxicity is a key factor limiting the use of CTA in diagnosing RAS in the azotemic patient.

The increased speed of acquisition that is obtained with the multidetector-row CTA allows for greater longitudinal coverage for a given scan duration and greater spatial resolution.[72] Although this may not be of as much importance for assessing renal artery disease, it has great advantages when assessing the thoracoabdominal, aortoiliac and lower extremity inflow and runoff, which may require up to 1400 mm of coverage.[56] The rapid acquisition of images allows for reduction in the amount of iodinated contrast material needed while maintaining excellent and uniform vascular enhancement.[67,70,71,73]

Beam collimation, rotational speed of the tube, and rate of table feed are key parameters in determining imaging protocols. The initial image output from all CT scans are sets of sequential or overlapping axial images. These should be interpreted in the same manner as any CT scan, with full attention to all nonvascular structures including bones, bowel, visceral organs, and lung. To create angiographic representations, post-processing of the volumetric data is necessary. The best post-processed images are created from overlapping images, usually 50% to 80% (Fig. 22-9). In the absence of overlap, the angiographic images may have a marked stair-step appearance.

The techniques used in the workstation post-processing of CT data are multiplanar reformation, maximal intensity projection (MIP), shaded surface display, and volumetric rendering.[73-75] These techniques allow the manipulation of raw data so as to optimize visualization of relevant lesions or disease processes. An important common pitfall is the selective visualization of the maximally opacified vascular lumen. Both automated and manual creations of post-processed images risk inadvertent rejection of critical vascular and nonvascular information. Post-processed images alone should *never* be used for interpretation of CT angiography.[56]

The sensitivity of CTA for RAS ranges from 89% to 100% and specificity from 82% to 100% (Table 22-6).[56,62,76-80] It is important to make sure the area of acquisition includes the area just proximal to the celiac artery to and including the iliac arteries. This will ensure that accessory renal arteries are detected and associated aortic and visceral artery pathologies are not overlooked.

The results obtained using duplex ultrasound, MRA, or CTA are not nearly as good for assessing RAS secondary to FMD, and catheter-based angiography remains the imaging modality of choice if FMD is suspected.[81]

Catheter-Based Angiography

Although duplex ultrasonography, MRA, and CTA have replaced catheter-based angiography in the diagnosis of RAS in most circumstances, catheter-based angiography remains the standard. It is the most accurate test to diagnose RAS secondary to both atherosclerosis and FMD. It can clearly visualize the branch vessels and cortical blood flow and is excellent for identifying accessory renal arteries.

Digital subtraction angiography (DSA) has replaced screen-film angiography in the majority of institutions for vascular applications. The resolution of DSA is less than that of screen film, but can approach 3 to 4 line pairs

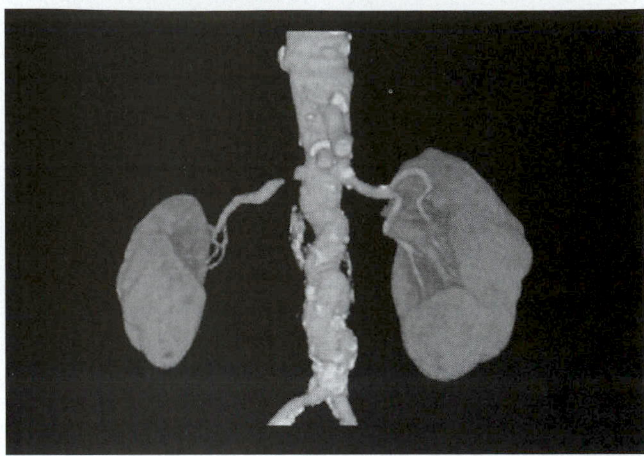

A

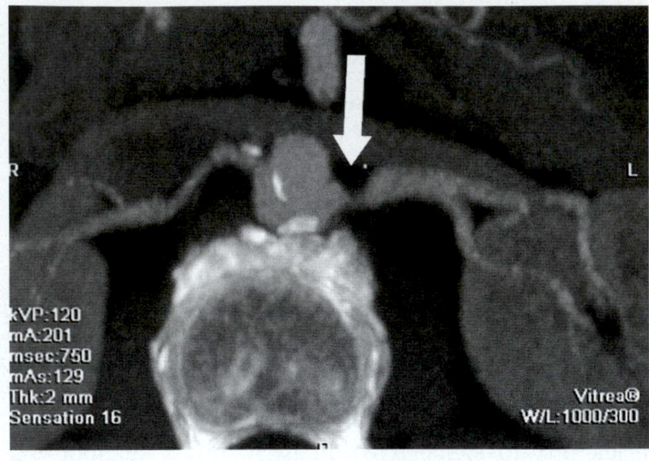

B

FIGURE 22-9. A, 3-D CT angiogram (reconstructed image) using a 16-slice CT scanner showing subtotal occlusion of the right renal artery with a smaller right kidney. Note the severe atherosclerosis of the aorta and diffuse calcium deposition most notable at the aortic bifurcation. **B,** Transverse view of a CT angiogram demonstrating severe stenosis of the left renal artery (*arrow*). This was found incidentally while investigating the patient for claudication. (**A,** Courtesy of Corey Goldman, MD, PhD, Department of Cardiovascular Medicine, Ochsner Clinic, New Orleans, LA.)

per millimeter with current equipment (see Fig. 22-1). The standard imaging matrix is now 1024 × 1024, with image intensifiers that range up to 16 inches in diameter. Flat-panel image intensifiers will soon become available. It is important to recognize that the renal arteries often come off the aorta posteriorly and, therefore, oblique views of the aorta may be needed to visualize their origin. Pressure gradients also should be obtained to confirm the physiologic significance of a given lesion.

New developments in hardware and software have led to greater diagnostic accuracy and better safety. Bolus chasing, rapid image acquisition, vessel diameter analysis, regional pixel shifting, image-stacking, 3-D reconstructions from rotational angiograms, and angioscopic representations of DSA data are now routinely available from manufacturers.[56,82-86] Lower concentrations of iodinated contrast, and non-nephrotoxic and nonallergenic alternative contrast agents, such as CO_2 gas and gadolinium chelates, can be used with DSA. This is particularly useful for patients with chronic renal insufficiency.

Carbon dioxide (CO_2) angiography provides an alternative to conventional angiography or DSA using iodinated contrast agents. This may be particularly useful in patients with renal insufficiency in whom contrast exposure may accelerate the decline of renal function. When compared with conventional angiography, CO_2 angiography demonstrates a sensitivity of 83% and a specificity of 99%.[87,88] CO_2 is rapidly eliminated via the lungs allowing repeated injections without increased risk of toxicity. The disadvantages of using CO_2 are related to the buoyancy, compressibility, and solubility of the gas. Because of its buoyancy, CO_2 does not optimally visualize posterior structures. The compressibility of the gas can make injection difficult and CO_2 dissolves rapidly in the blood and, thus, images degrade within a few seconds.[89] Although the use of CO_2 does prevent nephrotoxicity from contrast, the patient can still develop atheromatous embolization (from catheter manipulation in the aorta or renal artery) to the kidney. The major drawback of using CO_2 as a contrast agent is that the resolution and clarity are not as good as with iodinated contrast. The use of CO_2 angiography is not recommended as a screening test for RAS; however, once the diagnosis of RAS is made by a noninvasive imaging modality, CO_2 angiography is useful to identify the origins of the renal arteries. When using CO_2 alone or with a very small amount of contrast, one can perform an angioplasty and stent placement.[89,90] Gadolinamide as a contrast agent—either alone or with CO_2—in patients with renal insufficiency has been used in recent years.[91-95] Gadolinium provides excellent images and may supplant the use of CO_2 in the future.

TABLE 22-6 ACCURACY OF COMPUTED TOMOGRAPHIC ANGIOGRAPHY FOR ASSESSMENT OF VISCERAL AND RENAL ARTERY STENOSIS

Author	Year	Patients	Sensitivity (%)	Specificity (%)
Kaatee[80]	1997	71	92-100	96-100
Kim[79]	1998	50	90-100	97
Johnson[81]	1999	25	89-94	87-99
Qanadli[78]	2000	47	91	100
Willmann[77]	2003	46	91-92	99

The advantages of DSA are the high resolution compared with current cross-sectional imaging techniques, ability to selectively evaluate individual vessels, access direct physiological information such as pressure gradients, and use as a platform for intervention. The disadvantages are exposure to ionizing radiation, use of iodinated contrast agents (contrast-induced nephropathy), and risks related to vascular access (pseudoaneurysm, hematoma, retroperitoneal bleeding) and catheterization (atheromatous embolization). Nevertheless, until an alternative platform is developed for intervention, or completely MR-compatible devices become available,

DSA will continue to have a central role in the management of patients with vascular disease.

Renal Angiography at the Time of Cardiac Catheterization

This controversial subject has led to numerous debates over the most appropriate management strategy for patients with coronary artery disease and possible RAS. It has been demonstrated that patients with coronary artery disease have a higher prevalence of RAS than the general population. In addition, patients with RAS have a markedly increased mortality from cardiovascular disease. Conlon and colleagues demonstrated that the 4-year survival rate for patients with no RAS detected at the time of cardiac catheterization was 90% compared with survival rates of 70% for 50% to 75% stenosis, 68% for 75% to 95% stenosis, and 48% for greater than 95% stenosis.[25,96] The proponents of angiography at the time of catheterization state that the procedure can be preformed accurately with no added risk and provide the cardiologist with knowledge that the patient has RAS—so the patient can then be followed serially and treated with optimal secondary preventive measures.[26] Those against routine angiography claim that knowing that the patient has RAS adds nothing to the patient's overall management other than to tempt the angiographer to stent the stenotic lesion in the absence of accepted clinical indications.[97,98] This has been termed the *renal oculosten(t)otic reflex*.[99]

It is appropriate to perform renal angiography at the time of cardiac catheterization if acceptable indications for renal artery intervention are present. Further prospective natural history studies in this asymptomatic population are needed, however, to answer the question of whether routine screening should be performed at the time of cardiac catheterization.

Captopril Scintigraphy

Radionuclide imaging techniques are a noninvasive and safe way of evaluating renal blood flow and excretory function; however, the renal flow scan has unacceptably high false-positive and false-negative rates for diagnosing RAS.[100] When an ACE inhibitor such as captopril is added to isotope renography, the sensitivity and specificity of the test improve considerably, especially for patients with unilateral RAS. In most instances of unilateral RAS, the GFR of the stenotic kidney falls by approximately 30% after captopril administration.[101,102] In contrast, the contralateral normal kidney exhibits an increase in GFR, urine flow, and salt excretion despite a reduction in systemic blood pressure. These expected physiologic changes within the stenotic and contralateral kidneys are the basis of the asymmetry of renal function following ACE inhibition detected by renal scintigraphy (see Chapter 21).[103-105]

The Consensus Report on Captopril Renography suggested that both the scintigraphic images and computer-generated time-activity curves provide information about renal size, perfusion, and excretory capacity.[102] The diagnostic criteria that suggest RAS were:

- delayed time to maximal activity ($T_{MAX} > 11$ minutes after captopril);
- significant asymmetry of peak activity of each kidney;
- marked cortical retention of the radionuclide after captopril; and
- marked reduction in calculated GFR of the ipsilateral kidney after ACE.

Patients with normal renal function and unilateral disease demonstrate acceptable results with captopril renography with a sensitivity of approximately 85% to 90% (range 45 to 94) and specificity of approximately 93% to 98% (range 81 to 100).[97] However, the presence of significant azotemia or bilateral RAS may adversely affect the accuracy of captopril renography. Many investigators have excluded patients with a serum creatinine exceeding 2.5 to 3.0 mg/dL.[106] It is controversial whether the captopril renogram can predict which patients will exhibit a cure or improvement in blood pressure after revascularization.[107-109] There are no reliable data using the captopril renogram to predict whether revascularization will result in preservation or improvement in renal function. Although the captopril renogram was once the noninvasive diagnostic test of choice for patients with RAS, it is now relegated to a secondary screening modality because the quality of the images of duplex ultrasound, MRA, and CTA are excellent.

REFERENCES

1. Olin JW, Melia M, Young JR, et al: Prevalence of atherosclerotic renal artery stenosis in patients with atherosclerosis elsewhere. Am J Med 88:46N, 1990.
2. Harding MB, Smith LR, Himmelstein SI, et al: Renal artery stenosis: Prevalence and associated risk factors in patients undergoing routine cardiac catheterization. J Am Soc Nephrol 2:1608, 1992.
3. Safian RD, Textor SC: Renal-artery stenosis. N Engl J Med 344:431, 2001.
4. Olin JW: Atherosclerotic renal artery disease. Cardiol Clin 20:547, 2002.
5. Connolly JO, Higgins RM, Walters HL, et al: Presentation, clinical features and outcome in different patterns of atherosclerotic renovascular disease. QJM 87:413, 1994.
6. Mailloux LU, Napolitano B, Bellucci AG, et al: Renal vascular disease causing end-stage renal disease, incidence, clinical correlates, and outcomes: A 20-year clinical experience. Am J Kidney Dis 24:622, 1994.
7. Mailloux LU, Bellucci AG, Napolitano B, et al: Survival estimates for 683 patients starting dialysis from 1970 through 1989: Identification of risk factors for survival. Clin Nephrol 42:127, 1994.
8. Dustan HP, Humphries AW, DeWolfe VG, et al: Normal arterial pressure in patients with renal arterial stenosis. JAMA 187:1028, 1964.
9. Davis BA, Crook JE, Vestas RE, et al: Prevalence of renovascular hypertension in patients with grade III or IV hypertensive retinopathy. N Engl J Med 301:1273, 1979.
10. Chobanian AV, Bakris GL, Black HR, et al: The Seventh Report of the Joint National Committee on Prevention, Detection, Evaluation, and Treatment of High Blood Pressure: The JNC 7 report. JAMA 289:2560, 2003.
11. Gifford RW, Jr, McCormack LJ, Poutasse EF: The atrophic kidney: Its role in hypertension. Mayo Clin Proc 40:852, 1965.
12. Lawrie GM, Morris GC, Jr, Glaeser DH, et al: Renovascular reconstruction: Factors affecting long-term prognosis in 919 patients followed up to 31 years. Am J Cardiol 63:1085, 1989.
13. Textor SC, Tarazi RC, Novick AC, et al: Regulation of renal hemodynamics and glomerular filtration in patients with renovascular hypertension during converting enzyme inhibition with captopril. Am J Med 76:29, 1984.

14. Textor SC, Novick AC, Steinmuller DR, et al: Renal failure limiting antihypertensive therapy as an indication for renal revascularization: A case report. Arch Intern Med 143:2208, 1983.
15. Silas JH, Klenka Z, Solomon SA, et al: Captopril induced reversible renal failure: A marker of renal artery stenosis affecting a solitary kidney. Br Med J (Clin Res Ed) 286:1702, 1983.
16. Packer M, Lee WH, Medina N, et al: Functional renal insufficiency during long-term therapy with captopril and enalapril in severe chronic heart failure. Ann Intern Med 106:346, 1987.
17. Textor SC: Renal failure related to ACE inhibitors. Semin Nephrol 17:67, 1997.
18. Scoble JE, Maher ER, Hamilton G: Atherosclerotic renovascular disease causing renal impairment: A case for treatment. Clin Nephrol 31:119, 1989.
19. Scoble JE: Renal artery stenosis as a cause of renal impairment: Implications for treatment of hypertension and congestive heart failure. J R Soc Med 92:505, 1999.
20. Gray BH, Olin JW, Childs MB, et al: Clinical benefit of renal artery angioplasty with stenting for the control of recurrent and refractory congestive heart failure. Vasc Med 7:275, 2002.
21. Pickering TG, Herman L, Devereux RB, et al: Recurrent pulmonary oedema in hypertension due to bilateral renal artery stenosis: Treatment by angioplasty or surgical revascularisation. Lancet 2:551, 1988.
22. Diamond JR: Flash pulmonary edema and the diagnostic suspicion of occult renal artery stenosis. Am J Kidney Dis 21:328, 1993.
23. Khosla S, Kunjummen B, Manda R, et al: Prevalence of renal artery stenosis requiring revascularization in patients initially referred for coronary angiography. Catheter Cardiovasc Interv 58:400, 2003.
24. Scoble JE: The epidemiology and clinical manifestations of atherosclerotic renal artery disease. In Novick AC, Scoble J, Hamilton G (eds): Renal Vascular Disease. London, WB Saunders, 1996, p 303.
25. Conlon PJ, Little MA, Pieper K, et al: Severity of renal vascular disease predicts mortality in patients undergoing coronary angiography. Kidney Int 60:1490, 2001.
26. Rihal CS, Textor SC, Breen JF, et al: Incidental renal artery stenosis among a prospective cohort of hypertensive patients undergoing coronary angiography. Mayo Clin Proc 77:309, 2002.
27. Weber-Mzell D, Kotanko P, Schumacher M, et al: Coronary anatomy predicts presence or absence of renal artery stenosis: A prospective study in patients undergoing cardiac catheterization for suspected coronary artery disease. Eur Heart J 23:1684, 2002.
28. Louie J, Isaacson JA, Zierler RE, et al: Prevalence of carotid and lower extremity arterial disease in patients with renal artery stenosis. Am J Hypertens 7:436, 1994.
29. Conlon P, O'Riordan E, Kalra P: New insights into the epidemiologic and clinical manifestations of atherosclerotic renovascular disease. Am J Kidney Dis 35:573, 2000.
30. Dorros G, Jaff M, Mathiak L, et al: Four-year follow-up of Palmaz-Schatz stent revascularization as treatment for atherosclerotic renal artery stenosis. Circulation 98:642, 1998.
31. Eipper DF, Gifford RW, Jr, Stewart B, et al: Abdominal bruits in renovascular hypertension. Am J Cardiol 37:48, 1976.
32. Olin JW: Evaluation of the peripheral circulation. In Izzo JL, Black HR (eds): Hypertension Primer, 3rd ed. Dallas, American Heart Association, 2003, p 361.
33. Canzanello VJ, Textor SC: Noninvasive diagnosis of renovascular disease. Mayo Clin Proc 69:1172, 1994.
34. Emovon OE, Klotman PE, Dunnick NR, et al: Renovascular hypertension in blacks. Am J Hypertens 9:18, 1996.
35. Carman TL, Olin JW: Diagnosis of renal artery stenosis: What is the optimal diagnostic test? Curr Interv Cardiol Rep 2:111, 2000.
36. Radermacher J, Chavan A, Bleck J, et al: Use of Doppler ultrasonography to predict the outcome of therapy for renal-artery stenosis. N Engl J Med 344:410, 2001.
37. Olin JW, Piedmonte MR, Young JR, et al: The utility of duplex ultrasound scanning of the renal arteries for diagnosing significant renal artery stenosis. Ann Intern Med 122:833, 1995.
38. Olin JW: Role of duplex ultrasonography in screening for significant renal artery disease. Urol Clin North Am 21:215, 1994.
39. Carman TL, Olin JW, Czum J: Noninvasive imaging of the renal arteries. Urol Clin North Am 28:815, 2001.
40. Hansen KJ, Tribble RW, Reavis SW, et al: Renal duplex sonography: Evaluation of clinical utility. J Vasc Surg 12:227, 1990.
41. Hoffmann U, Edwards JM, Carter S, et al: Role of duplex scanning for the detection of atherosclerotic renal artery disease. Kidney Int 39:1232, 1991.
42. Kohler TR, Zierler RE, Martin RL, et al: Noninvasive diagnosis of renal artery stenosis by ultrasonic duplex scanning. J Vasc Surg 4:450, 1986.
43. Malatino LS, Polizzi G, Garozzo M, et al: Diagnosis of renovascular disease by extra- and intrarenal Doppler parameters. Angiology 49:707, 1998.
44. Miralles M, Cairols M, Cotillas J, et al: Value of Doppler parameters in the diagnosis of renal artery stenosis. J Vasc Surg 23:428, 1996.
45. Soulez G, Therasse E, Qanadli SD, et al: Prediction of clinical response after renal angioplasty: Respective value of renal Doppler sonography and scintigraphy. AJR Am J Roentgenol 181:1029, 2003.
46. Taylor DC, Moneta GL, Strandness DE, Jr: Follow-up of renal artery stenosis by duplex ultrasound. J Vasc Surg 9:410, 1989.
47. Hudspeth DA, Hansen KJ, Reavis SW, et al: Renal duplex sonography after treatment of renovascular disease. J Vasc Surg 18:381, 1993.
48. Bakker J, Beutler JJ, Elgersma OE, et al: Duplex ultrasonography in assessing restenosis of renal artery stents. Cardiovasc Intervent Radiol 22:475, 1999.
49. Soulez G, Oliva VL, Turpin S, et al: Imaging of renovascular hypertension: Respective values of renal scintigraphy, renal Doppler US, and MR angiography. Radiographics 20:1355, 2000.
50. Schoenberg SO, Knopp MV, Londy F, et al: Morphologic and functional magnetic resonance imaging of renal artery stenosis: A multireader tricenter study. J Am Soc Nephrol 13:158, 2002.
51. Aumann S, Schoenberg SO, Just A, et al: Quantification of renal perfusion using an intravascular contrast agent (part 1): Results in a canine model. Magn Reson. Med 49:276, 2003.
52. Prince MR, Chenevert TL, Foo TK, et al: Contrast-enhanced abdominal MR angiography: optimization of imaging delay time by automating the detection of contrast material arrival in the aorta. Radiology 203:109, 1997.
53. Zhang J, Pedrosa I, Rofsky NM: MR techniques for renal imaging. Radiol Clin North Am 41:877, 2003.
54. Saloner D: Determinants of image appearance in contrast-enhanced magnetic resonance angiography: A review. Invest Radiol 33:488, 1998.
55. Thornton J, O'Callaghan J, Walshe J, et al: Comparison of digital subtraction angiography with gadolinium-enhanced magnetic resonance angiography in the diagnosis of renal artery stenosis. Eur Radiol 9:930, 1999.
56. Olin JW, Kaufman JA, Bluemke DA, et al: Atherosclerotic Vascular Disease Conference. American Heart Association, Imaging, Writing Group IV. Circulation 109:2626, 2004.
57. Bakker J, Beek FJ, Beutler JJ, et al: Renal artery stenosis and accessory renal arteries: Accuracy of detection and visualization with gadolinium-enhanced breath-hold MR angiography. Radiology 207:497, 1998.
58. Schoenberg SO, Essig M, Bock M, et al: Comprehensive MR evaluation of renovascular disease in five breath holds. J Magn Reson Imaging 10:347, 1999.
59. Hahn U, Miller S, Nagele T, et al: Renal MR angiography at 1.0 T: Three-dimensional (3D) phase-contrast techniques versus gadolinium-enhanced 3D fast low-angle shot breath-hold imaging. AJR Am J Roentgenol 172:1501, 1999.
60. Tan KT, van Beek EJR, Brown PWG, et al: Magnetic resonance angiography for the diagnosis of renal artery stenosis: A meta-analysis. Clin Radiol 57:617, 2002.
61. De Cobelli F, Vanzulli A, Sironi S, et al: Renal artery stenosis: Evaluation with breath-hold, three-dimensional, dynamic, gadolinium-enhanced versus three-dimensional, phase-contrast MR angiography. Radiology 205:689, 1997.
62. Fain SB, King BF, Breen JF, et al: High-spatial-resolution contrast-enhanced MR angiography of the renal arteries: A prospective comparison with digital subtraction angiography. Radiology 218:481, 2001.
63. Hany TF, Debatin JF, Leung DA, et al: Evaluation of the aortoiliac and renal arteries: Comparison of breath-hold, contrast-enhanced, three-dimensional MR angiography with conventional catheter angiography. Radiology 204:357, 1997.
64. Rieumont MJ, Kaufman JA, Geller SC, et al: Evaluation of renal artery stenosis with dynamic gadolinium-enhanced MR angiography. AJR Am J Roentgenol 169:39, 1997.
65. Snidow JJ, Johnson MS, Harris VJ, et al: Three-dimensional gadolinium-enhanced MR angiography for aortoiliac inflow assessment plus renal artery screening in a single breath hold. Radiology 198:725, 1996.
66. Spuentrup E, Ruebben A, Stuber M, et al: Metallic renal artery MR imaging stent: Artifact-free lumen visualization with projection and standard renal MR angiography. Radiology 227:897, 2003.

67. Rubin GD: Three-dimensional helical CT angiography. Radiographics 14:905, 1994.
68. Rubin GD: MDCT imaging of the aorta and peripheral vessels. Eur J Radiol 45 Suppl 1:S42, 2003.
69. Rubin GD: 3-D imaging with MDCT. Eur J Radiol 45 Suppl 1:S37, 2003.
70. Rubin GD: Techniques for performing multidetector-row computed tomographic angiography. Tech Vasc Interv Radiol 4:2, 2001.
71. Bluemke DA, Chambers TP: Spiral CT angiography: An alternative to conventional angiography. Radiology 195:317, 1995.
72. Bluemke DA, Soyer PA, Chan BW, et al: Spiral CT during arterial portography: Technique and applications. Radiographics 15:623, 1995.
73. Zeman RK, Silverman PM, Vieco PT, et al: CT angiography. AJR Am J Roentgenol 165:1079, 1995.
74. Ibukuro K, Charnsangavej C, Chasen MH, et al: Helical CT angiography with multiplanar reformation: Techniques and clinical applications. Radiographics 15:671, 1995.
75. Addis KA, Hopper KD, Iyriboz TA, et al: CT angiography: In vitro comparison of five reconstruction methods. AJR Am J Roentgenol 177:1171, 2001.
76. Willmann JK, Wildermuth S, Pfammatter T, et al: Aortoiliac and renal arteries: Prospective intraindividual comparison of contrast-enhanced three-dimensional MR angiography and multi-detector row CT angiography. Radiology 226:798, 2003.
77. Qanadli SD, Mesurolle B, Coggia M, et al: Abdominal aortic aneurysm: Pretherapy assessment with dual-slice helical CT angiography. AJR Am J Roentgenol 174:181, 2000.
78. Kim TS, Chung JW, Park JH, et al: Renal artery evaluation: Comparison of spiral CT angiography to intra-arterial DSA. J Vasc Interv Radiol 9:553, 1998.
79. Kaatee R, Beek FJ, de Lange EE, et al: Renal artery stenosis: Detection and quantification with spiral CT angiography versus optimized digital subtraction angiography. Radiology 205:121, 1997.
80. Johnson PT, Halpern EJ, Kuszyk BS, et al: Renal artery stenosis: CT angiography: Comparison of real-time volume-rendering and maximum intensity projection algorithms. Radiology 211:337, 1999.
81. Slovut D, Olin JW: Fibromuscular dysplasia. N Engl J Med 350:1862, 2004.
82. Bosanac Z, Miller RJ, Jain M: Rotational digital subtraction carotid angiography: Technique and comparison with static digital subtraction angiography. Clin Radiol 53:682, 1998.
83. Seymour HR, Matson MB, Belli AM, et al: Rotational digital subtraction angiography of the renal arteries: Technique and evaluation in the study of native and transplant renal arteries. Br J Radiol 74:134, 2001.
84. Meijering EH, Niessen WJ, Bakker J, et al: Reduction of patient motion artifacts in digital subtraction angiography: Evaluation of a fast and fully automatic technique. Radiology 219:288, 2001.
85. Meijering EH, Niesssen WJ, Viergever MA: Retrospective motion correction in digital subtraction angiography: A review. IEEE Trans Med Imaging 18:2, 1999.
86. Ashleigh RJ, Hufton AP, Razzaq R, et al: A comparison of bolus chasing and static digital subtraction arteriography in peripheral vascular disease. Br J Radiol 73:819, 2000.
87. Schreier DZ, Weaver FA, Frankhouse J, et al: A prospective study of carbon dioxide-digital subtraction vs standard contrast arteriography in the evaluation of the renal arteries. Arch Surg 131:503, 1996.
88. Hawkins IF, Jr, Wilcox CS, Kerns SR, et al: CO_2 digital angiography: A safer contrast agent for renal vascular imaging? Am J Kidney Dis 24:685, 1994.
89. Caridi JG, Hawkins IF, Jr: CO_2 digital subtraction angiography: Potential complications and their prevention. J Vasc Interv Radiol 8:383, 1997.
90. Caridi JG, Stavropoulos SW, Hawkins IF, Jr: Carbon dioxide digital subtraction angiography for renal artery stent placement. J Vasc Interv Radiol 10:635, 1999.
91. Spinosa DJ, Matsumoto AH, Angle JF, et al: Safety of CO(2)- and gadodiamide-enhanced angiography for the evaluation and percutaneous treatment of renal artery stenosis in patients with chronic renal insufficiency. AJR Am J Roentgenol 176:1305, 2001.
92. Spinosa DJ, Matsumoto AH, Angle JF, et al: Use of gadopentetate dimeglumine as a contrast agent for percutaneous transluminal renal angioplasty and stent placement. Kidney Int 53:503, 1998.
93. Spinosa DJ, Matsumoto AH, Angle JF, et al: Gadolinium contrast agents: Their role in vascular and nonvascular diagnostic angiography and interventions. Tech Vasc Interv Radiol 4:45, 2001.
94. Spinosa DJ, Matsumoto AH, Angle JF, et al: Renal insufficiency: Usefulness of gadodiamide-enhanced renal angiography to supplement CO_2-enhanced renal angiography for diagnosis and percutaneous treatment. Radiology 210:663, 1999.
95. Spinosa DJ, Matsumoto AH, Angle JF, et al: Gadolinium-based contrast and carbon dioxide angiography to evaluate renal transplants for vascular causes of renal insufficiency and accelerated hypertension. J Vasc Interv Radiol 9:909, 1998.
96. Conlon PJ, Athirakul K, Kovalik E, et al: Survival in renal vascular disease. J Am Soc Nephrol 9:252, 1998.
97. Olin JW, Begelman SM: Renal Artery Disease. In Topol E (ed): Textbook of Cardiovascular Medicine, 2nd ed. Philadelphia, Lippincott Raven, 2002, p 2139.
98. Textor SC: Progressive hypertension in a patient with "incidental" renal artery stenosis. Hypertension 40:595, 2002.
99. White CJ: The renal oculosten(t)otic reflex. Cathet Cardiovasc Diagn 37:251, 1996.
100. Maxwell MH, Lupu AN, Taplin GV: Radioisotope renogram in renal arterial hypertension. J Urol 100:376, 1968.
101. Ploth DW: Angiotensin-dependent renal mechanisms in two-kidney, one-clip renal vascular hypertension. Am J Physiol 245:F131, 1983.
102. Nally JV, Barton DP: Contemporary approach to diagnosis and evaluation of renovascular hypertension. Urol Clin North Am 28:781, 2001.
103. Black HR, Bourgoignie JJ, Pickering T, et al: Report of the Working Party Group for Patient Selection and Preparation. Am J Hypertens 4:745S, 1991.
104. Setaro JF, Chen CC, Hoffer PB, et al: Captopril renography in the diagnosis of renal artery stenosis and the prediction of improvement with revascularization: The Yale Vascular Center experience. Am J Hypertens 4:698S, 1991.
105. Setaro JF, Saddler MC, Chen CC, et al: Simplified captopril renography in diagnosis and treatment of renal artery stenosis. Hypertension 18:289, 1991.
106. Fommei E, Ghione S, Hilson AJ, et al: Captopril radionuclide test in renovascular hypertension: A European multicentre study. European Multicentre Study Group. Eur J Nucl Med 20:617, 1993.
107. Geyskes GG, Oei HY, Puylaert CB, et al: Renography with captopril: Changes in a patient with hypertension and unilateral renal artery stenosis. Arch Intern Med 146:1705, 1986.
108. Mittal BR, Kumar P, Arora P, et al: Role of captopril renography in the diagnosis of renovascular hypertension. Am J Kidney Dis 28:209, 1996.
109. van Jaarsveld BC, Krijnen P, Derkx FH, et al: The place of renal scintigraphy in the diagnosis of renal artery stenosis: Fifteen years of clinical experience. Arch Intern Med 157:1226, 1997.

chapter 23

Treatment of Renal Artery Stenosis

Robert D. Safian
George Hanzel

The clinical diagnosis of renal artery stenosis relies on a high index of suspicion and confirmation by noninvasive imaging modalities. There are three distinct syndromes associated with renal artery stenosis: renin-dependent hypertension, essential hypertension, and ischemic nephropathy. Clinical features that heighten suspicion for renal artery stenosis include abrupt-onset or accelerated hypertension at any age, unexplained acute or chronic azotemia, azotemia induced by angiotensin-converting enzyme inhibitors (ACEIs), asymmetric renal dimensions, and congestive heart failure with normal left ventricular function. Therapeutic considerations, alone or in combination, include medical therapy, percutaneous revascularization with angioplasty (PTA) or stenting, and surgical revascularization with bypass surgery or endarterectomy (Table 23-1).

GENERAL CONSIDERATIONS ABOUT TREATMENT

Atherosclerosis accounts for greater than 90% of cases of renal artery stenosis, whereas the remaining 10% are associated with fibromuscular dysplasia (FMD) or other inflammatory diseases of the renal arterial circulation. Whereas FMD is typically a disease of young and middle-aged females and usually involves the distal two thirds of the renal artery and its branches, atherosclerotic renal artery stenosis (ARAS) is a disease of the elderly, particularly those with diabetes, aortoiliac occlusive disease, coronary artery disease, and hypertension. ARAS usually involves the ostium and proximal one third of the renal artery, and it is a common and progressive manifestation of atherosclerosis.

Despite the prevalence and progressive nature of ARAS, it is likely that many cases are never detected. Most patients with ARAS are identified during an evaluation for refractory hypertension or progressive renal failure, or fortuitously as part of angiographic evaluation for aneurysmal or occlusive diseases of the lower extremity arterial circulation. In general, decisions about treatment of patients with ARAS are usually based on arrest or reversal of systematic atherosclerosis, blood pressure control, and preservation of renal excretory function.

MEDICAL THERAPY FOR RENAL ARTERY STENOSIS

The risk of cardiovascular events in hypertensive adults is most dependent on the degree of hypertension rather than its cause. True renovascular hypertension (i.e., renin-dependent hypertension) is much more likely in young patients with FMD than in elderly patients with ARAS. In fact, most hypertensive patients with ARAS have essential hypertension, whereas those with accelerated or malignant hypertension may have a renovascular component superimposed on a background of essential hypertension.

Patients with FMD rarely have excretory dysfunction, and hypertension generally responds to ACEIs. In contrast, there are a number of issues concerning the medical management of patients with ARAS. First, although never specifically studied in patients with ARAS, it is reasonable to treat all patients with aggressive risk-factor modification to limit atherosclerosis. These measures include aspirin, lipid-lowering therapy, and smoking cessation.[1] Second, the medical therapy for hypertensive patients with ARAS is similar to that for patients with essential hypertension. In fact, even after renal artery revascularization, patients with ARAS typically have persistent hypertension, and continued medical therapy is necessary for blood pressure control. Third, patients with ischemic nephropathy represent a particularly high-risk group with a poor prognosis, and there are no studies demonstrating a benefit of medical therapy for reversing or stabilizing renal function. The impact of medical therapy on long-term renal function is controversial: One study reported a rise in serum creatinine concentration in 5% to 10% of patients,[2] whereas another showed a progressive rise in creatinine (despite excellent blood pressure control), which improved only after successful revascularization.[3]

Use of an ACEI or angiotensin-receptor blocker (ARB) is controversial in hypertensive patients with ARAS. Important considerations relate to the extent of renal artery stenosis and the degree of baseline renal impairment. Patients with hypertension, unilateral ARAS, and normal baseline renal function are good candidates for treatment with ACEIs or ARB. In fact, ACEIs appear to be more effective than other antihypertensive agents in this setting.[4] In patients with hypertension, unilateral renal artery stenosis (RAS), and abnormal baseline renal function, ACEIs exert a beneficial impact on survival without affecting renal function. In these patients, long-term renal function is influenced most by the degree of baseline renal dysfunction and proteinuria, not by pharmacologic treatment.[5] In diabetic patients with hypertension, unilateral renal artery stenosis, proteinuria, and normal or abnormal renal function, ACEIs and ARB are effective antihypertensive agents, and drug-induced reduction of intraglomerular

TABLE 23-1 THERAPEUTIC OPTIONS FOR PATIENTS WITH RENAL ARTERY STENOSIS

Treatment	Impact on Hypertension	Impact on Nephropathy	Comments
Medical therapy	Effective for control of hypertension	No confirmed benefit for reversing or stabilizing renal function	Mandatory for risk-factor modification (aspirin, lipid-lowering therapy, smoking cessation). Good randomized trials are needed to assess impact of medical therapy
PTA	Effective for refractory hypertension in patients with FMD; not superior to medical therapy in patients with ARAS	Uncertain role; complex relationship between revascularization vs. complications (distal embolization, contrast nephropathy)	Not useful for ostial ARAS because of suboptimal results
Stents	Not evaluated in patients with FMD; effective for achieving "statistical" improvement in blood pressure; not clearly superior to medical therapy	Same as for PTA. Anecdotal experience suggests benefit if patient does not have advanced nephropathy or parenchymal disease	Treatment of choice in most patients with ARAS if revascularization is needed
Bypass surgery	Not employed for FMD; not clearly useful in patients with ARAS	Anecdotal experience suggests possible benefit in the absence of advanced renal dysfunction	Used infrequently in patients with extensive aortic aneurysmal or occlusive disease; perioperative mortality rate is 2-6%

ARAS, atherosclerotic renal artery stenosis; FMD, fibromuscular dysplasia; PTA, percutaneous transluminal angioplasty.

capillary pressure decreases proteinuria and renal injury.[6] It is interesting to speculate whether renal revascularization in this subgroup of patients could offset the benefit of ACEI by increasing intraglomerular capillary pressure, proteinuria, and renal injury.

In contrast to patients with unilateral ARAS, patients with bilateral RAS (or stenosis in a single solitary kidney) may be especially sensitive to decline in intraglomerular pressure, leading to progressive renal failure. Such changes in intraglomerular pressure may occur in association with ACEIs or ARB (due to vasodilation of the efferent arterioles) and absolute or functional reduction in intravascular volume (due to diuretics, dehydration, bleeding, or congestive heart failure). In studies of thousands of patients with hypertension or congestive heart failure (many of whom may have had occult renal artery stenosis), discontinuation of ACEIs due to renal dysfunction was reported in 0.5% of patients, although mild-to-moderate increases in serum creatinine (> 0.5 mg/dL) were reported in 0.1% to 10%.[7,8] In contrast, discontinuation of an ACEI due to renal dysfunction was necessary in 5% to 20% of patients with bilateral ARAS or stenosis of a solitary kidney.[9-11] Taken together, available data suggest that most patients with unilateral ARAS and hypertension will benefit from an ACEI or ARB. Patients with bilateral ARAS (or stenosis of a solitary kidney) will also benefit from ACEIs or ARB, but renal function and serum potassium levels should be monitored closely during initiation of therapy, to identify those who may be intolerant.

INDICATIONS FOR RENAL ARTERY REVASCULARIZATION

Indications for renal artery revascularization are controversial and have not been established by any randomized trial. The decision to revascularize is usually based on the assumption that the stenosis is hemodynamically significant, and that revascularization will improve blood pressure control, preserve renal function, or have a favorable impact on cardiac or cerebrovascular manifestations of severe hypertension. Some physicians believe that renal preservation is a more important indication for renal revascularization than control of hypertension, but there is virtually no consensus about patient selection or timing of revascularization.

Patients with refractory hypertension and FMD should be treated with PTA; cure of hypertension is expected in more than 75% of such patients. In contrast, patients with refractory hypertension and ARAS are rarely cured by any form of surgical or percutaneous revascularization, although blood pressure may be easier to manage and medication requirements may decrease after revascularization.[12-20] Hypertension alone rarely should be considered a compelling indication for renal artery revascularization. Instead, renal revascularization is recommended for patients with unilateral or bilateral ARAS and functional impairment of the heart, brain, or kidneys. Manifestations of functional impairment include hypertensive crisis (nonischemic pulmonary edema, acute coronary syndrome, aortic dissection, or neurologic impairment) and renal insufficiency (rising creatinine due to ACEI, bilateral ARAS and rising creatinine or declining nuclear glomerular filtration rate [GFR], and unilateral ARAS and fractional GFR <40%) (Fig. 23-1). Revascularization of unilateral ARAS (when the contralateral renal artery is patent) in the setting of advanced renal dysfunction (serum creatinine >2.5 mg/dL) does not affect overall renal function because severe bilateral parenchymal disease is invariably present. Revascularization of isolated unilateral ARAS (without uncontrolled hypertension or elevated creatinine) may be reasonable if ipsilateral fractional GFR is equal to 40% because this is a manifestation of abnormal blood flow and functional impairment of the stenotic kidney.

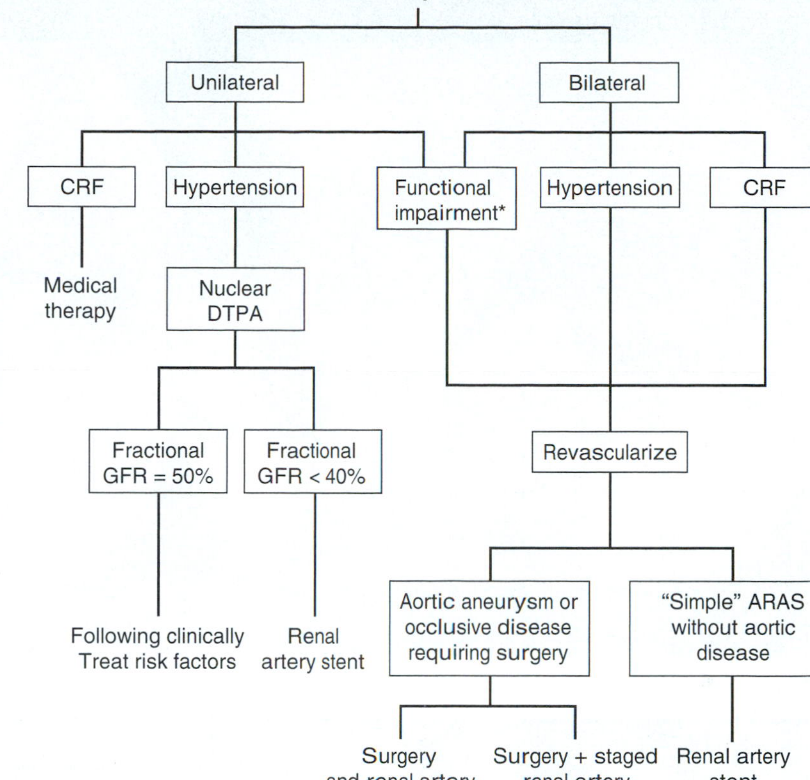

FIGURE 23-1. Management algorithm for patients with atherosclerotic renal artery stenosis. *Functional impairment includes hypertensive emergency with transient ischemic attack, stroke, intracranial hemorrhage, unstable angina, acute MI, pulmonary edema, aortic dissection, ACEI-induced renal failure, rising serum creatinine (bilateral ARAS or solitary kidney with ARAS), or fractional nuclear GFR of less than 40% (unilateral ARAS). ACEI, angiotensin-converting enzyme inhibitor; ARAS, atherosclerotic renal artery stenosis; CRF, chronic renal failure; DTPA, diethylene triamine pentaacetic acid; GFR, glomerular filtration rate.

TIMING OF RENAL ARTERY REVASCULARIZATION

Many physicians consider renal artery revascularization when there is bilateral renal artery stenosis (or severe stenosis affecting a solitary kidney) and serum creatinine is greater than 2 mg/dL. This bias for revascularization when the serum creatinine is elevated is unjustified because several observations suggest that earlier revascularization is better. It is crucial to recognize that the serum creatinine is insensitive to changes in GFR when baseline creatinine is less than 2 mg/dL, and that serum creatinine 1.5 to 2 mg/dL is associated with a 50% to 75% loss of renal mass and filtration function, consistent with advanced excretory dysfunction. Surgical revascularization is associated with a 1.5- to threefold higher risk of perioperative and late death for each 1.0 mg/dL increment in baseline creatinine, and the incidence and severity of postoperative renal failure are highly dependent on baseline creatinine. Late outcomes after surgical and percutaneous revascularization are better in patients with a baseline serum creatinine of less than 1.5 mg/dL.[18,21] Baseline creatinine of greater than 1.5 mg/dL is associated with a fivefold higher risk of death at 4 years after renal stenting, compared with patients with a baseline creatinine of less than 1.5 mg/dL.[22] Patients with critical bilateral renal artery stenosis or severe stenosis in a solitary kidney should be considered for renal revascularization if there is evidence for functional cardiac, neurological, or renal impairment. Because renal replacement therapy is a poor alternative for patients with potentially reversible ischemic nephropathy,[23] renal revascularization should be performed before the development of significant renal insufficiency. Patients with moderate renal insufficiency and ARAS may benefit from revascularization by stabilizing or reversing renal dysfunction.[15-17,19-22,24-27]

TYPE OF REVASCULARIZATION

Surgical revascularization for ARAS has evolved over the last 20 years. In the era before PTA and ACEI, the most common surgical technique was unilateral aortorenal bypass. In most centers, extra-anatomic bypass (where the bypass originates from the celiac or mesenteric vessels, rather than the aorta) and renal endarterectomy now account for more than 80% of renal vascular operations, with perioperative mortality rates of 2% to 6%.[20,22,28] In contrast, percutaneous renal stenting is routinely performed in patients with ARAS, with procedural success rates exceeding 95%, major complications in less than 5%, and restenosis in 10% to 15%. Although PTA achieves excellent results in patients with FMD, stenting is the endovascular procedure of choice in patients with ARAS. Prospective studies are underway to evaluate the benefit of embolic protection devices during renal stenting (Fig. 23-2).

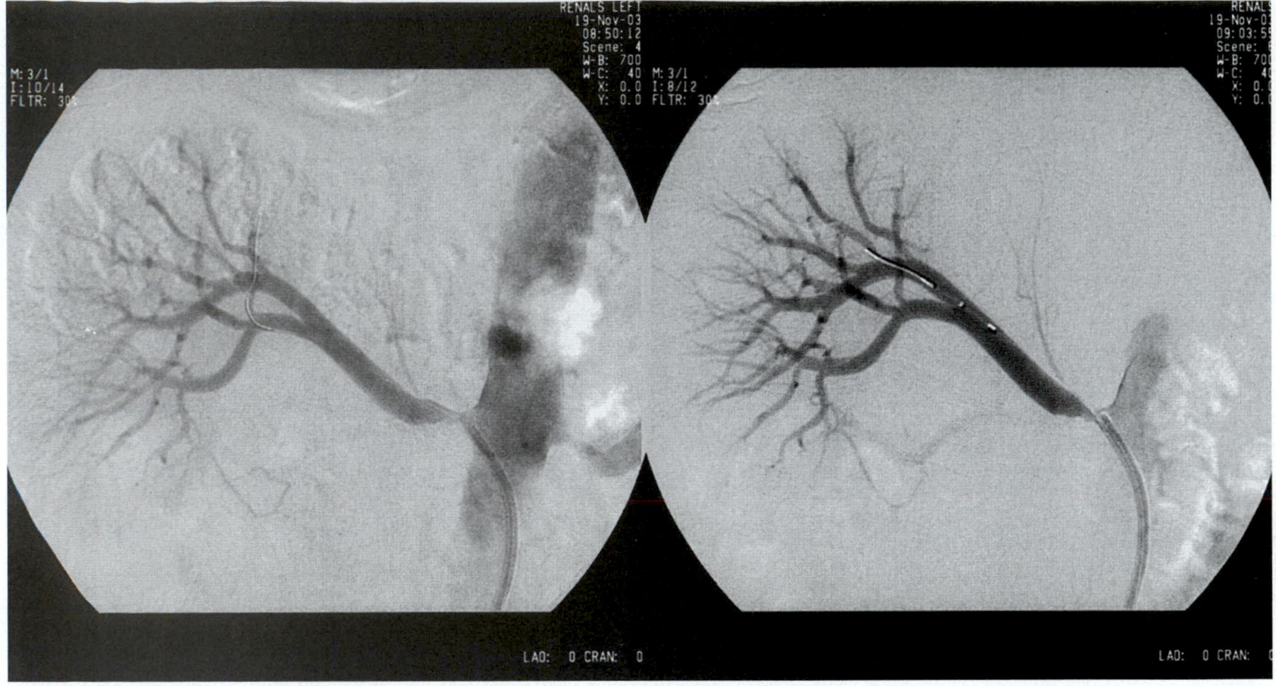

A

B

FIGURE 23-2. Percutaneous revascularization of the right renal artery using stent techniques and distal embolic protection. **A,** Baseline angiography shows severe stenosis of the ostium of the right renal artery (*left*). A short-tipped Angioguard protection device is positioned proximal to first bifurcation (*right*). **B,** The Angioguard filter is deployed (*left*; note three opaque markers proximal to the bifurcation, indicating filter deployment). After stenting, there is no residual stenosis or dissection (*right*); a small amount of debris was recovered in the filter.

IMPACT OF REVASCULARIZATION ON HYPERTENSION

Published studies on the impact of renal revascularization on hypertension have numerous limitations. Hypertension has been classified as "cured" (i.e., the blood pressure is normal without the need for medication), improved (the number or dose of medications is reduced, blood pressure is better controlled, or both), or unchanged. However, the ability to make direct comparisons among studies is limited because of differences in medical therapy, target blood pressure, and criteria for improvement. Interpretation of data is further limited by the uncertain clinical relevance of these classification groups because statistically significant differences in blood pressure and medications may not be clinically important. The effects of aggressive lipid-lowering therapy, risk-factor modification, antihypertensive therapy, and aspirin have not been studied in patients with ARAS.

Despite these limitations, it is apparent that hypertension is more likely to be cured after revascularization in patients with FMD than in those with ARAS (75% vs. < 20% percent), regardless of the type of revascularization.[20,21,29] Two small randomized trials of PTA and medical therapy for ARAS demonstrated a significant decrease in blood pressure and fewer medications after PTA, but cure of hypertension was rare.[29,30] A recent randomized trial in hypertensive patients with ARAS showed no difference in outcomes between PTA and medical therapy.[14] As with other means of revascularization, stenting is associated with a small but statistically significant decrease in blood pressure and medication requirements at 4 years.[12,18,27] The cure rates for hypertension after stenting are low and are similar to those after surgery and PTA.[18,19,26] One study suggested that improvement in hypertension after renal stenting was more likely in the presence of severe bilateral ARAS and severe baseline hypertension (mean arterial pressure > 110 mm Hg),[15] especially when parenchymal disease is absent.[27,30]

There are several potential reasons why renal artery revascularization may not result in dramatic improvement or cure of hypertension. First, most patients with ARAS have essential, not renovascular hypertension. Second, many patients with hypertension have intrarenal vascular disease and parenchymal disease, leading to hypertensive nephropathy and self-perpetuating hypertension. In hypertensive patients with or without ARAS, renal arteriography can identify patterns of progressive hypertensive nephropathy, including arteriolar narrowing, vascular pruning, and loss of cortical blood flow (Fig. 23-3). Correction of the main renal artery stenosis by surgery or stenting would have little or no impact on hypertension or renal function when severe intrarenal disease is present. Finally, some advocates of renal stenting suggest that randomized trials of PTA and medical therapy are invalid because of suboptimal lumen enlargement after PTA. However, most studies of renal revascularization report similar cure rates and improvement in hypertension, regardless of revascularization technique.

TREATMENT OF ISCHEMIC NEPHROPATHY

A common dilemma is the approach to the patient with ARAS and renal dysfunction. Several clinical and angiographic factors (renal dimensions, serum creatinine, presence of collaterals, and intact glomeruli by renal biopsy) have been proposed to suggest reversible renal failure, but the predictive values of these factors have not been validated. Factors that seem to identify irreversible dysfunction include severe diffuse intrarenal atherosclerosis (see Fig. 23-3), proteinuria greater than 1 gram/24 hours (especially in a diabetic patient), unilateral ARAS with a serum creatinine greater than 2.5 mg/dL, renal resistive index greater than 80, and marked atrophy of the renal cortex.[30] Renal resistive index is obtained by averaging values obtained in the upper, middle, and lower intrarenal segmental arteries, according to the formula $100 \times [1\text{-EDV/PSV}]$, where EDV and PSV are Doppler-derived end-diastolic and peak-systolic velocities, respectively.[30]

Most studies of renal artery revascularization describe serial changes in serum creatinine as lower than baseline, unchanged, or higher than baseline. Unfortunately, there is no consensus about which changes are clinically important, nor is there consensus about whether a lack of change in serum creatinine implies stabilization of renal function or lack of benefit. In considering the results of percutaneous and surgical revascularization, most studies have classified serum creatinine as improved in 55%, unchanged in 25%, and worse in 20%.[19,20,22,24,27,31] Some clinicians assess serial changes in reciprocal serum creatinine or calculated creatinine clearance using the Cockroft-Gault formula, which has been offered as evidence for the beneficial effect of renal revascularization on ischemic nephropathy.[24,25,27] When evaluating changes in reciprocal serum creatinine concentration over time, three different patterns (Fig. 23-4) suggest improvement in renal function (Fig. 23-5), stabilization, or decline in renal function. Analysis of the slope of reciprocal creatinine relationship suggests that most patients have stabilization or slower progression of renal dysfunction, and a minority have long-term improvement (Fig. 23-6). Potential explanations for failure of renal revascularization to improve renal function include underlying renal parenchymal disease that persists despite revascularization, percutaneous- or surgical-induced renal embolization, radiocontrast nephropathy, or acute tubular necrosis. Late decline in renal function might be due to progressive nephropathy, stent restenosis, or bypass graft failure.

IMPACT OF REVASCULARIZATION ON RENAL FUNCTION

In properly selected patients, renal artery revascularization can stabilize or improve renal function. In one study, surgical revascularization resulted in significant improvement in postoperative total- and single-kidney nuclear GFR.[32] Linear regression models suggested arrest of renal

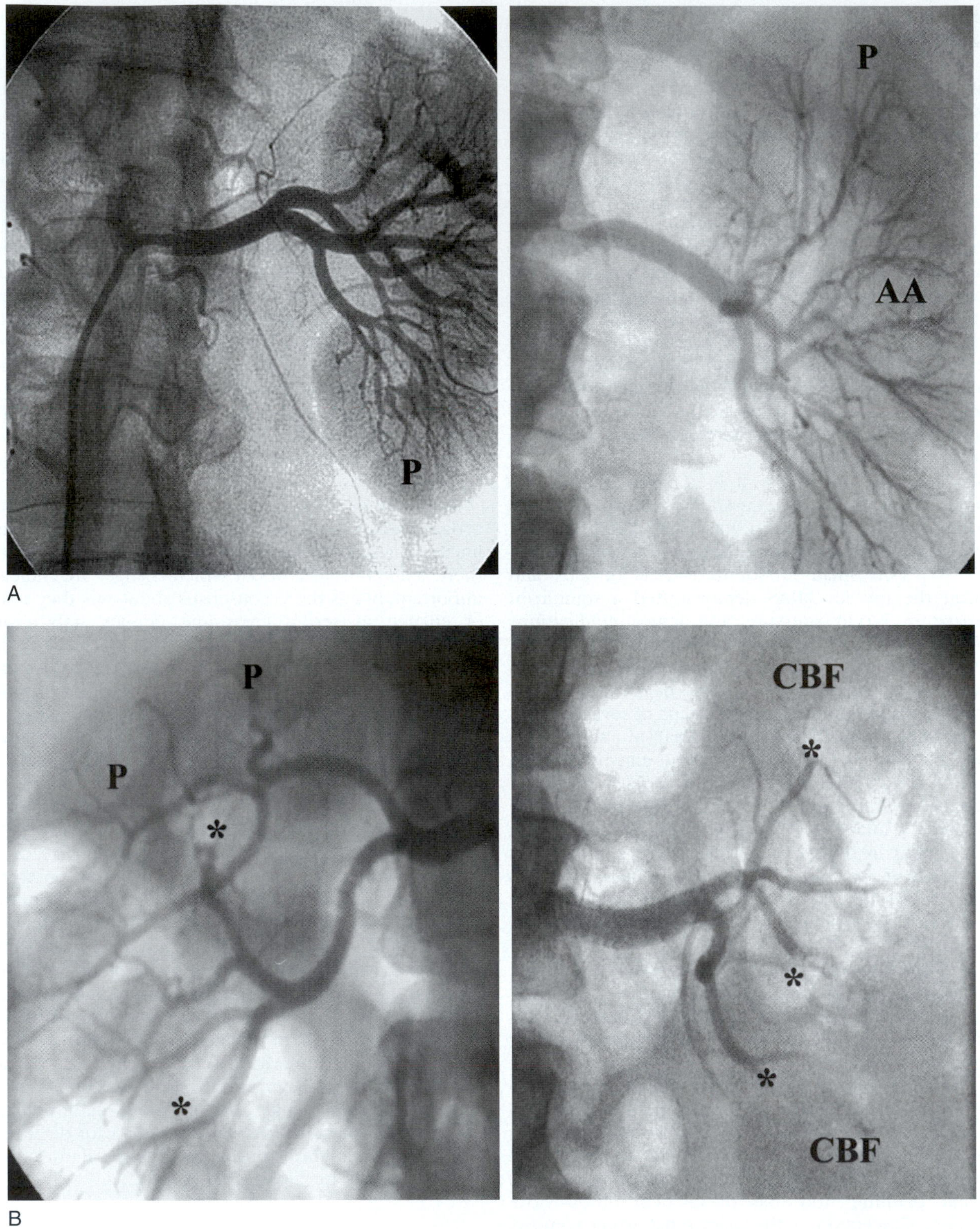

FIGURE 23-3. Arteriographic patterns of progressive hypertensive nephropathy. **A,** A normal renal arteriogram and nephrogram (*left*), showing excellent cortical blood flow extending into the renal pyramids. In mild hypertensive nephropathy (*right*), cortical blood flow into the renal pyramids is preserved, but there is diffuse intrarenal arteriolar narrowing (AA). **B,** This is a more advanced stage of hypertensive nephropathy (*left*), characterized by diminished cortical blood flow, some circulation to the renal pyramids (P), and pruning (*) of several lobar arteries. In end-stage hypertensive nephropathy (*right*), cortical blood flow is absent (CBF), and there is generalized pruning (*) of most lobar vessels.

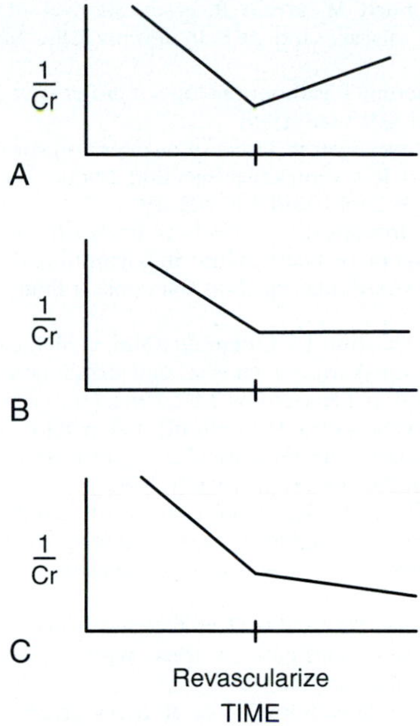

FIGURE 23-4. Patterns of change in renal function, before and after renal revascularization, using reciprocal serum creatinine concentrations. In all three patterns, serum creatinine rises over time before revascularization. After revascularization, pattern **A** shows improvement in renal function, manifested by a progressive fall in creatinine, and a positive slope in reciprocal creatinine. In pattern **B,** renal function stabilizes (does not improve or deteriorate), and the slope of the reciprocal serum creatinine relationship is zero. In pattern **C,** renal function continues to deteriorate, but the rate of decline may be slower than before revascularization.

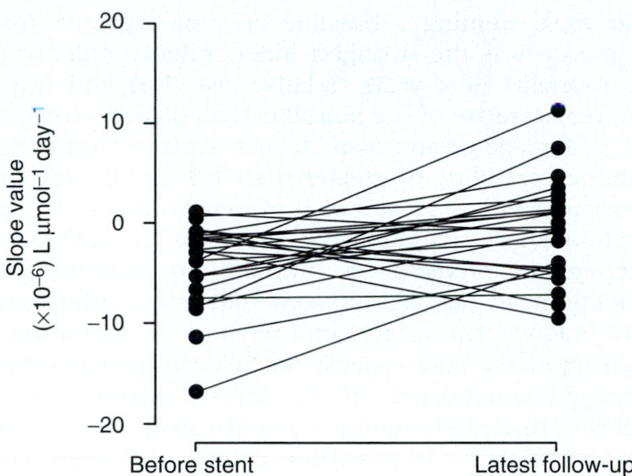

FIGURE 23-6. Slope of the relationship of reciprocal serum creatinine over time, measured before and after stenting, in 23 patients with ARAS ($P < .007$). Before stenting, virtually all patients had a negative slope, indicating progressive deterioration in renal function. After stenting, the slope improved in most patients, but was positive in only three patients with improvement in renal function. Most of the remaining patients had slower deterioration or stabilization of renal function. (Reproduced with permission from Harden PN, MacLeod MJ, Rodger RS, et al: Effect of renal-artery stenting on progression of renovascular renal failure. Lancet 349:1133, 1997.)

dysfunction manifested by a slower decline in GFR from 3.25% per week before surgery to 0.94% per week after surgery.[33] In other studies, stenting was associated with preservation of renal dimensions after 2 years,[25] and surgical revascularization resulted in significant improvements in renal dimensions, which correlated with improvements in total- and single-kidney GFR and hyperconcentration of urinary creatinine.[32] The most consistent predictor of improvement in renal function is the absence of parenchymal disease prior to intervention.[27,30] Baseline renal resistive index of greater than 80 is associated with poor outcomes (inadequate blood pressure control, worsening creatinine clearance, more frequent progression to dialysis, and higher mortality). Compared with patients with renal resistive index of less than 80, those greater than 80 were generally older, had more extensive atherosclerosis, and worse baseline renal function—suggesting that these patients had more parenchymal disease.[30]

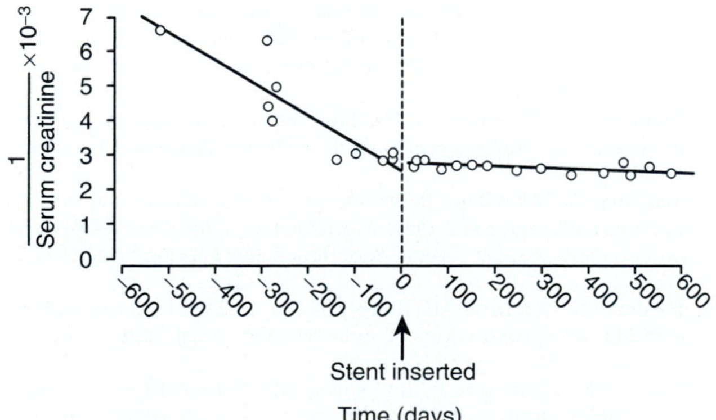

FIGURE 23-5. Relationship of reciprocal serum creatinine concentration over time, in a patient with ischemic nephropathy treated by stenting. In the 600 days prior to revascularization, renal function deteriorated progressively. After stenting, the slope of the reciprocal creatinine relationship is zero, suggesting stabilization of renal function. (Reproduced with permission from Harden PN, MacLeod MJ, Rodger RS, et al: Effect of renal-artery stenting on progression of renovascular renal failure. Lancet 349:1133, 1997.)

IMPACT OF RENAL REVASCULARIZATION ON CARDIOVASCULAR OUTCOME

Understanding the impact of renal revascularization on long-term survival is hampered by selection bias and the lack of carefully controlled randomized trials. The survival of medically-treated patients with ischemic nephropathy not requiring dialysis has not been defined. Survival at 3 to 5 years after surgical or percutaneous revascularization for these patients is approximately 70%, and most late deaths are due to cardiovascular events rather than progressive renal failure.[18,33] Although correction of ARAS may stabilize or improve renal function, the impact of renal artery revascularization on overall cardiovascular morbidity and mortality is uncertain. After surgical revascularization, predictors of 5- and 10-year mortalities include age greater than 60 years, coronary artery disease, and prior vascular surgery.[21] In patients with baseline renal insufficiency, persistent elevation of postoperative creatinine was associated with a poor long-term outcome and high mortality.[20]

After renal stenting, a baseline creatinine greater than 1.5 mg/dL was the strongest independent predictor of late mortality at 4 years (relative risk 5.0), and was a stronger correlate of late mortality than diabetes (relative risk 2.5) or age greater than 70 years (relative risk 1.9).[16] Baseline creatinine of greater than 1.5 mg/dL was also associated with a greater risk of deterioration in renal function after stenting.[26] The presence of ARAS is an independent predictor of mortality in patients with ischemic heart disease, and some data suggest improvement in long-term survival after renal revascularization.[23] Together, these data suggest that elderly patients with advanced generalized atherosclerosis, manifested by occlusive diseases in multiple vascular beds and baseline renal insufficiency, have a worse prognosis than patients with limited atherosclerosis and normal renal function.

Conclusion

Patients with true renin-dependent (renovascular) hypertension are typically young or middle-aged females with FMD. Initial therapy for renovascular hypertension associated with FMD is an ACEI; refractory hypertension responds readily to PTA without stenting. In contrast, ARAS is highly prevalent among elderly patients with other manifestations of atherosclerosis, and frequently results from in-growth of atherosclerotic plaque from the abdominal aorta, compromising the ostium of the renal artery. In elderly patients with generalized atherosclerosis and ARAS, hypertension is usually not renin-dependent (i.e., *essential hypertension*). Because renal revascularization rarely cures hypertension, these patients should be treated aggressively with antihypertensive medical therapy. Renal artery stenting may be considered for refractory severe hypertension to improve blood pressure control and modestly reduce medication requirements. Patients with ARAS, hypertension, and functional impairment of the heart, brain, or kidneys should be considered for renal revascularization. Patients with ischemic nephropathy should be treated before the development of advanced renal failure. The best candidates for revascularization are those with baseline serum creatinine levels of less than 2.0 mg/dL, bilateral ARAS, normal renal resistive indices, no proteinuria, and one or more manifestations of cardiac, cerebral, or renal functional impairment. In these patients, renal revascularization is best accomplished by stenting, although surgical revascularization may be considered in patients with concomitant severe aortic aneurysmal or occlusive disease.

REFERENCES

1. Safian RD, Textor SC: Renal-artery stenosis. N Engl J Med 344:431, 2001.
2. Caps MT, Zierler RE, Polissar NL, et al: Risk of atrophy in kidneys with atherosclerotic renal artery stenosis. Kidney Int 53:735, 1998.
3. Toto RD, Mitchell HC, Lee HC, et al: Reversible renal insufficiency due to angiotensin converting enzyme inhibitors in hypertensive nephrosclerosis. Ann Intern Med 115: 513, 1991.
4. Textor SC: ACE inhibitors in renovascular hypertension. Cardiovasc Drugs Therap 4:229, 1990.
5. Losito A, Gaburri M, Errico R, et al: Survival of patients with renovascular disease and ACE inhibition. Clin Nephrol 52:339, 1999.
6. Remuzzi G, Bertani T: Pathophysiology of progressive nephropathies. N Engl J Med 339:1448, 1998.
7. The SOLVD Investigators: Effect of enalapril on survival in patients with reduced left ventricular ejection fractions and congestive heart failure. N Engl J Med 325:293, 1991.
8. The SOLVD Investigators: Effect of enalapril on mortality and the development of heart failure in asymptomatic patients with reduced left ventricular ejection fractions. N Engl J Med 327:685, 1992.
9. Tillman DM, Malatino LS, Cumming AMM, et al: Enalapril in hypertension with renal artery stenosis: Long-term follow-up and effects on renal function. J Hypertens 2:93, 1984.
10. Jackson B, Matthews PG, McGrath BP, et al: Angiotensin converting enzyme inhibition in renovascular hypertension: Frequency of reversible renal failure. Lancet I:225, 1984.
11. Franklin SS, Smith RD: Comparison of effects of enalapril plus hydrochlorothiazide versus standard triple therapy on renal function in renovascular hypertension. Am J Med 79:14, 1985.
12. White CJ, Ramee SR, Collins TJ, et al: Renal artery stent placement: Utility in lesions difficult to treat with balloon angioplasty. J Am Coll Cardiol 30:1445, 1997.
13. Lossino F, Zuccala A, Busato F, et al: Renal artery angioplasty for renovascular hypertension and preservation of renal function: Long-term angiographic and clinical follow-up. AJR Am J Roentgenol 162: 853, 1994.
14. van Jaarsveld BC, Krijnen P, Pieterman H, et al: The effect of balloon angioplasty on hypertension in atherosclerotic renal artery stenosis. N Engl J Med 342:1007, 2000.
15. Rocha-Singh KJ, Mishkel GJ, Katholi RE, et al: Clinical predictors of improved long-term blood pressure control after successful stenting of hypertensive patients with obstructive renal artery atherosclerosis. Cathet Cardiovasc Intervent 47:167, 1999.
16. Rodriguez-Lopez JA, Werner A, Ray LI, et al: Renal artery stenosis treated with stent deployment: Indications, technique, and outcome for 108 patients. J Vasc Surg 29:617, 1999.
17. Henry M, Amor M, Henry I, et al: Stent placement in the renal artery: Three-year experience with the Palmaz stent. J Vasc Interv Radiol 7:343, 1996.
18. Dorros G, Jaff M, Mathiak L, et al: Four-year follow-up of Palmaz-Schatz stent revascularization as treatment for atherosclerotic renal artery stenosis. Circulation 98:642, 1998.
19. Iannone LA, Underwood PL, Nath A, et al: Effect of primary balloon expandable renal artery stents on long-term patency, renal function, and blood pressure in hypertensive and renal insufficient patients with renal artery stenosis. Cathet Cardiovasc Diagn 37: 243, 1996.
20. Hansen KJ, Starr SM, Sands RE, et al: Contemporary surgical management of renovascular disease. J Vasc Surg 16:319, 1992.
21. Steinbach F, Novick AC, Campbell S, et al: Long-term survival after surgical revascularization for atherosclerotic renal artery disease. J Urol 158:38, 1997.
22. Bredenberg CE, Sampson LN, Ray FS, et al: Changing patterns in surgery for chronic renal artery occlusive diseases. J Vasc Surg 15:1018, 1992.
23. Mailloux LU, Napolitano B, Bellucci AG, et al: Renal vascular disease causing end-stage renal disease: Incidence, clinical correlates and outcomes: A 20 year clinical experience. Am J Kidney Dis 24:622, 1994.
24. Harden PN, MacLeod MJ, Rodger RS, et al: Effect of renal-artery stenting on progression of renovascular renal failure. Lancet 349:1133, 1997.
25. Watson PS, Hadjipetrou P, Cox SV, et al: Effect of renal artery stenting on renal function and size in patients with atherosclerotic renovascular disease. Circulation 102:1671, 2000.
26. Dorros G, Jaff M, Jain A, et al: Follow-up of primary Palmaz-Schatz stent placement for atherosclerotic renal artery stenosis. Am J Cardiol 5:1501, 1995.
27. Zeller T, Ulrich F, Muller C, et al: Predictors of improved renal function after percutaneous stent-supported angioplasty of severe atherosclerotic ostial renal artery stenosis. Circulation 108: 2244, 2003.

28. Cambria RP, Brewster DC, L'Italien GJ, et al: The durability of different reconstructive techniques for atherosclerotic renal artery disease. J Vasc Surg 20:76, 1994.
29. Plouin PF, Chatellier G, Darne B, et al: Blood pressure outcome of angioplasty in atherosclerotic renal artery stenosis: A randomized trial. Hypertension 31: 823, 1998.
30. Radermacher J, Chavan A, Bleck J, et al: Use of Doppler ultrasonography to predict the outcome of therapy for renal-artery stenosis. N Engl J Med 344: 410, 2001.
31. van de Ven PJ, Beutler JJ, Kaatee, R, et al: Transluminal vascular stent for ostial atherosclerotic renal artery stenosis. Lancet 346:672, 1995.
32. Dean RH, Englund R, Dupert WD, et al: Retrieval of renal function by revascularization: Study of preoperative predictors. Ann Surg 202:367, 1985.
33. Dean RH, Tribble RW, Hansen KJ, et al: Evolution of renal insufficiency in ischemic nephropathy. Ann Surg 213:446, 1991.

chapter 24

Surgical Management of Atherosclerotic Renal Artery Disease

David B. Wilson
Matthew S. Edwards
Juan Ayerdi
Kimberley J. Hansen

The introduction of new, more potent antihypertensive agents and percutaneous endovascular techniques has influenced surgical intervention for atherosclerotic renovascular disease.[1] Many physicians currently limit surgical intervention to severe hypertension despite maximal medical therapy, failures, or disease patterns not amenable to percutaneous transluminal renal artery angioplasty (PTRA), or renovascular disease associated with excretory renal insufficiency (i.e., *ischemic nephropathy*). As a result, the patient population selected for operative management is characterized by ostial renal artery stenosis or occlusion (85%) superimposed on diffuse extrarenal atherosclerotic disease (95%) in combination with renal insufficiency (60%).[1-3]

Although there are several operative methods that can correct atherosclerotic renal artery disease, no single technique is clearly superior. Optimal methods of operative renal reconstruction vary with the patient, the pattern of renal artery disease, and the clinical significance of associated aortic lesions.

PREVALENCE, EVALUATION, AND DIAGNOSIS

Prevalence

The prevalence of renal artery disease has recently been estimated from a population-based sample of independent-living elderly men and women. Overall, the prevalence of hemodynamically significant renal artery stenosis and occlusion was 6.8%. Contrary to prior case series autopsy reports and nonrandomized clinical case series, renal artery stenosis demonstrated no significant associations with gender or ethnicity, but did increase with age.[4] Although renal artery disease demonstrated an association with increased serum creatinine, this relationship demonstrated significant interaction with the presence of hypertension.[5]

It has long been recognized that anatomic renal artery disease may be clinically silent. Conversely, the disease may account for 3% of hypertension within the general population. Of patients presenting for chronic renal replacement therapy, 10% to 20% have demonstrated renal artery disease.[6-8] Although its prevalence in patients with mild hypertension is low, renovascular disease is a frequent etiologic factor in patients with severe hypertension (diastolic blood pressure ≥95 mm Hg). Dietch and colleagues found that 50% of patients aged 60 years or older with diastolic blood pressure greater than or equal to 104 mm Hg demonstrated significant renal artery stenosis or occlusion.[7] When these characteristics were associated with serum creatinine (SCr) greater than 2.0 mg/dL, the prevalence of renovascular disease increased to 70%. One half of these latter patients demonstrated bilateral renal artery disease.

These data suggest that the probability of finding clinically significant renal artery disease correlates with the patient's age, the severity of hypertension, and the severity of renal insufficiency. With this in mind, we search for renovascular disease in all persons with severe hypertension, especially when severe hypertension is found in combination with excretory renal insufficiency.

Evaluation

A noninvasive screening test that accurately identifies renal artery disease in all individuals does not yet exist.[9] Currently available tests can be characterized broadly as functional or anatomic. With the exception of captopril renography, functional studies that rely on activation of the renin-angiotensin axis have been associated with an unacceptably high rate of false-negative results.[10] Current isotope renography uses a variety of radiopharmaceuticals before and after exercise or angiotensin-converting enzyme (ACE) inhibition. Suboptimal sensitivity and specificity have led to continuous modifications in technique and interpretation.[11]

Consequently, anatomic screening methods are preferable.[12] Although MRA, CTA, and other studies have been advocated, renal duplex sonography is the screening study of choice for both renovascular hypertension and ischemic nephropathy at our center. Through continued improvements in software and probe design, renal duplex has been proved an accurate and reliable method to identify hemodynamically significant renal artery occlusive disease.[13,14] The examination poses no risk to residual excretory renal function, and overall accuracy is not affected by concomitant aortoiliac disease. In addition, preparation is minimal (an overnight fast), and there is no need to alter antihypertensive medications.

When searching for renovascular renal insufficiency, a negative renal duplex effectively excludes ischemic nephropathy because the primary consideration is global renal ischemia based on main renal artery disease to both kidneys. When screening for renovascular hypertension, however, a negative duplex examination does not reliably exclude disease due to stenotic accessory or branch renal arteries.[13] Despite enhanced recognition of multiple arteries provided by Doppler color flow, only 40% of these accessory renal vessels are currently identified by renal duplex examination. Consequently, our group proceeds with conventional angiography when hypertension is severe or poorly controlled, despite a negative duplex result.

Diagnostic aortography and renal angiography may be indicated after a positive duplex study in select patients. As mentioned above, young patients with severe hypertension and negative duplex examinations or nondiagnostic studies should also undergo angiography. Diagnostic angiography can be performed with minimal risk in an outpatient setting. In planning open operative therapy, imaging for these patients includes lateral aortography to evaluate the mesenteric vessels. Concurrent mesenteric arterial disease was identified in 50% of patients with significant renal arterial stenosis in an angiographic case series of U.S. veterans.[15] In an elderly population-based cohort, the authors identified a significant association of mesenteric arterial stenosis with renal artery stenosis (P = .008, OR 2.9; 95% CI 1.31 to 6.21).[16] Concurrent mesenteric arterial disease has bearing on the use of splanchno-renal reconstruction.

Patients with elevated creatinine levels will require special preparation for angiography. Hydration before and after the procedure is essential. Low-osmolarity or isoosmolar iodinated contrast agents should be used routinely in this population. The use of mannitol or furosemide has not reliably demonstrated a clinical benefit.[17] Recent randomized controlled trials suggest protection from acute renal deterioration with oral[18] and intravenous[19] pretreatment with the antioxidant *N*-acetylcysteine. The use of CO_2 and gadolinium angiography may limit the nephrotoxic contrast load in selected cases.

Diagnosis

When a unilateral renal artery lesion is confirmed in a patient with severe hypertension, its functional significance should be defined. Both renal vein renin assays (RVRA) and split renal function studies have proved valuable in assessing the functional significance of renovascular disease. RVRA should demonstrate a ratio of renin activity exceeding 1.5:1.0 between involved and uninvolved sides before a presumptive diagnosis of renovascular hypertension is established.

Unfortunately, neither functional study has great value when severe bilateral disease or disease to a solitary kidney is present. Therefore, the decision for empiric intervention is based on the severity of the renal artery lesions, the severity of hypertension, and the degree of associated renal insufficiency. In the latter instance, issues determining recovery of excretory renal function in patients with ischemic nephropathy remain ill-defined. Our center's experience with over 240 patients with severe hypertension (mean 201/104 mm Hg) and a preoperative SCr greater than or equal to 1.8 mg/dL has demonstrated a significant association between an improved renal function response after operative intervention and the site of renal artery disease, the extent of renovascular repair, and the rate of decline in preoperative renal function.[1,2,20-23] Global renal ischemia submitted to complete renal artery repair after a rapid decline in excretory renal function is associated with the best opportunity for recovery of renal function.[20,21,23] Most importantly, improved renal function after operation was the primary determinant of dialysis-free survival among patients with preoperative ischemic nephropathy.[23]

Management of renal artery disease discovered incidentally during evaluation of cardiac, aortoiliac, or infrainguinal disease is controversial. In this setting, the decision must address the need for additional diagnostic tests and the decision of whether or not to perform combined intervention. The term *prophylactic repair* describes renal revascularization that is performed before any pathologic or clinical sequelae related to the lesion. By definition, therefore, the patient considered for prophylactic renal artery repair has neither hypertension nor reduced renal function. Correction of the renal artery lesion in this setting assumes that preemptive correction is necessary to prevent a clinically adverse event for which the patient either cannot be treated or for whom delayed treatment would be unduly hazardous or ineffective.

To consider this assumption, data regarding the frequency of anatomic progression of renovascular disease summarized in Table 24-1 are useful. In patients with hypertension, ipsilateral progression of renal artery lesions occurred in 11% to 53%. In the randomized trial by Dean and colleagues, 12% of those patients randomized to medical management progressed to renal artery occlusion, yet only one (3%) had loss of a previously reconstructible renal artery.[24] In the absence of hypertension, one must assume that the renal artery lesion will progress anatomically to become functionally significant (i.e., produce hypertension or renal dysfunction). Based on the preceding data, progression of an asymptomatic renal artery lesion to produce renovascular hypertension could be expected in approximately 44% of normotensive patients. If one also assumes that the subsequent development of renovascular hypertension is managed medically, 40% of patients with severe hypertension and lateralizing functional studies randomized to medical management demonstrated decreased estimated GFR at a follow-up period of 15 to 24 months.[24] These patients were considered failures of medical management and submitted to operative renal artery repair. Despite revascularization, 13% of these patients continued to exhibit progressive deterioration in renal function. Therefore, of the patients with renovascular hypertension randomized to medical management, only 36% had potentially preventable loss of renal function by means of an earlier operation. These results have been supported by the experience of Novick and colleagues.[25]

TABLE 24-1 NATURAL HISTORY STUDIES OF ATHEROSCLEROTIC RENAL ARTERY STENOSIS

Reference	Year	No. of Patients	No. of Renal Arteries	Mean Follow-Up (Months)	Anatomic Progression (% of Patients)	Progression to Occlusion (% of Arteries)	Anatomic Evaluation
Wollenweber[40]	1968	109	252	42	59	—	Angiography
Meaney[41]	1968	39	78	34	36	4	Angiography
Dean[28]	1981	41	—	44	17	12	Angiography
Schreiber[42]	1984	85	126	52	44	11	Angiography
Tollefson[43]	1991	48	—	54	53†	9*	Angiography
Zierler[44]	1996	76	132	32	20	7	Duplex ultrasound
Webster[29]	1998	30	—	—	13‡	0†	Angiography
Crowley[45]	1998	1178	—	30	11	0.3	Angiography
Caps[46]	1998	170	295	33	31	3	Duplex ultrasound
van Jaarsveld[30]	2000	50	100	12	20	5	Angiography

*Percent of renal arteries with baseline stenosis or stenosis in follow-up.
†Of eight patients with serial angiography.
From Edwards MS, Hansen KJ: Combined aortorenal reconstruction. In Green RM (ed): Complex Aortic Surgery. New York, Marcel Dekker (In press).

The relationship of these issues to prophylactic renal revascularization can be demonstrated by considering 100 hypothetical patients without hypertension who have an unsuspected renal artery lesion demonstrated (Table 24-2). If the renal artery lesion is not repaired prophylactically, 44 patients may eventually develop renovascular hypertension over 3 to 5 years of follow-up. Sixteen (36%) of these 44 patients may experience a preventable reduction in renal function during medical management. Delayed operation, however, would restore function in 11 (67%) of these 16 patients. In theory, therefore, only 5 of these 100 hypothetic patients would receive a *unique benefit* from prophylactic intervention. Based on available data, we find no justification for prophylactic renal artery surgery or percutaneous catheter-based procedures either independently or in combination with aortic repair or other percutaneous intervention.

TABLE 24-2 BENEFIT OF PROPHYLACTIC RENAL REVASCULARIZATION IN 100 HYPOTHETIC NORMOTENSIVE PATIENTS

Benefit/Risk	No. of Patients
Benefit	
Progression to RVH (44/100 or 44%)	44
RVH patients who lose renal function (16/44 or 36%)	16
Renal function restored by later operation (11/16 or 67%)	11
Renal function not restored by later operation (5/16 or 33%)	5
Unique Benefit	5 Patients
Risk	
Operative mortality (5.3%)	5
Early technical failure (0.8%)	1
Late failure of revascularization (3.6%)	4
Adverse Outcome	10 Patients

From Edwards MS, Hansen KJ: Combined aortorenal reconstruction. In Green RM (ed): Complex Aortic Surgery. New York, Marcel Dekker (In press).

These conclusions have been supported by the retrospective experience reported by Williamson and colleagues.[26]

In contrast to prophylactic renal revascularization, empiric renal artery repair is appropriate under select circumstances. The term *empiric repair* implies that severe hypertension and/or renal dysfunction are present, although a causal relationship between the renal artery lesion and these clinical sequelae has not been established by functional studies.

Repair of unilateral renal artery disease may be appropriate as a combined aortorenal procedure in the absence of functional studies (i.e., RVRA), when hypertension is severe, the patient is without significant risk factors for operation or catheter-based intervention, and the probability of technical success is certain (>99%). In these circumstances, correction of a renal artery lesion may be justified to eliminate all possible causes of hypertension and renal dysfunction. Because the probability of blood pressure benefit is lower in such a patient, morbidity from the procedure must also be predictably low.[3,12]

When a patient has bilateral renal artery stenoses and hypertension, the decision to intervene is based on the severity of the renovascular lesions and the degree of hypertension.[2,12] If the pattern of renal artery disease consists of severe stenoses on one side and only mild or moderate disease on the contralateral side, then the patient is treated as if only a unilateral lesion exists. If both renal arteries have only moderately severe disease (65% to 80% diameter-reducing stenosis), renal revascularization is undertaken only if the hypertension is severe. In contrast, if both renal artery lesions are severe (>80% stenosis) and the patient has drug-dependent hypertension, bilateral simultaneous renal revascularization is performed. Hypertension secondary to severe bilateral renal artery stenoses is often particularly severe and difficult to control. Furthermore, at least mild excretory renal insufficiency is often present. Because renal insufficiency usually parallels the severity of hypertension, a patient who presents with severe renal insufficiency but only mild hypertension usually has renal parenchymal disease. Characteristically, renovascular hypertension associated with severe renal insufficiency or dialysis-dependence is associated with very severe bilateral stenoses or total renal artery occlusions.[2,23] When considering repair of renal artery disease, one should evaluate the clinical status with respect to this characteristic presentation.

MANAGEMENT OPTIONS

No prospective, randomized clinical trial compares medical management, PTRA with endoluminal stenting, and surgical management. A recent meta-analysis, however, considers three prospective, randomized trials that compared medical management with PTRA and selective stenting.[27] Neither the individual reports nor the pooled data demonstrated a clear improvement in renal function or hypertension as a result of catheter-based intervention. Although each of these trials has been variously criticized, perhaps their greatest limitation was the failure to relate renal artery intervention to survival free of adverse cardiovascular events and progression to dialysis dependence.

Although data regarding medical therapy for renovascular hypertension suggest that a decrease in kidney size and renal function occur despite medical blood pressure control,[28] the value of medical management is suggested by these recent prospective randomized trials.[29-31] In the absence of level 1 data comparing the three modes of therapy, advocates of medical management, PTRA with endoluminal stenting, or operative management cite selective clinical data to support their views. In practice, a majority of the medical community evaluates patients for renovascular disease only when medications are not tolerated or hypertension remains severe and uncontrolled. The early study by Hunt and Strong[32] remains the most informative study available to assess the comparative value of medical therapy and operation. In their nonrandomized study, the results of operative treatment in 100 patients were compared with the results of drug therapy in 114 similar patients. After 7 to 14 years of follow-up, 84% of the operated group was alive, as compared with 66% in the drug therapy group. Of the 84 patients alive in the operated group, 93% were cured or significantly improved, compared with 16 (21%) of the patients alive in the drug therapy group. Death during follow-up was twice as common in the medically treated group as in the surgically managed group. Antihypertensive agents in current use provide improved blood pressure control compared with those in this earlier era. Consequently, these older data cannot be reliably applied to contemporary patient populations.

In patients with functionally significant renal artery lesions and severe hypertension, contemporary results of operative management argue for a selective attitude toward renal artery intervention.[1,2] Whether by open surgical repair or catheter-based methods, the indications for intervention are the same. These include all patients with severe or difficult-to-control hypertension, especially when associated with renal insufficiency. Patient age, type of lesion, medical comorbidity, and concomitant aortic disease must be considered in selecting patients for open surgical or endovascular management. In the complete absence of hypertension, renal artery intervention is not recommended by any method.

Percutaneous Transluminal Renal Angioplasty with and without Stenting

Experience with the liberal use of PTRA has helped to clarify its role as a therapeutic option in the treatment of renovascular hypertension. Like operative repair, accumulated data argue for its selective application. In this regard, PTRA of non-ostial atherosclerotic lesions and medial fibroplasia of the main renal artery yields blood pressure results comparable to the results of operative repair. In contrast, suboptimal lesions for PTRA include congenital lesions, fibrodysplastic lesions involving renal artery branches, ostial atherosclerotic lesions, and renal artery occlusions. In each instance, these lesions are associated with inferior results and increased risk of complications.

A review of published reports over the past 14 years documenting blood pressure and renal function after PTRA for atherosclerotic renovascular disease revealed angiographic success in 86% of cases and a beneficial blood pressure response in 65% of patients. Thirty-two percent of patients with preexisting renal insufficiency experienced improved excretory renal function, whereas 51% remained unchanged and 17% had worsened renal function. Major complications were observed in 12% of patients and restenosis was observed in 25% of treated arteries at 6- to 12-month follow-up intervals (Table 24-3).

In an effort to improve the outcome of angioplasty, endoluminal stenting has been combined with PTRA. Although no stent has been approved for renal use in the United States, the most common indications for the employment of such appear to be elastic recoil of the vessel immediately after angioplasty, renal artery dissection after angioplasty, and restenosis after angioplasty. Recently, primary stenting of atherosclerotic renal artery disease has been widely applied. Review of published reports of percutaneous renal artery stenting reveals no clinical improvement beyond PTRA alone, with 61% of atherosclerotic patients experiencing blood pressure benefit and 25% experiencing improvement in renal function. Restenosis was observed in 18% of patients at variable follow-up intervals (Table 24-4).

Review of PTRA and endoluminal stenting for ostial atherosclerosis of the renal artery demonstrated similar results. When renal artery stenting was applied to ostial atherosclerotic renal artery stenosis in patients with ischemic nephropathy, 18% of patients experienced improvement in excretory renal function, whereas 17% had worsened renal function. Restenosis was observed in 21% of patients (Table 24-5). These results are inferior to results reported in select patients treated surgically.[1,21,23] Because early renal function result has been the strongest predictor of dialysis-free survival, we believe operative repair remains the best treatment for ostial atherosclerotic renovascular disease associated with renal insufficiency. Nevertheless, the decision for interventional therapy for atherosclerotic renovascular disease must be individualized. In this regard, significant and independent predictors of accelerated death—regardless of renal

TABLE 24-3 RESULTS AFTER PRIMARY PERCUTANEOUS TRANSLUMINAL RENAL ARTERY ANGIOPLASTY FOR ATHEROSCLEROTIC RENAL ARTERY STENOSIS

Reference	Patients (n)	Technical Success (%)	Patients with Renal Dysfunction (n)	RENAL FUNCTION RESPONSE (%)			HYPERTENSION RESPONSE (%)			Restenosis (%)	Major Complications (%)
				Improved	Unchanged	Worsened	Cured	Improved	Failed		
Baert AL (1990)[47]	165	83	n/r	n/r	n/r	n/r	32	36	32	10	11
Tykarski A (1992)[48]	26	81	16	69	31	0	45	35	20	15	n/r
Weibull H (1993)[49]	29	83	n/r	21	75	4	13	71	17	25	17
Losinno F (1994)[50]	153	95	59	27	67	6	12	51	37	n/r	8
Rodriguez-Perez JC (1994)[51]	37	78	n/r		no change in mean SCr		3	80	17	11	8
Bonelli FS (1995)[52]	190	82	n/r		no change in mean SCr		8	62	30	10	23
Hoffman O (1998)[53]	50	58	36	44	23	33	3	64	32	27	14
Klow NE (1998)[54]	295	92	n/r		no change in mean SCr		5	59	31	40	8
Paulsen D (1998)[55]	135	90	79	23	56	21	6	41	53	45	9
Zuccala A (1998)[56]	99	92	33	39	50	11	18	44	48	17	8
van de Ven PJG (1999)[57]	41	57	22	18	55	27	5	44	51	48	29
Baumgartner I (2000)[58]	33	95	107	33	42	25	43	43	57	35	3
van Jaarsveld BC (2000)[30]	56	91	n/r		no change in mean SCr		7	61	32	48	5
Overall	**1543**	**86**	**418**	**32**	**51**	**17**	**11**	**54**	**35**	**25**	**12**

n/r, not reported; SCr, serum creatinine.

TABLE 24-4 RESULTS AFTER PRIMARY RENAL ARTERY STENT PLACEMENT FOR ATHEROSCLEROTIC RENAL ARTERY STENOSIS

Reference	Patients (n)	Technical Success (%)	Patients with Renal Dysfunction (n)	RENAL FUNCTION RESPONSE (%)			HYPERTENSION RESPONSE (%)			Restenosis (%)	Major Complication (%)
				Improved	Unchanged	Worsened	Cured	Improved	Failed		
Rees CR (1991)[59]	28	96	14	36	36	29	11	5	36	39	18
Wilms GE (1991)[60]	10	80	1	0	100	0	30	40	30	22	18
Kuhn FP (1991)[61]	8	92	n/r	n/r	n/r	n/r	22	34	44	17	13
Joffre F (1992)[62]	11	91	4	50	50	0	27	64	9	18	13
Hennequin LM (1994)[63]	15	100	6	20	40	40	7	93	0	27	19
Raynaud AC (1994)[64]	15	100	7	0	43	57	7	43	50	13	13
MacLeod M (1995)[65]	28	100	16	25	75	75	0	40	60	17	19
Dorros G (1995)[66]	76	100	29	28	28	45	6	46	48	25	11
Henry M (1996)[67]	55	100	10	20	80	80	18	57	24	9	3
Iannone LA (1996)[68]	63	99	29	36	46	18	4	35	61	14	32
Harden PN (1997)[69]	32	100	32	35	35	29	n/r	n/r	n/r	13	19
Blum U (1997)[70]	68	100	20	0	100	0	16	62	22	17	0
Boisclair C (1997)[71]	33	100	17	41	35	24	6	61	33	0	21
Rundback JH (1998)[72]	45	94	45	18	53	30	n/r	n/r	n/r	26	9
Fiala LA (1998)[73]	21	95	9	0	100	0	53	53	47	65	19
Dorros G (1998)[74]	163	99	63	No change in mean SCr			1	42	57	n/r	14
Tuttle KR (1998)[75]	120	98	74	16	75	9	2	46	52	14	4
Gross CM (1998)[76]	30	100	12	55	27	18	0	69	31	13	n/r
Henry M (1999)[77]	200	99	48	29	67	2	19	61	20	11	2
Rodriguez-Lopez JA (1999)[78]	108	98	32	No change in mean SCr			13	55	32	26	12
van de Ven PJ (1999)[57]	40	88	29	17	55	28	15	43	42	14	30
Baumgartner I (2000)[58]	64	95	n/r	33	42	25	43	43	57	28	9
Overall	**1257**	**98**	**497**	**25**	**56**	**19**	**10**	**51**	**39**	**18**	**11**

n/r, not reported; SCr, serum creatinine.

TABLE 24-5 RESULTS AFTER PRIMARY RENAL ARTERY STENT PLACEMENT FOR OSTIAL ATHEROSCLEROTIC RENAL ARTERY STENOSIS

Reference	Patients with Ostial Lesions (n)	Patients with Renal Dysfunction (n)	RENAL FUNCTION RESPONSE (%)			HYPERTENSION RESPONSE (%)			Restenosis (%)
			Improved	Unchanged	Worsened	Cured	Improved	Failed	
Rees CR (1991)[59]	28	14	36	35	29	11	54	36	39
Hennequin LM (1994)[63]	7	2	0	50	50	0	100	0	43
Raynaud AC (1994)[64]	4	3	0	33	67	0	50	50	33
MacLeod M (1995)[65]	22	13	15	85	85	0	31	69	20
Blum U (1997)[70]	68	20	0	100	0	16	62	22	17
Rundback JH (1998)[72]	32	32	16	53	31	n/r	n/r	n/r	26
Fiala LA (1998)[73]	21	9	0	100	0	53	53	47	65
Tuttle KR (1998)[75]	129	74	16	75	9	2	46	52	14
Gross CM (1998)[76]	30	12	55	27	18	0	69	31	12
Rodriguez-Lopez JA (1999)[78]	82	n/r	No change in mean SCr			13	55	32	26
van de Ven PJG (1999)[57]	40	29	17	55	28	15	43	42	14
Baumgartner I (2000)[58]	21	n/r	33	42	25	43	43	57	20
Overall	**508**	**208**	**18**	**65**	**17**	**7**	**53**	**40**	**21**

n/r, not reported; SCr, serum creatinine.
From Hansen KJ, Cherr GS, Edwards MS: Management of atherosclerotic renovascular disease. In Pearce WH, Yao JST (eds): Advances in Vascular Surgery. Chicago, Precept, 2001, p 209.

artery intervention (i.e., clinical congestive heart failure, long-standing diabetes mellitus, uncorrectable azotemia) are considered before intervention is chosen.[2,23]

Operative Management

General Issues

As discussed earlier, the authors consider the presence of hypertension a prerequisite for renal artery intervention. In general, functional studies are used to guide the management of unilateral lesions. Empirical renal artery repair is performed without functional studies when hypertension is severe, renal artery disease is bilateral, or the patient has ischemic nephropathy.[1,21,23] Accordingly, prophylactic renal artery repair in the absence of hypertension, whether as an isolated procedure or combined with aortic reconstruction, is not recommended. With the exception of disease requiring bilateral ex vivo reconstructions, which are staged, all hemodynamically significant renal artery disease is corrected in a single operation. Having observed beneficial blood pressure and renal function response regardless of kidney size or histologic pattern on renal biopsy, nephrectomy is reserved for unreconstructible renal artery disease to a non-functioning kidney (i.e., ≤10% function by renography).[3,20,21,23] Direct aortorenal reconstructions are preferred over indirect methods because concomitant disease of the celiac axis is present in 40% to 50% of patients and bilateral renal artery repair is required in one half.[1,3,15] Failed surgical repair is associated with a significantly increased risk of eventual dialysis dependence.[3] To minimize these failures, intraoperative duplex is used to evaluate the technical results of surgical repair.[33]

Preoperative Preparation

Antihypertensive medications are reduced during the preoperative period to the minimum necessary for blood pressure control. Patients requiring large doses of multiple medications will often have reduced requirements while hospitalized at bed rest. If continued therapy is required, vasodilators and selective β-adrenergic blocking agents are the agents of choice. If an adult's diastolic blood pressure exceeds 120 mm Hg, operative treatment is postponed until the pressure is brought under control. In this instance, intravenous therapy is administered in an intensive care setting.

Operative Techniques

A variety of operative techniques have been used to correct renal artery atherosclerosis. From a practical standpoint, the three basic operations that have been most frequently used are aortorenal bypass, renal artery thromboendarterectomy, and renal artery reimplantation. Although each method may have its proponents, no single approach provides optimal repair for all types of renal artery disease. Aortorenal bypass, preferably with saphenous vein, is probably the most versatile technique. However, thromboendarterectomy is especially useful for ostial atherosclerosis involving multiple renal arteries. When the artery is sufficiently redundant, reimplantation is probably the simplest technique and one particularly appropriate for combined repairs of aortic and renal pathology.

Certain measures are used in almost all renal artery operations. Mannitol is administered intravenously in 12.5 gm doses early, and repeated before and after periods of renal ischemia, up to a total dose of 1 gm per kilogram patient body weight. Just prior to renal artery occlusion, 100 units of heparin per kilogram body weight are given intravenously, and systemic anticoagulation is verified by activated clotting time. Unless required for hemostasis, protamine is not routinely administered for reversal of heparin at the completion of the operation.

Aortorenal Bypass

The most common method of revascularization is the aortorenal bypass (Fig. 24-1). Three types of material are available for conduit: autologous saphenous vein, autologous hypogastric artery, and prosthetic grafts. The choice of conduit depends on a number of factors. In adults, we use the saphenous vein preferentially. However, if the vein is small (<4 mm in diameter) or sclerotic, the hypogastric artery or a synthetic prosthesis may be preferable. A 6 mm, thin-walled polytetrafluoroethylene (PTFE) graft is satisfactory when the distal renal artery is of large caliber (≥4 mm) and provides long-term patency equivalent to that of saphenous vein.

Thromboendarterectomy

In cases of bilateral atherosclerosis of the renal artery origins, simultaneous bilateral endarterectomy may be the most appropriate procedure. Although endarterectomy may be performed in a transrenal fashion, the transaortic technique is used in the majority of instances. The transaortic method is particularly applicable in patients with multiple renal arteries that demonstrate orificial disease. Transaortic endarterectomy is performed through a longitudinal aortotomy with sleeve endarterectomy of the aorta and eversion endarterectomies of the renal arteries (Fig. 24-2). When combined aortic replacement is planned, the transaortic endarterectomy is performed through the transected aorta (Fig. 24-3). When using the transaortic technique, it is important to mobilize the renal arteries extensively, to allow eversion of the vessel into the aorta. This allows the distal endpoint to be completed under direct vision.

Renal Artery Reimplantation

After the renal artery has been dissected from the surrounding retroperitoneal tissue, the vessel may be somewhat redundant. When the renal artery stenosis is orificial and there is sufficient vessel length, the renal artery can be transected and reimplanted into the aorta at a slightly lower level. The renal artery must be spatulated and a portion of the aortic wall removed as in renal artery bypass.

Splanchnorenal Bypass

Splanchnorenal bypass and other indirect procedures have received increased use as an alternative method for

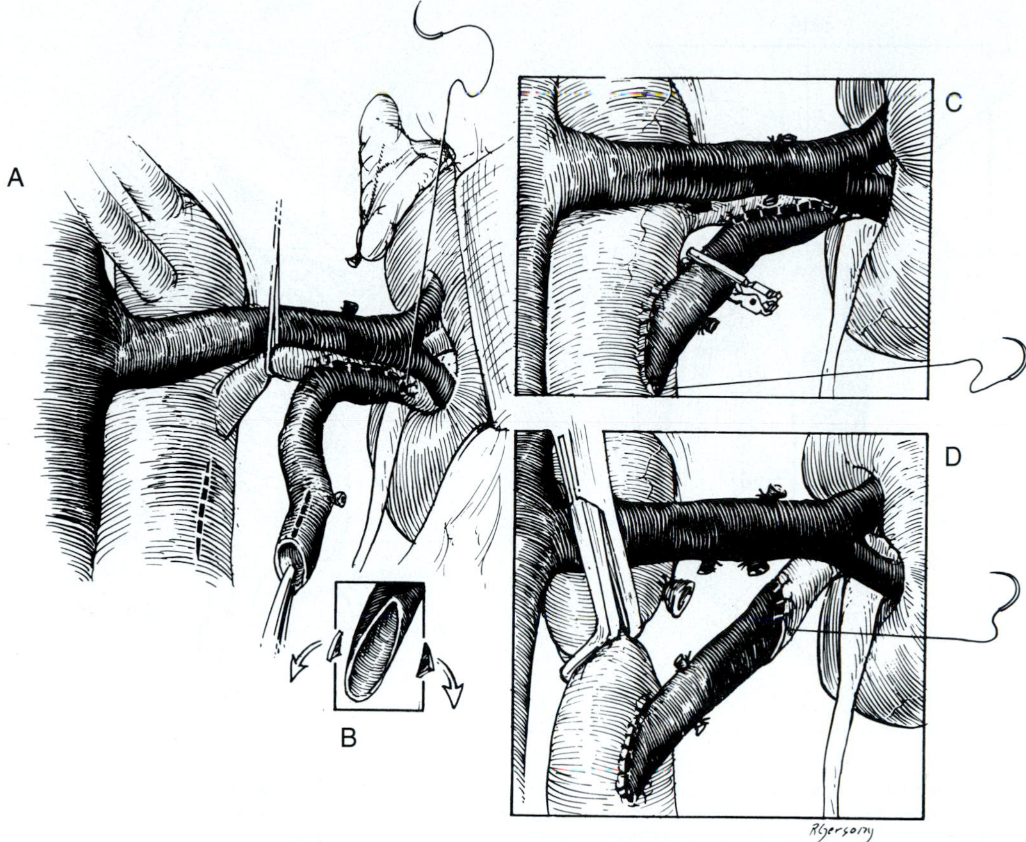

FIGURE 24-1. Technique for end-to-side (**A**, **B**, and **C**) and end-to-end (**D**) aortorenal bypass grafting. The length of arteriotomy is at least three times the diameter of the artery to prevent recurrent anastomotic stenosis. For the anastomosis, 6-0 or 7-0 monofilament polypropylene sutures are used in continuous fashion, under loupe magnification. If the apex sutures are placed too deeply or with excess advancement, stenosis can be created, posing a risk of late graft thrombosis. (From Benjamin ME, Dean RH: Techniques in renal artery reconstruction: Part I. Ann Vasc Surg 10[3]:306, 1996.)

renal revascularization.[34] In general, the authors do not believe that these procedures demonstrate equivalent long-term patency compared with direct aortorenal reconstructions, but they are useful in a select subgroup of high-risk patients. Subcostal incisions are used to perform splanchnorenal bypass.[34] The right and left renal arteries are exposed through medial visceral rotation. A greater saphenous vein graft is usually used to construct the bypass. Occasionally, the gastroduodenal artery on the right and splenic artery on the left can be transected and anastomosed directly to the renal artery.

Ex Vivo Reconstruction

In part, operative strategy for renal artery branch vessel repair is determined by the required exposure and anticipated period of renal ischemia. When reconstruction can be accomplished with less than 30 minutes of ischemia, an in situ repair is undertaken without special measures for renal preservation (Fig. 24-4). When longer periods of ischemia are anticipated, one of two techniques for hypothermic preservation of the kidney are considered. These techniques include renal mobilization without renal vein transection and ex vivo repair and anatomical replacement in the renal fossa. Ex vivo management is necessary when extensive exposure will be required for extended periods. For atherosclerotic renovascular disease, ex vivo techniques are most commonly required for branch renal artery repair after failed or complicated PTRA.

Intraoperative Duplex Sonography

Provided the best method of reconstruction is chosen for renal artery repair, the short course and high blood flow rates characteristic of renal reconstruction favor long-term patency. Consequently, flawless technical repair plays a dominant role in determining postoperative success. The negative impact of technical errors unrecognized and uncorrected at operation is implied by the fact that we have observed no late thromboses of renovascular reconstruction completely free of disease after 1 year.

Intraoperative duplex sonography provides a rapid, safe method of verifying technically flawless repair.[33] Because the ultrasound probe can be placed immediately adjacent to the vascular repair, high carrying frequencies may be used that provide excellent B-scan detail sensitive to less than 1 mm anatomical defects. Once imaged, defects can be viewed in a multitude of projections during conditions of uninterrupted, pulsatile blood flow. Intimal flaps not apparent during static conditions are easily imaged while avoiding the adverse

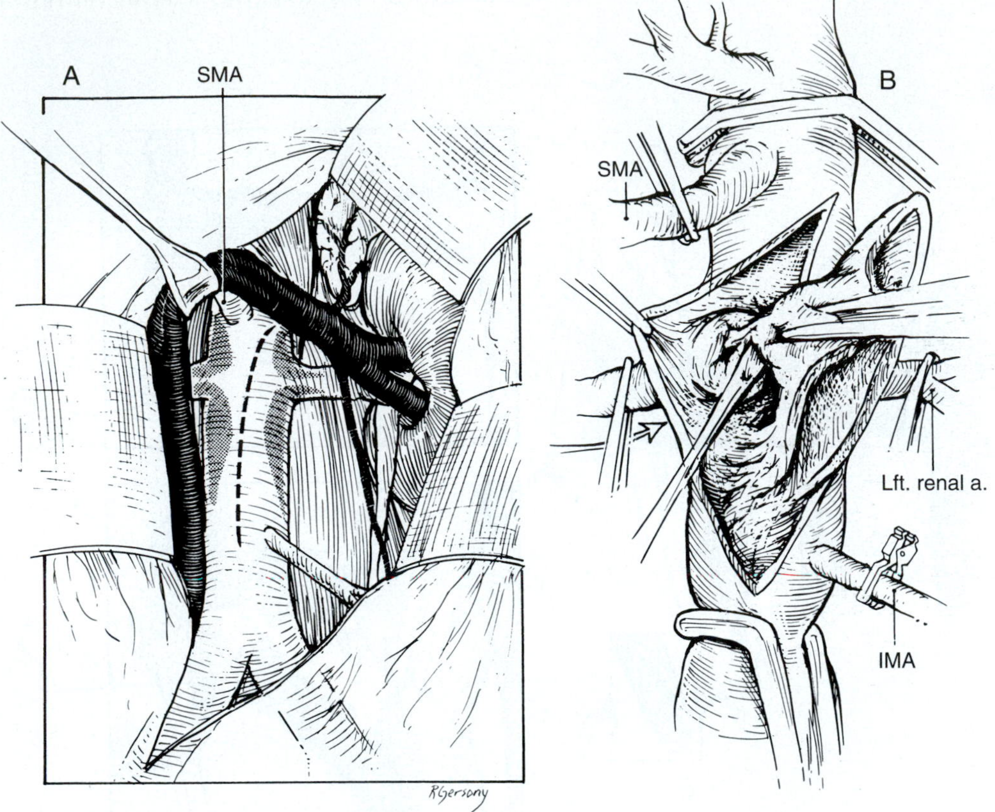

FIGURE 24-2. Exposure for a longitudinal transaortic endarterectomy is through the standard transperitoneal approach. The duodenum is mobilized from the aorta laterally in standard fashion or, for more complete exposure, the ascending colon and small bowel are mobilized. **A,** Dotted line shows the location of the aortotomy. **B,** The plaque is transected proximally and distally, and with eversion of the renal arteries, the atherosclerotic plaque is removed from each renal ostium. The aortotomy is typically closed with a running 4-0 or 5-0 polypropylene suture. IMA, inferior mesenteric artery; SMA, superior mesenteric artery. (From Benjamin ME, Dean RH. Techniques in renal artery reconstruction: Part I. Ann Vasc Surg 10[3]:306, 1996.)

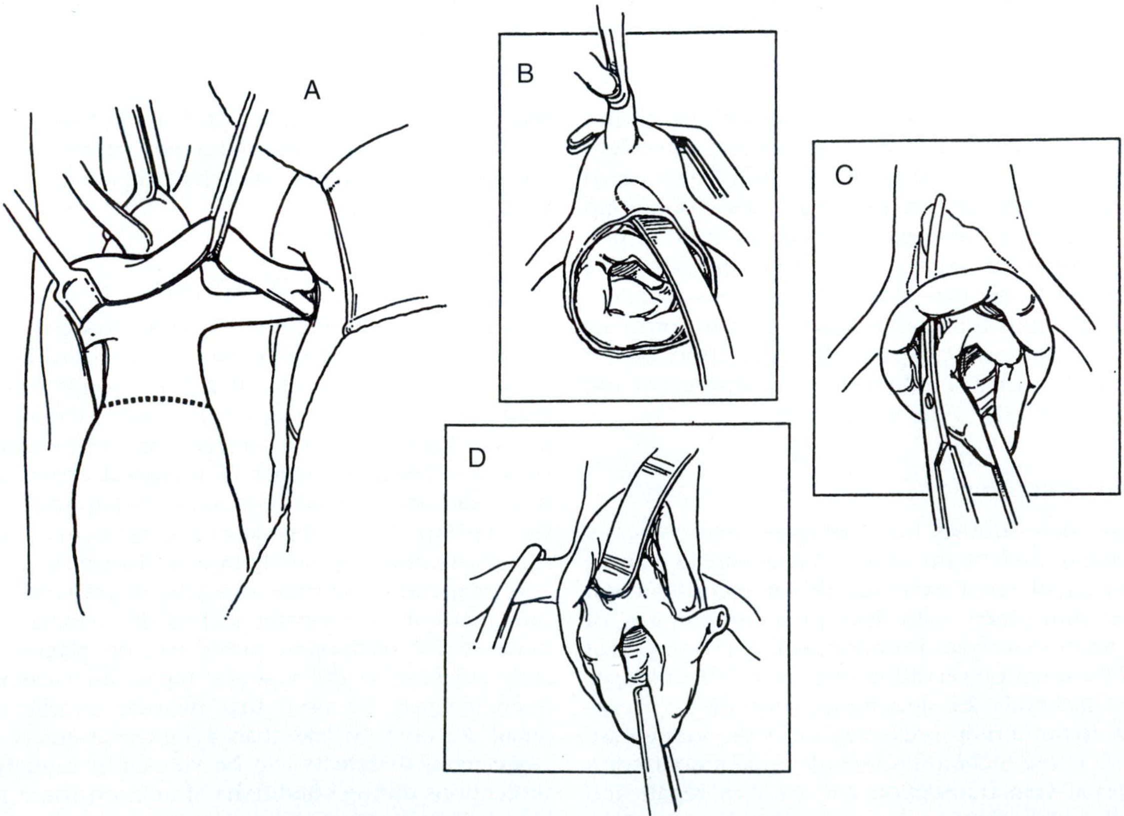

FIGURE 24-3. For aortic repair combined with bilateral ostial stenosis of the renal arteries, thromboendarterectomy is most commonly performed through the divided aorta. (With permission from Edwards MS, Cherr GS, Hansen KJ: Treatment of Renovascular Disease: Surgical Therapy. In Hallet JW, Mills JL, Earnshaw J, Reekers JA [eds]: Comprehensive Vascular and Endovascular Surgery, Edinburgh, Mosby, 2004.)

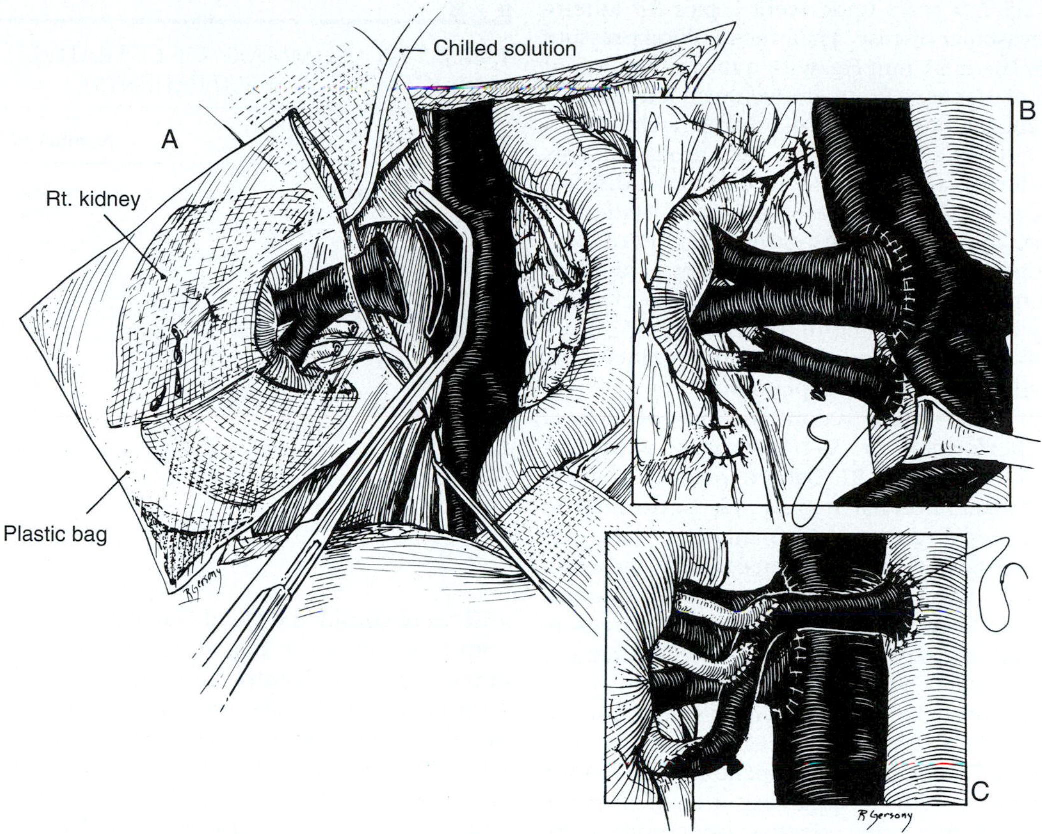

FIGURE 24-4. A, An ellipse of the vena cava containing the renal vein origin is excised by placement of a large, partially occluding clamp. After ex vivo branch repair, the renal vein can then be reattached without risk of anastomotic stricture. **B,** The kidney is repositioned in its native bed after ex vivo repair. Gerota fascia is reattached to provide stability to the replaced kidney. Arterial reconstruction can be accomplished via end-to-end anastomoses (as here) or occasionally with a combination of end-to-end and end-to-side anastomoses (**C**). (From Benjamin ME, Dean RH. Techniques in renal artery reconstruction: Part II. Ann Vasc Surg 10[4]:409, 1996.)

effects of additional renal ischemia. In addition to excellent anatomical detail, important hemodynamic information is obtained from the spectral analysis of the Doppler-shifted signal proximal and distal to the imaged defect.[33] Freedom from static projections, the absence of potentially nephrotoxic contrast material or additional ischemia, and the hemodynamic data provided by Doppler spectral analysis make duplex sonography a very attractive intraoperative method to assess renovascular repairs. Our technique of intraoperative assessment with the routine participation of a vascular technologist has yielded a scan time of 7 to 10 minutes and a 98% study completion rate.[35]

We have studied more than 600 renal artery repairs with anatomic follow-up evaluation and reported on a subgroup of 249 repairs.[36] Intraoperative assessment was normal in 157, whereas 84 (35%) repairs demonstrated one or more B-scan defect. Twenty-five of these defects (10%) had focal increases in estimated peak systolic velocity of greater than or equal to 2.0 msec with turbulent distal waveform and were defined as major. Each major B-scan defect prompted immediate operative revision, and in each case a significant defect was discovered. B-scan defects defined as minor were not repaired. At 12-month follow-up, renal artery patency free of critical stenosis was demonstrated in 97% of normal studies, 100% of minor B-scan defects, and 88% of revised major B-scan defects, providing an overall patency of 97%. Among the five failures with normal B-scan studies, three occurred after ex vivo branch renal artery repair.

RESULTS OF SURGICAL MANAGEMENT

Marone and colleagues have recently reported on operative management for ischemic nephropathy due to atherosclerotic renal artery disease.[37] Ninety-six patients underwent 104 renal artery revascularizations between 1990 and 2001. Perioperative mortality was 4.1%. Perioperative morbidity occurred in 5% of patients. After open surgical repair, 42% of their patients demonstrated improved early renal function, defined as a ≥20% decline in serum creatinine. Seventeen percent experienced a ≥20% increase in serum creatinine, and the remaining 41% exhibited no significant change. Improved renal function was durable among surgical survivors at a mean follow-up of 46 months, whereas 28% developed worsened function and 39% remained unchanged. These authors noted that early renal function response was an accurate predictor of long-term response. The results of Marone and colleagues are similar to those from the authors' center. From January 1987 through December 1999, 626 patients had operative renal artery repair at our center.[2] Overall, 254 women and 246 men, with a mean age of 65 ± 9 years underwent repair for atherosclerotic renovascular disease. Their mean blood pressure was 200 ± 35/104 ± 21 mm Hg, with a mean duration of hypertension of 10 years. Preoperative mean and median SCr was 2.6 mg/dL and 1.7 mg/dL, respectively, with a mean EGFR of 40.5 ± 23.2 ml/min/m^2. As a group, patients with atherosclerosis had widespread extrarenal disease, with 70% demonstrating at least one manifestation of cardiac disease and 32% demonstrating a history of cerebrovascular disease. Overall, 90% of patients exhibited some clinical manifestation of extrarenal atherosclerosis. Evidenced by a SCr of 1.8 mg/dL or greater, 49% were considered to have ischemic nephropathy, including 40 patients who were dialysis dependent.

Among 720 renal artery reconstructions, aortorenal bypass was performed in 384 instances, with 204 vein grafts, 159 PTFE, and 21 Dacron prosthetic grafts (Table 24-6). Splanchnorenal bypass was performed in 13 instances. Renal artery reimplantation was performed in 56 instances, whereas renal artery thromboendarterectomy was performed in 267 instances. Revascularization was combined with aortic or mesenteric reconstruction in 41% of patients. Of the 776 kidneys that were operated on, 56 required nephrectomy.

Perioperative mortality, defined as in-hospital death or death within 30 days of surgery, occurred in 23 patients (4.6%). Although this figure was comparable with reports from other centers with a large experience in renovascular disease,[38] few other elective operations carry such a high rate of mortality. All but one death occurred following bilateral renal artery reconstruction or renal reconstruction combined with simultaneous aortic or mesenteric artery repair. Mortality following isolated renal artery repair (0.8%) differed significantly from mortality following combined or bilateral repair (6.9%). Perioperative mortality demonstrated significant and independent associations with advanced age and clinical congestive heart failure.

Blood pressure measurements and medication requirements at least 1 month after operative intervention were used to define blood pressure response.[3] Among all surgical survivors, 85% were cured or improved, and 15% were considered failed (Table 24-7). When compared with blood pressure improved or failed, blood pressure cured was significantly and independently associated with an improved dialysis-free survival. Although improved blood pressure was associated with significant postoperative decreases in mean blood pressure and medication requirements (205/107 mm Hg versus 147/81 mm Hg and 2.8 versus 1.7), improved blood pressure was not associated with increased dialysis-free survival. Product-limit estimates of dialysis-free survival according to postoperative blood pressure response are depicted in Figure 24-5.

Considering all surgical survivors, renal function increased significantly after operation (preoperative versus postoperative mean EGFR, 41.1 ± 23.9 ml/min/m^2 versus 48.2 ± 25.5 ml/min/m^2 [P < .0001]). For individual patients, a significant change in excretory renal function was defined as a change in EGFR of greater than or equal to 20% obtained at least 3 weeks after repair. Fifty-eight percent of patients with ischemic nephropathy (preoperative SCr ≥ 1.8 mg/dL) were improved, including

TABLE 24-6 SUMMARY OF OPERATIVE MANAGEMENT (*N* = 500 PATIENTS)

Procedure	Number of Kidneys
Aortorenal bypass	384
Vein	204
PTFE	159
Dacron	21
Splanchnorenal bypass	13
Reimplantation	56
Endarterectomy	267
Nephrectomy	56
Primary	13
Contralateral	43
Total kidneys operated	776

PTFE, polytetrafluoroethylene.
From Cherr GS, Hansen KJ, Craven TE, et al: Surgical management of atherosclerotic renovascular disease. J Vasc Surg 35:236, 2002.

TABLE 24-7 BLOOD PRESSURE RESPONSE TO OPERATION (*N* = 472 PATIENTS)

Response*	No. of Patients (%)	Preoperative BP (mm Hg)	Postoperative BP (mm Hg)	Preoperative No. of Medications	Postoperative No. of Medications
Cured	57 (12)	195 ± 35 103 ± 22	137 ± 16† 78 ± 9†	2.0 ± 1.1	0 ± 0†
Improved	345 (73)	205 ± 35 107 ± 21	147 ± 21† 81 ± 11†	2.8 ± 1.1	1.7 ± 0.8†
Failed	70 (15)	182 ± 30 87 ± 13	158 ± 28† 82 ± 12‡	2.0 ± 0.9	2.0 ± 0.9
All	472 (100)	201 ± 35 104 ± 22	148 ± 22† 81 ± 11†	2.6 ± 1.1	1.6 ± 0.9*

*See text for definition.
†P < .0001 compared with preoperative value.
‡P .001 compared with preoperative value.
Blood pressure and medications are mean ± standard deviation.
From Cherr GS, Hansen KJ, Craven TE, et al: Surgical management of atherosclerotic renovascular disease. J Vasc Surg 35:236, 2002.

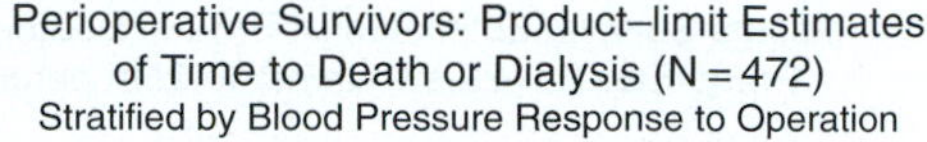

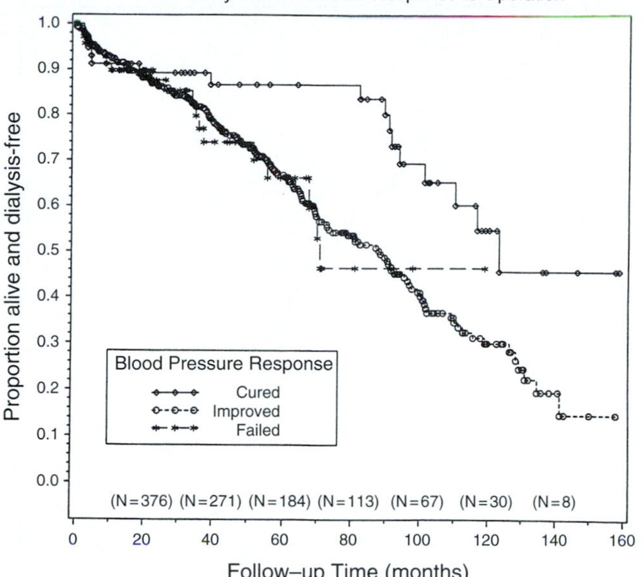

FIGURE 24-5. Product-limit estimates of time to death or dialysis according to blood pressure response to operation. (From Cherr GS, Hansen KJ, Craven TE, et al: Surgical management of atherosclerotic renovascular disease. J Vasc Surg 35:236, 2002.)

28 patients who were removed from dialysis. Thirty-five percent remained unchanged, whereas 7% had worsened renal function.[2,23,35] When patients were selected for surgery based on severe hypertension and rapidly deteriorating renal function, the proportion of patients improved increased with increasing severity of preoperative renal dysfunction. Seventy percent of dialysis-dependent patients were permanently removed from dialysis (Table 24-8). This association with increased preoperative SCr and improved postoperative renal function was significant ($P < .0001$).

Success after renal artery intervention is measured by survival free of dialysis dependence. Freedom from death or dialysis was significantly and independently associated with cured compared with improved or unchanged hypertension. Freedom from dialysis was also highly significantly and independently associated with improved compared with unchanged or worsened postoperative renal function. Preoperative factors significantly and independently associated with death or dialysis included diabetes mellitus, severe aortic occlusive disease, and poor preoperative renal function. The relationship between each category of renal function response and dialysis-free survival demonstrated significant interactions with preoperative renal function. For patients with renal function unchanged, an increased risk of death or dialysis was observed for patients with poor preoperative function (Fig. 24-6A). For patients with worsened renal function following surgery, an increased risk of death or dialysis was significantly associated with a preoperative renal function at median values of EGFR or greater. These significant and independent interactions are shown for predicted dialysis-free survival according to postoperative renal function response (see Fig. 24-6A and 24-6B).

These associations between renal function response and dialysis-free survival suggest that the designation of renal function unchanged after intervention as "preserved" may be misleading. Patients with ischemic nephropathy unchanged after open surgical repair remain at increased risk for death or dialysis. Similar data relating renal function response and survival free from dialysis after catheter-based intervention are not currently available.

CONSEQUENCES OF OPERATIVE FAILURES

Renal artery repairs failed in approximately 4% of patients on follow-up.[3] Blood pressure response after secondary operative intervention was equivalent to that observed after primary operative intervention. However, patients requiring secondary renal artery intervention had a significant and independent risk of eventual dialysis dependence (35% versus 4%).[3] To date, no peer-reviewed report has examined the dialysis risk associated with restenosis after catheter-based interventions.

Our experience with failed renal artery repairs reinforces two important issues. First, the irretrievable loss of excretory renal function observed after failed renal artery repair supports the view that renal revascularization should be performed for clear clinical indications, not as a "prophylactic" procedure in the absence of either hypertension or renal insufficiency.[2,19,22] Second, the direct aortorenal reconstructions in these patients are

TABLE 24-8 RENAL FUNCTION RESPONSE VERSUS PREOPERATIVE SERUM CREATININE (*N* = 469 PATIENTS)

	PREOPERATIVE SCr*				
Renal Function Response†	**<1.8 mg/dL**	**1.8-2.9 mg/dL**	**≥3.0 mg/dL**	**Dialysis Dependent**	**Total**
Improved (%)	71 (29)	75 (54)	29 (58)	28 (76)	203 (43)
No change (%)	142 (58)	52 (38)	17 (34)	9 (24)	220 (47)
Worse (%)	31 (13)	11 (8)	4 (8)	0 (0)	46 (10)

*$P < .0001$ for rate of improved response compared with preoperative serum creatinine.
†See text for definition.
SCr, Serum creatinine.
From Cherr GS, Hansen KJ, Craven TE, et al: Surgical management of atherosclerotic renovascular disease. J Vasc Surg 35:236, 2002.

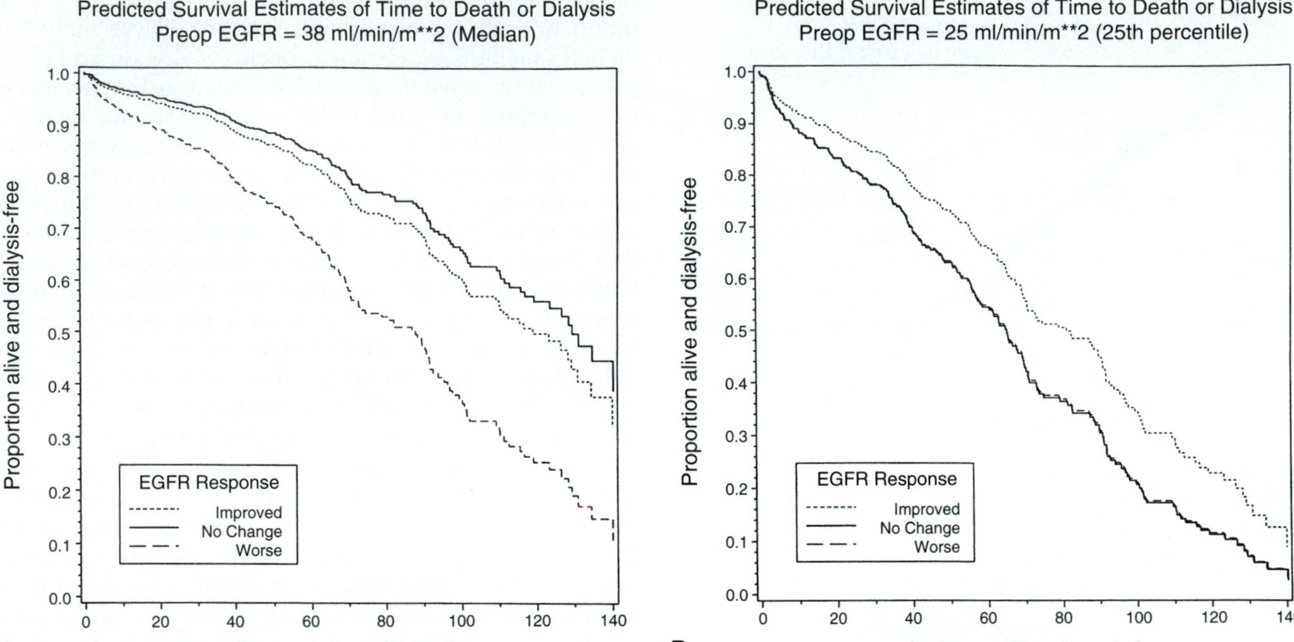

FIGURE 24-6. A and **B**, Predicted dialysis-free survival according to postoperative renal function response for patients with a preoperative EGFR of 25 ml/min/m² (25th percentile) or 39 ml/min/m² (median value). The interaction between preoperative EGFR and renal function response for dialysis-free survival was significant and independent. (From Cherr GS, Hansen KJ, Craven TE, et al: Surgical management of atherosclerotic renovascular disease. J Vasc Surg 35:236, 2002)

characterized by prolonged patency. Early failures of repair reflect errors in surgical technique or operative judgment.

SURGERY AFTER FAILED PTRA

We recently reviewed our experience with 32 consecutive atherosclerotic patients repaired after a failed PTRA (F-PTRA).[39] We examined the influence of failure of PTRA on methods of secondary surgical management, and blood pressure and excretory renal function response to operation.

Secondary operative repair was considered complicated by F-PTRA in more than half of patients. In all, four unnecessary nephrectomies were required. Unnecessary branch renal artery reconstruction was required in two thirds of patients. Hypertension after operative repair for F-PTRA was cured in 7%, improved in 50%, and considered unchanged in 43%. Compared with patients treated by operative repair only, F-PTRA was associated with significantly decreased blood pressure benefit (57% versus 89% benefited [$P < .001$]).

Summary

With proper patient selection, operative repair of atherosclerotic renovascular disease results in both blood pressure and renal function benefit. Improvement in renal function is associated with a significant increase in dialysis-free survival independent of all other comorbidities. The application of intraoperative duplex to assess renal artery reconstruction has resulted in long-term primary patency exceeding 96%. However, when failure of operative repair occurs, eventual renal function is worsened, culminating in an increased risk of dialysis dependence and death.

Percutaneous transluminal angioplasty with or without stenting offers similar blood pressure benefit as operative repair for non-ostial atherosclerotic lesions of the main renal artery. However, cumulative data for ostial lesions associated with ischemic nephropathy suggest that PTRA with or without endoluminal stenting yields inferior renal function benefit. The common practice of reporting unchanged renal function as "preserved" or "stabilized" after renal artery intervention may be misleading. Patients with ischemic nephropathy unchanged after open surgical repair remain at increased risk for eventual dialysis-dependence and death.[2,21,23] For these reasons, the authors recommend open operative repair of ostial atherosclerosis and renal artery occlusion associated with severe hypertension and renal insufficiency.

REFERENCES

1. Hansen KJ, Starr SM, Sands RE, et al: Contemporary surgical management of renovascular disease. J Vasc Surg 16:319, 1992.
2. Cherr GS, Hansen KJ, Craven TE, et al: Surgical management of atherosclerotic renovascular disease. J Vasc Surg 35:236, 2002.
3. Hansen KJ, Deitch JS, Oskin TC, et al: Renal artery repair: Consequence of operative failures. Ann Surg 227:678, 1998.
4. Hansen KJ, Edwards MS, Craven TE, et al: Prevalence of renovascular disease in the elderly: A population-based study. J Vasc Surg 36:443, 2002.
5. Edwards MS, Hansen KJ, Craven TE, et al: Relationships between renovascular disease, blood pressure, and renal function in the elderly: A population-based study. Am J Kidney Dis 41:990, 2003.
6. Appel RG, Bleyer AJ, Reavis S, et al: Renovascular disease in older patients beginning renal replacement therapy. Kidney Int 48:171, 1995.

7. Deitch JS, Hansen KJ, Craven TE, et al: Renal artery repair in African-Americans. J Vasc Surg 26:465, 1997.
8. Mailloux LU, Bellucci AG, Mossey RT, et al: Predictors of survival in patients undergoing dialysis. Am J Med 84:855, 1988.
9. Svetkey LP, Himmelstein SI, Dunnick NR, et al: Prospective analysis of strategies for diagnosing renovascular hypertension. Hypertension 14:247, 1989.
10. van Jaarsveld BC, Krijnen P, Derkx FH, et al: The place of renal scintigraphy in the diagnosis of renal artery stenosis: Fifteen years of clinical experience. Arch Intern Med 157:1226, 1997.
11. Nally JV, Jr, Chen C, Fine E, et al: Diagnostic criteria of renovascular hypertension with captopril renography: A consensus statement. Am J Hypertens 4:749S, 1991.
12. Dean RH, Benjamin ME, Hansen KJ: Surgical management of renovascular hypertension. Curr Probl Surg 34:209, 1997.
13. Hansen KJ, Tribble RW, Reavis SW, et al: Renal duplex sonography: Evaluation of clinical utility. J Vasc Surg 12:227, 1990.
14. Motew SJ, Cherr GS, Craven TE, et al: Renal duplex sonography: Main renal artery versus hilar analysis. J Vasc Surg 32:462, 2000.
15. Valentine RJ, Martin JD, Myers SI, et al: Asymptomatic celiac and superior mesenteric artery stenoses are more prevalent among patients with unsuspected renal artery stenoses. J Vasc Surg 14:195, 1991.
16. Hansen KJ, Wilson DB, Craven TE, et al: Mesenteric artery disease in the elderly. J Vasc Surg 40:45, 2004.
17. Solomon R, Werner C, Mann D, et al: Effects of saline, mannitol, and furosemide to prevent acute decreases in renal function induced by radiocontrast agents. N Engl J Med 331:1416, 1994.
18. Kay J, Chow WH, Chan TM, et al: Acetylcysteine for prevention of acute deterioration of renal function following elective coronary angiography and intervention: A randomized controlled trial. JAMA 289:553, 2003.
19. Baker CS, Wragg A, Kumar S, et al: A rapid protocol for the prevention of contrast-induced renal dysfunction: The RAPPID study. J Am Coll Cardiol 41:2114, 2003.
20. Dean RH, Tribble RW, Hansen KJ, et al: Evolution of renal insufficiency in ischemic nephropathy. Ann Surg 213:446, 1991.
21. Hansen KJ, Thomason RB, Craven TE, et al: Surgical management of dialysis-dependent ischemic nephropathy. J Vasc Surg 21:197, 1995.
22. Hansen KJ, Benjamin ME, Appel RG, et al: Renovascular hypertension in the elderly: Results of surgical management. Geriatr Nephrol Urol 6:3, 1996.
23. Hansen KJ, Cherr GS, Craven TE, et al: Management of ischemic nephropathy: Dialysis-free survival after surgical repair. J Vasc Surg 32:472, 2000.
24. Dean RH, Kieffer RW, Smith BM, et al: Renovascular hypertension: Anatomic and renal function changes during drug therapy. Arch Surg 116:1408, 1981.
25. Novick AC, Pohl MA, Schreiber M, et al: Revascularization for preservation of renal function in patients with atherosclerotic renovascular disease. J Urol 129:907, 1983.
26. Williamson WK, Abou-Zamzam AM Jr, Moneta GL, et al: Prophylactic repair of renal artery stenosis is not justified in patients who require infrarenal aortic reconstruction. J Vasc Surg 28:14, 1998.
27. Ives NJ, Wheatley K, Stowe RL, et al: Continuing uncertainty about the value of percutaneous revascularization in atherosclerotic renovascular disease: A meta-analysis of randomized trials. Nephrol Dial Transplant 18:298, 2003.
28. Dean RH, Kieffer RW, Smith BM, et al: Renovascular hypertension: Anatomic and renal function changes during drug therapy. Arch Surg 116:1408, 1981.
29. Webster J, Marshall F, Abdalla M, et al: Randomised comparison of percutaneous angioplasty vs. continued medical therapy for hypertensive patients with atheromatous renal artery stenosis. Scottish and Newcastle Renal Artery Stenosis Collaborative Group. J Hum Hypertens 12:329, 1998.
30. van Jaarsveld BC, Krijnen P, Pieterman H, et al: The effect of balloon angioplasty on hypertension in atherosclerotic renal-artery stenosis. N Engl J Med 342:1007, 2000.
31. Plouin PF, Chatellier G, Darne B, et al: Blood pressure outcome of angioplasty in atherosclerotic renal artery stenosis: A randomized trial. Essai Multicentrique Medicaments vs. Angioplastie (EMMA) Study Group. Hypertension 31:823, 1998.
32. Hunt JC, Strong CG: Renovascular hypertension. Mechanisms, natural history and treatment. Am J Cardiol 32:562, 1973.
33. Hansen KJ, O'Neil EA, Reavis SW, et al: Intraoperative duplex sonography during renal artery reconstruction. J Vasc Surg 14:364, 1991.
34. Moncure AC, Brewster DC, Darling RC, et al: Use of the splenic and hepatic arteries for renal revascularization. J Vasc Surg 3:196, 1986.
35. Messina LM: Operative evaluation of renal and visceral arterial reconstruction using duplex sonography. In Ernst CB and Stanley JC (eds): Current Therapy in Vascular Surgery, 4th Edition, Mosby, Philadelphia, 2001, pp 753–756.
36. Hansen KJ, Reavis SW, Dean RH: Duplex scanning in renovascular disease. Geriatr Nephrol Urol 6:89, 1996.
37. Marone LK, Clouse WD, Dorer DJ, et al: Preservation of renal function with surgical revascularization in patients with atherosclerotic renovascular disease. J Vasc Surg 39:322, 2004.
38. Stanley JC, David M: Hume memorial lecture: Surgical treatment of renovascular hypertension. Am J Surg 174:102, 1997.
39. Wong JM, Hansen KJ, Oskin TC, et al: Surgery after failed percutaneous renal artery angioplasty. J Vasc Surg 30:468, 1999.
40. Wollenweber J, Sheps SG, Davis GD: Clinical course of atherosclerotic renovascular disease. Am J Cardiol 21:60, 1968.
41. Meaney TF, Dustan HP, McCormack LJ: Natural history of renal arterial disease. Radiology 91:881, 1968.
42. Schreiber MJ, Pohl MA, Novick AC. The natural history of atherosclerotic and fibrous renal artery disease. Urol Clin North Am 11:383, 1984.
43. Tollefson DF, Ernst CB: Natural history of atherosclerotic renal artery stenosis associated with aortic disease. J Vasc Surg 14:327, 1991.
44. Zierler RE, Bergelin RO, Davidson RC, et al: A prospective study of disease progression in patients with atherosclerotic renal artery stenosis. Am J Hypertens 9:1055, 1996.
45. Crowley JJ, Santos RM, Peter RH, et al: Progression of renal artery stenosis in patients undergoing cardiac catheterization. Am Heart J 136:913, 1998.
46. Caps MT, Perissinotto C, Zierler RE, et al: Prospective study of atherosclerotic disease progression in the renal artery. Circulation 98:2866, 1998.
47. Baert AL, Wilms G, Amery A, et al: Percutaneous transluminal renal angioplasty: Initial results and long-term follow-up in 202 patients. Cardiovasc Intervent Radiol 13:22, 1990.
48. Tykarski A, Edwards R, Dominiczak AF, et al: Percutaneous transluminal renal angioplasty in the management of hypertension and renal failure in patients with renal artery stenosis. J Hum Hypertens 7:491, 1993.
49. Weibull H, Bergqvist D, Bergentz SE, et al: Percutaneous transluminal renal angioplasty versus surgical reconstruction of atherosclerotic renal artery stenosis: A prospective randomized study. J Vasc Surg 18:841, 1993.
50. Losinno F, Zuccala A, Busato F, et al: Renal artery angioplasty for renovascular hypertension and preservation of renal function: Long-term angiographic and clinical follow-up. AJR Am J Roentgenol 162:853, 1994.
51. Rodriguez-Perez JC, Plaza C, Reyes R, et al: Treatment of renovascular hypertension with percutaneous transluminal angioplasty: Experience in Spain. J Vasc Interv Radiol 5:101, 1994.
52. Bonelli FS, McKusick MA, Textor SC, et al: Renal artery angioplasty: Technical results and clinical outcome in 320 patients. Mayo Clin Proc 70:1041, 1995.
53. Hoffman O, Carreres T, Sapoval MR, et al: Ostial renal artery stenosis angioplasty: Immediate and mid-term angiographic and clinical results. J Vasc Interv Radiol 9:65, 1998.
54. Klow NE, Paulsen D, Vatne K, et al: Percutaneous transluminal renal artery angioplasty using the coaxial technique: Ten years of experience from 591 procedures in 419 patients. Acta Radiol 39:594, 1998.
55. Paulsen D, Klow NE, Rogstad B, et al: Preservation of renal function by percutaneous transluminal angioplasty in ischaemic renal disease. Nephrol Dial Transplant 14:1454, 1999.
56. Zuccala A, Losinno F, Zucchelli A, et al: Renovascular disease in diabetes mellitus: Treatment by percutaneous transluminal renal angioplasty. Nephrol Dial Transplant 13 Suppl 8:26, 1998.
57. van de Ven PJ, Kaatee R, Beutler JJ, et al: Arterial stenting and balloon angioplasty in ostial atherosclerotic renovascular disease: A randomised trial. Lancet 353:282, 1999.
58. Baumgartner I, von Aesch K, Do DD, et al: Stent placement in ostial and nonostial atherosclerotic renal arterial stenoses: A prospective follow-up study. Radiology 216:498, 2000.
59. Rees CR, Palmaz JC, Becker GJ, et al: Palmaz stent in atherosclerotic stenoses involving the ostia of the renal arteries: Preliminary report of a multicenter study. Radiology 181:507, 1991.

60. Wilms GE, Peene PT, Baert AL, et al: Renal artery stent placement with use of the Wallstent endoprosthesis. Radiology 179:457, 1991.
61. Kuhn FP, Kutkuhn B, Torsello G, et al: Renal artery stenosis: Preliminary results of treatment with the Strecker stent. Radiology 180:367, 1991.
62. Joffre F, Rousseau H, Bernadet P, et al: Midterm results of renal artery stenting. Cardiovasc Intervent Radiol 15:313, 1992.
63. Hennequin LM, Joffre FG, Rousseau HP, et al: Renal artery stent placement: Long-term results with the Wallstent endoprosthesis. Radiology 191:713, 1994.
64. Raynaud AC, Beyssen BM, Turmel-Rodrigues LE, et al: Renal artery stent placement: Immediate and midterm technical and clinical results. J Vasc Interv Radiol 5:849, 1994.
65. MacLeod M, Taylor AD, Baxter G, et al: Renal artery stenosis managed by Palmaz stent insertion: Technical and clinical outcome. J Hypertens 13:1791, 1995.
66. Dorros G, Jaff M, Jain A, et al: Follow-up of primary Palmaz-Schatz stent placement for atherosclerotic renal artery stenosis. Am J Cardiol 75:1051, 1995.
67. Henry M, Amor M, Henry I, et al: Stent placement in the renal artery: Three-year experience with the Palmaz stent. J Vasc Interv Radiol 7:343, 1996.
68. Iannone LA, Underwood PL, Nath A, et al: Effect of primary balloon expandable renal artery stents on long-term patency, renal function, and blood pressure in hypertensive and renal insufficient patients with renal artery stenosis. Cathet Cardiovasc Diagn 37:243, 1996.
69. Harden PN, MacLeod MJ, Rodger RS, et al: Effect of renal-artery stenting on progression of renovascular renal failure. Lancet 349:1133, 1997.
70. Blum U, Krumme B, Flugel P, et al: Treatment of ostial renal-artery stenoses with vascular endoprostheses after unsuccessful balloon angioplasty. N Engl J Med 336:459, 1997.
71. Boisclair C, Therasse E, Oliva VL, et al: Treatment of renal angioplasty failure by percutaneous renal artery stenting with Palmaz stents: Mid-term technical and clinical results. AJR Am J Roentgenol 168:245, 1997.
72. Rundback JH, Gray RJ, Rozenblit G, et al: Renal artery stent placement for the management of ischemic nephropathy. J Vasc Interv Radiol 9:413, 1998.
73. Fiala LA, Jackson MR, Gillespie DL, et al: Primary stenting of atherosclerotic renal artery ostial stenosis. Ann Vasc Surg 12:128, 1998.
74. Dorros G, Jaff M, Mathiak L, et al: Four-year follow-up of Palmaz-Schatz stent revascularization as treatment for atherosclerotic renal artery stenosis. Circulation 98:642, 1998.
75. Tuttle KR, Chouinard RF, Webber JT, et al: Treatment of atherosclerotic ostial renal artery stenosis with the intravascular stent. Am J Kidney Dis 32:611, 1998.
76. Gross CM, Kramer J, Waigand J, et al: Ostial renal artery stent placement for atherosclerotic renal artery stenosis in patients with coronary artery disease. Cathet Cardiovasc Diagn 45:1, 1998.
77. Henry M, Amor M, Henry I, et al: Stents in the treatment of renal artery stenosis: Long-term follow-up. J Endovasc Surg 6:42, 1999.
78. Rodriguez-Lopez JA, Werner A, Ray LI, et al: Renal artery stenosis treated with stent deployment: Indications, technique, and outcome for 108 patients. J Vasc Surg 29:617, 1999.

chapter 25

Epidemiology and Pathophysiology

Tara Karamlou
Gregory J. Landry
Lloyd M. Taylor
Gregory L. Moneta

Severe acute intestinal ischemia results from a sudden, symptomatic reduction in intestinal blood flow of sufficient magnitude to potentially result in intestinal infarction.[1] Acute ischemia of the small bowel and/or right colon may result from mesenteric arterial occlusion (embolus or thrombosis), mesenteric venous occlusion, and nonocclusive processes, especially vasospasm (Fig. 25-1). Isolated dissections of the superior mesenteric artery (SMA), either in association with cystic medial degeneration of the arteries, or, more commonly as progression of an existing dissection in the descending thoracic aorta into the SMA and celiac artery may also result in acute intestinal ischemia.

ACUTE ARTERIAL OCCLUSIVE MESENTERIC ISCHEMIA

Acute Mesenteric Arterial Embolism

Emboli to the SMA cause roughly 50% of all cases of acute mesenteric ischemia; 25% of cases are caused by thrombosis of preexisting atherosclerotic lesions, and the remaining 25% are from a variety of other etiologies.[2]

Mesenteric emboli can originate from left atrial or ventricular mural thrombi, or from cardiac valvular lesions.[1,3] These thrombi are most often associated with cardiac dysrhythmias such as atrial fibrillation, global myocardial dysfunction with poor ejection fraction, or discrete hypokinetic regions produced by previous myocardial infarction.[4] About 15% of emboli lodge at the origin of the SMA. The majority of SMA emboli, however, lodge 3 to 10 cm distally, in the tapered segment of the SMA just past the origin of the middle colic artery.[2] More than 20% of emboli to the SMA are associated with concurrent emboli to another arterial bed.[5] Intestinal ischemia due to embolic arterial occlusion can be compounded by reactive mesenteric vasospasm, further reducing collateral flow and exacerbating the ischemic insult.[2,6]

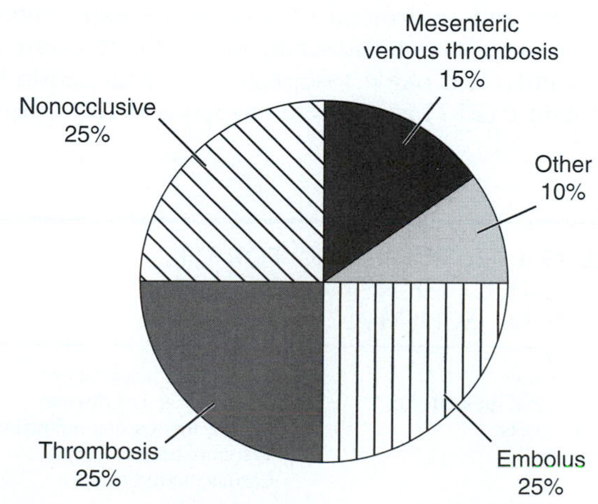

FIGURE 25-1. Etiology of acute mesenteric ischemia.

Acute Mesenteric Arterial Thrombosis

Thrombosis of the SMA or the celiac artery is usually associated with preexisting critical stenoses. Many of these patients have histories consistent with chronic mesenteric ischemia, including postprandial pain, weight loss, "food fear" and early satiety.[1,7] SMA thrombosis can be regarded as a complication of untreated chronic intestinal ischemia.[1] The SMA plaque likely slowly progresses to a critical stenosis over years until thrombosis occurs. Unlike embolic occlusions, thrombosis of the SMA generally occurs flush with the aortic origin of the vessel. Aortic dissection involving the visceral vessels, though rare, can cause acute mesenteric ischemia. The intimal flap of the dissection can extend, compress, or exclude the mesenteric orifice.[6] Acute mesenteric ischemia is also an uncommon (<1%), but serious complication, of cardiac surgery with a reported mortality rate of greater than 50% in most series.[6,8] Presumably, the nonpulsatile perfusion delivered by most extracorporeal circuits allows severely stenotic visceral vessels to occlude during the conduct of cardiopulmonary bypass.[9,10] Identified risk factors for this complication include prolonged cross-clamp times, use of intra-aortic balloon counterpulsation, low cardiac output syndromes, blood transfusion, triple-vessel disease, coronary artery disease, and peripheral arterial disease.[8]

Pathophysiology of Occlusive Acute Mesenteric Ischemia

Acute mesenteric ischemia, whether the underlying cause is embolic or thrombotic, may lead to eventual intestinal infarction. Hypoxia and hypercarbia that occur

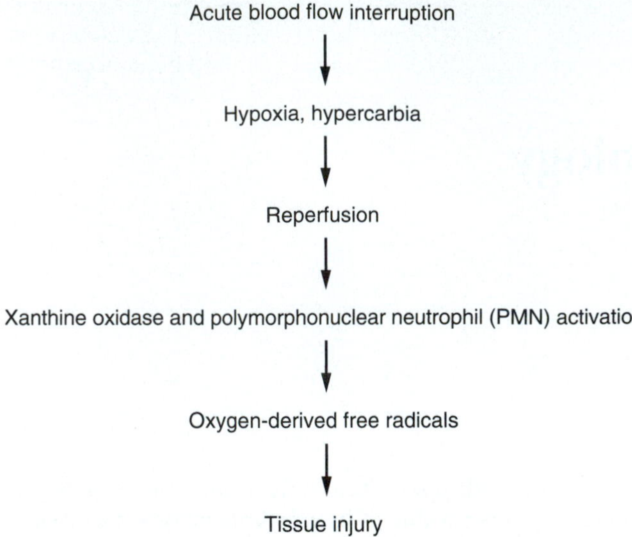

FIGURE 25-2. The pathophysiologic mechanism of acute occlusive mesenteric ischemia.

during flow interruption, and reperfusion injury once intestinal blood flow is restored all contribute to tissue loss (Fig. 25-2).[11] Reperfusion injury is believed to be principally mediated by the activation of the enzyme xanthine oxidase and the recruitment and activation of circulating neutrophils (PMNs).[12,13] The mechanism of injury likely involves the production of oxygen-derived free radicals by xanthine oxidase that then causes profound local tissue injury through lipid peroxidation, membrane disruption, and increased microvascular permeability.[6,12,13] The ischemic endothelium recruits PMNs in an autocrine and paracrine manner, by secreting chemotactic cytokines (tumor necrosis factor-α, interleukin-1, platelet-derived growth factor) that perpetuate further damage to the reperfused tissue.[14,15] PMNs, once activated, degranulate, releasing myeloperoxidase, collagenases, and elastases that further injure the already ischemic and vulnerable tissue.[6,16] The activation of this endogenous inflammatory cascade is not restricted to the injured organ, and may also have deleterious systemic effects, with cardiac, pulmonary, and other organ system dysfunction.[6]

Natural History of Acute Mesenteric Arterial Occlusive Disease

The mortality rate for occlusive acute mesenteric ischemia exceeds 70% in most series.[1,2,6,17,18] Occlusive acute intestinal ischemia secondary to SMA embolism has a more favorable prognosis than that resulting from SMA thrombosis.[1] Survival following acute intestinal ischemia due to SMA thrombosis is rare. The more favorable prognosis with embolism results from the fact that most emboli lodge distally in the SMA (beyond the origin of the middle colic artery), thus allowing perfusion of the proximal intestine via middle colic and jejunal artery branches.[1] Thrombotic occlusion of the SMA usually occurs proximal to the middle colic artery and, therefore, totally interrupts mid-gut arterial perfusion in patients with poorly developed celiac artery or inferior mesenteric artery (IMA) collateral flow.[1,4,7]

NONOCCLUSIVE MESENTERIC ISCHEMIA

Epidemiology

Nonocclusive mesenteric ischemia (NOMI) accounts for 25% of all episodes of acute intestinal ischemia.[1,6,19-21] In NOMI, microscopic arterial blood flow is inadequate to supply perfusion to the bowel. The result is intestinal ischemia and infarction in the presence of a patent macroscopic vasculature.[22] Previous reports have identified multiple risk factors for the development of NOMI (Table 25-1).[22-24] Mesenteric arterial vasospasm can also follow elective revascularization procedures for chronic SMA occlusion. In such cases, vasoconstriction of small- and medium-sized vessels is precipitated by early enteral feeding.[25] Without prompt intervention, NOMI may progress from localized intestinal ischemia to transmural infarction, peritonitis, and death.[26,27] Mortality is high irrespective of treatment due to the underlying serious medical conditions that precipitate NOMI, and the frequent delays in diagnosis.[6,19-22]

Pathophysiology

NOMI was first recognized following autopsies of patients with small intestinal gangrene in the absence of arterial or venous occlusion.[28,29] Virtually all patients with NOMI also have a severe coexisting illness, particularly severe cardiac failure.[19,30-32] It is postulated that hypoperfusion from primary cardiac failure, with resulting peripheral hypoxemia and paradoxic splanchnic vasoconstriction precipitates intestinal ischemia.[19-21] Investigation of the regulatory mechanisms of the mesenteric circulation has demonstrated that the pathophysiology of NOMI is multifactorial. Mesenteric vasoconstriction, intestinal hypoxia, and ischemia-reperfusion injury all play roles in the development of NOMI.

Mesenteric vasoconstriction is the hallmark of NOMI. It represents an exaggerated homeostatic mechanism, induced by excessive sympathetic activity during cardiogenic shock or hypovolemia, that attempts to maintain cardiac and cerebral perfusion at the expense of splanchnic and peripheral circulations.[19] Experimental evidence suggests that the mediators of this response are endothelin-1, nitric oxide, vasopressin, and angiotensin.[33,34] Endothelin-1 (ET-1) is a potent vasoconstrictor secreted

TABLE 25-1 RISK-FACTORS FOR THE DEVELOPMENT OF NONOCCLUSIVE MESENTERIC ISCHEMIA

Age > 50 years	Congestive heart failure
Atherosclerotic mesenteric arterial disease	Coronary artery disease
Digitalis use	Recent myocardial infarction
Sepsis	Vasoconstrictive drugs
Prior hypotensive episodes	Cardiac arrhythmias

from endothelial cells that, in concert with other vasoactive peptides, regulates myogenic cells in the vascular wall. Nitric oxide (NO) can have paradoxic effects on vascular tone depending on local concentration.[35] At low concentrations, it acts as a vasodilator, whereas at higher concentrations it acts as an oxygen-free radical, impairing mitochondrial energy production. The splanchnic autoregulatory system is effected by local arteriolar smooth muscle relaxation and vasodilation concomitant with increased cellular oxygen extraction.[19,36-39] Adequate oxygen delivery is maintained despite declining perfusion pressures until a finite threshold is reached. In experimental models, maximal extraction is reached at a critical pressure of 40 mm Hg. Beyond this point, oxygen consumption declines and ischemia ensues.[40] Neri and colleagues recently demonstrated that postoperative cardiac surgery patients who develop NOMI had persistent deficits between oxygen delivery (DO_2) and consumption (VO_2) because of poor circulatory reserve. In contrast, postoperative cardiac patients who did not develop NOMI were able to normalize their DO_2:VO_2 ratio by optimizing their cardiac output.[21]

In the presence of impaired perfusion, blood flow is not evenly distributed in the bowel wall. The mucosa retains its perfusion initially, at the expense of the serosal layers through the mucosal production of nitric oxide (NO), prostaglandins, and stimulation of dopamine-I receptors.[41] Therefore, histologic damage is first observed at the villous tip and progresses to the deeper muscularis, submucosa, and mucosa within a few hours.

Once set in motion, mesenteric vasospasm may persist despite correction of the precipitating event.[19-21] The etiology of persistent vasoconstriction once adequate blood flow is restored is unknown, but it may respond to direct intra-arterial papaverine infusion or other vasodilators, including iloprost.[42] This phenomenon of protracted vasoconstriction, however, plays an important role in the development and maintenance of occlusive and nonocclusive intestinal ischemia and also may complicate mesenteric revascularization.[25]

The use of vasoconstrictive agents and digitalis has been associated with the majority of cases of NOMI. Vasoactive agents, including α-adrenergic drugs and vasopressin, produce splanchnic vasoconstriction directly, whereas digoxin preparations alter mesenteric vasoreactivity by stimulating arterial and venous smooth muscle cell contraction.[41-43] This may enhance mesenteric arteriolar vasoconstriction in the setting of acute venous hypertension.[42]

Restoration of blood flow to ischemic intestine may be complicated by reperfusion injury. During critical ischemia, ATP levels are depleted, causing distortion of ATP-dependent cell membrane systems. This results in loss of cellular homeostasis, with cellular swelling and electrolyte imbalances.[41] The reduction in ATP levels also generates large amounts of adenosine, a precursor of hypoxanthine. Within the swollen cells, calcium accumulates and triggers the hydrolysis of the enzyme xanthine dehydrogenase into xanthine oxidase, which reacts with intracellular hypoxanthine to produce uric acid and toxic oxygen-free radicals.[6,19,41] These free radicals exert direct damage to cellular membranes causing capillary leak syndrome and incite endogenous inflammatory cascades that cause widespread tissue injury. The deleterious effects of free radicals are usually limited by endogenous scavengers such as glutathione, catalase, superoxide dismutase, and nitric oxide.[41] However, in cases of prolonged ischemia, the capacity of this scavenger system to eliminate reactive oxygen species is exceeded, and continued damage occurs. The degree of reperfusion injury is thus related to the frequency, as well as the duration, of the ischemic episodes. Clark and Gewertz demonstrated that two short 15-minute periods of low flow followed by reperfusion resulted in a more severe histologic injury than a single 30-minute period of ischemia.[44,45] In NOMI, a similar scenario exists: hypoperfusion may be partial and, occasionally, repetitive. It is believed that episodic reperfusion creates a local environment replete with primed neutrophils within the ischemic bed that are capable of degranulating and releasing superoxides. This concept is substantiated by recent experimental evidence that reperfusion injury may be attenuated by reperfusion with leuko-depleted blood or by blockade of endothelial cell surface receptors for leukocyte adherence.[46,47] In addition, several compounds, including *N*-acetylcysteine and vitamin E have been shown in animal models to reduce tissue damage caused by reactive oxygen species.[48] The application of these novel approaches in human NOMI awaits further study.

MESENTERIC VENOUS THROMBOSIS

Mesenteric venous thrombosis (MVT) refers to thrombosis of the veins draining the intestine (inferior mesenteric, superior mesenteric, splenic, and portal veins). The obstruction in venous return leads to edema, distention, and in some cases, infarction of the affected segments.[1,6]

Epidemiology

MVT is a comparatively rare form of mesenteric ischemia. The presentation may vary from asymptomatic to fulminant, with intestinal infarction and hemodynamic collapse. MVT was first described by Elliot in 1895 as "thrombosis of the porto-mesenteric venous system."[49] Warren and Eberhard in 1935 further characterized MVT as a distinct clinical entity. These authors reported a 34% mortality rate following intestinal resection for venous thrombosis.[50]

MVT currently comprises no more than 5% to 15% of all cases of acute mesenteric ischemia.[51] Only 372 patients with MVT were reported from 1911 to 1984.[52] MVT comprised only 6.2% of 1167 patients treated for mesenteric ischemia at the Mayo Clinic from 1972 to 1993.[53] Ottinger and Austen found that MVT comprised only 0.006% of hospital admissions.[54] It is estimated that intestinal infarction due to MVT is encountered in less than 1 in 1000 laparotomies for acute abdomen.[55]

Pathophysiology

MVT can be classified as primary or secondary. Primary MVT is defined as spontaneous, idiopathic thrombosis of mesenteric veins not associated with any other disease

TABLE 25-2 CAUSES OF SECONDARY MESENTERIC VENOUS THROMBOSIS

Trauma	Splenomegaly
Surgery	Pancreatitis
Cancer	Dehydration
Cirrhosis	Infection
Portal hypertension	Diverticular disease
Inflammatory bowel disease	Hypercoagulable states
Oral contraceptive use	

or etiologic factor.[1,6,51] The number of patients in this group has decreased substantially in the past decade because the ability to diagnose inherited thrombotic disorders and recognize hypercoagulable states has improved. Patients in whom an etiologic factor can be identified are said to have secondary MVT. Currently, however, a causative factor can be identified in only 35% of patients with MVT.[51,53] Known causes of secondary MVT are shown in Table 25-2. Oral contraceptive use accounts for 9% to 18% of episodes of MVT in young women.[56] Proteins C and S deficiencies, antithrombin III deficiency, dysfibrinogenemia, abnormal plasminogen, polycythemia vera, thrombocytosis, sickle-cell disease, and factor V Leiden mutation have all been associated with MVT.[1,6,51,56,57] Localized secondary MVT has also been reported, most commonly associated with volvulus, intussusception, or mechanical bowel strangulation.

The location of the thrombus may be predicted on the basis of the underlying cause. Thrombosis due to an intra-abdominal cause, such as inflammatory conditions or surgery, starts in the larger vessels at the site of compression and then propagates distally to involve the smaller venous arcades and arcuate channels.[56] In contrast, thrombosis due to an underlying hypercoagulable state usually begins in the small vessels and progresses to involve the larger vessels.[51,56] Occlusion of the venae rectae and the intramural vessels interferes with adequate venous drainage, with eventual hemorrhagic infarction of the involved bowel segment. The transition from ischemic to normal bowel is usually gradual, unlike that seen with acute embolic or thrombotic occlusion.

Natural History

The natural history of MVT is variable, depending on the etiology. In most cases, it usually does not result in gangrenous bowel.[1,6,56,57] Manifesting symptoms are diverse. Patients may present with a benign abdominal examination and few symptoms, or may present with profound hemodynamic collapse. Most patients have abdominal pain. The pain can be sudden in onset, but frequently begins insidiously and worsens over time. Approximately 50% of patients have pain from 5 to 30 days before seeking medical attention, and 27% report abdominal pain for more than 1 month.[58] In a recent review, only 16% of patients had severe peritonitis, and only 33% required bowel resection.[57] Despite improved diagnostic modalities and more aggressive treatment regimens, symptomatic acute MVT is an indicator of a poor prognosis with a 30-day mortality rate of about 25% and a 3-year survival rate of 35%.[57,59-63] Patients with evidence of chronic thrombosis fare somewhat better because collateral venous channels form that augment intestinal venous drainage.

CHRONIC MESENTERIC ISCHEMIA

Symptomatic chronic mesenteric arterial insufficiency is a well-described but infrequently encountered, clinical problem. The earliest report of chronic intestinal ischemia was by Councilman in 1894.[64] In 1918, Goodman credited Baccelli as the first individual to correctly associate postprandial pain with chronic mesenteric ischemia. Eighteen years later Dunphy suggested that the abdominal pain associated with chronic mesenteric arterial occlusion was a possible precursor of later intestinal infarction.[65] Later, Shaw and Maynard performed the first successful endarterectomy for chronic mesenteric ischemia.[66] Morris and colleagues described the technique of retrograde aortovisceral bypass in 1962.[67]

Epidemiology

Chronic mesenteric ischemia (CMI) is the result of atherosclerosis in 90% of cases.[1,6,68-72] The nonatherosclerotic causes of CMI are listed in Table 25-3. Nonatherosclerotic etiologies have been described in young adults and in children as young as 30 months of age.[68,69,70,72] Risk factors for atherosclerotic-associated CMI, in general, are similar to those of other atherosclerotic conditions, including a positive family history, sedentary lifestyle, hypertension, hypercholesterolemia, and smoking.[1,6,68-73] In contrast to other atherosclerotic vascular diseases, approximately 60% of patients with CMI are female. Nearly 50% of patients have a history of earlier cardiovascular surgery.[72,74] Symptomatic CMI generally manifests with a mean age of about 58 years.[1,6,68,74-81] More than one third of patients have hypertension, coronary artery disease, and/or cerebrovascular disease.[1,6,76-81] Nearly 20% have evidence of chronic renal insufficiency, and 10% have diabetes.[68,76-81]

TABLE 25-3 NONATHEROSCLEROTIC CONDITIONS ASSOCIATED WITH CHRONIC MESENTERIC ISCHEMIA

Neurofibromatosis	Polyarteritis nodosa
Middle aortic syndrome	Cogan's syndrome
Median arcuate ligament compression	Aortic coarctation repair
Visceral artery dissection	Radiation injury
Buerger's disease	Thrombosis associated with TAA repair
Rheumatoid arthritis	Mesenteric arteritis
Cocaine abuse	Congenital afibrogenemia
Ergot poisoning	
Systemic lupus erythematosus	

TAA, thoracic aortic aneurysm.

Although there is a high prevalence of mesenteric atherosclerosis, the clinical syndrome of symptomatic mesenteric ischemia is uncommon.[1,78,79,80] An autopsy series of unselected patients found significant stenoses in approximately 50% of celiac arteries, 30% of superior mesenteric SMAs, and 30% of inferior mesenteric arteries.[75] In a more recent series of 120 consecutive autopsies, however, rates of significant stenoses in the celiac, SMA, and IMA were not quite as high, with a 22%, 16%, and 10% incidence, respectively.[80] The prevalence of potentially flow-limiting stenosis within the mesenteric vessels increases with age, with up to 67% of those over 80 years of age having a greater than 50% stenosis in some mesenteric artery.[80] Aortograms performed for aortic aneurysmal or occlusive disease demonstrate significant stenosis of the celiac artery in 33% of cases and SMA lesions in nearly 20%.[78-81]

Pathophysiology and Natural History

CMI occurs when the blood supply is insufficient to meet the metabolic demands of the bowel, resulting from increased motility, secretion, and absorption after meals.[82] The infrequent occurrence of symptomatic disease may be explained, in part, by the extensive mesenteric collateral circulation, which includes both viscerovisceral (celiac artery-SMA—IMA), and parietovisceral (hypogastric—IMA) collateral blood flow.[1,6,76,80-82] The slow development of a chronic, high-grade stenosis or occlusion of one or more of the major mesenteric vessels may thus be fully compensated by collateral blood flow. In addition, recent evidence suggests that preexisting significant stenoses in even remote arterial beds may provide protective effects through the mechanism of ischemic preconditioning.[83-85]

It has been proposed that the pathophysiology of symptomatic CMI involves a regional vascular steal phenomenon.[86] Investigators have used tonometric assessment of splanchnic blood flow in dogs with 50% stenoses of both the celiac artery and SMA to show that food intake reduced intestinal perfusion by 50%. This reduction was associated with a significant decrease in intestinal intramural pH that was attributed to a steal from the intestinal to the gastric circulation stimulated by a food bolus within the stomach.[86]

Single-vessel disease of the SMA may produce symptoms characteristic of CMI. The vast majority of patients who present with symptomatic CMI, however, have arteriographic evidence of multivessel visceral artery disease.[1,6,68-72,74-76,80,81]

A variety of pain syndromes characterize patients with CMI. In general, the symptoms consist of upper abdominal crampy or aching pain beginning 20 to 30 minutes after eating. At first the pain may be of short duration but later it may become more persistent and last for 3 to 4 hours after eating. As the disease progresses, the amount of food that precipitates abdominal pain may decrease. Patients avoid eating to prevent the resulting abdominal pain. Most patients with CMI suffer weight loss secondary to diminished nutritional intake. Malabsorption is not the primary mechanism of weight loss.[82] No form of bowel activity is "classic" for CMI. Patients may have diarrhea that can potentially exacerbate their nutritional depletion, constipation, or normal bowel habits. Without intervention, such patients develop severe protein-calorie malnutrition and CMI can progress to visceral infarction.[68-72,76,80-82]

Most fatal cases of chronic mesenteric ischemia occur in patients with a prolonged history of chronic abdominal complaints.[1,68-72,76,80-82] Such cases are frequently characterized by months of abdominal complaints, multiple negative endoscopies, CT scans, and other diagnostic tests. In retrospect, the diagnosis is usually obvious. A high index of suspicion and prompt intervention are clearly indicated in cases of unexplained abdominal pain and weight loss. Early diagnosis may prevent acute thrombosis of stenotic vessels and the often fatal complication of intestinal infarction.[1,68-72,76,80-82]

REFERENCES

1. Moneta G: Acute mesenteric ischemia. In Rutherford RB (ed): Diagnosis of Intestinal Ischemia. Philadelphia, WB Saunders, 2000, p 2508.
2. McKinsey J, Gewertz BL: Acute mesenteric ischemia. Surg Clin North Am 77:307, 1997.
3. Vicente DC, Kazmers A: Acute mesenteric ischemia. Curr Opin Cardiol 14:453, 1999.
4. Park WM, Gloviczki P, Cherry KJ: Contemporary management of acute mesenteric ischemia: Factors associated with survival. J Vasc Surg 35:445, 2002.
5. Kaleya RN, Sammartano RJ, Boley SJ: Aggressive approach to acute mesenteric ischemia. Surg Clin North Am 72:157, 1992.
6. Schwartz LB, McKinsey JF, Gewertz BL: Visceral ischemic syndromes. In Moore WS (ed): Vascular Surgery: A Comprehensive Review, 6th ed. Philadelphia, WB Saunders, 2002, p 572.
7. Sreenarasimhaiah J: Diagnosis and management of intestinal ischemic disorders. BMJ 326:1372, 2003.
8. Ghosh S, Roberts N, Firmin RK, et al: Risk factors for intestinal ischemia in cardiac surgical patients. Eur J Cardiothorac Surg 21:411, 2002.
9. Schutz A, Eichinger W, Breuer M, et al: Acute mesenteric ischemia after open heart surgery. Angiology 49:267, 1998.
10. Klempnauer J, Grotheus F, Baktas H, et al: Acute mesenteric ischemia following cardiac surgery. J Cardiovasc Surg 38:639, 1997.
11. Schwartz LB, Oropello JM, Iberti TJ: Acute mesenteric ischemia: Pathophysiology, diagnosis, and treatment. Dis Mon 39:131, 1993.
12. Parks DA, Granger DN: Contributions of ischemia and reperfusion to mucosal lesion formation. Am J Physiol 250:G749, 1986.
13. Parks DA, Granger DN: Ischemia-induced vascular changes: Role of xanthine oxidase and hydroxyl radicals. Am J Physiol 245:G285, 1983.
14. Ali MH, Schlidt SA, Hynes KL, et al: Prolonged hypoxia alters endothelial barrier function. Surgery 124:491, 1998.
15. Marcus BC, Wyble CW, Hynes KL, et al: Cytokine-induced increases in endothelial permeability occur after adhesion molecule expression. Surgery 120:411, 1997.
16. Korthius RJ, Anderson DC, Granger DN: Role of neutrophil-endothelial cell adhesion in inflammatory disorders. J Crit Care 9:47, 1994.
17. Lock G: Acute mesenteric ischemia: Classification, evaluation and therapy. Acta Gastroenterol Belg 65:220, 2002.
18. Edwards MS, Cherr GS, Craven TE, et al: Acute occlusive mesenteric ischemia: Surgical management and outcomes. Ann Vasc Surg 17:72, 2003.
19. Bassiouny HS: Nonocclusive mesenteric ischemia. Surg Clin North Am 77:319, 1997.
20. Trompeter M, Brazda T, Remy CT, et al: Non-occlusive mesenteric ischemia: Etiology, diagnosis, and interventional therapy. Eur Radiol 12:1179, 2001.
21. Neri E, Sassi C, Massetti M, et al: Nonocclusive mesenteric ischemia in patients with acute aortic dissection. J Vasc Surg 36:738, 2002.

22. Howard TJ, Plaskon LA, Wiebke EA, et al: Nonocclusive mesenteric ischemia remains a diagnostic dilemma. Am J Surg 171:405, 1996.
23. Lock G, Scholmerich J: Non-occlusive mesenteric ischemia. Hepatogastroenterol 42:234, 1995.
24. Wilcox MG, Howard TJ, Plakson LA, et al: Current theories of pathogenesis and treatment of nonocclusive mesenteric ischemia. Dig Dis Sci 40:709, 1995.
25. Gewertz BL, Zarins CK: Postoperative vasospasm after antegrade mesenteric revascularization: A report of three cases. J Vasc Surg 14:382, 1991.
26. Patel A, Kaleya RN, Sammartano RJ: Pathophysiology of mesenteric ischemia. Surg Clin North Am 72:31, 1992.
27. Williams LF, Anastasia LF, Hasiotis CA, et al: Non-occlusive mesenteric infarction. Am J Surg 114:376, 1967.
28. Case records of the Massachusetts General Hospital (Case 35082). N Engl J Med 240:308, 1949.
29. Haglund U, Lundgren O: Nonocclusive acute intestinal vascular failure. Br J Surg 66:155, 1979.
30. Cohen EB: Infarction of the stomach. Am J Med 11:645, 1951.
31. Ende N: Infarction of the bowel in cardiac failure. N Engl J Med 25:879, 1958.
32. Wilson R, Qualheim RE: A form of acute hemorrhagic enterocolitis afflicting chronically ill individuals. Gastroenterol 27:431, 1954.
33. Bailey RW, Bulkey GB, Hamilton SR: Protection of the small intestine from nonocclusive mesenteric ischemia. Am J Surg 153:108, 1987.
34. McNeill JR, Stark RD, Greenway CV: Intestinal vasoconstriction after hemorrhage: Roles of vasopressin and angiotensin. Am J Physiol 219:1342, 1970.
35. Lamarque D, Whittle BJ: Increase in gastric intramucosal hydrogen ion concentration following endotoxin challenge in the rat and the actions of nitric oxide synthase inhibitors. Clin Exper Pharmacol Physiol 28:164, 2001.
36. Norris CP, Barnes GE, Smith EE, et al: Autoregulation of superior mesenteric flow in fasted and fed dogs. Am J Physiol 237:H174, 1979.
37. Shepherd AP: Myogenic responses of intestinal resistance and exchange vessels. Am J Physiol 233:H547, 1977.
38. Landow L: Splanchnic lactate production in cardiac surgery patients. Crit Care Med 21:884, 1993.
39. Grum CM: Tissue oxygenation in low flow states and during hypoxemia. Crit Care Med 21:844, 1993.
40. Mesh CL, Gewertz BL: The effect of hemodilution on blood flow regulation in normal and postischemic intestine. J Surg Res 48:183, 1990.
41. Kolkman JJ, Mensink PB: Non-occlusive mesenteric ischemia: A common disorder in gastroenterology and intensive care. Best Pract Res Clin Gastroenterol 17: 457, 2003.
42. Char D, Hines G: Chronic mesenteric ischemia: Diagnosis and treatment. Heart Dis 3:231, 2001.
43. Mikkelsen E, Andersson DK, Pedersen OL: Effects of digoxin on isolated human mesenteric vessels. Acta Pharm Tox 45:249, 1979.
44. Kim EH, Gewertz BL: Chronic digitalis administration alters mesenteric vascular reactivity. J Vasc Surg 5:382, 1987.
45. Clark ET, Gewertz BL: Intermittent ischemia potentiates intestinal reperfusion injury. J Vasc Surg 13:606, 1991.
46. Luscinskas FW, Brock AF, Araout MA, et al: Endothelial-leukocyte adhesion molecule-1-dependent and leukocyte (CD11/CD18)-dependent mechanisms contribute to polymorphonuclear leukocyte adhesion to cytokine-activated human vascular endothelium. J Immunol 1989:2257, 1989.
47. Mileski WJ, Winn R, Harlan JM, et al: Transient inhibition of neutrophil adherence with the anti-CD18 monoclonal antibody 60.3 does not increase mortality rates in abdominal sepsis. Surgery 109:497, 1991.
48. Dimakakos PB, Kotsis T, Kondi-Pafiti A, et al: Oxygen free radicals in abdominal aortic surgery: An experimental study. J Cardiovasc Surg 43:77, 2002.
49. Elliot JW: The operative relief of gangrene of intestine due to occlusion of the mesenteric vessels. Ann Surg 21:9, 1895.
50. Warren S, Eberhard TP: Mesenteric venous thrombosis. Surg Gynecol Obstet 61:102, 1935.
51. Rhee RY, Gloviczki P: Mesenteric venous thrombosis. Surg Clin North Am 77: 327, 1997.
52. Abdu R, Zakhour BJ, Dallis DJ: Mesenteric venous thrombosis—1911-1984. Surgery 101:383, 1987.
53. Rhee RY, Glovickzi P, Medonca CT, et al: Mesenteric venous thrombosis: Still a lethal disease in the 1990s. J Vasc Surg 20:688, 1994.
54. Ottinger LW, Austen WG: A study of 136 patients with mesenteric infarction. Surg Gynecol Obstet 124:251, 1967.
55. Kazmers A: Intestinal ischemia caused by venous thrombosis. In Vascular Surgery, Philadelphia, WB Saunders, 1995, p 526.
56. Kumar S, Sarr MG, Kamath PS: Mesenteric venous thrombosis. N Engl J Med 345:686, 2001.
57. Harward TR, Green D, Bergan JJ, et al: Mesenteric venous thrombosis. J Vasc Surg 9:328, 1989.
58. Morasch MD, Ebaugh JL, Chiou AC, et al: Mesenteric venous thrombosis: A changing clinical entity. J Vasc Surg 34:680, 2001.
59. Mathews JE, White RR: Primary mesenteric venous occlusive disease. Am J Surg 122:579, 1971.
60. Montany PF, Finley RK: Mesenteric venous thrombosis. Am Surg 54:161, 1988.
61. Clavien PA, Harder F: Mesenteric venous thrombosis. Helv Chir Acta 55:29, 1988.
62. Kaleya RN, Boley SJ: Mesenteric venous thrombosis. In Najarian JS, Delaney JP (eds): Progress in Gastrointestinal Surgery. Chicago, Year-Book, 1989, p 417.
63. Levy PJ, Krausz MM, Many J: The role of second-look procedure in improving survival time for patients with mesenteric venous thrombosis. Surg Gynecol Obstet 170:287, 1990.
64. Councilman WT: Three cases of occlusion of the superior mesenteric artery. Boston Medical and Surgical Journal 130:410, 1894.
65. Taylor LM, Porter JM: Treatment of chronic intestinal ischemia. Sem Vasc Surg 3:186, 1990.
66. Shaw RS, Maynard EP III: Acute and chronic thrombosis of the mesenteric arteries associated with malabsorption: A report of two cases successfully treated with thromboendarterectomy. N Engl J Med 258:874, 1958.
67. Morris GC, Crawford ES, Cooley DA, et al: Revascularization of the celiac and superior mesenteric arteries. Arch Surg 84:113, 1962.
68. Calderon M, Reul GJ, Gregoric ID, et al: Long-term results of the surgical management of symptomatic chronic intestinal ischemia. J Cardiovasc Surg 33:723, 1992.
69. Cunningham CG, Reilly LM, Stoney R: Chronic visceral ischemia. Three decades of progress. Ann Surg 214:276, 1991.
70. Sanders BM, Dalsing MC: Mesenteric ischemia affects young adults with predisposition. Ann Vasc Surg 17:270, 2003.
71. Stanton PE, Holiier PA, Seidel TW, et al: Chronic intestinal ischemia: Diagnosis and therapy. J Vasc Surg 4:338, 1986.
72. Moawad J, Gewertz BL: Chronic mesenteric ischemia: Clinical presentation and diagnosis. Surg Clin North Am 77:357, 1997.
73. Bech F, Loesberg A, Rosenblum J, et al: Median arcuate ligament compression syndrome in monozygotic twins. J Vasc Surg 19:934, 1994.
74. Schwartz LB, Gewertz BL: Chronic mesenteric arterial disease: Clinical presentation and diagnostic evaluation. In Perla BA, Becker GJ (eds): Vascular Intervention: A Clinical Approach. New York, Thieme Medical, 1998, p 517.
75. Crawford ES, Morris GC, Myhre HO, et al: Celiac axis, superior mesenteric artery, and inferior mesenteric artery occlusion: Surgical considerations. Surgery 82:856, 1977.
76. Hallett JW, James ME, Ahlquist DA, et al: Recent trends in the diagnosis and treatment of chronic intestinal ischemia. Ann Vasc Surg 4:126, 1990.
77. Shanley CJ, Ozaki CK, Zelenock GB: Bypass grafting for chronic mesenteric ischemia. Surg Clin North Am 77:381, 1997.
78. Jarvinen O, Laurikka J, Sisto T, et al: Atherosclerosis of the visceral arteries. Vasa 24:9, 1995.
79. Cleveland TJ, Nawaz S, Gaines PA: Mesenteric arterial ischemia: Diagnosis and therapeutic options. Vasc Med 7:311, 2002.
80. Chang JB, Stein T: Mesenteric ischemia: Acute and chronic. Ann Vasc Surg 17:323, 2003.
81. Chang JB, Stein TA: Mesenteric ischemia. Asian J Surg 26:55, 2003.
82. van Bockel JH, Geelkerken RH, Wasser MN: Chronic splanchnic ischemia. Best Prac Res Clin Gastroenterol 15:99, 2001.
83. Heusch G, Schulz R: Remote preconditioning. J Mol Cell Cardiol 34:1279, 2002.
84. Cinel I, Avlan D, Cinel L, et al: Ischemic preconditioning reduces intestinal apoptosis in rats. Shock 19:588, 2003.
85. Asoyek S, Cinel I, Avlan D, et al: Intestinal ischemic preconditioning protects the intestine and reduces bacterial translocation. Shock 18:476, 2002.
86. Poole JW, Sammartano RJ, Boley SJ: Hemodynamic basis of the pain of chronic mesenteric ischemia. Am J Surg 153:171, 1987.

chapter 26

Clinical Evaluation

Everett Y. Lam
Gregory L. Moneta

The clinical evaluation of possible mesenteric ischemia begins with a careful history and physical examination and, above all, an appropriate index of suspicion for the diagnosis. The major etiologies of mesenteric ischemia include mesenteric venous thrombosis, acute mesenteric ischemia, nonocclusive mesenteric ischemia, and chronic mesenteric ischemia. These differ in their underlying pathologies and in the clinical settings in which they occur; however, there may be significant overlap in their clinical presentation. The most crucial point is to understand the variety of clinical settings in which intestinal ischemia can occur and to include mesenteric ischemia in the differential diagnosis of patients presenting with abdominal pain. The goal is to achieve a diagnosis prior to the onset of bowel infarction. Without consideration of intestinal ischemia, the appropriate diagnostic evaluation is unlikely to be obtained with needless additional morbidity and mortality.

MESENTERIC VENOUS THROMBOSIS

Signs and Symptoms

Patients with mesenteric venous thrombosis present with a wide range of symptoms ranging from the asymptomatic state to the acute abdomen with peritoneal findings. Abdominal pain is the most common symptom and is present in approximately 80% of patients with documented mesenteric venous thrombosis.[1] Typically, patients present with prolonged abdominal discomfort associated with abdominal distention. With transmural bowel infarction, peritoneal findings may be present. Nausea, vomiting, and/or gastrointestinal bleeding may also be present in 20% to 30% of patients. Leukocytosis and metabolic acidosis may accompany mesenteric venous thrombosis that has resulted in bowel infarction.

Mesenteric venous thrombosis can be classified into primary or secondary thrombosis. Primary mesenteric venous thrombosis is associated with hereditary or acquired hypercoagulation disorders including factor V Leiden and deficiencies of protein C, protein S, and antithrombin III. Secondary mesenteric venous thrombosis can result from malignancy or inflammatory disorders. It is associated with trauma, cirrhosis, portal hypertension, or oral contraceptives.

Radiologic Diagnosis

Plain abdominal radiographs are usually obtained in patients with abdominal pain. Free air suggestive of a perforated viscus should be ruled out. In most patients with mesenteric venous thrombosis, plain abdominal radiographs show a nonspecific bowel gas pattern and are generally nondiagnostic.

In patients with minimal abdominal pain or who are asymptomatic, duplex ultrasonography may be used to evaluate the patency of the mesenteric veins. The examination is performed after a period of fasting and the blood flow velocities within the aorta, inferior vena cava, hepatic veins, portal vein, hepatic artery, splenic vein, and superior mesenteric vein are evaluated. Additional information that can be obtained from duplex ultrasonography include the presence or absence of ascites, recanalized umbilical vein and/or liver mass. Hepatopetal (toward the liver) or hepatofugal (away from the liver) flow within the portal vein can be determined.

Duplex ultrasonography is limited in the evaluation of the mesenteric veins when there is severe ascites, recent surgery or liver biopsy, and obesity. Occasionally, the liver is located high in the right upper quadrant and is obscured by ribs. In patients with peritoneal findings, duplex ultrasonography is difficult to perform secondary to patient discomfort and significant amounts of bowel gas.

Currently, contrast-enhanced abdominal CT scanning is the diagnostic study of choice in patients suspected of having mesenteric venous thrombosis. In addition to mesenteric venous thrombosis, CT scanning can accurately detect portal and ovarian vein thrombosis. Other suggestive findings include bowel wall thickening, pneumatosis intestinalis, or mesenteric edema. In one series, contrast-enhanced abdominal CT scanning was diagnostic for mesenteric venous thrombosis in 90% of patients.[1]

Arterioportography is indicated when associated arterial ischemia is suspected or when findings on abdominal CT scanning are equivocal. The mesenteric venous system cannot be directly punctured but is visualized indirectly through catheter-directed contrast injections into the superior mesenteric artery and the celiac artery followed by delayed filming (Fig. 26-1). Mesenteric venous thrombosis is demonstrated by a filling defect within the mesenteric veins.

ACUTE OCCLUSIVE MESENTERIC ISCHEMIA

Signs and Symptoms

Acute occlusive mesenteric ischemia is caused by embolism to the superior mesenteric artery (SMA) or from acute thrombotic occlusion of the SMA with a

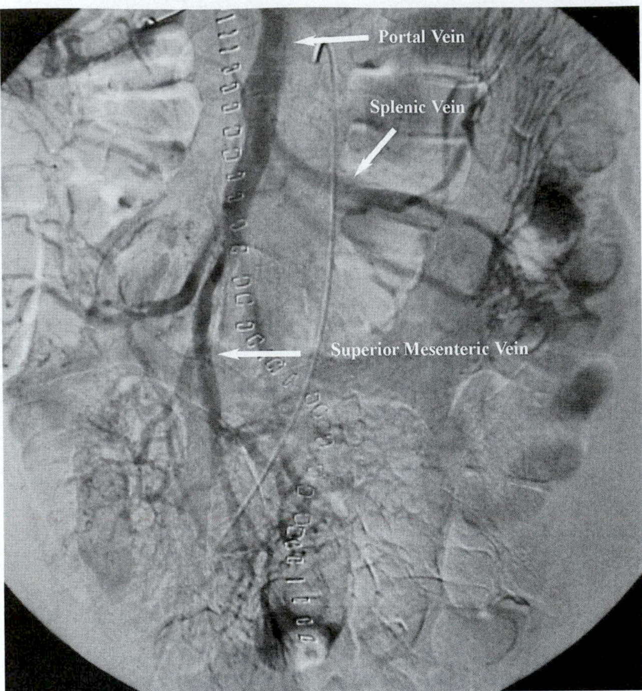

FIGURE 26-1. Aortoportography demonstrating patent portal vein, superior mesenteric vein, and splenic vein.

preexisting atherosclerotic lesion. The mortality rate exceeds 60%.[2,3] The majority of emboli to the SMA originate from the heart.

Thrombotic occlusion of the SMA carries a worse prognosis than embolism to the SMA. In thrombotic occlusion, the SMA occludes proximal to the middle colic artery and interrupts arterial flow to the entire small intestine. Emboli typically lodge in the SMA distal to the origin of the middle colic artery and some perfusion to the small intestine is maintained via the middle colic and jejunal artery branches.

Abdominal pain is the most common presenting symptom in patients with occlusive acute mesenteric ischemia and physical findings can range from nonspecific tenderness to an acute abdomen. Distention, rigidity, and rebound tenderness occur particularly when the diagnosis of acute mesenteric ischemia is delayed. The classic presentation is one of sudden onset of acute abdominal pain out of proportion to the physical findings. This reflects profound intestinal ischemia without associated bowel perforation and peritonitis. Vomiting, fever, and diarrhea are present in one third of patients with acute mesenteric ischemia. Patients with embolism tend to have a more acute presentation of abdominal pain, whereas patients with thrombosis of a stenotic SMA may have a more delayed presentation.[4]

Laboratory values are typically nonspecific. The majority of patients will have a moderate-to-marked leukocytosis. However, approximately 10% of patients will have a normal WBC count. Elevated serum amylase and metabolic acidosis may occur in patients with necrotic bowel.

Radiologic Diagnosis

Noninvasive imaging modalities have a limited role in the diagnosis of acute occlusive mesenteric ischemia. Duplex ultrasonography in the setting of an acute abdomen is limited by abdominal distention, excessive bowel gas, and patient discomfort.

An abdominal CT scan is often obtained during an evaluation of a patient with abdominal pain. In addition to other abdominal pathologies causing abdominal pain, CT scanning can detect late findings of acute mesenteric ischemia including bowel luminal dilation, bowel wall thickening, submucosal edema or hemorrhage, pneumatosis intestinalis, and portal venous gas with a sensitivity of 90%.[5] These findings are associated with some degree of intestinal infarction. Emboli tend to lodge distally and, thus, the sensitivity of CT scanning in detecting mesenteric arterial embolic occlusion is low and ranges from 37% to 80% (Fig. 26-2).[6,7] In patients with early ischemia, there may be minimal findings on CT scanning and these patients have the most benefit from early diagnosis and definitive mesenteric revascularization before the onset of intestinal infarction.

Mesenteric angiography remains the standard for the diagnosis of acute mesenteric ischemia. However, the use of mesenteric angiography is predicated on clinical judgment. In a patient with obvious peritoneal findings and signs of frankly necrotic bowel, such as hypotension and acidosis, an urgent exploratory laparotomy is required to resect necrotic bowel and perform revascularization. The preparation and performance of a mesenteric angiogram may delay definitive operative treatment and increase mortality.

In patients without peritoneal findings but who are clinically suspected to have mesenteric ischemia, angiography can be performed to make the definitive diagnosis and to plan operative therapy. Angiographically, an abrupt occlusion of the SMA distal to the origin of the middle colic artery is typically seen in patients with an embolus (Figs. 26-3, 26-4, and 26-5). In patients with thrombotic occlusion of a chronically stenotic SMA, the artery is occluded beginning at its origin at the aorta.

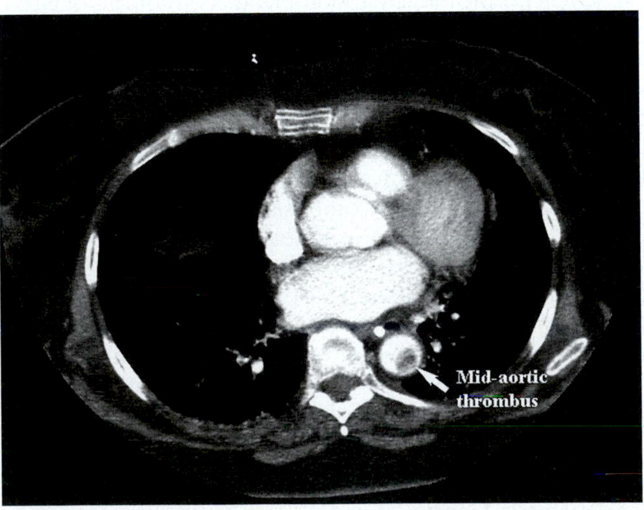

FIGURE 26-2. Axial CT scan demonstrating a mid-aortic thrombus that caused embolic occlusion of the superior mesenteric artery.

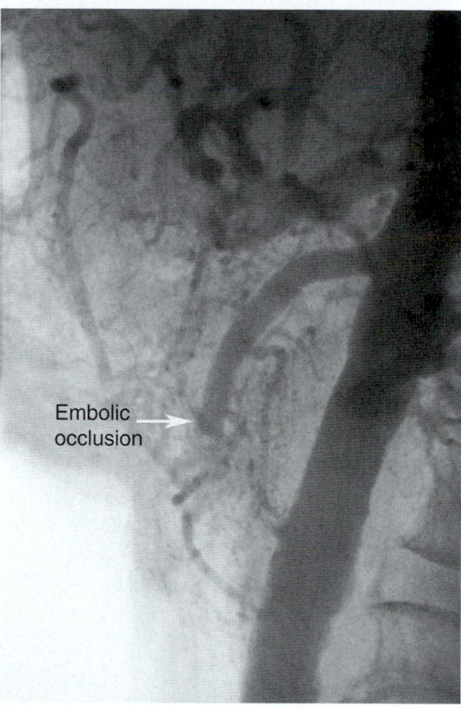

FIGURE 26-3. Lateral aortogram demonstrating abrupt embolic occlusion of the superior mesenteric artery.

ACUTE NONOCCLUSIVE MESENTERIC ISCHEMIA

Signs and Symptoms

Acute nonocclusive mesenteric ischemia (NOMI) occurs as a result of severe and prolonged mesenteric arterial vasospasm without evidence of arterial or venous obstruction. Twenty percent of patients with acute mesenteric ischemia have NOMI and mortality rates between 30% and 90% have been reported.[8] Patients with NOMI are often critically ill with decreased cardiac output and episodes of hypotension. They also tend to have significant comorbidities that can result in decreased intestinal perfusion. Early definitive diagnosis and treatment are essential for patient survival.

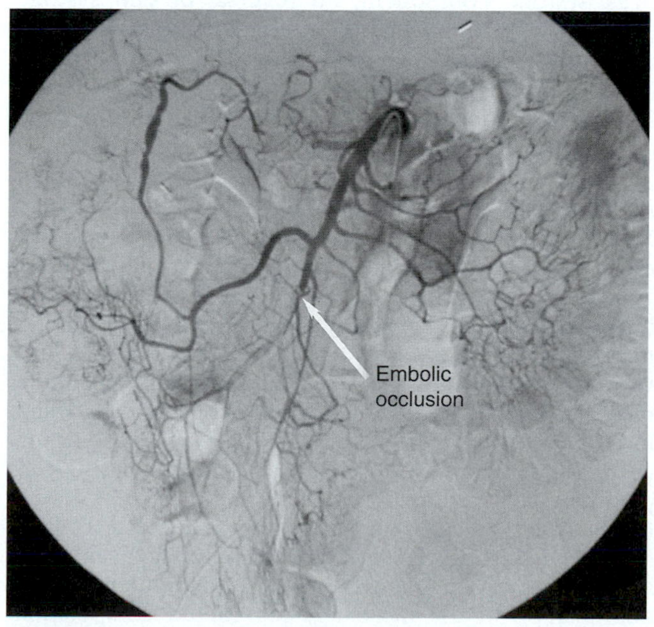

FIGURE 26-4. Anteroposterior angiogram of the superior mesenteric artery (SMA) demonstrating embolic occlusion of the distal SMA.

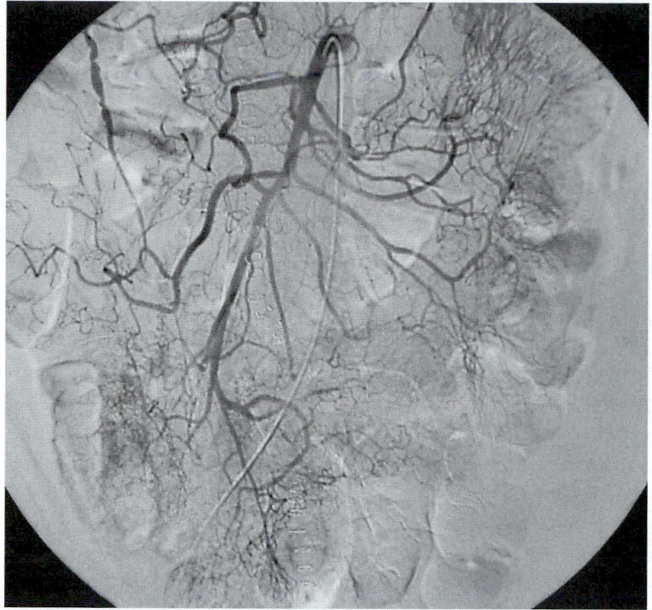

FIGURE 26-5. Anteroposterior angiogram of the superior mesenteric artery (SMA) after operative embolectomy demonstrating filling of the distal SMA.

The recognition of factors that are associated with NOMI is critical in the prompt diagnosis of NOMI. These factors include acute myocardial infarction, congestive heart failure, valvular heart disease, aortic dissection, cardiopulmonary bypass, renal failure requiring hemodialysis, and pharmacologic agents such as vasopressors and digitalis.[9-15] Digitalis can cause NOMI by altering mesenteric vaso-reactivity such that mesenteric arteriolar vasoconstriction increases with increases in portal venous pressure.

Findings on physical examination are varied and do not confirm the diagnosis of NOMI. Abdominal pain may be present and can vary widely in character, location, and intensity. Abdominal pain is absent in 20% to 25% of patients with NOMI.[10] Abdominal distention with occult or frank gastrointestinal bleeding may be present. As in occlusive acute mesenteric ischemia, laboratory values are nonspecific.

Radiologic Diagnosis

The radiologic evaluation of patients with NOMI is similar to that of patients with occlusive acute mesenteric ischemia. Plain abdominal films are obtained to rule out a perforated viscus. If technically feasible, duplex ultrasonography may detect persistent flow in the mesenteric arteries and exclude occlusive disease.

Patients suspected to have NOMI should undergo urgent mesenteric angiography to confirm the diagnosis because of the significant mortality associated with a delayed diagnosis. Images in the anterior-posterior and lateral planes are obtained. Findings of NOMI include patent mesenteric arterial trunks with tapered or spastic narrowing of visceral artery branches and impaired filling of intramural vessels.[10]

CHRONIC MESENTERIC ISCHEMIA

Signs and Symptoms

Patients with chronic mesenteric ischemia (CMI) are typically females (3:1 female to male ratio) between the ages of 40 and 70 years. A history of recurrent abdominal pain is the most critical factor in the diagnosis of CMI. The pain associated with CMI is mid-abdominal or epigastric in origin and is described as colicky or as a dull, intense ache that may radiate to the back. The pain is postprandial and generally begins 15 to 30 minutes after eating and lasts up to four hours. There are no signs of peritonitis and the degree of pain may be proportional to the volume of the ingested meal.

Patients may ingest some meals without pain early on in the course of CMI. Therefore, the pain may initially be attributed to cholelithiasis, peptic ulcer disease, or malignancy and patients often undergo an extensive evaluation including endoscopy, computed tomography, barium studies, and abdominal ultrasonography prior to reaching a diagnosis of CMI. As the disease progresses, patients begin to experience pain with each meal and may develop a fear of food. Weight loss, the hallmark of CMI, results from limited nutritional intake, not malabsorption. Therefore, patients with CMI will have normal tests of malabsorption.

Radiologic Diagnosis

Mesenteric Angiography

Contrast mesenteric angiography is the standard study to diagnose CMI. Radiographs are obtained in the lateral and anterior-posterior projections. Findings on angiography suggestive of CMI include stenosis or occlusion of the celiac artery (CA) and/or the SMA (Fig. 26-6). When the origins of the CA or SMA are occluded, the more distal vessels are often patent through filling by enlarged and easily visualized pancreaticoduodenal arterial collaterals. Not all patients, however, with mesenteric artery obstruction have mesenteric insufficiency. It is important to differentiate high-grade mesenteric artery stenosis from the clinical entity of CMI.

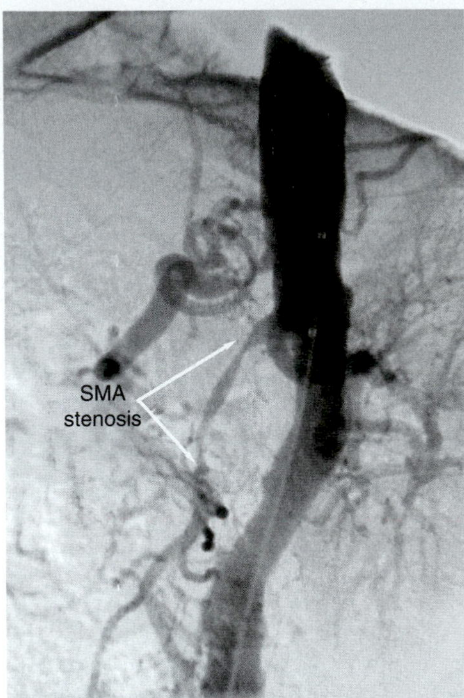

FIGURE 26-6. Lateral aortogram demonstrating long-segment stenosis of the superior mesenteric artery (SMA).

Duplex Ultrasonography

Duplex ultrasonography can serve as a valuable noninvasive screening test for splanchnic artery stenosis and for follow-up in patients with mesenteric artery reconstructions. Despite the accuracy of duplex detection of mesenteric artery stenoses, angiographic confirmation of high-grade stenoses or occlusion of the splanchnic vessels and appropriate history and physical examination are still required for the diagnosis of CMI. Duplex examination is technically difficult and should be performed by vascular technologists with extensive experience in intra-abdominal ultrasound techniques.

In healthy individuals, fasting blood flow velocity waveforms differ between the SMA and the CA. Arterial waveforms reflect end-organ vascular resistance. The liver and spleen have relatively high constant metabolic requirements and are, therefore, low-resistance organs. As a result, CA waveforms are generally biphasic, with a peak systolic component, no reversal of end systolic flow, and a relatively high EDV. The normal fasting SMA velocity waveform is triphasic, reflecting the high vascular resistance of the intestinal tract at rest. There is a peak systolic component, often an end-systolic reverse flow component, and a minimal diastolic flow component.

Changes in Doppler-derived arterial waveforms in response to feeding are also different in the CA and SMA. Because the liver and spleen basically have fixed metabolic demands, there is no significant change in CA velocity waveform after eating. Blood flow in the SMA, however, increases markedly after a meal—reflecting a marked decrease in intestinal arterial resistance. The waveform changes in the SMA postprandially include a near doubling of systolic velocity, tripling of the EDV, and loss of end-systolic reversal of blood flow. In addition, there is a detectable increase in the diameter of the SMA postprandially. The diameter of the SMA has been shown to be 0.60 ± 0.09 cm in the fasting state and 0.67 ± 0.09 cm after a meal. These changes are maximal at 45 minutes after ingestion of a test meal[16] and are dependent on the composition of the meal ingested. Mixed composition meals produce the greatest flow increase in the SMA when compared with equal caloric meals composed solely of fat, glucose, or protein.[17]

Detection of Splanchnic Arterial Stenosis

Duplex ultrasound can detect hemodynamically significant stenoses in splanchnic vessels. In 1986, investigators at the University of Washington found that flow velocities in stenotic SMA and CA were significantly increased when compared with normal SMA and CA.[18] Quantitative criteria for splanchnic artery stenosis were first developed and validated at Oregon Health & Science University.[19]

In a blinded prospective study of 100 patients who underwent mesenteric artery duplex scanning and lateral aortography, a peak systolic velocity (PSV) in the SMA of 275 cm/sec or more indicated a greater than or equal to 70% SMA stenosis with a sensitivity of 92%, a specificity of 96%, a positive-predictive value of 80%, and a negative-predictive value of 99% and an accuracy of 96% (Fig. 26-7).[20] In the same study, a PSV of greater than or equal to 200 cm/sec identified a greater than or equal to 70% angiographic celiac artery stenosis with a sensitivity of 87%, a specificity of 80%, a positive-predictive value of 63%, a negative-predictive value of 94%, and an accuracy of 82%.

Other duplex criteria for mesenteric artery stenoses are also in use. An SMA end-diastolic velocity (EDV) greater than 45 cm/sec correlates with a greater than or equal to 50% SMA stenosis with a specificity of 92% and a sensitivity of 100%; whereas a CA EDV of 55 cm/sec or greater predicts a greater than or equal to 50% CA stenosis with a sensitivity of 93%, specificity of 100%, and accuracy of 95%.[21,22]

Postprandial mesenteric duplex scanning may be as an adjunct to the diagnosis of mesenteric stenosis.[23] In patients with less than 70% SMA stenosis, the postprandial SMA PSV increases more than 20% over baseline. The percent increase in SMA PSV is less in patients with greater than or equal to 70% SMA stenosis. The specificity for the combination of fasting SMA PSVs and postprandial PSVs, however, is marginally improved over that provided by a fasting duplex scan alone. Therefore, although theoretically attractive, postprandial duplex scanning offers no significant improvement over fasting mesenteric duplex scanning and does not need to be routinely used as part of the ultrasound assessment of mesenteric artery stenosis. Postprandial examinations are, however, occasionally useful, in that if there is a postprandial response, the insonated vessel can be confirmed as being the SMA.

Duplex ultrasonography is best used as an initial screening study to evaluate for visceral artery stenosis in patients with chronic abdominal pain that may be consistent with CMI. Angiography is required to establish a definitive diagnosis.

Computed Tomography

Standard CT imaging is of limited value in the evaluation of mesenteric artery stenosis. Currently, no studies have compared the accuracy of spiral CT with angiography in the determination of visceral artery stenoses. CT angiography can detect proximal stenosis of the celiac and superior mesenteric arteries but is limited by lower resolution and bowel motion in its ability to detect lesions involving more distal branches.[24] CT scans are often obtained in the evaluation of patients with abdominal pain. Findings suggestive of mesenteric artery stenosis include calcification at the origin of the CA and SMA and lack of contrast enhancement within the vessel lumen (Fig. 26-8).

Magnetic Resonance Imaging

The development of fast breath-hold 3-D gadolinium-enhanced magnetic resonance angiography (Gd-enhanced MRA) has improved the ability of MRA to detect proximal splanchnic artery lesions. MRA is limited in its ability to image more distal visceral branches because of limited

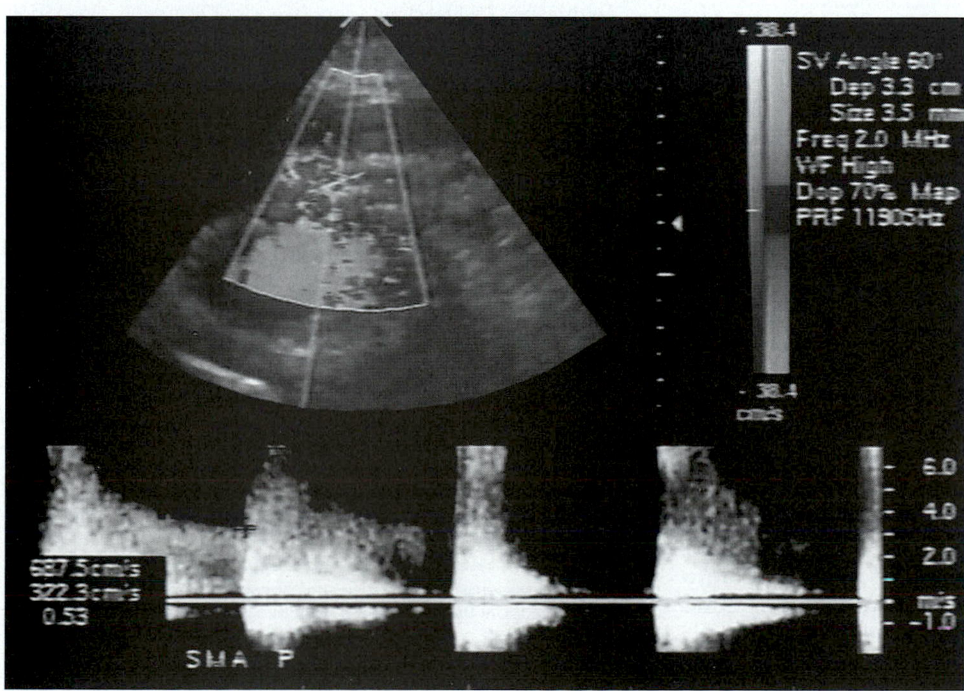

FIGURE 26-7. (See also Color Plate 26-7.) Duplex ultrasonography of the superior mesenteric artery (SMA) with a peak systolic velocity of 687 cm/sec signifying ≥ 70% stenosis of the SMA.

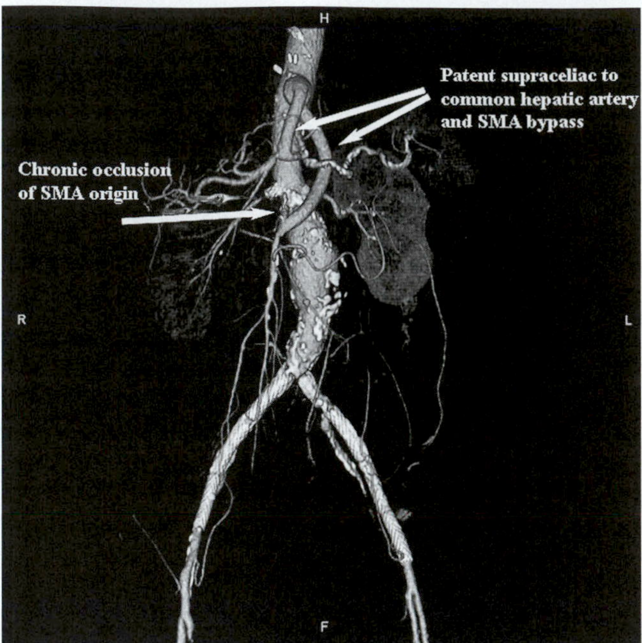

FIGURE 26-8. (See also Color Plate 26-8.) CT angiogram demonstrating a patent supraceliac aorta to common hepatic artery and superior mesenteric artery (SMA) bypass. The proximal SMA is occluded.

spatial resolution, peristaltic and respiratory motion, and chemical shift changes between the vessels and fat.[25] In a study by Meaney and colleagues,[26] the accuracy of 3-D Gd-enhanced MRA in detecting visceral artery stenosis in 14 patients suspected of having CMI was compared with that of contrast angiography or surgery. The celiac and superior mesenteric arteries were identified in all patients, whereas the inferior mesenteric artery was reliably detected in only 9 of 14 patients. The overall sensitivity and specificity for detecting greater than 75% stenosis or occlusion of the celiac, superior mesenteric, or inferior mesenteric arteries were 100% and 95%, respectively.

In addition to providing anatomic details, MR technology can quantify arterial flow using the phase-contrast MRI technique. This technique provides information about the presence, magnitude, and direction of blood flow and has been studied in patients with CMI.[27,28] In a study by Dalman and colleagues,[28] the fasting and postprandial flow in the SMA were compared in patients with documented atherosclerotic disease and normal volunteers. Mean fasting SMA fasting blood flow was higher in atherosclerotic patients than in volunteers. Postprandial hyperemia was reduced in patients with visceral stenoses, as determined by the mean percentage increase in superior mesenteric vein blood flow (270% in volunteers versus 70% in asymptomatic patients with visceral stenoses and 29% in symptomatic patients with visceral stenoses). Further validation studies correlating the degree of change in mesenteric blood flow with angiographic percentage stenosis will be needed before universal adoption of phase-contrast MRI as a routine noninvasive diagnostic method in patients with CMI.

REFERENCES

1. Morasch MD, Ebaugh JL, Chiou AC, et al: Mesenteric venous thrombosis: A changing clinical entity. J Vasc Surg 34:680, 2001.
2. Char DJ, Cuadra SA, Hines GL, et al: Surgical intervention for acute intestinal ischemia: Experience in a community teaching hospital. Vasc Endovasc Surg 37:245, 2003.
3. McKinsey JF, Gewertz BL: Acute mesenteric ischemia. Surg Clin North Am 77:307, 1997.
4. Eldrup-Jorgensen J, Hawkins R, Bredenberg C: Abdominal emergencies: Has anything changed? Surg Clin North Am 77:1306, 1997.
5. Sreenarasimhaiah J: Diagnosis and management of intestinal ischemic disorders. BMJ 326:1372, 2003.
6. Taourel PG, Deneuville M, Pradel JA, et al: Acute mesenteric ischemia: Diagnosis with contrast-enhanced CT. Radiology 199:632, 1996.
7. Klein HS, Lensing R, Klosterhalfen B, et al: Diagnostic imaging of mesenteric infarction. Rad 197:79, 1995.
8. Klotz S, Vestring T, Rotker J, et al: Diagnosis and treatment of nonocclusive mesenteric ischemia after open heart surgery. Ann Thor Surg 72:1583, 2001.
9. Diamond S, Emmett M, Henrich W: Bowel infarction as a cause of death in dialysis patients. JAMA 256:2545, 1986.
10. Bassiouny H: Nonocclusive mesenteric ischemia. Surg Clin North Am 77:319, 1997.
11. Valentine R, Whelan T, Meyers H: Non-occlusive mesenteric ischemia in renal patients: Recognition and prevention of intestinal gangrene. Am J Kidney Dis 15:598, 1990.
12. Zeier M, Weisel M, Ritz E. Non-occlusive mesenteric infarction in dialysis patients: Risk factors, diagnosis, intervention and outcome. Int J Art Org 15:387, 1992.
13. Niederhauser U, Genoni M, von Segesser LK, et al: Mesenteric ischemia after a cardiac operation: Conservative treatment with local vasodilatation. Ann Thor Surg 61:1817, 1996.
14. John A, Tuerff S, Kerstein M: Nonocclusive mesenteric infarction in hemodialysis patients. J Am Coll Surg 190:84, 2000.
15. Neri E, Sassi C, Masetti M, et al: Nonocclusive intestinal ischemia in patients with acute aortic dissection. J Vasc Surg 36:738, 2002.
16. Jager K, Bollinger A, Valli C, et al: Measurement of mesenteric blood flow by duplex scanning. J Vasc Surg 3:462, 1986.
17. Moneta GL, Taylor DC, Helton WS, et al: Duplex ultrasound measurement of postprandial intestinal blood flow: Effect of meal composition. Gastroenterology 95:1294, 1988.
18. Nicholls SC, Kohler TR, Martin RL, et al: Use of hemodynamic parameters in the diagnosis of mesenteric insufficiency. J Vasc Surg 3:507, 1986.
19. Moneta GL, Yeager RA, Dalman R, et al: Duplex ultrasound criteria for diagnosis of splanchnic artery stenosis or occlusion. J Vasc Surg 14:511, 1991.
20. Moneta GL, Lee RW, Yeager RA, et al: Mesenteric duplex scanning: A blinded prospective study. J Vasc Surg 17:79, 1993.
21. Bowersox JC, Zwolak RM, Walsh DB, et al: Duplex ultrasonography in the diagnosis of celiac and mesenteric artery occlusive disease. J Vasc Surg 14:780, 1991.
22. Zwolak RM, Fillinger MF, Walsh DB, et al: Mesenteric and celiac duplex scanning: A validation study. J Vasc Surg 27:1078, 1998.
23. Gentile AT, Moneta GL, Lee RW, et al: Usefulness of fasting and postprandial duplex ultrasound examinations for predicting high-grade superior mesenteric artery stenosis. Am J Surg 169:476, 1995.
24. Rubin GD, Walker PJ, Dake MD, et al: Three-dimensional spiral computed tomographic angiography: An alternative imaging modality for the abdominal aorta and its branches. J Vasc Surg 18:656, 1993.
25. Meaney JF. Non-invasive evaluation of the visceral arteries with magnetic resonance angiography. Eur Radiol 9:1267, 1999.
26. Meaney JF, Prince MR, Nostrant TT, et al: Gadolinium-enhanced MR angiography of visceral arteries in patients with suspected chronic mesenteric ischemia. J Magn Reson Imaging 7:171, 1997.
27. Li KC, Whitney WS, McDonnell CH, et al: Chronic mesenteric ischemia: Evaluation with phase-contrast cine MR imaging. Radiology190:175, 1994.
28. Dalman RL, Li KC, Moon WK, et al: Diminished postprandial hyperemia in patients with aortic and mesenteric occlusive disease: Quantification by magnetic resonance flow imaging. Circulation 94:II206, 1996.

■ ■ ■ chapter 27

Treatment

Mary E. Giswold
Gregory L. Moneta

With a few exceptions, as noted subsequently, surgery of some sort remains an integral part of the treatment of all etiologies of mesenteric ischemia.

CHRONIC AND ACUTE MESENTERIC OCCLUSIVE DISEASE

Because of the relatively few mesenteric revascularization procedures performed, the available literature includes no randomized or controlled clinical trials of surgical intervention. The published clinical reports include varied recommendations for treatment; and many do not include descriptions of operative methods. Others describe technically demanding procedures requiring extensive dissections in difficult areas.[1,2] Only recently has objective determination of postoperative graft patency been included in clinical series.[3-6] For all these reasons there is no current consensus regarding the surgical details of treatment for intestinal ischemia.

History

In 1936, Dunphy reviewed the medical records of twelve patients dying from intestinal ischemia and discovered that more than half (58%) had evidence of chronic abdominal pain.[7] This finding suggested that timely surgical intervention may have prevented progression to intestinal infarction and death. In 1957, Mikkelsen described the arteriographic appearance of the typical orificial atherosclerotic lesions affecting the mesenteric arteries.[8] During the same year, the first successful surgical procedure (SMA [superior mesenteric artery] endarterectomy) for treatment of chronic intestinal ischemia was performed by Maynard and Shaw.[9]

Since this time, numerous techniques have been developed to revascularize the mesenteric arteries. One debated issue is the optimal number of vessels to revascularize. Proponents of multiple vessel or "complete" revascularization have worried that although single vessel bypass is effective in relieving symptoms initially, there may be a higher incidence of recurrent symptoms secondary to graft failure.

Multiple Vessel Revascularization

Multiple vessel revascularization implies repair or bypass of all diseased or occluded vessels, most often the celiac and SMA. Most agree that bypass to the inferior mesenteric artery is unnecessary for successful revascularization, except in unusual cases. Grafts can be oriented antegrade from the supraceliac aorta or retrograde from the infrarenal aorta or an iliac artery.

An early report from the Mayo Clinic first suggested that "complete" revascularization resulted in decreased symptomatic recurrence.[10] A subsequent report including these patients and others indicated that graft patency and survival in patients with three vessel revascularization were improved compared to single vessel revascularization.[11] The authors speculated that this difference in outcome was a result of complete revascularization, which theoretically provides an additional measure of safety. These two studies, however, were limited to patients with chronic intestinal ischemia and did not use objective methods to determine postoperative graft patency. In the latter study, McAfee and colleagues[11] noted symptoms of recurrent ischemia were an unreliable measure of graft patency, because two of their three early occlusions were asymptomatic. The lack of symptoms may have resulted from the presence of additional patent grafts. Although these retrospective studies suggest that complete revascularization resulted in fewer recurrences and deaths, the results were not statistically significant.

Some believe that the antegrade orientation provides better inflow than the retrograde orientation because prograde flow is less turbulent, there may be less graft kinking, and the supraceliac aorta is usually less diseased than is the infrarenal aorta or an iliac artery. In the Mayo Clinic series published in 1981, the symptomatic recurrence rate was 26%; none of these grafts was antegrade.[10] In more current studies, in which the majority of grafts are positioned antegrade, the recurrence rate is lower.[12] Clearly the reduction in recurrence is multifactorial and cannot be attributed solely to graft orientation.

More recent data suggest the rate of symptomatic recurrence is unaffected by the number of vessels revascularized or the graft orientation. In a study of 91 patients treated for chronic mesenteric ischemia (CMI) with a bypass procedure, there were patients with both single and multiple vessel reconstructions and with grafts in either orientation. Survival was unaffected by the number of vessels revascularized. Patients with retrograde grafts had decreased survival but these patients were older than those with antegrade grafts.[12]

Single Vessel Revascularization

Proponents of single vessel revascularization have reported similar long-term results to multiple vessel revascularizations. Series from France have shown SMA reconstruction alone to be a durable form of treatment for intestinal ischemia.[13,14] Kieny and colleagues[13] performed 60 direct or indirect (using a short prosthetic segment) reimplantations of the SMA (10% of patients had additional vessels reconstructed) in patients with atherosclerotic lesions of the visceral arteries. Mean follow-up was 8.5 years; five patients (8.3%) developed recurrences, and one patient died as a result. The 5-year actuarial survival was 69.6%.

Favorable results for single vessel revascularization have also been reported in the United States.[15,16] Stanton and colleagues[15] performed 20 reconstructions in 17 patients and, at 60.9 months, they found no symptomatic recurrences. One method of mesenteric revascularization is transaortic endarterectomy (TEA), with antegrade aortoceliac bypass reserved for older or poor-risk patients.[17,18] TEA usually involves revascularization of both the celiac axis and the SMA. Similar recurrence rates have been observed between the two techniques with 86% of patients in both groups being asymptomatic at 5 years. Durable relief of symptoms did not appear to correlate with the number of visceral arteries repaired.[18]

At Oregon Health & Science University, the surgical approach to managing acute and chronic mesenteric ischemia has changed in the last 2 decades.[16,19] In 1984, Baur and colleagues[19] reported a series of 23 patients who underwent complete revascularization whenever possible. Perioperative mortality was 9%. During a mean follow-up of 2 years 9.5% of patients had graft failures. Since that initial report, the operative approach has been altered based on the patient population and newly available duplex ultrasound information. In 1994, Gentile and colleagues[16] reported 26 patients who had 29 isolated bypasses to the SMA for intestinal ischemia (23 chronic, 5 acute, 1 asymptomatic). Perioperative mortality was 10%. The mean follow-up was 40 months and the life-table determined 4-year primary graft patency rate and survival rate were 89% and 82%, respectively. This compared favorably with contemporary reports in the literature.[16] Based on this experience, revascularization of the SMA alone is recommended for most cases of intestinal ischemia.

Foley and colleagues recently reported a series of 50 SMA revascularizations employing objective means to determine graft postoperative patency.[6] This series differed from others with respect to the larger number of patients with previous attempts at revascularization (24%), the higher percentage of patients presenting with acute ischemia (42%), and the higher percentage of patients requiring simultaneous bowel resection (28%). The overall perioperative mortality (12%), however, was comparable to other recent series. Perioperative mortality was 3% for patients operated on electively. The incidence of perioperative graft occlusions (6%) was similar to other recent series, only one of which contains a significant number of patients presenting with acute intestinal ischemia. Three graft occlusions occurred during long-term follow-up and resulted in death in two patients, accounting for 22% of late deaths. In this series, the number of symptomatic late graft occlusions, number of deaths attributable to recurrent ischemia, and life-table determined survival were also comparable to other recent series employing more complete visceral revascularizations (Table 27-1). Mateo and colleagues[5] found significantly increased perioperative morbidity (including death) in patients who underwent complete revascularization for treatment of intestinal ischemia.

Although acute mesenteric ischemia is accompanied by a higher perioperative mortality rate, McMillan and colleagues[20] found no differences in long-term patency of bypass grafts between patients with acute or chronic ischemia. Two of the three late occlusions in this series occurred in patients whose initial graft was placed for chronic mesenteric ischemia; however, one of these occluded in the perioperative period and was replaced. Revascularization of the SMA alone continues to compare favorably with more complete mesenteric revascularizations.

Several authors have noted that symptoms are an insensitive measure of graft failure.[11,20] With improvements in duplex scanning, several studies have objective data for long-term graft patency.[21]

Indications for Operation

Revascularization is clearly indicated for symptomatic intestinal ischemia. Revascularization for asymptomatic high-grade SMA obstruction is recommended only in patients undergoing otherwise indicated aortic surgery for aneurysmal or occlusive disease. In this group of

TABLE 27-1 RECENT MESENTERIC REVASCULARIZATION OUTCOMES

Author	Patients (% Acute)	Perioperative Mortality (%)	Perioperative Occlusions (%)	Late Occlusions[a]	% Late Deaths from Ischemia	5 Yr. Survival[b] (%)
Foley 2000[6]	50 (42)	12	6	3	22	61
Mateo 1999[5d]	85(0)	8	3.5	16	21	64
Kihara 1999[4d]	42(0)	10	0	4	33	70
Moawad 1997[3d]	24(0)	4	4	2	25	71
McMillan 1995[20d]	25(36)	12	4	0	0	N/A[c]

[a]Symptomatic recurrences.
[b]Life-table determined.
[c]Not available.
[d]Included multiple vessel revascularizations.
From Foley MI, Moneta GL, Abou-Zamzam AM, et al: Revascularization of the superior mesenteric artery alone for treatment of intestinal ischemia. J Vasc Surg 32:37, 2000.

patients, acute intestinal ischemia following aortic surgery has been well documented, and SMA reconstruction seems prudent.[22]

Techniques of Superior Mesenteric Artery Bypass

Retrograde Grafting

The distal infrarenal aorta as an origin for an SMA bypass graft has advantages and disadvantages. This exposure is familiar and the risks of dissection and clamping are less than with more proximal aortic exposures. In addition, the procedure can be readily combined with other intra-abdominal vascular procedures. The primary disadvantage is that the infrarenal aorta and iliac arteries are frequently calcified, increasing the technical difficulty of the proximal anastomosis.

Prosthetic grafts are used most often in cases of mesenteric revascularization. The exceptions are cases complicated by bowel necrosis. For these patients, vein grafts are preferred to minimize the possibility of graft infection. Special attention to graft configuration must be paid to avoid graft kinking when the graft is placed in a retrograde configuration. A preference for the origin of the graft is from the area of the junction of the aorta and the right common iliac artery, although any suitable site on the infrarenal aorta or either common iliac artery is satisfactory. A single limb is cut from a bifurcation graft in the manner described by Wylie and colleagues which provides a "flange" for sewing and prevents anastomotic stricture[23] (Fig. 27-1). The ligament of Treitz is dissected. The proximal (inflow) anastomosis is completed first. The graft is then arranged, first cephalad, then turning anteriorly and inferiorly a full 180 degrees to terminate in an antegrade anastomosis to the anterior wall of the SMA—just beyond the inferior border of the pancreas (Fig. 27-2). The graft is excluded from the peritoneal cavity by closing the mesenteric peritoneum, reapproximating the ligament of Treitz, and closing the posterior parietal peritoneum.

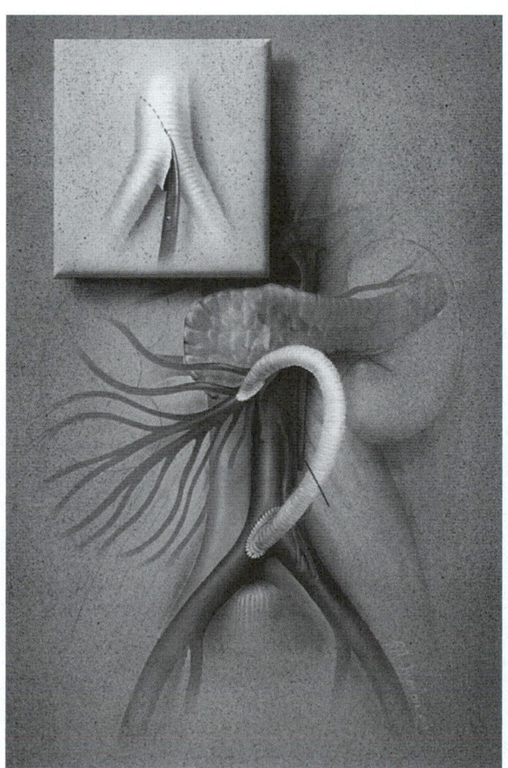

FIGURE 27-1. (See also Color Plate 27-1.) Artist's depiction of the technique of infrarenal aorta to superior mesenteric artery bypass. The graft is fashioned using one limb of a bifurcated graft.

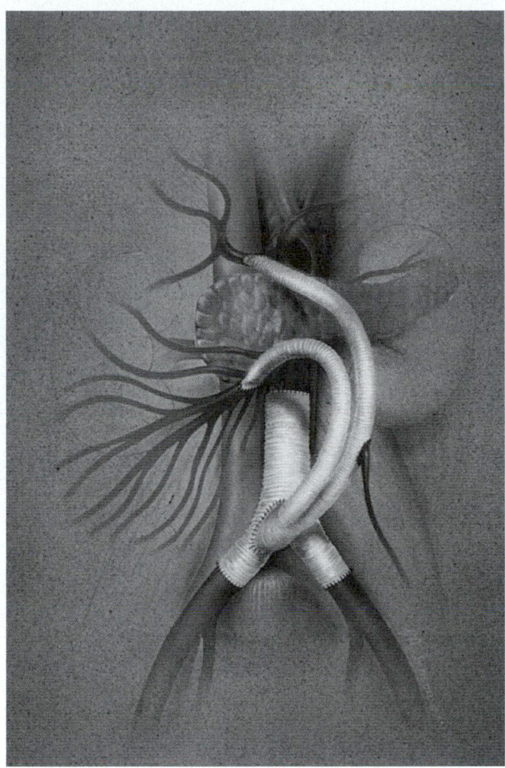

FIGURE 27-2. (See also Color Plate 27-2.) Artist's depiction of a retrograde mesenteric bypass to the celiac and superior mesenteric artery with reimplantation of the inferior mesenteric artery.

Antegrade Bypass

Antegrade bypasses originate from the anterior surface of the aorta proximal to the celiac artery. The proximal aorta is exposed through the upper midline (Fig. 27-3) or, when the intra-abdominal supraceliac aorta is calcified, using a low thoracoabdominal incision. Antegrade bypass provides prograde flow to the mesenteric vessels and is clearly the preferred approach in patients with contraindications to the use of the infrarenal aorta or an iliac artery as a bypass origin. Visceral bypass grafts can be constructed to many supraceliac aortas with partial-occlusion clamping of the aorta, although in most cases the "partial" occlusion is near total occlusion. Transient hepatic and renal ischemia is usually well tolerated but is a potential disadvantage to the antegrade approach. To minimize the risk associated with supraceliac aortic surgery, the procedure should be reserved for patients in whom this arterial segment is angiographically normal. Significantly diseased supraceliac aortas are dangerous origins for a visceral artery bypass.[23]

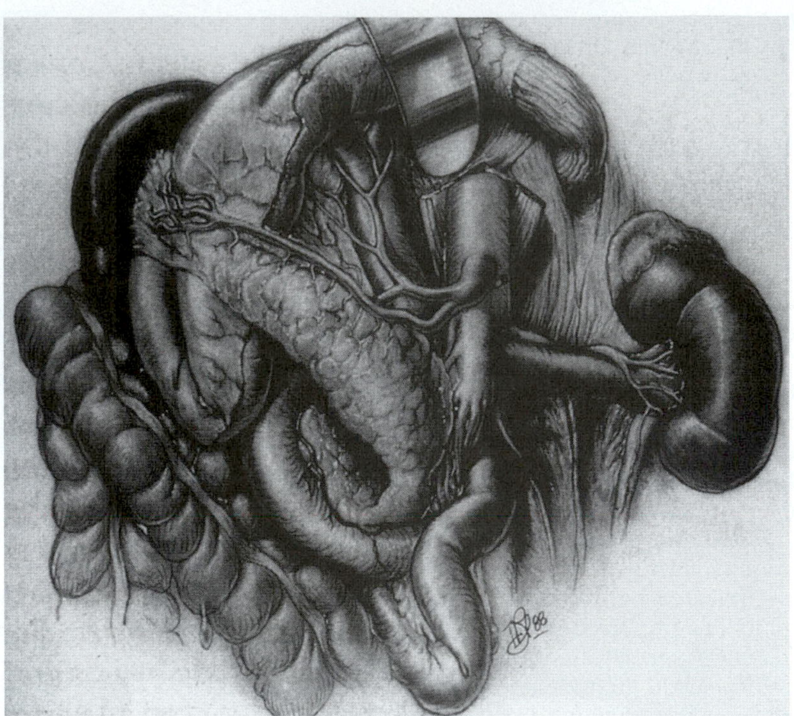

FIGURE 27-3. Artist's depiction of the exposure of the supraceliac aorta.

Antegrade grafts to the SMA are normally tunneled behind the pancreas and anastomosed to the anterior wall of the SMA in end-to-side fashion (Fig. 27-4). A disadvantage of antegrade bypass is that the retropancreatic space is limited and great care is necessary with tunneling the graft. Some surgeons advocate prepancreatic tunneling to avoid compression of the graft within the tunnel.[24] A prepancreatic tunnel, however, places the graft in opposition to the posterior wall of the stomach and theoretically increases the possibility of graft infection. Occasionally, in the setting of very focal SMA origin disease and an easily mobilized pancreas, the antegrade bypass can be constructed entirely superior to the pancreas, obviating the need for a retropancreatic tunnel.

Postoperative Monitoring of Graft Patency

The authors use sterilized Doppler probes to confirm normal flow signals in visceral artery bypass grafts and in the native mesenteric arteries distal to the anastomotic sites after graft completion. Arterial Doppler signals should be easily detected on the antimesenteric border of the revascularized bowel as well. It is important to repeat Doppler insonation after all packs and retractors have been removed and after the viscera have been returned to the peritoneum. This approach helps minimize technical failures from graft kinking.

In contrast to the situation with other vascular repairs, continuous monitoring of the patency of visceral artery repairs is impossible in the postoperative period. Postoperative graft thrombosis may be asymptomatic or confused with other causes of postoperative pain. When symptoms do occur with resumption of oral intake, reoperation may be difficult or impossible because of postoperative inflammatory scarring. Thus, routine imaging of the reconstruction 5 to 7 days postoperatively to confirm visceral revascularization patency is prudent (Figs. 27-5 and 27-6). If the graft is occluded or otherwise unsatisfactory, reoperation is mandatory.

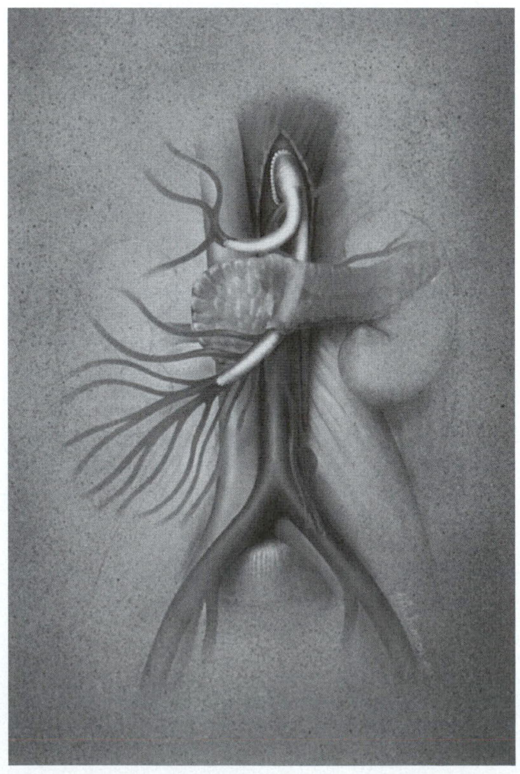

FIGURE 27-4. (See also Color Plate 27-4.) Artist's depiction of the technique of antegrade bypass from the supraceliac aorta to the celiac and superior mesenteric arteries.

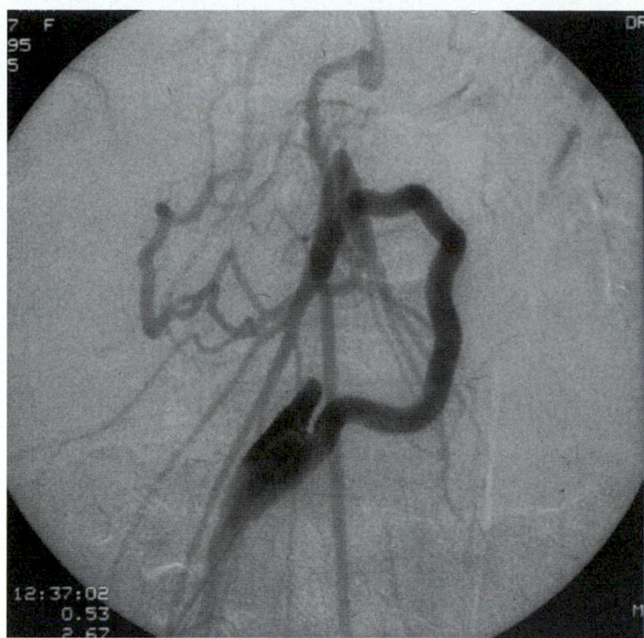

FIGURE 27-5. Postoperative arteriogram showing patent prosthetic graft from the iliac artery to the superior mesenteric artery.

Postoperative Care

Patients with chronic visceral ischemia often have significant ischemic bowel injury, which requires time for recovery. "Food fear" resulting from preoperative postprandial pain may persist at least temporarily. Prolonged periods of inability to achieve adequate oral nutrition are frequent following visceral revascularization. For this reason, total parenteral nutrition is used liberally.

Some patients with severe preoperative ischemia develop postoperative "revascularization syndrome." This syndrome consists of abdominal pain, tachycardia, leukocytosis and intestinal edema. It has been attributed to intestinal vasospasm after revascularization.[25] Any departure from a normal postoperative course should prompt arteriography, re-exploration, or both. Delayed diagnosis of graft occlusion or intestinal necrosis is usually fatal.

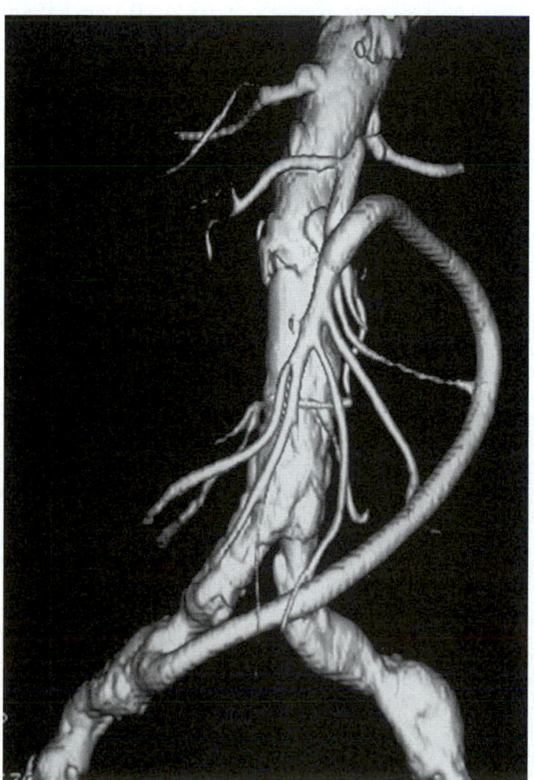

FIGURE 27-6. Postoperative CT angiogram of a patent prosthetic graft from the iliac artery to the superior mesenteric artery.

Endovascular Therapy for Mesenteric Occlusive Disease

Catheter-based therapy is becoming an accepted method for the treatment of mesenteric occlusive disease. The initial published series reported immediate technical success with endovascular therapy. The long-term success rates, however, were disappointing and inferior to open surgery.[26-28] The mortality and complication rates in these studies range from 0% to 6% and 0% to 32%, respectively. In a recent study by Sharafuddin and colleagues, 25 patients underwent angioplasty and stenting of the superior mesenteric or celiac artery.[29] Primary patency determined by ultrasound was 92% at 6 months. These series have established that endovascular treatment of mesenteric artery stenosis is technically feasible, but there are no data available with respect to long-term durability. At this point, catheter-based therapy for mesenteric occlusive disease is best reserved for patients with a limited life expectancy or significant medical comorbidities prohibiting surgery.

Summary

Symptomatic mesenteric ischemia remains uncommon. Recognition and treatment of the syndrome of chronic mesenteric ischemia may avoid progression to acute ischemia, alleviate symptoms, and provide durable long-term relief. This may be accomplished by a number of techniques. Single vessel bypass to the SMA compares favorably in terms of graft patency, death from recurrent ischemia, and survival to recent reports of intestinal revascularizations employing bypasses to multiple arteries.

With the small numbers of patients in previously published series, as well as differences in patient selection, it has been difficult to demonstrate a significant benefit of one technique over others. The technical issues involved in mesenteric revascularization are basic vascular surgical principles: choice of proximal anastomosis, distal target, and conduit. It is largely accepted that prosthetic grafts are effective for mesenteric revascularization. However, there has been considerable debate surrounding the choice of inflow vessel, the number of vessels revascularized, and the orientation of the graft. Surgeons should choose a revascularization procedure for chronic mesenteric ischemia that fits the patient. It is not necessary to rigidly adhere to a single approach. If operation is well planned and technically well performed, excellent results can be expected.

MESENTERIC VENOUS THROMBOSIS

Acute mesenteric ischemia occurs in 5% to 15% of patients as a result of mesenteric venous thrombosis (MVT).[30,31] Patients with MVT often have swelling of the intestine and have reduced intravascular volume. In addition to urgent anticoagulation, they often need fluid resuscitation. Ileus is present and bowel rest with insertion of a nasogastric tube is required.

Urgent laparotomy is undertaken in patients with peritoneal findings. Perioperative broad-spectrum antibiotics are administered. Findings at laparotomy consist of edema and cyanotic discoloration of the mesentery and bowel wall, with thrombus involving the distal mesenteric veins. Complete thrombosis of the superior mesenteric vein is rare, occurring in only 12% of patients undergoing laparotomy for suspected mesenteric vein thrombosis.[32] The arterial supply to the involved bowel is usually intact. Nonviable bowel is resected and primary anastomosis performed. If the viability of the remaining bowel is in question, a repeat, "second look," operation is performed in 24 to 48 hours. Thrombolytic therapy or surgical thrombectomy of mesenteric veins is not required; these interventions usually are not successful technically.

In patients without peritoneal findings, anticoagulation with intravenous unfractionated heparin is promptly initiated and the patient is observed with serial abdominal examinations while maintaining bowel rest. Ileus may be prolonged and hyperalimentation should be initiated early. Once the patient's clinical status improves, oral intake can be carefully started. A search for a predisposing primary or secondary hypercoagulable condition is required. The patient is transitioned to oral anticoagulation over 3 to 4 days, once intestinal function has returned. Lifelong anticoagulation is usually maintained, especially in cases of idiopathic MVT or when a primary hypercoagulable state has been identified.

NONOCCLUSIVE MESENTERIC ISCHEMIA

Acute intestinal ischemia may occur without actual occlusion of the mesenteric vessels, a condition termed nonocclusive mesenteric ischemia (NOMI). Infarction of the intestine in the absence of arterial or venous occlusion has been documented since 1943.[33] The etiology is severe and prolonged intestinal arterial spasm. Although a hypoperfusion state is present in most patients with NOMI, some patients have NOMI from visceral vasoconstriction alone, as is the case with cocaine or ergot intoxication.[34,35]

The primary treatment of NOMI is correction of the systemic condition leading to generalized hypoperfusion. The largest percentage of patients with NOMI have severe cardiac failure.[36-43] The etiology of the cardiac failure is not as important as optimization of blood pressure and cardiac output, with as little dependence as possible on agents that result in peripheral vasoconstriction.

In the past, digitalis was frequently used to treat congestive heart failure. Although digitalis is used much less frequently in modern practice, many patients remain on this drug or one of its derivatives. Patients treated with digitalis preparations are at risk for NOMI in the setting of worsening congestive heart failure.[38] Animal experiments indicate baseline intestinal arterial resistance is not altered by digitalis. Arterial resistance in animals treated with digitalis, however, does increase in response to intestinal venous hypertension when compared with that in controls.[44] Thus, patients who are treated with digitalis and who have increases in portal pressure, such as occur with worsening heart failure, may be more susceptible to the development of NOMI as a result of arterial mesenteric vasoconstriction. In patients with possible NOMI, digitalis preparations must be withdrawn and alternative medications used to treat underlying cardiac abnormalities.

Arteriography with selective catheterization of the SMA is required to confirm the diagnosis of NOMI and may also be used to administer therapy in many patients with NOMI.[45] For patients without overt peritonitis, transcatheter vasodilator therapy may be of benefit. In a retrospective case series, Boley and colleagues treated 15 patients with NOMI with intra-arterial infusions of papaverine.[45] Nine of fifteen patients survived. Another recent study of patients with NOMI after cardiac surgery demonstrated clinical improvement with administration of intra-arterial papaverine in 64% of patients.[46]

In patients with peritonitis, operation is required to determine bowel viability and for removal of any necrotic intestine. Catheter-based therapy alone is insufficient in patients with peritoneal findings. At operation, the bowel is inspected for viability and necrotic intestine removed. A hand-held Doppler instrument is used to assess the mesenteric vessels proximally and distally.[47] Intravenous fluorescein is also used to evaluate areas of possible ischemia. Absent, perivascular or patchy fluorescein patterns signify areas of ischemia.[48] A "second look" procedure at 24 to 48 hours allows for the reassessment of bowel viability. Further bowel resection can be performed at that time if necessary.

REFERENCES

1. Stoney RJ, Ehrenfeld EK, Wylie EJ: Revascularization methods in chronic visceral ischemia. Ann Surg 186:468, 1977.
2. Beebe HG, MacFarlane S, Raker EJ: Supraceliac aortomesenteric bypass for intestinal ischemia. J Vasc Surg 5:749, 1987.
3. Moawad J, McKinsey JF, Wyble CW, et al: Current results of surgical therapy for chronic mesenteric ischemia. Arch Surg 132:613, 1997.
4. Kihara TK, Blebea J, Anderson KM, et al: Risk factors and outcomes following revascularization for chronic mesenteric ischemia. Ann Vasc Surg 13:37, 1999.
5. Mateo RB, O'Hara PJ, Hertzer NR, et al: Elective surgical treatment of symptomatic chronic mesenteric occlusive disease: Early results and late outcomes. J Vasc Surg 29:821, 1999.
6. Foley MI, Moneta GL, Abou-Zamzam AM, et al: Revascularization of the superior mesenteric artery alone for treatment of intestinal ischemia. J Vasc Surg 32:37, 2000.
7. Dunphy JE: Abdominal pain of vascular origin. Am J Med Sci 192:109, 1936.
8. Mikkelsen WP: Intestinal angina: Its surgical significance. Am J Surg 94:262, 1957
9. Shaw RS, Maynard EP III: Acute and chronic thrombosis of the mesenteric arteries associated with malabsorption: A report of two cases successfully treated with thromboembolectomy. N Engl J Med 258:874, 1958.

10. Hollier LH, Bernatz PE, Pairolero PC, et al: Surgical management of chronic intestinal ischemia: A reappraisal. Surgery 90:940, 1991.
11. McAfee MK, Cherry KJ, Naessens JM, et al: Influence of complete revascularization on chronic mesenteric ischemia. Am J Surg 164:220, 1992.
12. Park WM, Cherry KJ Jr, Chua HK, et al: Current results of open revascularization for chronic mesenteric ischemia: A standard for comparison. J Vasc Surg 35:853, 2002.
13. Kieny R, Batellier J, Kretz J: Aortic reimplantation of the superior mesenteric artery for atherosclerotic lesions of the visceral arteries: Sixty cases. Ann Vasc Surg 4:122, 1990.
14. Cormier JM, Fichelle JM, Vennin J, et al: Atherosclerotic occlusive disease of the superior mesenteric artery: Late results of reconstructive surgery. Ann Vasc Surg 5:510, 1991.
15. Stanton PE Jr, Hollier PA, Seidel TW, et al: Chronic intestinal ischemia: Diagnosis and therapy. J Vasc Surg 4:338, 1986.
16. Gentile AT, Moneta GL, Taylor LM, Jr, et al: Isolated bypass to the superior mesenteric artery for intestinal ischemia. Arch Surg 129: 926, 1994.
17. Rapp JH, Reilly LM, Qvarfordt PG, et al: Durability of endarterectomy and antegrade grafts in the treatment of chronic visceral ischemia. J Vasc Surg 3:799, 1986.
18. Cunningham CG, Reilly LM, Rapp JH, et al: Chronic visceral ischemia: Three decades of progress. Ann Surg 214:276, 1991.
19. Baur GM, Millay DJ, Taylor LM Jr, et al: Treatment of chronic visceral ischemia. Am J Surg 148:138, 1984.
20. McMillan WD, McCarthy WJ, Bresticker M, et al: Mesenteric artery bypass: Objective patency determination. J Vasc Surg 21:729, 1995.
21. Moneta GL: Screening for mesenteric vascular insufficiency and follow-up of mesenteric bypass procedures. Semin Vasc Surg 14:186, 2001.
22. Connolly JE, Stemmer EA: Intestinal gangrene as the result of mesenteric arterial steal. Am J Surg 126:197, 1973.
23. Wylie EJ, Stoney RJ, Ehrenfeld WK: Manual of Vascular Surgery, New York, Springer-Verlag, 1980.
24. Cooley DA, Wukasch DC: Techniques in Vascular Surgery. Philadelphia, WB Saunders, 1979.
25. Gewertz BL, Zarins CK: Postoperative vasospasm after antegrade mesenteric revascularization: A report of three cases. J Vasc Surg 14:382, 1991.
26. Matsumoto AH, Tegtmeyer CJ, Fitzcharles EK, et al: Percutaneous transluminal angioplasty of visceral arterial stenoses: Results and long-term clinical follow-up. J Vasc Intervent Radiol 6:165, 1995.
27. Hallisey MJ, Deschaine J, Illescas FF, et al: Angioplasty for the treatment of visceral ischemia. J Vasc Intervent Radiol 6:785, 1995.
28. Allen T, Martin A, Rees C: Mesenteric angioplasty in the treatment of chronic intestinal ischemia. J Vasc Surg 24:415, 1996.
29. Sharafuddin MJ, Olson CH, Sun S, et al: Endovascular treatment of celiac and mesenteric arteries stenoses: Applications and results. J Vasc Surg 38:692, 2003.
30. Rhee RY, Gloviczki P, Jost C, et al: Acute mesenteric venous thrombosis. In Gloviczki P, Yao JST (eds): Handbook of Venous Disorders. New York, Arnold, 2001, p 321.
31. Morasch MD, Ebaugh JL, Chiou AC, et al: Mesenteric venous thrombosis: A changing clinical entity. J Vasc Surg 34:680, 2001.
32. Rhee RY, Gloviczki P, Mendonca CT, et al: Mesenteric venous thrombosis: Still a lethal disease in the 1990s. J Vasc Surg 20:688, 1994.
33. Thorek M, Smith HW: Surgical Errors and Safeguards. 4th ed. Philadelphia, JB Lippincott, 1943, p 478.
34. Green FL, Ariyan S, Stausel HC Jr: Mesenteric and peripheral vascular ischemia secondary to ergotism. Surgery 81:311, 1977.
35. Myers SI, Clagett GP, Valentine RJ, et al: Chronic intestinal ischemia caused by intravenous cocaine use: Report of two cases and review of the literature. J Vasc Surg 23:724, 1996.
36. Aldrete JS, Hansy SY, Laws HL, et al: Intestinal infarction complicating low cardiac output states. Surg Gynecol Obstet 144:371, 1977.
37. Williams LF, Anastasia LF, Hasiotis CA: Nonocclusive mesenteric infarction. Am J Surg 114:376, 1967.
38. Britt LG, Cheek RC: Nonocclusive mesenteric vascular disease: Clinical and experimental observations. Ann Surg 169:704, 1969.
39. Moneta GL, Misbach GA, Ivey TD: Hypoperfusion as a possible factor in the development of gastrointestinal complications after cardiac surgery. Am J Surg 149:648, 1985.
40. Rosemurgy AS, McAllister E, Karl RC: The acute surgical abdomen after cardiac surgery involving extracorporeal circulation. Ann Surg 207:323, 1988.
41. Allen KB, Salam AA, Lumsden AB: Acute mesenteric ischemia following cardiopulmonary bypass. J Vasc Surg 16:391, 1992.
42. Landreueau RJ, Fry WJ: The right colon as a target organ of nonocclusive mesenteric ischemia. Arch Surg 125:591, 1990.
43. Howard TJ, Plaskon LA, Wiebke EA, et al: Nonocclusive mesenteric ischemia remains a diagnostic dilemma. Am J Surg 171:405, 1996.
44. Kim EH, Gewertz BL: Chronic digitalis administration alters mesenteric vascular reactivity. J Vasc Surg 5:382, 1987.
45. Boley S, Sprayregan S, Siegelman S, et al: Initial results from an aggressive roentgenological and surgical approach to acute mesenteric ischemia. Surgery 82:848, 1977.
46. Klotz S, Vestring T, Rotker J, et al: Diagnosis and treatment of nonocclusive mesenteric ischemia after open heart surgery. Ann Thorac Surg 72:1583, 2001.
47. Hobson RW II, Wright CB, Rich NM, et al: Assessment of colonic ischemia during aortic surgery by Doppler ultrasound: J Surg Res 20:231, 1976.
48. Gloviczki P, Bergman RT, Stanson AW, et al: The role of intravenous fluorescein in the detection of colon ischemia during aortic reconstruction. Int Angiol 11:281,1992.

chapter 28

Erectile Dysfunction

Ricardo Munarriz
Noel N. Kim
Irwin Goldstein
Abdul M. Traish

This chapter will focus on the arousal aspect of male sexual function, which is uniquely characterized by a set of coordinated neurohormonal responses that lead to penile erection. Until recently, erectile dysfunction (ED) has been predominantly treated as a psychological condition and classified, along with other disorders leading to compromised sexual function, under the broad term of "impotence." In 1992, a panel at the National Institutes of Health Consensus Conference on Impotence identified that approximately 75% of erectile disorders originated from organic causes and defined ED as the persistent or repeated inability, for a duration of 6 months, to attain or maintain an erection sufficient for satisfactory sexual performance.[1]

EPIDEMIOLOGY OF ERECTILE DYSFUNCTION IN THE UNITED STATES AND WORLDWIDE

Erectile dysfunction is highly prevalent, estimated to affect 30 million men in the United States and more than 100 million men worldwide.[1-3] Erectile dysfunction adversely affects quality of life[4] and general well being. The population-based Massachusetts Male Aging Study (MMAS)[5] (1987 to 1989) included 1290 men between the ages of 40 and 70 who returned questionnaires about their sexual function. Erectile dysfunction of some degree was found in 52% of the volunteers and the age-adjusted prevalence of complete erectile dysfunction was 39% in men with coronary artery disease, 15% in men with hypertension, and 25% in men with diabetes.[5] A longitudinal evaluation of the original cohort was performed between 1995 and 1997. A total of 847 of the original 1290 men (average age 52.2 years) demonstrated an incidence rate during the follow-up of 25.9 cases per 1000 men per year (95% CI). The population projection for men between 40 and 69 years suggested that 617,715 new cases of erectile dysfunction are expected to occur in the United States every year. The incidence of erectile dysfunction was higher in those men with diabetes (50.7 cases per 1000 men per year), coronary artery disease (58.3 cases per 1000 men per year), and treated arterial hypertension (42.5 cases per 1000 men per year). It was predicted that the number of men affected by erectile dysfunction will increase in a constant manner as the world's population grows older.[6] A second population-based epidemiologic study, the National Health Social and Life Survey (NHSLS)[7] reported on the prevalence and predictive factors for erectile dysfunction and other sexual dysfunctions in American men. The overall prevalence of erectile dysfunction in 1410 men aged 18 to 59 years was 31%. The prevalence was 7% for the men aged 18 to 29 years, 9% for the group aged 30 to 39 years, 11% for those aged 40 to 49 years, and 18% for those aged 50 to 59 years. In 1993, Solstad and Hertoft[8] studied 411 men—a total of 4% reported erectile dysfunction on more than one occasion; 15% reported only occasional erectile dysfunction; and 7% considered erectile dysfunction a problem. Malmsten and colleagues[9] examined 10,458 men who presented with lower urinary tract symptoms. Erectile dysfunction was noted in 1.5% of 45-year-old men and in 17.8% of 80-year-old men. In 1997, Virag and colleagues[10] found an erectile dysfunction prevalence of 39% for the French population between 18 and 70 years of age. Fedele and colleagues[11] in 1998, found a prevalence of erectile dysfunction in Italy of 36%. In 2000, Ledda[12] demonstrated that diabetic patients presented with erectile dysfunction at an earlier age and with a higher prevalence (75%) than nondiabetic patients. Sandoica and colleagues[13] reported a 56% prevalence of erectile dysfunction in a Spanish population. Krimpen[14] recently studied 1604 men in the Netherlands from ages 50 to 75 years. For men between 50 and 54 years, the prevalence of erectile dysfunction was 21%. For men between 75 and 77 years, the prevalence of erectile dysfunction was 61%. An epidemiologic study (DENSA)[15] was carried out in men older than 40 years in various cities in Colombia, Ecuador, and Venezuela in South America. The prevalence of erectile dysfunction was 53%. Nicolosi and associates[16] estimated the prevalence rate of erectile dysfunction to be 34% in Japan, 22% in Malaysia, 17% in Italy, and 15% in Brazil. In this multinational study, the prevalence of erectile dysfunction was 9% in men between the ages of 40 and 44 years and 54% in men between the ages of 65 and 70 years.[16] Kongkanand[17] examined 1250 men in Thailand, in whom the prevalence of erectile dysfunction was 54%. In this study, the prevalence of erectile dysfunction increased with age, arterial hypertension, diabetes, coronary artery disease, cigarette smoking, and alcohol consumption.

ANATOMY OF THE PENIS

The penis consists of three cylindrical erectile bodies, the paired corpora cavernosa—the key structures mediating penile erection—and the corpus spongiosum. Each corpus cavernosum has a thick fibrous sheath, the tunica albuginea, which surrounds the whole cavernosal erectile tissue. Formation of local fibrous tissue plaques in the subtunical layer (Peyronie's disease) can result in low compliance of the tunica albuginea, penile curvature, and veno-occlusive dysfunction.[18] Bulbospongiosus muscles surround the corpus spongiosum in the bulbar region and facilitate ejaculation through rhythmic contractions. A thick elastic layer, Buck fascia, surrounds and is firmly attached to the tunica albuginea. Blood vessels and nerves run between Buck fascia and the tunica albuginea.

The blood supply to each corpus cavernosum is derived mainly from the internal pudendal artery, which feeds into the perineal artery in the Alcock canal. Along with the nerves that run in the Alcock canal, there are blood vessels in this region that are vulnerable to compression injuries, such as may occur during bicycle riding.[19] It has recently been demonstrated that the dorsal artery interconnects with the cavernosal artery, allowing arterial bypass surgery in the case of cavernosal artery obstruction.[20] Frequently, the accessory pudendal artery provides additional blood to the corpora cavernosa and has a critical role in men with reduced blood supply via ordinary pudendal arteries, especially those who have received radical pelvic surgery.[21]

Blood leaves the penis via three venous systems: superficial, intermediate, and deep. The superficial system (superficial dorsal veins) consists of small venous channels in the subcutaneous layer draining the skin and subcutaneous tissue above the Buck fascia. The intermediate system (deep dorsal vein and circumflex veins) drains blood from the glans, corpus spongiosum, and the distal two thirds of the corpora. Venous blood from the corporeal sinusoids drains initially into tiny subtunical venules that merge into emissary veins, penetrating the tunica albuginea, and empty into the deep dorsal vein, directly or via the circumflex veins.[22,23] Interestingly, the venous network connects the corpus spongiosum to the corpora cavernosa, allowing vasodilator substances absorbed through the urethral mucosa to transport into the erectile bodies. This anatomical arrangement enables the transurethral delivery of drugs used to treat men with ED. The deep system (cavernous and crural veins) are the main drainage system of the corpora cavernosa and a main source of leakage in venogenic impotence.

The sponge-like corpus cavernosum consists of bundles of smooth muscle cells embedded in a matrix of connective tissue and fibroblasts, forming trabeculated structures that define a series of blood-filled lacunar spaces lined with endothelium.[24] In the flaccid state, the trabecular smooth muscle and the central cavernosal and branching helicine arteries within each cavernosal body are constricted. During the transition to the erect state,

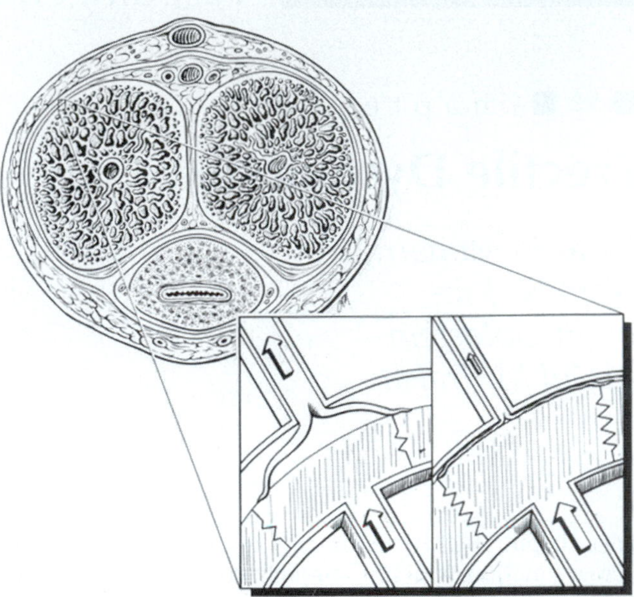

FIGURE 28-1. Schematic cross-section of the penis including two corporeal bodies and a corpus spongiosum. *Inserts:* Enlargements of the subtunical space between the trabeculae and the tunica albuginea. Drainage from erection tissue passes via subtunical venules into emissary veins that drain through the tunica. When the penis is in the flaccid state *(left insert),* the contracted corporeal smooth muscle allows blood to drain from the erectile tissue to the subtunical venules under conditions of low outflow resistance. When the penis is in the erect state *(right insert),* following activation of efferent autonomic nerves, the elevated pressure in the lacunar space expands the trabecular structures against the tunica albuginea. The expanded volume of the corporeal tissue both mechanically compresses and physically stretches the subtunical venules, greatly increasing the resistance to flow through these venous channels. The resultant restriction of venous outflow through the subtunical venules is called the *corporeal veno-occlusive mechanism.*

sacral parasympathetic stimulation causes the dilation of the cavernosal and helicine arteries, enabling a higher rate of blood flow into the penis. Concomitant relaxation of the trabecular smooth muscle greatly increases the compliance of the cavernosal bodies and allows the lacunar spaces to expand and accommodate the enhanced blood flow. Additionally, the outflow of blood must be reduced to achieve and maintain full tumescence and rigidity. The restriction of venous outflow from the cavernosal bodies is accomplished by elongation and compression of subtunical venules between the expanding trabecular structures and the tunica albuginea. This process is known as the veno-occlusive mechanism (Fig. 28-1). Somatic innervation is via the pudendal nerve, which is composed of efferent fibers innervating the striated musculature of the perineum and of afferent fibers from the penile and perineal skin.[25]

Cellular Organization and Mechanism of Trabecular Smooth Muscle Contraction and Relaxation

Trabecular smooth muscle constitutes approximately 50% of normal erectile tissue, as assessed by histomorphometric analysis. The bulk of the remaining tissue volume is occupied by extracellular matrix, which provides a fibroelastic framework. The trabecular smooth muscle cells of the corpus cavernosum form a functional syncytium by virtue of junctional plaques in the plasma membrane, similar to cardiac muscle. These plaques consist of numerous gap junction complexes or *connexons*. Each hexameric connexon assembly is formed by the self-association of connexin protein subunits. The major gap junction protein expressed by human cavernosal smooth muscle cells is connexin.

This continuity in the network of smooth muscle cells enables a coordinated response to various stimuli, which are not homogeneously distributed throughout the tissue. For example, neurotransmitters released from a limited number of nerve termini, as well as vasoactive substances secreted by the endothelium, are produced at discrete sites and may directly reach only a limited number of smooth muscle cells. The syncytial network allows smooth muscle cells, which are not directly stimulated, to respond in the same fashion as those that have been directly stimulated.

The contractile response of the smooth muscle cell is ultimately determined by the interaction between myosin cross bridges and actin filaments. The level of intracellular free Ca^{2+} is the principal factor in determining the activity of the actin-myosin complex. Vasoconstrictor agonists binding to specific plasma membrane receptors activate various intracellular signal transduction pathways to cause the release of Ca^{2+} from internal stores, elevating intracellular Ca^{2+} levels. One of these pathways involves the activation of G-proteins which may, in turn, activate phospholipase C. This membrane-bound enzyme hydrolyzes phosphatidylinositol 4,5-bisphosphate (PIP_2) to inositol 1,4,5-trisphosphate (IP_3) and 1,2-diacylglycerol (DAG). IP_3 binds to specific receptors on the sarcoplasmic reticulum to cause the release of calcium. Extracellular Ca^{2+} may also enter the cell through voltage-gated L-type Ca^{2+} channels, which are activated upon membrane depolarization during nonreceptor-mediated electromechanical coupling. Free Ca^{2+} binds calmodulin and promotes its association with myosin light-chain kinase (MLCK). Calmodulin activated MLCK phosphorylates the regulatory light chain of myosin (MLC) to initiate cross-bridge cycling and contraction.

Receptor-mediated smooth muscle relaxation is initiated by the generation of cyclic nucleotides (cGMP and cAMP) by guanylate and adenylate cyclases. Adenylate cyclase is localized in the plasma membrane and is activated by G proteins. Guanylate cyclase may exist as a particulate form, bound to the plasma membrane, or as a soluble form in the cytoplasm of the cell. Increases in cGMP and cAMP activate protein kinase G, which leads to the phosphorylation and inactivation of phospholamban. In its dephosphorylated and active state, phospholamban inhibits the sarcoplasmic reticulum Ca^{2+} ATPase (SERCA) pump. Thus, inhibition of phospholamban by cGMP and cAMP enables SERCA to become active and reduce intracellular Ca^{2+} by actively sequestering it within the sarcoplasmic reticulum. Protein kinases G and A have also been shown to phosphorylate and activate K^+ channels in the plasma membrane, causing hyperpolarization. This change in membrane potential inactivates L-type Ca^{2+} channels to inhibit Ca^{2+} influx. The importance of this mechanism in trabecular smooth muscle is not clear.

Central Mechanism of Erection

Penile erections are elicited by local sensory stimulation of the genital organs and by central psychogenic stimuli received by or generated within the brain.[25,26] Recently, specific regions of the brain (inferior temporal cortex, right insula, right inferior frontal cortex, and left anterior cingulated cortex) activated by visually evoked sexual arousal have been identified by positron emission tomography.[27] The medial preoptic area and the paraventricular nucleus within the hypothalamus appear to integrate visual (occipital area), tactile (thalamus), olfactory (rhinencephalon), and imaginative (limbic system) input and send neural projections to the thoracolumbar sympathetic and sacral parasympathetic centers of the spinal cord.[28] Dopamine and oxytocin are believed to play important roles in mediating the pre-erectile response in the medial preoptic area and the paraventricular nucleus, respectively.[29]

In contrast, the nucleus paragigantocellularis (nPGi) in the brain stem exerts an inhibitory effect on sexual arousal.[30] Nerves from the nPGi project to sacral segments of the spinal cord and release serotonin. This has been postulated as the reason specific serotonin reuptake inhibitors (SSRIs) depress sexual function. Interestingly, because men treated with SSRI drugs most commonly exhibit delayed or blocked ejaculation, cases of premature ejaculation have also been successfully managed with SSRI treatment. The locus caeruleus also exerts inhibitory input via sympathetic nerves that interface with hypothalamic nuclei as well as with the spinal cord. Withdrawal of sympathetic input due to suppressed activity of the locus caeruleus during rapid eye movement (REM) sleep is believed to lead to episodes of nocturnal penile tumescence.[29,31] The pudendal nerve, which is the afferent limb for reflexogenic erections, collects somatic sensation from the genital skin. The autonomic nerve fibers that arise from the sacral parasympathetic center (S2 to S4) make up the efferent limb for this reflex, innervating the penile smooth muscle. Reflexogenic and psychogenic erectile mechanisms probably act synergistically in the control of penile erection.[25,32-38]

Erection follows relaxation of arterial and trabecular smooth muscle.[39] Dilation of the cavernosal and helicine arteries increases blood flow into the lacunar spaces. Relaxation of the trabecular smooth muscle dilates the lacunar spaces, accommodating a larger volume of blood and thus engorging the penis. The expansion of the relaxed trabecular walls against the tunica albuginea compresses the plexus of subtunical venules.[40,41] This results in increased resistance to the outflow of blood with increased lacunar space pressure, making the penis rigid. The reduction of venous outflow by the mechanical compression of subtunical venules is known as the corporeal veno-occlusive mechanism.

Contraction of penile smooth muscle results in detumescence. Activation of sympathetic constrictor nerves causes an increase in the tone of the smooth muscle of the helicine arteries and the trabeculae, resulting in a reduction of arterial inflow, a collapse of the lacunar spaces with decompression of subtunical venules,[40,41] an increase in venous outflow from the lacunar space, and a return of the penis to the flaccid state.

Peripheral Mechanisms of Erection

Neurogenic Regulation of Penile Erection

Erectile function in the penis is regulated by autonomic (parasympathetic and sympathetic) and somatic (sensory and motor) pathways to the erectile tissues and perineal striated muscles (Fig. 28-2A). Three sets of peripheral nerves innervate the penis, the sympathetic nerves, the parasympathetic nerves, and the pudendal nerves.

The sympathetic nerves (T10 to L2), which are responsible for detumescence and maintenance of flaccidity, project to the corpora, as well as to the prostate and bladder neck via the hypogastric nerves. Postganglionic noradrenergic fibers pass posterolateral to the prostate in the so-called *nerves of Walsh* to enter the corpora cavernosa medially. Adrenergic tone is crucial in initiating detumescence and in maintaining the flaccid state of the penis because the smooth muscle of the arteries and cavernosal trabeculae must remain actively contracted. Contraction of cavernosal trabecular smooth muscle in response to norepinephrine is mediated by α_1-adrenergic receptors. Prejunctional α_2-adrenergic receptors on adrenergic nerves inhibit neurotransmission and provide a self-regulating negative feedback loop for secreted norepinephrine. Cholinergic nerves act on prejunctional muscarinic receptors to also inhibit adrenergic nerve activity. The role of α-adrenergic receptors in the physiology of penile erection is reviewed more completely elsewhere.[42,43]

The parasympathetic nerves, originating in the intermediolateral nuclei of the S2-S4 spinal cord segments, provide the major excitatory input to the penis. Exiting through the sacral foramina, these nerves pass forward lateral to the rectum as the pelvic nerve and synapse in the pelvic plexus with postganglionic nonadrenergic, noncholinergic (NANC) nerve fibers, which travel within the cavernous nerves to the corpora cavernosa. Vasoactive intestinal peptide (VIP) and nitric oxide (NO) are two NANC neurotransmitters that are often colocalized in the same nerves in penile tissue. The primary mediator of NANC parasympathetic input is NO. The ability of NO, a highly reactive and unstable gas, to regulate a wide array of physiologic functions in mammals has become evident only within the last 2 decades. Along with carbon monoxide, NO is a unique primary effector molecule with the characteristics of an intracellular second messenger that defies previous classification schemes. It is apparently synthesized on demand with little or no storage, and it directly activates a soluble enzyme (guanylate cyclase) rather than a "traditional" receptor molecule. NO is produced by nitric oxide synthase (NOS), which uses the amino acid L-arginine and molecular oxygen as substrates to produce NO and L-citrulline. NO can readily cross plasma membranes to enter target cells, where it binds the heme component of soluble guanylate cyclase. This activation of guanylate cyclase stimulates the production of cyclic guanosine monophosphate (cGMP), with the resultant activation of the cGMP-dependent protein kinase, which regulates the intracellular events, leading to relaxation of trabecular smooth muscle. The levels of cGMP also are regulated by phosphodiesterases, which break down cGMP and terminate signaling. Sildenafil is a reversible inhibitor of phosphodiesterase type 5, the major enzyme responsible for cGMP hydrolysis in penile erectile tissue.[44] Inhibition of this enzyme leads to the increase in levels of intracellular cGMP and enhancement of the relaxation of smooth muscle in response to stimuli that activate the NO/cGMP pathway. This activity may explain the success of sildenafil in the treatment of male ED.[45]

Recently, it has become evident that NO interacts directly with other cellular targets, including receptors, ion channels, and pumps, which may modulate the contractility of smooth muscle cells, independently of the cGMP pathway.[46-48] Thus, NO has intracellular targets in addition to guanylate cyclase that may play a role in the regulation of vascular and trabecular smooth muscle contractility.

The activity of NANC nerves may be modulated by cholinergic nerves, which facilitate NANC relaxation by stimulating the synthesis and release of NO and other vasodilatory neurotransmitters. Thus, the release of acetylcholine may coordinate withdrawal of adrenergic input and increase of NANC input by binding to prejunctional muscarinic receptors on adrenergic and NANC nerves.[31] In certain disease states, such as diabetes, the ability of the corpus cavernosum to synthesize and release acetylcholine is diminished.[49] Such processes may be responsible, in part, for the compromised erectile function associated with diabetes. Parasympathetic nerves are also vulnerable during surgical procedures such as abdominoperineal resection of the rectum and radical prostatectomy.[21,50]

Non-Neuronal Modulators of Penile Erection

In addition to neurogenic mechanisms, local paracrine/autocrine factors, with vasoactive and/or trophic effects, profoundly influence the function of the smooth muscle in the penis. These include endothelins, prostanoids, NO, and oxygen.

Endothelin-1 (ET-1) is one of the most potent vasoconstrictors known at this time. The release of endothelin from the intimal lining of vascular compartments can be induced by shear stress. It has also been suggested that endothelin may exert vasodilatory effects at low concentrations through a "super-high" affinity form of the ET_B receptor potentially by stimulating NO production. However, the significance of this mechanism in penile erection remains unclear.

Nitric oxide is synthesized and released not only by the NANC nerves but also by the vascular endothelium. Vasodilators such as acetylcholine and bradykinin act by binding their respective membrane receptors and increasing intracellular Ca^{2+} within endothelial cells. Physical stimuli, such as shear stress, are also known to enhance NO production in endothelium. In the penis, shear-induced NO production by endothelium is most likely to occur during the onset of erection, when blood flow into the cavernosal bodies is rapidly increased. The mode of

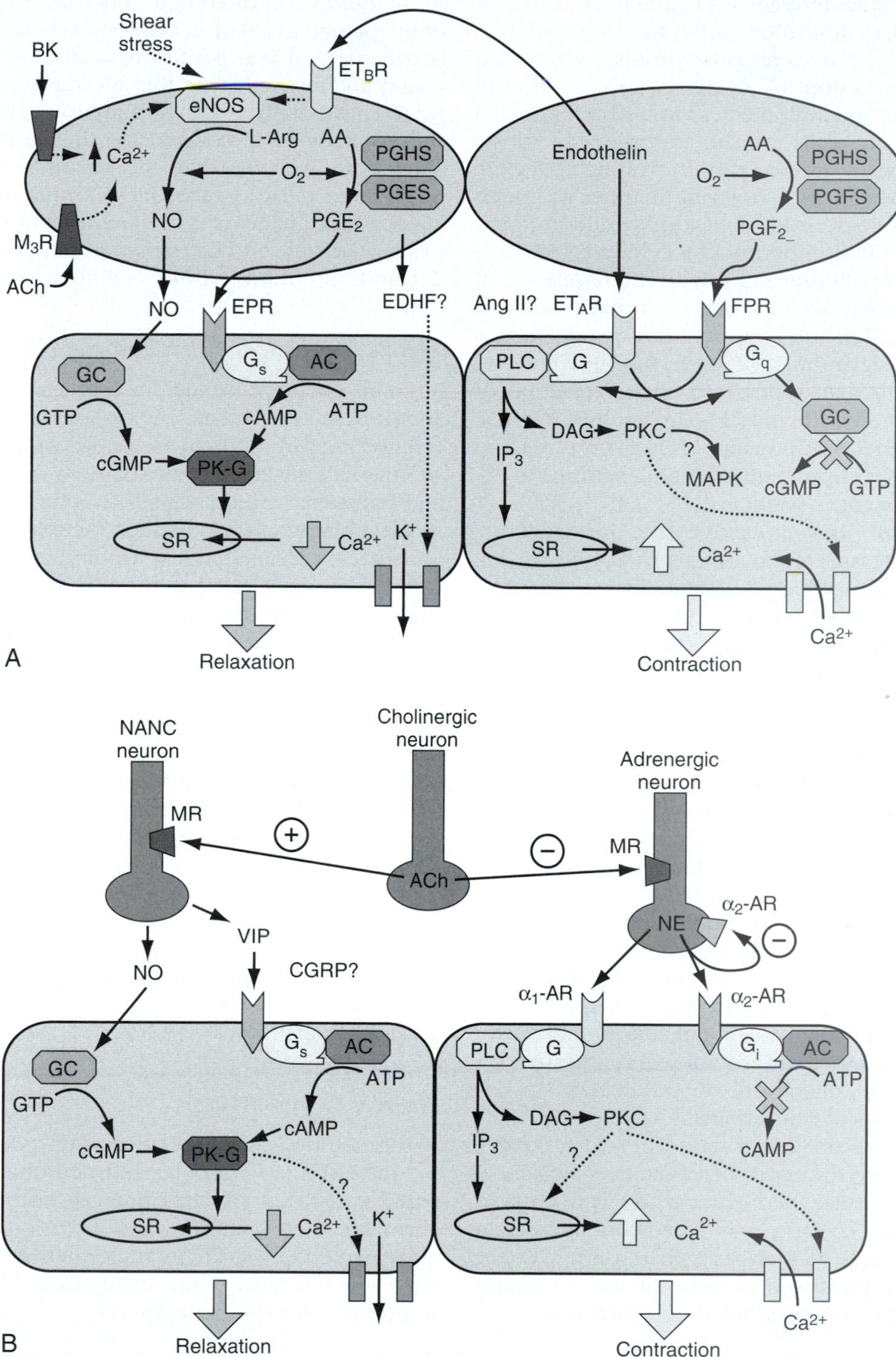

FIGURE 28-2. A, Endothelial regulation of penile trabecular smooth muscle contractility. **B,** Neurogenic regulation of penile trabecular smooth muscle contractility. AA, arachidonic acid; AC, adenylate cyclase; Ach, acetylcholine; AR, adrenergic receptor; BK, bradykinin; CGRP, calcitonin gene-related peptide; DAG, diacylglycerol; EDHF, endothelium-derived hyperpolarizing factor; eNOS, endothelial nitric oxide synthase; EPR, PGE receptor; ETR, endothelin receptor; FPR, PGF receptor; G, G-protein; GC, guanylate cyclase; L-Arg, L-arginine; MAPK, mitogen activated protein kinase; MR, muscarinic receptor; NANC, nonadrenergic-noncholinergic; NE, norepinephrine; NO, nitric oxide; PG, prostaglandin; PGFS, prostaglandin F synthase; PGHS, prostaglandin H synthase; PGES, prostaglandin E synthase; PKC, protein kinase C; PK-G, protein kinase G; PLC, phospholipase C; SR, sarcoplasmic reticulum; VIP, vasoactive intestinal polypeptide.

action of endothelium-derived NO is identical to that of nerve-derived NO, as described earlier (see Fig. 28-2B).

Prostaglandins (PGs) are prostanoids, which are produced by the action of cyclooxygenases on the common precursor arachidonic acid in both endothelial and smooth muscle cells of the corpora cavernosa. Prostanoids act locally and exert both trophic and tonic effects in an autocrine and paracrine manner. Although the precise physiologic role of PGs in penile erection remains poorly defined, experimental evidence indicates that they may play an important role in the regulation of the production of extracellular matrix. Prostanoids can induce both relaxation and contraction in penile corpus cavernosum. Prostaglandin E (PGE) is the only endogenous prostaglandin that appears to elicit relaxation of human trabecular smooth muscle. The multifunctional, dose-dependent effects of prostanoids may be explained by the coupling of receptor subtypes and isoforms to different second messenger systems.

Oxygen tension plays an active role in regulating penile erection. Measurements of cavernosal blood PO_2 in human volunteer subjects indicate that oxygen tensions change rapidly from venous (~35 mm Hg) to arterial (~100 mm Hg) levels during the transition of the penis from the flaccid to the erect state. Maintenance of constant oxygen tension is a critical imperative in most tissues of the body. This transition is the basis of a unique regulatory mechanism that takes advantage of key synthetic enzymes that use molecular oxygen as a co-substrate. NO synthase and prostaglandin synthase are two well-studied examples of a class of enzymes known as dioxygenases. At low oxygen tension, measured in the flaccid state of the penis, the synthesis of NO is inhibited, preventing relaxation of trabecular smooth muscle. This inhibition of NO production is probably necessary for the maintenance of penile flaccidity. Following vasodilation of the resistance arteries, the increase in arterial flow raises oxygen tension. In the oxygen-enhanced environment, autonomic dilator nerves and the endothelium are able to synthesize NO, thereby mediating relaxation of trabecular smooth muscle. The synthesis of prostanoids is similarly regulated in the flaccid versus the erect state. Therefore, oxygen tension may regulate the types of vasoactive substances present in the vascular bed. At low oxygen tension, norepinephrine- and endothelin-induced contraction may predominate, whereas at high oxygen tension, NO and prostaglandins are produced because of the availability of molecular oxygen required for their synthesis.

Management of Erectile Function

The process of care model for the evaluation and treatment of erectile dysfunction was developed with input from a multidisciplinary panel of experts to advance new guidelines for the diagnosis and treatment of ED.[51] These guidelines begin with the identification and diagnosis of the problem. ED is the persistent or repeated inability, for a duration of at least 3 months, to attain and/or maintain an erection sufficient for satisfactory sexual performance,[1] and the diagnosis is based on the patient's self-report in conjunction with a clinical evaluation. Validated sexual questionnaires, such as the International Index of Erectile Function (IIEF), may be helpful tools in the evaluation of erectile function.[52] The cornerstone of the patient evaluation is a comprehensive and detailed sexual, medical, and psychosocial history; physical examination; and focused laboratory testing. Specialized diagnostic tests, although not always indicated, may corroborate the impressions discovered on the initial evaluation. It should be stressed that the secondary psychological reaction to these organic factors must not be ignored. Successful management of the impotent patient who has primary organic and secondary psychological impotence demands attention to both dysfunctions.

Sexual, Medical, and Psychosocial History

A comprehensive sexual history should include past and present assessment of sexual desire (libido), orgasms, ejaculatory function, and erectile capabilities (rigidity, spontaneity, sustaining capabilities) during both sexual and nonsexual circumstances (nocturnal erections). The medical history should include focused questions on the patient's medical illness (chronic/medical illness (e.g., diabetes, anemia, renal failure), neurologic illness (e.g., spinal cord injury, multiple sclerosis, lumbosacral disc disease), endocrinologic illness (e.g., hypogonadism, hyperprolactinemia, thyroid disorders), atherosclerotic vascular risk factors (e.g., hypercholesterolemia, hypertension, diabetes, smoking, family history), medications/recreational drug use (e.g., antihypertensives, antidepressants, alcohol, cocaine), pelvic/perineal/penile trauma (e.g., bicycling injury), surgical (e.g., radical prostatectomy, laminectomy, vascular bypass surgery), and psychiatric history (e.g., depression, anxiety). Given the personal, interpersonal, social, and occupational implications of sexual problems, a brief psychosocial history is mandatory for every patient. Current psychological state, self-esteem, and history of sexual trauma/abuse, as well as past and present relationships and social and occupational performance, should be addressed.

Physical Examination

A routine physical examination with special emphasis on the genitourinary vascular and neurologic systems may confirm aspects of the medical history (e.g., penile curvature, neuropathies) and occasionally may reveal unsuspected physical findings, such as penile plaques (Peyronie's disease) and small testes (hypogonadism), responsible for the patient's ED.

Laboratory Testing

Laboratory testing is strongly recommended. Standard serum chemistries, complete blood cell count, and lipid profiles may elucidate vascular risk factors such as hypercholesterolemia, diabetes, and renal failure. The integrity of the hypothalamic-pituitary-gonadal axis should be examined in every patient with ED. It is unclear which testosterone assay (total, free, or bioavailable) is the best; however, there is a consensus that at least one of these assays should be performed. Although pituitary adenomas are a rare cause of sexual dysfunction, this potentially life-threatening disease and reversible cause of ED should not be forgotten. Abnormalities in any of these tests may correlate clinically with diminished sexual desire and with atrophic testes on physical examination.

Patient and Partner Education

Patient and partner education is a critical component in the diagnosis of ED and should be carried out whenever possible. The results of the history, physical examination, laboratory testing, and the need for additional diagnostic testing should be reviewed in detail with the patient and his partner, and if indicated, appropriate referrals should be made. Patient and partner education facilitates physician-patient-partner communication and enhances patient compliance and treatment adherence.

Specialized Diagnostic Testing

The introduction of sildenafil, in 1998, dramatically changed the need for specialized testing. Diagnostic modalities expand the physician's and patient's understanding of the pathophysiologic mechanisms, but disadvantages such as invasiveness, cost, and the associated risks and complications have reduced the indications for specialized testing.

Nocturnal penile tumescence testing is one of the most common diagnostic tests performed, but its ability to evaluate axial rigidity is poor. The use of this popular diagnostic tool should be limited to the discrimination between organic and psychogenic ED.[53]

Penile biothesiometry, a noninvasive diagnostic modality that measures vibratory thresholds, provides further understanding of the somatosensory pathway and has proved helpful in the management of diabetic patients with ED.

Noninvasive and invasive vascular testing of patients with ED has been reported in numerous series.[54,55] These include office intracavernosal injection testing, duplex ultrasound (Figs. 28-3 and 28-4), studies of the penile brachial index, penile plethysmography, cavernosal artery systolic occlusion pressure in the erect state,

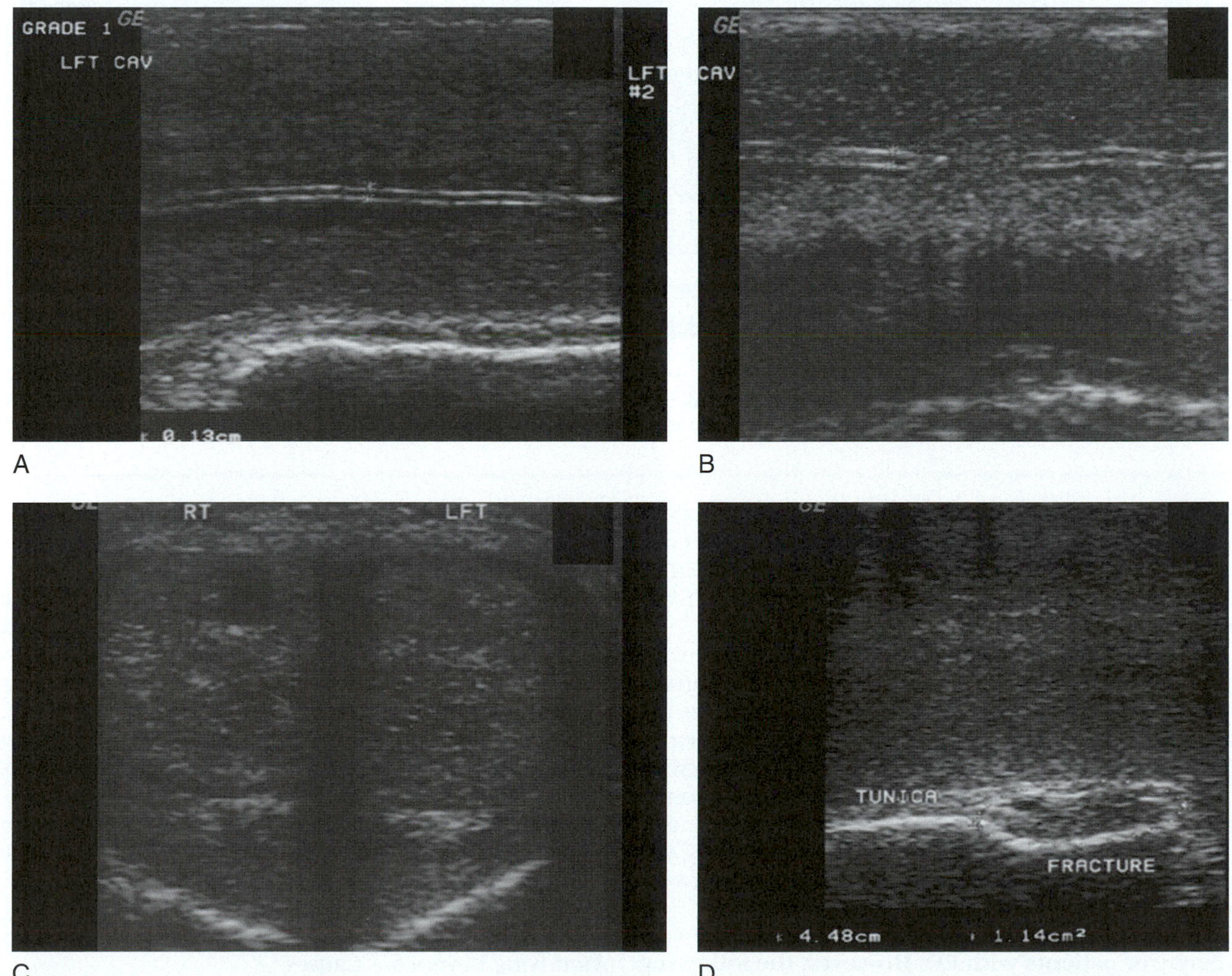

FIGURE 28-3. Penile gray scale ultrasound provides relevant clinical information on the integrity of the cavernosal arteries, tissues, and tunica. The authors have developed the following quantitative gray criteria. *CA integrity:* Grade I—continuous and smooth vessel wall (**A**), Grade II—smooth vessel wall but with short interruptions of CA continuity (**B**), and Grade III—ectatic walls with multiple or long luminal obstructions. *Erectile tissue integrity*: Normal—homogeneous throughout; fibrotic—patchy hypoechoic regions (moth-eaten appearance, **C**), or coalesced central hypoechoic defect (doughnut appearance); punctate—diffuse punctate hyperechoic regions. Calcified lesions—coalesced hyperechoic with back-shadowing. *Tunical integrity*: normal—smooth, continuous and with thickness less than 2 mm, consistent with Peyronie plaque—thickness (irregular-, camel-, or triangle-shaped, **D**); calcified plaque—coalesced hyperechoic with back-shadowing.

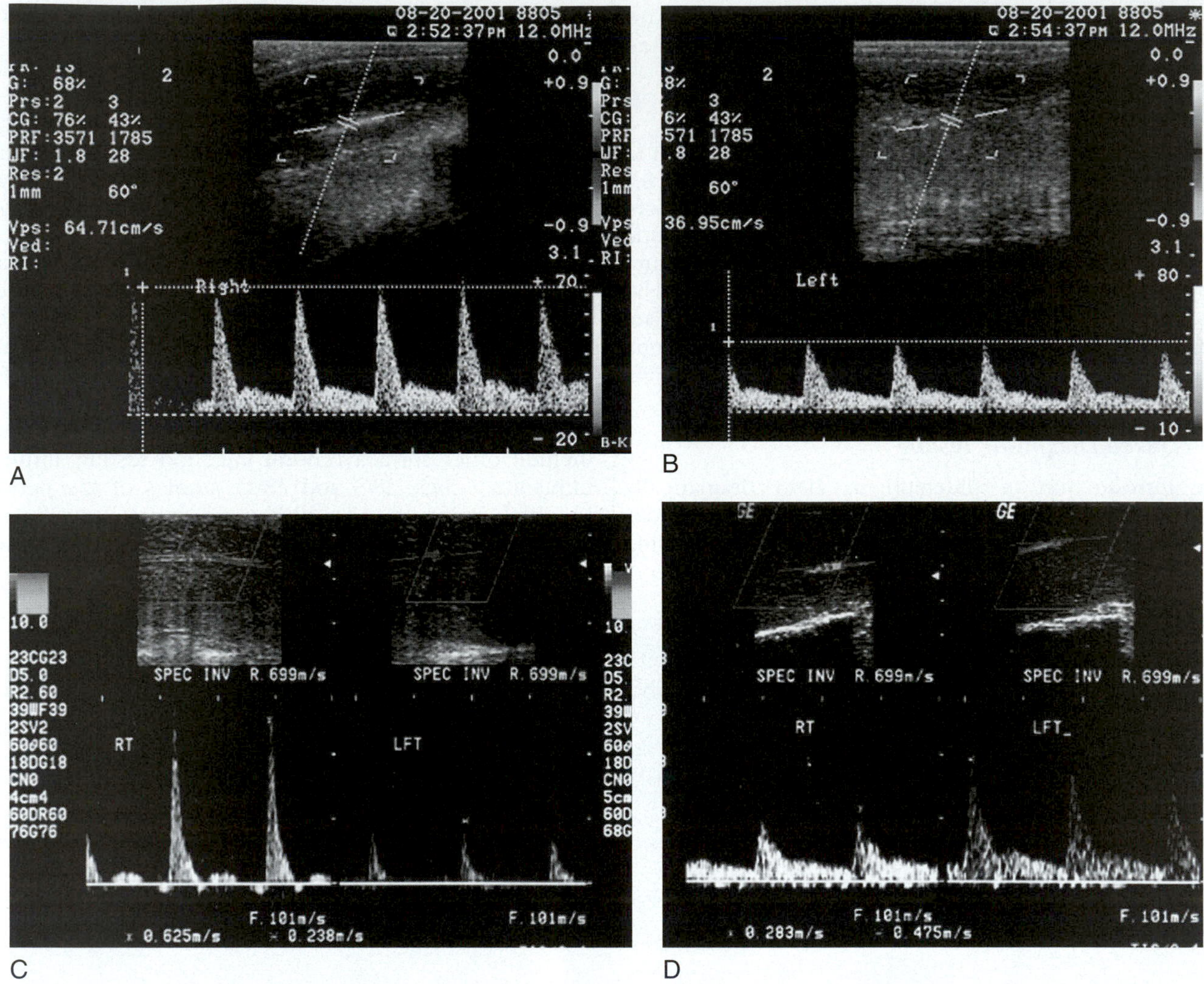

FIGURE 28-4. Penile duplex ultrasound after intracavernosal injection of vasoactive agents showing normal peak systolic velocities (**A** and **B**); abnormal left and right cavernosal peak systolic velocities consistent with cavernosal artery insufficiencies (**C** and **D**).

recordings of the change in the diameter of the cavernosal artery in the flaccid and erect states, and selective internal pudendal arteriography in the erect state. The incidence of suspected vascular pathology by such vascular testing has ranged from 33% to 87%.

Pharmacocavernosography (Fig. 28-5) of men with severe vasculogenic ED typically shows a diffuse pattern of venous leaking.[56,57] The diffuse diabetic pattern is different from the pharmacocavernosographic pattern of abnormal visualization of veins in impotent patients with Peyronie's disease,[58] following trauma, or as a consequence of a penile fracture.[59] The focal cavernosal pathology of these latter disorders is reflected by the focal site-specific abnormalities seen on pharmacocavernosography.

Primary care physicians should manage the vast majority of patients with ED. However, the following are indications for referrals:

- Young patients with presumed pure cavernosal artery insufficiency secondary to pelvic/perineal trauma. These patients may be candidates for curative vascular reconstruction.
- Patients with significant penile curvature (e.g., Peyronie's disease or congenital penile deformity). Surgical correction may be necessary to facilitate sexual intercourse.
- Patients with aortic aneurysm or bulbosacral disc disease that requires vascular or neurosurgical intervention.
- Patients with complicated endocrinopathies such as hypogonadism and pituitary adenoma.
- Patients with complicated psychiatric or psychosexual disorders (e.g., refractory depression, and transsexualism).
- Patient or physician request for specialized evaluation.
- Medical or legal reasons (occupational or iatrogenic injuries).

Modifying Reversible Causes

Health professionals should work with patients to modify reversible causes of ED, such as psychogenic ED, hypogonadism, and specific drug-related ED. Men with ED who are determined to be hypogonadotropic should receive hormonal therapy. In these cases, testosterone replacement is used to

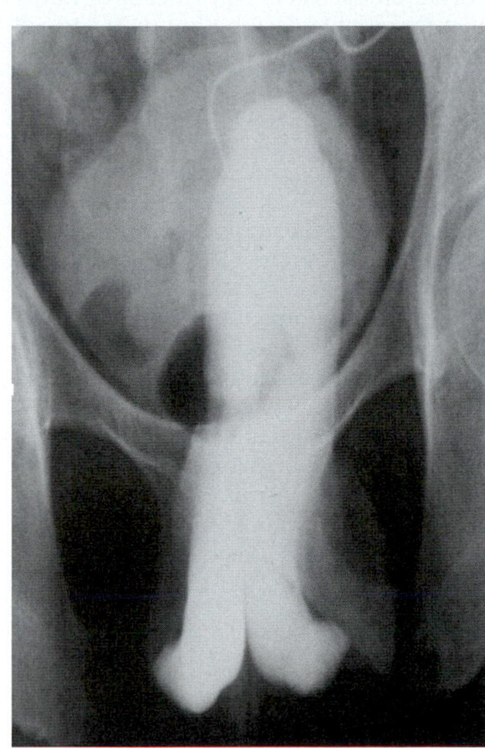
A

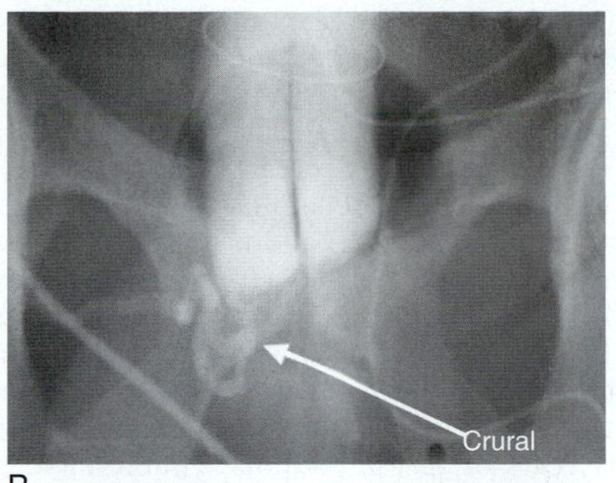

B

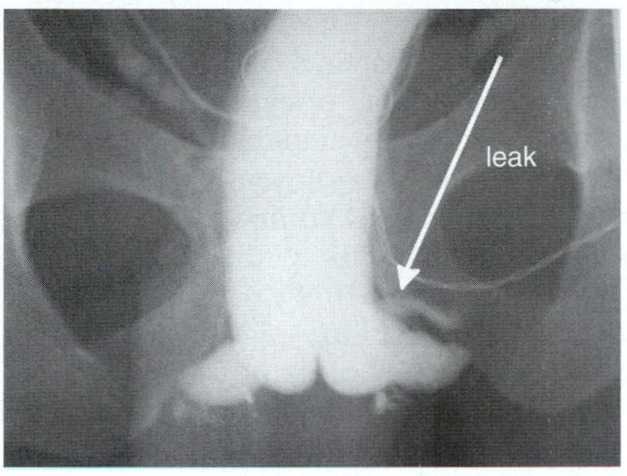

C

FIGURE 28-5. Pharmacocavernosography following administration of intracavernosal vasoactive agents in an impotent patient with normal corporeal veno-occlusion (**A**) and in an impotent patient with abnormal "crural" corporeal veno-occlusion following blunt perineal trauma (**B** and **C**).

maintain normal serum levels of testosterone and to restore potency and libido. Because of the relatively unpredictable serum levels of testosterone obtained following oral administration of testosterone and its poor efficacy and associated hepatic side effects,[60] testosterone enanthate administered intramuscularly in doses of 200 to 300 mg every 2 to 3 weeks is preferred. The amount and frequency of administration will vary with the individual and can be titrated.[61] Newer topical preparations (patch or gel) are better tolerated and more efficacious and have a significantly better side-effect profile. Testosterone is contraindicated in patients with adenocarcinoma of the prostate because testosterone may increase the rate of growth of the adenocarcinoma of the prostate.[62] In addition, testosterone replacement should be used with caution in patients with a history of bladder outlet obstruction. Before testosterone replacement therapy is initiated, it is recommended that a digital rectal examination be performed and that determinations of serum levels of prostate-specific antigen (PSA), liver function, and lipid profile be carried out. This practice should be repeated regularly.

The treatment of hyperprolactinemia consists of (1) the cessation of medication causing hyperprolactinemia (e.g., estrogens, α-methyldopa); (2) the administration of bromocriptine; or (3) the surgical ablation or extirpation of a pituitary prolactin-secreting tumor. Treatment with exogenous testosterone to supplement the diminished levels of serum testosterone usually seen with this disorder does not appear to reverse the ED.[63,64]

Thiazide diuretics and β-blockers are the antihypertensive agents most commonly associated with ED. α-Adrenergic blockers are perhaps least likely to cause erectile difficulties. Digoxin appears to be commonly associated with ED. Psychotropic agents have been associated with ED and with ejaculatory, orgasmic, and sexual desire difficulties. Luteinizing hormone-releasing hormone agonists and anti-androgens also are associated with ED and diminished sexual desire. Patients with destructive behaviors, alcoholism, cigarette smoking, and recreational drug use should be counseled on the potential etiologic role of these factors in ED.

Pure cavernosal artery insufficiency secondary to blunt perineal trauma, is a reversible cause of ED. In consequence, a small and select group of young patients may benefit from microvascular arterial bypass surgery.

First-line therapy is characterized by ease of administration, reversibility, noninvasive nature, and low cost; it includes oral erectogenics, vacuum erection devices, and psychosexual or couples therapy. The introduction of sildenafil, in 1998, revolutionized the management of men with ED. Sildenafil has allowed patients and health care professionals to openly discuss human sexuality, and has also increased the number of patients using other therapeutic modalities, such as intracavernosal injections and penile prostheses.

Sexual Therapy addressing relationship distress, sexual performance concerns, and dysfunctional communication patterns is likely to enhance sexual functioning.It is recommended that both patient and partner participate in the sexual therapy. Sexual therapy is also indicated and beneficial in patients or couples who desire to resume sexual activity after a prolonged period of abstinence. Last, sexual therapy is effective in addressing psychological reactions to the medical or surgical treatment.

Sildenafil citrate, a potent and selective inhibitor of phosphodiesterase type 5 (PDE 5), which blocks the hydrolysis of cGMP, enhances the accumulation of cGMP, and potentiates the relaxant effects of NO. Peak of plasma concentration is 60 minutes.[2,65,66] Fatty foods decrease the maximal concentration to 29%.[2,65,66] Sildenafil is metabolized in the liver by the cytochrome P450 and is excreted in feces (80%) and urine (13%).[2,65,66] Sildenafil is used on demand (prn), and the recommended initial dose is 50 mg taken 1 hour before sexual activity. The maximum recommended dose is 100 mg, no more than once per day, independent of the dosage used. The initial dose in patients older than 65 years of age, in patients with renal or liver insufficiency, or in patients receiving drugs that inhibit cytochrome P450 (erythomycin, cimetidine) is 25 mg. Sildenafil is contraindicated in patients taking nitroglycerin. The most recent package label update is recommended for use of sildenafil under careful medical supervision, in patients who have suffered a cardiovascular event, myocardial infarction, or severe arrhythmia within the previous 6 months; or in patients with hypotension (<90/50), severe hypertension (>170/110), cardiac insufficiency, unstable angina, or retinitis pigmentosa. The American College of Cardiology and the American Heart Association (ACC/AHA) also recommended the use of sildenafil with caution in patients receiving complex antihypertensive regimens; with coronary artery disease, borderline blood pressure, or renal or liver insufficiency; or who use drugs that inhibit cytochrome P450.[67] The rate of discontinuation of this agent is extremely low (0.4% to 1.2%),[68] most likely because of its low side-effect profile and high efficacy. The most common side effects of sildenafil are headaches (16%), facial flushing (10%), dyspepsia (7%), nasal congestion (4%), and diarrhea (3%).[2,68] Sildenafil is effective in treating ED caused by many different factors.[69-72] Two U.S. trials concerning sildenafil use in men with type 1 and type 2 diabetes mellitus reported that 51% to 56% of the sildenafil-treated patients showed improvement in erectile function compared with 10% to 12% of those treated with placebo.[73]

Vardenafil is also a highly potent and selective inhibitor of PDE 5 with a high bioavailability and rapid absorption.[74] The median time to maximum plasma concentration of vardenafil is 0.6 to 0.9 hours for all doses. Renal clearance of vardenafil is reduced by about 50% in patients with renal impairment but because only 5% of the administered dose appears in the urine, it is suggested that dose adjustment is not required in patients with renal impairment.[75] Vardenafil absorption is not altered by agents that affect stomach pH—such as aluminum hydroxide and magnesium hydroxide.[76] Cimetidine, a cytochrome P450 inhibitor, increases the bioavailablity of vardenafil by 12%. The metabolism of vardenafil is also affected by indinavir, ketoconazole, and erythromycin. These drugs produce 16-, 10-, and 4-fold increases in the area under the curve (AUC), respectively.[77] Adverse events associated with vardenafil are those commonly associated with PDE 5 inhibitors. There was no evidence of treatment-related changes in hematologic or biochemical parameters in a study of patients with erectile dysfunction receiving vardenafil.[79] Hellstrom and colleagues[80] reported on the safety and efficacy of vardenafil as a treatment for erectile dysfunction with a broad range of etiologies and severities in a double-blind, placebo-controlled, parallel-group, multi-center pivotal study in the United States and Canada. A total of 805 men were randomized to receive placebo or vardenafil at fixed doses of 5, 10, or 20 mg. Baseline mean erectile function domain scores were 13. At 12 weeks, relative to placebo, vardenafil 20 mg significantly improved erectile function domain scores (21 versus 15), per-patient successful penetration rates (80% versus 52%), and per patient rates of maintaining erections for successful intercourse (65% versus 32%). After 26 weeks of therapy, 85% of men receiving vardenafil 20 mg reported improved erections versus placebo (28%). A pivotal phase III study of the safety, tolerability, and efficacy of vardenafil as a treatment for erectile dysfunction in patients with diabetes mellitus, reported the final erectile function domain scores for the 20 mg and 10 mg doses of vardenafil were 19.0 and 17.1, respectively, compared with 12.6 for placebo.[81] Of interest, vardenafil treatment was effective in increasing intercourse success rates independently of HbA1c levels and of baseline erectile dysfunction severity in the men with erectile dysfunction and diabetes mellitus.[81] Vardenafil is also effective in the management of ED following radical prostatectomy.[82] Treatment with vardenafil 10 or 20 mg significantly improved erectile domain scores. Furthermore, the responder rate to the improved erectile function general assessment question and the successful penetration and intercourse rates were all significantly greater after 12 weeks of treatment with vardenafil 10 or 20 mg compared with placebo. The response rate to the general assessment question in those patients who had undergone the bilateral nerve-sparing procedure was significantly better with the 20-mg dose than with the 10-mg dose, whereas both doses were significantly better than placebo in this subgroup (71%, 60%, and 12%, respectively).[82]

Tadalafil is also a potent and selective PDE 5 inhibitor, but it has a long half-life (17.5 hrs). A European multicenter, double-blind, placebo-controlled study to assess the efficacy and safety of daily tadalafil in men with mild-to-moderate ED ($n = 294$) showed statistically significant increases in all domain scores of the IIEF.[83] Both the percentage of successful intercourse attempts and the number of satisfying intercourse attempts were increased with tadalafil. It was well tolerated with no significant changes in blood pressure, laboratory values, or electrocardiogram. The most common adverse events were headache, back pain, myalgia, and dyspepsia. Interestingly, no color vision alterations were observed.

Yohimbine hydrochloride, an α_2-adrenergic blocking agent, has long been considered an aphrodisiac. Reports of its efficacy in ED were first published 30 years ago.[84] In a prospective, double-blind, placebo-controlled study in patients with predominantly organic disease, the rate of response to yohimbine was not statistically increased over that to placebo.[85,86]

Phentolamine is an α_1- and α_2-adrenergic antagonist that decreases adrenergic tone, thus facilitating erectile function and delaying detumescence. Oral phentolamine is absorbed rapidly, with the peak plasma concentrations achieved in 30 to 60 minutes and a half-life of 5 to 7 hours.[87] A prospective, double-blind, placebo-controlled efficacy and safety trial of oral phentolamine (60 mg) reported a 36.7% success rate compared with 13.4% for placebo.[88] The most common side effects were nasal congestion (10%), headache (3%), dizziness (3%), tachycardia (3%), and nausea (1%).[87]

Apomorphine is a central dopamine agonist known to induce mild-to-moderate penile erection in men.[89] Two recent phase 3 clinical trials involving 977 men with mild-to-moderate ED treated with sublingual apomorphine reported the achievement of erections firm enough for sexual intercourse.[90] However, significant side effects such as nausea (25% to 44%), headache (12% to 19%), dizziness (5% to 16%), and yawning (10% to 16%) were reported during the first 4 weeks of treatment. The efficacy and tolerability of apomorphine in diabetic patients with ED were evaluated in a multicenter, double-blind, crossover study.[91] The percentage of attempts resulting in erections firm enough for sexual intercourse varied from 18% to 45% compared with 18% to 26% for placebo.

Topical alprostadil. A double-blind, placebo-controlled study of Topiglan (1% alprostadil in a formulation with 5% SEPA [soft enhancer of percutaneous absorption]) reported significant changes in penile rigidity with minimal side effects (skin erythema, mild warmth or burning) when applied to the glans penis in patients with mild-to-moderate ED in an office-based setting.[92]

Vacuum constrictive devices are a well-established noninvasive first-line therapy recently approved by the FDA for over-the-counter distribution.[93-95] While standing, the patient places his penis in the chamber, which is attached to a pump mechanism that can produce a negative pressure within the chamber. The negative pressure draws blood into the penis to produce an erection-like state. When adequate tumescence and rigidity have been achieved, the patient transfers a constrictor band at the base of the chamber to the base of the penis, thereby "trapping" blood within the penis. In most cases, manufacturers recommend that the vacuum-induced erection be maintained for less than 30 minutes. In monkeys, increases in cross-sectional corporeal area secondary to vacuum-induced erections were found to be only 50% of those induced by intracavernosal papaverine. This limited corporeal expansion may be secondary to the continued smooth muscle contraction of the corpora.[96] In humans, vacuum constrictive devices may induce an expansion of penile diameter equal to or greater than that attained during a physiologically induced erection, presumably secondary to the entrapment of blood in extracorporeal tissues. Venous drainage from the corpora proximal to the constrictor device is not altered.[97] Theoretically, in almost all men with ED, the vacuum constrictor devices should create penile rigidity sufficient for vaginal penetration. Men with diabetic ED who have had a penile prosthesis explanted may also be treated successfully with a vacuum constrictor device.[98] To date, the complications from the use of these devices have been minor and self-limited.[93-95,99] They have included difficulty with ejaculation, penile pain, ecchymoses, hematomas, and petechiae. Patients taking aspirin or warfarin are more likely to develop vascular complications. Many of the devices manufactured have a valve that limits the vacuum pressure (<250 mm Hg), a feature that might decrease the complication rate. Patient acceptance and satisfaction with vacuum constrictive devices in all types of impotence, including diabetic impotence, have been reported to be 68% to 83%. The reasons for discontinuation of this treatment have included premature loss of penile tumescence and rigidity, penile pain, pain during ejaculation, and inconvenience.[100]

Second-line therapy is indicated in cases of partial or minimal response to first-line therapy or when the associated side effects are not well tolerated. In addition, a small group of patients may prefer more invasive but efficacious or reliable therapies.

Intraurethral alprostadil is a relatively safe and moderately effective second-line therapy for the treatment of ED. A double-blind, placebo-controlled study of 1511 men showed that 65.9% of patients had erections sufficient for intercourse, and that 50% achieved successful intercourse in the home situation.[101] The most common side effect was penile pain (10.8%), with hypotension-related symptoms the next most common (3.3%).

Intracavernosal Self-Injection

One of the most important advances in the treatment of impotence during the past decade has been that of self-administration by intracavernosal injection of vasoactive agents that either relax the corporeal smooth musculature directly or block adrenergic tone of the corporeal smooth muscle.[102] The pioneering work in this area involved the use of papaverine hydrochloride,[103] a direct smooth-muscle relaxant, or phenoxybenzamine[104] or phentolamine mesylate,[105] both α-adrenergic blocking agents. More recently, the FDA approved two synthetic formulations of PGE_1: alprostadil sterile powder and alprostadil alfadex for intracavernosal administration. They are identical with respect to pharmacology, efficacy, and safety. The majority of responders (85%) required 20 μg or less. A variety of solutions containing the above agents are presently being used in clinical practice.[106,107]

Intracavernosal injections will work best in patients with ED whose arterial inflow and corporeal veno-occlusion mechanism are normal. Patients with ED caused by arterial insufficiency also may respond by virtue of the long-acting and maximal dilator effects provided by this therapy. Patients with ED caused by significant corporeal veno-occlusive dysfunction, however, would be those least likely to respond to such therapy. In general, intracavernosal pharmacotherapy, like vacuum constrictor therapy, can be offered to most patients with organic impotence. When patients are offered intracavernosal pharmacotherapy, they should be informed of the risks and complications of this form of therapy and informed that it will not affect orgasm or ejaculation and that it is used solely for restoration of erectile capabilities. The usual therapeutic goal is for the patient to achieve a rigid erection lasting 30 minutes to 1 hour that is rigid enough for satisfactory vaginal penetration.[108] A dosage-determination phase defines the lowest dose required for the achievement of an appropriate erectile response. To minimize pain and bleeding, an insulin syringe with a 30-gauge needle usually is used. Patients also are taught to compress the site of injection for 3 minutes following injection. Patients are told not to administer an injection more frequently than once a day.

Follow-up information has been obtained on approximately 4000 impotent patients throughout the world, including many with impotence, who have been treated with papaverine alone or in combination with phentolamine.[109] Reported side effects have included hematomas, burning pain after injection, urethral damage, cavernositis or local infections, fibrotic changes of the corpora cavernosa, curvature, and prolonged erections or priapism. Burning pain at the time of injection has been most common with PGE_1 and appears to be less of a problem when PGE_1 is mixed with other agents. The two most important complications are prolonged erections and localized fibrotic changes of the corpora cavernosum. Prolonged erections usually occur during the dosage-determination phase and have been reported in 2.3% to 15% of all patients treated. Patients must be cautioned to call their physician if an erection persists for 4 hours or longer. In the majority of patients, detumescence of these prolonged erections will occur without medical intervention; however, some patients will require an intracavernosal injection of an α-adrenergic agonist.[110]

Following the dosage-determination phase, the complication of prolonged erection is quite rare (less than 1% of injections) and, if treated according to the protocol described above, should not produce any permanent sequelae. The most frequent side effect (reported in 1.5% to 60% of patients treated for 1 year) of intracavernosal pharmacological therapy is the formation of painless fibrotic nodules within the corpora cavernosa, which sometimes leads to penile curvature. In one series, the development of fibrotic nodules was related to the frequency of injection and the duration of treatment.[111] The complications of corporeal fibrosis and prolonged erections have been seen less frequently in men treated with PGE_1 alone. The formation of cavernosal fibrotic nodules is to some extent secondary to trauma and bleeding within the corpus and for this reason the importance of application of compression over the injection site for 3 minutes is stressed. In addition, attempts to decrease the amount of fluid injected are encouraged. Theoretically, these patients should not respond to intracavernosal therapy, but there are several reports that document successful treatment of ED due to corporeal fibrosis with intracavernosal injection of a combination of papaverine and phentolamine.[112] In the first 201 patients treated by Padma-Nathan and colleagues, only three cases (1.5%) of abnormal liver function tests were reported during a mean follow-up period of 26 months.[108] Others have seen essentially no changes in liver function during this therapy, whereas one series reported at least one chemical abnormality of liver function in 40% of patients.

Forskolin, which directly activates the catalytic domain of adenylate cyclase, has demonstrated efficacy as an auxiliary vasoactive agent in a preliminary study of patients who had previously failed high-volume, high-concentration injection therapy.[113] Forskolin is especially useful in patients with diabetes or postradical prostatectomy ED who develop significant corporeal pain with the use of intracavernosal PGE_1 as FDA-approved Caverject and EDEX. Preliminary reports on the use of intracavernosal forskolin, papaverine, and phentolamine as a salvage tri-mix in the management of postradical prostatectomy ED when PGE_1 alone or standard three-agent pharmacotherapy results in clinically significant penile pain showed that 83% of patients had satisfactory and sustained axial rigidity for sexual intercourse. None of these patients experienced corporeal pain. Although penile self-injection therapy is highly effective (70% to 90%), the average dropout rate is 64% (range, 46% to 80%).[114,115] A recent study demonstrated that keeping the cost of therapy low and ensuring patient and partner education and continued support throughout treatment reduce dropout rates.[116]

Third-line therapy (penile prosthesis) should be viewed only as a last-resort therapy in patients with treatment-refractory ED. Despite their significant cost and potential invasiveness, penile prostheses have been associated with high rates of patient satisfaction in several studies.

The urologic subspecialty of ED was developed in the early 1970s, following the development of an intracorporeal penile prosthesis by Small and Carrion[117] and Scott and colleagues.[118] Through the 1970s and early 1980s, the development of penile prostheses proceeded along two distinct lines: the malleable or rigid prosthesis and the multicomponent inflatable prosthesis. Self-contained inflatable devices were introduced more recently. The inflatable devices, unlike the malleable devices, are based on hydraulic principles, thus allowing the patient to inflate and deflate the device to simulate tumescent and nontumescent phases. This provided an improved aesthetic result, especially in the "detumescent" phase, but initially was coupled with relative increases in component failure and reoperation. Activation of the multicomponent inflatable device allows for an increase in penile girth during the "tumescent" phase (Fig. 28-6). Self-contained inflatable devices have been designed to preserve the aesthetic qualities of an inflatable device and combine them with ease of surgical implantation and a potential decrease in component failure. Further ease of implantation of an inflatable device was attained with the introduction of two-piece inflatable devices. Data indicate that surgical success with inflatable penile prosthesis is 95% to 97%,[119,120] but surgical success does not always represent patient satisfaction. A phase 2, multi-institutional, retrospective study, with independently analyzed medical records and questionnaire data from consecutive eligible patients was carried out by seven physician investigators.[121] Among those who returned the questionnaire, 89% of patients with a Mentor Alpha-1, an inflatable device, answered that it fulfilled their expectations as a therapy for ED, including 28% who claimed fulfillment as expected, 31% better than expected, and 30% much better than expected. Satisfaction responses of 80% or greater were noted with regard to intercourse ability and confidence, device rigidity, and

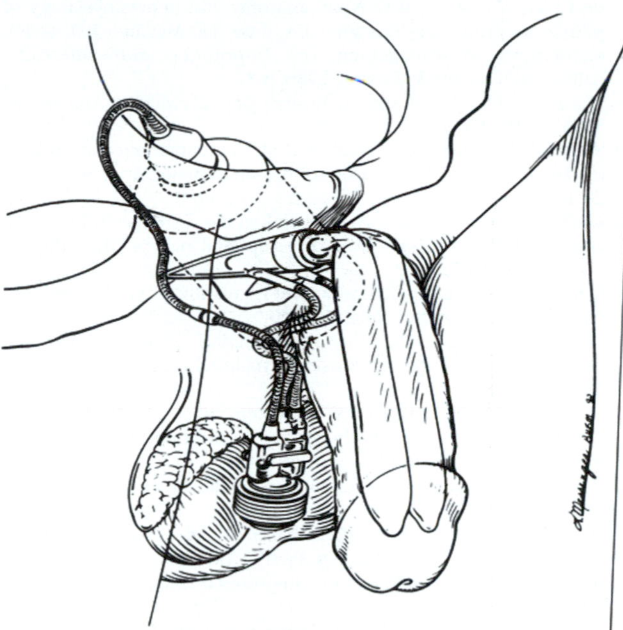

FIGURE 28-6. Inflatable devices are based on hydraulic principles, thus allowing the patient to inflate and deflate the device to simulate tumescent and nontumescent phases. The multicomponent device depicted, a Mentor Alpha-1, allows for an increase in penile girth during the simulated tumescent phase. The three components consist of a reservoir placed in the retropubic space, two penile cylinders placed in the corpora cavernosa, and a pump apparatus with inflate and deflate mechanisms placed in the scrotum. The advantage of this device is its lack of connectors or connector components between the pump and the cylinders, the known high-pressure portion of a hydraulic device.

function. Interestingly, implantation of inflatable penile prosthesis did not result in 80% or greater satisfaction responses in changes in partner relationship (as judged by the patient), feelings of the partner about the relationship (as judged by the patient), or increased confidence in social activities and work. Such information is important when providing preoperative counseling to patients so that postoperative expectations will be appropriate. The ability of the patient to ejaculate and have an orgasm is not altered by the implantation of a prosthesis but in some cases may be restored. The postoperative complications of penile implant surgery usually are relegated to those of component failure, postoperative infection, or device erosion. Probably the most significant complication of prosthetic surgery is infection. The incidence of infections following penile prosthetic surgery ranges between 1% and 9%.[122] Infections with more virulent and aggressive bacteria will manifest usually within the first few postoperative days, with the patient presenting with fever, pain, and swelling overlying the prosthesis, accompanied by purulent wound drainage. However, a group of patients will complain of prolonged pain overlying the device but will have no obvious purulent drainage from the wound. Prolonged pain, fixation of the pump or tubing to the overlying scrotal skin, elevated white blood cell count and sedimentation rate, and hyperglycemia in diabetic patients may all be helpful in diagnosing a possible infection by less virulent organisms. Duplex ultrasound may also be helpful in cases in which clinical findings are not conclusive.[123] The reoperative rate for penile prosthetic surgery has been reported to be between 3% and 44%, with newer series showing a markedly lower rate.[124]

Venous Surgery

At present, most patients who show evidence of corporeal veno-occlusive dysfunction by pharmacocavernosometry and cavernosography should not be considered for surgical and/or radiologic options to increase venous outflow resistance.[125,126] The available procedures have not demonstrated long-term success in impotent diabetic patients.[125,126]

Penile revascularization is currently the only modality of therapy that has the potential to permanently cure patients. The overall goal of penile revascularization surgery is to bypass obstructive arterial lesions in the hypogastric-cavernous arterial bed. Young men, without other vascular risk factors, who have erectile dysfunction of a pure arteriogenic nature represent the ideal patient population for this procedure. All young patients with a history suggestive of trauma-associated impotence (pelvic fractures and perineal trauma) undergo a comprehensive history and physical examination. They have a routine endocrinologic evaluation to ensure adequate circulating levels of testosterone. Duplex ultrasonography provides critical hemodynamic data. Finally, vascular assessment by dynamic infusion cavernosometry/cavernosography (DICC) is required to demonstrate arterial pressure gradients between the brachial artery and the cavernosal arteries and to further evaluate the veno-occlusive function. A selective internal pudendal arteriogram is performed to confirm the location of the obstructive lesion—which is generally in the common penile or cavernosal artery(ies)—and to select the best inferior epigastric artery (Fig. 28-7). The success of this operation is based on the selection of the correct candidate and the microsurgical capabilities of the surgeon. Complications are rare and may include penile pain and

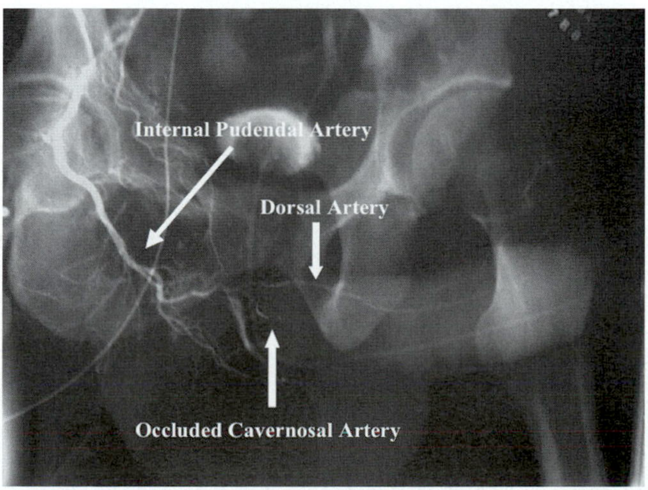

FIGURE 28-7. Selective internal pudendal arteriograms showing a focal cavernosal artery occlusion at the level of the Alcock canal.

diminished penile sensation from injury to the nearby dorsal nerve.[127] Glans hyperemia was a complication seen with inferior epigastric artery to deep dorsal vein anastomoses, a procedure that is no longer performed.[128]

REFERENCES

1. National Institutes of Health Consensus Statement. Development Panel on Impotence. JAMA 270:83, 1993.
2. Goldstein I, Lue T: Oral sildenafil in the treatment of erectile dysfunction. N Engl J Med 338:1397, 1998.
3. Melman A, Gingell J: The epidemiology and pathophysiology of erectile dysfunction. J Urol 161:5, 1999.
4. Krane RJ, Goldstein I, Saenz de Tejada I: Impotence. N Engl J Med 321:1648, 1989.
5. Feldman H, Goldstein I. Impotence and its medical and psychosocial correlates: Results of the Massachusetts Male Aging Study. J Urol 151:457, 1994.
6. Johannes C, Araujo A, Feldman H: Incidence of erectile dysfunction in men 40 to 69 years old: Longitudinal results of the Massachusetts Male Aging Study. J Urol 163:460, 2000.
7. Laumann E, Paik A, Rosen R: Sexual dysfunction in the United States: Prevalence and predictors. JAMA 281:537, 1999.
8. Solstad K, Hertoft P: Frequency of sexual problems and sexual dysfunction in middle-aged Danish men. Arch Sex Behav 22:51, 1993.
9. Malmsten U, Milsom I: Urinary incontinence and lower urinary tract symptoms: An epidemiological study of men aged 45 to 99 years. J Urol 158:1733, 1997.
10. Virag R, Beck-Ardilly L: Nosology, epidemiology and clinical quantification of erectile dysfunctions. Rev Med Interne 18(Suppl 1):S10, 1997.
11. Fedele D, Coscelli C: Incidence of erectile dysfunction in Italian men with diabetes. J Urol 166:1368, 2001.
12. Ledda A: Diabetes, hypertension and erectile dysfunction. Curr Med Res Opin 16(Suppl 1):S17, 1998.
13. Sandoica A, Sanchez E: Impotence in diabetic patients: Detection of prevalence and social/health implications. Aten Primaria 20:435, 1997.
14. Blanker M, Bosh R: Erectile and ejaculatory dysfunction in a community-based sample of men 50 to 78 years old: Prevalence, concern and relation to sexual activity. Urology 57:763, 2001.
15. DENSA Study Group: Prevalence of Male Erectile Dysfunction in Colombia, Ecuador and Venezuela and Epidemiologic Study Including Risk Factors Associated with Erectile Dysfunction. First International Consultation on Erectile Dysfunction and Sexual Dysfunctions. World Health Organization (WHO) and the Union Internationale Contre le Cancer (UICC), Paris, July 1-3, 1998.
16. Nicolosi A, Moreira ED Jr, Shirai M, et al: Epidemiology of erectile dysfunction in four countries: Cross-national study of the prevalence and correlates of erectile dysfunction. Urology 61:201, 2003.
17. Kongkanand A: Prevalence of erectile dysfuction in Thailand. Thai Erectile Dysfunction Epidemiological Study Group. Int J Androl 23(Suppl 2):77, 2000.
18. Akkus E, Carrier S, Baba K, et al: Structural alterations in the tunica albuginea of the penis: Impact of Peyronie's disease, ageing and impotence. Br J Urol 79:47, 1997.
19. Oberpenning F, Roth S, Leusmann DB, et al: The Alcock syndrome: Temporary penile insensitivity due to compression of the pudendal nerve within the Alcock canal. J Urol 151:423, 1994.
20. Hakim LS, Nehra A, Kulaksizoglu H, et al: Penile microvascular arterial bypass surgery. Microsurgery 16: 296, 1995.
21. Breza J, Aboseif SR, Orvis BR, et al: Detailed anatomy of penile neurovascular structures: Surgical significance. J Urol 141:437, 1989.
22. Lue TF, Tanagho EA: Functional anatomy and mechanism of penile erection. In Tanagho EA, Lue TF, McClue RD (eds): Contemporary Management of Impotence and Infertility. Baltimore, Williams & Wilkins, 1988, p 39.
23. Puech-Leao P, Reis JMSM, Glina S, et al: Leakage through the crural edge of corpus cavernosum: Diagnosis and treatment. Eur Urol 13: 163, 1987.
24. Goldstein AMB, Meehan JP, Zakhary R, et al: New observations on microarchitecture of corpora cavernosa in man and possible relationship to mechanism of erection. Urology 20:259, 1982.
25. de Groot WC, Steers WD: Neuroanatomy and neurophysiology of penile erection. In: Tanagho EA, Lue TF, McClue RD (eds): Contemporary Management of Impotence and Infertility. Baltimore, Williams & Wilkins, 1988, p 3.
26. Weiss HD: The physiology of human penile erection. Ann Intern Med 76:793, 1972.
27. Stoleru S, Gregoire MC, Gerard D, et al: Neuroanatomical correlates of visually evoked sexual arousal in human males. Arch Sex Behav 28:1, 1999.
28. Giuliano F, Bernabe J, Brown K, et al: Erectile response to hypothalamic stimulation in rats: Role of peripheral nerves. Am J Physiol 273:R1990, 1997.
29. Giuliano F, Rampin O: Central neural regulation of penile erection. Neurosci Biobehav Rev 24:517, 2000.
30. Marson L, McKenna KE: The identification of a brainstem site controlling spinal sexual reflexes in male rats. Brain Res 515:303, 1990.
31. Saenz de Tejada I, Kim NN, Goldstein I, et al: Regulation of pre-synaptic alpha adrenergic activity in the corpus cavernosum. Int J Impot Res 12(Suppl 1):S20, 2000.
32. Weiss HD: The physiology of human penile erection. Ann Intern Med 76:793, 1972.
33. Hart BL, Leedy MG: Neurological bases of male sexual behavior: A comparative analysis. In Adler N, Pfaff D, Goy RW (eds): Handbook of Behavioral Neurobiology, vol. 7. Reproduction. New York, Plenum, 1985, p 373.
34. MacLean PD, Ploog DW: Cerebral representation of penile erection. J Neurophysiol 25:29, 1962.
35. MacLean PD, Denniston RH, Dua S: Further studies on cerebral representation of penile erection: Caudal thalamus, midbrain, and pons. J Neurophysiol 26:274, 1963.
36. Dua S, MacLean PD: Localization for penile erection in medial frontal lobe. Am J Physiol 207:1425, 1964.
37. Saper CB, Loewy AD, Swanson LW, et al: Direct hypothalamo-autonomic connections. Brain Res 117:305, 1976.
38. Swanson LW, Sawchenko PE: Hypothalamic integration: Organization of the paraventricular and supraoptic nuclei. Annu Rev Neurosci 6:269, 1983.
39. Saenz de Tejada I, Goldstein I, Blanco R, et al: Smooth muscle of the corpora cavernosae: Role in penile erection. Surg Forum 36:623, 1985.
40. Blanco R, Saenz de Tejada I, Goldstein I, et al: Cholinergic neurotransmission in human corpus cavernosum. II. Acetylcholine synthesis. Am J Physiol 254:H468, 1988.
41. Ignarro LJ, Bush PA, Buga GM, et al: Nitric oxide and cyclic GMP formation upon electrical field stimulation cause relaxation of corpus cavernosum smooth muscle. Biochem Biophys Res Comm 170: 843, 1990.
42. Traish AM, Kim NN, Goldstein I, et al: Alpha adrenergic receptors in the penis. J Androl 20:671, 1999.
43. Traish AM, Kim NN, Moreland RB, et al: Proceedings of the International Symposium on Alpha Blockade in Sexual Dysfunction. Int J Impot Res 12(Suppl 1):S1, 2000.
44. Moreland RB, Goldstein I, Kim NN, et al: Sildenafil citrate, a selective phosphodiesterase type 5 inhibitor: Research and clinical implications in erectile dysfunction. Trends Endocrinol Metab 10:97, 1999.
45. Goldstein I, Lue TF, Padma-Nathan H, et al: Oral sildenafil in the treatment of erectile dysfunction. Sildenafil Study Group. N Engl J Med 338:1397, 1998.
46. Gupta S, Moreland RB, Munarriz R, et al: Possible role of Na^+-K^+-ATPase in the regulation of human corpus cavernosum smooth muscle contractility by nitric oxide. Br J Pharmacol 116:2201, 1995.
47. Stamler JS: Redox signaling: nitrosylation and related target interactions of nitric oxide. Cell 78:931, 1994.
48. Schmidt HH, Walter U: NO at work. Cell 78:919, 1994.
49. Blanco R, Saenz de Tejada I, et al: Dysfunctional penile cholinergic nerves in diabetic impotent men. J Urol 144:278, 1990.
50. Lue TF, Zeineh SJ, Schmidt RA, et al: Neuroanatomy of penile erection: Its relevance to iatrogenic impotence. J Urol 131:273, 1984.
51. The process of care model for the evaluation and treatment of erectile dysfunction. The Process of Care Consensus Panel. Int J Impot Res 11:59, 1999.
52. Rosen RC, Riley A, Wagner G, et al: The International Index of Erectile Function (IIEF): A multidimensional scale for assessment of erectile dysfunction. Urology 49:822, 1997.

53. Udelson D, Park K, Sadeghi-Nejad H, et al: Axial penile buckling forces vs. Rigidscan radial rigidity as a function of intracavernosal pressure: Why Rigidscan does not predict functional erections in individual patients. J Impot 11:327, 1999.
54. Abelson D: Diagnostic value of the penile pulse and blood pressure: A Doppler study of impotence in diabetics. J Urol 113:636, 1975.
55. Karacan I: Diagnosis of erectile impotence in diabetes mellitus: An objective and specific method. Ann Intern Med 92:334, 1980.
56. Goldstein I, Siroky MB, Krane RJ: Impotence in diabetes mellitus. In Krane RJ, Siroky MB, Goldstein I (eds): Male Sexual Dysfunction. Boston, Little, Brown, 1983, p 73.
57. Goldstein I, Krane RJ, Greenfield AJ, et al: Vascular diseases of the penis: Impotence and priapism. In Pollack HM (ed): Clinical Urography, vol 3. Philadelphia, WB Saunders, 1990, p 2231.
58. Gasior BL, Levine FJ, Howannesian A, et al: Plaque-associated corporal veno-occlusive dysfunction in idiopathic Peyronie's disease: A pharmacocavernosometric and pharmacocavernosographic study. World J Urol 8:90, 1990.
59. Penson DF, Seftel AD, Krane RJ, et al: The hemodynamic pathophysiology of impotence following blunt trauma to the erect penis. J Urol 148:1171, 1992.
60. Wilson JD, Griffin JE: The use and misuse of androgens. Metabolism 29:1278, 1980.
61. Snyder PJ, Lawrence DA: Treatment of male hypogonadism with testosterone enanthate. J Clin Endocrinol Metab 51:1335, 1980.
62. Jackson JA, Waxman J, Spiekerman AM: Prostatic complications of testosterone replacement therapy. Arch Intern Med 149:2365, 1989.
63. Carter JN, Tyson JE, Tolis G, et al: Prolactin-secreting tumors and hypogonadism in 22 men. N Engl J Med 299:847, 1978.
64. Franks S, Jacobs HS, Martin N, et al: Hyperprolactinaemia and impotence. Clin Endocrinol 8:277, 1978.
65. FDA submission. Viagra labeling information. New York, Pfizer, 1997.
66. Salonia A, Rigatti P, Montorsi F: Sildenafil in erectile dysfunction: A critical review. Curr Med Res Opin 19:241, 2003.
67. Cheitlin MD, Hutter AM, Jr, Brindis RG, et al: ACC/AHA expert document. Use of sildenafil (Viagra) in patients with clinical risk from cardiovascular disease. A report of the American College of Cardiology/American Heart Association Task Force. J Heart Valve Dis 7(6):672, 1998.
68. Moreira SG, Brannigan RE, Spitz A, et al: Side-effect profile of sildenafil citrate (Viagra) in clinical practice. Urology 56:474, 2000.
69. Carson CC, Burnett AL, Levine LA, et al: The efficacy of sildenafil citrate (Viagra) in clinical populations: An update. Urology 60(2 Suppl 2):12, 2002.
70. Fowler CJ, Miller J, Sharief M: ViagraÒ (sildenafil citrate) for the treatment of erectile dysfunction in men with multiple sclerosis. Ann Neurol 46:497, 1999.
71. Griffith ER, Tomoko MA, Timms RJ: Sexual function in spinal cord-injured patients: A review. Arch Phys Med Rehabil 54:539, 1973.
72. YenicerioGlu Y, Kefi A, Aslan G, et al: Efficacy and safety of sildenafil for treating erectile dysfunction in patients on dialysis. BJU Int 90:442, 2002.
73. Rendell MS, Rajfer J, Wicker PA, et al: Sildenafil for the treatment of erectile dysfunction in men with diabetes. JAMA 281:421, 1999.
74. Kim NN, Huang YH, Goldstein I, et al: Inhibition of cyclic GMP hydrolysis in human corpus cavernosum smooth muscle cells by vardenafil, a novel, selective phosphodiesterase type 5 inhibitor. Life Sci 69:2249, 2001.
75. Klotz T, Bauer R-J, Rohde G, et al: Effect of renal impairment on the single-dose pharmacokinetics of vardenafil 20 mg, a selective PDE5 inhibitor, for the treatment of erectile dysfunction. Pharmacotherapy 22:418, 2002.
76. Rohde G, Wensing G, Sachse R. The pharmacokinetics of vardenafil, a new selective PDE5 inhibitor, are not affected by the antacid, Maalox 70TM. Pharmacotherapy 21:1254, 2001.
77. Ormrod D, Easthope SE, Figgitt DP: Vardenafil. Drugs Aging 19:217, 2002.
78. Porst H, Rosen R, Padma-Nathan H, et al: Vardenafil Study Group. The efficacy and tolerability of vardenafil, a new oral selective phosphodiesterase type 5 inhibitor, in patients with erectile dysfunction: The first at-home clinical trial. Int J Impot Res 13:192, 2001.
79. Stark S, Sachse R, Leidl T, et al: Vardenafil increases penile rigidity and tumescence in men with erectile dysfunction after a single oral dose. Eur Urol 40:189, 2001.
80. Hellstrom WJ, Gittelman M, Karlin G, et al: Vardenafil for treatment of men with erectile dysfunction: Efficacy and safety in a randomized, double-blind, placebo-controlled trial. J Androl. 23(6):763, 2002.
81. Goldstein I, Young JM, Fischer J, et al: Vardenafil, a new phosphodiesterase type 5 inhibitor, in the treatment of erectile dysfunction in men with diabetes: A multicenter double-blind placebo-controlled fixed-dose study. Diabetes Care 26:777, 2003.
82. Brock G, Taylor T, Seger M: Efficacy and tolerability of vardenafil in men with erectile dysfunction following radical prostatectomy [abstract 598]. European Urology Supplements 1:152, 2002.
83. Porst H, Giuliano F, Meuleman E, et al: Daily IC 351 treatment of ED. In Program and Abstracts of the Second Fall Meeting of the Society for the Study of Impotence, Cleveland, OH, [abst B13], 2000.
84. Margolis R, Prieto P, Stein L, et al: Statistical summary of 10,000 male cases using Afrodex in treatment of impotence. Curr Ther Res 13:616, 1971.
85. Morales A, Condra M, Owen JA, et al: Is yohimbine effective in the treatment of organic impotence? Results of a controlled trial. J Urol 137:1168, 1987.
86. Morales A, Condra MS, Owen JE, et al: Oral and transcutaneous pharmacologic agents in the treatment of impotence. Urol Clin North Am 15:87, 1988.
87. Goldstein I, Carson C, Rosen R, et al: Vasomax for the treatment of male erectile dysfunction. World J Urol 19:51, 2001.
88. Becker AJ, Stief CG, Machtens S, et al: Oral phentolamine as treatment for erectile dysfunction. J Urol 159:1214, 1998.
89. Morales A, Heaton J, Johnston B, et al: Oral and topical treatment of erectile dysfunction: Present and future. Urol Clin North Am 22:879, 1995.
90. Padma-Natham H, Auerbach S, Lewis R, et al: Efficacy and safety of apomorphine SL vs. placebo for male erectile dysfunction. J Urol 161:214.
91. Dula E, Keating W, Siami PF, et al: Efficacy and safety of fixed-dose and dose-optimization regimens of sublingual apomorphine versus placebo in men with erectile dysfunction. The Apomorphine Study Group. Urology 56:130, 2000.
92. Goldstein I, Payton T, Schechter PJ: A double-blind, placebo-controlled, efficacy and safety study of topical gel formulation1% alprostadil (Topiglan) for the in-office treatment of erectile dysfunction. Urology 57:301, 2001.
93. Nadig PW, Ware JC, Blumoff R: Noninvasive device to produce and maintain an erection-like state. Urology 27:126, 1986.
94. Nadig PW: Vacuum erection devices: A review. World J Urol 8:114, 1990.
95. Witherington R: External penile appliances for management of impotence. Semin Urol 8:124, 1990.
96. Diederichs W, Kaula NF, Lue TF, et al: The effect of subatmospheric pressure on the simian penis. J Urol 142:1087, 1989.
97. Wespes E, Schulman CC: Hemodynamic study of the effect of vacuum device on human erection. Int J Impot Res 2:337, 1990.
98. Moul JW, McLeod DG: Negative pressure devices in the explanted penile prosthesis population. J Urol 142:729, 1989.
99. Witherington R: Vacuum constriction device for management of erectile impotence. J Urol 141:320, 1989.
100. Sidi AA, Becher EF, Zhang G, et al: Patient acceptance of and satisfaction with an external negative pressure device for impotence. J Urol 144:1154, 1990.
101. Padma-Natham H, Hellstrom WJ, Kaiser FE, et al: Treatment of men with erectile dysfunction with transurethral alprostadil. Medicated urethral system for erection. N Engl J Med 336:7, 1997.
102. Juenemann K-P, Lue TF, Fournier GR, Jr, et al: Hemodynamics of papaverine- and phentolamine-induced penile erection. J Urol 136:158, 1986.
103. Virag R: Intracavernous injection of papaverine for erectile failure (Letter). Lancet 2:938, 1982.
104. Brindley GS: Pilot experiments on the actions of drugs injected into the human corpus cavernosum penis. Br J Pharmacol 87:495, 1986.
105. Zorgniotti AW, Lefleur RS: Auto-injection of the corpus cavernosum with a vasoactive drug combination for vasculogenic impotence. J Urol 133:39, 1985.
106. Stackl W, Hasun R, Marberger M: Intracavernous injection of prostaglandin E1 in impotent men. J Urol 140:66, 1988.
107. Lee LM, Stevenson RWD, Szasz G: Prostaglandin E1 versus phentolamine/papaverine for the treatment of erectile impotence: A double-blind comparison. J Urol 141:549, 1989.
108. Padma-Nathan H, Goldstein I, Payton T, Krane RJ: Intracavernosal pharmacotherapy: The pharmacologic erection program. World J Urol 5:160, 1987.

109. Zentgraf M, Baccouche M, Jünemann KP: Diagnosis and therapy of erectile dysfunction using papaverine and phentolamine. Urol Int 43:65, 1988.
110. Padma-Nathan H, Goldstein I, Krane RJ: Treatment of prolonged or priapistic erections following intracavernosal papaverine therapy. Semin Urol 4:236, 1986.
111. Levine SB, Althof SE, Turner LA, et al: Side effects of self-administration of intracavernous papaverine and phentolamine for the treatment of impotence. J Urol 141:54, 1989.
112. Lakin MM, Montague DK: Intracavernous injection therapy in post-priapism cavernosal fibrosis. J Urol 140:828, 1988.
113. Mulhall JP, Daller M, Traish AM, et al: Intracavernosal forskolin: Role in management of vasculogenic impotence resistant to standard 3-agent pharmacotherapy. J Urol 1768, 1997.
114. Fallon B: Intracavernous injection therapy for male erectile dysfunction. Urol Clin North Am 22:833, 1995.
115. Mulhall JP: Intracavernosal injection therapy: A practical guide. Tech Urol 3:129, 1997.
116. Mulhall JP, Jahoda AE, Cairney M, et al: The causes of patient dropout from penile self-injection therapy for impotence. J Urol 162:1291, 1999.
117. Small MP, Carrion HM: A new penile prosthesis for treating impotence. Contemp Surg 7:29, 1975.
118. Scott FB, Bradley WE, Timm GW: Management of erectile impotence: Use of implantable inflatable prosthesis. Urology 2:80, 1973.
119. Merril DC: Mentro inflatable penile prosthesis. Urol Clin North Am 16:51, 1989.
120. Furlow WL, Motley RC: The inflatable penile prosthesis: Clinical experience with a new controlled expansion cylinder. J Urol 139:945, 1988.
121. Goldstein I, Newman L, Baum N, et al: Safety and efficacy outcome of Mentor Alpha-1 inflatable penile prosthesis implantation for impotence treatment. J Urol 157:833, 1997.
122. Carson CC: Infections in genitourinary prostheses. Urol Clin North Am 16:139, 1989.
123. Munarriz RM, McAuley I, Maitland S, et al: The diagnosis of penile prosthesis infection using duplex doppler ultrasound. In Program and Abstracts of the Second Fall Meeting of the Society for the Study of Impotence, [abstract A44]. Cleveland, Ohio, 2000.
124. Munarriz RM, Irwin Goldstein I: Experience with the Mentor Alpha-1. Urologic prosthetics. Humana, 2001, p. 101.
125. Sharlip ID: The role of vascular surgery in arteriogenic and combined arteriogenic and venogenic impotence. Semin Urol 8:129, 1990.
126. Bar-Moshé O, Vandendris M: Treatment of impotence due to perineal venous leakage by ligation of crura penis. J Urol 139:1217, 1988.
127. Zorgniotti AW, Lizza EF: Complications of penile revascularization. In Zorgniotti AW, Lizza EF (eds): Diagnosis and Management of Impotence. Philadelphia, BC Decker, 1991.
128. Hatzichristou DG, Goldstein I: Arterial bypass surgery for impotence. Curr Opin Urol 1:114, 1991.

chapter 29

Epidemiology of Cerebrovascular Disease*

Philip A. Wolf
William B. Kannel

More effective medical and surgical therapies to reduce the damage from impending or recent-onset stroke have recently emerged that are effective and continue to be pursued. Prevention, however, is the most effective strategy to reduce the disabling and economic consequences of cerebrovascular disease. Prevention of strokes requires knowledge of modifiable predisposing lifestyles, and personal attributes and identification of high-risk candidates for preventive treatment. Epidemiologic research has provided such information, and controlled clinical trials have demonstrated the effectiveness of modification of the identified predisposing factors in stroke prevention. In this chapter, data obtained from a number of prospective observational studies of populations will be presented. Assessment of predisposing risk factors measured systematically and prospectively in a variety of population samples prior to the appearance of disease provides an undistorted evaluation of the impact of these risk factors on stroke incidence.

Population-based epidemiologic research is also the best source of data on the prevalence, incidence, disability, and cost of cerebrovascular disease. It also provides valuable insights into the pathogenesis of the disease and secular trends in the magnitude of the problem.

SIZE OF THE PROBLEM

Stroke is the most common life-threatening neurologic disease and the third leading cause of death in the United States, exceeded only by heart disease and cancer. It is responsible for one of every 15 deaths. Despite being more often disabling than lethal, 167,660 deaths were attributed to stroke in 2000.[1] In 2000, the American Heart Association estimated that there were 500,000 initial strokes, 200,000 stroke recurrences, and 4,700,000 stroke survivors in the United States, many of whom required chronic care.[2] The problem is escalating in the United States, where in 1991 there were 3,060,000 stroke survivors.[1] Among the elderly, the segment of the population in which stroke occurs most frequently, it is a major cause of disability requiring long-term institutionalization. It is estimated that by 2015 the elderly population (>65 years) will increase to 14% of the population, up 2.3% from 1900. This growth in the elderly population will be a source of continuing disability from stroke unless vigorous effective preventive measures can be more aggressively implemented.

INCIDENCE OF STROKE

Valid stroke incidence data should be ascertained by systematic evaluation of a general population sample determined to be free of the disease at outset. Ideally, the population under study should be representative, allowing generalization of the findings. It is seldom feasible to recruit, and follow prospectively, a large sample of individuals who are representative of persons of an entire nation, state, or province. By accumulating data derived from a number of such general population samples, however, a more complete picture of the incidence and distribution of conditions such as stroke may be ascertained.

National data on stroke incidence are difficult to interpret because of incomplete case ascertainment, nonrepresentative samples, and failure to separate recurrent from initial strokes. A more accurate estimate of the true incidence is available from the Framingham Study. The incidence of stroke was ascertained from the Framingham prospective study of cardiovascular disease (CVD) over 55 years of follow-up of 5184 men and women, ages 30 to 62, who were free of stroke at entry to the study in 1950. The population sample has been reexamined every 2 years with approximately 85% of subjects participating in each examination. Since 1968, while hospitalized, suspected strokes were evaluated by the Framingham Study neurologist to confirm the cases. Prior to that year, hospital records (containing other neurologists' evaluations) provided confirmation. Since 1982, 91.5% of stroke victims had at least one CT scan or MRI scan of the brain and arteries. Confirmation by CT/MRI study was provided in 61% of cases. As a result, it has been possible to distinguish clearly hemorrhage from infarction and to classify the ischemic stroke events into lacunar, large artery, cardio-embolic, and infarct of undetermined cause subtypes with reasonable assurance using established criteria.[3] Follow-up of the population was satisfactory, with only about 7% lost to follow-up.

*This work was supported in part by the National Institute of Neurological Disorders and Stroke Grant No. 5R01 NS17950 and the National Heart, Lung, and Blood Institute's Framingham Heart Study Contract No. N01-HC-25195.

TABLE 29-1 ANNUAL INCIDENCE OF ATHEROTHROMBOTIC BRAIN INFARCTION (ABI) AND COMPLETED STROKES

	MEN		WOMEN		MEN/WOMEN COMBINED	
Age	*n*	Rate/ 1000	*n*	Rate/ 1000	*n*	Rate/ 1000
ABI						
35-44	1	0.12	1	0.1	2	0.11
45-54	15	0.97	13	0.67	28	0.81
55-64	37	1.94	35	1.4	72	1.64
65-74	80	5.14	68	3	148	3.87
75-84	79	9.06	119	7.52	198	8.07
85-94	16	8.64	72	13.79	88	12.44
Total	228	*3.60	308	*2.90	536	3.21
Completed Stroke						
35-44	3	0.37	3	0.3	6	0.33
45-54	25	1.61	20	1.04	45	1.29
55-64	60	3.15	60	2.41	120	2.73
65-74	127	8.16	115	5.08	242	6.33
75-84	126	14.45	203	12.83	329	13.41
85-94	30	16.21	121	23.18	151	21.35
Total	371	*5.89	522	*4.91	893	5.35

*Age-adjusted.
Unpublished data from the Framingham Heart Study: 55-year follow-up, PA Wolf, principal investigator.

During 55 years of follow-up, there were 893 cases of initial completed strokes and 152 instances of isolated transient ischemic attacks (TIA) observed to occur in the Framingham Study. The average annual stroke incidence (all varieties combined) approximately doubled with each successive age decade (Table 29-1). Overall, the annual age-adjusted (ages 35 to 94 years) total initial completed stroke event rates were 5.9/1000 in men and 4.9/1000 in women; a 20% excess in men (see Table 29-1). The annual age-adjusted incidence of isolated TIA also increased with age, and was 1.2/1000 in men and 0.71/1000 in women.

Comparing analogous myocardial infarction (MI) and ischemic stroke without a clear cardiac source for emboli atherothrombotic brain infarction (ABTI) provides some perspective (Fig. 29-1). In men, the age-adjusted average annual incidence rate of MI was 4 times that of ABTI; in women, MI incidence was only 1.6 times that of ABTI. In both sexes, rates doubled with each advancing decade, but the 20-year advantage of women over men in incidence of MI observed was not seen for ABTI, where age-specific rates were similar.

Recurrence of strokes is a major contributor to the disability, mortality, and cost of cerebrovascular disease.[4] Approximately 25% of persons hospitalized for a stroke have had a prior overt stroke. Of the 500,000 strokes that occur each year, 200,000 are recurrences. Risk of a second stroke is substantially increased in persons who have sustained an initial stroke or TIA. In the Framingham Study, the 5-year stroke recurrence rate after an ABTI was 42% for men and 24% for women.[5]

TIME OF ONSET

Stroke registries and prospective population studies indicate that there is a disproportionate rate of ischemic stroke occurrence after awakening between 6 AM and noon.[6] An increased rate of intracerebral hemorrhage has been reported in men who drink, possibly reflecting binge drinking on the weekend.[7]

STROKE PREVALENCE

From health interviews it is estimated that more than 3 million Americans have symptomatic cerebrovascular disease. National data indicate that stroke prevalence increases with age, and beyond age 65 years is more prevalent in men than in women. Its prevalence is much higher in blacks (2.6%) than in whites (1.6%) for ages 25 to 74 years (Fig. 29-2).[8]

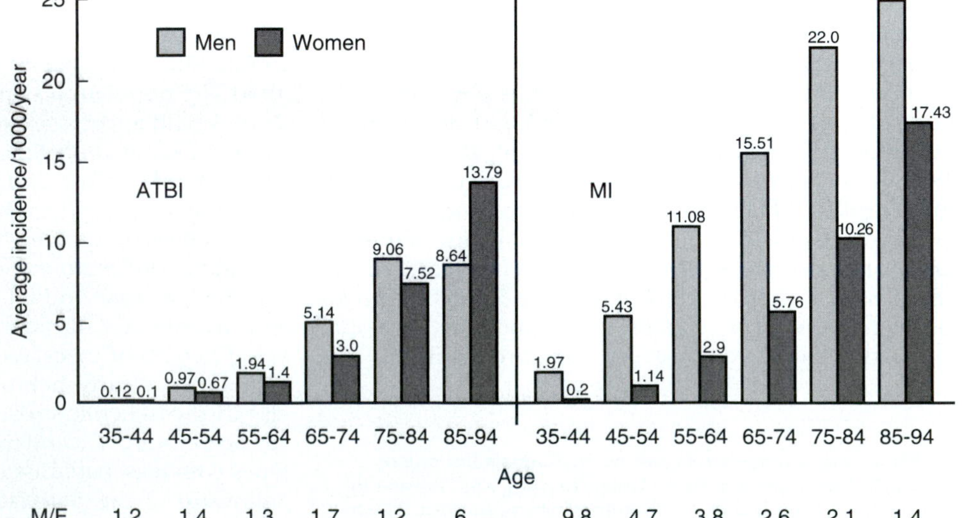

FIGURE 29-1. Incidence of atherothrombotic brain infarction (ABTI) and myocardial infarction (MI), 50-year follow-up. (Data from the Framingham Heart Study.)

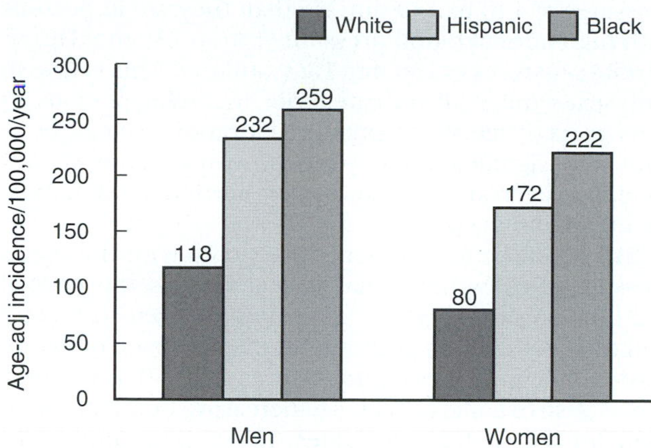

FIGURE 29-2. Stroke incidence—race/ethnicity. NOrthern MAnhattan Stroke Study (NOMASS). (Adapted from Sacco RL, Boden-Albala B, Gan R, et al: Stroke incidence among whites, blacks, and Hispanics from the same community of northern Manhattan. Am J Epidemiol 147:260, 1998.)

STROKE MORTALITY

Between 1962 and 1992, the CVD death rate declined 62% in sharp contrast to a modest 16% decline in noncardiovascular mortality.[9] About 70% of the decrease in total mortality was due to a decline in deaths from CVD. Coronary heart disease (CHD) and stroke mortality each declined about 65%. Declines in CVD mortality have continued since 1965, with an average annual percent decline in stroke mortality of 2.1%. Between 1990 and 1998, the stroke mortality decline was greater in blacks than in whites (same as above). In 1995 to 1997 stroke mortality was highest in the southeastern states that comprise the "stroke belt."

Hospital case-fatality rates for stroke declined substantially between 1971 and the mid-1980s and more modestly since that time.[10] The short-term, intermediate, and long-term adjusted mortality rates were investigated in the Department of Veterans Affairs care system in veterans who had experienced an initial hemorrhagic or ischemic stroke. These investigators found a 30-day mortality rate of 7.4% and 18.8% for ischemic and hemorrhagic strokes, respectively. The adjusted 90-day mortality rate for ischemic stroke was 11.4% and, for 1 year, 19.1%. The adjusted mortality rate for 30-day survivors of a hemorrhagic stroke was 5.6% for 30 to 90 days and 7.3% for 3 months to 1 year.[11] Between 1986 and 1996, 20 countries had greater declines in stroke mortality than the United States.[12]

STROKE FREQUENCY BY TYPE

In-hospital assessment of the strokes occurring in the Framingham Study by its neurologist provides credible data on subtypes of stroke. Diagnosis of lacunar infarction was based on clinical and brain CT- and MRI-scan findings. Criteria for embolic infarction required a definite cardiac source for embolism. Cerebral infarction from extracranial versus intracranial arterial disease was distinguished on clinical grounds—relying on noninvasive carotid studies

TABLE 29-2 FREQUENCY OF COMPLETE STROKE BY TYPE IN MEN AND WOMEN AGES 35-94 YEARS

Completed Stroke	Men	%	Women	%	Total	%
Atherothrombotic brain infarction	228	61.5	308	59	536	60
Cerebral embolus	87	23.5	137	26.2	224	25.1
Subarachnoid hemorrhage	20	5.4	28	5.4	48	5.4
Intracerebral hemorrhage	32	8.6	42	8	74	8.3
Other	4	1.1	7	1.3	11	1.2
Total	371	100	522	100	893	100

Unpublished data from the Framingham Heart Study: 55-Year follow-up, PA Wolf, principal investigator.

and magnetic resonance angiography. Contrast angiography was requested by the subjects' personal physicians, chiefly in cases of extracranial carotid stenosis prior to endarterectomy or with subarachnoid hemorrhage. TIA was systematically ascertained by routine questioning on each biennial examination and by scrutiny of physician records and hospital notes. Approximately 15% of ABTIs were preceded by TIAs, and isolated TIAs not followed by a stroke accounted for 14.8% of total cerebrovascular events in men and 12.7% of events in women.

The frequency of completed strokes by type was nearly identical in men and women (Table 29-2). ABTI (including infarction secondary to large vessel atherothrombosis, lacunar infarction, and infarct of undetermined cause) accounted for 61.5% of strokes in men and 60.0% in women. Extracranial large artery disease accounted for approximately 12% of stroke events. Intracranial hemorrhage, accounted for 14.0% of completed strokes in men and 13.4% in women. Age-adjusted annual incidence rates of IH were somewhat higher in men than in women (0.52 versus 0.38 per 1000), but rates of subarachnoid hemorrhage were not appreciably different (0.29 per 1000 in men and 0.28 in women). The relative frequency of intracranial hemorrhage and subarachnoid hemorrhage varies according to the age of the population sample studied, with subarachnoid hemorrhage predominating in those younger than age 65, but roughly the same at ages 65 to 74 years. At ages 75 to 84 years, intracranial hemorrhage predominated with an annual incidence of 1.26 per 1000 compared with 0.29 per 1000 for subarachnoid hemorrhage.

PREDISPOSING SYSTEMIC ATHEROSCLEROSIS

Having another clinical manifestation of CVD, such as peripheral arterial disease, MI or heart failure, substantially increases the risk of a stroke (see Table 29-2). For example, having peripheral arterial disease imposes a 20% 10-year probability of having a stroke. Carotid intima-media thickness is strongly associated with atheroma elsewhere in the carotid arteries, the coronary arteries, and the abdominal aorta, reflecting systemic atherosclerosis.[13]

The Framingham Study has shown that a carotid bruit predicts other atherosclerotic CVD events about as well as it predicts a stroke; and, when strokes occur, they are as likely to be brain infarcts on the contralateral as on the ipsilateral side.

RISK FACTORS FOR STROKE

Epidemiologic identification of risk factors for stroke, and assessment of their relative importance and of their interaction, can facilitate stroke prevention. Because the pathogenic process differs, it is reasonable to expect that risk factors for infarction differ from those for hemorrhage, and precursors of intraparenchymatous bleeding differ from those for subarachnoid hemorrhage. In addition, risk factors for stroke from atherosclerosis of the carotid and vertebral arteries may well differ in their impact when compared with stroke resulting from lacunar infarction. Precursors of embolic stroke are also likely to be different. Nevertheless, certain predisposing factors, particularly elevated blood pressure, are common to most stroke types.

Atherogenic Risk Factors

A number of modifiable atherogenic stroke risk factors were identified from the Framingham and other prospective epidemiologic studies. These risk factors include elevated blood pressure, diabetes mellitus, fibrinogen and other clotting factors, obesity, and several recently recognized factors, such as homocysteine and indices of inflammation. Ethnicity, age, and family history are cardinal nonmodifiable markers of increased vulnerability. Predisposing cardiac diseases include CHD, congestive heart failure, atrial fibrillation, left ventricular hypertrophy (LVH), and echocardiographic abnormalities.

Hypertension

Hypertension is the principal risk factor for ischemic stroke and intracerebral hemorrhage. It is commonly believed that hypertension is a stronger risk factor for hemorrhagic than for ischemic stroke; however, data from the Framingham Study and the large (17 studies; 115,757 participants and 1652 strokes) Eastern Stroke and CHD Project indicate an almost identical relationship of diastolic blood pressure risk ratios to ischemic and hemorrhagic strokes.[14] Hypertension also promotes stroke- predisposing cardiac conditions, notably MI and atrial fibrillation, inciting cerebral embolism. Thus, hypertension serves the unique role of being a prime risk factor for all major types of stroke.

Components and Level of Blood Pressure

Among hypertensive persons, the incidences of stroke and ABTI increase with the magnitude of the systolic blood pressure. Incidences of initial strokes, generally, and ABTI, in particular, are approximately 3 times greater in persons with systolic blood pressures greater than or equal to 160 mm Hg and 50% higher at systolic pressures of 140 to 159 mm Hg than they are in persons with high-normal blood pressure (130 to 139 mm Hg) or normal pressures (<130 mm Hg systolic).[15] This is true in both sexes and in all age categories, including persons 75 to 84 years of age. Blood pressure elevation makes a powerful and significant independent contribution to ABI incidence even after age and other pertinent risk factors are taken into account.

Risk of stroke increases incrementally with the blood pressure, even within what is regarded as the normal and high-normal range.[16,14] This applies even to carotid wall thickness which is greater in the presence of hypertension.[17] Framingham Study data indicate that the incidence of stroke increases with increasing blood pressure from lowest to highest values. There is a continuous graded epidemiologic link between blood pressure and risk of a stroke in that each 5-mm Hg increment in diastolic blood pressure confers a 33% increase in stroke incidence, and a 10- to 12-mm Hg increase in systolic blood pressure imposes a 38% increment in risk. Most initial stroke events, however, occur in persons with mild hypertension (systolic blood pressure 140 to 159 mm Hg). In fact, approximately one half of the initial stroke events in the Framingham cohort occurred in subjects with pressures in the high-normal or mild hypertension categories.

Traditionally, greater importance has been ascribed to the diastolic than to the systolic pressure component. Although most clinical trials of hypertension treatment have focused on diastolic blood pressure control, there is no evidence that the diastolic blood pressure exerts a greater influence on stroke rates than the systolic pressure. In fact, the systolic pressure exerts a greater influence, particularly in advanced age when most strokes occur.[18] With advancing age, systolic blood pressure continues to rise into the eighth decade, whereas diastolic pressure declines after reaching a plateau in the early 50s. This leads to isolated systolic hypertension and a widening pulse pressure that has been shown to be a hazard for the occurrence of stroke, particularly after age 65 years.

Isolated Systolic Hypertension

In the elderly, isolated systolic hypertension, (≥160/<90 mm Hg), becomes highly prevalent, affecting approximately 25% of persons older than 80 years. In fact, about 65% of the hypertension in the elderly is of this type. In the Framingham Study, men with isolated systolic hypertension had more than a doubled risk of stroke and women a 1.8-fold increased risk. The Physician's Health Study found that borderline isolated[19] systolic hypertension in healthy men confers an increased pulse pressure, which multivariable analysis of the SHEP data showed to be an important independent predictor of CVD in older persons, including stroke.[20] A 10-mm Hg increase in pulse pressure was associated with a 24% increase in the risk of a stroke—even after controlling for the systolic blood pressure.

Duration of Exposure

Stroke risk predictions are generally based on measurement of current blood pressure; however, the duration of the blood pressure elevation, as well as its magnitude contribute to cardiovascular risk. Using 50 years of Framingham blood pressure data, it was evident that elevated mid-life blood pressure during the prior 10 years increased the relative risk of stroke.[21] These data confirm clinical experience as well as prior prospective epidemiologic data that, at any current level of pressure, persons with evidence of prior elevated blood pressure are at increased risk of stroke.

Predisposition to Stroke Recurrence

Data from the Stroke Data Bank in 1989 showed that hypertension is a determinant of 30-day stroke recurrence,[22] but its influence on late stroke recurrence was not consistently found.[23-25] The United Kingdom Transient Ischemic Attack (UK-TIA) trial, however, provides compelling data supporting the importance of elevated blood pressure as a risk factor for a secondary stroke after a minor stroke or TIA.[26,27] A direct, continuous relationship between recurrent stroke and systolic and diastolic blood pressures was observed with no evidence to support the existence of a J-curve. Several recent clinical trials have demonstrated reduced stroke recurrence following reduction of blood pressure in stroke survivors. Indapamide, a thiazide diuretic, alone or in combination with the angiotensin-converting enzyme inhibitor, perindopril, in two randomized clinical trials, resulted in an approximate 28% risk reduction in stroke recurrence.[27,28]

BLOOD LIPIDS

For coronary artery disease, epidemiologic data indicate a stepwise increase in incidence in relation to the serum total cholesterol, a relationship that holds in both men and women and persists after accounting for other risk factors. The impact of total cholesterol, however, declines with advancing age. The total to HDL-cholesterol ratio, which best reflects the atherogenic lipid potential, has a significant impact on CHD incidence until age 80. For stroke, in general, and for nonembolic ischemic stroke, in particular, no consistent relationship to blood lipid levels has been found. The Atherosclerosis Risk in Communities Study found only weak and inconsistent associations between ischemic stroke and each of five lipid factors in 305 subjects developing ischemic strokes after 10 years of prospective follow-up.[29] These findings have been corroborated by analyses using Framingham Heart Study and Cardiovascular Health Study data.[30] Additionally, in a meta-analysis of 45 prospective epidemiologic studies comprising 450,000 subjects among whom 13,000 strokes occurred, no significant association between total serum cholesterol and total stroke incidence was seen.[31] Exceptions to these unexpected negative findings were noted, however, by the Honolulu Heart Study of Hawaiian men of Japanese ancestry and the Multiple Risk Factor Intervention Trial (MRFIT).[32] In Honolulu, total cholesterol measured years before was directly related to the incidence of cerebral thromboembolism.[33] In MRFIT, incidence of ischemic stroke, diagnosed on death certificates, was greater in those with the highest levels of serum total cholesterol obtained 6 years earlier.

In contrast to the inconsistent epidemiologic data on the impact of blood lipids on atherothrombotic stroke incidence, serum total cholesterol and LDL-cholesterol levels have been directly related to extent of extracranial carotid artery atherosclerosis with HDL-cholesterol exerting a protective effect. These relationships also apply to extracranial carotid artery wall thickness.[34-36]

In view of the equivocal association of blood lipids to incidence of ischemic stroke, the finding of a significant reduction in stroke incidence was unexpected in a series of trials of statins in patients with clinical CHD.[37-40] Trial data show a surprising benefit of treating dyslipidemia for prevention of stroke. The magnitude of the beneficial effect was 20% to 30%—little different from the benefit for CHD.[37,41,42] This has led to speculation that the benefit associated with statins is related to effects other than improving the lipid profile. These include the anti-inflammatory effects leading to plaque stabilization as well as a positive impact on the fibrinolytic system and platelet function. They clearly exert a salutary influence on endothelial function and may provide some degree of neuroprotection by upregulating eNOS activity.[43]

Low Cholesterol and Hemorrhage

Although reduction of serum cholesterol appears to reduce the risk of stroke, low total serum cholesterol has been associated with an increased incidence of intracerebral hemorrhage.[44,45] This was first noted in rural Japanese following World War II who had very low serum cholesterol levels by Western standards (i.e., less than 160 mg/dl).[46] As nutrition improved, intake of animal fat increased and sodium chloride intake fell, and an increase in total serum cholesterol was observed in this population.[46] Total serum protein levels and relative weight also rose significantly during these 20 years, whereas systolic and diastolic blood pressures declined. Accompanying these substantial changes in risk factor levels was a remarkable decline in the incidence of intracerebral hemorrhage, which fell 65% in men ($P < .05$) and 94% in women ($P < .001$) in the 15-year period from 1964 to 1968 to 1979 to 1983.[46]

An etiologic link has been suggested by the recent confirmation of this relationship in other Asian populations, in Hawaiian Japanese, and in white men in the United States. In 350,977 men screened for entry into the Multiple Risk Factor Intervention Trial (MRFIT), there were 83 deaths from intracerebral hemorrhage and 55 deaths from subarachnoid hemorrhage after 6 years of follow-up.[32] In the lowest serum cholesterol category, (<160 mg/dl), there was a significant excess occurrence of intracerebral hemorrhage. This adverse effect of a low serum cholesterol was confined to those with an elevated diastolic blood pressure.[32] An alteration in the cell membranes, which weakens the endothelium of intracerebral arteries, is the suggested mechanism. However, despite early concerns, no significant increases in intracerebral hemorrhage rates have been noted in the many trials using statins to reduce total and LDL-cholesterol levels.[47]

DIABETES

Diabetics have an increased susceptibility to coronary, femoral, and cerebral artery atherosclerosis—up to 80% of type 2 diabetics develop or die of macrovascular disease. Hypertension is twice as common in diabetics as in the normal population, affecting about 60% of them.[48,49] Approximately 80% of persons who have diabetes and hypertension are also obese.[50]

Surveys of stroke patients and prospective epidemiologic investigations confirm an increased risk of stroke in diabetics. The Honolulu Heart Program of Japanese men living in Hawaii found a quantitative relation of glucose intolerance to risk of thromboembolic stroke that was independent of other risk factors. There was, however, no relationship to hemorrhage (Fig. 29-3).[51] Evaluation of the impact of diabetes on stroke in a population-based cohort in Rancho Bernardo also disclosed a positive relationship. The relative risk of stroke was 1.8 in men and 2.2 in women—even after adjusting for the effects of other pertinent risk factors.[52]

In the Framingham Study, for ABTI, the impact of glucose intolerance (i.e., physician-diagnosed diabetes, glycosuria, or a blood sugar >150 mg/100 ml) was found at all ages in both men and women to approximately double the risk of ABI compared with nondiabetic men and women.[53] Whereas diabetes eliminated the female advantage over men for coronary disease, this was not the case for stroke.

The combination of hypertension and diabetes is particularly hazardous. Hypertensive diabetic persons have a sixfold greater risk of a stroke than the normal population and diabetics with hypertension are twice as likely to have a stroke as diabetics without hypertension.[54]

OBESITY

Obese persons have higher levels of blood pressure, blood glucose, and atherogenic serum lipids; and, on that account alone, could be expected to have an increased risk of stroke. Obesity, as expressed as relative weight 30% or more above average, is a significant independent contributor to ABI incidence in younger men and older women in the Framingham Study. In all age groups and in both sexes, however, obesity exerts an adverse influence on cardiovascular health status that is probably mediated through its promotion of elevated blood pressure, impaired glucose tolerance, and other mechanisms. In the Honolulu Heart Study, obesity was a risk factor for stroke that was independent of associated hypertension, glucose intolerance, and other covariates.[55] Also, in the Nurses Health Study, incidence of stroke increased directly with body mass index in women aged 30 to 55 years after adjustment for other risk factors.[56] However, no such independent relationship was seen in men, aged 40 to 75 years, in the Health Professionals Follow-Up Study.[57]

Abdominal obesity seems more closely related to adverse cardiovascular outcomes, including stroke, than elevated body mass index. In 28,643 male health professionals, the relative risk of stroke was significantly 2.3-fold greater in those men with a waist to hip ratio in the uppermost quintile. Obesity as reflected in the body mass index was less strongly related than waist circumference to stroke incidence possibly reflecting an influence of insulin resistance.[57]

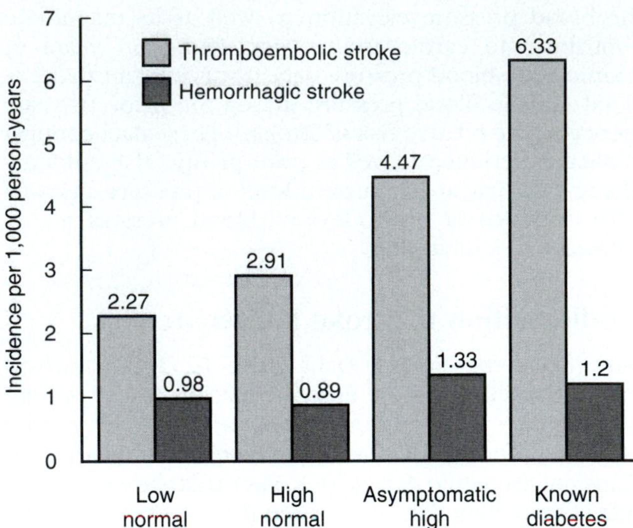

FIGURE 29-3. Incidence of stroke and glucose intolerance according to blood sugar levels. Honolulu Heart Study—22-year follow-up. (From Burchfiel CM, Curb JD, Rodgriquez BL, et al: Glucose intolerance and 22-year stroke incidence. The Honolulu Heart Program. Stroke 25:951, 1994.)

FIBRINOGEN, CLOTTING FACTORS, AND INFLAMMATION

It seems likely the atherogenic and procoagulant effects of inflammation are related to CVD incidence including stroke. Elevated fibrinogen has been implicated in atherogenesis and arterial thrombus formation. In a number of epidemiologic studies, a significant independent increase in CVD incidence, including stroke, was related to antecedent fibrinogen level. A prospective study of 54-year-old Swedish men found that increased fibrinogen, in combination with elevated systolic blood pressure, was a potent hazard for stroke.[58] Level of fibrinogen, measured on the tenth biennial examination in the Framingham Study, was also significantly related to incidence of CVD including stroke.[59] Fibrinogen was associated with many other risk factors for stroke including age, hypertensive status, hematocrit level, obesity, and diabetes.[60-62] In the Cardiovascular Health Study, fibrinogen and factor VIII were the only clotting factors associated with subclinical atherosclerotic disease.[63]

In the Framingham Original Cohort, C-reactive protein level (CRP) was found to be an independent risk marker for stroke and TIA incidence over 14 years of follow-up.[64] Men with CRP levels in the upper quartile had double the risk of stroke and TIA compared with men in the bottom quartile; for women, risk in the upper quintile was increased nearly threefold after other pertinent risk factors were taken into account.[64] CRP was also a potent independent risk marker for CVD in the Women's Health Study and was said to be a stronger predictor than the

LDL-cholesterol level, and made an independent contribution to CVD risk prediction above and beyond that provided by the Framingham risk score.[65]

BLOOD HOMOCYSTEINE LEVELS

In cross-sectional studies, case-control studies, and a meta-analysis, elevated plasma homocysteine was found to be associated with a higher incidence of CHD, and a 1.5-fold increased incidence of stroke.[66] Level of homocysteine is also directly related to many of the major components of cardiovascular risk profiles—including male sex, increasing age, cigarette smoking, increased blood pressure, elevated blood cholesterol level, and lack of exercise.[67] In the original Framingham cohort, however, even after taking these factors into account, risk of stroke is independently and significantly related to nonfasting homocysteine level after 10 years of follow-up with a relative risk in quartile four, compared with quartile one, of 1.82 and a highly significant linear trend across the quartiles ($P < 0.001$).[68]

A nested case-control study within the British Regional Heart Study cohort also demonstrated a powerful and independent relationship between nonfasting homocysteine level and stroke incidence.[69] There was a graded increase in risk with increasing levels of homocysteine over a 4.7-fold range. There was no threshold discernible and the relationship persisted after adjustments for serum creatinine (associated with increased tHcy levels), age, social class, blood pressure, and other pertinent risk factors.[69]

In other large population studies, however, such as the Atherosclerosis Risk in Communities Study, Physicians Health Study, the Finnish Study, and MRFIT, no statistically significant relationship was found.[70,71] Curiously, the Atherosclerosis Risk in Communities Study noted a strong independent relationship between fasting plasma total homocysteine concentrations and carotid artery intimal-medial wall thickening.[72] Increased levels of fasting plasma homocysteine were also related to ultrasound assessed extracranial common carotid artery stenosis of >25% in the Framingham cohort.[73] Furthermore, levels of homocysteine are inversely related to levels of dietary and plasma folic acid, and to vitamins B_{12} and B_6.[73,74] The *fasting* tHcy level may misclassify persons with impaired homocysteine metabolism because approximately 40% of persons with elevated homocysteine levels, in response to a methionine challenge, who are believed to be at increased cardiovascular risk, have normal fasting levels. Further, similar to other physiologic measures, such as blood pressure or serum cholesterol, the relation of homocysteine to CVD is continuous and graded without a threshold effect.

HEART DISEASE AND IMPAIRED CARDIAC FUNCTION

Cardiac diseases and impaired cardiac function predispose to stroke. Although hypertension is the pre-eminent risk factor for strokes of all types, at any blood pressure level, persons with impaired cardiac function or overt cardiac disease have a significantly increased stroke risk.[75] The prevalence of these cardiac contributors to stroke increases with age. The prevalence of CVD among stroke cases in the Framingham Study was high: 32.7% had prior CHD, 14.5% had prior congestive heart failure, and 14.5% had atrial fibrillation.

CORONARY HEART DISEASE

Coronary disease predisposes to stroke by a variety of mechanisms: as a source for embolism from the heart; by virtue of shared risk factors; as an untoward effect of medical and surgical treatments for coronary atherosclerotic disease; and, less commonly, as a consequence of pump failure. In the 2-week period after acute MI, stroke occurs at a rate estimated to be between 0.7% and 4.7%.[76] As expected, older age and ventricular dysfunction (chiefly decreased ejection fraction) increase stroke risk of MI.[76] Consistent with an embolic mechanism, treatment with aspirin, and particularly with warfarin anticoagulation, decreased the incidence of stroke in a large group of MI survivors.[76,77] Stroke occurs most frequently following *anterior* wall MI (2% to 6% of cases). The mechanism is often cerebral embolism, principally from left ventricular mural thrombus that is demonstrable on echocardiographic studies in 40% of cases. Inferior wall MI, however, is an infrequent basis for mural thrombus or stroke. Often, the mechanism of increased stroke risk in persons with CHD is less apparent, particularly in persons with uncomplicated angina pectoris (AP), non–Q-wave infarction, and clinically silent MI, who also have an increased incidence of ischemic stroke. Recent data from the Framingham Study suggest that silent or unrecognized MI survivors have a 10-year incidence of stroke of 17.8% in men and 17.3% in women, an incidence in men not much less than the 19.5%, seen following recognized MI. In women, the stroke rate following symptomatic MI is somewhat higher at 29.3%.

Atrial Fibrillation

Atrial fibrillation (AF) is the most prevalent persistent cardiac rhythm disturbance in the elderly. In the Framingham Study, AF incidence more than doubled in successive decades and rose from 0.2 per 1000 for ages 30 to 39 to 39.0 per 1000 for ages 80 to 89 years. The prevalence of this pernicious condition has increased alarmingly. Between 1982 and 1997, hospitalizations for AF increased 70% for persons ages 45 to 64 and more than doubled at age 65 and older.[10] In association with rheumatic heart disease and mitral stenosis, AF has always been acknowledged to predispose to stroke. Chronic AF without valvular heart disease was previously considered to be innocuous; it has now been shown to be associated with approximately a fivefold increase in stroke incidence.[78] AF as a stroke promoter is particularly important in the elderly because the proportion of total strokes associated with this arrhythmia increased steadily with age, reaching 36.2% for ages 80 to 89 years.[79] Although the prevalence of other cardiac contributors to stroke also increases with age, the increased incidence of stroke in persons with AF is more likely to be a consequence of the AF per se and not the associated CHD or congestive heart failure. This becomes apparent when age trends in risk of stroke are examined. Although risk of stroke attributable to AF increases with age, risk of stroke attributable to cardiac failure, CHD, and hypertension decline with age.[79] Notably, in the oldest age group 80 to 89 years, the percent of strokes attributable to AF was 23.5%—approaching that of hypertension (33.4%)—a far more prevalent disorder. A dispute as to whether AF is an independent risk factor or merely a risk marker for other conditions predisposing to stroke raged for several years.[80,81] This issue seems resolved by the six concordant randomized clinical trials of warfarin for stroke prevention in AF demonstrating a 68% stroke risk reduction on intention-to-treat analyses and over 80% on efficacy (on treatment).[82] The reduction in risk of stroke far outweighs the risk of serious and, particularly, intracranial bleeding. Aspirin has a far less potent impact and seems to prevent TIAs and milder, noncardioembolic strokes.[83]

Left Ventricular Hypertrophy

LVH by electrocardiogram increases in prevalence with age and blood pressure and is more common in diabetics. Risk of ABTI increased by more than fourfold in men and sixfold in women with this abnormal ECG pattern. The increased risk persists even after the influence of age and other atherogenic precursors, including systolic blood pressure, are taken into account.

A more sensitive and precise measure of cardiac muscle hypertrophy, left ventricular mass-to-height ratio, on echocardiography was shown to be directly related to incidence of stroke.[84] The hazard ratio for stroke and TIA, comparing the uppermost quartile of left ventricular mass-to-height ratio with the lowest, was 2.72 after adjusting for age, gender, and cardiovascular risk factors. There was a graded incremental risk with a hazard ratio of 1.45 for each quartile increment of left ventricular mass-to-height ratio. Thus, echocardiography and the ECG provide prognostic information beyond that provided by traditional stroke risk factors.

Host Factors

Race

Stroke mortality is highest in the southeastern United States where there is a high prevalence of blacks. At all ages, stroke mortality is appreciably higher in blacks than in whites (see Fig. 29-2).[85] This increased mortality appears to be due to a higher prevalence of hypertension, more severe grades of hypertension, and a greater adverse influence of blood pressure. In both blacks and whites, stroke rates are somewhat higher in men than in women.

Family History of Stroke

Family history of stroke has long been perceived to be an important marker of increased risk, but, until recently, confirmation by epidemiologic investigation has been lacking. In 1987, maternal history of death from stroke was shown to be significantly related to stroke incidence in a cohort of Swedish men born in 1913,[86] and this relationship persisted even after adjustment for other significant risk factors including hypertension, abdominal pattern of obesity, and fibrinogen level. In a study of familial predisposition to stroke in the original Framingham Study cohort in 1993, there was no relationship between a *history* of stroke *death* in parents and documented stroke in the subjects under surveillance. However, documented definite nonfatal and fatal strokes in these cohort members were related to the occurrence of observed stroke occurrence in their children who were members of the Framingham Offspring Study cohort. In these analyses, both maternal and paternal strokes were associated with approximately a 1.5-fold increased risk of stroke even after other risk factors were taken into account.[87] Thus, family history of stroke, so frequently acknowledged as a risk factor for stroke, has been identified only recently and documented by epidemiologic investigation.

Other Host Factors

Migraine

From clinical observations, case reports, and clinical series the notion evolved that migraine predisposes to stroke, particularly ischemic stroke. Complicated migraine with aura and migraine with neurologic concomitants appear to be most likely followed by stroke. Examples of the association between migraine and stroke occur in certain uncommon syndromes and instances. In CADASIL (cerebral autosomal dominant arteriopathy with subcortical infarcts and leukoencephalopathy), migraine headache is associated with white matter disease, dementia, and subcortical strokes.[88] Another syndrome of migraine and increased stroke risk is said to occur in the antiphospholipid antibody syndrome in which migraine is associated with a clearly elevated stroke risk and elevated titers of antiphospholipid antibodies.[88] Atypical migraine syndromes, such as hemiplegic migraine, are also associated with stroke but are quite rare.[89]

The relationship of stroke to the common migraine syndromes, encompassing migraine with aura and migraine without aura, has been investigated in two large case-control studies: the Italian National Research Council Study Group on Stroke in the Young,[90] and a substudy of the World Health Organization (WHO) Collaborative Study of CVD and Steroid Hormone Contraception.[12] Migraine as a predisposing factor for stroke was also investigated in the Physicians' Health Study. An increased risk of ischemic stroke was found in all of these aforementioned studies with relative risks or odds ratios ranging from 2.0 to 3.8.[91] The studies that distinguished between migraine with and without aura usually detected a higher risk for migraine with aura. The contribution of migraine to stroke risk decreases with increasing age.

Unruptured Intracranial Aneurysms

Unruptured intracranial aneurysms (UIAs) are an ominous genetic stroke risk factor. The prevalence of intracranial aneurysms in the general population is unknown. Detection of an unruptured intracranial aneurysm presents a therapeutic dilemma when risk of future rupture must be weighed against the hazard of intervention. Some guidance comes from data of the International Study of Unruptured Intracranial Aneurysms (ISHUA).[92] A retrospective cohort was assembled to permit examination of the outcome of UIAs in subjects with and without a history of subarachnoid hemorrhage. Another prospective cohort was formed to examine the morbidity and mortality of surgery for unruptured intracranial aneurysms. In the retrospective cohort, there were 727 subjects with unruptured intracranial aneurysms and no history of subarachnoid hemorrhage and 722 subjects with unruptured intracranial aneurysms with a history of SAH from another aneurysm.[92] For those with no history of previous SAH, aneurysm size was found to be the major predictor of rupture. The rupture rate for aneurysms less than 10 mm in size was only 0.05% per year, as compared with nearly 1% per year for aneurysms greater than or equal to 10 mm in size, and 6% in the first year for giant aneurysms (>25 mm). Location was another major predictor with posterior communicating, vertebrobasilar/posterior cerebral, and basilar tip aneurysms having higher rates of rupture.

For those with a history of subarachnoid hemorrhage, aneurysms less than10 mm in size had a rupture rate of 0.5% per year, 10 times higher than aneurysms of the same size in those without a history of subarachnoid hemorrhage. Aneurysms greater than or equal to 10 mm in size had a slightly higher hemorrhage rate of 0.65% per year. The only other clear predictor in this group was basilar tip location.

For subjects without a history of subarachnoid hemorrhage, the prospective component of ISHUA found a 30-day mortality rate for surgical treatment of unruptured intracranial aneurysms of 2.3%. ISHUA measured cognitive function as well as functional status to determine disability postsurgery and found that 12% of patients had cognitive or functional disability at 1 year postsurgery. This suggests a high toll for surgery in these subjects who were, for the most part, neurologically normal before surgery. Clearly, further study is needed, particularly in the face of the availability and increasing usefulness of neurovascular interventions that promise lower rates of death and disability.

Sleep Disturbance

Disordered breathing during sleep is often heralded by snoring and is an indication of obstructive sleep apnea that occurs in about 30% of the elderly. Snorers are reported to have more hypertension, and as many as 40% of hypertensive patients have sleep apnea.[93,94] Stroke incidence is reported to be increased by 50% in heavy snorers. The relationship is biologically plausible because there is a 50% reduction in blood flow to the brain in REM sleep in patients who snore heavily. The increased risk of stroke during sleep or shortly after awakening could be a result of sleep apnea.

Environmental Factors

Most ecologic and other analyses of vital statistics indicate that, for men in industrialized countries, lower socioeconomic status is associated with increased stroke mortality rates. For women, the relationship appears equivocal.[95] NHANES I epidemiologic follow-up data examining the relationship of education and poverty index to occurrence of initial strokes, showed a nonsignificant inverse trend of education with stroke occurrence. In women, there was a significantly lower age-adjusted rate in those with 12 or more years of education. In blacks, stroke incidence was significantly lower in those who had 8 or more years of education. There was a significant inverse graded age-adjusted rate associated with poverty index. However, after controlling for confounders and risk mediators, the association was diminished and no longer significant. It was concluded that much of the association appears to be mediated by other risk factors induced by or related to poverty and less education. However, that should not be taken to imply that these social influences are unimportant if poverty and lack of schooling are major determinants of powerful stroke risk factors.

Cigarette Smoking

Cigarette smoking, a powerful risk factor for MI and sudden death is also linked to brain infarction, intracranial hemorrhage, and subarachnoid hemorrhage.[96,97] In Hawaiian Japanese men of the Honolulu Heart Study, cigarette smoking made a significant independent contribution to cerebral infarction and intracranial hemorrhage risk.[98]

In the late 1970s, several studies of the connection between oral contraceptives and stroke in young women also identified cigarette smoking as an important risk factor. However, surprisingly, the association of cigarette smoking to stroke in oral contraceptive users was primarily to subarachnoid hemorrhage. These data from the Royal College of General Practitioners Study of oral contraceptive use found that the increased risk of subarachnoid hemorrhage occurred principally in current or former oral contraceptive users older than age 35 and those who smoked cigarettes.[99] The Nurses Health Study, of a cohort of almost 120,000 women followed prospectively for 8 years for development of stroke, not only confirmed this increased risk of subarachnoid hemorrhage, but also observed increased risk of thrombotic stroke in cigarette smokers. There was a dose-response relationship to subarachnoid hemorrhage from fourfold in light smokers to 9.8-fold in smokers of 25 or more cigarettes daily.[99] At any level of smoking, the relative risk of subarachnoid hemorrhage was twice as great as for thromboembolic stroke—even taking other risk factors into account (Table 29-3).

In case-control analysis, the association between cigarette smoking and subarachnoid hemorrhage was also found in men in the Framingham Study,[100] Finland,[101] and New Zealand.[102] In the Finland case-control study of 114 patients with subarachnoid hemorrhage, cigarette smokers were significantly more prevalent in cases than in controls matched for age, sex, and domicile.[101] Compared with nonsmokers, the relative risk of subarachnoid hemorrhage in smokers was 2.7 in men and 3.0 in women. The authors suggested that smoking promoted a temporary increase in blood pressure which, acting in concert with an emphysema effect, was responsible.

TABLE 29-3 AGE-ADJUSTED RELATIVE RISK (RR) OF STROKE (FATAL AND NONFATAL COMBINED), BY DAILY NUMBER OF CIGARETTES CONSUMED AMONG CURRENT SMOKERS

				No. of Cigarettes Smoked per Day Among Current Smokers			
Events	**Never Smoked**	**Former Smoker**	**Current Smoker**	**1-14**	**15-24**	**25-34**	**≥35**
Total stroke	1.00	1.35 (0.98-1.85)	2.73 (2.18-3.41)	2.02 (1.29-3.14)	3.34 (2.38-4.70)	3.08 (1.94-4.87)	4.48 (2.78-7.23)
Subarachnoid hemorrhage	1.00	2.26 (1.16-4.42)	4.85 (2.90-8.11)	4.28 (1.88-9.77)	4.02 (1.90-8.54)	7.95 (3.50-18.07)	10.22 (4.03-25.94)
Ischemic stroke	1.00	1.27 (0.85-1.89)	2.53 (1.91-3.35)	1.83 (1.04-3.23)	3.57 (2.36-5.42)	2.73 (1.49-5.03)	3.97 (2.09-7.53)
Cerebral hemorrhage	1.00	1.24 (0.64-2.42)	1.24 (0.64-2.42)	1.68 (0.34-5.28)	2.53 (0.71-6.05)	1.41 (0.39-5.05)	

Numbers in parentheses are 95% confidence intervals.
RR-Adjusted for age in 5-year intervals, follow-up period (1976-1978, 1978-1980, 1980-1982, 1982-1984, 1984-1986, or 1986-1988), history of hypertension, diabetes, high cholesterol levels, body mass index, past use of oral contraceptives, postmenopausal estrogen therapy, and age at starting smoking. Adapted from: Kawachi I, Colditz, GA, Stampfer MJ: Smoking cessation and decreased risk of stroke in women. JAMA 269; 233, 1993, with permission.

It is generally accepted that cigarette smoking increases risks of thrombotic stroke and subarachnoid hemorrhage, but the relationship of cigarette smoking to intracerebral hemorrhage is less well established. The Honolulu Heart Program data, however, firmly link cigarette smoking to both thromboembolic and hemorrhagic strokes, but it is not clear whether this applies to intracerebral hemorrhage per se.[98] Risk of "hemorrhagic" stroke was significantly greater (relative risk 2.5) in cigarette smokers than in nonsmokers and the excess risk persisted at a relative risk of 2.8 after the adjustments for other associated risk factors of age, diastolic blood pressure, serum cholesterol, alcohol consumption, hematocrit, and body mass.

A meta-analysis of 32 separate studies (including those cited) found cigarette smoking was a significant independent contributor to stroke incidence in both sexes and at all ages, conferring about a 50% increased risk overall compared with nonsmokers.[98,103] The risk of stroke generally, and of ABTI specifically, rose as number of cigarettes smoked per day increased, in both men and women.

Oral Contraceptive Use

In the 1970s, risk of stroke was estimated to be increased fivefold in women using oral contraceptives. This increased risk was most marked in older women, (older than age 35) and predominantly in those with other cardiovascular risk factors, particularly hypertension and cigarette smoking.[98,104] The relative risk of stroke was increased in oral contraceptive users and former users with risk concentrated in cigarette smokers older than 35 years of age.

The mechanism of stroke in oral contraceptive users is unclear. It is known that clotting is enhanced by the oral contraceptive-induced increased platelet aggregability and by its alteration of clotting factors to favor thrombogenesis. In young women with unexplained ischemic stroke, use of oral contraceptives is often presumed to be the "cause" of the brain infarct; however, the stroke was attributed to oral contraceptive use in no more than 10% of a series of carefully studied patients.[105]

No increase in stroke or other CVD was observed in the Nurses Health Study among former users of oral contraceptives.[106] An international ischemic stroke and oral contraceptive study assessed risk of stroke in women in Europe and in less developed countries.[107] Risk of stroke was increased, with an odds ratio of 2.99, and was lowest in younger women and nonsmokers without elevated blood pressure. Women with hypertension had an odds ratio of 10.7. In Europe, current use of low-dose oral contraceptives (<50 μg estrogen) was associated with a nonsignificant 1.53 odds ratio.[107]

In the United States, a population-based, case-control study of oral contraceptive use in women with stroke in whom the oral contraceptive preparations used contained the current low estrogen dose, was conducted using the California Kaiser-Permanente Medical Care Program.[108] Comparing current with former and never-users of oral contraceptives, the odds ratio for ischemic stroke was only a nonsignificant 1.18 after adjustments for other risk factors for stroke.[108] Thus, risk of ischemic stroke is quite low in women of childbearing age taking oral contraceptives and is not significantly increased in nonsmokers without hypertension.

A recent meta-analysis that addressed the relationship of oral contraceptive use and stroke included 16 studies published from 1960 to 1999. It found that the overall relative risk of ischemic stroke across all preparations and study designs was a statistically significant 2.75.[109] The relative risk in population-based studies of low-estrogen preparations controlling for both smoking and hypertension was also significantly elevated at 1.93. If these latter results are true, then low-dose oral contraceptive pills might lead to one stroke for every 24,000 women users, or 425 ischemic strokes in the United States each year. These results must be interpreted with caution because other studies did not find the same association between stroke and low-dose estradiol contraceptives.

Regarding subarachnoid hemorrhage, of particular interest is the interaction between the older preparations of oral contraceptives (containing high doses of estrogens) and cigarette smoking. Prospective observation of over 40,000 women, one half of whom were taking oral contraceptives, showed an increased risk of fatal subarachnoid hemorrhage (not cerebral infarction) in women taking oral contraceptives. Risk was increased fourfold in cigarette smokers older than age 35 with most cases confined to this group.[99] The odds ratio for hemorrhagic stroke in oral contraceptive users in the California Kaiser-Permanente Program study was not significantly increased.[108] There was a positive but nonsignificant interaction for hemorrhage in current users who smoked, with an odds ratio of 3.64 (95% CI 0.95 to 13.87).[108] In the WHO Collaborative Study, risk of hemorrhagic stroke was not increased in younger women and only slightly increased in older women.[110] The bulk of hemorrhages were subarachnoid, (200 of 248 in Europe), and risk was significantly increased in women aged more than 35 years. The odds ratio for hemorrhage among current oral contraceptive users, aged more than 35 years, who were current cigarette smokers was 3.91 (95% CI 1.54 to 9.89).[110]

Alcohol Consumption

As is the case for MI, the impact of alcohol consumption on stroke risk is related to the amount of alcohol consumed. Heavy alcohol use, either habitual daily heavy alcohol consumption or binge drinking, seems to be related to higher rates of CVD. Light or moderate alcohol consumption, on the other hand, is inversely related to incidence of CHD.[111] Light and moderate alcohol use tends to raise the HDL cholesterol, whereas high levels of alcohol intake are linked to hypertension and hypertriglyceridemia and may, in this way, predispose to fatal and nonfatal CHD.

The relationship of alcohol consumption to stroke occurrence is less clear.[112] Available evidence suggests a U-shaped relationship between level of alcohol consumption and ischemic stroke risk. Minimal consumption or total abstinence and heavy alcohol consumption seem to increase *ischemic* stroke occurrence, whereas moderate alcohol use is associated with the lowest risk. In addition, risk of stroke due to hemorrhage increases with the amount of alcohol consumed.[113] A powerful dose-response relationship between alcohol consumption and incidence of intracranial hemorrhage and subarachnoid hemorrhage was observed in the Honolulu Heart Study even after taking other pertinent risk factors into account. Increases in alcohol consumption were related to increasing levels of blood pressure, cigarette smoking, and to lower serum cholesterol levels, all risk factors for intracerebral hemorrhage. However, even after taking these factors into account, alcohol consumption was independently related to incidence of intracranial hemorrhage, both subarachnoid and intracerebral. No significant relationship was found between alcohol and thromboembolic stroke. Age-adjusted relative risk of intracerebral hemorrhage for light drinkers (1 to 14 oz per month), as compared with nondrinkers, was 2.1, for moderate drinkers (15 to 39 oz per month) 2.4, and for heavy drinkers (40+ oz per month) 4.0. After adjustment was made for the other associated risk factors, intracerebral hemorrhage was 2.0, 2.0, and 2.4 times as frequent, respectively, in these alcohol consumption categories.[113] However, recent data from the Framingham Study were also not supportive of a protective effect and suggested an increased incidence of brain infarction and stroke with increased levels of alcohol use.[112]

There are a number of mechanisms by which heavy alcohol consumption may predispose to, and moderate alcohol consumption protect from, stroke.[114] Cigarette smoking is more frequent in heavy drinkers, and contributes to the hemoconcentration accompanying heavy alcohol consumption, which increases hematocrit and viscosity.[115] In addition, rebound thrombocytosis during abstinence has been observed. Cardiac rhythm disturbances, particularly AF, occur with alcohol intoxication producing what has been termed "holiday heart."[116] Acute alcohol intoxication has been named as a precipitating factor in stroke in young people, both in thrombotic stroke and in subarachnoid hemorrhage.[115,117]

PHYSICAL ACTIVITY

Leisure-time and work-associated physical activity has been linked to lower CHD incidence. Regular exercise may exert a beneficial influence on risk factors for atherosclerotic disease reducing elevated blood pressure as a result of weight loss and by reducing the heart rate, raising the HDL and lowering the LDL cholesterol, improving glucose tolerance, and by promoting a lifestyle conducive to more favorable health habits. Only recently has physical activity been found to be associated with reduced stroke incidence.[118-122] In the Framingham Study, physical activity in subjects with a mean age of 65 years was associated with a reduced stroke incidence.[120] In men, the relative risk was 0.41 (95% CI 0.24 to 0.69, $P = 0.0007$) after taking other variables into account. However, there was no evidence of a protective effect of physical activity on risk of stroke in women. As in CHD, *moderate* physical activity conferred no less benefit than *heavy* activity levels. In a number of other population studies and in a series of case-control studies, low levels of physical activity were also found to be associated with increased incidence of stroke and, in these, a beneficial effect was also seen in women.[121]

The level of exercise required for protection has been disputed. A more graded response to exercise was reported in male British civil servants, aged 40 to 59, with the greatest reduction in stroke incidence derived from the most intense level of exercise and an intermediate protective effect from medium levels.[119] In the Honolulu Heart Study, a higher level of physical activity was associated with lower rates of both ischemic and hemorrhagic strokes even after adjustment for other risk factors.[118] In the NHANES 1 epidemiologic follow-up study, low levels of physical activity were associated with an increased incidence of stroke in women as well as men and in both blacks and whites.[120,122-124] Moderate levels of activity tended to provide an intermediate level of protection.[122]

DIET

Ample consumption of grains, fruits and vegetables, and fish in the diet appear to be associated with reduced incidence of stroke. In the Nurses Health Study (NHS), of more than 75,000 women, relative risk of ischemic stroke in the uppermost quintile of grain consumption was 0.69 relative to the lowest quintile, even adjusted for other stroke risk factors.[125] Whole grain consumption was also significantly associated with decreased risk of stroke; relative risk was 0.69. Women in the Nurses Health Study[126] who consumed five or more servings of fish per week had an adjusted relative risk for stroke of 0.38 compared with women consuming less than one serving per month. This suggests a protective effect of omega-3 fatty acids.[127] In the Health Professionals Follow-Up Study, consumption of fish once a week or more was associated with an approximate 50% reduced stroke incidence in women and in black men.[128] Incidence was reduced by a nonstatistically significant 15% in white men who consumed fish compared with those who never ate fish.[128]

Vitamin C or E levels have been related to stroke incidence, but the findings have been inconsistent. In the Shibata prospective cohort study, relative risk of stroke, adjusted for all other risk factors, was 0.71 in the subjects with the highest vitamin C levels relative to those with the lowest levels after 20 years of follow-up. The Health Professionals Follow-Up Study also looked at this issue, based on food frequency questionnaires administered to 43,738 men, aged 40 to 75 years. After 8 years of follow-up there were no significant relationships between consumption of vitamins C and E and the risk of stroke.[129]

In the randomized controlled clinical trial, the Heart Outcomes Prevention Trial (HOPE) 9541 patients, 55 years old or older with CHD, stroke, peripheral vascular disease, or diabetes mellitus and one other risk factor, received (in a 2 × 2 factorial design) either vitamin E, ramipril, neither, or both. There was no benefit from vitamin E intake on the composite outcome of MI, stroke, or vascular death.

MULTIVARIABLE RISK ESTIMATION TO IDENTIFY STROKE CANDIDATES

To identify persons at increased risk of stroke, a risk profile has been developed using data from 36 years of follow-up from the Framingham Study that allows physicians to determine a patient's probability of having a stroke.[130] This is accomplished from data collected from a medical history and physical examination and obtaining an ECG and laboratory tests for glucose and lipid assessments. Using a tabulated sex-specific point scoring system, stroke probability is determined depending on: age, systolic blood pressure, antihypertensive therapy use, presence of diabetes, cigarette smoking, history of CVD (CHD or congestive heart failure), and ECG abnormalities (LVH or AF). This index permits the physician to pull all the risk factor information together, to estimate each patient's probability of stroke, based on their risk profile, and to compare their absolute risk with that of an average person of the same age and sex.

The stroke risk profile aids in the identification of persons with stage 1 hypertension who are at increased probability of a stroke attributable to the presence of other risk factor abnormalities.[131] Comparing the risk profile of a man aged 70 years with systolic blood pressure levels in the 140 to 160 mm Hg range, it can be seen that, if all else is favorable, the risk is little different from average; whereas, if there are one or more additional risk factors, the risk rises well above average. In the presence of multiple risk factor abnormalities, the probability of stroke may be higher in the presence of a systolic blood pressure of 120 mm Hg than in a nonsmoking man with a pressure of 180 mm Hg who is free of diabetes, LVH, AF, and overt CVD (Fig. 29-4). This multivariable risk profile provides a quantitative assessment of the level of risk that is particularly helpful in the presence of seemingly innocuous multiple borderline risk factors values. The risk score provides the patient, and his physician, with a concrete estimate of how likely is the probability of a stroke in comparison with the average probability for a person of this age and gender. It also provides an illustration of how achieved risk factor modifications have altered the probability of having a stroke.[130]

Clearly there are other situations not considered here when a patient can be identified to be at substantially increased risk of stroke: recent TIA, particularly in the presence of internal carotid artery stenosis (>70%); recent onset AF; recent MI; during and immediately following cardiac surgery and cerebral angiography; and others discussed elsewhere in this chapter.

STROKE PREVENTION THROUGH RISK FACTOR MANAGEMENT

The rapid remarkable 60% decline in death rates from stroke since 1972 in the United States, and most other industrialized nations, demonstrates this condition is not an inevitable consequence of aging or genetic endowment. Part of the decline in death rate may be attributable to reduced severity or incidence of current strokes, but it is likely that improved detection and treatment of hypertension, as well as control of other cardiovascular risk factors, have also played roles.[132] Based on data from randomized clinical trials and from observational investigation, we can conclude that initial and recurrent strokes may be prevented by a number of risk factor interventions. These include reducing elevated blood pressure; cessation of cigarette smoking; warfarin anticoagulation in AF; increasing physical activity and promoting weight reduction; treating high-risk individuals with HMG CoA reductase inhibitors and the addition of angiotensin-converting enzyme inhibitors (ACE inhibitors) and angiotensin receptor blockers (ARBs). It is possible that by lowering plasma homocysteine and by achieving better control of blood sugar in diabetics, further reductions may be achieved. Ample intake of fruits, grains and vegetables, and fish appears to be warranted in a stroke prevention regimen. It is likely that prevention and treatment of predisposing cardiac diseases: coronary heart disease, congestive heart failure,

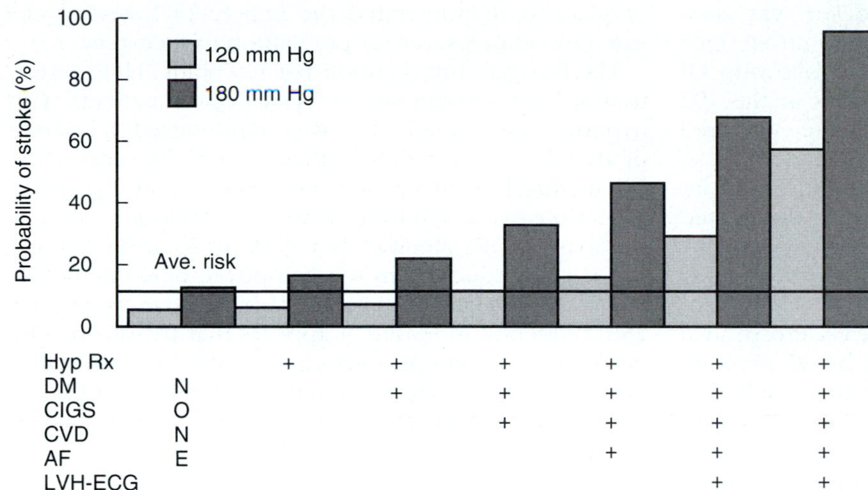

FIGURE 29-4. Probability of stroke in 10 years at two systolic bp levels: Impact of other risk factors—70-year-old man. AF, atrial fibrillation; CIGS, cigarette smoking; CVD, cardiovascular disease; DM, diabetes mellitus; Hyp Rx, hypertension treatment; LVH-ECG, left ventricular hypertrophy-electrocardiogram. (From Wolf PA, D'Agostino RB, Belanger AJ, Kannel WB: Probability of stroke: A risk profile from the Framingham Study. Stroke 22:312, 1991.)

AF, increased left ventricular mass, and valvular heart disease would also reduce stroke occurrence.

Nutritional Measures

Ample intake of increased amounts of fruits, grains and vegetables, and fish appears to be warranted in a stroke prevention regimen. Consumption of fish, once a week or more, appears to confer a 50% reduced stroke risk in women and black men[128] and possibly a 15% reduction in white men.[128]

There appears to be no support for taking C, E, folate, B_{12} or B_6 vitamin supplements. In the randomized controlled clinical trial, the Heart Outcomes Prevention Trial (HOPE), 9541 patients, 55 years or older with CHD, stroke, peripheral vascular disease, or diabetes mellitus and one other risk factor, received (in a 2 × 2 factorial design) either vitamin E, ramipril, neither, or both. There was no benefit from vitamin E intake on the composite outcome of MI, stroke, or vascular death.

Control of Hypertension and Stroke Prevention

Based on a combined analysis of nine major prospective (observational) studies of 420,000 individuals, a graded relationship between diastolic pressure and stroke and CHD incidence is evident.[133] There is no threshold level below which stroke risk gradients are flat, implying a steadily increasing risk with increasing diastolic pressure even in the normal range. The same continuous graded impact was also seen in a meta-analysis of drug treatment trials for hypertension.[133] The incidence of stroke increased 46% and CHD increased 29% with each 7.5 mm Hg increase in diastolic pressure.

These estimates were validated by randomized trials of blood pressure treatment that achieved comparable reductions in stroke occurrence.[134,135] Results of 14 treatment trials in 37,000 hypertensive subjects finally put to rest the long-standing fear that vigorous control of elevated blood pressure in hypertensives precipitates strokes. The average diastolic blood pressure reduction of 5.8 mm Hg resulted in a 42% reduction in stroke incidence—closely approximating that expected on the basis of prospective observational studies.[134,135] In these studies, the duration of blood pressure reduction was brief (from 2 to 5 years). Nevertheless, there was a dramatic impact on stroke incidence within this short period of time, suggesting that the treatment removed or reduced precipitating factors and reduced the progression of atherosclerosis. Presumably, more prolonged blood pressure control would have both effects.

Although stroke risk clearly is more directly related to systolic pressure, in virtually all of the older treatment trials, diastolic pressure was emphasized.[136] In the elderly, in whom isolated elevation of the systolic pressure is common, it was believed that treatment would be ineffective in reducing pressure, hazardous in terms of side effects, and unwarranted on the basis of available clinical data. In the Systolic Hypertension in the Elderly Program (SHEP Trial), 4736 persons, older than age 60, with systolic blood pressure levels above 160 mm Hg. and diastolic pressures below 90 mm Hg,[137] the treated group had a 36% reduction in stroke, and a 27% reduction in MI and coronary death after 4.5 years of follow-up. These findings have enormous importance because two thirds of all individuals with hypertension between the ages of 65 and 89 years have isolated systolic hypertension and the majority of strokes occur in this age group.[138]

It is clear from the SHEP Trial, and also from the European Working Party on Hypertension in the Elderly (EWPHE) study, that contrary to clinician concerns, antihypertensive medication is well tolerated by the elderly.[138-140] SHEP demonstrated that reduction of pressure was accomplished with relative ease; approximately one half were controlled with the thiazide diuretic, chlorthalidone, alone; it was well tolerated as evidenced by a 90% compliance rate in the active treatment group at 5 years. Because increased blood pressure is the most powerful risk factor for stroke, and because the benefits of treatment occur so promptly, control of increased blood pressure, systolic as well as diastolic levels, is the cornerstone of stroke prevention.

These findings were confirmed in the Syst-Eur Trial in 4695 persons with isolated systolic hypertension where a dihydropyridine calcium channel blocker was compared with placebo.[141] A 42% reduction in stroke incidence was seen after a mean of 2 years of follow-up. Of particular interest, cardiovascular outcomes in the 492 diabetic participants in the Syst-Eur Trial were compared to outcomes in the 4203 nondiabetic participants in post-hoc analyses.[142] The benefits in the diabetic group far exceeded those in the nondiabetic group. In the treated diabetic participants, overall mortality was reduced by 55%, mortality from CVD by 76%, all cardiovascular events by 69%, and risk of stroke by 73%. Consonant with these findings were the results of the UK Prospective Diabetes Study Group.[143] Tight diastolic blood pressure control in these elderly diabetic participants resulted in a 44% relative risk reduction in stroke compared with less stringent control.

Because increased blood pressure is the most powerful risk factor for stroke, and because the benefits of treatment occur so promptly, control of increased blood pressure, systolic as well as diastolic levels, is the cornerstone of stroke prevention. It would appear that diabetic patients benefit to a greater extent from antihypertensive therapy than nondiabetic patients.

EFFECTIVENESS OF CLASSES OF ANTIHYPERTENSIVE AGENTS

The effectiveness of the newer classes of antihypertensive agents, calcium channel blockers, and ACE inhibitors was compared with thiazide diuretics and β-blockers in the ALLHAT Study.[144] Results of this and other trials suggest all antihypertensive drugs have similar efficacy in the prevention of stroke with the degree of benefit proportional to the level of blood pressure control achieved. The medications also had similar safety profiles and earlier concerns regarding the safety of calcium channel blockers did not appear to be justified. However, recent trials of using ACE inhibitors and angiotensin receptor blockers suggest that these newer agents may have an effect on stroke prevention above and beyond their effect on blood pressure reduction.

ACE Inhibitors and Angiotensin Receptor Antagonists

In the Heart Outcomes Prevention Evaluation (HOPE) Trial, 9297 subjects with CVD or diabetes plus one other risk factor were randomized to 10 mg/day of the ACE inhibitor ramipril or to placebo.[145,146] The ramipril arm experienced a 26% reduction in cardiovascular death, a 20% reduction in MI, and a 32% reduction in stroke compared with placebo. It was suggested the degree of risk reduction achieved could not be explained by the amount of blood pressure reduction. It would appear that much of the protective effect of ramipril is attributable to other mechanisms such as beneficial effects on endothelial function, fibrinolysis, and smooth muscle proliferation.[146,147] The Perindopril Protection Against Recurrent Stroke Study (PROGRESS) of hypertensive and nonhypertensive subjects with a prior stroke or TIA, randomized to either a perindopril-based treatment protocol or placebo, demonstrated the benefit of lowering elevated blood pressures for prevention of recurrences.[27]

The Losartan Intervention For Endpoint (LIFE) reduction in hypertension study[148] investigated patients with hypertension and LVH who were randomized to losartan or atenolol.[149] After a mean follow-up of 4.8 years, virtually identical mean systolic and diastolic blood pressure reductions were achieved in the two treatment groups. Compared with atenolol, subjects on losartan therapy had a 13% reduction in the composite outcome of cardiovascular mortality, stroke, and MI, and an impressive 25% reduction in stroke. It appears that treatment with ramipril or losartan produces a level of stroke risk reduction greater than that expected from the degree of blood pressure reduction alone.

PREVENTION OF CARDIOVASCULAR SEQUELAE OF DIABETES

Despite the increased risk of stroke in a diabetic populace, tight diabetic control in type-1 and type-2 diabetes patients in the recent UK Prospective Diabetes Study Group and in the earlier Diabetes Control and Complications Trial was not found to decrease stroke incidence over 9 years of follow-up.[150] Given that even tight diabetic control is not sufficient in this high-risk population to prevent cardiovascular events such as stroke, some of the focus has shifted to other strategies for primary prevention in type-2 diabetes.

Many diabetic people have coexisting hypertension, and this combination is particularly hazardous in terms of elevated stroke risk. As in the Syst-Eur Trial, however, diabetic subjects experienced a more marked risk reduction as a result of control of hypertension than did nondiabetic subjects. Thus, aggressive blood pressure control in diabetic patients is a proven strategy for risk reduction and is a major strategy for stroke prevention in patients with diabetes.[48,131]

Intensive Diabetes Therapy

Intensive therapy with insulin, three or more doses per day, to achieve tight control of hyperglycemia in recent onset insulin-dependent diabetic subjects was shown to reduce microvascular complications, nephropathy, and retinopathy, as well as peripheral neuropathy.[151] This demonstration that improved glycemic control reduces some complications is the first clear evidence of what was previously believed likely but was not proved before the publications by the Diabetes Control and Complications Trial Research Group (DCCT).[151] Whether improved glycemic control will reduce the risk of stroke and other macrovascular diseases in diabetics, remains to be demonstrated.

STATUS OF BLOOD PRESSURE CONTROL

Only a small portion of the potential benefits derived from the treatment of elevated blood pressure has been achieved to date. There are an estimated 50 million Americans who have elevated blood pressure (systolic

TABLE 29-4 AWARENESS, TREATMENT, AND CONTROL AMONG PARTICIPANTS WITH HYPERTENSION IN THE U.S. POPULATION, 1988-2000*

	Prevalence, % (SE)			Change, 1988 to 2000	
	1988-1991 (*n* = 3045)	**1991-1994 (*n* = 3017)**	**1999-2000 (*n* = 1565)**	**% (95% CI)**	***P* Value**
Awareness	69.2 (1.3)	67.8 (1.8)	68.9 (1.5)	−0.3 (−4.2 to 3.6)	0.58
Treatment	52.4 (1.4)	52.0 (1.0)	58.4 (2.0)	6.0 (1.2 to 10.8)	0.01
Control					
Among those treated	46.9 (2.2)	43.6 (1.7)	53.1 (2.4)	6.2 (0 to 12.6)	0.03
Among all with hypertension	24.6 (1.4)	22.7 (1.1)	31.0 (2.0)	6.4 (1.6 to 11.2)	0.00
<140/90 mm Hg (Among treated hypertensive diabetic individuals)	53.1 (4.5)	41.6 (5.8)†	46.9(4.7)	−6.2 (−19.0 to 6.6)	0.83
<130/85 mm Hg (Among treated hypertensive diabetic individuals)	28.5 (4.2)	17.2 (4.2)†	25.4 (4.0)	−3.1 (−14.5 to 8.3)	0.70

*Data are weighted to the U.S. population.
†Estimates are unreliable because of National Health and Nutrition Examination Survey minimum sample size criteria or coefficient of variation of at least 0.30.
CI, confidence interval.

blood pressure 140 mm Hg or greater and/or diastolic blood pressure 90 mm Hg or greater) or are taking antihypertensive medication.[131,152] Although 70% of these 50 million are aware that their blood pressure is elevated, and 59% are on treatment, in only 34% has blood pressure control been achieved. Thus, using the ≥140/≥90 mm Hg level in the JNC7 report, approximately two thirds of Americans are unaware, untreated, or uncontrolled (Table 29-4).[131]

Evidence incriminating systolic blood pressure as the dominant determinant of cardiovascular events in hypertension, has not greatly influenced clinical practice. Most uncontrolled hypertension is concentrated in those with systolic hypertension. The Framingham Study found that although 90% of hypertensive persons on treatment have their diastolic pressure reduced to below 90 mm Hg, only 48% have their systolic pressure controlled to below 140 mm Hg.[153] A general practice survey noted that isolated systolic hypertension was the least likely to be treated.[154]

CESSATION OF CIGARETTE SMOKING

Based on data from the Framingham Study, it is clear that stroke risk in cigarette smokers is reduced about 60% by stopping.[96,155] This reduction in risk occurs in a remarkably short time and is similar to the reduction in CHD risk, which decreases by approximately 50% within 1 year of smoking cessation and reaches the level of those who never smoked within 5 years. In Framingham, in both men and women, risk of stroke in former cigarette smokers did not differ from that of persons who never smoked by the end of 5 years.[96] There was no interaction with age suggesting that cigarette smoking exerted a precipitating effect on stroke regardless of age or duration of smoking. Similar findings from the Nurses Health Study show a sizable reduction of risk within 2 years and a reduction to a relative risk of 0.4 (same as women who never smoked) from a referent level for current smokers of 1.0 (Fig. 29-5).[155] Because smoking confers an increase in stroke risk of 40% in men and 60% in women, after all other pertinent risk factors have been taken into account, cessation may be expected to significantly reduce risk of stroke.

PHYSICAL ACTIVITY

Physical activity exerts a beneficial influence on risk factors for atherosclerotic disease by reducing blood pressure and weight, by reducing the heart rate, by raising the high-density lipoprotein cholesterol and lowering

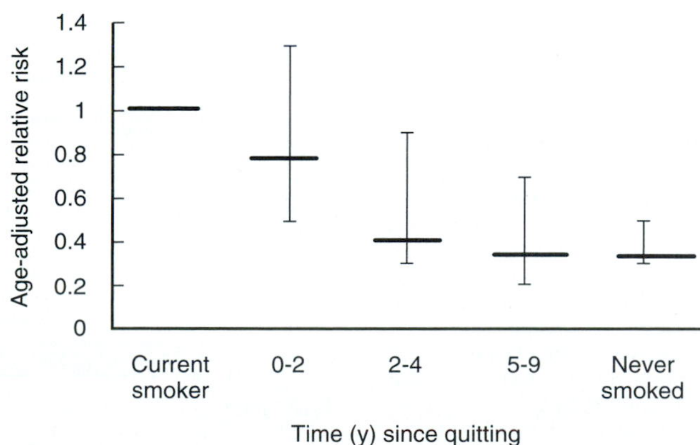

FIGURE 29-5. Smoking cessation and risk of stroke in women. (From Kawachi I, Colditz GA, Stampfer MJ, et al: Smoking cessation and decreased risk of stroke in women. JAMA 269:232, 1993.)

the low-density lipoprotein cholesterol, by decreasing platelet aggregability, and by increasing insulin sensitivity and improving glucose tolerance. Increased physical activity levels have now been convincingly associated with reduced incidence of stroke. Moderate levels of recreational and nonrecreational physical activity provide substantial benefit and may be recommended as a sensible lifestyle modification to reduce the risk of CVD, including stroke.

As with cigarette smoking, recently published data from observational studies strongly suggest an association between increased levels of physical activity and longer life span, and reduced CVD, including CHD and stroke. Whether benefit accrues from physical fitness and training over and above that achieved from weight reduction, blood pressure reduction, improved glucose tolerance, and other physiologic effects on clotting factors is unknown. There are conflicting data on the benefit of intensive versus moderate exercise. No randomized clinical trial data are likely to appear to bolster these data, but better measures of physical activity, recreational and nonrecreational, and physical fitness may help to clarify these issues. Nevertheless, the beneficial effects on vigor, feeling of well being, as well as the positive effects on cardiovascular risk factors are compelling. It is clear that regular, moderate physical activity should be an integral part of a lifestyle, which will help to reduce the risks of stroke and other CVDs.

WARFARIN ANTICOAGULATION IN ATRIAL FIBRILLATION

Prophylactic anticoagulation with warfarin is indicated in all persons with AF with the possible exception of persons younger than age 65 who have no history of hypertension, diabetes, TIA, or stroke, and who are free of structural heart disease. Persons in whom anticoagulants are contraindicated may be placed on aspirin. Aspirin has a far less potent impact and seems to prevent milder noncardioembolic strokes.[83] From a pooled analysis of the five primary prevention trials, four risk factors were shown to increase AF stroke risk (i.e., increasing age, a history of prior stroke or TIA, diabetes, or hypertension).[82] Warfarin reduces the incidence of stroke in persons with each of these risk factors at all ages past 65 years (Fig. 29-6).[82] In the presence or absence of these risk factors, warfarin anticoagulation reduces the fourfold increased incidence of stroke to approximately 1%. In persons younger than age 65 who have no risk factors, the stroke incidence without warfarin is only 1%, and it is only in this age group that anticoagulation is not currently indicated. In addition, persons having "lone AF" may be treated with aspirin alone, but this conclusion is based on sparse data and will require more studies to refine who may safely be followed without warfarin prophylaxis.

The relative lack of efficacy of aspirin in patients with a stroke or TIA was clearly demonstrated in a large secondary prevention trial, the European Atrial Fibrillation Trial. Aspirin (300 mg/per day) did not significantly reduce the annual stroke rate of 12%.[156] No case of intracranial bleeding was seen in those more effectively treated with warfarin. In this high risk group of elderly persons with AF and a prior cerebrovascular event, 90 events (mostly strokes) would be prevented in 1 year for every 1000 patients anticoagulated. The authors suggested that a target INR of 3.0 would produce the lowest rates of ischemic stroke without an increase in the risk of serious hemorrhage.[157] In another study, the risk of stroke rose steeply below an INR of 2.0.[158] Also, combinations of subtherapeutic doses of warfarin combined with aspirin provided little protection. Rates of hemorrhage were no lower and stroke prevention was far less effective than therapeutic levels of warfarin anticoagulation.[159]

Despite the evidence, physicians and patients are reluctant to use warfarin, particularly in elderly patients.[160] Patients 80 years or older were least likely to be given warfarin. In 1992 to 1993, only 19% of eligible octogenarians were treated. On the positive side, overall, warfarin use for stroke prevention in AF has increased from 7% between 1980 and 1981 to 32% between 1992 and 1993.[160]

Warfarin anticoagulation requires dosage adjustment and monitoring of the INR, an index of prothrombin activity. There is a narrow therapeutic window beyond

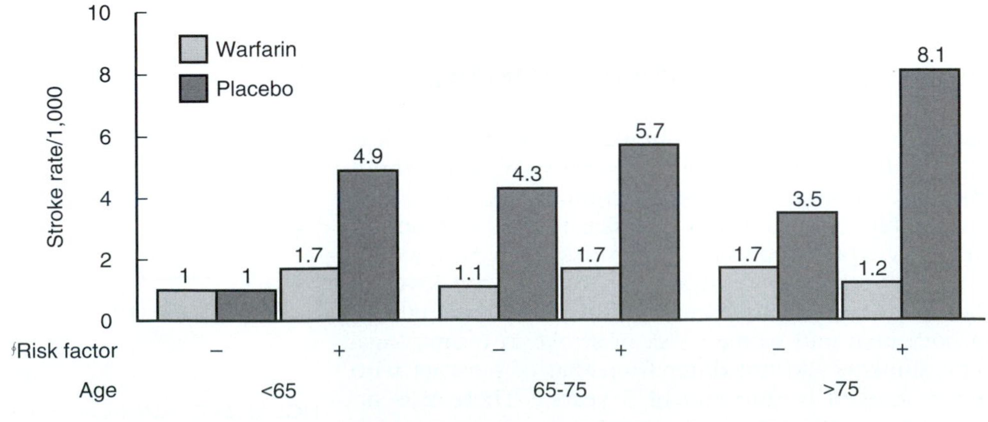

FIGURE 29-6. Efficacy of warfarin by risk category (hypertension, diabetes, prior stroke, or TIA), pooled analysis of AF trials. (From Atrial Fibrillation Investigators: Risk factors for stroke and efficacy of antithrombotic therapy in atrial fibrillation: Analysis of pooled data from five randomized controlled trials. Arch Intern Med 154, 1449, 1994.)

which embolic stroke occurs on the low side and bleeding, including intracranial bleeding with INRs above 4.5. Results of the SPORTIF III trial of the oral direct thrombin inhibitor, ximelagatran, in fixed-dose 36 mg, twice daily demonstrated a 29% relative risk reduction of stroke and systemic embolism on intention to treat analysis.[161] On treatment analysis, results showed a 41% relative risk reduction in the ximelagatran group, which was superior to warfarin. There was no significant difference in major or minor bleeding and, particularly, no increase in intracranial hemorrhage with ximelagatran (0.2% per year in the ximelagatran group versus 0.5% per year for the subjects given warfarin). If these preliminary findings are reproduced, this drug (or others in this class) offers promise for a greater likelihood of physician prescription and improved patient compliance facilitating stroke prevention in patients with AF.

Based on currently available information, anticoagulation may be safely administered to persons older than age 75 years, should be continued indefinitely, and at an intensity of INR greater than 2.0, with a target INR of 3.0.[157,158,162] Because there appears to be no lower risk of stroke in the presence of paroxysmal AF, warfarin is indicated in these patients as well.

STROKE PREVENTION WITH STATINS

A meta-analysis of older cholesterol-lowering trials showed a definite benefit in reduction in MI but no significant impact on stroke occurrence.[163] The recent evidence, from trials of HMG CoA reductase inhibitors in men with elevated LDL-cholesterol and usually with preexisting CHD, that treatment reduced stroke incidence, opens a new area for stroke prevention.[40,164] Pravastatin was shown to reduce carotid artery plaque progression or to promote regression in an early study, and these findings have been corroborated with other statins.[165] In the Cholesterol and Recurrent Events Trial, pravastatin and placebo were randomly allocated to 4159 survivors of an MI with total cholesterol levels below 240 mg/dl and low-density lipoprotein cholesterol levels of 115 to 174 mg/dl (mean 139).[38] Stroke occurred in 3.8% of the placebo group and 2.6% of the pravastatin group, a statistically significant relative risk reduction of 31% ($P < .05$).[41] It was estimated that 25 strokes would be prevented by treating 1000 such patients, ≥60 years of age, with pravastatin for 5 years. Similar benefit in stroke prevention was seen in the Long-Term Intervention with Pravastatin in Ischaemic Disease (LIPID) Study Group Trial.[39] All of these trials enrolled CHD patients, a small percentage of whom had sustained a cerebral infarct. More recently, The Heart Protection Study randomized 20,536 high-risk individuals, ages 40 to 80 years with total cholesterol levels of 3.5 mol/L (135 mg/dl) to simvastatin 40 mg or placebo daily. A 30% relative risk reduction in ischemic stroke was seen. In 7150 participants without diagnosed coronary disease, 1820 had prior cerebrovascular disease. The benefit in these persons was an approximate 25% relative risk reduction in overall event rate occurrence—suggesting the simvastatin benefit occurred in the absence of prior CHD.[40] The issue of stroke prevention with statins was recently supported in the Anglo-Scandinavian Cardiac Outcomes Trial-Lipid Lowering Arm (ASCOT-LLA).[164] After 3.3 years' mean follow-up, the trial was stopped with fatal and nonfatal strokes occurring in 89 atorvastatin assignees versus 121 placebo subjects (hazard ratio 0.73 [0.56 to 0.96], $P = .024$) (Fig. 29-7).[164] This significant benefit for stroke prevention occurred in the absence of CHD in otherwise high-risk individuals, strongly suggesting an indication for statins in the primary prevention of ischemic stroke.

It seems likely that the significant reductions in stroke and MI in these trials did not result from the fraction of a hundredth of a millimeter reduction in plaque thickness or intimal medial thickness in the arterial wall observed in subjects in the statin arm of a number of clinical trials.[34-36,166,167] Reversal of the lipid atherogenesis alone is not sufficient to account for the 20% to 30% relative risk reduction in ischemic stroke events seen in the statin trials, where benefits occur soon after institution of statins, often within 1 or 2 years.[40,164] It has been

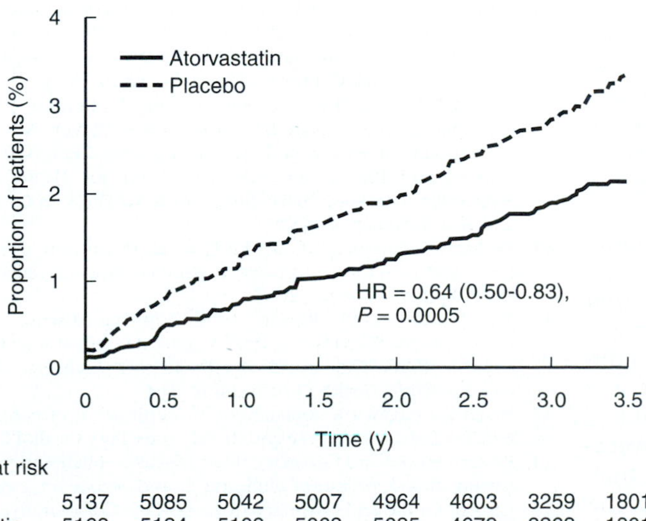

FIGURE 29-7. Cumulative incidence for primary endpoint of nonfatal myocardial infarction and fatal coronary heart disease. (From Sever PS, Dahlof B, Poulter NR, et al: Prevention of coronary and stroke events with atorvastatin in hypertensive patients who have average or lower-than-average cholesterol concentrations, in the Anglo-Scandinavian Cardiac Outcomes Trial—Lipid Lowering Arm (ASCOT-LLA): A Multicentre Randomised Controlled Trial. Lancet 361:1149, 2003.)

suggested the statin drugs acted by altering the lipid composition of the plaque, reducing the tendency to rupture or fissure, reducing inflammation, and evoking antiplatelet effects.[168]

PREVENTION AND TREATMENT OF HEART DISEASE

Because CHD, congestive heart failure, and AF predispose to stroke, prevention of these cardiovascular contributors can be anticipated to reduce the incidence of stroke.[81] On the basis of current knowledge of the epidemiology of congestive heart failure, prevention of obesity and treatment of hypertension, LVH, and diabetes may be beneficial. Reduction of CHD risk requires, in addition to hypertension control and smoking cessation, dietary or pharmacologic treatment to reduce elevated total and LDL cholesterol and to increase the HDL-cholesterol fraction. Prevention of AF might best be accomplished by preventing the appearance of the major precursor of AF, which is heart disease, particularly CHD.

Folic Acid to Reduce Total Plasma Homocysteine Levels

A number of clinical trials using folic acid supplements, along with vitamins B_6 and B_{12}, to prevent MI and stroke recurrence have been undertaken.[169,170] The Vitamin Intervention for Stroke Prevention (VISP) trial of 3600 patients with mild nondisabling stroke and TIA found no benefit for stroke, MI, or CVD prevention by vitamin supplementation with folic acid, B_6, and B_{12}.

Such supplementation will reduce homocysteine levels even in persons with adequate dietary intake and normal plasma vitamin levels.[45,171] Evidence of benefit for such supplementation is currently lacking; however, during the VISP trial, there appeared to be no risk resulting from supplementation and the cost of these vitamins is minimal. Adding 1 mg of cyanocobalamin should alleviate concerns about masking pernicious anemia or B_{12} deficiency.

Hormone Replacement Therapy

Hormonal replacement therapy (HRT) was believed to be protective against CVD. The presumed estrogen benefits include activation of endothelial nitric oxide synthase, leading to arterial vasodilation; modulation of the response to injury and atherosclerosis; favorable effects on lipids and fibrinolytic proteins; and favorable influences on endothelial function.[172]

Observational studies have either shown no influence of HRT on stroke or a weak protective effect. The Women's Estrogen for Stroke Trial (WEST) randomized 652 postmenopausal women, aged 46 to 91 years, to placebo or estradiol within 90 days of a TIA or nondisabling stroke. After a mean 2.7 year follow-up, there was no difference in the outcome of nonfatal stroke or death.[173] This was consistent with previous findings of no protective impact of HRT on stroke incidence. The largest trial, to date, examining the issue of HRT and CVD was the Women's Health Initiative Randomized Controlled Trial which randomized 16,608 subjects to conjugated estrogens plus progesterone or placebo.[174] The trial was stopped after 5.2 years because of a significant increase in breast cancer in the treatment group and because a global statistic indicated that the risks of treatment exceeded the benefit. Women taking HRT had an increased risk of stroke with a relative risk of 1.41 (1.07 to 1.85).[174] Despite a large body of observational evidence supporting a preventive effect of HRT on CHD, women on treatment also had a significantly increased risk of CHD and stroke. Pending further evidence to the contrary, HRT increases stroke and other negative outcomes and cannot be recommended as a measure to prevent CVD.

Summary

Understanding of the risk factors for stroke has increased substantially and new therapies for stroke prevention are now available. Identification of those persons at greatest risk for stroke is key to prevention. With an aging population of increasing size, it is apparent that stroke will be an increasing cause of death and disability in the future. Despite improvements in diagnosis and treatment of persons with acute stroke, it is certain that *prevention* holds the key to control of stroke.

REFERENCES

1. American Heart Association: Heart and Stroke Facts. Dallas, 1994.
2. American Heart Association: Heart and Stroke Facts Statistics: 1997 Statistical Supplement. Dallas, 1997.
3. Sacco RL, Ellenberg JH, Mohr JP, et al: Infarcts of undetermined cause: The NINCDS Stroke Data Bank. Ann Neurol 25:382, 1989.
4. Hankey GJ, Warlow CP: Treatment and secondary prevention of stroke: Evidence, costs, and effects on individuals and populations. Lancet 354:1457, 1999.
5. Sacco RL, Wolf PA, Kannel WB, et al: Survival and recurrence following stroke: The Framingham Study. Stroke 13:290, 1982.
6. Marler JR, Price TR, Clark GL, et al: Morning increase in onset of ischemic stroke. Stroke 20:473, 1989.
7. Kelly-Hayes M, Wolf PA, Kase CS, et al: Temporal patterns of stroke onset: The Framingham Study. Stroke 26:1343, 1995.
8. NHLBI, NHANES 1971-1994 public date release file documentation. National Center for Health Statistics 1999.
9. National Center for Health Statistics Preliminary Mortality Statistics for 1998, Public Mortality data 1950-1996 division of Vital Statistics for 1998. Public Mortality data 1950-1996 division of Vital Statistics. National Center for Health Statistics, 1998.
10. National Hospital Discharge Survey: Annual Summary, 1997. Series 13: Data from the National Health Care Survey No. 144. U.S. Department of Health and Human Services. Centers for Disease Control and Prevention. National Center for Health Statistics. Hyattsville, Maryland. DHHS Publication No. (PHS) 2000-1715. Vital and Health Statistics, 1999.
11. Collins TC, Petersen NJ, Menke TJ, et al: Short-term, intermediate-term, and long-term mortality in patients hospitalized for stroke. J Clin Epidemiol 56:81, 2003.
12. The World Health Report 1996. Fighting disease, Fostering Development. WHO World Health Statistics annual selected issues, Geneva 1996. The World Health Report Archives 1995-2000. Geneva, World Health Organization, 1996.
13. Nagai Y, Kitagawa K, Matsumoto M: Implication of earlier carotid atherosclerosis for stroke and its subtypes. Prev Cardiol 6:99, 2003.
14. Eastern Stroke and Coronary Heart Disease Collaborative Research Group: Blood pressure, cholesterol, and stroke in eastern Asia. Eastern Stroke and Coronary Heart Disease Collaborative Research Group. Lancet 352:1801, 1998.

15. JNC-VI: The sixth report of the Joint National Committee on prevention, detection, evaluation, and treatment of high blood pressure [erratum appears in Arch Intern Med 158:573, 1998] Arch Intern Med 157:2413, 1997.
16. MacMahon S, Sharpe N, Gamble G, et al: Effects of lowering average of below-average cholesterol levels on the progression of carotid atherosclerosis: Results of the LIPID Atherosclerosis Substudy. LIPID Trial Research Group. Circulation 97:1784, 1998.
17. Gamble G, MacMahon S, Culpan A, et al: Atherosclerosis and left ventricular hypertrophy: Persisting problems in treated hypertensive patients. J Hypertens 16:1389, 1998.
18. Hajjar I, Kotchen TA: Trends in prevalence, awareness, treatment, and control of hypertension in the United States, 1988-2000. JAMA 290:199, 2003.
19. O'Donnell CJ, Ridker PM, Glynn RJ, et al: Hypertension and borderline isolated systolic hypertension increase risks of cardiovascular disease and mortality in male physicians. Circulation 95:1132, 1997.
20. Vaccarino V, Berger AK, Abramson J, et al: Pulse pressure and risk of cardiovascular events in the systolic hypertension in the elderly program. Am J Cardiol 88:980, 2001.
21. Seshadri S, Wolf PA, Beiser A, et al: Elevated midlife blood pressure increases stroke risk in elderly persons: The Framingham Study. Arch Intern Med 161:2343, 2001.
22. Sacco RL, Foulkes MA, Mohr JP, et al: Determinants of early recurrence of cerebral infarction: The Stroke Data Bank. Stroke 20:983, 1989.
23. Sacco RL, Shi T, Zamanillo MC, et al: Predictors of mortality and recurrence after hospitalized cerebral infarction in an urban community: The Northern Manhattan Stroke Study. Neurology 44:626, 1994.
24. Chalmers J: Trials on blood pressure-lowering and secondary stroke prevention. Am J Cardiol 91:3G, 2003.
25. Solzi P, Ring H, Najenson T, et al: Hemiplegics after a first stroke: Late survival and risk factors. Stroke 14:703, 1983.
26. Rodgers A, MacMahon S, Gamble G, et al: Blood pressure and risk of stroke in patients with cerebrovascular disease: The United Kingdom Transient Ischaemic Attack Collaborative Group. Br Med J 313:147, 1996.
27. Progress Collaborative Group: Randomised trial of a perindopril-based blood-pressure-lowering regimen among 6,105 individuals with previous stroke or transient ischaemic attack. Lancet 358:1033, 2001.
28. PATS Collaborating Group: Post-stroke antihypertensive treatment study: A preliminary result. PATS Collaborating Group. Chin Med J (Engl) 108:710, 1995.
29. Shahar E, Chambless LE, Rosamond WD, et al: Plasma lipid profile and incident ischemic stroke: The Atherosclerosis Risk in Communities (ARIC) study. Stroke 34:623, 2003.
30. Wolf PA, D'Agostino RB, Belanger AJ, et al: Are blood lipids risk factors for stroke [abstract]? Stroke 22:26,1991.
31. Prospective Studies Collaboration: Cholesterol, diastolic blood pressure and stroke: 13,000 strokes in 450,000 people in 45 prospective cohorts. Lancet 346:1647, 1995.
32. Iso H, Jacobs DR, Jr, Wentworth D, et al: Serum cholesterol levels and six-year mortality from stroke in 350,977 men screened for the multiple risk factor intervention trial. N Engl J Med 320:904, 1989.
33. Benfante R, Yano K, Hwang LJ, et al: Elevated serum cholesterol is a risk factor for both coronary heart disease and thromboembolic stroke in Hawaiian Japanese men. Implications for shared risk. Stroke 25:814, 1994.
34. Fine-Edelstein JS, Wolf PA, O'Leary DH, et al: Precursors of extracranial carotid atherosclerosis in the Framingham Study. Neurology 44:1046, 1994.
35. Wilson PWF, Hoeg JM, Belanger AJ, et al: Cholesterol-years, blood pressure-years, pack-years and carotid stenosis [abstract]. Circulation 92:I-519,1995.
36. O'Leary DH, Polak JF, Kronmal RA, et al: Thickening of the carotid wall: A marker for atherosclerosis in the elderly? Stroke 27:224, 1996.
37. Scandinavian Simvastatin Survival Study Group: Randomised trial of cholesterol lowering in 4444 patients with coronary heart disease: The Scandinavian Simvastatin Survival Study (4S). Lancet 344:1383, 1994.
38. Sacks FM, Pfeffer MA, Moye LA, et al: The effect of pravastatin on coronary events after myocardial infarction in patients with average cholesterol levels: Cholesterol and Recurrent Events Trial investigators. N Engl J Med 335:1001, 1996.
39. LIPID Study Group: Prevention of cardiovascular events and death with pravastatin in patients with coronary heart disease and a broad range of initial cholesterol levels: The Long-Term Intervention with Pravastatin in Ischaemic Disease (LIPID) Study Group. N Engl J Med 339:1349, 1998.
40. Heart Protection Study Collaborative Group: MRC/BHF Heart Protection Study of cholesterol lowering with simvastatin in 20,536 high-risk individuals: A randomised placebo-controlled trial. Lancet 360:7, 2002.
41. Plehn JF, Davis BR, Sacks FM, et al: Reduction of stroke incidence after myocardial infarction with pravastatin: The Cholesterol And Recurrent Events (CARE) study. The CARE Investigators. Circulation 99:216, 1999.
42. Shepherd J, Cobbe SM, Ford I, et al: Prevention of coronary heart disease with pravastatin in men with hypercholesterolemia: West of Scotland Coronary Prevention Study Group. N Engl J Med 333: 1301, 1995.
43. Amarenco P, Lavallee P, Touboul P: Stroke prevention, blood cholesterol, and statins. Lancet Neurol 3:271, 2004.
44. Yano K, Reed DM, MacLean CJ: Serum cholesterol and hemorrhagic stroke in the Honolulu Heart Program. Stroke 20: 1460, 1989.
45. Selhub J, Jacques PF, Wilson PWF, et al: Vitamin status and intake as primary determinants of homocysteinemia in an elderly population. JAMA 270:2693, 1993.
46. Shimamoto T, Komachi Y, Inada H, et al: Trends for coronary heart disease and stroke and their risk factors in Japan. Circulation 79: 503, 1989.
47. Tomlinson B, Chan P, Lan W: How well tolerated are lipid-lowering drugs? Drugs Aging 18:665, 2001.
48. Vijan S, Hayward RA: Treatment of hypertension in type 2 diabetes mellitus: Blood pressure goals, choice of agents, and setting priorities in diabetes care. Ann Intern Med 138:593, 2003.
49. Kannel WB, McGee DL: Diabetes and cardiovascular risk factors: The Framingham Study. Circulation 59:8, 1979.
50. Statement on hypertension in diabetes mellitus: Final report. The Working Group on Hypertension in Diabetes. Arch Intern Med 147:830, 1987.
51. Burchfiel CM, Curb JD, Rodriguez BL, et al: Glucose intolerance and 22-year stroke incidence: The Honolulu Heart Program. Stroke 25:951, 1994.
52. Barrett Connor E, Khaw KT: Diabetes mellitus: An independent risk factor for stroke? Am J Epidemiol 128:116, 1988.
53. Kannel WB, McGee DL: Diabetes and cardiovascular disease. The Framingham Study. JAMA 241:2035, 1979.
54. Kuller LH, Dorman JS, Wolf PA: Cerebrovascular disease and diabetes. National Diabetes Data Group, Diabetes in America, Diabetes Data Compiled 1984. NIH Publication No.85-1468. US Department of Health and Human Services 1486, XVIII-1-XVIII-18. 1985. Public Health Service, National Institutes of Health, National Institute of Arthritis, Diabetes, and Digestive and Kidney Diseases. National Diabetes Data Group.
55. Curb JD, Marcus EB: Body fat, coronary heart disease, and stroke in Japanese men. Am J Clin Nutr 53:1612S, 2004.
56. Rexrode KM, Hennekens CH, Willett WC, et al: A prospective study of body mass index, weight change, and risk of stroke in women. JAMA 277:1539, 1997.
57. Walker SP, Rimm EB, Ascherio A, et al: Body size and fat distribution as predictors of stroke among U.S. men. Am J Epidemiol 144:1143, 1996.
58. Wilhelmsen L, Svardsudd K, Korsan Bengtsen K, et al: Fibrinogen as a risk factor for stroke and myocardial infarction. N Engl J Med 311:501, 1984.
59. Kannel WB, Wolf PA, Castelli WP, et al: Fibrinogen and risk of cardiovascular disease: The Framingham Study. JAMA 258:1183, 1987.
60. Kannel WB, D'Agostino RB, Belanger AJ: Fibrinogen, cigarette smoking, and risk of cardiovascular disease: Insights from the Framingham Study. Am Heart J 113:1006, 1987.
61. Folsom AR, Qamhieh HT, Flack JM, et al: Plasma fibrinogen: Levels and correlates in young adults. Am J Epidemiol 138:1023, 1993.
62. Lee AJ, Lowe GD, Woodward M, et al: Fibrinogen in relation to personal history of prevalent hypertension, diabetes, stroke, intermittent claudication, coronary heart disease, and family history: The Scottish Heart Health Study. Br Heart J 69:338, 1993.

63. Tracy RP, Arnold AM, Ettinger W, et al: The relationship of fibrinogen and factors VII and VIII to incident cardiovascular disease and death in the elderly: Results from the cardiovascular health study. Arterioscler Thromb Vasc Biol 19:1776, 1999.
64. Rost NS, Wolf PA, Kase CS, et al: Plasma concentration of C-reactive protein and risk of ischemic stroke and transient ischemic attack: The Framingham Study. Stroke 32:2575, 2001.
65. Ridker PM, Rifai N, Rose L, et al: Comparison of C-reactive protein and low-density lipoprotein cholesterol levels in the prediction of first cardiovascular events. N Engl J Med 347:1557, 2002.
66. Boushey CJ, Beresford SAA, Omenn GS, et al: A quantitative assessment of plasma homocysteine as a risk factor for vascular disease: Probable benefits of increasing folic acid intakes. JAMA 274:1049, 1995.
67. Nygard O, Vollset SE, Refsum H, et al: Total plasma homocysteine and cardiovascular risk profile: The Hordaland Homocysteine Study. JAMA 274:1526, 1995.
68. Bostom AG, Rosenberg IH, Silbershatz H, et al: Nonfasting plasma total homocysteine levels and stroke incidence in elderly persons: The Framingham Study. Ann Intern Med 131:352, 1999.
69. Perry IJ, Refsum H, Morris RW, et al: Prospective study of serum total homocysteine concentration and risk of stroke in middle-aged British men. Lancet 346:1395, 1995.
70. Stampfer MJ, Malinow MR, Willett WC, et al: A prospective study of plasma homocyst(e)ine and risk of myocardial infarction in U.S. physicians. JAMA 268:877, 1992.
71. Verhoef P, Hennekens CH, Malinow MR, et al: A prospective study of plasma homocyst(e)ine and risk of ischemic stroke. Stroke 25: 1924, 1994.
72. Malinow MR, Nieto FJ, Szklo M, et al: Carotid artery intimal-medial wall thickening and plasma homocyst(e)ine in asymptomatic adults: The Atherosclerosis Risk in Communities Study. Circulation 87:1107, 1993.
73. Selhub J, Jacques PF, Bostom AG, et al: Association between plasma homocysteine concentrations and extracranial carotid-artery stenosis. N Engl J Med 332:286, 1995.
74. Selhub J, Jacques PF, Bostom AG, et al: Relationship between plasma homocysteine, vitamin status and extracranial carotid-artery stenosis in the Framingham Study population. J Nutr 126:1258S, 1996.
75. Wolf PA, Kannel WB, McNamara PM, et al: The role of impaired cardiac function in atherothrombotic brain infarction: The Framingham Study. Am J Public Health 63:52, 1973.
76. Loh E, Sutton MSJ, Wun CC, et al: Ventricular dysfunction and the risk of stroke after myocardial infarction. N Engl J Med 336:251, 1997.
77. Smith P, Arnesen H, Holme I: The effect of warfarin on mortality and reinfarction after myocardial infarction. N Engl J Med 323: 147, 1990.
78. Wolf PA, Dawber TR, Thomas HE, Jr, et al: Epidemiologic assessment of chronic atrial fibrillation and risk of stroke: The Framingham Study. Neurology 28:973, 1978.
79. Wolf PA, Abbott RD, Kannel WB: Atrial fibrillation: A major contributor to stroke in the elderly: The Framingham Study. Arch Intern Med 147:1561, 1987.
80. Chesebro JH, Fuster V, Halperin JL: Atrial fibrillation: Risk marker for stroke. N Engl J Med 323:1556, 1990.
81. Wolf PA, Abbott RD, Kannel WB: Atrial fibrillation as an independent risk factor for stroke: The Framingham Study. Stroke 22:983, 1991.
82. Atrial Fibrillation Investigators: Risk factors for stroke and efficacy of antithrombotic therapy in atrial fibrillation: Analysis of pooled data from five randomized controlled trials. Arch Intern Med 154:1449, 1994.
83. Miller VT, Rothrock JF, Pearce LA, et al: Ischemic stroke in patients with atrial fibrillation: Effect of aspirin according to stroke mechanism. Neurology 43:32, 1993.
84. Bikkina M, Levy D, Evans JC, et al: Left ventricular mass and risk of stroke in an elderly cohort. JAMA 272:33, 1994.
85. Sacco RL, Boden-Albala B, Gan R, et al: Stroke incidence among white, black, and Hispanic residents of an urban community: The Northern Manhattan Stroke Study. Am J Epidemiol 147:259, 1998.
86. Welin L, Svardsudd K, Wilhelmsen L, et al: Analysis of risk factors for stroke in a cohort of men born in 1913. N Engl J Med 317:521, 1987.
87. Kiely DK, Wolf PA, Cupples LA, et al: Familial aggregation of stroke: The Framingham Study. Stroke 24:1366, 1993.
88. Chabriat H, Vahedi K, Iba-Zizen MT, et al: Clinical spectrum of CADASIL: A study of 7 families. Lancet 346:934, 1995.
89. Tanne D, Triplett DA, Levine SR: Antiphospholipid-protein antibodies and ischemic stroke: Not just cardiolipin any more. Stroke 29:1755, 1998.
90. Carolei A, Marini C, De Matteis G: History of migraine and risk of cerebral ischaemia in young adults: The Italian National Research Council Study Group on Stroke in the Young. Lancet 347:1503, 1996.
91. Buring JE, Hebert P, Romero J, et al: Migraine and subsequent risk of stroke in the Physicians' Health Study. Arch Neurol 52:129, 1995.
92. International Study of Unruptured Intracranial Aneurysms Investigators: Unruptured Intracranial Aneurysms—Risk of Rupture and Risks of Surgical Intervention. N Engl J Med 339:1725, 1998.
93. Spriggs DA, French JM, Murdy JM, et al: Snoring increases the risk of stroke and adversely affects prognosis. Q J Med 83:555, 1992.
94. Palomaki H: Snoring and the risk of ischemic brain infarction. Stroke 22:1021, 1991.
95. Gillum RF, Mussolino ME: Education, poverty, and stroke incidence in whites and blacks: The NHANES I Epidemiologic Follow-Up Study. J Clin Epidemiol 56:188, 2003.
96. Wolf PA, D'Agostino RB, Kannel WB, et al: Cigarette smoking as a risk factor for stroke: The Framingham Study. JAMA 259:1025, 1988.
97. Colditz GA, Bonita R, Stampfer MJ, et al: Cigarette smoking and risk of stroke in middle-aged women. N Engl J Med 318:937, 1988.
98. Abbott RD, Yin Y, Reed DM, et al: Risk of stroke in male cigarette smokers. N Engl J Med 315:717, 1986.
99. Royal College of General Practitioners' Oral Contraception Study: Further analyses of mortality in oral contraceptive users. Lancet 1:541, 1981.
100. Sacco RL, Wolf PA, Bharucha NE, et al: Subarachnoid and intracerebral hemorrhage: Natural history, prognosis, and precursive factors in the Framingham Study. Neurology 34:847, 1984.
101. Fogelholm R, Murros K: Cigarette smoking and subarachnoid haemorrhage: A population-based case-control study. J Neurol Neurosurg Psychiatry 50:78, 1987.
102. Bonita R: Cigarette smoking, hypertension and the risk of subarachnoid hemorrhage: A population-based case-control study. Stroke 17:831, 1986.
103. Shinton R, Beevers G: Meta-analysis of relation between cigarette smoking and stroke. Br Med J 298:789, 1989.
104. Stadel BV: Oral contraceptives and cardiovascular disease (second of two parts). N Engl J Med 305:672, 1981.
105. Adams HP, Jr, Butler MJ, Biller J, et al: Nonhemorrhagic cerebral infarction in young adults. Arch Neurol 43:793, 1986.
106. Stampfer MJ, Willett WC, Colditz GA, et al: A prospective study of past use of oral contraceptive agents and risk of cardiovascular diseases. N Engl J Med 319:1313, 1988.
107. WHO Collaborative Study of Cardiovascular Disease and Steroid Hormone Contraception. Ischaemic stroke and combined oral contraceptives: Results of an international, multicentre, case-control study. Lancet 348:498, 1996.
108. Petitti DB, Sidney S, Bernstein A, et al: Stroke in users of low-dose oral contraceptives. N Engl J Med 335:8, 1996.
109. Gillum LA, Mamidipudi SK, Johnston SC: Ischemic stroke risk with oral contraceptives: A meta-analysis. JAMA 284:72, 2000.
110. WHO Collaborative Study of Cardiovascular Disease and Steroid Hormone Contraception. Haemorrhagic stroke, overall stroke risk, and combined oral contraceptives: Results of an international, multicentre, case-control study. Lancet 348:505, 1996.
111. Stampfer MJ, Colditz GA, Willett WC, et al: A prospective study of moderate alcohol consumption and the risk of coronary disease and stroke in women. N Engl J Med 319:267, 1988.
112. Djoussé L, Ellison R, Beiser A, et al: Alcohol consumption and risk of ischemic stroke: The Framingham Study. Stroke 33:907, 2002.
113. Donahue RP, Abbott RD, Reed DM, et al: Alcohol and hemorrhagic stroke: The Honolulu Heart Program. JAMA 255:2311, 1986.
114. Camargo CA, Jr: Moderate alcohol consumption and stroke: The epidemiologic evidence. Stroke 20:1611, 1989.
115. Hillbom M, Kaste M, Rasi V: Can ethanol intoxication affect hemocoagulation to increase the risk of brain infarction in young adults? Neurology 33:381, 1983.

116. Ettinger PO, Wu CF, De La Cruz C, Jr, et al: Arrhythmias and the "Holiday Heart:" Alcohol-associated cardiac rhythm disorders. Am Heart J 95:555, 1978.
117. Taylor JR, Combs Orme T: Alcohol and strokes in young adults. Am J Psychiatry 142:116, 1985.
118. Abbott RD, Rodriguez BL, Burchfiel CM, et al: Physical activity in older middle-aged men and reduced risk of stroke: The Honolulu Heart Program. Am J Epidemiol 139:881, 1994.
119. Wannamethee G, Shaper AG: Physical activity and stroke in British middle-aged men. Br Med J 304:597, 1992.
120. Kiely DK, Wolf PA, Cupples LA, et al: Physical activity and stroke risk: The Framingham Study. Am J Epidemiol 140:608, 1994.
121. Manson J, Stampfer M, Willett W, et al: Physical activity and incidence of coronary heart disease and stroke in women [abstract]. Circulation 91:927, 1995.
122. Gillum RF, Mussolino ME, Ingram DD: Physical activity and stroke incidence in women and men. The NHANES I Epidemiologic Follow-Up Study. Am J Epidemiol 143:860, 1996.
123. Lee IM, Hennekens CH, Berger K, et al: Exercise and risk of stroke in male physicians. Stroke 30:1, 1999.
124. Hu FB, Stampfer MJ, Colditz GA, et al: Physical activity and risk of stroke in women. JAMA 283:2961, 2000.
125. Liu S, Manson JE, Stampfer MJ, et al: Whole grain consumption and risk of ischemic stroke in women: A prospective study. JAMA 284:1534, 2000.
126. Joshipura K J, Ascherio A, Manson J E, et al: Fruit and vegetable intake in relation to risk of ischemic stroke. JAMA 282:1233, 1999.
127. Iso H, Rexrode KM, Stampfer MJ, et al: Intake of fish and omega-3 fatty acids and risk of stroke in women. JAMA 285:304, 2001.
128. Gillum RF, Mussolino ME, Madans JH: The relationship between fish consumption and stroke incidence. The NHANES I Epidemiologic Follow-Up Study (National Health and Nutrition Examination Survey). Arch Intern Med 156:537, 1996.
129. Ascherio A, Rimm EB, Hernan MA, et al: Relation of consumption of vitamin E, vitamin C, and carotenoids to risk for stroke among men in the United States. Ann Intern Med 130:963, 1999.
130. Wolf PA, D'Agostino RB, Belanger AJ, et al: Probability of stroke: A risk profile from the Framingham Study. Stroke 22(3):312, 1991.
131. Chobanian AV, Bakris GL, Black HR, et al: The Seventh Report of the Joint National Committee on Prevention, Detection, Evaluation, and Treatment of High Blood Pressure: The JNC 7 report. JAMA 289:2560, 2003.
132. Bonita R, Beaglehole R: The enigma of the decline in stroke deaths in the United States: The search for an explanation. Stroke 27:370, 1996.
133. MacMahon S, Rodgers A: The epidemiological association between blood pressure and stroke: Implications for primary and secondary prevention. Hypertens Res 17:S23, 1994.
134. Collins R, Peto R, MacMahon S, et al: Blood pressure, stroke, and coronary heart disease. Part 2, Short-term reductions in blood pressure: Overview of randomised drug trials in their epidemiological context. Lancet 335:827, 1990.
135. MacMahon S, Peto R, Cutler J, et al: Blood pressure, stroke, and coronary heart disease. Part 1, Prolonged differences in blood pressure: Prospective observational studies corrected for the regression dilution bias. Lancet 335:765, 1990.
136. Kannel WB, Dawber TR, Sorlie P, et al: Components of blood pressure and risk of atherothrombotic brain infarction: The Framingham Study. Stroke 7:327, 1976.
137. SHEP Cooperative Research Group: Prevention of stroke by antihypertensive drug treatment in older persons with isolated systolic hypertension: Final results of the Systolic Hypertension in the Elderly Program (SHEP). JAMA 265:3255, 1991.
138. Wilking SV, Belanger A, Kannel WB, et al: Determinants of isolated systolic hypertension. JAMA 260:3451, 1988.
139. Amery A, Birkenhager W, Brixko P, et al: Mortality and morbidity results from the European Working Party on High Blood Pressure in the Elderly trial. Lancet 1:1349, 1985.
140. Staessen J, Amery A, Birkenhager W, et al: Syst-Eur: A multicenter trial on the treatment of isolated systolic hypertension in the elderly: First interim report. J Cardiovasc Pharmacol 19:120, 1992.
141. Staessen JA, Fagard R, Thijs L, et al: Randomised double-blind comparison of placebo and active treatment for older patients with isolated systolic hypertension: The Systolic Hypertension in Europe (Syst-Eur) Trial Investigators. Lancet 350:757, 1997.
142. Curb JD, Pressel SL, Cutler JA, et al: Effect of diuretic-based antihypertensive treatment on cardiovascular disease risk in older diabetic patients with isolated systolic hypertension. Systolic Hypertension in the Elderly Program Cooperative Research Group. JAMA 276:1886, 1996.
143. UK Prospective Diabetes Study Group: Tight blood pressure control and risk of macrovascular and microvascular complications in type 2 diabetes: UKPDS 38. UK Prospective Diabetes Study Group. Br Med J 317:703, 1998.
144. The ALLHAT Officers and Coordinators for the ALLHAT Collaborative Research Group: Major Outcomes in High-Risk Hypertensive Patients Randomized to Angiotensin-Converting Enzyme Inhibitor or Calcium Channel Blocker vs. Diuretic: The Antihypertensive and Lipid-Lowering Treatment to Prevent Heart Attack Trial (ALLHAT). JAMA 288:298, 2002.
145. Yusuf S, Sleight P, Pogue J, et al: Effects of an angiotensin-converting-enzyme inhibitor, ramipril, on cardiovascular events in high-risk patients: The Heart Outcomes Prevention Evaluation Study Investigators. N Engl J Med 342:145, 2000.
146. Bosch J, Yusuf S, Pogue J, et al: Use of ramipril in preventing stroke: Double blind randomised trial. Br Med J 324:699, 2002.
147. Lonn E, Yusuf S, Dzavik V, et al: Effects of ramipril and vitamin E on atherosclerosis: The study to evaluate carotid ultrasound changes in patients treated with ramipril and vitamin E (SECURE). Circulation 103:919, 2001.
148. Kjeldsen SE, Dahlof B, Devereux RB, et al: Effects of losartan on cardiovascular morbidity and mortality in patients with isolated systolic hypertension and left ventricular hypertrophy: A Losartan Intervention For Endpoint Reduction (LIFE) substudy. JAMA 288: 1491, 2002.
149. Dahlof B, Devereux RB, Kjeldsen SE, et al: Cardiovascular morbidity and mortality in the Losartan Intervention For Endpoint reduction in hypertension study (LIFE): A randomised trial against atenolol. Lancet 359:995, 2002.
150. The Diabetes Control and Complications Trial Research Group: The effect of intensive treatment of diabetes on the development and progression of long-term complications in insulin-dependent diabetes mellitus. N Engl J Med 329:977, 1993.
151. Diabetes Control and Complications Trial Research Group: The effect of intensive diabetes therapy on the development and progression of neuropathy: The Diabetes Control and Complications Trial Research Group. Ann Intern Med 122:561, 1995.
152. JNC V. The Fifth Report of the Joint National Committee on Detection, Evaluation, and Treatment of High Blood Pressure. NIH Publication No.93-1088, 1993.
153. Lloyd-Jones DM, Evans JC, Larson MG, et al: Differential control of systolic and diastolic blood pressure: Factors associated with lack of blood pressure control in the community. Hypertension 36: 594, 2000.
154. Coppola WG, Whincup PH, Walker M, et al: Identification and management of stroke risk in older people: A national survey of current practice in primary care. J Hum Hypertens 11:185, 1997.
155. Kawachi I, Colditz GA, Stampfer M J, et al: Smoking cessation and decreased risk of stroke in women. JAMA 269:232, 1993.
156. European Atrial Fibrillation Trial Study Group (EAFT): Secondary prevention in non-rheumatic atrial fibrillation after transient ischaemic attack or minor stroke. Lancet 342:1255, 1993.
157. European Atrial Fibrillation Trial Study Group: Optimal oral anticoagulant therapy in patients with nonrheumatic atrial fibrillation and recent cerebral ischemia: The European Atrial Fibrillation Trial Study Group. N Engl J Med 333:5, 1995.
158. Hylek EM, Skates SJ, Sheehan MA, et al: An analysis of the lowest effective intensity of prophylactic anticoagulation for patients with nonrheumatic atrial fibrillation. N Engl J Med 335:540, 1996.
159. Stroke Prevention in Atrial Fibrillation Investigators: Adjusted-dose warfarin versus low-intensity, fixed-dose warfarin plus aspirin for high-risk patients with atrial fibrillation: Stroke Prevention in Atrial Fibrillation III randomized clinical trial. Lancet 348:633, 1996.
160. Stafford RS, Singer DE: National patterns of warfarin use in atrial fibrillation. Arch Intern Med 156:2537, 1996.
161. Verheugt FW: Can we pull the plug on warfarin in atrial fibrillation? Lancet 362:1686, 2003.
162. Laupacis A, Albers G, Dalen J, et al: Antithrombotic therapy in atrial fibrillation. Chest 114:579S, 1998.
163. Atkins D, Psaty BM, Koepsell TD, et al: Cholesterol reduction and the risk for stroke in men: A meta-analysis of randomized, controlled trials. Ann Intern Med 119:136, 1993.

164. Sever PS, Dahlof B, Poulter NR, et al: Prevention of coronary and stroke events with atorvastatin in hypertensive patients who have average or lower-than-average cholesterol concentrations, in the Anglo-Scandinavian Cardiac Outcomes Trial—Lipid Lowering Arm (ASCOT-LLA): A multicentre randomised controlled trial. Lancet 361:1149, 2003.
165. Furberg CD, Adams HP, Jr, Applegate WB, et al: Effect of lovastatin on early carotid atherosclerosis and cardiovascular events. Asymptomatic Carotid Artery Progression Study (ACAPS) Research Group. Circulation 90:1679, 1994.
166. Tell GS, Crouse JR, Furberg CD: Relation between blood lipids, lipoproteins, and cerebrovascular atherosclerosis: A review. Stroke 19:423, 1988.
167. O'Leary DH, Anderson KM, Wolf PA, et al: Cholesterol and carotid atherosclerosis in older persons: The Framingham Study. Ann Epidemiol 2:147, 1992.
168. Vaughan CJ, Murphy MB, Buckley BM: Statins do more than just lower cholesterol. Lancet 348:1079, 1996.
169. Stampfer MJ, Malinow MR: Can lowering homocysteine levels reduce cardiovascular risk? N Engl J Med 332:328, 1995.
170. Stampfer MJ, Rimm EB: Folate and cardiovascular disease. Why we need a trial now. JAMA 275:1929, 1996.
171. Stampfer MJ, Willett WC: Homocysteine and marginal vitamin deficiency: The importance of adequate vitamin intake. JAMA 270:2726, 1993.
172. Mendelsohn ME: Protective effects of estrogen on the cardiovascular system. Am J Cardiol. 89:12E, 2002.
173. Viscoli CM, Brass LM, Kernan WN, et al: A Clinical Trial of Estrogen-Replacement Therapy after Ischemic Stroke. N Engl J Med 345:1243, 2001.
174. Writing Group for the Women's Health Initiative Investigators: Risks and benefits of estrogen plus progestin in healthy postmenopausal women: Principal results from the women's Health Initiative Randomized Controlled Trial. JAMA 288:321, 2002.

chapter 30

Cerebrovascular Disease: Clinical Presentation and Diagnosis

Louis R. Caplan

OVERVIEW OF DIAGNOSIS

Cerebrovascular disease is heterogeneous in etiology and clinical presentation.[1] Management of individual patients depends on the type, location, and severity of the cerebrovascular lesions and the presence, severity, and location of the resulting brain injury. A question-driven approach is suggested in arriving at a diagnosis.

Does the Patient Have Cerebrovascular Disease or a Mimic?

Many conditions can cause clinical symptoms and signs that closely resemble cerebrovascular disease syndromes. Syncope, migraine, and seizures may be misdiagnosed as transient ischemic attacks (TIAs). TIAs and strokes represent focal brain injuries. Table 30-1 lists important mimics and their tendency to produce focal or generalized brain dysfunction. Table 30-2 lists differential diagnostic features of syncope, seizures, migraine, and TIAs. Brain tumors can cause the sudden onset of symptoms, as can some toxic and metabolic disorders. Diagnosis is based on the presence of vascular disease risk factors, the tempo of onset, the presence of concurrent conditions, and the clinical course of development of neurologic symptoms and signs. In many patients, recognition that the disorder is not cerebrovascular is based on neuroimaging or blood and spinal fluid testing consistent with traumatic, neoplastic, toxic, metabolic, or infectious processes rather than brain infarction or hemorrhage.

TABLE 30-1 CAUSES OF TRANSIENT ISCHEMIC ATTACKS ("TURNS") AND THEIR TENDENCY TO CAUSE FOCAL OR NONFOCAL SYMPTOMS

Conditions	Focal Symptoms	Nonfocal Symptoms
Common Disorders		
Seizures	++	++
TIAs	++++	Occasionally
Migraine	++++	
Syncope		++++
Less Common Conditions		
Vestibulopathy	++	++
Metabolic	+	+++
"Tumor attacks"	+++	+
Multiple sclerosis	++++	
Psychiatric	++	++
Nerves and nerve root	++++	
TGA	++++	

TIA, transient ischemic attacks; TGA, transient global amnesia.

If the Disorder Is Cerebrovascular, Is the Problem Hemorrhage or Ischemia?

Differentiation into hemorrhagic and ischemic conditions is an important initial step.[1] These two etiologies are diametrically opposite. In hemorrhage, there is too much blood in the head, whereas in ischemia, there is too little blood and energy supply. In patients with brain ischemia, the aim is to deliver more blood-containing nutrients, whereas in patients with hemorrhage the aim is to limit bleeding and prevent further hemorrhages. About 80% of strokes are ischemic, whereas 20% are hemorrhagic. Separation between bleeding and ischemia is based on the clinical history and examination, but collaboration is always necessary by brain imaging that shows subarachnoid and/or intraparenchymatous blood, or a brain infarct. In some patients, spinal puncture is necessary to document bleeding into the subarachnoid space because brain imaging in these patients may not show blood, especially if the hemorrhage was small or occurred days before imaging. The absence of bleeding, or important nonvascular pathology on brain neuroimaging in patients with acute onset focal brain symptoms is usually sufficient evidence that the problem is brain ischemia, especially when the patient has stroke risk factors and cardiac or cerebrovascular lesions shown by vascular imaging and cardiac evaluation.

What If the Problem Is Hemorrhage? Is the Bleeding Subarachnoid or Intracerebral?

Hemorrhage should be separated into subarachnoid hemorrhage (SAH) and intracerebral hemorrhage (ICH). These two subtypes of hemorrhage have different etiologies, different clinical findings, and different treatment strategies. About 10% of strokes are due to SAH and about 10% to ICH, depending on the age, sex, educational and social status, and race of the patients studied. Patients with SAH have the sudden onset of severe, usually diffuse, headache. Vomiting, cessation of activity, and decreased level of consciousness are often present. Ordinarily there are no focal signs. CT and MRI show subarachnoid blood,

TABLE 30-2 DIFFERENTIAL DIAGNOSTIC FEATURES AMONG SEIZURES, MIGRAINE, TRANSIENT ISCHEMIC ATTACKS, AND SYNCOPE

	Seizures	TIAs	Migraine	Syncope
Demography	Any age youths; common among the young	Older patients with stroke risks; Men > women	Younger age Women > men	Any age; Often younger Women > men
CNS Symptoms	*Positive Symptoms—* Limb jerking, head turning; loss of consciousness; negative symptoms may develop and remain	*Negative Symptoms—* Numbness, visual loss, paralysis ataxia; all sensory modalities affected at same time	*First positive, then negative symptoms—in same modality;* scintillations and paresthesias most common; 2nd sensory modality after the first clears	Light-headedness, dim vision, noises distant, decreased alertness; transient loss of consciousness
Timing	20-180 sec; absence, atonic seizures, and myoclonic jerks shorter; spells occur over years	Usually minutes; mostly <1 hr; spells during days, weeks, or months not usually years	Usually 20-30 minutes; sporadic attacks over years	Usually a few seconds; sporadic attacks during years
Associated Symptoms	Tongue biting, incontinence, muscles sore, headache after attack	Headaches may occur during time of the TIAs	Headache after; nausea, vomiting, photophobia	Sweating, pallor, nausea

and the spinal fluid is under increased pressure and shows blood or xanthochromia.

Patients with intracerebral hemorrhage develop focal neurologic signs that increase gradually over minutes, sometimes hours. After the focal signs increase, headache, vomiting, and decrease in level of consciousness may develop if the ICH is large.[2] The patient often has risk factors for hemorrhage such as hypertension, use of amphetamines or cocaine, or an iatrogenic or intrinsic bleeding diathesis (most often prescription anticoagulants). CT and MRI scans show a localized collection of blood within the brain, an intracerebral "hematoma."

What If the Hemorrhage is Subarachnoid?

SAH is most often due to leakage of blood from an aneurysm. Less often, arteriovenous malformations that abut on pial surfaces bleed. Amyloid angiopathy, bleeding disorders, drugs, and occult trauma are other etiologies. Evaluation attempts to define an aneurysm or other bleeding lesion. Vascular imaging, usually including cerebral dye contrast angiography, is usually needed. CTA and MRA are sometimes used for preliminary screening but may not be definitive.[3] Treatment of patients with aneurysms is aimed at destroying the potential of the aneurysm to bleed again, either by direct surgery or by endovascular techniques that contain and thrombose the aneurysmal sac. Because the subarachnoid blood often induces vasoconstriction that can cause secondary brain ischemia, another aim of therapy is to use drugs and strategies that decrease vasoconstriction and maximize cerebral blood flow after the aneurysm is treated.

What If the Hemorrhage Is Intracerebral?

The most common and important cause of ICH is uncontrolled hypertension. Hypertensive hemorrhages most often are located in the lateral ganglionic region (putamen and internal capsule), thalamus, caudate nucleus, pons, and cerebellum.[2] Some hypertensive hematomas are located in the cerebral lobes. Treatment includes control of hypertension without overzealous reduction in brain perfusion pressure. Hemorrhages due to bleeding disorders are treated by reversing the bleeding diathesis. Some lobar hematomas in older patients are caused by amyloid angiopathy. Drugs, trauma, and vascular malformations (arteriovenous and cavernous angiomas) are less frequent causes of ICH. Surgical, radiotherapeutic, and endovascular control of vascular malformations are considered in appropriate patients.

In some patients with large hemorrhages that have not adequately decompressed themselves by bleeding into the CSF, surgical drainage is considered, especially hematomas that are lobar and cerebellar and cause mass effects. Drugs that decrease intracranial pressure are considered in patients with increased intracranial pressure. Ventricular drainage is considered in some patients with hydrocephalus caused by obstruction of CSF pathways.

What If the Problem Is Ischemia? Is the Ischemia Due to Systemic Hypoperfusion, Embolism, or In-Situ Vascular Occlusive Disease?

There are three quite different mechanisms of brain ischemia (1) diffusely diminished blood flow to the brain caused by a systemic process; (2) blockage of an artery supplying the brain related to a local in-situ process within that artery or vein (usually referred to as *thrombosis*); and (3) embolic occlusion of arteries feeding the brain. Thrombosis and embolism are not mutually exclusive because a thrombus that forms in-situ in an artery can embolize to a distal artery (artery-to-artery brain embolism). Differentiation into global hypoperfusion and thromboembolism is usually quite easy but separation of thrombosis from embolism is difficult without extensive brain and vascular imaging.[1,3]

Patients with systemic hypoperfusion report lightheadedness, visual blurring, dampened and distant sounding auditory stimuli, and difficulty thinking and concentrating. They feel faint especially when standing. They do not have promontory TIAs. Blood pressure may be low and the pulse may be fast. The usual cause is cardiac arrest or arrhythmia. Pulmonary embolism, gastrointestinal bleeding, and hypovolemia can also produce the same syndrome. There are usually no lateralized neurologic deficits. When present, signs are symmetric and emphasize visual, cognitive, and behavioral abnormalities. Brain imaging may be normal or show infarcts in the border-zone territories between the major cervicocranial arteries.

Thromboembolism is characterized by the sudden or rapid onset of focal neurologic signs. There are often preceding TIAs. Neurologic examination shows signs attributable to a brain region supplied by single arteries and CT or MRI usually shows brain infarcts in patients with persistent neurologic signs or lengthy (>6 hours) TIAs. Rapid vascular imaging (CTA, MRA, or transcranial Doppler [TCD] ultrasound) often shows occlusion of an intracranial artery.

What If the Cause of the Ischemia Is Systemic Hypoperfusion?

The aim is to correct the cause and to maximize brain blood flow quickly. Cardiac disease should be treated. Blood pressure should be restored. Transfusion and intravenous fluids are important in patients with systemic bleeding and hypovolemia.

What If the Cause of Ischemia Is Thromboembolism?

Thromboembolism is by far the most important cause of brain ischemia. The initial evaluation should be rapid, efficient, and thorough. Neurologic signs should be determined and quantified. Standard stroke scales should be used whenever possible to quantify the neurologic deficit. Brain imaging (CT or MRI) should be performed quickly to determine the presence, location, and extent of brain infarction. Vascular imaging should also be performed quickly to identify occlusive lesions. Is all of the territory of the brain supplied by the occluded artery already infarcted, normal, or somewhere in between, that is, nonfunctioning but not yet infarcted ("stunned")? Table 30-3 lists the information needed to optimally treat patients with brain ischemia. If there is considerable brain tissue still at risk, and the brain infarct is not too large, an effort should be made to recanalize the obstructed artery. This is most often done using thrombolytic agents administered either intravenously or intra-arterially. Mechanical means (angioplasty, stenting, or mechanical removal or break-up of the thrombus) or surgery are sometimes used to open or bypass the blockage. Maximizing brain circulation helps to increase blood flow to ischemic zones by opening occluded arteries and increasing flow through collateral vascular channels.

TABLE 30-3 DATA NEEDED TO TREAT A PATIENT WITH BRAIN ISCHEMIA

The nature, location, and severity of causative cardiac, aortic, and cervicocranial lesions
Hematologic and serologic factors that alter blood coagulability, blood viscosity, and delivery of nutritionally adequate blood to the brain
The mechanism of ischemia: hypoperfusion, embolism, or a combination?
State of the brain: normal, infarcted, or "stunned"?

An important aim is to prevent a recurrence of stroke. Definitions of the causative vascular lesions and any other cardio-cerebrovascular-hematologic disorders that pose a threat for future brain injury are important in order to choose an appropriate prophylactic regimen. Recognition and treatment of risk factors such as hypertension, diabetes, smoking, obesity, inactivity, and hyperlipidemia are important. In most patients with thromboembolism, prescription of agents that decrease the formation of platelet-fibrin "white thrombi" or erythrocyte-fibrin "red thrombi" is indicated. So-called platelet antiaggregants (aspirin, clopidogrel, modified-release dipyridamole—alone or in combination with aspirin) are used to prevent the formation of white thrombi and standard anticoagulants (heparin, low-molecular-weight heparin, or warfarin) are used to prevent red thrombi.[1] At times, it is appropriate to use both of these types of agents. Correctible cardiac, aortic, and cervicocranial lesions are sought. Lesions that cause severe stenosis of cervicocranial arteries are sometimes treatable by surgical or endovascular techniques.

HISTORY, PHYSICAL, AND NEUROLOGIC EXAMINATIONS

History—Strategies and Important Factors

The patient's history is crucial. Begin by letting the patient tell their story uninterrupted.[4] This practice offers insight into the intelligence, language, and organizing skills of the patient as well as their concerns. As the story unfolds, aided by accompanying family or significant others, the clinician should begin to generate *what* (pathology and pathophysiology of the brain and vascular lesions) and *where* (location of the brain and vascular lesions) hypotheses and to test them actively as the history is taken.[1,4] Table 30-4 lists information used for *what* (etiologic) diagnosis and Table 30-5 lists information used in determining *where* (localization) diagnosis.

The patient's sex, age, and past illnesses give initial clues. For example, suppose the patient is an elderly hypertensive man who developed a slight left hemiplegia 4 days earlier. Hypertension raises the possibility of intracerebral hemorrhage (ICH). His age also favors some types of hemorrhage (e.g., amyloid angiopathy or minor trauma). Alternatively, hypertension may have caused penetrating artery disease (the cause of lacunar infarcts) or have accelerated the development of large artery

TABLE 30-4 DATA USED FOR THE *"WHAT"* (ETIOLOGY) DIAGNOSIS

Etiology—demography and medical conditions known in the past and/or recognized now (age, race, sex, hypertension, angina pectoris, diabetes, hypercholesterolemia, rheumatic heart disease, etc.)
Past cerebrovascular events—transient ischemic attacks and past strokes: distribution, nature, and cause
Activity at onset of cerebrovascular event
Course—maximal at outset, fluctuating from normal to abnormal, stepwise, gradually progressive, or rapid improvement
Associated symptoms—headache, vomiting, loss of consciousness, seizures
Neuroimaging—computed tomography or magnetic resonance imaging of the brain and cervicocranial vessels

extracranial and intracranial atherosclerosis. I have listed three hypotheses about stroke type (*what* diagnosis). As the account of the course of development of the deficit is pursued, the physician mentally decides whether the patient's and family's accounts of the early symptoms and their subsequent course favor one of these hypotheses or suggest a different possibility.[5] The generation and testing of *what* (etiologic) hypotheses should continue throughout the entire patient encounter.

At the same time, the physician also should be thinking about *where* diagnoses, the localization of the lesion in the nervous system and the arteries that supply these regions. The patient's description of neurologic symptoms should generate anatomic hypotheses. A pattern-matching strategy is used attempting to match the patient's reports of neurologic symptoms (and later the neurologic signs found on examination) with common location patterns.[5] In most patients the findings conform to one of six general patterns (1) left anterior circulation—non lacunar (left internal carotid artery [ICA], middle cerebral artery [MCA]); (2) right anterior circulation—nonlacunar—(right ICA-MCA); (3) vertebrobasilar arteries (brain stem and cerebellum); (4) right posterior cerebral artery (PCA); (5) Left PCA; and (6) lacunar. The usual findings in patients with each of these patterns are listed in Table 30-6. If a homonymous visual-field defect is present, the lesion must be supratentorial and posteriorly located in the contralateral cerebral hemisphere, most often in the territory of the posterior cerebral artery.[1,6] An arm monoparesis or a great discrepancy in

TABLE 30-5 DATA USED FOR THE *"WHERE"* (LOCALIZATION) DIAGNOSIS

Neurologic symptoms described by patient
Neurologic signs found on neurologic examination
Vascular examination
Brain neuroimaging—CT and MRI
Vascular diagnostic tests—ultrasound (extracranial and intracranial), MRA, CTA, standard angiography

CT, computed tomography; CTA, computed tomography angiography; MRA, magnetic resonance angiography; MRI, magnetic resonance imaging.

TABLE 30-6 COMMON PATTERNS OF FINDINGS ACCORDING TO STROKE LOCATION

1. Left anterior circulation (left ICA-MCA)—nonlacunar; right hemiparesis, hemisensory loss, hemianopia, aphasia
2. Right anterior circulation (right ICA-MCA)—nonlacunar; left hemiparesis, hemisensory loss, hemianopia; left neglect, decreased awareness of the deficit, abnormal drawing and copying, abnormal visual-spatial abilities
3. Vertebro-basilar system (brain stem and cerebellum); vertigo, diplopia, crossed motor and/or sensory signs (one side of the face and the contralateral body), ataxia; bilateral motor and/or sensory signs
4. Left PCA; right hemianopia, alexia without agraphia; right hemisensory symptoms
5. Right PCA; left hemianopia, left hemisensory symptoms; topographical disorientation
6. Lacunar infarction: weakness of face, arm, and leg on one side of the body without other signs; sensory symptoms in face, arm, and leg on one side of the body without other symptoms and signs; weakness with ataxia on one side of the body; dysarthria and clumsiness of one hand

ICA, internal carotid artery; MCA middle cerebral artery; PCA posterior cerebral artery.

the severity of weakness in the patient's face, arm, hand, and leg suggests a cortical, paracentral localization. As the history taking proceeds, physicians should construct hypotheses of the location of the brain lesion.

Demographics, Past Illnesses, and Comorbid Conditions

Age, sex, race, family history, and the patient's medical history strongly affect the probability of the various stroke mechanisms. Some illnesses heavily favor only one mechanism (e.g., rheumatic mitral stenosis with atrial fibrillation strongly suggests embolism of cardiac origin). Others, such as hypertension, predispose to a number of possibilities. Factors such as race and sex affect the likelihood of particular vascular occlusive lesions. In general, white men have more extracranial occlusive disease of the internal carotid (ICA) and vertebral artery origins in the neck; women, blacks, and Asians have more intracranial large artery occlusive disease.[7] Blacks and Asians have a higher frequency of ICH. Table 30-7 estimates the relative weights attributable to various risk factors. Knowledge of risk factors also helps physicians assess the chances of future vascular disease—stroke, coronary artery disease, and peripheral vascular occlusive disease.

Past Cerebrovascular Events

A history of a stroke or TIA can yield important clues to the present cerebrovascular event. As arteries gradually occlude, there are often brief periods of intermittent reduced distal blood flow and embolization of white platelet-fibrin aggregates, red fibrin-dependent thrombi, and plaque material into the intracranial branches supplied by that artery. About 50% of patients with large artery occlusive lesions and one fourth of patients with penetrating artery disease have preceding TIAs in the

TABLE 30-7 WEIGHING OF ETIOLOGIC FACTORS

	Thrombosis	Lacune	Embolus	ICH	SAH
Hypertension	++	+++		++	+
Hypertension	+++	+		++++	++
Coronary disease	+++		++		
Claudication	+++		+		
Atrial fibrillation			++++		
Sick sinus syndrome			++		
Valvular heart disease			+++		
Diabetes	+++	+	+		
Bleeding diathesis				++++	+
Smoking	+++		+		+
Cancer	++		++		
Old age	+++	+	+	+	
Black or Asian origin	+	+		++	

Hypertension +++, severe hypertension; ICH, intracerebral hemorrhage; SAH, subarachnoid hemorrhage.

same vascular territory as their stroke. In large artery lesions (e.g., the ICA in the neck), attacks are spread over a long interval and are often heterogeneous, with, for example, transient monocular blindness in one attack, hand and face numbness in a second attack, and aphasia with hand weakness in a third spell. In penetrating artery disease, attacks usually, but not always, occur during a shorter time span and closer to the time of the stroke. Attacks are often similar in their features and reflect the subcortical blood supply (e.g., tingling on the left side of the body in each attack is most often due to disease of a thalamogeniculate branch artery supplying the lateral thalamus).

Patients whose present stroke is a small deep infarct caused by penetrating artery or branch atheromatous disease have often had past lacunar strokes in different regions. Similarly, patients with emboli originating from the heart have often also had prior embolic strokes or unrecognized brain infarcts in other vascular territories.[8] These past lacunar and embolic brain infarcts may be detectable clinically but sometimes are shown only on CT and MRI images. Patients with lobar ICHs may have had other smaller bleeds detectable by susceptibility-weighted (T2*) MRI images.

The nature of prior attacks or recent TIAs as revealed by the history provides a clue to the nature of the present event. Unfortunately, most individuals are naive about the workings of their bodies, especially their nervous systems. Patients may attribute temporary hand numbness and weakness to a local lesion in the limb and may not think of reporting it. Similarly, most patients are unlikely to report having white sparkles in the left visual field 10 days earlier, thinking it is a symptom for the eye doctor. To elicit the history of prior TIAs or strokes, the physician must doggedly and tenaciously ask and ask again about specific functions. Did you ever have your foot or leg go temporarily limp… your vision fade temporarily in one eye… your speech fail you or come out garbled, slurred, or wrong… and so forth? Family members may remember spells that patients did not recognize or recall. The patient may not recall symptoms the first time questions are asked but may remember them later.

Onset and Course of Stroke

Most strokes and TIAs occur during activities of daily living. Emboli can be precipitated by a cough, sneeze, suddenly rising from bed during the night to go to the bathroom, or sexual intercourse (especially paradoxical emboli). SAH and ICH can be precipitated by intercourse or emotional stress. In patients with large artery occlusive disease, standing or rising after bending can precipitate brief ischemic attacks. Vigorous turning or neck stretching can cause extracranial arterial dissections. Always inquire what the patient was doing before and during the attack. Was there any unusual or vigorous physical activity or emotional duress in the minutes, hours, or days before the attack?

Each stroke subtype has its usual common signature of development and evolution.[1,4,5] Emboli most often (more than 80%) occur suddenly and create deficits that are maximal immediately. Patients suddenly slump in their chair with a hemiplegia. In contrast, ICHs grow gradually over minutes, and the signs gradually increase. If the hematoma becomes large, then headache, vomiting, and decreased consciousness ensue—after the initial signs of focal brain dysfunction. SAH also begins suddenly, but the blood released into the cerebrospinal fluid under arterial pressure causes severe headache, vomiting, and transient interruption in posture or activities. Unlike ICH, focal symptoms of brain dysfunction are not usually present at outset. In patients with large artery occlusive disease, fluctuations in the symptoms and signs are characteristic, with stepwise increases in deficits, temporary improvements or return to normal function, and the gradual but erratic progression of symptoms and signs during a few days. These fluctuations and changes are due to changes in the systemic circulation affecting collateral blood flow and propagation and embolization of thrombi distally into downstream branches. Few patients can give an accurate account of the development of symptoms. Those with right hemisphere strokes may not recognize any deficit. Family and friends can supply useful data. Have the patient *walk through* the events before and after the stroke began. One patient whom I recall reported that she gradually developed a left-sided paralysis that morning. When she described the events in more detail, she said, "During breakfast, my left hand and arm went weak and clumsy, and I dropped a coffee cup from my hand. I went upstairs to my bedroom, and walked OK on the stairs. I rested for a half hour, and then when I came downstairs my hand was alright. I cleaned the room without trouble. An hour later, my hand and arm went weak again. This time I stumbled on the steps and had to limp with my left leg. When I called my daughter, my words were slurred. I laid down again, but this time, when I tried to get up, I couldn't use my left side." This fluctuating pattern of development of the deficit is characteristic of occlusion of a feeding artery with distal hypoperfusion. In her case, the symptoms fit the pattern of a pure motor hemiparesis most likely caused by penetrating artery disease.

Accompanying Symptoms

Headache, loss of consciousness, vomiting, and seizures all provide clues to the cause of the stroke. Headaches, unusual for the patient before the stroke, may signify large artery occlusive disease or recent elevation in blood pressure. Headache at stroke onset is invariable in SAH and sometimes occurs in brain embolism. In ICH, headache usually follows the onset of other symptoms and signs. Vomiting is very frequent near the onset of SAH and is common in large supratentorial and infratentorial ICHs. Vomiting is also frequent in patients with cerebellar and medullary infarcts. Seizures are slightly more common in patients with embolic infarcts and lobar ICHs than in patients with other stroke subtypes. Loss of consciousness is common in patients with SAH, large ICHs, and brain stem infarcts that affect the tegmentum bilaterally.

The General and Neurologic Examinations

The general and neurologic examinations[4,9] should be planned ahead of time, after taking the history. One must ask what features could be found during the examination that would clarify the stroke mechanism and the anatomy. For example, in a patient with left hemiparesis, visual field testing, tests for neglect, drawing, and copying, somatosensory testing, and careful cranial nerve examination should allow more precise localization. The neck should be auscultated with a stethoscope for carotid and vertebral artery bruits, and a careful cardiac and peripheral vascular examination is warranted. Are there any signs of systemic bleeding or head injury? At times, the examination uncovers findings completely unsuspected from the history. For example, the patient with left hemiparesis might have additional right-sided weakness and a bilateral Babinski sign or nystagmus suggesting a brain stem (pontine) localization or an enlarged nodular liver that may indicate metastatic cancer. As the examination proceeds, the physician should continue to weigh *what* and *where* hypotheses and their probabilities. Cardiac, ophthalmologic, and vascular examinations are important in all patients suspected of having cerebrovascular disease.

Clinical localization of the brain lesion is primarily determined from the findings on neurologic examination.[4,9] The most important and most frequently missed signs of brain dysfunction involve abnormalities of (1) higher cortical function; (2) level of alertness; (3) the visual and oculomotor systems; and (4) gait. These are parts of the examination most often overlooked by non-neurologists, that provide key clues to anatomical localization.

IMAGING AND LABORATORY EVALUATIONS

After completing the history and examination and constructing a list of *what* and *where* (etiologic and localization) differential diagnoses, the physician is ready to plan the appropriate investigations.[1,3] Often the patient has already had some studies. It is best to obtain the history and examine the patient before reviewing the images and accompanying information. The nature and speed of the evaluation depend on the circumstances. Imaging and laboratory testing should also be planned to answer sequential queries.

Is the Brain Lesion Caused by Ischemia or Hemorrhage, or Is It due to a Nonvascular Stroke Mimic?

Computed Tomography (CT)

CT is readily available in most hospitals and can reliably show ICH. When the mechanism is ischemic, CT may show infarction as a low-density lesion or may initially be normal. The signs of infarction on CT scans can be quite subtle in patients who are imaged within several hours of the onset of symptoms. Loss of distinction between gray and white matter, obscuring of the basal ganglia density, loss of definition of the insula, and slight hypodensity within the infarcted zone are often visible in patients with very acute brain infarcts.

Contrast enhancement is not very helpful. During the first days after stroke onset, infarcts are usually round or oval and have poorly defined margins. Later, infarcts become more hypodense and darker and are more wedge-like and more circumscribed. Some infarcts that had been hypodense become isodense during the second and third weeks after stroke onset. This so-called "fogging" effect may obscure the lesion for some time. Later, infarcts again become hypodense. Edema begins to develop within the first days in patients with large infarcts and is manifested by low density surrounding the lesion and mass effect with displacement of adjacent structures.

Immediately after the onset of bleeding, intracerebral hematomas are seen on CT as well-circumscribed high-density areas with smooth borders. Sequential scans in some patients show continued bleeding with enlargement of hematomas in later scans. Occasionally, a blood-fluid level is seen within acute hematomas. Edema develops within the first days and is seen as a dark rim around the white hematoma. As absorption of blood proceeds, the white image becomes more irregular and hypodense, and edema subsides. In patients with low hematocrits, or those scanned initially weeks after stroke onset, hematomas can appear solely as hypodense lesions.

SAH is not as reliably diagnosed by CT, especially if the bleeding is minor or has occurred days earlier.[10] Increased density caused by SAH is in the CSF adjacent to bone, where it is difficult to separate from bone density. Because contrast infusions make this meningeal area bright on CT, SAH is particularly difficult to diagnose if there has not been an unenhanced scan.

Magnetic Resonance Imaging

MRI is more sensitive than CT in detecting very early ischemic changes. MRI can also accurately show ICH especially when echo-planar and gradient-echo susceptibility-weighted (T2*) images are performed (Fig. 30-1).[11] MRI shows tomographic sections in multiple planes. Infarction prolongs the T1 and T2 relaxation constants and appears as a dark, hypointense image on T1-weighted sequences and as a bright hyperintense lesion on T2-weighted films.[12] Fluid-attenuated inversion recovery (FLAIR) images and diffusion-weighted images[13] are especially sensitive for detection of acute brain infarcts. T1-weighted MR images performed during the first day show infarcts as a loss of gray-white contrast and decreased image intensity (darkness). T2-weighted sequences show hyperintensive, bright foci of ischemia. During the next days, lesions become darker on T1-weighted and brighter on T2-weighted images. Increased signals on T2-weighted images may be evident years after the stroke. Even in patients with TIAs and no residual symptoms or signs at the time of scanning, MRI imaging often shows a brain infarct.

The appearances of ICH are quite different from ischemia but are complex and depend on the time since the bleed and the choice of MRI technique. Hemoglobin derivatives have paramagnetic effects. Imaging appearance depends on the nature of the compound, oxyhemoglobin, methemoglobin, hemosiderin, or ferritin, and whether the substances are present inside cells or in the interstitial extracellular spaces.[14] During the first 12 hours after intracerebral bleeding, hematomas contain mostly oxyhemoglobin, which is not paramagnetic. Hematoma appearance during that time reflects mostly protein and water content. On T1-weighted images, the acute hematoma is isointense or slightly hypointense (dark), with a surrounding hypointense darker rim. T2-weighted images are often hyperintense (bright) very acutely, reflecting water content. Between 12 and 48 hours after the onset of hemorrhage, deoxyhemoglobin is formed within extravascular RBCs, especially within the depth of the hematoma. During the next week, oxidation to methemoglobin occurs, beginning at the periphery of the lesion. By day 5 or 6, T1-weighted images show a central area of bright signal due to short T1, and a darker signal around the hematoma due to edema. On T2-weighted images, the center becomes dark and is surrounded by bright images. Chronic bleeds contain hemosiderin within macrophages and tissues and show as bright, intense areas on T2-weighted images. Susceptibility-weighted gradient echo images are particularly sensitive to blood and calcium and can show even very hyperacute hemorrhages.

Patients with SAH are not easily studied by MRI. Restless, ill patients often have difficulty holding still for the time required for high-quality images. The relaxation times of blood admixed with CSF approximate the signal from normal brain parenchyma, especially in T1-weighted images. T2 images often do show a bright signal. FLAIR images can show SAHs as a bright signal adjacent to the low-signal intensity cerebrospinal fluid.

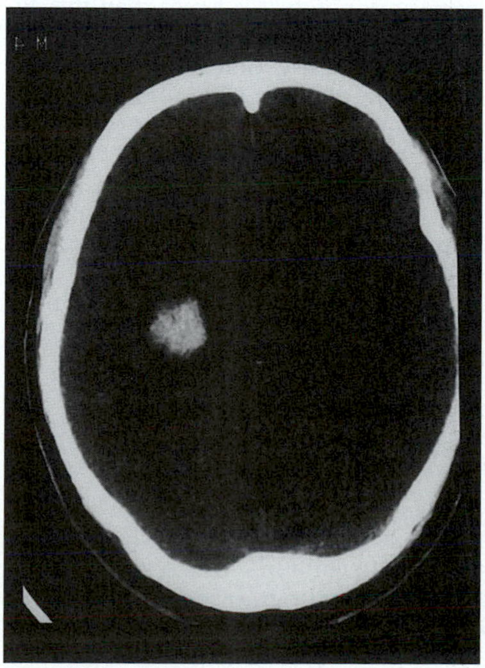

A

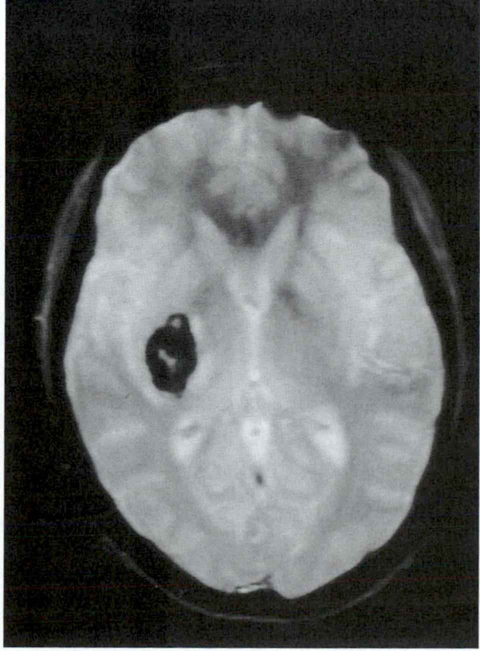

B

FIGURE 30-1. Acute intracerebral hemorrhage imaged by CT and MRI. **A,** CT shows a recent putaminal hemorrhage on the left of the scan as a well circumscribed hyperdense lesion surrounded by a small dark rim that represents edema. **B,** is a susceptibility-weighted (T2*) MRI that shows the same lesion now imaged as a black area. (With permission from Caplan LR: Caplan's Stroke: A Clinical Approach, 3rd ed. Boston, Butterworth-Heinemann, 2000.)

Lumbar Puncture

Lumbar puncture (LP) is especially important in the diagnosis and management of patients with SAH. CT and MRI are not very sensitive for the detection of SAH, especially if bleeding is minor and occurred days before scanning.[10] The accuracy of CT in documenting subarachnoid blood diminishes after 24 hours. Large SAHs are often preceded by small, warning leaks that are easily overlooked by CT but readily diagnosed by LP. By definition, subarachnoid blood rapidly disseminates and is present in the lumbar theca within minutes. *The absence of blood on LP excludes the diagnosis of SAH.* When blood is present, the quantity of blood and the pressure of CSF can also be measured and followed by later LPs. Counting the number of erythrocytes in the first and third or fourth tubes of CSF and measurement of the CSF hematocrit and spectrophotometric CSF analysis give an accurate quantitative database. LP is also useful in patients with brain infarcts and hemorrhages related to various infectious and neoplastic diseases.

What Is the Nature, Location, and Morphology of the Brain Lesion?

The next important questions the clinician should ask concern the characteristics of the brain lesion found. Where is the lesion? How large is it? What is its extent? What is the effect of the lesion on intracranial structures? Do the location and characteristics of the lesion correlate well with the clinical findings and explain the patient's symptoms and signs? Are there other lesions, and, if so, are they similar or different from the symptomatic lesion?

Delineation of the morphology of the brain process usually comes from neuroimaging with CT and/or MRI. Clinicians are fortunate to have available clinical data from the neurologic examination before neuroimaging. Having made hypotheses about lesion localization, clinicians can match these hypotheses with the imaging. Does the location of the lesion(s) on CT or MRI explain the clinical signs? Could the lesion(s) be asymptomatic, an incidental finding not related to the recent event? Are the clinical signs more severe than expected from imaging? A discrepancy might indicate that some tissue, although not damaged enough to show on scans, is not functioning normally.

What If the Lesion Is an Infarct

What Vascular Territory Is Involved?

Identification of the vessels supplying an area of symptomatic infarction is the first step toward identifying the causative vascular lesion. Ultrasound and vascular-imaging tests can then be planned to study the vessels involved. Once a plumber has pinpointed a blocked sink, the plumber can examine the water tank, the pump, and the pipes that lead to that sink, knowing that the problem must be located within that water delivery system. Suppose an infarct involves the right paramedian frontal lobe cortex in the supply region of the anterior cerebral artery (ACA). The causative lesion must lie within the pathway of the heart, aorta, right innominate, extracranial and intracranial carotid, ACA pathway. In a patient with quadriparesis, in whom MRI shows an infarct in the paramedian basis pontis and a small infarct is found in the right cerebellum in the territory of the anterior inferior cerebellar artery (AICA), then the lesion must involve the basilar artery proximal to the AICA branches.[6] The vascular process could be an in situ occlusive lesion within the basilar artery or an embolus to this region arising from the heart, the aorta, the innominate or subclavian arteries, or the cervical or intracranial portion of one of the vertebral arteries (VAs). If the cerebellar lesion had involved the PICA territory, the clinician would know that the vascular lesion must have affected the intracranial VA from which the PICA branches.[6] Knowledge of vascular distribution and supply is essential to localizing the vascular abnormality.

How Large Is the Infarct?

The size of the lesion is helpful in the prognosis. Although the severity of the clinical deficit is not directly proportional to infarct size, bigger lesions in the same anatomic area cause more severe deficits than smaller lesions in the same location. The infarct size, as shown on CT or MRI, should be matched in the clinician's mind with the size of the vascular territory involved. The noninfarcted tissue (entire vascular territory minus the infarct) represents tissue at risk for further ischemia. To determine the at-risk tissue, the vascular lesion must be known. For example, a small infarct in the territorial supply of a lenticulostriate branch might represent the entire supply of that small penetrating branch, but if the vascular lesion were in the MCA proximal to that lenticulostriate branch, a large area of brain tissue would still be at risk for infarction. Diffusion-weighted and perfusion MRI studies can give more direct information about the brain tissue at risk for infarction by a given vascular lesion. When the perfusion defect is larger than the diffusion-weighted zone of infarction, then the remainder of the brain that shows the perfusion deficit is at imminent risk if the blood flow to that zone is not improved.[15] Figure 30-2 shows an example of modern MR evaluation of a patient. Large lesions often exert mass effect and displace normal intracranial contents, especially if edema develops. Large lesions are also more often accompanied by reduced alertness. Mass effect and stupor often dictate treatment strategies. Large infarcts also represent a relative contraindication for anticoagulant treatment because parenchymatous brain hemorrhage develops more often in large infarcts than in small ones.

Do the Location and Extent of the Infarct Correlate with the Clinical Findings? Are Other Ischemic Lesions Present?

Clinicians should decide if the lesion found is appropriate to the patient's clinical symptoms and signs. In some patients, especially those with TIAs and minor clinical symptoms and signs, and those patients with minor or equivocal brain imaging findings, it may be difficult to know if a brain imaging lesion relates to the clinical findings.

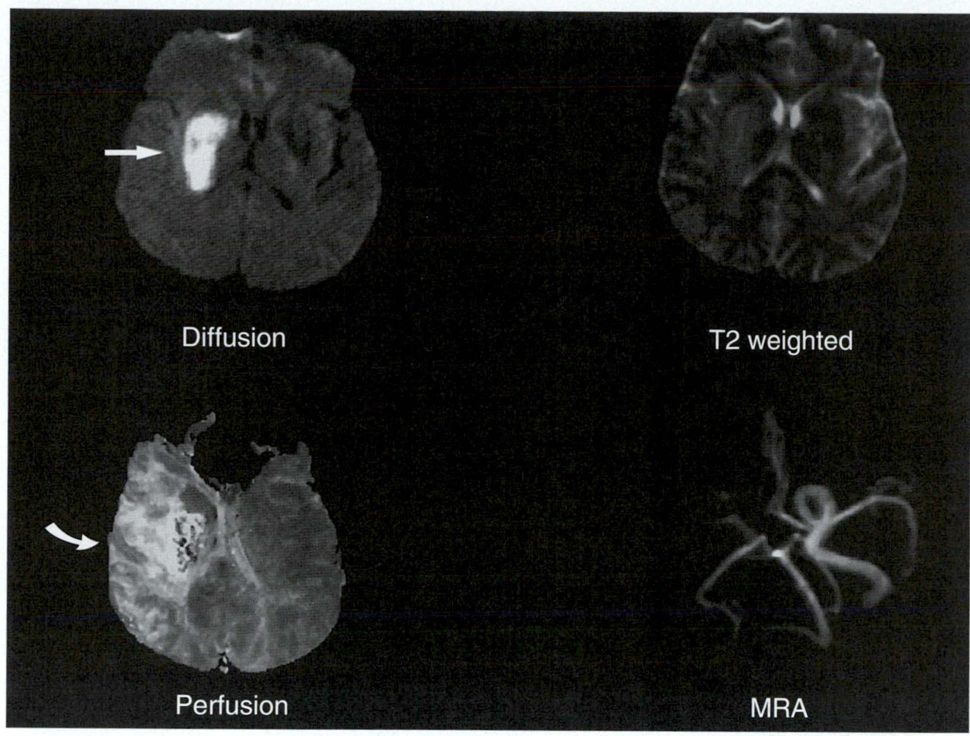

FIGURE 30-2. Magnetic resonance studies a few hours after symptom onset in a patient with a left internal carotid artery occlusion. The left cerebral hemisphere is on the left of these figures. The diffusion-weighted MRI (*top left*) shows a large striatocapsular abnormality (*white arrow*). The perfusion-weighted scan below shows a much larger area of decreased perfusion involving both the deep and superficial blood supply of the left middle cerebral artery. The T2-weighted MRI (*upper right*) shows the deep infarct but the abnormality is less intense than on the diffusion scan. The MRA (*lower right*) shows no image of the left internal carotid and middle cerebral arteries. This patient worsened after these acute images were performed. (With permission from Caplan LR: Caplan's Stroke: A Clinical Approach, 3rd ed. Boston, Butterworth-Heinemann, 2000.)

It is also useful to match the extent of the infarct with the severity of neurologic signs. When the clinical findings outweigh the brain imaging lesion, there may be considerable brain tissue that is not functioning normally but is not yet infarcted. This "stunned" brain often retains the ability to return to normal when reperfused.

Is Edema or Mass Effect Present?

Edema can develop around infarcts and may even be potentiated by reperfusion of a blocked artery. Sometimes the zone of actual infarction is small, but the surrounding edema zone is large. In young patients, edema is more threatening than in geriatric patients in whom brain atrophy allows room for brain expansion. Displacement of midline structures, effacement of gyri, encroachment on cisternal spaces, and brain stem displacement can often be judged well on diagnostic-quality CT and MRI scans.

What If Imaging Shows an Intracerebral Hemorrhage? Does the Location Provide Clues to Etiology of the Hemorrhage?

Hypertensive brain hemorrhages are usually deep and are most often located in the lateral ganglionic region, subcortex, thalamus, caudate nucleus, pons, and cerebellum. In a hypertensive patient with a hematoma confined to one of these regions, the likelihood of an etiology other than hypertension is quite low. Angiography in patients with hypertension and deep hematomas has a very low yield for showing aneurysms, arteriovenous malformations (AVMs), or other vascular lesions. Hematomas resulting from aneurysms, so-called *meningocerebral bleeds,* are contiguous to the aneurysms at the brain base or surface. In amyloid angiopathy, hemorrhages are lobar and are often multiple and can be accompanied by small infarcts. Anticoagulant-related ICHs are most often lobar or cerebellar, evolve gradually, and enlarge.[2] AVMs occur anywhere in the brain, especially in subependymal areas. Calcifications and heterogeneity in hematomas raise suspicion of an underlying AVM.

How Large Is the Hematoma? Is There Mass Effect?

Large size correlates with poor outcome in hematomas at any location. Both mass effect and displacement of adjacent structures are readily analyzed on CT and MR images.

Does the Hematoma Drain into CSF Pathways? Is the Hemorrhage Causing Hydrocephalus?

Hematomas decompress themselves by draining into the CSF on the surface of the brain and into the ventricles. Ventricular drainage was once considered an ominous sign, but now is recognized as not always adverse. The alternative to drainage is an increase in the mass of blood in the brain parenchyma. Nature might have already accomplished decompression of the lesion, a goal that surgeons hope to gain by operative drainage. Mass effect and blood in the ventricular system can obstruct the flow of CSF. Blockage of the ventricular system is most common at the foramen of Munro (putaminal bleeds) and at the level of the third (thalamic hemorrhage) and fourth ventricles (cerebellar hemorrhage). Hydrocephalus augments the mass effect of the hematoma and is often amenable to surgical decompression by temporary drainage or permanent shunting of CSF fluid.

What If Imaging Studies Show Subarachnoid Hemorrhage?

Where is the blood? Blood may accumulate around a bleeding aneurysm or in the adjacent subarachnoid spaces and cisterns, thus yielding a clue to the site of bleeding. Blood in the suprasellar cisterns and frontal interhemispheric fissure predicts an anterior communicating artery aneurysm. Blood predominantly in one sylvian fissure suggests an MCA bifurcation aneurysm on that side. Thick blood in the pontine and cerebellopontine angle cisterns predicts a posterior fossa aneurysm. Nonaneurysmal hemorrhages often are found in the cisterns around the brain stem.[16]

How much bleeding has occurred generally or locally? The thickness of blood on CT or MRI correlates roughly with the amount of blood. Large subarachnoid bleeds are more often complicated by hydrocephalus and delayed brain infarction due to vasoconstriction than are smaller leaks. Vertical layers of blood clot more than 1 mm thick, or local clots larger than 5×3 mm in size are often associated with angiographically documented vasoconstriction.

Are There Regions of Infarction? Is Hydrocephalus Present?

SAH is often complicated by vasoconstriction and delayed ischemic damage. Infarction is most often localized to the territory supplied by the artery harboring the aneurysm but can be located elsewhere. The presence of acute ischemia suggests that vasoconstriction is present. Vasoconstriction can also produce generalized brain ischemia without focal infarction. Blood within the subarachnoid space can diminish the absorptive capability of the arachnoid granulations. Communicating hydrocephalus develops because CSF production exceeds absorption.

What If Computed Tomography and Magnetic Resonance Imaging Are Negative?

Normal neuroimaging is common in patients with transient ischemia. In those patients who have only transient ischemia or persistent ischemia without infarction, the clinical symptoms and signs provide localization clues.

What Are the Nature, Site, and Severity of the Vascular Lesion(s)?

Having localized and quantified the process in the brain, clinicians are now ready to identify the vascular lesion(s). The clinical findings and brain neuroimaging studies usually have isolated the vascular region of interest in the individual stroke patient. *Remember that stroke is a* ***cerebrovascular disease*** *and that treatment and prophylaxis depend on the nature of that vascular disease.*

What If the Stroke Mechanism Is Ischemia?

New technology and improvements in older techniques now provide clinicians with a menu of different strategies for brain and vascular studies in patients with ischemia. All investigations—MRI, MRA, diffusion and perfusion MRI—can be performed using magnetic resonance technology within a few minutes.[15] Alternatively, if MR is not readily available or cannot be used, spiral CT can be used to create brain images and CTA of the cervicocranial arteries. Extracranial and TCD can be used as the diagnostic vascular tests in patients who have only had brain imaging and is used to corroborate and quantify the blood flow effects of vascular lesions found by CTA and MRA. Ultrasound is also used to monitor the progression and regression of vascular occlusive lesions once they are identified.

Ultrasound

During the 1970s, amplitude modulation (A-mode) and brightness modulation (B-mode) pulse echo ultrasounds were introduced into clinical examinations of the extracranial arteries. During the 1980s, Duplex scanning that includes B-mode images of the extracranial artery being insonated combined with a pulsed Doppler spectrum analysis became widely used. Ultrasonic information is received through a probe or transducer held over an artery, and the information is converted into electrical energy to develop images and Doppler curves of blood-flow velocity.

B-Mode Imaging

High-resolution B-mode ultrasound scanning of the neck provides images in several planes of the neck arteries. B-mode scanning is quite accurate at the carotid bifurcation in the neck and at the origin of the VA from the subclavian artery. Lesions higher in the neck and more proximally located are technically harder to image well. Figure 30-3 shows a composite of B-mode images of the innominate artery of a patient. B-mode imaging can

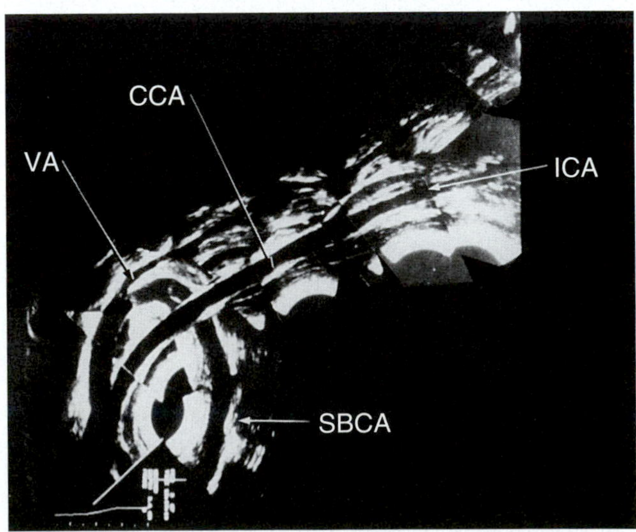

FIGURE 30-3. Composite B-mode ultrasound image showing the innominate artery and its subclavian, carotid, and vertebral artery branches in the neck. CCA, common carotid artery; ICA, internal carotid artery; SBCA, subclavian artery; VA, vertebral artery. (With permission from Caplan LR: Caplan's Stroke: A Clinical Approach, 3rd ed. Boston, Butterworth-Heinemann, 2000.)

show the severity of luminal narrowing, ulcerations and intraplaque hemorrhages, the surface-wall characteristics of the carotid arteries. However B-mode performed by itself has limitations. The large size of the ultrasound probe and sharp angulation of the vessels sometimes prevent adequate display of some vessels, especially at the VA origin. Calcifications and clots are not imaged. B-mode is accurate at separating normal arteries and those with minor plaques from those arteries with severe stenosing lesions (>70% stenosis). Analysis of B-mode images requires experience and familiarity with vascular anatomy. Arteries can be misidentified, especially from analyzing only one view. Experience has shown that B-mode imaging is enhanced by the addition of a multigated pulsed-Doppler apparatus (*duplex systems*). The pulsed-Doppler in this duplex system helps identify the arteries and orientation of B-mode images. The analysis of flow-velocity patterns by Doppler, recorded from different positions within the arterial lumen, provides qualitative and quantitative information abouthemodynamic changes. The B-mode images help show the location of the velocity changes.

Doppler Sonography Systems

Continuous-Wave and Pulsed-Doppler Systems Continuous wave (CW) Doppler measures an average velocity for blood moving through an artery or vein beneath the probe. *Pulsed-Doppler* is range gated to measure the velocity of blood in small volumes at specific selected arterial sites. The CW Doppler device shows mean flow velocities of the carotid arteries in the neck, and the VAs at their origins and at the cervical region near the skull base. Moving the Doppler probe along the course of the carotid and vertebral arteries allows identification of the bifurcation of the carotid arteries and major changes in audible blood-flow signals. Doppler curves can be analyzed using fast Fourier transform spectral analysis to detect peak frequencies and spectral broadening.

Severity of stenosis is estimated by the increase in peak systolic frequency, the presence and severity of poststenotic turbulence, and an increase in diastolic blood-flow velocity.[17] In regions of luminal narrowing, blood velocity increases in an inverse proportion to the size of the lumen until a critical reduction in lumen size severely limits flow.

Color Doppler Flow Imaging and Power Doppler

Color Doppler flow imaging (CDFI) represents a recent technology advance. In this technique, the spatial and temporal distribution of color-coded Doppler signals are visualized in real time and displayed as color images superimposed on gray-scale images of the surrounding tissues.[18] This technique shows changes in blood-flow near small plaques, and has a high sensitivity and accuracy for detecting minor, moderate, and severe degrees of carotid artery stenosis. Real-time images are easier to see and interpret than are velocity curves. Power Doppler improves assessment of the severity of stenosis and plaque morphology compared with CDFI.[19]

Transcranial Doppler Ultrasound

Introduction of TCD was a major advance. This system permits study of intracranial arteries. Extracranial ultrasound examinations use pulse frequencies ranging from 3 to 10 MHz. These ultrasound frequencies cannot penetrate bone sufficiently to reflect signals from the intracranial arteries; however, signals can be obtained from intracranial arteries using 2-MHz probes. Three windows are used for probe placement, taking advantage of natural skull foramina and soft-tissue regions. Figure 30-4A shows the TCD probe at these windows. The temporal window is used to insonate the MCA and its major branches, the proximal ACA, the ICA bifurcation, and the posterior cerebral arteries. A transorbital probe is placed near the eye and is used to study blood velocities in the ICA siphon and ophthalmic arteries. A suboccipital window through the foramen magnum allows recording from the intracranial VAs and the proximal basilar artery. Figure 30-4B shows Doppler spectra from TCD in a patient with an intracranial VA stenosis. TCD has improved study of stroke patients at the bedside. TCD can accurately detect important lesions in the major basal cerebral arteries: the intracranial ICAs, MCAs, intracranial VAs and the proximal and middle basilar artery. TCD is also helpful in showing the hemodynamic effects of extracranial occlusive lesions on velocities in the intracranial branches. The combination of continuous-wave Doppler, color-flow Doppler, and TCD is very effective in screening for major occlusive lesions in the extracranial and intracranial arteries. Vascular narrowing due to vasoconstriction and augmented flow through collateral channels and through AVMs all increase blood flow velocity. TCD can be used to monitor vasoconstriction in patients with SAH.

Emboli can be detected as sudden alterations in flow with characteristic sound signals.[20] Figure 30-5 shows a microembolic signal. Emboli monitoring can be used to study the origin and quantity of emboli and also to study the effects of various treatments.

Computed Tomography and Magnetic Resonance Imaging and Angiography

Some information about the brain vessels can often be gleaned from careful scrutiny of CT and MRI scans, especially after contrast enhancement (see Chapters 11 and 12). On plain CT, an acutely thrombosed artery can sometimes be seen as a hyperdense image that has the shape and distribution of an artery or vein. The MCA is the most frequently involved artery. The hyperdense MCA sign is virtually diagnostic of the presence of a clot in the MCA. Occasionally the intracranial ICA, the basilar artery, and the PCAs can show similar hyperdensity on unenhanced scans indicating thromboembolic occlusion of these vessels. Calcific particles arising from calcific material in heart valves or a calcified atherostenotic plaque can also sometimes be identified in brain arteries on plain CT scans. Contrast enhancement can show large berry aneurysms and dolichoectatic fusiform aneurysms; absence of opacification of an artery can indicate the high probability of occlusion of that vessel. CT can also suggest dural sinus thrombosis by showing thrombosed

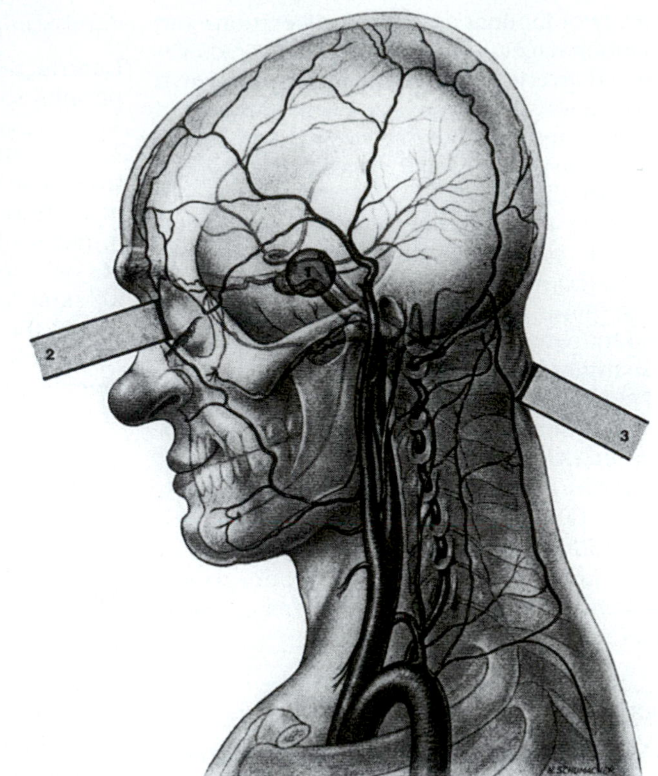

A

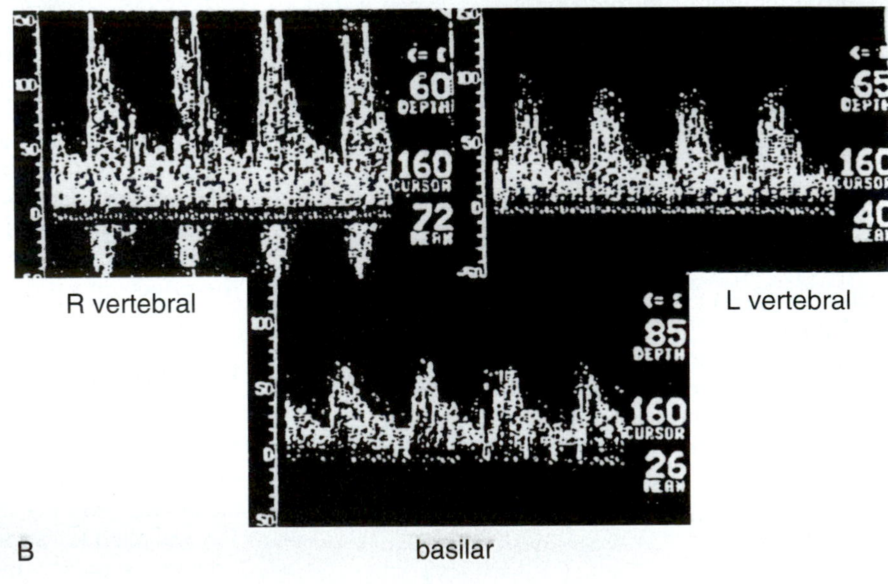

FIGURE 30-4. A, Diagram showing locations for TCD probes: (1) temporal window; (2) orbital window; (3) suboccipital foramen magnum window. **B,** TCD spectra: The velocities in the right intracranial VA are much higher than in the left VA and the basilar artery. Arteriography showed a region of severe stenosis in the intracranial right VA. TCD, transcranial Doppler; VA, vertebral artery. (With permission from Caplan LR: Caplan's Stroke: A Clinical Approach, 3rd ed. Boston, Butterworth-Heinemann, 2000.)

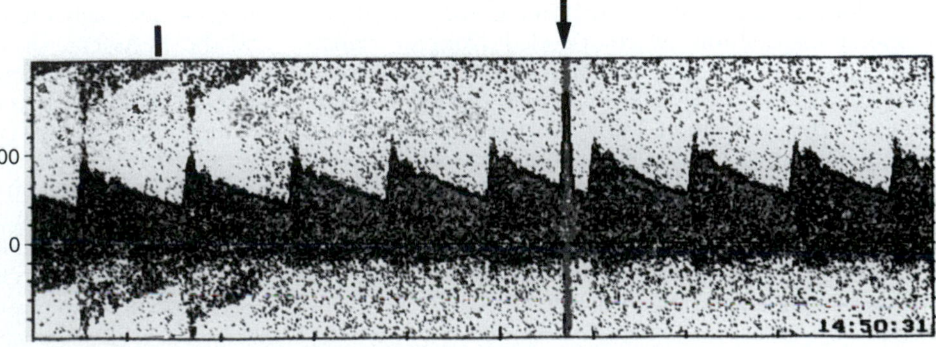

FIGURE 30-5. TCD recording over a middle cerebral artery (MCA) showing a microembolic signal (*black arrow*).

serpiginous cortical veins or the superior sagittal or other sinuses as high-density thrombi on plain CT scans. After contrast enhancement, CT may show a filling defect, representing a thrombus in the sagittal sinus, the so-called empty delta sign. Flow in brain arteries can also be studied with MRI. Vessels with high-velocity flow appear black (signal void) on MRI images, whereas arteries with slower flow may appear white. Occlusions can be inferred when a flow void is not seen on images that show cross-section views of arteries. Aneurysms and dissections can also frequently be identified and followed by MRI scanning. Cross-sectional views of dissections often show intramural hematomas.

Magnetic resonance angiography (MRA) offers many advantages over other noninvasive methods of vascular imaging. MRA films can be acquired with MRI and are noninvasive and safe. High-quality MRAs of the extracranial and intracranial arteries can be achieved by using gradient-echo techniques and short echo times. Figure 30-6 shows an MRA of the neck arteries. Veins can also be studied; the imaging of veins is referred to as MR venography (MRV). MRA can be performed using a variety of different techniques including 2-D and 3-D time-of-flight, and phase-contrast imaging. MRA is a functional process that creates an image of flow in blood vessels. Unlike standard contrast injection angiograms, the images do not show anatomy. At times, contrast infusion of gadolinium solutions (Gd-DTPA) are needed to obtain better arterial images. MRA has proved to be an excellent screening technique for occlusive disease. Standard catheter angiography may still be needed in some patients to better delineate the vascular lesions.

Advances in MR technology have made it possible to acquire a great deal of information about brain ischemia and brain perfusion, safely and quickly. In acute stroke patients, diffusion-weighted MRI shows regions of increased brain water content that usually represent regions that will become infarcted.[15,21] Brain perfusion can also be imaged using dynamic contrast-enhanced MR scans. Ultrafast imaging after Gd-DTPA injection is used to calculate regional cerebral blood volume and rCBF. and to produce so-called perfusion-weighted images.[15,21] Comparison of the region of probable infarction on diffusion-weighted scans with the region of reduced perfusion shows brain regions that are underperfused but not yet infarcted (the presumed ischemic penumbra). When the region of reduced perfusion matches the zone of infarction, progression of infarction and progression of neurologic signs are rare. When this information is supplemented by vascular imaging, usually MRA which is acquired at the same time as the diffusion-weighted and perfusion MRI scans, treating physicians have the information needed to facilitate a logical decision about the likely usefulness of acute treatments such as thrombolysis. A patient with an occluded MCA shown by MRA, who has a large zone of reduced perfusion in the MCA territory shown by perfusion MR, and a relatively small region of infarction shown by diffusion-weighted MR represents the ideal candidate for thrombolysis. A large zone of infarction on diffusion-weighted MR, open ICA and MCA on MRA, and perfusion deficits that match or are less than the zone of infarction on diffusion-weighted scans are characteristics of candidates in whom thrombolysis has little likely usefulness. Figures 30-2 and 30-6 illustrate acute modern magnetic resonance studies.

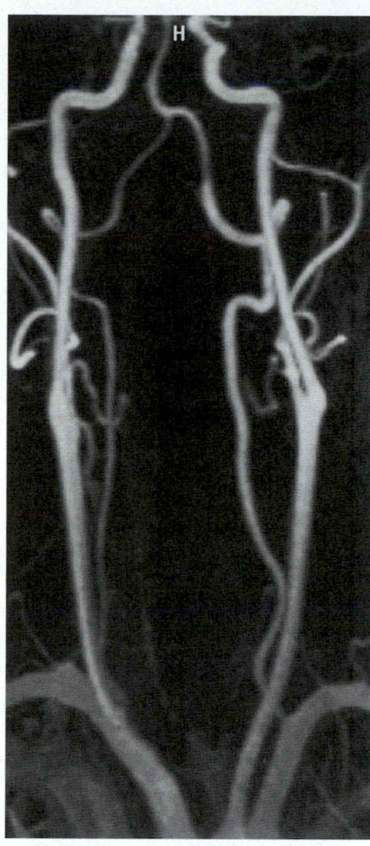

FIGURE 30-6. Gadolinium-enhanced MRA image of the neck and proximal intracranial arteries. The innominate, subclavian, carotid, and vertebral arteries are shown quite well. (With permission from Caplan LR: Caplan's Stroke: A Clinical Approach, 3rd ed. Boston, Butterworth-Heinemann, 2000.)

The development of more rapid spiral (helical) CT scanners has enabled the development of computed tomography angiography (CTA). This technique involves intravenous injection of a bolus of dye followed by helical scanning. Volumetric data acquisition and improved computerized image manipulation have improved the CTA image display into 3-D reformations. CTA is based on anatomic imaging and, when blood flow is severely reduced, CTA has theoretical advantages over MRA, which is a functional imaging technique. Bolus injection of contrast followed by sequential imaging using helical CT can yield rapid information about regions of brain ischemia and blockage of intracranial arteries.[22] Occlusion of the MCA or its branches can be detected from the images even without reformation, allowing rapid decisions about thrombolysis. The contrast dye infusion also enhances the brain CT images yielding a perfusion CT scan that is somewhat comparable with an MR perfusion scan.[23]

Standard Contrast Catheterization Cerebral Angiography

MRA and CTA have the advantages of being able to be performed at the same time as brain imaging and of being noninvasive. The advent of high-quality CTA,

MRA, and cervical and TCD ultrasound have led to a marked decrease in the indications for standard catheter angiography. Standard catheter angiography is indicated when the preliminary tests do not satisfactorily clarify the nature of vascular lesions and when treatment depends on the nature and severity of those vascular lesions. For example, angiography is used in patients in whom carotid artery stenosis has been shown by MRA and duplex sonography, but these two tests give conflicting estimates of the severity of stenosis. Angiography is often required to better define cerebral aneurysms and vascular malformations. Catheter angiography is used as a prelude to intravascular interventions, such as intra-arterial thrombolysis and angioplasty, because treatment is given directly in the artery. In experienced hands, angiography reveals valuable information and has a low incidence of serious complications.

Cardiac Evaluation

Cardioembolic ischemic strokes are common. The proportion of ischemic strokes considered to originate from cardioembolic sources has increased dramatically with the development of sophisticated technology that can define cardiac, aortic, and vascular lesions. A wide variety of different cardiac lesions are now known to be potential sources of embolism, whereas formerly only acute myocardial infarction and rheumatic mitral stenosis with atrial fibrillation were generally accepted cardiac sources. Atrial fibrillation is the most common and most important heart condition that predisposes to brain embolism. Anticoagulation and control of the cardiac rate are very important in preventing embolism in patients with atrial fibrillation.

Cardiac emboli arise from an assortment of diseases that affect the heart valves, heart rhythm, endocardial surface, and myocardium. In addition, many patients with brain ischemia due to atherosclerosis have coexisting coronary artery disease. Late deaths in patients with ischemic stroke are often due to coronary artery disease and myocardial infarction rather than cerebrovascular disease. These facts should direct attention to the stroke patient's heart, as well as the brain and its vascular supply.

A discussion of the technical aspects of echocardiography to diagnose intracardiac sources of embolism is beyond the scope of this chapter. Transesophageal echocardiography (TEE) yields important information about the proximal aorta. The aorta is an important potential source of embolism especially during angiography and cardiac surgery. Presently TEE is the most effective method of imaging the aorta. The ascending aorta can also be insonated using a Duplex ultrasound probe placed in the right supraclavicular fossa and the arch and proximal descending thoracic aorta can be imaged using a left supraclavicular probe.[24] Most plaques are located in the curvature of the arch from the distal ascending aorta to the proximal descending aorta, regions shown by B-mode ultrasound.

The usefulness of monitoring for cardiac rhythm disturbances is not clear. In patients suspected of brain embolism, the yield is probably high enough to dictate the use of monitoring. In patients with lacunar infarcts and those with a well-defined atherosclerotic extracranial vascular cause for their stroke, the yield is low. Cardiac rhythm monitoring should be done in any patient whose initial ECG suggests a cardiac rhythm abnormality.

Are Abnormalities in the Blood Causing or Adding to Brain Ischemia or Hemorrhage?

Once clinicians have determined the nature, site, and severity of the vascular lesion, it is important to know whether abnormalities of blood constituents are causing or contributing to brain ischemia or hemorrhage. *Clinicians must not forget the blood.* Abnormalities of the clotting system can lead to hypercoagulability and thrombosis. Even in patients with lesions known to predispose to thromboembolism and brain ischemia, the acute event is often precipitated by a change in the blood and its coagulability. Infections, cancer, and inflammatory bowel disease are associated with release of acute phase reactants that may alter coagulability sufficiently to promote thromboembolism especially in the presence of a preexisting lesion that affects an endothelial surface. Bleeding diatheses often cause intracranial bleeding. Increased blood viscosity can alter blood flow, especially in small brain arterioles and capillaries, and in patients with occlusive lesions. Increased viscosity can cause or contribute to regional decreases in cerebral blood flow and potentiate ischemia. Autoimmunity, which can be detected and monitored by blood tests, can lead to occlusive cerebrovascular disease.

What If the Problem Is Ischemia?

The formed cellular elements of the blood, (erythrocytes, leukocytes, and platelets) should always be studied. Screening tests of coagulation functions should also be a part of the routine evaluation of patients with brain ischemia. Other blood components may also be analyzed, such as serum proteins, coagulation factors, blood viscosity, and antiphospholipid antibodies.

Erythrocytes

Quantitative and qualitative RBC abnormalities can affect blood flow and clotting. The level of the *hematocrit* affects blood viscosity and the rheologic properties of blood. In older patients with preexisting atherosclerosis and small-vessel disease, high hematocrits that are still within the normal range can compound the vascular disease and limit perfusion. The hematocrit has a heavy impact on blood viscosity. Lowering of the hematocrit from 45 to 32 results in doubling of cerebral blood flow (CBF).

Sickle-cell disease and other hemoglobinopathies can lead to altered flow and hypercoagulability. Sickle-cell disease and spherocytosis are associated with multifocal brain infarcts. Very severe anemia also can compound brain ischemia.

Leukocytes

The WBC is often elevated in patients with myocardial infarction and is also often slightly elevated in patients with brain infarcts. Leukemia with very high WBC counts can cause packing of capillaries and small arterioles with aggregates of large WBCs, causing multiple small infarcts and hemorrhages. This happens when the leukocrit is high in the capillary tube used to measure the hematocrit. Measurement of WBC count is usually a routine part of a complete blood count (CBC), which should be ordered on each stroke patient.

Platelets

Quantitative and qualitative platelet abnormalities can cause hypercoagulability and bleeding. Thrombocytosis, especially with platelet counts over 1 million/μl, can cause hypercoagulability. Platelet counts should be a routine part of the initial evaluation of patients with ischemic stroke because thrombocytosis can potentiate thrombosis, and low platelet counts can suggest the presence of other disorders, such as the antiphospholipid antibody syndrome, consumptive coagulopathies, lupus erythematosus, and thrombotic thrombocytopenic purpura, all of which are often complicated by brain ischemia. Platelet counts can fall during the course of illness (e.g., after use of heparin) so that a baseline count before treatment is useful for later comparison. Some patients with platelet counts in the normal range have increased aggregability or secretory function of their platelets, or have qualitative abnormalities of platelet morphology and function.

Serum Proteins

Fibrinogen is a very important part of the coagulation system because fibrinogen is converted to fibrin monomers by the action of thrombin. Fibrin is an essential component of both red and white thrombi. Fibrinogen also contributes to blood viscosity. The hematocrit and fibrinogen levels are the two most important single predictors of whole blood viscosity. High levels of fibrinogen have been shown to be risk factors for stroke in several prospective studies.[25] Fibrinogen levels can also rise as acute-phase reactants in the early period after stroke.

Studies of Coagulation Factors and Coagulation

The prothrombin time (PT), INR, and activated partial thromboplastin time (aPTT) are excellent screening tests of coagulation function and are routinely available. Measurement of the INR and the aPTT should be a part of the evaluation of all stroke patients. Other tests are ordered if a hypercoagulable state is suspected by acceleration of the PT or aPTT, the presence of multiple vascular occlusions, a past history of recurrent thrombophlebitis or miscarriages, or the presence of known neoplastic, collagen vascular, rheumatologic, or inflammatory diseases. Some serum proteins—such as antithrombin III, protein C, and protein S—are natural inhibitors of coagulation. A decrease in the level of these substances because of a familial inherited disorder or due to acquired disease can cause hypercoagulability. Prothrombin gene mutations, and the presence of resistance to activated protein C (factor V Leiden) can cause hypercoagulability. The risk of arterial events in patients with these genetic abnormalities is low compared with the risk of venous occlusions.

The level of coagulation factors VII, VIII, IX, and X can be measured in most hematologic laboratories but have not been well studied in large groups of stroke patients. Abnormally high levels of factor VIII can cause hypercoagulability and recurrent strokes. Factor VIII elevation can be chronic, can precede and predispose to stroke, can be elevated as an acute-phase reactant in systemic illnesses such as ulcerative colitis, and can be elevated secondary to thrombosis. In the latter case it is a marker and not the cause of the thrombosis.

Hemostatic markers of coagulation activity have been used to detect and monitor hypercoagulability. Thrombin acts as a catalyst of the proteolysis of fibrinogen to fibrin. During this reaction, fibrinopeptide A (FPA) is generated. The level of fibrin D-dimer is also an index of fibrin generation. The level of the prothrombin activation fragment F1.2 is a measure of in vivo thrombin generation. Increasing intensity of anticoagulation is accompanied by decreasing thrombin generation as measured by the F1.2 levels.[26] Fibrinolysis involves the dissolution of fibrin by endogenous fibrinolytic mechanisms. Fibrinolytic activity can be estimated by the levels of fibrinopeptide B-B1-42 (FPB) and of tissue plasminogen activator (tPA) and its inhibitor (PAI-1). Thrombosis is favored when thrombin proteolysis of fibrinogen (increased FPA and D-dimer levels) and its conversion to fibrin exceeds plasmin proteolysis of fibrin (increased FPB and tPA/tPAI ratio).[27]

Antiphospholipid Antibodies

Antiphospholipid antibodies (APLA) are usually IgG or IgM antibodies that bind to negatively charged phospholipids and associated membrane proteins. Phospholipids are important constituents of vascular endothelium, heart proteins, platelets, and other cells. The two most commonly measured APLAs are anticardiolipin antibody and the so-called *lupus anticoagulant* (LA). LAs are acquired immunoglobins associated clinically with thrombosis, not bleeding; most patients with LA do not have systemic lupus erythematosus. The laboratory hallmark of LA is a prolonged aPTT that does not correct when normal plasma is added. This indicates the presence of an inhibitor of clotting rather than a deficiency of a necessary coagulation factor.

Patients with the APLA syndrome have an increased frequency of spontaneous abortions, thrombophlebitis, pulmonary embolism, and large- and small-artery occlusions. In addition to the presence of LA and/or anticardiolipins, laboratory abnormalities include positive VDRL, thrombocytopenia, and antinuclear antibodies. Mitral and aortic valve abnormalities and ocular ischemia are also common. The coagulopathy and valvular abnormalities probably relate to immune-related endothelial and valve-surface injuries. Patients with high-positive IgG APLA have a high incidence of subsequent vascular occlusive lesions. Angiography in patients with APLA syndrome shows a high frequency of intracranial occlusive disease and venous and dural sinus occlusions.

APLAs should be measured in patients with clinical features that suggest the APLA syndrome and in patients who do not have the usual risk factors for ischemic stroke, and in patients with livedo reticularis and strokes (Sneddon's syndrome).[28,29]

REFERENCES

1. Caplan LR: Caplan's Stroke, A Clinical Approach, 3rd ed. Boston, Butterworth-Heinemann, 2000.
2. Kase CS, Caplan LR: Intracerebral hemorrhage. Boston, Butterworth-Heinemann, 1994, p 117.
3. Caplan LR, Dewitt LD, Breen JC. Neuroimaging in patients with cerebrovascular disease. In Greenberg JO (ed): Neuroimaging, 2nd ed. New York, McGraw-Hill, 1999, p 493.
4. Caplan LR, Hollander J: The Effective Clinical Neurologist, 2nd ed. Butterworth Heinemann, Boston, 2001.
5. Caplan, LR: Course-of-illness graphs. Hosp Pract 20:125, 1985.
6. Caplan LR: Posterior Circulation Disease: Clinical Findings, Diagnosis, and Management. Boston, Blackwell Science, 1996.
7. Caplan LR, Gorelick PB, Hier DB: Race, sex, and occlusive cerebrovascular disease: A review. Stroke 17:649, 1986.
8. Caplan LR: Significance of unexpected (silent) brain infarcts. In Caplan LR, Shifrin EG, Nicolaides AN, Moore WS (eds): Cerebrovascular Ischaemia: Investigation and Management. London, Med-Orion, 1996, p 423.
9. Caplan LR: The neurological examination. In Fisher M, Bogousslavsky J (eds): Textbook of Neurology. Boston, Butterworth-Heinemann, 1998, p 3.
10. Edlow JA, Caplan LR: Primary care: Avoiding pitfalls in the diagnosis of subarachnoid hemorrhage. N Engl J Med 342:29, 2000.
11. Linfante I, Llinas RH, Caplan LR, Warach S: MRI features of intracerebral hemorrhages within two hours from symptom onset. Stroke 30:2263, 1999.
12. Meuli RA, Maeder P, Uske A: Magnetic resonance imaging. In Ginsberg MD, Bogousslavsky J (eds): Cerebrovascular Disease: Pathophysiology, Diagnosis, and Management, vol 2. Boston, Blackwell Science, 1998, p 1265.
13. Schellinger PD, Fiebach JB, Jansen O, et al: Stroke magnetic resonance imaging within 6 hours after onset of hyperacute cerebral ischemia. Ann Neurol 49:460, 2001.
14. Dul K, Drayer BP: CT and MR imaging of intracerebral hemorrhage. In Kase CS, Caplan LR: Intracerebral Hemorrhage, Boston, Butterworth-Heinemann, 1994, p 73.
15. Schellinger PD, Fiebach JB, Hacke W. Imaging-based decision making in thrombolytic therapy for ischemic stroke: Present status. Stroke 34:575, 2003.
16. Rinkel GJ, Wijdicks EF, Vermeulen M, et al: Outcome in perimesencephalic (non-aneurysmal) subarachnoid hemorrhage: A follow-up study in 37 patients. Neurology 40:1130, 1990.
17. von Reutern GM, von Budingen HJ: Ultrasound Diagnosis of Cerebrovascular Disease. New York, Georg Thieme, 1993.
18. Bartels E: Color-coded Duplex ultrasonography of the cerebral vessels. Stuttgart, Schattauer, 1998.
19. Steinke W, Ries S, Artemis N, et al: Power Doppler imaging of carotid artery stenosis: Comparison with color Doppler flow imaging and angiography. Stroke 28:1981, 1997.
20. Sliwka U, Lingnau A, Stohlmann W-D, et al: Prevalence and time course of microembolic signals in patients with acute strokes: A prospective study. Stroke 28:358, 1997.
21. Baird AE, Warach S: Magnetic resonance imaging of acute stroke. J Cereb Blood Flow Metab 18:583, 1999.
22. Na DG, Byun HS, Lee KH, et al: Acute occlusion of the middle cerebral artery: Early evaluation with triphasic helical CT— preliminary results. Radiology 207:113, 1998.
23. Wintermark M, Reichhart M, Thiran J-P, et al: Prognostic accuracy of cerebral blood flow measurement by perfusion computed tomography, at the time of emergency room admission, in acute stroke patients. Ann Neurol 51:417, 2002.
24. Weinberger J, Azhar S, Danisi F, et al: A new noninvasive technique for imaging atherosclerotic plaque in the aortic arch of stroke patients by transcutaneous real-time B-mode ultrasonography. Stroke 29:673, 1998.
25. Ernst E, Resch KL: Fibrinogen as a cardiovascular risk factor: A meta-analysis and review of the literature. Ann Int Med 118: 956, 1993.
26. Feinberg WM, Cornell ES, Nightingale SD, et al: Relationship between prothrombin activation fragment F1.2 and International Normalized Ratio in patients with atrial fibrillation. Stroke 28: 1101, 1997.
27. Feinberg WM: Coagulation in brain ischemia: Basic concepts and clinical relevance. In Caplan LR (ed): Brain Ischemia: Basic Concepts and Clinical Relevance. London, Springer-Verlag, 1995, p 85.
28. Bailey DP, Coull BM, Goodnight SH: Neurological disease associated with antiphospholipid antibodies. Ann Neurol 25:221, 1989.
29. Markus HS, Hambley H: Neurology and the blood: Haematological abnormalities in ischaemic stroke. J Neurol Neurosurg Psychiatry 64:150, 1998.

■ ■ ■ chapter 31

Antithrombotic Approaches in Cerebrovascular Disease

Gregory J. del Zoppo

Stroke is a syndrome of cerebral vascular disorders with neurologic sequelae (see Chapters 29 and 30). For this reason, antithrombotic agents play a central role in the treatment of ischemic cerebrovascular disease. Stroke consists of fixed or transient neurologic deficits resulting from atherothrombotic events, embolism, lacunar events, subarachnoid hemorrhage, intracerebral hemorrhage, and other causes. The vascular anatomy, thrombotic or embolic source, and timing of the stroke are critical features of cerebrovascular ischemia. Thrombotic and thromboembolic events account for 60% to 80% of ischemic strokes in the carotid artery territory (Fig. 31-1). These often arise from platelet-fibrin thrombi on atheromata within the extracranial portion of the internal carotid artery (ICA, at the carotid artery bifurcation), the aortic arch, or the middle cerebral artery (MCA). Thromboemboli also originate from the left ventricular wall along dyskinetic segments formed during myocardial ischemia, atrial thrombi formed in association with (nonvalvular) atrial fibrillation, and valvular injury caused by rheumatic disease or from prosthetic valves. Occlusion of small, penetrating cerebral arteries from lipohyalinosis leads to the formation of lacunae in the cerebral hemispheres, which relate in part to hypertension. In the basilar system, thrombi may form at the subclavian-vertebral artery junction and embolize into the basilar artery. In situ thrombosis of the basilar artery can occur independently, which can cause obstruction of penetrating arterioles, thereby producing brain stem ischemia.

In both the carotid and vertebral-basilar territories, the development of the infarction observed in stable stroke involves local inflammatory processes. Experimental work

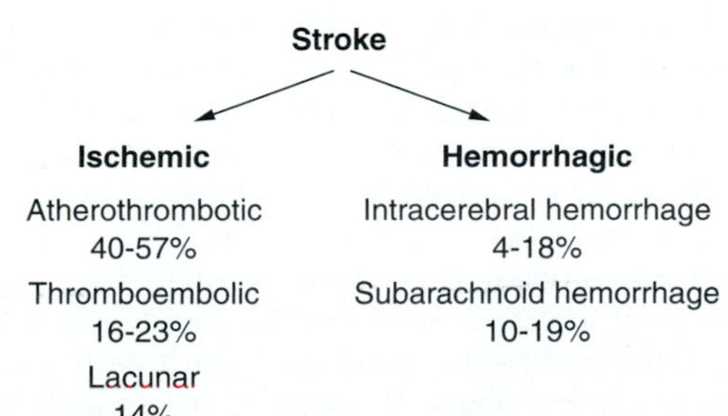

FIGURE 31-1. Classifications of stroke (stroke subtypes). Approximately 80% of strokes are of the ischemic subtype, and 10% result from lacunes.

supports the clinical premise that the ischemic lesion stabilizes as an infarct by 24 hours after arterial occlusion.[1-6] Other experimental studies have indicated that metastable, potentially reversible zones of neuron injury occur in the ischemic vascular territory supplied by the occluded cerebral artery.[7,8] This concept is the basis for contemporary acute interventional strategies.

Knowledge of the specific vascular anatomy and occlusion location has been valuable to understanding the fate of symptomatic occlusions and to defining clinical outcome. Studies employing angiography during the early hours of stroke have shown a high frequency of arterial occlusions in individuals who present within 6 hours of onset of carotid artery territory symptoms.[9-12]

CLASSIFICATION OF CEREBROVASCULAR DISEASE

A clinical classification of cerebrovascular ischemic events (see Chapter 29) divides the neurologic presentation broadly into transient ischemic attacks (TIAs), reversible ischemic neurologic deficits (RINDs) or minor stroke, stroke in progression, and completed stroke. TIAs refer to episodes of focal cerebral dysfunction of short duration often lasting only minutes, but not more than 24 hours, and leaving no detectable residual neurologic deficit. Experimental studies suggest that transient MCA occlusion of short duration produces permanent cell injury. Approximately 64% of individuals with TIAs show evidence of cerebral infarction on their initial CT scan.[13] On that basis, revised criteria for TIAs have been proposed.[14] In contrast, completed strokes are cerebral ischemic events that produce focal neurologic deficits of varying severity that are fixed and persistent. Generally, however, symptom severity gradually improves without intervention. Full recovery depends on stroke subtype—with atheroembolic strokes having the least likelihood of complete symptom resolution.[15] Patients with lacunar strokes fare better than those suffering thromboembolic events.

Initial symptoms depend on the regions of arterial occlusion. A review of the functions of the cortex, subcortex (striatum), and brain stem regions is beyond the scope of this chapter, but their vascular supply and cell functions are central to their ischemic vulnerability. As an example, proximal middle carotid artery MCA occlusion

(MI segment) produces significant striatal injury and cortical dysfunction in the downstream territory. The severity, injury volume, and location are dependent on the integrity of the collateral arterial supply formed by the circle of Willis and pial arterial anastomoses, which protect the cerebral hemispheres. The striatum does not have an obvious vascular protection that has been defined so far, and is differentially sensitive to ischemia. Experimental studies have demonstrated that thrombosis of the microvessel bed occurs in the ischemic regions, marked by accumulation of fibrinogen and activated platelets.[16,17] Antithrombotic interventions can reduce occlusion formation and the volume of cerebral injury in the ischemic territory.

NATURAL HISTORY OF CEREBRAL ARTERY THROMBOSIS

TIAs have prognostic significance. In the carotid artery territory, completed stroke occurs in 40% to 75% of individuals with one or more TIAs,[18,19] with a prevalence of approximately 30% per year. Of individuals with a premonitory TIA, about 50% may have a stroke within the first year.[20] Stroke-related death and cardiac death have been reported to occur in 28% and 37% of TIA patients, respectively, indicating that cardiovascular mortality is significant in the stroke population.[20] More recent evaluations, which have included data from placebo groups in large trials of antithrombotic efficacy, suggest a lower mortality. For example, 14% of placebo-treated individuals displayed the combined outcome events of stroke, myocardial infarction (MI), and death over 2 years in the UK-TIA Study Group Trial.[21]

Patients presenting with a stroke are at risk for recurrence, often within the same vascular territory. The 5-year cumulative incidence of secondary stroke was 42% among males in one prospective study. A separate study noted a 32% 7-year cumulative incidence for recurrent stroke.[22] The highest recurrence rates for stroke are within the first year following the initial event.

Mortality alone, however, is not considered a suitable outcome in stroke intervention trials because of its low incidence and many causes. Cerebral edema from large, hemispheric ischemic lesions leads to transtentorial herniation and death in nearly 80% of individuals who succumb within 7 days of a stroke.[23]

HEMOSTASIS AND CEREBROVASCULAR ISCHEMIA

Thrombosis and thromboembolism are frequent causes of ischemic stroke. Migrating retinal arterial thromboemboli and refractile bodies, and thrombi in cortical arteries during cerebral ischemia support a pathogenic role for these thrombotic events.[24-28] The frequency of occlusions of a cerebral artery in the carotid territory that causes symptom decreases from 81% within 8 hours of symptom onset to 59% at 24 hours, and in 41% at 1 week.[9-12,29]

Indirect evidence for the involvement of thrombi in cerebrovascular ischemia derives from studies of platelet, coagulation, and fibrinolytic system activation in patients with thrombotic stroke and with TIAs.[30-41] Experimental studies have confirmed the deposition of fibrin and activated platelets in microvessels of the ischemic regions shortly after MCA occlusion.[17,42-46] Those observations implicate local activation of hemostasis by ischemia.

HEMORRHAGIC TRANSFORMATION IN CEREBRAL ISCHEMIA

Hemorrhage accounts for approximately 10% of all strokes. Hemorrhagic transformation of the ischemic lesion occurs naturally during thromboembolic stroke. Hemorrhage within the infarct may result from fragmentation and distal migration of thromboemboli that expose ischemic vessels to arterial pressure.[47] Angiographic studies of thrombolytic agents in patients with thrombotic stroke have broadened this notion[11,48-50] and have suggested that hemorrhage in the absence of reperfusion can occur from other vascular sources (e.g., collateral channels).[47,51,52] Localized (petechial) hemorrhage is associated with loss of the basal lamina of microvessels.[53] Hemorrhagic transformation of the evolving injury is classified as hemorrhagic infarction (HI), parenchymal hematoma (PH), or both.[51,54-56] Postmortem studies have described HI as a spectrum, from scattered petechiae to more confluent hemorrhage within a region of infarction in 50% to 70% of ischemic stroke patients.[47,51,55] Most commonly, HI occurs in association with cardioembolic stroke, but not with in situ atherothrombotic vascular occlusion.[57] Radiographically, PH is a homogeneous, discrete circumscribed mass of blood, often associated with shifts of midline structures and ventricular extension. Many reports of PH in patients with cerebral embolism are associated with anticoagulant treatment.[58,59]

The frequency of hemorrhage in the neuraxis can be affected by the use of antithrombotic agents (Fig. 31-2).[11,12,60-67] The risk of symptomatic hemorrhage within the ischemic lesion in stroke patients increases with exposure to antiplatelet agents, anticoagulants, and plasminogen activators. Normal platelet function appears to be necessary to maintain the integrity of the cerebrovascular bed and to prevent detectable hemorrhage. With anticoagulant use, the increased risk of intracerebral hemorrhage is related to advanced age (>75 years), the intensity of anticoagulation, and the concomitant use of other antithrombotics.[68] The International Stroke Trial (IST) demonstrated a significant 0.1% increase in the incidence of symptomatic intracerebral hemorrhage in the aspirin (ASA) arms.[63,64,69] The UK-TIA Study in the European Stroke Prevention Study-2 (ESPS-2) trial demonstrated that ASA increases the incidence of symptomatic intracerebral hemorrhage.[70] Although a recent, prospective, open phase II study of abciximab within 24 hours of stroke onset produced no apparent difference in the risk of brain hemorrhage from controls,[71]

Hemorrhagic transformation

Hemorrhagic infarction (HI)	
Post-mortem	**~51-67%**
Non-anticoagulated*	**5-43%**
Cardiogenic embolism	**~53-71%**
Parenchymal hematoma (PH)	
No intervention*	**0.6-10.6%**
Antiplatelet agents*	**0.9-1.1%**
Anticoagulants*	**1.2-6.4%**
Plasminogen activators*	**6.4-19.8%**

FIGURE 31-2. Hemorrhagic transformation of ischemic stroke. Postmortem studies have shown that hemorrhagic transformation, mostly hemorrhagic infarction, occurs in up to 67% of stroke patients who succumb. Separate studies suggest that these are mostly associated with cardiogenic thromboembolism. Antithrombotic agents can increase the frequency of parenchymal hematoma (PH), although the incidence depends on the individual agent. Ranges derive from a compilation of studies (see text). *Refers to data derived from studies using computed tomography.

experimental studies of two different integrin $\alpha_{IIb}\beta_3$ inhibitors demonstrated a significant increase in major hemorrhage.[43,46]

ANTITHROMBOTIC INTERVENTIONS IN CEREBRAL ISCHEMIA

Antiplatelet agents and anticoagulants have been used to limit the consequences of recent transient ischemia or the fixed neurologic deficits associated with stroke (Table 31-1). They also have been used as prophylaxis against secondary ischemic events (i.e., secondary prevention). In addition, anticoagulants have been used for the treatment of venous sinus thrombosis and the prevention of systemic and CNS thromboembolic events accompanying atrial fibrillation (AF), acute MI, or cardiac valve injury. Fibrinolytic agents are, thus far, the only antithrombotics successfully used to treat acutely symptomatic focal cerebral ischemia. The literature concerning the use of antithrombotic agents in cerebrovascular disease is extensive, and the reader is referred to reviews examining various aspects of this problem.[67,72-74] Here, the use of antithrombotic agents is based on clinical trials according to "rules of evidence," which distinguish prospective placebo-controlled studies (level I) from descriptive case reports (level V).[75] Updated recommendations for the use of antithrombotics in ischemic stroke are made at regular intervals by the ACCP based on similar criteria.[67,74]

TRANSIENT CEREBRAL ISCHEMIA

TIAs are focal neurologic events lasting not more than 24 hours, but typically of shorter duration. TIAs can be a manifestation of ongoing activation of platelets and coagulation, and vascular injury in brain-supplying arteries.[9-12,24,29,34,39,53,76] Nearly all clinical trials have employed the more conservative definition of transient ischemia.

TABLE 31-1 SUMMARY OF ANTITHROMBOTIC INTERVENTIONS IN CEREBROVASCULAR DISEASE

	INTERVENTION		
Indication	*Antiplatelet Agents*	*Anticoagulants*	*Plasminogen Activators*
Acute Intervention			Intravenous: rt-PA (100 mg) Intra-arterial: on protocol only
Primary Prevention			
TIA or completed stroke			
Nonvalvular atrial fibrillation		Warfarin, INR 2.0-3.0 (2.5)	
Acute myocardial infarction		Warfarin (see text)	
Mechanical prosthetic valves		Warfarin, INR 2.0-3.5† (± dipyridamole 400 mg)	
Xenograft prosthetic valves		Warfarin, INR 2.0-3.0 (2.5) for 3 months postoperatively	
Secondary Prevention			
TIA or minor stroke*	ASA (50-325 mg/day) ASA (25 mg)/SR dipyridamole (200 mg) Clopidogrel (75 mg/day)		
Stroke (completed)	ASA (50-325 mg/day) ASA (25 mg)/SR dipyridamole (200 mg) Clopidogrel (75 mg/day)		
Deep venous thrombosis			Heparin 5000 U × 2, or LMWH
Cerebral venous sinus thrombosis			Heparin, treatment acute warfarin, long-term
Carotid endarterectomy stroke	ASA (81-325 mg/day)		

*Noncardioembolic events.
†INR recommendation dependent on prosthetic valve type (see ref. 201)
ASA, aspirin; INR, International Normalized Reagent; LMWH, low-molecular-weight heparin; rt-PA, recombinant tissue plasminogen activator; SR, sustained release; TIA, transient ischemic attack.

Antiplatelet Agents

Aspirin

Antiplatelet agents have become a central therapeutic approach in patients with transient cerebral ischemia (see Tables 31-1and 31-2). Among antiplatelet agents, ASA can reduce the incidence of vascular events following TIAs, including completed stroke. The Aspirin in TIA (AITIA) study demonstrated a reduced incidence of stroke and vascular death at 6 months in the ASA group, and a significant reduction in the combined outcome events of recurrent TIAs, cerebral/retinal infarction, and death.[77] At the 24-month follow-up; however, there was no difference in the incidence of stroke. The Canadian Cooperative Study Group trial, a randomized, double-blind (level I), four-arm study, demonstrated that ASA (130 mg/day) significantly reduces the incidence of stroke and death after a mean follow-up of 2.2 years.[78] Similarly, ASA decreased the incidence of stroke, MI, and death in the double-blind (level I) "AICLA" trial in patients presenting with a history of TIAs (990 mg/day).[79]

The question of ASA dose was addressed by the UK-TIA aspirin trial, which randomized patients with TIAs or minor ischemic stroke to "high dose" ASA (1200 mg/day), "low dose" ASA (300 mg/day), or placebo.[21] The incidence of nonfatal MI, nonfatal major stroke, and vascular or non-vascular death was significantly reduced among patients receiving ASA at a mean follow-up of 4 years. Nine deaths were attributed to intracranial hemorrhage in the ASA-treated group. Although the incidence of stroke was lower in the ASA-treated groups, there was no difference in outcome between the ASA-dose groups. The Swedish Aspirin Low-Dose Trial (SALT) Collaborative Group reported an 18% reduction in risks of stroke and death among patients with TIA who began a lower dose of ASA (75 mg/day) within 1 to 4 months of their initial symptoms, confirming the benefit of low-dose ASA after signal TIAs.[80]

Thus, the results of four level I trials indicate a benefit from ASA (even at low dose) on early stroke and vascular mortality in patients with a history of TIAs or minor ischemic events. The pathophysiologic basis for the relative benefit seen among ASA-treated individuals, however, is not settled. Also, recently the possibility that some patients may have recurrent TIAs or stroke because of "resistance to ASA" has been raised. The attributes of this condition are undefined.

Dipyridamole

To enhance this effect, ASA has been used in combination with other antiplatelet agents. Based on positive interactions between the agents in both preclinical experiments and in clinical platelet survival studies, ASA has been combined with dipyridamole.[81-84] The efficacy of this combination, however, has been challenged.[82,83]

Dipyridamole (400 to 800 mg/day) alone does not alter the incidence of stroke or related mortality compared with placebo[85]; however, the combination of ASA (975 mg/day) and dipyridamole (225 mg/day) conferred a benefit over placebo in the European Stroke Prevention Study (ESPS).[86] A 33% reduction in the risk of stroke and death was seen after a mean follow-up of 2 years. In the "AICLA" study, the combination of ASA with dipyridamole showed benefit over placebo for TIA patients when the outcome events of stroke, MI, and mortality were combined.[79] In contrast, neither the American-Canadian Cooperative Study Group,[87] nor a smaller prospective study[88] found benefit with the combination.

TABLE 31-2 ANTIPLATELET AGENTS FOR TRANSIENT ISCHEMIC ATTACKS (MINOR STROKE)

Study	Agent	Dose (per day)	Patients (n)	Stroke (n)
AITIA Study[77]	ASA	1300 mg	88	10
	Placebo	—	90	12
Canadian Cooperative Study Group[78]	ASA/placebo 1	1300 mg/—	144	22
	Sulfinpyrazone/placebo 2	800 mg/—	156	29
	ASA/sulfinpyrazone	1300 mg/800 mg	146	14
	Placebo1/placebo 2	—/—	139	20
AICLA	ASA/dipyridamole	990 mg/225 mg	202	18
	ASA	990 mg	198	17
	Placebo	—	204	31
UK-TIA Study Group[21]	ASA	1200 mg	815	66
	ASA	300 mg	806	68
	Placebo	—	814	88
SALT[80]	ASA	75 mg	676	93
	Placebo	—	684	112
European Stroke Prevention Study Group[86]	ASA/dipyridamole	975 mg/225 mg	1250	114[1]
	Placebo	—	1250	184[1]
European Stroke Prevention Study-2[70]	ASA/dipyridamole*	400 mg/50 mg	1650	157
	Dipyridamole	400 mg	1654	211
	ASA	50 mg	1649	206
	placebo	—	1649	250
Hass, et al.[89]	Ticlopidine	500 mg	1529	172
	ASA	1300 mg	1540	212

[1]Intention-to-treat analysis.
ASA, aspirin; dipyridamole*, extended release dipyridamole.

More recently, the ESPS-2 from the European Stroke Prevention Working Group compared sustained release dipyridamole (200 mg) and ASA (25 mg) in a single tablet twice a day with placebo in a study to limit stroke, death—or both—in patients suffering TIAs or stroke. Low dose ASA alone, dipyridamole alone, and the combination were superior to placebo at 2-year follow-up.[70] For individuals with a history of TIAs or recent stroke, the combination was superior to no treatment, but not substantially different from ASA alone.

Thienopyridines

Ticlopidine has benefit in patients suffering TIAs or minor stroke, and as secondary stroke prophylaxis of completed stroke (see later). Ticlopidine (500 mg/day) was associated with a significant 12% reduction in the risk of stroke and death from any cause in one level I trial, and with a similar 21% reduction in the risk of secondary outcomes of stroke and stroke-related death compared with ASA (1300 mg/day).[89] The use of ticlopidine has been substantially curtailed because of the incidence of reversible leukopenia, thrombocytopenia, and the concerns about the frequency of thrombotic thrombocytopenic purpura (TTP). Clopidogrel, a related thienopyridine, has supplanted ticlopidine because of these concerns, although no equivalency study in stroke has been performed for ischemic stroke. Several studies examining the benefits of combination clopidogrel/ASA are underway.

Other Antiplatelet Agents

Other antiplatelet agents have also been tested. The Canadian Cooperative Study Group compared ASA, sulfinpyrazone, and placebo in patients with episodes of amaurosis fugax and TIAs, but no significant differences in the incidence of stroke and mortality were observed between sulfinpyrazone (800 mg/day) and placebo.[78] Two other studies suggested a nonsignificant reduction in TIAs or stroke and mortality at 4 months' follow-up[90] and an even higher incidence of stroke, MI, and vascular death.[91] Hence, sulfinpyrazone has not found a role in the treatment of cerebrovascular disease.

In summary, ASA reduces the risk of stroke, MI, and mortality in patients with a history of TIAs or minor stroke (see Table 31-1). This risk reduction is not obviously dose dependent.[21] The fixed combination of low-dose ASA/sustained-release dipyridamole also produces a substantial risk reduction.[92,70] Although ticlopidine was more effective than ASA in preventing stroke and mortality after TIAs in one study, it is seldom used now because of untoward side-effects. When used alone, dipyridamole and sulfinpyrazone have little demonstrated benefit. Clopidogrel has been used in this patient group, instead of ticlopidine, although efficacy has yet to be tested.

Anticoagulation

Until recently, no properly randomized, blinded, level I study had evaluated the long-term consequences of anticoagulation in patients with a history of TIA or minor stroke. Several uncontrolled reports suggested that heparin can decrease the incidence of basilar artery TIAs[93,94]; however, small level II studies were unable to demonstrate a benefit of anticoagulation in the outcome of TIAs.[95-97]

Among 10 studies enrolling patients with TIAs or stroke, patients receiving anticoagulant therapy fared significantly worse than controls in prevention of subsequent death or stroke.[98] Only the Cerebral Embolism Study Group trial suggested a benefit from immediate anticoagulation for cardiogenic embolism.[99]

Among the few controlled, level I studies, the recently completed Warfarin-Aspirin Recurrent Stroke Study (WARSS) found no difference in outcome between TIA and stroke patients treated with tightly controlled oral anticoagulation or aspirin.[100] The ongoing European/Australian Stroke Prevention in Reversible Ischaemia Trial (ESPRIT) compares patients with a TIA or minor ischemic stroke randomized with oral anticoagulation (INR = 2.0 to 3.0), the combination ASA (25 mg)/dipyridamole (200 mg), or ASA alone for the outcomes of vascular death, nonfatal stroke, nonfatal MI, or major hemorrhage. At interim analysis, oral anticoagulation at an INR range of 2.0 to 3.0 was found to be safe.[101]

The use of anticoagulants in transient ischemia may carry an increased risk of intracerebral hemorrhage.[102,103] The risk of symptomatic intracranial hemorrhage among patients with TIAs receiving anticoagulants under the conditions of these studies, however, is also in accord with the increased incidence of fatal hemorrhagic complications observed among elderly individuals receiving anticoagulation.[104] The results of the International Stroke Trial (IST) suggested an increase in symptomatic hemorrhage in patients given subcutaneous heparin (at doses not usually associated with hemorrhage)[63]; however, in the WARSS experience there was no increase in intracerebral hemorrhage in the anticoagulated group. This result suggests that the risk of cerebral hemorrhage in the population could be limited by rigid management of anticoagulation.[100]

In summary, excluding individuals with atrial fibrillation or cardiac valvular prostheses, the results of a number of small studies do not conclusively support a role for anticoagulation in patients with TIAs or minor stroke. The risk of intracerebral hemorrhage is increased for patients receiving oral anticoagulants at INRs in excess of 3.0 to 4.5.

Plasminogen Activators

There is no rationale for the use of fibrinolytic agents in patients with TIAs or cerebral ischemic episodes of limited extent, and there is, perhaps, increased risk. Treatment of patients with fibrinolytics acutely after the onset of ischemic stroke (see later), however, does not necessarily exclude patients with TIAs.

STROKE-IN-PROGRESSION

Early symptom progression in ischemic stroke has been attributed to (1) anterograde extension of in situ thrombus to occlude critical arterial branches; (2) recurrent embolism; or (3) edema and tissue swelling. Although unproved, the possibility of thrombus extension led to the early enthusiasm for the antithrombotic approaches in patients with progressively severe stroke. Presently, there is uncertainty regarding the pathogenesis of "evolving stroke." Lack of proof that this entity can be defined clinically, and the absence of properly controlled, randomized trials with adequate power to test the concept have proved limited.[105-107]

Only one level I prospective comparison of anticoagulation for stroke in progression has been undertaken. The Trial of Org 10172 in Acute Stroke Treatment (TOAST) compared the heparinoid danaparoid with placebo in patients with early stroke.[108-110] Initially, patients with stroke in progression were randomized, but the recruitment was opened to all patients with hemispheric stroke symptoms ≤24 hours' duration.[108] Favorable outcomes were more frequent in the danaparoid group than placebo at 7 days in a post-hoc analysis[108]; however, no difference in clinical outcome or mortality at 3 months was observed. In general, there was no advantage of danaparoid over placebo. Intracerebral hemorrhage of a serious nature occurred in 14 patients who received danaparoid, but in only 4 patients who received placebo.[111] A significant advantage for prevention of deep venous thrombosis (DVT) confirmed the anticoagulant effect of danaparoid in TOAST (see later).

COMPLETED STROKE

It has been proposed that antithrombotic interventions beyond 24 to 72 hours after symptom onset in carotid artery territory ischemic stroke are unlikely to have a beneficial impact, and are likely to be associated with an increased risk of hemorrhage. Antithrombotic agents, particularly antiplatelet agents, do play a role in prevention of secondary strokes (see Table 31-1). In patients suffering an initial ischemic stroke, the rate of these subsequent ischemic events, MI, or death is 10% to 12% per year.[112-114]

Antiplatelet Agents

Aspirin

Several large meta-analyses have suggested that antiplatelet agents can be beneficial in patients presenting with TIAs or stroke[111,115]; however, the impact of these agents on the natural history of the first stroke is variable. The Swedish Cooperative Study found no difference in the outcomes of recurrent stroke or death between patients treated within 3 weeks of completed stroke with ASA (1500 mg/day) or placebo.[113] Similarly, suloctidil (600 mg/day) and sulfinpyrazone (800 mg/day) did not have a beneficial effect on secondary stroke events.

Two large level I trials have examined the relative effects of simple antithrombotic regimens in patients with completed stroke (Table 31-3). IST randomized 19,436 patients with presumed ischemic stroke within 48 hours of symptom onset to receive placebo, ASA (300 mg/day), subcutaneous heparin (low dose, 10,000 IU/day; or medium dose, 25,000 IU/day), or both ASA and heparin for 14 days in a 3 × 2 factorial design.[63] ASA was associated with an overall significant reduction in total recurrent ischemic strokes within 14 days, but a significant 0.1% increase in symptomatic intracranial hemorrhage. At 6 months, a modest decrease in the risk of death or dependency was seen. The Chinese Acute Stroke Trial (CAST) demonstrated similar outcomes.[116] IST and CAST together indicated that the use of ASA within 2 days of ischemic stroke is associated with a small reduction in the incidence of recurrent stroke and mortality in the first weeks after the signal stroke; however, those benefits did not persist.

TABLE 31-3 ANTIPLATELET AGENTS FOR COMPLETED STROKE

Study	Agent	Dose (per day)	Patients (n)	Stroke (n)
Canadian-American Ticlopidine Study[112]	Ticlopidine	500 mg	525	54
	Placebo		528	89
CAPRIE[117]*	Clopidogrel	75 mg	3233	315
	ASA	325 mg	3198	338
IST[63]	ASA†	300 mg	9720	362‡
	No ASA†	—	9715	452‡
CAST[69]	ASA	160 mg	10554	335
	No ASA	—	10552	351

*Stroke subgroup.
†Factorial design (include heparin ± ASA).
‡14-day outcomes.
ASA, aspirin.

Dipyridamole

As noted earlier, the combination of ASA/sustained release dipyridamole significantly reduced the incidence of second stroke and/or death in patients presenting with a history of TIAs or stroke compared with ASA or dipyridamole alone.[92]

Thienopyridines

After a mean follow-up of 2 years, patients who suffered a signal thromboembolic stroke and received ticlopidine (500 mg/day) within 1 to 16 weeks had significant decreases in the combined outcomes of stroke, MI, and vascular mortality compared with placebo in the Canadian-American Ticlopidine Study (CATS).[112] Side effects related to ticlopidine, principally reversible leukopenia, diarrhea, or rash, occurred in 8% of the treated patients. The Clopidogrel versus Aspirin in patients at Risk of Ischaemic Events (CAPRIE) study prospectively compared clopidogrel (75 mg/day) with ASA (325 mg/day) in patients with thrombotic disease, ischemic stroke (including lacunar disease), MI of less than 35 days, or symptomatic atherosclerotic peripheral arterial disease (PAD) in a blinded, randomized fashion.[117] A significant 8.7% reduction in relative risk in favor of clopidogrel for the combined outcomes of ischemic stroke, MI, and vascular-related death at 1 year was demonstrated. The overall benefit associated with clopidogrel was driven by the outcome for peripheral arterial disease; however, no independent significant difference in outcome within the stroke cohort was detected. In the setting of coronary artery revascularization, clopidogrel is often given with ASA. The Management of Atherothrombosis with Clopidogrel in High-risk patients (MATCH) trial compared the efficacy of daily clopidogrel (75 mg)/ASA (75 mg) with clopidogrel (75 mg) alone for ischemic vascular events including stroke. No added benefit to clopidogrel by ASA at these doses was seen, although initial data assessment indicates an increase in intracerebral hemorrhage for the combination. The impact of these results in practice is not yet clear. Clopidogrel is now often substituted for ticlopidine for secondary stroke prevention.

Platelet-Fibrin Interaction Inhibitors

Platelet glycoprotein IIb/IIIa (integrin $\alpha_{IIb}\beta_3$) antagonists have been proposed as agents in stroke treatment; however, the target is unspecified. One phase II study of abciximab given within 24 hours of stroke onset did not produce significant improvement or intracerebral hemorrhage in 74 patients at the doses tested.[71] This is in contrast to published experimental studies with polypeptide or organic integrin $\alpha_{IIb}\beta_3$ inhibitors in acute middle cerebral artery occlusion.[43,46]

On the basis of its beneficial effects on outcome in patients with recent TIAs or completed stroke, ASA is the first choice for secondary prevention. ASA/extended release dipyridamole is superior to ASA alone (see Table 31-1). Ticlopidine was shown to produce a significant reduction in subsequent stroke, MI, or vascular-related death over ASA, but clopidogrel has been substituted by some physicians in practice. Supportive data are still pending. Current ACCP recommendations for secondary prevention in noncardioembolic ischemic stroke are management with ASA (50 to 325 mg/day), ASA/extended release dipyridamole, or clopidogrel (75 mg/day).[67]

Anticoagulants

For many years, impressions about the salutary effect of heparin or long-term oral anticoagulation on the outcome of presumed atherothrombotic stroke were based on three randomized, controlled trials[102,118,119] and clinical impression[120-122]; however, the evidence was conflicting. An increase in symptomatic (fatal) intracerebral hemorrhage was often associated with excessive anticoagulation. Design weaknesses also plagued those studies. More recent approaches have focused on the potential for benefit in large, prospectively controlled trials (Table 31-4).

Heparin

IST and CAST tested the effects of subcutaneous unfractionated heparin (5000 IU or 10,000 IU) on recurrent ischemic stroke.[63,64,71] In IST, low-dose heparin was associated with a significant reduction in recurrent stroke compared with placebo, but in that trial, the associated significant increase in symptomatic intracerebral hemorrhage nullified the benefits on recurrent stroke.[63,64,71] Major concerns about those trials have been patient selection, medication delivery, and the management of hemorrhage. The form of anticoagulation tested in those studies is not routinely used for cerebrovascular disease.

Low-Molecular-Weight Heparins

In view of their superior bioavailability and lower relative incidence of intracerebral hemorrhage,[123,124] low-molecular-weight heparins (LMWHs) have also been tested. In the Fraxiparin in Stroke Study (FISS), patients were randomized within 48 hours after stroke onset to either subcutaneous "high-dose" nadroparin (8200 IU of antifactor Xa per day), "low-dose" nadroparin (4100 IU/day), or placebo for 10 days.[125] A significant dose-dependent reduction in 6-month mortality and dependence was observed favoring nadroparin, but the benefit was seen only after 3 months. A second trial of nadroparin in completed stroke, FISS-bis, tested the same hypothesis, but the outcomes contradicted the results of FISS. No difference in combined outcome or

TABLE 31-4 ANTICOAGULATION FOR COMPLETED STROKE

Study	Agent	Dose (per day)	Patients (n)	Stroke (n)	Death/Stroke (n)
FISS[125]	Nadroparin*	8200 aFXa	100	1	13
	Nadroparin*	4100 aFXa	101	2	17
	Placebo*	—	105	5	20
FISS-bis	Nadroparin*	172 aFXa/kg	245	16	145
	Nadroparin*	86 aFXa/kg	272	15	156
	Placebo*	—	250	11	142
HAEST[126]	Dalteparin	200 IU/kg	224	19†	—
	ASA	160 mg	225	17†	—
TOPAS[127]	Certoparin	16,000 aFXa	97	13‡	—
	Certoparin	10,000 aFXa	103	10‡	—
	Certoparin	6000 aFXa	102	6‡	—

aFXa, anti-factor Xa activity.
*Death or dependency at 6-month follow-up.
†at 14 days.
‡including TIAs.

mortality was seen in that unpublished trial. The TOAST results, when interpreted as a reflection of the outcome of completed stroke, also showed no sustained benefit from danaparoid.[108]

In the HAEST study, dalteparin, delivered early following symptom onset of ischemic stroke, produced no significant improvement in favorable outcome compared with placebo.[126] There was also no difference in detectable intracerebral hemorrhage between the groups. The effect of certoparin on ischemic stroke outcome was examined in a level II dose-finding trial. In dose steps ranging from 3000 U to 16000 U/day, no significant difference in outcome was detected, although there was a modest increase in the number of patients suffering symptomatic hemorrhage.[127] Overall, the experience with LMWHs for stroke treatment has been disappointing; most studies tested the LMWH beginning 24 to 48 hours after symptom onset.

Warfarin

The Warfarin-Aspirin Recurrent Stroke Study (WARSS) examined the differential effect of warfarin or ASA on the frequency of secondary cerebral ischemic events in patients presenting within 30 days of the signal stroke.[100] No difference in outcomes was observed between the warfarin and the aspirin groups. Importantly, warfarin was not associated with an increase in intracerebral hemorrhage, due probably to the tight monitoring of anticoagulation. ESPRIT, an ongoing trial, compares therapeutic oral anticoagulation with combination ASA/dipyridamole, or ASA alone.[101] It would appear that there is no advantage to the use of anticoagulants for the purposes of secondary prevention following completed stroke.[128,129] None of those studies instituted the anticoagulant acutely (see Table 31-1).

Plasminogen Activators

Plasminogen activators are contraindicated for use in patients with completed stroke. Early studies, most often uncontrolled, failed to demonstrate efficacy when symptomatic improvement and death were considered as the primary outcomes. Most studies were associated with an increase in symptomatic intracerebral hemorrhage.[130] A central question about those studies was whether, given the long interval to treatment after stroke symptom onset, neurologic deficits were caused by undiagnosed hemorrhage. Low doses of plasminogen activators were not felt to be efficacious.

ACUTE INTERVENTIONS IN STROKE

Two concepts that address injury reduction are now applied to stroke patients: (1) to salvage tissue, recanalization of the occluded artery must occur immediately; and (2) the incidence/severity of hemorrhage can be limited with early acute intervention (<6 to 8 hours from symptom onset).[131] Consequently, intervention with plasminogen activators in patients selected by strict CT and clinical criteria has shown evidence of benefit (see Tables 31-1 and 31-5).[11,65]

Antiplatelet Agents and Anticoagulants

Experimental studies of focal ischemia have suggested that interventions with antiplatelet agents and anticoagulants, as well as agents active on nonvascular cells, could be associated with microvascular recanalization and tissue salvage.[43,46] As of this time, there are no clinical studies of acute intervention of either antiplatelet agents or anticoagulants in ischemic stroke patients. When to start these agents after the use of a plasminogen

TABLE 31-5 PLASMINOGEN ACTIVATORS FOR ACUTE INTERVENTION IN STROKE

Study[1]	Agent	Patients (n)	Δ(T-0) (hours)[2]	Clinical Improvement (%)	HEMORRHAGE nil	HI	PH	%
MAST-E[145]	SK	156	<6.0	35.0	88	25	24	17.5
	C	154		18.1	116	13	4	0.3
ASK[146]	SK	106	<4.0	43.4	—	—	—	—
	C	122		22.1	—	—	—	—
MAST-I[147]	SK	313	<6.0	26.5	232	60	21	6.7
	C	309		11.7	280	27	2	0.7
NINDS (Part 1)[11]	rt-PA	144	≤1.5, ≤3.0	1.2[3]	—	—	13	5.6
	C	147			—	—	3	0.0
NINDS (Part 2)[11]	rt-PA	168	≤1.5, ≤3.0	50[4] 31[5]	—	—	21	7.1
	C	165		38[4] 20[5]	—	—	8	2.1
ECASS[65]	rt-PA	313	<6.0	35.9	179	72	62	19.8
	C	307		29.3	184	93	30	6.5
ECASS-2[136]	rt-PA	409	<6.0	40.3[4]	217	142	48	11.8
	C	391		36.6[4]	233	141	12	3.1

[1]Randomized studies without vascular diagnosis.
[2]Time from symptom onset to treatment.
[3]Relative risk reduction.
[4]Modified Rankin scale (mRS) scores 0 and 1.
[5]National Institutes of Health Stroke Scale (NIHSS).
C, control; HI, hemorrhagic infarction; PH, parenchymatous hematoma; rt-PA, recombinant tissue-type plasminogen activator; SK, streptokinase.

activator has been debated. Usually, it has been no earlier than 24 hours after the administration of the plasminogen activator.

Plasminogen Activators

The contributions of local vascular anatomy and collateral vascular protection to tissue perfusion, as well as the predominantly thrombotic basis for focal cerebral ischemia, underlie attempts to achieve early recanalization with fibrinolytic agents.[9]

Intravenous Systemic Infusion

Recanalization of carotid artery territory occlusions by intravenous infusion techniques has been achieved in 34% to 59% of patients treated within 8 hours of symptom onset[11,50,132,133]; however, recanalization of ICA occlusions is unusual (0% to 25%), possibly because of the low flow in the occluded arterial segment, the length of the thrombus, and compromised distal run-off.[11,50,133] One prospective, open, multicenter dose-rate study of intravenous recombinant tissue plasminogen activator (rt-PA [duteplase]) demonstrated that early reperfusion of MCA division and branch occlusions occurred more frequently than ICA occlusions.[11] Mori and colleagues first demonstrated that patients treated with rt-PA (duteplase) had improved recanalization and a significantly better clinical improvement at 30 days than those treated with placebo.[50] Hemorrhagic transformation occurred in 29% to 53% of treated patients in those studies.[11,50,132,133] Those studies demonstrated both the feasibility and safety of exposure to plasminogen activators and set the stage for larger phase III intervention trials of safety and efficacy.

The National Institute of Neurological Disorders and Stroke (NINDS) undertook a two-part, four-armed, placebo-controlled outcome study of rt-PA in patients entered within 3 hours from ischemic stroke symptom onset (see Table 31-5).[11] In the second part of the study, rt-PA recipients displayed a significant 11% to 13% absolute increase over placebo in the number of patients with no or minimal disability/deficit in Barthel index, modified Rankin scale (mRS) score, Glasgow outcome scale score, and NIHSS, at 3 months and at 12 months. The frequency of symptomatic hemorrhage was significantly greater among those patients receiving rt-PA (6.4%) than among those who received placebo (0.6%) at 3 months. Although mortality was unchanged, intracerebral hemorrhage contributed to demise in the rt-PA group.[11,134] That study supported the current acute use of rt-PA in ischemic stroke.

Three further phase III prospective, randomized safety and efficacy studies of intravenous rt-PA (alteplase) broadened these impressions (see Table 31-5). The European Cooperative Acute Stroke Study (ECASS) compared rt-PA with placebo within 6 hours of symptom onset. There was, at 3 months, no significant difference between the two groups in disability outcome.[65] A post hoc analysis of the "target population" suggested an 11% to 12% absolute improvement in no or minimal disability (mRS = 0 and 1) in the rt-PA-treated group over the placebo group. In that study, too, there was a significantly higher proportion of patients with serious intracerebral hemorrhage (PH2, parenchymal hemorrhage with clinical deterioration) in those who received rt-PA (6.1%) compared with placebo (2.6%). The subgroup of patients with early evidence of ischemia on CT scans had increased mortality, which was further increased by treatment with rt-PA. To reduce the number of patients at risk of intracerebral hemorrhage, careful review of the baseline CT scans for "early signs of ischemia" was performed for the follow-up study.[135,136] In ECASS-II, a favorable outcome (mRS = 0 or 1) was seen in 40.3% of rt-PA patients compared with 36.6% of placebo patients.[137] Cerebral hemorrhage causing death or deterioration (PH2) was significantly more frequent in the rt-PA group than the placebo group (11.7% versus 3.1%). Although the outcome differences were not statistically significant, the trends (in ECASS and ECASS-II) and benefits (NINDS) are consistent. The STARS group completed a further prospective phase IV evaluation of rt-PA use in ischemic stroke and confirmed the NINDS results. Significant beneficial outcome was associated with age ≤75 years and the absence of "early signs" of ischemic injury.[138]

These and other studies have also suggested significant contributors to the risk of hemorrhage from intravenous plasminogen activators. Contributors include excessive time from the onset of symptoms to treatment, low body mass index, diastolic hypertension, older age, and the use of rt-PA.[139-141] The appearance of "early signs of ischemia" on the initial CT scan is also associated with increased risks of hemorrhage and demise.[65,141-144] Taken together, the results of the ECASS and NINDS studies indicate the enormous importance of patient selection to reduce the hemorrhagic risk accompanying the use of plasminogen activators in acute stroke.[11,65,66]

In contrast, experience with streptokinase (SK) in patients with ischemic stroke has been problematic. Three symptom-based, randomized, placebo-controlled trials of acute intravenous delivery were terminated because of unacceptable outcomes.[145-147] The Multicenter Acute Stroke Trial Europe (MAST-E) and the Australia Streptokinase (ASK) trials were terminated because of excessive early mortality and symptomatic intracranial hemorrhage,[145,146] whereas the Multicentre Acute Stroke Trial-Italy (MAST-I) was terminated because of excessive early casefatality.[147] No dose-finding study preceded those trials, so a safe SK dose was not determined.[148,149]

In summary, rt-PA (alteplase) is approved for treatment of ischemic stroke in appropriately selected individuals within 3 hours of symptom onset in North America and select other countries. SK by intravenous delivery is not used in ischemic stroke.

Intra-Arterial Direct Infusion

Intra-arterial infusion studies have provided considerable information about both cerebrovascular anatomy and treatment outcomes with thrombolytic agents. Early studies using flow-directed and guidewire-directed catheters reported recanalization of symptomatic carotid artery territory occlusions in 46% to 90% of patients treated with intra-arterial infusion of SK or urokinase plasminogen activator (u-PA) within 8 hours.[48,49,150] In those studies, hemorrhagic transformation in the ischemic territory occurred in 18% to 33% of treated patients.[48,49,150] Clinical improvements were observed in a substantial number of those patients, although outcomes were not quantitatively assessed.

Occlusions in the vertebrobasilar artery territory can produce significant ischemia-related disability. A retrospective comparison of clinical outcome indicated that stroke patients who received direct intra-arterial u-PA or SK infusion had apparent survival benefit over those who received conventional therapy (i.e., heparin) when recanalization was documented.[151] Hemorrhagic transformation occurred in four patients treated with u-PA or SK, of whom two deteriorated and died from the hemorrhage.

Until recently, no randomized, controlled studies of intra-arterial direct infusion had been undertaken. Two prospective level I studies of intra-arterial plasminogen activator delivery in patients with acute thrombotic stroke have now been reported.[12,152] A phase II, placebo-controlled level I study (Prourokinase in Acute Cerebral Thromboembolism, PROACT) compared recombinant single chain u-PA (scu-PA or pro-UK, 6 mg) with placebo in patients treated within 6 hours of symptom onset for recanalization of M1 and M2 segment MCA occlusions and safety outcomes.[12] A significant increase in MCA recanalization was observed in the scu-PA group, which was accompanied by an increase in hemorrhagic transformation. The increases in recanalization and hemorrhage were heparin dependent. PROACT-2 prospectively tested the effect of intra-arterial recombinant scu-PA (9 mg) against no intervention for recanalization and disability outcome. Patients with proximal MCA occlusion were openly randomized, but both groups received intravenous heparin, and no instrumentation was performed on placebo patients.[152] Recanalization was significantly increased with recombinant scu-PA (65.7%) compared with no intervention (18.0%), and the frequency of symptomatic intracerebral hemorrhage also increased. Disability outcome measured as mRS = 0 to 2 improved in the scu-PA cohort, but was not significantly different from the control group when measured as mRS = 0 to 1. Hence, both recanalization and hemorrhage appear to be dependent on the use of both plasminogen activator and the anticoagulant in those studies.

In summary, two controlled trials of direct intra-arterial infusion plasminogen activators indicate the feasibility and relative safety of this approach. The agent under study is not available, and no plasminogen activator is approved for the intra-arterial approach in thrombotic stroke patients. Local infusion thrombolysis is performed at centers with expertise, where safety is paramount, a well-formed interventional/clinical team is in place, and appropriate, approved protocols are followed (see Table 31-1).

Defibrinogenating Agents

Certain snake venoms can induce defibrinogenation when infused intravenously into humans.[153] Ancrod infused acutely has been shown to be relatively safe in patients with ischemic stroke, when a reduction in fibrinogen of 100 mg/dl was maintained.[154] According to prespecified covariate-adjusted analysis (taking into account baseline stroke severity), favorable outcomes were observed significantly more frequently in the ancrod group (42.2%) than in the placebo group (34.4%).[154,155] Severe disability was less frequent and mortality was unchanged. Intracranial hemorrhage was moderately more frequent in the ancrod group. The novel design of the Stroke Treatment with Ancrod Trial (STAT) has demonstrated that careful intervention with this agent could produce a favorable benefit-risk profile.[155] In contrast, no advantage to ancrod was observed in the European Stroke Treatment with Ancrod Trial (ESTAT), whose study design and patient recruitment were unlike STAT.[156]

RETINAL VASCULAR THROMBOSIS

Fibrinolytic agents have been used successfully in patients with retinal artery and retinal vein occlusion.[157] In the few reports available, partial visual recovery was observed when retinal vein occlusion was treated with intravenous SK within 2 weeks of symptom onset. Partial recovery of form vision was possible in some patients with retinal artery occlusion with acute intervention.[158,159] Neither approach has been tested prospectively, however.

CAROTID ARTERY ATHEROTHROMBOTIC DISEASE

The carotid artery bifurcation has complex flow dynamics and is a predilection site for atheroma formation. As such, it can be a source of cerebral ischemic symptoms, due to platelet-fibrin thromboemboli. It has long been debated whether medical or surgical management of the symptomatic artherothrombotic lesions might be beneficial in patients with TIAs. Endarterectomy of the extracranial portion of the carotid artery, with or without patch angioplasty, can resolve local vascular flow abnormalities, but cerebral ischemic symptoms can recur. Results of both the North American Symptomatic Carotid Endarterectomy Trial (NASCET) and the MRC European Carotid Surgery Trial (ECST) demonstrated significant survival benefit and symptom relief from endarterectomy over medical therapy (i.e., antiplatelet agents) for carotid stenoses of 70% to 99%.[160,161] Further analyses indicated that ipsilateral stroke is reduced in patients undergoing endarterectomy for symptomatic stenosis of intermediate extent (50% to 69%), but the benefit depends partly on surgical risk.[162]

Adjunctive antiplatelet treatment might further decrease the incidence of stroke and death, or the incidence of carotid restenosis after carotid endarterectomy; however, controlled clinical trials have not supported this notion. In one prospective, double-blind trial of carotid endarterectomy, patients randomized to ASA (1300 mg/day) or to placebo within 5 days of the procedure, the incidence of stroke or death at 6 months was marginally greater in those receiving placebo.[163] No significant differences in the outcomes of stroke, MI, or vascular death were seen between patients receiving ASA (50 to 100 mg/day) or placebo within 1 to 12 weeks of carotid endarterectomy in a separate trial.[164] In another prospective comparison of presurgical ASA (1000 mg/day) with no treatment, survival was prolonged in the ASA-treated group, although cerebral events occurred equally in both.[165,166] All three trials were small, which may have obscured any potential benefit to cerebrovascular outcome in the active arms.

Thus, there are no level I trials that support any recommendation for specific adjunctive antiplatelet therapy after carotid endarterectomy; however, both in trials and the clinic, the practice has been to continue patients undergoing endarterectomy on ASA alone after the procedure. There is little information regarding a role for anticoagulants after endarterectomy, and fibrinolytic agents are contraindicated. Current practice is to treat patients with antiplatelet agents, usually with ASA (81 to 325 mg/day), prior to and following endarterectomy.

CARDIAC SOURCE CEREBRAL EMBOLISM

Mural thrombi associated with left ventricular dyskinesia after MI, prosthetic valves and rheumatic valvular vegetations, and atrial thrombi that arise during atrial fibrillation can embolize and lead to focal cerebral ischemia. Anticoagulation has found a role for both the primary and secondary prevention of most cardioembolic events (see Tables 31-1 and 31-6).

Acute Myocardial Infarction

The incidence of systemic thromboembolism, including stroke, after MI varies from 1% to 3% per year without adjunctive therapy, but may be as high as 3.7% during the first month after an MI.[167-172] Evidence that antiplatelet agents might be effective in decreasing the incidence of post-MI cerebral events is limited. The CAPRIE study suggested that clopidogrel could reduce the combined events of second MI, stroke, or vascular death following an initial MI, although the benefit for the MI group was marginal.[117]

Anticoagulation during acute in-hospital phase and in the chronic post-hospitalization phase reduces the number of cerebrovascular events.[167-173] Secondary prevention trials designed to determine the incidence of recurrent MI as the main outcome event have also examined the relative effect of long-term anticoagulation on the incidence of stroke. Among patients randomized within 21 days of acute MI to long-term oral anticoagulation or placebo in the Veterans Administration Cooperative Study, no difference in the stroke incidence over 1 to 5 years was observed.[167] There was, however, a significant overall reduction in the combined outcomes of stroke, second MI, and death. A similar trend was noted in a double-blind, randomized trial of long-term phenprocoumon versus placebo when treatment was initiated at least 12 months after the acute MI[169]; however, serious hemorrhage was more frequent in the anticoagulant group. The open German-Austrian Aspirin Trial (GAAT) reported a decreased incidence of stroke in individuals receiving phenprocoumon compared with placebo when treatment began within 42 days of MI.[170] In the Sixty Plus Reinfarction Study, patients older than 60 years were randomized to oral anticoagulation or placebo in a double-blind fashion after recovery from the signal MI.[171] A trend toward a lower incidence of stroke with anticoagulation was evident at 2-year follow-up; however, an increased incidence of serious hemorrhagic complications was seen in all four level II studies, which contributed to morbidity or mortality in the anticoagulated group.[167,169-171]

Two level I trials demonstrated that anticoagulation significantly reduced stroke incidence in patients surviving

TABLE 31-6 ANTIPLATELET AGENTS AND ANTICOAGULANTS FOR ATRIAL FIBRILLATION (NON-VALVULAR)

Study	Agent	Dose (per day)	Patients (n)	Stroke (n)[1]	Total Mortality (n)
AFASAK[185]	Warfarin	INR = 2.8-4.2	335	5	—
	ASA	75 mg	336	17 (3)	—
	Placebo	—	336	19 (2)	—
SPAF[185]	1. Warfarin/ASA	INR = 2.0-3.5/325 mg	393	7	14
	Placebo	—	195	17 (1)	8
	2. ASA	325 mg	517	18 (1)	31
	Placebo	—	528	34 (4)	39
BAATAF[233]	Warfarin	INR = 1.5-2.7	212	2	11
	Placebo	—	208	13	26
CAFA[234]	Warfarin	INR = 2.0-3.0	187	4 (1)	7
	Placebo	—	191	9 (2)	6
SPAF-2[190]	Warfarin[2]	INR = 2.0-4.5	358	13 (1)	36
	ASA	325 mg	357	19 (2)	41
	Warfarin[3]	INR = 2.0-4.5	197	13 (1)	26
	ASA	325 mg	188	18 (0)	24
SPAF-3[191]	Warfarin	INR = 2.0-3.0	523	11 (0)	35
	Warfarin	INR = 1.2-1.5	521	43 (1)	42

[1]Numbers in parentheses indicate systemic embolic events.
[2]Patients < 75 years.
[3]Patients > 75 years.
ASA, aspirin; INR, international normalized ratio.

an MI. One placebo-controlled trial based in Copenhagen reported a significantly decreased incidence of stroke during a mean 3-year follow-up in those MI patients who received anticoagulation.[168] The Warfarin Reinfarction Study (WARIS) also reported a significant decrease in the incidence of cerebrovascular accidents (a secondary endpoint) at the 3.1-year follow-up in patients receiving warfarin over those receiving placebo.[172] The incidence of death and reinfarction (MI) was also reduced by warfarin in that study. In both trials, hemorrhage was more common in the anticoagulant group. ASA was not used in WARIS, unlike current practices.

A decreased incidence of stroke in the acute (i.e., in-hospital) phase of myocardial ischemia was noted in four trials of anticoagulation[174-177]; however, in two of the studies, there was no effect on the combined outcomes of stroke, second MI, and death.[175,177] In the third study, there was a significant decrease in the incidence of systemic embolism.[176] Interestingly, both the incidence and severity of hemorrhagic complications accompanying anticoagulation during the acute phase of MI in those trials were quite low.

The question of anticoagulant dose and incidence of intracerebral hemorrhage is an important one. Only one study indicated a correlation between the frequency of hemorrhagic events and the degree of anticoagulation[174]; however, there was no difference in the number of intracerebral hemorrhages between the low-dose and high-dose regimens (one each) in that study.

Hence, long-term anticoagulation can lead to a decrease in the number of cerebrovascular events after recovery from MI.[167-169,171-173,178] In practice, however, concerns about the higher incidence of serious hemorrhagic events, including intracerebral hemorrhage, have limited routine use of anticoagulants in this setting.

Cardioembolic Stroke in Atrial Fibrillation

Cerebral embolism occurs with rheumatic valvular disease, mechanical or xenograft prosthetic cardiac valves, and calcified mitral annuli. The risk of cerebral embolism is greatly increased by concurrent atrial fibrillation (AF).[179-181] AF is classified either as nonvalvular (i.e., nonrheumatic) or as associated with valvular dysfunction. Atrial fibrillation is a significant risk factor for thromboembolic stroke and stroke recurrence; the two-year incidence of stroke in patients with chronic nonvalvular AF is 6.2% to 7.6%.[182,183]

Oral anticoagulants are indicated for primary prevention in nonvalvular AF (see Tables 31-1 and 31-6). The Stroke Prevention in Atrial Fibrillation (SPAF) study randomized patients to warfarin, ASA, or placebo (group 1) if they were eligible for warfarin, or to ASA or placebo (group 2, double-blind) if they were not.[184] SPAF was terminated when the warfarin and ASA arms of group 1 were shown to have a significant combined risk reduction of 81% for the outcomes of ischemic stroke and systemic embolism. Although the relative benefit of warfarin over ASA was not reported, 10.9% of the warfarin patients were withdrawn because of drug intolerance. There were, however, insignificant differences between the outcomes of nonvalvular patients in the ASA treatment and control arms in the Atrial Fibrillation Aspirin and Anticoagulation (AFASAK)-1 study, the European Atrial Fibrillation Trial (EAFT), and ESPS-2.[70,185,186] ASA was associated with a 21% relative risk reduction (RRR) in annual stroke events (ASA treated = 6.3, control = 8.1%, $P = .05$) in an individual patient combined analysis of AFASAK-1, EAFT, and SPAF-1.[187] That conclusion was supported by a broader meta-analysis,[188] but heterogeneity in the results could not be excluded.[189]

Concern about the risk of intracranial hemorrhage associated with warfarin stimulated other approaches using ASA or adjusted low-dose oral anticoagulation.[190,191] The SPAF-2 trial tested the relative efficacies of warfarin and ASA in patients with nonvalvular AF and suggested a modest, but not significant, decrease in ischemic stroke events with warfarin over ASA in the less than 75-year group (33%) and greater than 75-year group (27%). There Zwas a significantly greater frequency of major hemorrhagic events with warfarin in the older cohort (>75 years). However, both AFASAK-1 and the EAFT demonstrated that warfarin could significantly reduce the annual stroke rate compared with ASA.[185]

In the SPAF-3 trial, patients received either adjusted dose warfarin (INR = 2.0 to 3.0) or low-intensity warfarin with ASA (325 mg/day) to maintain an INR of 1.2 to 1.5.[191] SPAF-3 was terminated because the annual disabling stroke rate in the low-intensity warfarin/ASA combination group exceeded that of adjusted-dose warfarin. This result led to the early termination of the AFASAK-2 study of moderate-risk patients.[192,193] A further examination of antiplatelet agents in AF has not taken place. But, a meta-analysis suggests that patients who are at low risk for complications of AF could benefit from ASA alone.[194]

A recent study reported that the direct antithrombin ximelagatran appears as safe as warfarin in patients with nonvalvular AF,[195] and is not inferior to well-managed warfarin in patients with nonvalvular AF who are at high-risk for embolization to the systemic circulation or CNS.[196,197]

Nonetheless, for high-risk AF patients (with a prior TIA/stroke or systemic embolus, history of hypertension, poor left ventricular function, age >75 years, rheumatic mitral valve disease, or a prosthetic valve), the recommended therapy is adjusted-dose warfarin anticoagulation at a target INR of 2.5 (range 2.0 to 3.0), rather than ASA.[74]

Cardiac Valve Disease

Coulshed and colleagues recorded a 3.7% and 1.9% yearly incidence of systemic embolism from untreated rheumatic mitral stenosis and mitral insufficiency, respectively.[198] Recurrent embolism is frequent, most often occurring within 6 to 12 months after the signal embolism.[179,199] The incidence of systemic embolism from prosthetic cardiac valves is greater for mechanical devices than for xenograft prostheses. Antiplatelet agents and anticoagulants have been used as prophylaxis against the embolic complications of mechanical valves.[181,200,201] The use of nonmechanical prostheses, however, has altered the approach to prophylaxis with anticoagulants.

Mechanical Prosthetic Cardiac Valves

A group of level III studies indicated significant reductions in the frequency of systemic emboli in anticoagulated patients compared with those receiving placebo.[202-204] This decrease was often greatest for patients with mechanical prostheses in the aortic position. Barnhorst and colleagues confirmed that long-term warfarin in patients with Starr-Edwards prostheses in the aortic or mitral position was associated with a significant reduction in the rate of systemic embolism.[199]

Generally, all individuals with mechanical prosthetic valves should be treated with long-term anticoagulation (see Table 31-1). Current recommendations depend on the valve type.[205-207] A comparison of high intensity warfarin (INR = 9) with moderate intensity warfarin (INR = 2.65) showed a significant increase in hemorrhagic episodes with the high-intensity regimen, without further reduction in thromboembolic events.[205] Loeliger suggested that a target INR of 4.0 for mechanical valves and 3.5 for tissue valves produces an acceptable reduction in hemorrhagic risk.[206]

Antiplatelet agents can increase the protection afforded by anticoagulants alone, but the hemorrhagic risk may also increase. Two level I studies demonstrated reduced thromboembolic risk in individuals with aortic or mitral mechanical prostheses receiving combination anticoagulation with ASA over anticoagulation alone.[207,208] However, ASA is known to add hemorrhagic risk to oral anticoagulation, and is seldom used as the primary approach in this setting.

Given the lower rate of gastrointestinal side effects with non-ASA antiplatelet agents, studies using those agents are of interest. In one prospective, randomized, double-blind trial, the addition of dipyridamole (400 mg/day) to warfarin produced a significant reduction in thromboembolism or death over warfarin and placebo.[209,210] Two separate trials of patients with mechanical prostheses demonstrated that those who received anticoagulation and dipyridamole had fewer thrombotic events than those receiving anticoagulation alone[211] or with ASA.[212] The frequency of major hemorrhage was also lower. A meta-analysis of trials combining dipyridamole with oral anticoagulation suggests a decrease in the frequency of fatal and nonfatal thromboemboli.[213,214] In general, both the use of dipyridamole with warfarin in level II and III studies, and the combination of warfarin and ASA in level I studies have been associated with a reduction in cerebral thromboembolism from mechanical cardiac valve prostheses, whereas dipyridamole has been associated with fewer hemorrhagic events.[181]

An additional challenge is provided by individuals who are pregnant and require valve replacement. Anticoagulation with warfarin, subcutaneous heparin, or standard intravenous heparin during pregnancy each has significant risks that must be weighed against the thromboembolic risk of the valve itself.[215,216]

Xenograft (Bio) Prosthetic Cardiac Valves

The incidence of systemic thromboembolic events associated with bioprostheses at 3 years is 16% in patients with atrial fibrillation,[218] and 4% in those with sinus rhythm abnormalities.[219] The greatest risk of thromboembolism appears to occur during the first 3 months after placement of the bioprosthesis.[220,221] In one study, patients with porcine biosynthetic valves treated with dicumarol postoperatively for 6 to 12 weeks had a lower frequency of major embolic events at 3 years.[218] Turpie and colleagues found no significant difference in the incidence of systemic emboli in patients with xenograft prostheses randomized to oral anticoagulation at an INR of 2.0 to 2.25, or at an INR of 2.5 to 4.0 (standard anticoagulation) for the first 3 postoperative months.[222] In that study, clinically significant hemorrhagic events were more frequent in the group receiving standard anticoagulation. An advantage of the use of bioprostheses is that they can significantly reduce the incidence of systemic thromboembolic events originating from the aortic valve.

The lower incidence of thromboembolic events with xenograft valve prostheses compared with mechanical prostheses implies that antiplatelet prophylaxis may have some benefit with lower hemorrhagic risk. Experience from two prospective, nonrandomized trials of warfarin versus ASA (1000 or 500 mg/day) suggested that with mitral valve bioprostheses, ASA alone can provide some protection against embolic events[223,224]; however, that conclusion has not been rigorously tested. Generally accepted clinical practice requires the anticoagulation of patients with a bioprosthesis for the initial 3 postoperative months, when the thromboembolic risk is greatest (see Table 31-1).

DEEP VENOUS THROMBOSIS IN STROKE

Deep venous thrombosis (DVT) commonly complicates the course of stroke patients during the recuperation phase.[225] Both heparinoids and low-molecular-weight heparins have been tested in an attempt to improve the effects of prophylactic unfractionated heparin. Early experience with two low-molecular-weight heparin preparations as prophylaxis was mixed.[226-228] Twice daily subcutaneous treatment with one preparation was associated with a significant reduction in the frequency of DVT.[228] Turpie and colleagues demonstrated an advantage to twice daily subcutaneous treatment with a low-molecular-weight heparinoid compared with low-dose subcutaneous heparin in decreasing DVT.[229] In the TOAST trial, danaparoid produced a significant reduction in the frequency of post-stroke DVT, compared with placebo.[109,110,230-232] It is standard practice to use an anticoagulant as prophylaxis against DVT in patients suffering stroke.

Conclusions

The contributions of atherothrombotic occlusions and thromboembolism to cerebrovascular disease have supported the enthusiasm for using antithrombotic agents to preserve flow in the central nervous system. Antithrombotic approaches have been relatively successful, with modest-to-significant contributions to benefit in acute interventions (plasminogen activators), prevention of second strokes (antiplatelet agents), and prophylaxis of systemic emboli from valvular injury, valve prosthesis, and nonvalvular atrial fibrillation (anticoagulants ± antiplatelet agents). Hence, treatments of arterial occlusions, which can compromise the supply to the brain, whether from presumed thromboembolism or in situ thrombosis, are mainstays of stroke treatment and prophylaxis at this time.

REFERENCES

1. Garcia JH, Liu K-F, Ho K-L: Neuronal necrosis after middle cerebral artery occlusion in Wistar rats progresses at different time intervals in the caudoputamen and the cortex. Stroke 26:636, 1995.
2. Tagaya M, Liu K-F, Copeland B, et al: DNA scission after focal brain ischemia. Temporal differences in two species. Stroke 28:1245, 1997.
3. Zülch K-J: The Cerebral Infarct: Pathology, Pathogenesis, and Computed Tomography. Springer-Verlag, Berlin, 1:74, 1985.
4. Baron JC, von Kummer R, del Zoppo GJ: Treatment of acute ischemic stroke: Challenging the concept of a rigid and universal time window. Stroke 26:2219, 1995.
5. von Kummer R, Meyding-Lamade U, Forsting M, et al: Sensitivity and prognostic value of early CT in occlusion of the middle cerebral artery trunk. Am J Neuronadiol 15:9, 1994.
6. Warach S, Gaa J, Siewert B, et al: Acute human stroke studied by whole brain echo planar diffusion-weighted magnetic resonance imaging. Ann Neurol 37:231, 1995.
7. Astrup J, Siesjö BK, Symon L: Thresholds in cerebral ischemia: The ischemic penumbra. Stroke 12:723, 1981.
8. Baron JC: Perfusion thresholds in human cerebral ischemia: Historical perspective and therapeutic implications. Cerebrovasc Dis 11:2, 2001.
9. Solis OJ, Roberson GR, Taveras JM, et al: Cerebral angiography in acute cerebral infarction. Revist Interam Radiol 2:19, 1977.
10. Fieschi C, Argentino C, Lenzi GL, et al: Clinical and instrumental evaluation of patients with ischemic stroke within the first six hours. J Neurol Sci 91:311, 1989.
11. The National Institutes of Neurological Disorders and Stroke rt-PA Stroke Study Group: Tissue plasminogen activator for acute ischemic stroke. N Engl J Med 333:1581, 1995.
12. del Zoppo GJ, Higashida RT, Furlan AJ, et al: PROACT: A phase II randomized trial of recombinant pro-urokinase by direct arterial delivery in acute middle cerebral artery stroke. Stroke 29:4, 1998.
13. Caplan LR: Are terms such as completed stroke or RIND of continued usefulness? Stroke 14:431, 1983.
14. Albers GM, Caplan LR, Easton JD, et al: Transient ischemic attack: Proposal for a new definition. N Engl J Med 347:1713, 2002.
15. Wityk RJ, Pessin MS, Kaplan RF, et al: Serial assessment of acute stroke using the NIH Stroke Scale. Stroke 25:362, 1994.
16. Okada Y, Copeland BR, Mori E, et al: P-selectin and intercellular adhesion molecule-1 expression after focal brain ischemia and reperfusion. Stroke 25:202, 1994.
17. Okada Y, Copeland BR, Fitridge R, et al: Fibrin contributes to microvascular obstructions and parenchymal changes during early focal cerebral ischemia and reperfusion. Stroke 25:1847, 1994.
18. Marshall J: The natural history of transient ischemic cerebrovascular attacks. Quarterly J Med 33:309, 1964.
19. Wolf PA, Kannel WB, McGee DL, et al: Duration of atrial fibrillation and imminence of stroke: The Framingham Study. Stroke 14:664, 1983.
20. Whisnant JP, Matsumoto N, Elveback LR: Transient cerebral ischemic attacks in a community, Rochester, Minnesota, 1955 through 1969. Mayo Clin Proc 48:194, 1973.
21. UK-TIA Study Group: United Kingdom Transient Ischemic Attack (UK-TIA) Aspirin Trial: Interim results. Br Med J 296:316, 1988.
22. Schmidt EV, Smirnov VE, Ryabova VS: Results of the seven-year prospective study of stroke patients. Stroke 19:942, 1988.
23. Shaw C-M, Alvord EC, Jr, Berry RG: Swelling of the brain following ischemic infarction with arterial occlusion. Arch Neurol 1:161, 1959.
24. Denny-Brown D: Recurrent cerebrovascular episodes. Arch Neurol 2:194, 1960.
25. Russell RWR: Atheromatous retinal embolism. Lancet 2:1354, 1963.
26. Hollenhorst RW: Vascular status of patients who have cholesterol emboli in the retina. Am J Ophthalmol 77:1159, 1966.
27. Barnett HJM: The pathophysiology of transient cerebral ischemic attacks: Therapy with platelet antiaggregants. Med Clin North Am 63:649, 1979.
28. Marshall J: The Management of Cerebrovascular Diseases. Blackwell Scientific Publications, Oxford, UK, 1976, p 57.
29. Irino T, Taneda M, Minami T: Angiographic manifestations in postrecanalized cerebral infarction. Neurology 27:471, 1977.
30. Dougherty JH, Levy DE, Weksler BB: Platelet activation in acute cerebral ischemia: Serial measurements of platelet function in cerebrovascular disease. Lancet 3:821, 1977.
31. Mettinger KL, Nyman D, Kjellin K-G, et al: Factor VIII related antigen, anti-thrombin III, spontaneous platelet aggregation and plasminogen activator in ischemic cerebrovascular disease: A study of stroke before 55. J Neurol Sci 41:31, 1979.
32. de Boer AC, Turpie AG, Butt RW, et al: Plasma beta thromboglobulin and serum fragment E in acute partial stroke. Br J Haematol 50: 327, 1982.
33. Cella G, Zahavi J, de Haas HA, et al: β-Thromboglobulin, platelet production time, and platelet function in vascular disease. Br J Haematol 43:127, 1979.
34. Feinberg WM, Bruck DC, Ring ME, et al: Hemostatic markers in acute stroke. Stroke 20:592, 1989.
35. van Kooten F, Ciabattoni G, Patrono C, et al: Evidence for episodic platelet activation in acute ischemic stroke. Stroke 25:278, 1994.
36. Feinberg WM, Pearce LA, Hart RG, et al: Markers of thrombin and platelet activity in patients with atrial fibrillation: Correlation with stroke among 1531 participants in the stroke prevention in atrial fibrillation III study. Stroke 30:2547, 1999.
37. Fisher M, Zipser R: Increased excretion of immunoreactive thromboxane B2 in cerebral ischemia. Stroke 16:10, 1985.
38. van Kooten F, Ciabattoni G, Koudstaal PJ, et al: Increased platelet activation in the chronic phase after cerebral ischemia and intracerebral hemorrhage. Stroke 30:546, 1999.
39. Iwamoto T, Kubo H, Takasaki M: Platelet activation in the cerebral circulation in different subtypes of ischemic stroke and Binswanger's disease. Stroke 26:52, 1995.
40. Shah AB, Beamer N, Coull BM: Enhanced in vivo platelet activation in subtypes of ischemic stroke. Stroke 16:643, 1985.
41. Booth WJ, Berndt MC, Castaldi PA: An altered platelet granule glycoprotein in patients with essential thrombocythemia. J Clin Invest 73:291, 1984.
42. del Zoppo GJ, Copeland BR, Harker LA, et al: Experimental acute thrombotic stroke in baboons. Stroke 17:1254, 1986.
43. Abumiya T, Fitridge R, Mazur C, et al: Integrin $\alpha_{IIb}\beta_3$ inhibitor preserves microvascular patency in experimental acute focal cerebral ischemia. Stroke 31:1402, 2000.
44. del Zoppo GJ, Schmid-Schönbein GW, Mori E, et al: Polymorphonuclear leukocytes occlude capillaries following middle cerebral artery occlusion and reperfusion in baboons. Stroke 22:1276, 1991.
45. Garcia JH, Liu KF, Yoshida Y, et al: Influx of leukocytes and platelets in an evolving brain infarct (Wistar rat). Am J Pathol 144:188, 1994.
46. Choudhri TF, Hoh BL, Zerwes HG, et al: Reduced microvascular thrombosis and improved outcome in acute murine stroke by inhibiting GP IIb/IIIa receptor-mediated platelet aggregation. J Clin Invest 102:1301, 1998.
47. Fisher CM, Adams RD: Observations on brain embolism with special reference to the mechanism of hemorrhagic infarction. J Neuropathol Exp Neurol 10:92, 1951.
48. Mori E, Tabuchi M, Yoshida T, et al: Intracarotid urokinase with thromboembolic occlusion of the middle cerebral artery. Stroke 19:802, 1988.
49. del Zoppo GJ, Ferbert A, Otis S, et al: Local intra-arterial fibrinolytic therapy in acute carotid territory stroke: A pilot study. Stroke 19: 307, 1988.
50. Mori E, Yoneda Y, Tabuchi M, et al: Intravenous recombinant tissue plasminogen activator in acute carotid artery territory stroke. Neurology 42:976, 1992.
51. Fisher CM, Adams RD: Observations on brain embolism with special reference to hemorrhage infarction. In Furlan AJ (ed): The Heart

and Stroke: Exploring Mutual Cerebrovascular and Cardiovascular Issues. New York, Springer-Verlag, 1987, p 17.

52. Ogata J, Yutani C, Imakita M, et al: Hemorrhagic infarct of the brain without a reopening of the occluded arteries in cardioembolic stroke. Stroke 20:876, 1989.
53. Hamann GF, Okada Y, del Zoppo GJ: Hemorrhagic transformation and microvascular integrity during focal cerebral ischemia/reperfusion. J Cereb Blood Flow Metab 16:1373, 1996.
54. Fisher M, Adams RD: Observations on brain embolism with special reference to the mechanism of hemorrhagic infarction. Neuropathol Exp Neurol 10:92, 1951.
55. Jörgensen L, Torvik A: Ischaemic cerebrovascular diseases in an autopsy series. Part 2. Prevalence, location, pathogenesis, and clinical course of cerebral infarcts. J Neurol Sci 9:285, 1969.
56. Kwa VI, Franke CL, Verbeeten B, Jr, et al: Silent intracerebral microhemorrhages in patients with ischemic stroke. Amsterdam Vascular Medicine Group. Ann Neurol 44:372, 1998.
57. Yamaguchi T, Minematsu K, Choki J, et al: Clinical and neuroradiological analysis of thrombotic and embolic cerebral infarction. Jpn Circ J 48:50, 1984.
58. Cerebral Embolism Study Group: Immediate anticoagulation of embolic stroke: Brain hemorrhage and management options. Stroke 15:779, 1984.
59. Babikian VL, Kase CS, Pessin MS, et al: Intracerebral hemorrhage in stroke patients anticoagulated with heparin. Stroke 29:1500, 1989.
60. Mohr JP, Caplan LR, Melski JW, et al: The Harvard Cooperative Stroke Registry: A prospective registry. Neurology 28:754, 1978.
61. Bogousslavsky J, Van Melle G, Regli F: The Lausanne Stroke Registry: Analysis of 1,000 consecutive patients with first stroke. Stroke 19:1083, 1988.
62. Foulkes MA, Wolf PA, Price TR, et al: The stroke data bank: Design, methods, and baseline characteristics. Stroke 19:547, 1988.
63. International Stroke Trial Collaborative Group: The International Stroke Trial (IST): A randomised trial of aspirin, subcutaneous heparin, both, or neither among 19,435 patients with acute ischaemic stroke. Lancet 349:1569, 1997.
64. Chen ZM, Sandercock P, Pan HC, et al: Indications for early aspirin use in acute ischemic stroke: A combined analysis of 40,000 randomized patients from the Chinese acute stroke trial and the international stroke trial. On behalf of the CAST and IST collaborative groups. Stroke 31:1240, 2000.
65. Hacke W, Kaste M, Fieschi C, et al: Intravenous thrombolysis with recombinant tissue plasminogen activator for acute hemispheric stroke. The European Cooperative Acute Stroke Study (ECASS). JAMA 274:1017, 1995.
66. del Zoppo GJ: Acute stroke—On the threshold of a therapy? N Engl J Med 333:1632, 1995.
67. Albers GW, Amarenco P, Easton JD, et al: Antithrombotic and thrombolytic therapy for ischemic stroke. Chest 119:300S, 2001.
68. Levine MN, Raskob G, Landefeld S, et al: Hemorrhagic complications of anticoagulant treatment. Chest 119:108S, 2001.
69. CAST (Chinese Acute Stroke Trial) Collaborative Group: CAST: A randomised placebo-controlled trial of early aspirin use in 20,000 patients with acute ischaemic stroke. Lancet 349:1641, 1997.
70. Diener H, Cunha L, Forbes C, et al: European Stroke Prevention Study 2. Dipyridamole and acetylsalicylic acid in the secondary prevention of stroke. J Neurol Sci 143:1, 1996.
71. The Abciximab in Ischemic Stroke Investigators: Abciximab in acute ischemic stroke: A randomized, double-blind, placebo-controlled, dose-escalation study. Stroke 31:601, 2000.
72. Barnett HJ: Antithrombotic therapy in cerebral vascular disease; antispasmodics and fibrinolysis. In Barnett HJM, Mohr JP, Stein BM, Yatsu EM (eds): Stroke: Pathophysiology, Diagnosis, and Management. New York, Churchill-Livingstone, 1986, p 989.
73. Sherman DG, Dyken ML, Fisher M, et al: Antithrombotic therapy for cerebrovascular disorders. Chest 95:140S, 1989.
74. Albers GW, Dalen JE, Laupacis A, et al: Antithrombotic therapy in atrial fibrillation. Chest 119:194S, 2001.
75. Sackett DL: Rules of evidence and clinical recommendations on the use of antithrombotic agents. Chest 89:2S, 1989.
76. Russell RW: Observations on the retinal blood vessels in monocular blindness. Lancet 2:1422, 1961.
77. Fields WS, Lemak NA, Frankowski RF, et al: Controlled trial of aspirin in cerebral ischemia. Stroke 8:301, 1977.
78. The Canadian Cooperative Study Group: A randomized trial of aspirin and sulfinpyrazone in threatened stroke. N Engl J Med 299:53, 1978.
79. Bousser MG, Eschwege E, Haguenau M, et al: "AICLA" controlled trial of aspirin and dipyridamole in the secondary prevention of athero-thrombotic cerebral ischemia. Stroke 14:5, 1983.
80. The SALT Collaborative Group: Swedish Aspirin Low-Dose Trial (SALT) of 75 mg aspirin as secondary prophylaxis after cerebrovascular ischemic events. Lancet 338:1345, 1991.
81. Harker LA: Antiplatelet drugs in the management of patients with thrombotic disorders. Semin Thromb Hemost 12:134, 1986.
82. Fitzgerald GA: Dipyridamole. N Engl J Med 316:1247, 1987.
83. Fitzgerald GA: Dipyridamole. N Engl J Med 317:1734, 1987.
84. Harker LA, Slichter SJ: Arterial and venous thromboembolism: Kinetic characterization and evaluation of therapy. Thromb Diath Haemorrh 31:188, 1974.
85. Acheson J, Danta G, Hutchinson EC: Controlled trial of dipyridamole in cerebral vascular disease. Br Med J 1:614, 1969.
86. European Stroke Prevention Study Group: The European Stroke Prevention Study (ESPS). Principal end-points. Lancet 2:1351, 1987.
87. American-Canadian Cooperative Study Group: Persantine aspirin trial in cerebral ischemia. Part II. Endpoint results. Stroke 16:406, 1985.
88. Matias-Guiu J, Davalos A, Pico M, et al: Low-dose acetylsalicylic acid (ASA) plus dipyridamole versus dipyridamole alone in the prevention of stroke in patients with reversible ischemic attacks. Acta Neurol Scand 76:413, 1987.
89. Hass WK, Easton JD, Adams HP, Jr, et al: A randomized trial comparing ticlopidine hydrochloride with aspirin for prevention of stroke in high-risk patients. Ticlopidine Aspirin Stroke Study Group. N Engl J Med 321:501, 1989.
90. Roden S, Low-Beer T, Carmalt M, et al: Transient cerebral ischemic attacks: Management and prognosis. Postgrad Med J 57:275, 1981.
91. Candelise L, Landi G, Perrone P, et al: A randomized trial of aspirin and sulfinpyrazone in patients with TIA. Stroke 13:175, 1982.
92. ESPS-2 Working Group: Second European Stroke Prevention Study. J Neurol 239:299, 1992.
93. Campbell MH: Basilar artery syndrome. Can Med Assoc J 69:314, 1953.
94. Millikan CH, Siekert RG, Shick RM: Studies in cerebrovascular disease: III. The use of anticoagulant drugs in the treatment of insufficiency or thrombosis within the basilar arterial system. Mayo Clin Proc 30:116, 1955.
95. Estol CJ, Pessin MS: Anticoagulation: Is there still a role in atherothrombotic stroke? Stroke 21:820, 1990.
96. Putnam SF, Adams HP, Jr: Usefulness of heparin in initial management of patients with recent transient ischemic attacks. Arch Neurol 42:960, 1985.
97. Biller J, Bruno A, Adams HP, Jr, et al: A randomized trial of aspirin and heparin in hospitalized patients with recent transient ischemic attacks: A pilot study. Stroke 20:441, 1989.
98. Jones S: Anticoagulant therapy in cerebrovascular disease: Review and meta-analysis. Stroke 19:1043, 1988.
99. Cerebral Embolism Study Group: Immediate anticoagulation of embolic stroke: A randomized trial. Stroke 14:668, 1983.
100. Albers GW: Antithrombotic agents in cerebral ischemia. Am J Cardiol 75:34B, 1995.
101. ESPRIT: Oral anticoagulation in patients after cerebral ischemia of arterial origin and risk of intracranial hemorrhage. Stroke 34:e45, 2003.
102. Baker RN, Broward JA, Fang HC, et al: Anticoagulant therapy in cerebral infarction. Neurology 12:823, 1962.
103. Siekert RG, Whisnant JP, Millikan CH: Surgical and anticoagulant therapy of occlusive cerebrovascular disease. Ann Intern Med 58:637, 1963.
104. Walker AM, Jick H: Predictors of bleeding during heparin therapy. JAMA 244:1209, 1980.
105. Millikan CH: Anticoagulant therapy in cerebrovascular disease. In Millikan CH, Siekert RG, Whisnant JP (eds): Cerebral Vascular Diseases. New York, Grune and Stratton, 1965, p 183.
106. Carter AB: Anticoagulant treatment in progressing stroke. Br Med J 2:70, 1961.
107. Marshall J, Shaw DA: Anticoagulant therapy in acute cerebrovascular accidents: A controlled trial. Lancet 1:995, 1960.

108. The Publications Committee for the Trial of ORG 10172 in Acute Stroke Treatment (TOAST) Investigators: Low molecular weight heparinoid, ORG 10172 (danaparoid), and outcome after acute ischemic stroke: A randomized controlled trial. JAMA 279:1265, 1998.
109. Adams HP, Jr, Bendixen BH, Leira E, et al: Antithrombotic treatment of ischemic stroke among patients with occlusion or severe stenosis of the internal carotid artery: A report of the Trial of Org 10172 in Acute Stroke Treatment (TOAST). Neurology 53:122, 1999.
110. Hassaballa H, Gorelick PB, West CP, et al: Ischemic stroke outcome: Racial differences in the trial of danaparoid in acute Stroke (TOAST). Neurology 57:691, 2001.
111. Gubitz G, Sandercock P, Counsell C: Antiplatelet therapy for acute ischaemic stroke. Cochrane Database of Systematic Reviews (computer file) CD000029 CD000029. 2000.
112. Gent M, Blakely JA, Easton JD, et al: The Canadian-American Ticlopidine Study (CATS) in thromboembolic stroke. Lancet 1:1215, 1989.
113. [No authors listed] High-dose acetylsalicylic acid after cerebral infarction: A Swedish Cooperative Study. Stroke 18:325, 1987.
114. Gent M, Blakeley JA, Hachinski V, et al: A secondary prevention, randomized trial of suloctidil in patients with a recent history of thromboembolic stroke. Stroke 16:416, 1985.
115. Fisher M, Sandler R, Weiner JM: Delayed cerebral ischemia following arteriography. Stroke 16:431, 1985.
116. Chen ZM, Xie JX, Peto R, et al: Chinese Acute Stroke Trial (CAST): Rationale, design and progress. Cerebrovasc Dis 6:23, 1996.
117. CAPRIE Steering Committee: A randomised, blinded, trial of clopidogrel versus aspirin in patients at risk of ischaemic events (CAPRIE). Lancet 348:1329, 1996.
118. Fisher CM: Anticoagulant therapy in cerebral thrombosis and cerebral embolism: A national cooperative study, interim report. Neurology 11:119, 1961.
119. Hill AB, Marshall J, Shaw DA: Cerebrovascular disease: Trial of long-term anticoagulant therapy. Br Med J 2:1003, 1962.
120. McDowell F, McDevitt E: Treatment of the completed stroke with long-term anticoagulant. Six and one-half years' experience. In Siekert RH, Whisnant JR (eds): Cerebral Vascular Diseases, Fourth Princeton Conference. New York, Grune and Stratton, 1965, p 185.
121. Enger E, Boyesen S: Long-term anticoagulant therapy in patients with cerebral infarction: A controlled clinical study. Acta Med Scand 179:1, 1965.
122. Baker RN: An evaluation of anticoagulant therapy in the treatment of cerebrovascular disease: Report of the Veterans Administration Cooperative Study of Atherosclerosis, Neurology Section. Neurology 11:132, 1961.
123. Cosmi B, Hirsh J: Low molecular weight heparins. Curr Opin Cardiol 9:612, 1994.
124. Hoppensteadt D, Walenga JM, Fareed J: Low molecular weight heparins: An objective overview. Drugs and Aging 2:406, 1992.
125. Kay R, Wong KA, Yu YL, et al: Low-molecular weight heparin in the treatment of acute ischemic stroke. N Engl J Med 333:1588, 1995.
126. Berge E, Abdelnoor M, Nakstad PH, et al: Low-molecular-weight heparin versus aspirin in patients with acute ischemic stroke and atrial fibrillation: A double-blind randomised study. Lancet 355:1205, 2000.
127. Diener HC, Ringelstein EB, von Kummer R, et al: Treatment of acute ischemic stroke with the low-molecular-weight heparin certoparin: Results of the TOPAS trial. Stroke 32:22, 2001.
128. Liu M, Counsell C, Sandercock P: Anticoagulants for preventing recurrence following ischaemic stroke or transient ischaemic attack. Cochrane Database of Systematic Reviews (2):CD000248 2000.
129. Gubitz G, Counsell C, Sandercock P, et al: Anticoagulants for acute ischaemic stroke. Cochrane Database of Systematic Reviews (2): CD000024, 2000.
130. Fletcher AP, Alkjaersig N, Lewis M, et al: A pilot study of urokinase therapy in cerebral infarction. Stroke 7:135, 1976.
131. del Zoppo GJ, Zeumer H, Harker L: Thrombolytic therapy in stroke: Possibilities and hazards. Stroke 17:595, 1986.
132. von Kummer R, Forsting M, Sartor K, Hacke W: Intravenous recombinant tissue plasminogen activator in acute stroke. In Hacke W, del Zoppo GJ, Hirschberg M (eds): Thrombolytic Therapy in Acute Ischemic Stroke. Heidelberg, Springer, 1991, p 161.
133. Yamaguchi T: Intravenous rt-PA in acute embolic stroke. In Hacke W, del Zoppo GJ, Hirschberg M (eds): Thrombolytic Therapy in Acute Ischemic Stroke. Heidelberg, Springer, 1991, p 168.
134. Kwiatkowski TG, Libman RB, Frankel M, et al: Effects of tissue plasminogen activator for acute ischemic stroke at one year. National Institute of Neurological Disorders and Stroke Recombinant Tissue Plasminogen Activator Stroke Study Group. N Engl J Med 340:1781, 1999.
135. von Kummer R, Allen KL, Holle R, et al: Acute stroke: Usefulness of early CT findings before thrombolytic therapy. Radiology 205:327, 1997.
136. Hacke W, Kaste M, Fieschi C, et al: Randomised double-blind placebo-controlled trial of thrombolytic therapy with intravenous alteplase in acute ischaemic stroke (ECASS II). The Lancet 352: 1245, 1998.
137. Hacke W, Bluhmki E, Steiner T, et al: Dichotomized efficacy end points and global end-point analysis applied to the ECASS intention-to-treat data set: Post hoc analysis of ECASS I. Stroke 29:2073, 1998.
138. Albers GW, Bates VE, Clark WM, et al: Intravenous tissue-type plasminogen activator for treatment of acute stroke: The Standard Treatment with alteplase to reverse stroke (STARS) study. JAMA 283:1145, 2000.
139. del Zoppo GJ, Poeck K, Pessin MS, et al: Recombinant tissue plasminogen activator in acute thrombotic and embolic stroke. Ann Neurol 32:78, 1992.
140. Levy DE, Brott TG, Haley EC, Jr, et al: Factors related to intracranial hematoma formation in patients receiving tissue-type plasminogen activator for acute ischemic stroke. Stroke 25:291, 1994.
141. Larrue V, von Kummer R, del Zoppo GJ, et al: Hemorrhagic transformation in acute ischemic stroke: Potential contributing factors in the European Cooperative Acute Stroke Study. Stroke 28:957, 1997.
142. Larrue V, von Kummer RR, Muller A, et al: Risk factors for severe hemorrhagic transformation in ischemic stroke patients treated with recombinant tissue plasminogen activator: A secondary analysis of the European-Australasian Acute Stroke Study (ECASS II). Stroke 32(2):438, 2001.
143. Dubey N, Bakshi R, Wasay M, et al: Early computed tomography hypodensity predicts hemorrhage after intravenous tissue plasminogen activator in acute ischemic stroke. J Neuroimaging 11:184, 2001.
144. Kalafut MA, Schriger DL, Saver JL, et al: Detection of early CT signs of >1/3 middle cerebral artery infarctions: Interrater reliability and sensitivity of CT interpretation by physicians involved in acute stroke care. Stroke 31:1667, 2000.
145. Hommel M, Boissel JP, Cornu C, et al: Termination of trial of streptokinase in severe acute ischemic stroke (Letter). MAST Study Group. Lancet 345:578, 1995.
146. Donnan GA, Davis SM, Chambers BR, et al: Trials of streptokinase in severe acute ischaemic stroke. Lancet 345:578, 1995.
147. Multicentre Acute Stroke Trial-Italy (MAST-I) Group: Randomised controlled trial of streptokinase, aspirin, and combination of both in treatment of acute ischaemic stroke. Lancet 346:1509, 1995.
148. Gruppo Italiano Per Lo Studio Della Streptochinasi Nell'Infarto Miocardico (GISSI): Effectiveness of intravenous thrombolytic treatment in acute myocardial infarction. Lancet 1:397, 1986.
149. Gruppo Italiano Per Lo Studio Della Streptochinasi Nell'Infarto Miocardico (GISSI): GISSI-2: A factorial randomized trial of alteplase versus streptokinase and heparin versus no heparin among 12,490 patients with acute myocardial infarction. Lancet 336:65, 1990.
150. Matsumoto K, Satoh K: Topical intraarterial urokinase infusion for acute stroke. In Hacke W, del Zoppo GJ, Hirschberg M (eds): Thrombolytic Therapy in Acute Ischemic Stroke. Heidelberg, Springer-Verlag, 1991, p 207.
151. Hacke W, Zeumer H, Ferbert A, et al: Intra-arterial thrombolytic therapy improves outcome in patients with acute vertebrobasilar occlusive disease. Stroke 19:1216, 1988.
152. Furlan A, Higashida R, Wechsler L, et al: Intra-arterial prourokinase for acute ischemic stroke. The PROACT II Study: A randomized controlled trial. JAMA 282:2003, 1999.
153. Bell WR, Jr: Defibrinogenating enzymes. Drugs 54 3:18, 2001.
154. The Ancrod Stroke Study Investigators: Ancrod for the treatment of acute ischemic brain infarction. Stroke 25:1755, 1994.

155. Sherman DG, Atkinson RP, Chippendale T, et al: Intravenous ancrod for treatment of acute ischemic stroke. The STAT study: A randomized controlled trial. Stroke Treatment with Ancrod Trial. JAMA 283:2395, 2000.
156. Orgogozo JM, Verstraete M, Kay R, et al: Outcomes of ancrod in acute ischemic stroke. Independent Data and Safety Monitoring Board for ESTAT. Steering Committee for ESTAT. European Stroke Treatment with Ancrod Trial. JAMA 284:1926, 2000.
157. Kwaan HC: Thromboembolic disorders of the eye. In Comerota AC (ed): Thrombolytic Therapy. Orlando, Grune and Stratton, 1988, p 153.
158. Freitag H-J, Zeumer H, Knospe V: Acute central retinal artery occlusion and the role of thrombolysis. In del Zoppo GJ, Mori E, Hacke W (eds): Thrombolytic Therapy in Acute Ischemic Stroke II. Heidelberg, Springer, 1993, p 103.
159. Schmidt D, Schumacher M, Wakhloo AK: Microcatheter urokinase infusion in central retinal artery occlusion. Am J Ophthalmol 113:429, 1992.
160. Northern American Symptomatic Carotid Endarterectomy Trial Collaborators: Beneficial effect of carotid endarterectomy in symptomatic patients with high-grade carotid stenosis. N Engl J Med 325:445, 1991.
161. European Carotid Surgery Trialists' Collaborative Group: MRC European Carotid Surgery Trial: Interim results for symptomatic patients with severe (70-99%) or with mild (0-29%) carotid stenosis. Lancet 337:1235, 1991.
162. Barnett HJ, Taylor DW, Eliasziw M, et al: Benefit of carotid endarterectomy in patients with symptomatic moderate or severe stenosis. North American Symptomatic Carotid Endarterectomy Trial Collaborators. N Engl J Med 339:1415, 1998.
163. Fields WS, Lemak NA, Frankowski RF, et al: Controlled trial of aspirin in cerebral ischemia. Part II. Surgical group. Stroke 9:309, 1978.
164. Boysen G, Sorensen PS, Juhler M, et al: Danish very low dose aspirin after carotid endarterectomy trial. Stroke 19:1211, 1988.
165. Kretschmer G, Pratschner T, Prager M, et al: Antiplatelet treatment prolongs survival after carotid bifurcation endarterectomy: Analysis of the clinical series followed by a controlled trial. Ann Surg 211:317, 1990.
166. Pratschner T, Kretschmeter G, Prager M, et al: Antiplatelet therapy following carotid bifurcation endarterectomy: Evaluation of a controlled clinical trial. Prognostic significance of histologic plaque examination on behalf of survival. Eur J Vasc Surg 4:285, 1990.
167. Cooperative Study: Long-term anticoagulant therapy after myocardial infarction. JAMA 193:929, 1965.
168. Harvald B, Hilden T, Lund E: Long-term anticoagulant therapy after myocardial infarction. Lancet 2:626, 1962.
169. Loeliger EA, Hensen A, Kroes F, et al: A double blind trial of long-term anticoagulant treatment after myocardial infarction. Acta Med Scand 182:549, 1967.
170. Breddin K, Loew D, Lechner K, et al: The German-Austrian Aspirin Trial: A comparison of acetylsalicylic acid, placebo, and phenprocoumon in secondary prevention of myocardial infarction. On behalf of the German-Austrian Study Group. Circulation 62:V63. 1980.
171. Report of the Sixty-Plus Reinfarction Study Research Group: A double-blind trial to assess long-term anticoagulant therapy in elderly patients after myocardial infarction. Lancet 2:989, 1980.
172. Smith P, Arnesen H, Holme I: The effect of warfarin on mortality and reinfarction after myocardial infarction. N Engl J Med 323:147, 1990.
173. Breddin K, Loew D, Lechner K, et al: Secondary prevention of myocardial infarction: A comparison of acetylsalicylic acid, placebo, and phenprocoumon. Haemostasis 9:325, 1980.
174. Medical Research Council: An assessment of long-term anticoagulant administration after cardiac infarction. Br Med J 2:837, 1964.
175. Veterans Administration Hospital Investigators: Anticoagulants in acute myocardial infarction. Results of a cooperative clinical trial. JAMA 225:724, 1973.
176. Medical Research Council: Assessment of short-term anticoagulant administration after cardiac infarction. Br Med J 8:335, 1969.
177. Drapkin RL, Gee TS, Dowling MD, et al: Prophylactic heparin therapy in acute promyelocytic leukemia. Cancer 41:2484, 1978.
178. Anand SS, Yusuf S: Oral anticoagulant therapy in patients with coronary artery disease: A meta-analysis. JAMA 282:2058, 1999.
179. Szekely P: Systemic embolism and anticoagulant prophylaxis in rheumatic heart disease. Br Med J 1:1209, 1964.
180. Levine HJ, Pauker SG, Salzman EW: Antithrombotic therapy in valvular heart disease. Chest 95 (suppl):98S, 1989.
181. Stein PD, Kantrowitz A: Antithrombotic therapy in mechanical and biological prosthetic heart valves and saphenous vein bypass grafts. Chest 95:107S, 1989.
182. Wolf PA, Abbott RD, Kannel WB: Atrial fibrillation: A major contributor to stroke in the elderly. The Framingham Study. Arch Intern Med 147:1561, 1987.
183. Sherman DG, Goldman L, Whiting RB, et al: Thromboembolism in patients with atrial fibrillation. Arch Neurol 41:708, 1984.
184. Stroke Prevention in Atrial Fibrillation Study Group Investigators: Preliminary report of the Stroke Prevention in Atrial Fibrillation Study. N Engl J Med 322:863, 1990.
185. Petersen P, Boysen G, Godtfredsen J, et al: Placebo-controlled randomized trial of warfarin and aspirin to prevention of thromboembolic complications in chronic atrial fibrillation. The Copenhagen AFASAK Study. Lancet 1:175, 1989.
186. EAFT European Atrial Fibrillation Trial Study Group: Secondary prevention in non-rheumatic atrial fibrillation after transient ischaemic attack or minor stroke. Lancet 342:1255, 1993.
187. Atrial Fibrillation Investigators: The efficacy of aspirin in patients with atrial fibrillation: Analysis of pooled data from three randomized trials. Arch Intern Med 157:1237, 1997.
188. Hart RG, Benavente O, McBride R, et al: Antithrombotic therapy to prevent stroke in patients with atrial fibrillation: A meta-analysis. Ann Intern Med 131:492, 1999.
189. Segal JB, McNamara RL, Miller MR, et al: Prevention of thromboembolism in atrial fibrillation: A meta-analysis of trials of anticoagulants and antiplatelet drugs. J Gen Intern Med 15:56, 2000.
190. Stroke Prevention in Atrial Fibrillation Investigators: Warfarin versus aspirin for prevention of thromboembolism in atrial fibrillation: Stroke Prevention in Atrial Fibrillation II Study. Lancet 343:687, 1994.
191. Stroke Prevention in Atrial Fibrillation Investigators: Adjusted-dose warfarin versus low-intensity, fixed-dose warfarin plus aspirin for high-risk patients with atrial fibrillation: Stroke prevention in atrial fibrillation III randomised clinical trial. Lancet 348:633, 1996.
192. Gullov AL, Koefoed BG, Petersen P, et al: Fixed mini-dose warfarin and aspirin alone and in combination versus adjusted-dose warfarin for stroke prevention in atrial fibrillation: Second Copenhagen Atrial Fibrillation, Aspirin, and Anticoagulation Study (the AFASAK-2 study). Arch Intern Med 158:1513, 1998.
193. Gullov AL, Koefoed BG, Petersen P: Bleeding during warfarin and aspirin therapy in patients with atrial fibrillation: The AFASAK-2 Study. Atrial Fibrillation Aspirin and Anti-coagulation. Arch Intern Med 159:1322, 1999.
194. Hart RG, Benavente O, McBride R, Pearce LA: Antithrombotic Therapy to Prevent Stroke in Patients with Atrial Fibrillation: A Meta-Analysis. Ann Intern Med 133: 492, 1999.
195. Petersen P, Grind M, Adler J, et al: Ximelagatran versus warfarin for stroke prevention in patients with nonvalvular atrial fibrillation. SPORTIF II: A dose-guiding, tolerability, and safety study. J Am Coll Cardiol 41:1445, 2003.
196. Halperin JL: Ximelagatran compared with warfarin for prevention of thromboembolism in patients with nonvalvular atrial fibrillation: Rationale, objectives, and design of a pair of clinical studies and baseline patient characteristics: SPORTIF III and V. Am Heart J 146:431, 2003.
197. Olsson SB: Executive Steering Committee on behalf of the SPORTIF III Investigators. Stroke prevention with the oral direct thrombin inhibitor ximelagatran compared with warfarin in patients with non-valvular atrial fibrillation: SPORTIF III: Randomised controlled trial. Lancet 362:1691, 2003.
198. Coulshed N, Epstein EJ, McKendrick CS, et al: Systemic embolism in mitral valve disease. Br Med J 32:26, 1970.
199. Daley R, Mattingly TW, Holt CI, et al: Systemic arterial embolism in rheumatic heart disease. Am Heart J 42:566, 1981.
200. Salem DN, Levine HJ, Pauker SG, et al: Antithrombotic therapy in valvular heart disease. Chest 114:590S, 1998.
201. Stein PD, Alpert JS, Bussey HI, et al: Antithrombotic therapy in patients with mechanical and biological prosthetic heart valves. Chest 119:220S, 2001.

202. Barnhorst DA, Oxman HA, Connolly DC, et al: Long-term follow-up of isolated replacement of the aortic or mitral valve with the Starr-Edwards prosthesis. Am J Cardiol 35:233, 1975.
203. Moggio RA, Hammond GL, Stansel HL, Jr, et al: Incidence of emboli with cloth-covered Starr-Edwards value without anticoagulation and with varying forms of anticoagulation. Analysis of 183 patients followed for 31/2 years. J Thorac Cardiovasc Surg 75: 299, 1978.
204. Akbarian M, Austen WG, Yurchak PM, et al: Thromboembolic complications of prosthetic cardiac valves. Circulation 37:826, 1986.
205. Saour JN, Sieck JO, Mamo LA, et al: Trial of different intensities of patients with prosthetic heart valves. N Engl J Med 322:428, 1990.
206. Loeliger EA: Therapeutic target values in oral anticoagulation: Justification of Dutch policy and a warning against the so-called moderate-intensity regimens. Ann Hematol 64:60, 1992.
207. Dale J, Myhre E, Storstein O, et al: Prevention of arterial thromboembolism with acetylsalicylic acid: A controlled clinical study in patients with aortic ball valves. Am Heart J 94:101, 1977.
208. Altman R, Boullon F, Rouvier J, et al: Aspirin and prophylaxis of thromboembolic complications in patients with substitute heart valves. J Thorac Cardiovasc Surg 72:127, 1976.
209. Sullivan JM, Harken DE, Gorlin R: Effect of dipyridamole on the incidence of arterial emboli after cardiac valve replacement. Circulation 39/40:I149, 1969.
210. Sullivan JM, Harken DE, Gorlin R: Pharmacologic control of thromboembolic complications of cardiac valve replacement. N Engl J Med 284:1391, 1971.
211. Hassouna A, Allam H, Awad A, et al: Standard versus low-level anticoagulation combined to low-dose dipyridamole after mitral valve replacement. Cardiovasc Surg 8:491, 2000.
212. Chesebro JH, Fuster V, Elveback LR, et al: Trial of combined warfarin plus dipyridamole or aspirin therapy in prosthetic heart valve replacement: Danger of aspirin compared with dipyridamole. Am J Cardiol 51:1537, 1983.
213. Pouleur H, Buyse M: Effects of dipyridamole in combination with anticoagulant therapy on survival and thromboembolic events in patients with prosthetic heart valves: A meta-analysis of the randomized trials. J Thorac Cardiovasc Surg 110:463, 1995.
214. Massel D, Little SH: Risks and benefits of adding anti-platelet therapy to warfarin among patients with prosthetic heart valves: A meta-anaylsis. J Am Coll Cardiol 37:569, 2001.
215. Ferraris VA, Klingman RR, Dunn L, et al: Home heparin therapy used in a pregnant patient with a mechanical heart valve prosthesis. Ann Thorac Surg 58:1168, 1994.
216. Thomas D, Boubrit K, Darbois Y, et al: Pregnancy in patients with heart valve prosthesis: Retrospective study apropos of 40 pregnancies (French). Ann Cardiol Angeiol (Paris) 43:313, 1994.
217. Reimold SC, Rutherford JD: Clinical practice: Valvular heart disease in pregnancy. N Engl J Med 349:52, 2003.
218. Williams JB, Karp RB, Kirklin JW, et al: Considerations in selection and management of patients undergoing valve replacement with glutaraldehyde-fixed porcine bioprostheses. Ann Thorac Surg 30:247, 1980.
219. Cohn LH, Allred EN, DiSesa VJ, et al: Early and late risk of aortic valve replacement: A 12-year concomitant comparison of the porcine bioprosthetic and tilting disc prosthetic aortic valves. J Thorac Cardiovasc Surg 88:695, 1984.
220. Oyer PE, Stinson EB, Griepp RB, et al: Valve replacement with the Starr-Edwards and Hancock prostheses: Comparative analysis of late morbidity and mortality. Ann Surg 186:301, 1977.
221. Ionescu MI, Smith DR, Hasan SS, et al: Clinical durability of the pericardial xenograft valve: Ten years experience with mitral replacement. Ann Thorac Surg 34:265, 1982.
222. Turpie AG, Gunstensen J, Hirsh J, et al: Randomized comparison of two intensities of oral anticoagulant therapy after tissue heart valve placement. Lancet 1:1242, 1988.
223. Nuñez L, Gil Aguado MG, Celemin D, et al: Aspirin or coumadin as the drug of choice for valve replacement with porcine bioprosthesis. Ann Thorac Surg 33:354, 1982.
224. Nuñez L, Gil Aguado MG, Larrea JL, et al: Prevention of thromboembolism using aspirin after mitral valve replacement with porcine bioprosthesis. Ann Thorac Surg 37:84, 1984.
225. Oczkowski WJ, Ginsberg JS, Shin A, et al: Venous thromboembolism in patients undergoing rehabilitation for stroke. Arch Phys Med Rehabil 73:712, 1992.
226. Sandset PM, Dahl T, Stiris M, et al: A double-blind and randomized placebo-controlled trial of low molecular weight heparin once daily to prevent deep-vein thrombosis in acute ischemic stroke. Semin Thromb Hemost 16:25, 1990.
227. Elias A, Milandre L, Lagrange G, et al: Prevention des thromboses veineuses profondes des membres inferieurs par une fraction d'heparine de tres bas poids moleculaire (CY 222) chez des patients porteurs d'une hemiplegie secondaire a un infarctus cerebral: Etude pilote randomisee (30 patients). Revue de Medecine Interne 11:95, 1990.
228. Prins MH, Gelsema R, Sing AK, et al: Prophylaxis of deep vein thrombosis with a low-molecular-weight heparin (Kabi 2165/Fragmin) in stroke patients. Haemostasis 19:245, 1989.
229. Turpie AG, Gent M, Cote R, et al: A low-molecular weight heparinoid compared with unfractionated heparin in the prevention of deep vein thrombosis in patients with acute ischemic stroke: A randomized, double-blind study. Ann Intern Med 117: 353, 1992.
230. Adams HP, Jr, Woolson RF, Biller J, et al: Studies of Org 10172 in patients with acute ischemic stroke. TOAST Study Group. Haemostasis 22:99, 1992.
231. Madden KP, Karanjia PN, Adams HP, Jr, et al: Accuracy of initial stroke subtype diagnosis in the TOAST study. Trial of ORG 10172 in Acute Stroke Treatment. Neurology 45:1975, 1995.
232. Davis PH, Clarke WR, Bendixen BH, et al: Silent cerebral infarction in patients enrolled in the TOAST study. Neurology 46:942, 1996.
233. The Boston Area Anticoagulation Trial/Atrial Fibrillation Investigators: The effect of low-dose warfarin on the risk of stroke in patients with non-rheumatic atrial fibrillation. N Engl J Med 323:1505, 1990.
234. Connolly SJ, Laupacis A, Gent M, et al: Canadian Atrial Fibrillation Anticoagulation (CAFA) Study. J Am Coll Cardiol 18: 349, 1991.

chapter 32

Carotid Artery Stenting

Giora Weisz
Gary S. Roubin
Jiri J. Vitek
Sriram S. Iyer

Carotid artery stenting is rapidly becoming the standard of care for treatment of atherosclerotic carotid disease (Fig. 32-1). In many respects, it represents one of the last arterial territories to be approached by vascular interventionalists. The necessary path through technical development and scientific discovery has been extremely difficult.

Similar to the skepticism faced by Dotter and Gruentzig in the peripheral arteries and Gruentzig and others in the coronaries, interventional endeavors in the carotid arteries were initially met with disbelief. In addition, the brain was rightly or wrongly viewed as a more vulnerable end organ for stenting than were the heart and certainly the lower extremities. Finally, carotid stenting did not fit easily under the purview of any of the existing medical specialties.

Cardiologists had the technical skills, equipment, and clinical expertise to accomplish the work safely, but no traditional experience in working cephalad to the aortic arch. Neuroradiologists lacked experience with large-vessel stenting, embolic protection, and clinical management, and vascular surgeons, for the most part, lacked the refined endovascular skills and the clinical imperative to find a less invasive alternative to carotid endarterectomy. In the end, the difficult task of establishing carotid stenting as a viable treatment option was left to a small cadre of cardiologists assisted by a number of neuroradiologists who accepted that other specialists might be able to provide techniques, insight, and solution to the challenges ahead. In this chapter, we will review the development and current "state of the art" in carotid stenting, including current technique and clinical trial data, that support the growth of the procedure.

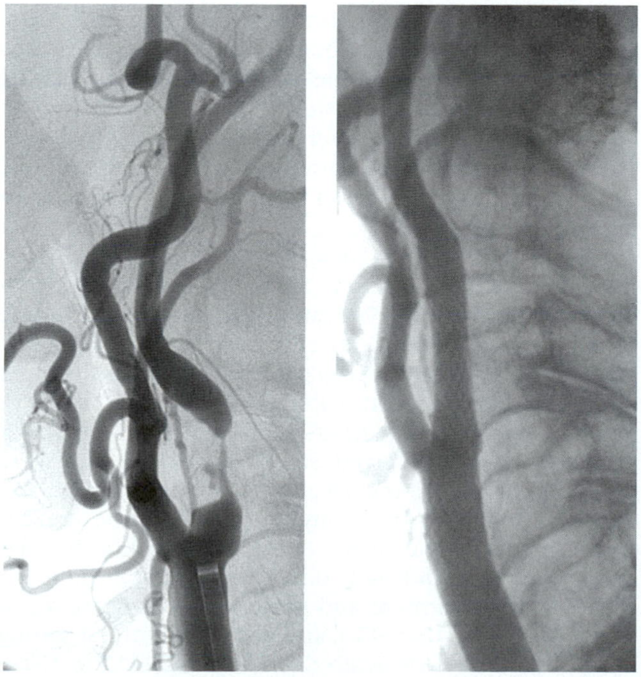

A B

FIGURE 32-1. A, An ideal lesion for carotid artery bifurcation stenting; **B,** after stent placement.

HISTORICAL PERSPECTIVE

Surgical treatment for carotid stenoses was introduced in the early 1950s. Prospective observational data suggested benefit for surgery over medical therapy, but large prospective randomized trials investigating the effect of carotid endarterectomy (CEA) on stroke reduction were not completed until the late 1980s and early 1990s. Studies such as the North American Symptomatic Carotid Endarterectomy Trial (NASCET),[1-5] the European Carotid Surgery Trial (ECST),[6] and the Asymptomatic Carotid Atherosclerosis Study (ACAS),[7] confirmed the short- and long-term superiority of surgery over medical management, in symptomatic and asymptomatic patients with significant carotid stenosis. CEA surgery is comprehensively discussed in Chapter 33.

The CEA studies excluded patients who were at high risk for this surgery. Thus excluded were patients with previous ipsilateral endarterectomy, intracranial stenosis that was more severe than the surgically accessible lesion, unstable angina pectoris, recent myocardial infarction, recent contralateral CEA, progressive neurologic dysfunction, recent surgical procedure, long-term anticoagulation therapy, and surgically inaccessible lesions.[2,7]

Cardiovascular complications of surgery, such as myocardial infarction and congestive heart failure, are well recognized, and a significant number of patients have been reported to have transient myocardial ischemia and occult infarction, associated with adverse cardiac events.[8] CEA has significant surgical complications, not always reported (as the case with the ESCT study), but should be acknowledged. In the NASCET, perioperative wound complications (9.3%) and cranial nerve damage (8.6%) emphasized the adverse events associated with an open surgical procedure.[4] Medical complications were common (8.1%), largely of cardiovascular origin (7.1%), including myocardial infarction (1.2%) and congestive heart failure (1.2%).[5]

The mission to develop safer, percutaneous solutions to arterial stenosis was pioneered by Dotter[9] and Gruentzig[10] in the 1960s and 1970s, and by 1980, interventional radiologists were cautiously approaching the brachiocephalic and carotid arteries. Mathias and colleagues first reported balloon angioplasty of the carotid bifurcation,[11] followed by case reports of successful carotid angioplasty preformed in the surgical suite.[12,13] In 1984, Vitek[14] reported angioplasty of the innominate artery with distal occlusion balloon protection of the common carotid artery. The progress with angioplasty of the supra-aortic vessel was slow—due to concerns of local injury and risk of distal embolization. Balloon angioplasty of the carotid artery was widely practiced, but only small series of patients were reported.[15] In 1986, Rabkin[16] reported the use of primitive nitinol stents in the carotid artery, and Theron[17] began pivotal work with distal balloon protection during carotid bifurcation angioplasty. In 1994, Roubin and his group at the University of Alabama began routine carotid stenting under rigorous institutional protocols.[18] Later, the use of distal protection devices was recognized as an integral part of carotid artery dilatation and stenting.[19-30] The high technical success rate noted in the early works and the progress made over the years have led to an exponential growth in the number of cases around the world.[31]

Initially, several authors reported early acceptable results with direct percutaneous carotid arterial puncture.[32] This approach, however, was associated with technical difficulties and potentially severe complications, including cervical hematomas, thrombosis, and significant patient discomfort. This approach was rapidly abandoned and the femoral approach became the standard of care, with brachial arterial access becoming a rare option for special cases.[33]

Early Results of Balloon Angioplasty for Carotid Artery Stenosis

Several early studies with balloon angioplasty alone were published. Most included small numbers of patients from single institutions, and only four reports included more than 40 patients.[34-37] Kachel and colleagues summarized the case reports of carotid angioplasty in the literature through 1995. Of 523 cases reported, 503 (96.2%) were technically successful. No deaths occurred. Major strokes were reported in 2.1%, and minor complications were uncommon (6.3%).[36]

Gil-Peralta reported his experience in 85 procedures of balloon angioplasty in a 4-year period.[35] All patients were symptomatic with greater than 70% stenosis of the internal carotid artery. Periprocedural transient cardiovascular effects were frequent: hypotension (54.1%), bradycardia (67.1%), asystole (25.9%), and syncope (16.5%). Transient ischemic attack occurred in 3 of 82 patients (3.7%), and disabling stroke occurred in 4 (4.9%), and no mortality. After a mean follow-up period of 18.7 months, four patients died, one died of fatal stroke. The overall probability of surviving any stroke or death was 86.7%. Restenosis (>70%) was seen in six cases (7.4%).

Kachel[36] reported balloon angioplasty in 220 symptomatic patients with 245 stenosed or occluded supra-aortic arteries; among these were 74 carotid stenoses. Balloon angioplasty was successful in 69 patients. He used temporary balloon occlusion to avoid cerebral embolization. There was no mortality, and only one patient had a major stroke and another had a transient ischemic attack.

Theron and colleagues published their extensive experience of carotid angioplasty in 259 patients.[34] In 69 patients, stents were placed when images obtained immediately after angioplasty showed signs of dissection or insufficient arterial opening. No procedure-related complications occurred in the 71 patients who had nonatherosclerotic stenotic lesions (most of them with restenosis after endarterectomy). Among the 38 patients with atherosclerotic lesions that underwent balloon angioplasty without cerebral protection, embolic complication occurred in 8% during the procedure. Their first generation distal protection balloon (triple coaxial catheter) was used in 136 of the cases. None of these patients had any embolic complication during the balloon angioplasty, but two had strokes during or after the stent was deployed without the distal protection; this was the first series that underscored the importance of distal protection. Unfortunately, this primitive distal protection balloon could be used only for angioplasty, but not with stent placement (given the primitive stent delivery systems at the time). Although these operators thought that the main embolic burden came from the angioplasty, this early body of experience indicated the risk of emboli during the stenting and post-dilatation phases. The addition of stents to balloon dilatation, however, did ensure a safer and more reliable result. These results were comparable with CEA reports, but one could argue that publication bias influenced the success rates in these reports.

The multicenter Carotid and Vertebral Artery Transluminal Angioplasty Study (CAVATAS-I)[38] was conducted between 1992 and 1997, in an era before suitable carotid stent devices were widely available. Essentially, balloon angioplasty was compared in a randomized fashion with CEA. In this UK-based study of 504 patients, only 55 patients (26%) of the endovascular treatment group received stents. Initially, stents were used only as a bail-out treatment, with increased use toward the end of the study; distal protection devices were not used. The major event rates within 30 days after treatment did not differ significantly between endovascular treatment and surgery: disabling stroke or death (6.4% versus 5.9%), and any major stroke lasting more than 7 days or death (10.0% versus 9.9%). These relatively high rates of neurologic complication can be related to most patients not receiving stents and the execution of the treatment without distal embolic protection.

This study demonstrated, however, that endovascular techniques were superior to surgery in avoiding risks related to the incision in the neck and the use of general anesthesia. Cranial neuropathy was reported in 8.7% of the surgical patients, but in none after endovascular treatment ($P < .0001$). Major groin or neck hematomata occurred less often after endovascular treatment than after surgery (1.2% versus 6.7%, $P < .0015$).

The introduction by Roubin, Iyer, and Vitek[18,39-42] of elective carotid stenting as the technique of choice for carotid intervention and the rapid adoption of this technique by the cardiology community heralded the modern era for the treatment of carotid bifurcation disease.

CAROTID STENTING

Indications and Contraindications

The indications for intervention with carotid stenting are similar to those of carotid surgery with respect to symptomatic status and severity of carotid stenosis. The AHA/SVS guidelines for CEA[43] logically should apply to stenting and, accordingly, individual operator experience and documented 30-day outcomes must be known before an informed decision on a treatment option can be made.

This approach to patient management is based on documented, prospective outcome assessments from many experienced operators and centers and will be discussed later in this chapter. Many operators are now providing credible outcome data to support such an approach. In intracenter analysis, if prospective, independent neurologic audit shows, for example, that in a group of surgically eligible symptomatic or asymptomatic patients, the 30-day death rate is less than 1% and total 30-day stroke events are less than 3%, then stenting should be an attractive therapeutic option.

There are notable exceptions to these therapeutic principles. Subsets of patients are emerging as better candidates for stenting and other patients as better candidates for CEA. It is, therefore, now becoming important for the medical community to understand the relative indications and contraindications (Table 32-1). Patients who have comorbid medical conditions that increase their risk from an open surgical approach or the use of general anesthesia are one important group that should be primary candidates for stenting. Based on the results of the recently presented SAPPHIRE Trial,[44] these conditions include advanced age, cardiac and pulmonary disease, and a variety of other medical disabilities.

Any condition that increases the risk of operative exposure also represents a clear indication for stenting. These conditions include prior ipsilateral endarterectomy, prior neck dissection or radiation, high lesions that need extensive cephalad dissection, and low lesions that require thoracic exposure. Patients with contralateral occlusion also should be included in this group, given their inclusion in the SAPPHIRE Trial and the documented 14% and 30-day mortality and stroke rates in this subset of patients in the NASCET Study. Even the most facile surgeon takes a few minutes to shunt lesions during CEA. For patients with isolated hemispheres, neurologic consequences are not unexpected. The use of embolic protection filters during stenting facilitates constant perfusion of the brain. Balloon inflations used during stenting are necessary only for 10 seconds to 20 seconds. Another advantage of stenting is that the anatomical status (anatomy, collaterals, intact circle of Willis, intracranial lesions, and flow characteristics) is usually well defined during or before the stenting procedure. For experienced operators, the risk of angiography is minimal and, as stent use increases, so too will the angiographic skills and experience in the interventional community increase.

Although not emphasized in the carotid surgery trials, the incidence of cranial nerve damage, wound hematoma, and infection were significant and need to be considered before referring patients for neck surgery. Additionally, the complications from the general anesthesia that is still being used in 90% of endarterectomies done in the United States need to be carefully considered. In the SAPPHIRE Trial,[29] although the risk of stroke or death favored stenting in all categories, the initial overall number of events did not yield statistically significant differences between groups. Perioperative procedural myocardial infarction, however, was twice as common for surgery patients compared with stented patients, and overall complications significantly favored stenting. One-year stroke, myocardial infarction, and all-cause mortality showed incremental benefit for stenting over time.

Carotid stenting also has a number of notable relative contraindications. The experience with stenting over the last decade has defined circumstances that increase the risk of the procedure. First, patients who are intolerant of, or are allergic to, a combination of antiplatelet agents, may be more safely managed with endarterectomy.

TABLE 32-1 CONTRAINDICATIONS FOR STENTING

Absolute Contraindications

Medical

Hemodynamic instability

Anatomic

Inability to selectively access the common carotid artery
Occluded common, or internal, carotid artery

Relative Contraindications

Medical

Intolerance/allergy to aspirin and thienopyridines
Need for antiplatelet therapy cessation in 3-4 weeks following stenting
Advanced age (>80 years)
Renal failure
Recent (<14 days) cerebral infarction

Anatomic

Inability to get femoral artery access
Aortic arch calcification and atherosclerosis
Severe common carotid tortuosity
Severe internal carotid tortuosity distal to the stenosis
String sign
Acute take-off of the internal carotid artery
Heavy calcification of the carotid artery bifurcation
Inability to deploy embolic protection device

Experience has shown that a combination of aspirin and clopidogrel or aspirin and ticlopidine is mandatory adjunctive therapy to prevent platelet activation and embolization during and for at least 3 to 4 weeks after stenting. The details of how these agents should be administered will be discussed later in this chapter.

Similarly, if the patient has a compelling reason to undergo a major surgical procedure within 3 to 4 weeks that will require the cessation of antiplatelet therapy, endarterectomy may be a better option. The most common clinical situation in which this is encountered is in the patient with critical carotid disease and critical coronary disease requiring coronary artery bypass graft (CABG). Given the risks of endarterectomy in this setting or the risks of a combined procedure (CABG and CEA), careful consideration is required. For the vast majority of patients, stenting followed by CABG after cessation of antiplatelet therapy 3 to 4 weeks later is the option of choice. There are very few coronary patients who cannot be safely managed for 3 to 4 weeks on aggressive antiplatelet therapy and anti-ischemic cardiac medical therapy. In rare instances, (e.g., critical left main disease in combination with critical bilateral carotid disease), patients must proceed to CABG soon after stenting. Carotid stenting may still be the initial procedure of choice in such patients. Stenting needs to be done with optimal modulation of blood pressure and heart rate support, and, possibly, the use of intra-aortic balloon pump support. Many cardiothoracic surgeons are able to operate successfully in the presence of aggressive antiplatelet therapy, but the increased use of blood and blood products is usually required. Of note, cessation of antiplatelet therapy soon after stenting and in combination with cardiac surgery has been associated with stent thrombosis.

Age and gender are important considerations when selecting a patient for carotid revascularization. For less experienced operators, advancing age appears to be an important predictor of an adverse outcome. In the NINDS-NIH-sponsored CREST randomized trial (lead in/credentialing registry), an increasing proportion of patients had stroke or death with increasing age. In patients younger than 60 years, it was 1.1%; 61 to 69 years, 0.6%; 70 to 79 years, 4.7%; and 80 years or greater, 11.9% ($P = .0005$). These outcomes differ dramatically from those reported by very experienced operators. Roubin and colleagues have shown that the use of embolic protection devices dramatically reduced the periprocedural risk in octogenarians.[45] Others have also reported excellent outcomes in the elderly.[46] Patient selection based on anatomy and general comorbid status probably plays an important role in ensuring safe results in octogenarians. Elderly patients tend to have greater degrees of carotid tortuosity, calcification, and aortic arch atherosclerosis. In addition, elderly patients have less "cerebral reserve" with a higher incidence of intra-cranial disease, microangiopathy, prior symptomatic and asymptomatic strokes, and general dementia. Of note, advanced age is also an established risk for CEA.[47] A meta-analysis of more than 30 studies revealed that CEA surgery in patients older than 75 years was associated with a 36% increased risk of perioperative stroke/death.[47]

Alternatively, female gender appears to favor stenting over endarterectomy. In the trials of CEA versus medical management, female gender was a predictor of an adverse surgical outcome.[7,48] In the authors' experience in more than 1400 procedures, gender has no effect on short- or long-term outcomes.[30,42]

Chronic renal failure is another relative contraindication to carotid stenting, although this condition has also been shown to increase the risk of endarterectomy. Experienced operators, stenting patients with good anatomy, can complete the procedure with 50 ml to 75 ml of contrast. If the patient is well hydrated and managed with mitigating adjunctive therapy, acceleration of renal failure is usually not a concern. If, however, the patient has complex anatomy that may prolong the procedure and necessitate the use of large volumes of contrast, endarterectomy may be a safer option.

An important relative contraindication is the presence of an extremely high-grade stenosis and a recent (<14 day) cerebral infarction. The more critical the stenosis, particularly in a hypertensive patient, the larger the size of the cerebral infarction and the closer the time to the index event, the greater is the risk of hemorrhagic conversion after relieving the stenosis. Of course, this may also apply to CEA, but the risk is increased in the presence of the large doses of antiplatelet agents and the anticoagulation necessary for the stenting procedure. In addition, lesions that have recently embolized are typically more likely to shower debris from the unstable plaque and could potentially overwhelm embolic protection systems. Medical therapy for a period of 10 to 14 days allows the plaque and cerebral tissue to "heal" before intervention. The risk of cerebral hemorrhage has been mitigated in recent years by the use of minimal doses of antithrombin therapy during the procedure (i.e., heparin 4000 IU) (activated clotting time [ACT] 200 to 300 seconds) or use of newer antithrombin agents (e.g., bivalirudin). This drug has demonstrated lower hemorrhagic complications in other types of interventions. Critical management of hypertension at the time of opening the stenosis is also of importance in avoiding this devastating complication. It is noteworthy that in elective carotid stenting using the protocol described in this chapter, the risk of cerebral hemorrhage is less than 3 in 1000.

Anatomic Considerations

There are important relative anatomic contraindications that increase the risk of stenting and make alternative medical or surgical therapies better options. The first is difficult vascular access. Stenting can be done from a brachial approach but requires advanced skills.[33] The procedure is generally much more straightforward with femoral access, and, if this is not possible because of severe occlusive vascular disease, other options should be explored. Similarly, severe, diffuse disease, calcification, and tortuosity of the proximal great vessels and aortic arch make access to the carotid bifurcation difficult and dangerous (Figs. 32-2 and 32-3). Discrete lesions at the origin of the great vessels can be treated safely, and this is usually best done in a separate index procedure before approaching the bifurcation lesion.

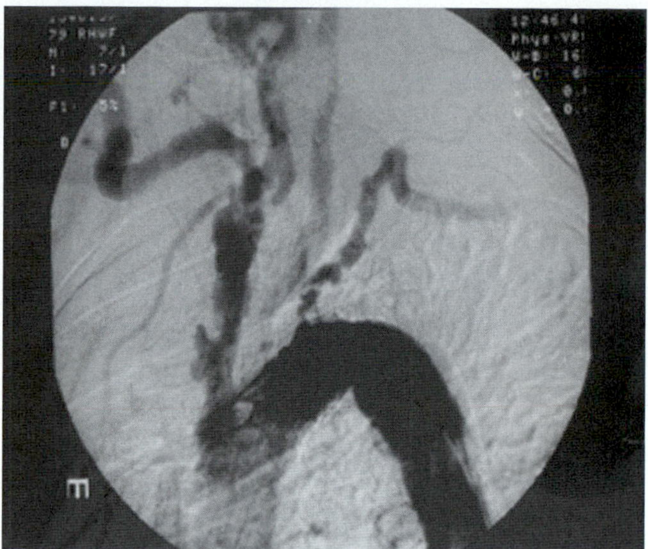

FIGURE 32-2. Atheromatous aortic arch and proximal great vessels are contraindications for carotid stenting due to the high risk of emboli.

Severe tortuosity and or angulation in the region of the carotid bifurcation is another high-risk anatomic finding for stenting (Fig. 32-4). It cannot be overemphasized that given the limitations of current technology, tortuosity represents an important contraindication to stenting.

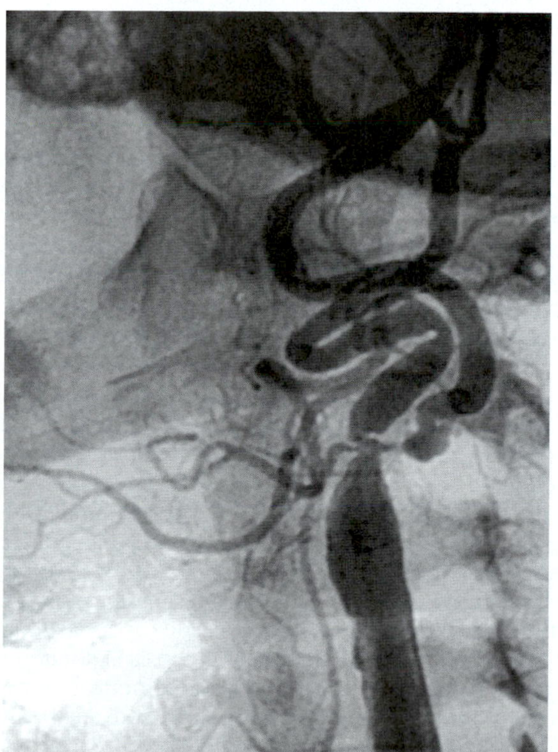

FIGURE 32-3. This carotid artery with a significant lesion in the origin of the internal carotid artery manifests five adverse morphologic features for carotid artery stenting (1) significant extension of the lesion into the common carotid artery; (2) 90-degree take-off of the internal carotid artery (ICA); (3) severe tortuosity of the ICA; (4) severe concentric calcification; (5) luminal filling defect that may represent mobile thrombus. Two or more of these morphologic features may make the lesion unsuitable or at high risk for stenting.

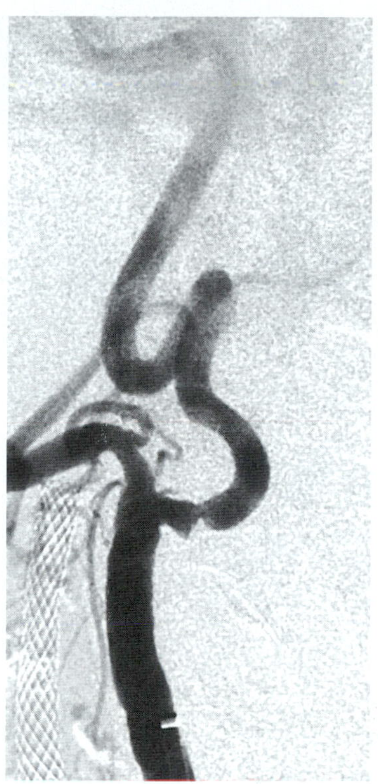

FIGURE 32-4. Severe tortuosity/angulation at the bifurcation of the carotid artery.

The placement of embolic protection systems, wire guides, and stents is much more complicated in such anatomy. Heavy calcification amplifies the technical complexity in such lesions. The degree of tortuosity may increase substantially after the placement of a carotid access sheath or guiding catheter (Fig. 32-5). Accordingly, the final decision to proceed with carotid stenting is always made after placement of the guiding sheath and final assessment of angiographic anatomy.

Other relative anatomic contraindications are the presence of high grade, complex multiple lesions in a bifurcation with an acute take-off of the internal carotid artery and severe tortuosity distal to the lesion. If the disease involves the common carotid artery and the external carotid origin, the risks are enhanced. Access to a disease-free external carotid branch can be important in securing a wire guide for successful sheath placement. Severe calcifications further complicate the procedure. Individually, all of these features can be handled by experienced operators, but if all contraindications are present, the patient may be better treated by other therapies.

The ideal lesion is a discrete subcritical stenosis in an "up going," straight internal carotid segment (see Fig. 32-1) Using embolic protection, severe ulceration is not a contraindication, but the presence of a large, mobile thrombus should direct the patient to surgery or 3 weeks of combination antiplatelet therapy and anticoagulation with warfarin (Coumadin) or subcutaneous heparin prior to stenting.

Fibromuscular dysplasia with severe stenosis, spontaneous dissection, high lesions, and diffuse disease are not contraindications. "String sign" lesions can be treated

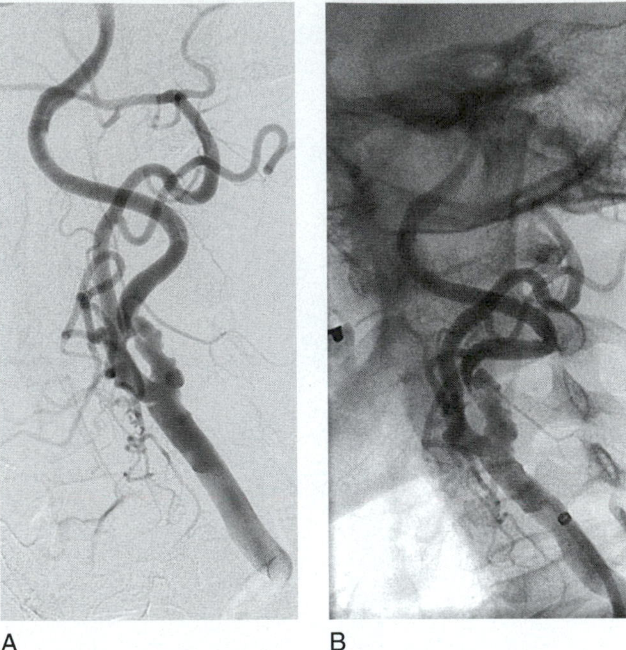

FIGURE 32-5. A, Moderate tortuosity on the initial diagnostic angiogram. **B,** Increase in tortuosity after placement of the guiding sheath in the common carotid artery (CCA). This may result in difficulty in crossing the lesion, or in advancing or placement of the embolic protection device.

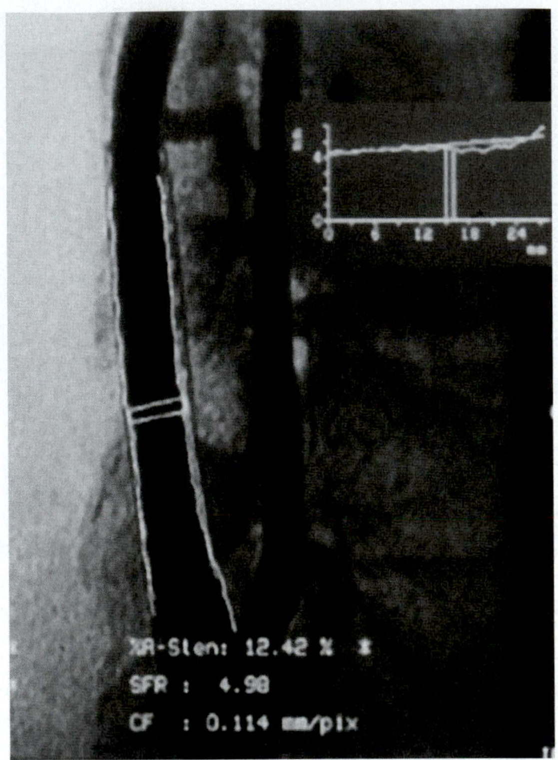

FIGURE 32-6. Carotid angiography will reduce unnecessary carotid endarterectomy. This patient was referred for carotid artery stenting, based on a duplex study demonstrating a "critical" internal carotid stenosis: systolic velocity was 268 mm/sec, diastolic 100 mm/sec (ratio of 2.68), indicating ICA stenosis of 70% to 90%. Carotid angiography revealed 43% stenosis (minimal luminal diameter of 4.29 mm). No intervention was performed.

if the distal vessel reconstitutes to a good vessel well below the entry into the skull base and there is a clear segment to place an embolic protection device once the lesion is crossed. Intracranial stenoses are not a contraindication nor are arteriovenous malformations (AVMs) or stable aneurysmal disease. With the latter, critical control of hypertension and modulation of anticoagulation are mandatory.

Preprocedure Evaluation and Management

The majority of patients are referred after clinical evaluation, and duplex ultrasonography has demonstrated the presence of a significant stenosis at the carotid bifurcation. Good quality magnetic resonance angiography (MRA) studies may be helpful in assessing the severity of the lesion and presence of other disease in the extracranial and intracranial vessels. Computerized tomographic angiography (CTA) is also evolving into an important noninvasive diagnostic procedure. After assessing the relative benefits and risks of alternative strategies, patients are scheduled for carotid angiography and stenting. Patients are informed that providing the angiographic severity of the lesions merits intervention and if the lesion is anatomically suitable; stenting will proceed in the same session. Angiography usually takes 15 to 20 minutes and stenting takes an additional 15 to 20 minutes.

For experienced operators, the angiography required for carotid stenting is associated with minimal risk of a neurologic complication.[49-51] Alternatively, and of note, a sizable percentage of patients referred with significant lesions documented by duplex and/or MRA are found to have insignificant stenoses by angiographic NASCET criteria (Fig. 32-6).[52] The large majority of these patients are asymptomatic. They are discharged the same day on optimal medical therapy and they are at no short- or intermediate-term risk of stroke. Of importance, had these patients been referred to a vascular surgeon and no angiography performed, most would have received an unnecessary operation with its attending risks. Of those patients with angiographically critical stenosis, approximately 5% to 10% (depending on age) have anatomy not suitable for stenting (usually vessel tortuosity). These patients are taken off the angiography table and discharged for elective endarterectomy at an appropriate time.

General clinical assessment preprocedure includes assessments of peripheral vascular and cardiovascular status. If iliac and coronary anatomy needs evaluation, this can be simply done at the time of carotid angiography, particularly when the interventionalist is a cardiologist. Not infrequently, critical coronary stenosis is documented. If this is the case, a relative risk assessment is done and coronary intervention can be prioritized as the index procedure and patients rescheduled for carotid intervention. Alternatively, the carotid stenosis is treated and the patient is rescheduled for subsequent coronary intervention. This type of coordinated cardiovascular assessment leads to efficient and better management of the patient's problems. Combined carotid and coronary or carotid and iliac interventions can be performed in the same setting,[53,54] but for a variety of reasons, particularly procedure time and contrast load, they are best done in separate procedures. Bilateral carotid stenoses can be treated in the same procedure,[55] but if both lesions are critical, there is a risk of inducing a hyperperfusion syndrome and prolonged hypotension. Procedure time and contrast load are also relevant in this situation.

Patients with renal dysfunction require special care. Contrast load should be minimized and angiography focused on ipsilateral extracranial and intracranial evaluation. If embolic filter devices are to be used, evaluation of collateral supply is not mandatory. If distal or proximal occlusion embolic protection systems are to be used, assessment of the contralateral and or posterior circulation and documentation of a functioning circle of Willis may be necessary. In general, experienced operators with access to good digital angiographic equipment can perform carotid stenting with minimal volumes of contrast. All patients with chronic renal impairment should be well hydrated and pretreated with *N*-acetylcysteine.[56-58]

Antiplatelet therapy preprocedure is an important element of the intervention. Ideally, patients should receive a combination of aspirin 325 mg plus clopidogrel 75 mg daily for 5 days to 7 days preprocedure. A loading dose can be used, but it must be given at least 6 hours prior to stenting. Studies[59] have shown that 600 mg and 450 mg of clopidogrel are superior to 300 mg in producing effective platelet inhibition. A recent study in coronary intervention demonstrated that clopidogrel significantly reduces ischemic events, but only if given in sufficient doses preprocedure.[60] The potential for platelet clumping on the large metallic stents placed in the carotid bifurcation is marked and the use of antiplatelet therapy cannot be overemphasized. For patients taking warfarin, this agent should be stopped 5 days prior to intervention and replaced with 5 days of aspirin plus clopidogrel therapy.

Because stenting of the carotid bifurcation "pressurizes" the carotid baroreceptors and induces hypotension, patients on large doses of antihypertensive medication should have these agents withheld on the morning of the procedure. If necessary, blood pressure can be controlled during preparation of the patient with intravenous nitroglycerin but this should be stopped 10 minutes before stenting and postdilatation of the stent.

Mild sedation may be offered to anxious patients before the procedure but for the most patients, gentle reassurance is all that is necessary to facilitate the continuous, accurate neurologic monitoring preprocedure, during, and postprocedure. Conscious sedation is not necessary for carotid stenting. Intraprocedural neurologic monitoring can be accomplished by talking to the patient and having the patient count and intermittently use a squeeze toy in the contralateral hand.

Hemodynamic and Anticoagulation Management

Careful hemodynamic monitoring and management are essential elements of carotid stenting and can alleviate significant cerebral hemorrhage, hyperperfusion events, and cerebral ischemia. Pulse oximetry, intra-arterial pressure monitoring, and heart rate monitors are essential. Atropine, 0.6 mg to 1 mg should be administered to all patients at the start of the procedure. If the blood pressure remains elevated after the stenosis has been relieved, it should be rapidly lowered using intravenous nitroglycerin, nitroprusside, or other appropriate rapidly acting agents. If an occlusion balloon embolic protection system is being used, blood pressure should be lowered before deflating the balloon.

Usually, substantial hypotension is noted after postdilatation of the stent, particularly in elderly patients with highly calcified stenoses. This hypotension is invariably quite benign and does not require aggressive treatment. However, in patients with other critical disease in intracranial, extracranial, or coronary vessels treatment is necessary. Phenylephrine 100 mcg boluses intravenously, hydration, and, occasionally, dopamine infusions are necessary.

Bradycardia and, rarely, asystole observed with balloon inflations is abolished or blunted by atropine. Severe bradycardia or asystole resolves immediately on balloon deflation. In elderly patients with preclinical conduction system disease, bradycardia may be seen postprocedure for 3 to 5 days. Intraprocedural temporary pacing is rarely, if ever, necessary. On rare occasions, carotid stenting will precipitate the need for permanent pacing postprocedure.

With optimal antiplatelet therapy per procedure, only ACT (200 seconds to 300 seconds) is necessary for stenting. Excessive anticoagulation may induce intracranial hemorrhage. Activated clotting times must be monitored during the intervention. Heparin, 4000 IU, is used depending on body weight. Bivalirudin is a new antithrombin agent that has a very short half-life, and requires a bolus and infusion depending on the length of the case. It is an extremely reliable antithrombin agent with the potential to limit cerebral and femoral access bleeding. In the usual case completed in 10 to 15 minutes, only the bolus is required; this should be administered just before placing the guiding sheath or catheter. Intravenous glycoprotein IIbIIIa receptor antagonists are not routinely used and, in the presence of the other oral and intravenous agents administered, may predispose the patient to disastrous intracranial hemorrhage.

Clinical Management Postprocedure

Intensive care monitoring postprocedure is not necessary. Patients should be managed in a step-down, monitored bed with nursing staff familiar with postinterventional patients, and groin observations and care. If sheaths are not removed in the interventional suite with femoral closure systems, they should be removed as soon as possible by experienced personnel once the ACT has fallen below 150 seconds.

Prolonged anticoagulation is not indicated, and if the access site is stable, patients do not require bed rest, sedation, or narcotics. All of these exacerbate hypotension and act against rapid ambulation and recovery. Hypotension may continue for up to 3 days. Patients' families and nursing staff should be reassured. Patients, particularly the elderly, should be assisted with ambulation if there are additional postural effects. If necessary, standard oral pseudoephedrine will increase the blood pressure as a temporary intervention. All patients with hypotension should be well hydrated, have routine hemoglobin and hematocrit checks, and have the inguinal puncture site examined. It is important that other important causes of hypotension such as retroperitoneal bleeding not be overlooked. Patients who have an uncomplicated case and femoral anatomy suitable for a percutaneous closure device can be discharged on the same day as the procedure. Al Murbarak and colleagues[61] reported the results in 98 consecutive patients that met these criteria and were able to be safely discharged without any untoward consequences.

Discharge Management

Patients should be discharged on a combination of clopidogrel 75 mg, and aspirin, 325 mg, for 1 month. After this time, either aspirin or clopidogrel should be continued indefinitely depending on other indications for antiplatelet therapy and patient tolerance. Aggressive antiplatelet regimens are important in preventing stent thrombosis, and this therapy should not be stopped for elective surgery for at least 3 to 4 weeks. If this drug combination cannot be tolerated, alternatives may include aspirin plus ticlopidine, clopidogrel plus dipyridamole, or greater doses of aspirin and dipyridamole. In addition to antiplatelet therapy, all patients should be discharged on a lipid-lowering agent (preferably a statin), optimal blood pressure control medication (preferably an angiotensin-converting-enzyme inhibitor and a thiazide diuretic), and advice on smoking, diet, and exercise. In diabetic patients, optimal management of blood glucose levels should be emphasized. Depending on arterial puncture site considerations, patients may travel or return to work immediately. Some patients notice mild neck stiffness for a period of 2 weeks, and may need mild analgesic support.

Baseline duplex ultrasound studies are performed within 1 month, and may serve as a reference for future follow-up evaluations. Not infrequently, despite documented good angiographic results, velocities assessed by Doppler ultrasound are elevated post-stenting. Evidence suggests this finding neither predicts excessive progression of neointimal proliferation nor an adverse clinical outcome. Such early measurements, however, do clarify later readings recorded at 6- and 12-month follow-ups. Angiographic follow-up correlations[62] have shown that although low velocity measurements denote favorable angiographic findings, moderately elevated velocities are not well correlated with significant restenoses. In correlative studies, 80% of patients undergoing follow-up angiography because of high duplex velocities had less than 50% stenosis. Only a small minority, 5%, had greater than 80% stenosis.[63] Efforts to redefine the optimal methodology (velocity plus B-mode analysis) to examine the carotid bifurcation are undergoing intensive investigation. The problem appears to relate to a relatively long 3-cm length of the stented vessel that develops a moderate layer of intimal proliferation to cover the stent. Although this layer of tissue effectively sequesters the underlying atheromatous plaque and appears to bestow a favorable clinical outcome, it may confound the duplex ultrasound follow-up surveillance. Importantly, the neointimal layer is maximal at 4 months to 6 months, and does not appear to progress over time.

Magnetic resonance angiography is not useful for follow-up purposes due to signal dropout associated with the metallic stent. Computerized tomographic angiography has shown some promise and may prove to be the follow-up modality of choice. Significant angiographic restenosis greater than 80% is an uncommon finding and is rarely associated with clinical symptoms. Cases of restenosis are seen more commonly in patients with disease associated with radiation-induced injury. Patients who have been stented for recurrent stenosis after CEA also tend to have increased recurrence after stenting. Should restenosis after stenting occur, it can be managed by repeat balloon dilatation and, occasionally, additional stenting.

Procedural Technique

Details of the stenting technique (Fig. 32-7) have been covered in many interventional texts.[64-66] In principle, the intervention should be as brief as possible and done with minimal manipulation of the lesion and the vessel. If at any point during guiding sheath placement, or attempts to initially pass a guidewire or embolic protection device, significant difficulty is encountered, the decision to proceed must be reassessed. Owing to the availability of an alternative surgical option for many patients, operators must be aware of their technical limitations and additional risks associated with the patient's particular anatomy. The procedure can safely be terminated at any time before predilatation of the lesion and the patient referred for elective surgery. Emergency surgical back-up has never been required or used for carotid stenting. Surgery should be scheduled for a later date when the antiplatelet effects have decreased.

In experienced centers, transcranial Doppler (TCD) studies have shown that few particles are generated during sheath placement or crossing the lesion with an embolic protection system.[22,67,68] TCD studies done before the use of embolic protection showed that predilatation (low profile 3-mm to 4-mm coronary balloons) caused release of only a modest number of particles. The largest number of particles were released during stent release and, most importantly, post-dilatation of the stent. These findings support the view that if an embolic protection system cannot be easily passed through the lesion in a safe, expeditious manner, the procedure should be abandoned. Operators should be reassured that in tortuous anatomy, inability to deploy the embolic protection device may be encountered by even the most experienced carotid interventionalists. Although aggressive techniques such as use of a "buddy wire" can accomplish the task of negotiating tortuous anatomy, this maneuver can present additional risk to the patient. The use of proximal occlusion, flow reversal embolic protection systems, can be used in these patients if they have an intact circle of Willis and, thus, good collateral supply, and, suitable iliac and proximal carotid anatomy to facilitate

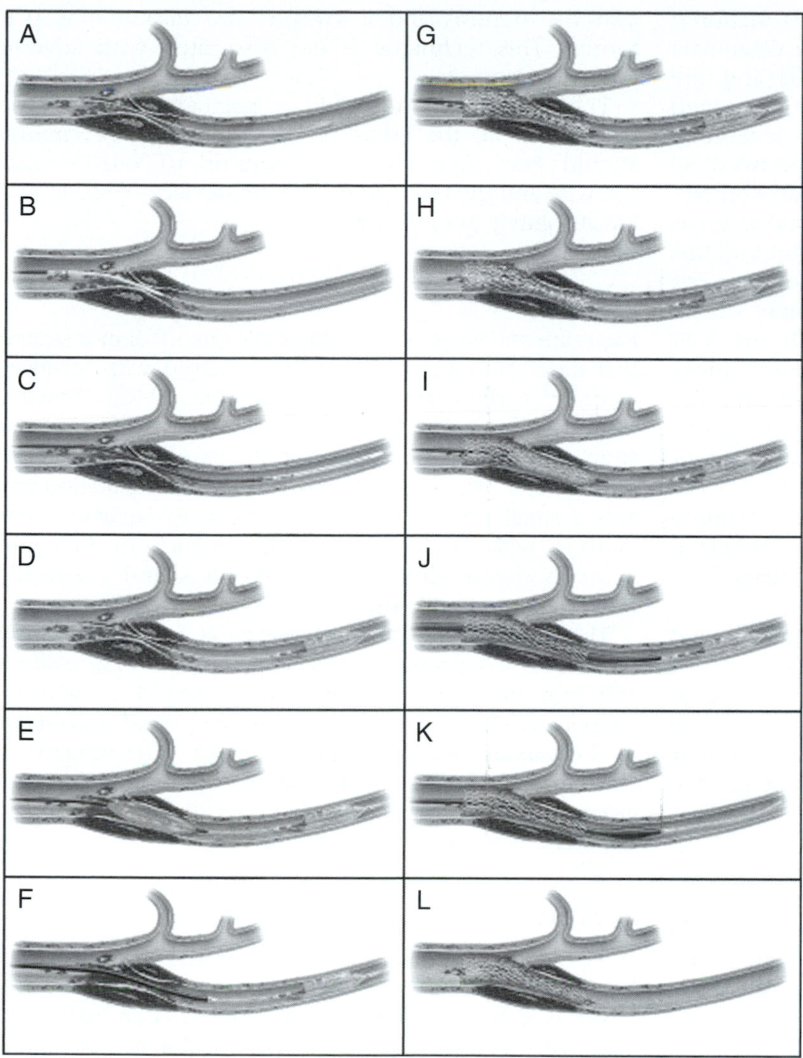

FIGURE 32-7. (See also Color Plate 32-7.) Carotid artery stenting technique using a filter for distal protection. **A,** After placement of a guiding catheter in the common carotid artery, the lesion is crossed with a guidewire. **B** and **C,** Specially designed filter guidewire. The lesion is crossed with the distal protection filter delivery catheter, which can be advanced easily over the guidewire by means of a rapid-exchange system (**D**), opening the filter (**E**). Balloon predilatation before stent placement (**F**), positioning of the stent (**G**), deployment of self-expanding stent (**H**). The self-expanding stent is deployed, but the vessel still is stenosed (**I**). Balloon postdilatation after stent placement allows further dilatation of the stenosed segment (**J**). Advancement of the retrieval catheter (**K**) and retrieval of the filter that contains the embolic debris into the retrieval catheter (**L**). Stent is fully deployed with good apposition to the vessel wall.

placement of this higher profile device. Transcranial Doppler studies also demonstrated the importance of minimal manipulation of the lesion with balloon dilatation and stent placement.

The procedure usually begins with varying degrees of diagnostic carotid angiography that can be tailored to the anatomic information gained from preceding noninvasive duplex and MRA or CT angiographic studies. It should be performed by experienced angiographers who are familiar with the use of low-profile, atraumatic, and safe neuroradiology diagnostic catheters and coated guidewires. The Vitek catheter (Cook, Inc.) and 0.038″ angle-tipped Glide wire (Meditech, Inc.) are recommended.[49] The minimal information required are the severity and anatomy of the bifurcation lesion to be treated, ipsilateral intracranial anatomy in anterior-posterior (AP) cranial and lateral views, and an assessment of disease and tortuosity that involve the common carotid. The latter is important in determining safe access with a guiding sheath. If an occlusion type embolic protection system is to be used, it is useful to have an assessment of collateral supply from the contralateral internal carotid artery and/or the posterior circulation and complete cerebral angiography is recommended.

The stenting procedure has seven components: (1) a neurodiagnostic catheter is used to safely access the common carotid artery and subsequently the external carotid artery and a glide wire is placed to allow tracking of a long sheath; (2) a 6 Fr-guiding sheath is placed into the distal common carotid artery; (3) the embolic protection device is deployed in a distal segment of the cervical internal carotid artery; (4) the lesion is predilated; (5) a self-expandable stent is placed; (6) the stent is postdilated with a conservatively sized, low-profile, balloon; (7) the embolic protection system is removed and final extracranial and intracranial angiography is performed. Using contemporary, rapid exchange (monorail) filters, balloons, and stent systems, the entire process can take as little as 15 to 20 minutes.

Access Sheath Placement

Following the diagnostic study, the 5 Fr catheter is advanced, using the 0.038-inch glide wire, into the external carotid artery. The glide wire is then replaced with an extra stiff 0.35-inch or 0.038-inch exchange wire. The catheter is withdrawn, and the 6 Fr 90-cm guiding sheath (Shuttle; Cook, Inc.) is advanced into the common carotid artery over the exchange wire, which is anchored in the external carotid artery. If brachiocephalic diagnostic angiography has previously been performed and the target lesion identified, the procedure can be shortened by placing the 6 Fr 90-cm Shuttle sheath, via the femoral approach, into the upper thoracic aorta, followed by introducing a 125-cm 5 Fr catheter (VTK Thorocon NB, Cook, Inc.) into the sheath. The common carotid artery is then catheterized with the 125-cm 5 Fr catheter, and this catheter is advanced into the external carotid artery, which serves as an anchor. If the advancement of the sheath over the 5 Fr catheter is not smooth, the 5 Fr catheter is removed, replaced with the sheath's inner introducer, and then the sheath is advanced into the common carotid artery. There are modifications of this technique, especially if the stenosis is located in mid- or distal segments of the common carotid artery or if the external carotid artery cannot be catheterized. Gaining access to the common carotid artery is the preferred point at which to administer anticoagulation (heparin or direct thrombin inhibitor).

Sheath placement is done without distal protection and should be performed with special caution. The common carotid artery may have atherosclerotic disease. In case of angiographically demonstrated atherosclerotic plaque in the common carotid artery, the operator may consider bringing the procedure to an end and sending the patient for surgery.

Crossing the Stenosis

Placement of the stiffer sheath in the common carotid artery (CCA) changes the anatomy of the bifurcation, which is usually distorted cephalad and tortuosity of the internal carotid artery (ICA) exaggerated. Therefore, repeat baseline angiograms are acquired through the sheath. The angiographic view should open the carotid bifurcation. The operator should have a clear image of the lesion location in relationship to the bony landmarks because this will facilitate accurate stent placement.

All currently available distal protection devices include a 0.014-inch wire system. With the currently available devices, the guidewire is an unchangeable integral part of the protection system. The wire tip is shaped appropriately and the device is negotiated through the stenosis (see Fig. 32-7A).

Embolic Protection Device Deployment

The device has to be placed at least ≥2 cm cephalad to the stenosis to have adequate distance to accommodate the tip of the stent delivery system and satisfactory coverage of the lesion with the stent (see Fig. 32-7C, D). In complex cases of high-grade stenoses, heavily calcified or eccentric lesions, and severe tortuosity of the ICA (especially when ICA take-off is significantly angulated), it can be technically difficult and sometimes impossible to advance the embolic protection system into the distal ICA. In these situations, a buddy wire, especially a hydrophilic one, may enhance gliding the device distal to the lesion. Another option is a "gentle predilatation" with a low profile angioplasty balloon (2.0 to 2.5 mm), which is advanced into the stenosis and a low-pressure dilatation is performed. This technique is not associated with adverse embolic events.[69]

The tip of this wire should be angiographically visible throughout all the steps of the procedure; precaution should be taken by the operator to ensure that the wire and the embolic protection device are stable, and are absolutely not moving.

Predilatation

Experimental work of Ohki and colleagues[70] demonstrated that more embolic debris can be released with "primary stenting" without predilatation (see Fig. 32-7E). "Primary stenting" is associated with more "scissoring effect" of the stent struts on the plaque during the latter post dilatation, with greater risk of embolization. Balloon predilatation creates a small passage within the lesion to facilitate stent delivery without "forceful crossing," which might cause major occlusive dissections in the ICA and eventually release large embolic shower.

The predilatation of the stenosis is performed using 0.014-inch low-profile coronary balloons. A long balloon (40 mm in length) is generally preferred to achieve balloon stability during the inflation and avoid movement of the balloon during inflation. A single brief inflation is all that is required. Again, before stenting, a control arteriogram is performed to reestablish the relationship of the stenosis to the bony landmarks.

Stent Placement

Self-expanding stents are routinely used. The self-expanding nature of the stent allows it to cover and appose the vessel wall without inducing the trauma often associated with balloon dilatation. Balloon-expandable stents can be subject to external compression and deformation. The only indications for using balloon-expandable stents in the carotid circulation are to treat ostial common carotid artery stenosis, to treat distal cervical or intracranial ICA stenoses, in the rare case when the self-expanding stent cannot be advanced through the stenosis, despite adequate balloon predilatation. In the latter case, a balloon-expandable stent is first deployed within the stenosis to prevent recoil at the lesion site—followed by a self-expanding stent that will prevent late compression of the balloon-expandable stent by constant radial force (see Fig. 32-7G, F).

The diameter of the self-expanding stent should be at least 1 to 2 mm larger than the largest vessel segment to be covered by the stent (almost always the CCA). A 10-mm diameter stent is recommended in all cases except when the stent is placed exclusively in the internal carotid artery. Thus, a large stent has larger and denser area coverage in the ICA lesion, effectively trapping the plaque material against the arterial wall and reducing the risk of embolization postdilatation. Oversizing the stent to the diameter of the ICA doesn't have any ill-effect on the stented vessel. The stent is deployed to cover the entire length of the carotid lesion that is typically located at the origin or the very proximal segment of the ICA (see Fig. 32-1). The stent is deployed "from normal to normal," from the healthy looking segment of the ICA distal to the lesion into the CCA, covering the origin of the ECA. If a nitinol stent is selected, a 30- or 40-mm long stent (9 to 10 mm in diameter) is typically required to cover the lesion completely. The stent is deployed using the vertebral bodies as landmarks (road-mapping is also helpful). Covering the origin of the ECA with the stent is usually not associated with adverse clinical consequences. Follow-up arteriograms have shown that, with rare exceptions, the ECA remains patent.

Postdilatation

The size of the postdilatation balloon is matched to the diameter of the ICA and the dilatation should be limited to the stent margins (see Fig. 32-7I). Typically, the self-expanding stent is postdilated with a low-profile 5.0- or 5.5-mm balloon. The stent postdilatation is a critical step and requires careful attention. It is the time of the procedure when embolic neurologic events are most likely to develop.[22,71] The balloon should not be inflated more than once because a second inflation in the same position has the effect of "shearing off" large amounts of plaque through the stent struts. It is safer to under dilate than over dilate the self-expanding stent, and a residual stenosis of 10% to 20% is acceptable. Minor residual stenosis following carotid artery stenting is acceptable and does not cause any hemodynamic problems. Over dilatation may potentially squeeze the atherosclerotic material through the stent mesh and result in emboli. The self-expanding stent has the tendency for late, progressive expansion, slowly reducing the residual stenosis. In some cases, continued flow via the stent struts into an ulcer crater is visualized at the end of the procedure (Fig. 32-8). An attempt to obliterate this communication by using larger balloons or higher pressures should be avoided because this communication usually seals off in the ensuing few days and is of no clinical consequence.

Embolic Protection Device Removal

At the completion of the procedure, the embolic protection device (see Fig. 32-7J, K, L) is retrieved, according to the specific device used. Guidewire removal and partial retrieval of the guiding sheath to the proximal CCA will assist in relieving the spasm as it relaxes the artery, and also helps the operator get a better assessment of the stented segment. The authors practice is to obtain repeat assessment of intracranial vasculature to compare with prestenting angiography to exclude "silent" emboli and to assess improvement in intracranial blood supply.

Access site hemostasis can be achieved at the end of the procedure using a vascular closure device. This vascular sealing approach is particularly valuable for those patients who can be discharged on the same day. It allows rapid ambulation with enhanced restoration of normal blood pressure regulation. In the authors' experience, the combined use of anticoagulation with a direct thrombin inhibitor and closure device was associated with less vascular complications, bleeding events, and need for blood transfusions.

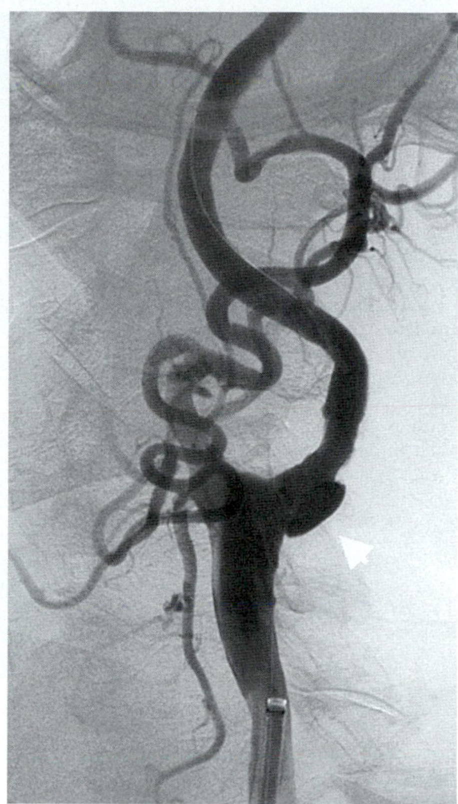

FIGURE 32-8. After stenting, an ulcer crater can still be seen (*arrowhead*). This is benign without any adverse events. There is no need for further dilatation of the stent.

Embolic Protection Devices

Embolic protection devices come in two formats (Fig. 32-9). The first groups have "umbrella," or "windsock," like micropore filters that are compressed in low profile sheaths and deployed distal to the lesion. Appropriate sizing and positioning of these devices provide good wall apposition and filtration efficiency. Numerous studies have documented the ability of these devices to capture plaque, thrombus, and even cholesterol crystals in sizes larger than 100 μm.[24,72-77] After dilatation of the stent, they are collapsed using a variety of innovative technologies and removed from the artery and patient.

The advantages of the filters are that they provide continuous perfusion to the brain. The disadvantages include somewhat higher profile than distal balloon occlusion systems; for some systems difficulty in tracking more angulated bifurcations and tortuous vessels; and the theoretical issue of not capturing very small particles. A number of these devices will be available in the near future with FDA approvals likely for both coronary saphenous vein graft labeling and high-risk CEA carotid stent indications.

Balloon occlusion devices are available in two systems. The most commonly used system is a very low profile, soft latex balloon that occludes the distal ICA below the siphon. Blood containing any debris is aspirated after the stent has been dilated. The balloon is then deflated and removed. This device has a very low profile and is

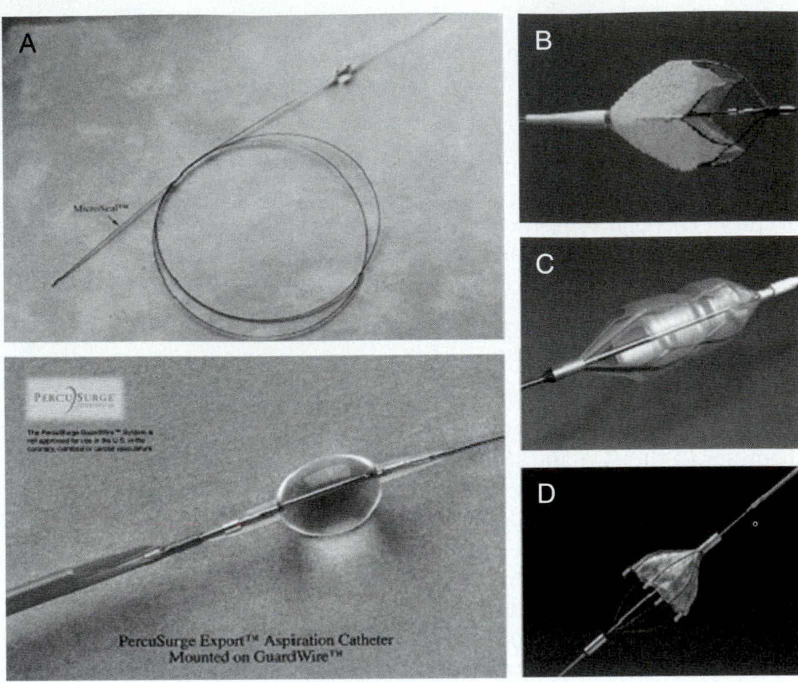

FIGURE 32-9. Some of the embolic protection devices available. **A,** The GuardWire (Medtronic) balloon distal occlusion. Wire and balloon are placed distal to the lesion. Inflation of the balloon results in occlusion of the distal vessel. All the debris that is dislodged from the lesion is then aspirated by the Export aspiration catheter. With the filters, the embolic material is caught in the filter umbrella. Retrieval with a special retrieval catheter closes the filter, thus entrapping the debris inside the filter. **B,** The Accunet filter (Guidant); **C,** Emboshield filter (Abbott); **D,** Angioguard (Cordis, Johnson & Johnson).

trackable through tortuous vessels. Theoretically the aspiration removes all particles. The principle disadvantage of the device is that 5% to 10% of patients do not tolerate the vessel occlusion. To be certain that a patient will tolerate the device, a complete cerebral angiogram is necessary. In addition, particles can be diverted up the external carotid and reach the cerebral tissue via ophthalmic or vertebral collaterals. Retinal infarction has also been noted. Rarely, significant dissection of the distal ICA has occurred. Second generation distal occlusion systems employing CO_2-filled balloons, and active "flush and extract" mechanisms appear more user friendly because of shorter occlusion times and more complete particle removal.

An alternative proximal occlusion system uses a more complicated device that features a cuff balloon surrounding the guiding sheath. The sheath occludes the distal CCA. A side port allows placement of a latex balloon that occludes the external carotid artery. In patients with a collateralization from the circle of Willis, flow in the ICA is reversed. Blood is shunted back through the guiding sheath and via a filter to a small catheter placed in the femoral vein. The theoretical advantage of this approach is removal of all particles—even those that may be produced when crossing the lesion. The disadvantages include the large profile of the guiding catheter that necessitates an 11 Fr sheath in the femoral artery and the somewhat more complicated set-up procedure. Again, 5% to 10% of patients with "isolated hemispheres" do not have the physiology to promote reversal of flow and do not tolerate the absence of cerebral perfusion.

From a practical perspective, all of the devices described have been studied in well-conducted prospective trials involving hundreds, even thousands, of patients. When used by experienced operators in the correct anatomical situation, all of the embolic protection approaches have demonstrated excellent recovery of debris and excellent procedural outcomes. By comparing distal occluding balloon with the various filters, Weisz and colleagues found no differences between the two groups. Device placement success, as well as the procedural success and 30-day outcomes were similar.[78] When there will be several protection systems approved and available, the operator will choose a specific device according to the patients extra- and intracranial anatomy, as well as the lesion characteristics.

RESULTS

Results of Carotid Stenting Without Embolic Protection

Stenting of arterial stenosis is safer than simple balloon angioplasty. Plaque rupture, arterial dissection, and acute occlusion are less likely to occur. Stents "wall off" or sequestrate the atherosclerotic plaque from the lumen with reduced adverse consequences of plaque rupture. Laminar flow is maintained. Improved dilatation achieved by stenting may also reduce the restenosis rate.

As was the case with other arterial percutaneous intervention sites, the evolution and availability of arterial stents transformed Gruentzig's less predictable balloon procedure, and by the early 1990s prospective observational studies of carotid stenting had been initiated.[39,41] Careful patient selection and technique minimized neurologic complications and from the outset carotid stenting performed by experienced operators produced acceptable outcomes in terms of disabling stroke and death. Nondisabling neurologic events (7%) were evident and clustered in patients with advanced age and more complex and severe stenoses.[42,79]

Carotid stenting studies were all initiated with prospective 24-hour pre- and postevaluations of patients by a board-certified neurologist and completion of an objective NIH (National Institute of Health) stroke scale data form. This level of rigorous adjudication had never been applied to CEA. The NASCET and ACAS trials had independent prospective neurologic evaluations of patients at 30 days postsurgery. In addition, early carotid stent studies were heavily biased toward patients at high risk of an adverse event due to their general medical status and risk profile for CEA. It became clear early in the development of carotid stenting that comparable patient selection and equivalent documentation of adverse events would be necessary for a fair comparison to CEA.

Numerous case reports and clinical series of carotid stenting without embolic protection have been published.[31,40,42,72,80-92] An early report of 117 carotid stenting procedures by Diethrich and colleagues[80] highlighted a high rate (6.4%) of periprocedural neurologic events; however, most of them were transient ischemic events or minor strokes with eventual full recovery. A high rate of local adverse events was related to direct common carotid cervical access, a technique that is no longer performed.

Naylor and associates reported a "randomized trial" of only 15 patients that was prematurely terminated.[93] Of the eight patients who were stented, six had a neurologic event. These results suggest that the operators lacked the knowledge and skill to perform carotid intervention.

The series that followed reported encouraging results from experienced centers.[31,34,40,42,72,81-92] These were mixed series of symptomatic and asymptomatic patients, with varying degrees of stenosis. Asymptomatic patients were largely required to have more severe stenosis or additional evidence of compromised cerebral circulation.[18,34,42,80,88] Some of the reports also included CCA lesions, which are not easily accessible by surgical measures.[18,42,80,81,88] These studies reported very high rates of procedural and stenting successes, usually higher than 95%, with periprocedural minor stroke rates of 1.6% to 4.8%, major stroke rates of 0.9% to 1.0%, and mortality rates of 0% to 1.6%.

Wholey published repeated updates of the global status of carotid artery stent placement before the introduction of embolic protection devices.[31,92] These observational and unaudited data provided an overall worldwide reflection on the status of stenting at that time. In 36 centers included in the survey, 5210 stenting procedures had a technical success rate of 98.4%. The 30-day rates of transient ischemic attacks (TIAs), minor strokes, major strokes, and mortality were 2.6%, 2.5%, 1.4%, and 0.8%, respectively.[31] Technical failures were usually related to inability to access the CCA (2% to 7% of patients) with excessive catheter manipulation that could result in catastrophic embolic events. Furthermore, prolonged procedural time was associated with increased morbidity.[92] These results in a series of patients at high surgical risk were very encouraging. The rates of adverse outcomes were highly competitive with lower risk patients treated with surgery.

The Wallstent study was the first multicenter randomized study that compared carotid stenting (using the primitive tracheobronchial self-expanding Wallstent system with no neuroprotection) with CEA surgery in patients with severe (NASCET criteria) carotid stenosis.[94] The primary endpoint was vascular death (procedural, myocardial, or stroke-related) and ipsilateral stroke at 1 year. Study design intended to show equivalence, with an anticipated sample size of 700 patients over 2 to 3 years. Patient enrollment was slower than expected, and after 2.5 years, only 219 patients (107 stenting, 112 endarterectomy) were randomized. The company that acquired the Wallstent technology decided to stop the study because an interim analysis suggested the statistical endpoint equivalence between the groups would not be achieved by further patient recruitment, although there were no prespecified stopping criteria. At 1 year, there was a tendency for higher incidence of combined vascular death and ipsilateral stroke in the stent group than in the surgery group (12% versus 4%), a difference that reached borderline significance ($P = .05$) owing to the small sample size. Closer examination of the data[95] revealed one death in the stent group was really procedure related. The periprocedural complication rate was 7.5% for stents and 1.8% for CEA ($P = .055$). The event-free survival from fatal or major stroke was identical during the follow-up period. It should be stressed that this study had significant methodologic weaknesses. There was no primary investigator to provide trial oversight and to make management and scientific decisions. There was no "lead-in" phase to evaluate operator technique and equipment. Preprocedure antiplatelet therapy was suboptimal. Importantly, most of the operators in the study were inexperienced. In summary, no conclusions regarding safety or efficacy of carotid stenting versus CEA can be based on the analysis of this trial.

Another small randomized trial from a single community hospital compared carotid stenting without embolic protection with endarterectomy surgery.[96] A total of 104 symptomatic patients were randomized to either of the above procedures and followed for 2 years. One death occurred in the surgical group (1/51) and one TIA occurred in the stent group (1/53). There were no strokes. The perception of procedurally related pain/discomfort was similar, but the stent group tended to be discharged earlier (1.8 versus 2.7 days). Return to full activity was achieved within 1 week by 80% of the stent group and 67% of the surgical group.

Results of Carotid Stenting Using Embolic Protection

Because of the nature of the carotid lesion, the incidence of embolic nondisabling neurologic events was not entirely unexpected. Transcranial Doppler studies have shown that few particles are generated during sheath placement or crossing the lesion with an embolic protection system.[22,67] Transcranial Doppler studies performed before use of embolic protection showed that predilatation caused release of a modest number of particles, followed by stent deployment. The largest number of particles were released during the postdilatation phase.

Later, histologic findings confirmed that material is dislocated from the atheromatous plaque during the procedure.[75,77] The embolic particles include plaque debris, lipid or cholesterol vacuoles, and calcium fragments.[27] The median number of particles, their maximal diameter, and their maximal area were found to be higher in aspirates obtained during procedures associated with neurological complications than in aspirates obtained during procedures not associated with complications.[76] However, the marked overlap in the distributions of the number and maximal diameter of particles preclude any predictive assumptions. By contrast, a maximal particle area greater than 0.8 mm^2 was found to be associated with a 60% chance of having periprocedural neurologic events.[76] These findings provided important justification and support for the routine use of embolic protection systems during carotid stenting; when the device cannot be easily passed through the lesion in a safe, expeditious manner, the procedure should be abandoned.

Increasing expertise over time might have influenced the favorable complication rates attributed to embolic protection. An improvement over time was noted even before the introduction of protection devices.[42,97] This possible effect on outcome must be taken into account when the favorable results of carotid stenting with embolic protection are interpreted, particularly when one considers that these new protective devices were tested primarily in highly experienced centers.[98]

The understanding of the potential embolic risk during the intervention and the desire to further improve the safety of the stenting procedure led to the development of embolic protection techniques and devices. The first step was to use a balloon, occluding the artery distal to the lesion. Theron[17,19] began pivotal work with distal balloon protection during carotid bifurcation angioplasty, later supplemented by stenting. Later, Henry and Amour[72] perfected Theron's technique with a low-profile occlusion balloon system for embolic protection. Independently, Roubin, Iyer, Gilson, and Yadav developed various distal embolic filter devices, a concept earlier proposed by Wholey. Parodi and others focused on proximal occlusion devices that facilitated embolic protection by temporarily reversing flow in the internal carotid artery.[74] Following the availability of embolic protection systems, many single-center studies and multicenter registries confirmed the ability of experienced operators to achieve good results from carotid stenting with remarkably low risks of stroke and death.

Single Center Experiences

The authors of this chapter have recently presented their prospective long-term experience (1994-2003) in 1268 patients who had 1397 carotid stenting procedures, with or without embolic protection.[30] All patients had National Institutes of Health (NIH) stroke-scale examinations performed before and within 24 hours, and at 30 days after the procedure, by an independent neurologist. The selection of the specific embolic protection device was based mainly on research protocol availability. Comparisons of the groups with or without embolic protection (Table 32-2) show significant reductions in the rate of stroke (mainly minor stroke) and the combined endpoint of stroke or death. Multivariate regression analysis confirmed that no use of embolic protection was the strongest predictor of periprocedural stroke. The subgroup of octogenarians demonstrated even more striking reduction of events associated with carotid stenting (Table 32-3; see subsequent discussion). These results highlight the importance of patient selection, use of embolic protection, and extra-cautious care of elderly patients. No differences in outcomes were found when the distal balloon temporary occlusion and aspiration system or various filter-based distal protection devices were used.[78]

These results from a highly experienced group of operators are important because they provide insight into what can be expected from many other operators who have received training and are rapidly gaining experience with the technique. Embolic protection devices, even in their early stage of development, improve outcomes. The results are most dramatic in patients at higher risk of events (i.e., elderly, recently symptomatic, severe stenoses, and long, bulky lesion). Compared with historical surgical controls, stenting leads to equivalent outcomes without the risks of operation, general anesthesia, and the attending complications. In patients at higher risk for CEA, the stent procedure is clearly a safer option. In low-CEA risk patients, the stent

TABLE 32-2 COMPARISON OF GROUPS WITH OR WITHOUT EMBOLIC PROTECTION

N = 1397 Procedures	No Embolic Protection (%) *N* = 809	Embolic Protection (%) *N* = 588	*P* Value
Minor stroke	33 (4.1)	7 (1.2)	<.001
Major stroke	8 (1.0)	2 (0.3)	ns
Fatal stroke	4 (0.5)	2 (0.3)	ns
All strokes	45 (5.6)	11 (1.9)	<.001
All deaths	9 (1.1)	5 (0.9)	ns
Nonstroke death	5 (0.6)	3 (0.5)	ns
All strokes + deaths	50 (6.2)	14 (2.4)	<.001

ns, not significant.

TABLE 32-3 COMPARISON OF OCTOGENARIANS WITH OR WITHOUT EMBOLIC PROTECTION

N = 220 Procedures	No Embolic Protection (%) *N* = 91	Embolic Protection (%) *N* = 129	*P* Value
Minor stroke	7 (7.7)	2 (1.6)	<.05
Major stroke	6 (6.6)	1 (0.8)	.02
Fatal stroke	1 (1.1)	0	ns
All strokes	14 (15.4)	3 (2.3)	<.001
All deaths	2 (2.2)	0	ns
Nonstroke death	1 (1.1)	0	ns
All strokes + deaths	15 (16.5)	3 (2.3)	<.001

procedure is as effective and much more acceptable to the patient.

Another, large, single-center experience is also worth discussing in detail. The group of Mathias and associates in Dortmund, Germany, were also early investigators of percutaneous, carotid intervention and have accumulated an extensive and powerful dataset for analysis. These results are entirely concordant with the author's experience. From 1984 to 1998, they treated 1222 arteries (hemispheres) with carotid angioplasty and more recently stenting without embolic protection.[99] In this population, minor stroke was 2.1%, major stroke 1.1%, and death 0.5%; and a total 30-day combined death and stroke rate of 3.8%. Since 1998, an additional 577 patients have been treated with the inclusion of embolic protection devices, demonstrating a minor stroke rate of 0.9%, a major stroke rate of 0.4%, and a 30-day mortality rate of 0.2%. Overall, this group also observed a dramatic reduction in stroke events associated with the introduction of embolic protection systems. Of importance to patients and neurologists alike, the incidence of major, disabling stroke has been 0.35% in this large series. This finding is similar to that observed in our series and suggests a dramatic departure from that observed from endarterectomy surgery where stroke events are most frequently disabling. The Dortmund group reported a procedure-related stroke and death rate in symptomatic patients of 2.8% and in asymptomatic patients of 1.75%.

A large body of evidence confirms the premise that experienced operators using contemporary equipment, including embolic protection systems, can produce results comparable with, even superior to, CEA (Table 32-4). Henry and colleagues[72] were the first to report results from a large series using a commercially available balloon

TABLE 32-4 RESULTS OF CAROTID ARTERY STENTING WITH EMBOLIC PROTECTION: 30-DAY OUTCOMES

Study	Year	No. of Patients	No. of Procedures	Embolic Protection System	Embolic Protection Device Success	Procedural Success (%)	Minor Stroke (%)	Major Stroke (%)	Mortality (%)	All Strokes and Deaths (%)
Theron[34]	1996	NA	65	Theron device	NA	NA	NA	NA	NA	NA
Henry[21]	1999	48	53	GuardWire[†]	NA	NA	1-1.9	0	1-1.9	2-3.8
Henry[72]	2000	NA	150	GuardWire[†] Theron device[19]	NA	98	NA	NA	NA	NA
Parodi[74]	2000	25	25	GuardWire[†] AngioGuard[‡] Parodi[¶]	NA	100	0	0	0	0
D'Audiffret[124]	2001	15	15	GuardWire[†]	NA	100	0	0	0	0
Dietz[90]	2001	43	43	GuardWire[†]	72		0	0	1-2.5	2-5
Yaeger[73]	2001	20	20	AngioGuard[‡]	75	93	0	0	0	0
Reimers[75]	2001	84	88	AngioGuard[‡] NeuroShild[§] FilterWire[&]	97	98	1-1.2	0	0	1-1.2
Tubler[76]	2001	54	58	GuardWire[†]	NA	NA	0	1-1.7	0	1-1.7
Café USA[125]	2001	125	125	GuardWire[†]	98	100	0.8	2.4	0.8	4.0
Angelini[77]	2002	36	38	AngioGuard[‡]	100	97	0	0	2.6	2.6
Whitlow[27]	2002	75	75	GuardWire[†]	NA	NA	0	0	0	0
Adami[126]	2002	30	30	Parodi[¶]	93	NA	0	0	0	0
Al-Mubarak[24]	2002	162	164	NeuroShild[§]	94	99	1.2	0	1.2	2.4
Guimaraens[100]	2002	164	194	Theron device[19] GuardWire[†]	NA	98	0	1	1.8	2.6
Cremonesi[127]	2003	442	442	AngioGuard[‡] FilterWire[&] Microvena[Ψ] NeuroShild[§] Parodi[¶] MO.MA[∉]	99	99	0.9	0.2	0	1.1
Weisz[30*]	2003	551	588	GuardWire[†] NeuroShild[§] AngioGuard[‡] FilterWire[&] Accunet[#] Parodi[¶]	98	99	1.2	0.3	0.9	14-2.4

NA, not available.
[†]GuardWire, PercuSurge, Medtronic
[‡]Angioguard, Johnson & Johnson
[¶]Arteria
[§]MedNova, Abbott
[&]EPI, Boston Scientific
[#]Guidant
[Ψ]EV3
Microvena Trap Filter
[∉]Invatec

distal occlusion system (Percusurge-Medtronic Inc., Minneapolis, MN). In a consecutive series of 150 patients, they observed a 1.3% nondisabling stroke rate, a 1.6% disabling stroke rate, and 1 fatal stroke (0.75%) at 30 days. Parodi and colleagues,[74] in 46 consecutive procedures, reported a 9.5% complication rate in the first 23 patients in the series in which no embolic protection was used and 0% complications in a subsequent 23 patients treated with the benefit of embolic protection. Reimers and colleagues[75] reported 84 consecutive patients treated with three different embolic protection systems with a 1.2% nondisabling stroke rate and no disabling strokes. Guimaraens and colleagues[100] reported on 164 patients with 194 procedures (hemispheres treated). In this group 92% were symptomatic. They demonstrated a stroke rate of 1.3% and a 30-day mortality of 1.9%. These investigators concluded that stenting results with embolic protection produced salutary results and that its application should probably not be restricted to symptomatic patients.

Multicenter Registries

There now exist numerous prospective, multicenter studies that support the results from single operator and single center reports; the results are summarized in Table 32-5. The German Quality Assurance Program (Prospective Registry) reported their results in 2002, from 35 centers in Germany, Austria, and Switzerland.[101] During 30 months, 2142 planned carotid interventions were registered, in 98%, stents were used. Embolic protection systems became available in the last half of the series, and were used in 55% of interventions since that time. The overall stroke and death rate was 3.0%. They reported a mortality rate of 0.7%, a major stroke rate of 1.4%, and a minor stroke rate of 0.8%. Al-Mubarak and colleagues[24] reported the combined outcomes from three experienced centers in the United States, United Kingdom, and Italy using a single embolic protection filter device. Of 162 patients studied, 48% were symptomatic. The overall 30-day stroke and death rate was 2%. There were no major strokes; there were two minor strokes, one death from cerebral hemorrhage, and one nonrelated cardiac death.

The ARCHeR (Acculink for Revascularization of Carotids in High Risk patients) trial also showed favorable 30-day results, demonstrating that carotid stenting with filter protection can be safely performed in high-risk surgical patients in a multicenter trial.[102] The ARCHeR trial was a prospective, nonrandomized, multi-center clinical study that was designed to show equivalency in safety and performance of the combined use of the Accunet embolic protection filter, combined with the nitinol, self-expanding Acculink carotid stent (both, Guidant Corporation, Santa Clara, CA) in the treatment of high-risk surgical and nonsurgical patients with internal carotid artery stenosis (at least 50% in symptomatic patients and at least 80% in asymptomatic patients). A total of 76 patients were enrolled in the lead-in phase and 437 in the registry. The study filter device was successfully delivered, placed, and retrieved in 92.7% of the cases, and embolic material was captured in 57%. The 30-day event rates are summarized in Table 32-5. The composite death/stroke rate was 7.8%. Of note, patients with restenosis after CEA had significantly lower event rates (composite death/stroke 1.4%), whereas patients who were dialysis dependent had 28.6% event rates. Contralateral occlusion, or the presence of two or more comorbidities, has no prognostic weight. A second phase of this study (ARCHeR RX) will evaluate the use of "rapid exchange" versions of the devices.

The SECURITY (Study to Evaluate the NeuroShield Bare Wire Cerebral Protection System and Xact Stent in Patients at High Risk for Carotid EndarTerectomY) also examined the outcome from stenting high-risk surgical patients in a prospective, multicenter study.[103] Entry criteria were similar to the ARCHeR, but this trial recruited a large number of octogenarians (28.2%) with and without a variety

TABLE 32-5 RESULTS OF MULTICENTER REGISTRIES

	NeuroShield[24] (%)	German Program[101] (%)	ARCHeR[102] (%)	SECURITY[103] (%)
Number of Patients	*N = 162*	*N = 2142*	*N = 437*	*N = 305*
Stroke				
Minor stroke	1.2	0.8	3.7	4.6
Major stroke	0	1.4	1.6	1.6
All strokes	1.2	2.2	5.3	6.2
Death				
Stroke related	0.6	NA	0.7	0.7
Nonstroke related	0.6	NA	1.6	0.3
All deaths	1.2	0.7	2.3	1.0
Composite Endpoint				
Stroke/Death	2.0	3	6.6	7.2

ARCHeR, Acculink for Revascularization of Carotids in High Risk patients; NA, not available; SECURITY, Study to Evaluate the NeuroShield Bare Wire Cerebral Protection System and Xact Stent in Patients at High Risk for Carotid EndarTerectomY.

of additional high surgical risk comorbidities and less patients with CEA restenosis. As with the ARCHeR and SAPPHIRE studies, this trial was completed with first-generation devices. Of the 305 patients entered in this registry, 28.5% had a history of stroke and 29.5% a history of TIA. The study filter device was able to be placed in 97%. The 30-day event rates are summarized in Table 32-5. The composite death/stroke rate was 7.2%. A second phase of this trial is in progress with a 4th generation filter and stent with a rapid exchange delivery system.

Special Patient Subsets

Octogenarians

No comparison from randomized CEA trials can be made in the elderly subset of patients because age of 80 years or older was one of the exclusion criteria.[1,6,104] Observational data reported from surgical series, however, demonstrated an increased risk of stroke for elderly patients.[105,106] Gupta and colleagues[87] reported results of stenting on 100 elderly (>65 years) patients. Most (85%) were symptomatic, 24% were women, and 80% had concomitant coronary artery disease. This series was completed without the use of embolic protection devices. There were five nondisabling strokes (5%) and one disabling stroke (1%), and all were reversed within 30 days. There were no deaths in the first 30 days. Before the introduction and use of embolic protection devices, the best predictor of stroke and death was age older than 80 years.[42] In the authors' last analysis of 220 procedures in patients older than 80 years, the use of embolic protection device, as compared with no protection, reduced the risks of minor and major strokes (2.3% versus 15.4%, $P < .001$), as well as the combined outcome of any stroke and death (2.3% versus 16.5%, $P < .001$) (Table 32-3). Thus, the use of an embolic protection device is mandatory in all procedures performed in the elderly population. These data are in marked contradistinction to the outcomes in the CREST lead-in study (see later) and emphasize the importance of patient selection and expertise in treating this group.

Post Carotid Endarterectomy Restenosis

Restenosis after CEA is a known phenomenon. Restenosis that occurs within the first 2 years after CEA has been attributed to intimal hyperplasia. Later than 2 years, recurrence and progression of the atherosclerotic process are responsible for recurrent stenosis. Restenosis was reported in 10% of the patients during the first year after surgery (range 1.9% to 25.9%)[107] and is associated with 0% to 11% risk of ipsilateral stroke,[107] especially in patients with late (>12 months) occlusion.[108] Smoking has been associated with increased risk for restenosis after CEA.[109] Due to the relative risk for neurologic events associated with recurrent stenosis after CEA, treatment of high-grade restenosis is indicated. New and colleagues[110] examined outcomes in patients with prior ipsilateral CEA and restenosis. A total of 358 arteries were stented in 14 centers in the United States. The overall 30-day stroke and death rate was 3.7%. The minor stroke rate was 1.7%; major disabling stroke rate was 0.8%; and the fatal stroke rate was 0.3%. Nonstroke related death rate at 30 days was 0.9%. Overall 3-year freedom from all fatal and nonfatal strokes was 96 ± 1%. In the ARCHeR trial, there were 141 patients with restenosis at a prior CEA site. At 30 days, the composite event rate of stroke/death was 0.7%.

Carotid Artery Stenting versus Carotid Endarterectomy Surgery

In North America, three recent studies deserve consideration, (SAPPHIRE), CREST; (lead-in credentialing registry), and the Carotid Revascularization with Endarterectomy or Stenting Systems (CARESS; phase I, clinical registry).

The SAPPHIRE study was the first randomized, multicenter trial that compared carotid stenting with embolic protection with endarterectomy surgery and showed a definitive advantage of stenting in the group of patients classified as high risk.[29] The SAPPHIRE study was conducted in 29 U.S. centers, and was planned to enroll at least 600 randomized patients, but due to the slow rate of enrollment, it was concluded earlier than designed. Eligibility required that, asymptomatic patients had at least 80% stenosis and symptomatic patients had at least 50% stenosis, as assessed by ultrasound-Doppler examination, and at least one high-risk feature. Excluded were patients with prior stent in the target lesion, or total occlusion. In cases with angiographic/ultrasound evidence of thrombus, the recommendation was to exclude the patient, but if already randomized, the patient was treated after 1 month of anticoagulation. Patients with acute or recent (<48 hours) stroke or intracranial mass were excluded. Two primary endpoints were prechosen; the composite of major adverse events including death, and stroke, and/or myocardial infarction at 30-days' postprocedure, and the composite of the above adverse events plus death and/or ipsilateral stroke between 31 days and 1 year postprocedure. Eligible patients were screened by a team that included a neurologist, an interventionalist, and a vascular surgeon. Consensus that patients were good candidates for either procedure was required for randomization (stenting = 159, CEA = 151); those rejected from surgery underwent stenting (stenting registry, 406 patients); and those rejected from endovascular intervention entered the surgical registry (seven patients). This diversity shows that only a few patients are rejected from stenting, in contrast to almost 50% of the patients rejected from surgery by the vascular surgeons. The interventional equipment used were the Precise nitinol stent (Cordis, Johnson & Johnson, Warren, NJ), and the Angioguard XP, filter-based distal protection device (Cordis, Johnson & Johnson, Warren, NJ). This combination of devices demonstrated a high procedural success rate (88%) with the combined use of stent and filter-based distal protection placement (90%). In the randomized patients (Table 32-6), the superiority of carotid artery stenting in high-risk patients was clearly recognized by comparing the primary composite endpoint of death/stroke/MI at 30-days postprocedure (5.8% versus 12.6%, $P < .05$). Despite higher baseline rates of coronary artery disease, and prior revascularization procedures, the stented group had a significantly lower event rate of

TABLE 32-6 THE SAPPHIRE STUDY, RANDOMIZED ARM: 30-DAY RESULTS

N = 310 **Procedures**	**Stent (%)**	**Endarterectomy (%)**	***P* Value**
	N = 159	*N* = 151	
Death	0.6	2.0	.36
All strokes	3.8	5.3	.59
Minor stroke (ipsilateral)	3.2	3.3	>.99
Minor stroke (contralateral)	0.6	0	>.99
Major stroke (ipsilateral)	0	1.3	.24
Major stroke (contralateral)	0.6	0.7	>.99
Myocardial infarction	2.6	7.3	.07
Q-wave MI	0	1.3	.24
Non-Q wave MI	2.6	6.0	.16
Death/stroke	4.5	6.6	.46
Death/stroke/MI*	5.8	12.6	.047

*primary endpoint.
MI, myocardial infarction.

myocardial infarction (2.6% versus 7.3%, $P = .07$). The stenting outcomes were similar in the randomized and the stenting registry groups, confirming the low event rate and the safety of carotid stenting in a wide range of patients. This study demonstrated the high complication rate of CEA surgery in high-risk patients excluded from previous CEA trials. The particular high rate of myocardial infarction in the surgical group highlights the determinable outcomes of patients with medical comorbidities, especially coronary artery disease, a disease that is so frequent in patient with carotid stenosis. The improved outcomes with stenting as compared with CEA were most striking among the patients with medical comorbidities as compared with those with anatomic risk factors.[44]

The NIH-NINDS supported Carotid Revascularization Endarterectomy versus Stent Trial (CREST) is a prospective randomized multicenter trial comparing carotid stenting with embolic protection to CEA in symptomatic patients with a 70% or greater stenosis by duplex ultrasound studies or a greater than or equal to 50% stenosis by angiography. The trial includes a "lead-in" credentialing phase to establish the clinical technical skills of interventionalists before entering the "blinded" randomized phase of the trial. The interventionalists in the trial include a large number of cardiologists, radiologists, and vascular surgeons with a broad spectrum of prior interventional experience. Prior carotid stenting experience varied from as few as six procedures as primary operators to more than 100 cases (average 26 cases). The lead-in/credentialing phase of the trial was designed to familiarize the operators with the stent embolic protection system to be used and to assess operator efficacy before starting randomization. As of December, 2003, 691 patients had carotid stents.[111] In the lead-in phase, the combined 30-day stroke and death rate was 3.3% for asymptomatic patients, and 4.2% (0.7% mortality, and 3.5% stroke) for symptomatic patients. Myocardial infarction occurrence was less than 0.9%. The initial event rate represents a relatively early experience of some of the operators, and it should be remembered that in the first 81 patients, stenting had been performed without embolic protection. Thus, the investigators expect the event rate to decline with time.

The Carotid Revascularization with Endarterectomy or Stenting Systems trial (CARESS) was designed as a prospective, comparative cohort trial that has two phases, feasibility and pivotal, recruiting consecutive patients who are candidates for either carotid stenting or endarterectomy. The choice of treatment, and consequently, treatment arm, is based solely on physician and patient preference. The objective of the study was to compare carotid stenting with embolic protection to CEA in both high-risk (symptomatic = 50% stenosis) and low-risk (asymptomatic = 75% stenosis) populations consistent with current clinical practice for the broadest possible indication. By allowing the use of more than one available stent protection system, it will be possible to assess aggregate performance in a real setting. In the first feasibility phase,[112] 397 patients with carotid stenosis had endarterectomy surgery (254 patients) or stenting (143 patients, using the GuardWire embolic protection and the monorail Wallstent). The primary endpoints were all-cause mortality and nonfatal stroke at 30 days. The event rates were similar and extremely low in both treatment groups: 2.4% in the surgical group, and 2.1% in the stent with protection group. In the second phase of the study, 3000 patients will be enrolled in a 2:1 ratio to surgery or stenting. Up to six carotid stent systems (including protection devices) will be used, with randomization between the carotid stent systems.

Long-Term Results of Carotid Stenting

The Carotid and Vertebral Artery Transluminal Angioplasty Study (CAVATAS) is most noteworthy because of its extremely valuable late outcome results. No substantial difference in the rate of ipsilateral stroke was noted with survival analysis up to 3 years after randomization. Carotid endovascular treatment was shown to be effective at prevention of subsequent stroke. Of note—there were no strokes in the patients treated with stenting.[38]

The SAPPHIRE study was not only the first randomized, multicenter trial to show the superiority of carotid stenting with embolic protection to endarterectomy surgery in terms of procedural safety and short-term (30 days) results, but also demonstrated favorable long-term (1 year) outcomes.[113] In the randomized arm of the study, the cumulative events rate continued to diverge over time, reaching the composite primary endpoint in 11.9% of the stented patients versus 19.9% of the CEA patients. The particular event rates are summarized in Table 32-7. Patients who had carotid stenting as compared with CEA had lower rates of stroke (5.7% versus 7.3%), especially major ipsilateral stroke (0% versus 3.3%, $P = .03$). Cumulative myocardial infarction at 1-year postprocedure was also lower in the stented group (2.5% versus 7.9%, $P = .04$).

The largest and longest follow-up was published by Roubin and colleagues, reporting 604 carotid stenting procedures, done without embolic protection.[42] After the 30-day period, at 5-years follow-up, the incidence

TABLE 32-7 THE SAPPHIRE STUDY, RANDOMIZED ARM: 1-YEAR RESULTS

N = 310 Procedures	Stent (%)	Endarterectomy (%)	*P* Value
	N = 159	*N* = 151	
Deaths	6.9	12.6	.12
All strokes	5.7	7.3	.65
Minor stroke (ipsilateral)	3.8	2.0	.50
Minor stroke (contralateral)	1.9	2.0	>.99
Major stroke (ipsilateral)	0	3.3	.03
Major stroke (contralateral)	0.6	0.7	>.99
Myocardial infarction	2.5	7.9	.04
Q-wave MI	0	1.3	.24
Non-Q wave MI	2.5	6.6	.10
Death/ipsilateral stroke/MI*	11.9	19.9	.048

*primary endpoint.
MI, myocardial infarction.

of fatal and nonfatal stroke was 3.2%. Among those who survived the 30-day periprocedural period, the overall 3-year freedom from fatal and nonfatal stroke was 95%. There were no differences in freedom from stroke between men and women and symptomatic and asymptomatic patients. Late non-neurologic deaths were mainly attributed to cardiac disease and cancer. These results are better than those reported in the 5-year follow-up of the NASCET participants (15.7%).

Restenosis

In-stent restenosis is the main long-term limitation of coronary angioplasty and stenting.[114-117] In-stent restenosis is defined as stenosis greater than 50% of the vessel lumen diameter. The occurrence of in-stent restenosis is related mainly to proliferation of smooth muscle cells with neointima formation.[118,119] In the coronary artery, there is a high rate of in-stent restenosis,[116,117,120] which reaches angiographic significance with reduced blood flow within 3 to 6 months following intervention.[121] In the CAVATAS study, severe (>70%) restenosis was more prevalent after balloon angioplasty (without stenting) than after surgery (14% versus 4%, $P < .001$).[38] With carotid artery stenting, various series found that the rate of in-stent restenosis is in the range of 2% to 5%.* In these series, the follow-up method differed (clinical, duplex ultrasound, or angiography), with various follow-up periods reported (6 months to 5 years). Few case reports of stent deformity have been reported.[31,88,92] The rate of stent deformity in the world global survey was 2.5%, occurring exclusively with the balloon-expandable Palmaz stent.[31]

Treatment of in-stent restenosis is usually done by dilatation with a noncompliant balloon. Learning from previous experience from treating coronary in-stent restenosis, Bendok and colleagues implemented the use of a cutting balloon in cases of carotid in-stent restenosis.[123] In one of the three patients reported, an additional stent was required due to some recoil. These authors speculate that due to the controlled trauma of this balloon, its use may result in lower occurrence of in-stent restenosis as compared with a conventional angioplasty balloon.

Operator Experience

As with any interventional procedure, outcomes are predicated on operator expertise and experience. There is a steep learning curve for physicians beginning carotid stenting.[89,97] Authors of this chapter involved in the development of the current technique since the first days of carotid stenting, have experienced constant increase in the safety of the procedure with reduction in the periprocedural event rate. Similar observations were reported by others,[89] and are being observed again in the roll-in phase of CREST. In the worldwide global survey there was a J-curve of learning experience. Those centers with fewer than 50 cases had a significantly higher rate of 30-day strokes and death than the centers that performed 50 to 100 cases, or 200 to 300 procedures (6.8% versus 4.6 versus 4.0%, respectively). Interestingly, adverse events (combined strokes and deaths) among centers that performed more than 300 procedures had higher rates (5.5%).[31] This phenomenon can be attributed to patient selection that is probably more "daring" with increasing experience. These observations suggest that, to be certified in carotid stenting and to be active researchers in randomized trials and registries, a learning phase of approximately 20 to 30 carotid stent cases may be required, depending on previous interventional experience of the individual operator.

Future Directions

Based on the current updated results of the recent published registries and the SAPPHIRE randomized trial, the interventional community expects the FDA to approve the use of a vascular stent combined with a filter embolic protection device for carotid stenting in patients at high surgical risk. By demonstration of comparable safety and efficacy, approval of additional stents and protection systems will follow.

Ongoing international studies such as the CAVATAS II, EVA-3S, SPACE, and ALLSTAR trials are designed to have similar endpoints as prior registries and trials. The results of the largest randomized study, CREST, are expected in the next few years. Further studies will focus on asymptomatic, low surgical-risk patients. To prove the safety and efficacy of carotid stenting in this patient population, the periprocedural event rate (safety) will need to be very small, and lower than the natural history of the disease. Recently published single and multicenter studies (CARESS) suggest that this will certainly be the case. Ultimately, it may be necessary to compare carotid stenting plus optimal contemporary medical management (antiplatelet agents, statin drugs, and optimal

*See references 31,34,42,72,80,87,88,92,100,122.

blood-pressure control) with medical management alone. Superiority of carotid stenting to medical management in low-risk patients will result in the need for better screening of the general population for carotid disease.

The near future will bring dramatic technical and device improvements. Most of the manufacturers of the current stents and embolic protection devices are developing rapid-exchange (monorail) systems. The second-, third-, and fourth-generation embolic protection devices are expected to be more "user-friendly" with better guidewire tractability and deliverability. Moreover, the next generation of protection devices will have lower crossing profile—further simplifying the procedure. Emboli capture efficiency will also improve with next-generation devices. New occlusion balloons will have more favorable balloon profiles. Newer proximal occlusion balloons are currently being evaluated. All of these devices enable reduced risk of embolization while crossing the lesion with the wire. Similarly, the next generation of self-expanding stents will have more reliable placement characteristics, with lower crossing profile and better tractability and deliverability.

Although restenosis is not a major issue in carotid stenting it is likely that future stents will have antiproliferative coatings and likely, coatings that will inhibit platelet and thrombin accumulation. There are no current imaging techniques that provide reliable tools for follow-up after stent placement. Duplex ultrasound studies have high false-positive rates, and there is not enough data regarding the use and limitations of CT after stent placement. Further research and experience are needed to find the best accurate noninvasive imaging tool for long-term follow-up of the patients after stenting.

Adjunctive pharmacology has provided increased safety of stenting. The combined use of aspirin and clopidogrel, the current standard, will be further enhanced and new thienopyridines, including a short-term intravenous preparation, will be studied. As discussed earlier in this chapter, anticoagulation with heparin has many limitations, and the use of direct thrombin inhibitors has emerged as a safe alternative for coronary and carotid interventions. Anticoagulation with bivalirudin during carotid stenting (with various types of embolic protection devices) is now being tested by the authors of this chapter with excellent preliminary results.

Since introduced in 1994, carotid artery stenting has progressed dramatically as a treatment for carotid stenoses. Technical expertise and device improvements have underpinned the progress. The procedure has been shown repeatedly in rigorous studies to be safe and effective in reducing embolic strokes that originate from carotid stenosis. The increased acceptance of this procedure, combined with widespread practice by a variety of disciplines, has proved carotid stenting to be an established medical treatment modality.

REFERENCES

1. North American Symptomatic Carotid Endarterectomy Trial Collaborators: Beneficial effect of carotid endarterectomy in symptomatic patients with high-grade carotid stenosis. N Engl J Med 325:445, 1991.
2. National Institute of Neurological Disorders and Stroke Stroke and Trauma Division. North American Symptomatic Carotid Endarterectomy Trial (NASCET) Investigators: Clinical alert: Benefit of carotid endarterectomy for patients with high-grade stenosis of the internal carotid artery. Stroke 22:816, 1991.
3. Barnett HJ, Taylor DW, Eliasziw M, et al: Benefit of carotid endarterectomy in patients with symptomatic moderate or severe stenosis: North American Symptomatic Carotid Endarterectomy Trial Collaborators. N Engl J Med 339:1415, 1998.
4. Ferguson GG, Eliasziw M, Barr HW, et al: The North American Symptomatic Carotid Endarterectomy Trial: Surgical results in 1415 patients. Stroke 30:1751, 1999.
5. Paciaroni M, Eliasziw M, Kappelle LJ, et al: Medical complications associated with carotid endarterectomy: North American Symptomatic Carotid Endarterectomy Trial (NASCET). Stroke 30: 1759, 1999.
6. No authors listed: Randomised trial of endarterectomy for recently symptomatic carotid stenosis: Final results of the MRC European Carotid Surgery Trial (ECST). Lancet 351:1379, 1998.
7. Executive Committee for the Asymptomatic Carotid Atherosclerosis Study: Endarterectomy for asymptomatic carotid artery stenosis. JAMA 273:1421, 1995.
8. Landesberg G, Shatz V, Akopnik I, et al: Association of cardiac troponin, CK-MB, and postoperative myocardial ischemia with long-term survival after major vascular surgery. J Am Coll Cardiol 42:1547, 2003.
9. Dotter C: Transluminal angioplasty: A long view. Radiology 35:561, 1980.
10. Gruentzig A, Hopff H: Percutane rekanalisation chronischer arterieller verschlusse mit einem neven dilatationskatheter. Dtsch Med Wochenschr 99:2502, 1974.
11. Mathias K: Ein neuariges katheter-system zur perkutanen transluminalen angioplastie von karotisstenosen. Fortschr Med 95:1007, 1977.
12. Kerber CW, Cromwell LD, Loehden OL: Catheter dilatation of proximal carotid stenosis during distal bifurcation endarterectomy. AJNR Am J Neuroradiol 1:348, 1980.
13. Mullan S, Duda EE, Patronas NJ: Some examples of balloon technology in neurosurgery. J Neurosurg 52:321, 1980.
14. Vitek JJ, Raymon BC, Oh SJ: Innominate artery angioplasty. Am J Neuroradiol 5:113, 1984.
15. Bockenheimer SA, Mathias K: Percutaneous transluminal angioplasty in arteriosclerotic internal carotid artery stenosis. AJNR Am J Neuroradiol 4:791, 1983.
16. Rabkin I, Germashev VG: Five-year experience with roentgenologically controlled endovascular nitinol prosthesis [In Russian]. Kardiologiia 30:11, 1990.
17. Theron J, Raymond J, Casasco A, et al: Percutaneous angioplasty of atherosclerotic and postsurgical stenosis of carotid arteries. AJNR Am J Neuroradiol 8:495, 1987.
18. Yadav JS, Roubin GS, Iyer S, et al: Elective stenting of the extracranial carotid arteries. Circulation 95:376, 1997.
19. Theron J, Courtheoux P, Alachkar F, et al: New triple coaxial catheter system for carotid angioplasty with cerebral protection. AJNR Am J Neuroradiol 11:869, 1990.
20. Theron JG: Protected angioplasty and stenting of atherosclerotic stenosis at the carotid artery bifurcation. Philadelphia, WB Saunders, 1998.
21. Henry M, Amor M, Henry I, et al: Carotid stenting with cerebral protection: First clinical experience using the PercuSurge GuardWire system. J Endovasc Surg 6:321, 1999.
22. Al-Mubarak N, Roubin GS, Vitek JJ, et al: Effect of the distal-balloon protection system on microembolization during carotid stenting. Circulation 104:1999, 2001.
23. Henry M, Henry I, Klonaris C, et al: Benefits of cerebral protection during carotid stenting with the PercuSurge GuardWire system: Midterm results. J Endovasc Ther 9:1, 2002.
24. Al-Mubarak N, Colombo A, Gaines PA, et al: Multicenter evaluation of carotid artery stenting with a filter protection system. J Am Coll Cardiol 39:841, 2002.
25. Sievert H, Rabe K: Role of distal protection during carotid stenting. J Interv Cardiol 5:499, 2002.
26. Iyer SS, Roubin GS, Vitek JJ, et al: Carotid artery stenting with neuroprotection. Circulation 39:30A, 2002.
27. Whitlow PL, Lylyk P, Londero H, et al: Carotid artery stenting protected with an emboli containment system. Stroke 33:1308, 2002.

28. Parodi JC, Schonholz C, Ferreira LM, et al: "Seat belt and air bag" technique for cerebral protection during carotid stenting. J Endovasc Ther 9:20, 2002.
29. Yadav J: Stenting and angioplasty with protection in patients at high risk for endarterectomy: The SAPPHIRE Study. Circulation 106:2, 2002.
30. Weisz G, Iyer S, Vitek J, et al: Distal protection devices improve the safety of carotid artery stenting: Analysis of over 1350 procedures. Circulation 108:IV-605, 2003.
31. Wholey MH, Wholey M, Mathias K, et al: Global experience in cervical carotid artery stent placement. Catheter Cardiovasc Interv 50:160, 2000.
32. Bergeon P, Rudondy P, Benichou H, et al: Transluminal angioplasty for recurrent stenosis after carotid endarterectomy: Prognostic factors and indications. Int Angiol 12:256, 1993.
33. Al-Mubarak N, Vitek JJ, Iyer SS, et al: Carotid stenting with distal-balloon protection via the transbrachial approach. J Endovasc Ther 8:571, 2001.
34. Theron JG, Payelle GG, Coskun O, et al: Carotid artery stenosis: Treatment with protected balloon angioplasty and stent placement. Radiology 201:627, 1996.
35. Gil-Peralta A, Mayol A, Marcos JR, et al: Percutaneous transluminal angioplasty of the symptomatic atherosclerotic carotid arteries: Results, complications, and follow-up. Stroke 27:2271, 1996.
36. Kachel R: Results of balloon angioplasty in the carotid arteries. J Endovasc Surg 3:22, 1996.
37. Munari LM, Belloni G, Perretti A, et al: Carotid percutaneous angioplasty. Neurol Res 14:156, 1992.
38. Endovascular versus surgical treatment in patients with carotid stenosis in the Carotid and Vertebral Artery Transluminal Angioplasty Study (CAVATAS): A randomised trial. Lancet 357: 1729, 2001.
39. Yadav SS, Roubin GS, Iyer SS, et al: Application of lessons learned from cardiac interventional techniques to carotid angioplasty. J Am Coll Cardiol 25:380A, 1995.
40. Yadav JS, Roubin GS, King P, et al: Angioplasty and stenting for restenosis after carotid endarterectomy: Initial experience. Stroke 27:2075, 1996.
41. Roubin GS, Yadav S, Iyer SS, et al: Carotid stent-supported angioplasty: A neurovascular intervention to prevent stroke. Am J Cardiol 78:8, 1996.
42. Roubin GS, New G, Iyer SS, et al: Immediate and late clinical outcomes of carotid artery stenting in patients with symptomatic and asymptomatic carotid artery stenosis: A 5-year prospective analysis. Circulation 103:532, 2001.
43. Biller J, Feinberg WM, Castaldo JE, et al: Guidelines for carotid endarterectomy: A statement for healthcare professionals from a Special Writing Group of the Stroke Council, American Heart Association. Circulation 97:501, 1998.
44. Yadav J, Ouriel K: Impact of medical vs. anatomic risk factors on 30-day and 1-year outcomes in the SAPPHIRE trial. Circulation 108:IV-603, 2003.
45. New G, GS R, Iyer S, et al: Distal protection improves outcomes from carotid stenting in octogenarians. Circulation 106:II-714, 2002.
46. Shawl FA: Carotid artery stenting: Acute and long-term results. Curr Opin Cardiol 17:671, 2002.
47. Rothwell PM, Slattery J, Warlow CP: Clinical and angiographic predictors of stroke and death from carotid endarterectomy: Systematic review. Br Med J 315:1571, 1997.
48. Goldstein LB, Samsa GP, Matchar DB, et al: Multicenter review of preoperative risk factors for endarterectomy for asymptomatic carotid artery stenosis. Stroke 29:750, 1998.
49. Vitek JJ: Femoro-cerebral angiography: Analysis of 2,000 consecutive examinations: Special emphasis on carotid arteries catheterization in older patients. Am J Roentgenol Radium Ther Nucl Med 118:633, 1973.
50. Vitek JJ, Powel DF, Anderson RD: Damage of the brachiocephalic vessels due to catheterization. Neurology 9:63, 1975.
51. Davies KN, Humphrey PR: Complications of cerebral angiography in patients with symptomatic carotid territory ischaemia screened by carotid ultrasound. J Neurol Neurosurg Psychiatry 56:967, 1993.
52. New G, Roubin GS, Oetgen ME, et al: Validity of duplex ultrasound as a diagnostic modality for internal carotid artery disease. Catheter Cardiovasc Interv 52:9, 2001.
53. Mathur A, Roubin GS, Yadav JS, et al: Combined coronary and bilateral carotid stenting: A case report. Cathet Cardiovasc Diagn 40:202, 1997.
54. Shawl FA: Carotid stenting in patients with symptomatic coronary artery disease: A preferred approach. J Invasive Cardiol 10:432, 1998.
55. Al-Mubarak N, Roubin GS, Vitek JJ, et al: Simultaneous bilateral carotid stenting for restenosis after endarterectomy. Cathet Cardiovasc Diagn 45:11, 1998.
56. Tepel M, van der Giet M, Schwarzfeld C, et al: Prevention of radiographic-contrast-agent-induced reductions in renal function by acetylcysteine. N Engl J Med 343:180, 2000.
57. Kay J, Chow WH, Chan TM, et al: Acetylcysteine for prevention of acute deterioration of renal function following elective coronary angiography and intervention: A randomized controlled trial. JAMA 289:553, 2003.
58. Birck R, Krzossok S, Markowetz F, et al: Acetylcysteine for prevention of contrast nephropathy: Meta-analysis. Lancet 362:598, 2003.
59. Muller I, Seyfarth M, Rudiger S, et al: Effect of a high loading dose of clopidogrel on platelet function in patients undergoing coronary stent placement. Heart 85:92, 2001.
60. Steinhubl SR, Berger PB, Mann I, et al: Early and sustained dual oral antiplatelet therapy following percutaneous coronary intervention. JAMA 288:2411, 2002.
61. Al-Mubarak N, Roubin GS, Vitek JJ, et al: Procedural safety and short-term outcome of ambulatory carotid stenting. Stroke 32:2305, 2001.
62. Robbin ML, Lockhart ME, Weber TM, et al: Carotid artery stents: Early and intermediate follow-up with Doppler US. Radiology 205:749, 1997.
63. Roffi M, Mukherjee D, Chan A, et al: Can ultrasound accurately predict restenosis after carotid artery stenting? [Abstract], Circulation 104:II-583, 2001.
64. Roubin GS, Vitek JJ, Iyer SS, et al: Carotid Artery Intervention. In: Stack RS, Roubin GS, O'Neill WW (eds): Interventional Cardiovascular Medicine. 2nd ed. Philadelphia, Churchill Livingstone, 2002, p 959.
65. Henry M, Amor M, Theron J, et al: Carotid Angioplasty and Stenting. Essey-les-Nancy: Groupe Composer, 1998.
66. Vitek JJ, Roubin GS, Al-Mubarek N, et al: Carotid artery stenting: Technical considerations. AJNR Am J Neuroradiol 21:1736, 2000.
67. Al-Mubarak N, Roubin GS, Vitek JJ, et al: Microembolization during carotid stenting with the distal-balloon antiemboli system. Int Angiol 21:344, 2000.
68. Beebe HG, Archie JP, Baker WH, et al: Concern about safety of carotid angioplasty. Stroke 27:197, 1996.
69. Weisz G, Vitek JJ, Brennan C, et al: Predilatation before distal protection device placement in stenting carotid arteries is successful and not associated with adverse outcome. J Am Coll Cardiol 43:90A, 2004.
70. Ohki T, Marin ML, Lyon RT, et al: Ex vivo human carotid artery bifurcation stenting: Correlation of lesion characteristics with embolic potential. J Vasc Surg 27:463, 1998.
71. Al-Mubarak NR, Vitek J, Iyer S: Microembolization during carotid stenting with the distal-balloon antiemboli system. Int Angiol 21:344, 2000.
72. Henry M, Amor M, Klonaris C, et al: Angioplasty and stenting of the extracranial carotid arteries. Tex Heart Inst J 27:150, 2000.
73. Jaeger H, Mathias K, Drescher R, et al: Clinical results of cerebral protection with a filter device during stent implantation of the carotid artery. Cardiovasc Intervent Radiol 24:249, 2001.
74. Parodi JC, La Mura R, Ferreira LM, et al: Initial evaluation of carotid angioplasty and stenting with three different cerebral protection devices. J Vasc Surg 32:1127, 2000.
75. Reimers B, Corvaja N, Moshiri S, et al: Cerebral protection with filter devices during carotid artery stenting. Circulation 104:12, 2001.
76. Tubler T, Schluter M, Dirsch O, et al: Balloon-protected carotid artery stenting: Relationship of periprocedural neurological complications with the size of particulate debris. Circulation 104:2791, 2001.
77. Angelini A, Reimers B, Della Barbera M, et al: Cerebral protection during carotid artery stenting: Collection and histopathologic analysis of embolized debris. Stroke 33:456, 2002.
78. Weisz G, Iyer S, Vitek J, et al: Comparison of filter (flow) vs. balloon (occlusion) distal protection devices in carotid artery stenting. Circulation 108:IV-605, 2003.
79. Mathur A, Roubin GS, Iyer SS, et al: Predictors of stroke complicating carotid artery stenting. Circulation 97:1239, 1998.

80. Diethrich EB, Ndiaye M, Reid DB. Stenting in the carotid artery: Initial experience in 110 patients. J Endovasc Surg 3:42, 1996.
81. Wholey MH, Jarmolowski CR, Eles G, et al: Endovascular stents for carotid artery occlusive disease. J Endovasc Surg 4:326, 1997.
82. Al-Mubarak N, Gomez CR, Vitek JJ, et al: Stenting of symptomatic stenosis of the intracranial internal carotid artery. AJNR Am J Neuroradiol 19:1949, 1998.
83. Bergeron P, Becquemin JP, Jausseran JM, et al: Percutaneous stenting of the internal carotid artery: The European CAST I Study. Carotid Artery Stent Trial. J Endovasc Surg 6:155, 1999.
84. Lanzino G, Mericle RA, Lopes DK, et al: Percutaneous transluminal angioplasty and stent placement for recurrent carotid artery stenosis. J Neurosurg 90:688, 1999.
85. New G, Roubin GS, Iyer SS, et al: Carotid artery stenting: Rationale, indications, and results. Compr Ther 25:438, 1999.
86. Qureshi AI, Luft AR, Janardhan V, et al: Identification of patients at risk for periprocedural neurological deficits associated with carotid angioplasty and stenting. Stroke 31:376, 2000.
87. Gupta A, Bhatia A, Ahuja A, et al: Carotid stenting in patients older than 65 years with inoperable carotid artery disease: A single-center experience. Catheter Cardiovasc Interv 50:1, 2000.
88. Shawl F, Kadro W, Domanski MJ, et al: Safety and efficacy of elective carotid artery stenting in high-risk patients. J Am Coll Cardiol 35:1721, 2000.
89. Ahmadi R, Willfort A, Lang W, et al: Carotid artery stenting: Effect of learning curve and intermediate-term morphological outcome. J Endovasc Ther 8:539, 2001.
90. Dietz A, Berkefeld J, Theron JG, et al: Endovascular treatment of symptomatic carotid stenosis using stent placement: Long-term follow-up of patients with a balanced surgical risk/benefit ratio. Stroke 32:1855, 2001.
91. Fox DJ, Jr., Moran CJ, Cross DT III, et al: Long-term outcome after angioplasty for symptomatic extracranial carotid stenosis in poor surgical candidates. Stroke 33:2877, 2002.
92. Wholey MH, Wholey M, Bergeron P, et al: Current global status of carotid artery stent placement. Cathet Cardiovasc Diagn 44:1, 1998.
93. Naylor AR, Bolia A, Abbott RJ, et al: Randomized study of carotid angioplasty and stenting versus carotid endarterectomy: A stopped trial. J Vasc Surg 28:326, 1998.
94. Alberts M: Results of a multicenter prospective randomized trial of carotid artery stenting vs. carotid endarterectomy. Stroke 32:325, 2001.
95. Gray WA: The Carotid Wallstent Trial: Do the results really favor endarterectomy? Presented at Transcatheter Cardiovascular Therapeutics (TCT), Washington D.C., 2002.
96. Brooks W, McClure RR, Jones MR, et al: Carotid angioplasty and stenting versus carotid endarterectomy: Randomized trial in a community hospital. J Am Coll Cardiol 38:1589, 2001.
97. New G, Roubin GS, Iyer S, et al: Outcomes from carotid artery stenting in over 1000 cases from a single group of operators. J Am Coll Cardiol 41:6, 2003.
98. Kastrup A, Groschel K, Krapf H, et al: Early outcome of carotid angioplasty and stenting with and without cerebral protection devices: A systematic review of the literature. Stroke 34:813, 2003.
99. Mathias K: IPSdSK, Dortmund, Germany. (Personal communication). 2002.
100. Guimaraens L, Sola MT, Matali A, et al: Carotid angioplasty with cerebral protection and stenting: Report of 164 patients (194 carotid percutaneous transluminal angioplasties. Cerebrovasc Dis 13:114, 2002.
101. Theiss W, Hermanek P, Mathias K, et al: Pro-CAS: A prospective registry of carotid angioplasty and stenting. Publication of the German Societies of Angiology and Radiology, Munich, 2002, p19.
102. Wholey M: Personal cummunication, 2003.
103. Whitlow P: Personal communication, 1993.
104. MRC European Carotid Surgery Trial: Interim results for symptomatic patients with severe (70-99%) or with mild (0-29%) carotid stenosis. European Carotid Surgery Trialists' Collaborative Group. Lancet 337:1235, 1991.
105. McCrory DC, Goldstein LB, Samsa GP, et al: Predicting complications of carotid endarterectomy. Stroke 24:1285, 1993.
106. O'Hara PJ, Hertzer NR, Mascha EJ, et al: Carotid endarterectomy in octogenarians: Early results and late outcome. J Vasc Surg 27:860, 1998.
107. Frericks H, Kievit J, van Baalen JM, et al: Carotid recurrent stenosis and risk of ipsilateral stroke: A systematic review of the literature. Stroke 29:244, 1998.
108. Carballo RE, Towne JB, Seabrook GR, et al: An outcome analysis of carotid endarterectomy: The incidence and natural history of recurrent stenosis. J Vasc Surg 23:749, 1996.
109. Ricotta JJ, O'Brien-Irr MS: Conservative management of residual and recurrent lesions after carotid endarterectomy: Long-term results. J Vasc Surg 26:963, 1997.
110. New G, Roubin GS, Iyer SS, et al: Safety, efficacy, and durability of carotid artery stenting for restenosis following carotid endarterectomy: A multicenter study. J Endovasc Ther 7:345, 2000.
111. Roubin GS: Personal communication, 2004.
112. White A: Carotid revascularization with endarterectomy or stenting systems (CARESS): Feasibility results. Circulation 108:IV-687, 2003.
113. Yadav J: SAPPHIRE: A prospective, randomized trial of carotid stenting vs. endarterectomy in high-risk patients. Presented at Transcatheter Cardiovascular Therapeutics (TCT), September 2003, Washington D.C.
114. Roubin GS, King SB III, Douglas JS, Jr: Restenosis after percutaneous transluminal coronary angioplasty: The Emory University Hospital experience. Am J Cardiol 60:39B, 1987.
115. Fischman DL, Leon MB, Baim DS, et al: A randomized comparison of coronary-stent placement and balloon angioplasty in the treatment of coronary artery disease. Stent Restenosis Study Investigators. N Engl J Med 331:496, 1994.
116. Mehran R, Dangas G, Abizaid AS, et al: Angiographic patterns of in-stent restenosis: Classification and implications for long-term outcome. Circulation 100:1872, 1999.
117. Leon MB, Teirstein PS, Moses JW, et al: Localized intracoronary gamma-radiation therapy to inhibit the recurrence of restenosis after stenting. N Engl J Med 344:250, 2001.
118. Hoffmann R, Mintz GS, Dussaillant GR, et al: Patterns and mechanisms of in-stent restenosis: A serial intravascular ultrasound study. Circulation 94:1247, 1996.
119. Kearney M, Pieczek A, Haley L, et al: Histopathology of in-stent restenosis in patients with peripheral artery disease. Circulation 95:1998, 1997.
120. Teirstein PS, Massullo V, Jani S, et al: Catheter-based radiotherapy to inhibit restenosis after coronary stenting. N Engl J Med 336:1697, 1997.
121. Kimura T, Nosaka H, Yokoi H, et al: Serial angiographic follow-up after Palmaz-Schatz stent implantation: Comparison with conventional balloon angioplasty. J Am Coll Cardiol 21:1557, 1993.
122. Vitek J, Iyer S, Roubin G: Carotid stenting in 350 vessels: Problems faced and solved. J Invasive Cardiol 10:311, 1998.
123. Bendok BR, Roubin GS, Katzen BT, et al: Cutting balloon to treat carotid in-stent stenosis: Technical note. J Invasive Cardiol 15: 227, 2003.
124. d'Audiffret A, Desgranges P, Kobeiter H, et al: Technical aspects and current results of carotid stenting. J Vasc Surg 33:1001, 2001.
125. Mehran R, Roubin GS, New G, et al: Neurologic events after carotid stenting with distal protection using an occlusion balloon: Final results from the CAFE-USA trial. Circulation 104:367, 2001.
126. Adami CA, Scuro A, Spinamano L, et al: Use of the Parodi anti-embolism system in carotid stenting: Italian trial results. J Endovasc Ther 9:147, 2002.
127. Cremonesi A, Manetti R, Setacci F, et al: Protected carotid stenting: Clinical advantages and complications of embolic protection devices in 442 consecutive patients. Stroke 34:1936, 2003.

chapter 33

Cerebrovascular Disease: Carotid Endarterectomy

Robert W. Hobson II

Carotid endarterectomy (CEA) has become the principal technique for cerebral revascularization in symptomatic[1-3] and asymptomatic[4,5] patients with extracranial carotid occlusive disease. Simultaneously, CEA has become the most commonly performed vascular operation and the most comprehensively studied procedure in the practice of vascular surgery. More than 140,000 operations are performed annually in the United States[6] and efficacy for the procedure has been established by rigorous randomized clinical trial methodology.[1-5]

Cerebrovascular disease constitutes the third leading cause of death in this country, resulting in over 150,000 deaths per year among nearly 700,000 strokes.[7-9] Thromboembolic disease accounts for the largest number of new strokes. Of these, carotid occlusive disease is probably the single most important causal factor in the development of cerebrovascular ischemia. Transient monocular blindness (TMB) or amaurosis fugax and transient ischemic attack (TIA) constitute important warning signs of impending stroke, and stroke prevention includes the recognition of these events during a careful history and interpretation of important physical findings. Medical management of identifiable risk factors including hypertension, hypercholesterolemia, cigarette smoking, diabetes, and history of coronary artery disease or atrial fibrillation contributes to optimal medical care, and should be used in patients selected for CEA.

HISTORICAL REVIEW

The ancient Greeks understood the importance of the carotid arteries because the term *carotid* is derived from the Greek word *karoo*, which means to stupefy. Compression of the carotid arteries was known to cause "sudden sleep."[10] Occlusive disease of the carotid and vertebral arteries was recognized and described by John James Wepner as a postmortem finding in 1658.[10] His contemporary Thomas Willis encountered similar findings in postmortem examinations and described communications between the carotid and vertebral arteries (Circle of Willis) which would provide for cerebral collateralization. For the next 200 years, strokes were attributed to intracranial rather than extracranial vascular disease.

In 1913, Ramsay Hunt[11] emphasized the relationship between extracranial carotid occlusive disease and stroke. He urged that, in all cases of cerebral symptoms of vascular origin, the main arteries of the neck be carefully examined for diminution or absence of pulsations. The definitive antemortem diagnosis of cerebrovascular disease became possible when Egaz Moniz of Lisbon developed cerebral angiography as a method for localizing cerebral tumors in 1927.[12]

In 1951, Fisher performed 373 postmortem examinations of the brain from patients who had died of cerebrovascular disease.[13] He made several salient observations. Hemorrhagic infarcts were present in fewer than 20% of his specimens; he therefore concluded that most cases of stroke were ischemic infarcts. Fisher also reported that atheroma tended to form at the extracranial carotid bifurcation, and he observed that arteries distal to the cervical carotid disease were frequently spared. He correctly indicated that extracranial carotid disease was an important cause of stroke, and speculated that vascular surgeons would find a way to bypass the occluded carotid segment in the neck by direct vascular anastomosis of the internal and external carotid systems above the area of stenosis.

Carrea, Molins, and Murphy,[14] three Argentinean surgeons, acknowledged the importance of Fisher's speculations. On cerebral angiography, they diagnosed a 41-year-old man who had recently developed aphasia and right hemiparesis as having a severe left internal carotid stenosis. On October 20, 1951, they performed the first successful vascular reconstruction for cerebral ischemia. Carrea and his colleagues resected the diseased portion of the left internal carotid and performed an end-to-end anastomosis between the external and distal internal carotid arteries. Their report was not published until the patient had made an uneventful recovery and after a 39-month follow-up that showed him to be neurologically intact. On January 28, 1953, Strully and colleagues[15] attempted a thromboendarterectomy of a totally occluded internal carotid artery without success, but these authors predicted that endarterectomy would be feasible prior to thrombosis if the distal vasculature were patent. The first successful CEA was performed in this country by Michael DeBakey on August 7, 1953.[16] The patient was a 53-year-old bus driver with a 30-month history of intermittent weakness in the right arm and leg. A thromboendarterectomy of the common and internal carotid arteries was undertaken and the arteriotomy closed primarily. An intraoperative arteriogram confirmed patency of the distal circulation. The patient survived

19 more years without recurrence of symptoms. However, it was the report in 1954 by Eastcott, Pickering, and Rob[17] that captured the imagination of vascular surgeons. Their patient was a 60-year-old housewife with recurrent ocular and cerebral TIAs. On angiography, a near occlusion of the internal carotid was observed. She underwent resection of the left internal carotid, ligation of the external carotid artery, and an end-to-end anastomosis between the common and internal carotid arteries. Twenty-six years after her operation, she was still symptom free.

The success of these early operations accompanied by long symptom-free periods of survival has made CEA one of the most commonly performed vascular operations in the United States. Data from randomized clinical trials resolved controversy over the efficacy of CEA combined with best medical care versus optimal medical therapy alone in the management of extracranial carotid occlusive disease. With the acceptance of uniform indications for operation[18,19] and expected results, CEA can be recommended for the treatment of symptomatic and asymptomatic extracranial carotid occlusive disease.

PATHOGENESIS

The pathophysiology of stroke as a result of carotid artery disease is a subject of ongoing clinical research. A detailed understanding of the pathogenesis of cerebral ischemia is as essential as an accurate knowledge of the natural history of carotid artery stenosis in developing a rational therapeutic program for extracranial vascular occlusive disease.

In the early 1950s, Fisher[13] described a variety of pathologic changes occurring in the carotid arteries of patients dying of stroke. He recognized the two basic mechanisms by which a carotid artery lesion produced ischemia (1) embolization from irregular luminal surfaces, usually but not exclusively associated with an ulcerated plaque; and (2) decreased flow from a narrowed or occluded internal carotid artery. These observations were verified clinically in the 1968 report of the Joint Study of Extracranial Arterial Occlusions,[20] which reported that approximately 75% of the more than 4000 patients studied had significant extracranial arterial lesions, producing greater than 30% stenosis as shown by aortic arch and cerebral angiography. Stenosis occurred more frequently than did occlusion, and the carotid arterial bifurcation was the most frequently involved site (34%), followed by origins in the vertebral artery (20%). These findings, together with the then newly recognized significance of cholesterol emboli to the retina (Hollenhorst plaques),[21] confirmed that cerebral ischemia could occur from either mechanism.

Atherosclerosis, the most common cause of extracranial carotid artery stenosis in humans, is an intimal disease, with secondary changes occurring in the media of the artery. Several theories concerning the formation of these plaques have been proposed and modified during the last century. Ross and Glomset[22] postulated a "reaction-to-injury hypothesis," which proposed that injury to the endothelium was the initiating event in atherogenesis. They reported that the endothelium responds to injury in a variety of ways, including endothelial desquamation, with loss of its nonthrombogenic character and local secretion of growth factors with minimal or no morphologic alteration of the involved endothelium. Platelets adhere to the exposed subendothelial connective tissue and release the contents of their granules. Chemotactic and mitogenic factors such as platelet-derived growth factor (PDGF), epidermal growth factor (EGF) and other cytokines induce the proliferation of smooth muscle cells and their migration from the media to the intima.

Atherosclerosis also shows a predilection for developing in specific vascular sites, including the Circle of Willis and the extracranial carotid artery system. In particular, these sites include bifurcations and areas of anatomic arterial curvature. Hydrogen bubble flow visualization and velocity profile studies (Fig. 33-1) have demonstrated that flow in the common carotid artery is laminar.[23] Decrease in the velocity of blood flow from the core to periphery is known as the velocity gradient. Because each fluid lamina travels at its own speed, it exerts a force on an immediately adjacent lamina traveling at a different speed; this force is referred to as *shear stress.* When a column of blood traveling with laminar flow reaches the carotid bifurcation, it separates at the flow divider formed by the internal and external carotid branches (Fig. 33-2). Flow laminae are compressed toward the flow divider, and flow remains laminar, with a high-velocity profile and an associated high wall shear stress.

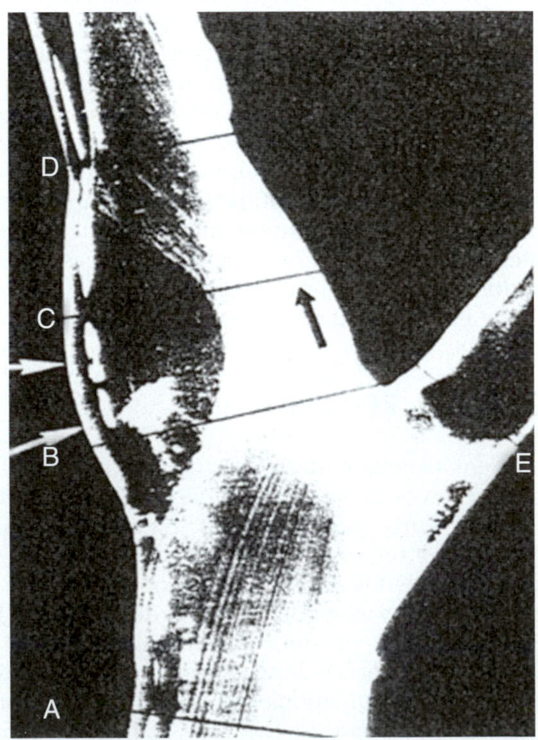

FIGURE 33-1. Hydrogen bubble flow visualization technique in a glass model human carotid bifurcation shows laminar flow in the inner wall of the bulb (*arrow*) and area of flow separation in the outer wall where the atherosclerotic plaque localizes (**B-D**). (Reproduced, with permission, from. Zarins CK, Giddens DP, Bharadvaj BK, et al: Carotid bifurcation atherosclerosis: Quantitative correlation of plaque localization with flow velocity profiles and wall shear stress. Circ Res 53:502, 1983.)

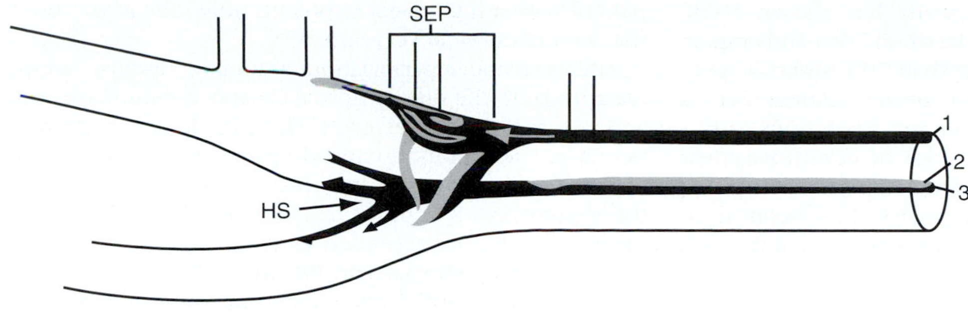

FIGURE 33-2. Dye flow visualization technique in an acrylic model human carotid bifurcation at the flow divider (HS) shows boundary layer separation (SEP) at the level of the outer wall of the bulb where the atherosclerotic plaque localizes. Laminar flow (2-3) is observed centrally, which is disrupted at the arterial wall laterally (1). (Reproduced, with permission, from LoGerfo FW, Nowak MD, Quist WC: Structural details of boundary layer separation in a model human carotid bifurcation under steady and pulsatile flow conditions. J Vasc Surg 2:263, 1985.)

Flow patterns, nonetheless, retain their axial and unidirectional alignment. Along the outer wall of the widened carotid bulb, however, flow patterns become complex and include areas of flow separation and reversal with the development of counter-rotating helical trajectories. In this region, the wall shear stress is low. In the distal bulb and the distal internal carotid, flow resumes laminar conditions linked to a high velocity and high wall shear stress.[24] Contrast media washout and particle tracking studies have also shown decreased clearance of particles opposite to the flow divider in the region of low velocity and shear stress. These flow properties are thus associated with an increased residence time for atherogenic blood-borne cellular elements that are given an increased probability of adhering, interacting, and possibly injuring the endothelium, leading to atherogenic plaque formation. Hemodynamic changes secondary to the unique geometry of the carotid bifurcation result in the creation of an environment susceptible to atherogenic plaque formation.

These factors contribute to the formation of an atherosclerotic plaque at the carotid bifurcation, which leads to a variety of complications, depending on whether the plaque ulcerates and creates emboli or hemorrhages or fractures, leading to increasingly severe arterial stenosis and possible thrombosis. Imparato and colleagues[25] analyzed the histologic and gross morphology characteristics of 69 carotid plaques from 50 symptomatic patients; these investigators reported that although great variability in plaque morphology was found, 65% of the specimens exhibited some degree of intraplaque hemorrhage. A prospective study of 376 carotid plaques (275 symptomatic, 101 asymptomatic) obtained as endarterectomy specimens in 280 patients demonstrated a correlation between plaque morphology and symptoms. Ulceration was found to be the most frequent gross morphologic characteristic, but hemorrhage was the only gross characteristic that was significantly more frequent in plaques from symptomatic patients than in those from asymptomatic patients. Intraplaque hemorrhage also correlated significantly with the degree of stenosis present.[26] Other studies in asymptomatic patients with greater than 60% carotid stenosis have reported intraplaque hemorrhages in nearly all specimens and ulcerations and/or recent mural thrombi in half of them.[27] Atherosclerotic stenosis—with or without plaque ulceration, rupture, and hemorrhage—remains the greatest risk factor for carotid atheroemboli or thrombosis. Recently, analysis of carotid plaques by pixel distribution analysis of B-mode ultrasonograms has demonstrated its potential to identify plaque components more characteristic of asymptomatic or symptomatic plaques.[28]

ANGIOGRAPHY

Cerebral angiography is the most complete preoperative study for anatomic delineation of the carotid arteries and their intracranial branches. In the patient considered a candidate for CEA, angiographic examination includes bilateral visualization of the extracranial arteries, evaluation of hemispheric blood flow, and aortic arch imaging. Selective views are added to aid in the diagnosis of ulcerative lesions and provide additional information on the vertebrobasilar system. Angiography can also help rule out other causes of neurologic symptoms, such as siphon and branch stenoses, cerebral aneurysms, tumors, and arteriovenous malformation.

The invasive nature of cerebral angiography coupled with its reported 1.2% risk of stroke,[5] and high cost has led to increasing use of duplex ultrasound for the selection of patients for CEA. Angiography also requires needle puncture of an artery which may be diseased in many of these patients, making the procedure painful and technically difficult. The injection of a contrast medium can cause transient renal dysfunction or lead to dependency on renal dialysis in high-risk patients.[29] Mechanical injury from catheter manipulation can result in acute arterial occlusion, distal embolization, arterial dissection, and hematoma formation. Furthermore, neurovascular complications such as TIAs and strokes have also been reported.[30] Carotid artery thrombosis can occur in patients with plaque dissection or a "string sign" (greater than 90% luminal narrowing) at the time of angiography. The overall incidence of complications following angiography ranges from 0.2% to 2%.

Magnetic resonance angiography (MRA) has been introduced to overcome the limitations seen with duplex scanning. It is not operator-dependent, it can assess the intracranial circulation and aortic arch, and calcified vessels do not obstruct its signals. A comparison study of

MRA, duplex scan, and angiography has shown 100% sensitivity and 92% specificity between MRA and angiography when lesions with greater than 70% stenosis were studied.[31] The greater cost and limited patient access associated with MRA are the principal objections to this test being used as a screening tool of cerebrovascular disease rather than duplex scanning. Recently, computed tomographic angiography (CTA) also has been used effectively to measure arterial cross-sectional reduction and characterize plaque composition.[32]

DESCRIPTION OF CAROTID ENDARTERECTOMY

Preparation of the patient for CEA includes the establishment of an adequate intravenous route for fluid replacement, and strict pharmacologic control of blood pressure. An intraarterial catheter in the radial artery is employed for continuous monitoring of arterial blood pressure. The systolic arterial blood pressure is regulated within the 20 to 30 mm Hg of the patient's baseline pressure to prevent hypo- or hypertension. General anesthesia is preferred by the author; however, local anesthesia or cervical block anesthesia may be employed based on the preference of the surgeon or anesthesiologist.

The skin incision may follow the anterior border of the sternocleidomastoid; alternatively, a transverse incision may be considered. The incision is extended through the platysma and superficial cervical fascia, and the sternocleidomastoid is mobilized along its anterior border. Next, the anteromedial border of the internal jugular vein is mobilized for its length, and the common facial vein, which usually marks the carotid bifurcation, is ligated and divided along with any other medial venous tributaries. A self-retaining retractor is used to displace the sternomastoid muscle and the internal jugular vein laterally and posteriorly, which allows unobstructed visualization of the bulb and surrounding sheath (Fig. 33-3A). Division of the ansa hypoglossi which supplies the strap muscles of the neck may be unavoidable and produces no residual weakness. It also becomes useful in retracting the hypoglossal nerve atraumatically in cases requiring higher exposure of the internal carotid artery. The common, external, and internal carotid arteries are isolated by sharp dissection. Manipulation of the carotid bulb and proximal internal carotid artery is avoided to preclude dislodging intraluminal debris. Should bradycardia or hypotension be observed during the dissection of the carotid bulb, 0.5 to 1.0 ml of 1.0% lidocaine is injected at the bifurcation into the area of the carotid body nerve.[33] Generally, dissection is carried superiorly on the internal carotid artery until the hypoglossal nerve is identified. Surgical dissection is more difficult when the bifurcation of the common carotid is anatomically high in the neck and distal exposure of the internal carotid artery is restricted by the overlying ramus of the mandible. Division of the posterior belly on the digastric muscle and gentle downward traction of the internal carotid are also used to facilitate its exposure. Mandibular subluxation, accompanied by nasotracheal intubation, can be used in the unusual patient with a high distal exposure, generally at or above the second cervical vertebra.[34,35]

After systemic heparinization, atraumatic vascular clamps are applied to the distal internal carotid, common carotid, and external carotid arteries. The carotid arteriotomy is begun in the common carotid artery in its anterolateral location and continued into the internal carotid artery for approximately 3 to 4 cm, (see Fig. 33-3B). The arteriotomy should be extended beyond all grossly visible disease in the internal carotid artery. When a shunt is used, the distal end is first inserted into the proximal internal carotid artery and backbleeding expels air or atheromatous debris from the shunt before its insertion into the common carotid artery. The shunt is secured using an appropriate atraumatic vascular clamps or Rummel tourniquets.

The endarterectomy is begun at the site of greatest disease, generally the posterolateral carotid bulb, using a Freer elevator, and carried distally into the internal carotid artery. A plane is developed between the diseased intima and the circular medial fibers to achieve a feathering of the plaque at its distal end on the internal carotid artery (see Fig. 33-3C). If the observed endpoint is irregular or associated with an intimal flap, the arteriotomy must be extended beyond the limit of the established endpoint and a new endpoint established. The distal intima can also be secured by use of interrupted tacking sutures. Proximally, the plaque is transected sharply with Pott scissors in the common carotid artery. The plaque is extracted from the external carotid artery by eversion endarterectomy. The endarterectomized surface of the carotid artery is inspected carefully, irrigated with heparinized saline, and shreds of residual tissue removed by gentle teasing in a transverse direction. Primary arterial closure can be performed using fine monofilament vascular suture (6-0 or 7-0) from each direction. However, during the last 15 years, patch closure with saphenous vein or synthetic materials (see Fig. 33-3D) has been recommended for the purposes of reducing perioperative stroke and death,[36,37] as well as restenosis.[38,39] AbuRahma[40] reported a randomized clinical trial in which CEA with patch angioplasty (vein or PTFE) was less likely than primary closure to cause perioperative stroke. Although his group[41] has expressed concern about the higher incidence of perioperative stroke and recurrent stenosis observed with use of Dacron patches, O'Hara and colleagues[42] recently reported no significant differences in patch closure with vein or Dacron. The shunt is then removed, the arteries are flushed with heparinized saline, vascular clamps are reapplied, and the closure is completed expeditiously.

If satisfactory hemostasis is achieved, heparin reversal with protamine is unnecessary prior to closure of the skin incision.[43] Reversal of heparin by protamine sulfate has also been reported to increase the incidence of postendarterectomy stroke.[44] Consequently, care must be exercised in deciding to reverse the effects of heparin. Intraoperative Doppler assessment of the internal carotid artery is performed to check adequacy of flow. If there is any doubt about the adequacy of flow, intraoperative ultrasonography or arteriography is recommended. Any unsuspected technical defect visible on

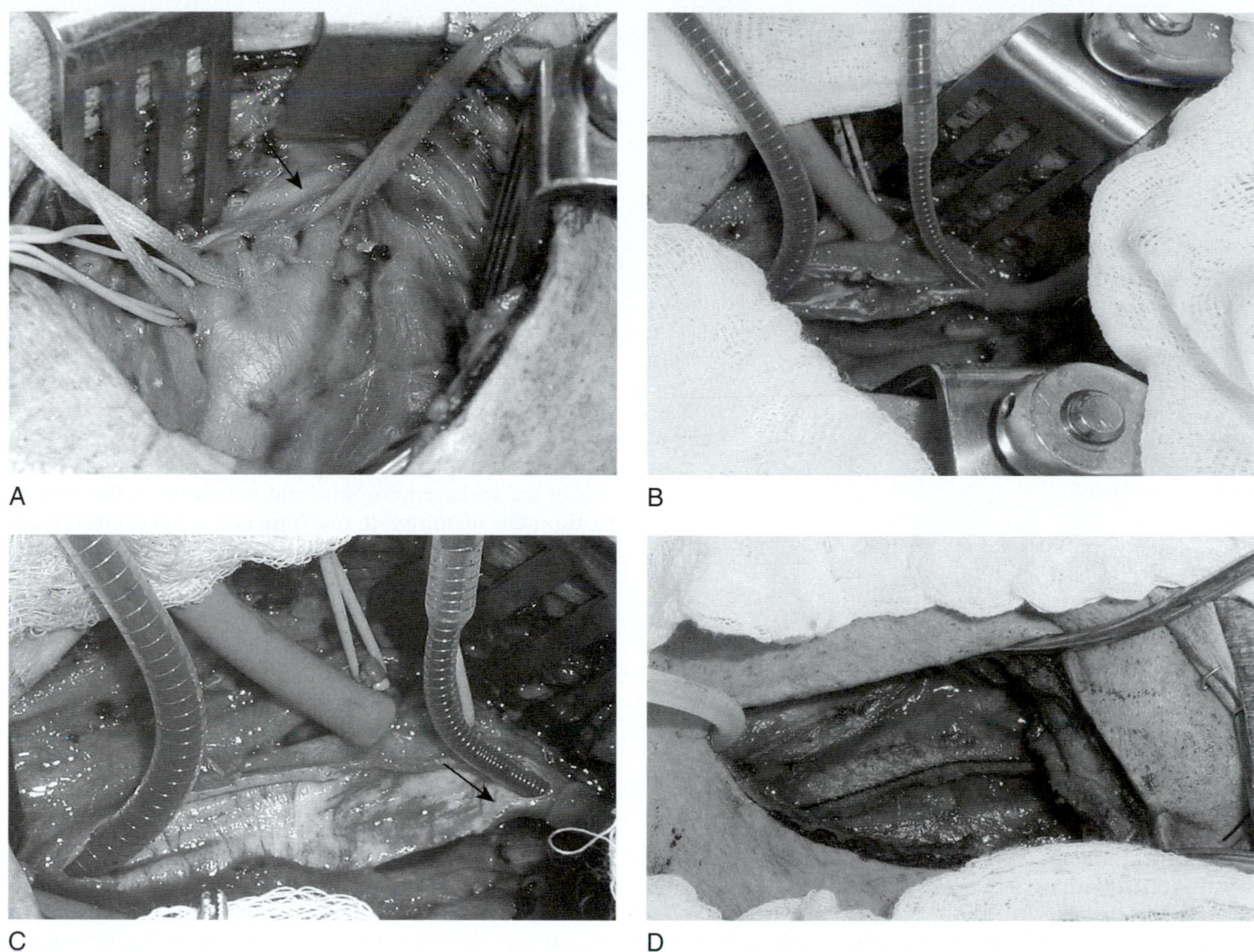

FIGURE 33-3. (See also Color Plate 33-3.) **A,** Exposure of the carotid bifurcation. The hypoglossal nerve (*arrow*) is seen superiorly crossing the internal carotid artery. **B,** An arteriotomy has been made exposing an ulcerative plaque and shunt placement. **C,** The operative site illustrates the fine tapering of the distal plaque (*arrow*) removed from the internal carotid artery. **D,** Patch angioplasty using Dacron.

arteriogram must be repaired, which generally then indicates patch closure, if primary closure was used initially. The skin incision is closed in layers using interrupted sutures to reapproximate the platysma muscle and a continuous subcuticular suture is used to close the skin. A closed suction drain is routinely employed and removed the next morning postoperatively. On completion of the operation, the patient is monitored in the recovery unit or intensive care unit for abnormalities in blood pressure, arrhythmias, or the development of neurological deficits. If stable after 3 to 4 hours, the patient may be transferred to a surgical floor without need for further intensive care. Antiplatelet therapy (aspirin) is begun perioperatively and maintained postoperatively. Most patients are discharged on the first (80%) or second postoperative day.[45,46]

Cerebral embolization of platelet aggregates or atheromatous material from the carotid plaque is probably the most important cause of neurological deficits or strokes in the postoperative period (Table 33-1). Rough or excessive handling of the carotid bifurcation, inadequate removal of loose medial fibers after endarterectomy, and the technically improper use of a shunt all increase the likelihood of emboli. The second cause of operative neurologic deficits is cerebral ischemia from inadequate or impaired collateral circulation. Cerebral ischemia may also result from hypotension during the operative procedure, leading to arterial thrombosis of intracerebral arteries. A reliable method to ensure adequate cerebral blood flow during carotid clamping is the use of a temporary indwelling shunt. However, most patients can tolerate temporary carotid clamping without deleterious effects, as has been reported by judging the patient's conscious response to carotid clamping during endarterectomies performed under local anesthesia.[47] To maximize benefits and minimize complications, a temporary shunt may be used routinely or selectively based on neurologic testing with the patient under local anesthesia, when the internal carotid artery back pressure is low (less than 50 mmHg), or when electroencephalographic changes occur following carotid clamping.[48] However, patients with a history of stroke, bilateral carotid disease, or contralateral occlusion are generally considered shunt candidates.

TABLE 33-1 COMPLICATIONS OF CAROTID ENDARTERECTOMY

Wound

Hematoma
Infection

Surgical Technique

Carotid artery
- Disruption
- False aneurysm
- Carotid-cavernous arteriovenous fistula
- Graft infection

Cranial nerve injury
Embolism
Cerebral ischemia

Postoperative Period

Stroke
- Thrombosis of endarterectomized segment
- Hypotension
- Hypertension
- Intracranial hemorrhage—reperfusion syndrome

Myocardial infarction
Recurrent stenosis

From Wilson SE, Hobson RW II: Extracranial carotid occlusive disease. In Hobson RW II, Wilson SE, Veith SJ (eds): Vascular Surgery: Principles and Practice, Marcel Dekker, New York, 2004.

Technical errors, cerebral emboli, and carotid thrombosis—not inadequate collateral flow—account for most of the neurologic deficits after CEA. Therefore, in the patient who awakens with a neurologic deficit or a suspected stroke in the early postoperative period, surgical re-exploration may be indicated.[47] Noninvasive carotid artery assessment is less reliable postoperatively, and angiography delays the potential therapeutic correction of cerebral ischemia. At reoperation, carotid blood flow is assessed using Doppler examination. If the internal carotid is found to be patent, an arteriogram is obtained through a common carotid puncture proximal to the endarterectomy site. If a pulseless thrombosed carotid is found or significant irregularities are noted on operative angiography, the patient is heparinized, and the endarterectomy site explored. The arteriotomy is opened and the internal carotid is allowed to backbleed to remove any thrombus that may have formed distally. If no backbleeding is observed, a Fogarty catheter may be introduced and a thrombectomy restricted to the extracranial cervical carotid artery is performed. Once backbleeding is established, a temporary shunt is inserted to ensure restoration of cerebral blood flow. If technical errors are observed, revision of the operative site is indicated. Patch angioplasty with saphenous vein is recommended and a completion arteriogram is obtained to confirm a technically satisfactory result. An algorithm[49] for the management of stroke after CEA (Fig. 33-4) has been helpful. Thrombosis is the most common cause of postoperative stroke following CEA, and prompt re-exploration is associated with neurologic improvement in many patients.[50]

Transient postoperative dysfunction of the hypoglossal, recurrent laryngeal, or marginal mandibular branch of the facial nerve has also been reported following CEA.[51] Injury to either the vagus nerve or recurrent laryngeal nerve produces paralysis of the ipsilateral vocal cord, hoarseness, and loss of an effective cough mechanism. In the patient with a history of prior CEA or thyroidectomy, preoperative laryngoscopy is useful to evaluate vocal cord function. Bilateral recurrent laryngeal *or* vagal nerve injuries may be life threatening because of airway obstruction, and tracheostomy may be required. Vagal nerve injury may also occur during dissection of the carotid artery or by entrapment of the nerve by incorrect placement of a clamp or retractor at the time of common carotid occlusion. Because of its proximity to the carotid bifurcation, the hypoglossal nerve is also at high risk for injury. Trauma to this nerve results in paralysis of the ipsilateral tongue and deviation of the tongue to the side of injury. If the injury is severe, clumsiness during speech and mastication can occur. The marginal mandibular branch lies between the platysma and the deep cervical fascia, and may be injured due to pressure from a self-retaining retractor or a poorly placed incision. Injury to the nerve is associated with a temporary or, at times, a permanent drooping of the corner of the mouth on the operated side.

Alterations of blood pressure after CEA are associated with transient and permanent neurologic deficits as well as myocardial infarction. Hypertension and hypotension have been reported in up to 66% of patients following CEA,[52] making their management an important overall aspect of patient care. Transient hypotension and bradycardia are occasionally observed owing to stimulation of the carotid body nerve[53] and can be controlled with injection of 0.5 to 1.0 ml of 1% lidocaine into the nerve at the bifurcation. Persistent postoperative hypotension usually responds to fluid administration if the patient's central venous pressure is low, but a few patients require administration of a vasoconstrictor such as Neo-Synephrine or phenylephrine. Careful cardiac monitoring is a must if vasopressors are employed. Postoperative hypertension probably occurs secondary to a loss or alteration of cerebrovascular autoregulation. Cerebral hyperperfusion, subclinical cerebral edema, and elevated intracranial pressure, alone or in combination, lead to an increase of central and peripheral norepinephrine levels and a subsequent elevation of the systemic blood pressure.[54] Good preoperative blood pressure control aids in the prevention of postoperative hypertension; but if the systolic blood pressure rises above 180 mm Hg or the diastolic pressure exceeds 100 mm Hg, intravenous vasodilators or short-acting β-blockers must be used to bring the blood pressure into the range of 140 to 160 mm Hg. Oral preoperative antihypertensive agents should be restarted as soon as the patient can tolerate them. Postoperative hypertension is associated with as high as a 10% incidence of neurologic deficits, which are prolonged with permanent deficits in 20% of patients.[55]

Headaches and seizures are unusual neurologic complications associated with CEA. Although minor headaches are occasionally encountered in the postoperative period, severe headaches are rare. They may be attributed to increased flow following endarterectomy

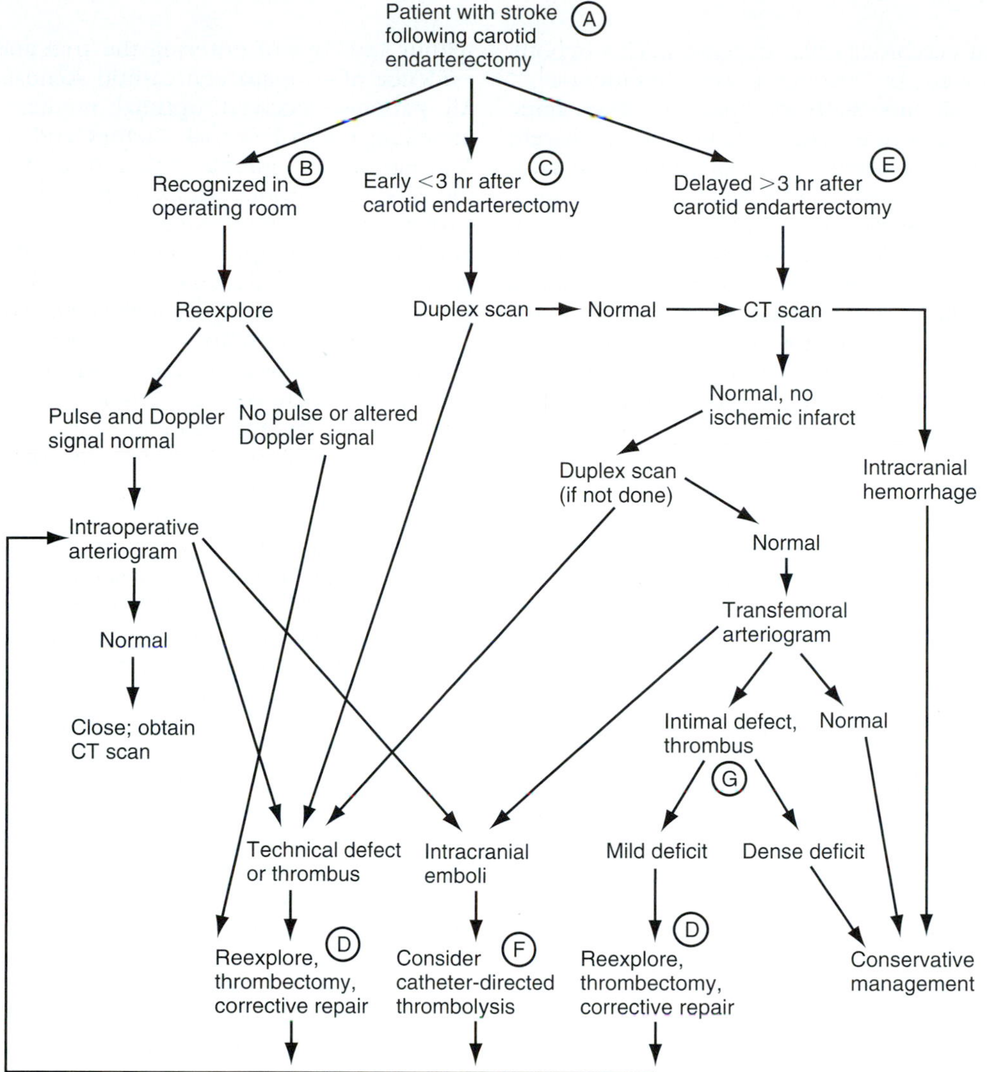

FIGURE 33-4. Mechanisms responsible for postoperative stroke have been classified in great detail by Riles and colleagues. Most of these events could be assigned to three broad etiologic categories: (1), stroke resulting from inadequate cerebral perfusion or embolization during the carotid endarterectomy; (2) stroke due to embolization or fresh thrombus or thrombotic occlusion after restoration of flow in the carotid artery; and (3) stroke from intracerebral hemorrhage—probably associated with reperfusion injury. **A,** More than 50% of the postendarterectomy neurologic events are related to the first two of these three categories. On careful review of the VA Study, four of five postoperative strokes were associated with technical errors at the endarterectomy site. The mechanism of stroke will obviously influence postoperative management, but at the outset, the cause may be suspected but is unknown. Therefore, clinical decisions are best keyed initially to the time of stroke discovery and to the findings of appropriate imaging studies. **B,** If general anesthesia is used, patients should be awakened in the operating room so that neurologic status can be assessed. If it is apparent that the patient has experienced a postoperative stroke, we recommend reintubation and exploration of the wound. If there is no carotid artery pulse or if the Doppler signal is abnormal, the arteriotomy is reopened and appropriate corrective measures are carried out. If the pulse and Doppler interrogation are normal, an intraoperative arteriogram is performed including intracranial views. The management of specific findings is discussed subsequently. If the arteriogram is normal, the arteriotomy and neck incision are closed and a CT scan of the brain is obtained later. If ambiguity exists concerning the presence or absence of lateralizing signs or symptoms, the patient is transferred to the recovery room. **C,** If a stroke occurs or is discovered during the first 1 to 3 hours postoperatively, a duplex ultrasound scan is obtained expeditiously. If the scan reveals occlusion, stenosis, or low flow, re-exploration is performed. If the scan is negative, a CT scan is performed to evaluate the presence or absence of intracerebral hemorrhage, which, if present, would indicate medical management. If the CT scan is negative, percutaneous (transfemoral) arteriography is recommended to direct further therapy. **D,** The details of immediate or early re-exploration for a thrombosed or technically defective carotid endarterectomy are beyond the scope of these comments, but briefly they involve (1) gentle removal of any thrombus present; (2) correction of technical defects; and (3) closure with vein patch angioplasty. A completion arteriogram is indicated to confirm a good result and to exclude distal emboli. **E,** For delayed strokes, a CT scan is obtained to evaluate the presence or absence of intracerebral hemorrhage, which for delayed stroke is generally a part of the reperfusion injury syndrome. If no hemorrhage is found, a duplex scan is performed to direct further therapy. If a technical defect or significant thrombus is found, it can be dealt with by reoperation if the evaluation has been expeditious, as it may be for an early in-hospital event. If the delay exceeds 3 hours after the occurrence of stroke, however, observation becomes appropriate. If the CT and duplex scans are normal, transfemoral arteriography is recommended to exclude an intimal flap, intracranial embolism, or other cause. **F,** Arteriographic evidence of an intracranial carotid branch occlusion should stimulate consideration for selective thrombolytic therapy delivered to the area of thrombus distal to the endarterectomy via microcatheter. With the decision to proceed with thrombolytic therapy, it should be recognized that its value in the postoperative patient versus its associated complications has not been rigorously evaluated and its use is based on anecdotal case experience. However, in institutions with rapid response evaluation of stroke victims within 3 hours of the event, this option can be considered. **G,** Most agree that operating in the presence of a dense neurologic deficit may be associated with higher risk. The area between a mild and severe deficit will continue to be unclear in the absence of better early markers of ischemic damage to the cerebral microcirculation and definitive comparative studies. Elapsed time after a stroke may also influence the choice of operative or conservative therapy. Beyond a certain short interval (~3 hours), the risk of operation on acute strokes and exacerbation of the ischemic injury or risk of intracranial hemorrhage escalates.

and subsequent cerebrovascular distention. This hypothesis is supported by the increased incidence of headaches in patients with preoperative high-grade carotid stenosis or severe hypertension postoperatively. Severe headaches localized to the operated side have also been found to correlate with the onset of seizures. Seizures are also observed with increased incidence in patients with high-grade carotid stenosis or presence of prior strokes. CT scans are usually normal or unchanged and carotid repairs are patent in these patients. Furthermore, an increase of more than 100% in cerebral blood flow has been documented in patients with postoperative seizures following CEA.[56] The patient with a high-grade stenosis or prior stroke who develops a severe ipsilateral headache following CEA should be started prophylactically on phenytoin. The patient who develops seizures should also be started on anticonvulsants, and CT scan or MRI of the head must be obtained to rule out the presence of cerebral hemorrhage.[57]

RANDOMIZED CLINICAL TRIALS

The key issue is whether the risks of stroke and stroke/death are reduced after CEA in patients also receiving optimal medical care versus optimal medical management alone. Before 1991, the only large randomized prospective study that compared operative and medical treatment appeared in 1970.[20] This study demonstrated that although patients randomized to CEA had a lower incidence of stroke and death during long-term follow-up, this benefit was offset by a high perioperative stroke rate of 12%. Previously, the appropriateness of CEA was criticized when the Rand Corporation randomly reviewed 1302 Medicare claims received for the performance of this operation in three different geographic areas in 1981.[58] Two thirds of the patients were judged to have had the operation for equivocal or inappropriate reasons. Equally alarming was the finding that 9.8% of the patients suffered a major complication: stroke with residual deficit at the time of discharge or death within 30 days of surgery. These authors concluded that CEA was overused in this country and that the procedure should be limited to the hospitals and surgeons with highest standards and lowest rates of complications. These concerns led to the initiation of multicenter randomized trials evaluating the efficacy of CEA combined with best medical care versus medical therapy alone in the prevention of stroke and death. Results of these clinical trials have determined indications for CEA and its role in the prevention of stroke.

SPECIFIC TRIALS

The NASCET (North American Symptomatic CEA Trial) trial was conducted at centers primarily located in the United States and Canada.[1] Participating surgeons reported a less than 6%, 30-day perioperative morbidity and mortality (the average for participating surgeons was 3.4% by their audited past records). Patients were eligible for the trial if they were younger than 80 years of age with a hemispheric TIA or a nondisabling stroke within 180 days of entering the trial and angiographic evidence of an ipsilateral carotid stenosis 30% to 99%. All patients received optimal medical management, including control of risk factors and aspirin therapy. A group of 659 patients with a 70% to 99% stenosis of the internal carotid artery and either a nondisabling stroke (32%) or one or more TIAs (68%) underwent randomization into optimal medical therapy alone (331 patients) or medical management combined with operative intervention (328 patients). The perioperative stroke morbidity and mortality rate was 5.8% for the surgical group, with a mortality rate of less than 1%. During a period of similar duration, there was just over a 3% stroke morbidity and mortality for the medical group. After a 2-year follow-up by life-table analysis, 26% of the medically treated patients but only 9% of the surgical patients had experienced a fatal or nonfatal ipsilateral stroke. An absolute risk reduction of 17% at 2 years for any ipsilateral stroke was observed for patients who underwent CEA.[1] A secondary analysis of these patients with high-grade stenosis showed that those with less severe stenosis (70% to 79%) had a lower risk of stroke; therefore their gains from surgical intervention were smaller than those of patients with more severe stenoses (90% to 99%).

Among patients with stenoses of 50% to 69%, efficacy of CEA was also confirmed.[59] The 5-year rate of any ipsilateral stroke (failure rate) was 15.7% among patients treated surgically and 22.2% among those treated medically ($P = 0.045$). CEA was less effective in this group of patients with moderate stenoses. Conversely, among patients with less than 50% stenosis, CEA was not effective with a reported failure rate in the surgical group (14.9%) which was not significantly different than the medically treated group (18.7%, $P = 0.16$).

Complementary beneficial results were observed in the European Carotid Surgery Trial (ECST)[2] and the Veterans Administration symptomatic endarterectomy trial.[3] The ECST was initiated in 1981 and involved 80 centers in 14 European countries. It was designed to randomize patients who had experienced a TIA, transient monocular blindness, or nondisabling ischemic stroke attributable to ipsilateral proximal carotid occlusive disease to CEA combined with best medical care (60% of the patients) versus best medical care alone. Best medical care included aspirin administration, treatment of any essential hypertension, and advice to quit smoking. The patients were stratified into three groups: mild (less than 30%); moderate (30% to 69%); or severe (70% to 99%) carotid stenosis.

An interim report issued in 1991,[2] 10 years after the initiation of this trial, showed that 778 symptomatic patients with severe (70% to 99%) carotid stenosis underwent randomization into immediate operative intervention (455 patients) or medical therapy alone (323 patients). The total risk of surgical death, surgical stroke, ipsilateral ischemic stroke, or any other stroke was 12.9% for the surgical group and 21.9% for the medical group at a follow-up of 3 years ($P < 0.05$), thus, confirming the efficacy of CEA, despite a 30-day stroke and death rate of 7.5%.

In the same report, 374 patients who had mild carotid stenosis (0% to 29%) were randomized into surgical (219 patients) or medical (155 patients) therapy. At a

3-year follow-up, there was little risk of ipsilateral stroke in the medical or surgical group; the perioperative stroke morbidity and mortality rate of CEA erased any benefit that surgical intervention provided to this cohort of patients.[58]

The Veterans Administration (VA) Symptomatic Trial Cooperative Studies Program was designed to determine the role of CEA in preventing stroke from symptomatic carotid stenosis and was initiated at 13 VA medical centers in 1986.[3] Only men presenting within 120 days of onset of symptoms that were consistent with TIAs, transient monocular blindness, or recent nondisabling strokes were medically screened. Patients with ischemic symptoms attributed to a greater than 50% stenosis of the ipsilateral carotid artery were randomized to either CEA plus best medical care versus best medical care alone. Best medical care in this study included daily aspirin administration and treatment of all coexisting medical disorders. The primary endpoints selected as evidence of treatment failure included cerebral or retinal infarction, crescendo TIAs, or death from any cause within 30 days of randomization.

A total of 189 patients were entered into the trial after initial screening of nearly 5000 patients.[3] CEA was performed in 90 of the 91 patients randomized to surgical treatment; one patient suffered a stroke prior to operation. The trial was terminated early because of the NASCET and ECST results. However, at a mean follow-up of 11.9 months, there was a significant reduction in the combined incidence of stroke and crescendo TIAs in the patients who underwent CEA (7.7%) versus nonsurgical patients (19.4%). Among the 129 patients with carotid artery stenosis greater than 70%, the benefit of CEA was even more pronounced. The surgical group had a stroke and crescendo TIA rate of 7.9%, versus 25.9% for the medical group. Discounting the one preoperative stroke, CEA was performed with a perioperative stroke and mortality rate of 5.5% in multiple centers and among relatively high-risk patients.

CLINICAL TRIALS ON EFFICACY OF CAROTID ENDARTERECTOMY FOR ASYMPTOMATIC STENOSIS

This VA Asymptomatic Trial Cooperative Studies Program was initiated at 11 VA medical centers in 1982 to assess the effect of CEA on the combined incidence of neurologic events, TIA, and stroke, in patents with asymptomatic carotid stenosis.[4] The trialists randomized 444 male patients with documented angiographic diameter-reducing stenoses of 50% or greater which, when coupled with positive ocular pneumoplethysmography (OPG) or duplex scan, constituted area-reducing stenoses greater than 75%. Patients were randomized to optimal medical management and CEA (211 patients) versus optimal medical management alone (233 patients). The 30-day post-randomization permanent stroke and death rate was 4.3% for the surgical group[60] and 9.7% including neurologic complications of angiography for the entire group. The combined incidence of all neurologic events was 24.5% for the medical group, which was reduced significantly ($P < .002$) in the surgical group to 12.8%. If only ipsilateral events were considered (75% of all neurologic events), the incidence was 20.6% in the medical group and 8.0% in the surgical group ($P < 0.001$). Reduction in ipsilateral stroke alone favored the surgical group by a trend of 2:1, however, the trial was not powered to evaluate stroke alone and the data lacked statistical significance.

The Asymptomatic Carotid Atherosclerosis Study (ACAS), sponsored by the National Institutes of Health,[5] investigated patients with asymptomatic carotid stenosis in a trial with many similarities to the VA trial. The threshold stenosis for randomization was a 60% diameter-reducing lesion. In addition, precise Doppler velocity criteria permitted randomization without arteriography. A total of 1662 patients with asymptomatic carotid stenosis were randomized to aspirin therapy and best medical care versus aspirin, best medical care, and CEA. After a median follow-up of 2.7 years, the aggregated risk over 5 years of ipsilateral stroke and any perioperative stroke or death in the surgical group was estimated to be 11.0% for patients treated with medical therapy alone as compared with 5.1% for patients treated with medical therapy plus CEA. Although this represented a relative risk reduction of 53%, absolute risk reduction in stroke was noted to be approximately 1.2% per year. The overall 30-day stroke and death rate for the surgical cohort was 2.3%. However, of the 414 patients in this surgical cohort who underwent arteriography prior to CEA, the arteriographic stroke complication rate was 1.2%, which was included in the overall perioperative complication rate of 2.3%. These data have formed the basis for modern recommendations on the use of CEA in asymptomatic patients in this country. The VA trial established that overall neurologic events including TIA and stroke could be reduced significantly after CEA,[4] whereas the larger ACAS trial established this goal for stroke alone.[5] Some clinicians are cautious in the selection of patients for operation, particularly in the 60% to 79% stenosis category, owing to the anticipated absolute benefit of only 1.2% per year.[5] Unfortunately, the ACAS investigators did not have adequate arteriographic data from the medical treatment arm of the study to categorize differential neurologic event rates in patients with 60% to 79% stenosis as compared with 80% to 99%. Nevertheless, our current recommendation favors endarterectomy, particularly in patients with stenoses of 80% to 99% in institutions that have audited 30-day stroke and death rates of less than 3%.

In studying the natural history of asymptomatic stenosis, it should be acknowledged that only one fifth of the patients in the medical group developed neurologic symptoms. Although presence of a high-grade stenosis (arteriographic diameter reduction of >50% or a calculated area reduction of >75% in the VA trial and 60% diameter stenosis angiographically in ACAS), the degree of stenosis may be only one of several factors determining incidence of stroke. The current clinical challenge is to identify factors such as ultrasonic plaque morphology, incidence of silent CT-confirmed cerebral infarction, status of collateral cerebral circulation, and combinations of clinical risk factors such as hypertension, coronary artery disease, smoking, and peripheral vascular disease, which when superimposed on a high-grade threshold stenosis will result in an increased risk of stroke as a first event. These data support the selective use of CEA in centers with low complication rates[61] among better-risk patients whose life expectancy is 5 or more years.

INDICATIONS FOR CAROTID ENDARTERECTOMY: SPECIAL CONSIDERATIONS

Recommendations regarding the use of CEA have been carefully reviewed by consensus panels of the American Heart Association in 1995[18] and again in 1998.[19] Indications were categorized into the following groups: proven, acceptable but not proven, uncertain, and proven inappropriate. For patients with symptomatic disease, including recent TIA and nondisabling stroke who are good risks with a surgeon whose surgical morbidity and mortality is less than 6%, the following conditions are indications for CEA:

1. Proven: One or more TIAs in the past 6 months and carotid stenosis greater than 70% or mild stroke within 6 months and a carotid stenosis of greater than or equal to 70%. Recent recommendations from the NASCET trialists have also included patients with moderate carotid stenosis, 50% to 69% in this group of indications for CEA.[59]
2. Acceptable but not proven: Ipsilateral CEA combined with CABG in a symptomatic patient in the presence of stenosis greater than or equal to 50%.
3. Proven inappropriate: Moderate stroke with stenosis less than 50%, not on antiplatelet therapy; single TIA with less than 50% stenosis, not on antiplatelet therapy; high-risk patient with multiple TIAs not on antiplatelet therapy, stenosis less than 50%; high-risk patient, mild or moderate stroke, stenosis less than 50%, not on antiplatelet therapy; global ischemic symptoms with stenosis of less than 50%; acute dissection, asymptomatic on heparin.

For patients with asymptomatic carotid occlusive disease whose surgical risk is less than 3% and whose life expectancy exceeds 5 years, the following indications are recommended:

1. Proven: Ipsilateral CEA is acceptable for stenotic lesions (greater than or equal to 60% diameter reduction) with or without ulceration and with or without antiplatelet therapy, regardless of contralateral disease status.
2. Acceptable but not proven: Unilateral CEA simultaneously with coronary artery bypass grafting for stenotic lesions (≥60%) with or without ulceration and with or without antiplatelet therapy, regardless of contralateral artery status.
3. Uncertain indications: unilateral CEA for stenosis greater than 50% with B or C ulcers,[61] irrespective of contralateral internal carotid artery status.
4. Proven inappropriate: Patients with stenoses less than 60% or patients whose risk of operation exceeds 3% or whose life expectancy is greater than 5 years.

Crescendo TIAs are defined by a change in symptom pattern in the patient with symptomatic carotid disease. There must be an increase in the frequency of symptoms over a period of one to several days, an increase in the duration of symptoms with episodes lasting longer than the primary event, and/or increased severity of ischemia with the development of increased or new transient motor, sensory, or visual defects. An evaluation of 12 of the 189 patients in the VA symptomatic trial[3] identified as having an internal carotid stenosis greater than 50% developed crescendo TIAs. All 12 of these patients were in the medical group, and were treated with intravenous heparin and underwent emergent CEA within 24 hours of onset of symptom progression. None suffered a postoperative complication. Other reports in the surgical literature of patients with crescendo symptoms have also shown that CEA can be undertaken with good results.[62,63] The patient with crescendo TIAs constitutes a neurologic emergency and should undergo immediate anticoagulation and prompt CEA by an experienced surgical team.

Completed stroke with recovery and a minimal to modest neurologic deficit is an indication for operation if accompanied by appropriate ipsilateral carotid disease, as confirmed in the symptomatic trials.[1-3] Other potential sources of infarction such as intracranial small or large arterial disease, emboli arising from the heart or aortic arch, and other systemic disorders must be ruled out. CT scan or MRI is also indicated to determine the extent of the infarct, whether it is hemorrhagic or ischemic in nature, and to exclude tumors or vascular malformations as their cause. In the presence of a fixed neurologic deficit or larger central cerebral infarct (CT/MRI), operative intervention generally is delayed 4 to 6 weeks or until the patient's neurologic improvement reaches baseline. The use of a shunt is also recommended because the status of cerebral flow autoregulation is difficult to determine at the time of operation. A preoperative angiogram (contrast or MRA) may be obtained after noninvasive tests have been performed and the patient is considered to be a good surgical candidate. The operative team must be able to perform an endarterectomy in this group of higher-risk patients with a morbidity and mortality rate of less than 6%.

Stroke in evolution or progressive stroke occurs when an acute neurologic deficit progresses within hours or days in a sequential series of acute exacerbations to a major stroke.[62] In Mentzer's series,[63] 12 of 17 patients who underwent emergent CEA for fluctuating and progressive neurologic deficits improved, but only 3 of 26 patients treated medically improved. Furthermore, only 1 patient in the surgical group deteriorated, compared to 14 patients in the medical group. At 6 months, 80% of the nonoperated patients had some degree of neurologic deficit versus 53% of the operated patients. Moderate or severe deficits were considerably more common in the nonoperated group. Patients should undergo a rapid diagnostic work-up, which should include a carotid duplex scan to document the presence of a high-grade carotid stenosis or an irregular plaque with soft thrombus, followed by CT scan or MRI to exclude a hemorrhagic stroke. Prompt anticoagulation and operative intervention should follow if the patient is medically fit. Angiography carries a higher risk in these patients and further delays the initiation of surgical therapy.

An *acute stroke* due to acute occlusion and associated with a neurologic deficit lasting longer than 24 hours continues to be a challenging problem in surgical management. Patients are generally considered neurologically unstable, morbidity or mortality is high, and reperfusion of ischemic tissue can result in hemorrhagic transformation of an originally ischemic stroke. CEA may be applicable only under extremely limited circumstances, depending on the time of onset of the deficit and the timeliness of surgical intervention.[64]

Concurrent *CEA and coronary artery bypass* are performed in patients with existing comorbid factors, and each procedure carries its own set of risks. As originally presented by Bernhard and associates,[65] the combined procedure has been associated during more recent years with a somewhat higher combined stroke, myocardial infarction, and mortality than when either procedure is performed alone.[66] Brener[67] performed a meta-analysis on three operative strategies: simultaneous carotid and coronary artery bypass grafting (CABG), carotid surgery followed by CABG, and CABG followed by carotid surgery. The analysis reported that perioperative stroke rate was similar if the carotid and coronary procedures were combined or if CEA preceded CABG. However, the frequency of stroke was significantly greater if CABG preceded the carotid operation. Conversely, the frequency of myocardial infarction ($P = 0.01$) and death ($P = 0.02$) were greater when CEA preceded CABG. In the absence of a randomized clinical trial comparing these various options, each institution and surgical group must audit their results and determine the best mode of operative intervention. More recent publications on the combined procedure[68] have demonstrated moderately reduced 30-day stroke and death rates. If an institution audits its results appropriately and is able to achieve complications in the 5% to 7% range, combined procedures are appropriate if both are clinically indicated. This would be particularly true for a patient with a high-grade symptomatic carotid lesion. This procedure is routinely recommended in our service as well as for the patient with bilateral high grade asymptomatic lesions or unilateral occlusion and contralateral asymptomatic high grade stenoses. The exception to the combined procedure would be the unilateral high grade asymptomatic stenosis with a more normal contralateral artery which could be treated by CABG and then a delayed CEA well after recovery from the cardiac surgical procedure. In the future, a cooperative trial to evaluate these various options will become essential. It is also possible that carotid artery stenting may be used in this group if stenting is proved to be efficacious in its randomized trials.

Operation on patients with *tandem extracranial and intracranial lesions* may carry an increased risk.[69] The course of the internal carotid artery in the neck extends from its bifurcation to the base of the skull, where it continues intracranially as the petrous segment through the carotid canal in the petrous portion of the temporal bone; the cavernous segment follows the sphenoid bone to emerge intradurally at the Circle of Willis. In the cerebral circulation, the carotid siphon is said to be the second site, after the carotid bulb, most likely to develop atherosclerotic changes. Roederer and colleagues[70] have concluded that patients with severe carotid bulb lesions should be referred for CEA. Accompanying siphon stenoses did not result in greater risk for recurrent symptoms. Thus, nonoperative management should be considered only when the degree of siphon stenosis exceeds that of the lower carotid bulb lesion.

External CEA has specialized indications. The combined stroke and TIA rate for those patients with an ipsilateral occluded internal carotid artery is as high as 20%.[71] In the presence of an internal carotid artery occlusion, the external carotid artery supplies blood flow to the ipsilateral hemisphere from a rich source of collaterals originating through the internal maxillary artery.[72] Tributaries from these collaterals provide a route for emboli. Strokes may occur due to emboli originating from external carotid arterial plaque, from the stump of the occluded internal carotid artery, or because of decreased flow from the available collateral circulation. In Gertler and Cambria's[72] collective review, 48 of 52 patients who had external carotid endarterectomies for amaurosis fugax or hemispheric TIAs in the presence of an occluded internal carotid artery but a patent external carotid artery became asymptomatic; the other four were improved. There were no deaths and no perioperative strokes. Zarins and associates[73] have also reported increased ipsilateral and contralateral cerebral blood flow in patients who had undergone external CEA. In the symptomatic patient with an occluded internal carotid artery and a diseased external carotid artery, endarterectomy of the external carotid artery can be undertaken with good results. The more complex extracranial-intracranial bypass (EC-IC) previously had been recommended in selected patients with symptomatic internal carotid occlusions or distal occlusive disease. However, the cooperative trial results[74] demonstrated no benefit in stroke prevention over optimal medical management. In recent years, selection of patients using positron emission (PET) scanning has identified a subset of patients who may benefit from EC-IC bypass.[75]

REFERENCES

1. North American Symptomatic Carotid Endarterectomy Trial Collaborators: Beneficial effect of carotid endarterectomy in symptomatic patients with high-grade carotid stenosis. N Engl J Med 325:445, 1991.
2. European Carotid Surgery Trialist's Collaborative Group: MRC European carotid surgery trial: Interim results for symptomatic patients with severe (70-99%) or with mild (0-29%) carotid stenosis. Lancet 337:1235, 1991.
3. Mayberg MR, Wilson SE, Yatsu F, et al: Carotid endarterectomy and prevention of cerebral ischemia in symptomatic carotid stenosis. Veterans Affairs Cooperative Studies Program. JAMA 266:3289, 1991.
4. Hobson RW II, Weiss DG, Fields WS, et al: Efficacy of carotid endarterectomy for asymptomatic carotid stenosis. Veterans Affairs Cooperative Studies Program. N Engl J Med 328:221, 1993.
5. Toole JF, Baker WH, Castaldo JE, et al: Executive Committee for the Asymptomatic Carotid Atherosclerosis Study: Endarterectomy for asymptomatic carotid artery stenosis. JAMA 273:1421, 1995.
6. Cronenwett JL, Birkmeyer JD: Carotid artery disease. In The Dartmouth Atlas of Vascular Health Care. Chicago, AHA Press, 2000, p 41.
7. Broderick J: Feinberg Lecture, International Stroke Conference, AHA, 2003.

8. Wolf PA, Cobb JL, D'Agostino RB: Epidemiology of stroke. In Barnett HJM, Mohr JP, Stein BM, Yatsu FM (eds): Stroke: Pathophysiology, Diagnosis, and Management. New York, Churchill Livingstone, 1992, p 3.
9. Sacco RL: Clinical Practice. Extracranial carotid stenosis. N Engl J Med 345:1113, 2001.
10. Friedman SG: A history of vascular surgery. New York, Futura, 1989.
11. Hunt JR: The role of the carotid arteries in the causation of vascular lesions of the brain, with remarks on certain special features of symptomatology. Am J Med Sci 147:704, 1914.
12. Moniz E, Lima A, de Lacerda R: Hemiplegies par thrombose de la carotide interne. Presse Med 45:977, 1937.
13. Fisher M: Occlusion of the internal carotid artery. Arch Neurol Psychiatry 65:346, 1951.
14. Carrea R, Molins M, Murphy G: Surgical treatment of spontaneous thrombosis of the internal carotid artery in the neck: Carotid-carotideal anastomosis—Report of a case. Acta Neurol Latinoamer 1:17, 1955.
15. Strully KJ, Hurwitt ES, Blankenberg HW: Thrombo-endarterectomy for thrombosis of the internal carotid artery in the neck. J Neurosurg 10:474, 1953.
16. DeBakey ME: Successful carotid endarterectomy for cerebrovascular insufficiency: Nineteen-year follow-up. JAMA 233:1083, 1975.
17. Eastcott HH, Pickering GW, Rob C: Reconstruction of internal carotid artery in patients with intermittent attacks of hemiplegia. Lancet 2:944, 1954.
18. Moore WS, Barnett HJ, Beebe HG, et al: Guidelines for carotid endarterectomy: A multidisciplinary consensus statement from the Ad Hoc Committee, American Heart Association. Stroke 26:188, 1995.
19. Biller J, Feinberg WM, Castaldo JE, et al: Guidelines for carotid endarterectomy: A statement for healthcare professionals from a special writing group of the Stroke Council, American Heart Association. Stroke 29:554, 1998.
20. Fields WS, Maslenikov V, Meyer JS, et al: Joint study of extracranial arterial occlusion: V. Progress report of prognosis following surgery or non-surgical treatment for transient cerebral ischemic attacks and cervical carotid lesions. JAMA 211:1993, 1970.
21. Hollenhorst RW: Significance of bright plaques in the retinal arterioles. JAMA 178:23, 1961.
22. Ross R, Glomset JA: The pathogenesis of atherosclerosis (first of two parts). N Engl J Med 295:369, 1976.
23. Zarins CK, Giddens DP, Bharadvaj BK, et al: Carotid bifurcation atherosclerosis: Quantitative correlation of plaque localization with flow velocity profiles and wall shear stress. Circ Res 53: 502, 1983.
24. LoGerfo FW, Nowak MD, Quist WC: Structural details of boundary layer separation in a model human carotid bifurcation under steady and pulsatile flow conditions. J Vasc Surg 2:263, 1985.
25. Imparato AM, Riles TS, Gostein F: The carotid bifurcation plaque: Pathological findings associated with cerebral ischemia. Stroke 10:238, 1979.
26. Imparato AM, Riles TS, Mintzer R, et al: The importance of hemorrhage in the relationship of gross morphological characteristics and cerebral symptoms in 376 carotid artery plaques. Ann Surg 197:195, 1983.
27. Svindland A, Torvik A: Atherosclerotic carotid disease in asymptomatic individuals: A histological study of 53 cases. Acta Neurol Scand 78:506, 1988.
28. Lal BK, Hobson RW II, Pappas PJ, et al: Pixel distribution analysis of B-mode ultrasound scan images predicts histologic features of atherosclerotic carotid plaques. J Vasc Surg 35:1210, 2002.
29. Martin-Paredero V, Dixon SM, Baker JD, et al: Risk of renal failure after major angiography. Arch Surg 118:1417, 1983.
30. Mani RL: Complications of catheter cerebral angiography: Analysis of 5000 procedures: I. Criteria and Incidence. AJR Am J Roentgenol 131:861, 1978.
31. Mattle HP, Kent KC, Edelman RR, et al: Evaluation of extracranial carotid arteries: Correlation of magnetic resonance angiography, duplex ultrasonography, and conventional angiography. J Vasc Surg 13:838, 1991.
32. Cinat M, Lane CT, Pham H, et al: Helical CT angiography in the preoperative evaluation of carotid artery stenosis. J Vasc Surg 28: 290, 1998.
33. Crawford ES, DeBakey ME, Blaisdell FW, et al: Hemodynamic alterations in patients with cerebral insufficiency before and after operation. Surgery 48:76, 1960.
34. Fisher DF Jr, Clagett GP, Parker JI, et al: Mandibular subluxation for high carotid exposure. J Vasc Surg 1:727, 1984.
35. Simonian GT, Pappas PJ, Padberg FT, Jr, et al: Mandibular subluxation for distal internal carotid exposure: Technical considerations. J Vasc Surg 30:1116, 1999.
36. Archie JP: Prevention of early restenosis and thrombosis-occlusion after carotid endarterectomy by saphenous vein patch angioplasty. Stroke 17:901, 1986.
37. Hertzer NR, Beven EG, O'Hara PJ, et al: A prospective study of vein patch angioplasty during carotid endarterectomy. Three year results for 801 patients and 917 operations. Ann Surg 206:628, 1987.
38. Nicholls SC, Phillips DJ, Bergelin RO, et al: Carotid endarterectomy: Relationship of outcome to early restenosis. J Vasc Surg 2:375, 1985.
39. Eikelboom BC, Ackerstaff RG, Hoeneveld H, et al: Benefits of carotid patching: A randomized study. J Vasc Surg 7:240, 1988.
40. AbuRahma AF, Robinson PA, Saiedy S, et al: Prospective randomized trial of carotid endarterectomy with primary closure and patch angioplasty with saphenous vein, jugular vein, and polytetrafluoroethylene: Long-term follow-up. J Vasc Surg 27:222, 1998.
41. AbuRahma AF, Robinson PA, Hannay RS, et al: Prospective controlled study of carotid endarterectomy with hemashield patch: Is it thrombogenic? J Vasc Surg 35:167, 2001.
42. O'Hara PJ, Hertzer NR, Mascha EJ, et al: A prospective, randomized study of saphenous vein patching versus synthetic patching during carotid endarterectomy. J Vasc Surg 35:324, 2002.
43. Rhee RY, Donayre CE, Ouriel K, et al: Low dose heparin therapy: In vitro verification of antithrombotic effect. J Vasc Surg 14:628, 1991.
44. Gupta SK, Veith FJ, Ascer E, et al: Anaphylactoid reactions to protamine: An often lethal complication in insulin-dependent diabetic patients undergoing vascular surgery. J Vasc Surg 9:342, 1989.
45. Collier PE: Do clinical pathways for major vascular surgery improve outcomes and reduce cost? J Vasc Surg 26:179, 1997.
46. Sheehan MK, Baker WH, Littooy FN, et al: Timing of postcarotid complications: A guide to safe discharge planning. J Vasc Surg 34: 13, 2001.
47. Connolly JE: Carotid endarterectomy in the awake patient. Am J Surg 150:159, 1985.
48. Moore WS: Shunting during carotid endarterectomy: Always, never, sometimes? Semin Vasc Surg 2:28, 1989.
49. Simonian G, Hobson RW: Stroke following carotid endarterectomy. In Cronenwett J, Rutherford R (eds): Decision Making in Vascular Surgery. Philadelphia, WB Saunders, p 70.
50. Koslow AR, Ricotta JJ, Ouriel K, et al: Reexploration for thrombosis in carotid endarterectomy. Circulation 80: III73, 1989.
51. Hertzer NR, Feldman BJ, Beven EG, et al: A prospective study of incidence of injury to the cranial nerves during carotid endarterectomy. Surg Gynecol Obstet 151:781, 1980.
52. Bove EL, Fry WJ, Gross WS, et al: Hypotension and hypertension as consequences of baroreceptor dysfunction following carotid endarterectomy. Surgery 85:633, 1971.
53. Tarlov E, Schmidek H, Scott RW, et al: Reflex hypotension following carotid endarterectomy: Mechanism and management. J Neurosurg 39:323, 1973.
54. Ahn SS, Marcus DR, Moore WS: Post-carotid endarterectomy hypertension: Association with elevated cranial norepinephrine. J Vasc Surg 9:351, 1989.
55. Towne JB, Bernhard VM: The relationship of postoperative hypertension to complications following carotid endarterectomy. Surgery 88:575, 1980.
56. Sundt TM, Sharbrough FW, Piepgras DG, et al: Correlation of cerebral blood flow and electroencephalographic changes during carotid endarterectomy with results of surgery and hemodynamics of cerebral ischemia. Mayo Clin Proc 56:533, 1981.
57. Youkey JR, Clagett GP, Jaffin JH, et al: Focal motor seizures complicating carotid endarterectomy. Arch Surg 119:1080, 1984.
58. Winslow CM, Solomon DH, Chassin MR, et al: The appropriateness of carotid endarterectomy. N Engl J Med 318:721, 1988.
59. Barnett HJ, Taylor DW, Eliasziw M, et al: Benefit of carotid endarterectomy in patients with symptomatic moderate or severe stenosis. North American Symptomatic Carotid Endarterectomy Trial Collaborators. N Engl J Med 339:1415, 1998.
60. Towne JB, Weiss DG, Hobson RW II: First phase report of Veterans Administration asymptomatic carotid stenosis study—Operative morbidity and mortality. J Vasc Surg 11:252, 1990.

61. Moore WS, Boren C, Malone JM, et al: Natural history of non-stenotic, asymptomatic ulcerative lesions of the carotid artery: A further analysis. Arch Surg 113:1352, 1978.
62. Goldstone J, Moore WS: Emergency carotid surgery in neurological unstable patients. Arch Surg 111:1284, 1976.
63. Mentzer RM, Finkelmeiser BA, Crosby IK, et al: Emergency carotid endarterectomy for fluctuating neurological deficits. Surgery 89:60, 1981.
64. Callow AD: Fact or fancy: A twenty-year personal perspective on the detection and management of carotid occlusive disease. J Cardiovasc Surg 21:21, 1980.
65. Bernhard VM, Johnson WD, Peterson JJ: Carotid artery stenosis: Association with surgery for coronary artery disease. Arch Surg 105:837-840, 1972.
66. Reul GJ Jr, Cooley DA, Duncan JM, et al: The effect of coronary bypass on the outcome of peripheral vascular operations in 1093 patients. J Vasc Surg 3:788, 1986.
67. Brener BJ, Brief DK, Alpert J, et al: The risk of stroke in patients with asymptomatic carotid stenosis undergoing cardiac surgery: A follow-up study. J Vasc Surg 5:269, 1987.
68. Char D, Cuadra S, Ricotta J, et al: Combined coronary artery bypass and carotid endarterectomy: Long-term results. Cardiovasc Surg 10:111, 2002.
69. Schuller JJ, Flanigan DP: The effect of carotid siphon stenosis on stroke rate, death, and relief of symptoms following elective carotid endarterectomy. Surgery 92:1058, 1982.
70. Roederer GO, Langlois YE, Chan ARW, et al: Is siphon disease important in predicting outcome of carotid endarterectomy? Arch Surg 118:1177, 1983.
71. Nicholls SC, Bergelin R, Strandness DE: Neurologic sequelae of unilateral carotid artery occlusion: Immediate and late. J Vasc Surg 10:542, 1989.
72. Gertler JP, Cambria RP: The role of external carotid endarterectomy in the treatment of ipsilateral internal carotid artery occlusion: Collective review. J Vasc Surg 6:158, 1987.
73. Zarins CK, Del Beccaro EJ, Johns L, et al: Increased cerebral blood flow after external artery revascularization. Surgery 89:730, 1981.
74. The EC/IC Bypass Study Group. Failure of extracranial-intracranial arterial bypass to reduce the risk of ischemic stroke: Results of an international randomized trial. N Engl J Med 313:1191, 1985.
75. Derdeyn CP, Gage BF, Grubb RL Jr, Powers WJ: Cost-effectiveness analysis of therapy for symptomatic carotid occlusion: PET screening before selective extracranial-to-intracranial bypass versus medical treatment. J Nuclear Med 41:800, 2000.

chapter 34

Pathophysiology, Clinical Evaluation, and Medical Management

Patrick O'Gara

Acute aortic dissection is an uncommon but life-threatening medical and surgical emergency that requires prompt recognition, rapid triage, and expeditious treatment. Continuing advances in noninvasive imaging, surgical techniques, and endovascular therapies have led to improved patient outcomes. More widespread awareness of the acute aortic syndromes is a critical first step in establishing care pathways to reduce the persistently high rates of death and disability associated with this disease.

EPIDEMIOLOGY

The incidence of aortic dissection in the general population has been difficult to ascertain. Aortic dissection may account for a small percentage (3% to 5%) of sudden deaths; up to 30% to 40% of cases may escape diagnosis.[1-3] Aortic dissection had been considered the most common acute aortic catastrophe requiring urgent surgical therapy, although recent studies suggest that ruptured abdominal aortic aneurysm is a significantly more frequent indication.[3] Population-based studies from Hungary and Olmsted County, Minnesota, estimate an annual incidence rate of 2 to 5 acute aortic dissections per 100,000 persons.[2,3] Incidence rates increase with age and are higher for men than for women. In the Olmsted County survey, 39 residents from among an average population of 100,000 people were identified with aortic dissection between 1980 and 1994. Fifteen patients (38%) were diagnosed at autopsy, and the 5-year survival rate among the remaining 24 patients managed with the medical and surgical therapies available during that time period was only 51% (expected survival 77% among age- and gender-matched controls, $p < .001$).[3] By comparison, the landmark natural history study reported by Hirst and colleagues in 1958 established mortality rates of 1% per hour for the first 24 hours, 37% at 48 hours, 74% at 2 weeks, and 90% at 3 months for patients with untreated aortic dissection.[4]

CLASSIFICATION

The classification of aortic dissection based on anatomic location and time from onset of symptoms has provided a useful tool for both prognosis and treatment (Fig. 34-1). The Stanford classification, currently the most widely used, designates dissections that involve the ascending aorta as type A (regardless of the site of entry) and those that involve the aorta distal to the origin of the left subclavian artery as type B.[5] This distinction is important, as involvement of the ascending aorta is associated with a much higher risk of early death and major morbidity. Aortic dissections limited to the arch are considered separately. In the older DeBakey classification, a type I dissection begins in the ascending aorta and extends for a variable distance beyond the origin of the innominate artery, whereas a type II dissection is confined to the ascending aorta. A type III dissection originates in the descending thoracic aorta, stopping above (type IIIA) or extending below (type IIIB) the level of the diaphragm.[6] Dissections involving the ascending aorta have also been referred to as "proximal," and those restricted to the descending thoracic aorta as "distal." The Stanford classification is used throughout this chapter. The terms "communicating" and "noncommunicating" refer to the presence or absence, respectively, of blood flow between the true and false lumens of the aorta.

Aortic dissection is termed acute if presentation occurs within 14 days of the onset of symptoms and chronic if more than 2 weeks have elapsed. Morbidity and

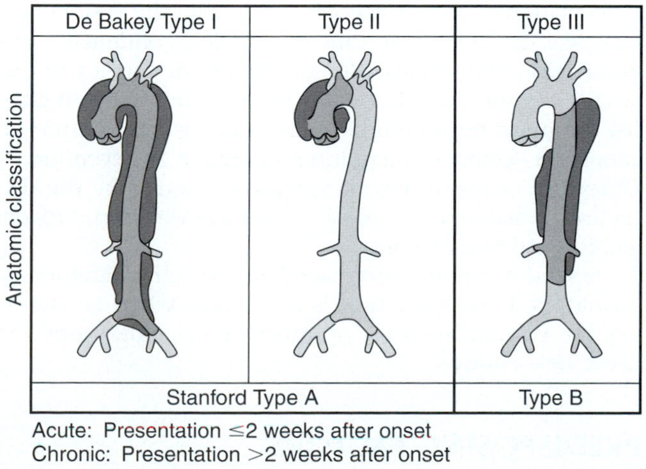

FIGURE 34-1. Stanford and DeBakey anatomic classifications of aortic dissection (see text). (From Nienaber CA, Eagle KA: Aortic dissection: New frontiers in diagnosis and management. Circulation 108:630, 2003.)

mortality are highest within the acute phase; patients who have survived without treatment for 2 weeks are self selected for better short-term outcomes.

PATHOGENESIS

In classic acute aortic dissection, the initiating event is an intimal tear through which blood surges into the media under systolic pressure, splitting the layers of the aortic wall and creating an intimal flap that separates the true from the false lumen. The primary entry tear is located in the ascending aorta, usually just a few centimeters from the aortic valve along the right anterolateral wall, in 60% of cases. Because of its proximity to the heart, this area of the aorta is exposed to relatively greater hemodynamic, shear, and torsional forces. The second most common entry site (30% of cases) is located in the descending thoracic aorta just beyond the insertion of the ligamentum arteriosum, where the relatively mobile arch meets the fixed descending thoracic aorta. Arch (7%) and abdominal (3%) aortic entry sites are distinctly less common.[4] The dissecting hematoma usually propagates in an anterograde direction, although retrograde extension can occur. By this mechanism, as many as 20% of dissections that originate in the distal arch or descending thoracic aorta may involve the ascending aorta.[7]

Blood within the false lumen may reenter the true lumen anywhere along the length of the dissection. Reentry may be a mechanism for spontaneous decompression of the false lumen with attenuation of the possible early consequences of rupture or malperfusion syndromes, or both, from aortic branch vessel compromise. The site of rupture is usually dictated by the location of the primary intimal tear. Rupture into the pericardial space with tamponade occurs in type A dissection, whereas rupture into the left pleural space is usually encountered with type B dissection. Branch vessel involvement occurs as a result of compression by the hematoma, continuation of the dissection across the ostium of the vessel, or dynamic obstruction caused by the oscillating flap. Compromise of the coronary, brachiocephalic, mesenteric, renal, spinal, and iliac circulations can occur and result in a myriad of clinical presentations. Thrombosis of blood within the false lumen may seal the entry tear, thus eliminating continued communication with the true lumen. Persistent patency of the false lumen, on the other hand, is associated with a higher risk of longer-term complications, such as late rupture or aneurysm formation requiring operative intervention.[8,9] Distortion or disruption of the aortic annulus by the dissecting hematoma may result in acute severe aortic regurgitation and heart failure.

Dissection of the aorta need not result in aneurysm formation. This distinction is important when considering the natural histories of and surgical indications for these two entities.

PREDISPOSING FACTORS

As is true for aneurysm disease, any process that leads to the destruction or degeneration of the major supporting elements of the aortic media (elastin, collagen, smooth muscle cells [SMCs]) can predispose to the development of dissection. The histopathologic term, cystic medial degeneration (CMD), refers to the noninflammatory destruction or fragmentation of elastic lamellar units, dropout of SMCs, and accumulation of mucopolysaccharide ground substances and characterizes the final common pathway for various processes that affect the integrity of the aortic media (Fig. 34-2). Both genetic and acquired disorders are associated with an increased risk for aortic dissection (Table 34-1).

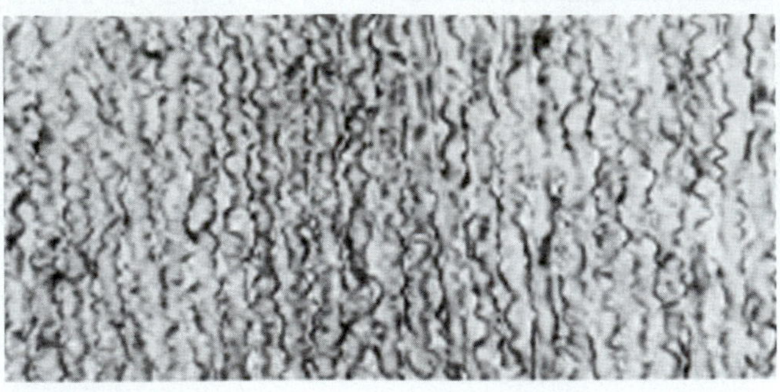

A

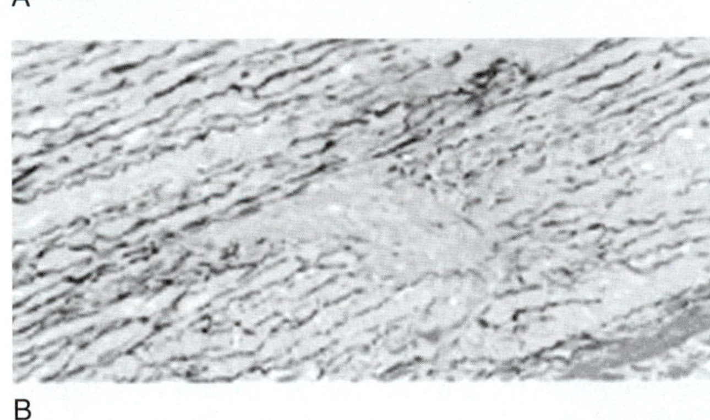

B

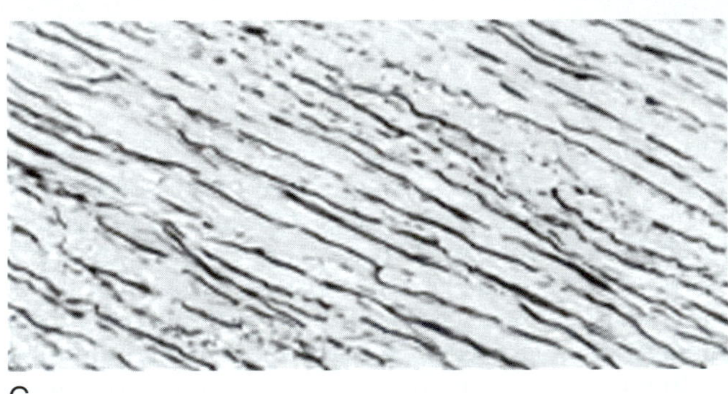

C

FIGURE 34-2. (See also Color Plate 34-2.) Cystic medial degeneration. Representative cross sections of a control ascending aorta **(A)**, an aortic aneurysm associated with Marfan's syndrome **(B)**, and an aneurysm associated with bicuspid aortic valve **(C)**, stained with Alcian blue and Verhoeff van Gieson (magnification ×250). In the control aorta, the elastic lamellae form dense, parallel sheets. In the Marfan and bicuspid aortic valve specimens, there are areas of elastic lamellar degradation and fragmentation with variable accumulation of mucoid substances. No inflammatory cells are present. (From Nataatmadja M, West M, West J, et al: Abnormal extracellular matrix protein transport associated with increased apoptosis of vascular smooth muscle cells in Marfan syndrome and bicuspid aortic valve thoracic aortic aneurysm. Circulation 108:II-329, 2003.)

TABLE 34-1 AORTIC DISSECTION PREDISPOSING FACTORS

Genetic	Acquired
Marfan's syndrome	Hypertension
Ehlers-Danlos syndrome	Iatrogenic
Familial thoracic aortic aneurysm disease	Pregnancy
Bicuspid aortic valve disease	Inflammatory aortitis
Aortic coarctation	Cocaine
Noonan's syndrome	
Turner's syndrome	
Polycystic kidney disease	

Genetic Disorders

Marfan's syndrome (MFS) is the most common inherited disorder of connective tissue with an estimated incidence of 1 affected individual per 7 to 10,000 population. MFS is an autosomal dominant disorder with variable penetrance; up to 25% of cases, however, are sporadic. Phenotypic expression can involve the skin (inguinal hernia), eyes (ectopia lentis, myopia), heart (mitral valve prolapse), aorta (annulo-aortic ectasia, aneurysm, dissection), skeleton (scoliosis, pectus carinatum/excavatum, arachnodactyly, dolichostenomelia), and central nervous system (dural ectasia, attention deficit disorder). More limited organ system involvement ("forme fruste") is frequently encountered, such as mitral valve prolapse with gracile body habitus, and overlap syndromes have been described. The clinical criteria for the diagnosis of MFS were revised in 1996.[10] Mutations in the gene encoding fibrillin-1 *(FBN1),* a critical component of extracellular microfibrils, are responsible for the disease.[11] The variability in clinical phenotype is not entirely explained on the basis of the more than 100 mutations described to date, and the existence of a second gene *(MFS2)* has been demonstrated.[12] Investigators have established that a minority of patients (7% to 16%) with MFS have normal fibrillin metabolism.[13,14] Enhanced expression of tissue metalloproteinases 2 and 9 in vascular SMCs (VSMCs) from Marfan patients with thoracic aortic aneurysms has been reported.[15] In addition, the qualitative severity of cystic medial degeneration seen in Marfan patients with annulo-aortic ectasia may be related in part to the upregulation of PPAR-γ in VSMCs.[16] The interrelationships among fibrillin defects, enhanced elastolysis, and VSMC apoptosis remain under active investigation.

Ehlers-Danlos syndrome (EDS) comprises a heterogeneous group of disorders characterized clinically by articular hypermobility, hyperextensile skin, and tissue fragility, with a predisposition to spontaneous vascular rupture. Its estimated incidence is 1 in 5000 births; there is no ethnic predisposition. Aortic involvement occurs in EDS type IV, an autosomal dominant disorder attributed to structural defects in the proα1 (III) chain of type III collagen, encoded by the *COL3A1* gene on chromosome 2q31.[17,18]

Familial thoracic aortic aneurysm disease has been mapped to other genetic loci, including 5q13-14 and 11q23.2-q24, that are not associated with abnormalities of fibrillin or collagen.[19,20] Reported patterns of inheritance have included autosomal dominant, autosomal recessive, and sex linked.[21] More than five mutations in the fibrillin-1 gene have been identified in patients with familial or spontaneous thoracic aortic aneurysm and dissection, with histopathologic changes characteristic of cystic medial degeneration, yet no demonstrable abnormalities of collagen or fibrillin in fibroblast culture.[22,23] Familial abdominal aortic aneurysm disease is often accompanied by thoracic involvement, but specific candidate genes have not been identified. Clearly, there is significant genetic heterogeneity and important genomic investigation remains to be done.

Patients with bicuspid aortic valve (BAV) disease often demonstrate ascending aortic enlargement out of proportion to the associated hemodynamic change imposed by the valve lesion itself. Cystic medial degeneration of the type seen in fibrillin-1–deficient murine models and patients with MFS underlies this dilatation and predisposes to dissection or aneurysm formation, or both.[24-26] Similar changes have been described in patients with aortic coarctation, independent of an association with BAV disease. Aortic dissection has also been reported in patients with Noonan's syndrome,[27] Turner's syndrome,[28] and polycystic kidney disease.[29]

Acquired Disorders

Systemic hypertension is the most common treatable risk factor for aortic dissection and is present in approximately 75% of patients.[30] Hypertension accelerates the normal aging process and leads to intimal thickening, SMC apoptosis, fibrosis, loss of elasticity, and compromise of nutritive blood supply. Increased aortic stiffness and vulnerability to pulsatile forces predispose to injury and create the substrate for dissection.

Iatrogenic dissection that occurs as a result of diagnostic or therapeutic catheterization or prior cardiac surgery is more common than previously appreciated.[31] Risk factors for late dissection after aortic valve replacement surgery include regurgitant valve lesions and thinning and fragility of the aortic wall.[32] Retrograde dissections created at the time of catheterization usually seal spontaneously upon withdrawal of the catheter. Aortic atherosclerosis itself is not generally considered a predisposing risk factor for spontaneous dissection. Indeed, in contrast to the lengthy and unimpeded intimal tears observed in patients with Marfan's syndrome, the atherosclerotic plaque presents a barrier that limits the longitudinal extent of dissection. Aortic dissection is a recognized complication of balloon dilatation for treatment of coarctation. Dissections arising from sites where the aorta has been incised or cross-clamped may occur intraoperatively or at any time following surgery. Deceleration injury from high-speed accidents results in aortic transection with false aneurysm formation and rupture, most commonly in the region of the aortic isthmus just beyond the origin of the left subclavian artery. Transection results in a transmural tear that is different both pathologically and etiologically from aortic dissection.

Previous reports suggested that up to 50% of all dissections in women younger than age 40 occurred in temporal relationship to pregnancy, specifically in the last trimester or early puerperium.[4,33] Although this relationship has been questioned by some investigators, there is a reasonable body of evidence to attest to its clinical and biologic plausibility. Histopathologic changes affecting the aortic media of pregnant women have been described, including alterations in elastic fibers and SMCs.[34] Both estrogen and relaxin are associated with alterations in matrix metalloproteinase homeostasis and contribute to vascular remodeling and a susceptibility to injury, independent of the hemodynamic stress of labor and delivery. Similar changes likely contribute to the predisposition to spontaneous coronary artery dissection described among pregnant women. Aortic root size greater than 4 cm is considered a contraindication to pregnancy in women with MFS or BAV disease due to the increased maternal risk for spontaneous rupture or dissection.

Inflammatory diseases of the aorta can lead to destruction of extracellular matrix proteins and SMCs, with subsequent aneurysm formation or dissection, or both. Aortic dissection has been reported in patients with Takayasu's arteritis,[35] giant cell aortitis,[36] Behçet's disease,[37] relapsing polychondritis,[38] systemic lupus erythematosus,[39] and the aortitis associated with inflammatory bowel disease.[40] Syphilitic aortitis, on the other hand, does not predispose to dissection, perhaps because of the intense medial scarring and fibrosis that occur in response to the spirochetal infection.

β-Amino propionitrile fumarate, the active ingredient in animal sweat pea meal that inhibits the activity of lysyl oxidase, an enzyme responsible for elastin polymerization, has been used to create an animal model of aortic dissection.[41] In humans there are now several reports of cocaine-related aortic dissection (predominantly type B) among urban, African-American young men with hypertension.[42] The presumed mechanisms of injury with cocaine involve a weakened aortic media, endothelial dysfunction, and extreme catecholamine-induced shear forces with abrupt hypertension and tachycardia.

CLINICAL PRESENTATION

The most important element of any diagnostic algorithm for suspected acute aortic syndrome is a high clinical index of suspicion, based foremost on the presenting history and physical examination. Absent an appreciation for the cardinal features of dissection, the diagnosis can be missed in a substantial number of patients. Simple clinical prediction rules have been developed to estimate the probability of acute aortic dissection.[43]

History

Most case series of patients with aortic dissection show a 2 to 3:1 male predominance with average age at presentation in the seventh decade. A history of hypertension is present in approximately 75% of patients; atherosclerotic vascular disease in a third; prior cardiac surgery or catheterization in as many as 20%; and MFS in roughly 5%.[30]

Chest pain is the dominant feature of the clinical presentation and occurs in more than 90% of patients.[30] It is qualitatively severe, abrupt in onset and of maximal intensity at its inception. The pain is described as sharp more often than tearing or ripping in nature. Anterior chest pain is more common with type A dissection, whereas patients with type B dissection usually report interscapular, lower back, or abdominal pain. Substantial overlap exists. The pain may migrate from its initial location to other sites as the dissecting hematoma migrates along the course of the aorta. Ischemic visceral or limb pain may accompany branch vessel compromise. As has been reported for acute myocardial infarction, stroke, and sudden cardiac death, acute aortic dissection displays a chronobiologic pattern with both circadian and seasonal variations. Acute dissection occurs more frequently between 6 A.M. and 10 A.M. and in the early afternoon and is more common in the winter than at other times of the year.[44]

Neurologic complications develop in 15% to 20% of patients and are frequently established at the time of presentation. Syncope may occur as a consequence of rupture with pericardial tamponade, hypoperfusion of brainstem structures, or via vagally mediated mechanisms in response to the intense pain of the dissection. Stroke is due to compromise of the carotid or vertebral circulations. Paraplegia may develop if there is critical impairment of flow to the anterior spinal artery, thoracic intercostals, or the artery of Adamkiewicz. Ischemic peripheral neuropathy with asymmetric motor and sensory deficits is indicative of complete inflow obstruction.

Patients with type A dissection and involvement of the aortic valve/annulus may present with heart failure symptoms if acute severe aortic regurgitation is present. The dyspnea is usually profound, given the magnitude and rate of rise of left ventricular end-diastolic pressure. For the extremely rare patient with type A dissection and ST segment elevation myocardial infarction from coronary artery ostial (right > left) compromise, the chest pain may be crescendo in nature and intensify more slowly over time. Severe oliguria or anuria may signify renal artery involvement. Numerous other uncommon manifestations of aortic dissection have been reported including Horner's syndrome (compression of the superior cervical ganglion), hoarseness (pressure against the recurrent laryngeal nerve), hemoptysis (rupture into a bronchus), hematemesis (perforation into the esophagus), ischemic enterocolitis (mesenteric artery compromise), and fever of undetermined source (pyrogens released from the false lumen).

Physical Examination

Patients with acute aortic dissection appear ill, uncomfortable, and apprehensive. Hypertension is present in more than two thirds of type B patients and in approximately one third of type A patients.[30] Rarely, with renal artery involvement, the hypertension is severe and refractory to medical therapy. Hypotension or shock, or both, are particularly ominous and more common among patients with ascending aortic involvement. These signs may reflect pericardial tamponade, coronary artery compression, acute severe aortic regurgitation, or rupture. Pseudo-hypotension can result from the inability to measure the central aortic pressure when bilateral subclavian or femoral artery compromise, or both, are present.

A murmur of aortic regurgitation can be heard in approximately 40% of patients with type A dissection.[30] It is usually of shorter duration, lower pitch, and lesser intensity than the diastolic murmur of chronic severe aortic regurgitation. Its acoustic characteristics derive from the rapid equilibration of aortic and left ventricular diastolic pressures in the acute setting. Aortic regurgitation results from annular widening, leaflet prolapse, or flail. Additional auscultatory findings include a soft first heart sound and a grade 1 or 2 midsystolic murmur at the base or along the left sternal border. Patients with acute severe aortic regurgitation are invariably tachycardic. Signs of severe diastolic runoff, such as bounding peripheral pulses, are absent.

Pulse deficits are less common than previously appreciated. In the International Registry of Acute Aortic Dissection (IRAD), pulse deficits were reported in approximately 20% of type A patients and 9% of type B patients. The pulse examination can change over time, and serial assessment is required. Pulse deficits are predictive of an increased risk of major in-hospital complications and early mortality.[45]

Elevation of the jugular venous pressure may indicate pericardial involvement or right heart failure. A careful screen for pulsus paradoxus and auscultation for a pericardial friction rub are important. Marked elevation of the jugular venous pressure without inspiratory change and cervico-facial plethora may indicate superior vena cava syndrome from localized compression. Thoracic dullness with decreased breath sounds suggests pleural effusion, which is more common in the left chest, and is not necessarily indicative of rupture. In fact, pleural effusions are quite frequent with both types A and B dissections and are usually sympathetic in nature, reflective of the intense inflammation associated with the acute tear.

LABORATORY TESTING

The chest radiograph is abnormal in 80% to 90% of patients with aortic dissection, though the findings may be nonspecific. Sensitivity is limited when pathology is confined to the ascending aorta.[46] Whenever possible, postero-anterior, lateral, and oblique films should be acquired and comparison with previous films performed. Such testing is not always appropriate in an emergency department setting, and too much time spent with the performance of chest x-rays is ill advised. Findings suggestive of aortic dissection include mediastinal widening; a disparity in the caliber of the ascending and descending thoracic aortic segments; a localized bulge or angulation along the normally smooth contour of the aorta; displacement of intimal calcium, especially in the region of the aortic knob; and a double-density appearance of the aorta. Associated findings might include cardiomegaly (pericardial effusion) and pleural effusion (left > right). Effusions that occupy more than 50% of the chest cavity may be indicative of rupture with hemothorax.

Nonspecific electrocardiographic repolarization abnormalities are present in approximately 40% of dissection patients, left ventricular hypertrophy in 25%, and evidence of an old myocardial infarction in about 10%.[30] Changes indicative of active ischemia may be found in 15% of patients, and findings suggestive of acute myocardial infarction (new Q waves, ST segment elevation) are present in a small minority (3%) of cases.[30] Acute reperfusion therapy, either fibrinolytic or catheter based, can be extremely hazardous in these unusual circumstances.

Serologic markers specific for the diagnosis of acute aortic dissection are not available for routine clinical use. Suzuki and colleagues have reported elevated levels of circulating smooth muscle myosin heavy chain protein among type A patients presenting within 3 hours of symptom onset.[47] Shinohara and colleagues measured elevated levels of soluble elastin fragments among aortic dissection patients with patent false lumens.[48] Others have proposed that elevated D-dimer levels should provide predictive value, though their presence has also been reported in various disease states with intrinsic fibrinolytic activation (e.g., acute coronary syndromes, venous thromboembolism, cancer).[49] Other nonspecific laboratory findings observed among patients with aortic dissection include mild anemia, leukocytosis, and thrombocytopenia; elevations of lactic dehydrogenase and indirect bilirubin; and microscopic hematuria. Disseminated intravascular coagulation has been rarely reported.

DIAGNOSTIC IMAGING

The diagnosis of aortic dissection depends on the demonstration of an intimal flap with separation of true and false lumens. In type A dissection, the true lumen is usually displaced along the inner curvature of the aortic arch and continues caudally along the medial aspect of the descending thoracic aorta. Aortic branch vessel blood flow may derive from either lumen, and the dissection flap may extend into and continue peripherally along the length of any branch for a variable distance. Alternatively, flow may be sluggish or absent within the false lumen, or branch vessels may be completely occluded at or near their origins. Over the past two decades, continuous advances in noninvasive imaging with transesophageal echocardiography (TEE), computed tomographic angiography (CTA), and MRI/MRA have led to the rapid and accurate diagnosis of the disease and virtually eliminated the need for contrast aortography in more than 95% of patients. At present, the relative sensitivities and specificities of these three noninvasive techniques are essentially equivalent and exceed 90% in most series. The choice of imaging technique depends chiefly on availability, speed, safety, and local expertise in performance and interpretation. Worldwide, CTA is the most frequently performed diagnostic test, followed by TEE. Experience has shown, however, that a second test is frequently necessary for clarification when the first study is abnormal but nondiagnostic. In the IRAD series, an average of 1.8 imaging studies per patient were performed.[30,50] Regardless of the diagnostic sequence employed, an institutional commitment to rapid imaging of critically ill patients is critical. The essential features to be defined for both treatment and prognosis include: the presence or absence of ascending aortic involvement, entry and reentry sites, pericardial and aortic valve involvement, the extent of the dissection, major branch vessel compromise, and the potential for malperfusion syndrome(s).

Transesophageal Echocardiography (Fig. 34-3)

A complete TEE study can be performed at the bedside or in the operating room within 15 to 20 minutes. Oropharyngeal anesthesia and conscious sedation are required with simultaneous monitoring of the heart rate, rhythm, blood pressure, and oxygen saturation. TEE provides information regarding: (1) entry and reentry sites; (2) the longitudinal extent and oscillation of the intimal flap; (3) flow velocity and direction within the true and false lumens; (4) spontaneous contrast or thrombus within the false lumen; (5) aortic valve competence and the mechanism of regurgitation; (6) ostial coronary artery involvement; (7) pericardial effusion; and (8) global and regional left ventricular function. Even with omni-plane probes, difficulty is sometimes encountered in visualizing the ascending aorta and proximal arch within the TEE "blind spot," which lies anterior to the trachea and left main stem bronchus. Artifacts due to reverberations within the ascending aorta may create difficulty for the less experienced observer. A "quick look" transthoracic echocardiogram (TTE) can be obtained but should not delay performance of the TEE. The assembly of the TEE team should not require more than 30 minutes even during off hours.

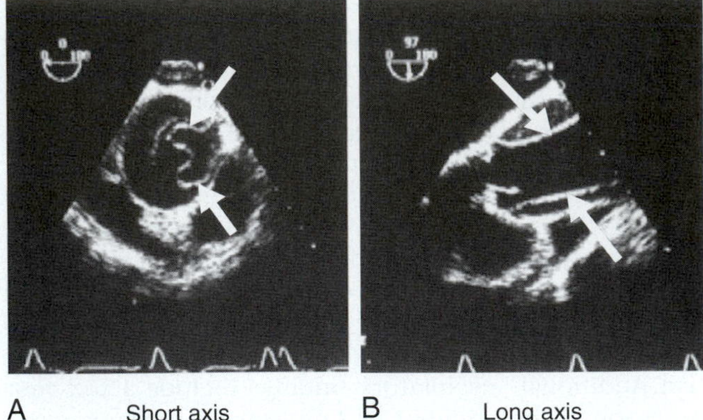

FIGURE 34-3. Transesophageal echocardiographic images of type A dissection in short-axis **(A)** and long-axis **(B)** planes. The intimal flap *(arrows)* is clearly seen in these still frames. (From Pineiro DJ, Bellido CA: Circumferential dissection of the aorta. N Engl J Med 340:1553, 1999.)

Computed Tomographic Angiography (Fig. 34-4)

Multislice CTA using rapid acquisition protocols and postprocessing of the volumetric data (multiplanar reformation, maximum intensity projection, shaded surface display, volumetric rendering) provides highly detailed and visually familiar anatomic images (also see Chapter 12). The initial CT images consist of a series of overlapping transverse sections that are interpreted according to standard protocols with attention to soft tissue, pulmonary, and bony structures. The intimal flap appears as a thin, low attenuation, linear or spiral structure that separates the true and false lumens. Additional findings include luminal displacement of intimal calcium, delayed contrast enhancement of the false lumen, and aortic widening. Branch vessel involvement anywhere along the course of the aorta to the level of the iliac arteries can be precisely displayed. In addition, CTA can visualize the proximal third of the coronary arteries. While information regarding pericardial involvement is readily apparent, neither aortic valve nor left ventricular function can be appreciated. CTA requires intravenous contrast and exposure to ionizing radiation. Postprocessed images may have a "stairstep" appearance when the initial transverse images are acquired without adequate overlap. Dedicated emergency department scanners are now widespread, and studies can be obtained,

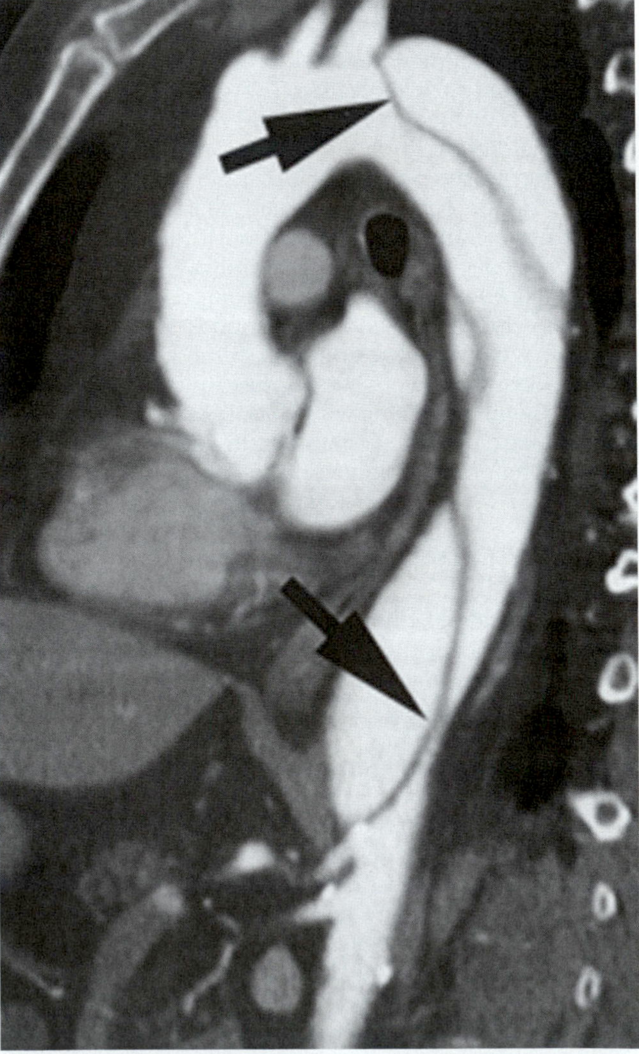

FIGURE 34-4. Reformatted oblique sagittal computed tomographic angiography demonstrating a type B dissection *(arrows)*. (From Olin JW, Kaufman JA, Bluemke DA, et al: Atherosclerotic vascular disease conference. Writing Group IV: Imaging. Circulation 109:2626, 2004.)

reconstructed, and interpreted within 15 to 20 minutes. CTA has several advantages relative to MRA including wider availability, higher spatial resolution, absence of arterial flow-related artifacts, and the capability to visualize calcification and metallic implants.

Magnetic Resonance Imaging/Angiography

MRI is infrequently used as the initial imaging study of patients with suspected acute aortic syndromes (also see Chapter 11).[50] Many hospitals do not have 24-hour availability. The magnet is usually located at a distance from the emergency department, operating rooms, and intensive care units. Monitoring and treatment of an acutely ill and hemodynamically unstable patient within the magnet can be difficult. In addition, implanted cardiac devices and certain metallic clips are contraindications to MRI. Nevertheless, rapid imaging protocols using single breath hold have been established at regional centers with an interest in aortic diseases, and accurate diagnoses can be rendered in less than 30 minutes. Contrast enhancement with a nonnephrotoxic agent, gadolinium, and three-dimensional multiplanar reconstruction provide superior detail. Ionizing radiation is not used. Precise information regarding the dissection flap, entry/reentry sites, true and false lumen blood flow, branch vessel involvement, and aortic size is provided (Fig. 34-5). MRI also allows for the assessment of pericardial involvement, aortic regurgitation, proximal coronary artery involvement, and left ventricular function. No other single test provides such comprehensive anatomic and physiologic information. This technique is particularly well suited to the long-term surveillance of patients with aortic disease after hospital-based treatment.

Contrast Aortography

Contrast aortography, the previous gold standard, is less sensitive than currently available noninvasive cross-sectional imaging techniques for the diagnosis of aortic dissection and its variants. In the IRAD experience, aortography was used as the initial study in only 4% of patients, though it was chosen more frequently when a second or even third test was required for diagnosis.[50] Its chief limitations include its invasive nature, the time required to assemble the angiographic team in an emergency situation, the need for contrast and ionizing radiation, and the incidence of false-negative studies (up to 23%).[54] The diagnosis of dissection may be missed when the intimal flap is not visualized in the projection chosen, when there is thrombosis of the false lumen with sealing of the entry tear and lack of communication with the true lumen, when the injection is incorrectly made in the false lumen, or when there is equal and rapid opacification of the true and false lumens without obvious aortic dilatation. Direct evidence of dissection includes visualization of the intimal flap and two lumens; indirect evidence consists of true lumen compression and deformation, aortic wall thickening, branch vessel compromise, and aortic regurgitation. Svensson and coworkers reported the usefulness of aortography for the identification of discrete, limited aortic dissection (healed intimal tear) when cross-sectional techniques were nondiagnostic.[55] Contrast aortography is a requisite for any catheter-based intervention.

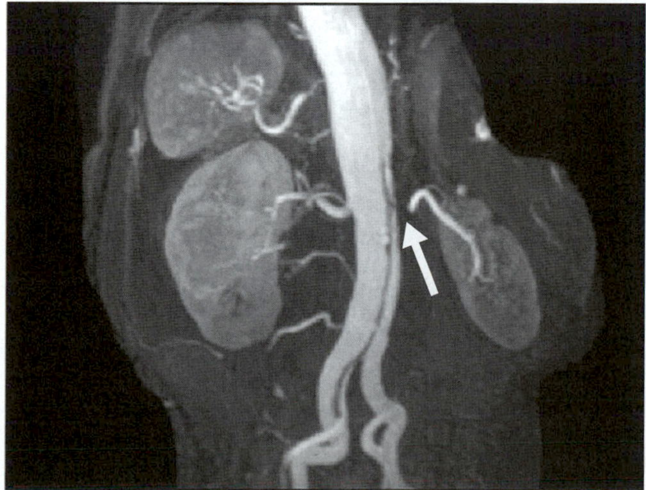

FIGURE 34-5. Magnetic resonance angiogram (posterior oblique view) of aortic dissection with extension of the intimal flap into the left common iliac artery and involvement of the origin of the right renal artery *(arrow)*.

Intravascular Ultrasound

Intravascular ultrasound (IVUS) can provide clear delineation of the intimal flap; its pulsatile movement; longitudinal and circumferential extent; luminal dimensions and contour; the mechanism of branch vessel compromise; and the presence of thrombus, fibrin strands, or spontaneous contrast in the false lumen. Sensitivities and specificities of nearly 100% have been reported.[56] Doppler assessment is not routinely feasible, and the entire aorta cannot be displayed in areas of significant aneurysmal enlargement. It is quite accurate for the detection of intramural hematoma and complicated aortic atherosclerotic plaque with medial hemorrhage. IVUS is often used during the performance of catheter-based fenestration procedures in which access is achieved either via retrograde femoral artery insertion or via placement in the common femoral vein with advancement to the inferior vena cava.[57]

Coronary Angiography

Coronary angiography is neither indicated nor advisable in anticipation of emergency surgery for type A dissection.[58] Operative mortality is generally not related to myocardial ischemia, but rather to aortic rupture, and the performance of angiography consumes valuable time before life-saving surgery. Angiography may be indicated in special circumstances, however, such as in the evaluation of a patient with a chronic type A dissection following previous coronary artery bypass graft surgery or in the type B patient with unstable angina before planned aortic or coronary intervention, or both. Other clinical exigencies may pertain that require surgical judgment, but these are infrequent.

DIFFERENTIAL DIAGNOSIS

Other Acute Aortic Syndromes (Box 34-1)

Aortic transection from deceleration injury and traumatic aortic valve disruption with acute severe aortic regurgitation occur in the setting of high-speed vehicular accidents or vertical falls. The nontraumatic acute aortic syndromes, however, are often not distinguishable from classic dissection on clinical grounds alone.

BOX 34-1 Acute Aortic Syndromes

Aortic dissection
Intramural hematoma
Penetrating aortic ulcer
Rapid aneurysm expansion
Trauma

Aortic Intramural Hematoma (Fig. 34-6)

Evidence of medial hemorrhage without an identifiable intimal flap, entry tear, or double lumen is observed clinically in 10% to 30% of cases of suspected acute aortic dissection.[58] In autopsy studies, intramural hematoma (IMH) accounts for up to 5% to 13% of cases of acute aortic syndromes.[59] The radiologic differentiation of IMH from noncommunicating aortic dissection with thrombosis of the false lumen, sealing of the entry tear, and reapposition of the intimal flap can be difficult, although unlikely to affect patient treatment. IMH is thought to result from rupture of the nutrient vasa vasorum and can extend both circumferentially and longitudinally, though branch vessel compromise is less likely. Some investigators have postulated that the inciting event is an intimal tear that is too limited to be visualized by noninvasive imaging techniques.[60] Predisposing factors and clinical presentation are similar to those described in patients with classic aortic dissection.[61] TEE criteria for diagnosis include crescentic or circumferential wall thickening of greater than 0.7 cm with displacement of intimal calcium. Echolucency implies a more active hematoma; flow is absent by Doppler criteria. IMH is seen as an area of high attenuation thickening on noncontrast CT images without enhancement after contrast bolus. Acute IMH has iso-dense signal intensity on T1-weighted MR images and high signal intensity on T2-weighted MR images. As the hematoma matures with time, and more oxyhemoglobin is converted to methemoglobin, the T1-weighted images show high signal intensity in the area of wall thickening. IMH may also be difficult to distinguish from aneurysm with mural thrombus, severe atherosclerosis, and aortitis with medial inflammation and edema.

IMH has a variable natural history, and controversy exists regarding its management.[62-68] Longitudinal studies with clinical and radiologic follow-ups have demonstrated spontaneous resorption, evolution to classic dissection, rupture, aneurysm formation, and false aneurysm development. Factors associated with risk of death and major complications include ascending aortic involvement, maximal aortic diameter greater than 5 cm

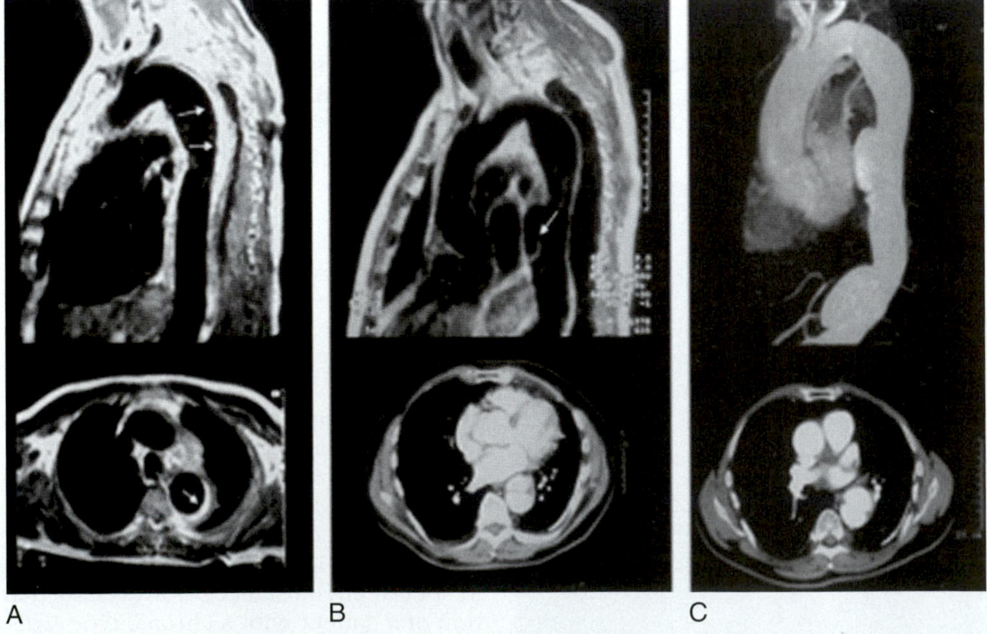

FIGURE 34-6. Type B intramural hematoma (IMH) with evolution to dissection and false aneurysm formation over 4 years. In the acute phase **(A, top and bottom),** MRI shows the IMH as a high-signal intensity lesion within the wall of the aorta. At 6 months, there is a localized dissection at the site of the IMH. The intimal flap is clearly seen in the computed tomographic angiography **(B, lower panel).** At 4 years, there are two pseudoaneurysms, one at the site of the localized dissection and another in the abdominal aorta **(C, upper panel gradient echo MRI, lower panel CTA).** (From Evangelista A, Dominguez R, Sebastia C, et al: Long-term follow-up of aortic intramural hematoma. Predictors of outcome. Circulation 108:583, 2003.)

on initial study, a progressive increase in aortic wall thickness on serial studies, the coexistence of an active, penetrating atherosclerotic ulcer, and age. Most authorities advise treating IMH and classic aortic dissection in the same way, with emergency surgery for type A disease and initial medical management for type B disease.[58,69]

Penetrating Aortic Ulcer (Fig. 34-7)

Erosion of the internal elastic membrane beneath an inflamed, atherosclerotic plaque allows luminal blood to burrow into the media of the aorta. The extent, severity, and fate of the accompanying intramural hemorrhage vary widely among patients. Such lesions are observed most commonly in the distal segment of the descending thoracic aorta in older individuals with hypertension and evidence of systemic atherosclerosis. Severe chest or back pain is the hallmark of presentation; signs of branch vessel compromise are distinctly uncommon. Diagnosis with TEE consists of the demonstration of deep ulcerations with jagged edges in association with complex atheromatous plaques and inward displacement of intimal calcium. CT/MRA criteria for diagnosis include ulcerative projections of contrast beyond the lumen of the aorta, aortic wall thickening with medial hemorrhage, inward displacement of intimal calcium, and the absence of an intimal flap. Periaortic hemorrhage of variable magnitude, atelectasis of neighboring lung parenchyma, and pleural effusion are commonly present. The penetrating aortic ulcer (PAU) may stabilize with conservative therapy or progress to formation of an aneurysm, pseudo-aneurysm, classic dissection, or rupture. Risk factors for disease progression include refractory pain, location in the proximal segment of the descending thoracic aorta, maximal ulcer diameter greater than 2 cm, and maximal ulcer depth greater than 1 cm.[66] Medical management with vigilant clinical and radiologic follow-up is advised for the initially uncomplicated descending thoracic PAU. Surgery or endovascular stent grafting when feasible can be undertaken for failed medical therapy, false aneurysm, or rupture.

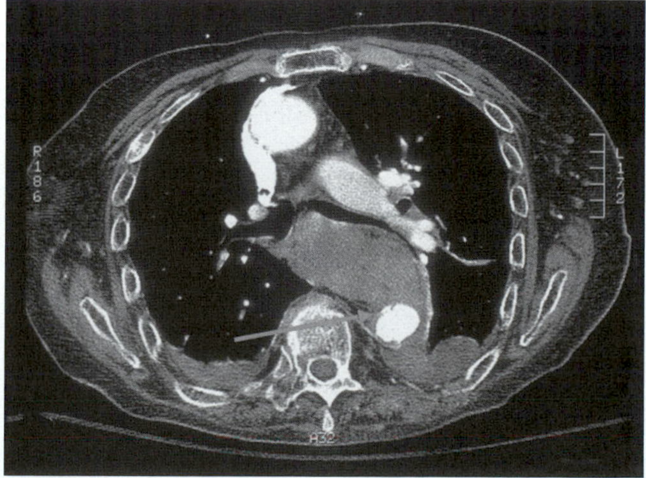

FIGURE 34-7. Computed tomographic angiography of type B penetrating aortic ulcer with large periaortic hematoma formation. The aortic lumen is irregular with spiculated borders *(arrows)*.

Acute Aneurysm Expansion

Acute, painful expansion of a previously established aortic aneurysm may herald impending rupture. Compression of contiguous anatomic structures may cause various associated symptoms, such as hoarseness (recurrent laryngeal nerve), dysphagia (esophagus), wheezing (bronchus), and facial edema (superior vena cava). Expansion can occur with aneurysm due to atherosclerosis (especially abdominal or descending thoracic in location), aortitis (giant cell), or cystic medial degeneration. Imaging studies may reveal wall thickening and periaortic stranding or hematoma, as well as a measurable increase in aortic dimensions when compared with available past studies. Urgent surgical management is indicated.

Nonaortic Diseases

Chest or back pain may be the presenting symptom of various conditions including acute myocardial infarction, unstable angina, pericarditis, musculoskeletal pain, pulmonary embolism, pneumonia, pleuritis, and cholecystitis.[70] Attention to the patient's description of the nature and quality of the pain, the presence of predisposing factors, the physical examination, and the initial laboratory studies should allow early differentiation.

INITIAL MEDICAL TREATMENT (Fig. 34-8)

Patients with acute aortic syndromes should be treated with IV medications to lower the arterial blood pressure and its rate of rise (dP/dT) as expeditiously as possible, even as imaging studies are being organized. Concomitant analgesia for pain control is essential. The blood pressure should be reduced to the lowest level possible without compromise of vital organ perfusion, usually in the range of 90 to 100 mm Hg systolic, and the heart rate to 50 to 60 beats/min. The mainstay of medical therapy is treatment with a β-adrenoreceptor antagonist, either alone or in combination with a potent vasodilator such as sodium nitroprusside. The use of propranolol (up to 0.15 mg/kg intravenously over 20 to 30 minutes) has largely been replaced by the reliance on metoprolol in doses similar to those provided to patients with acute coronary syndromes (5 mg bolus every 5 minutes for 3 doses). Esmolol, an ultra-short acting cardioselective agent, can be given by continuous infusion (50 mcg/kg/min) after a bolus dose of 0.5 mg/kg but is expensive and obligates a fluid load for administration. Alternatively, labetalol, an agent with both α- and nonselective β-blocking properties, can be used. The drug is initiated as an IV bolus of 10 to 20 mg with repeat doses of 20 to 40 mg every 10 to 15 minutes as needed to a total dose of 300 mg. An infusion of 1 to 2 mg/min can then be given for maintenance control. The standard contraindications to β-adrenoreceptor antagonists include known allergy, severe reactive airway disease, significant bradycardia (heart rate less than 50 beats/min), marked first-degree or advanced heart block, hypotension, and decompensated heart failure. A rate-slowing calcium channel blocker, such as diltiazem or verapamil, can be substituted as indicated.

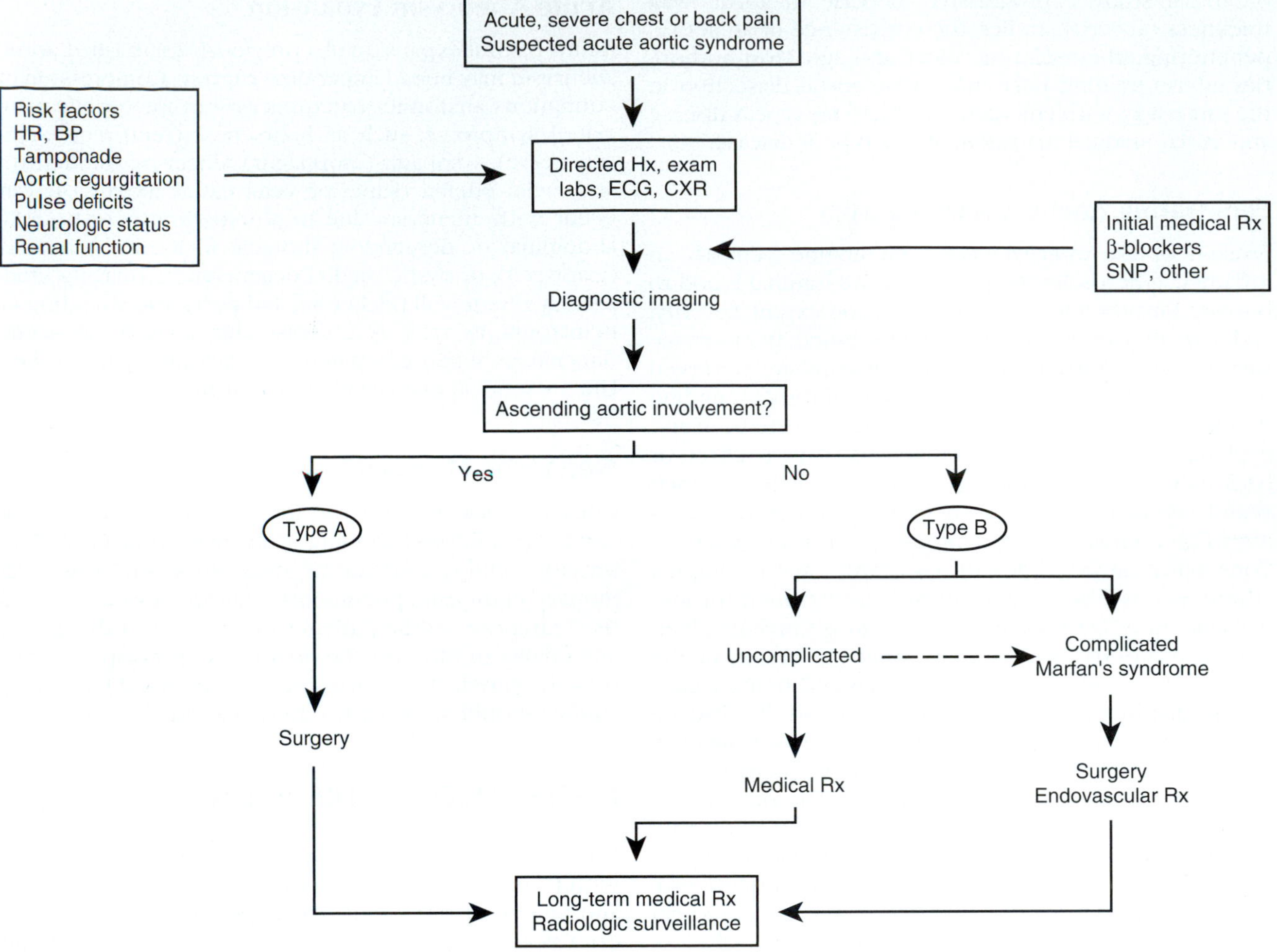

FIGURE 34-8. Clinical decision making in acute aortic syndromes. Hx, history; CXR, chest x-ray; Rx, therapy, HR, heart rate; BP, blood pressure; SNP, sodium nitroprusside.

Sodium nitroprusside should not be initiated without adequate heart rate control, as reflex tachycardia would be deleterious. The starting dose is 25 mcg/min by continuous infusion. Dose adjustments are usually made in increments of 10 to 25 mcg, and continuous intra-arterial blood pressure monitoring is required. Measurement of thiocyanate levels is especially indicated in patients with renal insufficiency. Other IV vasodilators available for use in the acute setting include enalaprilat and hydralazine. Sublingual nifedipine is no longer approved.

INDICATIONS FOR SURGERY

(Table 34-2, Fig. 34-8)

The definitive treatment of acute aortic dissection has evolved empirically over the past 50 years, predicated largely on continued improvements in surgical and anesthetic techniques, the advent of endovascular stent grafting, the application of percutaneous fenestration and branch vessel stenting, and the adoption of standardized protocols for medical therapy. Prospective randomized controlled trials are lacking and not likely to be undertaken. Nevertheless, strong consensus has been achieved regarding the initial approach to aortic dissection.

Early mortality following aortic dissection varies inversely as a function of the distance of the entry tear from the aortic valve. Emergency surgery is indicated for all type A dissections, regardless of the site of entry.[58,71]

TABLE 34-2 INDICATIONS FOR SURGERY

Acute Dissection	Chronic Dissection
• All Type A • Complicated Type B	• Type A Maximal dimension ≥ 5-5.5 cm Marfan's syndrome, dimension ≥ 4.5-5 cm Increase in dimension ≥ 1 cm/yr Severe aortic regurgitation Symptoms related to expansion or compression
Rupture Recurrent/Refractory pain Extension Rapid aneurysm expansion Malperfusion syndrome Marfan's syndrome	• Type B Maximal dimension ≥ 6 cm Increase in dimension > 1 cm/yr Symptoms related to expansion or compression

Surgery is performed to prevent rupture with exsanguination or tamponade and to relieve aortic regurgitation when present. The extent and complexity of surgery (resection/grafting of the ascending aorta, valve resuspension or replacement, coronary artery reimplantation) depends on the radiologic and intraoperative findings (see Chapter 35). Incorporation of the aortic arch in the primary repair is indicated when the tear traverses this segment of the aorta or when it has become acutely aneurysmal. Uncomplicated type B dissection is treated medically. Surgery for acute type B dissection is reserved for those patients who have failed initial conservative therapy as indicated by refractory or recurrent pain; continued extension; early aneurysmal expansion, rupture, or malperfusion syndrome; and for patients with Marfan's syndrome. Surgery is also recommended when dissection occurs within a previously known aneurysmal aortic segment. The indications for endovascular stent grafting, percutaneous fenestration, and branch vessel stenting, as alternatives to surgery, are evolving and likely to assume more prominent roles at an earlier treatment stage in the management of type B dissection (see Chapter 36).[58,71]

Surgery for chronic aortic dissection is indicated for the treatment of severe, aortic regurgitation when present, as dictated by symptoms or signs of left ventricular dysfunction, or for the management of aneurysm disease according to conventional size criteria (≥5 cm for ascending aortic aneurysm, ≥6 cm for descending thoracic aneurysm, ≥5 to 5.5 cm for abdominal aortic aneurysm, or ≥1 cm/yr increase in maximal dimension). Aneurysmal enlargement and recurrent dissection are more likely with long-term patency of the false lumen.[8,9]

PROGNOSIS

Survival and functional outcomes have clearly improved over the past four to five decades, but much progress remains to be made. In the original IRAD report comprising 464 patients from 12 international referral centers, the overall hospital mortality rate was 27.4%.[30] As noted previously, clear distinctions between types A and B dissection have informed clinical decision making.

With medical management of type A dissection, mortality rates approach 20% at 24 hours after presentation, 30% at 48 hours, 40% at day 7, and 50% by 1 month (Fig. 34-9).[30] In contrast, surgical repair of type A dissection is associated with mortality rates of 10% at 24 hours, 13% at 1 week, and 20% at 1 month. The overall hospital mortality rate for type A patients is approximately 35%.[30] The most common causes of death include rupture, tamponade, low-output syndrome, stroke, and malperfusion syndromes. Multivariate predictors of death identified by logistic regression include: age 70 years and older (odds ratio [OR] 1.7, 95% confidence interval [CI] 1.05-2.77); abrupt onset of chest pain (OR 2.6, 95% CI 1.22-5.54); hypotension/shock/tamponade (OR 2.97, 95% CI 1.83-4.81); renal failure (OR 4.77, 95% CI 1.80-12.6); pulse deficit (OR 2.03, 95% CI 1.25-3.29), and abnormal ECG (OR 1.77, 95% CI 1.06-2.95).[72] A bedside risk prediction tool for in-hospital mortality incorporating these variables offers clinicians, patients, and families a useful method by which to understand the complexities and hazards of the acute dissection process (Fig. 34-10).[72]

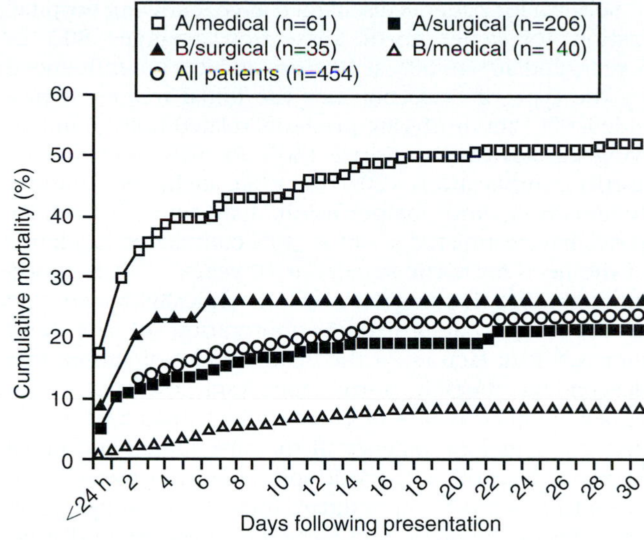

FIGURE 34-9. Thirty-day survival for patients with acute aortic dissection in the International Registry of Acute Aortic Dissection. Note differences in survival as a function of type of dissection and surgical versus medical treatment. (From Hagan PG, Nienaber CA, Isselbacher EM, et al: The international registry of acute aortic dissection (IRAD): New insights into an old disease. JAMA 283:897-903, 2000.)

For type B dissection, overall in-hospital mortality rates approach 15%.[30] For patients with uncomplicated type B dissection managed medically, 1 month survival is 90%, whereas for patients who require surgical intervention for the indications listed previously, 1 month survival is only 75%. Independent predictors of early mortality include advanced age, rupture, and malperfusion syndromes.[58] The excess mortality risk imposed by early complications necessitating surgical treatment, and thus operation on acutely sicker patients, has prompted investigation of the prophylactic use of endovascular stent grafting for select patients.[58,73]

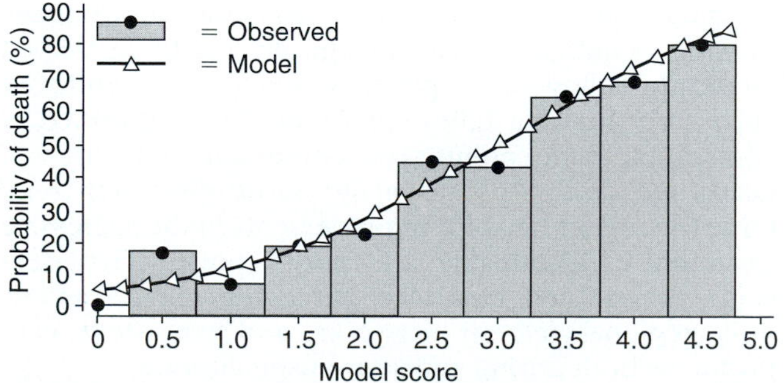

FIGURE 34-10. Observed versus predicted mortality rate for patients with acute type A dissection in the International Registry of Aortic Dissection. Both predicted and observed mortality rates increase as a function of the number of validated risk factors. Variables used in the risk model include age, female gender, abrupt onset of pain, abnormal ECG, pulse deficit, renal failure, and hypotension/shock/tamponade. (From Mehta RH, Manfredini R, Hassan F, et al: Predicting death in patients with acute type A aortic dissection. Circulation 105:200-206, 2002.)

Survival for patients discharged alive following hospitalization for acute aortic dissection averages 80% at 5 years and 40% to 60% at 10 years, and it is not influenced by the type of dissection nor the initial treatment provided.[58,71] Late deaths are primarily related both to underlying cardiovascular disease (30% to 50%) and to fatal aortic complications (20% to 40%), including rupture, redissection, and malperfusion syndromes.[74,75] Older series have estimated a 10% to 30% cumulative incidence of the need for aortic surgery at 10 years.[76,77] It is important to realize that less than 10% of surgically treated type A dissections demonstrate obliteration of the false lumen.[58] Risk factors for the development of subsequent descending thoracic aortic aneurysm formation, with either operated type A or conservatively managed type B dissection, include patency of the false lumen and initial maximal descending thoracic aortic diameter greater than or equal to 4 cm.[8,9] The standard indications for operation or endovascular stent grafting of aortic aneurysm disease include maximal dimension, change in dimension over time (≥1cm/yr), associated symptoms (chiefly pain), and, in the case of ascending aortic involvement, severe aortic regurgitation. Size criteria are more restricted for patients with Marfan's disease (see Table 34-2).

LONG-TERM SURVEILLANCE

Because of the life-long risk of subsequent aortic and cardiovascular complications, vigilant clinical and radiologic follow-up is mandatory for all hospital survivors. Medical management remains targeted to strict blood pressure (≤130/80 mm Hg) and heart rate (≤70 beats/min) goals, as tolerated by an individual patient. β-Adreno-receptor antagonists are the cornerstone of medical therapy; additional antihypertensive medications are used as needed and as indicated by other medical conditions (such as diabetes, heart failure, chronic kidney disease, or systemic atherosclerotic disease). Strenuous exercise is discouraged. Imaging of the entire aorta is recommended before discharge and at 1, 3, 6, 9, and 12 months, then annually thereafter.[71] The choice of imaging modality should again reflect local availability, expertise, and individual patient attributes. CTA and MRA are most commonly used. These protocols apply equally to patients initially managed surgically and those treated medically. Follow-up of patients after primary endovascular stent grafting relies chiefly on CTA performed at comparable time points. The continued high rates of death and disability from acute aortic dissection reinforce the urgent need for improvements in the aggressive treatment of identifiable risk factors (notably, hypertension), genetic and biomarker screening, clinical awareness, regional referral networks, and consistent care protocols both during and after hospitalization.

REFERENCES

1. Anagnostopoulos C: Acute Aortic Dissections. Baltimore, University Park Press, 1975.
2. Meszaros I, Morocz J, Szlavi J, et al: Epidemiology and clinicopathology of aortic dissection. Chest 117:1271, 2000.
3. Clouse WD, Hallett JW Jr, Schaff HV, et al: Acute aortic dissection: Population-based incidence compared with degenerative aortic aneurysm rupture. Mayo Clin Proc 79:176, 2004.
4. Hirst AE Jr, Johns VJ Jr, Kime SW Jr: Dissecting aneurysm of the aorta: A review of 505 cases. Medicine (Baltimore) 37:217, 1958.
5. Daily PO, Trueblood HW, Stinson EB, et al: Management of acute aortic dissections. Ann Thorac Surg 10:237, 1970.
6. DeBakey ME, Beall AC Jr, Cooley DA, et al: Dissecting aneurysms of the aorta. Surg Clin North Am 46:1045, 1966.
7. Lansman SL, McCullough JN, Nguyen KH, et al: Subtypes of acute aortic dissection. Ann Thorac Surg 67:1975, 1999.
8. Nataatmadja M, West M, West J, et al: Abnormal extracellular matrix protein transport associated with increased apoptosis of vascular smooth muscle cells in Marfan syndrome and bicuspid aortic valve thoracic aortic aneurysm. Circulation 108(Suppl 1):II329, 2003.
9. De Paepe A, Devereux RB, Dietz HC, et al: Revised diagnostic criteria for the Marfan syndrome. Am J Med Genet 62:417, 1996.
10. Sakai LY, Keene DR, Engvall E: Fibrillin, a new 350-kD glycoprotein, is a component of extracellular microfibrils. J Cell Biol 103:2499, 1986.
11. Boileau C, Jondeau G, Babron MC, et al: Autosomal dominant Marfan-like connective-tissue disorder with aortic dilation and skeletal anomalies not linked to the fibrillin genes. Am J Hum Genet 53:46, 1993.
12. Milewicz DM, Pyeritz RE, Crawford ES, et al: Marfan syndrome: Defective synthesis, secretion, and extracellular matrix formation of fibrillin by cultured dermal fibroblasts. J Clin Invest 89:79, 1992.
13. Aoyama T, Francke U, Dietz HC, et al: Quantitative differences in biosynthesis and extracellular deposition of fibrillin in cultured fibroblasts distinguish five groups of Marfan syndrome patients and suggest distinct pathogenetic mechanisms. J Clin Invest 94:130, 1994.
14. Segura AM, Luna RE, Horiba K, et al: Immunohistochemistry of matrix metalloproteinases and their inhibitors in thoracic aortic aneurysms and aortic valves of patients with Marfan's syndrome. Circulation 98:II331, 1998.
15. Sakomura Y, Nagashima H, Aoka Y, et al: Expression of peroxisome proliferator-activated receptor-gamma in vascular smooth muscle cells is upregulated in cystic medial degeneration of annuloaortic ectasia in Marfan syndrome. Circulation 106:I259, 2002.
16. Dalgleish R: The human collagen mutation database 1998. Nucleic Acids Res 26:253, 1998.
17. Dalgleish R: The human type I collagen mutation database. Nucleic Acids Res 25:181, 1997.
18. Guo D, Hasham S, Kuang SQ, et al: Familial thoracic aortic aneurysms and dissections: Genetic heterogeneity with a major locus mapping to 5q13-14. Circulation 103:2461, 2001.
19. Vaughan CJ, Casey M, He J, et al: Identification of a chromosome 11q23.2-q24 locus for familial aortic aneurysm disease, a genetically heterogeneous disorder. Circulation 103:2469, 2001.
20. Coady MA, Davies RR, Roberts M, et al: Familial patterns of thoracic aortic aneurysms. Arch Surg 134:361, 1999.
21. Glesby MJ, Pyeritz RE: Association of mitral valve prolapse and systemic abnormalities of connective tissue. A phenotypic continuum. JAMA 262:523, 1989.
22. Furthmayr H, Francke U: Ascending aortic aneurysm with or without features of Marfan syndrome and other fibrillinopathies: New insights. Semin Thorac Cardiovasc Surg 9:191, 1997.
23. Pereira L, Lee SY, Gayraud B, et al: Pathogenetic sequence for aneurysm revealed in mice underexpressing fibrillin-1. Proc Natl Acad Sci U S A 96:3819, 1999.
24. Bunton TE, Biery NJ, Myers L, et al: Phenotypic alteration of vascular smooth muscle cells precedes elastolysis in a mouse model of Marfan syndrome. Circ Res 88:37, 2001.
25. Roberts CS, Roberts WC: Dissection of the aorta associated with congenital malformation of the aortic valve. J Am Coll Cardiol 17:712, 1991.
26. Shachter N, Perloff JK, Mulder DG: Aortic dissection in Noonan's syndrome (46 XY Turner). Am J Cardiol 54:464, 1984.
27. Lie JT: Aortic dissection in Turner's syndrome. Am Heart J 103:1077, 1982.
28. Biagini A, Maffei S, Baroni M, et al: Familiar clustering of aortic dissection in polycystic kidney disease. Am J Cardiol 72:741, 1993.
29. Hagan PG, Nienaber CA, Isselbacher EM, et al: The international registry of acute aortic dissection (IRAD): New insights into an old disease. JAMA 283:897, 2000.
30. Januzzi JL, Sabatine MS, Eagle KA, et al: Iatrogenic aortic dissection. Am J Cardiol 89:623, 2002.

31. von Kodolitsch Y, Simic O, Schwartz A, et al: Predictors of proximal aortic dissection at the time of aortic valve replacement. Circulation 100:II287, 1999.
32. Mandel W, Evans EW, Walford RL: Dissecting aortic aneurysm during pregnancy. N Engl J Med 251:1059, 1954.
33. Manalo-Estrella P, Barker AE: Histopathologic findings in human aortic media associated with pregnancy. Arch Pathol 83:336, 1967.
34. Garret R: Chronic diffuse giant cell mesaortitis, with dissecting aneurysm and rupture. Am J Clin Pathol 38:406, 1962.
35. Harris M: Dissecting aneurysm of the aorta due to giant cell arteritis. Br Heart J 30:840, 1968.
36. Nuenninghoff DM, Hunder GG, Christianson TJ, et al: Incidence and predictors of large-artery complication (aortic aneurysm, aortic dissection, and/or large-artery stenosis) in patients with giant cell arteritis: A population-based study over 50 years. Arthritis Rheum 48:3522, 2003.
37. Ando M, Okita Y, Tagusari O, et al: A surgically treated case of Takayasu's arteritis complicated by aortic dissections localized in the ascending and abdominal aortae. J Vasc Surg 31:1042, 2000.
38. Hainer JW, Hamilton GW: Aortic abnormalities in relapsing polychondritis: Report of a case with dissecting aortic aneurysm. N Engl J Med 280:1166, 1969.
39. Walts AE, Dubois EL: Acute dissecting aneurysm of the aorta as the fatal event in systemic lupus erythematosus. Am Heart J 93:378, 1977.
40. Kim MH, Abrams GD, Pernicano PG, et al: Sudden death in a 55-year-old woman with systemic lupus erythematosus. Circulation 98:271, 1998.
41. Harris ED, Rayton JK, DeGroot JE: A critical role for copper in aortic elastin structure and synthesis. Adv Exp Med Biol 79:543, 1977.
42. Hsue PY, Salinas CL, Bolger AF, et al: Acute aortic dissection related to crack cocaine. Circulation 105:1592, 2002.
43. von Kodolitsch Y, Schwartz AG, Nienaber CA: Clinical prediction of acute aortic dissection. Arch Intern Med 160:2977, 2000.
44. Mehta RH, Manfredini R, Hassan F, et al: Chronobiological patterns of acute aortic dissection. Circulation 106:1110, 2002.
45. Bossone E, Rampoldi V, Nienaber CA, et al: Usefulness of pulse deficit to predict in-hospital complications and mortality in patients with acute type A aortic dissection. Am J Cardiol 89:851, 2002.
46. von Kodolitsch Y, Nienaber CA, Dieckmann C, et al: Chest radiography for the diagnosis of acute aortic syndrome. Am J Med 116:73, 2004.
47. Suzuki T, Katoh H, Tsuchio Y, et al: Diagnostic implications of elevated levels of smooth-muscle myosin heavy-chain protein in acute aortic dissection: The smooth muscle myosin heavy chain study. Ann Intern Med 133:537, 2000.
48. Shinohara T, Suzuki K, Okada M, et al: Soluble elastin fragments in serum are elevated in acute aortic dissection. Arterioscler Thromb Vasc Biol 23:1839, 2003.
49. Weber T, Hogler S, Auer J, et al: D-dimer in acute aortic dissection. Chest 123:1375, 2003.
50. Moore AG, Eagle KA, Bruckman D, et al: Choice of computed tomography, transesophageal echocardiography, magnetic resonance imaging, and aortography in acute aortic dissection: International Registry of Acute Aortic Dissection (IRAD). Am J Cardiol 89:1235, 2002.
51. Bansal RC, Chandrasekaran K, Ayala K, et al: Frequency and explanation of false negative diagnosis of aortic dissection by aortography and transesophageal echocardiography. J Am Coll Cardiol 25:1393, 1995.
52. Svensson LG, Labib SB, Eisenhauer AC, et al: Intimal tear without hematoma: An important variant of aortic dissection that can elude current imaging techniques. Circulation 99:1331, 1999.
53. Yamada E, Matsumura M, Kyo S, et al: Usefulness of a prototype intravascular ultrasound imaging in evaluation of aortic dissection and comparison with angiographic study, transesophageal echocardiography, computed tomography, and magnetic resonance imaging. Am J Cardiol 75:161, 1995.
54. Chavan A, Hausmann D, Dresler C, et al: Intravascular ultrasound-guided percutaneous fenestration of the intimal flap in the dissected aorta. Circulation 96:2124, 1997.
55. Nienaber CA, Eagle KA: Aortic dissection: New frontiers in diagnosis and management: Part I: From etiology to diagnostic strategies. Circulation 108:628, 2003.
56. Nienaber CA, Eagle KA: Aortic dissection: New frontiers in diagnosis and management: Part II: Therapeutic management and follow-up. Circulation 108:772, 2003.
57. Mohr-Kahaly S: Aortic intramural hematoma: From observation to therapeutic strategies. J Am Coll Cardiol 37:1611, 2001.
58. Cambria RP: Regarding "Analysis of predictive factors for progression of type B aortic intramural hematoma with computed tomography." J Vasc Surg 35:1295, 2002.
59. Nienaber CA, von Kodolitsch Y, Petersen B, et al: Intramural hemorrhage of the thoracic aorta: Diagnostic and therapeutic implications. Circulation 92:1465, 1995.
60. Kang DH, Song JK, Song MG, et al: Clinical and echocardiographic outcomes of aortic intramural hemorrhage compared with acute aortic dissection. Am J Cardiol 81:202, 1998.
61. Maraj R, Rerkpattanapipat P, Jacobs LE, et al: Meta-analysis of 143 reported cases of aortic intramural hematoma. Am J Cardiol 86:664, 2000.
62. Sawhney NS, DeMaria AN, Blanchard DG: Aortic intramural hematoma: An increasingly recognized and potentially fatal entity. Chest 120:1340, 2001.
63. Song JK, Kim HS, Song JM, et al: Outcomes of medically treated patients with aortic intramural hematoma. Am J Med 113:181, 2002.
64. Ganaha F, Miller DC, Sugimoto K, et al: Prognosis of aortic intramural hematoma with and without penetrating atherosclerotic ulcer: A clinical and radiological analysis. Circulation 106:342, 2002.
65. von Kodolitsch Y, Csosz SK, Koschyk DH, et al: Intramural hematoma of the aorta: Predictors of progression to dissection and rupture. Circulation 107:1158, 2003.
66. Evangelista A, Dominguez R, Sebastia C, et al: Long-term follow-up of aortic intramural hematoma: Predictors of outcome. Circulation 108:583, 2003.
67. Nienaber CA, Sievers HH: Intramural hematoma in acute aortic syndrome: More than one variant of dissection? Circulation 106:284, 2002.
68. Eagle KA, Quertermous T, Kritzer GA, et al: Spectrum of conditions initially suggesting acute aortic dissection but with negative aortograms. Am J Cardiol 57:322, 1986.
69. Erbel R, Alfonso F, Boileau C, et al: Diagnosis and management of aortic dissection. Eur Heart J 22:1642, 2001.
70. Bernard Y, Zimmermann H, Chocron S, et al: False lumen patency as a predictor of late outcome in aortic dissection. Am J Cardiol 87:1378, 2001.
71. Yeh CH, Chen MC, Wu YC, et al: Risk factors for descending aortic aneurysm formation in medium-term follow-up of patients with type A aortic dissection. Chest 124:989, 2003.
72. Mehta RH, Suzuki T, Hagan PG, et al: Predicting death in patients with acute type A aortic dissection. Circulation 105:200, 2002.
73. Bortone AS, Schena S, D'Agostino D, et al: Immediate versus delayed endovascular treatment of post-traumatic aortic pseudoaneurysms and type B dissections: Retrospective analysis and premises to the upcoming European trial. Circulation 106:I234, 2002.
74. DeSanctis RW, Doroghazi RM, Austen WG, et al: Aortic dissection. N Engl J Med 317:1060, 1987.
75. Glower DD, Fann JI, Speier RH, et al: Comparison of medical and surgical therapy for uncomplicated descending aortic dissection. Circulation 82:IV39, 1990.
76. DeBakey ME, McCollum CH, Crawford ES, et al: Dissection and dissecting aneurysms of the aorta: Twenty-year follow-up of five hundred twenty-seven patients treated surgically. Surgery 92:1118, 1982.
77. Svensson LG, Crawford ES, Hess KR, et al: Dissection of the aorta and dissecting aortic aneurysms: Improving early and long-term surgical results. Circulation 82:IV24, 1990.
78. Pineiro DJ, Bellido CA: Images in clinical medicine: Circumferential dissection of the aorta. N Engl J Med 340:1553, 1999.
79. Olin JW, Kaufman JA, Bluemke DA, et al: Atherosclerotic vascular disease conference: Writing Group IV: Imaging. Circulation 109:2626, 2004.

chapter 35

Surgical Therapy

Scott A. LeMaire
Robert W. Thompson

Aortic dissection can produce a wide variety of life-threatening sequelae, including aortic rupture, pericardial tamponade, acute aortic valve insufficiency, and branch vessel malperfusion causing myocardial infarction, stroke, mesenteric ischemia, renal failure, or limb-threatening ischemia (Fig. 35-1). The potential for these acute complications, combined with severe physiologic derangement and extreme tissue fragility, make aortic dissection one of the most challenging conditions faced by cardiovascular surgeons.

Several aspects of surgical management—including the indications for operation and the strategies employed during repair—are based largely on when the dissection occurred and which parts of the aorta are involved. Within the first 14 days following the initial tear in the aortic wall, the dissection is considered *acute*. After 14 days, the dissection is described as *chronic*. Although arbitrary, the distinction between acute and chronic distal aortic dissections has important implications in perioperative management strategies, operative techniques, and surgical results. A guiding principle in the management of aortic dissection is that surgical repair becomes safer as the dissection becomes older and the aorta becomes less fragile. Dissections are also categorized based on anatomical location and extent in order to guide treatment. Borst and associates have advocated a simplified, descriptive classification of aortic dissection in favor of the traditional DeBakey and Stanford classifications (Fig. 35-2).[1] In this system the *proximal* (ascending and transverse arch) and *distal* (descending thoracic and thoracoabdominal) aortic segments are considered independently. This is useful because treatment strategies—detailed as follows—are based on which of these segments are involved.

ACUTE PROXIMAL DISSECTION

Without treatment, nearly one half of patients with acute proximal aortic dissection die within 48 hours.[2] Therefore aggressive pharmacologic reduction is initiated immediately once the diagnosis is suspected. Once pharmacologic treatment has started, the focus can shift to confirming the diagnosis and assessing treatment options (see Chapter 34).

Indications for Operation

Proximal aortic repairs performed in the chronic phase uniformly have better outcomes than those performed in the acute phase. Unfortunately, the high risk associated with early operation is outweighed by the even higher risk of a fatal complication, such as aortic rupture, during medical management. Therefore, the presence of an acute proximal aortic dissection has traditionally been considered an absolute indication for emergency surgical repair. Many authors continue to advocate this approach.[3-5] Although controversial, recent data suggest that specific patient groups—including the elderly, patients with severe malperfusion, and patients who have had previous cardiac operations—may benefit from nonoperative management or delayed operation.

Elderly Patients

In the wake of improving cardiac surgical outcomes in an aging population, recent attention has focused on the surgical treatment of elderly patients with acute proximal aortic dissection.[6] On the basis of discouraging outcomes in octogenarians who underwent emergency surgical repair of acute proximal dissection, Neri and colleagues[7] concluded that surgical treatment is not warranted in the elderly, because "it does not reverse the unfavorable prognosis of the disease." In response to this conclusion, other authors have reported more acceptable outcomes in the elderly, cautioned against generalizing Neri's data, and argued in favor of creating local policies based on institutional results and community input.[8,9] In their reply, Neri and colleagues proposed that the elderly be treated medically during the acute phase followed by elective repair during the subacute phase.[10] The interval essentially selects patients with the potential to recover from a second physiologic insult (i.e., surgery) and allows their medical optimization. Using this approach in eight elderly patients, the authors reported substantial improvements in survival. With such limited data from a single report, it is difficult to justify applying this strategy to patients on the basis of age alone; however, this approach does deserve consideration in elderly patients with substantial comorbidity. The recovery from an emergency operation in the setting of an acute dissection certainly requires more physiologic reserve than the recovery from an elective operation performed in the chronic phase. Therefore, patients who are poor candidates for emergency aortic repair may be reasonable candidates for elective surgery.

Severe Malperfusion

Branch vessel obstruction due to dissection creates a spectrum of malperfusion that ranges from mild

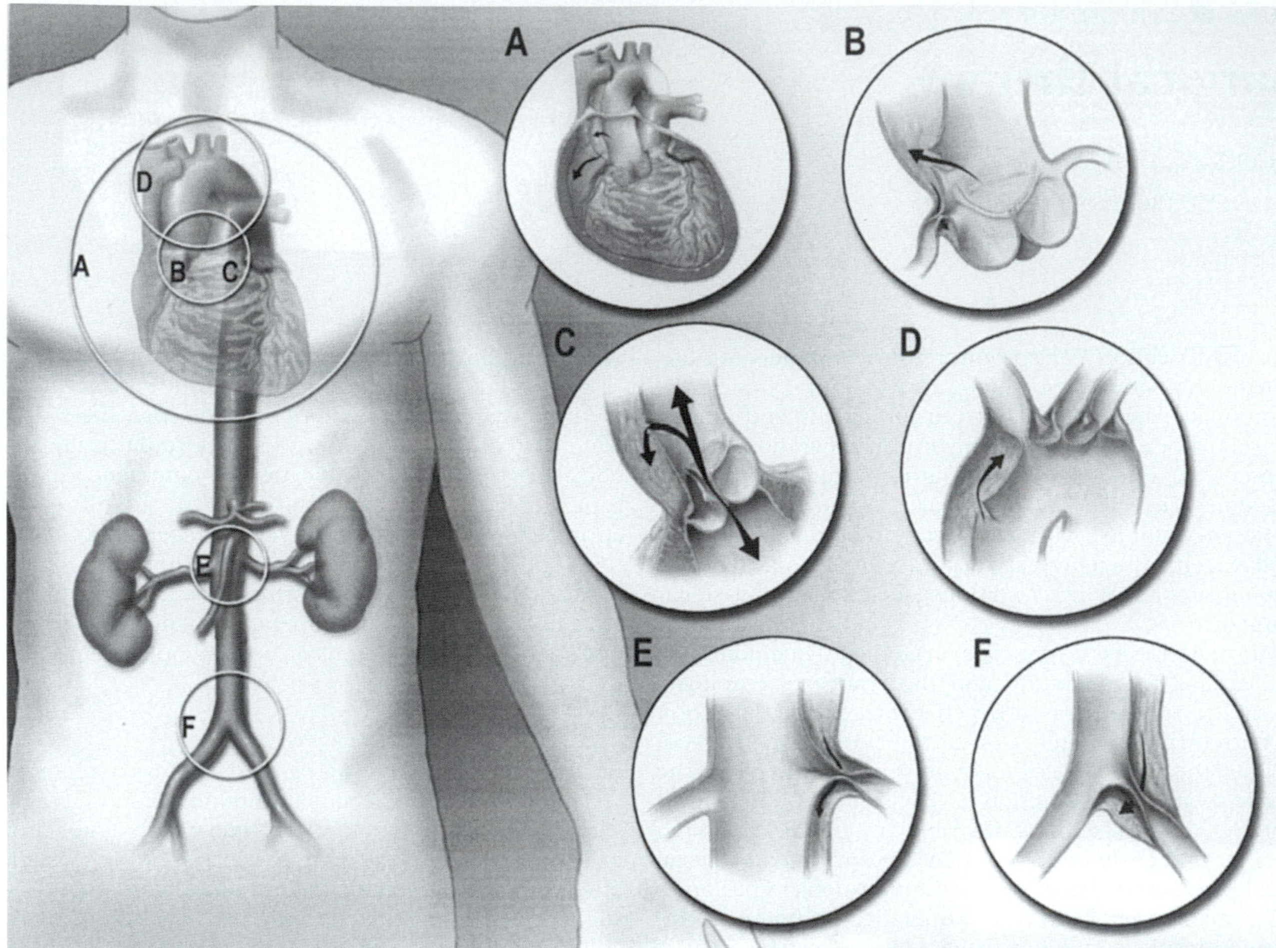

FIGURE 35-1. Common life-threatening sequelae of aortic dissection. The weakened aortic wall can rupture at any location and often results in fatal exsanguination. Rupture of the ascending aorta into the pericardial space **(A)** causes cardiac tamponade. Aortic dissection can lead to acute cardiac failure via **(B)** extension into the coronary ostia causing myocardial ischemia and **(C)** disruption of the aortic valve commissures causing valvular insufficiency. Complications of branch vessel malperfusion include **(D)** stroke or upper extremity ischemia when the brachiocephalic branches are involved; paraplegia when the segmental intercostal and lumbar arteries are compromised; **(E)** renal failure or mesenteric ischemia when the visceral vessels are disrupted; and **(F)** lower limb ischemia when the iliac arteries are occluded. The authors gratefully acknowledge Scott Weldon and Carol Larson for creating the artwork used throughout this chapter.

(e.g., diminished pulse in an extremity) to severe (e.g., bowel infarction). In most cases of mild to moderate malperfusion, surgical repair of the proximal aorta redirects flow into the true lumen and restores adequate peripheral blood flow; however, patients in whom ischemia has caused severe end-organ dysfunction—such as those with acute severe stroke or mesenteric ischemia—are unlikely to benefit from immediate aortic repair.[11] Deeb and colleagues[12] reported that eight of nine patients who underwent early proximal aortic repair in the setting of severe malperfusion, as defined in Box 35-1, died before discharge from the hospital. All of the deaths were attributed to irreversible organ damage from ischemia and severe reperfusion injury following cardiopulmonary bypass. On the basis of these results, these surgeons initiated a policy of delayed surgical management in patients with severe malperfusion; this strategy consisted of aggressive pharmacologic treatment to reduce dP/dT, confirmatory arteriography, percutaneous fenestration or stenting (if needed) to restore flow to compromised branch vessels, and elective operation after complete recovery from malperfusion. Of the 20 patients managed with this strategy, 17 underwent delayed operation an average of 20 days after presentation.[12] To reduce selection bias, the authors' analysis included all patients, including the three patients who died without operation (one due to rupture and two due to reperfusion injury) and the two patients who died after delayed surgery. The overall survival for these patients treated without immediate operation (15/20, 75%) was a significant improvement compared with the dismal survival obtained with a strategy of immediate surgery. Fabre and colleagues[13] have also advocated percutaneous intervention before operation in patients with severe ischemic sequelae.

Dissection after Cardiac Operations

Another group of patients who may benefit from early medical stabilization and delayed elective operation are those who have had cardiac surgery in the remote past. Surgical treatment of proximal dissection is aimed at

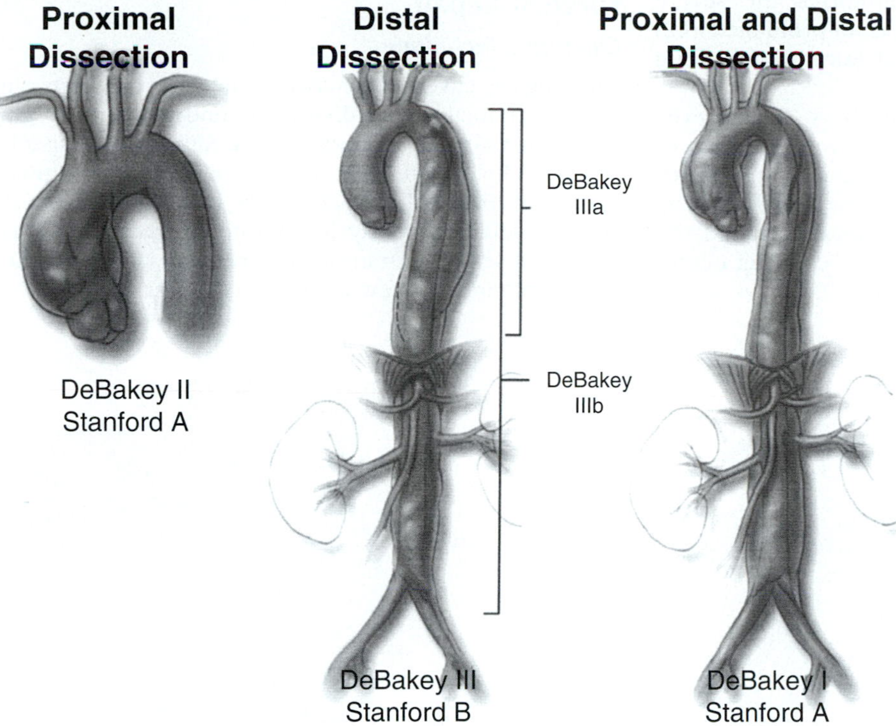

FIGURE 35-2. This simplified, descriptive classification scheme categorizes aortic dissection based on the involvement of the proximal aorta, the distal aorta, or both segments. The corresponding traditional classifications are included for comparison. The primary limitation of the Stanford classification is that it is based solely on the presence (type A) or absence (type B) of ascending aortic involvement; it does not provide information about distal aortic involvement, a factor that has important management and prognostic implications.

preventing aortic rupture, valvular dehiscence, and coronary occlusion. In the setting of a previous cardiac operation—especially previous aortic valve replacement—the risks of these complications are substantially reduced. Existing coronary bypass grafts or a previous aortotomy (as used for aortic valve replacement) can prevent coronary malperfusion. Ascending aortic rupture and tamponade are prevented by local postoperative changes including aortic wall thickening, adjacent scarring, and adhesions that obliterate the pericardial space. When the ascending aorta does rupture in this setting, the rupture is usually either contained by adjacent adhesions or it occurs through the lateral wall, into the right pleural space. As a caveat, it must be emphasized that the reduced risk of rupture does not apply to dissections that occur during the initial three weeks after cardiac surgery.[14] In fact, acute dissection during the early postoperative period carries a high risk of rupture and tamponade; these patients should undergo early operation.[15]

BOX 35-1 Definitions of Severe Malperfusion[12]

Severe myocardial malperfusion
Acute infarction diagnosed by electrocardiographic changes or elevated myocardial-specific enzyme levels associated with new-onset ventricular dysfunction
Severe cerebral malperfusion
Generalized nonresponsiveness or severe localized neurologic deficit lasting >48 hours
Severe visceral malperfusion
Abdominal pain, physical findings consistent with an acute abdomen, and associated abnormal laboratory findings
Severe extremity malperfusion
New-onset absence of pulse for more than 4 hours associated with pain, neurologic symptoms, and physical findings consistent with threatened limb function

Transport to Specialized Centers

The successful shift in management paradigm from immediate surgery to delayed operation in select patients has provided support for another evolving trend: transport to high-volume centers. Patients diagnosed with dissection in hospitals without cardiothoracic surgery are, of course, routinely transferred to centers that can provide surgical treatment. Accumulating evidence supports the intuitive notion that outcomes following many aortic and cardiac operations are best when performed by surgeons who have the most experience with the procedure in question.[16-18] Therefore, cardiac surgeons often transfer hemodynamically stable patients with acute proximal aortic dissection to regional high-volume centers that specialize in thoracic aortic operations.

The patient's condition is optimized before proceeding with transport. Aggressive pharmacologic management is initiated, and metabolic disturbances are corrected. The reliable delivery and titration of vasoactive medications during transport are facilitated by central venous and arterial catheters, respectively. Inotropes and diuretics are administered to patients with low cardiac output and acute ventricular distention due to aortic valvular insufficiency and volume overload. If a patient with pericardial tamponade must be transferred to receive surgical treatment, a pericardial drain is placed to allow intermittent drainage during transport.[19] Whenever possible, patients with limb-threatening ischemia should undergo revascularization—usually via a femoral-to-femoral artery bypass—before transport. This minimizes the severe metabolic derangements that result from prolonged limb ischemia and improves chances of survival following aortic repair.[12]

Standardized treatment protocols have been developed to optimize the hemodynamic management of patients with acute aortic dissection during transport. Implementation of the protocol developed by the Stanford Health Care Life Flight program reduced the number of patients who arrived at the receiving center with inadequate blood pressure control.[20]

Surgical Repair

Operative Techniques

Granting the caveats discussed earlier, most patients with acute proximal aortic dissection undergo urgent graft replacement of the ascending aorta. Although the specific strategies for accomplishing the repair vary substantially based on patient characteristics and surgeon preferences, a detailed description of one approach (Fig. 35-3) illustrates several common features and provides background regarding a few areas of controversy.

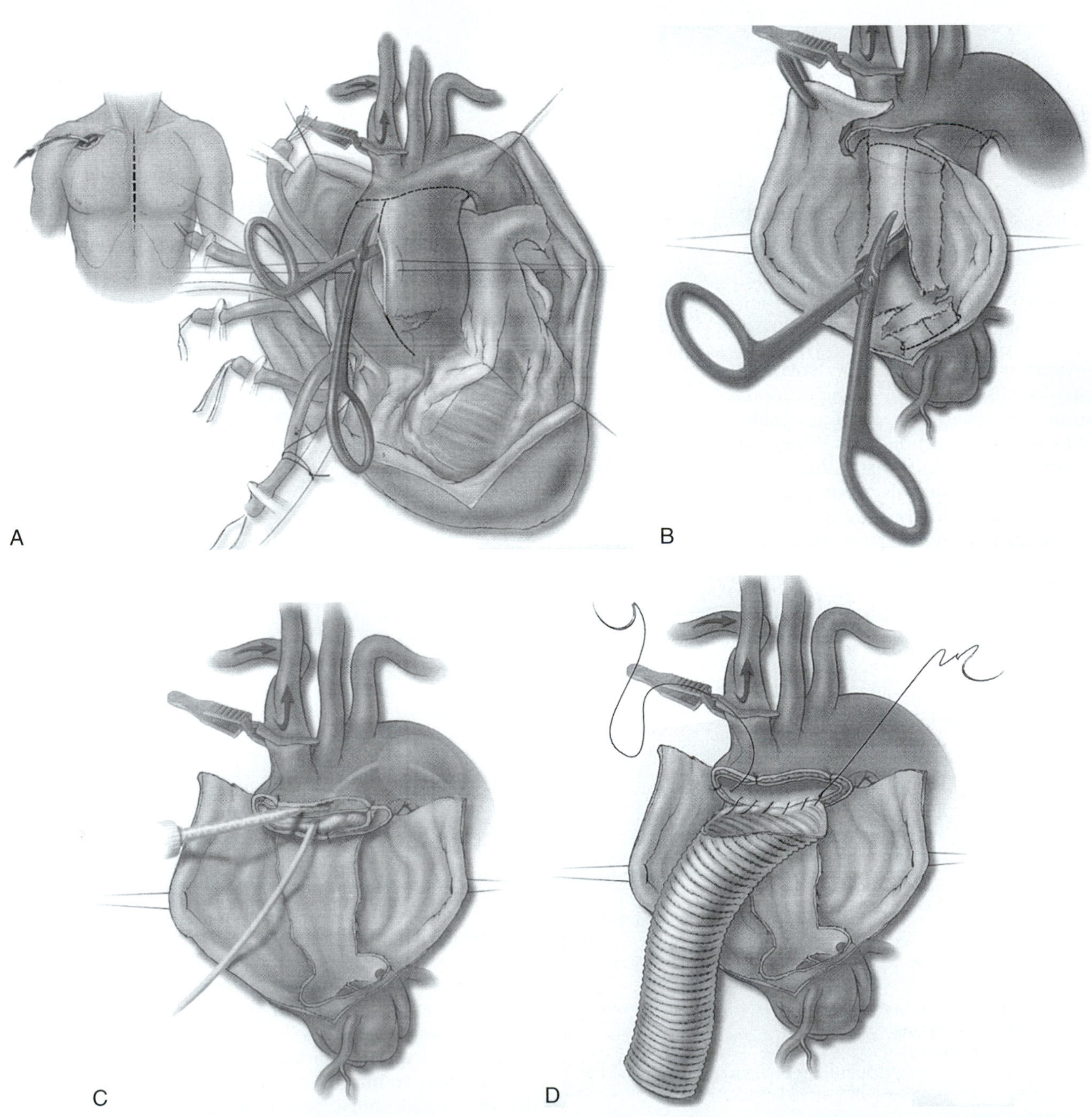

FIGURE 35-3. Graft repair of the ascending aorta and proximal transverse aortic hemiarch with concomitant aortic valve resuspension. **(A),** The operation is performed via a median sternotomy. Cardiopulmonary bypass is established via cannulas placed in the right axillary artery (arterial inflow) and the superior and inferior vena cavae (venous drainage). After initiating circulatory arrest and antegrade cerebral perfusion, the ascending aorta is opened and **(B),** the dissecting membrane is excised. **(C),** The distal aortic cuff is prepared using surgical adhesive; a balloon catheter in the descending aorta prevents distal migration of the adhesive. **(D),** The open distal anastomosis between the graft and the aorta is completed and reinforced with additional adhesive.

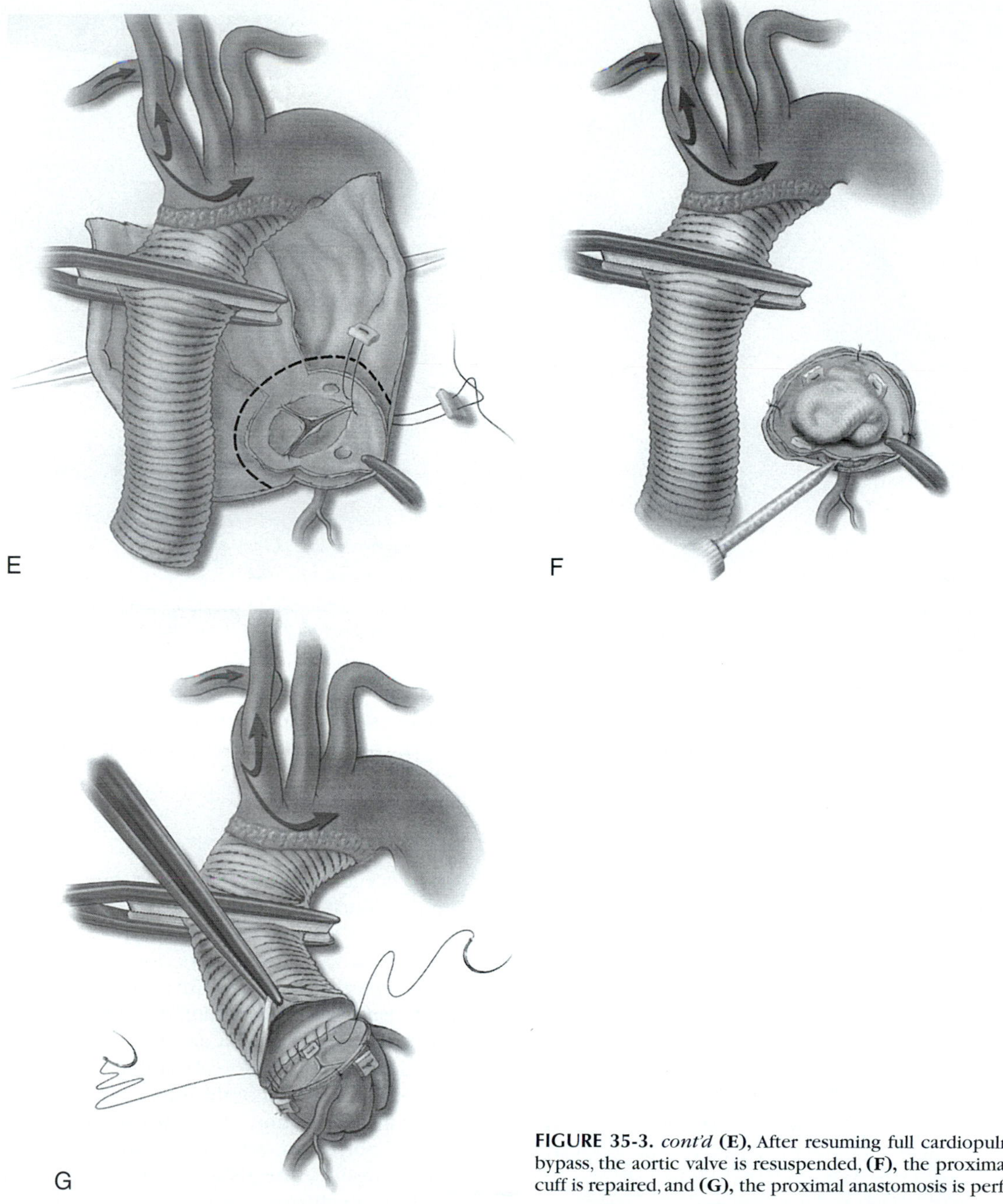

FIGURE 35-3. *cont'd* **(E),** After resuming full cardiopulmonary bypass, the aortic valve is resuspended, **(F),** the proximal aortic cuff is repaired, and **(G),** the proximal anastomosis is performed.

The operation is performed via a median sternotomy with cardiopulmonary bypass and hypothermic circulatory arrest (Fig. 35-3*A*). In preparation for circulatory arrest, cannulas are placed in the right axillary artery (arterial inflow) and the superior and inferior vena cavae (venous drainage). After initiating cardiopulmonary bypass, the patient is cooled until electroencephalographic monitoring demonstrates electrocerebral silence; this usually occurs when the patient's nasopharyngeal temperature falls below 20°C.[21] Cardiopulmonary bypass is then stopped, and the ascending aorta is opened. After occluding the innominate artery with a clamp or balloon catheter, flow from the axillary artery cannula is used to provide antegrade cerebral perfusion. The dissecting membrane that separates the true and false lumens is completely excised (see Fig. 35-3*B*). The transverse aortic arch—the segment from which the brachiocephalic branches arise—is carefully inspected. Replacement of the entire arch (Fig. 35-4) is performed only if a primary tear is located in the arch or if the full arch is aneurysmal; in most cases, a less extensive beveled "hemiarch" repair is adequate. The distal aortic cuff is prepared by tacking the inner and outer walls together and using surgical adhesive to obliterate the false lumen and strengthen the tissue (see Fig. 35-3*C*).[11,22-25] A polyester tube graft is sutured to the distal aortic cuff (see Fig. 35-3*D*). The anastomosis between the graft and the aorta is fashioned so that blood flow is directed into the true lumen; this often alleviates mild distal malperfusion problems that were present preoperatively.

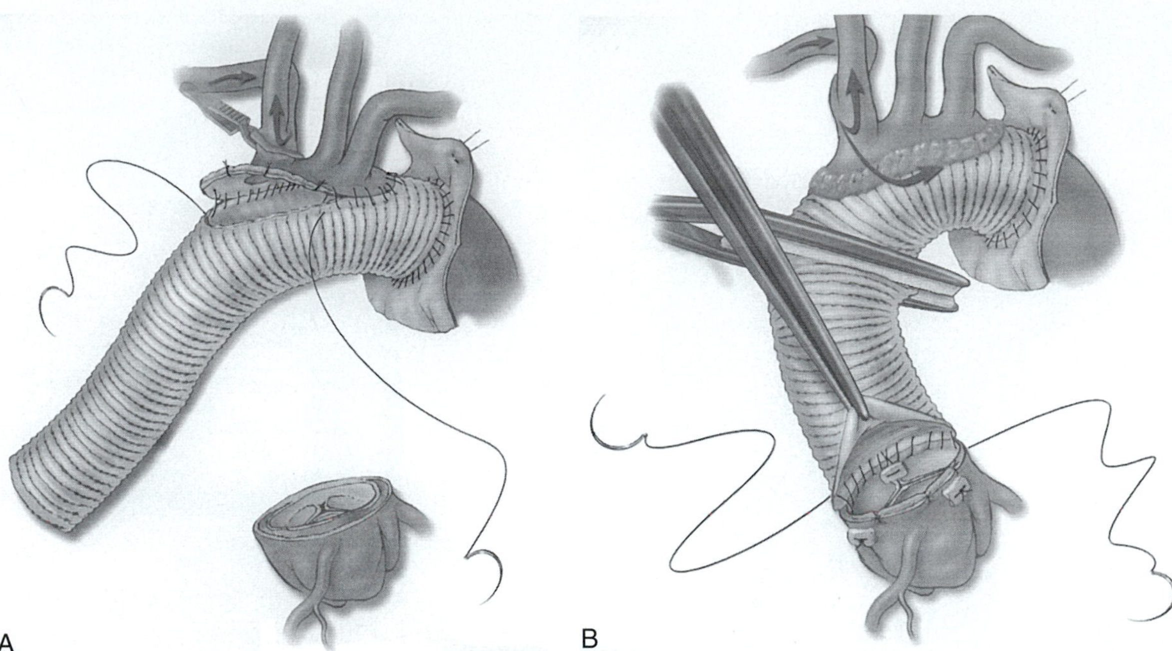

FIGURE 35-4. Graft replacement of the entire transverse aortic arch involves a distal anastomosis to the descending thoracic aorta and separate reattachment of the brachiocephalic branches. This approach is generally reserved for patients with primary tears within the arch or large aortic arch aneurysms.

After reinforcing the distal anastomosis with additional adhesive, retrograde cerebral perfusion is briefly delivered via the superior vena caval cannula, the graft is deaired and clamped, full cardiopulmonary bypass is resumed, rewarming is initiated, and the proximal portion of the repair is started (see Fig. 35-3*E*). In the absence of annuloaortic ectasia or Marfan's syndrome, aortic valve insufficiency can be corrected by resuspending the commissures onto the outer aortic wall (Fig. 35-5). The proximal aortic cuff is prepared with tacking sutures and surgical adhesive (see Fig. 35-3*F*) before performing the proximal aortic anastomosis (see Fig. 35-3*G*).

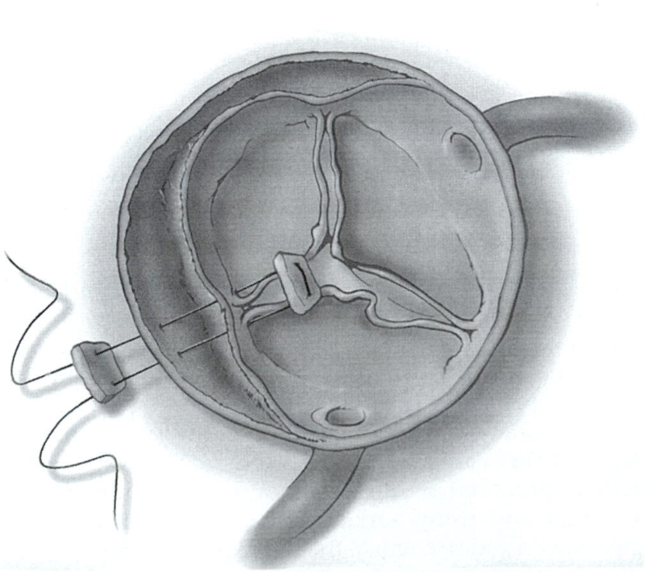

FIGURE 35-5. This cross-sectional drawing of the aortic root illustrates dehiscence of two aortic valve commissures, which causes acute valvular insufficiency. Resuspending the commissures onto the outer aortic wall restores valve competency.

Options for Perfusion

Most surgeons perform proximal aortic dissection repairs during a period of hypothermic circulatory arrest.[4,11,23,25-40] This strategy allows an "open distal anastomosis" with direct inspection of the entire arch and avoids creating additional tears that can result from placing a clamp across the fragile aorta. Although brief periods of circulatory arrest are generally well tolerated, this technique does have substantial limitations. The well recognized risks of brain injury and death increase dramatically as the time of circulatory arrest increases.[41]

Two perfusion strategies have been developed in order to reduce the risks of circulatory arrest: retrograde cerebral perfusion and selective antegrade cerebral perfusion. Retrograde cerebral perfusion delivers cold, oxygenated blood from the pump into a cannula placed in the superior vena cava.[26,28,38,42-44] The initial hope was that the retrograde delivery of blood would provide oxygen to the brain. Unfortunately, accumulating evidence suggests that this technique does not provide cerebral oxygenation.[39,45,46] The apparent benefits of this technique are more likely due to maintenance of cerebral hypothermia and retrograde flushing of air and debris. Selective antegrade cerebral perfusion delivers blood directly into the brachiocephalic arteries while circulatory arrest is maintained in the rest of the body. This technique originally required cumbersome bypass grafts and cannulas and, consequently, fell out of favor. Recent improvements in technology and new strategies for delivery, however, have resulted in a resurgence of interest in this adjunct.[29,47,48] One common way of delivering antegrade cerebral perfusion employs small, flexible, balloon perfusion catheters that are inserted into one or more of the branch arteries. Another method, which is rapidly gaining popularity due to its relative simplicity, involves cannulation of the right axillary artery (see Fig. 35-3).[49-51] After initiating circulatory arrest and occluding the proximal innominate artery, the axillary artery cannula delivers blood flow into the cerebral circulation via the right common carotid artery. Because antegrade and retrograde cerebral perfusion have distinct mechanisms of providing cerebral protection, combining them may be beneficial. In the combined approach, antegrade perfusion is delivered during the arch reconstruction and a brief period of terminal retrograde perfusion is used to provide flushing immediately before resuming full cardiopulmonary bypass. The relative efficacy of these different perfusion strategies has never been established via an appropriately designed clinical trial.

Options for Managing the Aortic Arch

In each case, a major technical decision relates to whether the arch needs to be replaced and, if so, how much (Box 35-2). Most patients require at least graft replacement of the entire tubular segment of the ascending aorta, between the sinotubular junction and the origin of the innominate artery. In the setting of acute dissection, increasingly aggressive repairs of the aortic arch are associated with increasing early morbidity and mortality.[52] Therefore, the repair is generally only extended into the arch if the arch is aneurysmal or if the primary tear in located within the arch. When only the proximal portion of the arch is involved in the disease process (a common scenario), a beveled graft replacement of the lower curvature (hemiarch) is performed (see Fig. 35-3). Extensive aneurysms involving the entire arch usually require total replacement, with a distal anastomosis created at the proximal descending thoracic aorta and separate reattachment of the brachiocephalic branches (see Fig. 35-4). The brachiocephalic vessels can be reattached to one or more openings made in the graft or replaced with separate smaller grafts if they are aneurysmal or damaged by the dissection. In the most extreme cases, the aneurysm extends past the arch and into the descending thoracic aorta. This can be managed using Borst's elephant trunk technique for total arch replacement.[53,54] The distal anastomosis is constructed so that a portion of the graft is left suspended within the true lumen of the proximal descending thoracic aorta. In addition to directing flow into the true lumen, this "trunk" can be used to assist repair of the descending thoracic aorta during a subsequent operation.

Options for Managing the Aortic Valve

Another major technical decision relates to how the aortic valve and root are managed (Box 35-3). Many patients undergoing proximal aortic dissection repair require concomitant correction of aortic valve pathology. The majority of these patients have separation of one or more commissures from the outer aortic wall; the resulting valve insufficiency can be corrected by resuspending the commissures into their normal position (see Fig. 35-5).[55] Many surgeons use surgical adhesive within the false channel to strengthen this aortic root reconstruction.[23,24,26,56,57] If there is mild to moderate annular dilatation, a commissural plication annuloplasty helps to restore and maintain effective leaflet coaptation. By preserving the aortic valve, long-term anticoagulation is often avoided; this is believed to favor thrombosis of the false lumen and thereby prevent subsequent dilatation of the thoracoabdominal aorta. Another advantage of these valve-sparing techniques is that they only require a few stitches (usually between one and six) and can be performed quickly. Limiting the extent of repair reduces cardiac ischemic time, cardiopulmonary bypass time, and overall operative time; this translates into lower postoperative morbidity and mortality. Therefore, although more extensive procedures can reduce the risk of reoperation, limited repairs are performed whenever possible in order to optimize the chance of survival after the initial operation.[36,40,58]

Occasionally, the valvular damage caused by the dissection is too severe to repair. In this case, separate replacement of the valve and graft replacement of the tubular segment of the ascending aorta are performed. This is also an option for patients who have significant preexisting aortic valvular disease (unrelated to the dissection).

The preceding options are generally not applicable to patients with annuloaortic ectasia or Marfan's syndrome because progressive dilatation of the remaining sinus segment eventually leads to complications

BOX 35-2 Options for Managing the Aortic Arch During Proximal Aortic Dissection Repair

Ascending replacement only
Beveled hemiarch replacement
Total arch replacement with reattachment of brachiocephalic branches
Total arch replacement with separate bypass grafts to each brachiocephalic branch
Elephant trunk technique

BOX 35-3 Options for Managing the Aortic Valve During Proximal Aortic Dissection Repair

- Aortic valve repair
  - Commissural resuspension
  - Commissural plication annuloplasty
  - Resuspension and annuloplasty
- Aortic valve replacement with mechanical or biologic prosthesis
- Aortic root replacement
  - Composite valve graft
  - Aortic homograft
  - Stentless porcine root
  - Valve sparing techniques (controversial)

requiring reoperation. Therefore, these patients usually require some form of aortic root replacement. Full aortic root replacement employs a mechanical or biologic graft that has both valve and aortic conduit components. Three commercially available graft options are: (1) composite valve grafts, which consist of a mechanical valve attached to a polyester tube graft; (2) aortic root homografts, which are harvested from cadavers and cryopreserved; and (3) stentless porcine aortic root grafts. Valve-sparing aortic root reimplantation is an alternative to full root replacement that involves excision of the aortic sinuses, attachment of a prosthetic graft to the patient's annulus, and resuspension of the native aortic valve inside the graft. The superior hemodynamics of the native valve and the avoidance of anticoagulation are major advantages to this approach. Experienced centers have performed valve-sparing root replacements in patients with acute dissection and have obtained mixed results.[59-62] Due to the substantial technical demands and lack of long-term outcome data, the role of valve-sparing root replacement in patients with acute aortic dissection remains controversial, especially in patients with Marfan's syndrome.[36,63]

Outcomes

The outcomes following surgical repair of acute proximal aortic dissection vary substantially.* In recent reports, early mortality ranges from 5% to 36%; it exceeds 15% in most centers. Reported risk factors for operative mortality include increasing patient age, cardiac tamponade, preoperative shock, preoperative neurologic deficits, delay in diagnosis, repair of the aortic arch, coronary artery disease, acute myocardial infarction, concomitant coronary artery bypass, and malperfusion. The reported risks of stroke (3% to 18%), bleeding requiring reoperation (4% to 15%), and renal failure (2% to 9%) demonstrate similar variation. The variability in results reflects differences in patient populations, referral mechanisms, selection practices, management strategies, outcome definitions, and reporting methods. Despite the substantial risks involved, the contemporary results of surgical treatment are excellent compared with the lethality of unrepaired acute proximal aortic dissection.[67] The International Registry of Acute Aortic Dissection documented a 58% hospital mortality rate in patients who received medical treatment alone.[65]

Survival 1 year after surgical repair of proximal aortic dissection ranges from 60% to 85%; survival drops to 37% to 71% at 10 years.[27,28,30,32,52,56,66,68] Rupture of the dilated distal aorta is the most common cause of late death. In the majority of patients who have undergone proximal repairs, the dissection persists beyond the site of the initial repair and the false lumen remains patent. Therefore, after the proximal aorta is repaired, most patients require aggressive management of the remaining distal dissection, including anti-impulse therapy and careful surveillance with imaging studies (see Chapter 34). Patients who develop extensive dilatation of the distal aortic segment undergo graft repair to prevent aneurysm rupture.

*See references 4,6,11,23,25,27-33,44,52,56,64-66.

CHRONIC PROXIMAL DISSECTION

Occasionally, patients with proximal aortic dissection present for repair in the chronic phase. With rare exceptions, the mere presence of proximal aortic dissection continues to warrant surgical repair in order to prevent aortic rupture. In most regards, the operation is conducted in a manner similar to acute dissection repair; however, the improved tissue strength in the chronic setting makes it easier to obtain secure, hemostatic suture lines. Additionally, instead of obliterating the false lumen at the distal anastomosis, the dissecting membrane is fenestrated into the arch to assure blood flow in both lumens and prevent postoperative peripheral ischemia. The absence of both acute inflammation and malperfusion simplifies the perioperative management considerably. These factors partially account for the substantial differences in outcomes between patients who undergo surgery in the acute setting and those who are repaired in the chronic phase. Compared with patients who underwent repairs in the acute phase, those who have repairs of chronic dissection have lower incidences of death and stroke. Contemporary series report both early mortality and stroke rates below 8%.[34,35,47,69]

ACUTE DISTAL DISSECTION

In most centers, nonoperative management of acute distal aortic dissection results in significantly lower morbidity and mortality rates than surgical treatment.[65] These patients, therefore, are primarily managed with pharmacologic treatment (see Chapter 34). Because aortic rupture and end-organ ischemia are the most common causes of death during the acute phase, however, patients are continually reassessed for the development of complications, which are managed directly.[70,71]

Indications for Operation

Surgical repair of the descending thoracic or thoracoabdominal aorta in the setting of acute aortic dissection is associated with high morbidity and mortality. Therefore, during the acute phase, surgery is reserved for patients who experience complications. Interventions are aimed at preventing fatal aortic rupture and correcting ischemia from malperfusion. Specific indications for operative treatment include aortic rupture, rapid aortic expansion, uncontrolled hypertension, and persistent pain despite aggressive pharmacologic therapy. Acute dissection superimposed on a preexisting aneurysm is considered a life-threatening condition and is also an indication for operation. Most patients with acute distal dissections have a serosanguineous left pleural effusion; this does not indicate impending rupture and is not a sole indication for surgery. However, increasing periaortic or pleural fluid associated with other worrisome findings, such as aortic expansion, warrants consideration of aortic repair. Finally, surgical treatment should be considered in patients who are noncompliant with medical therapy, provided they are otherwise satisfactory operative candidates.

Intervention is also required for acute renal, visceral, or limb ischemia. Previously, visceral and renal malperfusion were considered indications for surgical treatment. Advances in percutaneous interventions, however, have largely replaced open surgery for these complications.[3,23,70,72,73] Therefore, patients who develop evidence of visceral or renal malperfusion undergo urgent aortography. Percutaneous fenestration of the dissecting membrane or placement of stents into obstructed branch vessels can restore organ perfusion. When this approach is unavailable or unsuccessful, surgical options—including graft replacement of the aorta, open aortic fenestration, and branch artery bypass—can be applied.[71,74] Lower limb ischemia has also been managed with percutaneous techniques but is often corrected by performing extra-anatomic revascularization, such as femoral-to-femoral crossover bypass.

Surgical Repair

Operative Techniques

In the acute setting, the primary goals of surgery are to prevent fatal rupture and restore branch artery blood flow. A limited graft repair of the life-threatening segment achieves these objectives while minimizing risks.[68] Because the most common site of rupture is in the upper third of the descending thoracic aorta, the replacement usually extends from the level of the left subclavian artery to the mid-descending level. The distal portion of the descending thoracic aorta is also replaced if it is aneurysmal. Graft replacement of the entire thoracoabdominal aorta is only considered if there is a large coexisting aneurysm. Similarly, the repair is not extended proximally into the arch, even if the primary tear is located there, unless the arch is substantially enlarged.

Because surgery for acute distal aortic dissection carries an increased risk of postoperative paraplegia, adjuncts that provide spinal cord protection (discussed later in detail) are used liberally. Cerebrospinal fluid drainage and left heart bypass are often used, even when the planned repair is limited to the upper descending thoracic aorta. Proximal control is usually obtained by placing a clamp between the left common carotid and left subclavian arteries. Manipulation of mediastinal hematoma around the proximal descending thoracic aorta is avoided until proximal control is established. The aorta is opened, and the dissecting membrane is removed from the segment being replaced. The proximal and distal anastomoses incorporate all layers of the aortic wall, thereby obliterating the false lumen with the suture lines and directing all blood flow into the true lumen.[24] Although there are usually multiple patent intercostal arteries, the extreme tissue fragility often precludes their reattachment.

Outcomes

Aggressive pharmacologic management has led to a substantial decrease in the mortality rate for patients with acute distal aortic dissection. Still, approximately 10% to 20% of medically treated patients die during the initial treatment phase.[65,70,75] The primary causes of death during nonoperative management include rupture, malperfusion, and cardiac failure. Risk factors associated with medical treatment failure—defined as death or need for surgery—include an enlarged aorta, persistent hypertension despite maximal treatment, oliguria, and peripheral ischemia.

Patients undergoing surgery for acute distal aortic dissection comprise a high-risk group that includes patients with rupture, neurologic dysfunction, renal failure, and peripheral ischemia. Therefore, it is not surprising that results following surgery for acute aortic dissections are often worse than those of medical therapy. Contemporary reports on acute distal dissection repairs document mortality and paraplegia rates of up to 32%.[64,65,69,70,75-79]

Despite the early survival advantage with nonoperative management compared with surgical treatment, long-term results are similar in patients in both groups. The reported actuarial survival rates with nonoperative management are 58% to 76% at 5 years and 25% to 56% at 10 years.[67,70,71] Five- and 10-year survival rates after repair range from 63% to 80% and 39% to 55%, respectively.[70,77]

CHRONIC DISTAL DISSECTION

Chronic aortic dissection is a progressive disease that requires life-long management. The rationale for careful surveillance lies in the natural history of the disease. Surgical intervention is eventually required in 25% to 35% of patients. Rupture and ischemic events related to the dissection are responsible for 15% to 30% of late deaths.[70,80]

Indications for Operation

In general terms, indications for surgical repair of distal aortic dissection include (1) aneurysms with symptoms or significant dilatation and (2) ischemia due to malperfusion. The acuity of presentation is a major factor when deciding the logistics of operation. Emergent surgery is reserved for patients with rupture. Urgent operations are considered for patients presenting with symptoms. Patients with symptomatic aneurysms are at increased risk of rupture and deserve expeditious evaluation and treatment. The onset of new pain in a patient with a known aneurysm is particularly concerning and may herald significant expansion, leakage, or impending rupture. In contrast, many patients are asymptomatic at the time of presentation and can undergo thorough preoperative evaluation and optimization. Elective operation is considered when the aneurysmal segment has reached 5 to 6 cm or when it has enlarged more than 1 cm during a 1-year period. A lower threshold is often used for patients with Marfan's syndrome.

Preoperative Assessment

Given the influence of preexisting comorbidity on surgical outcomes, a careful preoperative assessment of physiologic reserve is critical. Most patients undergo a thorough evaluation before undergoing elective operation. The preoperative assessment focuses on cardiovascular, pulmonary, and renal status.

Cardiovascular Status

Coronary artery occlusive disease is common in patients with thoracic aortic aneurysms and contributes to a substantial proportion of early and late postoperative deaths. Additionally, valvular pathology and myocardial dysfunction have important implications when planning anesthetic management and strategies for aortic repair. Transthoracic echocardiography is routinely obtained to evaluate both valvular and ventricular functions. Nuclear stress tests or comparable imaging studies are used selectively to identify reversible myocardial ischemia. Cardiac catheterization with coronary arteriography should be considered in patients who have evidence of coronary disease—on the basis of history or noninvasive studies—or an ejection fraction of 30% or less. Patients who have asymptomatic distal aortic aneurysms and severe coronary artery occlusive disease may undergo percutaneous angioplasty or surgical revascularization before aneurysm repair.

The hemodynamic changes that occur during thoracic aortic repair can precipitate stroke in patients with significant cerebrovascular disease. Therefore, carotid duplex ultrasound studies are also routinely obtained to detect occult carotid artery stenosis. It is recommended that significant carotid artery stenosis is corrected with an endarterectomy before proceeding with the aortic operation.

Pulmonary Status

The most common complication following descending thoracic and thoracoabdominal aortic repairs is pulmonary dysfunction.[81] Therefore, pulmonary function testing, including arterial blood gases and spirometry, is also routinely obtained before surgery to assess risk and allow optimization of the patient's pulmonary status. Patients with an FEV_1 exceeding 1 liter and a P_{CO_2} below 45 mm Hg are considered candidates for elective surgery. In select patients, borderline pulmonary function can be improved with a 1- to 3-month regimen that includes smoking cessation, exercise, weight loss, and treatment of bronchitis. In most cases, operation is not withheld in patients with symptomatic aneurysms and poor pulmonary reserve. Surgical techniques, however, can be modified to improve the chance of recovery in these high-risk patients. For example, precautions can be taken to assure preservation of the left recurrent laryngeal and phrenic nerves. Diaphragm-sparing techniques may also be helpful in such patients.[82]

Renal Status

Preoperative renal status is evaluated on the basis of serum electrolytes, blood urea nitrogen, and creatinine measurements. The computed tomography or magnetic resonance imaging studies obtained to evaluate the aorta also provide information regarding kidney size and perfusion. Accurate information regarding baseline renal function has important prognostic and therapeutic implications. For example, patients with severely impaired renal function frequently require at least temporary hemodialysis after operation; these patients are also at increased risk of death.[83] Additionally, perfusion strategies and perioperative medications are adjusted based on renal function. Finally, patients with poor renal function due to renal malperfusion from a dissection flap or occlusive disease can undergo renal endarterectomy, stenting, or bypass grafting during thoracoabdominal aortic aneurysm repair.

Surgical Repair

Operative Techniques

Patients with chronic dissection who require emergency repair due to acute pain or rupture undergo limited graft replacement of the symptomatic segment. Although the entire thoracoabdominal aorta may be dissected and aneurysmal (Fig. 35-6), typically a relatively localized segment is the cause of the symptoms. Limited repair minimizes early postoperative morbidity; however, it leaves the patient with a segment of dissected aorta that can potentially expand and rupture in the future. Therefore, in appropriate surgical candidates, elective repairs replace the entire descending thoracic aorta and often extend to include the thoracoabdominal aorta (Fig. 35-7).

Several aspects of the surgical strategy are based on the extent of the aneurysm being repaired.[84,85] Descending thoracic aortic aneurysms are confined to the chest and, therefore, are repaired through a left thoracotomy. In patients with thoracoabdominal aortic aneurysms, this incision is extended across the costal margin and into the abdomen (Fig. 35-8*A*). A double-lumen endobronchial tube is used to allow selective right lung ventilation and left lung deflation. Transperitoneal exposure of the thoracoabdominal aorta is achieved by dividing the diaphragm and performing medial visceral rotation. Aortic repair usually is performed during a period of aortic clamping. The clamp is often placed between the left common carotid artery and the left subclavian artery. In patients who have undergone previous coronary artery bypass surgery using the left internal thoracic artery, clamping proximal to the left subclavian artery can precipitate severe myocardial ischemia and cardiac arrest. When clamping at this location is anticipated in these patients, a left common carotid to subclavian bypass is performed to avoid cardiac complications.

In select situations, hypothermic circulatory arrest is required; the primary indication for this approach is the inability to clamp the aorta due to rupture, an extremely large aneurysm, or extension of the aneurysm into the distal transverse aortic arch.[76] Regardless of the technique, once proximal control is established, the aneurysmal segment of aorta is replaced with a polyester tube graft (see Fig. 35-8*B-J*). Because of the periaortic inflammation caused by the dissection, the vagus and left recurrent laryngeal nerves are often adherent to the aortic wall and susceptible to injury during repair of the proximal descending segment. Careful separation of the proximal descending thoracic aorta from the underlying esophagus before performing the proximal anastomosis minimizes the risk of a secondary aortoesophageal fistula. Wedges of dissecting membrane are excised proximally and distally from within the aortic cuffs, allowing blood to flow through both true and false channels after the

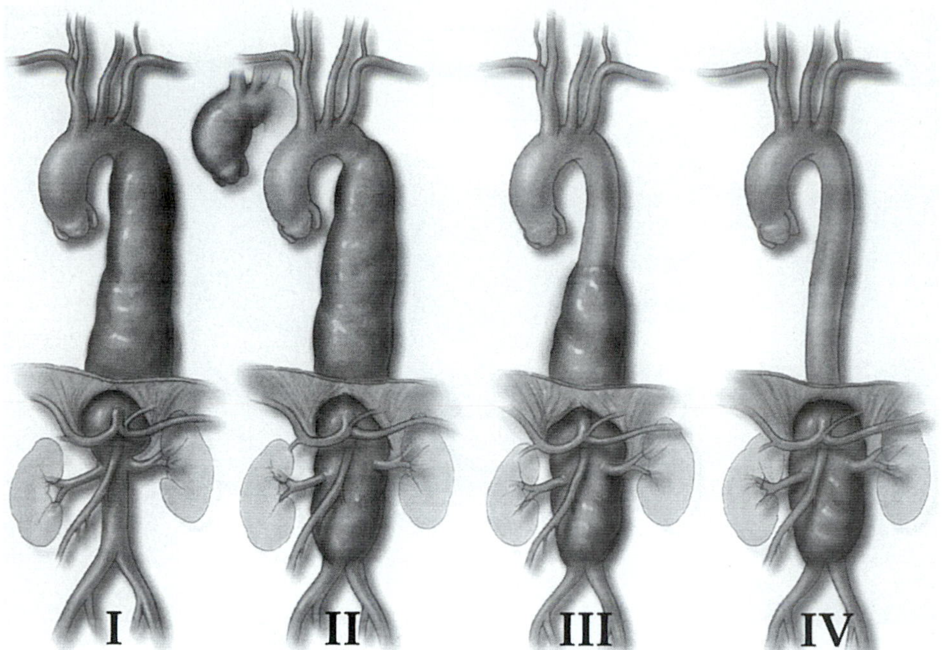

FIGURE 35-6. Crawford's classification categorizes thoracoabdominal aortic aneurysms based on the extent of aorta involved. Extent I aneurysms begin in the upper descending thoracic aorta, often near the left subclavian artery, and extend to the region of the visceral and renal arteries. Extent II aneurysms also involve the upper descending thoracic aorta but extend distally beyond the renal arteries, often to the aortic bifurcation. Extent III aneurysms begin in the lower descending thoracic aorta (below the sixth rib) and extend into the abdominal segment. Extent IV aneurysms begin at the diaphragmatic crura and extend distally, often involving the entire abdominal aorta.

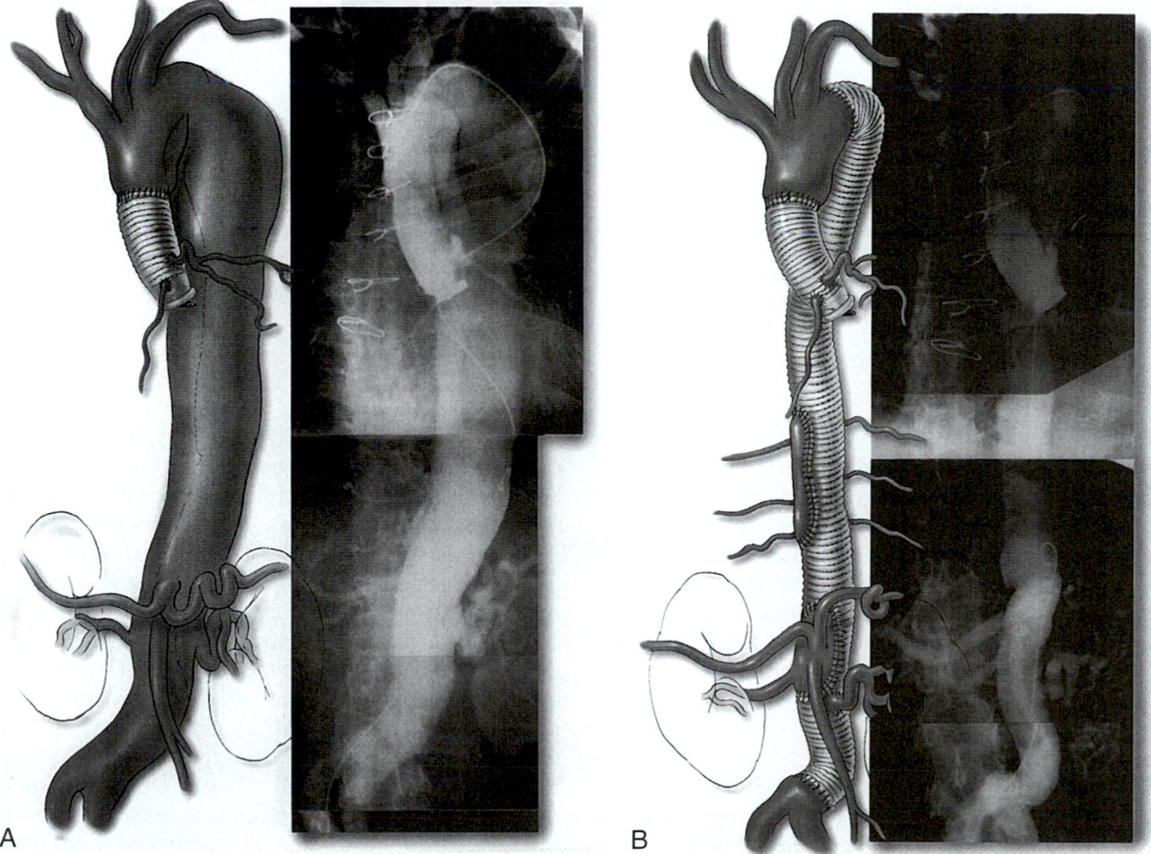

FIGURE 35-7. These drawings and aortograms illustrate the presentation **(A)** and repair **(B)** of an extent II thoracoabdominal aortic aneurysm that developed due to chronic distal aortic dissection. The patient had previously undergone repair of a proximal aortic dissection.

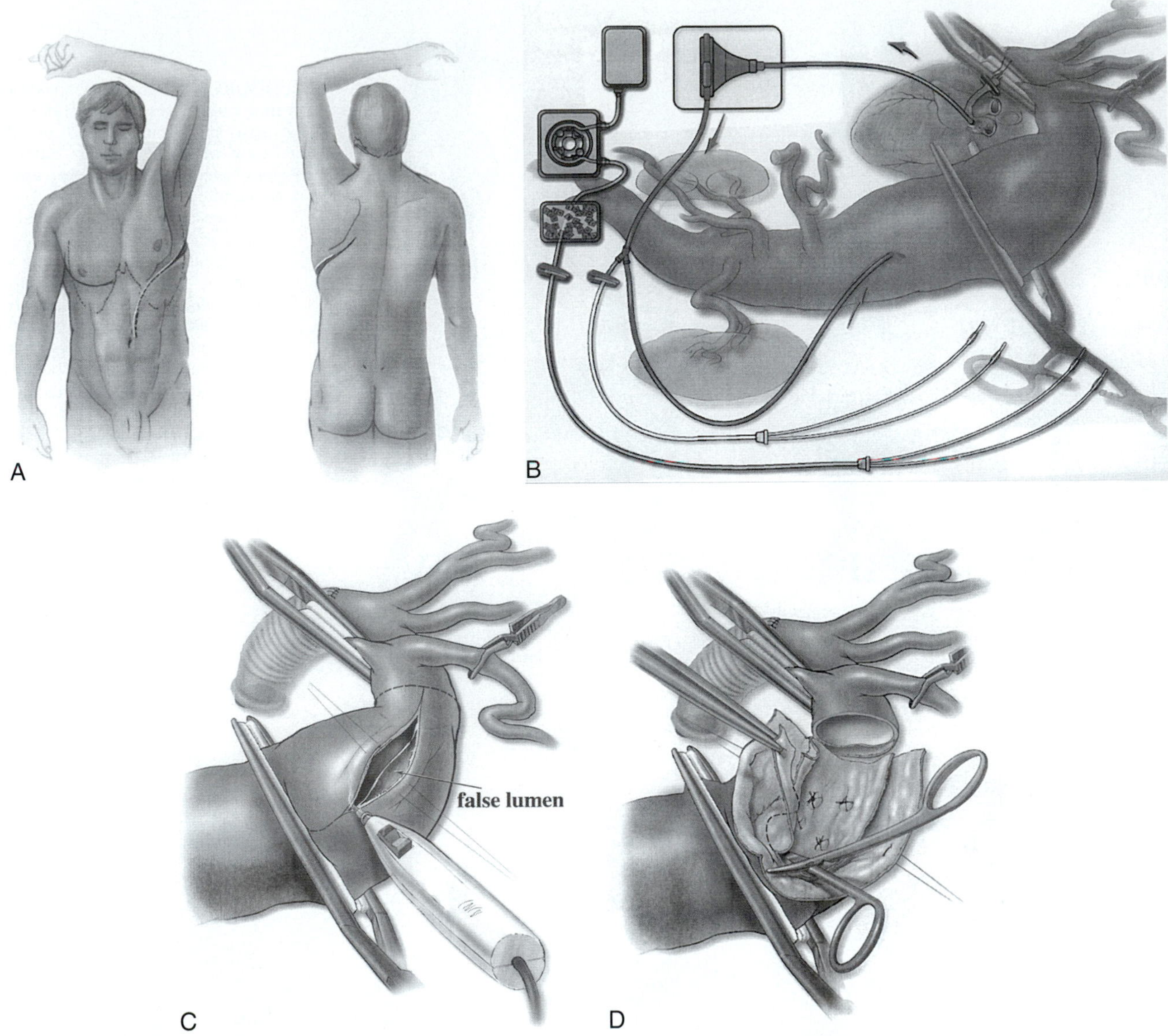

FIGURE 35-8. Surgical techniques involved in repairing an extent II thoracoabdominal aortic aneurysm related to chronic aortic dissection. The repair is performed through a left thoracoabdominal incision **(A)**. Aortic clamps are applied after establishing distal aortic perfusion via a left heart bypass circuit **(B)**. The segment of aorta isolated between the clamps is opened **(C)**, the dissecting membrane is excised, and intercostal arteries are ligated **(D)**.

reconstruction is completed. Important branch vessels—including the intercostal, celiac, superior mesenteric, renal, and lumbar arteries—are reattached to openings made in the graft. When the dissection extends into the visceral or renal arteries, the membrane can be fenestrated or the false lumen can be obliterated using sutures or intraluminal stents.[86] Asymmetric expansion of the false lumen often displaces the left renal artery laterally enough to require separate reattachment or use of a side branch graft.

Organ Protection

Clamping the descending thoracic aorta creates ischemia of the spinal cord and abdominal viscera. Clinically significant postoperative manifestations of hepatic, pancreatic, and bowel ischemia are relatively uncommon. Acute renal failure and spinal cord injury, however, are major causes of morbidity and mortality after these operations. Therefore, several aspects of the operation are devoted to minimizing spinal and renal ischemia (Box 35-4).[85] A multimodality approach to spinal cord protection includes: expeditious repair to minimize aortic clamp time, moderate systemic heparinization to prevent small vessel thrombosis, mild permissive hypothermia (32°C to 34°C, nasopharyngeal), and reattachment of segmental intercostal and lumbar arteries. As the aorta is replaced from proximal to distal, the aortic clamp is moved sequentially to lower positions along the graft to restore perfusion to newly reattached branch vessels. During extensive thoracoabdominal aortic repairs (i.e., extents I and II), cerebrospinal fluid drainage is used. The benefits of this adjunct, which improves spinal perfusion by reducing cerebrospinal fluid pressure, have been confirmed by a

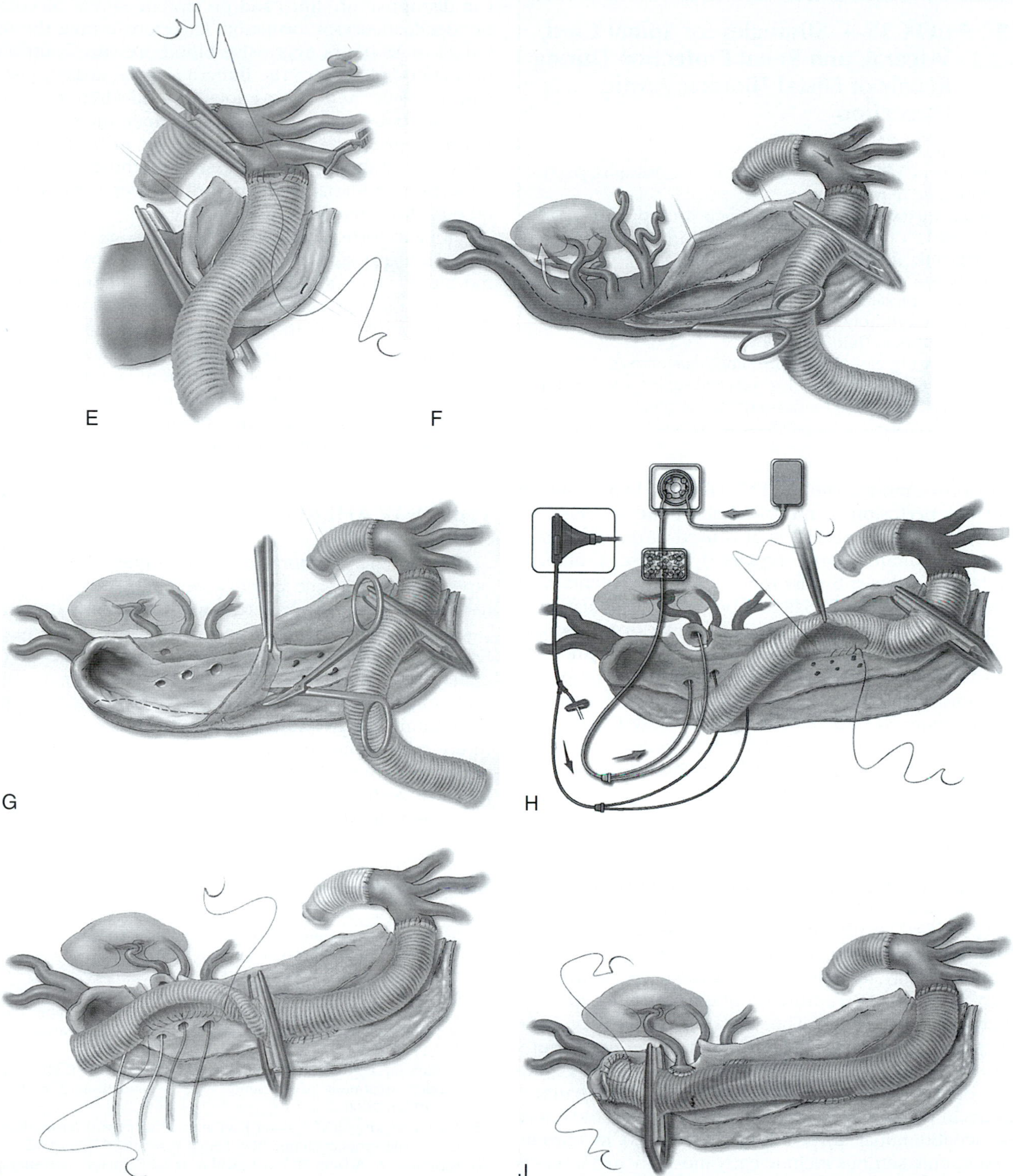

FIGURE 35-8. *cont'd* After the graft is sutured to the proximal descending thoracic aorta **(E)**, clamps are repositioned to restore perfusion of the left subclavian artery, left heart bypass is stopped, and the remainder of the aneurysm is opened **(F)**. The dissecting membrane is removed to allow identification of patent segmental arteries and the origins of the visceral and renal arteries **(G)**. Blood from the left heart bypass circuit is delivered to the celiac axis and superior mesenteric artery via balloon perfusion catheters **(H)**. Cold crystalloid is delivered to the kidneys through catheters placed in the renal arterial ostia. Critical intercostal arteries are attached to an opening in the graft. Reattachment of the visceral branches **(I)** and the distal aortic anastomosis **(J)** complete the repair. Courtesy of Scott Weldon and Carol Larson.

BOX 35-4 Strategies for Spinal Cord, Visceral, and Renal Protection During Repair of Distal Thoracic Aortic Dissection

All extents
- Permissive mild hypothermia (32°C-34°C, nasopharyngeal)
- Moderate heparinization
- Aggressive reattachment of segmental arteries (especially T8-L1)
- Sequential aortic clamping when possible
- Perfusion of renal arteries with 4°C crystalloid solution when possible

Extent I and II thoracoabdominal repairs
- Cerebrospinal fluid drainage
- Left heart bypass during proximal anastomosis
- Selective perfusion of celiac axis and superior mesenteric artery during intercostal and visceral/renal anastomoses

prospective randomized trial.[87] Left heart bypass, which provides perfusion of the distal aorta and its branches during the clamp period, is also used during extensive thoracoabdominal aortic repairs.[88] Because it unloads the heart, left heart bypass is also useful in patients with poor cardiac reserve. Balloon perfusion cannulas connected to the left heart bypass circuit can be used to deliver blood directly to the celiac axis and superior mesenteric artery during their reattachment. The potential benefits of reducing hepatic and bowel ischemia include reduced risks of postoperative coagulopathy and bacterial translocation, respectively. Whenever possible, renal protection is enhanced by perfusing the kidneys with cold (4°C) crystalloid.[89]

Outcomes

When performed in specialized centers, these operations achieve excellent survival with acceptable morbidity.[69,75,78,79,90,91] Early mortality rates for chronic distal dissection repairs range from 6% to 10%. Predictors of operative mortality include increasing age, congestive heart failure, aortic rupture (contained or free), and preoperative renal failure. The risk of paraplegia or paraparesis is 3% to 9%. These outcomes are significantly better than those obtained in patients who undergo surgery during the acute phase. For example, comparative results in patients who require replacement of the entire thoracoabdominal aorta (extent II repairs) in chronic versus acute settings include early mortality in 5% versus 10%, paraplegia/paraparesis in 5% versus 11%, and renal failure in 13% versus 20%, respectively.[91]

POSTOPERATIVE CONSIDERATIONS

Two specific considerations regarding postoperative management apply to all thoracic aortic repairs. Aortic anastomoses are often extremely fragile during the early postoperative period, especially following acute dissection repair. Even brief episodes of postoperative hypertension can disrupt suture lines and precipitate severe bleeding or pseudoaneurysm formation. Therefore, during the initial 24 to 48 hours, aggressive blood pressure control is maintained to protect the integrity of the anastomoses. Nitroprusside and intravenous (IV) β-adrenoreceptor antagonists are routinely used to maintain the mean arterial blood pressure at 80 to 90 mm Hg. In patients with extremely friable aortic tissue, such as those with acute dissection or Marfan's syndrome, a lower target (70 to 80 mm Hg) is used.

Thoracic aortic graft infections are a threat to anastomotic integrity and are associated with extremely high morbidity and mortality.[92] Definitive treatment often requires complete removal of the graft and complex vascular reconstruction. In an attempt to prevent this complication, administration of IV antibiotics is recommended until all drains, chest tubes, and central venous lines are removed. Similarly, all postoperative infections are treated aggressively with parenteral antibiotics to minimize the risk of secondary graft infection.

THE VIEW AHEAD

The landscape of thoracic aortic surgery is changing rapidly. As patient age and disease complexity continue to increase, the new challenges are being met with innovative treatment strategies and technological advances. Experience with endovascular thoracic aortic stent-grafts is accruing (see Chapter 36); stent-grafts will undoubtedly become a major tool in the surgical armamentarium for treating aortic dissection in the near future. Improvements in the understanding of the molecular mechanisms of dissection may lead to novel forms of medical treatment aimed at reducing the rate of aortic expansion and the risk of fatal rupture.

REFERENCES

1. Borst HG, Heinemann MK, Stone CD: Surgical Treatment of Aortic Dissection. New York, Churchill Livingston, 1996.
2. Fann JI, Miller DC: Aortic dissection. Ann Vasc Surg 9:311, 1995.
3. Slonim SM, Miller DC, Mitchell RS, et al: Percutaneous balloon fenestration and stenting for life-threatening ischemic complications in patients with acute aortic dissection. J Thorac Cardiovasc Surg 117:1118, 1999.
4. Ehrlich MP, Ergin MA, McCullough JN, et al: Results of immediate surgical treatment of all acute type A dissections. Circulation 102:III248, 2000.
5. Estrera AL, Huynh TTT, Porat E, et al: Is acute type A aortic dissection a true surgical emergency? Semin Vasc Surg 15:75, 2002.
6. Kawahito K, Adachi H, Yamaguchi A, et al: Early and late surgical outcomes of acute type A aortic dissection in patients aged 75 years and older. Ann Thorac Surg 70:1455, 2000.
7. Neri E, Toscano T, Massetti M, et al: Operation for acute type A dissection in octogenarians: Is it justified? J Thorac Cardiovasc Surg 121:259, 2001.
8. McKneally MF: "We don't do that here:" Reflections on the Siena experience with dissecting aneurysms of the thoracic aorta in octogenarians. J Thorac Cardiovasc Surg 121:202, 2001.
9. Fehrenbacher J, Halbrook H, Siderys H: Operation for acute type A dissection in octogenarians: Is it justified? (letter) J Thorac Cardiovasc Surg 123:393, 2002.
10. Neri E: Operation for acute type A dissection in octogenarians: Is it justified? (reply) J Thorac Cardiovasc Surg 123:393, 2002.

11. Westaby S, Saito S, Katsumata T: Acute type A dissection: Conservative methods provide consistently low mortality. Ann Thorac Surg 73:707, 2002.
12. Deeb GM, Williams DM, Bolling SF, et al: Surgical delay for acute type A dissection with malperfusion. Ann Thorac Surg 64:1669, 1997.
13. Fabre O, Vincentelli A, Willoteaux S, et al: Preoperative fenestration for type A acute aortic dissection with mesenteric malperfusion. Ann Thorac Surg 73:950, 2002.
14. Gillinov AM, Lytle BW, Kaplon RJ, et al: Dissection of the ascending aorta after previous cardiac surgery: Differences in presentation and management. J Thorac Cardiovasc Surg 117:252, 1999.
15. Murphy DA, Craver JM, Jones EL, et al: Recognition and management of ascending aortic dissection complicating cardiac surgical operations. J Thorac Cardiovasc Surg 85:247, 1983.
16. Pearce WH, Parker MA, Feinglass J, et al: The importance of surgeon volume and training in outcomes for vascular surgical procedures. J Vasc Surg 29:768, 1999.
17. Cowan JAJ, Dimick JB, Henke PK, et al: Surgical treatment of intact thoracoabdominal aortic aneurysms in the United States: Hospital and surgeon volume-related outcomes. J Vasc Surg 37:1169, 2003.
18. Birkmeyer JD, Stukel TA, Siewers AE, et al: Surgeon volume and operative mortality in the United States. N Engl J Med 349:2117, 2003.
19. Garcia-Jimenez A, Peraza Torres A, Martinez Lopez G, et al: Cardiac tamponade by aortic dissection in a hospital without cardiothoracic surgery. Chest 104:290, 1993.
20. Perez L, Wise L: A standardized treatment protocol for blood pressure management in transport patients with a reported diagnosis of acute aortic dissection or symptomatic aortic aneurysm. Air Med J 18:111, 1999.
21. Coselli JS, Crawford ES, Beall AC Jr, et al: Determination of brain temperatures for safe circulatory arrest during cardiovascular operation. Ann Thorac Surg 45:638, 1988.
22. Bachet J, Goudot B, Dreyfus GD, et al: Surgery for acute type A aortic dissection: The Hopital Foch experience (1977-1998). Ann Thorac Surg 67:2006, 1999.
23. Bavaria JE, Brinster DR, Gorman RC, et al: Advances in the treatment of acute type A dissection: An integrated approach. Ann Thorac Surg 74:S1848, 2002.
24. Coselli JS, LeMaire SA, Köksoy C: Thoracic aortic anastomoses. Operative Tech Thorac Cardiovasc Surg 5:258, 2000.
25. Nguyen B, Muller M, Kipfer B, et al: Different techniques of distal aortic repair in acute type A dissection: Impact on late aortic morphology and reoperation. Eur J Cardiothorac Surg 15:496, 1999.
26. Deeb GM, Williams DM, Quint LE, et al: Risk analysis for aortic surgery using hypothermic circulatory arrest with retrograde cerebral perfusion. Ann Thorac Surg 67:1883, 1999.
27. Kazui T, Washiyama N, Bashar AH, et al: Surgical outcome of acute type A aortic dissection: Analysis of risk factors. Ann Thorac Surg 74:75, 2002.
28. Ehrlich MP, Grabenwoger M, Kilo J, et al: Surgical treatment of acute type A dissection: Is rupture a risk factor? Ann Thorac Surg 73:1843, 2002.
29. Tan ME, Dossche KM, Morshuis WJ, et al: Operative risk factors of type A aortic dissection: Analysis of 252 consecutive patients. Cardiovasc Surg 11:277, 2003.
30. Lai DT, Robbins RC, Mitchell RS, et al: Does profound hypothermic circulatory arrest improve survival in patients with acute type A aortic dissection? Circulation 106:I-218, 2002.
31. Di Eusanio M, Tan ME, Schepens MA, et al: Surgery for acute type A dissection using antegrade selective cerebral perfusion: Experience with 122 patients. Ann Thorac Surg 75:514, 2003.
32. Moon MR, Sundt TM III, Pasque MK, et al: Does the extent of proximal or distal resection influence outcome for type A dissections? Ann Thorac Surg 71:1244, 2001.
33. Ohtsubo S, Itoh T, Takarabe K, et al: Surgical results of hemiarch replacement for acute type A dissection. Ann Thorac Surg 74:S1853, 2002.
34. Kazui T, Yamashita K, Washiyama N, et al: Impact of an aggressive surgical approach on surgical outcome in type A aortic dissection. Ann Thorac Surg 74:S1844, 2002.
35. Kouchoukos NT, Masetti P, Rokkas CK, et al: Single-stage reoperative repair of chronic type A aortic dissection by means of the arch-first technique. J Thorac Cardiovasc Surg 122:578, 2001.
36. Elefteriades JA: What operation for acute type A dissection? J Thorac Cardiovasc Surg 123:201, 2002.
37. Svensson LG, Nadolny EM, Kimmel WA: Multimodal protocol influence on stroke and neurocognitive deficit prevention after ascending/arch aortic operations. Ann Thorac Surg 74:2040, 2002.
38. Coselli JS, LeMaire SA, Walkes JC: Surgery for acute type A dissection. Operative Tech Thorac Cardiovasc Surg 4:13, 1999.
39. Moon MR, Sundt TM III: Influence of retrograde cerebral perfusion during aortic arch procedures. Ann Thorac Surg 74:426, 2002.
40. Sabik JF, Lytle BW, Blackstone EH, et al: Long-term effectiveness of operations for ascending aortic dissections. J Thorac Cardiovasc Surg 119:946, 2000.
41. Svensson LG, Crawford ES, Hess KR, et al: Deep hypothermia with circulatory arrest: Determinants of stroke and early mortality in 656 patients. J Thorac Cardiovasc Surg 106:19, 1993.
42. David TE, Armstrong S, Ivanov J, et al: Surgery for acute type A dissection. Ann Thorac Surg 67:1999, 1999.
43. Coselli JS, LeMaire SA: Experience with retrograde cerebral perfusion during proximal aortic surgery in 290 patients. J Card Surg 12:232, 1997.
44. Estrera AL, Miller CC III, Huynh TT, et al: Replacement of the ascending and transverse aortic arch: Determinants of long-term survival. Ann Thorac Surg 74:1058, 2002.
45. Wong CH, Bonser RS: Retrograde cerebral perfusion: Clinical and experimental aspects. Perfusion 14:247, 1999.
46. Hagl C, Khaladj N, Karck M, et al: Hypothermic circulatory arrest during ascending and aortic arch surgery: The theoretical impact of different perfusion techniques and other methods of cerebral protection. Eur J Cardiothorac Surg 24:371, 2003.
47. Matalanis G, Hata M, Buxton B: A retrospective comparative study of deep hypothermic circulatory arrest, retrograde, and antegrade cerebral perfusion in aortic arch surgery. Ann Thorac Cardiovasc Surg 9:174, 2003.
48. Kazui T, Yamashita K, Washiyama N, et al: Usefulness of antegrade selective cerebral perfusion during aortic arch operations. Ann Thorac Surg 74:S1806, 2002.
49. Sabik JF, Lytle BW, McCarthy PM, et al: Axillary artery: An alternative site of arterial cannulation for patients with extensive aortic and peripheral vascular disease. J Thorac Cardiovasc Surg 109: 885, 1995.
50. Neri E, Massetti M, Campannini G, et al: Axillary artery cannulation in acute type A aortic dissection operations. J Thorac Cardiovasc Surg 118:324, 1999.
51. Pasic M, Schubel J, Bauer M, et al: Cannulation of the right axillary artery for surgery of acute type A aortic dissection. Eur J Cardiothorac Surg 24:231, 2003.
52. Crawford ES, Kirklin JW, Naftel DC, et al: Surgery for acute dissection of ascending aorta: Should the arch be included? J Thorac Cardiovasc Surg 104:46, 1992.
53. Borst HG, Frank G, Schaps D: Treatment of extensive aneurysms by a new multiple-stage approach. J Thorac Cardiovasc Surg 95:11, 1988.
54. Schepens MA, Dossche KM, Morshuis WJ, et al: The elephant trunk technique: Operative results in 100 consecutive patients. Eur J Cardiothorac Surg 21:276, 2002.
55. Fann JI, Glower DD, Miller DC, et al: Preservation of aortic valve in type A aortic dissection complicated by aortic regurgitation. J Thorac Cardiovasc Surg 102:62, 1991.
56. Casselman FP, Tan MESH, Vermeulen FEE, et al: Durability of aortic valve preservation and root reconstruction in acute type A aortic dissection. Ann Thorac Surg 70:1227, 2000.
57. Murashita T, Kunihara T, Shiiya N, et al: Is preservation of the aortic valve different between acute and chronic type A aortic dissections? Eur J Cardiothorac Surg 20:967, 2001.
58. Kirsch M, Soustelle C, Houel R, et al: Risk factor analysis for proximal and distal reoperations after surgery for acute type A aortic dissection. J Thorac Cardiovasc Surg 123:318, 2002.
59. von Segesser LK, Lorenzetti E, Lachet M, et al: Aortic valve preservation in acute type A dissection: Is it sound? J Thorac Cardiovasc Surg 111:381, 1996.
60. Leyh RG, Fischer S, Kallenbach K, et al: High failure rate after valve-sparing aortic root replacement using the "remodeling technique" in acute type A aortic dissection. Circulation 106(Suppl):I-229, 2002.
61. Erasmi AW, Stierle U, Bechtel JFM, et al: Up to 7 years' experience with valve-sparing aortic root remodeling/reimplantation for acute type A dissection. Ann Thorac Surg 76:99, 2003.

62. Kallenbach K, Pethig K, Leyh RG, et al: Acute dissection of the ascending aorta: First results of emergency valve sparing aortic root reconstruction. Eur J Cardiothorac Surg 22:218, 2002.
63. Bachet J: Acute type A dissection: Can we dramatically reduce surgical mortality? Ann Thorac Surg 73:701, 2002.
64. Coselli JS, LeMaire SA: Thoracic aortic aneurysms and aortic dissection. In Brunicardi FC, Andersen DK, Billiar TR, et al (eds): Schwartz's Principles of Surgery. New York, McGraw-Hill, 2005:691-715.
65. Hagan PG, Nienaber CA, Isselbacher EM, et al: The International Registry of Acute Aortic Dissection (IRAD): New insights into an old disease. JAMA 283:897, 2000.
66. Pansini S, Gagliardotto PV, Pompei E, et al: Early and late risk factors in surgical treatment of acute type A aortic dissection. Ann Thorac Surg 66:779, 1998.
67. Masuda Y, Yamada Z, Morooka N, et al: Prognosis of patients with medically treated aortic dissections. Circulation 84 (Suppl):III-7, 1991.
68. Fann JI, Smith JA, Miller DC, et al: Surgical management of aortic dissection during a 30-year period. Circulation 92:II113, 1995.
69. Safi HJ, Miller CC III, Reardon MJ, et al: Operation for acute and chronic aortic dissection: Recent outcome with regard to neurologic deficit and early death. Ann Thorac Surg 66:402, 1998.
70. Umana JP, Lai DT, Mitchell RS, et al: Is medical therapy still the optimal treatment strategy for patients with acute type B aortic dissections? J Thorac Cardiovasc Surg 124:896, 2002.
71. Elefteriades JA, Hartleroad J, Gusberg RJ, et al: Long-term experience with descending aortic dissection: The complication specific approach. Ann Thorac Surg 53:11, 1992.
72. Chavan A, Lotz J, Oelert F, et al: Endoluminal treatment of aortic dissection. Eur Radiol 13:2521, 2003.
73. Vedantham S, Picus D, Sanchez LA, et al: Percutaneous management of ischemic complications in patients with type-B aortic dissection. J Vasc Interv Radiol 14:181, 2003.
74. Panneton JM, Teh SH, Cherry KJ Jr, et al: Aortic fenestration for acute or chronic aortic dissection: An uncommon but effective procedure. J Vasc Surg 32:711, 2000.
75. Gysi J, Schaffner T, Mohacsi P, et al: Early and late outcome of operated and non-operated acute dissection of the descending aorta. Eur J Cardiothorac Surg 11:1163, 1997.
76. Kouchoukos NT, Masetti P, Rokkas CK, et al: Hypothermic cardiopulmonary bypass and circulatory arrest for operations on the descending thoracic and thoracoabdominal aorta. Ann Thorac Surg 74:S1885, 2002.
77. Lansman SL, Hagl C, Fink D, et al: Acute type B aortic dissection: Surgical therapy. Ann Thorac Surg 74:S1833, 2002.
78. Coselli JS, LeMaire SA, Poli de Figueiredo L, et al: Paraplegia following thoracoabdominal aortic aneurysm repair: Is dissection a risk factor? Ann Thorac Surg 63:28, 1997.
79. Svensson LG, Crawford ES, Hess KR, et al: Dissection of the aorta and dissecting aortic aneurysms: Improving early and long-term surgical results. Circulation 82(Suppl IV):24, 1990.
80. Glower DD, Speier RF, White WD, et al: Management and long-term outcome of aortic dissection. Ann Surg 214:31, 1991.
81. Svensson LG, Hess KR, Coselli JS, et al: A prospective study of respiratory failure after high-risk surgery on the thoracoabdominal aorta. J Vasc Surg 14:271, 1991.
82. Engle J, Safi HJ, Miller CC III, et al: The impact of diaphragm management on prolonged ventilator support after thoracoabdominal aortic repair. J Vasc Surg 29:150, 1999.
83. LeMaire SA, Miller CC III, Conklin LD, et al: A new predictive model for adverse outcomes after elective thoracoabdominal aortic aneurysm repair. Ann Thorac Surg 71:1233, 2001.
84. Coselli JS, LeMaire SA: Surgical techniques: Thoracoabdominal aorta. Cardiol Clin 17:751, 1999.
85. Coselli JS, Conklin LD, LeMaire SA: Thoracoabdominal aortic aneurysm repair: Review and update of current strategies. Ann Thorac Surg 74:S1881, 2002.
86. LeMaire SA, Jamison AL, Carter SA, et al: Deployment of balloon expandable stents during open repair of thoracoabdominal aortic aneurysms: A new strategy for managing renal and mesenteric artery lesions. Eur J Cardiothorac Surg 26:599, 2004.
87. Coselli JS, LeMaire SA, Köksoy C, et al: Cerebrospinal fluid drainage reduces paraplegia after thoracoabdominal aortic aneurysm repair: Results of a randomized clinical trial. J Vasc Surg 35:635, 2002.
88. Coselli JS, LeMaire SA: Left heart bypass reduces paraplegia rates following thoracoabdominal aortic aneurysm repair. Ann Thorac Surg 67:1931, 1999.
89. Köksoy C, LeMaire SA, Curling PE, et al: Renal perfusion during thoracoabdominal aortic operations: Cold crystalloid is superior to normothermic blood. Ann Thorac Surg 73:730, 2002.
90. Estrera AL, Miller CC III, Huynh TT, et al: Preoperative and operative predictors of delayed neurologic deficit following repair of thoracoabdominal aortic aneurysm. J Thorac Cardiovasc Surg 126:1288, 2003.
91. Coselli JS, LeMaire SA, Conklin LD, et al: Morbidity and mortality after extent II thoracoabdominal aortic aneurysm repair. Ann Thorac Surg 73:1107, 2002.
92. Coselli JS, Köksoy C, LeMaire SA: Management of thoracic aortic graft infections. Ann Thorac Surg 67:1990, 1999.

■ ■ ■ chapter 36

Endovascular Therapy

Sunita D. Srivastava
Matthew J. Eagleton
Gilbert R. Upchurch Jr.

The diagnosis and treatment of aortic dissection has undergone considerable transformation since Italian anatomist and pathologist Giovanni Morgagni first described it in the 1700s. The term *aortic dissection* is credited to Laënnec in 1826. Along with his colleagues, Laënnec proposed that the intimal tear was the initial event that resulted in propagation of blood flow into the media of the aorta. Developments in imaging modalities to assist early diagnosis, as well as the emergence of percutaneous-based therapies, may alter the otherwise morbid course of the disease.

The recognition of the impact of the ischemic complications of aortic dissection on morbidity and mortality has resulted in the emergence of alternative percutaneous-based therapies. The early and judicious use of endovascular therapy may be used as definitive therapy for aortic branch compromise or to optimize branch perfusion before aortic repair. Early intervention can alter potentially reversible ischemia and preserve organ function, especially with respect to intestinal viability and kidney function.

Catheter-based endovascular therapy for the treatment of aortic dissection encompasses a wide range of treatment options. Techniques such as percutaneous fenestration, endoluminal stent placement in aortic branch vessels or fenestrated septum, and covered endovascular stent grafts have expanded the therapeutic options in aortic dissection. This chapter reviews the relevant pathophysiology, indications, technical considerations, and results regarding endovascular therapy for acute aortic dissection.

PATHOPHYSIOLOGY

Ischemic complications from dissection have been classically described in two ways. Williams and colleagues[1] categorize obstructions as those caused by the dissection flap and those that are not. Three mechanisms of obstructions are described as a result of the flap (Fig. 36-1). The first is a static/fixed obstruction from the flap

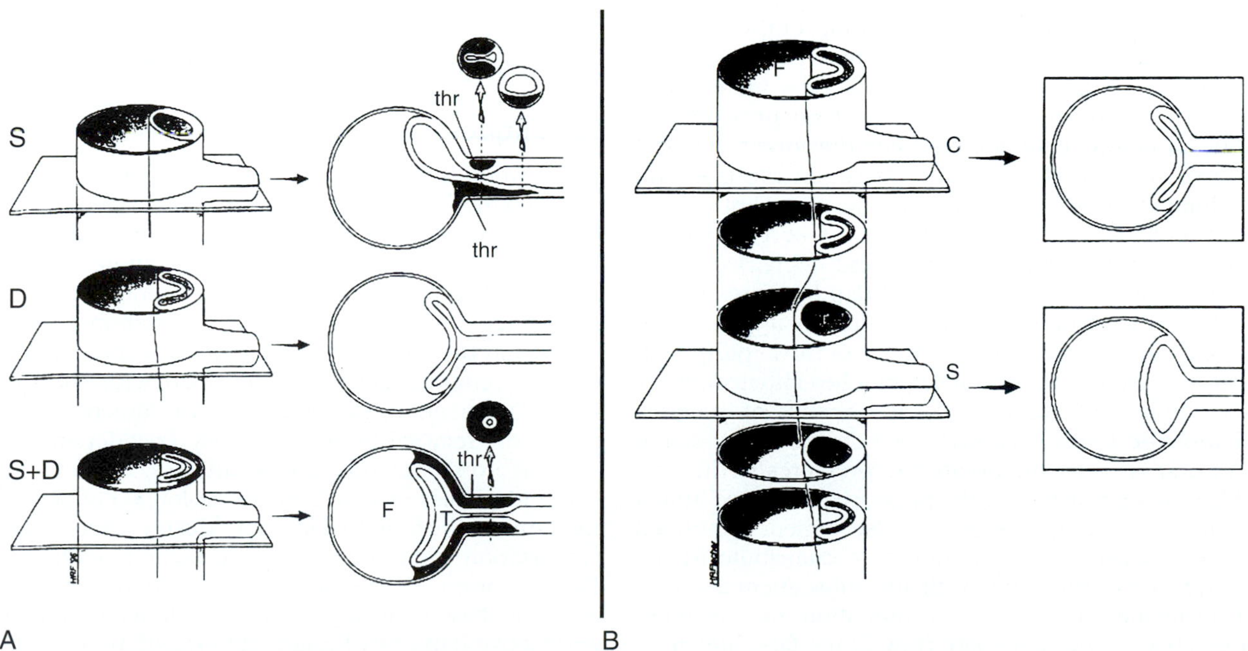

FIGURE 36-1. A, Demonstration of dynamic and static forces in obstruction. In static obstruction (*S*), the dissected flap enters the origin of the vessel causing compromised flow. In dynamic (*D*) obstruction, the dissected flap in the aorta prolapses into the vessel origin, causing branch obstruction. In the mixed obstruction (*S+D*), both elements contribute to branch vessel compromise. **B,** Mechanisms of obstruction in the visceral vessels caused by dynamic obstruction in the thoracic aorta despite adequate flow channel in the abdominal aorta. C, celiac artery; S, superior mesenteric artery; thr, thrombus. (From Williams DM, LePage MA, Lee DY: The dissected aorta. Part I. Early anatomic changes in an in vitro model. Radiology 203:26, 1997 and Williams DM, Lee DY, Hamilton BH, Marx MV: The dissected aorta. Part III. Anatomy and radiologic diagnosis of branch-vessel compromise. Radiology 203:39, 1997.)

entrance into the lumen and resultant narrowing of the vessel origin. The second is a dynamic obstruction where the flap is prolapsed across the vessel covering the origin, and the third is a combination of the two.

Static obstruction can be diagnosed with cross-sectional imaging demonstrating the flap at the origin of the vessel or with invasive methods showing a pressure difference between the vessel in question and the aorta. In addition, angiography may exhibit luminal scalloping, narrowing or linear defect (as seen with a concomitant reentry tear in the vessel showing contrast in both true and false lumens). In dynamic obstruction, cross-sectional imaging indicates true lumen collapse above the branch vessel and pressure gradients between the aorta and the vessel or between the true and false lumens. The angiographic appearance of dynamic obstruction has been called the "floating viscera" sign, demonstrating little to no filling of the aortic true lumen and contrast filling of the branch vessels seemingly from nowhere.[2,3] In surgical inspection or at autopsy, dynamic obstructions may not be appreciated because of an unpressurized aorta causing the flap to lose its prolapsing configuration and seemingly spare the branch vessel.[1]

Other mechanisms of compromised flow include embolic and thrombotic complications of the aortic dissection. Luminal thrombosis can occur in both lumens as a result of obstructing flaps in the case of true lumen thrombosis or from the thrombogenic surface of the false lumen. In this setting the length of ischemia and chances of end-organ salvage need to be addressed as local thrombolytic therapy, or thrombectomy can be initiated in conjunction with fenestration and stenting.

In a review of branch vessel compromise in the dissected aorta by Williams and colleagues,[1,2] several features have been characterized. Compromised branch vessels tend to originate from the true lumen or have flow from both false and true lumens. False lumen pressures usually are higher than true lumen pressures. In addition, pressure gradients between the aorta and vessel may exist even if the pressures between the true and false lumens are no different.[1] The development of true lumen collapse can be attributed to several factors including: cardiovascular collapse and decreased aortic inflow; compression of the intimal flap by a pressurized false lumen; obstruction of the true lumen at the level of the tear; and a physiologic state of low peripheral vascular resistance in the aortic branches initiated by the vasodilation of the vessel as a consequence of ischemia and antihypertensive medications.[4] The goal of creating a fenestration is to equilibrate the pressures in the true and false lumen by raising the pressure in the true lumen and not by decompressing the false lumen. Continued false lumen pressure over time may contribute to the degeneration of the vessel wall and subsequent aneurysmal formation. It may be a limitation of treatment options that do not eliminate flow in the false lumen.

In ischemic patients relegated to medical management or those too ill to undergo surgical repair, minimally invasive options such as fenestration and stent placement have played an important role in revascularization of essential organ beds. The treatment paradigms vary depending on the type of obstruction responsible for the ischemia. The most common presentation of ischemic complications is a peripheral pulse deficit that can be successfully treated with prosthetic repair of the thoracic aorta. Resolution of 90% of static and dynamic obstructions encountered in DeBakey type 1 dissections with aortic reconstruction alone has been reported.[1] Static obstructions caused by extension of the dissection into the origin of the branch vessel are treated with stent placement within the lumen of the vessel. These lesions are resistant to angioplasty alone because of the elastic nature of the intravascular septum created by the dissection. This is similar to the reported elastic recoil seen in vessels after angioplasty.

Prolapse of the dissection flap into the origin of the branch vessel, as seen in dynamic obstruction, is best treated by measures that restore flow in the true lumen and eliminate the flap in the true lumen. Fenestration and aortic stent placement are used for these reasons, respectively. Ischemia attributed to thrombosis of the false lumen or compromised true lumen can be addressed with local thrombolysis or thrombectomy (Fig. 36-2) especially if a vital organ bed is in jeopardy. Iliac obstruction resulting in limb ischemia has been characterized as having both static and dynamic components.[1,5] The limb with the weak femoral pulse has typically been felt to be continuous with the aortic true lumen, while that with the strong pulse is associated with the false lumen. This pathophysiology has implications for all percutaneous techniques involving femoral access, as false lumen catheterization is most effectively accessed from the groin with the stronger pulse. In addition, organ ischemia may result from the initial propagation of the dissection and subsequent reperfusion injury instead of from arterial obstruction.

ENDOVASCULAR FENESTRATION

Technique

Fenestration is the creation of a communicating channel between the false and true lumen, as described later. The patient is prepared for intervention with IV hydration, analgesics, and antihypertensive medications, usually in the ICU. The procedure is done in a fluoroscopy suite with fixed imaging equipment and monitoring. Both groins and the left arm are typically available for access. Bilateral femoral access is established with sheath and wire placements in the true and false lumens. As noted earlier, the femoral pulse status may vary depending on iliac involvement, true lumen collapse, and continuity with either false or true lumens. Prolonged injections in each lumen with multisided hole flush catheters enable visualization and evaluation of the aortic branch vessels. The compromised vascular territory is determined to be ischemic based on angiographic demonstration of an obstructive flap or by luminal stenosis of more than 50% and the presence of thrombus in the branch lumen. Additional indications of ischemia include a hemodynamic pressure gradient of 10 mm Hg in the lumen or branch vessel.[4]

Fenestrations exist naturally within dissections and can also be created to improve true lumen blood flow.

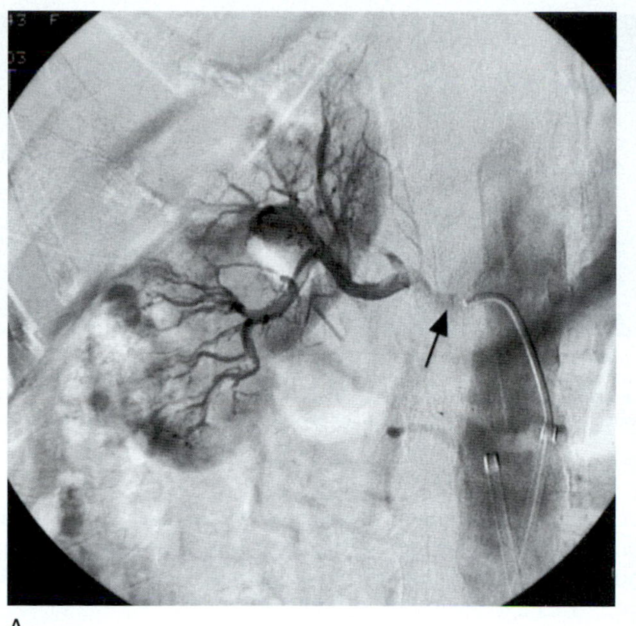
A

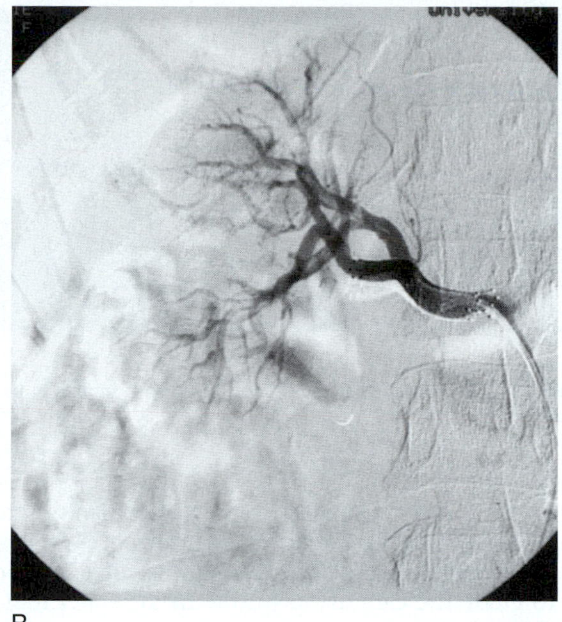
B

FIGURE 36-2. A, Selective injection of right renal artery with evidence of static obstruction of the origin with dissection extending into lumen (*arrow*). **B,** Result after local thrombolytic injection and placement of self-expanding stent.

Preexisting fenestrations can be cannulated and treated with balloon angioplasty to allow flow to a malperfused vessel. The creation of a fenestration to allow equilibration of flow and pressure within the two lumens can be performed with either fluoroscopic or intravascular ultrasound (IVUS) guidance. Typically, access is obtained in both the true and false lumens. The IVUS probe is placed in the false lumen through an 8-French (Fr) sheath, while the true lumen is accessed with a 7-Fr sheath to allow insertion of a Rosch-Uchida cannula (COOK, Bloomington, Ind.) or a Colapinto needle (COOK) (Fig. 36-3). With fluoroscopy or IVUS, the needle/cannula is placed in the area requiring fenestration, typically above the compromised aortic branch vessel (Fig. 36-4).

FIGURE 36-3. Depiction of the Rosch-Uchida cannula and the Colapinto needle.

The position is confirmed with IVUS visualization of the cannula or needle. If a cannula is used, a small needle is then passed through the intimal flap into the other lumen. If the Colapinto needle is used, it is guided in the same fashion. Care is taken not to pass the devices toward the free wall of the aorta, and IVUS assistance is crucial in this step. IVUS confirmation of the needle tip in the second lumen verifies successful penetration of the septum. Wire passage through the needle is then followed by catheter placement. Next, contrast injection is done to verify the position. Following this, the balloon of appropriate size is then passed to dilate and create the fenestration. Flush aortography in addition to IVUS imaging after injection of a mixture of saline and 1 ml of air in the area of the fenestration is used to assess the outcome.

IVUS evaluation of the dissection flap and branch orifices and the relationship between the two is often helpful to determine the cause of ischemic compromise. IVUS also enables real-time evaluation along the length of the aorta and supplements the anatomic detail provided by angiography without the morbidity of contrast infusion. It is helpful in the assessment of flap orientation and phasic response with the cardiac cycle. IVUS plays a critical role in the visual guidance during fenestration and stent placement.[6,7-12] In addition, the identification of thrombus, visualization of the dissection septum, phasic flow differences in the two channels with the cardiac cycle, as well as evaluation of luminal compromise, have contributed to the value of IVUS in the percutaneous treatment of aortic dissection. Williams and colleagues[2] evaluated 32 patients with dissections using IVUS and found a sensitivity and specificity of 97% and 100%, respectively, in its ability to distinguish the intact true lumen wall from the single-layered appearance of the outer wall.

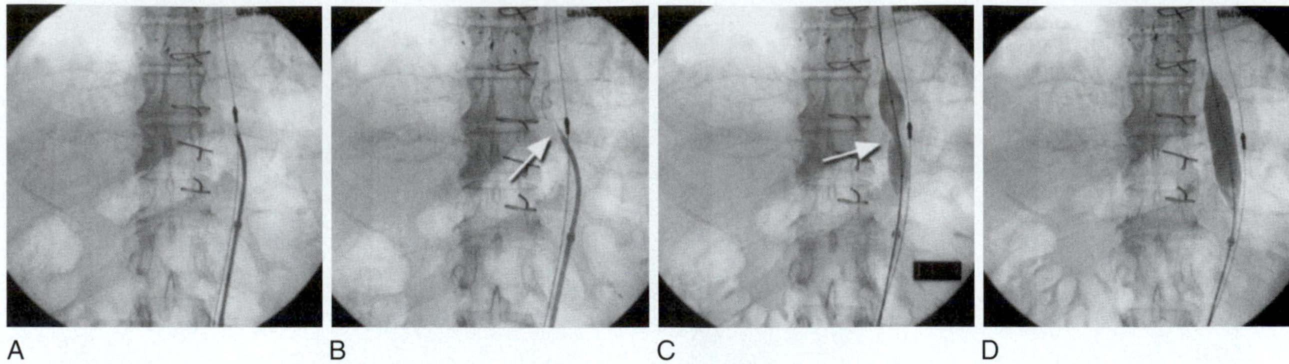

FIGURE 36-4. A, Intravascular ultrasound probe and cannula in false and true lumen, respectively. **B,** Arrow demonstrates placement of needle and wire into false lumen. **C,** Arrow points to balloon expansion with waist demonstrating tear. **D,** Full expansion of balloon for fenestration creation.

When IVUS is not available or not a physician's preference, fluoroscopic guidance is maximized. A balloon catheter is placed in the larger lumen (usually false) and used to guide the cannula or needle in the other lumen toward it. Multiplanar fluoroscopic visualization confirms needle passage through the intimal flap and not the free wall. Following this, the dilation of the fenestration is performed in the same fashion as described previously. Flush aortography, IVUS interrogation, and manometry are then performed to assure distal perfusion and relief of pressure gradients between the two lumens.

Another technique has been described to create a channel between the two lumens and is called the endovascular "scissor" method. This method is used to treat multiple ischemic vascular beds resulting from the dynamic compression of the aortic true lumen. This procedure is initiated with the placement of two rigid wires through a single 8-Fr sheath. One wire is in the true lumen, while the other is placed in the false lumen. The guidewires are then held firmly together while the sheath is advanced to the exit site of the dissection. The sheath and guidewires function as a pair of scissors as they are advanced several centimeters along the dissection and the flap is torn. Flush aortography is performed after this and can demonstrate three possible outcomes as described by Beregi and colleagues,[13] who are proponents of the intravascular scissor technique. The first possible result, which is ideal, is a tear in the middle of the dissection flap. A second, less favorable configuration is that of a free-floating dissection flap resulting from a tear created at an area of attachment of the dissection septum to the aortic wall. The third potential outcome is an intact flap but extension of the dissection in a circumferential manner, allowing the true lumen to float within the false lumen. All three mechanisms of decompression enable pressure equalization, but long-term results of this technique are not known and the published series are small.[9,13]

Decompression with fenestration alone may not permit adequate flow in the true lumen because of continued dynamic compromise. Relief of symptoms or equalization of pressures may not occur despite initial fenestration. Several options are then available. The first is to create a second fenestration further downstream to improve local flow at that point. Another option is to stent across the channel created to permit better flow and maintain patency. The stent can buttress the flap and prevent collapse of the fenestrated septum (Fig. 36-5).[14,15]

Outcomes

Deeb and colleagues[16] reported a decrease in mortality rate from 89% to 15% when percutaneous fenestration was performed before aortic surgery. Slonin and colleagues[11,12] reported their experience in a series of 40 patients, 10 with type A dissections and 30 with type B dissections, who had clinical symptoms of ischemic compromise and were referred for endovascular management. Of these patients, 14 were treated with stenting of either true or false lumen in addition to fenestration, 24 were treated with stents only, and 2 with fenestration only. Successful restoration of flow was established in 37 of the 40 patients (93%), and many patients had multiple stents placed. The majority of the type A dissections (9 of 10) underwent surgical repair before percutaneous intervention. Procedural-related complications occurred in 9 of 40 patients (23%) and represent the challenging nature of fenestration and stent placement in dissected and abnormal vessels.

Williams and colleagues[5] evaluated 24 patients in their series, including 11 patients who had type 1 dissections. In contrast to the Stanford series, surgical reconstruction was postponed in seven patients because of profound ischemia. Of this group, three patients died before aortic replacement could be performed secondary to complications from ischemia. Restoration of flow occurred in 93% of the vessels treated with fenestration and stent placement both alone and in combination.

Complications of fenestration and stent placement have been well documented.[6,8-12,14,17-19] They include intussusception of the flap distal to the fenestration, resulting in occlusions of other branch origins and diffuse embolization from catheter and balloon manipulations in an abnormal aorta. Altered flow dynamics from fenestrations may also occur and impair perfusion. This can be avoided by careful assessment of the flow characteristics with contrast angiography and IVUS, as well as pressure measurements before the decision to create a fenestration. Technical complications such as perforation of the aorta, dissection propagation, and distal vessel

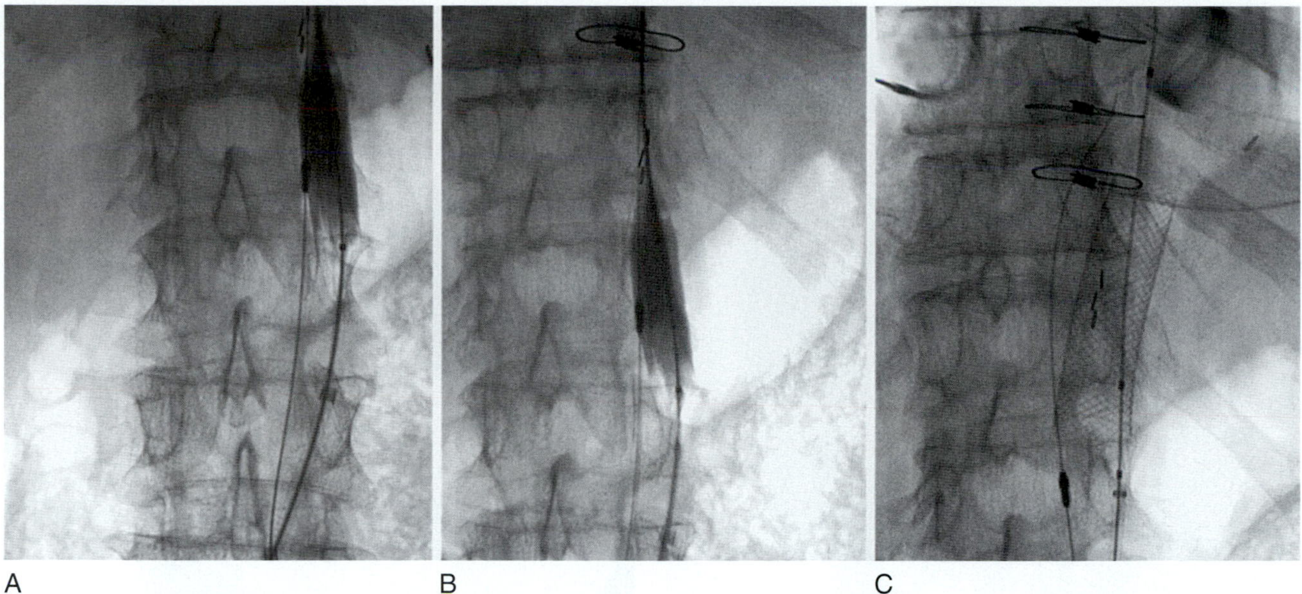

FIGURE 36-5. Various stages of balloon angioplasty of large self-expanding stent through fenestration within the true lumen to maintain patency. **A,** Passage of balloon across channel. **B,** Inflation of angioplasty balloon. **C,** Complete expansion of self-expanding stent.

occlusion can occur. Difficulty in stent sizing and determining appropriate diameters in abnormal vessels that have static and dynamic influences, as well as accuracy in deployment in these elastic vessels, also contribute to the challenges encountered by this percutaneous approach.

Although fenestration and stenting are valuable techniques to minimize and treat acute ischemic complications from dissections, continued investigation of the long-term results is warranted. Persistent flow in the false lumen, as created by a reentry tear from fenestration, may result in dilation of the lumen and resultant aneurysmal formation in the future. The impact of the bare aortic stents through these reentry channels has yet to be evaluated.

ENDOVASCULAR STENT GRAFTS

Stent graft technology and applications have widened since the common use of such devices for the treatment of both thoracic aortic and abdominal aortic aneurysms. The use of a covered stent graft, with its ability to seal an entry tear and promote thrombosis in the false lumen, may prevent the future degeneration of the aorta and improve long-term survival.[20-35] The use of the stent graft also promotes perfusion to branch vessels distally. Dake and colleagues[23] reported distal flow improvement and revascularization to obstructed vessels by sealing the primary tear (Figs. 36-6 and 36-7).

The goals of treatment with stent graft placement are twofold. The first is to reverse ischemic complications from the dissection, and the second is to prevent aneurysmal dilation over time. The advantages of endovascular stent graft include the avoidance of a thoracotomy, cardiopulmonary bypass, aortic cross clamping, and blood loss. The average time for graft insertion is typically less than 2 hours.[36] Anesthetic considerations are similar for both open and endovascular repair, as both are performed under general anesthesia and require careful hemodynamic monitoring intraoperatively.

The anatomic criteria include the following: suitable proximal and distal attachment zones of at least 1 cm and 2 cm, respectively. This can be evaluated using CT, MRI, or calibrated angiography. The aortic diameters are difficult to assess in aortic dissection. Typically, the diameter of the nondissected aorta proximal to the tear is the measurement used to plan for device size. The distal graft is sized to the combined lumens (true and false) in the descending thoracic aorta or supraceliac abdominal aorta. Tears just at the subclavian artery may require coverage of that vessel and carotid-subclavian artery bypass for revascularization. This can be done preoperatively, particularly in patients with coronary bypass grafts, using the internal mammary artery. Test occlusion of the left subclavian artery can be performed to assess symptoms before coverage of the vessel. Devices with bare proximal stents may afford fixation proximal to the subclavian and coverage of the tear simultaneously. As fenestrated and side branch devices are developed, more proximal deployment of the devices within the arch may become feasible. Iliac artery pathology such as stenosis, dissection, and tortuosity influence suitability for stent graft repair, as the iliac artery serves as access vessels for device delivery and deployment.

The initial devices used were homemade and consisted of self-expanding Gianturco Z stents (COOK, Bloomington, Ind.) and woven polyester material.[23,37,38] These devices were then loaded into 20- to 24-Fr Keller-Timmerman sheaths (COOK) via femoral cutdown or iliac exposure. The successful use of homemade devices led to the development of manufactured stent grafts. These devices are in various phases of clinical trials in the United States. They include the Talent Thoracic Endograft (Medtronic, Santa Rosa, Calif.), the GORE Excluder

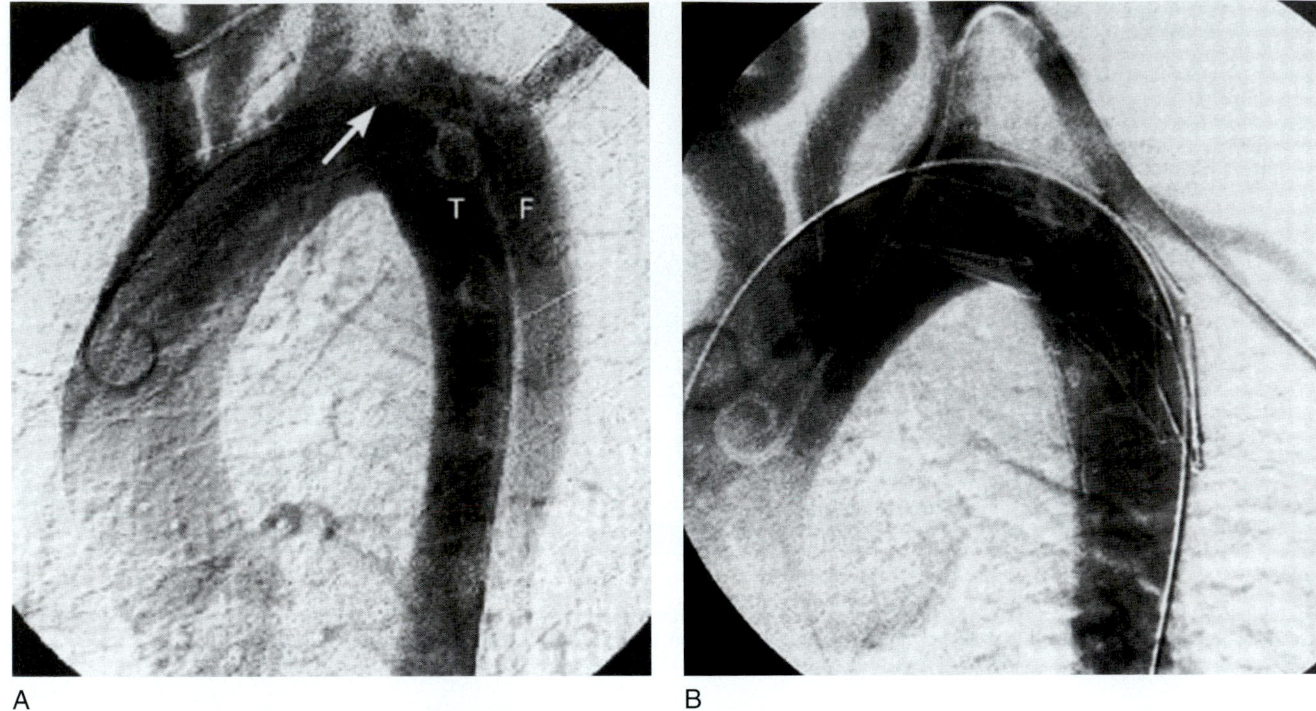

FIGURE 36-6. Thoracic aortograms before and immediately after stent-graft placement over the primary entry tear. Before stent-graft deployment **(A)**, there is flow of contrast medium from the true lumen (*T*) across the entry tear (*arrow*) into the false lumen (*F*). After stent-graft placement **(B)**, only the true lumen is evident. (From Dake M, Kato N, Mitchell R, et al: Endovascular stent-graft placement for the treatment of acute aortic dissection. N Engl J Med 340:1546, 1999.)

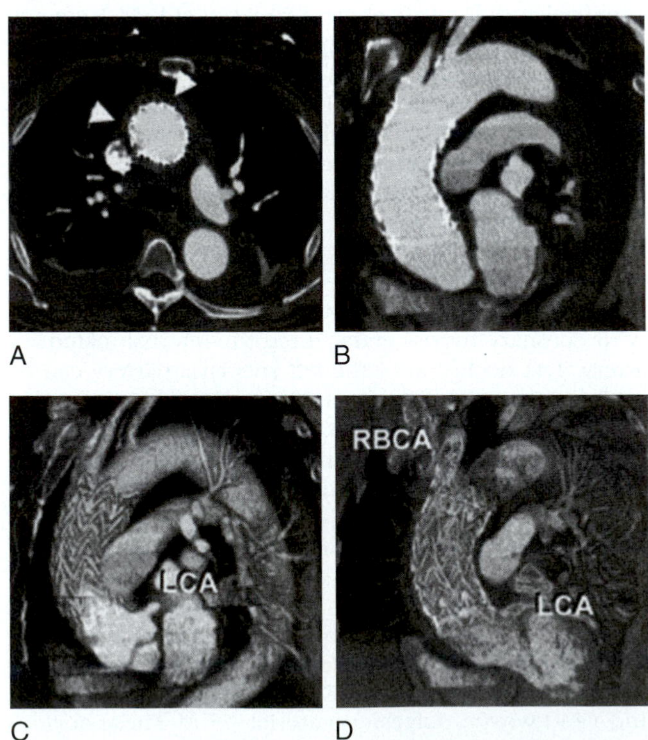

FIGURE 36-7. (See also Color Plate 36-7.) CT angiography after treatment of ascending aortic dissection with a stent graft (*arrow*). Axial **(A)** and oblique-sagittal **(B)** CT images confirm coverage of intimal tear with aortic stent graft. Volume-rendered views **(C, D)** show relationship of stent graft to left coronary artery (*LCA*) and right brachiocephalic artery (*RBCA*). (From Ihnken K, Sze D, Dake MD, et al: Successful treatment of a Stanford type A dissection by percutaneous placement of a covered stent graft in the ascending aorta. J Thorac Cardiovasc Surg 127:1809, 2004.)

(WL Gore, Flagstaff, Ariz.), and the Zenith Thoracic Endograft (COOK). The manufactured grafts offer better construction, smaller and more flexible delivery systems, as well as additional prostheses and balloons for implantation.

Technique

General anesthesia and cardiovascular monitoring is performed during the procedure. Bilateral femoral cutdowns or retroperitoneal iliac exposure is obtained. Left brachial artery catheterization is performed with the placement of a multisided hole flush catheter for aortic injections at the level of the left subclavian artery. Full heparinization based on weight is administered. After passage of stiff wires via the iliac artery into the arch, the device is loaded onto a delivery system and followed by fluoroscopy to the site of the tear. The mean arterial pressure is lowered to 50 mm Hg pharmacologically, and the stent graft is deployed. The proximal and distal sites of the stent graft are then balloon-expanded to ensure an appropriate seal. Completion angiography or IVUS is performed to evaluate the proximal fixation and to assess the false and true lumens for size and flow patterns. Transesophageal echocardiographic guidance can also be used to assist stent graft deployment.

A team of interventionalists and cardiovascular surgeons perform the procedure. High-quality imaging is essential for precise device deployment. Depending on the location of suitable imaging equipment, the procedure can be performed in cardiology catheterization suites, interventional radiology suites, or the operating room.

Outcomes

Excellent results with stent grafting have been reported. The procedure was 100% technically successful in the series by Dake and colleagues.[23] Their report, including 19 cases of dissection, showed complete thrombosis of the aortic false lumen in 15 patients (79%) and partial thrombosis in 4 patients (21%).[23,39] Seventy-six percent of obstructed vascular beds were reperfused with stent graft insertion. There were no deaths or aortic ruptures. Nienaber and associates[36] prospectively evaluated stent grafts in 12 patients versus open repair in matched patients with aortic dissection. Endovascular grafting was successful in all patients, and thrombosis of the false lumen was confirmed on MRI. No deaths or complications occurred in the stent graft group. The open cohort did not fare as well, with four deaths and five adverse events within a year. No paraplegia was reported in the stent graft group. The authors attributed this to careful use of short stents and deployment far from T8-L2.

Shimono and colleagues[34] performed endovascular stent graft procedures on 37 patients with dissections in the descending thoracic aorta. The survival rate and freedom from cardiovascular events at 2 years were 97.3% and 78.3%, respectively. Thrombosis of the false lumen occurred in 35 out of 36 cases by the first postoperative CT scan results.

Palma and colleagues,[40] who treated 70 patients with type B dissections, reported the largest series. Procedural success was demonstrated in 65 patients (92%), and only 2 deaths were reported. Twenty percent of patients had residual flow in the false lumens after endografting due to more distal fenestrations. The rate of survival at 29 months was 91%. Continued perfusion of the false channel and multiple reentry tears in the abdominal aorta may be a limitation of this therapy and eventually lead to aneurysmal degeneration despite adequate seal of the entry tear in the thoracic aorta. This lack of remodeling is more commonly seen in the treatment of chronic dissections with stent grafts. Dake and colleagues[23] reported false lumen thrombosis in only 5% of patients. In the series by Won and associates,[41] 12 patients with chronic type B dissections were treated with stent graft repair, and successful occlusion of the primary tear was seen in all but 2 patients. Although a CT scan confirmed thrombosis of the thoracic false lumen, persistent flow in the false lumen channel of the abdominal aorta remained. In this series, the abdominal aortic dissections did not progress during a mean follow-up of 22 months.

Aortic wall remodeling and stability is induced by false lumen thrombosis and occurs with stent graft placement. True lumen expansion with improved flow, downstream perfusion, and reduction in false lumen flow has been demonstrated by Nienaber and colleagues.[36] These observed occurrences are associated with improved survival and fewer adverse events in the long term. Acute type B dissections are the most suitable for stent graft treatment because of the apposition of the intimal tear and closure of the false lumen. In chronic type B dissections, the septum may be fibrosed and less likely to collapse with false lumen thrombosis. In addition, multiple reentry tears may continue to perfuse the false channel from below and maintain pressure within the lumen.

Complications related to stent grafts include technical failure, stent graft migration, the creation of new tears from stent graft placement, aneurysmal degeneration, postimplantation syndrome, and neurologic complications. Technical failure secondary to the inability to deploy the stent graft is seen most frequently in patients with severe atherosclerotic disease of the distal aorta and common iliac arteries.[29] The large delivery systems may fail to traverse tortuous and stenotic vessels despite adjunctive measures, such as balloon angioplasty and retroperitoneal exposure for iliac access. The more flexible introducer systems, which have lower profile sheaths, have improved the ease of device delivery. Problems with the deployment of stent grafts can occur, with resultant migration and failure of proximal seal. This may result from the behavior and alignment of the stents in the aorta. Mitchell and colleagues[22] noted improved radial force of the self-expanding stents in the straight segment of the aorta as compared with the curved portion. The curve of the arch may hamper the ability of the graft to seal circumferentially. Shorter stents and more flexible stent graft design may be required to maintain position in the arch.[33] Precise stent graft placement in the arch can be challenging, and guidewire length can be limited near the great vessel origins. Saccular aneurysmal development may occur in the proximal portion of the aorta at the level of the stent graft. In the series by Kato and colleagues,[42] 4 of 14 patients developed saccular aneurysms in the proximal descending thoracic aorta. Aneurysmal dilation and the creation of new entry tears have been attributed to the force of the stent graft on the aortic wall with resultant weakening, and they may also be caused by the rigidity and oversizing of the grafts.[33,42]

Several investigators have described postimplantation syndrome. This typically includes fever, leukocytosis, and elevation of C-reactive protein.[26,41] Lopera and colleagues[29] observed this transient syndrome in 55 (81%) of 68 patients. Back pain of unknown etiology was also seen in 30 (44%) of patients but resolved within a few days. Life-threatening complications such as rupture, leak, and visceral/renal ischemia need to be considered in the differential diagnosis when evaluating the postoperative stent graft patient.

Neurologic complications include stroke and paraplegia. The manipulation of rigid wires in the aorta, particularly if diseased, can be associated with strokes. Avoidance of frequent catheter and wire manipulations may minimize this devastating outcome. Paraplegia can be caused by many factors including emboli, hemodynamic instability, malperfusion of intercostal vessels, and obliteration of a false lumen that supplies the T8-T12 intercostal vessels. Other factors that may contribute include the length of thoracic aorta covered by the stent graft in patients with previous prosthetic replacement of the abdominal aorta, as this causes the loss of both thoracic and lumbar branch arteries. The incidence of paraplegia after open repair has been reported to be as low as 2.9% in patients with chronic dissection and as high as 19% in those with acute aortic dissection, whereas the incidence of paraplegia has been reported to be 1% to 3% in the setting of graft placement for aortic dissection.[22-24,26,40,43] This lower incidence of paraplegia with stent grafts as compared with open repair may result from the lack of an aortic cross-clamp and consequent reperfusion injury with stent grafts.

Long-term exclusion and thrombosis of the false lumen to prevent aneurysmal dilation and degeneration of the aorta is hampered by the existence of reentry tears in the abdominal aorta. These reentry channels maintain perfusion and pressurization of the false channel with the potential for aneurysmal expansion. Dake and colleagues[23] reported thrombosis of the false lumen in the thoracic aorta and sealing of the tear after stent grafting in 15 out of 19 patients. Only one patient had thrombosis of the false lumen in the abdominal aorta. Palma and associates[40] demonstrated residual flow in the false lumen below the diaphragm in 20% of their patients because of distal fenestrations. Stent graft obliteration of the false lumen was evaluated in acute and chronic dissections by Shimono and colleagues.[34] Complete obliteration of the false lumen was seen in 21 of 36 acute dissection cases (58.3%) and in only 5 of 13 patients with chronic dissection. Maximum size of the thrombosed false lumen decreased in all patients with acute dissections but not in 15.4% of chronic dissections. The effectiveness of stent graft repair on the treatment of dissections and thrombosis of the false lumen may be limited by distal reentry tears, which allow retrograde flow into the false channel.[33,42,44] The small series of patients reported and insufficient data make it difficult to draw any definitive conclusions.

Stent graft therapy for the treatment of aortic dissections offers several advantages. It avoids the morbidity of open aortic surgery while providing an effective means to perfuse ischemic beds, seal the entry tear, allow false lumen thrombosis, and perform favorable aortic wall remodeling. Long-term data are not available to determine the ultimate fate of the stented aorta with respect to aneurysmal formation.

REFERENCES

1. Williams D, Lee D, Hamilton B, et al: The dissected aorta. Part III: Anatomy and radiologic diagnosis of branch-vessel compromise. Radiology 203:37, 1997.
2. Lee D, Williams D, Abrams G: The dissected aorta. Part II: Differentiation of the true from the false lumen with intravascular US. Radiology 203:32, 1997.
3. Williams D, LePage M, Lee D: The dissected aorta. Part I: Early anatomic changes in an in vitro model. Radiology 203:23, 1997.
4. Vedantham S, Picus D, Sanchez L, et al: Percutaneous management of ischemic complications in patients with type-B aortic dissection. J Vasc Interv Radiol 14:181, 2003.
5. Williams D, Lee D, Hamilton B, et al: The dissected aorta: Percutaneous treatment of ischemic complications—principles and results. J Vasc Interv Radiol 8:605, 1997.
6. Chavan A, Hausman D, Dresler C, et al: Intravascular ultrasound-guided percutaneous fenestration of the intimal flap in the dissected aorta. Circulation 96:2124, 1997.
7. Lee D, Williams D, Abrams G: The dissected aorta: Part II: Differentiation of the true from the false lumen with intravascular ultrasound. Radiology 203:32, 1997.
8. Clair D: Aortic dissection with branch vessel occlusion: percutaneous treatment with fenestration and stenting. Semin Vasc Surg 15:116, 2002.
9. Fabre O, Vincentelli A, Willoteaux S, et al: Preoperative fenestration for type A acute aortic dissection with mesenteric malperfusion. Ann Thorac Surg 73:950, 2002.
10. Reber D, Aebert H, Manke M, et al: Percutaneous fenestration of the aortic dissection membrane in malperfusion syndrome. Eur J Cardiothorac Surg 15:91, 1999.
11. Slonim S, Nyman U, Semba C, et al: Aortic dissection: Percutaneous management of ischemic complications with endovascular stents and balloon fenestration. J Vasc Surg 23:241, 1996.
12. Slonim S, Miller D, Mitchell R, et al: Percutaneous balloon fenestration and stenting for life-threatening ischemic complications in patients with acute aortic dissection. J Thorac Cardiovasc Surg 117:1118, 1999.
13. Beregi J-P, Prat A, Gaxotte V, et al: Endovascular treatment for dissection of the descending aorta. Lancet 356:482, 2000.
14. Nienaber C, Eagle K: Aortic dissection: New frontiers in diagnosis and management. Part II: Therapeutic management and follow-up. Circulation 108:772, 2003.
15. Walker P, Dake M, Mitchell R, et al: The use of endovascular techniques for the treatment of complications of aortic dissection. J Vasc Surg 18:1042, 1993.
16. Deeb G, Williams D, Bolling S, et al: Surgery delay for acute type A dissection with malperfusion. Ann Thorac Surg 64:1669, 1997.
17. Lookstein R, Mitty H, Falk A, et al: Aortic intimal dehiscence: a complication of percutaneous balloon fenestration for aortic dissection. J Vasc Interv Radiol 12:1347, 2001.
18. Nienaber C, Eagle K: Aortic dissection: New frontiers in diagnosis and management. Part I: From etiology to diagnostic strategies. JAMA 108:628, 2003.
19. Nienaber C, Ince H, Petzsch M, et al: Endovascular treatment of acute aortic syndrome. Endovasc Today Nov/Dec(suppl):12, 2003.
20. Bortone A, Schena S, Mannatrizio G, et al: Endovascular stent-graft treatment for diseases of the descending thoracic aorta. Eur J Cardiothorac Surg 20:514, 2001.
21. Czermak B, Waldenberger P, Perkmann R, et al: Placement of endovascular stent-grafts for emergency treatment of acute disease of the descending thoracic aorta. Am J Roent 179:337, 2002.
22. Dake M, Miller D, Mitchell R, et al: The "first generation" of endovascular stent-grafts for patients with aneurysms of the descending thoracic aorta. J Thorac Cardiovasc Surg 116:689, 1998.
23. Dake M, Kato N, Mitchell R, et al: Endovascular stent-graft placement for the treatment of acute aortic dissection. N Engl J Med 340:1546, 1999.
24. Doss M, Balzer J, Martens S, et al: Emergent endovascular stent grafting for perforated acute type B dissections and ruptured thoracic aortic aneurysms. Ann Thorac Surg 76:493, 2003.
25. Ehrlich M, Grabenwoger M, Cartes-Zumelzu F, et al: Endovascular stent graft repair for aneurysms on the descending thoracic aorta. Ann Thorac Surg 66:19, 1998.
26. Fattori R, Napoli G, Lovato L, et al: Descending thoracic aortic diseases: Stent-graft repair. Radiology 229:176, 2003.
27. Grabenwoger M, Fleck T, Czerny M, et al: Endovascular stent graft placement in patients with acute thoracic aortic syndromes. Eur J Cardiothorac Surg 23:788, 2003.
28. Kang S-G, Lee D, Maeda M, et al: Aortic dissection: Percutaneous management with a separating stent-graft—preliminary results. Radiology 220:533, 2001.
29. Lopera J, Patino J, Urbina C, et al: Endovascular treatment of complicated type-B aortic dissection with stent-grafts: Midterm results. J Vasc Interv Radiol 14:195, 2003.
30. Mitchell R: Stent grafts for the thoracic aorta: A new paradigm? Ann Thorac Surg 74:S1818, 2002.
31. Miyairi T, Ninomiya M, Endoh M, et al: Conventional repair and operative stent-grafting for acute and chronic aortic dissection. Ann Thorac Surg 73:1621, 2002.
32. Palma J, de Souza J, Rodrigues Alves C, et al: Self-expandable aortic stent-grafts for treatment of descending aortic dissections. Ann Thorac Surg 73:1138, 2002.
33. Quinn S, Duke D, Baldwin S, et al: Percutaneous placement of a low-profile stent-graft device for aortic dissections. J Vasc Interv Radiol 13:791, 2002.
34. Shimono T, Kato N, Yasuda F, et al: Transluminal stent-graft placements for the treatments of acute onset and chronic aortic dissections. Circulation 106(suppl):I241, 2002.
35. Umana J, Miller D, Mitchell R: What is the best treatment for patients with acute type B aortic dissections—medical, surgical, or endovascular stent-grafting? Ann Thorac Surg 74:S1840, 2002.

36. Nienaber C, Fattori R, Lund G, et al: Nonsurgical reconstruction of thoracic aortic dissection by stent-graft placement. N Engl J Med 340:1539, 1999.
37. Kato N, Hirano T, Takeda K, et al: Treatment of acute aortic dissection with expandable metallic stents: Experimental study. J Vasc Interv Radiol 5:417, 1994.
38. Kato N, Hirano T, Shimono T, et al: Treatment of chronic aortic dissection by transluminal endovascular stent-graft placement: Preliminary results. J Vasc Interv Radiol 12:835, 2001.
39. Chung J, Elkins C, Sakai T, et al: True-lumen collapse in aortic dissection. Part I: Evaluation of causative factors in phantoms with pulsatile flow. Radiology 214:87, 2000.
40. Palma J, Marcos y Robles J, Amparo E, et al: Self-expanding aortic stent-grafts for treatment of descending aortic dissections. Ann Thorac Surg 73:1138, 2002.
41. Won J, Lee D, Shim W, et al: Elective endovascular treatment of descending thoracic aortic aneurysms and chronic dissections with stent-grafts. J Vasc Interv Radiol 12:575, 2001.
42. Kato M, Hirano T, Kawaguchi T: Aneurysmal degeneration of the aorta after stent-graft repair of acute aortic dissection. J Vasc Surg 34:513, 2001.
43. Coselli J, LeMaire S, Figueiredo L, et al: Paraplegia after thoracoabdominal aortic aneurysm repair: Is dissection a risk factor? Ann Thorac Surg 63:28, 1997.
44. Kato M, Matsuda T, Kaneko M, et al: Outcomes of stent-graft treatment of false lumen in aortic dissection. Circulation 98 (suppl):II305-II311, 1998.

chapter 37

Pathophysiology, Epidemiology, and Prognosis

Joshua A. Beckman

Aortic aneurysms account for more than 15,000 deaths and 63,000 hospital discharges per year in the United States.[1] Aneurysms may affect any part of the aorta from its root to the abdominal segment. The prognosis and outcome of aortic aneurysm vary based on the location and etiology. Appropriate intervention may improve the natural history of the disease process. This chapter reviews the pathophysiology, epidemiology, and prognosis of aortic aneurysms.

THE NORMAL AORTA

The aorta is the conduit through which the heart delivers blood that is ejected from the left ventricle to the body. Coursing through the thorax and abdomen, the aorta terminates in bifurcation to the common iliac arteries. It can be subdivided into three compartments in the thorax and one in the abdomen. The sections of the thoracic aorta include the ascending aorta, the portion arising from the base of the heart to the innominate artery; the transverse aorta or aortic arch, which includes the great vessels; and the descending aorta, which begins at the distal edge of the subclavian artery and ends at its junction with the abdominal aorta at the level of the diaphragm (Fig. 37-1).

Composed of three layers—the tunica intima, tunica media, and adventitia—the aorta contains elastic fibers and is therefore characterized as an elastic artery. At the innermost surface of the aorta, at the blood-aorta interface, lies a single-cell-thick layer of endothelial cells. The intima is bound by the internal elastic lamina. The tunica media comprises smooth muscle cells, collagen, fibroblasts, elastin fibers, and ground substance. The presence of elastin fibers in the media defines the aorta as an elastic artery and provides the tensile strength permitting the aorta to withstand pulsatile delivery of blood by the heart. Elastin content gradually decreases with distance from the heart.[2] Left ventricular contraction distends the aorta, thereby storing some of the ejected blood during systole and creating potential energy within the vessel. This is expended during diastole as the aorta recoils and propels blood to the coronary arteries and other systemic vascular beds. The outermost layer, the adventitia, is a thin layer that contains connective tissue, fibroblasts, and the nutritive vasa vasorum.

The aging process is associated with changes in aortic structure, which may make the aorta prone to aneurysm formation. The most prominent process is a stiffening of the vessel as a result of fragmentation of the elastin fibers, deposition of glycated proteins, and replacement of vascular smooth muscle cells by collagen.[3-5] Each layer of the aorta changes with aging and increases the stiffness of the vessel. In the intima, extracellular matrix increases in thickness while there is a decrease in endothelium-derived nitric oxide.[6] In the media, collagen content, collagen crosslinking, fibronectin deposition, and glycosaminoglycans all increase.[6] Each process increases aortic rigidity, decreases the vessel's ability to distend normally with left ventricular contraction, and weakens the vessel wall, thus increasing the tendency for deformation and ectasia.[7]

DEFINITION OF AORTIC ANEURYSM

In adults, the diameter of the aorta is approximately 3 cm at the origin, 2.5 cm in the descending portion in the

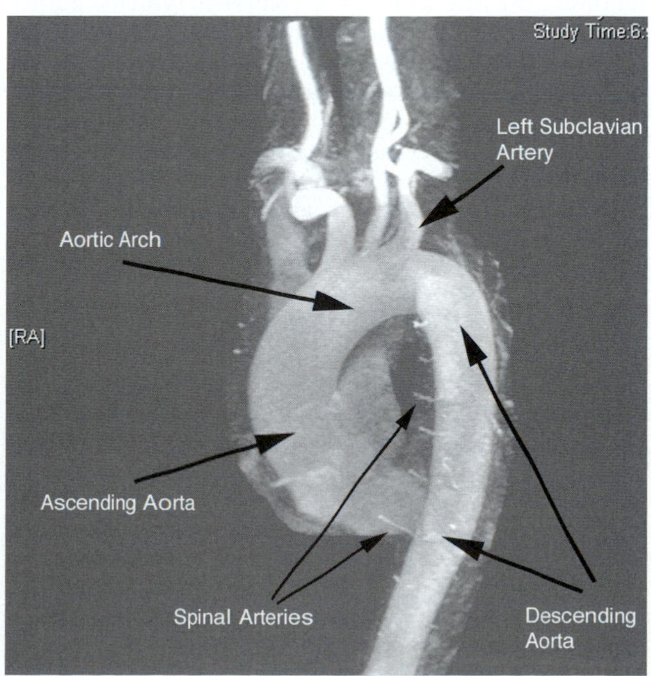

FIGURE 37-1. MRA of the thoracic aorta. Note the different segments of the aorta including the ascending aorta, aortic arch, and descending aorta. The left subclavian artery separates the aortic arch from the descending aorta.

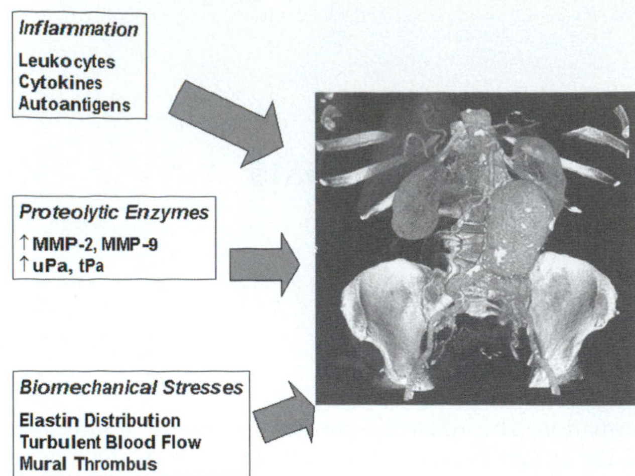

FIGURE 37-2. (See also Color Plate 37-2.) Three pathophysiologic mechanisms best characterize the process of aneurysm formation. Aortic aneurysm specimens reveal an increase in leukocyte infiltration, cytokine concentration, and leukocyte adhesion molecules. Both elastin-related and collagen-related autoantigens have been identified and may participate in the initiation of the process. Once the process has begun, proteolytic enzymes, particularly matrix metalloproteinases-2 and -9, increase in concentration and break down elastin and collagen. Increases in enzyme coactivators, such as urokinase plasminogen activator (uPa) and tissue plasminogen activator (tPa), further augment matrix breakdown. This increase in proteolysis is not accompanied by a change in inhibitors of this process, yielding a degenerative environment. Finally, the abdominal aorta is predisposed to aneurysm formation because of its relative lack of elastin and vascular smooth muscle compared with the thoracic aorta and adverse blood flow patterns. (Volumetric rendering CT image of the abdominal aortic aneurysm used with permission of Joseph Schoepf, MD.)

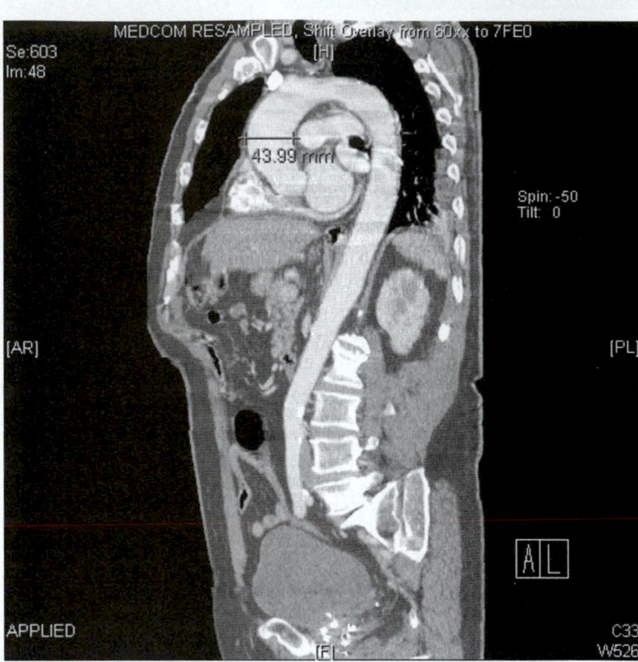

FIGURE 37-3. CT angiogram of an ascending aortic aneurysm. Notice that the proximal descending portion of the aorta is ectatic as well. The aneurysm involves the entire circumference of the aorta and is thus fusiform. The normal size for the ascending aorta is less than 3 cm.

thorax, and 1.8 to 2 cm in the abdomen. Modest expansion results in ectasia; the definition of an aneurysm requires a 50% increase in size compared with the normal segment proximal to the aneurysm. True aneurysms can be classified on the basis of morphology into two major groups: fusiform (Figs. 37-2 and 37-3), which represents circumferential expansion of the aorta, and saccular, which is an outpouching of a segment (Fig. 37-4). The former are more common. In contrast to true aneurysms, pseudoaneurysms are not aneurysms but contained ruptures of the aorta.

PATHOPHYSIOLOGY OF AORTIC ANEURYSMS

A wide variety of pathologic states are associated with aortic aneurysms (Box 37-1). These include degenerative diseases, developmental (inherited) diseases, infections, vasculitis, and trauma. The specific disorders associated with aortic aneurysms are discussed later in this chapter. Important determinants of aortic aneurysm formation include inflammation, biomechanical forces, and proteolytic degradation of connective tissue.[8] Pathologic expansion of the aorta was formerly ascribed to a process akin to atherogenesis.[9] Although advances in basic and clinical investigation in both lesion types have revealed some common themes, these studies suggest that aneurysm formation is fundamentally different from atherosclerosis.

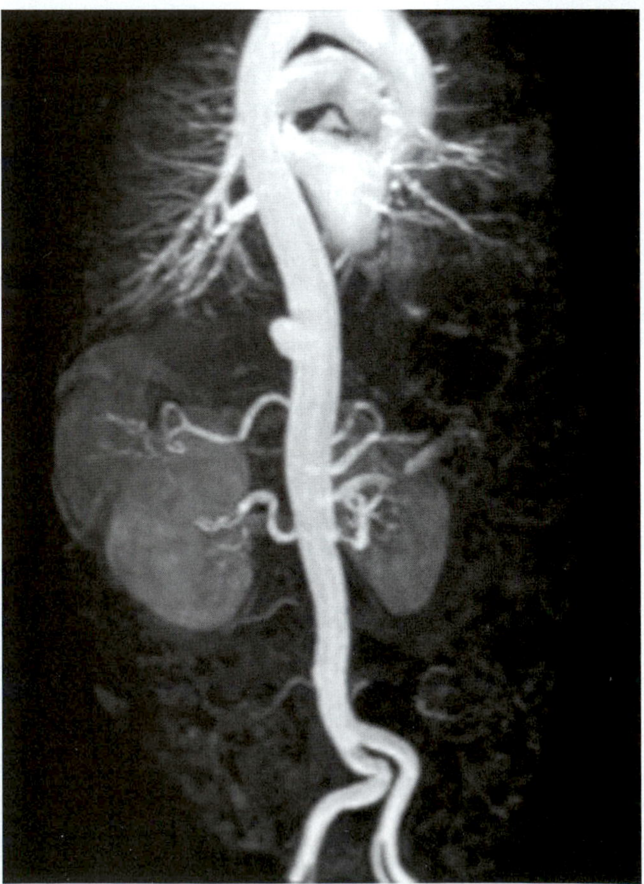

FIGURE 37-4. Maximal intensity projection of an MRI of a saccular aneurysm. Notice the outpouching of an otherwise normal aorta. This pattern of aneurysm is more common in infectious aneurysms.

BOX 37-1 Disorders Associated with Aortic Aneurysms

Degenerative
Cystic medial necrosis
Aortic dissection

Developmental
Marfan's syndrome
Ehlers-Danlos syndrome
Bicuspid aortic valve
Turner's syndrome
Aortic coarctation

Infectious
Tuberculosis
Syphilis
Staphylococcus
Salmonella

Vasculitis
Takayasu's arteritis
Giant cell arteritis
Ankylosing spondylitis
Rheumatoid arthritis
Systemic lupus erythematosus
Sarcoidosis
Reiter's syndrome
Behçet's disease
Relapsing polychondritis
Cogan's syndrome

Trauma

The preferential weakening of the adventitia and media, instead of an intimal proliferative process as in atherosclerosis, results in diminished aortic resilience and tensile strength, culminating in aortic wall thinning, dilation, and increased wall stress, all of which may result in rupture.

When studied histologically, aneurysms are characterized by the destruction of elastin and collagen in the media, neovascularization, a reduction in vascular smooth muscle cell mass, and infiltration of inflammatory cells.[10] Yet the pathology of aortic aneurysms varies in different segments of the aorta and in different predisposing diseases. In thoracic aneurysms, there is often cystic medial necrosis, mucoid infiltration, and cyst formation in the setting of elastin necrosis and vascular smooth muscle apoptosis. In patients with either Marfan's syndrome, bicuspid aortic valve, or Turner's syndrome, inflammation is not as prominent as in abdominal aortic aneurysms (AAAs).[11-13] Cystic medial necrosis usually is not observed in AAAs, where there may be deficiency in glycosaminoglycan production.[14] These aneurysms typically have disrupted elastin fibers, variable inflammation, and a decrease in vascular smooth muscle cell density.[10,15] The inflammatory cells include T cells, B cells, and macrophages at the junction of the media and adventitia.[15] Elastin fragmentation occurs adjacent to the inflammatory cells. Moreover, there is an increase in the rate of vascular smooth muscle cell apoptosis compared with normal aorta.[16] Nonetheless, the formation of all aortic aneurysms likely involves the processes described as follows, but not uniformly.

The development of aneurysms is associated with the loss of two aortic structural elements, elastin and collagen. The former is thought to have a half-life of 40 to 70 years,[17] so that breakdown of elastin in adults represents pathologic destruction with inadequate regeneration. Elastin provides radial and longitudinal support, enabling the aorta to respond to pulsatile flow while maintaining arterial proportions. The relevance of elastin breakdown can be seen in experimental animal studies of elastase infusion, which yields aortic aneurysms.[18] The loss of elastin is seen on histologic examination[19]; however, breakdown of elastin alone does not seem sufficient to cause aneurysmal expansion and rupture. Early in aneurysm formation, the aorta compensates for the loss of elastin by increasing production of collagen,[20] the other important structural element; however, as elastin content decreases, collagen, as the major source of tensile strength, is overwhelmed and aortic expansion occurs. With another undefined signal, collagenases are produced, promoting collagen destruction. As collagen degrades, aneurysm rupture becomes possible.[21] Three pathophysiologic processes have been characterized as mechanisms important in aneurysm formation: inflammation, proteolytic degradation of structural elements, and increases in biomechanical stress (see Fig. 37-2).

Inflammation

In 1981 Rose and Dent[22] evaluated 51 consecutively removed AAAs and reported mild chronic inflammation in 72.5% and moderate inflammation in 15.7%. Populations of B and T lymphocytes and macrophages are found in greater quantity in the adventitia and media of AAAs than of atherosclerotic or normal aortas.[23,24] Ocana and colleagues[25] demonstrated that B and T lymphocytes that infiltrate aortic aneurysms act as activated memory cells, express molecules of B-T costimulation, and occasionally give rise to the formation of lymphoid structures and germinal centers within the aneurysm wall. These characteristics differentiate aneurysm-based lymphocytes from those in the peripheral blood, making extravasation into the arterial wall an unlikely mechanism of accrual.

Once activated within the vessel wall, the inflammatory cells create an environment permissive for the progression of disease and further recruitment of inflammatory cells. Surgical explant specimens from patients with aortic aneurysms demonstrate higher levels of adhesion molecules, including intracellular adhesion molecule (ICAM)-1 and vascular cell adhesion molecule (VCAM)-1, than in atherosclerotic and normal aortas.[26,27] Similarly, tissue levels of cytokines in aneurysms, including tumor necrosis factor alpha (TNF-α), interleukin-1 beta (IL-1-β), IL-8, monocyte chemoattractant protein-1 (MCP-1), interferon gamma (IFN-γ), and IL-6, have all been noted to be elevated when compared with control subjects.[28-30] Interestingly, cytokine levels are higher in ruptured aortic aneurysms than in asymptomatic aortic aneurysms, suggesting that an increasing level of inflammation is associated with worse outcome.[31] Other acute phase proteins, including C-reactive protein and ceruloplasmin, are present at increased levels within the vessel wall as well.[32]

The source of these inflammatory mediators is largely the infiltrating macrophages; however, lymphocytes and aortic endothelial and smooth muscle cells also contribute to the inflammatory milieu.[29] Thus, immune cells invade the aortic wall, become activated, and create an inflammatory environment that engages the activity of local stabilizing cells, initiating the process of elastin and collagen breakdown and aneurysm formation.

The signal that drives inflammatory cell recruitment remains unclear. Several proposed antigens have been identified as possible initiators of aneurysm formation. These include infectious causes, such as cytomegalovirus and *Chlamydia pneumonia*, although the data are mixed and limited.[24,33,34] *C. pneumoniae*, in particular, has been detected in both the blood and aorta of patients with aneurysms. Patients with aneurysms are more likely to have been exposed to *C. pneumoniae* than control subjects, and antibody titer positivity has been correlated with aneurysm expansion,[35-42] although the data are not uniform.[43,44]

A second possible basis for inflammatory cell recruitment is the presence of an aortic wall autoantigen. Two have been described, one of which is associated with elastin fibers and the other with collagen fibers. In 1996 Tilson and colleagues[45] extracted IgG from aneurysm specimens and applied them as a probe to normal human aortas. They described an immunoreactive protein that colocalizes with elastin-associated microfibers, predominantly in the aorta, called aortic aneurysm associated protein (AAAP)-40. Further experiments to characterize the protein suggest it may be a human homologue to the aorta-specific, microfibril-associated glycoprotein (MAGP)-36 of pigs and cows.[46] This protein has regions of substantial homology with sequences in the α- and β-chains of fibrinogen, vitronectin, and Ig-κ.[47,48] Although present throughout the aorta, binding was strongest in the abdominal segment.[49] More recently, this same group has described an 80 kDa protein that localized to collagen fibers in the aneurysm wall.[50] The relative importance of each antigen, its normal distribution, and the presence of other antigens remain undefined. Moreover, whether or not these are true initiators of the disease is also unclear. Because breakdown products of elastin promote inflammatory cell recruitment,[51] these epitopes may only become exposed after tissue breakdown and cellular immune system activation has begun.

Supporting the concept of an autoantigenic mechanism is the greater than 100-fold increase in IgG and complement found in human aneurysm tissue when compared with normal aortas.[52,53] Moreover, the presence of immunoglobulin aggregated within the vessel wall suggests an immune-mediated destruction of aortic wall supporting elements.[23,45] Why autoimmunity develops is unclear, although there is evidence that inherited variations of HLA-DR B1 may predispose to or protect from aneurysm formation.[54]

Proteolytic Degradation

Although the signal that initiates the development of an inflammatory environment and causes engagement of local cells in aneurysm formation remains unclear, the means by which these cells degrade the supportive elements of the aortic wall have been better characterized. Matrix metalloproteinases (MMPs) are endopeptidases that degrade one or more components of the extracellular matrix. Thus far, at least six classes of MMPs, comprising nearly 30 individual proteinases, have been characterized, including collagenases, gelatinases, stromelysins, matrilysins, membrane-type (MT-) MMPs, and other MMPs.[55] Metalloproteinases are normally secreted by endothelial cells, vascular smooth muscle cells, and adventitial fibroblasts, thereby participating in arterial remodeling. Macrophages and lymphocytes can produce these enzymes in greater quantities in pathologic settings.

Typically produced as a proenzyme, MMPs may be activated both intracellularly and extracellularly. Extracellular regulation of activation may occur as a result of an MMP–MT-MMP interaction or via interaction with plasmin or reactive oxygen species.[56-58] The inhibitors of MMPs are the tissue inhibitors of matrix metalloproteinases (TIMPs) and plasminogen activator inhibitors (PAI) 1 and 2. TIMPs bind MMPs in stoichiometric proportions to inactivate them.[55]

Increased local production of MMPs in aortic aneurysm was reported more than 10 years ago.[59-61] Although elevations of several MMPs have been noted, MMP-1 (collagenase) and MMP-3 (stromelysin), MMP-2 (gelatinase A), and MMP-9 (gelatinase B) represent the principal elastases in aortic aneurysms.[62,63] MMP-2 and -9 are primarily derived from infiltrating macrophages; however, they are also made by resident aortic vascular smooth muscle cells.[64,65] MMP-9, as a gelatinase, can also break down collagen. MMP-9 is most typically found in the adventitia, near the vasa vasorum, localizing to infiltrating macrophages.[66] MMP-2 can act exclusively as an elastase and collagenase for fibrillar collagen. It is synthesized constitutively by vascular smooth muscle cells[67] but can also be synthesized by infiltrating leukocytes. Interestingly, MMP-2 production is increased in the vasculature remote from the aorta, suggesting a systemic underlying disease process that manifests with aortic aneurysmal disease.[68]

The centrality of these enzymes in aneurysm formation has been demonstrated in experimental models. MMP-9 and MMP-2 knockout mice do not form aortic aneurysms after abluminal exposure to calcium chloride.[69] Reinfusion of competent macrophages from wild-type mice into MMP-9 knockout mice enables aneurysm formation, whereas similar reinfusion into MMP-2 knockout mice does not. These results suggest that macrophages are an important source of MMP-9, whereas mesenchymal production of MMP-2 may be more important.[69] Adding another layer of complexity, expression of these proteolytic enzymes may vary based on the stage of aneurysm formation. An early study of human aortic aneurysm specimens demonstrated increased gelatinase A (MMP-2) expression in smaller aneurysms, while expression of gelatinase B (MMP-9) is greater in large aneurysms.[70] More recent studies, however, have demonstrated no relationship or increment in levels of MMP-2 in aneurysms based on size.[71-74] Most studies do show an increase in MMP-9 expression as aneurysm size increases, and MMP-9

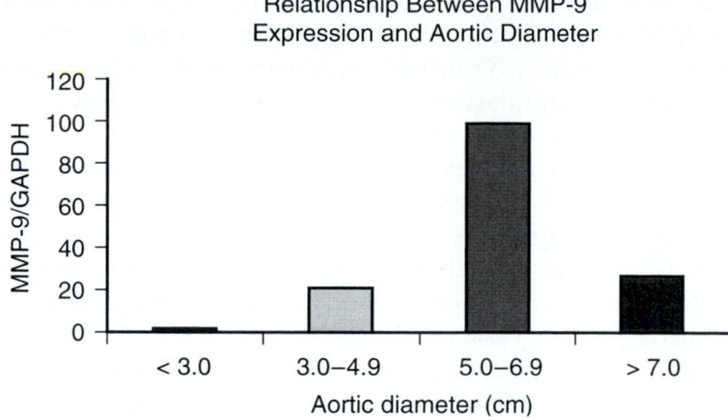

FIGURE 37-5. Relationship between MMP-9 expression and aortic diameter. Matrix metalloproteinase-9 expression increases as aortic diameter increases until the aorta becomes large. (Adapted from Petersen and colleagues.[71])

content has been associated with aneurysm rupture (Fig. 37-5).[75]

Other proteolytic enzymes are increased as well, including interstitial collagenase-1 (MMP-1), human macrophage metalloelastase (MMP-12), and membrane type-1 metalloproteinase (MT1-MMP). Akin to MMP-2, MMP-1 expression is increased in aneurysms and is derived primarily from mesenchymal cells.[76] It can degrade types 1 and 3 collagen, but its contribution to aneurysm formation remains unknown. As made clear by its name, expression of MMP-12 is increased in aortic aneurysms as a result of macrophage infiltration. Its relevance to aneurysm formation has been attenuated by the finding that MMP-12 knockout mice are not protected from aneurysm formation.[77] MT1-MMP is a collagenase that is produced by macrophages and increased in aortic aneurysms. It likely has its greatest effect as an activator of the proenzyme form of MMP-2.[78,79]

In addition to the increased expression of matrix metalloproteinases, aneurysm formation is characterized by alterations in proteolytic enzyme agonist and antagonist balance. As discussed earlier, components of inflammation, including plasminogen activators and oxidative stress, activate MMPs. Indeed, urokinase-type plasminogen activator (uPA) and tissue-type plasminogen activator (tPA) expression are increased in aortic aneurysms but not in healthy aortic specimens.[56,64] Plasminogen activators have been demonstrated to be specific physiologic regulators of gelatinase (MMP-2 and MMP-9) activation.[80] Reactive oxygen species can also convert proenzyme MMPs to their active form.[81,82] Compared with nonaneurysmal sections of aorta, superoxide anion and markers of oxidative stress are increased in aneurysmal segments. One key source of increased oxidative stress is activation of NAD(P)H oxidases.[83]

Not only are MMP levels increased in aortic aneurysms, but MMP antagonist expression and activity is reduced. Although early work has reported decreased concentration of tissue inhibitors of metalloproteinases (TIMPs) in aneurysmal tissue,[60,84] most investigators report no difference in TIMP concentration between aneurysmal and healthy aortic tissue.[75,78,85-87] However, remembering that TIMPs inhibit MMPs stoichiometrically, the relative increase in MMPs above that of TIMPs serves to alter the ratio and create a proteolytic environment.[76] The relevance of TIMPs has been demonstrated experimentally. Local overexpression of TIMP-1 prevented aneurysm formation in a rat model of aortic aneurysm,[88] while TIMP knockout mice had increased MMP activity and aneurysm formation.[89] Similar to expression of TIMPs, plasminogen activator inhibitor (PAI)-1 expression has been described as similar to or lower than healthy aortic controls.[56,84,90] Increases in expression of plasminogen activators without reciprocal changes in their inhibitors alters the balance toward fibrinolysis, MMP activation, and tissue degradation. Experimental overexpression of PAI-1 prevents aneurysm formation in a rat model of aortic aneurysm,[57] confirming the importance of relative instead of absolute concentrations.

As the understanding of the process of aneurysm formation has increased, several therapeutic interventions have been tested and reinforce the mechanisms outlined earlier. The best studied treatment to date is doxycycline. Tetracyclines have long been recognized as generalized inhibitors of metalloproteinases.[91,92] Their potential value in aortic aneurysmal disease has been demonstrated in reducing aneurysm formation in both organ culture and rodent models of aneurysm,[77,93,94] as well as the ability to achieve the same therapeutic plasma levels of the medications in humans.[95] In human aneurysm specimens, doxycycline limits the activity of both gelatinases: it reduces macrophage MMP-9 mRNA expression and diminishes activation of the proenzyme form of MMP-2.[96] When administered to patients with AAAs, doxycycline decreases plasma levels of MMP-9.[97] Finally, in a small, randomized phase 2 trial, doxycycline decreased the aneurysm expansion rate.[98] Although these data await confirmation in a larger trial, they do support the conceptual framework of aneurysm formation and the importance of proteolytic enzymes in that context.

Other therapies that are in development and may shed light on the pathogenesis of aneurysm formation include indomethacin and hydroxymethyl glutaryl (HMG) CoA reductase inhibitors, or statins. Indomethacin prevents aortic aneurysm formation in a rat model.[99] The mechanism seems to be inhibition of cyclooxygenase 2, prostaglandin E2, and then MMP-9.[100-102] Prostaglandin E2 (PGE2) expression is upregulated more than 30-fold in aortic aneurysms. PGE2 localizes to infiltrating macrophages and its expression is dependent on cyclooxygenase activity.[103] Prostaglandin E2, via activation of IL-6, may increase vascular smooth muscle cell apoptosis, further weakening the structural elements of the aorta.[102,104,105] More recently, statins have shown some antianeurysm properties experimentally via reductions in oxidative stress and macrophage production of MMPs.[106,107]

Increases in Biomechanical Wall Stress

The overwhelming frequency of aneurysm formation in the abdominal aorta suggests a predisposition in this area. Biomechanical factors were among the first noted relevant variations among the regions of the aorta. Relative deficiencies in vessel-wall-stabilizing elements combine with adverse blood flow patterns to make the abdominal aorta more likely to develop an aneurysm. Compensatory mechanisms occur after aneurysm formation have developed, but they do not stop the process. Thus an imbalance of biomechanical forces and reactions promotes aneurysm formation.

Classification of the aorta as an elastic artery arises from the elastin contained in the vessel wall. Elastin is organized into circumferential plates or lamellae to respond to the pulsatile load created by the heart. Each lamellar unit consists predominantly of two elastin bundles and vascular smooth muscle.[2] Deposition of elastin is not uniform within the aorta. The thoracic aorta incorporates 35 to 56 lamellar units, while the abdominal aorta incorporates 28.[108] Thus the abdominal aorta may be more susceptible to elastin breakdown because of the relative increase in pressure withstood per lamellar unit compared with the rest of the vessel. In addition, the abdominal aorta has a decreased concentration of nutritive vasa vasorum when compared with more proximal aortic segments.[109] Reductions in aortic tissue perfusion stiffen the vessel, reducing compliance and the ability to withstand pulsatile stress.[110,111]

Another factor that may make the abdominal segment of the aorta more prone to aneurysm formation is blood flow patterns specific to that segment. In experimental models, the infrarenal segment of the aorta is subject to much higher levels of oscillating flow and reflected pressure waves compared with the suprarenal segment[112]; this results in higher levels of aortic wall tension. Indeed, turbulence and pressure are exacerbated by the aneurysm morphology, which promotes vortex and turbulent flow patterns.[113-116] Excluding these flow patterns from the aneurysm through placement of an aortic endograft rapidly reduces plasma MMP-9 levels in patients.[117,118] In animal models of aortic aneurysm, changing the flow characteristics in the aorta can change the structure of the aorta. In a rodent elastase-infusion model of aortic aneurysm, flow conditions were examined via the creation of a left femoral arteriovenous fistula or left iliac artery ligation. Increases in shear stress as a result of fistula formation resulted in a more stable aortic phenotype with decreased oxidative stress, decreased macrophage density in the media, increased aortic endothelial and vascular smooth muscle cells, and reduced apoptosis when compared with the ligation arm of the study.[119-121] Indeed, the increase in flow decreased aortic expansion by 26%.[119]

In addition to the adverse biomechanical forces creating an environment permissive for aneurysm formation, effective and ineffective compensatory mechanisms to slow aneurysm expansion are present, specifically thrombus formation and elastin production, respectively. The role of intraluminal thrombus has recently come under study. Using finite element analysis in a 3-D model of the aorta derived from CT scans, intraluminal thrombus reduced peak wall stress up to 38%,[122] relatively independent of the thrombus constituents.[123] The thrombus decreases the transmission of luminal pressure to the aneurysm wall and may prevent aneurysm rupture by reducing wall strain.[124] Intraluminal thrombus may also contribute to aneurysm formation. Intraluminal thrombus has been demonstrated to have higher levels of proteolytic enzymes and enzyme activators than the aneurysm itself.[125] Thus it may act as a proteolytic enzyme reservoir through polymorphonuclear leukocytes, and enzyme accumulation provides a ready source of destructive elements for the adjacent aneurysm.[125]

Interestingly, the vascular cells in the aorta attempt to restore elastin content in the setting of elastin degradation to compensate for the reductions in tensile and radial strength. Human AAA samples show a fourfold to sixfold increase in tropoelastin protein compared with control arteries.[126] The elastin is produced by smooth muscle cells and macrophages. In areas of macrophage infiltration, elastin deposition is not organized into mature, effective bundles. Indeed, the aneurysm specimens have a ninefold reduction in desmosine, a marker for mature elastin crosslinking, compared with normal specimens.[126] Thus attempts at elastin replacement are disordered and do not improve aortic compliance.

EPIDEMIOLOGY AND PROGNOSIS OF AORTIC ANEURYSMS

Abdominal Aortic Aneurysms

Aortic aneurysms are typically defined as an increase in diameter of 50% compared with the adjacent normal segment of the aorta. The upper limit of normal for the abdominal aorta is 3 cm. The absolute size definition for AAA is preferable, for body size and baseline diameter may vary on the basis of height, sex, weight, and the presence of a thoracoabdominal aortic aneurysm. Infrarenal AAAs represent approximately 90% of all aortic aneurysms.

Prevalence

The prevalence of aneurysms of the abdominal aorta has been determined on the basis of several large screening studies and autopsy series (Table 37-1). In one series of 24,000 consecutive autopsies performed over 23 years, 1.97% of the subjects were found to have an AAA during postmortem examination.[127] Of the 473 aneurysms found, 58% were larger than 4 cm in diameter, nearly three quarters of the patients were men, and one fourth of the aneurysms had ruptured. The incidence of aortic aneurysms has been reported to range between 40.6 and 49.3 per 100,000 men and 6.8 and 12.3 per 100,000 women during a 6-year follow-up period.[128]

The highest reported frequency of AAA derives from a Dutch study of 2419 men aged 60 to 80 years.[129] These investigators reported that 8.1% of the men had an AAA greater than or equal to 3 cm, and 1.7% had an AAA greater than or equal to 4 cm. Indeed, in studies with more than 1000 subjects, using a definition of aneurysm as greater than 29 mm, the prevalence ranged from 0.7% to 8.4%.[129-135] Subsequently, large screening programs in targeted populations have further evaluated the prevalence. The largest screening program was performed in the Aneurysm Detection and Management (ADAM) Study Screening Program, which studied 126,196 veterans aged 50 to 79 years.[136] In this cohort of American veterans, 3.6% of the subjects had an infrarenal aortic diameter

TABLE 37-1 PREVALENCE OF AORTIC ANEURYSM

Author	N	Gender	Age (yr)	Aneurysm Frequency (%)	Nation
Boll[129]	2149	M	60-80	8.1	Netherlands
Kullman[130]	1256	M	≥60	7.3	Norway
Pleumeekers[131]	5419	42% M	>55	4.1 M, 0.7 W	Netherlands
Lucarotti[132]	4232	M	65	7.1	United Kingdom
Morris[133]	3030	M	>50	50-64 yr 0.3 65-79 yr 2.5	United Kingdom
Smith[135]	2669	M	65-75	8.4	United Kingdom
Lederle[136]	126,196	97% M	50-79	1.3	United States
Ashton[137]	27147	M	65-74	4.9	United Kingdom
Singh[139]	2998	F	25-84	2.2	Norway
Lederle[140]	3450	F	50-79	1.0	United States
Scott[147]	9342	F	65-80	1.3	United Kingdom

greater than 3 cm, while an AAA greater than or equal to 4 cm was found in 1.2%. This population was 97% men, as expected in a veteran population. The Multicentre Aneurysm Screening Study (MASS) screened 27,147 of 33,830 invited men aged 65 to 74 years and reported that 4.9% of the subjects had an AAA greater than or equal to 3 cm.[137]

The prevalence of AAAs in women has been determined in smaller studies. Among 4237 subjects aged 65 to 80 years who participated in a screening study among general practitioners in West Sussex, United Kingdom, 2290 women agreed to undergo abdominal ultrasonography.[138] Only 1.4% of the women had an AAA greater than or equal to 3 cm, while 0.3% had an AAA greater than or equal to 4 cm. This dramatically lower prevalence in women has been seen in two studies subsequently. In the Dutch Rotterdam study, 3143 women aged 55 years or older were screened.[131] The prevalence in these women was 0.7%. Correspondingly, in the Norwegian Tromso study, only 2% of 2943 women aged 55 to 84 years had an AAA greater than or equal to 3 cm and 0.5% had an abdominal aneurysm greater than or equal to 4 cm.[139] Even among female American veterans, the prevalence of an AAA greater than or equal to 3 cm was just 1%.[140]

Risk Factors

Three risk factors predict the vast majority of AAAs: age, gender, and cigarette smoking. Aneurysms usually affect the elderly, seldom occurring in subjects younger than 60 years old. In a Norwegian population-based study of 6386 men and women aged 25 to 84 years, the incidence of AAA in men increased from 0% in ages 25 to 44 to 6% in ages 55 to 64 and to 18.5% in subjects aged 75 to 84 years.[139] Large North American epidemiologic studies have demonstrated an increase in AAA risk ranging from 58% to 300% with each additional decade of life.[141,142] Indeed, all studies have demonstrated an age dependence, with the incidence increasing dramatically after age 60 and peaking in the oldest age group studied, even when limiting the study group to older subjects.[133,143-145]

In addition to age, gender is an important predictor of AAA formation. At all age groups, the risk of AAA in men is increased twofold to sixfold compared with women.[131,139,140,146-148] In the Chicago Heart Association Detection Project in Industry cohort, 10,574 men and 8700 women aged 40 to 64 years were screened.[146] Men had more than a doubling of risk, even in this relatively young cohort. Similar findings were noted in European patients.[147]

Cigarette smoking is the most potent modifiable risk factor. Smoking increases the risk of AAA by 60% to 850%.[149-155] In the ADAM and Edinburgh Artery Study, the risk of an aneurysm increased threefold with any smoking history.[136,156] The risk of an AAA lessens with smoking cessation, such that former smokers have a lower risk than current smokers.[142,157,158] Furthermore, the risk of AAA development increases with the number of cigarettes smoked, the duration of smoking, and the lack of filtration, indicating a dose-response relationship.[157] In the Whitehall study of 18,403 male civil servants examined at age 40 to 64 years, aneurysm frequency increased from sixfold with manufactured cigarettes with filters to 25-fold with hand-rolled cigarettes.[159]

In addition to the strong relationships of the risk factors mentioned earlier, risk factors for cardiovascular disease in general also increase the risk of AAA formation. The data on hypertension are inconsistent in small- and moderate-sized studies,[146,160] but aneurysm formation seems to correlate best with diastolic blood pressure[161] or use of an antihypertensive medication.[148] The association between cholesterol and AAA is stronger.[131,145,162] The risk of AAA formation increased 30% per 40 mg/dL total cholesterol in the Chicago Heart Association Detection Project in Industry cohort.[146] For specific components of the lipid profile, higher levels of low-density lipoprotein and lower levels of high-density lipoprotein cholesterol are both associated with aneurysm formation.[143,162] Similarly, the presence of atherosclerosis also increases the risk of aneurysm formation.[131,143,144] In the ADAM study of more than 100,000 subjects, hypertension, elevated cholesterol, and the presence of other vascular disease increased the risk of aneurysm formation by 15%, 44%, and 66%, respectively.[136] In contrast, diabetes and black race appear protective against formation of an aneurysm.[136,140,142,163] Diabetes decreases the risk of aneurysm formation by 30% to 50%.[136,161]

A dramatic increase in the frequency of AAA formation in the relatives of patients with aortic aneurysm demonstrates a genetic component to disease formation. Cigarette smoking accounts for the vast majority of AAAs in the population,[142] but the most potent risk factor for aneurysm formation is an aneurysm in a first-degree relative. This relationship has been demonstrated for more than 20 years. Norgaard and colleagues[164] identified an 18% incidence of aneurysms in first-degree relatives of patients with AAA. In the ADAM study, family history doubled the risk of AAA but was found in only 5.1% of the more than 100,000 participants.[165] Investigations specific to the impact of family history demonstrate a larger risk. Several studies have demonstrated that a family history of AAA increased the risk of AAA fourfold to fivefold compared with those without a family history.[161,166] Indeed, a family history of AAA caused AAA formation to occur earlier and rupture nearly a decade sooner.[167] The rate of rupture was nearly fourfold higher in patients with a family history than in sporadic AAA patients. Frydman and colleagues[168] recently screened the siblings of 400 AAA patients, finding an AAA in 43% of male siblings and 16% of female siblings. Indeed, coning down the family subgroups, the risk of AAA formation consistently rises above 20% for men above the age of 50 with a first-degree relative with AAA.[164,169-172] Using segregation analysis, Majumder and colleagues[173] reported that the relative risk of developing an AAA is 3.97 and 4.03 with paternal and maternal involvement, respectively. The risk increases to 9.92-fold with an affected male sibling and 22.93-fold when a female sibling is affected.[173] Thus an inherited component of AAA seems clear.

Despite the wealth of data demonstrating family-associated genes, no single candidate gene has been identified. Associations have been made with blood types, haptoglobin variations, α_1-antitrypsin, and human leukocyte antigen class II (HLA-II) immune response genes[54,174-177]; however, no one defect can be singled out. Confirming this, even the mode of inheritance remains unclear. There is evidence of both sex-linking and autosomal dominant patterns of inheritance.[178]

Prognosis

The natural history of AAA is one of silent coexistence and sudden, lethal rupture. In a large autopsy study performed over a quarter of a century, one fourth of the abdominal aneurysms were ruptured on postmortem examination.[127] The frequency of rupture was size dependent in this study population, ranging from 9.5% in aneurysms smaller than 4 cm to 45.6% in aneurysms 7.1 to 10 cm in diameter. Actuarial analysis has borne out this relationship.[179] In a comparison of patients with aortic aneurysms divided into two groups at a cut-off point of 6 cm, survival was markedly decreased in the patients with larger aneurysms.[180] Indeed, the patients with smaller aneurysms had a 5-year survival of 48%, while those with the larger aneurysms had a 1-year survival of 48%. In a single-center study that included 60 AAA ruptures over a 30-year period, only two occurred with an aneurysm diameter below 5 cm.[181] Similarly, in a study in Rochester, Minnesota, over the course of follow-up, no ruptures occurred in aneurysms smaller than 5 cm, while 25% of the AAAs larger than 5 cm ruptured.[182] In 198 patients with aneurysms 5.5 cm in diameter or larger but who were deemed too risky for surgery, 23% had probable rupture over a mean follow-up of 1.6 years.[183] Mortality rates as high as 64% are observed in patients who present with a ruptured aortic aneurysm.[184]

On the basis of these data, two large trials have been conducted to determine the optimal strategy to affect the natural history of AAA. The U.K. Small Aneurysm Trial randomized 1090 patients aged 60 to 76 years, with symptomless AAA 4 to 5.5 cm in diameter to undergo early elective open surgery or ultrasonographic surveillance.[185] In the surveillance group surgery was performed when the aneurysm reached 5.5 cm. Early surgery did not affect overall mortality. At 3 years, nearly 20% of both groups had died, although abdominal aneurysms accounted for only a quarter of the deaths in both groups. Cardiovascular mortality unrelated to the aneurysm accounted for 40% of total mortality, and cancer caused slightly more than 20% of the deaths. In a similar study performed by the Veterans Administration in the United States, 1136 subjects aged 50 to 79 years with asymptomatic AAA 4 to 5.5 cm in diameter were randomized to undergo early elective open surgery or ultrasonographic surveillance (Fig. 37-6).[186] After 5 years there was no significant difference in survival between the groups, each with a near-25% mortality rate. In this study, aneurysm-related deaths accounted for only 3% of total mortality.

Several factors may be taken into account to predict the likelihood of expansion and rupture of AAAs to identify which patients require surgery. The factor most predictive of rupture is initial size of the aneurysm.[179,181] In one recent study of patients too ill for surgery, aneurysm rupture rates ranged from 9.4% for AAA of 5.5 to 5.9 cm to 32.5% for AAA of 7 cm or more.[183] In the U.K. Small Aneurysm Study,

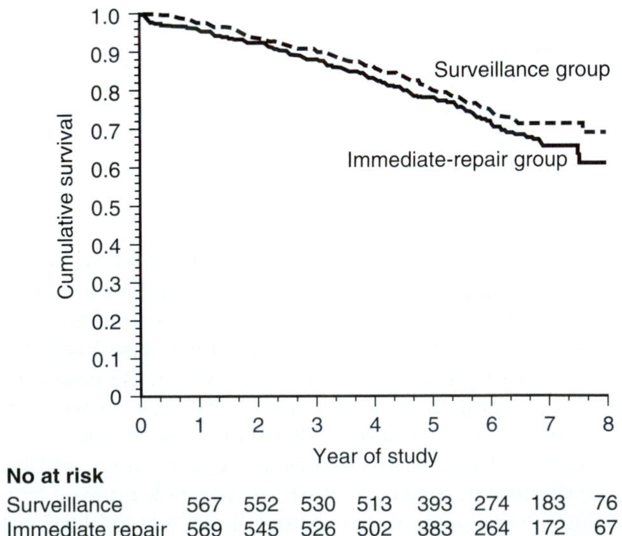

FIGURE 37-6. Survival curves in the early surgery group compared with the ultrasound surveillance group in the Aneurysm Detection and Management Veterans Affairs Cooperative Study. No significant difference in mortality was found between the two. (From Lederle FA, Wilson SE, Johnson GR, et al: Immediate repair compared with surveillance of small abdominal aortic aneurysms. N Engl J Med 346:1437, 2002.)

rate of rupture was 0.9% in aneurysms 3 to 3.9 cm, 2.7% in aneurysms 4 to 5.5 cm, and 27.8% in aneurysms 5.6 cm and larger.[187] Indeed, this may occur because larger aneurysm size also predicted a more rapid increase in diameter.[188] Similar to factors that predispose the development of AAA, cigarette smoking and higher blood pressure increase the risks of rapid expansion and rupture. In contrast to the decreased risk of AAA development in women, female gender increases the risk of rupture and the risk of death with rupture in those with established AAA.[187,190,191] In the U.K. Small Aneurysm Study, women had a threefold higher risk of AAA rupture than men.[187]

Thoracic Aortic Aneurysm

Prevalence

The prevalence of thoracic aortic aneurysms (TAA) is poorly defined. The relative infrequency of TAA in comparison to AAA is reflected in the extent of medical literature devoted to the topic. Autopsy records were reported from 63% of 70,368 deaths in the city of Malmo, Sweden between 1958 and 1985.[192] TAAs were diagnosed in 205 subjects, 53% of whom were men. More than half of the thoracic aneurysms involved the descending aorta, while only 17% involved the ascending aorta. Among the 44,332 autopsies performed, 63 patients, or 0.14%, died of a ruptured TAA. The relative infrequency of TAA is confirmed by a retrospective analysis in Rochester, Minnesota.[193] Over 30 years, of approximately 45,000 residents, 72, or 0.16%, were diagnosed with a TAA. Of these, 61% were women. Sixty-seven patients had thoracic aortic involvement only. Most studies, however, suggest that men are twice as likely to develop a TAA as women.[193-195] Involvement of the ascending aorta is most common and found in 51%, while the descending aorta is affected in 38%. A similar prevalence is found in Asian populations. In a chest CT screening program for lung cancer and tuberculosis in Chiba, Japan, using a mobile unit, 6971 subjects (3847 men) with a mean age of 60 years were studied.[196] Only 11 subjects, or 0.16%, had TAAs.

Similar to AAA, the development of TAA is an age-dependent phenomenon. Both the Swedish and Japanese studies noted previously and an earlier study[197] reported a relative absence of TAA in persons younger than 50 and a peak in incidence at age 70 years for men and more than 80 years for women. The median age for presentation varies from 64 to 69 years.[193,194,198]

The most common etiology underlying TAA development is a degenerative aneurysmal process found in 82% of patients, followed by aortic dissection in 17%, an inherited abnormality of collagen in 9%, infection in 2%, and aortitis in 1.2%.[199] Although important historically, even by the early 1980s, syphilis was becoming an oddity and found in only 4% of aneurysms.[193] Rarer causes of TAA include coarctation of the aorta and trauma.[200]

Prognosis

The natural history of TAA depends on the rate of expansion. The factor most related to expansion and rupture is the size of the aneurysm at diagnosis.[201,202] The survival rates for TAA range from 39% to 87% at 1 year and from 13% to 46% at 5 years.[193,198,201,203,204] In a study of 67 patients with TAA with a mean age of 65 years, subjects with an aortic diameter less than 5 cm had a 90% 3-year survival rate compared with 60% for patients with a TAA larger than 5 cm.[204] Similarly, in a Japanese population, patients with TAAs greater than or equal to 6 cm had a higher mortality rate than subjects with smaller aneurysms.[205] In 1964 the 5-year survival of TAA patients was 50%, compared with 71% in 1997.[197,206]

Coady and colleagues[206] evaluated the factors associated with expansion and rupture in 79 patients. They demonstrated that annual growth rates increased as the aortic diameter increased. At the sample mean of 5.2 cm, the rate of growth was 0.12 cm per year. The presence of a chronic aortic dissection was associated with a much greater rate of growth of 0.37 cm per year and worse survival.[207] Descending TAAs tend to increase in size more rapidly than ascending TAAs[208] and are similarly associated with a worse survival.[207] A study of 67 TAA patients confirmed the prognostic importance of baseline aortic diameter on aneurysm growth rates.[204] Moreover, this study found that in subjects who smoked, the rate of TAA expansion was twofold greater than in nonsmoking subjects. Based on the limited literature, referral for surgery typically occurs when the aneurysm reaches 5.5 to 6 cm in the ascending segment and 6.5 to 7 cm in the descending segment of the thoracic aorta.[208] Other factors reported to increase significantly the rate of rupture or need for surgery include older age, a history of chronic obstructive pulmonary disease, pain possibly related to the aneurysm, higher blood pressure, and extension of the aneurysm into the abdomen.[209,210]

Thoracoabdominal Aortic Aneurysms

Thoracoabdominal aortic aneurysms (TAAAs), defined by contiguous involvement of the descending thoracic aorta and the abdominal aorta, comprise less than 5% of all aortic aneurysms.[192-194] Of the 44,332 people to undergo necropsy in Malmo, Sweden, merely 10 had a TAAA.[192] Another autopsy study reported 7 TAAAs among 7642 studies.[211] In the Rochester, Minnesota, experience the incidence was 0.37 per 100,000 person-years of follow-up.[193]

Because of the relatively small sample sizes reported in the literature, risk factors for TAAA development are less well defined. Risk factors currently associated with the development of TAAA include smoking, hypertension, and atherosclerotic vascular disease.[194,212-215]

The natural history for these aneurysms is poor. The extension of a TAA into the abdomen is associated with a 50% relative increase in the risk of rupture compared with those limited to the thoracic aorta alone.[216] In a study of 94 patients with TAAAs who did not undergo operative repair accumulated over 25 years, 76% died within 2 years of follow-up, with half of the deaths resulting from aneurysm rupture.[217] A more recent experience with 57 TAAA patients managed without operation revealed a 69% 2-year survival.[201] Rupture was responsible for 19% of the deaths. Features associated with aneurysm expansion and rupture include smoking, chronic obstructive pulmonary disease, and renal insufficiency.[210]

Dissection as an underlying cause of aneurysm formation is also associated with a greater risk of rupture compared with degenerative causes.[218]

OTHER CONDITIONS ASSOCIATED WITH AORTIC ANEURYSMS

Although most aortic aneurysms occur as a result of the degenerative processes in the aortic wall as described earlier, certain disease states including vasculitis, infection, and inherited abnormalities of structural proteins predispose patients to aortic aneurysm formation (see Box 37-1).

Vasculitides

Giant Cell Arteritis (also see Chapter 43)

Giant cell (temporal) arteritis (GCA) is a medium vessel, chronic inflammatory vasculitis that affects the aorta and its branches. It most commonly occurs in patients older than the age of 55 years and is twice as common in women compared with men.[219] Of GCA patients, 1% to 20% develop aneurysms, most commonly in the thoracic aorta.[220-222] In a series of 41 patients with GCA-related TAAs, 16 developed an aortic dissection, 15 had valvular annular expansion causing symptomatic aortic valve insufficiency, and 18 required surgery.[220] In a series of 168 patients with GCA, 18% of the subjects developed aortic aneurysm or dissection, and these occurrences were inversely associated with the development of intracranial disease manifestations.[222] Aneurysmal disease was not associated with an increase in mortality.[223] The mechanism of aneurysm formation seems to be similar to patients without GCA with increases in matrix metalloproteinase 2- and 9-associated destruction of the vessel wall.[224,225]

Takayasu's Arteritis (also see Chapter 42)

Named for a Japanese professor of ophthalmology, Takayasu's arteritis (TA) is a large vessel vasculitis that typically has its onset between ages 10 and 30 years. The most common vascular presentation is occlusive disease, which is found in 80% to 94% of patients; however, aortic aneurysms may be found in up to one fourth of patients with TA.[226,227] The development of aneurysmal disease has been associated with worse outcome in a series of 120 Japanese patients followed for 13 years.[228] Blood levels of MMP-2 and -9 are elevated in TA; however, the mechanism of aneurysm formation remains unknown.[232]

Behçet's Disease (also see Chapter 41)

Originally a set of three symptoms characterized Behçet's disease: aphthous stomatitis, genital ulcers, and uveitis.[229] Small vessel vasculitis, augmented neutrophil function, and increased inflammation comprise the typical pathology in Behçet's disease. Larger vessels are affected by vasculitis of the vasa vasorum.[230] Vascular lesions, including aneurysms, can be found in 7% to 38% of patients and should be treated with corticosteroids.[229,231]

Seronegative Spondyloarthropathies (also see Chapter 41)

The diseases characterized as spondyloarthropathies are grouped by inflammation of the spine and sacroiliac joints, an association with HLA-B27, and the absence of rheumatoid factor and are associated with aortic aneurysm formation. The disorders include ankylosing spondylitis, Reiter's syndrome, and relapsing polychondritis. Ankylosing spondylitis is an HLA-B27 disease that requires the presence of four of the five following features: onset younger than 40 years old; back pain for more than 3 months; insidious onset of symptoms; morning stiffness; and improvement with exercise. Aortic root and valve disease is present in up to 80% of patients.[232] In a series of 44 outpatients, aortic root disease and valve disease were found in 82%; thickening of the aortic valve was noted in 41% of patients. The aortic valve thickening manifested as nodularities of the aortic cusps, forming a characteristic subaortic bump.[232] Valvar regurgitation was seen in almost half of the patients, and 40% had moderate lesions.

Reiter's syndrome is a reactive arthritis, which affects the lower limbs, causing an asymmetric oligoarthritis. To make the diagnosis, patients must have evidence of a preceding infection, diarrhea, or urethritis 4 weeks preceding the syndrome.[233] Less than 1% of Reiter's syndrome patients develop cardiovascular complications. Among this group, aortic insufficiency is a late finding.[234] Relapsing polychondritis[235] is a paroxysmal and progressive inflammatory disease of the cartilaginous structures, affecting the ear, nose, and hyaline cartilage of the tracheobronchial tree. Cardiovascular disease, including aortic aneurysms, is found in 25% to 50% of patients.

Infectious Aortic Aneurysms (also see Chapter 61)

Mycotic Aneurysms

Also known as infective endarteritis, mycotic aneurysms are rare phenomena. Two large necropsy studies including 22,000 and 20,000 patients, respectively, revealed a combined incidence of 0.03% in the United States.[236,237] More common in older patients, the average age of patients with mycotic aneurysms is 65 years old. Men are threefold more likely to develop mycotic aneurysms than women.[238,239] Hematogenous seeding, such as occurs in patients with endocarditis, affects a vessel "at risk" because of atherosclerosis or previous damage and represents the most common cause of mycotic aneurysms.[240] Indeed, as many as 15% of patients with endocarditis developed mycotic aneurysm before the antibiotic era.[241] Other etiologies include septic microemboli, contiguous extension, and trauma with direct contamination.[242] In contrast to the typical degenerative or vasculitic fusiform expansion, mycotic aneurysms are more likely to be saccular outpouchings (see Fig. 37-4).[243] The outpouching may range in size from 1 mm to 10 cm and include components of acute and chronic inflammation, hemorrhage, abscess formation, and necrosis.

Clinical manifestations resulting from mycotic aneurysm most commonly include pain and fever and, if related to a new aneurysm, should prompt directed investigation. The organisms that most commonly cause mycotic aneurysms include *Staphylococcus* and *Salmonella* species, which cause 40% and 20% of mycotic aneurysms, respectively.[244,245] Surgery should be prompt, for rupture occurs in up to 80%.[246,247] Prognosis for cerebral vascular infection is dire, with 1-year mortality for patients who have cerebral vascular mycotic aneurysms reaching as high as 90%.[247]

Tuberculous Aneurysms

Aortic aneurysms resulting from tuberculosis are quite rare. In a series of more than 22,000 autopsies performed at one urban medical center in the first half of the twentieth century, only 1 of 308 aortic aneurysms had tuberculous aneurysms,[236] whereas there were no tuberculous aneurysms of 20,000 autopsies performed in a rural setting.[237] Three mechanisms have been postulated to facilitate tuberculous adhesion and endarteritis. It is thought that direct extension from a contiguous source, such as the spine or lung, may cause 75% of tuberculous aneurysms.[248] Other possibilities include adhesion to a vessel damaged by atherosclerosis or by infiltration of the inner layers of the aorta via the vasa vasorum.[248] The abdominal and thoracic portions of the aorta are affected similarly. The presentation of the patient with a tuberculous aneurysm varies significantly. The patient may be asymptomatic, have a palpable or radiologically visible para-aortic mass, complain of chest or abdominal pain, or present with aortic rupture and hypovolemic shock.[248] Tuberculous aneurysms that are symptomatic or rapidly expanding and pseudoaneurysms typically require surgical repair.

Syphilitic Aneurysms

Antibiotics have greatly diminished the incidence of syphilitic aortic aneurysms, such that fewer than 50 cases have been reported in the antibiotic era.[249] Central nervous system and cardiovascular complications denote the tertiary stage of syphilis. Syphilitic aortitis may occur in up to 10% of patients with tertiary syphilis. Interruption of the elastic lamina occurs as a result of a lymphoplasmacytic infiltrate around the vasa vasorum. The histologic changes are not specific, and the diagnosis must be made serologically. Luetic aortic aneurysms commonly involve the ascending aorta and are saccular.[250] Involvement of the coronary ostia may result in anginal symptoms. The diagnosis may be suggested by linear calcification of the ascending aorta on chest radiography. When the diagnosis is made, survival is worse than the general population.[251]

Inherited Disorders of Connective Tissue

Marfan's Syndrome

In Marfan's syndrome, there is a defect in the synthesis of fibrillin because of a mutation in chromosome 15. Abnormalities in fibrillin synthesis may affect multiple tissues in patients with Marfan's syndrome: the eye (ectopia lentis), the skeleton (dolichostenomelia), ligamentous redundancy, the mitral valve (regurgitation), and the ascending aorta (aneurysm). As patients with Marfan's syndrome have been living longer, abnormalities in skin, fascia, skeletal muscle, and adipose tissue have been reported as well.

Medial changes in the elastic arteries include fragmentation and disarray of elastic fibers, a paucity of smooth muscle cells, and the separation of muscle fibers by collagen and glycosaminoglycans.[252] The pooling of glycosaminoglycans resembles cysts; this entity was previously described as cystic medial necrosis, although no walled vesicles occur. The changes are not pathognomonic for Marfan's syndrome and can be demonstrated as a result of aging or hypertension. Dilation of the aortic root has been demonstrated early in childhood in patients with Marfan's syndrome.[253]

Ehlers-Danlos Syndrome

Ehlers-Danlos syndrome is a rare congenital defect in the synthesis of type 3 collagen.[254] Patients with Ehlers-Danlos syndrome typically present with acrogeria (distinctive facial appearance), bruising, thin skin, and vascular or visceral rupture. Histologic examination reveals a thinned, fragmented internal elastic lamina.[255] Moreover, deposition of glycosaminoglycans in the media of major arteries and in the intima of smaller arteries with intimal thickening has been noted.[256] Abnormalities in type 3 collagen fiber formation reduce the stability or prevent the formation of collagen, decreasing vascular wall stability.[255] In a study of 199 patients with confirmed Ehlers-Danlos syndrome, 25% of patients suffered a ruptured vessel or viscus by age 20 and 80% by age 40.[257] The mean survival was 48 years. There were 131 deaths, 103 of which were due to vascular rupture. Complications of pregnancy caused the death of 15% of the women who became pregnant.

Bicuspid Aortic Valve

The presence of a bicuspid aortic valve (BAV) increases the risk of ascending aortic aneurysm formation. The ascending aorta tends to be larger in patients with a bicuspid valve than those without one.[258] The aortic expansion occurs independent of valvular dysfunction, severity, age, and body morphology.[259,260] In one study of 118 consecutive patients with bicuspid aortic valve, the diameter of the ascending aorta was not correlated with the severity of aortic stenosis.[261] Indeed, the valve itself is only a marker for the aortic abnormality. Replacement of the valve does not change the rate of aortic expansion.[262]

Patients with bicuspid aortic valves (BAVs) may be predisposed to aneurysm formation. Aorta and pulmonary artery specimens were compared between patients with BAV and tricuspid aortic valve (TAV) disease. The BAV patients had decreased fibrillin-1 concentrations in both the aortic and pulmonary specimens, suggesting a systemic disorder.[263] Indeed, the vascular smooth muscle cells from patients with BAV showed intracellular accumulation and reduction of extracellular distribution of several structural elements including fibrillin, fibronectin, and tenascin.[13] Moreover, aggravating impaired production of structural proteins, vascular smooth muscle cells demonstrate increased rates of apoptosis.[264] Indeed, the process of aneurysm formation may be similar to that of idiopathic aneurysm formation. Surgical specimens demonstrate greater amounts of inflammation and increased expression of MMP-2 and MMP-9 in patients with BAV compared with TAV.[265,266]

Patients with Turner's syndrome also exhibit an increased rate of aneurysm formation. These patients commonly have bicuspid aortic valves and are more likely than healthy matched subjects to have increased aortic root diameters.[11,267-269]

Aortic Coarctation

Coarctation of the aorta represents 5% of congenital heart disease. Its severity ranges from life threatening in infancy to unappreciated until adulthood.[270] It has been associated with aortic aneurysm through two mechanisms. First, a bicuspid aortic valve is found in approximately 15% of patients with aortic coarctation.[271,272] Second, aortic aneurysm formation is not an uncommon complication at the coarctation repair site. Surgical repair has been associated with rates of aneurysm formation up to 20%, with patch-angioplasty repair specifically predisposing to this outcome.[273,274] Intermediate follow-up studies suggest that percutaneous balloon angioplasty repair results in a 2% to 5% rate of repair-site aortic aneurysm formation.[275,276]

Trauma

Aneurysms related to trauma are discussed in Chapter 63.

REFERENCES

1. American Heart Association: Heart Disease and Stroke Statistics—2005. Dallas, AHA, 2005.
2. Wolinsky H, Glagov S: A lamellar unit of aortic medial structure and function in mammals. Circ Res 20:99, 1967.
3. Movat HZ, More RH, Haust MD: The diffuse intimal thickening of the human aorta with aging. Am J Pathol 34:1023, 1958.
4. Kawasaki T, Sasayama S, Yagi S, et al: Non-invasive assessment of the age related changes in stiffness of major branches of the human arteries. Cardiovasc Res 21:678, 1987.
5. Breithaupt-Grogler K, Belz GG: Epidemiology of the arterial stiffness. Pathol Biol (Paris) 47:604, 1999.
6. Lakatta EG: Arterial and cardiac aging: Major shareholders in cardiovascular disease enterprises: Part III: Cellular and molecular clues to heart and arterial aging. Circulation 107:490, 2003.
7. Groenink M, Langerak SE, Vanbavel E, et al: The influence of aging and aortic stiffness on permanent dilation and breaking stress of the thoracic descending aorta. Cardiovasc Res 43:471, 1999.
8. Wassef M, Baxter BT, Chisholm RL, et al: Pathogenesis of abdominal aortic aneurysms: A multidisciplinary research program supported by the National Heart, Lung, and Blood Institute. J Vasc Surg 34:730, 2001.
9. Creager MA, Halperin JL, Whittemore AD: Aneurysmal Disease of the Aorta and Its Branches. In Dzau VJ (ed): Vascular Medicine: A Textbook of Vascular Biology and Diseases. Boston, Little, Brown & Company, 1996, p 901.
10. Lopez-Candales A, Holmes DR, Liao S, et al: Decreased vascular smooth muscle cell density in medial degeneration of human abdominal aortic aneurysms. Am J Pathol 150:993, 1997.
11. Lin AE, Lippe BM, Geffner ME, et al: Aortic dilation, dissection, and rupture in patients with Turner syndrome. J Pediatr 109:820, 1986.
12. de Sa M, Moshkovitz Y, Butany J, et al: Histologic abnormalities of the ascending aorta and pulmonary trunk in patients with bicuspid aortic valve disease: Clinical relevance to the ross procedure. J Thorac Cardiovasc Surg 118:588, 1999.
13. Nataatmadja M, West M, West J, et al: Abnormal extracellular matrix protein transport associated with increased apoptosis of vascular smooth muscle cells in Marfan syndrome and bicuspid aortic valve thoracic aortic aneurysm. Circulation 108(suppl 1):II329, 2003.
14. Tamarina NA, Grassi MA, Johnson DA, et al: Proteoglycan gene expression is decreased in abdominal aortic aneurysms. J Surg Res 74:76, 1998.
15. Zhang J, Schmidt J, Ryschich E, et al: Increased apoptosis and decreased density of medial smooth muscle cells in human abdominal aortic aneurysms. Chin Med J (Engl) 116:1549, 2003.
16. Henderson EL, Geng YJ, Sukhova GK, et al: Death of smooth muscle cells and expression of mediators of apoptosis by T lymphocytes in human abdominal aortic aneurysms. Circulation 99:96, 1999.
17. Rucker RB, Tinker D: Structure and metabolism of arterial elastin. Int Rev Exp Pathol 17:1, 1977.
18. Halpern VJ, Nackman GB, Gandhi RH, et al: The elastase infusion model of experimental aortic aneurysms: Synchrony of induction of endogenous proteinases with matrix destruction and inflammatory cell response. J Vasc Surg 20:51, 1994.
19. Campa JS, Greenhalgh RM, Powell JT: Elastin degradation in abdominal aortic aneurysms. Atherosclerosis 65:13, 1987.
20. Baxter BT, Davis VA, Minion DJ, et al: Abdominal aortic aneurysms are associated with altered matrix proteins of the nonaneurysmal aortic segments. J Vasc Surg 19:797, 1994.
21. Dobrin PB, Mrkvicka R: Failure of elastin or collagen as possible critical connective tissue alterations underlying aneurysmal dilatation. Cardiovasc Surg 2:484, 1994.
22. Rose AG, Dent DM: Inflammatory variant of abdominal atherosclerotic aneurysm. Arch Pathol Lab Med 105:409, 1981.
23. Koch AE, Haines GK, Rizzo RJ, et al: Human abdominal aortic aneurysms: Immunophenotypic analysis suggesting an immune-mediated response. Am J Pathol 137:1199, 1990.
24. Satta J, Laurila A, Paakko P, et al: Chronic inflammation and elastin degradation in abdominal aortic aneurysm disease: An immunohistochemical and electron microscopic study. Eur J Vasc Endovasc Surg 15:313, 1998.
25. Ocana E, Bohorquez JC, Perez-Requena J, et al: Characterisation of T and B lymphocytes infiltrating abdominal aortic aneurysms. Atherosclerosis 170:39, 2003.
26. Szekanecz Z, Shah MR, Pearce WH, et al: Intercellular adhesion molecule-1 (ICAM-1) expression and soluble ICAM-1 (sICAM-1) production by cytokine-activated human aortic endothelial cells: A possible role for ICAM-1 and sICAM-1 in atherosclerotic aortic aneurysms. Clin Exp Immunol 98:337, 1994.
27. Davis CA III, Pearce WH, Haines GK, et al: Increased ICAM-1 expression in aortic disease. J Vasc Surg 18:875, 1993.
28. Newman KM, Jean-Claude J, Li H, et al: Cytokines that activate proteolysis are increased in abdominal aortic aneurysms. Circulation 90:II224, 1994.
29. Koch AE, Kunkel SL, Pearce WH, et al: Enhanced production of the chemotactic cytokines interleukin-8 and monocyte chemoattractant protein-1 in human abdominal aortic aneurysms. Am J Pathol 142:1423, 1993.
30. Szekanecz Z, Shah MR, Pearce WH, et al: Human atherosclerotic abdominal aortic aneurysms produce interleukin (IL)-6 and interferon-gamma but not IL-2 and IL-4: The possible role for IL-6 and interferon-gamma in vascular inflammation. Agents Actions 42:159, 1994.
31. Treska V, Kocova J, Boudova L, et al: Inflammation in the wall of abdominal aortic aneurysm and its role in the symptomatology of aneurysm. Cytokines Cell Mol Ther 7:91, 2002.
32. Vainas T, Lubbers T, Stassen FR, et al: Serum C-reactive protein level is associated with abdominal aortic aneurysm size and may be produced by aneurysmal tissue. Circulation 107:1103, 2003.
33. Meijer A, van Der Vliet JA, Roholl PJ, et al: *Chlamydia pneumoniae* in abdominal aortic aneurysms: Abundance of membrane components in the absence of heat shock protein 60 and DNA. Arterioscler Thromb Vasc Biol 19:2680, 1999.
34. Yonemitsu Y, Nakagawa K, Tanaka S, et al: In situ detection of frequent and active infection of human cytomegalovirus in inflammatory abdominal aortic aneurysms: Possible pathogenic role in sustained chronic inflammatory reaction. Lab Invest 74:723, 1996.

35. Juvonen J, Juvonen T, Laurila A, et al: Demonstration of *Chlamydia pneumoniae* in the walls of abdominal aortic aneurysms. J Vasc Surg 25:499, 1997.
36. Lindholt JS, Ostergard L, Henneberg EW, et al: Failure to demonstrate *Chlamydia pneumoniae* in symptomatic abdominal aortic aneurysms by a nested polymerase chain reaction (PCR). Eur J Vasc Endovasc Surg 15:161, 1998.
37. Petersen E, Boman J, Persson K, et al: *Chlamydia pneumoniae* in human abdominal aortic aneurysms. Eur J Vasc Endovasc Surg 15:138, 1998.
38. Halme S, Juvonen T, Laurila A, et al: *Chlamydia pneumoniae* reactive T lymphocytes in the walls of abdominal aortic aneurysms. Eur J Clin Invest 29:546, 1999.
39. Blanchard JF, Armenian HK, Peeling R, et al: The relation between *Chlamydia pneumoniae* infection and abdominal aortic aneurysm: Case-control study. Clin Infect Dis 30:946, 2000.
40. Karlsson L, Gnarpe J, Naas J, et al: Detection of viable *Chlamydia pneumoniae* in abdominal aortic aneurysms. Eur J Vasc Endovasc Surg 19:630, 2000.
41. Lindholt JS, Ashton HA, Scott RA: Indicators of infection with *Chlamydia pneumoniae* are associated with expansion of abdominal aortic aneurysms. J Vasc Surg 34:212, 2001.
42. Maraha B, den Heijer M, Wullink M, et al: Detection of *Chlamydia pneumoniae* DNA in buffy-coat samples of patients with abdominal aortic aneurysm. Eur J Clin Microbiol Infect Dis 20:111, 2001.
43. Petersen E, Boman J, Wagberg F, et al: Presence of *Chlamydia pneumoniae* in abdominal aortic aneurysms is not associated with increased activity of matrix metalloproteinases. Eur J Vasc Endovasc Surg 24:365, 2002.
44. Porqueddu M, Spirito R, Parolari A, et al: Lack of association between serum immunoreactivity and *Chlamydia pneumoniae* detection in the human aortic wall. Circulation 106:2647, 2002.
45. Gregory AK, Yin NX, Capella J, et al: Features of autoimmunity in the abdominal aortic aneurysm. Arch Surg 131:85, 1996.
46. Tilson MD, Ozsvath KJ, Hirose H, et al: A genetic basis for autoimmune manifestations in the abdominal aortic aneurysm resides in the MHC class II locus DR-beta-1. Ann N Y Acad Sci 800:208, 1996.
47. Xia S, Ozsvath K, Hirose H, et al: Partial amino acid sequence of a novel 40-kDa human aortic protein, with vitronectin-like, fibrinogen-like, and calcium binding domains: Aortic aneurysm-associated protein-40 (AAAP-40) [human MAGP-3, proposed]. Biochem Biophys Res Commun 219:36, 1996.
48. Ozsvath KJ, Hirose H, Xia S, et al: Expression of two novel recombinant proteins from aortic adventitia (kappafibs) sharing amino acid sequences with cytomegalovirus. J Surg Res 69:277, 1997.
49. Chew DK, Knoetgen J III, Xia S, et al: Regional distribution in human of a novel aortic collagen-associated microfibrillar protein. Exp Mol Pathol 66:59, 1999.
50. Chew DK, Knoetgen J, Xia S, et al: The role of a putative microfibrillar protein (80 kDa) in abdominal aortic aneurysm disease. J Surg Res 114:25, 2003.
51. Cohen JR, Sarfati I, Danna D, et al: Smooth muscle cell elastase, atherosclerosis, and abdominal aortic aneurysms. Ann Surg 216:327, 1992.
52. Capella JF, Paik DC, Yin NX, et al: Complement activation and subclassification of tissue immunoglobulin G in the abdominal aortic aneurysm. J Surg Res 65:31, 1996.
53. Pasquinelli G, Preda P, Gargiulo M, et al: An immunohistochemical study of inflammatory abdominal aortic aneurysms. J Submicrosc Cytol Pathol 25:103, 1993.
54. Monux G, Serrano FJ, Vigil P, et al: Role of HLA-DR in the pathogenesis of abdominal aortic aneurysm. Eur J Vasc Endovasc Surg 26:211, 2003.
55. Visse R, Nagase H: Matrix metalloproteinases and tissue inhibitors of metalloproteinases: structure, function, and biochemistry. Circ Res 92:827, 2003.
56. Louwrens HD, Kwaan HC, Pearce WH, et al: Plasminogen activator and plasminogen activator inhibitor expression by normal and aneurysmal human aortic smooth muscle cells in culture. Eur J Vasc Endovasc Surg 10:289, 1995.
57. Allaire E, Hasenstab D, Kenagy RD, et al: Prevention of aneurysm development and rupture by local overexpression of plasminogen activator inhibitor-1. Circulation 98:249, 1998.
58. Reilly JM, Sicard GA, Lucore CL: Abnormal expression of plasminogen activators in aortic aneurysmal and occlusive disease. J Vasc Surg 19:865, 1994.
59. Vine N, Powell JT: Metalloproteinases in degenerative aortic disease. Clin Sci (Colch) 81:233, 1991.
60. Brophy CM, Marks WH, Reilly JM, et al: Decreased tissue inhibitor of metalloproteinases (TIMP) in abdominal aortic aneurysm tissue: A preliminary report. J Surg Res 50:653, 1991.
61. Herron GS, Unemori E, Wong M, et al: Connective tissue proteinases and inhibitors in abdominal aortic aneurysms. Involvement of the vasa vasorum in the pathogenesis of aortic aneurysms. Arterioscler Thromb 11:1667, 1991.
62. Newman KM, Malon AM, Shin RD, et al: Matrix metalloproteinases in abdominal aortic aneurysm: Characterization, purification, and their possible sources. Connect Tissue Res 30:265, 1994.
63. Newman KM, Ogata Y, Malon AM, et al: Identification of matrix metalloproteinases 3 (stromelysin-1) and 9 (gelatinase B) in abdominal aortic aneurysm. Arterioscler Thromb 14:1315, 1994.
64. Newman KM, Jean-Claude J, Li H, et al: Cellular localization of matrix metalloproteinases in the abdominal aortic aneurysm wall. J Vasc Surg 20:814, 1994.
65. Patel MI, Melrose J, Ghosh P, et al: Increased synthesis of matrix metalloproteinases by aortic smooth muscle cells is implicated in the etiopathogenesis of abdominal aortic aneurysms. J Vasc Surg 24:82, 1996.
66. Thompson RW, Holmes DR, Mertens RA, et al: Production and localization of 92-kilodalton gelatinase in abdominal aortic aneurysms: An elastolytic metalloproteinase expressed by aneurysm-infiltrating macrophages. J Clin Invest 96:318, 1995.
67. Davis V, Persidskaia R, Baca-Regen L, et al: Matrix metalloproteinase-2 production and its binding to the matrix are increased in abdominal aortic aneurysms. Arterioscler Thromb Vasc Biol 18:1625, 1998.
68. Goodall S, Crowther M, Hemingway DM, et al: Ubiquitous elevation of matrix metalloproteinase-2 expression in the vasculature of patients with abdominal aneurysms. Circulation 104:304, 2001.
69. Longo GM, Xiong W, Greiner TC, et al: Matrix metalloproteinases 2 and 9 work in concert to produce aortic aneurysms. J Clin Invest 110:625, 2002.
70. Freestone T, Turner RJ, Coady A, et al: Inflammation and matrix metalloproteinases in the enlarging abdominal aortic aneurysm. Arterioscler Thromb Vasc Biol 15:1145, 1995.
71. Petersen E, Gineitis A, Wagberg F, et al: Activity of matrix metalloproteinase-2 and -9 in abdominal aortic aneurysms: Relation to size and rupture. Eur J Vasc Endovasc Surg 20:457, 2000.
72. Papalambros E, Sigala F, Georgopoulos S, et al: Immunohistochemical expression of metalloproteinases MMP-2 and MMP-9 in abdominal aortic aneurysms: Correlation with symptoms and aortic diameter. Int J Mol Med 12:965, 2003.
73. Nishimura K, Ikebuchi M, Kanaoka Y, et al: Relationships between matrix metalloproteinases and tissue inhibitor of metalloproteinases in the wall of abdominal aortic aneurysms. Int Angiol 22:229, 2003.
74. Petersen E, Wagberg F, Angquist KA: Serum concentrations of elastin-derived peptides in patients with specific manifestations of atherosclerotic disease. Eur J Vasc Endovasc Surg 24:440, 2002.
75. Petersen E, Wagberg F, Angquist KA: Proteolysis of the abdominal aortic aneurysm wall and the association with rupture. Eur J Vasc Endovasc Surg 23:153, 2002.
76. Tamarina NA, McMillan WD, Shively VP, et al: Expression of matrix metalloproteinases and their inhibitors in aneurysms and normal aorta. Surgery 122:264, 1997.
77. Pyo R, Lee JK, Shipley JM, et al: Targeted gene disruption of matrix metalloproteinase-9 (gelatinase B) suppresses development of experimental abdominal aortic aneurysms. J Clin Invest 105:1641, 2000.
78. Annabi B, Shedid D, Ghosn P, et al: Differential regulation of matrix metalloproteinase activities in abdominal aortic aneurysms. J Vasc Surg 35:539, 2002.
79. Crowther M, Goodall S, Jones JL, et al: Localization of matrix metalloproteinase 2 within the aneurysmal and normal aortic wall. Br J Surg 87:1391, 2000.
80. Mazzieri R, Masiero L, Zanetta L, et al: Control of type IV collagenase activity by components of the urokinase-plasmin system: A regulatory mechanism with cell-bound reactants. EMBO J 16:2319, 1997.
81. Henrotin YE, Bruckner P, Pujol JP: The role of reactive oxygen species in homeostasis and degradation of cartilage. Osteoarthritis Cartilage 11:747, 2003.

82. Siwik DA, Colucci WS: Regulation of matrix metalloproteinases by cytokines and reactive oxygen/nitrogen species in the myocardium. Heart Fail Rev 9:43, 2004.
83. Miller FJ Jr, Sharp WJ, Fang X, et al: Oxidative stress in human abdominal aortic aneurysms: A potential mediator of aneurysmal remodeling. Arterioscler Thromb Vasc Biol 22:560, 2002.
84. Defawe OD, Colige A, Lambert CA, et al: TIMP-2 and PAI-1 mRNA levels are lower in aneurysmal as compared to athero-occlusive abdominal aortas. Cardiovasc Res 60:205, 2003.
85. Elmore JR, Keister BF, Franklin DP, et al: Expression of matrix metalloproteinases and TIMPs in human abdominal aortic aneurysms. Ann Vasc Surg 12:221, 1998.
86. Saito S, Zempo N, Yamashita A, et al: Matrix metalloproteinase expressions in arteriosclerotic aneurysmal disease. Vasc Endovascular Surg 36:1, 2002.
87. Ailawadi G, Knipp BS, Lu G, et al: A nonintrinsic regional basis for increased infrarenal aortic MMP-9 expression and activity. J Vasc Surg 37:1059, 2003.
88. Allaire E, Forough R, Clowes M, et al: Local overexpression of TIMP-1 prevents aortic aneurysm degeneration and rupture in a rat model. J Clin Invest 102:1413, 1998.
89. Silence J, Collen D, Lijnen HR: Reduced atherosclerotic plaque but enhanced aneurysm formation in mice with inactivation of the tissue inhibitor of metalloproteinase-1 (TIMP-1) gene. Circ Res 90:897, 2002.
90. Falkenberg M, Holmdahl L, Tjarnstrom J, et al: Abnormal levels of urokinase plasminogen activator protein and tissue plasminogen activator activity in human aortic aneurysms. Eur J Surg 167:10, 2001.
91. Golub LM, Ramamurthy N, McNamara TF, et al: Tetracyclines inhibit tissue collagenase activity: A new mechanism in the treatment of periodontal disease. J Periodontal Res 19:651, 1984.
92. Thompson RW, Liao S, Curci JA: Therapeutic potential of tetracycline derivatives to suppress the growth of abdominal aortic aneurysms. Adv Dent Res 12:159, 1998.
93. Boyle JR, McDermott E, Crowther M, et al: Doxycycline inhibits elastin degradation and reduces metalloproteinase activity in a model of aneurysmal disease. J Vasc Surg 27:354, 1998.
94. Manning MW, Cassis LA, Daugherty A: Differential effects of doxycycline, a broad-spectrum matrix metalloproteinase inhibitor, on angiotensin II-induced atherosclerosis and abdominal aortic aneurysms. Arterioscler Thromb Vasc Biol 23:483, 2003.
95. Prall AK, Longo GM, Mayhan WG, et al: Doxycycline in patients with abdominal aortic aneurysms and in mice: Comparison of serum levels and effect on aneurysm growth in mice. J Vasc Surg 35:923, 2002.
96. Curci JA, Mao D, Bohner DG, et al: Preoperative treatment with doxycycline reduces aortic wall expression and activation of matrix metalloproteinases in patients with abdominal aortic aneurysms. J Vasc Surg 31:325, 2000.
97. Baxter BT, Pearce WH, Waltke EA, et al: Prolonged administration of doxycycline in patients with small asymptomatic abdominal aortic aneurysms: Report of a prospective (phase II) multicenter study. J Vasc Surg 36:1, 2002.
98. Mosorin M, Juvonen J, Biancari F, et al: Use of doxycycline to decrease the growth rate of abdominal aortic aneurysms: A randomized, double-blind, placebo-controlled pilot study. J Vasc Surg 34:606, 2001.
99. Holmes DR, Petrinec D, Wester W, et al: Indomethacin prevents elastase-induced abdominal aortic aneurysms in the rat. J Surg Res 63:305, 1996.
100. Franklin IJ, Walton LJ, Greenhalgh RM, et al: The influence of indomethacin on the metabolism and cytokine secretion of human aneurysmal aorta. Eur J Vasc Endovasc Surg 18:35, 1999.
101. Miralles M, Wester W, Sicard GA, et al: Indomethacin inhibits expansion of experimental aortic aneurysms via inhibition of the cox2 isoform of cyclooxygenase. J Vasc Surg 29:884, 1999.
102. Walton LJ, Franklin IJ, Bayston T, et al: Inhibition of prostaglandin E2 synthesis in abdominal aortic aneurysms: Implications for smooth muscle cell viability, inflammatory processes, and the expansion of abdominal aortic aneurysms. Circulation 100:48, 1999.
103. Holmes DR, Wester W, Thompson RW, et al: Prostaglandin E2 synthesis and cyclooxygenase expression in abdominal aortic aneurysms. J Vasc Surg 25:810, 1997.
104. Bayston T, Ramessur S, Reise J, et al: Prostaglandin E2 receptors in abdominal aortic aneurysm and human aortic smooth muscle cells. J Vasc Surg 38:354, 2003.
105. Reilly JM, Miralles M, Wester WN, et al: Differential expression of prostaglandin E2 and interleukin-6 in occlusive and aneurysmal aortic disease. Surgery 126:624, 1999.
106. Nagashima H, Aoka Y, Sakomura Y, et al: A 3-hydroxy-3-methylglutaryl coenzyme A reductase inhibitor, cerivastatin, suppresses production of matrix metalloproteinase-9 in human abdominal aortic aneurysm wall. J Vasc Surg 36:158, 2002.
107. Ejiri J, Inoue N, Tsukube T, et al: Oxidative stress in the pathogenesis of thoracic aortic aneurysm: Protective role of statin and angiotensin II type 1 receptor blocker. Cardiovasc Res 59:988, 2003.
108. Wolinsky H, Glagov S: Comparison of abdominal and thoracic aortic medial structure in mammals: Deviation of man from the usual pattern. Circ Res 25:677, 1969.
109. Benjamin HB, Becker AB: Etiologic incidence of thoracic and abdominal aneurysms. Surg Gynecol Obstet 125:1307, 1967.
110. Heistad DD, Marcus ML, Larsen GE, et al: Role of vasa vasorum in nourishment of the aortic wall. Am J Physiol 240:H781, 1981.
111. Stefanadis C, Vlachopoulos C, Karayannacos P, et al: Effect of vasa vasorum flow on structure and function of the aorta in experimental animals. Circulation 91:2669, 1995.
112. Moore JE Jr, Ku DN, Zarins CK, et al: Pulsatile flow visualization in the abdominal aorta under differing physiologic conditions: Implications for increased susceptibility to atherosclerosis. J Biomech Eng 114:391, 1992.
113. Egelhoff CJ, Budwig RS, Elger DF, et al: Model studies of the flow in abdominal aortic aneurysms during resting and exercise conditions. J Biomech 32:1319, 1999.
114. Peattie RA, Asbury CL, Bluth EI, et al: Steady flow in models of abdominal aortic aneurysms. Part II: Wall stresses and their implication for in vivo thrombosis and rupture. J Ultrasound Med 15:689, 1996.
115. Peattie RA, Schrader T, Bluth EI, et al: Development of turbulence in steady flow through models of abdominal aortic aneurysms. J Ultrasound Med 13:467, 1994.
116. Schrader T, Peattie RA, Bluth EI, et al: A qualitative investigation of turbulence in flow through a model abdominal aortic aneurysm. Invest Radiol 27:515, 1992.
117. Sangiorgi G, D'Averio R, Mauriello A, et al: Plasma levels of metalloproteinases-3 and -9 as markers of successful abdominal aortic aneurysm exclusion after endovascular graft treatment. Circulation 104:I288, 2001.
118. Lorelli DR, Jean-Claude JM, Fox CJ, et al: Response of plasma matrix metalloproteinase-9 to conventional abdominal aortic aneurysm repair or endovascular exclusion: Implications for endoleak. J Vasc Surg 35:916, 2002.
119. Nakahashi TK, Hoshina K, Tsao PS, et al: Flow loading induces macrophage antioxidative gene expression in experimental aneurysms. Arterioscler Thromb Vasc Biol 22:2017, 2002.
120. Hoshina K, Sho E, Sho M, et al: Wall shear stress and strain modulate experimental aneurysm cellularity. J Vasc Surg 37:1067, 2003.
121. Sho E, Sho M, Hoshina K, et al: Hemodynamic forces regulate mural macrophage infiltration in experimental aortic aneurysms. Exp Mol Pathol 76:108, 2004.
122. Wang DH, Makaroun MS, Webster MW, et al: Effect of intraluminal thrombus on wall stress in patient-specific models of abdominal aortic aneurysm. J Vasc Surg 36:598, 2002.
123. Di Martino ES, Vorp DA: Effect of variation in intraluminal thrombus constitutive properties on abdominal aortic aneurysm wall stress. Ann Biomed Eng 31:804, 2003.
124. Thubrikar MJ, Robicsek F, Labrosse M, et al: Effect of thrombus on abdominal aortic aneurysm wall dilation and stress. J Cardiovasc Surg (Torino) 44:67, 2003.
125. Fontaine V, Jacob MP, Houard X, et al: Involvement of the mural thrombus as a site of protease release and activation in human aortic aneurysms. Am J Pathol 161:1701, 2002.
126. Krettek A, Sukhova GK, Libby P: Elastogenesis in human arterial disease: A role for macrophages in disordered elastin synthesis. Arterioscler Thromb Vasc Biol 23:582, 2003.
127. Darling RC, Messina CR, Brewster DC, et al: Autopsy study of unoperated abdominal aortic aneurysms. The case for early resection. Circulation 56:II161, 1977.

128. Lilienfeld D, Baxter J, Sprafka J: Prevalence of AA in the Twin Cities Metropolitan Area, 1979-84. Public Health Reports 108:506, 1993.
129. Boll AP, Verbeek AL, van de Lisdonk EH, et al: High prevalence of abdominal aortic aneurysm in a primary care screening programme. Br J Surg 85:1090, 1998.
130. Kullmann G, Wolland T, Krohn CD, et al: [Ultrasonography for early diagnosis of abdominal aortic aneurysm]. Tidsskr Nor Laegeforen 112:1825, 1992.
131. Pleumeekers HJ, Hoes AW, van der Does E, et al: Aneurysms of the abdominal aorta in older adults. The Rotterdam Study. Am J Epidemiol 142:1291, 1995.
132. Lucarotti M, Shaw E, Poskitt K, et al: The Gloucestershire Aneurysm Screening Programme: the first 2 years' experience. Eur J Vasc Surg 7:397, 1993.
133. Morris GE, Hubbard CS, Quick CR: An abdominal aortic aneurysm screening programme for all males over the age of 50 years. Eur J Vasc Surg 8:156, 1994.
134. Scott RA, Wilson NM, Ashton HA, et al: Influence of screening on the incidence of ruptured abdominal aortic aneurysm: 5-year results of a randomized controlled study. Br J Surg 82:1066, 1995.
135. Smith FC, Grimshaw GM, Paterson IS, et al: Ultrasonographic screening for abdominal aortic aneurysm in an urban community. Br J Surg 80:1406, 1993.
136. Lederle FA, Johnson GR, Wilson SE, et al: The aneurysm detection and management study screening program: Validation cohort and final results. Aneurysm Detection and Management Veterans Affairs Cooperative Study Investigators. Arch Intern Med 160:1425, 2000.
137. Ashton HA, Buxton MJ, Day NE, et al: The Multicentre Aneurysm Screening Study (MASS) into the effect of abdominal aortic aneurysm screening on mortality in men: A randomised controlled trial. Lancet 360:1531, 2002.
138. Scott RA, Ashton HA, Kay DN: Abdominal aortic aneurysm in 4237 screened patients: prevalence, development and management over 6 years. Br J Surg 78:1122, 1991.
139. Singh K, Bonaa KH, Jacobsen BK, et al: Prevalence of and risk factors for abdominal aortic aneurysms in a population-based study: The Tromso Study. Am J Epidemiol 154:236, 2001.
140. Lederle FA, Johnson GR, Wilson SE: Abdominal aortic aneurysm in women. J Vasc Surg 34:122, 2001.
141. Blanchard JF: Epidemiology of abdominal aortic aneurysms. Epidemiol Rev 21:207, 1999.
142. Lederle FA, Johnson GR, Wilson SE, et al: Prevalence and associations of abdominal aortic aneurysm detected through screening. Aneurysm Detection and Management (ADAM) Veterans Affairs Cooperative Study Group. Ann Intern Med 126:441, 1997.
143. Alcorn HG, Wolfson SK Jr, Sutton-Tyrrell K, et al: Risk factors for abdominal aortic aneurysms in older adults enrolled in The Cardiovascular Health Study. Arterioscler Thromb Vasc Biol 16:963, 1996.
144. Kurvers HA, van der Graaf Y, Blankensteijn JD, et al: Screening for asymptomatic internal carotid artery stenosis and aneurysm of the abdominal aorta: Comparing the yield between patients with manifest atherosclerosis and patients with risk factors for atherosclerosis only. J Vasc Surg 37:1226, 2003.
145. Tornwall ME, Virtamo J, Haukka JK, et al: Life-style factors and risk for abdominal aortic aneurysm in a cohort of Finnish male smokers. Epidemiology 12:94, 2001.
146. Rodin MB, Daviglus ML, Wong GC, et al: Middle age cardiovascular risk factors and abdominal aortic aneurysm in older age. Hypertension 42:61, 2003.
147. Scott RA, Bridgewater SG, Ashton HA: Randomized clinical trial of screening for abdominal aortic aneurysm in women. Br J Surg 89:283, 2002.
148. Vardulaki KA, Walker NM, Day NE, et al: Quantifying the risks of hypertension, age, sex and smoking in patients with abdominal aortic aneurysm. Br J Surg 87:195, 2000.
149. Rogot E, Murray JL: Smoking and causes of death among U.S. veterans: 16 years of observation. Public Health Rep 95:213, 1980.
150. Hammond EC: Smoking in relation to the death rates of one million men and women. Natl Cancer Inst Monogr 19:127, 1966.
151. Weir JM, Dunn JE Jr: Smoking and mortality: A prospective study. Cancer 25:105, 1970.
152. Doll R, Peto R, Wheatley K, et al: Mortality in relation to smoking: 40 years' observations on male British doctors. BMJ 309:901, 1994.
153. Nilsson S, Carstensen JM, Pershagen G: Mortality among male and female smokers in Sweden: A 33 year follow up. J Epidemiol Community Health 55:825, 2001.
154. Tang JL, Morris JK, Wald NJ, et al: Mortality in relation to tar yield of cigarettes: A prospective study of four cohorts. BMJ 311:1530, 1995.
155. Goldberg RJ, Burchfiel CM, Benfante R, et al: Lifestyle and biologic factors associated with atherosclerotic disease in middle-aged men: 20-year findings from the Honolulu Heart Program. Arch Intern Med 155:686, 1995.
156. Lee AJ, Fowkes FG, Carson MN, et al: Smoking, atherosclerosis and risk of abdominal aortic aneurysm. Eur Heart J 18:671, 1997.
157. Wilmink TB, Quick CR, Day NE: The association between cigarette smoking and abdominal aortic aneurysms. J Vasc Surg 30:1099, 1999.
158. Lederle FA, Nelson DB, Joseph AM: Smokers' relative risk for aortic aneurysm compared with other smoking-related diseases: A systematic review. J Vasc Surg 38:329, 2003.
159. Strachan DP: Predictors of death from aortic aneurysm among middle-aged men: The Whitehall Study. Br J Surg 78:401, 1991.
160. Franks PJ, Edwards RJ, Greenhalgh RM, et al: Risk factors for abdominal aortic aneurysms in smokers. Eur J Vasc Endovasc Surg 11:487, 1996.
161. Blanchard JF, Armenian HK, Friesen PP: Risk factors for abdominal aortic aneurysm: Results of a case-control study. Am J Epidemiol 151:575, 2000.
162. Hobbs SD, Claridge MW, Quick CR, et al: LDL cholesterol is associated with small abdominal aortic aneurysms. Eur J Vasc Endovasc Surg 26:618, 2003.
163. Gillum RF: Epidemiology of aortic aneurysm in the United States. J Clin Epidemiol 48:1289, 1995.
164. Norrgard O, Rais O, Angquist KA: Familial occurrence of abdominal aortic aneurysms. Surgery 95:650, 1984.
165. Lederle FA: Ultrasonographic screening for abdominal aortic aneurysms. Ann Intern Med 139:516, 2003.
166. Baird PA, Sadovnick AD, Yee IM, et al: Sibling risks of abdominal aortic aneurysm. Lancet 346:601, 1995.
167. Verloes A, Sakalihasan N, Koulischer L, et al: Aneurysms of the abdominal aorta: Familial and genetic aspects in three hundred thirteen pedigrees. J Vasc Surg 21:646, 1995.
168. Frydman G, Walker PJ, Summers K, et al: The value of screening in siblings of patients with abdominal aortic aneurysm. Eur J Vasc Endovasc Surg 26:396, 2003.
169. Adams DC, Tulloh BR, Galloway SW, et al: Familial abdominal aortic aneurysm: Prevalence and implications for screening. Eur J Vasc Surg 7:709, 1993.
170. Cole CW, Barber GG, Bouchard AG, et al: Abdominal aortic aneurysm: Consequences of a positive family history. Can J Surg 32:117, 1989.
171. Webster MW, St Jean PL, Steed DL, et al: Abdominal aortic aneurysm: Results of a family study. J Vasc Surg 13:366, 1991.
172. Webster MW, Ferrell RE, St Jean PL, et al: Ultrasound screening of first-degree relatives of patients with an abdominal aortic aneurysm. J Vasc Surg 13:9, 1991.
173. Majumder PP, St Jean PL, Ferrell RE, et al: On the inheritance of abdominal aortic aneurysm. Am J Hum Genet 48:164, 1991.
174. Norrgard O, Cedergren B, Angquist KA, et al: Blood groups and HLA antigens in patients with abdominal aortic aneurysms. Hum Hered 34:9, 1984.
175. Wiernicki I, Gutowski P, Ciechanowski K, et al: Abdominal aortic aneurysm: Association between haptoglobin phenotypes, elastase activity, and neutrophil count in the peripheral blood. Vasc Surg 35:345, 2001.
176. St Jean P, Hart B, Webster M, et al: Alpha-1-antitrypsin deficiency in aneurysmal disease. Hum Hered 46:92, 1996.
177. Schardey HM, Hernandez-Richter T, Klueppelberg U, et al: Alleles of the alpha-1-antitrypsin phenotype in patients with aortic aneurysms. J Cardiovasc Surg (Torino) 39:535, 1998.
178. Tilson MD, Seashore MR: Fifty families with abdominal aortic aneurysms in two or more first-order relatives. Am J Surg 147:551, 1984.
179. Cronenwett JL, Murphy TF, Zelenock GB, et al: Actuarial analysis of variables associated with rupture of small abdominal aortic aneurysms. Surgery 98:472, 1985.

180. Szilagyi DE, Elliott JP, Smith RF: Clinical fate of the patient with asymptomatic abdominal aortic aneurysm and unfit for surgical treatment. Arch Surg 104:600, 1972.
181. Bickerstaff LK, Hollier LH, Van Peenen HJ, et al: Abdominal aortic aneurysms: The changing natural history. J Vasc Surg 1:6, 1984.
182. Nevitt MP, Ballard DJ, Hallett JW Jr: Prognosis of abdominal aortic aneurysms: A population-based study. N Engl J Med 321:1009, 1989.
183. Lederle FA, Johnson GR, Wilson SE, et al: Rupture rate of large abdominal aortic aneurysms in patients refusing or unfit for elective repair. JAMA 287:2968, 2002.
184. Harris LM, Faggioli GL, Fiedler R, et al: Ruptured abdominal aortic aneurysms: Factors affecting mortality rates. J Vasc Surg 14:812, 1991.
185. Mortality results for randomised controlled trial of early elective surgery or ultrasonographic surveillance for small abdominal aortic aneurysms. The UK Small Aneurysm Trial Participants. Lancet 352:1649, 1998.
186. Lederle FA, Wilson SE, Johnson GR, et al: Immediate repair compared with surveillance of small abdominal aortic aneurysms. N Engl J Med 346:1437, 2002.
187. Brown LC, Powell JT: Risk factors for aneurysm rupture in patients kept under ultrasound surveillance. UK Small Aneurysm Trial Participants. Ann Surg 230:289, 1999.
188. Brown PM, Sobolev B, Zelt DT: Selective management of abdominal aortic aneurysms smaller than 5.0 cm in a prospective sizing program with gender-specific analysis. J Vasc Surg 38:762, 2003.
189. Chang JB, Stein TA, Liu JP, et al: Risk factors associated with rapid growth of small abdominal aortic aneurysms. Surgery 121:117, 1997.
190. Powell JT, Brown LC: The natural history of abdominal aortic aneurysms and their risk of rupture. Acta Chir Belg 101:11, 2001.
191. Evans SM, Adam DJ, Bradbury AW: The influence of gender on outcome after ruptured abdominal aortic aneurysm. J Vasc Surg 32:258, 2000.
192. Svensjo S, Bengtsson H, Bergqvist D: Thoracic and thoracoabdominal aortic aneurysm and dissection: An investigation based on autopsy. Br J Surg 83:68, 1996.
193. Bickerstaff L, Pairolero P, Hollier L, et al: Thoracic aortic aneurysms: A population-based study. Surgery 92:1103, 1982.
194. Svensson LG, Crawford ES, Hess KR, et al: Experience with 1509 patients undergoing thoracoabdominal aortic operations. J Vasc Surg 17:357, 1993.
195. Vaccaro PS, Elkhammas E, Smead WL: Clinical observations and lessons learned in the treatment of patients with thoracoabdominal aortic aneurysms. Surg Gynecol Obstet 166:461, 1988.
196. Itani Y, Watanabe S, Masuda Y, et al: Measurement of aortic diameters and detection of asymptomatic aortic aneurysms in a mass screening program using a mobile helical computed tomography unit. Heart Vessels 16:42, 2002.
197. Joyce JW, Fairbairn JF 2nd, Kincaid OW, et al: Aneurysms of the thoracic aorta: A clinical study with special reference to prognosis. Circulation 29:176, 1964.
198. Crawford ES, Crawford JL, Safi HJ, et al: Thoracoabdominal aortic aneurysms: Preoperative and intraoperative factors determining immediate and long-term results of operations in 605 patients. J Vasc Surg 3:389, 1986.
199. Panneton JM, Hollier LH: Nondissecting thoracoabdominal aortic aneurysms: Part I. Ann Vasc Surg 9:503, 1995.
200. Beckman JA, O'Gara PT: Diseases of the aorta. Adv Intern Med 44:267, 1999.
201. Cambria RA, Gloviczki P, Stanson AW, et al: Outcome and expansion rate of 57 thoracoabdominal aortic aneurysms managed nonoperatively. Am J Surg 170:213, 1995.
202. Masuda Y, Yamada Z, Morooka N, et al: Prognosis of patients with medically treated aortic dissections. Circulation 84:III7, 1991.
203. Pressler V, McNamara JJ: Aneurysm of the thoracic aorta: Review of 260 cases. J Thorac Cardiovasc Surg 89:50, 1985.
204. Dapunt OE, Galla JD, Sadeghi AM, et al: The natural history of thoracic aortic aneurysms. J Thorac Cardiovasc Surg 107:1323, 1994.
205. Masuda Y, Takanashi K, Takasu J, et al: Unoperated thoracic aortic aneurysms: Survival rates of the patients and determinants of prognosis. Intern Med 31:1088, 1992.
206. Coady MA, Rizzo JA, Hammond GL, et al: What is the appropriate size criterion for resection of thoracic aortic aneurysms? J Thorac Cardiovasc Surg 113:476, 1997.
207. Davies RR, Goldstein LJ, Coady MA, et al: Yearly rupture or dissection rates for thoracic aortic aneurysms: Simple prediction based on size. Ann Thorac Surg 73:17, 2002.
208. Elefteriades JA: Natural history of thoracic aortic aneurysms: Indications for surgery, and surgical versus nonsurgical risks. Ann Thorac Surg 74:S1877, 2002.
209. Juvonen T, Ergin MA, Galla JD, et al: Prospective study of the natural history of thoracic aortic aneurysms [published erratum appears in Ann Thorac Surg 64:594, 1997]. Ann Thorac Surg 63:1533, 1997.
210. Griepp RB, Ergin MA, Galla JD, et al: Natural history of descending thoracic and thoracoabdominal aneurysms. Ann Thorac Surg 67:1927, 1999.
211. Fomon JJ, Kurzweg FT, Broadaway FK: Aneurysms of the aorta: A review. Ann Surg 165:557, 1967.
212. Hollier LH, Symmonds JB, Pairolero PC, et al: Thoracoabdominal aortic aneurysm repair: Analysis of postoperative morbidity. Arch Surg 123:871, 1988.
213. Cambria RP, Brewster DC, Moncure AC, et al: Recent experience with thoracoabdominal aneurysm repair. Arch Surg 124:620, 1989.
214. Golden MA, Donaldson MC, Whittemore AD, et al: Evolving experience with thoracoabdominal aortic aneurysm repair at a single institution. J Vasc Surg 13:792, 1991.
215. Lynch DR, Dawson TM, Raps EC, et al: Risk factors for the neurologic complications associated with aortic aneurysms. Arch Neurol 49:284, 1992.
216. Juvonen T, Ergin MA, Galla JD, et al: Prospective study of the natural history of thoracic aortic aneurysms. Ann Thorac Surg 63:1533, 1997.
217. Crawford ES, DeNatale RW: Thoracoabdominal aortic aneurysm: Observations regarding the natural course of the disease. J Vasc Surg 3:578, 1986.
218. Pitt MP, Bonser RS: The natural history of thoracic aortic aneurysm disease: An overview. J Card Surg 12:270, 1997.
219. Beckman JA: Giant cell arteritis. Curr Treat Options Cardiovasc Med 2:213, 2000.
220. Evans JM, Bowles CA, Bjornsson J, et al: Thoracic aortic aneurysm and rupture in giant cell arteritis: A descriptive study of 41 cases [published erratum appears in Arthritis Rheum 38:290, 1995]. Arthritis Rheum 37:1539, 1994.
221. Evans JM, O'Fallon WM, Hunder GG: Increased incidence of aortic aneurysm and dissection in giant cell (temporal) arteritis: A population-based study. Ann Intern Med 122:502, 1995.
222. Nuenninghoff DM, Hunder GG, Christianson TJ, et al: Incidence and predictors of large-artery complication (aortic aneurysm, aortic dissection, and/or large-artery stenosis) in patients with giant cell arteritis: A population-based study over 50 years. Arthritis Rheum 48:3522, 2003.
223. Nuenninghoff DM, Hunder GG, Christianson TJ, et al: Mortality of large-artery complication (aortic aneurysm, aortic dissection, and/or large-artery stenosis) in patients with giant cell arteritis: A population-based study over 50 years. Arthritis Rheum 48:3532, 2003.
224. Nikkari ST, Hoyhtya M, Isola J, et al: Macrophages contain 92-kd gelatinase (MMP-9) at the site of degenerated internal elastic lamina in temporal arteritis. Am J Pathol 149:1427, 1996.
225. Tomita T, Imakawa K: Matrix metalloproteinases and tissue inhibitors of metalloproteinases in giant cell arteritis: An immunocytochemical study. Pathology 30:40, 1998.
226. Subramanyan R, Joy J, Balakrishnan KG: Natural history of aortoarteritis (Takayasu's disease). Circulation 80:429, 1989.
227. Kerr GS, Hallahan CW, Giordano J, et al: Takayasu arteritis. Ann Intern Med 120:919, 1994.
228. Ishikawa K, Maetani S: Long-term outcome for 120 Japanese patients with Takayasu's disease: Clinical and statistical analyses of related prognostic factors. Circulation 90:1855, 1994.
229. Sakane T, Takeno M, Suzuki N, et al: Behçet's disease. N Engl J Med 341:1284, 1999.
230. Yazici H, Yurdakul S, Hamuryudan V: Behçet disease. Curr Opin Rheumatol 13:18, 2001.
231. Ehrlich GE: Vasculitis in Behçet's disease. Int Rev Immunol 14:81, 1997.
232. Roldan CA, Chavez J, Wiest PW, et al: Aortic root disease and valve disease associated with ankylosing spondylitis. J Am Coll Cardiol 32:1397, 1998.
233. Amor B: Reiter's syndrome: Diagnosis and clinical features. Rheum Dis Clin North Am 24:677, 1998.

234. Cosh JA, Barritt DW, Jayson MI: Cardiac lesions of Reiter's syndrome and ankylosing spondylitis. Br Heart J 35:553, 1973.
235. Letko E, Zafirakis P, Baltatzis S, et al: Relapsing polychondritis: A clinical review. Semin Arthritis Rheum 31:384, 2002.
236. Parkhurst GF, Dekcer JP: Bacterial aortitis and mycotic aneurysm of the aorta: A report of twelve cases. Am J Pathol 31:821, 1955.
237. Sommerville RL, Allen EV, Edwards JE: Bland and infected arteriosclerotic abdominal aortic aneurysms: A clinicopathologic study. Medicine (Baltimore) 38:207, 1959.
238. Bennett DE, Cherry JK: Bacterial infection of aortic aneurysms: A clinicopathologic study. Am J Surg 113:321, 1967.
239. Sedwitz MM, Hye RJ, Stabile BE: The changing epidemiology of pseudoaneurysm: Therapeutic implications. Arch Surg 123:473, 1988.
240. Mansur AJ, Grinberg M, Leao PP, et al: Extracranial mycotic aneurysms in infective endocarditis. Clin Cardiol 9:65, 1986.
241. Anderson CB, Butcher HR, Jr., Ballinger WF: Mycotic aneurysms. Arch Surg 109:712, 1974.
242. Jarrett F, Darling RC, Mundth ED, et al: The management of infected arterial aneurysms. J Cardiovasc Surg (Torino) 18:361, 1977.
243. Vogelzang RL, Sohaey R: Infected aortic aneurysms: CT appearance. J Comput Assist Tomogr 12:109, 1988.
244. Jarrett F, Darling RC, Mundth ED, et al: Experience with infected aneurysms of the abdominal aorta. Arch Surg 110:1281, 1975.
245. Goldberg MB, Rubin RH: The spectrum of Salmonella infection. Infect Dis Clin North Am 2:571, 1988.
246. Taylor LM Jr, Deitz DM, McConnell DB, et al: Treatment of infected abdominal aneurysms by extraanatomic bypass, aneurysm excision, and drainage. Am J Surg 155:655, 1988.
247. Johansen K, Devin J: Mycotic aortic aneurysms: A reappraisal. Arch Surg 118:583, 1983.
248. Long R, Guzman R, Greenberg H, et al: Tuberculous mycotic aneurysm of the aorta: Review of published medical and surgical experience. Chest 115:522, 1999.
249. Pugh PJ, Grech ED: Syphilitic aortitis. N Engl J Med 346:676, 2002.
250. Kampmeier RH: Saccular aneurysms of the thoracic aorta: A clinical study of 633 cases. Ann Intern Med 12:624, 1938.
251. Rich C Jr, Webster B: The natural history of uncomplicated syphilitic aortitis. Am Heart J 43:321, 1952.
252. Saruk M, Eisenstein R: Aortic lesion in Marfan syndrome: The ultrastructure of cystic medial degeneration. Arch Pathol Lab Med 101:74, 1977.
253. Sisk HE, Zahka KG, Pyeritz RE: The Marfan syndrome in early childhood: Analysis of 15 patients diagnosed at less than 4 years of age. Am J Cardiol 52:353, 1983.
254. Germain DP: Clinical and genetic features of vascular Ehlers-Danlos syndrome. Ann Vasc Surg 16:391, 2002.
255. Arteaga-Solis E, Gayraud B, Ramirez F: Elastic and collagenous networks in vascular diseases. Cell Struct Funct 25:69, 2000.
256. Nishiyama Y, Manabe N, Ooshima A, et al: A sporadic case of Ehlers-Danlos syndrome type IV: Diagnosed by a morphometric study of collagen content. Pathol Int 45:524, 1995.
257. Pepin M, Schwarze U, Superti-Furga A, et al: Clinical and genetic features of Ehlers-Danlos syndrome type IV, the vascular type. N Engl J Med 342:673, 2000.
258. Pachulski RT, Weinberg AL, Chan KL: Aortic aneurysm in patients with functionally normal or minimally stenotic bicuspid aortic valve. Am J Cardiol 67:781, 1991.
259. Hahn RT, Roman MJ, Mogtader AH, et al: Association of aortic dilation with regurgitant, stenotic and functionally normal bicuspid aortic valves. J Am Coll Cardiol 19:283, 1992.
260. Nistri S, Sorbo MD, Marin M, et al: Aortic root dilatation in young men with normally functioning bicuspid aortic valves. Heart 82:19, 1999.
261. Keane MG, Wiegers SE, Plappert T, et al: Bicuspid aortic valves are associated with aortic dilatation out of proportion to coexistent valvular lesions. Circulation 102:III35, 2000.
262. Yasuda H, Nakatani S, Stugaard M, et al: Failure to prevent progressive dilation of ascending aorta by aortic valve replacement in patients with bicuspid aortic valve: Comparison with tricuspid aortic valve. Circulation 108(suppl 1):II291, 2003.
263. Fedak PW, de Sa MP, Verma S, et al: Vascular matrix remodeling in patients with bicuspid aortic valve malformations: Implications for aortic dilatation. J Thorac Cardiovasc Surg 126:797, 2003.
264. Schmid FX, Bielenberg K, Schneider A, et al: Ascending aortic aneurysm associated with bicuspid and tricuspid aortic valve: Involvement and clinical relevance of smooth muscle cell apoptosis and expression of cell death-initiating proteins. Eur J Cardiothorac Surg 23:537, 2003.
265. Schmid FX, Bielenberg K, Holmer S, et al: Structural and biomolecular changes in aorta and pulmonary trunk of patients with aortic aneurysm and valve disease: Implications for the Ross procedure. Eur J Cardiothorac Surg 25:748, 2004.
266. Boyum J, Fellinger EK, Schmoker JD, et al: Matrix metalloproteinase activity in thoracic aortic aneurysms associated with bicuspid and tricuspid aortic valves. J Thorac Cardiovasc Surg 127:686, 2004.
267. Sybert VP: Cardiovascular malformations and complications in Turner syndrome. Pediatrics 101:E11, 1998.
268. Mutinelli MR, Nizzoli G, Chiumello G, et al: Echocardiographic diagnosis of congenital bicuspid aortic valve in gonadal dysgenesis. G Ital Cardiol 16:496, 1986.
269. Miller MJ, Geffner ME, Lippe BM, et al: Echocardiography reveals a high incidence of bicuspid aortic valve in Turner syndrome. J Pediatr 102:47, 1983.
270. Jenkins NP, Ward C: Coarctation of the aorta: Natural history and outcome after surgical treatment. QJM 92:365, 1999.
271. Scovil JA, Nanda NC, Gross CM, et al: Echocardiographic studies of abnormalities associated with coarctation of the aorta. Circulation 53:953, 1976.
272. Tawes RL Jr, Berry CL, Aberdeen E: Congenital bicuspid aortic valves associated with coarctation of the aorta in children. Br Heart J 31:127, 1969.
273. Knyshov GV, Sitar LL, Glagola MD, et al: Aortic aneurysms at the site of the repair of coarctation of the aorta: A review of 48 patients. Ann Thorac Surg 61:935, 1996.
274. Bergdahl L, Ljungqvist A: Long-term results after repair of coarctation of the aorta by patch grafting. J Thorac Cardiovasc Surg 80:177, 1980.
275. Rao PS, Galal O, Smith PA, et al: Five- to nine-year follow-up results of balloon angioplasty of native aortic coarctation in infants and children. J Am Coll Cardiol 27:462, 1996.
276. Fletcher SE, Nihill MR, Grifka RG, et al: Balloon angioplasty of native coarctation of the aorta: Midterm follow-up and prognostic factors. J Am Coll Cardiol 25:730, 1995.

chapter 38

Clinical Evaluation

Joshua A. Beckman
Mark A. Creager

The vast majority of aortic aneurysms are asymptomatic, accounting for a much higher disease prevalence than hospitalization and mortality statistics would suggest (see Chapter 37). These data underscore the central challenge in aortic aneurysmal disease: a common clinical problem that is silent until rupture and death. Aortic aneurysms typically increase in size slowly over years or decades with few warning signs. The management of aortic aneurysmal disease, therefore, requires suspicion and diligence to avoid adverse outcomes. This chapter focuses on the history, physical examination, and diagnostic tests important to the management of aortic aneurysms.

CLINICAL HISTORY

Thoracic Aortic Aneurysms

Aneurysms of the thoracic aorta typically produce no symptoms, but various symptom complexes may arise, related to the size of the aneurysm and its location within the thorax.

Patients with aneurysmal dilatation of the ascending thoracic aorta may develop clinical manifestations of congestive heart failure as a consequence of aortic valvular regurgitation. Enlargement of the sinuses of Valsalva may cause myocardial ischemia or infarction due to direct compression of the coronary arteries or coronary arterial thromboembolism.[1] Right ventricular outflow tract obstruction and tricuspid regurgitation may result from aneurysmal deformation of the noncoronary sinus.[1] Aneurysms of the sinuses of Valsalva may rupture directly into the right ventricular cavity, right atrium, or pulmonary artery, causing heart failure associated with a continuous murmur.[2-6] Chest pain may occur when the aneurysm compresses surrounding structures or erodes into adjacent bone, such as the ribs or sternum. Compression of the superior vena cava may produce venous congestion of the head, neck, and upper extremities. Symptoms are frequently a harbinger of rupture or death. Rupture may occur into the left pleural space, pericardium, pulmonary artery, or superior vena cava.[3,7,8]

Aneurysms of the aortic arch may produce symptoms by compression of contiguous structures, but most are asymptomatic. Dyspnea or cough may be caused by compression of the trachea or main stem bronchi, dysphagia by compression of the esophagus, or hoarseness secondary to left vocal cord paralysis related to compression of the left recurrent laryngeal nerve.[9-11] The superior vena cava syndrome and pulmonary artery stenosis result when these vessels are compressed.[9,12-15] Chest pain, related either to compression of adjacent structures or to erosion of ribs or vertebrae, is typically positional. Aneurysms of the aortic arch may rupture into the mediastinum, pleural space, tracheobronchial tree (causing hemoptysis), or esophagus (causing hematemesis). Arteriovenous fistulas may result from rupture into the superior vena cava or pulmonary artery. Tuberculous aneurysms, akin to other causes of thoracic aortic aneurysms (TAAs), may present with pain but are commonly asymptomatic. They may also present with hypovolemic shock as a consequence of rupture.[16]

Symptoms of descending TAAs include chest pain from compression of surrounding soft tissues or erosion of vertebrae. Irritation of the recurrent laryngeal nerve may produce hoarseness.[17-19] Dyspnea may result from bronchial compression, and hemoptysis from direct erosion into the lung parenchyma.[20-22] Dysphagia and hematemesis are features of esophageal compression or erosion. Rupture may occur into the mediastinum or left pleural space.

Thoracoabdominal Aortic Aneurysms

Although most patients with thoracoabdominal aortic aneurysms (TAAAs) are asymptomatic, discomfort occasionally develops in the epigastrium or left upper quadrant of the abdomen. Back or flank pain may occur when the patient lies in left lateral decubitus position. Erosion of the anterior surfaces of the vertebral bodies may occur, leading to radiculopathy.[23] Visceral artery occlusion may occur, but frank ischemia and infarction are infrequent.[24,25] Patients who complain of claudication also may have occlusive atherosclerotic disease of the aorta, iliac, or more distal arteries. Because mural thrombosis is so common in atherosclerotic aneurysms, they may be the source of peripheral atheroembolism, causing occlusion of distal vessels.[26-28] Rupture of the thoracic component of these aneurysms generally occurs into the left pleural space, producing a hemothorax; the abdominal component may rupture into the retroperitoneum, inferior vena cava, or duodenum.

Abdominal Aortic Aneurysms

Most patients with abdominal aortic aneurysms (AAAs) are asymptomatic, yet symptoms may take the form of abdominal discomfort or back pain; some patients become aware of abdominal pulsation.[29,30] Less frequently, pain may occur in the legs, chest, or groin; anorexia, nausea, vomiting, constipation, or dyspnea may develop.[31-33] Compression of the left iliac vein may cause left leg swelling, just as compression of the left ureter may cause hydronephrosis or compression of testicular veins may cause varicocele. As the aneurysm expands and compresses vertebrae and lumbar nerve roots, pain may develop in the lower back and may radiate to the posterior aspects of the legs. Flank pain radiating to the anterior left thigh or scrotum may reflect compression of the left genitofemoral nerve. Nausea and vomiting may occur as the aneurysm compresses the duodenum. Bladder compression may cause urinary frequency or urgency.

Occasionally, nascent or frank rupture occurs and causes symptoms indicating a life-threatening emergency. The mortality rate of patients with AAA rupture is 60%; thus patients with symptoms suggestive of rupture require emergent surgical referral.[34-36] The classic triad associated with AAA rupture includes hypotension, back pain, and a pulsatile abdominal mass; however, less than 50% of the patients have all components of this triad.[37] Diverticulitis, renal colic, and gastrointestinal hemorrhage represent common disorders in the differential diagnosis in these patients.[38]

In the absence of patient complaints, physicians must infer the presence of aneurysm on the basis of the clinical characteristics of the patient. Risk factors for aortic aneurysm disease (see Chapter 37) can be used to guide directed physical examination and, if necessary, diagnostic testing.

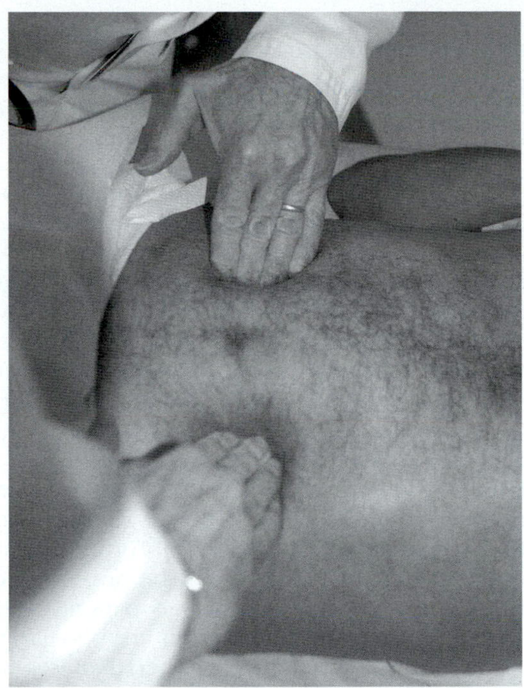

FIGURE 38-1. As depicted, determining the lateral borders of an aortic aneurysm should be performed with the fingertips of both hands. The aneurysm should expand laterally with each heartbeat. Aortic aneurysm transverse diameter may be estimated as the distance between the closest fingers.

PHYSICAL EXAMINATION

The key physical finding is a pulsatile abdominal mass. The patient should be positioned supine with the knees flexed. A pulsatile epigastric or periumbilical mass may be visible, as well as palpable. To distinguish an AAA from para-aortic masses requires that the examiner's hands address the lateral borders (Fig. 38-1). An aneurysm *expands* laterally with each systole. This technique also permits estimation of the transverse diameter of the aneurysm.[39] Auscultation may reveal a bruit over the mass, but abdominal bruits are not specific for aneurysm formation, and only about 40% of such aneurysms are associated with bruits. Proper physical examination of the abdomen may detect the presence of an AAA in 30% to 48% of the patients with AAA.[40,41] In a review of 15 studies, the sensitivity of abdominal examination for aneurysm detection was 49% (Table 38-1).[42] Several factors limit the potential for AAA diagnosis.

TABLE 38-1 SENSITIVITY AND SPECIFICITY OF THE PHYSICAL EXAMINATION FOR ABDOMINAL AORTIC ANEURYSM

Source	Age Range	No. Screened	All AAA	Sensitivity	4-4.9 cm AAA	Sensitivity	≥5 cm AAA	Sensitivity
Cabellon[100]	43-79	73	9	22%	NA	NA	NA	NA
Ohman[101]	50-88	50	3	0%	1	0%	0	NA
Twomey[102]	>50	200	14	64%	3	100%	4	75%
Allen[103]	>65	168	3	0%	0	NA	1	0%
Allardice[104]	39-90	100	15	33%	3	100%	2	100%
Lederle[44]	60-75	201	20	45%	5	20%	5	80%
Collin[105]	65-74	426	23	35%	NA	NA	NA	NA
Shapira[106]	31-83	101	4	0%	0	NA	2	0%
Andersson[107]	38-86	288	14	29%	NA	NA	NA	NA
Spiridonov[108]	17-67	163	10	70%	4	100%	3	100%
MacSweeney[109]	NA	200	55	24%	16	44%	6	100%
Karanja[110]	55-82	89	9	100%	5	100%	2	100%
Molnar[111]	65-83	411	7	43%	3	33%	2	50%
al Zahrani[112]	60-80	392	7	57%	4	50%	2	100%
Arnell[113]	55-81	96	1	100%	0	NA	0	NA
Fink[43]	51-88	200	99	68%	44	69%	14	82%
Summary		3155	293	49%				

AAA, abdominal aortic aneurysm; NA, not available.
Modified from Lederle FA, Simel DL: The rational clinical examination: Does this patient have abdominal aortic aneurysm? JAMA 281:77, 1999.

First, palpation for an aneurysm requires that one consider the diagnosis before examination. Routine physical examination decreases the sensitivity of the examination. Second, size matters; as the size of the aneurysm increases, so does the likelihood of diagnosis. The sensitivity of palpation increased to 75% in patients with aneurysms greater than 5 cm in diameter.[42] Third, increasing abdominal girth decreases the likelihood of discovery.[43] In one study of 201 patients, all six aneurysms present were diagnosed in patients with an abdominal girth of less than 100 cm; however, only 3 of 12 were picked up when the abdominal girth exceeded 100 cm.[44] Thus, although the directed physical examination has a moderate sensitivity and specificity for AAA diagnosis, routine examination misses the diagnosis more commonly than making it.

The finding of a pulsatile mass in the groin, suggesting an iliac artery aneurysm, or in the popliteal fossa, suggesting a popliteal artery aneurysm, further raises the index of suspicion that an AAA may be present, because multiple aneurysms often coexist in patients. Physical signs may reflect atherosclerosis of other vessels, including carotid bruits or diminished arterial pulses in the lower extremities.

Rupture of an AAA usually produces the clinical picture of extreme distress as a result of abdominal catastrophe. Despite surgical advances, mortality is still the rule because of the abrupt nature of circulatory collapse, which prevents timely intervention in most cases. Patients frequently have severe abdominal or back pain, but the pattern of pain varies considerably and may be either persistent or intermittent, sharp or dull, constricting or burning. The aneurysm may rupture into the retroperitoneum or into the peritoneal or pleural cavities. Patients may develop hypotension, tachycardia, pallor, diaphoresis, or shock, depending on the extent of rupture and associated blood loss into the extravascular space. On occasion, rupture occurs directly into the duodenum, causing an aortoduodenal fistula and acute gastrointestinal bleeding. This possibility should be considered when gastrointestinal bleeding is evident along with signs of an aneurysm on physical examination. Rupture may also occur into the inferior vena cava or iliac veins, producing an arteriovenous fistula; this is suggested by rapid development of leg swelling or "high-output" congestive heart failure in the presence of an AAA.

The physical examination is usually not helpful in the diagnosis of TAAs because the rib cage precludes palpation of the aorta. Physical examination may demonstrate right sternoclavicular lift or tracheal deviation. Dilation of the aortic root may cause aortic valve regurgitation.

SCREENING AND SURVEILLANCE OF AORTIC ANEURYSMS

Currently, there are no guidelines to direct patient screening for aortic aneurysm. Several trials have evaluated the possibility of reducing AAA event rates as a result of screening. In a study from Chichester, United Kingdom, 15,775 men and women aged 65 to 80 years were divided into two groups and one half were invited for a screening abdominal ultrasound.[45] Nearly 70% of the subjects accepted the invitation, and aneurysm was detected in 4% of the subjects. A 55% reduction in aneurysm rupture (2.8 per 1000 vs. 6.2 per 1000 subjects) and a 42% reduction in AAA-related mortality in men only (3 per 1000 vs. 5.3 per 1000 male subjects) was noted in the screening group compared with the control subjects. A similar study in Denmark offered 12,658 males aged 65 to 73 a screening invitation; 9620 accepted, and 3038 declined.[46] There was a tenfold reduction in AAA-related death in the group that accepted the invitation compared with those who did not (.006% vs. .06%). Only one trial has assessed the impact of screening on total mortality. The Multicentre Aneurysm Screening Study (MASS) assessed the impact of AAA screening in 67,800 men aged 65 to 74 years.[47] Half of the men were invited for AAA screening, and the others were not. Long-term mortality was monitored in both groups. In the screened group, there was a 42% relative risk reduction in aneurysm-related mortality from 0.33% to 0.19%, representing 48 fewer deaths. The reduction in absolute mortality, however, was a statistically insignificant 0.27%.

Some clinical features exist to suggest which patients should definitely undergo screening for aortic aneurysm, and AAA in particular. These include patients with a family history for aneurysm, those with inherited disorders of connective tissue, such as Marfan's disease, and those with arteritis, such as Takayasu's arteritis and giant cell arteritis. Siblings of patients with AAA have a 25% chance of having an aneurysm.[48] Diagnostic screening should also be considered for male smokers older than age 60. The threshold for women is higher because men are much more likely to develop an aortic aneurysm. Also, those with a connective tissue disorder are at markedly increased risk for aneurysm formation.

DIAGNOSTIC TESTING

Diagnostic testing is indicated for screening patients at high risk for aneurysm, such as patients with Marfan's disease, bicuspid aortic valve, and those with a family history of aneurysm for aneurysm diagnosis. Routine screening should also be considered for men older than age 60 who smoke. Data are insufficient to make any definitive recommendation about routine screening for elderly women, even those who smoke. Imaging studies are also indicated for longitudinal surveillance of known aneurysms, or for anatomic definition before endovascular or surgical repairs. The major objectives of imaging studies include identification of the aorta and its branches, diagnosis and characterization of the type of aneurysm (fusiform or saccular), determination of the transverse and longitudinal dimensions of the aneurysm, and detection of associated pathology that may affect treatment. An understanding of the benefits and limitations of the several imaging modalities enables appropriate test selection (Table 38-2).

Chest roentgenography may provide the first indication of a TAA (Fig. 38-2). Aneurysms of the ascending aorta are usually evident on the right side of the mediastinum.

TABLE 38-2 ABDOMINAL AORTIC ANEURYSM IMAGING MODALITIES: STRENGTHS AND WEAKNESSES*

Modality	Advantages	Disadvantages	Optimal Use
Ultrasound	Highly accurate sizing Inexpensive	Unable to discern longitudinal extent Cannot define branch artery anatomy	Initial diagnosis Follow-up until repair
CT	Highly accurate sizing Defines branch artery involvement well	Ionizing radiation Contrast required	Prerepair assessment Stent graft follow-up
MRA	Highly accurate sizing No ionizing radiation Defines branch artery involvement well	Cannot image some stent grafts	Prerepair assessment
Contrast angiography	Defines branch artery involvement well	Cannot size aneurysm Invasive Ionizing radiation Contrast required	Stent-graft implantation

*The sensitivity and specificity of each examination exceed 95% for the diagnosis of an abdominal aortic aneurysm.

Aneurysms of the aortic arch widen the mediastinal shadow and may project more toward the left. These aneurysms may displace or compress the trachea or left mainstem bronchus. Descending TAAs typically appear as mediastinal masses extending into the left hemithorax. Assessment of the aorta by chest roentgenography requires both posteroanterior and lateral projections. Failure to detect an ascending TAA roentgenographically, however, does not exclude the diagnosis, as aneurysms may not become apparent until considerable dilatation has occurred.

Similarly, plain roentgenography frequently discloses an unsuspected AAA.[49] Anteroposterior and lateral views of the abdomen may disclose a curvilinear rim of calcification in the wall of the aneurysm, and the diameter of the aneurysm may be estimated when such calcification is visible in two opposing walls.[39,49-52] In 25% to 50% of suspected cases, however, the walls of the aneurysm are not sufficiently calcified to permit radiographic identification.[49,51,53,54] Furthermore, it may underestimate anteroposterior aneurysm size by 15%.[39]

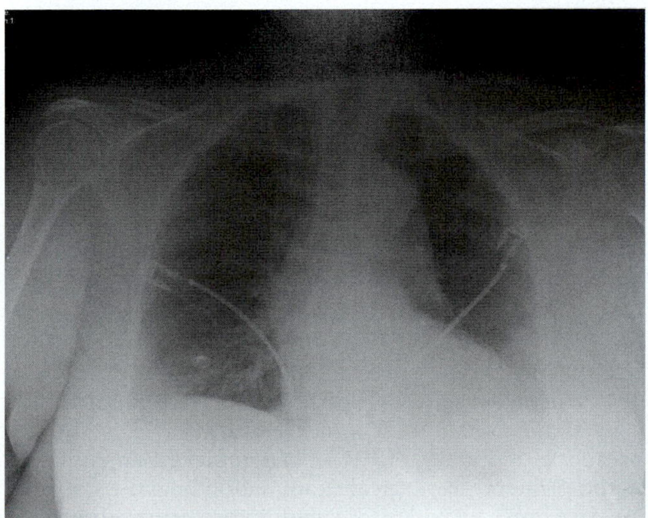

FIGURE 38-2. Posterior-anterior chest radiograph demonstrating a widened mediastinum in a patient with a 5-cm ascending aortic aneurysm.

Ultrasound

Duplex ultrasonography is the most commonly used method for the identification and characterization of AAA. It is the least expensive modality, does not expose the patient to ionizing radiation, and can accurately determine the anterior-posterior, transverse, and longitudinal dimensions of an AAA (Fig. 38-3). The sensitivity for the diagnosis of an AAA 3 cm or larger approaches 100%.[55] The examination is rapid and easily performed. The abdominal aorta is subject to anteroposterior, transverse, and longitudinal evaluations. Sonographic classification of AAA begins when the maximum diameter exceeds 3 cm, in either anteroposterior or transverse dimensions. Care must be taken to image the aorta perpendicularly to its longitudinal axis to avoid eccentricity, which may lead to overestimation of the true diameter. Thrombus is identified frequently within the lumen, and echodense calcification may be present in or adjacent to the aortic wall. Beyond determining the size of an aneurysm, ultrasound imaging may help define the relation of major arterial branches and adjacent organs. Certain ultrasound characteristics have potential value in predicting rupture. Intramural hematoma, appearing as a hypoechoic soft-tissue mass surrounding the aorta, which may silhouette the psoas muscle, appears to represent such a sign.[56] This may be indistinguishable from periaortic fibrosis, which appears on ultrasound examination as a hypoechoic mantle surrounding the aortic wall in patients with inflammatory aortic aneurysms.

Recently, several groups have demonstrated the reliability of a "quick screen" in emergency departments.[57,58] In a prospective study of 125 emergency department patients, quick evaluations did not miss an AAA. Emergency department testing reported 100% sensitivity and 98% specificity rates.[59] Indeed, accuracy is maintained at 100% when the "quick screen" and classic examination approaches are compared within a noninvasive vascular laboratory.[60]

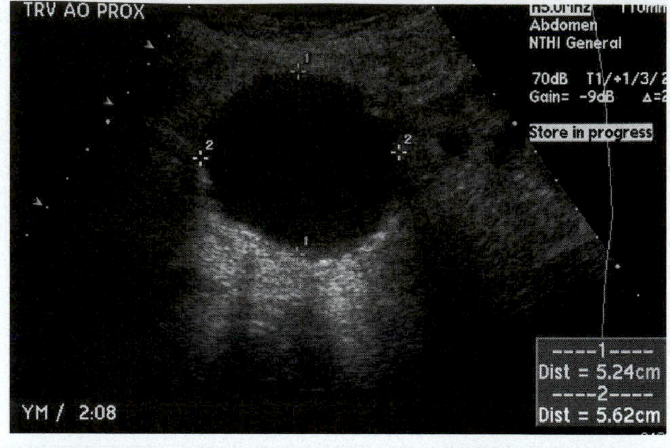

A

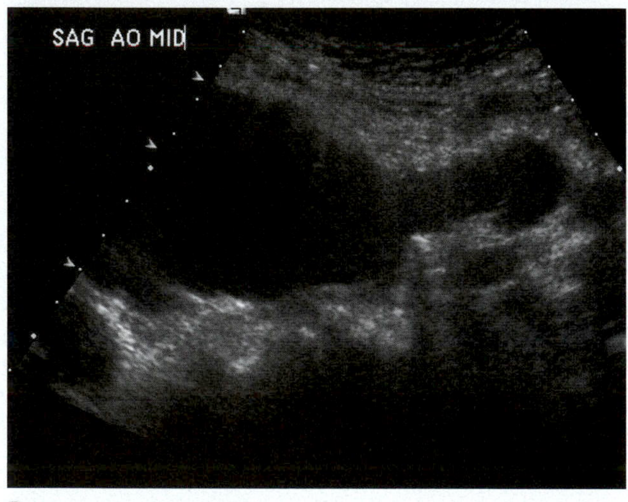

B

FIGURE 38-3. A, Transverse B-mode ultrasound image of the widest portion of the abdominal aorta. Electronic calipers have been applied and demonstrate a 5.6-cm transverse diameter and 5.2-cm anterior-posterior diameter. **B,** Sagittal view of the same vessel demonstrating the transition from normal to aneurysmal aorta.

The accuracy of ultrasonography should be considered in respect to other imaging modalities (see later). In the Abdominal Aortic Aneurysm Detection and Management Veterans Administration Cooperative Study Group (ADAM) study, CT and ultrasound were compared. Although both techniques demonstrated sizing variabilities between local and central reading sites,[61] in one third of subjects the variation between ultrasound and CT was 0.5 cm or more. Ultrasonographic evaluation undersized the aneurysm by a mean of 0.27 cm compared with CT measurements. Similarly, in 334 patients participating in an aneurysm endograft study, CT reported a greater aneurysm diameter than ultrasound 95% of the time.[62] The correlation between the two measurements was strong, but in nearly one half the patients, the aortic diameter varied by a centimeter or more between the ultrasound and CT studies. Smaller studies confirm both the high sensitivity yet consistent undersizing by ultrasound.[63,64]

Despite these observations, two large clinical trials suggest that ultrasonography is an appropriate method to evaluate and follow AAA. The United Kingdom Small Aneurysm Trial[65] and the Aneurysm Detection and Management Trial[66] used ultrasonographic monitoring to determine the time of surgical repair in the group of patients randomized to surveillance. In the absence of any clinical data suggesting the inadequacy of ultrasound, it remains the primary tool for diagnosis and follow-up.

Postoperatively, duplex ultrasound can evaluate important ongoing clinical issues including peri-aneurysm aortic size, and anastomotic aneurysm and pseudoaneurysm formation.[67] Ultrasonography, however, is not an ideal imaging test following aortic stent grafting. It has a wide range of sensitivity and specificity for the various problems encountered after endovascular grafting including endoleaks and device migration or thrombosis and, therefore, should not be used as the primary method of follow-up.[68] Improvements in technique, including contrast agents and three-dimensional imaging, are currently in development and will likely improve the ultrasound's accuracy to diagnose complications of endografts.[69-71]

Ultrasound also can be employed to diagnose and monitor TAA. Transthoracic echocardiography visualizes the aortic root and a portion of the ascending aorta. Transesophageal echocardiography (TEE) images much of the thoracic aorta well with sensitivity and specificity both above 95%,[72] except where obscured by the trachea. The limitation of TEE for routine diagnostic purposes is that it requires sedation and is relatively invasive compared with other techniques to evaluate TAA, such as CT and MRI examinations (see later).

Computed Tomography (also see Chapter 12)

Rapid advances in technology have put computed tomographic angiography (CTA) in the forefront of aortic imaging. Multidetector-row CTA currently acquires 16 simultaneous helices creating high-resolution images, providing better sensitivity and specificity than could be obtained previously with single-detector–row technology (Fig. 38-4) (also see Fig. 12-20 in Chapter 12). Yet even with single-detector scanners, CT determined aortic aneurysm size to within 0.2 mm.[73]

CTA is now a preferred imaging modality for preoperative definition of acute aneurysms because of its accuracy. CT can define the proximal and distal extensions of AAAs[73,74] and determine the relationship of the aneurysm to branch arteries.[75,76] In a study of 30 patients undergoing AAA repair, both spiral CT and conventional contrast angiography were performed. Spiral CT had a 100% sensitivity for determining aneurysm extent and better sized the aneurysm than angiography but revealed only 2 of 9 accessory renal arteries.[77] In one study comparing CTA with conventional angiography, CTA had a 93% sensitivity and 96% specificity in determining clinically significant branch vessel stenoses (≥85%) and the presence of aneurysm.[78] CTA has replaced angiography as the primary presurgical examination because it is noninvasive and provides detailed information about the vessel walls, such as inflammation, mural thrombus, and vascular calcification. Moreover, CTA creates a better anatomical definition through the use of the various three-dimensional visualization techniques (Fig. 38-5).[79]

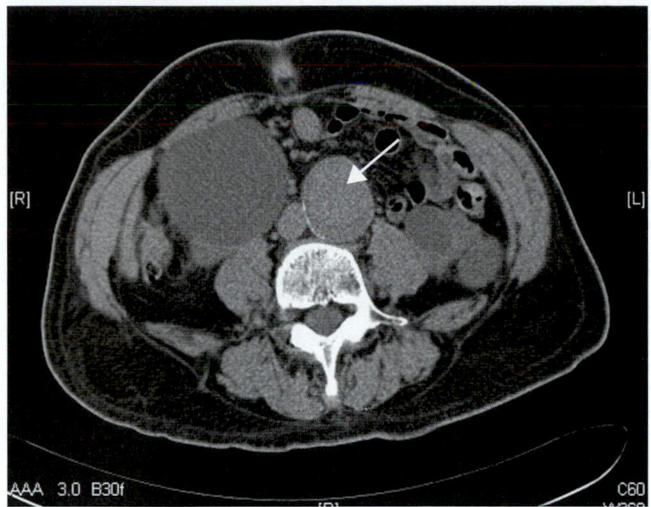

FIGURE 38-4. Coronal section of an x-ray multidetector computed tomographic scan of the abdomen. The large white arrow indicates the abdominal aortic aneurysm.

Also, it can diagnose abnormalities in adjacent structures. Recent data suggest that multidetector CTA has a similar image quality and diagnostic accuracy as MRA, with a sensitivity of 91% and a specificity of 98%.[80]

CTA also can demonstrate mural calcification and, with three-dimensional reconstruction, show aortic angulation.[81] The placement of aortic stent grafts for AAA requires the acquisition of specific anatomic information before the procedure. The most important parameter measured before the placement of an endograft is the diameter of the neck. Modalities that create a cross-sectional image, including CT, can accurately determine vessel diameter.[82,83] Helical CT, MRA, and digital subtraction angiography were compared in a prospective study of 61 patients planned for aortic stent-graft placement.[84] MRA and helical CT were similar in their abilities to determine the proximal aneurysm extent and aortic diameter. Yet CT performed better at imaging accessory renal arteries and detecting renal artery stenosis.

Postoperatively, CT imaging is directed at the primary complications of stent-grafts including endoleaks, device failure, aneurysm expansion, and aneurysm rupture. Determining the type of endoleak has important prognostic implications. In a study of 40 aortic stent-graft patients, CTA was superior to digital subtraction angiography in determining the presence of endoleak with a sensitivity of 92% for CTA and only 63% for angiography. CTA also is effective in the determination of stent-graft migration, distortion, and destruction. Thus CT imaging is indicated for preprocedural planning and post-endograft surveillance. After the implantation, imaging typically is performed at 3, 6, and 12 months and yearly thereafter.[83]

CTA also is useful to image the thoracic aorta for diagnosis, follow-up, and perioperative management of TAA (Fig. 38-6).[85] CT can be used to follow aneurysm growth,[87] detecting changes as small as a millimeter. The use of contrast permits the evaluation of aneurysms from any angle and the creation of three-dimensional images.[76] In one study of 49 patients, CT accurately assessed the spinal cord circulation and predicted the requirement for hypothermic circulatory arrest 94% of the time.[88] CT may also play an important role in follow-up of thoracic endovascular grafts by demonstrating volumetric changes in the aneurysm and thrombus suggestive of a successful repair.[89] CTA accurately assesses the thoracic

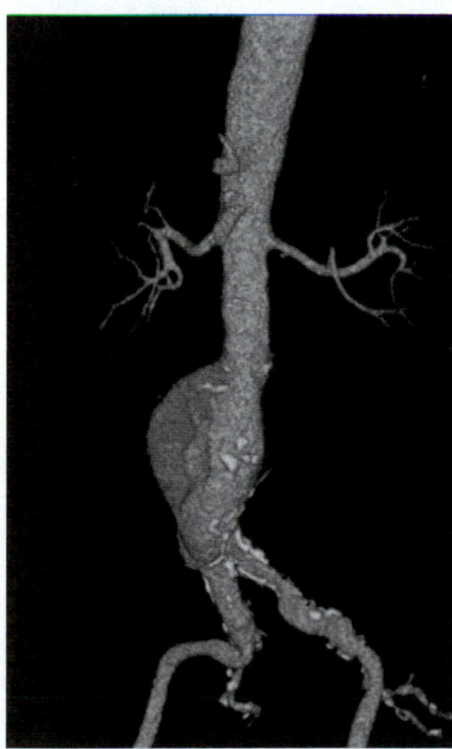

FIGURE 38-5. (See also Color Plate 38-5.) Three-dimensional reconstruction of an abdominal aortic aneurysm from a multidetector computed tomographic angiographic scan. Note the infrarenal location of the aneurysm, the vascular calcification in white, and the tortuosity of the iliac arteries.

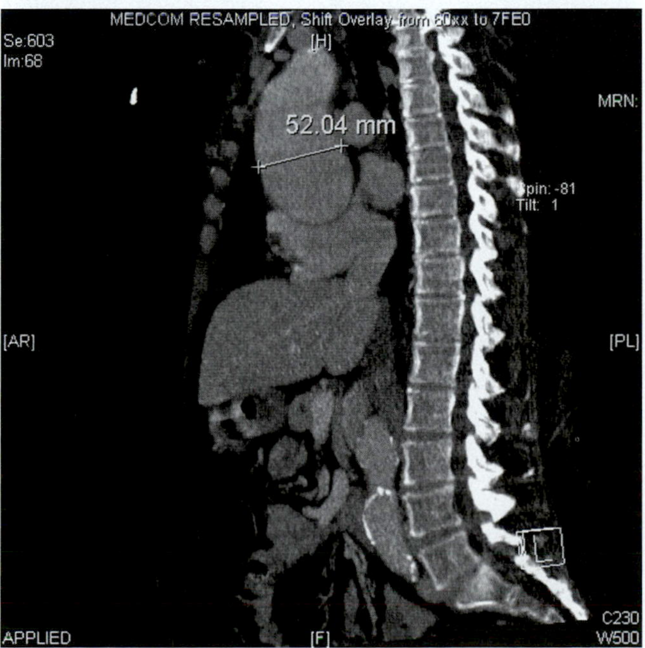

FIGURE 38-6. Sagittal view of a computed tomographic scan of the thorax demonstrating an ascending aortic aneurysm measuring more than 5 cm in diameter.

aorta before operation, assists in operative planning, and is the standard imaging modality for follow-up.

Magnetic Resonance Imaging

(also see Chapter 11)

MRI and MRA are also used to image and characterize aortic aneurysms. The technique has been used for the diagnosis of AAA for 20 years[90] and is quite acceptable for preoperative evaluation (Fig. 38-7).[91] MRA can determine aneurysm diameter, longitudinal extent, involvement of branch vessels, and proximity to the renal arteries.[79] Both MRI and gadolinium-enhanced MRA have a greater than 90% sensitivity and specificity for the determination of TAA.[92] Moreover, MRA has a greater than 90% sensitivity and specificity for the detection of concordant stenoses in splanchnic, renal, or iliac branches.[93]

MRA is an accurate method to define aortic anatomy required before aortic endograft and is superior to duplex ultrasonography.[82,94] MRA may have advantages over CT for postprocedural surveillance of stent grafts. In a study of 31 patients, MRA diagnosed 18 of 19 endoleaks compared with 10 of 19 by helical CT.[95] Cine MRA can show the pulsatility of the aneurysm and quantify AAA wall motion before and after endovascular graft placement to help identify endoleaks.

One of the more important issues associated with repair of the thoracic aorta is the identification of the artery of Adamkiewicz. This artery arises most commonly from the left side of the aorta between T8 and L4 and supplies perfusion to the lower two thirds of the spinal cord. Both CT and MRA, with their high spatial resolution, visualize the artery well.[96,97] In a series of 30 patients with TAA, both MRA and CTA provided clear visualization of the artery of Adamkiewicz via a clear identification of the vascular anatomy.[98]

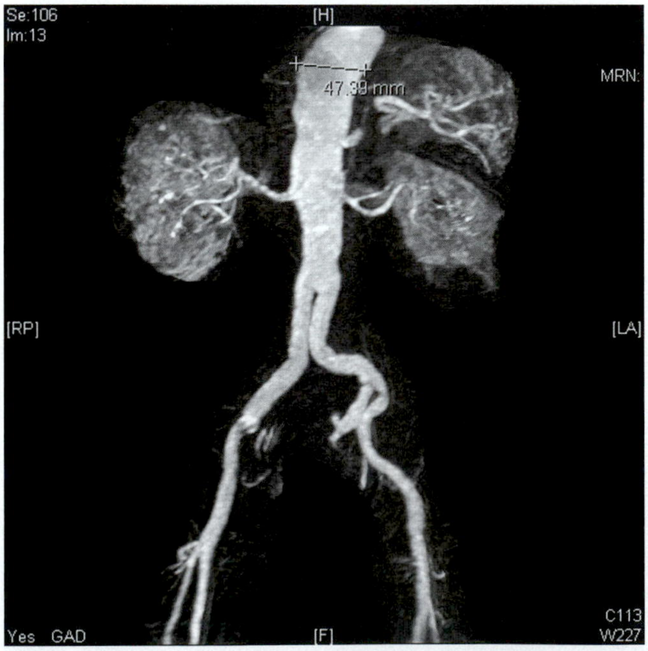

FIGURE 38-7. Maximal intensity projection of a magnetic resonance angiogram demonstrating a 4.7 cm suprarenal abdominal aortic aneurysm.

Contrast Angiography

Contrast angiography is useful to define branch vessel anatomy and the longitudinal extent of aortic aneurysms (Fig. 38-8). Angiography, which provides information about the aortic lumen, cannot accurately size an aneurysm because it does not visualize the vessel wall or aneurysm thrombus. Digital subtraction angiography (DSA) has similar accuracy to MRA and CTA in defining aneurysm length and aortic anatomy before endograft placement.[99] In a study of 20 patients before endograft placement, length and diameter measurements were similar between MRA and CT but superior to DSA.[94] Contrast angiography is less commonly performed than noninvasive imaging studies because of its invasive nature, the nephrotoxicity of contrast, and the lack of diagnostic superiority.

Recommendations

Once an acute aneurysm is diagnosed, serial imaging studies should be performed every 3 to 12 months until the rate of expansion is greater than 1 cm per year or the diameter increases to that which merits surgical or endovascular repair (see Chapters 39 and 40).

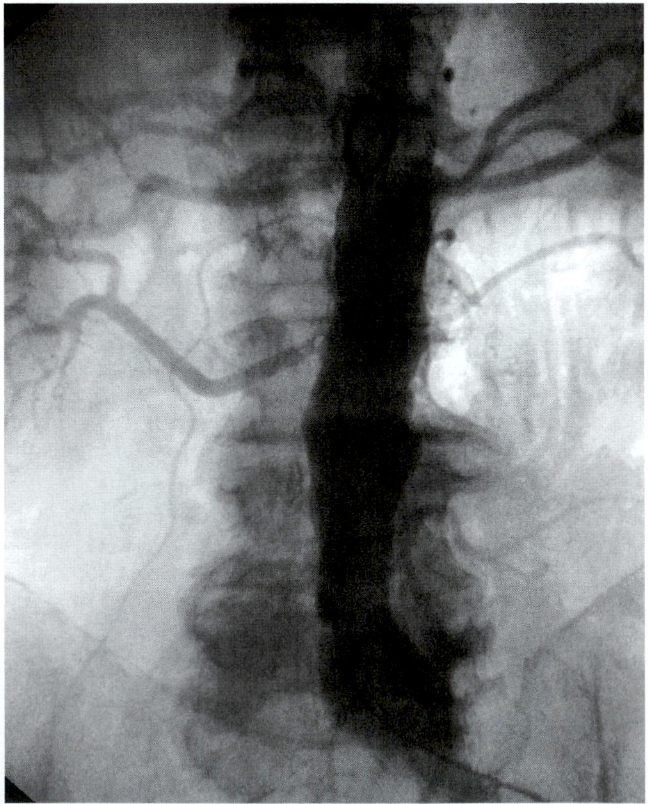

FIGURE 38-8. Contrast abdominal aortography revealing an infrarenal abdominal aortic aneurysm. Of note is that the angiogram cannot determine aneurysm size but can show that the renal arteries are not involved.

REFERENCES

1. Bulkley BH, Hutchins GM, Ross RS: Aortic sinus of Valsalva aneurysms simulating primary right-sided valvular heart disease. Circulation 52:696, 1975.
2. Erdol C, Gokce M, Baykan M, et al: Rupture of the right sinus of Valsalva into the right ventricle: Echocardiographic and angiographic imaging. J Invasive Cardiol 12:435, 2000.
3. Kar AK, Bhattacharya S, Ray D, et al: Rupture of the sinus of Valsalva into the pulmonary artery. Indian Heart J 54:415, 2002.
4. Budts W, Moons P, Mertens L, Van de Werf F: Ruptured aneurysm of the sinus of Valsalva into the right atrium: An uncommon congenital heart defect. Acta Clin Belg 58:120, 2003.
5. Blieden LC, Edwards JE: Anomalies of the thoracic aorta: Pathologic considerations. Prog Cardiovasc Dis 16:25, 1973.
6. Davies GJ, Watt J, Muir JR: Ruptured sinus of Valsalva aneurysm with aortic-left atrial fistula. Eur J Cardiol 3:213, 1975.
7. Brabham KR, Roberts WC: Fatal intrapericardial rupture of sinus of Valsalva aneurysm. Am Heart J 120:1455, 1990.
8. Kaye GC, Edmonson SJ, Caplin JL, Tunstall-Pedoe DS: Rupture of an aneurysm of the sinus of Valsalva into the superior vena cava. Thorax 39:475, 1984.
9. Gorman RB, Merritt WT, Greenspun H, et al: Aneurysmal compression of the trachea and right mainstem bronchus complicating thoracoabdominal aneurysm repair. Anesthesiology 79:1424, 1993.
10. Stoob K, Alkadhi H, Lachat M, et al: Resolution of hoarseness after endovascular repair of thoracic aortic aneurysm: A case of Ortner's syndrome. Ann Otol Rhinol Laryngol 113:43, 2004.
11. Rabago G, Martin-Trenor A, Lopez-Coronado JL: Chronic aneurysm of the descending thoracic aorta presenting with right pleural effusion and left phrenic paralysis. Tex Heart Inst J 26:96, 1999.
12. Moreno AJ, Carpenter AL, Pacheco EJ, Turnbull GL: Large thoracic aortic aneurysm seen on equilibrium blood pool imaging. Clin Nucl Med 19:1113, 1994.
13. Seymour J, Emanuel R, Pattinson N: Acquired pulmonary stenosis. Br Heart J 30:776, 1968.
14. Drachler DH, Willis PW III: Acquired right ventricular outflow tract obstruction. Am Heart J 82:536, 1971.
15. Banker VP, Maddison FE: Superior vena cava syndrome secondary to aortic disease. Dis Chest 51:656, 1967.
16. Long R, Guzman R, Greenberg H, et al: Tuberculous mycotic aneurysm of the aorta: Review of published medical and surgical experience. Chest 115:522, 1999.
17. Benzaquen BS, Therrien J: Thoracic aortic aneurysm occurring at a coarctation repair site. Can J Cardiol 19:561, 2003.
18. Fujita T, Fukushima N, Taketani S, et al: Late true aneurysm after bypass grafting for long aortic coarctation. Ann Thorac Surg 62:1511, 1996.
19. Edwards JE: Aneurysms of the thoracic aorta complicating coarctation. Circulation 48:195, 1973.
20. Cramer M, Foley WD, Palmer TE, et al: Compression of the right pulmonary artery by aortic aneurysms: CT demonstration. J Comput Assist Tomogr 9:310, 1985.
21. Nagamine S, Kamada M, Ohsaka K, Kakihata H: Left pulmonary artery occlusion due to compression by aortic aneurysm. Jpn J Thorac Cardiovasc Surg 50:481, 2002.
22. Varkey B, Tristani FE: Compression of pulmonary artery and bronchus by descending thoracic aortic aneurysm. Perfusion and ventilation changes after aneurysmectomy. Am J Cardiol 34:610, 1974.
23. Forutan H, Herdmann J, Huber R, et al: Paraparesis due to pressure erosion of the thoracic spine by an aortic aneurysm: Remission of symptoms following resection of the aneurysm and vertebral reconstruction. Acta Neurochir (Wien) 146:303; discussion 308, 2004.
24. Kochi K, Sueda T: Inflammatory aortic arch aneurysm with total occlusion of cervical branches. Ann Thorac Cardiovasc Surg 10:51, 2004.
25. Fomon JJ, Kurzweg FT, Broadaway FK: Aneurysms of the aorta: A review. Ann Surg 165:557, 1967.
26. Williams HC, Pembroke AC: Livedo reticularis and massive thoracoabdominal aneurysm. Clin Exp Dermatol 19:353, 1994.
27. van der Heyde M, Zwaveling A: Resection of an abdominal aortic aneurysm in a patient with Marfan's syndrome. J Cardiovasc Surg (Torino) 2:359, 1961.
28. DeBakey ME, Crawford ES, Garrett HE, et al: Surgical considerations in the treatment of aneurysms of the thoraco-abdominal aorta. Ann Surg 162:650, 1965.
29. Edwards JZ, Weiner SD: Chronic back pain caused by an abdominal aortic aneurysm: Case report and review of the literature. Orthopedics 26:191, 2003.
30. Rose J, Civil I, Koelmeyer T, et al: Ruptured abdominal aortic aneurysms: Clinical presentation in Auckland 1993-1997. ANZ J Surg 71:341, 2001.
31. Lynch RM: Ruptured abdominal aortic aneurysm presenting as groin pain. Br J Gen Pract 52:320, 2002.
32. Iosca A, Dell'Abate P, Galimberti A, et al: Aortic graft in the jejunum without bleeding: A real surprise at endoscopy. Surg Endosc 15:1226, 2001.
33. Victor DW Jr, Werdick GM, Proudfoot RW: Internal iliac artery aneurysm presenting as severe constipation. J Ky Med Assoc 85:310, 1987.
34. Piotrowski JJ, Akhrass R, Alexander JJ, et al: Rupture of known abdominal aortic aneurysms: An ethical dilemma. Am Surg 61:556, 1995.
35. Ottinger LW: Ruptured arteriosclerotic aneurysms of the abdominal aorta. Reducing mortality. JAMA 233:147, 1975.
36. Johnson G Jr, McDevitt NB, Proctor HJ, et al: Emergent or elective operation for symptomatic abdominal aortic aneurysm. Arch Surg 115:51, 1980.
37. Cates JR: Abdominal aortic aneurysms: Clinical diagnosis and management. J Manipulative Physiol Ther 20:557, 1997.
38. Ernst CB: Abdominal aortic aneurysm. N Engl J Med 328:1167, 1993.
39. Hall AD, Zubrin JR, Moore WS, Thomas AN: Surgical treatment of aortic aneurysm in the aged: A review of 100 patients. Arch Surg 100:455, 1970.
40. Karkos CD, Mukhopadhyay U, Papakostas I, et al: Abdominal aortic aneurysm: The role of clinical examination and opportunistic detection. Eur J Vasc Endovasc Surg 19:299, 2000.
41. Kiev J, Eckhardt A, Kerstein MD: Reliability and accuracy of physical examination in detection of abdominal aortic aneurysms. Vasc Surg 31:143, 1997.
42. Lederle FA, Simel DL: The rational clinical examination: Does this patient have abdominal aortic aneurysm? JAMA 281:77, 1999.
43. Fink HA, Lederle FA, Roth CS, et al: The accuracy of physical examination to detect abdominal aortic aneurysm. Arch Intern Med 160:833, 2000.
44. Lederle FA, Walker JM, Reinke DB: Selective screening for abdominal aortic aneurysms with physical examination and ultrasound. Arch Intern Med 148:1753, 1988.
45. Scott RA, Wilson NM, Ashton HA, Kay DN: Influence of screening on the incidence of ruptured abdominal aortic aneurysm: 5-year results of a randomized controlled study. Br J Surg 82:1066, 1995.
46. Lindholt JS, Juul S, Fasting H, Henneberg EW: Hospital costs and benefits of screening for abdominal aortic aneurysms: Results from a randomised population screening trial. Eur J Vasc Endovasc Surg 23:55, 2002.
47. Ashton HA, Buxton MJ, Day NE, et al: The Multicentre Aneurysm Screening Study (MASS) into the effect of abdominal aortic aneurysm screening on mortality in men: A randomised controlled trial. Lancet 360:1531, 2002.
48. Frydman G, Walker PJ, Summers K, et al: The value of screening in siblings of patients with abdominal aortic aneurysm. Eur J Vasc Endovasc Surg 26:396, 2003.
49. Friedman SA, Hufnagel CA, Conrad PW, et al: Abdominal aortic aneurysms: Clinical status and results of surgery in 100 consecutive cases. JAMA 200:1147, 1967.
50. Romano CC, Blaudeau E, Neitzschman HR: Radiology case of the month: Calcified mass and indistinct retroperitoneal landmarks on abdominal radiograph: Ruptured abdominal aortic aneurysm. J La State Med Soc 149:267, 1997.
51. Brewster DC, Darling RC, Raines JK, et al: Assessment of abdominal aortic aneurysm size. Circulation 56(Suppl):II164, 1977.
52. Winsberg F, Cole-Beuglet C, Mulder DS: Continuous ultrasound "B" scanning of abdominal aortic aneurysms. Am J Roentgenol Radium Ther Nucl Med 121:626, 1974.
53. Janower ML: Ruptured arteriosclerotic aneurysms of the abdominal aorta: Roentgenographic findings on plain films. N Engl J Med 265:12, 1961.

54. Boyd DP, McCann JC Jr: Abdominal aneurysm. Surg Clin North Am 45:675, 1965.
55. LaRoy LL, Cormier PJ, Matalon TA, et al: Imaging of abdominal aortic aneurysms. AJR Am J Roentgenol 152:785, 1989.
56. Cumming MJ, Hall AJ, Burbridge BE: Psoas muscle hematoma secondary to a ruptured abdominal aortic aneurysm: Case report. Can Assoc Radiol J 51:279, 2000.
57. Kuhn M, Bonnin RL, Davey MJ, et al: Emergency department ultrasound scanning for abdominal aortic aneurysm: Accessible, accurate, and advantageous. Ann Emerg Med 36:219, 2000.
58. Salen P, Melanson S, Buro D: ED screening to identify abdominal aortic aneurysms in asymptomatic geriatric patients. Am J Emerg Med 21:133, 2003.
59. Tayal VS, Graf CD, Gibbs MA: Prospective study of accuracy and outcome of emergency ultrasound for abdominal aortic aneurysm over two years. Acad Emerg Med 10:867, 2003.
60. Lee TY, Korn P, Heller JA, et al: The cost-effectiveness of a "quick-screen" program for abdominal aortic aneurysms. Surgery 132:399, 2002.
61. Lederle FA, Wilson SE, Johnson GR, et al: Variability in measurement of abdominal aortic aneurysms. Abdominal Aortic Aneurysm Detection and Management Veterans Administration Cooperative Study Group. J Vasc Surg 21:945, 1995.
62. Sprouse LR II, Meier GH III, Lesar CJ, et al: Comparison of abdominal aortic aneurysm diameter measurements obtained with ultrasound and computed tomography: Is there a difference? J Vasc Surg 38:466; discussion 471, 2003.
63. Wilmink AB, Forshaw M, Quick CR, et al: Accuracy of serial screening for abdominal aortic aneurysms by ultrasound. J Med Screen 9:125, 2002.
64. Thomas PR, Shaw JC, Ashton HA, et al: Accuracy of ultrasound in a screening programme for abdominal aortic aneurysms. J Med Screen 1:3, 1994.
65. Mortality results for randomised controlled trial of early elective surgery or ultrasonographic surveillance for small abdominal aortic aneurysms. The UK Small Aneurysm Trial Participants. Lancet 352:1649, 1998.
66. Lederle FA, Wilson SE, Johnson GR, et al: Immediate repair compared with surveillance of small abdominal aortic aneurysms. N Engl J Med 346:1437, 2002.
67. Bastounis E, Georgopoulos S, Maltezos C, Balas P: The validity of current vascular imaging methods in the evaluation of aortic anastomotic aneurysms developing after abdominal aortic aneurysm repair. Ann Vasc Surg 10:537, 1996.
68. Teodorescu VJ, Morrissey NJ, Olin JW: Duplex ultrasonography and its impact on providing endograft surveillance. Mt Sinai J Med 70:364, 2003.
69. van Essen JA, Gussenhoven EJ, Blankensteijn JD, et al: Three-dimensional intravascular ultrasound assessment of abdominal aortic aneurysm necks. J Endovasc Ther 7:380, 2000.
70. Leotta DF, Paun M, Beach KW, et al: Measurement of abdominal aortic aneurysms with three-dimensional ultrasound imaging: Preliminary report. J Vasc Surg 33:700, 2001.
71. Bendick PJ, Bove PG, Long GW, et al: Efficacy of ultrasound scan contrast agents in the noninvasive follow-up of aortic stent grafts. J Vasc Surg 37:381, 2003.
72. Chirillo F, Cavallini C, Longhini C, et al: Comparative diagnostic value of transesophageal echocardiography and retrograde aortography in the evaluation of thoracic aortic dissection. Am J Cardiol 74:590, 1994.
73. Todd GJ, Nowygrod R, Benvenisty A, et al: The accuracy of CT scanning in the diagnosis of abdominal and thoracoabdominal aortic aneurysms. J Vasc Surg 13:302, 1991.
74. Simoni G, Perrone R, Cittadini G Jr, et al: Helical CT for the study of abdominal aortic aneurysms in patients undergoing conventional surgical repair. Eur J Vasc Endovasc Surg 12:354, 1996.
75. Cohan RH, Siegel CL, Korobkin M, et al: Abdominal aortic aneurysms: CT evaluation of renal artery involvement. Radiology 194:751, 1995.
76. Posacioglu H, Islamoglu F, Apaydin AZ, et al: Predictive value of conventional computed tomography in determining proximal extent of abdominal aortic aneurysms and possibility of infrarenal clamping. Tex Heart Inst J 29:172, 2002.
77. Errington ML, Ferguson JM, Gillespie IN, et al: Complete pre-operative imaging assessment of abdominal aortic aneurysm with spiral CT angiography. Clin Radiol 52:369, 1997.
78. Raptopoulos V, Rosen MP, Kent KC, et al: Sequential helical CT angiography of aortoiliac disease. AJR Am J Roentgenol 166:1347, 1996.
79. Prokop M, Schaefer-Prokop C, Galanski M: Spiral CT angiography of the abdomen. Abdom Imaging 22:143, 1997.
80. Willmann JK, Wildermuth S, Pfammatter T, et al: Aortoiliac and renal arteries: Prospective intraindividual comparison of contrast-enhanced three-dimensional MR angiography and multi-detector row CT angiography. Radiology 226:798, 2003.
81. Broeders IA, Blankensteijn JD: Preoperative imaging of the aortoiliac anatomy in endovascular aneurysm surgery. Semin Vasc Surg 12:306, 1999.
82. Lutz AM, Willmann JK, Pfammatter T, et al: Evaluation of aortoiliac aneurysm before endovascular repair: Comparison of contrast-enhanced magnetic resonance angiography with multidetector row computed tomographic angiography with an automated analysis software tool. J Vasc Surg 37:619, 2003.
83. Whitaker SC: Imaging of abdominal aortic aneurysm before and after endoluminal stent-graft repair. Eur J Radiol 39:3, 2001.
84. Thurnher SA, Dorffner R, Thurnher MM, et al: Evaluation of abdominal aortic aneurysm for stent-graft placement: Comparison of gadolinium-enhanced MR angiography versus helical CT angiography and digital subtraction angiography. Radiology 205:341, 1997.
85. Costello P, Ecker CP, Tello R, Hartnell GG: Assessment of the thoracic aorta by spiral CT. AJR Am J Roentgenol 158:1127, 1992.
86. Costello P, Gaa J: Spiral CT angiography of abdominal aortic aneurysms. Radiographics 15:397, 1995.
87. Masuda Y, Takanashi K, Takasu J, et al: Expansion rate of thoracic aortic aneurysms and influencing factors. Chest 102:461, 1992.
88. Quint LE, Francis IR, Williams DM, et al: Evaluation of thoracic aortic disease with the use of helical CT and multiplanar reconstructions: Comparison with surgical findings. Radiology 201:37, 1996.
89. Czermak BV, Fraedrich G, Schocke MF, et al: Serial CT volume measurements after endovascular aortic aneurysm repair. J Endovasc Ther 8:380, 2001.
90. Amparo EG, Hoddick WK, Hricak H, et al: Comparison of magnetic resonance imaging and ultrasonography in the evaluation of abdominal aortic aneurysms. Radiology 154:451, 1985.
91. Petersen MJ, Cambria RP, Kaufman JA, et al: Magnetic resonance angiography in the preoperative evaluation of abdominal aortic aneurysms. J Vasc Surg 21:891, discussion 899, 1995.
92. Krinsky GA, Rofsky NM, DeCorato DR, et al: Thoracic aorta: Comparison of gadolinium-enhanced three-dimensional MR angiography with conventional MR imaging. Radiology 202:183, 1997.
93. Prince MR, Narasimham DL, Stanley JC, et al: Gadolinium-enhanced magnetic resonance angiography of abdominal aortic aneurysms. J Vasc Surg 21:656, 1995.
94. Engellau L, Albrechtsson U, Dahlstrom N, et al: Measurements before endovascular repair of abdominal aortic aneurysms: MR imaging with MRA vs. angiography and CT. Acta Radiol 44:177, 2003.
95. Haulon S, Lions C, McFadden EP, et al: Prospective evaluation of magnetic resonance imaging after endovascular treatment of infrarenal aortic aneurysms. Eur J Vasc Endovasc Surg 22:62, 2001.
96. Yamada N, Okita Y, Minatoya K, et al: Preoperative demonstration of the Adamkiewicz artery by magnetic resonance angiography in patients with descending or thoracoabdominal aortic aneurysms. Eur J Cardiothorac Surg 18:104, 2000.
97. Kudo K, Terae S, Asano T, et al: Anterior spinal artery and artery of Adamkiewicz detected by using multi-detector row CT. AJNR Am J Neuroradiol 24:13, 2003.
98. Yoshioka K, Niinuma H, Ohira A, et al: MR angiography and CT angiography of the artery of Adamkiewicz: Noninvasive preoperative assessment of thoracoabdominal aortic aneurysm. Radiographics 23:1215, 2003.
99. Nasim A, Thompson MM, Sayers RD, et al: Role of magnetic resonance angiography for assessment of abdominal aortic aneurysm before endoluminal repair. Br J Surg 85:641, 1998.
100. Cabellon S Jr, Moncrief CL, Pierre DR, Cavanaugh DG: Incidence of abdominal aortic aneurysms in patients with atheromatous arterial disease. Am J Surg 146:575, 1983.
101. Ohman EM, Fitzsimons P, Butler F, Bouchier-Hayes D: The value of ultrasonography in the screening for asymptomatic abdominal aortic aneurysm. Ir Med J 78:127, 1985.

102. Twomey A, Twomey E, Wilkins RA, Lewis JD: Unrecognised aneurysmal disease in male hypertensive patients. Int Angiol 5:269, 1986.
103. Allen PI, Gourevitch D, McKinley J, et al: Population screening for aortic aneurysms. Lancet 2:736, 1987.
104. Allardice JT, Allwright GJ, Wafula JM, Wyatt AP: High prevalence of abdominal aortic aneurysm in men with peripheral vascular disease: Screening by ultrasonography. Br J Surg 75:240, 1988.
105. Collin J, Araujo L, Walton J, Lindsell D: Oxford screening programme for abdominal aortic aneurysm in men aged 65 to 74 years. Lancet 2:613, 1988.
106. Shapira OM, Pasik S, Wassermann JP, et al: Ultrasound screening for abdominal aortic aneurysms in patients with atherosclerotic peripheral vascular disease. J Cardiovasc Surg (Torino) 31:170, 1990.
107. Andersson AP, Ellitsgaard N, Jorgensen B, et al: Screening for abdominal aortic aneurysm in 295 outpatients with intermittent claudication. Vasc Surg 25:516, 1991.
108. Spiridonov AA, Omirov Sh R: [Selective screening for abdominal aortic aneurysms by using the clinical examination and ultrasonic scanning]. Grud Serdechnososudistaia Khir (9-10):33, 1992.
109. MacSweeney ST, O'Meara M, Alexander C, et al: High prevalence of unsuspected abdominal aortic aneurysm in patients with confirmed symptomatic peripheral or cerebral arterial disease. Br J Surg 80:582, 1993.
110. Karanjia PN, Madden KP, Lobner S: Coexistence of abdominal aortic aneurysm in patients with carotid stenosis. Stroke 25:627, 1994.
111. Molnar LJ, Langer B, Serro-Azul J, et al: [Prevalence of intraabdominal aneurysm in elderly patients]. Rev Assoc Med Bras 41:43, 1995.
112. al-Zahrani HA, Rawas M, Maimani A, et al: Screening for abdominal aortic aneurysm in the Jeddah area, western Saudi Arabia. Cardiovasc Surg 4:87, 1996.
113. Arnell TD, de Virgilio C, Donayre C, et al: Abdominal aortic aneurysm screening in elderly males with atherosclerosis: The value of physical exam. Am Surg 62:861, 1996.

chapter 39

Surgical Treatment of Abdominal Aortic Aneurysms

Eva M. Rzucidlo
Jack L. Cronenwett

Abdominal aortic aneurysms (AAAs) are a leading cause of death in the elderly. In the United States, ruptured AAAs are the 15th leading cause of death overall and the 10th leading cause of death in men older than age 55.[1] In 1991 AAAs caused more than 8500 hospital deaths in the United States,[2] which underestimates their true number, as 30% to 50% of all patients with ruptured AAAs die before they reach a hospital.[3] In addition, 30% to 40% of patients with ruptured AAAs die after reaching a hospital but without operation.[3] When combined with an operative mortality rate of 40% to 50%,[4-8] this results in an overall mortality rate of 80% to 90% for AAA rupture.[9-11] Unfortunately, this high mortality rate has not changed over the past 20 years despite improvements in operative technique and perioperative management that have reduced the elective surgical mortality rate to less than 5% in most series.[4] Unfortunately, ruptured aneurysms also impose a substantial financial burden on overall health care costs. One report estimated that $50 million and 2000 lives could have been saved if AAAs had been repaired before they ruptured.[12] Another study showed that emergency operations for AAAs resulted in a mean financial loss to the hospital of $24,655 per patient.[13] For all of these reasons, AAAs remain a central focus for vascular surgeons and a common health care problem for all physicians.

DEFINITION

Most aortic aneurysms are true aneurysms, which involve all layers of the aortic wall and are infrarenal in location. As shown by Pierce and colleagues,[14] normal aortic diameter gradually decreases from the thorax (28 mm in men) to the infrarenal location (20 mm in men). At all levels, normal aortic diameter is approximately 2 mm larger in men than in women and increases with age and increased body surface area.[14] Because the average infrarenal aortic diameter was 2 cm for these patients, using a 3-cm definition for an infrarenal AAA was recommended, without the need to consider a more complicated definition based on factors such as gender or body surface area. Although such definitions are useful for large patient groups, in clinical practice with individual patients it is more common to define an aneurysm based on a greater than or equal to 50% enlargement compared with the diameter of the adjacent, non-aneurysmal artery diameter.[15] This is particularly true for patients with unusually small arteries, in whom even a 2.5-cm local dilation of the infrarenal aorta might be aneurysmal if the adjacent aorta was only 1.5 cm in diameter.

DECISION-MAKING FOR ELECTIVE ABDOMINAL AORTIC ANEURYSM REPAIR

The choice between observation and elective surgical repair of an AAA for an individual patient at any given point should take into account (1) the rupture risk under observation, (2) the operative risk of repair, (3) the patient's life expectancy, and (4) the personal preferences of the patient.[16,17] Two recent randomized trials have provided substantial information to assist with this decision-making process. The United Kingdom (UK) Small Aneurysm Trial was the first randomized trial to compare early surgery with surveillance for AAAs 4 to 5.5 cm in diameter in 1090 patients aged 60 to 76 who were enrolled.[18] Those undergoing surveillance underwent repeat ultrasound every 6 months for AAAs 4 to 4.9 in diameter cm and every 3 months for those 5 to 5.5 cm. If AAA diameter exceeded 5.5 cm, the expansion rate was more than 1 cm per year, the AAA became tender, or repair of an iliac or thoracic aneurysm was necessary, elective surgical repair was recommended. At the initial report in 1998, after a mean 4.6 years' follow-up, there was no difference in survival between the two groups. After 3 years, patients who had undergone early surgery had better late survival, but the difference was not significant. It was notable that more than 60% of patients randomized to surveillance eventually underwent surgery at a median time of 2.9 years. The rupture risk among those undergoing careful surveillance was 1% per year.

In 2002 the UK Trial participants published results of long-term follow-up.[19] At 8 years there was a small survival advantage in the early surgery group (7.2% improved survival). However, the proportion of deaths caused by rupture of an unrepaired AAA was low (6%). The early surgery group had a higher rate of smoking cessation, which may have contributed to a reduction in overall mortality. An additional 12% of surveillance patients underwent surgical repair during extended follow-up to bring the total to 74%. Fatal rupture occurred in only 5% of men but 14% of women. Risk of rupture was more than four times as high for women than for men. This prompted the participants to recommend a lower diameter threshold for elective AAA repair in women.

The Aneurysm Detection and Management (ADAM) study conducted at U.S. Department of Veterans Affairs (VA) hospitals was published in 2002.[20] In this trial 1163 veterans (99% male) aged 50 to 79 with AAAs 4 to 5.4 cm were randomized to early surgery versus surveillance. Surveillance entailed ultrasound or CT scan every 6 months with elective surgery for expansion to 5.5 cm, expansion of greater than 0.7 cm in 6 months or greater than 1 cm in 1 year, or development of symptoms attributable to the AAA. CT was used for the initial study with the AAA diameter defined as the maximal cross-sectional measurement in any plane that was perpendicular to the aorta. Ultrasound was used for the majority of surveillance visits, but CT was used when the diameter reached 5.3 cm. Patients with severe heart or lung disease were excluded, as were those who were not likely to comply with surveillance. As in the UK Trial, there was no survival difference after a mean follow-up of 4.9 years. Similarly, greater than 60% of patients in the surveillance arm underwent repair. Initial AAA diameter predicted subsequent surgical repair in the surveillance group, as 27% of those with AAAs initially 4 to 4.4 cm underwent repair during follow-up, compared with 53% of those with 4.5 to 4.9 cm, and 81% of those with 5- to 5.4-cm diameter AAAs. Operative mortality was 2.7% in the early surgery group and 2.1% in the surveillance group. Rupture risk in those undergoing surveillance was 0.6% per year. This trial confirmed the results of the UK Trial demonstrating the lack of benefit of early surgery for AAAs 4 to 5.5 cm even if operative mortality is low. Compliance with surveillance was high in both trials.

Taken together, these two randomized trials indicate that it is generally safe to wait for AAA diameter to reach 5.5 cm before performing surgery in select men who are compliant with surveillance, even if their operative mortality is predicted to be low. However, compliance in these carefully monitored trials of select patients was high. In another VA population, Valentine and colleagues[21] reported that 32 of 101 patients undergoing AAA surveillance were not compliant despite several appointment reminders, and 3 or 4 of these 32 patients experienced rupture. Additionally, the increased rupture risk for women seen in the UK Trial highlights the need to individualize treatment on the basis of a careful assessment of individual patient characteristics (rupture risk, operative risk, life expectancy, and patient preferences).

RUPTURE RISK (also see Chapter 37)

The importance of diameter in determining AAA rupture risk is universally accepted, initially on the basis of a pivotal study reported by Szilagyi and associates in 1966.[22] These authors compared the outcome of patients with large (>6 cm by physical examination) and small (<6 cm) AAAs who were managed nonoperatively, even though at least one half were considered fit for surgery in that era. During follow-up, 43% of the larger AAAs ruptured, compared with only 20% of the small AAAs, although the actual size at the time of rupture is unknown. This difference in rupture rate contributed to a 5-year survival of only 6% for patients with large AAAs compared with 48% for patients with small AAAs. These results were confirmed by Foster and colleagues in 1969,[23] who reported rupture in 16% of AAAs less than 6 cm in diameter, compared with 51% for AAAs greater than 6 cm in patients managed nonoperatively. Modern imaging techniques were not available to accurately measure these aneurysms. Therefore, it is likely that diameter was overestimated by physical examination, such that the "large" 6-cm AAAs in these studies were closer to 5 cm by today's standards. Nonetheless, the influence of size on AAA rupture risk was firmly established and has provided a sound basis for recommending elective repair for large AAAs, especially because both these studies demonstrated a marked improvement in survival after operative repair.[23,24]

Autopsy studies have also demonstrated that larger AAAs are more prone to rupture. In an influential study from 1977, Darling and colleagues[25] analyzed 473 consecutive patients who had an AAA at autopsy, of which 25% had ruptured. Probability of rupture increased with diameter: less than 4 cm, 10%; 4 to 7 cm, 25%; 7 to 10 cm, 46%; and greater than 10 cm, 61%. Sterpetti and associates[26] confirmed these results in a more recent autopsy series of 297 patients with AAAs in which rupture had occurred in 5% of AAAs less than or equal to 5 cm in diameter; in 39% of 5- to 7-cm diameter AAAs; and in 65% of greater than or equal to 7-cm diameter AAAs.[26] Although these autopsy studies have clearly shown the impact of relative AAA size on rupture rate, absolute diameter measurements at autopsy likely underestimate actual size because the aorta is no longer pressurized. Following rupture, size measurement is even more difficult because the AAA is not intact. Furthermore, autopsy series are biased toward patients with larger AAAs that rupture and more likely lead to autopsy than smaller AAAs in asymptomatic patients who die of other causes. Thus, the rupture rates assigned to specific aneurysm diameters by autopsy studies almost certainly overestimate true rupture risk.

The simple observation that not all AAAs rupture at a specific diameter indicates that other patient-specific and aneurysm-specific variables must also influence rupture. Several studies have employed multivariate analyses to examine the predictive value of various clinical parameters on AAA rupture risk. The UK Small Aneurysm Trialists followed 2257 patients over the 7-year period of the trial, including 1090 randomized patients and an additional 1167 patients who were ineligible for randomization.[18] There were 103 documented ruptures. Predictors of rupture using proportional hazards modeling (adjusted hazard ratio in parentheses) were: female gender (3), initial AAA diameter (2.9 per cm), smoking status (never smokers 0.65, former smokers 0.59—both vs. current smokers), mean blood pressure (1.02 per mm Hg), and lower FEV_1 (0.62 per L). The mean diameter for ruptures was 1 cm lower for women (5 cm) compared with men (6 cm). By comparing patients with ruptured and intact AAAs at autopsy, Sterpetti and colleagues also concluded that larger initial AAA size, hypertension, and bronchiectasis were independently associated with AAA rupture.[27] Patients with ruptured AAAs had significantly larger aneurysms (8 vs. 5.1 cm), more frequently had hypertension (54% vs. 28 %), and more frequently had both emphysema (67% vs. 42 %) and bronchiectasis (29% vs. 15%). Thus, in addition to AAA size, these reports strongly implicate hypertension, chronic pulmonary disease, female gender, and current smoking status as important risk factors for AAA rupture.

Women are known to have smaller aortas than men.[28] Intuitively, a 4-cm AAA in a small woman with a 1.5-cm diameter native aorta would be at greater rupture risk than a comparable 4-cm AAA in a large man with a native aortic diameter of 2.5 cm. The validity of this concept, however, has not been proved. Ouriel and colleagues[29] have suggested that a relative comparison between aortic diameter and the diameter of the third lumbar vertebra may increase the accuracy for predicting rupture risk, by adjusting for differences in body size. The improvement in prediction potential was minimal, however, when compared with absolute AAA diameter and the relative risk of gender.

Although a positive family history of AAA is known to increase the prevalence of AAAs in other first-degree relatives (FDRs), it also appears that familial AAAs have a higher rupture risk. Darling and colleagues[30] reported that the frequency of ruptured AAAs increased with the number of FDRs who have AAAs: 15% with 2 FDRs, 29% with 3 FDRs, and 36% with greater than or equal to 4 FDRs. Women with familial aneurysms were more likely (30%) to present with rupture than men with familial AAAs (17%). Verloes and colleagues[31] found that the rupture rate was 32% in patients with familial versus 9% in patients with sporadic aneurysms and that familial AAAs ruptured 10 years earlier (65 vs. 75 years of age). These observations suggest that patients with a strong family history of AAA may have an individually higher risk of rupture, especially if they are female. However, these studies did not consider other potentially confounding factors, such as AAA size, which might have been different in the familial group. Thus, further epidemiologic research is required to determine whether a positive family history is an independent risk factor for AAA rupture in addition to a risk factor for increased AAA prevalence.

In summary, AAA rupture risk requires more precise definition. Currently available data suggest the following estimates for rupture risk as a function of diameter: less than 4-cm AAAs, 0% per year; 4- to 5-cm AAAs, 0.5% to 5% per year; 5- to 6-cm AAAs, 3% to 15% per year; 6- to 7-cm AAAs, 10% to 20% per year; 7- to 8-cm AAAs, 20% to 40% per year; and greater than 8-cm AAAs, 30% to 50% per year. For a given-sized AAA, gender, hypertension, COPD, current smoking status, and wall stress appear to be independent risk factors for rupture. Family history and rapid expansion are probably risk factors for rupture, whereas the influences of thrombus content and diameter ratio are less certain.

EXPANSION RATE

Estimating expected AAA expansion rate is important to predict the likely time when a given AAA will reach the individual threshold diameter for elective repair. Expansion rate is most accurately represented as an exponential rather than a linear function of initial AAA size. Limet and colleagues[32] calculated the median expansion rate of small AAAs to be $e^{0.106t}$, where t equals years. For a 1-year time interval, this formula predicts an 11% increase in diameter per year, nearly identical to the 10% per year calculation reported by Cronenwett and colleagues[33] in 1990. Several more recent studies have confirmed this estimate of approximately 10% per year for clinically relevant AAAs in the size range of 4 to 6 cm in diameter.[6,34-36] In particular, a recent literature review by Hallin and colleagues[6] found mean expansion rates of 0.33 cm/year for AAAs 3 to 3.9 cm, 0.41 cm/year for AAAs 4 to 5 cm, and 0.51 cm/year for AAAs greater than 5 cm. Studies that have identified small AAAs, usually through screening, suggest that the expansion rate may be less than 10% a year for AAAs smaller than 4 cm.[6,37-39]

Although average AAA expansion rate can be estimated for a large population, it is important to realize that individual AAAs behave in a more erratic fashion. Periods of rapid expansion may be interspersed with periods of slower expansion.[40,41] Chang and colleagues[41] found that in addition to large initial AAA diameter, rapid expansion is independently associated with advanced age, smoking, severe cardiac disease, and stroke. The influence of smoking has been confirmed by others.[42-44] The UK Trialists showed that current smoking is predictive of more rapid expansion whereas former smoking is not.[45] In addition to these factors, hypertension and pulse pressure have been identified as independent predictors of a more rapid expansion rate.[6,33,38,46] Finally, Krupski and others[47,48] have shown that increased thrombus content within an AAA and the extent of the aneurysm wall in contact with the thrombus are associated with more rapid expansion.

β blockade has been postulated to decrease the rate of AAA expansion. This was first demonstrated in animal models.[49-53] Subsequent retrospective analyses in humans appeared to corroborate this.[35,54,55] However, two subsequent randomized trials failed to demonstrate any reduction in growth rate with β blockade.[56,57] Furthermore, the randomized trial from Toronto demonstrated that patients taking β blockers had worse quality of life and did not tolerate the drug well.[56] Even when they analyzed only those who tolerated their medication, there was no effect of propranolol on AAA expansion rate.

Doxycycline, 150 mg daily, was shown to slow the rate of AAA expansion in one small randomized trial, whereas roxithromycin, 30 mg daily, was shown to reduce expansion rate in another.[58,59] These antibiotics have activity against *Chlamydia pneumoniae,* which has been shown to be present in many AAAs.[60,61] Vammen and colleagues[62] showed that antibodies to *C. pneumoniae* predicted expansion in small AAAs and suggested that antibody-positive patients may benefit from anti-*C. pneumoniae* treatment. Doxycycline has also been shown to suppress MMP expression in human AAAs and to reduce aneurysm formation in animal models.[63-65] Further research in this exciting area is necessary before routine treatment with these antibiotics can be recommended, but the low incidence of side effects has stimulated some clinicians to use doxycycline treatment for patients with small AAAs under surveillance, especially those at high operative risk.

ELECTIVE OPERATIVE RISK

As expected, considerable variation in operative risk occurs among individual patients and depends on specific risk factors. A meta-analysis by Steyerberg and colleagues[66] identified seven prognostic factors that were independently predictive of operative mortality after elective AAA repair and calculated the relative risk for these factors (Table 39-1). The most important risk factors for increased operative mortality were renal dysfunction (creatinine >1.8 mg/dL), congestive heart failure (CHF) (cardiogenic pulmonary edema, jugular vein distension, or the presence of a gallop rhythm), and ischemic changes on resting ECG (ST depression >2 mm). Age had a limited effect on mortality when corrected for the highly associated comorbidities of cardiac, renal, and pulmonary dysfunction (mortality increased only 1.5-fold per decade). This explains the excellent results reported in multiple series in which select octogenarians have undergone elective AAA repair with mortality comparable with younger patients.[67]

On the basis of their analysis, Steyerberg and colleagues[66] developed a clinical prediction rule to estimate the operative mortality for individual patients undergoing elective AAA repair (Table 39-2). This scoring system takes into account the seven independent risk factors plus the average overall elective mortality for a specific center. To demonstrate the impact of the risk factors on a hypothetical patient, it can be seen that the predicted operative mortality for a 70-year-old man in a center with an average operative mortality of 5% could range from 2% if no risk factors were present to more than 40% if cardiac, renal, and pulmonary comorbidities were all present. Obviously, this would have a substantial impact on the decision to perform elective AAA repair. A similar Bayesian model for perioperative cardiac risk assessment in vascular patients has been reported by L'Italien and colleagues,[68] which demonstrated the added predictive value of dipyridamole-thallium studies in patients with intermediate risk for cardiac death. This study also demonstrated the protective effect of coronary artery bypass surgery within the previous 5 years, which reduced the risk of myocardial infarction or death following AAA repair by 2.2-fold. Although this type of statistical modeling cannot substitute for experienced clinical judgment, it helps identify high-risk patients who might benefit from further evaluation, risk factor reduction, or medical management instead of surgery if AAA rupture risk is not high.

TABLE 39-1 INDEPENDENT RISK FACTORS FOR OPERATIVE MORTALITY AFTER ELECTIVE AAA REPAIR[66]

Risk Factor	Odds Ratio*	95% CI
Creatinine >1.8 mg/dl	3.3	1.5-7.5
Congestive heart failure	2.3	1.1-5.2
ECG ischemia	2.2	1-5.1
Pulmonary dysfunction	1.9	1-3.8
Older age (per decade)	1.5	1.2-1.8
Female gender	1.5	0.7-3

*Indicates relative risk compared with patients without that risk factor.
AAA, abdominal aortic aneurysm; CI, confidence interval.

TABLE 39-2 PREDICTING OPERATIVE MORTALITY AFTER ELECTIVE AAA REPAIR[66]

1. Surgeon-specific average operative mortality:

Mortality (%):	3	4	5	6	8	12	
Score:	−5	−2	0	+2	+5	+10	______

2. Individual patient risk factors:

Age (yr):	60	70	80
Score:	−4	0	+4
Gender:	Female	Male	
Score:	+4	0	
Cardiac comorbidity:	MI	CHF	ECG Ischemia
Score:	+3	+8	+8
Renal comorbidity:	Creatinine >1.8 mg/dl		
Score:	+12		
Pulmonary comorbidity:	COPD, Dyspnea		
Score:	+7		

3. Estimated individual surgical mortality **Total Score:** _____

Total Score:	−5	0	5	10	15	20	25	30	35	40
Mortality (%):	1	2	3	5	8	12	19	28	39	51

Based on total score from sum of scores for each risk factor (line 2), including surgeon-specific average mortality for elective AAA repair (line 1), estimate patient-specific mortality from the table (line 3).
AAA, abdominal aortic aneurysm; CHF, congestive heart failure; COPD, chronic obstructive pulmonary disease; ECG, electrocardiogram; MI, myocardial infarction.

The review of Hallin and colleagues[6] supports the findings of Steyerberg that renal failure is the strongest predictor of mortality with a four- to ninefold increased mortality risk. Cardiac disease (a history of either coronary artery disease, CHF, or prior myocardial infarction) was associated with a 2.6- to 5.3-fold greater operative mortality risk. Older age and female gender appeared to be associated with increased risk, but the evidence was not as strong. Valuable data regarding predictors of operative risk have been generated by prospective trials. In the Canadian Aneurysm Study, overall operative mortality was 4.8%.[69] Preoperative predictors of death were ECG evidence of ischemia, chronic pulmonary disease, and renal insufficiency. The randomized UK Small Aneurysm Trial found older age, lower forced expiratory volume in 1 second (FEV_1), and higher creatinine to be associated with mortality on univariate analysis.[70] With multivariate analysis the effect of age was diminished, whereas renal disease and pulmonary disease remained strong predictors of operative mortality. The predicted mortality ranged from 2.7% for younger patients with below-average creatinine and above-average FEV_1 to 7.8% in older patients with above-average creatinine and below-average FEV_1. The UK Trial participants noted that the Steyerberg prediction rule did not work well for the UK Trial patients. However, they did not gather information on a history of CHF (one of the strongest predictors in Steyerberg's analysis) in the randomized UK Trial. Female gender has also been found to be associated with higher operative risk in several population-based studies using administrative data.[4,66,71,72] However, these databases may suffer from inaccurate coding of comorbidities and thereby lack of ability to fully adjust for comorbid conditions.[73] Gender has not been found to be associated with operative mortality in prospective trials.[69,70]

LIFE EXPECTANCY

Assessment of life expectancy is crucial to determine if an individual patient will benefit from prophylactic repair of an AAA. Most patients with AAAs have been long-term smokers. Most AAA patients also have extensive comorbid disease, particularly coronary artery disease, chronic obstructive pulmonary disease, hypertension, hyperlipidemia, cerebrovascular disease, and cancer.[74-79] Many of these chronic conditions increase operative risk, as noted earlier. In addition, these factors shorten life expectancy. Patients who survive elective AAA repair have a reduced life expectancy compared with the age- and gender-matched population.[80-82] In 2001, Norman and colleagues[83] reviewed 32 publications over 20 years that described long-term survival after AAA repair. They found that the mean 5-year survival after AAA repair was 70%, compared with 80% in the age- and gender-matched population without AAA. Predictors of late death after successful AAA repair include age, cardiac disease, chronic pulmonary disease, renal insufficiency, and continued smoking.[80,84,85] The UK Trial participants found (after adjustment for age, gender, and AAA diameter, but not cardiac disease) that both FEV_1 and current smoking status (plasma cotinine) predicted late death.[85] Table 39-3 shows U.S. census data from 1998 that has been adjusted to reflect the life expectancy of an average patient surviving elective AAA repair. These numbers should be adjusted according to the relative severity of comorbid disease but may be used to guide clinical decision-making.

SURGICAL DECISION-MAKING

In patients with symptomatic AAAs, operative repair is nearly always appropriate because of the high mortality associated with rupture or thrombosis and the high likelihood of limb loss associated with peripheral embolism. Occasionally, high-risk patients or those with short life expectancies may choose to forego emergency repair of symptomatic AAAs, but in general, surgical decision-making for symptomatic AAAs is straightforward.

For those with asymptomatic AAAs the recent randomized trials have provided assurance that the typical male patient can generally be safely monitored with careful ultrasound surveillance until the AAA reaches 5.5 cm, at which time elective repair can be performed. However, decision analyses and cost-effectiveness modeling have previously demonstrated that individual patient rupture risk, operative risk, and life expectancy need to be considered to determine the optimal threshold for intervention.[16,17,86,87] Both the UK and ADAM Trials excluded patients who were considered "unfit" for repair, highlighting the fact that those with high operative risk and short life expectancy should have a threshold diameter greater than 5.5 cm. In the UK Trial, the rupture risk for women was 4.5-fold higher than for men, prompting the authors to recommend a lower threshold for women than men. It seems logical to consider other factors that may make rupture more likely during surveillance as well. In both randomized trials, 60% to 75% of patients undergoing surveillance eventually underwent AAA repair.[20,88] In the UK Trial, 81% of those with initial diameters 5 to 5.4 cm eventually underwent repair. Clearly, for many patients with this size AAA, the question is not *whether* to perform AAA repair but *when*. Therefore, in patients with AAA diameters approaching 5.5 cm whose life expectancy is expected to be more than 5 years and whose operative risk is estimated to be low, the patient should be informed that AAA repair would likely be required within the next few years. This subgroup of patients could be offered surgery at a time when it is convenient for them, with the understanding that waiting for expansion to 5.5 cm has little risk. In these cases patient preference should weigh heavily in the decision-making process. For those with multiple risk factors for rupture, long life expectancy, and low operative risk, it would seem prudent to recommend AAA repair at less than 5.5 cm. Additionally, the ability of the patient to comply with careful surveillance should be considered. Although the recent randomized trials have provided a great deal of information to guide decision-making, clinicians should not adopt a "one-size-fits-all" policy for treating patients with AAA.

TABLE 39-3 LIFE EXPECTANCY (YEARS) FOR PATIENTS WITH AAA BY AGE, GENDER, AND RACE

		MALE		FEMALE	
Age (yr)	Total	White	Black	White	Black
60	13	12	11	14	13
65	11	11	10	12	11
70	10	9	8	10	10
75	8	8	7	9	8
80	6	6	6	7	6
85 and older	5	4	4	5	5

AAA, abdominal aortic aneurysm.

PREOPERATIVE ASSESSMENT

Patient Evaluation

A careful history, physical examination, and basic laboratory data are the most important factors for estimating perioperative risk and subsequent life expectancy. These factors may not only influence the decision to perform elective AAA repair, but they may focus preoperative management to reduce modifiable risk. Assessments of activity level, stamina, and stability of health are important and can be translated into metabolic equivalents to help assess both cardiac and pulmonary risks.[89] As COPD is an independent predictor of operative mortality,[69,70] it should be assessed by pulmonary function studies, as well as room air arterial blood gas measurement in patients who have apparent pulmonary disease. In some cases, preoperative treatment with bronchodilators and pulmonary toilet can reduce operative risk.[90] In more extreme cases, pulmonary risk may substantially reduce life expectancy, and in these cases, formal pulmonary consultation may be helpful to estimate survival. Serum creatinine is one of the most important predictors of operative mortality[69] and must be assessed. The impact of other diseases, such as malignancy, on expected survival should also be carefully considered.

It is well established that patients with AAAs have a high prevalence of coronary artery disease (CAD). By performing routine preoperative coronary arteriography at the Cleveland Clinic, Hertzer and colleagues,[91] in 1979, reported that only 6% of patients with AAAs had normal arteries; 29% had mild to moderate CAD; 29% had advanced compensated CAD; 31% had severe correctable CAD; and 5% had severe uncorrectable CAD. Furthermore, this study established that clinical prediction of the severity of CAD was imperfect, because 18% of patients without clinically apparent CAD had severe correctable CAD on arteriography, compared with 44% of patients whose CAD was clinically apparent. This pivotal study has led to intense efforts to identify risk factors and algorithms that more accurately predict the presence of severe CAD that would justify its correction before AAA repair, or would lead to avoiding AAA repair. A number of clinical parameters, such as angina, history of myocardial infarction, Q-wave on ECG, ventricular arrhythmia, CHF, diabetes, and increasing age have been reported to increase the risk of postoperative cardiac events.[92] Various combinations of these risk factors have been used to generate prediction algorithms for perioperative cardiac morbidity.[89] In general, these algorithms identify low-risk, high-risk, or intermediate-risk patients. For high-risk patients, such as those with unstable angina, more sophisticated cardiac evaluation is required, whereas low-risk patients may undergo elective AAA repair without further testing. For intermediate-risk patients, who comprise the vast majority with AAAs, decision-making is more difficult and may be assisted by additional cardiac testing.[92]

ANEURYSM EVALUATION

Most surgeons recommend a preoperative imaging study using either CT scanning, MRI or MRA, or arteriography. Contrast-enhanced CT scanning appears to be the most useful study for preoperative AAA evaluation when considering information obtained, invasiveness, and cost (also see Chapter 12). This is particularly true for spiral CT scanning, with thin "slices" in the region of interest. This allows not only accurate size measurements but also accurate definition of the relationship of an AAA to visceral and renal arteries. Furthermore, CT scanning aids in the identification of venous anomalies, such as a retroaortic left renal vein or a duplicated vena cava, or renal abnormalities, such as horseshoe or pelvic kidney, which would influence operative techniques and approach. CT scanning is the technique of choice to identify suspected inflammatory aneurysms and may reveal unsuspected abdominal pathology, such as associated malignancy or gallbladder disease. In centers with experience with these techniques, CT angiography has made percutaneous intra-arterial angiography unnecessary in the vast majority of AAA patients.

MRI is comparable with CT scanning in terms of AAA measurement accuracy and other preoperative planning issues (also see Chapter 11). It avoids IV contrast, which may represent an advantage over CT scanning for select patients. Because it is more expensive and time consuming, it also is not as widely used as CT scanning. When MRA is included with this technique, however, it can significantly increase the value in patients where arteriography would otherwise be required.

SURGICAL TREATMENT

For the past 40 years, AAAs have been repaired using the technique of endoaneurysmorrhaphy with intraluminal graft placement, as described by Creech.[93] This procedure is described later in the section on transperitoneal approach. The development of this technique was based in part on the failure of previous "nonresective" operations including aneurysm ligation, wrapping, and attempts at inducing aneurysm thrombosis that yielded uniformly dismal results. AAA thrombosis by iliac ligation combined with axillobifemoral bypass enjoyed a brief resurgence in popularity for high-risk patients but demonstrated a high complication rate, including late aneurysm rupture, and an operative mortality rate comparable with conventional repair in similar patients.[94-98] Thus this technique was similarly abandoned. As an alternative to standard open AAA repair, Shah and Leather and colleagues[99] proposed exclusion of an AAA with bypass to reduce operative blood loss. However, this group has recently published long-term follow-up and no longer recommends this procedure due to persistent flow in the excluded AAA sac and rupture in rare cases.[100] In another attempt to reduce the invasiveness of AAA repair, the use of laparoscopy has been suggested to assist AAA repair. This approach uses laparoscopic techniques to dissect the aneurysm neck and iliac arteries followed by a standard endoaneurysmorrhaphy through a mini-laparotomy. Cohen and colleagues[101] have reported their results in 20 patients to demonstrate the feasibility of this approach, but a clear benefit has not been shown, because the intraoperative, intensive care unit and total hospital duration appear comparable with conventional AAA repair. Further experience with this technique may identify a subgroup of patients for which a laparoscopic-assisted AAA repair is advantageous.

Endovascular AAA (see Chapter 40) repair was introduced by Parodi in 1991 and has rapidly gained in popularity in the United States after reports of clinical trials and subsequent FDA approval.[102] Endovascular AAA repair has been shown to reduce operative morbidity, mortality, length of stay, and disability after surgery.[103-106]

Recovery time is shorter after endovascular repair than open repair.[104,107] However, endovascular repair may not be as durable as open repair.[108-113] Frequent and lifelong surveillance is required after endovascular repair along with reintervention or conversion to open repair in some. There appears to be a small ongoing risk of rupture after endografting as well. Decision analysis suggests that there is little difference between open and endovascular repair for most patients.[111] However, endovascular AAA repair may be preferred for those who are at high operative risk for open surgery. Open surgery may be preferred for younger, healthier patients in whom there is little difference in operative risk between the two strategies, and for whom long-term durability is a concern. For the vast majority of patients, however, patient preference should weigh heavily in the decision-making process. Randomized trials comparing open with endovascular surgery have been completed or are currently under way in Europe and in the VA system in the United States. The DREAM trial group reported lower 30-day mortality and severe complications with endovascular compared with open repair, but the survival difference was not sustained after the first postoperative year.[111a,111b] An additional European trial is under way comparing endovascular repair with observation in high-risk patients. These trials will provide much more information for planning AAA repair in individual patients. However, rapid advances continue to be made in stent-graft technology, and they will need to be considered.

PERIOPERATIVE MANAGEMENT

Preoperative IV antibiotics are administered to reduce the risk of prosthetic graft infection.[114] Ample IV access, intra-arterial pressure recording, and Foley catheter monitoring of urine output are routine. For patients with significant cardiac disease, pulmonary artery catheters are frequently used to guide volume replacement and vasodilator or inotropic drug therapy, both intraoperatively and in the early postoperative period. Mixed venous oxygen tension measuring, available with these catheters, can provide an additional estimate of global circulatory function. Transesophageal echocardiography can be useful in select patients to monitor ventricular volume and cardiac wall motion abnormalities and to guide fluid administration and the use of vasoactive drugs. Despite the frequent usage of pulmonary artery catheters, studies examining their use during AAA surgery have been unable to easily demonstrate added value.[115,116] However, these studies have usually excluded high-risk patients, who are most likely to benefit from such monitoring. As these techniques are not without risk, selective use is probably more appropriate than routine application.

The volume of blood lost during AAA repair often requires blood replacement. Therefore, intraoperative auto-transfusion as well as preoperative autologous blood donation has become popular, primarily to avoid the infection risk associated with allogeneic transfusion. Studies of the cost-effectiveness of such procedures, however, question their routine use.[117-119] Autologous blood donation is less important for elderly patients in whom life expectancy is shorter than the usual time for development of transfusion associated viral illness. Autologous blood donation does not appear to be cost effective in elderly cardiovascular patients because the allogenic blood pool has become safer and the transfusion requirement for elective AAA repairs lower.[117] Intraoperative auto-transfusion during AAA repair is widely used because of the documented safety of this technique.[120] Because it is usually difficult to predict the volume of blood loss during AAA repair, most surgeons employ auto-transfusion in case blood loss becomes extensive. Optimizing oxygen delivery to patients with reduced cardiac output by maintaining an adequate hematocrit appears beneficial in patients undergoing AAA repair. One study has shown that a postoperative hematocrit of less than 28% was associated with significant cardiac morbidity in vascular surgery patients.[121]

Maintenance of normal body temperature during aortic surgery is important to prevent coagulopathy, allow extubation, and maintain normal metabolic function. In a review of patients undergoing elective AAA repair, Bush and colleagues[122] noted significantly more organ dysfunction (53% vs. 29%) and higher mortality (12% vs. 1.5%) in hypothermic patients (temperature <34.5°C) compared with normothermic patients. The only predictor of intraoperative hypothermia was female gender, whereas prolonged hypothermia was related to initial hypothermia, indicating the difficulty in rewarming cold patients. A recent randomized trial found significantly reduced cardiac morbidity (1.4% vs. 6.3%) in patients who were normothermic (36.7°C) versus hypothermic (35.4°C) intraoperatively.[123] To prevent hypothermia, a recirculating warm forced-air blanket should be placed in contact with the patient and IV fluids, including any blood returned from an auto-transfusion device, should be warmed before administration.

ANESTHESIA

Nearly all patients undergo general anesthesia for AAA repair. The supplemental use of continuous epidural anesthesia, begun immediately preoperatively and continued for postoperative pain control, is increasing in popularity.[124] This technique allows a lighter level of general anesthesia to be maintained, while controlling pain through the epidural blockade. Additional benefits may include a reduction in the sympathetic-catecholamine stress response, which might decrease cardiac complications. One randomized trial comparing general anesthesia with combined general-epidural anesthesia demonstrated decreased deaths, cardiac events, infection, and overall complications.[125] However, these benefits were not observed in another randomized trial,[126] suggesting that the details of perioperative management and patient selection may determine the impact of epidural anesthesia. Furthermore, it is possible that the major benefit of epidural anesthesia accrues in the postoperative period, rather than intraoperatively.[127]

Preoperative β-adrenergic blockade is an important adjunct to reduce left ventricular work by decreasing heart rate, blood pressure, and cardiac contractility. This will decrease myocardial oxygen demand to reduce or prevent ischemia. Pasternack and colleagues[128] demonstrated that patients who underwent vascular surgery and received metoprolol immediately before operation had significantly lower heart rates and less intraoperative myocardial ischemia than untreated controls. Mangano and colleagues[129] performed the first randomized, placebo-controlled trial to assess the effect of atenolol (given intravenously immediately before and after surgery and orally during that hospitalization) in patients at risk for coronary artery disease who underwent noncardiac surgery. A significant reduction in mortality extending 2 years after discharge was observed in the atenolol-treated patients (3% vs. 14% 1-year mortality) due to a reduction in death from cardiac causes. In a separate analysis they noted that atenolol-treated patients had a 50% lower incidence of myocardial ischemia during the first 48 hours after surgery and a 40% lower incidence during postoperative days 0 to 7.[130] Patients with perioperative myocardial ischemia were significantly more likely to die within 2 years after surgery. Poldermans and colleagues[131] performed a randomized trial of perioperative β blockade with bisoprolol in patients with abnormal dobutamine echocardiograms undergoing aortic or lower extremity arterial reconstruction. They found that perioperative cardiac death was significantly reduced from 17% (placebo) to 3% (bisoprolol). Additionally, nonfatal myocardial infarction occurred in 17% of those given placebo versus none of those given bisoprolol. A subsequent publication from the same authors demonstrated that during a mean follow-up of 22 months, cardiac events were significantly lower in those who had received perioperative β blockade (12% vs. 32%).[132]

Given this knowledge, it has been suggested that β blockers are underused, likely due to fears about use in patients with COPD or prior heart failure. However, chronic β blocker usage is now known to improve outcomes in patients with heart failure.[133,134] Additionally, Gottlieb and colleagues[133] demonstrated that COPD should not be considered a contraindication for β blockade. They found a 40% reduction in risk of death after myocardial infarction in patients with COPD who were taking β blockers compared with those who were not. In Mangano's trial, the only exclusion criteria were preexisting ECG abnormalities that would preclude detection of new ischemic events. β Blockers were withheld during the trial only for a heart rate of less than 55 beats/min, systolic blood pressure less than 100 mm Hg, acute bronchospasm, current evidence of CHF, or third-degree heart block. The weight of evidence supports the routine use of β blockers for nearly all patients undergoing AAA repair.

CHOICE OF INCISION

AAA repair can be accomplished through an anterior transperitoneal incision (midline or transverse) (Fig. 39-1) or through a retroperitoneal approach (Fig. 39-2). Midline, transperitoneal incisions can be performed rapidly and provide wide access to the abdomen, but they may be associated with more pulmonary complications due to postoperative splinting from upper abdominal pain. Transverse abdominal incisions, just above or below the umbilicus, require more time to open and close but may be associated with fewer pulmonary complications and late incisional hernias, although this has not yet been proved. Retroperitoneal incisions, from the lateral rectus margin extending into the 10th or 11th intercostal space, afford good exposure of both the infrarenal and suprarenal aorta but limit exposure of the contralateral renal and iliac arteries. In addition, this exposure does not allow access to intra-abdominal organs unless the peritoneum is purposely opened so that associated abdominal disease can remain undetected. The left retroperitoneal approach is usually favored over the right for exposure of the upper abdominal aorta because the spleen is easier to mobilize and retract than the liver. The right retroperitoneal approach is used when specific abdominal problems, such as a stoma, preclude the left-sided approach.[135]

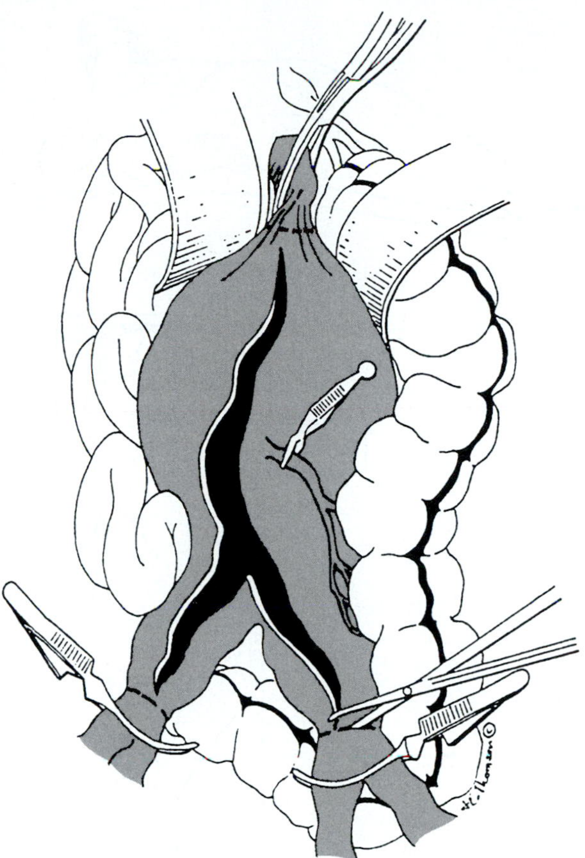

FIGURE 39-1. Transperitoneal abdominal aortic aneurysm exposure, vascular clamps in place, incising the aneurysm.

In recent years the left retroperitoneal approach has enjoyed a resurgence in popularity due to suggestions that pulmonary morbidity, ileus, and IV fluid requirements are decreased postoperatively. Randomized trials have reached different conclusions about the potential advantages of retroperitoneal over transabdominal incisions, however. Sicard and colleagues[136] reported more prolonged ileus, small bowel obstruction, and overall

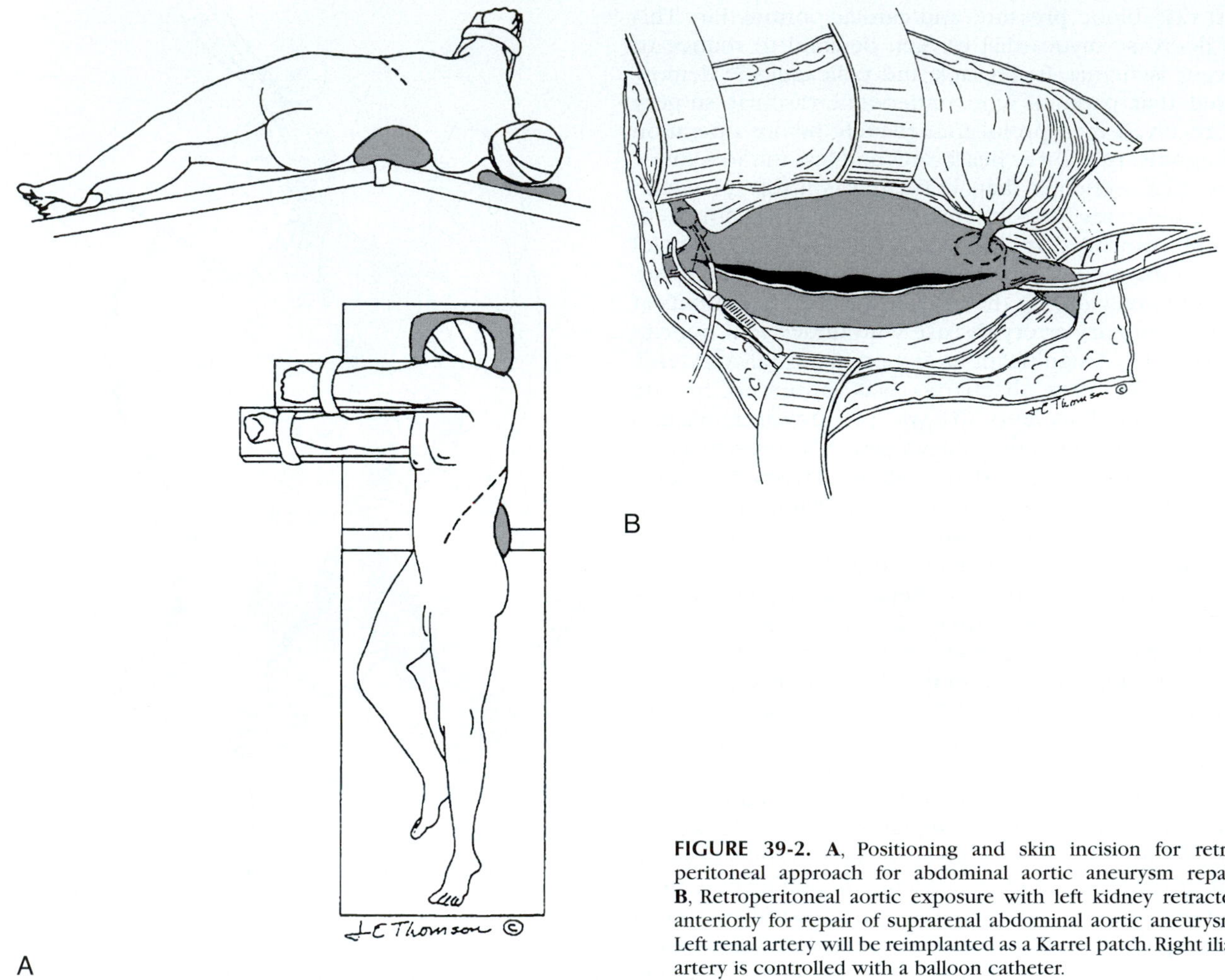

FIGURE 39-2. **A**, Positioning and skin incision for retroperitoneal approach for abdominal aortic aneurysm repair. **B**, Retroperitoneal aortic exposure with left kidney retracted anteriorly for repair of suprarenal abdominal aortic aneurysm. Left renal artery will be reimplanted as a Karrel patch. Right iliac artery is controlled with a balloon catheter.

complications after transabdominal compared with retroperitoneal aortic surgery, although pulmonary complications were similar. Cambria and colleagues[137] found no differences in these incisions in terms of pulmonary complications, fluid or blood requirements, or other postoperative complications, except for slightly prolonged return to oral intake after the transperitoneal approach.

In the most recent randomized trial, Sieunarine and colleagues[138] found no differences in operating time, cross-clamp time, blood loss, fluid requirement, analgesia requirement, gastrointestinal function, intensive care unit stay, or hospital stay for transperitoneal versus retroperitoneal approaches for aortic surgery. In long-term follow-up, however, there were significantly more wound problems (hernias, bulging, and pain) in the retroperitoneal group. These results suggest that in most cases, the choice of incision for AAA repair is a matter of personal preference. However, both the transperitoneal and retroperitoneal approaches have advantages in certain patients. Relative indications for retroperitoneal exposure include a "hostile" abdomen due to multiple previous transperitoneal operations, an abdominal wall stoma, a horseshoe kidney, an inflammatory aneurysm, or anticipated need for suprarenal endarterectomy or anastomosis. Relative indications for a transperitoneal approach include a ruptured AAA, coexistent intra-abdominal pathology, uncertain diagnosis, left-sided vena cava, large bilateral iliac aneurysms, or need for access to both renal arteries. The advantages of each approach make it advisable for surgeons to become proficient with both techniques.

Transperitoneal Approach

After entering the abdomen through a transperitoneal incision, the abdomen is thoroughly explored to exclude other pathology and to assess the extent of the aneurysm. The transverse colon is then retracted superiorly, and the ligament of Treitz is divided to allow retraction of the small bowel to the right. Exposure is greatly assisted using a fixed, self-retaining retractor. A longitudinal incision is made in the peritoneum just to the left of the base of the small bowel mesentery to expose the aneurysm. This incision extends from the inferior border of the pancreas proximally to the level of normal iliac arteries distally. Care must be taken to avoid the ureters, especially if exposure includes the iliac bifurcation where the ureters normally cross. Autonomic nerves to the pelvis course anterior to the proximal left common iliac artery and should be retracted with associated retroperitoneal tissue rather than incised, to prevent sexual dysfunction in men. The left renal vein should be identified and retracted superiorly if necessary to fully expose the neck of the aneurysm. Care must be taken not to avulse renal vein tributaries, particularly a descending lumbar vein, frequently encountered to the left of the aorta, which must be divided before the left renal vein is mobile enough to allow upward retraction. Rarely, proximal exposure cannot be obtained without division of the left renal vein. In such cases, this should be done at its junction with the vena cava to maintain patency of collateral drainage via adrenal and gonadal branches. In most cases reanastomosis is not required but can be performed if renal vein engorgement suggests inadequate collateral drainage.

After obtaining adequate aorto-iliac exposure, the normal aorta and iliac arteries are dissected sufficiently to place a vascular clamp proximal and distal to the aneurysm. Regardless of the proximal extent of an infrarenal AAA, it is desirable to construct the proximal aortic anastomosis near the renal arteries, in order to avoid subsequent aneurysmal degeneration of residual infrarenal aorta. When an AAA approaches or involves the renal arteries, it can be safer to apply the cross-clamp proximal to the celiac artery, rather than between the renal arteries and the superior mesenteric artery (SMA). Green and colleagues[139] demonstrated much higher operative mortality (32% vs. 3%) and renal failure requiring dialysis (23% vs. 3%) after infrarenal AAA repair when clamping was performed between the SMA and renal arteries versus proximal to the celiac artery. They attributed this to the greater likelihood of dislodging atherosclerotic debris in the pararenal aorta as opposed to the supraceliac aorta, which is usually less diseased. Complications resulted from atheroembolization to the kidneys, legs, and intestine or injury to the aorta or renal arteries. Others have also noted the relative safety of clamping the supraceliac aorta, which can easily be accessed by dividing the gastro-hepatic ligament and the diaphragmatic crus.[140] However, aortic clamping between the renal arteries and the SMA is also safe when performed in properly selected patients without extensive plaque in this region.[141] Occasionally it is possible to obtain distal control of an AAA on the aorta, but usually aneurysmal changes or calcification in this location make iliac clamping preferred. A disease-free area of proximal aorta and iliac arteries should be identified for clamping to minimize the possibility of clamp injury or embolization of arterial debris. Some iliac arteries may be so diffusely calcified that clamping without injury is impossible. In such cases internal occlusion with a balloon catheter or extension of the graft to the femoral arteries is required. In most cases it is unnecessary to completely encircle the aorta and iliac arteries, as vascular clamps can be placed in the anterior-posterior direction, leaving the back wall undissected. This minimizes the likelihood of injury to both lumbar and iliac veins. Sometimes posterior arterial plaque necessitates placement of a vascular clamp transversely on either the aorta or iliac arteries, which then require careful posterior dissection precisely on the plane of the artery to avoid venous injury.

AAA repair can be accomplished with a straight ("tube") graft in 40% to 50% of patients, without extension onto the iliac arteries.[142,143] Although concern has been raised about the potential for future aneurysm development in the iliac arteries after tube graft repair of AAAs, late follow-up has shown that this is not clinically significant if the iliac arteries were not aneurysmal at the time of AAA repair.[144] Extension to the iliac arteries with a bifurcated graft for AAA repair is necessary in the remaining 50% to 60% of patients due to aneurysmal involvement of the iliac arteries or to severe calcification of the aortic bifurcation. Extension of the graft to the femoral level is indicated for severe concomitant iliac occlusive disease or rarely because of technical difficulties associated with a deep pelvic anastomosis. Iliac anastomoses are preferred, however, due to decreased infection and pseudoaneurysm complications compared with femoral anastomoses. Prosthetic grafts available for AAA repair include knitted Dacron, knitted Dacron impregnated with collagen or gelatin to decrease porosity, woven Dacron, and polytetrafluoroethylene (PTFE). There is no clear evidence that any of these graft types provides superior outcome. In a prospective randomized comparison of PTFE and Dacron, long-term patency was equivalent, but PTFE had a higher incidence of early graft failure and graft sepsis.[145] In contrast, in a smaller trial with shorter follow-up, PTFE was found to be superior.[146] Most surgeons prefer an impervious graft to avoid the need for preclotting and thus select impregnated knitted Dacron, PTFE, or woven Dacron.[147] This not only saves time and more reliably prevents bleeding through the graft but also allows graft selection to be delayed until the aneurysm is opened so that a graft diameter corresponding to the inner diameter of the normal proximal aorta can be selected. It also allows delayed selection of a straight versus bifurcated graft that may not always be obvious before the aneurysm is open and the distal aorta can be carefully inspected.

Most surgeons use heparin anticoagulation during aortic cross-clamping to reduce lower-extremity thrombotic complications. Heparin dosage varies from 50 to 150 units per kg, based on personal preference. Activated clotting time (ACT) measurement is useful to determine the need for supplemental heparin in prolonged cases and the appropriate dose of protamine sulfate to reverse anticoagulation after declamping.[148] The sequence for applying proximal and distal vascular clamps is selected to apply the initial clamp in the area of least atherosclerotic disease in order to reduce the risk of distal embolization. The aneurysm is opened longitudinally along its anterior surface, away from the inferior mesenteric artery (IMA) in case this requires later reimplantation. The proximal aorta is then incised horizontally at the level selected for proximal anastomosis (see Fig. 39-1). To avoid potential injury to posterior veins, this incision does not need to extend through the back wall of the aorta, although some surgeons prefer complete transection for better exposure. Intraluminal thrombotic material and atherosclerotic debris are extracted from the aneurysm, which usually discloses several backbleeding lumbar artery orifices that require suture ligation. If the IMA is patent, it should be controlled temporarily with a small vascular clamp (see Fig. 39-1) so that its need for reimplantation can be assessed after the

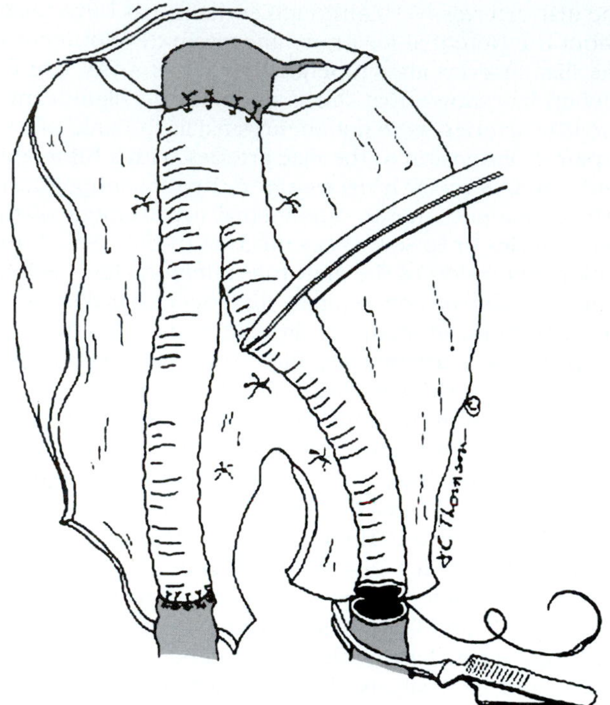

FIGURE 39-3. Completing the iliac anastomosis of an abdominal aortic aneurysm repair. Lumbar artery orifices have been suture ligated. Flow has already been established through the right graft limb.

revascularization is completed. IMA revascularization may be advised if the hypogastric arteries are diseased or if one requires ligation for technical reasons.

Once hemostasis within the opened aneurysm sac has been achieved, the proximal anastomosis is performed. There is often a distinct ring at the aneurysm neck that defines the appropriate level for this anastomosis. Usually polypropylene suture is used, taking large aortic "bites" and incorporating a double thickness of posterior aortic wall for added strength. If the aortic wall is friable, pledgets of Teflon or Dacron can be incorporated into the suture line. After completing the proximal anastomosis, the graft is clamped and the proximal aortic clamp is released briefly to check for and correct any suture line bleeding. If the distal anastomosis is to the aorta, a similar technique is used just above its bifurcation, suturing from within the lumen and encompassing both iliac artery orifices within the suture line. If iliac artery aneurysms exist, these are incised anteriorly so that the limbs of a bifurcated graft can be sutured to the normal iliac artery beyond these aneurysms (Fig. 39-3). Often this requires graft extension to the common iliac bifurcation, including the orifices of both the internal and external iliac arteries within the distal anastomosis. In rare instances, aneurysmal involvement of the distal common iliac artery may preclude anastomosis to both the internal and external iliac artery orifices because these are widely separated. In such cases, an external iliac artery anastomosis can be constructed, but care must be taken to preserve adequate pelvic blood flow, which may mean direct revascularization of at least one internal iliac artery. The need for internal iliac revascularization is usually assessed by the extent of back-bleeding, as discussed later in this chapter (isolated iliac aneurysms). For large aneurysms of the left iliac artery, medial reflection of the sigmoid mesocolon assists a retroperitoneal approach to the distal common iliac artery and prevents unnecessary dissection of autonomic nerves crossing the proximal left common iliac artery. Before completing the distal anastomoses, arterial clamps are carefully removed and vigorous irrigation is used to flush out any thrombus or debris.

When the first iliac (or distal aortic) anastomosis is completed, flow into that extremity should be restored, releasing the clamp slowly to minimize "declamping" hypotension. Declamping shock is rare if adequate IV fluid replacement has been administered. However, sudden restoration of blood flow into a dilated distal vascular bed and the associated venous return of vasoactive substances that have accumulated in the ischemic limbs usually causes some hypotension. Declamping should therefore be gradual and carefully coordinated with the anesthesia team, because additional volume administration can be required. In some cases the clamp must be intermittently reapplied to allow adequate volume resuscitation and prevent hypotension. After restoration of lower-extremity and pelvic blood flow, the IMA and sigmoid colon are inspected.

The IMA can be ligated with a transfixing suture applied to its internal orifice if it is small and not associated with known SMA occlusive disease; if it has good backflow on release of its vascular clamp; if the sigmoid color and arterial pulsations are good; and if at least one internal iliac artery is patent. In questionable cases Doppler signals from the sigmoid colon or an assessment of IMA stump pressure[149] may be necessary to determine the need for IMA reimplantation. In the rare circumstances when sigmoid colon perfusion appears marginal, a circular cuff of the aortic wall around the IMA orifice is excised (Karrel patch) and anastomosed to the left side of the graft (Fig. 39-4). Next, the adequacy of lower-extremity blood flow is determined by visual inspection of the feet, palpation of distal pulses, or more sophisticated

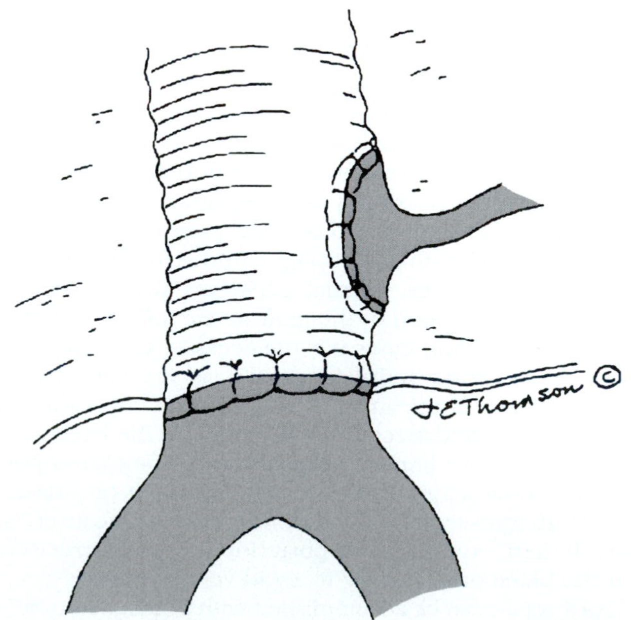

FIGURE 39-4. Reimplanting inferior mesenteric artery with a Karrel patch technique after abdominal aortic aneurysm repair with tube graft.

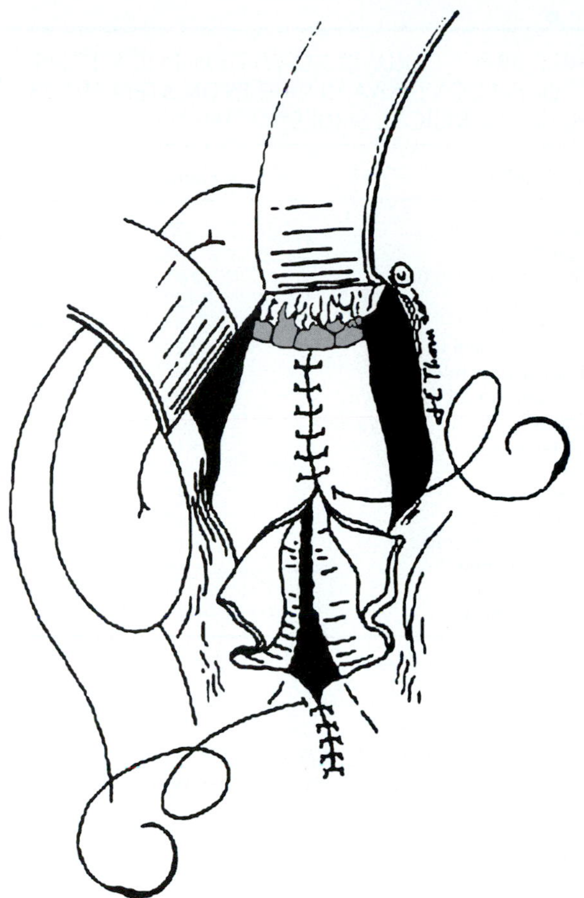

FIGURE 39-5. Closing aneurysm sac and retroperitoneum between graft and duodenum.

Doppler or pulse volume recording. If reduced blood flow is detected, intraoperative arteriography can differentiate thrombosis or embolism from peripheral vasoconstriction, which is relatively common if the procedure is prolonged and the patient is cold. Embolism or thrombosis requires prompt surgical correction, whereas vasoconstriction requires correction of any volume deficit and rewarming. After assuring adequate intestinal and lower-extremity circulation, heparin is reversed with protamine sulfate if sufficient heparin has been given to justify reversal, and hemostasis is achieved. The aneurysm wall and retroperitoneum are then closed over the graft to provide a tissue barrier between the prosthesis and the adjacent intestine (Fig. 39-5). The aortic prosthesis and upper anastomosis must be isolated from the overlying duodenum during closure; if necessary, a pedicle of greater omentum can be interposed to achieve this purpose. The small bowel should be inspected carefully and replaced in its normal position before abdominal closure.

Retroperitoneal Approach

Proper patient positioning is essential to achieve optimal exposure using the retroperitoneal approach. For most infrarenal AAAs a left retroperitoneal incision centered on the 11th or 12th rib is employed. The patient's left shoulder is elevated at a 45- to 60-degree angle relative to the table while the pelvis is positioned relatively flat. The table is flexed with the break positioned at a level midway between the iliac crest and the costal margin (see Fig. 39-2*A*). An air-evacuating "bean bag" is helpful to maintain proper positioning. Beginning at the lateral border of the left rectus muscle midway between the pubis and umbilicus, the skin incision is carried superiorly and then curved laterally up to the tip of the 11th or 12th rib. If extensive exposure of the right iliac artery is required, the incision can be extended inferolaterally into the right lower quadrant, or a separate right lower quadrant retroperitoneal incision can be used. The underlying lateral abdominal wall muscles are divided, exposing the underlying peritoneum and the anterior edge of the properitoneal fat layer at the lateral aspect of this exposure. Dissection in the retroperitoneal plane is then developed, either anterior or posterior to the left kidney, until the aorta is encountered.

For infrarenal aneurysm exposure, it is often sufficient to proceed anteriorly and leave the left kidney in its normal position. For juxtarenal or suprarenal aneurysms that require more cephalad exposure, the kidney is mobilized anteriorly to approach the aorta from behind the left renal artery (see Fig. 39-2*B*). If the need for higher exposure is anticipated, the incision should be directed more cephalad over the 9th or 10th rib and the shoulders positioned as perpendicularly as possible to the table. In this case, more table flexion is required to open the space between the pelvis and ribs and the trunk is twisted so that the angle between the pelvis and the table is about 30 degrees. When approaching the aorta from behind the left renal artery, it is necessary to divide a large lumbar branch of the left renal vein to mobilize the kidney and renal vein anteriorly. The ureter must be identified and retracted medially with the kidney, taking care to separate it from the iliac bifurcation distally.

Medial mobilization of the peritoneal contents exposes the IMA, which usually is divided for more complete exposure of the aortic bifurcation and right renal artery, depending on the size of the AAA. Exposure is greatly assisted by using a fixed, self-retaining retractor. If necessary, exposure of the right iliac artery and right renal artery is easier after opening and decompressing the AAA. Right iliac artery control is often best accomplished by using a balloon occlusion catheter after entering the aneurysm (see Fig. 39-2*B*). After achieving adequate exposure, repair of the AAAs is usually carried out as described earlier for the transperitoneal approach. The retroperitoneal technique does not normally afford an opportunity to inspect colonic and intestinal viability, but the peritoneum can be opened to accomplish this if any concern exists.

Associated Arterial Disease

Indications for concomitant mesenteric or renal artery revascularization during elective AAA repair are comparable with those used for isolated disease in these arteries. Occasionally, patients with asymptomatic, high-grade stenoses of these arteries warrant "prophylactic" concomitant reconstruction, if the patient is at low operative risk and the AAA repair proceeds uneventfully. Although the natural history of asymptomatic mesenteric artery stenosis is not well characterized, it appears that patients with critical disease of all three mesenteric arteries are at sufficiently high risk for future complications of mesenteric ischemia that concomitant revascularization is justified.[150] Progression of renal artery stenosis has been better documented,[151,152] but the ultimate clinical impact of such progression appears minimal in nonhypertensive patients with normal renal function.[153] The adjacency of the renal arteries to the operative field for AAA repair has led some to recommend prophylactic repair of critical but asymptomatic renal artery stenoses.[154] Although this may be appropriate in younger, good-risk patients, it adds morbidity and mortality to the AAA repair, leading others to recommend the combined procedure only for standard indications of hypertension or ischemic nephropathy.[155,156]

COMPLICATIONS OF AAA REPAIR

Despite major improvements in the outcome of elective AAA repair, major complications occur and must be correctly managed or avoided to maintain the low mortality necessary to justify prophylactic AAA repair. Myocardial infarction is the leading single-organ cause of both early and late mortality in patients undergoing AAA repair[69] and must be carefully assessed and managed to reduce mortality. In a recent review of patients undergoing elective AAA repair, however, Huber and colleagues[119] found that multisystem organ failure (MSOF) caused more deaths (57%) than cardiac events (25%). Visceral organ dysfunction was the most common cause of MSOF, followed by postoperative pneumonia. However, most patients with MSOF had associated cardiac dysfunction, which may have aggravated visceral ischemic injury. Several factors may be responsible for the emergence of MSOF as a more prominent cause of death following elective AAA repair. First, with modern techniques of intensive care, it is uncommon for patients to die with single-system failure (even cardiac) following AAA repair. Second, strict attention to cardiac risk in these patients may have reduced the relative impact of cardiac complications. Finally, older patients with more associated visceral and renal artery disease underwent AAA repair in this series and had the highest likelihood of MSOF postoperatively. The relative frequency of single system complications following elective AAA repair is listed in Table 39-4.

TABLE 39-4 EARLY (30-DAY) COMPLICATIONS AFTER ELECTIVE AAA REPAIR ESTIMATED FROM RECENT SURGICAL SERIES[69,142,143,183-185]

Complication	Frequency
Death	<5%
All cardiac	15%
Myocardial infarction	2-8%
All pulmonary	8-12%
Pneumonia	5%
Renal insufficiency	5-12%
Dialysis dependent	1-6%
Deep vein thrombosis	8%
Bleeding	2-5%
Ureteral injury	<1%
Stroke	1%
Leg ischemia	1-4%
Colon ischemia	1%
Spinal cord ischemia	<1%
Wound infection	<5%
Graft infection	<1%
Graft thrombosis	<1%

AAA, abdominal aortic aneurysm.

Cardiac Complications

The majority of cardiac ischemic events occur within the first 2 days following surgery, during which time intensive care monitoring is appropriate for high-risk patients. Maximizing myocardial function with adequate preload, controlling oxygen consumption by the reduced heart rate and blood-pressure product, ensuring adequate oxygenation, and establishing effective analgesia are important techniques for preventing myocardial ischemia postoperatively. Patients with cardiac dysfunction have a greater risk of myocardial infarction when the postoperative hematocrit is less than 28%, even though this is well tolerated by normal individuals.[157] Postoperative epidural analgesia, in addition to providing excellent pain control, may reduce myocardial complications by decreasing the catecholamine stress response.[125]

Hemorrhage

Intraoperative or postoperative hemorrhage usually results from difficulties with the proximal aortic anastomosis or from iatrogenic venous injury. Proximal suture line bleeding, particularly when posterior, can be difficult to control, especially if the proximal anastomosis is juxtarenal. Venous bleeding usually results from injury to the iliac or left renal veins during initial exposure. Often the distal aortic aneurysm or common iliac aneurysm is densely adherent to the associated iliac vein, making circumferential arterial dissection hazardous. In such cases, vascular clamps can usually be applied successfully without complete dissection of the posterior wall of the iliac artery, or vascular control obtained with balloon occlusion catheters. A posterior left renal vein or a large lumbar vein may pose similar hazards during the proximal dissection. If undetected by preoperative CT scanning, such anomalies pose a high risk for venous injury. Diffuse bleeding after substantial intraoperative blood loss is usually due to exhausted coagulation factors and platelets, combined with hypothermia. Aggressive rewarming with platelet and coagulation factor replacement is required to overcome this complication.

Renal Failure

Although once common after infrarenal AAA repair, renal failure is now rare, due to adequate volume replacement and maintenance of normal cardiac output and renal blood flow. Precautions are still required, however, to reduce the risk of this complication. Because of the renal toxicity of IV contrast, it is prudent to delay AAA repair following arteriography or contrast-enhanced CT scanning to be certain that renal dysfunction has not been induced. A more likely cause of renal failure following infrarenal AAA repair is embolization of aortic atheromatous debris into the renal arteries during proximal aortic cross-clamping. Preoperative CT scanning may reveal pararenal atheromatous debris or thrombus, which should prompt temporary supraceliac cross-clamping until the infrarenal aorta is open. As preoperative renal insufficiency is the best predictor of postoperative renal failure,[69,158] special precautions are appropriate in such patients. Some evidence supports a beneficial effect of IV mannitol when given before aortic cross-clamping (≈25 g).[158] Although some have advocated maintenance of higher urine volume using furosemide, the efficacy of this approach has not been proved and may hinder the assessment of fluid balance by artificially increasing urine output.

Gastrointestinal Complications

Some degree of bowel dysfunction occurs after any major abdominal procedure. However, the paralytic ileus that follows evisceration and dissection of the base of the mesentery during transperitoneal AAA repair often lasts longer than that occurring after other procedures. Consequently, one must use caution in reinstituting oral feeding postoperatively. Anorexia, periodic constipation, or diarrhea is commonly seen in the first few weeks following aneurysm surgery.

Sigmoid colon ischemia following AAA repair is a rare but devastating complication that occurs after approximately 1% of elective AAA repairs.[159,160] This may result from embolization into, or ligation of, the inferior mesenteric artery (IMA) or internal iliac arteries. Although the IMA is often chronically occluded, ligation too far from the aneurysm wall can obliterate important SMA collaterals. Fortunately, the abundance of collateral flow to the sigmoid colon usually prevents ischemia. Sigmoid ischemia is three to four times more likely following ruptured AAA repair, presumably due to the associated hypotension and shock added to the usual risk of this complication.[159-161] Careful inspection of the sigmoid colon following graft placement is important and may be facilitated by Doppler insonation of the bowel wall and mesentery. Preoperatively, patent IMAs should be carefully inspected for back bleeding following the aortic reconstruction and ligated only when back bleeding is pulsatile and colon viability is assured. In questionable circumstances, IMA reimplantation or direct internal iliac revascularization is indicated.[162] Postoperatively, colon ischemia should be suspected in the presence of early diarrhea, usually containing blood; left lower quadrant abdominal pain; unexplained fever or leukocytosis; or excessive IV fluid requirement. This should prompt immediate flexible sigmoidoscopy or colonoscopy. In most cases patchy, partial-thickness mucosal necrosis and sloughing are detected and often resolve with antibiotic therapy and bowel rest. In more severe cases of transmural infarction, however, early reexploration is indicated to avoid the high mortality rate associated with delayed treatment of this complication. Treatment requires sigmoid resection and colostomy, rarely combined with aortic graft excision followed by extra-anatomic bypass if substantial graft contamination has occurred.

Distal Embolization

Lower-extremity ischemia may occur after AAA repair, usually from embolization of aneurysmal debris that occurs during aneurysm mobilization or aorto-iliac clamping. Usually such emboli are small (termed microemboli) and not amenable to surgical removal, and they result in transient, patchy areas of dusky skin or "blue toes" (also see Chapter 48). This can result in persistent pain or skin loss, occasionally necessitating amputation. Some have recommended treatment with low-molecular weight dextran or even sympathectomy for such microembolic lesions, but their management is largely expectant. Occasionally, larger emboli or distal intimal flaps, particularly in diseased iliac arteries, may require operative intervention. For this reason, the legs should be carefully inspected intraoperatively for ischemia after AAA repair while the incision is still open, and arterial access can be easily obtained if necessary.

Paraplegia

Paraplegia due to spinal cord ischemia is rare following infrarenal AAA repair. It can result when important spinal artery collateral flow via the internal iliac arteries or an abnormally low origin of the accessory spinal artery (arterial magna radicularis or artery of Adamkiewicz) is obliterated or embolized during AAA repair.[163] As the accessory spinal artery normally originates from the descending thoracic or upper abdominal aorta, this complication is much more common following thoracoabdominal aneurysm repair.

Impaired Sexual Function

Impotence or retrograde ejaculation may result after AAA repair due to injury of autonomic nerves during para-aortic dissection.[164] The incidence of this complication is difficult to determine due to the multiple causes of impotence in this age group and frequent underreporting. In the recent ADAM Trial in U.S. VA hospitals, 40% of men had impotence before AAA repair.[165] Contrary to most other reports that asked patients retrospectively if they had impotence before AAA repair, in the ADAM Trial, less than 10% developed new impotence in the first year after repair. However, the proportion reporting new impotence increased over time such that by 4 years after AAA repair, more than 60% reported having impotence, which underscores the multifactorial etiology of impotence in this age group. Careful preservation of nerves, particularly as they course along the left side of the infrarenal aorta, around the IMA, and cross the proximal left common iliac artery has been shown to substantially reduce this complication, which has reportedly occurred in up to 25% of patients.[166,167] Other possible causes of postoperative impotence include reduction in pelvic blood flow due to internal iliac occlusion or embolization.

Venous Thromboembolism

Pulmonary embolism and deep vein thrombosis are less common after AAA repair than after other abdominal operations, perhaps due to intraoperative anticoagulation. Unrecognized deep vein thrombosis, however, can occur in up to 18% of untreated patients.[168] Therefore, perioperative prophylaxis with intermittent pneumatic compression stockings or subcutaneous heparin is appropriate.

FUNCTIONAL OUTCOME

Williamson and colleagues[169] recently reviewed their experience with open AAA repair with regard to functional outcome. They found that two thirds of patients experienced complete recovery at an average time of 4 months, whereas one third had not fully recovered at an average time of nearly 3 years. Additionally, 18% said they would not undergo AAA repair again after knowing the recovery process, despite appearing to understand the implications of AAA rupture. Eleven percent were initially discharged to a skilled nursing facility with an average stay of 3.7 months. This is similar to a 9% rate of discharge to a facility other than home, as reported in a review of national administrative data by Huber and colleagues.[170] Although all patients in Williamson's review were ambulatory preoperatively, at a mean of 25 months' follow-up, only 64% were fully ambulatory, whereas 22% required assistance and 14% were nonambulatory. Although it is difficult to determine the extent of this disability that is due to the AAA repair, this report highlights the high rate of disability after open AAA repair. More research into long-term functional outcomes is clearly necessary.

LONG-TERM SURVIVAL

As noted previously, the early (30-day) mortality after elective AAA repair in properly selected patients is less than or equal to 5%, whereas the early mortality after ruptured AAA repair averages 54% (not including patients who died from rupture before repair).[6,16] Five-year survival after successful AAA repair in modern series is approximately 70% compared with approximately 80% in the age- and gender-matched general population.[83,84,143,171-176] Ten-year survival after AAA repair is approximately 40%. Although survival is similar in men and women, women without AAA have longer survival than men. Therefore survival relative to gender-specific norms is lower in women after AAA repair than men.[174] Survival after successful ruptured AAA repair versus successful elective repair was similar in one report[177] but reduced in others.[178,179] In a population-based analysis from Western Australia, survival after ruptured or elective AAA repair was similar for men but significantly reduced for women with ruptured AAA.[174] Overall, survival after AAA repair is reduced compared with an age- and sex-matched population because of greater associated comorbidity in patients with aneurysms.[75,180] Not surprisingly, systemic complications of atherosclerosis cause most late deaths after AAA repair in this predominately elderly, male population. The cause of late deaths after AAA repair are cardiac disease (44%), cancer (15%), rupture of another aneurysm (11%), stroke (9%), and pulmonary disease (6%).[171,180,181] Combining cardiac causes, aneurysmal disease, and stroke indicates that vascular complications account for two thirds of the late deaths following AAA repair.

When outcome is stratified according to these risk factors, the 5-year survival rate improves to 84% in patients without heart disease, which is substantially better than the 54% survival rate observed in patients with known heart disease.[171] Hypertension also reduces 5-year survival after AAA repair, from 84% to 59%.[171] In patients without hypertension or heart disease, late survival after AAA repair is identical to normal, age-matched controls.[172] Multivariate analysis indicates that uncorrected coronary artery disease is the most significant variable associated with late mortality after AAA repair, but that age, renal dysfunction, COPD, and peripheral occlusive disease also contribute.[83,84,143,182] One analysis of coronary artery bypass grafting performed in preparation for AAA repair indicates that it may improve long-term survival in patients younger than age 70 but that older patients do not benefit from this aggressive approach.[182] A recent prospective, multi-centered study identified not only age, cardiac, carotid, and renal disease as independent predictors of late mortality following elective AAA repair but also aneurysm extent, as judged by size, suprarenal extension, and external iliac involvement.[173]

REFERENCES

1. Silverberg E, Boring CC, Squires TS: Cancer statistics, 1990. Cancer 40:9, 1990.
2. Gillum RF: Epidemiology of aortic aneurysm in the United States. J Clin Epidemiol 48:1289, 1995.
3. Bengtsson H, Nilsson P, Bergqvist D: Natural history of abdominal aortic aneurysm detected by screening. Br J Surg 80:718, 1993.
4. Heller J, Weinberg A, Arons R, et al: Two decades of abdominal aortic aneurysm repair: Have we made any progress? J Vasc Surg 32:1091, 2000.
5. Adam DJ, Mohan IV, Stuart WP, et al: Community and hospital outcome from ruptured abdominal aortic aneurysm within the catchment area of a regional vascular surgical service. J Vasc Surg 30:922, 1999.
6. Hallin A, Bergqvist D, Holmberg L: Literature review of surgical management of abdominal aortic aneurysm. Eur J Vasc Endovasc Surg 22:197, 2001.
7. Bown MJ, Sutton AJ, Bell PR, Sayers RD: A meta-analysis of 50 years of ruptured abdominal aortic aneurysm repair. Br J Surg 89:714, 2002.
8. Ernst CB: Abdominal aortic aneurysm. N Engl J Med 328:1167, 1993.
9. Heikkinen M, Salenius JP, Auvinen O: Ruptured abdominal aortic aneurysm in a well-defined geographic area. J Vasc Surg 36:291, 2002.
10. Kantonen I, Lepantalo M, Brommels M, et al: Mortality in ruptured abdominal aortic aneurysms. The Finnvasc Study Group. Eur J Vasc Endovasc Surg 17:208, 1999.
11. Bengtsson H, Bergqvist D: Ruptured abdominal aortic aneurysm: A population-based study. J Vasc Surg 18:74, 1993.
12. Pasch AR, Ricotta JJ, May AG, et al: Abdominal aortic aneurysm: The case for elective resection. Circulation 70:I-1, 1984.
13. Breckwoldt WL, Mackey WC, O'Donnell TF Jr: The economic implications of high-risk abdominal aortic aneurysms. J Vasc Surg 13:798, 1991.

14. Pearce WH, Slaughter MS, LeMaire S, et al: Aortic diameter as a function of age, gender, and body surface area. Surgery 114:691, 1993.
15. Johnston KW, Rutherford RB, Tilson MD, et al: Suggested standards for reporting on arterial aneurysms. Subcommittee on Reporting Standards for Arterial Aneurysms, Ad Hoc Committee on Reporting Standards, Society for Vascular Surgery and North American Chapter, International Society for Cardiovascular Surgery. J Vasc Surg 13:452, 1991.
16. Katz DA, Littenberg B, Cronenwett JL: Management of small abdominal aortic aneurysms: Early surgery vs watchful waiting. JAMA 268:2678, 1992.
17. Brewster DC, Cronenwett JL, Hallett JW Jr, et al: Guidelines for the treatment of abdominal aortic aneurysms: Report of a subcommittee of the Joint Council of the American Association for Vascular Surgery and Society for Vascular Surgery. J Vasc Surg 37:1106, 2003.
18. Brown LC, Powell JT: Risk factors for aneurysm rupture in patients kept under ultrasound surveillance. UK Small Aneurysm Trial Participants. Ann Surg 230:289, 1999; discussion 296.
19. Mortality results for randomised controlled trial of early elective surgery or ultrasonographic surveillance for small abdominal aortic aneurysms. The UK Small Aneurysm Trial Participants. Lancet 352:1649, 1998.
20. Lederle FA, Wilson SE, Johnson GR, et al: Immediate repair compared with surveillance of small abdominal aortic aneurysms. N Engl J Med 346:1437, 2002.
21. Valentine RJ, Decaprio JD, Castillo JM, et al: Watchful waiting in cases of small abdominal aortic aneurysms—appropriate for all patients? J Vasc Surg 32:441, 2000; discussion 448.
22. Szilagyi DE, Smith RF, DeRusso FJ, et al: Contribution of abdominal aortic aneurysmectomy to prolongation of life. Ann Surg 164:678, 1966.
23. Foster JH, Bolasny BL, Gobbel WG Jr, Scott HW Jr: Comparative study of elective resection and expectant treatment of abdominal aortic aneurysm. Surg Gynecol Obstet 129:1, 1969.
24. Szilagyi DE, Smith RF, DeRusso FJ, et al: Contribution of abdominal aortic aneurysmectomy to prolongation of life. Ann Surg 164:678, 1966.
25. Darling RC, Messina CR, Brewster DC, Ottinger LW: Autopsy study of unoperated abdominal aortic aneurysms: The case for early resection. Circulation 56:II161, 1977.
26. Sterpetti AV, Cavallaro A, Cavallari N, et al: Factors influencing the rupture of abdominal aortic aneurysms. Surg Gynecol Obstet 173:175, 1991.
27. Sterpetti AV, Cavallaro A, Cavallari N, et al: Factors influencing the rupture of abdominal aortic aneurysm. Surg Obstet Gynecol 173:175, 1991.
28. Sonesson B, Lanne T, Hansen F, Sandgren T: Infrarenal aortic diameter in the healthy person. Eur J Vasc Surg 8:89, 1994.
29. Ouriel K, Green RM, Donayre C, et al: An evaluation of new methods of expressing aortic aneurysm size: Relationship to rupture. J Vasc Surg 15:12, 1992; discussion 19.
30. Darling RC III, Brewster DC, Darling RC, et al: Are familial abdominal aortic aneurysms different? J Vasc Surg 10:39, 1989.
31. Verloes A, Sakalihasan N, Koulischer L, Limet R: Aneurysms of the abdominal aorta: Familial and genetic aspects in three hundred thirteen pedigrees. J Vasc Surg 21:646, 1995.
32. Limet R, Sakalihassan N, Albert A: Determination of the expansion rate and incidence of rupture of abdominal aortic aneurysms. J Vasc Surg 14:540, 1991.
33. Cronenwett JL, Sargent SK, Wall MH, et al: Variables that affect the expansion rate and outcome of small abdominal aortic aneurysms. J Vasc Surg 11:260, 1990; discussion 268.
34. Hirose Y, Hamada S, Takamiya M: Predicting the growth of aortic aneurysms: A comparison of linear vs exponential models. Angiology 46:413, 1995.
35. Englund R, Hudson P, Hanel K, Stanton A: Expansion rates of small abdominal aortic aneurysms. Aust NZ J Surg 68:21, 1998.
36. Bengtsson H, Ekberg O, Aspelin P, et al: Ultrasound screening of the abdominal aorta in patients with intermittent claudication. Eur J Vasc Surg 3:497, 1989.
37. Guirguis EM, Barber GG: The natural history of abdominal aortic aneurysms. Am J Surg 162:481, 1991.
38. Santilli SM, Littooy FN, Cambria RA, et al: Expansion rates and outcomes for the 3.0-cm to the 3.9-cm infrarenal abdominal aortic aneurysm. J Vasc Surg 35:666, 2002.
39. Vardulaki KA, Prevost TC, Walker NM, et al: Growth rates and risk of rupture of abdominal aortic aneurysms. Br J Surg 85:1674, 1998.
40. Sterpetti AV, Schultz RD, Feldhaus RJ, et al: Factors influencing enlargement rate of small abdominal aortic aneurysms. J Surg Res 43:211, 1987.
41. Chang JB, Stein TA, Liu JP, et al: Risk factors associated with rapid growth of small abdominal aortic aneurysms. Surgery 121:117, 1997.
42. Brady AR, Thompson RW, Greenhalgh RM, Powell JT: Cardiovascular risk factors and abdominal aortic aneurysm expansion: Only smoking counts [abstract]. Br J Surg 90:492, 2003.
43. Lindholt JS, Heegaard NH, Vammen S, et al: Smoking, but not lipids, lipoprotein(a) and antibodies against oxidised LDL, is correlated to the expansion of abdominal aortic aneurysms. Eur J Vasc Endovasc Surg 21:51, 2001.
44. MacSweeney ST, Ellis M, Worrell PC, et al: Smoking and growth rate of small abdominal aortic aneurysms. Lancet 344:651, 1994.
45. Brown PM, Zelt DT, Sobolev B: The risk of rupture in untreated aneurysms: The impact of size, gender, and expansion rate. J Vasc Surg 37:280, 2003.
46. Schewe CK, Schweikart HP, Hammel G, et al: Influence of selective management on the prognosis and the risk of rupture of abdominal aortic aneurysms. Clin Invest 72:585, 1994.
47. Wolf YG, Thomas WS, Brennan FJ, et al: Computed tomography scanning findings associated with rapid expansion of abdominal aortic aneurysms. J Vasc Surg 20:529, 1994; discussion 535.
48. Krupski WC, Bass A, Thurston DW, et al: Utility of computed tomography for surveillance of small abdominal aortic aneurysms. Arch Surg 125:1345, 1990.
49. Brophy CM, Tilson JE, Tilson MD: Propranolol stimulates the crosslinking of matrix components in skin from the aneurysm-prone blotchy mouse. J Surg Res 46:330, 1989.
50. Ricci MA, Slaiby JM, Gadowski GR, et al: Effects of hypertension and propranolol upon aneurysm expansion in the Anidjar/Dobrin aneurysm model. Ann N Y Acad Sci 800:89, 1996.
51. Simpson CF: Sotalol for the protection of turkeys from the development of aminopropionitrile-induced aortic ruptures. Br J Pharmacol 45:385, 1972.
52. Simpson CF, Boucek RJ: The B-aminopropionitrile-fed turkey: A model for detecting potential drug action on arterial tissue. Cardiovasc Res 17:26, 1983.
53. Simpson CF, Boucek RJ, Noble NL: Influence of d-, l-, and dl-propranolol, and practolol on beta-amino-propionitrile-induced aortic ruptures of turkeys. Toxicol Appl Pharmacol 38:169, 1976.
54. Leach SD, Toole AL, Stern H, et al: Effect of beta-adrenergic blockade on the growth rate of abdominal aortic aneurysms. Arch Surg 123:606, 1988.
55. Gadowski GR, Pilcher DB, Ricci MA: Abdominal aortic aneurysm expansion rate: Effect of size and beta-adrenergic blockade. J Vasc Surg 19:727, 1994.
56. Propranolol for small abdominal aortic aneurysms: Results of a randomized trial. J Vasc Surg 35:72, 2002.
57. Wilmink AB, Hubbard CS, Day NE, Quick CR: Effect of propranolol on the expansion of abdominal aortic aneurysms: A randomized study. Br J Surg 87:499, 2000.
58. Vammen S, Lindholt JS, Ostergaard L, et al: Randomized double-blind controlled trial of roxithromycin for prevention of abdominal aortic aneurysm expansion. Br J Surg 88:1066, 2001.
59. Mosorin M, Juvonen J, Biancari F, et al: Use of doxycycline to decrease the growth rate of abdominal aortic aneurysms: A randomized, double-blind, placebo-controlled pilot study. J Vasc Surg 34:606, 2001.
60. Petersen E, Boman J, Persson K, et al: Chlamydia pneumoniae in human abdominal aortic aneurysms. Eur J Vasc Endovasc Surg 15:138, 1998.
61. Juvonen J, Juvonen T, Laurila A, et al: Demonstration of Chlamydia pneumoniae in the walls of abdominal aortic aneurysms. J Vasc Surg 1997;25:499, 1997.
62. Vammen S, Lindholt JS, Andersen PL, et al: Antibodies against Chlamydia pneumoniae predict the need for elective surgical intervention on small abdominal aortic aneurysms. Eur J Vasc Endovasc Surg 22:165, 2001.
63. Petrinec D, Liao S, Holmes DR, et al: Doxycycline inhibition of aneurysmal degeneration in an elastase-induced rat model of abdominal aortic aneurysm: Preservation of aortic elastin associated with suppressed production of 92 kD gelatinase. J Vasc Surg 23:336, 1996.

64. Curci JA, Petrinec D, Liao S, et al: Pharmacologic suppression of experimental abdominal aortic aneurysms: A comparison of doxycycline and four chemically modified tetracyclines. J Vasc Surg 28:1082, 1998.
65. Curci JA, Mao D, Bohner DG, et al: Preoperative treatment with doxycycline reduces aortic wall expression and activation of matrix metalloproteinases in patients with abdominal aortic aneurysms. J Vasc Surg 31:325, 2000.
66. Steyerberg EW, Kievit J, de Mol Van Otterloo JC, et al: Perioperative mortality of elective abdominal aortic aneurysm surgery: A clinical prediction rule based on literature and individual patient data. Arch Intern Med 155:1998, 1995.
67. Kazmers A, Perkins AJ, Jacobs LA: Outcomes after abdominal aortic aneurysm repair in those > or = 80 years of age: Recent Veterans Affairs experience. Ann Vasc Surg 12:106, 1998.
68. L'Italien GJ, Paul SD, Hendel RC, et al: Development and validation of a Bayesian model for perioperative cardiac risk assessment in a cohort of 1,081 vascular surgical candidates. J Am Coll Cardiol 27:779, 1996.
69. Johnston KW: Multicenter prospective study of nonruptured abdominal aortic aneurysm. Part II. Variables predicting morbidity and mortality. J Vasc Surg 9:437, 1989.
70. Brady AR, Fowkes FG, Greenhalgh RM, et al: Risk factors for postoperative death following elective surgical repair of abdominal aortic aneurysm: Results from the UK Small Aneurysm Trial. On behalf of the UK Small Aneurysm Trial participants. Br J Surg 87:742, 2000.
71. Katz DJ, Stanley JC, Zelenock GB: Gender differences in abdominal aortic aneurysm prevalence, treatment and outcome. J Vasc Surg 25:561, 1997.
72. Katz DA, Cronenwett JL: The cost-effectiveness of early surgery versus watchful waiting in the management of small abdominal aortic aneurysms. J Vasc Surg 19:980, 1994; discussion 990.
73. Iezzoni LI: Assessing quality using administrative data. Ann Intern Med 127:666, 1997.
74. Lederle FA, Johnson GR, Wilson SE, et al: The aneurysm detection and management study screening program: Validation cohort and final results. Aneurysm Detection and Management Veterans Affairs Cooperative Study Investigators. Arch Intern Med 160:1425, 2000.
75. Newman AB, Arnold AM, Burke GL, et al: Cardiovascular disease and mortality in older adults with small abdominal aortic aneurysms detected by ultrasonography: The cardiovascular health study. Ann Intern Med 134:182, 2001.
76. Rodin MB, Daviglus ML, Wong GC, et al: Middle age cardiovascular risk factors and abdominal aortic aneurysm in older age. Hypertension 42:61, 2003.
77. Singh K, Bonaa KH, Jacobsen BK, et al: Prevalence of and risk factors for abdominal aortic aneurysms in a population-based study: The Tromso Study. Am J Epidemiol 154:236, 2001.
78. Tornwall ME, Virtamo J, Haukka JK, et al: Life-style factors and risk for abdominal aortic aneurysm in a cohort of Finnish male smokers. Epidemiology 12:94, 2001.
79. Wilmink AB, Quick CR: Epidemiology and potential for prevention of abdominal aortic aneurysm. Br J Surg 85:155, 1998.
80. Johnston KW: Nonruptured abdominal aortic aneurysm: Six-year follow-up results from the multicenter prospective Canadian aneurysm study. J Vasc Surg 20:163, 1994.
81. Batt M, Staccini P, Pittaluga P, et al: Late survival after abdominal aortic aneurysm repair. Eur J Vasc Endovasc Surg 17:338, 1999.
82. Aune S, Amundsen SR, Evjensvold J, Trippestad A: Operative mortality and long-term relative survival of patients operated on for asymptomatic abdominal aortic aneurysm. Eur J Vasc Endovasc Surg 9:293, 1995.
83. Norman PE, Semmens JB, Lawrence-Brown MM: Long-term relative survival following surgery for abdominal aortic aneurysm: A review. Cardiovasc Surg 9:219, 2001.
84. Hertzer NR, Mascha EJ, Karafa MT, et al: Open infrarenal abdominal aortic aneurysm repair: The Cleveland Clinic experience from 1989 to 1998. J Vasc Surg 35:1145, 2002.
85. Smoking, lung function and the prognosis of abdominal aortic aneurysm. The UK Small Aneurysm Trial Participants. Eur J Vasc Endovasc Surg 19:636, 2000.
86. Michaels JA: The management of small abdominal aortic aneurysms: A computer simulation using Monte Carlo methods. Eur J Vasc Surg 6:551, 1992.
87. Schermerhorn ML, Birkmeyer JD, Gould DA, Cronenwett JL: Cost-effectiveness of surgery for small abdominal aortic aneurysms on the basis of data from the United Kingdom small aneurysm trial. J Vasc Surg 31:217, 2000.
88. Long-term outcomes of immediate repair compared with surveillance of small abdominal aortic aneurysms. N Engl J Med 346:1445, 2002.
89. Eagle KA, Berger PB, Calkins H, et al: ACC/AHA guideline update for perioperative cardiovascular evaluation for noncardiac surgery—executive summary, a report of the American College of Cardiology/American Heart Association Task Force on Practice Guidelines (Committee to Update the 1996 Guidelines on Perioperative Cardiovascular Evaluation for Noncardiac Surgery). Circulation 105:1257, 2002.
90. Fagevik Olsen M, Hahn I, Nordgren S, et al: Randomized controlled trial of prophylactic chest physiotherapy in major abdominal surgery. Br J Surg 84:1535, 1997.
91. Hertzer NR, Young JR, Kramer JR, et al: Routine coronary angiography prior to elective aortic reconstruction: Results of selective myocardial revascularization in patients with peripheral vascular disease. Arch Surg 114:1336, 1979.
92. Eagle KA, Coley CM, Newell JB, et al: Combining clinical and thallium data optimizes preoperative assessment of cardiac risk before major vascular surgery. Ann Intern Med 110:859, 1989.
93. Creech O Jr: Endo-aneurysmorrhaphy and treatment of aortic aneurysm. Ann Surg 164:935, 1966.
94. Hollier LH, Reigel MM, Kazmier FJ, et al: Conventional repair of abdominal aortic aneurysm in the high-risk patient: A plea for abandonment of nonresective treatment. J Vasc Surg 3:712, 1996.
95. Inahara T, Geary GL, Mukherjee D, et al: The contrary position to the nonresective treatment for abdominal aortic aneurysm. J Vasc Surg 2:42, 1985.
96. Karmody AM, Leather RP, Goldman M, et al: The current position of nonresective treatment for abdominal aortic aneurysm. Surgery 94:591, 1983.
97. Lynch K, Kohler T, Johansen K: Nonresective therapy for aortic aneurysm: Results of a survey. J Vasc Surg 4:469, 1986.
98. Schwartz RA, Nichols WK, Silver D: Is thrombosis of the infrarenal abdominal aortic aneurysm an acceptable alternative? J Vasc Surg 3:448, 1986.
99. Shah DM, Chang BB, Paty PS, et al: Treatment of abdominal aortic aneurysm by exclusion and bypass: An analysis of outcome. J Vasc Surg 13:15, 1991; discussion 20.
100. Darling RC III, Ozsvath K, Chang BB, et al: The incidence, natural history, and outcome of secondary intervention for persistent collateral flow in the excluded abdominal aortic aneurysm. J Vasc Surg 30:968, 1999.
101. Kline RG, D'Angelo AJ, Chen MH, et al: Laparoscopically assisted abdominal aortic aneurysm repair: First 20 cases. J Vasc Surg 27:81, 1998; discussion 88.
102. Parodi JC, Palmaz JC, Barone HD: Transfemoral intraluminal graft implantation for abdominal aortic aneurysms. Ann Vasc Surg 5:491, 1991.
103. Moore WS, Brewster DC, Bernhard VM: Aorto-uni-iliac endograft for complex aortoiliac aneurysms compared with tube/bifurcation endografts: Results of the EVT/Guidant trials. J Vasc Surg 33:S11, 2001.
104. Matsumura JS, Brewster DC, Makaroun MS, Naftel DC: A multicenter controlled clinical trial of open versus endovascular treatment of abdominal aortic aneurysm. J Vasc Surg 37:262, 2003.
105. Zarins C, White R, Schwarten D, et al: AneuRx stent graft versus open surgical repair of abdominal aortic aneurysms: Multicenter prospective clinical trial. J Vasc Surg 29:292, 1999.
106. Lee WA, Carter JW, Upchurch G, et al: Perioperative outcomes after open and endovascular repair of intact abdominal aortic aneurysms in the United States during 2001. J Vasc Surg 39:491, 2004.
107. Aquino RV, Jones MA, Zullo TG, et al: Quality of life assessment in patients undergoing endovascular or conventional AAA repair. J Endovasc Ther 8:521, 2001.
108. Bernhard VM, Mitchell RS, Matsumura JS, et al: Ruptured abdominal aortic aneurysm after endovascular repair. J Vasc Surg 35:1155, 2002.
109. Harris P, Vallabhaneni S, Desgranges P, et al: Incidence and risk factors of late rupture, conversion, and death after endovascular repair of infrarenal aortic aneurysms: The EUROSTAR experience. J Vasc Surg 32:739, 2000.

110. Holzenbein TJ, Kretschmer G, Thurnher S, et al: Midterm durability of abdominal aortic aneurysm endograft repair: A word of caution. J Vasc Surg 33:S46, 2001.
111. Schermerhorn ML, Finlayson SR, Fillinger MF, et al: Life expectancy after endovascular versus open abdominal aortic aneurysm repair: Results of a decision analysis model on the basis of data from EUROSTAR. J Vasc Surg 36:1112, 2002.
111a. Prinssen M, Verhoeven EL, Buth J, et al: A randomized trial comparing conventional and endovascular repair of abdominal aortic aneurysms. N Engl J Med 351:1607, 2004.
111b. Blankensteijn JD, de Jong SE, Prinssen M, et al: Two-year outcomes after conventional or endovascular repair of abdominal aortic aneurysms. N Engl J Med 352:2398, 2005.
112. Zarins C, White R, Fogarty T: Aneurysm rupture after endovascular repair using the AneuRx stent graft. J Vasc Surg 31:960, 2000.
113. Ohki T, Veith FJ, Shaw P, et al: Increasing incidence of midterm and long-term complications after endovascular graft repair of abdominal aortic aneurysms: A note of caution based on a 9-year experience. Ann Surg 234:323, 2001; discussion 334.
114. Kaiser AB, Clayson KR, Mulherin JL Jr, et al: Antibiotic prophylaxis in vascular surgery. Ann Surg 188:283, 1978.
115. Bender JS, Smith-Meek MA, Jones CE: Routine pulmonary artery catheterization does not reduce morbidity and mortality of elective vascular surgery: Results of a prospective, randomized trial. Ann Surg 226:229, 1997; discussion 236.
116. Ziegler DW, Wright JG, Choban PS, Flancbaum L: A prospective randomized trial of preoperative "optimization" of cardiac function in patients undergoing elective peripheral vascular surgery. Surgery 122:584, 1997.
117. Birkmeyer JD, AuBuchon JP, Littenberg B, et al: Cost-effectiveness of preoperative autologous donation in coronary artery bypass grafting. Ann Thorac Surg 57:161, 1994; discussion 168.
118. Goodnough LT, Monk TG, Sicard G, et al: Intraoperative salvage in patients undergoing elective abdominal aortic aneurysm repair: An analysis of cost and benefit. J Vasc Surg 24:213, 1996.
119. Huber TS, McGorray SP, Carlton LC, et al: Intraoperative autologous transfusion during elective infrarenal aortic reconstruction: A decision analysis model. J Vasc Surg 25:984, 1997; discussion 993.
120. Ouriel K, Shortell CK, Green RM, DeWeese JA: Intraoperative autotransfusion in aortic surgery. J Vasc Surg 18:16, 1993.
121. Nelson AH, Fleisher LA, Rosenbaum SH: Relationship between postoperative anemia and cardiac morbidity in high-risk vascular patients in the intensive care unit. Crit Care Med 21:860, 1993.
122. Bush HL Jr, Hydo LJ, Fischer E, et al: Hypothermia during elective abdominal aortic aneurysm repair: The high price of avoidable morbidity. J Vasc Surg 21:392, 1995; discussion 400.
123. Frank SM, Fleisher LA, Breslow MJ, et al: Perioperative maintenance of normothermia reduces the incidence of morbid cardiac events. A randomized clinical trial. JAMA 277:1127, 1997.
124. Mason RA, Newton GB, Cassel W, et al: Combined epidural and general anesthesia in aortic surgery. J Cardiovasc Surg (Torino) 31:442, 1990.
125. Yeager MP, Glass DD, Neff RK, et al: Epidural anesthesia and analgesia in high-risk surgical patients. Anesthesiology 66:729, 1987.
126. Baron JF, Bertrand M, Barre E, et al: Combined epidural and general anesthesia versus general anesthesia for abdominal aortic surgery. Anesthesiology 75:611, 1991.
127. Raggi R, Dardik H, Mauro AL: Continuous epidural anesthesia and postoperative epidural narcotics in vascular surgery. Am J Surg 154:192, 1987.
128. Pasternack PF, Grossi EA, Baumann FG, et al: Beta blockade to decrease silent myocardial ischemia during peripheral vascular surgery. Am J Surg 158:113, 1989.
129. Mangano DT, Layug EL, Wallace A, Tateo I: Effect of atenolol on mortality and cardiovascular morbidity after noncardiac surgery. Multicenter Study of Perioperative Ischemia Research Group. N Engl J Med 335:1713, 1996.
130. Wallace A, Layug B, Tateo I, et al: Prophylactic atenolol reduces postoperative myocardial ischemia. McSPI Research Group. Anesthesiology 88:7, 1998.
131. Poldermans D, Boersma E, Bax JJ, et al: The effect of bisoprolol on perioperative mortality and myocardial infarction in high-risk patients undergoing vascular surgery. Dutch Echocardiographic Cardiac Risk Evaluation Applying Stress Echocardiography Study Group. N Engl J Med 341:1789, 1999.
132. Poldermans D, Boersma E, Bax JJ, et al: Bisoprolol reduces cardiac death and myocardial infarction in high-risk patients as long as 2 years after successful major vascular surgery. Eur Heart J 22:1353, 2001.
133. Gottlieb SS, McCarter RJ, Vogel RA: Effect of beta-blockade on mortality among high-risk and low-risk patients after myocardial infarction. N Engl J Med 339:489, 1998.
134. Cleland JG, McGowan J, Clark A, Freemantle N: The evidence for beta blockers in heart failure. BMJ 318:824, 1999.
135. Chang BB, Paty PS, Shah DM, et al: The right retroperitoneal approach for abdominal aortic surgery. Am J Surg 158:156, 1989.
136. Sicard GA, Reilly JM, Rubin BG, et al: Transabdominal versus retroperitoneal incision for abdominal aortic surgery: report of a prospective randomized trial. J Vasc Surg 21:174, 1995; discussion 181.
137. Cambria RP, Brewster DC, Abbott WM, et al: Transperitoneal versus retroperitoneal approach for aortic reconstruction: A randomized prospective study. J Vasc Surg 11:314, 1990.
138. Sieunarine K, Lawrence-Brown MM, Goodman MA: Comparison of transperitoneal and retroperitoneal approaches for infrarenal aortic surgery: Early and late results. Cardiovasc Surg 5:71, 1997.
139. Green RM, Ricotta JJ, Ouriel K, DeWeese JA: Results of supraceliac aortic clamping in the difficult elective resection of infrarenal abdominal aortic aneurysm. J Vasc Surg 9:124, 1989.
140. Breckwoldt WL, Mackey WC, Belkin M, O'Donnell TF Jr: The effect of suprarenal cross-clamping on abdominal aortic aneurysm repair. Arch Surg 127:520, 1992.
141. Nypaver TJ, Shepard A, Reddy DJ, et al: Repair of pararenal abdominal aortic aneurysms: An analysis of operative management. Arch Surg 128:803, 1993.
142. Johnston KW, Scobie TK: Multicenter prospective study of nonruptured abdominal aortic aneurysms. I. Population and operative management. J Vasc Surg 7:69, 1988.
143. Olsen PS, Schroeder T, Agerskov K, et al: Surgery for abdominal aortic aneurysms: A survey of 656 patients. J Cardiovasc Surg (Torino) 32:636, 1991.
144. Provan JL, Fialkov J, Ameli FM, St Louis EL: Is tube repair of aortic aneurysm followed by aneurysmal change in the common iliac arteries? Can J Surg 33:394, 1990.
145. Polterauer P, Prager M, Holzenbein T, et al: Dacron versus polytetrafluoroethylene for Y-aortic bifurcation grafts: A six-year prospective, randomized trial. Surgery 111:626, 1992.
146. Lord RS, Nash PA, Raj BT, et al: Prospective randomized trial of polytetrafluoroethylene and Dacron aortic prosthesis. I. Perioperative results. Ann Vasc Surg 2:248, 1988.
147. Piotrowski JJ, McCroskey BL, Rutherford RB: Selection of grafts currently available for repair of abdominal aortic aneurysms. Surg Clin North Am 69:827, 1989.
148. Mabry CD, Thompson BW, Read RC: Activated clotting time (ACT) monitoring of intraoperative heparinization in peripheral vascular surgery. Am J Surg 138:894, 1979.
149. Ernst CB, Hagihara PF, Daugherty ME, Griffen WO Jr: Inferior mesenteric artery stump pressure: A reliable index for safe IMA ligation during abdominal aortic aneurysmectomy. Ann Surg 187:641, 1978.
150. Thomas J, Blake K, Pierce G, et al: The clinical course of asymptomatic mesenteric arterial stenosis. J Vasc Surg 27:840, 1998.
151. Tollefson DF, Ernst CB: Natural history of atherosclerotic renal artery stenosis associated with aortic disease. J Vasc Surg 14:327, 1991.
152. Zierler RE, Bergelin RO, Davidson RC, et al: A prospective study of disease progression in patients with atherosclerotic renal artery stenosis. Am J Hypertens 9:1055, 1996.
153. Dean RH, Benjamin ME, Hansen KJ: Surgical management of renovascular hypertension. Curr Probl Surg 34:209, 1997.
154. Cambria RP, Brewster DC, L'Italien G, et al: Simultaneous aortic and renal artery reconstruction: Evolution of an eighteen-year experience. J Vasc Surg 21:916, 1995; discussion 925.
155. Benjamin ME, Hansen KJ, Craven TE, et al: Combined aortic and renal artery surgery: A contemporary experience. Ann Surg 223:555, 1996; discussion 565.
156. Williamson WK, Abou-Zamzam AM Jr, et al: Prophylactic repair of renal artery stenosis is not justified in patients who require infrarenal aortic reconstruction. J Vasc Surg 28:14, 1998; discussion 20.

157. Nenhaus HP, Javid H: The distinct syndrome of spontaneous aortic-caval fistula. Am J Med 44:464, 1968.
158. Miller DC, Myers BD: Pathophysiology and prevention of acute renal failure associated with thoracoabdominal or abdominal aortic surgery. J Vasc Surg 5:518, 1987.
159. Jarvinen O, Laurikka J, Salenius JP, Lepantalo M: Mesenteric infarction after aortoiliac surgery on the basis of 1752 operations from the National Vascular Registry. World J Surg 23:243, 1999.
160. Bast TJ, van der Biezen JJ, Scherpenisse J, Eikelboom BC: Ischaemic disease of the colon and rectum after surgery for abdominal aortic aneurysm: A prospective study of the incidence and risk factors. Eur J Vasc Surg 4:253, 1990.
161. Welling RE, Roedersheimer LR, Arbaugh JJ, et al: Ischemic colitis following repair of ruptured abdominal aortic aneurysm. Arch Surg 120:1368, 1985.
162. Ernst CB: Prevention of intestinal ischemia following abdominal aortic reconstruction. Surgery 93:102, 1983.
163. Szilagyi DE, Hageman JH, Smith RF, et al: Spinal cord damage in surgery of the abdominal aorta. Surgery 83:38, 1978.
164. DePalma R, Levine SB, Feldman S: Preservation of erectile function after aortoiliac reconstruction. Arch Surg 113:958, 1978.
165. Lederle FA, Johnson GR, Wilson SE, et al: Quality of life, impotence, and activity level in a randomized trial of immediate repair versus surveillance of small abdominal aortic aneurysm. J Vasc Surg 38:745, 2003.
166. Flanigan DP, Schuler JJ, Keifer T, et al: Elimination of iatrogenic impotence and improvement of sexual function after aortoiliac revascularization. Arch Surg 117:544, 1982.
167. Weinstein MH, Machleder HI: Sexual function after aorto-lliac surgery. Ann Surg 181:787, 1975.
168. Olin JW, Graor RA, O'Hara P, Young JR: The incidence of deep venous thrombosis in patients undergoing abdominal aortic aneurysm resection. J Vasc Surg 18:1037, 1993.
169. Williamson WK, Nicoloff AD, Taylor LM Jr, et al: Functional outcome after open repair of abdominal aortic aneurysm. J Vasc Surg 33:913, 2001.
170. Huber TS, Wang JG, Derrow AE, et al: Experience in the United States with intact abdominal aortic aneurysm repair. J Vasc Surg 33:304, 2001; discussion 310.
171. Crawford ES, Saleh SA, Babb JW 3rd, et al: Infrarenal abdominal aortic aneurysm: Factors influencing survival after operation performed over a 25-year period. Ann Surg 193:699, 1981.
172. Hollier LH, Plate G, O'Brien PC, et al: Late survival after abdominal aortic aneurysm repair: Influence of coronary artery disease. J Vasc Surg 1:290, 1984.
173. Koskas F, Kieffer E: Long-term survival after elective repair of infrarenal abdominal aortic aneurysm: Results of a prospective multicentric study: Association for Academic Research in Vascular Surgery (AURC). Ann Vasc Surg 11:473, 1997.
174. Norman PE, Semmens JB, Lawrence-Brown MM, Holman CD: Long term relative survival after surgery for abdominal aortic aneurysm in western Australia: Population based study. BMJ 317:852, 1998.
175. Soreide O, Lillestol J, Christensen O, et al: Abdominal aortic aneurysms: Survival analysis of four hundred thirty-four patients. Surgery 91:188, 1982.
176. Vohra R, Reid D, Groome J, et al: Long-term survival in patients undergoing resection of abdominal aortic aneurysm. Ann Vasc Surg 4:460, 1990.
177. Stonebridge PA, Callam MJ, Bradbury AW, et al: Comparison of long-term survival after successful repair of ruptured and non-ruptured abdominal aortic aneurysm. Br J Surg 80:585, 1993.
178. Kazmers A, Perkins AJ, Jacobs LA: Aneurysm rupture is independently associated with increased late mortality in those surviving abdominal aortic aneurysm repair. J Surg Res 95:50, 2001.
179. Cho JS, Gloviczki P, Martelli E, et al: Long-term survival and late complications after repair of ruptured abdominal aortic aneurysms. J Vasc Surg 27:813, 1998; discussion 819.
180. Hollier LH, Plate G, O'Brien PC, et al: Late survival after abdominal aortic aneurysm repair: Influence of coronary artery disease. J Vasc Surg 1:290, 1984.
181. Hertzer NR: Fatal myocardial infarction following abdominal aortic aneurysm resection. Ann Surg 192:667, 1980.
182. Reigel MM, Hollier LH, Kazmier FJ, et al: Late survival in abdominal aortic aneurysm patients: The role of selective myocardial revascularization on the basis of clinical symptoms. J Vasc Surg 5:222, 1987.
183. AbuRahma AF, Robinson PA, Boland JP, et al: Elective resection of 332 abdominal aortic aneurysms in a southern West Virginia community during a recent five-year period. Surgery 109:244, 1991.
184. Diehl JT, Cali RF, Hertzer NR, et al: Complications of abdominal aortic reconstruction: An analysis of perioperative risk factors in 557 patients. Ann Surg 197:49, 1983.
185. Richardson JD, Main KA: Repair of abdominal aortic aneurysm: A statewide experience. Arch Surg 126:614, 1991.

■ ■ ■ chapter 40

Endovascular Grafts

Matthew J. Eagleton
Sunita D. Srivastava
Gilbert R. Upchurch Jr.

The surgical treatment of abdominal aortic aneurysms (AAAs) dates back centuries. Some of the initial approaches involved techniques similar, in some fashion, to modern endovascular techniques. In 1684, Moore reported on the use of large quantities of wire placed intraluminally into the aneurysm sac in order to induce thrombosis of AAA.[1] Later, electrical currents were passed through the wire to further promote thrombosis. A self-expanding endoluminally placed umbrella device was reported by Colt in the early 1900s to treat AAA.[2] In the mid-1900s, the use of endoluminally placed wire with the passage of electricity through it was revived and remained the procedure of choice until conventional operative therapy of AAA was introduced.[3] Operative repair of AAA evolved during the second half of the 1900s. Early techniques ranged from simple aortic ligation to aortic wrapping with cellophane.[4,5] Neither was successful. In 1951, the first replacement of an aortic aneurysm with an aortic homograft was described by Dubost.[6] Homografts, however, became aneurysmal over time, and the procedure evolved to the use of prosthetic material to reconstruct the aorta.[7,8] This technique was later modified by Creech, who reported on endoaneurysmorrhaphy with intraluminal graft placement, leaving the aneurysm sac in situ[9]; this has become the mainstay of treatment.

Although excellent results have been obtained with conventional aneurysm repair, it remains a complex, challenging operation that initiates great physiologic stress for patients. The pursuit of a less invasive approach to AAA repair has subsequently evolved. Parodi and colleagues[10] reported the first clinical use of endovascular AAA repair. This approach allowed for the intraluminal exclusion of an aneurysm with the placement, through the femoral arteries, of an endograft. The hope was that this would decrease the morbidity and mortality of aneurysm repair and allow repairs to be performed in patients with significant comorbidities. The original endograft was constructed as a Dacron tube sutured to a Palmaz stent. Several generations of endografts have since been developed, tested, and put into general clinical use. With the evolution of aortic endografting, our knowledge of the pathophysiology of AAA has changed. Our understanding of the complexities of this mode of treatment is only just being realized and examined. This chapter reviews what is currently understood about endograft repairs of aortic aneurysms, with the main focus on AAA.

INDICATIONS

The indications for endovascular repair of an AAA remain the same as conventional repair with regard to the size of the aneurysm and its rate of growth. The classic teaching is that rupture rates for aneurysms depend on the size of the aneurysm. Rupture rates of 5% to 7% per year are estimated for aneurysms between 5 and 7 cm in diameter, and a greater than 20% rupture rate per year is estimated for larger aneurysms.[11] Surgical treatment for patients with these larger aneurysms significantly improves mortality compared with observation.[12] Although it is known that small aneurysms do have the potential to rupture, the U.K. Small Aneurysm Trial, which randomized patients with AAAs between 4.5 and 5.5 cm to either surgery or operation, suggested that early repair did not improve survival.[13] The operative arm of this study, however, had a mortality rate of 5.8%, which is high compared with other, large series of elective open AAA repair.[14] Perhaps with lower mortality rates in the operative arm, the conclusions of the study would have been reversed.[15]

Endovascular AAA repair is a "less-invasive" technique than open surgery and offers several potential benefits over conventional AAA repair. It requires small femoral incisions instead of a large abdominal incision, which may decrease the incidence of postoperative pulmonary complications. There is the avoidance of extensive retroperitoneal dissection, which decreases the risk for perioperative bleeding. The period of aortic occlusion is minimal and accounts for the lower incidence of intraoperative hemodynamic changes and metabolic stress compared with patients undergoing open surgery.[16] Given these differences, endovascular aneurysm repair may be ideal in patients who are "unfit" for conventional AAA surgery.[17] Proving its durability as a replacement for conventional surgery in relatively healthy patients is the aim of many clinical trials, and is discussed next.

ANATOMIC REQUIREMENTS

The exact anatomic requirements for placing an aortic endograft vary with device design. There are key aspects of each device and aortic anatomy to be aware of when assessing a patient as a potential candidate for endograft repair. Preprocedural imaging is paramount in order to assess properly the proximal and distal sites of fixation, as well as to assess the path the endograft will traverse before taking its postdeployment position.

Imaging

Successful endograft placement is completely dependent on adequate and accurate preoperative planning. One of the major elements distinguishing preoperative planning in open aneurysm repair from endovascular repair is the latter's increased dependency on imaging to provide information necessary for clinical decisions. Preprocedural imaging allows the surgeon to determine whether a patient is an acceptable candidate for endovascular aortic grafting and which device is best suited for a particular patient; this ultimately allows for determining the proper size of the endograft.

Spiral CT of the abdomen and pelvis is the mainstay of aorto-iliac imaging. The imaging protocol is different from the standard protocol for most abdominal CT scans. Acquisition should use a 1:1.5 helical pitch and 3 to 5 mm collimation.[18] Two- to 3-mm slices are ideal for providing adequate information for stent graft planning. The 2-D images, however, can often be misinterpreted. The axial images may "cut" vessels at an angle, particularly iliac arteries that have some degree of tortuosity—thus creating an ellipse as opposed to visualization of the true lumen diameter. Due to this problem, some physicians recommend 3-D image processing as a better method to evaluate aorto-iliac anatomy for endograft therapy.[19] Although it was common initially to perform an angiogram in addition to CT scan, recent evaluations suggest that high-quality 3-D CT scans alone may provide sufficient data for endovascular graft planning.[20,21] Currently, proprietary products for CT postprocessing provide the ability to evaluate the 3-D reconstruction of the aorto-iliac system rapidly, rotate the images on the screen to obtain better vessel diameter measurements, and provide "virtual endograft" simulation.

Diagnostic angiography, although it may be replaced by developing technologies, still provides a great deal of information regarding aorto-iliac anatomy. It is not, however, useful for luminal diameter measurements. Aneurysms are often lined with thrombus, and thus the image visualized by angiography only represents the flow channel and not the true arterial diameter. Marker catheters can aid in length measurements, although magnification artifacts can vary from 16% to 35%, depending on body habitus, making measurements obtained in this fashion inaccurate.[18] If the aorta or iliac vessels are tortuous, multiple views must be taken in order to obtain an accurate visualization of these arteries.

MRA can provide information similar to that of a CT scan. It, too, can provide thin slice reconstructions and 3-D postprocessing. Its usefulness, however, is often limited by availability and physician expertise. MRA may provide a useful modality in patients with chronic renal insufficiency in order to avoid the use of iodinated contrast agents. Intravascular ultrasound (IVUS) is not routinely used in the preoperative evaluation of an endograft candidate. It is an invasive procedure, often performed at the time of angiography. Images produced by IVUS have a similar problem as viewing axial images on a 2-D CT scan. Unless the catheter remains centerline within the aorta, the images produced will be elliptical, which may also provide shorter than required length measurements. Its primary use is at the time of stent graft placement to assess graft position relative to the renal artery ostia; this can help to diminish the amount of contrast agent required.

Aortic Neck

The aortic neck is defined as the area of the aorta cephalad to the aneurysm in which the aortic endograft is placed (Fig. 40-1). This zone of the aorta is important for two reasons during aortic endografting. First, it is the site of proximal fixation that will prevent the device from migrating distally. Second, a circumferential seal must be obtained between the graft and the aorta in this area in order to prevent leakage of blood into the aneurysm sac. The exact length of aortic neck required is somewhat device dependent, but most commercially available devices require a 15-mm length of aortic neck below the level of the most caudal renal artery. Some investigational devices may allow for shorter necks. Several devices employ the use of a suprarenal, uncovered (or bare) stent to provide additional protection against graft migration. Suprarenal stent fixation may be useful, particularly in patients who have a shorter aortic neck, as it transfers protection against migration to a more normal segment of aorta. The suprarenal stent, however, does not provide any function with regard to creating a circumferential seal.

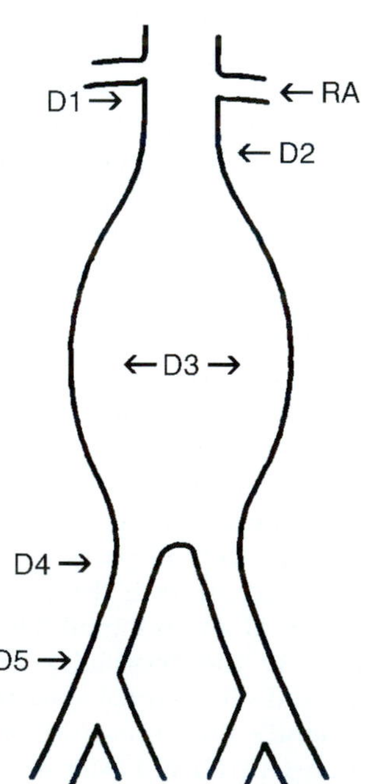

FIGURE 40-1. Diagram representing an abdominal aortic aneurysm. *D1* represents the diameter at the proximal aspect of the aortic neck, and *D2* represents the diameter at the distal aspect of the aortic neck. The distance between *D1* and *D2,* in general, must be 15 mm in order to adequately place an endograft. In addition, the difference between the diameter at *D1* and *D2* should not exceed 10%. *D3* represents the aortic diameter. *D4* and *D5* represent the diameter within the common iliac artery where the distal fixation point of the aortic endograft occurs. The distance between *D4* and *D5* should also exceed 15 mm. *RA* is the left and, in this case, most caudal renal artery.

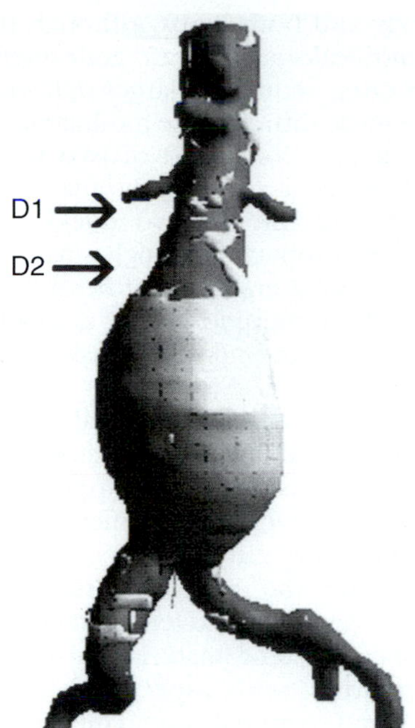

FIGURE 40-2. A three-dimensional reconstruction from a spiral CT scan of an abdominal aortic aneurysm. This is representative of a conical neck. The distance between *D1* and *D2* is 15 mm. The diameter at *D1* is 23 mm and at *D2* is 28 mm, representing a greater than 10% increase. This patient was not a suitable endograft candidate.

In addition to the length of the neck, other anatomic characteristics are important when determining whether patients are suitable candidates for endovascular aneurysm repair. These include aortic neck angulation, the shape of the neck, and the quality of the neck. Neck angulation refers to an alteration in the direction the aorta takes with regard to the centerline pathway. Acute angulation of the aortic neck can greatly affect the endograft's ability to obtain a proximal seal. Aortic neck angulation of greater than 60 degrees compared with the centerline is often considered prohibitive for endovascular aneurysm repair. The shape of the aortic neck also affects the ability of the graft to obtain a seal as well as fixation. A conical-shaped neck (Fig. 40-2) is generally felt to be unstable and predisposes to distal migration.[22] An increase in diameter from the top of the neck to the bottom of greater than 10% is often believed to be a contraindication to routine aortic endografting. The presence of circumferential thrombus or aortic calcification can also negatively affect an endograft's ability to obtain a proximal seal.

Iliac Arteries

The iliofemoral arterial system is important in endograft placement for two reasons. First, most endografts are placed through the common femoral artery and must traverse the iliofemoral system to reach the aorta. Iliac artery diameter and tortuosity can adversely affect the ease with which the endograft traverses this course. This topic is covered in more detail later. Certainly, the presence of significant atherosclerotic disease can cause arterial narrowing that inhibits the placement of the device. In addition, tortuosity of the iliac arteries can hinder placement of the grafts (Fig. 40-3). Second, the

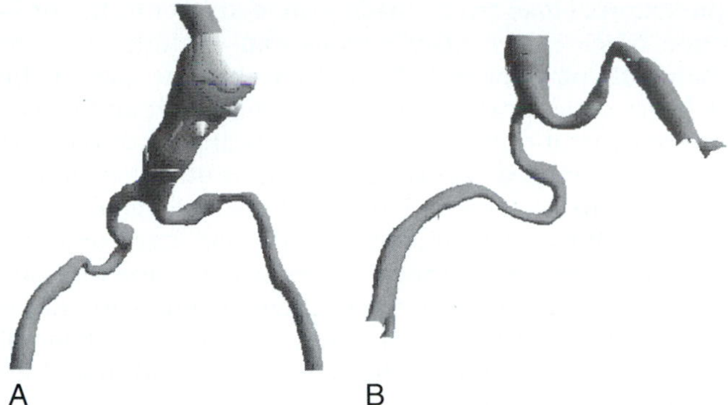

FIGURE 40-3. A three-dimensional reconstruction from a spiral CT scan of an abdominal aortic aneurysm. Note the tortuous iliac arteries **(A)**. The degree of tortuosity may be underestimated in the direct anterior-posterior view, but on a more oblique angle **(B)** a more significant degree of tortuosity is visible.

iliofemoral system is important because it is the site of the distal seal between the endograft and the iliac artery, preventing retrograde flow of blood into the aneurysm sac. Many of the features necessary for an adequate aortic neck are also necessary for the distal landing zone. The presence of thrombus, calcification, and tortuosity can significantly hinder the iliac limb seal. Ectatic or aneurysmal iliac arteries obviously affect the ability of the graft to seal against the iliac limb. Most available endograft systems require at least a 15-mm segment of iliac artery to be of adequate caliber and free of significant disease in order to obtain a distal seal. If this is not present, adjunct interventions can be performed to assist in placing the device (i.e., iliac artery conduit placement or coil embolization of the internal iliac artery). Management of these complicated situations is discussed in more detail later.

ENDOGRAFT DESIGN

Endograft design can greatly affect the ability of the device to be placed in patients, particularly in patients with complex anatomy. Alterations in the characteristics of the grafts are what distinguish one manufacturer's device from another. Some of the key elements in endograft design are outlined as follows.

Delivery System

Standard endograft insertion involves placement of the device through an arteriotomy in the common femoral artery, from where the graft traverses the external iliac and common iliac arteries. The ability to deliver the endograft safely and effectively in this fashion is a prerequisite for effective repair. Three factors are important determinants of device delivery.[23]

Delivery System Size

With the placement of most endografts through the iliofemoral arterial system, any site along this pathway can represent a size limitation, the most common of which is the external iliac artery. Inadequate diameter or the presence of extensive calcifications can exclude standard endograft placement. It is intuitive that the size of the delivery system cannot be larger than the size of the iliac arteries that it traverses. Most sheaths are sized based on inner diameter, so knowledge of the outer diameter of the sheaths is therefore required for safe graft placement.[24] Different manufacturer's devices have different size measurements for the delivery systems, and thus one device may be suitable for placement, whereas another is not. Most delivery systems easily traverse an iliofemoral segment of 7 to 8 mm in diameter (or a sheath that does not exceed 21 French [Fr]).

Flexibility

Another anatomic variant, other than arterial narrowing, that can affect the ability to deliver adequately the endograft system is the presence of tortuous vessels. Tortuous iliac vessels can be "straightened" with the use of stiff guidewires, but this is not always possible or desirable. The ideal delivery system easily traverses these arteries on the basis of an intrinsic degree of flexibility. Again, different delivery systems have different abilities to track through tortuous iliacs, and thus some may be more successfully placed than others in this anatomic variant. Delivery systems composed of long, flexible, tapered tips pass more easily than those with short, stiff, blunt tips.[24] In addition, other aspects of device construction, such as metallic struts that provide columnar strength, increase device rigidity.[23]

Deliverability

A number of features have been noted to affect the deliverability of endograft devices. As stated previously, long, flexible, tapered tips pass more easily than short, blunt, stiff ones. This allows for easier maneuverability through tortuous vessels, as well as past sites of narrowing. Larger-caliber devices are also more difficult to deliver, particularly in patients with smaller-diameter arteries.[23] Some delivery systems allow for the placement of the endograft system through alternate sheaths, whereas other systems necessitate the use of the manufacturer's own delivery system. This can greatly affect the placement of specific endografts in specific anatomic variants. A thorough understanding of the patient's arterial anatomy and the limitations of several different endograft systems are important. The complexity of the delivery system also affects the ease with which it is placed.[23] Some devices generally provide a simple maneuver to deploy the graft, whereas others have several complicated steps.

Endograft Features

The ideal endograft should be flexible enough to maneuver through tortuous and angulated vessels but also rigid enough to prevent kinking. It should have a low profile (having a small external diameter) that would allow it to be placed through as small of an arteriotomy as possible. Two general classifications of endografts exist: unibody and modular. A unibody device is a single-piece graft—including the main body and both limbs. Although this decreases the risk of endoleaks at the graft-graft interface, the unibody design often requires a larger delivery system and sizing can be more difficult. The modular system includes endografts that are composed of two to three pieces. Generally, there is a main body that may have one attached limb and one or two docking limbs. These devices can be introduced through smaller delivery systems and offer a greater degree of flexibility with regard to placement. With multiple sites of graft-graft interface, however, there is an increased risk of endoleak, as explained later.

Graft material is variable from graft to graft and can range from thin-walled polytetrafluorethylene to polyester. The graft material is typically supported by a metal framework, which generally is stainless steel; its modified version, Elgiloy; or nitinol. The graft support can be placed inside the graft material (endoskeleton) or outside the graft (exoskeleton). Grafts can be fully supported, having stent material throughout, or only partially supported, with aspects of the device composed only of graft material and no metal. The graft skeleton provides several key elements to endograft make-up. First, it assists in graft fixation and in obtaining a seal. These stents provide some degree of radial force that helps to provide a seal, as well as providing a point of fixation. Some devices have hooks or barbs in the proximal aspect of the skeleton that help to anchor the graft onto the aortic wall and prevent migration. In addition, some devices employ metal framework that extends above the fabric and is used to engage the aorta in the pararenal or suprarenal location. Although the long-term effects of endovascular manipulation of the aorta in the pararenal location are not known, intermediate results suggest there is no significant development of renal dysfunction or renal artery occlusion.[25] The second function of the skeleton is to provide columnar strength, which may prevent graft migration. The skeleton can also prevent kinking and occlusion of limbs as they traverse the aorto-iliac anatomy. The lack of stents, however, may allow a graft to adapt more readily to morphological changes without dislocation of attachment sites. The interplay of the stent and fabric materials can lead to eventual erosion of the fabric.

Specific Grafts

Various endografts are currently commercially available or in clinical trials in the United States. A brief description of some of these endograft systems is outlined in Table 40-1 and depicted in Figure 40-4.

GRAFT PLACEMENT AND POSTOPERATIVE MANAGEMENT

Once the patient is deemed an endograft candidate, the best graft has been chosen, and the device properly sized, the patient can undergo implantation. The majority of endografts are placed through the femoral arteries that have been operatively exposed. Experience is growing with percutaneously placed endografting; this is discussed

TABLE 40-1 CHARACTERISTICS OF ENDOGRAFT USED TO TREAT ABDOMINAL AORTIC ANEURYSMS

Company	Device	Design	Stent Material	Graft Material	Limb Support
Cook	Zenith	Modular	Stainless steel exoskeleton/ endoskeleton	Woven polyester	Supported
Cordis	Fortron	Modular	Nitinol endoskeleton	Polyester	Supported
Edwards	Lifepath	Unibody	Stainless steel endoskeleton	Thin-walled PTFE	Supported
Endologix	Powerlink	Modular	Elgiloy endoskeleton	Woven polyester	Supported
Gore	Excluder	Modular	Nitinol exoskeleton	ePTFE	Supported
Guidant	Ancure	Unibody	Elgiloy endoskeleton	Woven polyester	Unsupported
Medtronic	AneuRx	Modular	Nitinol exoskeleton	Woven polyester	Supported
Medtronic	Talent	Modular	Nitinol endoskeleton	Woven polyester	Supported

ePTFE, expanded polytetrafluoroethylene; PTFE, polytetrafluoroethylene.

in more detail later. The aorta is then cannulated with a guidewire and catheter. Small boluses of contrast agent are delivered to further define the anatomy and localize the renal arteries. With an angulated aorta, it is important to remember that the best view of the renal arteries and visualization of the fixation zone may not be in a direct anterior-posterior plane but at a more cranial-caudal angle. The device is then generally advanced over a stiff guidewire and correctly positioned to allow the most extensive coverage within the aortic neck without

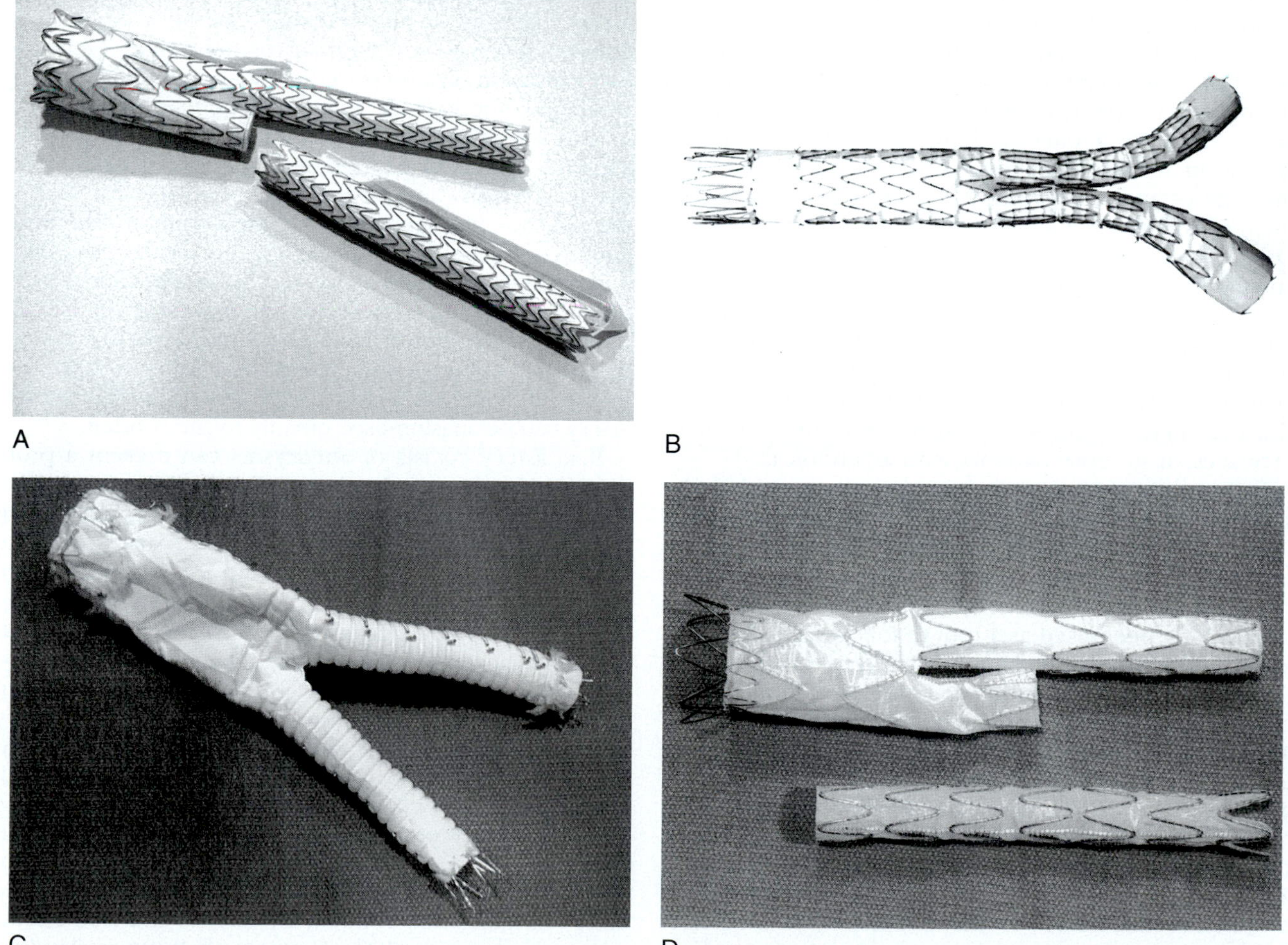

FIGURE 40-4. Several endograft systems illustrating different features. **A,** The Excluder endograft (WL Gore and Associates, Flagstaff, Ariz.), which represents a two-piece modular system. The graft is constructed from expanded polytetrafluoroethylene and is fully supported by a nitinol exoskeleton. **B,** The Zenith endograft (Cook, Inc., Bloomington, Ind.) represents a three-piece modular system with a main body and separate bilateral limbs. This graft design uses a bare suprarenal stent and internal stents at the sealing zones and is otherwise supported by a stainless steel Z-stent exoskeleton. **C,** The Ancure endograft (Guidant, Menlo Park, Calif.) represents a one-piece design and lacks stent support throughout the body of the graft. **D,** The Talent endograft system (Medtronic AVE, Santa Rosa, Calif.) represents a two-piece modular system that is composed of a suprarenal bare stent and then a nitinol endoskeleton.

intruding on the orifice of the renal arteries. Each device has its own unique instruction for actual deployment. Once the main body and ipsilateral limb have been placed, the contralateral limb needs to be placed. The sequence of events for this varies depending on graft design—whether unibody or modular.

Postoperative surveillance is extremely important in patients undergoing endovascular AAA repair. Complications may be asymptomatic at first but may subsequently result in aneurysm rupture, despite having had an endovascular graft in place.[27,28] This complication may not become apparent for years after graft deployment; thus patients require careful lifelong evaluation.[29] Protocols for graft surveillance vary from institution to institution, but most entail four-view abdominal plain radiographic evaluation and CT scanning. Major imaging generally occurs at 1 month, 3 months, 6 months, 12 months, and then yearly. CT scanning is performed with IV contrast and in a similar format as in preoperative scanning. From these images assessments can be made as to graft location, and an evaluation made for evidence of migration, aneurysm size, and the presence of endoleaks.

Another adjunct used to track aneurysms following endograft repair is by calculation of aneurysm volume. Aneurysm volume can be determined from 3-D reconstructions of spiral CT scans. Morphologic changes in the aorta after endograft repair include changes in aorto-iliac and aneurysm lengths.[30] Because of this change in morphology, some physicians believe that a measure of aneurysm volume is a more accurate assessment of changes in aneurysm morphology after endovascular repair. Wolf and colleagues[31] reported that aneurysm volume decreases after endovascular repair and parallels that of maximal aortic diameter. Wolf and colleagues, however, suggest that although in most patients diameter assessment is adequate, volumetric analysis appears to be helpful in patients who do not show aneurysm regression, in whom the aortic diameter increases, or in those patients with an endoleak.[31]

Duplex ultrasound (US) has been suggested to be a less invasive means of following aortic aneurysms following endovascular exclusion. US provides a less expensive alternative to routine CT scanning and does not require the addition of iodinated contrast. Although US has long been used as a tool to follow small AAAs for expansion, the real question is whether it is effective at detecting the development of endoleaks or significant changes in the aortic and endograft morphology. Wolf and colleagues compared US with CT for postoperative evaluation of patients having undergone aortic endografting.[32] US was found to have a sensitivity and specificity of 81% and 95%, respectively, when compared with CT scanning for the detection of endoleaks.[32] Golzarian and colleagues,[33] however, reported that although US may detect substantial perigraft endoleaks, CT is superior for detecting the origin of the perigraft leak, the outflow vessels, and the detection of complications related to the endografting procedure. The use of US contrast agents to augment duplex studies may increase the sensitivity and specificity of this modality. Although it still may represent a less expensive, less invasive method of endograft surveillance, at this point its use is not routine.[34,35]

PROBLEMS WITH ENDOGRAFTING AND MANAGEMENT

Various problems can arise in the planning and placement of abdominal aortic endografts. Once the grafts are in place, several complications can arise over time that may require intervention to prevent the subsequent expansion and possible rupture of the previously excluded aneurysm. In the following paragraphs, several of the more common problems that occur following endograft placement are outlined.

Iliac Artery Disease

When iliac artery disease is present, whether it be aneurysmal disease, atherosclerotic disease, or severe tortuosity, the use of an iliac conduit can provide a safe route to deliver the endograft.[36] In the cases of iliac artery lumen narrowing secondary to atherosclerotic disease or increased vessel tortuosity, advancement of the device, despite the presence of resistance, can result in rupture of the iliac artery. Iliac artery rupture has been reported in 1% to 2% of cases.[37,38] To circumvent prohibitive iliac artery anatomy, an iliac conduit can be used. An iliac conduit involves suturing a prosthetic graft (generally 8 to 10 mm in diameter) to the mid-common iliac artery, even if it is aneurysmal. This can be done in an end-to-end or end-to-side fashion, although the latter often provides a greater lumen for passage of the device.[24] The device is placed through the prosthetic graft, and the iliac limb of the endovascular graft traverses the common iliac artery and anastomosis and seals within the conduit. The distal end of the graft is tunneled along the natural course of the iliac artery and anastomosed to the femoral artery. The distal end of the common iliac artery is oversewn to allow retrograde flow through the external iliac artery to supply the ipsilateral hypogastric artery. Alternatively, the hypogastric artery can be anastomosed directly to the conduit.

Iliac artery ectasia or aneurysms can present a problem in obtaining a distal seal. Enlarged common iliac arteries are present in up to 30% of patients presenting for endovascular aneurysm repair.[39-42] As many available endografts do not allow for ectatic or aneurysmal common iliac arteries, the distal seal may need to be obtained within the external iliac artery, which is often of normal caliber. If the distal seal occurs in the external iliac artery, the hypogastric artery is generally sacrificed using coil embolization. The presence of a hypogastric artery aneurysm would necessitate the same approach. Rarely, bilateral hypogastric artery embolization is required. Hypogastric artery embolization can occur before aneurysm repair or concurrently. If bilateral embolization is planned, it is generally performed in a staged fashion, although its occlusion is not always planned. Hypogastric artery embolization is not without risk, and side effects can occur in up to 50% of patients.[40] Buttock claudication is the predominant complaint after hypogastric artery occlusion. This occurs in 12% to 50% of the patients, but in most it generally resolves after several months.[39-43] Five to 25% of men complain of new-onset erectile dysfunction.[42,43] Buttock ischemia and bowel ischemia requiring resection are of theoretical concern, but they have not been described in any of the larger series. Patients requiring embolization in the more distal branches of the hypogastric artery (as might be done with the presence of an internal iliac artery aneurysm) and those in whom coil placement was not adequately controlled are at higher risk of developing pelvic symptoms.[44] Bilateral hypogastric artery embolization has not been associated with increased symptoms when compared with unilateral occlusion.[40,41,43] Coil embolization of the internal iliac artery is not necessary if it is not aneurysmal. In the face of common iliac artery aneurysms, Wyers and colleagues[45] have shown that if there is a 5-mm neck of iliac artery proximal to the hypogastric artery in addition to a 15-mm neck in the external iliac artery, coil embolization of the hypogastric artery is not necessary to obtain a distal seal. This may be possible in up to two thirds of patients requiring coverage of the hypogastric artery.

Endoleaks

An endoleak is the persistence of blood flow outside the endograft, but in the aneurysm sac.[46] Endoleaks are classified according to their etiology, and currently five types have been described (Table 40-2).[47,48] A type 1 endoleak (Fig. 40-5) arises from inadequate sealing at either the proximal aortic (allowing antegrade flow) or distal iliac (allowing retrograde flow) attachment sites. Type 2 endoleaks (Fig. 40-6) arise from patent branch vessels off of the aortic sac that allow for retrograde flow into the aneurysm. Such branches may include a patent lumbar or inferior mesenteric artery. Type 3 endoleaks develop from defects in the fabric of the graft or at the junction zone between modular components. Type 4 endoleaks develop secondary to diffuse "leaking" of blood between the interstices of the fabric or where the graft is sutured to a stent. Type 5 endoleaks describe a scenario in which the aneurysm sac remains pressurized and the aneurysm enlarges, but no demonstrable flow of blood into the sac can be visualized on current imaging modalities. These may be due to imaging that is not sophisticated enough to discern these leaks or due to intermittent episodes of leakage.[49] The pressure applied to the aneurysm sac causing it to continue to expand, in this situation, has been termed "endotension."[50,51] Controversy with regard to this concept exists, in particular with the ability of the thrombus to transmit pressure to the aneurysm wall. It is argued that these merely represent a type 1, 2, or 3 endoleak in which the defect is large enough to allow blood to flow into the sac and transmit pressure to the sac, but the exit site is not present or too small to be detected.[24]

TABLE 40-2 ENDOLEAK CLASSIFICATION

Endoleak	Cause	Blood Flow into Sac
Type 1	Inadequate seal at aortic or iliac attachment sites	Antegrade or retrograde
Type 2	Patent branches off aneurysm sac	Retrograde
Type 3	Fabric defects or component junctions	Antegrade
Type 4	Leak at fabric interstices	Antegrade
Type 5	Endotension	No clear leak

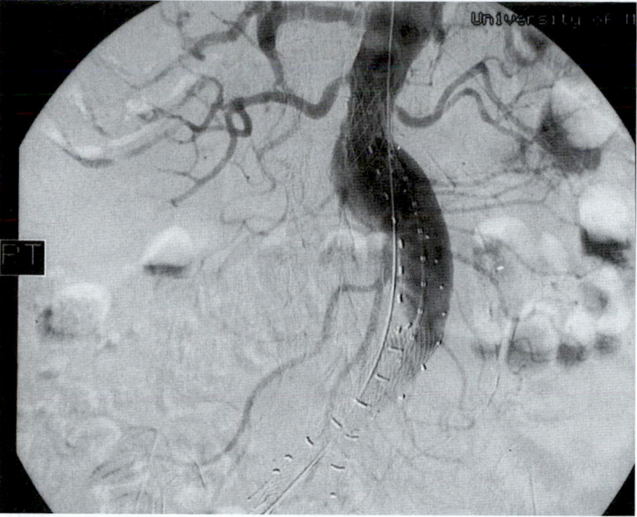

FIGURE 40-5. This is an angiogram demonstrating a type 1 endoleak. The contrast can be seen "leaking" around the proximal part of the graft and filling the aneurysm sac. The patient subsequently had a giant Palmaz stent placed in the aortic neck, and this ameliorated the endoleak.

Types 1 and 3 endoleaks are associated with significant risks of aneurysm enlargement and possible rupture, and these should be treated.[52,53] This may be accomplished with the placement of an extension cuff limb over the site of the leak. If the leak is a type 1 and the graft is juxtaposed to the inferior border of the renal arteries, a large balloon-expandable stent can be placed in the proximal aspect of the endograft. This provides increased radial force, causing better juxtaposition of the graft and aortic wall and thus ameliorating the leakage. If this is unsuccessful, open repair and graft explantation are generally indicated. Fabric tears are easily managed if the site of the leak is localized. In these situations, the

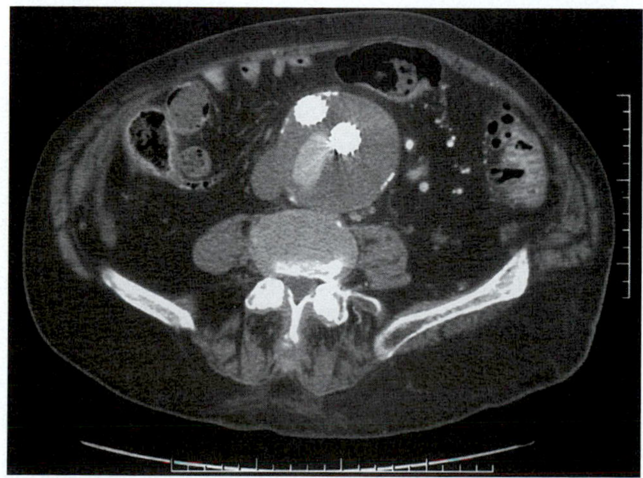

FIGURE 40-6. CT scan representative of a type 2 endoleak. There is contrast within the aneurysm sac but outside of the limbs of the endograft. This aneurysm had continued expansion until the patient underwent embolization of the inferior mesenteric artery.

tear can be covered with a cuff or extension. When it is more diffuse, the entire endograft can be relined with a second endograft, or the device can be removed and the aneurysm repaired in an open fashion.

Type 2 endoleaks are rarely associated with aneurysm rupture.[54] At least 10% to 15% of patients are identified with a type 2 endoleak during follow-up.[55-58] Warfarin treatment is not associated with an increased incidence of early or delayed postoperative endoleak, but type 2 endoleaks are less likely to undergo spontaneous resolution in these patients.[59] Type 2 endoleaks are generally observed unless they are associated with an increase in aneurysm size or are associated with aortic pulsatility on physical examination. In these situations, arteriography is the next step in order to identify the source of the endoleak. Superior mesenteric artery injection reveals retrograde inferior mesenteric artery flow as the source, whereas selective hypogastric artery injection demonstrates a lumbar artery filling the aneurysm. Super-selective arterial canalization can then be performed with embolization of the feeding vessels. Another approach is through direct aneurysm sac puncture.[60] With direct sac puncture, one can measure sac pressure and inject the sac directly with contrast agent to precisely identify the leak. The systolic sac pressure is related to the size of the leak, and the pulse amplitude is related to the resistance of the outflow vessels and sac compliance.[61] After localization of the leak, feeding vessels can be directly accessed and embolized.[62] In addition, the sac can be filled with substances such as coils, glue, or gel foam in order to further prevent flow.

Measurement of intrasacral pressures may help determine if an endoleak is present at the time of the original surgery or if an endoleak has been adequately treated if it has been approached through direct sac puncture. In an ex vivo model of endoleaks, Parodi and colleagues[63] evaluated the pressure changes in the aortic sac with various types and sizes of endoleaks. In this model, sac pressures were significantly higher than systemic pressures in the presence of all endoleaks. This obviously places the aneurysm at significant risk for rupture. The presence of patent side branches significantly reduced the pressure within the sac, particularly the mean pressure and diastolic pressure. Clinically, persistent side branches augment the development of type 2 endoleaks and influence early sac behavior.[64,65] Gawend and colleagues[66] evaluated the use of sac pressure monitoring and found it helpful in the detection and treatment of endoleaks. They noted, however, that intrasacral pressure measurements did not correlate with AAA size change over ensuing follow-up. This may be an effective modality for monitoring aneurysms after endograft exclusion once less invasive methods of pressure measurement are developed.

Structural Failure

Material failure represents one of the most concerning problems for potential failure of endograft placement. This is a difficult event to identify, as patients are often asymptomatic and may not present with any acute changes in their endograft evaluation. Three modes of structural failure have been described in aortic endografting and involve fabric erosion, suture disruption, and metal fracture.[67]

The development of endoleaks secondary to graft erosion has been documented with some first-generation endograft devices (Fig. 40-7).[68,69] It has been speculated that the areas of graft erosion are secondary to friction between the stent material and the fabric, which can be confounded by the pulsation of the aorta. Predicting the incidence of fabric fatigue is difficult, and although this does occur in grafts placed by conventional open aneurysm repair, it occurs much more rapidly and more commonly in the endograft systems.[70,71] In several device designs, the graft fabric is attached to the metal skeleton through the use of sutures. Disruption of these sutures is believed to explain graft failure in some instances.[72-74] The mechanism for suture failure is believed to be the same as for fabric erosion. Namely, motion of the stents with aortic pulsations causes friction and wear of the sutures with subsequent suture fracture.

The most common structural problem identified in aortic endograft systems has been metallic stent fractures.[71] Stent and hook fractures in the phase 1 trial of the Endovascular Technologie's graft resulted in suspension of the program and redesign of the metallic attachment system.[75] In a review of 686 patients who underwent endovascular aneurysm repair, Jacobs and colleagues identified 60 patients who had material failure.[71] Forty-three (72%) of these failures were due to metallic stent fractures and occurred in various different

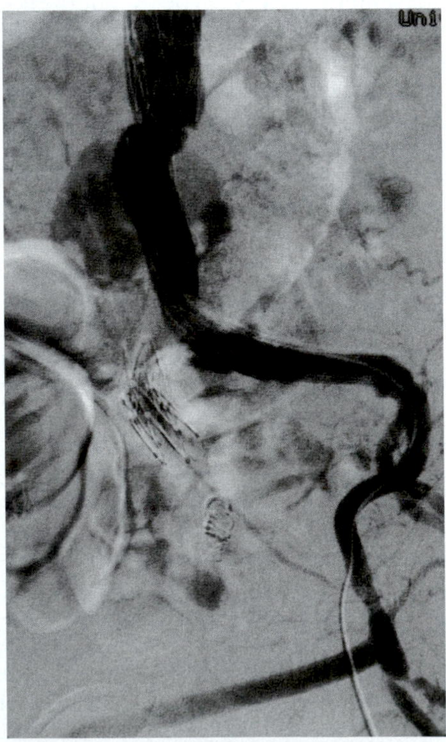

FIGURE 40-7. Angiogram revealing a type 3 endoleak that developed at the site of a tear in the graft fabric. This was a "homemade" aortouniiliac graft that had been in place for approximately 5 years. The patient presented with new onset abdominal pain and had a CT scan that revealed an aneurysm sac that had significantly expanded in diameter. The tear was sealed by placement of a new endograft.

endografts with different stent composition. The cause of metal failure has been attributed to stress fatigue and metal corrosion, particularly in nitinol stents.[76] Corrosion has not been seen in next-generation endografts and may reflect improved nitinol processing.[77-79] Tortuosity of the arterial system can also stress the stent graft system and lead to metal fracture. This has been reported in the longitudinal bar of the Talent and Gore stent graft devices.[71,80]

Limb Thrombosis

Endograft limb thrombosis after endovascular repair of infrarenal AAA is a recognized complication occurring in up to 11% of patients.[81-86] Various underlying factors have been purported to place patients at increased risk for limb thrombosis. One reported risk factor is the lack of device support. Although Carroccio and colleagues[82] reported on the results of 351 bifurcated grafts with no significant association between the use of unsupported devices and graft thrombosis, others have suggested there is a significant relationship. Baum and colleagues[83] specifically evaluated the rates of graft limb kinking and thrombosis between supported and unsupported abdominal aortic stent grafts. In total, 12% of the limbs in their series required an intervention for kinking. In the supported limbs, 5% required subsequent placement of arterial stents. Two percent required these for evidence of kinking at the time of the initial operation, whereas 3% required stenting in the postoperative period after the patients presented with limb thrombosis. In the unsupported grafts, there was an intervention rate of 44%. Approximately one half of these had an additional stent placed at the time of the initial procedure, whereas the remainder had a subsequent stent placed in the postoperative follow-up period secondary to limb thrombosis or severe stenosis.

Another factor increasing the risk of limb thrombosis is oversizing of the iliac limb. Oversizing causes the graft material to have a significant amount of infolding, reducing the intraluminal diameter.[84] Along these lines, significant intraluminal vessel narrowing secondary to underlying atherosclerotic disease or tortuosity can result in flow abnormalities and eventually cause graft limb thrombosis.[82] Extension of the graft limb into the external iliac artery has also been described as a risk factor for developing limb thrombosis.[82] It was believed that transition into the external iliac artery caused both a significant reduction in arterial diameter, as well as a kink in the graft due to acute angulation of the limb as it passed through the pelvis. Damage to the distal iliac or femoral artery, such as dissection during graft placement, can subsequently cause outflow obstruction and graft limb thrombosis.[81]

Management of patients presenting with limb thrombosis depends on the severity of the patient's symptoms. In the series by Carroccio and colleagues,[82] nearly one third of the patients presenting with symptoms had such mild symptoms that no intervention was required. Most patients, however, underwent a femoral–femoral bypass to restore flow to the affected extremity. Few patients are successfully treated with thrombolysis or graft thrombectomy followed by endovascular repair of the underlying problem. In most series, patients with limb problems generally present early, within the first 6 months following endograft repair.[81-83,87-89] In fact, Sampram and colleagues[87] reported that no limb occlusions presented after 30 months of follow-up.

Migration

Distal stent-graft migration after abdominal aortic endografting has been reported to occur in 9% to 45% of patients.[22,28,58,90,91] Migration certainly has been identified as a risk for the development of a type 1 endoleak and delayed aneurysm rupture or late conversion to open repair.[91] The pathophysiology behind aortic endograft migration is complex, and various factors contribute to its development.[92] A number of forces are at play within the aortic endograft, but blood flow acts as the main displacing force. As the tube of the aortic graft curves, there is a change in the velocity of the blood resulting in an increased displacement force. For many endografts, the forces providing protection against migration are friction forces of the graft against the aortic wall and the columnar strength of the graft. The friction forces depend on the apposition of the graft fabric and the aortic wall and obviously can be affected by the aortic wall composition (thrombus, calcifications), the size of the aorta, the radial force of the stent, and the nature of the graft fabric. It has been suggested that the presence of barbs or hooks in the proximal portion of the stent graft may provide additional protection.[93]

The infrarenal aortic neck length and its maximum diameter, shape, and angulation have all been implicated as causes of stent graft migration.[22,90,91,94] All of these work to decrease the friction between the stent graft and aortic wall. Albertini and colleagues[90] evaluated the development of proximal perigraft endograft leak and device migration following endovascular aneurysm repair. Fifteen patients had graft migration, and 31 of 184 repairs developed a proximal endoleak. Neck angulation was the only factor found to be significant in the development of device migration, whereas neck angulation and neck diameter were the two factors important in developing a proximal perigraft endoleak.[90] Lee and colleagues,[95] however, were not able to identify any specific anatomical correlate and device migration. They did observe, however, that any device that migrated distally by more than 1 cm subsequently required an intervention.

Other hypotheses as to the cause of device migration have focused on the morphologic changes in the aneurysm and the aortic neck after endovascular AAA repair. Specifically, aortic neck dilation, longitudinal sac shrinkage, and graft shortening have been described.[22,30,96,97] One of the more widely accepted hypotheses is aortic neck dilation following aortic endografting. After endovascular aneurysm repair, the aneurysm neck has been documented to dilate significantly, mostly in the first 2 years after graft placement.[98] In a review by Cao and colleagues,[91] 17(15%) of 148 patients had an episode of device migration. The only two independent risk factors for device migration were neck dilation postoperatively and an AAA diameter of greater than 55 mm. Others have argued that neck dilation is not a significant event provided adequate graft oversizing was performed at initial endograft placement.[95] The amount the aortic neck dilated to did not exceed the size of the original aortic endograft placed. Larger aneurysms have also been noted to have increased risks of developing type 1 endoleak, graft migration, and the subsequent need for open surgical conversion compared with larger aneurysms.[99]

OUTCOMES

Results of Aortic Endografting

Endograft AAA repair generally has a low mortality rate (1% to 3%) compared with open repair, and subsequent rates of aneurysm rupture after endovascular repair are reduced to 1% per year.[53,58,87,100] Endograft placement is not free of adverse events, however, and there is not an infrequent need for secondary interventions. Naslund and colleagues[101] reported technical complications in 26% of 34 endografts placed. Fairman and colleagues evaluated the occurrence of critical events during the deployment of their initial 75 endografts, and patients were divided into three groups corresponding to the time period in which the graft was placed.[88] Critical events were defined as unanticipated technical difficulties that occurred during the course of operation that threatened the success of the procedure. Difficulty in obtaining access occurred in nearly one quarter of all patients. Although it would be expected that the latter 25 patients should not have experienced as great a difficulty in obtaining access, these patients had increased complexity of their aorto-iliac anatomy compared with endograft patients earlier in their experience. This group had a greater frequency of iliac artery balloon angioplasty, as well as the use of iliac artery conduits. Deployment difficulties existed and were composed mostly of graft foreshortening, necessitating the placement of additional distal covered extensions. Other deployment issues encountered included suprarenal graft displacement, infrarenal graft displacement, and device-related issues such as iliac limb kinking or twisting. Malplacement of the graft did not correlate with anatomic complexity.

The need for subsequent secondary procedures has been evaluated by several large series of patients who had an abdominal aortic endograft placed.[85,87,102,103] The Eurostar registry reported the results of 1023 patients with a follow-up of 12 months or longer.[102] Overall, 186 (18%) patients required a secondary intervention. The majority of these interventions (76%) involved a transfemoral procedure, whereas the remaining patients required transabdominal (12%) or extra-anatomic (11%) surgery. The rates of freedom from intervention at 1, 3, and 4 years were 89%, 67%, and 62%, respectively. The transfemoral procedures performed most frequently were aortic or iliac limb extension for graft migration or endoleak. Late death was more frequent in those patients requiring a secondary intervention (85%) compared with those who did not (90%) and was more frequently associated with those requiring a transabdominal procedure.

Montefiore Medical Center and the Cleveland Clinic Foundation have published their single institution results on the durability of aortic endografting. Montefiore reported on 239 endografts placed over 9 years, with a technical success rate of 88.7%.[85] The 5-year survival rate in this group was only 37%. Secondary interventions were required in 10% of the patients, with more than one half of the secondary procedures being performed for the presence of an endoleak. Sampram and colleagues[87] reported the results from the Cleveland Clinic Foundation on 703 patients undergoing endovascular aortic endografting with follow-up averaging 1 year. Survival in this group was 90% at 1 year and declined to 70% at 3 years. Overall, 128 secondary interventions were performed in 105 patients (15%). Freedom from intervention mirrored that of the Eurostar registry with freedom from intervention rates of 88%, 76%, and 65% at 1, 2, and 3 years, respectively. Mortality related to the secondary procedure was 8% but rose to 18% in those requiring a transabdominal procedure. Univariate analysis revealed that secondary procedures were more common in patients with larger major and minor sac axes, in patients who received a large aortic stent because of a proximal endoleak present at initial aneurysm repair, and in patients who received treatment later in the course of the review. This latter finding is felt to be secondary to the increased complexity of cases approached in an endovascular fashion.

The Cleveland Clinic Foundation review included the use of six different devices, which included two Zenith grafts—one that was part of the multicenter national trial and one group that was part of a sponsor-investigator investigational device exemption trial.[23] The overall freedom from risk of rupture was 98.7% at 2 years. The results of this review reveal that there are significant differences in outcomes between groups with different endovascular devices, in particular with regard to limb occlusion and rate of endoleak. Limb occlusion occurred most frequently with the Ancure device at a rate of 11% at 2 years. Endoleak of any kind was most common with the Excluder device at a rate of 64% at 1 year. Modular separations were the most frequent with the Zenith graft at 3.5%. Aneurysm sac shrinkage correlated directly with the frequency of endoleaks, and aneurysm sac shrinkage was most common in the Zenith and Talent groups but least common in the Excluder group. There were no differences with regard to rate of secondary procedures, conversion to open repair, or migration. Sternbergh and colleagues[104] have reported similar findings. Outcomes were compared between the Zenith device and the AneuRx device, and it was determined that the Zenith graft was associated with fewer endoleaks and a higher rate and amount of aneurysm sac shrinkage. Bertges and associates[105] also reported similar findings in their evaluation. Regression of AAA size after endograft placement was more significant after placement of the Talent and Ancure endografts compared with the AneuRx or Excluder devices. During the first 2 years of follow-up the initial size of the AAA, the presence of an endoleak, and the type of graft used were significant predictors of sac shrinkage. After 2 years, however, only graft type was significant. Ouriel and colleagues[99] have additionally concluded that the outcome after endovascular AAA repair depends on the initial size of the aneurysm.

Comparison with Open Surgery

Several studies have attempted to compare endograft repair with open AAA repair.[37,38,106-110] None has been a randomized, prospective trial. The majority of trials compare outcomes with historical controls or a series of patients who have undergone conventional AAA repair during the same time period. One problem with these comparisons to open AAA repair is that the long-term outcome of aortic endografting is not known. Only recently are data being obtained from patients who have had the grafts implanted for several years—at least sufficient enough data to make reasonable statistical comparisons with open repair. Several reports have compared the results of endovascular aneurysm repair with open surgical repair, despite these limitations (Table 40-3). The majority of these studies contained fairly large numbers of patients. Some include reports from single institutions, whereas others involve multicenter, nonrandomized but clinically controlled trials.

Moore and colleagues[106] evaluated data from two prospective multicenter, nonrandomized but clinically controlled studies. The implantation of these devices and performance of open surgery occurred at multiple sites. A total of 573 patients underwent endograft placement and were compared with 111 patients who were excluded from endovascular repair secondary to anatomic reasons. The combined morbidity and mortality for the endovascular group was nearly one half that of the open surgical group. There were higher rates of bleeding requiring transfusion, cardiac complications, and respiratory problems in those patients undergoing open repair. In addition, those patients undergoing endovascular repair had significantly shorter hospital stays, less blood loss, and less intensive care unit use. There were no differences in 30-day mortality rates. In long-term follow-ups, there were no differences in survival and no patients experienced aneurysm rupture. Nearly one fourth of the patients in the endograft group, however, had a detectable endoleak, and one third of the patients required a secondary procedure to treat compromised limb flow. However, there was only a 2% conversion to open repair over the long-term follow-up.

Some generalizations with regard to outcome compared with open surgery can be drawn from these reports. Hospital stay is shorter for patients undergoing endovascular repair. Carpenter and colleagues,[110] however, reported that although the initial length of stay was shorter for those undergoing endovascular repair, patients undergoing endovascular AAA repair were more likely to be readmitted during the follow-up interval compared with those undergoing open surgical repair. The readmission-free rate after AAA repair at 12 months was 95% for patients undergoing open AAA repair compared with 71% for those undergoing endovascular AAA repair. If total hospital days were compared, including the initial stay and then subsequent stays related to AAA repair, there was no significant difference in total length of stay. Patients undergoing endovascular AAA repair were most commonly readmitted for treatment of endoleak (31/337), wound infection (12/337), and graft limb thrombosis (9/337).

Major morbidity is generally lower in patients undergoing endovascular AAA repair. Zarins and colleagues[37] reported that the rate of complications requiring reoperation was the same between the two groups. The magnitude of the complications, however, was significantly different. Ten percent of the surgical group required major abdominal operations, whereas in the stent graft group only 1% of the patients required a major abdominal operation. Most systemic sequelae in both groups are cardiac in nature. Pulmonary and bleeding complications tend to be higher in the open surgical groups. Late secondary procedures for graft-related complications were similar between the two groups. It is interesting to note, however, that major morbidity following secondary intervention is much greater in those undergoing conventional AAA repair approaching 22%.[107] Most secondary interventions following endovascular AAA repair are managed in an endovascular fashion and have minimal morbidity and mortality. Patient survival has been shown

TABLE 40-3 ENDOVASCULAR ABDOMINAL AORTIC ANEURYSM REPAIR VERSUS OPEN SURGERY

	NO. PATIENTS		PERIOPERATIVE MORTALITY		LENGTH OF STAY (DAYS)		MAJOR MORBIDITY		TECHNICAL SUCCESS*	
Author	Endo	Open	Endo	Open	Endo	Open	Endo	Open	Endo	Open
Zarins et al. 1999	190	60	3%	0% (NS)	3.9	9.4 ($P < .05$)	12%	23% ($P < .05$)	79%	100% ($P < .05$)
Carpenter et al. 2002	174	163	4%	4.4% (NS)	5	8 ($P < .05$)	NR	NR	NR	NR
Arko et al. 2002	200	255	0.5%	3.4% ($P < .05$)	2.8	8.3 ($P < .05$)	7.5%	14.5% ($P < .05$)	NR	NR
Moore et al. 2003	573	111	10%	3% (NS)	2	6 ($P < .05$)	28.8%	44.1% ($P < .05$)	92.7%	100% (NS)
Matsumura et al. 2003	334	99	1%	0% (NS)	2	10 ($P < .05$)	14%	57% ($P < .05$)	100%	100% (NS)

*Definitions of technical success differ among the studies.
NR, not reported; NS, not significant.

to favor endovascular repair. May and colleagues[38] reported survival curves that were significantly different between endovascular repair and open surgical repair, favoring endovascular repair. Three-year survival for the endovascular group was 96% and only 85% for the open arm.

Zarins and colleagues[37] reported a procedural success rate in the surgery group as 98% and only 77% in the endovascular group. It was felt, however, that the reporting standard did not take into full account the complications that may accompany stent graft and open AAA procedures. Instead, they defined primary procedural success as those patients alive at 30 days with a patent graft, excluded aneurysm (no endoleaks), no need for reoperation or secondary procedures, and no major complication. With this definition, the primary procedure success was 77% in the open surgical group and 78% in the stent graft group. A secondary procedural success was defined as patients who were alive and home from the hospital at 30 days with an excluded aneurysm and a patent graft. This measure excludes complications but includes the benefits derived from a secondary intervention. There was no significant difference in secondary procedural success between the open surgical group and the endovascular surgical group (95% vs. 89%, respectively).

In the majority of the studies, endovascular groups exhibit more comorbidities. This may cause a selection bias toward the open surgical arms as patients were "less sick." On the other hand, many patients receiving open surgical therapy were not candidates for endovascular repair due to the aneurysm morphology. In order to overcome this aspect of bias, Hill and colleagues[108] evaluated the outcomes of patients who underwent endovascular AAA repair with a group of open surgical AAA repairs that were morphologically able to have had an endovascular repair. This was a retrospective review with a 30-day mortality rate similar between the two groups (2.5% vs. 2.9%). More complications occurred in the surgical group (40%) compared with the endovascular group (24%), but the number of major complications was similar between the two cohorts. Due to complications, 5.7% of the surgical arm and 6.3% of the endograft arm required reoperation. As expected, blood loss was less and hospital stays were shorter in the endovascular group. No long-term graft complications were noted in the open surgical group, whereas 15% of the endovascular group had an endoleak detected. In all studies, however, the degree of graft-related complications may be underestimated in the open AAA group, as these patients do not typically undergo the intense radiographic surveillance that endovascular AAA repairs do.

Shermerhourn and colleagues[111] evaluated quality-adjusted life expectancy after endovascular AAA repair compared with open surgical repair using a Markov decision-analysis model. Data with regard to the endograft patients were derived from the Eurostar database. This database began in 1996 as a voluntary, broad-based, multicenter evaluation of endovascular AAA repair outcomes as it is broadly applied across the continent of Europe ($n = 3222$). The open surgical outcome data were derived from the 1995 Medicare claims for elective repair of nonruptured AAA ($n = 24{,}386$). There was a base-case analysis of 70-year-old men. Life expectancy after endovascular AAA repair was 7.09 quality-adjusted life years compared with open AAA repair of 7.03 quality-adjusted life years. This represents an insignificant difference of approximately 3 weeks. Sensitivity analysis, however, revealed that at younger than 64 years of age, open surgical repair resulted in a greater quality-adjusted life expectancy, but the difference was small (<3 months) across the entire range of ages studies (60 to 85 years). By this assessment, open surgical repair may be preferred in young patients with a low operative risk, and endovascular repair is favored in older patients at higher operative risk.

To effectively compare the outcomes in patients undergoing open and endovascular repair of AAA, a randomized prospective trial is necessary. Currently, the U.S. Department of Veterans Affairs is conducting a randomized prospective trial to address this issue. Patients who are candidates for both endovascular and open AAA repair are randomly assigned to one procedure method. Two European trials have a two-year follow-up showing endovascular and open AAA are equal in terms of mortality and morbidity.[111a,111b]

Endovascular Abdominal Aortic Aneurysm Repair in Women

Women represent a small minority of patients in whom endovascular aneurysm repair is undertaken. They present with unique problems, mostly secondary to their smaller stature. Overall, women comprise between 8% and 17% of endovascular AAA repairs.[38,100,106,109,110,112] Despite the smaller number presenting for repair, equivalent percentages are deemed anatomically suitable to undergo graft placement. Women, however, were found to have smaller aortic neck diameters, shorter aortic neck lengths, smaller common iliac artery diameters, and smaller external iliac artery diameters when compared with males.[112] In fact, it is the short aortic neck that has accounted for the exclusion of women from endovascular therapy. In addition, women tend to have a greater incidence of complications during endovascular aneurysm repair compared with men. The majority of these complications are related to arterial access and the need for more frequent arterial reconstruction, up to 42% in some series compared with only 21% in men.[112] The incidence of endoleak also appears to be higher in women than men.[56]

FUTURE DIRECTIONS

Percutaneous Placement

With the development of lower-profile devices, the ability to place endografts through an entirely percutaneous approach will become readily available. Presently, this approach is being investigated with some success. Using various percutaneous closure devices placed preprocedurally allows for the percutaneous placement of endografts through sheaths of sizes ranging from 14 Fr to 25 Fr.[113-116] Howell and colleagues[116] report successful percutaneous placement of the iliac limb of an endograft system placed through a 16-Fr sheath. Successful percutaneous deployment was possible in 136 (94.4%) of 144 patients. Hemostasis was obtained at the puncture site using a percutaneous closure device. No complications were noted with follow-ups extending to 1 year in one third of the patients. Torsello and colleagues[114] have performed a randomized, prospective trial evaluating endovascular suture versus cutdown for endovascular AAA repair. A total of 30 patients, involving 55 femoral arteries, were included. The duration of surgery and the time to ambulation were significantly shorter in those patients undergoing percutaneous treatment. Complications were equivalent between the two groups, and no cost benefit could be attributable to percutaneous graft placement. With the advent of new, smaller profile devices and improved delivery systems, the use of percutaneous endograft treatment of AAA will likely increase.[117]

Thoracic Aortic Grafts

At first glance it may seem that the concept of a thoracic endograft system would be easily manufactured and deployed as a simple tube graft system. The placement would appear to lack the complexities of the aortic bifurcation and be able to avoid placement near the visceral vessels. Early experience with these systems has proved this not to be the case. Several properties of thoracic aneurysms complicate the effective placement of these grafts.[24] The first problem involves the anatomical location of the aneurysm with regard to the left subclavian artery, often providing only a few millimeters of "normal" aorta after this branch point before the aneurysm begins. This adds a great deal of complexity to obtaining a proximal fixation point and seal.

The hemodynamics of the thoracic aorta are also significantly different than those of the infrarenal abdominal aorta.[24] The increased force in this region can hinder accurate graft placement and may provide increased stress on the graft over time, which may lead to excessive material wear and damage, as well as promote graft migration. In addition, although lumbar arteries can be occluded with little sequelae, disruption of flow to the intercostal arteries may result in paraplegia.[24,118-120] Finally, due to the increased size of the thoracic aorta, the sizes of the stent grafts and their delivery systems are also increased. This makes them significantly more difficult to maneuver and place with the same accuracy as that experienced with abdominal aortic endografting.[24]

It is generally understood that a 2-cm neck is required in the proximal and distal aspect of the aorta for graft placement.[121] In some instances, in order to obtain adequate fixation in the proximal aorta, the orifice of the left subclavian artery is covered. This has been reported as being well tolerated with few patients requiring a carotid-subclavian bypass for ischemic complications or ligation of the proximal left subclavian artery due to the development of an endoleak.[122,123] Occasionally, more complex brachiocephalic reconstruction is necessary, allowing stent graft fixation to occur up to the level of the innominate artery (Fig. 40-8). This entails providing inflow to the left carotid artery and left subclavian artery from the right carotid artery with a bypass.[121] Long-term outcomes from these maneuvers are not known.

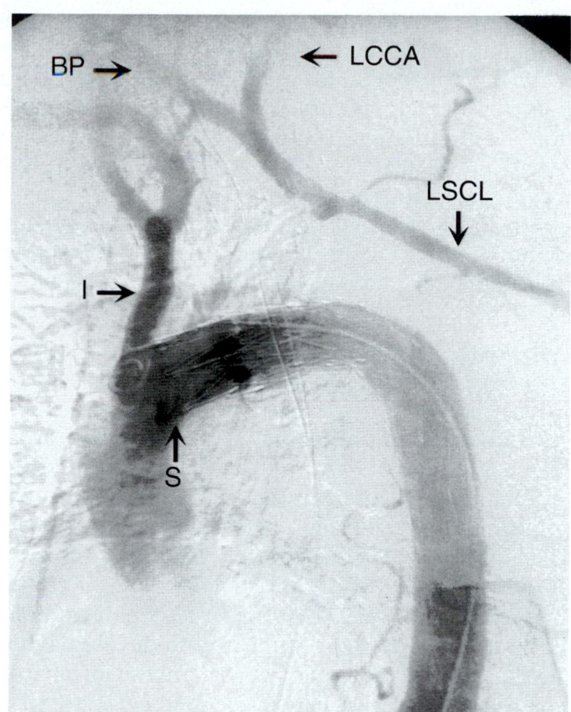

FIGURE 40-8. Completion angiogram after deployment of a thoracic endograft. The patient had presented with hemoptysis due to erosion of a thoracic aortic aneurysm. The endograft required placement up to the innominate artery in order to obtain an adequate proximal seal. Before endograft placement, the patient underwent a right carotid to left carotid artery bypass and a left carotid to left subclavian artery bypass. *S* is the proximal aspect of the endograft at the origin of the innominate artery; *I* is the innominate artery; *LCCA* and *LSCL* are the left common carotid artery and left subclavian artery now arising from a bypass graft *(BP)*.

In addition to proximal fixation, distal fixation may encroach on the origins of the mesenteric arteries—the celiac artery in particular. The coverage of the celiac artery without subsequent visceral ischemia has been described, but an extensive experience does not exist and long-term outcomes are not known.[24]

At the time of writing this chapter, no commercially available, FDA-approved thoracic aorta stent graft systems were available in the United States. Presently, Gore TAG endovascular thoracic graft is available to treat thoracic aneurysms.[123a] Several manufacturers including Gore, Medtronic, and Cook have devices that are in clinical trials. Most reported experiences entail anecdotal experiences or retrospective reviews and evaluate the use of "homemade" grafts in the treatment of thoracic aneurysms, ruptured thoracic aneurysms, and aortic dissections.[124-131] Many of these studies were for mixed pathology of aneurysms and dissections together. A recent review involving only repair of descending thoracic aortic aneurysms using manufactured devices was reported by Ellozy and colleagues.[132] The authors performed thoracic stent-graft repair of thoracic aortic aneurysms in 84 patients using the Gore TAG stent graft and the Talent thoracic stent graft as part of three distinct U.S. Food and Drug Administration trials. Successful aneurysm exclusion occurred in 69 (82%) patients. There was a 38% incidence of major procedure-related or device-related complications including problems with proximal attachment failures (8%), distal attachment failures (6%), and intergraft attachment failures (1%). The periprocedural mortality rate was 6%, and there were five late aneurysm ruptures. The overall survival at 40 months was 67%, and freedom from rupture or type 3 endoleak was 74%. These results suggest that improvements in thoracic stent graft systems are required and additional evaluation is necessary before determining whether this is a durable option for patients with thoracic aortic aneurysms.

Treatment of Ruptured Abdominal Aortic Aneurysm with Endografts

Despite advances in prehospital care, operative care, and critical care, patients presenting with ruptured AAAs continue to have a significant mortality, approaching 70% in some series.[133-136] Aortic endografting may offer a unique approach to this difficult problem. Initial concerns with the use of endovascular repair of ruptured AAA involved the ability to obtain adequate radiologic studies in a short period of time and to develop a device that would be suitable for a broad range of anatomic sizes. Several device designs have been described that generally entail an aorto-uniiliac system.[137-139] The system described by the Nottingham and Eindhoven groups used a modular design and allows for various "tops" and "bottoms" that can be placed together to allow placement in a number of different aortic and iliac diameters, as well as different lengths.[139-141] This configuration allows for as few as eight components to be kept in stock to meet the needs of the full spectrum of aortic morphology. The graft design of the Montefiore group is different and is described as "one-size fits all" (Fig. 40-9). The graft is cut to length as it emerges from the common femoral artery. This requires occlusion of the ipsilateral hypogastric artery. Both grafts then require a subsequent femoral-femoral bypass and the placement of an occluder device in the contralateral common iliac artery to prevent retrograde flow into the aneurysm. Opinions differ on whether to occlude the aorta during repair. The groups in the United Kingdom generally prefer swift deployment of the graft, whereas others have used a balloon occluder placed through the brachial artery to temporarily occlude the aorta during endograft placement.

Endovascular repair of ruptured AAA is feasible. The published series to date has been relatively small, describing the outcomes of 20 to 30 patients.[139-142] The group at Montefiore reported the repair of 25 patients with ruptured AAA using their endograft system.[142] In all patients the graft was successfully deployed and the ruptured aneurysm excluded. The 30-day mortality rate from this experience was only 9.7%. Two patients required subsequent laparotomy and evacuation of a large retroperitoneal hematoma causing an abdominal compartment syndrome. The Eindhoven group reported on 24 patients presenting with ruptured AAA who underwent endovascular repair.[141] The 30-day mortality rate was 24%, which was not significantly different from the mortality rate in control patients (41%) undergoing standard open repair for ruptured AAA. In the endovascular group, significantly less blood was lost and hospital stays were shorter. Similarly, the Nottingham group reported endovascular repair of ruptured AAA in 20 patients as part of a feasibility study. Their perioperative mortality rate was 45% with a number of postoperative complications that required both endovascular and open surgical repair.

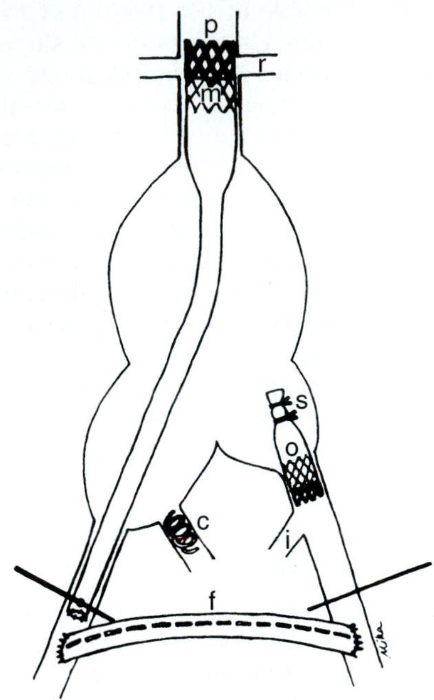

FIGURE 40-9. Diagram of the Montefiore repair device for the endovascular treatment of ruptured abdominal aortic aneurysm. The aorto-uniiliac graft seals in the aortic neck with a Palmaz stent *(p)*; a bare portion of the stent may overlap the renal arteries *(r)*. The distal aspect is sutured into the proximal common femoral/distal external iliac artery. The ipsilateral hypogastric artery undergoes occlusion by coil embolization *(c)*. An occluder device is placed in the contralateral common iliac artery *(o)*. A femoral-femoral bypass is performed to provide blood flow to the contralateral leg and pelvis *(f)*. (Reprinted from Ohki T, Veith FJ, Sancez LA, et al: Endovascular graft repair of ruptured aortoiliac aneurysms. J Am Coll Surg 189:102, 1999; with permission from The American College of Surgeons.)

Although the results of endovascular repair of ruptured AAA cannot be adequately assessed on the basis of these small case series, it suggests that endovascular AAA repair may hold promise as a better procedure for patients presenting with this devastating problem. No endovascular rupture systems are currently available in the United States, but several individual centers have investigational trials under way.

Branch Vessel Grafts

The application of endovascular technology is advancing. Two areas currently being investigated that would significantly expand the application of this technology involve the use of fenestrated aortic grafts to accommodate visceral vessels and endografts that contain branch vessels. In order to treat patients with short aortic necks (<15 mm) and pararenal aneurysms, endografts need to obtain their anchorage and point of seal in a more proximal area of the aorta above the level of the aneurysm. This becomes difficult in that the renal and mesenteric arteries hinder graft placement. In order to accommodate these vessels, endografts that contain areas of fenestration (or holes) in order to allow blood flow into these visceral segments have been constructed. Several reports from Australia have been published evaluating the outcomes of a modification of the Zenith endograft incorporating fenestrations for the renal and visceral vessels.[143,144] Anderson and colleagues[144] describe the placement of fenestrated grafts in 13 patients with unsuitable infrarenal aortic necks. Flow to 33 renal and superior mesenteric arteries was maintained. It was determined that transgraft renal artery stenting is necessary to maintain patency of the renal arteries. These grafts are under evaluation at several centers in the United States.

In addition to fenestrations to treat pararenal AAA, branches have been incorporated into endovascular grafts in order to treat thoracoabdominal aortic aneurysms (TAAAs). This technology is in the early stages of development, but its application has progressed to the clinical arena. Chuter and colleagues[145] described the use of a multi-branched stent graft to treat a TAAA. They used a complex system with 10 components placed through the femoral and brachial arteries. The graft allows branches for the celiac, superior mesenteric, and each renal artery. Distally it was a bifurcated system landing in each iliac artery. The patient required interventions postoperatively to correct kinking in the visceral branches and developed paraplegia on postoperative day 2. Bleyn and associates[146] likewise describe a case report of deploying a branched endograft system to treat a TAAA. Unlike the Chuter device, this one required only one branch vessel to perfuse the celiac artery while the distal aspect of the graft was landed above the level of the superior mesenteric artery.

SUMMARY

Aortic endografting provides a less invasive method of treating AAA. It provides a beneficial way of treating aneurysms in patients who are at high risk for conventional open surgical repair. The durability of this procedure, however, and its application to young patients or those with complicated anatomy is still in question. As technology advances, results with new devices must be carefully reassessed.

REFERENCES

1. Criado FJ, Barnatan MF, Lingelbach JM, et al: Abdominal aortic aneurysm: Overview of stent-graft device. J Am Coll Surg 194:S88, 2002.
2. Power D: Palliative treatment of aneurysms by wiring with Colt's apparatus. Br J Surg 9:27, 1927.
3. Blakemore AH, King BG: Electrothermic coagulation of aortic aneurysms. JAMA 111:1821, 1938.
4. Matas R: Ligation of the abdominal aorta: Report of the ultimate result. 1 year, 5 months and 9 days after the ligation of the abdominal aorta for aneurysm of the bifurcation. Ann Surg 81:457, 1925.
5. Rea CE: Surgical treatment of aneurysm of the abdominal aorta. Minn Med 31:153, 1948.
6. Dubost C, Allary M, Oeconomos N: Resection of an aneurysm of the abdominal aorta: Resection of the continuity by a preserved arterial graft, with result after five months. Arch Surg 64:405, 1952.
7. Voorhees AB, Jaretski A, Blakemore AH: Use of tubes constructed from Vinyon "N" cloth in bridging arterial defects: A preliminary report. Ann Surg 135:322, 1952.
8. Edwards WS, Tapp JS: Chemically treated nylon tubes as arterial grafts. Surgery 38:61, 1955.
9. Creech O: Endo-aneurysmorrhaphy and treatment of aortic aneurysm. Ann Surg 164:935, 1966.
10. Parodi JC, Palmaz JC, Barone HD: Transfemoral intraluminal graft implantation for abdominal aortic aneurysms. Ann Vasc Surg 5:491, 1991.
11. Ernst CB: Abdominal aortic aneurysm. N Engl J Med 328:1167, 1993.
12. Szilagyi DE, Smith RF, DeRusso FJ, et al: Contributions of abdominal aortic aneurysmectomy to prolongation of life. Ann Surg 164:678, 1966.
13. United Kingdom Small Aneurysm Trial Participants: Long-term outcomes of immediate repair compared with surveillance of small abdominal aortic aneurysms. N Engl J Med 346:1445, 2002.
14. Hertzer NR, Mascha EJ, Karafa MT, et al: Open infrarenal abdominal aortic aneurysm repair: The Cleveland Clinic experience from 1989 to 1998. J Vasc Surg 35:1145, 2002.
15. Cronenwett JL, Johnston KW: The United Kingdom Small Aneurysm Trial: Implications for surgical treatment of abdominal aortic aneurysms. J Vasc Surg 29:191, 1999.
16. Baxendale BR, Baker DM, Hutchinson A, et al: Haemodynamic and metabolic response to endovascular repair of infra-renal aortic aneurysms. Br J Anesth 77:581, 1996.
17. Laheij RJF, van Marrewijk CJ, on behalf of the Eurostar group: Endovascular stenting of abdominal aortic aneurysm in patients unfit for elective open surgery. Lancet 356:832, 2000.
18. Beebe HG, Kritpracha B: Imaging of abdominal aortic aneurysm: Current status. Ann Vasc Surg 17:111, 2003.
19. Beebe HG, Jackson T, Pigott JP: Aortic aneurysm morphology for planning endovascular aortic grafts: Limitations of conventional imaging methods. J Endovasc Surg 2:139, 1995.
20. Beebe HG, Kritpracha B, Serres S, et al: Endograft planning without preoperative arteriography: A clinical feasibility study. J Endovasc Ther 7:8, 2000.
21. Fillinger MF: New imaging techniques in endovascular surgery. Surg Clin North Am 79:451, 1999.
22. Resch T, Ivancev K, Brunkwall J, et al: Distal migration of stent-grafts after endovascular repair of abdominal aortic aneurysms. J Vasc Interv Radiol 10:257, 1997.
23. Ouriel K: Endovascular repair of abdominal aortic aneurysms: The Cleveland Clinic experience with five different devices. Semin Vasc Surg 16:88, 2003.
24. Ouriel K, Greenberg RK, Clair DG: Endovascular treatment of aortic aneurysm. Curr Probl Surg 39:233, 2002.
25. Lau LL, Hakaim AG, Oldenburg WA, et al: Effect of suprarenal versus infrarenal aortic endograft fixation on renal function and renal artery patency: A comparative study with intermediate follow-up. J Vasc Surg 37:1162, 2003.
26. White RA: Clinical and design update on the development and testing of one-piece, bifurcated, polytetrafluoroethylene endovascular graft for abdominal aortic aneurysm exclusion: The Endologix device. J Vasc Surg 33:S154-S156, 2001.
27. White RA, Donayre CE, Walot I, et al: Abdominal aortic aneurysm rupture following endoluminal graft deployment: Report of a predictable event. J Endovasc Ther 7:257, 2000.
28. Harris PL, Vallavhaneni SR, Desgranges P, et al: Incidence and risk factors of late rupture, conversion, and death after endovascular repair of infrarenal aortic aneurysms: The EUROSTAR experience. J Vasc Surg 32:739, 2000.
29. Whitaker SC: Imaging of abdominal aortic aneurysm before and after endoluminal stent-graft repair. Eur J Radiol 39:3, 2001.
30. Harris P, Brennan J, Martin J, et al: Longitudinal aneurysm shrinkage following endovascular aortic aneurysm repair: A source of intermediate and late complications. J Endovasc Surg 6:11, 1999.
31. Wolf YG, Tillich M, Lee WA, et al: Changes in aneurysm volume after endovascular repair of abdominal aortic aneurysm. J Vasc Surg 36:305, 2002.
32. Wolf YG, Johnson BL, Hill BB, et al: Duplex ultrasound scanning versus computed tomographic angiography for postoperative evaluation of endovascular abdominal aortic aneurysm repair. J Vasc Surg 32:1142, 2000.
33. Golzarian J, Murgo S, Dussaussois L, et al: Evaluation of abdominal aortic aneurysm after endoluminal treatment: Comparison of color Doppler sonography with biphasic helical CT. Am J Roent 178:623, 2002.

34. Bendick PJ, Bove PG, Long GW, et al: Efficacy of ultrasound scan contrast agents in the noninvasive follow-up of aortic stent grafts. J Vasc Surg 37:381, 2003.
35. Bendick PJ, Zelenock GB, Bove PG, et al: Duplex ultrasound imaging with an ultrasound contrast agent: The economic alternative to CT angiography for aortic stent graft surveillance. Vasc Endovasc Surg 37:165, 2003.
36. Yao OJ, Faries PL, Morrissey N, et al: Ancillary techniques to facilitate endovascular repair of aortic aneurysms. J Vasc Surg 34:69, 2001.
37. Zarins CK, White RA, Schwarten D, et al: AneuRx stent graft versus open surgical repair of abdominal aortic anuerysms: Multicenter prospective clinical trial. J Vasc Surg 29:292, 1999.
38. May J, White GH, Waugh R, et al: Improved survival after endoluminal repair with second-generation prostheses compared with open repair in the treatment of abdominal aortic aneurysms: A 5-year concurrent comparison using life table method. J Vasc Surg 33:S21, 2001.
39. Lee WA, O'Dorisio J, Wolf YG, et al: Outcome after unilateral hypogastric artery occlusion during endovascular aneurysm repair. J Vasc Surg 33:921, 2001.
40. Wolpert LM, Dittrich KP, Hallisey MJ, et al: Hypogastric artery embolization in endovascular abdominal aortic aneurysm repair. J Vasc Surg 33:1193, 2001.
41. Criado FJ, Wilson EP, Velazequez OC, et al: Safety of coil embolization of the internal iliac artery in endovascular grafting of abdominal aortic aneurysms. J Vasc Surg 32:684, 2000.
42. Schoder M, Zaunbauer L, Holzenbein T, et al: Internal iliac artery embolization before endovascular repair of abdominal aortic aneuryms: Frequency, efficacy, and clinical results. Am J Radiol 177:599, 2001.
43. Mehta M, Veith FJ, Ohki T, et al: Unilateral and bilateral hypogastric artery interruption during aortoiliac aneurysm repair in 154 patients: A relatively innocuous procedure. J Vasc Surg 33:S27-S32, 2001.
44. Kritpracha B, Pigott JP, Price CI, et al: Distal internal iliac artery embolization: A procedure to avoid. J Vasc Surg 37:943, 2003.
45. Wyers MC, Shermerhorn ML, Fillinger MF, et al: Internal iliac occlusion without coil embolization during endovascular abdominal aortic aneurysm repair. J Vasc Surg 36:1138, 2002.
46. White GH, Yu W, May J: Endoleak: A proposed new terminology to describe incomplete aneurysm exclusion by an endoluminal graft. J Endovasc Surg 3:124, 1996.
47. White GH, May J, Waugh RC, et al: Type I and type II endoleaks: A more useful classification for reporting results of endoluminal AAA repair. J Endovasc Surg 5:189, 1998.
48. White GH, May J, Waugh RC, et al: Type III and type IV endoleaks: Toward a complete definition of blood flow in the sac after endoluminal AAA repair. J Endovasc Surg 5:305, 1998.
49. Schurink GW, Aarts NJ, Wilde J, et al: Endoleakage after stent-graft treatment of abdominal aneurysm: Implications on pressure and imaging: An *in vitro* study. J Vasc Surg 28:234, 1998.
50. White GH, May J, Petrasek P, et al: Endotension: An explanation for continued AAA growth after successful endoluminal repair. J Endovasc Surg 6:308, 1999.
51. Gilling-Smith G, Brennan J, Harris P, et al: Endotension after endovascular aneurysm repair: Definition, classification, and strategies for surveillance and intervention. J Endovasc Surg 6:305, 1999.
52. Zarins CK, White RA, Hodgson KJ, et al: Endoleak as a predictor of outcome after endovascular aneurysm repair: AneuRx multicenter clinical trial. J Vasc Surg 32:90, 2000.
53. Holzenbein T, Kretschmer G, Thurnher S, et al: Midterm durability of abdominal aortic aneurysm endograft repair: A word of caution. J Vasc Surg 33:S46-S54, 2001.
54. Buth J, Harris PL, van Marrewijk C, et al: The significance and management of different types of endoleaks. Semin Vasc Surg 16:95, 2003.
55. Chuter TAM, Faruqi RM, Sawhney R, et al: Endoleak after endovascular repair of abdominal aortic aneurysm. J Vasc Surg 34:98, 2001.
56. Buth J, Laheji RJF: Early complications and endoleaks after endovascular abdominal aortic aneurysm repair: Report of a multicenter study. J Vasc Surg 31:134, 2000.
57. Dattilo JB, Brewster DC, Fan C-M, et al: Clinical failures of endovascular abdominal aortic aneurysm repair: Incidence, causes, and management. J Vasc Surg 35:1137, 2002.
58. Zarins CK: The US AneuRx clinical trial: 6-year clinical update 2002. J Vasc Surg 37:904, 2003.
59. Fairman RM, Carpenter JP, Baum RA, et al: Potential impact of therapeutic warfarin treatment on type II endoleaks and sac shrinkage rates on midterm follow-up examination. J Vasc Surg 35:679, 2002.
60. Baum RA, Carpenter JP, Cope C, et al: Aneurysm sac pressure measurements after endovascular repair of abdominal aortic aneurysms. J Vasc Surg 33:32, 2001.
61. Marty B, Sanchez LA, Ohki T, et al: Endoleak after endovascular graft repair of experimental aortic aneurysms: Does coil embolization with angiographic "seal" lower intraaneurysmal pressure? J Vasc Surg 27:454, 1998.
62. Baum RA, Cope C, Fairman RM, et al: Translumbar embolization of type 2 endoleaks after endovascular repair of abdominal aortic aneurysms. J Vasc Interv Radiol 12:111, 2001.
63. Parodi JC, Berguer R, Ferreira LM, et al: Intra-aneurysmal pressure after incomplete endovascular exclusion. J Vasc Surg 33:909, 2001.
64. Back MR, Bowser AN, Johnson BL, et al: Patency of infrarenal aortic side branches determines early aneurysm sac behavior after endovascular repair. Ann Vasc Surg 17:27, 2003.
65. Fan C-M, Rafferty EA, Geller SC, et al: Endovascular stent-graft in abdominal aortic aneurysms: The relationship between patent vessels that arise from the aneurysmal sac and early endoleak. Radiology 218:176, 2001.
66. Gawenda M, Heckenkamp J, Zaehringer M, et al: Intra-aneurysm sac pressure—the holy grail of endoluminal grafting of AAA. Eur J Vasc Endovasc Surg 24:139, 2002.
67. Jacobs T, Teodorescu V, Morrissey N, et al: The endovascular repair of abdominal aortic aneurysm: An update analysis of structural failure modes of endovascular grafts. Semin Vasc Surg 16:103, 2003.
68. Stelter W, Umscheid T, Ziegler P: Three-year experience with modular stent-graft devices for endovascular AAA treatment. J Endovasc Surg 4:362, 1997.
69. Beebe HG, Cronenwett JL, Katzen BT, et al: Results of an aortic endograft trial: Impact of device failure beyond 12 months. J Vasc Surg 33:S55-S63, 2001.
70. Riepe G, Loos J, Imig H, et al: Long-term in vivo alterations of polyester vascular grafts in humans. Eur J Endovasc Surg 13:540, 1997.
71. Jacobs TS, Won J, Graveraux EC, et al: Mechanical failure of prosthetic human implants: A 10-year experience with aortic stent graft devices. J Vasc Surg 37:16, 2003.
72. Alimi YS, Chakfe N, Rivoal E, et al: Rupture of an abdominal aortic aneurysm after endovascular graft placement and aneurysm size reduction. J Vasc Surg 28:178, 1998.
73. Riepe G, Heilberger P, Umschield T, et al: Frame dislocation of body middle rings in endovascular stent tube grafts. J Endovasc Surg 17:28, 1999.
74. Krajcer Z, Howell M, Dougherty K: Unusual case of AneuRx stent-graft failure two years after AAA exclusion. J Endovasc Ther 8:465, 2001.
75. Moore WS, Rutherford RB: Transfemoral endovascular repair of abdominal aortic aneurysm: Results of the North American EVT phase I trial. J Vasc Surg 34:353, 1996.
76. Heintz C, Riepe G, Birken L: Corroded nitinol wires in explanted aortic endografts: An important mechanism of failure? J Endovasc Ther 8:248, 2001.
77. Trepanier C, Tabrizian M, Yahia L, et al: Effect of modification of oxide layer on NiTi stent corrosion resistance. J Biomed Mater Res (Appl Biomater) 43:433, 1998.
78. Duerig TW, Pelton AR, Stockel D: An overview of nitinol medical applications. Mater Sci Eng A273-275:149, 1999.
79. Starosvetsky E, Gotman I: Corrosion behavior of titanium nitride coated Ni-Ti shape memory surgical alloy. Biomaterials 22:1853, 2001.
80. Umschied T, Stelter W: Time-related alterations in shape, position, and structure of self-expanding modular aortic stent-grafts: A 4 year single center follow-up. J Endovasc Surg 6:17, 1999.
81. Fairman RM, Baum RA, Carpenter JP, et al: Limb interventions in patients undergoing treatment with an unsupported bifurcated aortic endograft system: A review of the Phase II EVT Trial. J Vasc Surg 36:118, 2002.
82. Carroccio A, Faries PL, Morrissey NJ, et al: Predicting iliac limb occlusion after bifurcated aortic stent grafting: Anatomic and device-related causes. J Vasc Surg 36:679, 2002.
83. Baum RA, Shetty SK, Carpenter JP, et al: Limb kinking in supported and unsupported abdominal aortic stent-grafts. J Vasc Interv Radiol 11:1165, 2000.

84. Amesur NB, Zajko AB, Orons PD, et al: Endovascular treatment of iliac limb stenoses or occlusion in 31 patients treated with the Ancure endograft. J Vasc Interv Radiol 11:421, 2000.
85. Ohki T, Veith FJ, Shaw P, et al: Increasing incidence of midterm and long-term complications after endovascular graft repair of abdominal aortic aneurysms: A note of caution based on a 9-year experience. Ann Surg 234:323, 2001.
86. Carpenter JP, Neschis DG, Fairman RM, et al: Failure of endovascular abdominal aortic aneurysm graft limbs. J Vasc Surg 33:296, 2001.
87. Sampram ES, Karafa MT, Mascha EJ, et al: Nature, frequency, and predictors of secondary procedures after endovacular repair of abdominal aortic aneurysm. J Vasc Surg 37:930, 2003.
88. Fairman RM, Velazequez OC, Baum RA, et al: Endovascular repair of aortic aneurysms: Critical events and adjunctive procedures. J Vasc Surg 33:1226, 2001.
89. Conners III MS, Sternbergh III WC, Carter G, et al: Secondary procedures after endovascular aortic aneurysm repair. J Vasc Surg 36:992, 2002.
90. Albertini J-N, Kalliafas S, Travis S, et al: Anatomical risk factors for proximal perigraft endoleak and graft migration following endovascular repair of abdominal aortic aneurysms. Eur J Vasc Endovasc Surg 19:308, 2000.
91. Cao P, Verzini F, Zannetti S, et al: Device migration after endoluminal abdominal aortic aneurysm repair: Analysis of 113 cases with a minimum follow-up period of 2 years. J Vasc Surg 35:229, 2002.
92. Lawrence-Brown MMD, Semmens JB, Hartley D, et al: How is durability related to patient selection and graft design with endoluminal grafting for abdominal aortic aneurysm? In Greenlaugh R (ed): The Durability of Vascular and Endovascular Surgery. London, WB Saunders, 1999:375.
93. Resch T, Malina M, Lindblad B, et al: The impact of stent design on proximal stent-graft fixation in the abdominal aorta: An experimental study. Eur J Vasc Endovasc Surg 20:190, 2000.
94. Malina M, Lindblad B, Ivancev K, et al: Endovascular AAA exclusion: Will stents with hooks and barbs prevent stent-graft migration? J Endovasc Ther 6:4, 1998.
95. Lee JT, Lee J, Aziz I, et al: Stent-graft migration following endovascular repair of aneurysms with large proximal necks: Anatomical risk factors and long-term sequelae. J Endovasc Ther 9:652, 2002.
96. White GH, May J, Waugh R, et al: Shortening of endografts during deployment in endovascular AAA repair. J Endovasc Ther 6:4, 1999.
97. Prinssen M, Wever JJ, Mali WPTM, et al: Concerns for the durability of the proximal abdominal aortic aneurysm endograft fixation from a 2-year and 3-year longitudinal computed tomography angiography study. J Vasc Surg 33:S64-S69, 2001.
98. Badran MF, Gould DA, Raza I, et al: Aneurysm neck diameter after endovascular repair of abdominal aortic aneurysms. J Vasc Interv Radiol 13:887, 2002.
99. Ouriel K, Srivastava SD, Sarac TP, et al: Disparate outcome after endovascular treatment of small versus large abdominal aortic aneurysm. J Vasc Surg 37:1206, 2003.
100. Becker GJ, Kovacs M, Mathison MN, et al: Risk stratification and outcomes of transluminal endografting for abdominal aortic aneurysm: 7-year experience and long-term follow-up. J Vasc Interv Radiol 12:1033, 2003.
101. Naslund TC, Edwards WH, Neuzil DF, et al: Technical complications of endovascular abdominal aortic aneurysm repair. J Vasc Surg 26:502, 1997.
102. Laheji RJF, Buth J, Harris PL, et al: Need for secondary interventions after endovascular repair of abdominal aortic aneurysms: Intermediate-term follow-up results of a European collaborative registry (EUROSTAR). Br J Surg 87:1666, 2000.
103. May J, White GH, Waugh R, et al: Life-table analysis of primary and assisted success following endoluminal repair of abdominal aortic aneurysms: The role of supplementary endovascular intervention in improving outcome. Eur J Vasc Endovasc Surg 19:648, 2000.
104. Sternbergh III WC, Conners MS, Tonnessen BH, et al: Aortic aneurysm sac shrinkage after endovascular repair is device-dependent: A comparison of Zenith and AneuRx endografts. Ann Vasc Surg 17:49, 2003.
105. Bertges DJ, Chow K, Wyers MC, et al: Abdominal aortic aneurysm size regression after endovascular repair is endograft dependent. J Vasc Surg 37:716, 2003.
106. Moore WS, Matsumura JS, Makaroun MS, et al: Five-year interim comparison of the Guidant bifurcated endograft with open repair of abdominal aortic aneurysm. J Vasc Surg 38:46, 2003.
107. Arko FR, Hill BB, Olcott IV C, et al: Endovascular repair reduces early and late morbidity compared to open surgery for abdominal aortic aneurysm. J Endovasc Ther 9:711, 2002.
108. Hill BB, Wolf YG, Lee A, et al: Open versus endovascular AAA repair in patients who are morphological candidates for endovascular treatment. J Endovasc Ther 9:255, 2002.
109. Matsumura JS, Brewster DC, Makaroun MS, et al: A multicenter controlled clinical trial of open versus endovascular treatment of abdominal aortic aneurysm. J Vasc Surg 37:262, 2003.
110. Carpenter JP, Baum RA, Barker CF, et al: Durability of benefits of endovascular versus conventional abdominal aortic aneurysm repair. J Vasc Surg 35:222, 2002.
111. Shermerhorn ML, Finlayson S, Fillinger MF, et al: Life expectancy after endovascular versus open abdominal aortic aneurysm repair: Results of a decision analysis model on the basis of data from EUROSTAR. J Vasc Surg 36:1112, 2002.
111a. Blankensteijn JD, de Jong SE, Prinssen M, et al: Two-year outcomes after conventional or endovascular repair of abdominal aortic aneurysms. N Engl J Med 352:2398, 2005.
111b. EVAR Trial participants: Endovascular aneurysm repair versus open repair in patients with abdominal aortic aneurysms (EVAR trial 1): Randomised controlled trial. Lancet 365:2179, 2005.
112. Wolf YG, Arko FR, Hill BB, et al: Gender differences in endovascular abdominal aortic aneurysm repair with the AneuRx stent graft. J Vasc Surg 35:882, 2002.
113. Krajcer Z, Howell M: A novel technique using the percutaneous vascular surgery device to close the 22 French femoral artery entry site used for percutaneous abdominal aortic aneurysm exclusion. Catheter Cardiovasc Interv 50:356, 2000.
114. Torsello GB, Kasprzak B, Klenk E, et al: Endovascular suture versus cutdown for endovascular aneurysm repair: A prospective randomized pilot study. J Vasc Surg 38:78, 2003.
115. Traul DK, Clair DG, Gray B, et al: Percutaneous endovascular repair of infrarenal abdominal aortic aneurysms: A feasibility study. J Vasc Surg 32:770, 2000.
116. Howell M, Villareal R, Krajcer Z: Percutaneous access and closure of femoral artery access sites associated with endoluminal repair of abdominal aortic aneurysms. J Endovasc Ther 8:68, 2001.
117. Kerr A, Marsan B, Lyon R: Slimgraft: A percutaneous endovascular graft system. J Endovasc Ther 7:41, 2000.
118. Dake MD: Endovascular stent-graft management of thoracic aortic diseases. Eur J Radiol 39:42, 2001.
119. Mitchell RS, Miller DC, Dake MD, et al: Thoracic aortic aneurysm repair with an endovascular stent graft: The "first generation." Ann Thorac Surg 67:1971, 1999.
120. Kasirajan K, Dolmatch B, Ouriel K, et al: Delayed onset of ascending paralysis after thoracic aortic stent graft deployment. J Vasc Surg 31:196, 2000.
121. Criado FJ, Barnatan MF, Rizk Y, et al: Technical strategies to expand stent-graft applicability in the aortic arch and proximal descending thoracic aorta. J Endovasc Ther 9:II32-II38, 2002.
122. Burks Jr JA, Faries PL, Graveraux EC, et al: Endovascular repair of thoracic aortic aneurysms: Stent-graft fixation across the aortic arch vessels. Ann Vasc Surg 16:24, 2002.
123. Gorich J, Asquan Y, Seifarth H, et al: Initial experience with intentional stent-graft coverage of the subclavian artery during endovascular thoracic aortic repairs. J Endovasc Ther 9:II39, 2002.
123a. Makaroun MS, Dillavou ED, Kee ST, et al: Endovascular treatment of thoracic aortic aneurysms: Results of the phase II multicenter trial of the GORE TAG thoracic endoprosthesis. J Vasc Surg 41:1, 2005.
124. Dake MD, Miller DC, Semba CP, et al: Transluminal placement of endovascular stent-grafts for the treatment of descending thoracic aortic aneurysms. N Engl J Med 331:1729, 1994.
125. Won JY, Lee DY, Shim WH, et al: Elective endovascular treatment of descending thoracic aortic aneurysms and chronic dissections with stent-grafts. J Vasc Interv Radiol 12:575, 2001.
126. Faries PL, Lang E, Ramdev P, et al: Endovascular stent-graft treatment of a ruptured thoracic aortic ulcer. J Endovasc Ther 9:II-20, 2002.
127. Alric P, Berthet J-P, Branchereau P, et al: Endovascular repair for acute rupture of the descending thoracic aorta. J Endovasc Ther 9:II-51-II-59, 2002.

128. Nio D, Vos PM, de Mol BAJM, et al: Emergency endovascular treatment of thoracic aortic rupture in three accident victims with multiple injuries. J Endovasc Ther 9:II-60-II-66, 2002.
129. Woody JA, Walot I, Donayre CE, et al: Endovascular exclusion of leaking thoracic aortic aneurysms. J Endovasc Ther 9:II-79-II-83, 2002.
130. White RA, Donayre CE, Walot I, et al: Endovascular exclusion of descending thoracic aortic aneurysms and chronic dissection: Initial clinical results with the AneuRx device. J Vasc Surg 33:927, 2001.
131. Criado FJ, Clark NS, Barnatan MF: Stent graft repair in the aortic arch and descending thoracic aorta: A 4-year experience. J Vasc Surg 36:1121, 2002.
132. Ellozy SH, Carroccio A, Minor M, et al: Challenges of endovascular tube graft repair of thoracic aortic aneurysm: Midterm follow-up and lessons learned. J Vasc Surg 38:676, 2003.
133. Wakefield TW, Whitehouse WM, Wu SC, et al: Abdominal aortic aneurysm rupture: Statistical analysis of factors affecting outcome of surgical treatment. Surgery 91:586, 1982.
134. Marty-Ane CH, Alric P, Picot MC, et al: Ruptured abdominal aortic aneurysm: Influence of intraoperative management on surgical outcome. J Vasc Surg 22:780, 1995.
135. Lazarides MK, Arvantis DP, Drista H, et al: POSSUM and APACHE II scores do not predict the outcome of ruptured infrarenal aortic aneurysms. Ann Vasc Surg 11:155, 1997.
136. Dardik A, Burleyson GP, Bowman H, et al: Surgical repair of ruptured abdominal aortic aneruysms in the state of Maryland: Factors influencing outcome among 527 recent cases. J Vasc Surg 28:413, 1998.
137. Greenberg RK, Srivastava SD, Ouriel K, et al: An endoluminal method of hemorrhage control and repair of ruptured abdominal aortic aneurysms. J Endovasc Ther 7:1, 2000.
138. Ohki T, Veith FJ, Sanchez LA, et al: Endovascular graft repair of ruptured aortoiliac aneurysms. J Am Coll Surg 189:102, 1999.
139. Hinchliffe RJ, Braithwaite BD, Hopkinson BR: The endovascular management of ruptured abdominal aortic aneurysms. Eur J Vasc Endovasc Surg 25:191, 2003.
140. Hinchcliffe RJ, Yusuf SW, Macierewicz JA, et al: Endovascular repair of ruptured abdominal aortic aneurysms—a challenge to open repair? Results of a single centre experience in 20 patients. Eur J Endovasc Surg 22:528, 2001.
141. Yilmaz N, Peppelenbosch N, Cuypers PWM, et al: Emergency treatment of symptomatic or ruptured abdominal aortic aneurysms: The role of endovascular repair. J Endovasc Ther 9:449, 2002.
142. Veith FJ, Ohki T: Endovascular approaches to ruptured infrarenal aortoiliac aneurysms. J Cardiovasc Surg 43:369, 2002.
143. Stanley BM, Semmens JB, Lawrence-Brown MMD, et al: Fenestration in endovascular grafts for aortic aneurysm repair: New horizons for preserving blood flow in branch vessels. J Endovasc Ther 8:16, 2001.
144. Anderson J, Berce M, Hartley DE: Endoluminal aortic grafting with renal and superior mesenteric artery incorporation by graft fenestration. J Endovasc Ther 8:3, 2001.
145. Chuter TAM, Gordon RL, Reilly LM, et al: Multi-branched stent-graft for type III thoracoabdominal aortic aneurysm. J Vasc Interv Radiol 12:391, 2001.
146. Bleyn J, Schol F, Vanhandenhove I, et al: Side-branched modular endograft system for thoracoabdominal aortic aneurysm repair. J Endovasc Ther 9:838, 2002.

chapter 41

Overview of Vasculitis

Peter A. Merkel

The vasculitides are a group of rare diseases linked by the pathologic consequences of vascular inflammation, including bleeding, ischemia, and infarction of downstream organs (Table 41-1). However, the clinical spectrum of these diseases is wide ranging and includes a myriad of clinical and pathologic findings. Not all disease phenotypes that occur in the vasculitides are due to true "vasculitis" (i.e., inflammation of vascular structures). Some damage in vasculitis occurs due to nonvascular inflammation. For example, arthritis, uveitis, and pulmonary nodules are parts of different vasculitides but are not due to interruption of vascular flow. The pathophysiology of vasculitis is covered in Chapter 7 and in individual chapters on Takayasu's arteritis (Chapter 42), giant cell arteritis (GCA) (Chapter 43), and Kawasaki disease (Chapter 45).

The diseases outlined in this chapter are rare, and all are considered "orphan" diseases, with fewer than 200,000 cases in the United States at any time. As with most rare diseases, few well-controlled clinical treatment trials have been performed for this group of disorders. Much of the clinical investigation stems from studies of patient cohorts at large referral centers. In the past decade, however, increasing international cooperation among vasculitis centers has resulted in several important randomized controlled treatment trials that have had significant impacts on the care and management of patients with vasculitis. Similarly, advances in diagnostic imaging and laboratory testing have improved clinicians' ability to diagnose and evaluate patients with vasculitis.

This chapter reviews the major types of vasculitis, discusses the evaluation of suspected cases of vasculitis, and outlines the approach to treatment and management of these disorders. There is a focus on differentiating inflammatory from noninflammatory disease as it relates to the types of patients that physicians specializing in vascular medicine are likely to encounter in a consultative practice (Table 41-2). The newest advances in diagnosis and treatment are also reviewed briefly.

CLASSIFICATION OF VASCULITIS

The classification and nomenclature of vasculitis can be unnecessarily confusing. The most important first step in approaching these disorders is for clinicians to consider the possibility of "some sort of vasculitis" and, once clinical proof is found, to narrow down the specific type. Nevertheless, knowledge of the classification criteria is quite useful when considering treatment and clinical follow-up. Establishing a treatment plan for a case of vasculitis relies on both an understanding of the prognosis of a specific type and applying results of clinical trials that always include patients who meet specific classification criteria. For example, a patient with arthritis, purpura, and abdominal pain might well be treated with glucocorticoids alone if believed to have Henoch-Schönlein purpura (HSP) but would also receive an additional immunosuppressive drug, such as methotrexate or cyclophosphamide, if determined to have Wegener's granulomatosis (WG).

TABLE 41-1 CLASSIFICATION OF VASCULITIS BY PREDOMINANT SIZE OF VESSEL INVOLVEMENT

Most of these diseases can involve vessels of varying sizes but are listed here by the size of the most commonly affected arteries for convenience purposes. This is not an exhaustive list of vasculitides.

Large Vessel	Medium Vessel	Small Vessel
Giant cell arteritis	Polyarteritis nodosa	Henoch-Schönlein purpura
Takayasu's arteritis	Wegener's granulomatosis	Cryoglobulinemic vasculitis
Behçet's disease	Microscopic polyangiitis	Primary angiitis of the CNS
Relapsing polychondritis	Churg-Strauss syndrome	Goodpasture's syndrome
Cogan's syndrome	Kawasaki disease	Rheumatoid arthritis (rheumatoid vasculitis)
Aortitis associated with spondyloarthropathies		Sjögren's syndrome
Retroperitoneal fibrosis		Systemic lupus erythematosus
Idiopathic aortitis		Systemic sclerosis (scleroderma)
		Drug-induced vasculitis

TABLE 41-2 MANIFESTATIONS OF VASCULITIS THAT MIMIC NONINFLAMMATORY CARDIOVASCULAR DISEASE

Type of Vasculitis	Thoracic Aortic Disease	Abdominal Aortic Disease	Carotid/Vertebral Arterial Disease	Stroke Due to Small or Medium Arterial Disease	Upper and Lower Extremity Arterial Stenosis	Renal Arterial Disease	Coronary Artery Disease	Mesenteric Arteritis	Myocarditis	Pericarditis
Giant cell arteritis	++[*]	+[†]			+	+	Rare[‡]	Rare		
Takayasu's arteritis	+++[§]	++			+++	++	+	+	Rare	Rare
Behçet's disease	+	++	Rare	Rare	+	Rare	Rare		+	
Other large vessel diseases (RPC, CS, RPF, IA)	++	+	+	Rare	+	+	Rare	+	Rare	Rare
Polyarteritis nodosa				+	+	+	Rare	+++	+	+
Wegener's granulomatosis	Rare			Rare	+	Rare	Rare	+	Rare	+
Microscopic polyangiitis				Rare		Rare	Rare	+	Rare	+
Churg-Strauss syndrome				Rare			Rare	+	++	++
Kawasaki disease			Rare	Rare			+++		++	+
Henoch-Schönlein purpura								+++		
Cryoglobulinic vasculitis				Rare			Rare	Rare	+++	
Primary angiitis of CNS			++	++						
Small vessel vasculitis of RA SS, SLE, or SSc			Rare	+	Rare	+	+	++	+	+++

*Moderately common manifestation.
†Well described but relatively uncommonly seen.
‡Reported but quite rare.
§Common manifestation.
CNS, Central nervous system; CS, Cogan's syndrome; IA, idiopathic aortitis; RPC, relapsing polychondritis; RA, rheumatoid arthritis; RPF, retroperitoneal fibrosis; SLE, systemic lupus erythematosus; SS, Sjögren's syndrome; SSc, systemic sclerosis (scleroderma).

Similarly, the nature of follow-up visits, examinations, and subsequent evaluations are also heavily influenced by the specific type of vasculitis. For example, new-onset hemoptysis in a patient believed to be in remission after treatment for GCA would be concerning for infection or malignancy, whereas the same finding in a patient with WG would usually prompt immediate reinstitution of high-dose glucocorticoids to treat potential alveolar hemorrhage while further evaluations, including for infection, are put in place.

Two major classification systems for vasculitis exist: the American College of Rheumatology (ACR) system[1] and the Chapel Hill Consensus conference definitions.[2] These systems were not meant to be strictly *diagnostic* systems but rather *classification* systems. These are definitions to apply to established vasculitis and to use to differentiate one vasculitis from another. The main use of these systems has been for clinical trials and other types of clinical research. Nevertheless, these systems have been adapted for use by clinicians as helpful guides to practice. Not all types of vasculitis are included in the ACR or Chapel Hill systems.

The practice of differentiating among the inflammatory vasculitides by associated diagnostic antibodies is at this time limited to the use of antineutrophil cytoplasmic antibodies (ANCA). Specifically, some authors speak of "ANCA-positive" (or "ANCA-associated") versus "ANCA-negative" diseases. The ANCA-associated disorders include WG, microscopic polyangiitis, renal-limited pauci-immune glomerulonephritis, and the Churg-Strauss syndrome (CSS). Although it is convenient to refer to these related diseases as *ANCA positive,* the term excludes so many other types of vasculitis that it has limited usefulness.

Perhaps the simplest method of sorting out the vasculitides, albeit also incomplete and not fully accurate, is to list them according to the size of artery *predominantly*, but not necessarily exclusively, involved (see Table 41-1). This results in considering *small vessel, medium vessel*, and *large vessel* vasculitides. This system, although not applied for clinical trials or even clinically for treatment purposes, is an easy one to use as a first approach to describing the diseases and their major manifestations. This size-based system is used to outline the descriptions of the vasculitides in this chapter; however, when specific diseases and results of treatment trials are mentioned, the ACR and Chapel Hill Consensus systems are applied.

LARGE VESSEL VASCULITIS

The large vessel vasculitides include those disorders in which the aorta and its main branches are affected, including the subclavian, carotid, vertebral, renal, mesenteric, and iliac arteries (see Fig. 41-1).[3] Because such vessels are so frequently involved in noninflammatory vascular diseases and patients with these diseases are frequently encountered by specialists in vascular medicine, these

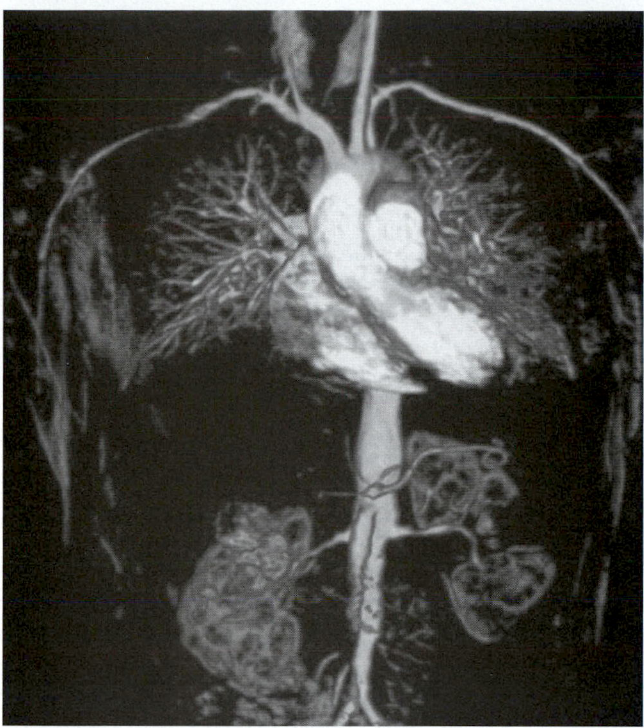

FIGURE 41-1. (See also Color Plate 41-1.) Large vessel vasculitis with stenotic lesions of abdominal aorta and the left subclavian, left carotid, and bilateral renal arteries as imaged using three-dimensional, dynamic, gadolinium-enhanced MRA.

disorders are particularly highlighted in this textbook. Also included are individual chapters on Takayasu's arteritis (Chapter 42), giant cell (temporal) arteritis (Chapter 43), and Kawasaki disease (Chapter 45). The vasculitides involving large arteries are briefly described in this section. Although these vasculitides involve large arteries and are thus listed in this section, it is important to realize that many of them also involve smaller-sized vessels.

Giant Cell Arteritis

GCA, also commonly known as temporal arteritis, is the most common of the idiopathic vasculitides.[3,4] GCA affects men and women aged 50 and older but is especially prevalent after age 70. Many vascular and systemic manifestations are seen in this disease. Vascular disease occurs in the aorta and its branches with predilection to the branches of the carotid arteries, especially the ophthalmic artery, with resulting headaches, jaw claudication, and visual impairment. Rapid-onset irreversible monocular blindness is the most feared complication, but stroke, limb ischemia, and aortic disease can occur, the latter more common than generally appreciated, especially several years after the initial presentation. Common systemic manifestations include fever, anemia, proximal arthralgias (polymyalgia rheumatica), and fatigue. Diagnosis is often established on finding arteritis on temporal artery biopsy, but this is not required for a diagnosis. Elevated acute phase reactants are seen in 90% of cases. Treatment with high-dose glucocorticoids is highly effective but often results in significant drug-related morbidity.

GCA is described in detail in Chapter 43 of this text.

Takayasu's Arteritis

Takayasu's arteritis is a vasculitis that involves the aorta and all its major branches and the pulmonary arteries, including, but not limited to, the brachiocephalic, carotid, vertebral, subclavian, renal, femoral, and coronary arteries, often resulting in stenoses and occlusions with ischemic damage to end organs and limbs.[3,5] Stroke, myocardial infarction, limb claudication, and severe renovascular hypertension are all complications well known to occur in this disease. The disease is mostly seen in women and usually first presents clinically in the second or third decade, but it can occur at older ages. Many patients have associated systemic symptoms of fever, arthralgias, and malaise. The disease has a waxing and waning course, and delay in diagnosis is common. Treatment involves glucocorticoids in almost all patients and often the addition of immunosuppressive medications. Surgical bypass procedures may be necessary in select cases.

Takayasu's arteritis is described in detail in Chapter 42 of this text.

Behçet's Disease

Behçet's disease is a systemic inflammatory disease with multiple mucocutaneous manifestations, especially including genital and oral ulcers and often severe sight-threatening inflammatory eye disease.[6] Arthritis, gastrointestinal disease including mucosal lesions, epididymitis, and secondary amyloidosis can also occur. Although the prevalence is markedly increased in countries in the Eastern Mediterranean, Middle East, and East Asia and descendents of people from these regions, Behçet's disease is found in populations worldwide.

Vasculitis occurs in up to one third of patients with Behçet's disease and is unique among the inflammatory vasculitides for the relatively common clinical involvement of *venous* disease. Both arterial and venous manifestations may occur in the same patients. Venous involvement includes superficial phlebitis, varices, and thromboses of deep veins, vena cava, cerebral sinuses, and other major veins.

The arterial lesions in Behçet's disease are often in large vessels and frequently result in aneurysms, stenoses, or rupture. The most common sites of arteritis are the aorta and its branches and the pulmonary arteries; however, Behçet's disease may also involve medium and small vessels.

Behçet's disease can involve a huge range of different types of histopathologies consistent with the protean disease manifestations. The oral and genital ulcers do not have specific pathognomonic features. Similarly, biopsy specimens of the gastrointestinal lesions cannot differentiate Behçet's disease from inflammatory bowel disease. Although the vascular lesions can include large and small arteries as well as veins, these lesions are similar to those of other vasculitides.

Treatment of Behçet's disease varies with the manifestation being addressed and may range from colchicine and topical glucocorticoids for aphthous ulcers to large doses of glucocorticoids for many problems including mucocutaneous, vascular, and eye lesions. The uveitis is treated with long-term immunosuppressive agents, including cyclosporine, azathioprine, chlorambucil, and cyclophosphamide. The usefulness of inhibitors of tumor necrosis factor-alpha (TNF-α) is currently being investigated for this disorder. Many treatment protocols are based on expert opinion, but in recent years an increasing number of controlled clinical trials have been performed, especially involving eye disease. Behçet's disease can be a highly aggressive form of vasculitis that frequently results in significant morbidity and mortality.

Relapsing Polychondritis

Relapsing polychondritis is a rare connective tissue disease that predominantly affects the cartilaginous structures of the eyes, ears, nose, and subglottis/trachea but may also affect a wide variety of other organ systems and is associated with vasculitis, especially of large vessels.[7] The cardinal feature of polychondritis is auriculitis, inflammation of the outer ear, usually sparing the noncartilaginous lobe. Auriculitis, which is also a feature of WG but virtually of no other diseases, is readily treated with glucocorticoids and can result in disfigurement if allowed to go untreated. Other common manifestations include inflammatory eye disease that can lead to blindness, destruction of nasal cartilage leading to internal derangement and external disfigurement, sensorineural hearing loss and vertigo, arthritis, and subglottic inflammation with resulting stenosis, a life-threatening condition. Each of these features can also be seen in WG, although auriculitis is rare in this disease and relapsing polychondritis is not associated with pulmonary manifestations.

The vasculitis seen in relapsing polychondritis can affect vessels of any size, but large vessel vasculitis is the most common. Aortitis with associated aortic valvular dysfunction and accompanied by thoracic or abdominal aortic aneurysms is fairly common and can lead to heart failure, aneurysmal rupture or dissection, and involvement of branch arteries. Small vessel disease can affect nerves, eyes, kidneys, and other systems.

The histopathology of relapsing polychondritis includes destructive inflammation of various types of cartilage, necrotizing aortitis, vasculitis small vessels (e.g., skin, glomeruli), and direct inflammatory infiltration of eye structures, heart valves, pericardium, skin, and other tissues.

Relapsing polychondritis has been associated with various other primary autoimmune diseases, such as inflammatory bowel disease, lupus, and others. The rarity of this syndrome has precluded comprehensive research that might help both better differentiate cases from other conditions and learn more about the pathophysiology. Treatment almost always involves systemic glucocorticoids, and immunosuppressive agents are frequently prescribed for this often rapidly progressive disease.

Cogan's Syndrome

Cogan's syndrome is a rare disorder characterized by inflammatory eye and inner ear/vestibular disease that can also involve inflammatory vasculitis.[8] It is a disease of young adults, usually first affecting patients before age 40, although both children and older patients have also been affected.

The characteristic clinical manifestations of Cogan's syndrome are interstitial keratitis, sensorineural hearing loss, and vestibulatory dysfunction. Although interstitial keratitis is the most common eye problem in Cogan's syndrome, uveitis, scleritis, and many other types of ophthalmologic inflammation can occur. The eye and ear damage is often permanent and can be quite debilitating. The diagnosis of Cogan's syndrome necessitates the combination of inflammatory eye disease and inner ear problems, but these findings can occur in other diseases, including various infections, malignancies, sarcoidosis, and various autoimmune diseases, including other vasculitides, such as WG, relapsing polychondritis, and Behçet's disease. Other organ systems are less commonly involved, as well.

Vasculitis occurs in up to 15% of patients with Cogan's syndrome and is mostly large vessel disease with some medium-vessel manifestations reported. The large vessel disease in Cogan's syndrome is similar to that of Takayasu's arteritis and includes aortitis with aortic insufficiency, stenoses of the carotid and subclavian and other aortic branch arteries, and even coronary artery disease. Treatment of Cogan's syndrome includes both glucocorticoids and immunosuppressive drugs, appropriate rehabilitation such as vestibular retraining, surgical correction of eye damage, and use of hearing aides or surgical correction of hearing loss.

Idiopathic Aortitis

Aortitis may be found in the absence of any other manifestations of a systemic inflammatory disease.[9] These cases often come to the attention of vascular medicine specialists when patients undergoing surgical repair of aortic aneurysms and dissections are found to have inflammation on the pathologic specimens consistent with aortitis. Autopsies and studies of large numbers of surgical specimens have demonstrated that noninfectious aortitis occurs in 4% to 15% of cases. Although on detailed investigation, many of these patients are found to have had evidence of GCA, Takayasu's arteritis, relapsing polychondritis, WG, or another definable vasculitis retrospectively, it is not uncommon among these cases to find no evidence of more systemic inflammatory disease. The majority of cases of so-called idiopathic aortitis involve thoracic lesions in contrast to the overall predominance of abdominal aortic lesions for noninflammatory disease.

It is possible that cases of isolated inflammatory aortic aneurysms will be increasingly identified earlier as MRI technology continues to improve and helps demonstrate inflammations in the arterial wall. It can, however, be difficult to differentiate inflammation due to true idiopathic aortitis and vasculitis from the vascular and periaortic inflammations' seen in association with atherosclerotic disease. Currently, in the absence of pathologic specimens or other evidence of a vasculitis, MRI alone is not diagnostic for inflammation. The emergence of PET scanning for large vessel disease may also help in the evaluation of such patients.

The approach to treatment of idiopathic aortitis is unclear, as many patients never develop other findings of vasculitis; however, new aneurysms and significant vascular disease do occur in some cases. Comprehensive evaluation of evidence of systemic disease is necessary and should include a detailed physical examination, diagnostic imaging, laboratory studies, and other approaches outlined later in this chapter. Appropriate treatment should be given if inflammatory disease other than that seen in the surgical specimen is found; however, not all patients require glucocorticoids, especially in the postoperative period. Furthermore, regular follow-up of such patients by a specialist knowledgeable about vasculitis is imperative, as lesions may develop subtly and only years after the initial pathologic diagnosis is made.

Miscellaneous Forms of Large Vessel Vasculitis

Although large vessel vasculitis is only rarely seen with other systemic inflammatory conditions, it is important to recognize these potential associations. Aortitis is rarely associated with long-standing *seronegative spondyloarthropathies* (ankylosing spondylitis, reactive arthritis, psoriatic arthritis, and inflammatory bowel disease) and can result in aortic insufficiency. *Retroperitoneal fibrosis,* a rare disease of proliferating fibroblasts usually causing ureteral obstruction and at times aortic stenosis and periaortitis, is also associated with true inflammatory aortitis. There have been a few case reports of large vessel vasculitis in patients with rheumatoid arthritis, systemic lupus erythematosus (SLE), and WG.

MEDIUM VESSEL VASCULITIS

Among the inflammatory vasculitides, the medium vessel diseases have the greatest variety of clinical manifestations, which result from the broad range of vessel sizes actually involved in the process. As stated earlier, classifying the vasculitides by affected vessel size is problematic, but no more so than with the "medium vessel" disorders.

Specialists in vascular medicine need to be aware of protean presentations of active medium vessel disease and the lasting damage they can cause. As with large vessel disease, these disorders can mimic noninflammatory cardiac, renal, cerebral, and other vascular problems. This fascinating set of diseases is also the vasculitides for which the highest quality and quantity of clinical trial data are available to help guide therapy.

Polyarteritis Nodosa

Polyarteritis nodosa (PAN) is among the "purer" vasculitides in that most of its manifestations are due to true vascular inflammation.[10] With the identification of other types of vasculitis, the spectrum of what is now diagnosed as PAN has narrowed over the past 50 years. Although characterized as a medium vessel disease, PAN may also involve small vessels such as those in the skin. PAN frequently involves inflammation leading to multiple small aneurysms that often appear angiographically as a "string of beads." Ischemia and infarction of kidneys,

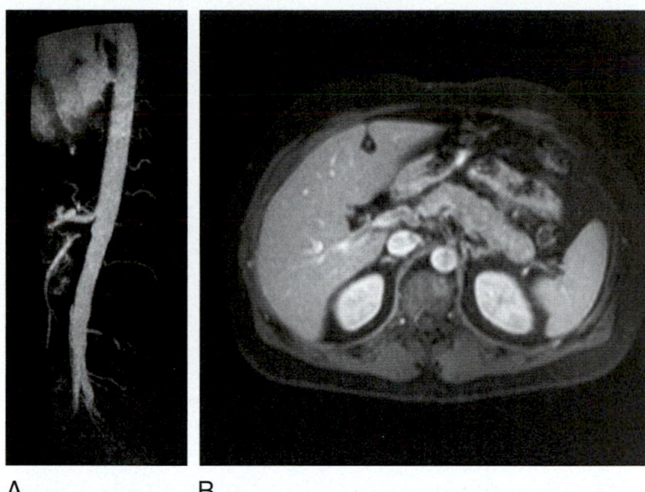

FIGURE 41-2. Polyarteritis nodosa with stenotic lesions **(A)** and wall thickening and enhancement **(B)** of celiac and superior mesenteric arteries as imaged using three-dimensional, dynamic, gadolinium-enhanced MRA.

intestines, and skin are common in PAN with arthralgias, myalgias, and fevers also frequently seen. Diagnosis is based on angiographic appearance (Fig. 41-2) or tissue pathology, often from surgical specimens such as a resected ischemic bowel segment. Interestingly, PAN in one subset of patients is associated with either hepatitis B or hepatitis C infections.[10,11] Importantly, there is a difference between hepatitis C–associated PAN and hepatitis C–associated cryoglobulinemic vasculitis (CV, see later section). Cardiac manifestations of PAN are due to coronary arteritis or malignant hypertension (secondary to renal arterial disease) and include myocardial ischemia, heart failure, and arrhythmias.

Treatment of PAN almost always involves high-dose glucocorticoids followed by a slow tapering of the dose. In more severe cases, an immunosuppressive agent is added. Hepatitis-associated PAN is now often treated with short courses of glucocorticoids and prolonged courses of antiviral agents. The rate of disease relapse in PAN is lower than that for many other types of vasculitis, and this relatively good prognosis is another important factor to take into consideration when deciding on a therapeutic regimen. Due to the rarity of the disease, controlled clinical trials for PAN are unlikely to occur and treatment is based on case series and expert opinion.

Wegener's Granulomatosis

WG is characterized by the triad of inflammation and destruction of tissue in the upper airway and sinuses (Fig. 41-3), lower airway (Fig. 41-4), and kidneys (Fig. 41-5), as well as the development of antineutrophil cytoplasmic autoantibodies (ANCAs).[12,13] Approximately 70% of patients with WG are positive for ANCA at diagnosis, although some will develop the antibodies later in the course of their illness. Among patients with WG and glomerulonephritis, more than 90% are positive for ANCA. Although the combination of these features is common in WG, many patients present with only a subset of these findings and WG also frequently involves

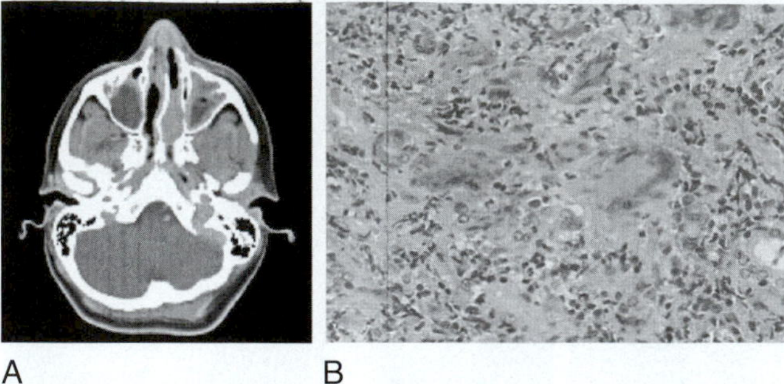

A B

FIGURE 41-3. (See also Color Plate 41-3.) Severe sinusitis in a patient with Wegener's granulomatosis. **A,** CT scan during an acute flare of disease. **B,** H&E stain of a sinus biopsy from this patient demonstrating characteristic inflammation, including a giant cell.

many other organ systems. The upper airway lesions include destructive rhinitis, often leading to nasal bridge collapse and the "saddle nose" deformity, sinusitis, and subglottic inflammation that can lead to life-threatening tracheal stenosis. The most severe form of pulmonary disease in WG is alveolar hemorrhage, and this is a common cause of early death. Other common pulmonary lesions include nodules, with or without cavitation, and tracheobronchitis. Other common features of WG are retro-orbital pseudotumor with resulting proptosis, conductive and sensorineural hearing loss, mononeuritis multiplex, arthritis, and purpura. Peripheral vascular involvement with gangrene is seen in WG and may be the presenting feature (Fig. 41-6).

Inflammatory cardiac disease is rare in WG but can include myocarditis and pericarditis. Aortic or large vessel involvement in WG is extremely uncommon; however, a recent report indicates that venous thromboses, including both deep vein thromboses and pulmonary emboli, occur frequently in WG and may be associated with active disease.[14]

Although some of the pathology in WG is, indeed, granulomatous with histiocytes, piecemeal necrosis, and occasional giant cells and eosinophils, other manifestations of inflammation are also seen in the disease. True vasculitis occurs and includes capillaritis. The renal disease of WG is identical to other ANCA-positive diseases, and the pathology is that of rapidly progressive glomerulonephritis.

Untreated, WG most often almost leads to death or serious damage.[15] Glucocorticoids are always used for

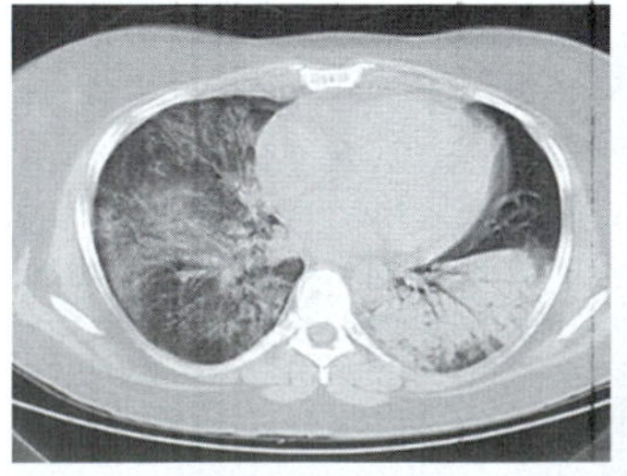

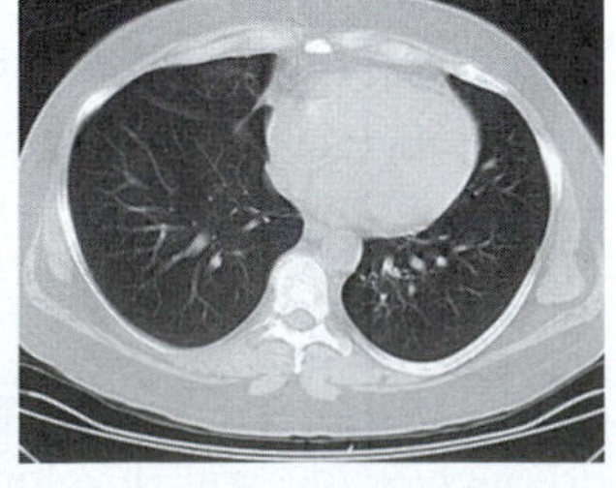

A B

FIGURE 41-4. Pulmonary hemorrhage in a patient with Wegener's granulomatosis as seen on chest CT scans. **A,** During the acute flare of disease, and **(B)** the same patient after treatment with glucocorticoids and cyclophosphamide. The patient's dyspnea and plain radiographic changes mostly resolved within 2 weeks of starting glucocorticoids.

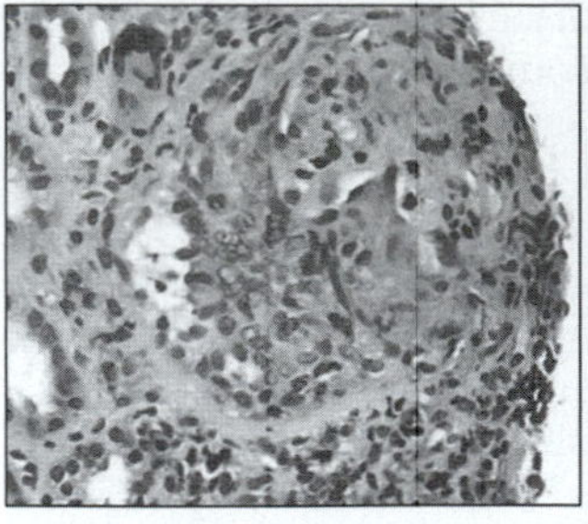

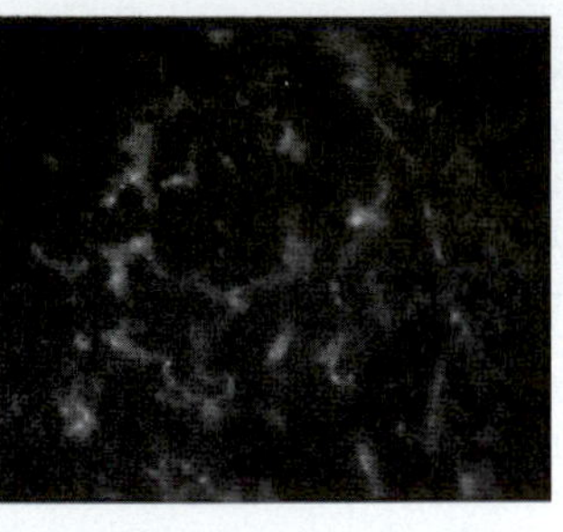

A B

FIGURE 41-5. (See also Color Plate 41-5.) Renal biopsy in a patient with Wegener's granulomatosis (same patient as in Fig. 41-4) with rapidly progressive glomerulonephritis. **A,** (H&E stain) demonstrates marked glomerular destruction as well as a multinucleated giant cell *(upper left).* **B,** demonstrates the characteristic "pauci-immune" immunofluorescent staining seen in Wegener's granulomatosis and microscopic polyangiitis.

treatment, but the prognosis of WG changed considerably when a protocol using cyclophosphamide was introduced in the 1970s at the National Institutes of Health. The morbidity and mortality of WG was markedly improved by cytotoxic therapy: 1-year mortality changed from more than 80% to less than 20%.[12,15,16] However, serious side effects are common with the use of cyclophosphamide and the rate of recurrent disease in WG after therapy is greater than 50%. In recent years new treatment protocols have been tested in open and control trials that incorporate less toxic immunosuppressive drugs, including methotrexate and azathioprine.[17-19]

Microscopic Polyangiitis

With the publication of the Chapel Hill Consensus Conference Classification system, the recognition of microscopic polyangiitis (MPA) as a separate entity gained acceptance.[2,10] MPA is a mostly small vessel to medium vessel, ANCA-associated vasculitis with manifestations that strongly overlap with WG. Its key features include glomerulonephritis, alveolar hemorrhage, skin lesions, and mononeuritis multiplex, but many other organ systems may be involved as well. Unlike WG, the pathology of MPA is nongranulomatous and does not involve the type of nonvascular disease seen in WG or CSS. The glomerulonephritis of MPA is identical to that seen in WG. Most patients with MPA are positive for ANCA, and the predominant ANCA antigen specificity is myeloperoxidase (MPO). Cardiac manifestations of MPA are uncommon, but peripheral arterial disease and gangrene are seen and may be confused with noninflammatory vascular disease. MPA should be differentiated from classic polyarteritis nodosa (PAN). PAN is more of a medium-vessel disease and does not include glomerulonephritis or pulmonary capillaritis. MPA does not produce the microaneurysms seen in PAN. Treatment of MPA is essentially identical to that for WG.

Churg-Strauss Syndrome

CSS, also known as *allergic granulomatous angiitis*, is a rare disease characterized by the triad of asthma,

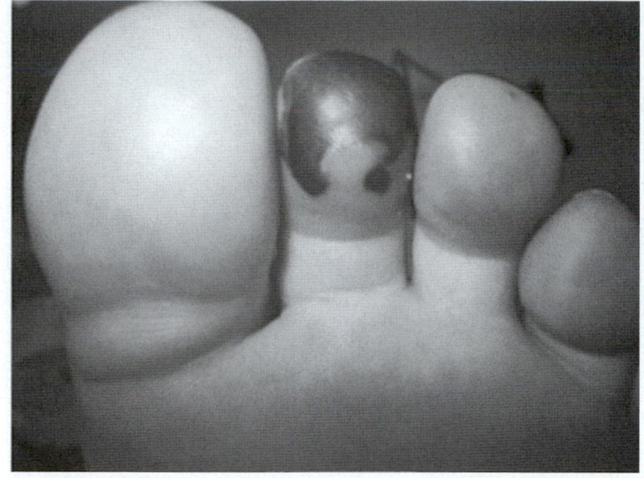

A

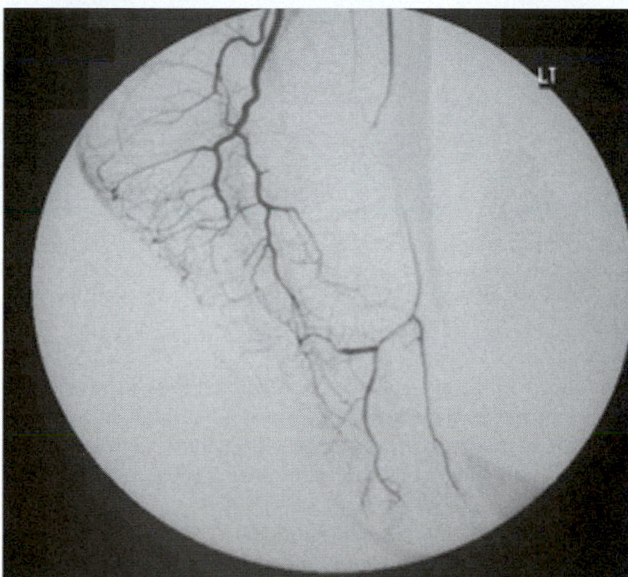

B

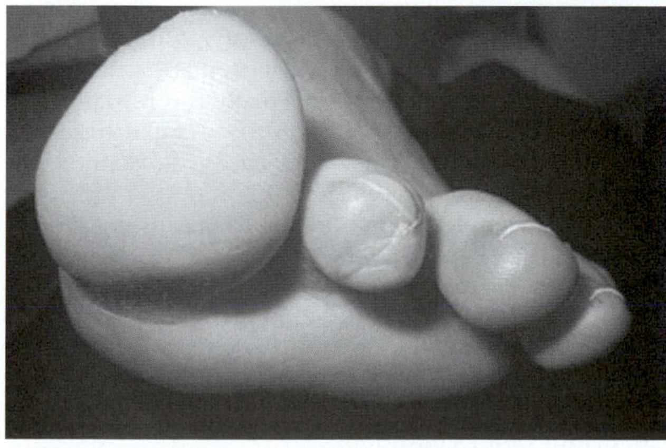

C

FIGURE 41-6. (See also Color Plate 41-6.) Gangrenous toe in a patient with Wegener's granulomatosis. **A,** Gangrenous left fourth toe pretreatment. **B,** Conventional angiogram of left foot at time of gangrene seen in **A** demonstrating marked stenosis/occlusion of dorsal pedal artery and runoff. **C,** Same toe months after initiation of glucocorticoids and cyclophosphamide. Only minimal tissue loss resulted, and toe is now well perfused.

pulmonary infiltrates, and hypereosinophilia.[20,21] CSS can, however, involve almost all of the clinical features seen in WG including the presence of ANCA in some cases. As with WG, much of the pathology seen in CSS is due to inflammation that is not "vasculitis" per se but is every bit as damaging as vascular inflammation. Tissue eosinophilia, although seen in other types of vasculitis, is particularly common in CSS and often striking. More than 90% of patients have asthma, often severe; the hypereosinophilia may be a marker of disease activity for some patients but is not always present. The pulmonary manifestations include dense infiltrates that rapidly clear with glucocorticoid therapy. Additionally, neuropathies, especially mononeuritis multiplex and gastrointestinal ischemia, are common features and quite damaging. The diagnosis is based on the combination of clinical findings, hypereosinophilia, and pathology specimens that often show granulomatous and eosinophilic inflammation.

Cardiovascular manifestations of CSS are fairly common and include myocarditis with resultant congestive heart failure and pericarditis. Angina is rare in CSS. Cardiac involvement in CSS may be rapid in onset and fatal.

The mainstay of treatment for CSS is glucocorticoids, but immunosuppressive agents are increasingly being used for more severe cases and to help wean patients from glucocorticoids. It is important to avoid overtreating the asthma component of the syndrome, as asthma is not in itself a reason to start cytotoxic medications.

Kawasaki Disease

Kawasaki disease, a vasculitis of young children involving medium and small arteries, is a leading cause of acquired coronary artery disease in children.[22] The disease manifests as a systemic illness with high fevers, conjunctival injection, erythematous oropharyngeal lesions, erythematous rashes and skin desquamation, lymphadenopathy, and other signs and symptoms. Cardiac involvement is frequent in Kawasaki disease and can result in long-term morbidity. Myocarditis and pericarditis are common and can be serious, but coronary artery aneurysms are the most feared aspect of the disease. Both panarteritis and granulomas can be seen in the vessels with subsequent scarring and aneurysm formation. Treatment includes aspirin and intravenous immunoglobin (IVIG), and such regimens have been shown to reduce the incidence of coronary complications markedly. Kawasaki disease is described in detail in Chapter 45 of this text.

SMALL VESSEL VASCULITIS

Henoch-Schöenlein Purpura

HSP is a small vessel vasculitis that classically involves the clinic triad of inflammatory arthritis, ischemic abdominal pain, and purpura, although not all cases exhibit all three manifestations.[23] The most feared manifestation of HSP is glomerulonephritis, which can lead to renal failure. Cardiac disease is not a feature of HSP, but hypertension from renal insufficiency can be severe.

The lesions in HSP often involve leukocytoclasia and IgA deposition. An elevated serum IgA level is commonly seen in patients with HSP.

HSP is much more common among young children and is probably the most common type of vasculitis among children. Nevertheless, HSP is also seen in adults. The disease is more often self-limited among children and more likely to lead to chronic renal insufficiency in adults. Relapse is common in all age groups. Treatment of HSP varies from watchful waiting in some cases of pediatric HSP to high-dose glucocorticoids to the addition of immunosuppressive agents.

Cryoglobulinemic Vasculitis

CV occurs when cryoglobulins, any of various types of immunoglobulins that precipitate from serum at temperatures below body temperature, induce an immune complex–mediated inflammatory process in any organ.[24] Several types of cryoglobulins can occur, and cryoglobulinemia is subclassified based on the mix of IgG and IgM antibodies that make up the cryoglobulin portion of serum (the "cryocrit") and whether the excess cryoproteins are polyclonal or monoclonal.

CV was previously considered to be a quite rare phenomenon sometimes seen in chronic inflammatory diseases such as lupus or rheumatoid arthritis or associated with lymphoproliferative disorders. Once the association between hepatitis C infection and type 2 mixed CV was established, however, it became apparent that coincident with the worldwide rise in hepatitis C infection, CV has been increasingly identified as a cause of vasculitis. The vast majority of cases of CV now seen are associated with hepatitis C infection.

The major clinical manifestations of CV include cutaneous vasculitis (purpura), arthralgias, peripheral neuropathy, and nephropathy with associated renal insufficiency or nephrotic syndrome, or both. Cardiovascular manifestations of CV include Raynaud's phenomenon, hypertension, and congestive heart failure. The hypertension in CV, which is often associated with renal disease, can be severe and lead to cardiac failure.

The histopathology of CV includes necrotizing vasculitis but may also involve immunoglobulin and complement deposition detected by immunofluorescence staining.

Treatment of CV is controversial and may include glucocorticoids, cytotoxic agents, and plasmapheresis. Considering CV in the differential diagnosis of patients with vasculitis is extremely important, as is identifying hepatitis C virus infection, because not only do most of these patients require treatment of their liver disease, but treatment of hepatitis C–associated CV now often includes antiviral therapy regardless of the extent or type of liver disease.

Primary Angiitis of the Central Nervous System

The term *primary angiitis of the central nervous system (PACNS)* actually describes a series of related vasculopathies limited to the central nervous system.[25,26] True vasculitis can occur and is frequently associated with subacute, nonfocal neurologic deficits, although strokes and hemorrhage can also be seen. A subset of patients has a more vasospastic presentation characterized by the acute-onset of severe headache and a focal neurological event.

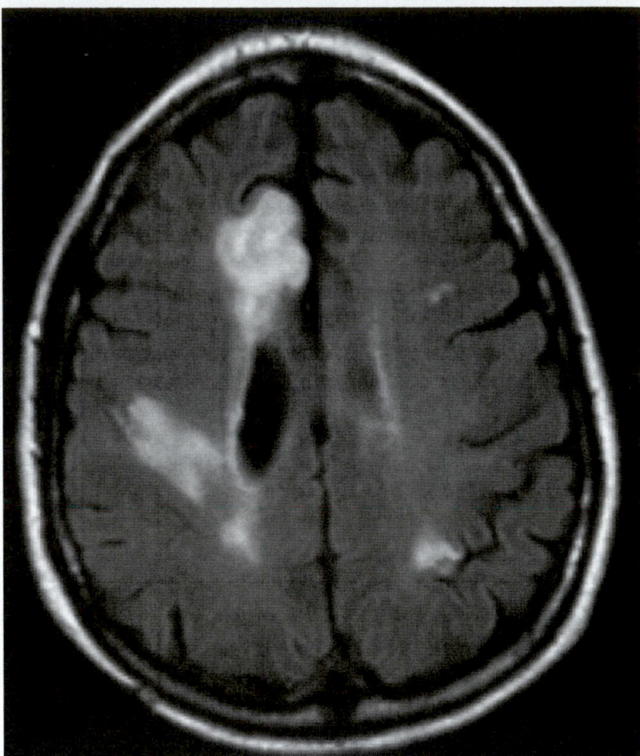

FIGURE 41-7. Multiple areas of brain infarction secondary to primary angiitis of the CNS as seen on gadolinium-enhanced MRA. The cerebral angiogram on this patient was unremarkable, but brain biopsy demonstrated small vessel vasculitis.

Diagnosis of PACNS necessitates first suspecting this rare disease. Conventional angiography may be helpful in identifying other entities, such as aneurysms and emboli, but is often not diagnostic for vasculitis for several reasons (Fig. 41-7). First, in older patients the endothelial changes of atherosclerosis may mimic those of vasculitis. Second, vasospasm can be confused with stenosis from either atherosclerosis or inflammation. Finally, the resolution of conventional angiography is such that small arteries are not well visualized, and thus many cases of vasculitis may be missed by this technique. Leptomeningeal biopsies or larger tissue samples from affected brain areas are often necessary to demonstrate PACNS and provide the level of evidence necessary to institute therapy. The histopathology is that of vasculitis, but granulomas and giant cells are not always seen; there may be no inflammation in the vasospastic variant. Tests of CSF are often normal in patients with PACNS but are important in evaluating patients for other conditions.

Experts in vascular medicine need to be aware of the various types and presentations of PACNS, because it can easily be mistaken for atherosclerotic disease with multiple infarcts. PACNS is extremely rare, but the approach to treatment is quite different from atherosclerotic disease.

Treatment recommendations are based solely on case series and an incomplete understanding of the pathophysiology. The "benign" form of PACNS may be treated with aggressive vasodilators, including calcium channel blockers and strict avoidance of smoking and vasoconstricting drugs and substances, including caffeine, cocaine, sympathomimetics, and serotonin receptor agonists (e.g., sumatriptan). The inflammatory forms of PACNS are treated with glucocorticoids, with immunosuppressive agents often added.

Vasculitis Secondary to Autoimmune/ Connective Tissue Diseases

Vasculitis, especially of small arteries, can be seen in various systemic autoimmune diseases, including SLE, rheumatoid arthritis, Sjögren's syndrome, and systemic sclerosis (scleroderma). In these diseases vasculitis usually accompanies evidence of severe disease in other organs or with long-standing disease (rheumatoid arthritis). Skin vasculitis is common, but mesenteric and central nervous system vasculitis are the most feared and dangerous vascular manifestations seen in these diseases.

Although coronary arteritis is rarely seen in these systemic autoimmune disorders, there is an increased recognition of early, accelerated atherosclerotic coronary artery disease among patients with SLE, rheumatoid arthritis, and other chronic inflammatory diseases. The pathophysiology of this problem is under active investigation and parallels the increased attention that vascular biologists are paying to the contribution of inflammation to atherosclerosis. When vasculitis occurs in SLE or rheumatoid arthritis, it is frequently severe and often necessitates treatment with high-dose glucocorticoids and cyclophosphamide.

Drug-Induced Vasculitis

Many drugs or other toxins have been implicated as causing inflammatory vasculitis involving vessels of all sizes, especially small arteries. A full list of drugs considered to be causative for vasculitis and details regarding the clinical syndromes of drug-induced vasculitis are available in recent reviews.[27,28] There is an interesting subset of patients with ANCA-associated vasculitis whose disease is caused by exposure to certain medications.[29]

The clinical manifestations of drug-induced vasculitis range from skin-only disease to widespread, life-threatening multisystemic disease. No clinical, laboratory, or pathologic findings differentiate drug-induced from other types of vasculitis. Given that agents from most classes of drugs have been implicated in vasculitis, it is imperative that clinicians consider the possible contribution to a case of vasculitis of not only every medication the patient was taking at the time of clinical presentation but also medications, supplements, and illegal drugs used in the previous year. The temporal association between drug exposure and disease combined with the pattern of illness and evidence for or against a different vasculitic process are helpful in establishing a diagnosis of drug-induced vasculitis.

Management of drug-induced vasculitis always includes discontinuation of the putative causative agent when possible but may also involve treatment with clinical observation alone, glucocorticoids, or immunosuppressive agents. It is also imperative that patients be followed for an extended period, even after apparent disease resolution, to ensure the diagnosis of drug-induced vasculitis rather than waxing and waning idiopathic vasculitis.

EVALUATION AND DIAGNOSIS OF POSSIBLE VASCULITIS

When evaluating cases of potential vasculitis, the clinician's first challenge is to consider that one of these rare diseases is a possibility. Rather than quickly focusing on a specific type of vasculitis, it is best to consider first whether "some sort of" vasculitis is present and determine the specific type once more information becomes available. It is common that when clinicians are evaluating patients for vasculitis, they are also conducting parallel evaluations for nonvasculitic diseases, an appropriate approach given the rarity of vasculitis and the urgency to diagnose and treat conditions that mimic vasculitis, such as infection.

Due to the protean potential manifestations of the vasculitides, clinicians must be comprehensive in their evaluation of patients for possible inflammatory vascular disease. By "looking everywhere" at all organ systems with complete history-taking, physical examinations, and selective laboratory and radiographic diagnostic tests, evidence is sought both for the presence of vasculitis and the size of vessel involved. Finding the "worst" manifestation of any new diagnosis or flare of disease is important; however, the goal is to both determine the diagnosis of a vasculitis and to ensure that all manifestations are documented, as treatment protocols differ based on the extent of disease and later assessment of response depends on accurate baseline evaluation of all features of disease.

With the exception of tissue pathology, no single test is fully diagnostic for vasculitis. A comprehensive initial medical evaluation including medical history, physical examination, and routine laboratory studies can provide most of the information clinicians need either to dismiss the diagnosis of vasculitis or to focus on more specific diagnostic testing. Finally, it is imperative that clinicians continually reconsider a diagnosis of vasculitis or consider a coexisting problem when either the clinical course changes or treatment response is not characteristic for vasculitis.

Medical History

Medical history and physical examination remain key elements of evaluation for vasculitis. A comprehensive review of systems is essential, and the potential queries related to vasculitis are numerous. Examples of symptoms to inquire about include any visual changes or eye symptoms, changes in hearing, nasal discharge or epistaxis, sinusitis, headaches, any mental status change, any neurologic symptom, stridor, wheezing, cough, hemoptysis, pleuritic chest pain, jaw or limb claudication, abdominal pain, any skin lesion, arthralgias, arthritis, myalgias, weakness, fevers, weight loss, and many other symptoms.

A full and accurate medication and drug use history is mandatory and should include any prescription drugs, over-the-counter products, illegal drugs, and alternative/herbal products taken within the prior 6 to 12 months, as well as accurate stop and start dates. If patients have been prescribed medications to address specific symptoms that may be vasculitic, documenting the response to these treatments may be important.

Physical Examination

A full physical examination is required whenever a patient is evaluated for potential vasculitis, and several examination findings should always prompt consideration of vasculitis in any patient. Blood pressure should be measured in both arms for discrepancies. Obtaining pressures in the legs may be appropriate if lower extremity stenoses are suspected. Hypertension may result from renal arterial stenoses from vasculitis, and similar physiology occurs with some tight suprarenal aortic stenoses. A full examination of bilateral pulses should include the radial, ulnar, brachial, carotid, femoral, popliteal, posterior tibial, and dorsalis pedis pulses. Bruits should be listened for over the aorta and the carotid, femoral, axillary, subclavian, and renal arteries.

Careful examination of skin and mucosal surfaces can reveal many clues to vasculitis. Although palpable purpura is the classic vasculitis skin lesion, not all purpura is vasculitis and not all skin vasculitis manifests as purpura. Macular lesions, both flat and raised, as well as bullae and nonerythematous lesions, can all occur in vasculitis. Livedo reticularis may be a clue to vasculitis or vasospasm. One should examine the patients for oral or genital aphthous ulcers. Extremity cyanosis and pallor may be seen and may be variable depending on the ambient temperature and limb positioning. Ulcerations and crusting should be sought in the nasopharynx. Nailfold capillary changes can be seen on bedside microscopical examination with an ophthalmoscope. Signs of capillary fragility, especially over sites of blood pressure cuff or tourniquet application, may be seen.

The rest of a full physical examination is also essential in evaluating for vasculitis. Lung examination may reveal any of the many abnormalities commonly seen in vasculitis including rhonchi, pleural rubs, dullness due to effusions, and wheezing. Careful cardiac auscultation might reveal evidence of aortic regurgitation as seen in aortitis or pericardial rubs. Gross inspection of the eyes may reveal signs of inflammation, and funduscopic examinations may show retinal pallor or other signs of ischemia. A full ophthalmologic examination including slit lamp is necessary for any patient suspected of vasculitis with eye symptoms. A full joint examination may reveal even asymptomatic effusions. Detailed neurologic examination is essential, as subtle cranial and peripheral neuropathies often go unnoticed by both patients and physicians but are clues to severe disease.

Laboratory Studies

Acute Phase Reactants

Acute phase reactants, including the Westergren erythrocyte sedimentation rate (ESR), C-reactive protein, and others are perhaps the most misunderstood and misused tests in the evaluation of vasculitis. ESR should never be considered a screening test for vasculitis, as acute phase reactants are neither highly sensitive nor specific *diagnostically* for any type of vasculitis. There is good evidence that a normal ESR can be found in active Takayasu's arteritis, GCA, WG, PACNS, drug-induced vasculitis, and other vasculitides. Although ESR is most helpful in evaluating patients for possible GCA, even in that disease up to 10% of patients with documented GCA have normal sedimentation rates at the time of diagnosis. Furthermore, an elevated ESR can be seen in most of the disorders usually considered in the differential diagnosis of patients with possible vasculitis, notably infections and malignancies, thus emphasizing the lack of diagnostic usefulness of this test. Acute phase reactants are somewhat useful for monitoring disease *activity* and therefore in some cases may be supportive of a disease flare.

Renal Function Tests

Laboratory tests of renal function are an essential part of evaluating patients for possible vasculitis. A properly performed urinalysis is mandatory. Glomerulonephritis is a major feature of many small and medium vessel vasculitides and may manifest first as subtle findings on urinalysis, including proteinuria and hematuria. If the urine dipstick is abnormal, clinicians need to examine the urinary sediment. Clinicians must *not* count on hospital or reference laboratories to perform a manual urine sediment analysis, as urinary casts are often dissolved by the time laboratory personnel run the test. If clinicians are not comfortable examining the sediment themselves, they should consult a nephrologist or another provider expert in this key test. Creatinine elevations may reflect both acute renal disease and longstanding damage and scarring from prior flares of disease, and knowing a patient's "baseline" value is always important. Furthermore, the doses of many drugs used for patients with vasculitis are modified based on renal function, including cyclophosphamide, methotrexate, cyclosporine, and NSAIDs. Hematuria may also be a clue to bladder toxicity from cyclophosphamide, including hemorrhagic cystitis and transitional cell carcinoma.

Complete Blood Counts and White Blood Cell Differential Counts

No findings from a blood count and review of a blood smear are diagnostic for vasculitis, but the tests may provide clues to other diagnoses. Many, but certainly not all, patients with systemic vasculitis are anemic at initial presentation. Although eosinophilia is frequently present in CSS, WG, drug-induced disease, and other vasculitides, this finding is also neither sensitive nor specific enough for diagnosis. Significant eosinophilia does, however, help narrow the potential diagnoses and may help in classifying patients with established vasculitis. Additionally, it is not uncommon for patients with CSS to have an increase in their total eosinophil count before or during a flare of disease.

Antineutrophil Cytoplasmic Autoantibodies Testing

The discovery of antineutrophil cytoplasmic autoantibodies (ANCAs) and their association with WG, microscopic polyangiitis, CSS, and renal-only pauci-immune glomerulonephritis was extremely important in the evolution of diagnostic testing for vasculitis.[30] ANCA testing, when performed properly, is highly specific for these syndromes, and in the correct clinical setting may be the last piece of data necessary to establish a diagnosis, even in the absence of a tissue biopsy. Additionally, the finding of a positive test for ANCA in a patient with already established vasculitis essentially narrows the diagnosis to one of four ANCA-associated diseases.

Currently the methodology for conducting ANCA testing is not standardized, which leads to problems with reliability and interpretation of test results. At a minimum, a laboratory should perform both immunofluorescence testing to identify the cytoplasmic ("C") ANCA pattern or the perinuclear ("P") pattern, as well as conduct ELISA testing for antibodies to proteinase 3 (anti-PR3) and antibodies to myeloperoxidase (anti-MPO). The antigen-specific ELISA tests are less prone to false-positive results (for the diagnosis of vasculitis) than the somewhat subjective immunofluorescence tests. Positive ANCA testing by the combined presence of C-pattern/anti-PR3 or P-pattern/anti-MPO is extremely specific for vasculitis, with other types of ANCA not helpful diagnostically.

The specificity of properly performed ANCA testing is greater than 90% and may be closer to 99% in certain laboratories.[30,31] The sensitivity of ANCA testing varies with the type of disease and clinical manifestations. Although greater than 90% of patients with WG who have renal involvement are ANCA positive, this rate drops to approximately 70% for patients without renal disease. Most patients with microscopic polyangiitis and renal-limited pauci-immune glomerulonephritis are ANCA positive, but the rate of ANCA positivity among patients with CSS varies in the literature from 50% to 80%. Thus, although ANCA is highly specific for vasculitis when present, a negative test by no means excludes the diagnosis.

Other Immunology Tests

Antinuclear antibodies (ANAs) and rheumatoid factor should be tested only in select cases. ANA is a useful screening test for SLE, as 99% of patients with SLE have a positive ANA test, especially if they have vasculitis; however, a positive ANA is by no means specific for any autoimmune disease. In the absence of arthritis, a test for rheumatoid factor is rarely useful diagnostically, because it can be seen in various infections and in type 2 cryoglobulinemia. Also, the test often has false-positive results. Furthermore, it is not diagnostic in itself for rheumatoid arthritis but is almost always positive in patients with rheumatoid vasculitis.

Testing for the presence of cryoglobulins is important, as their presence may not only help make the diagnosis, but treatment may be different and include plasmapheresis or antiviral agents, or both, in cases of hepatitis C–associated disease. Testing for cryoglobulins is not simple and is frequently done incorrectly. The blood specimen must be kept at body temperature (37°C) from the moment it is drawn through transport to the laboratory, where it must be allowed to clot in a warm water bath or heated box. Once the clot forms at 37°C, further special processing is required. From a Bayesian perspective, it is not unreasonable to repeat testing for cryoglobulins when the likelihood of their presence is medium to high, especially if the patient is infected with hepatitis C virus.

Microbiologic Testing

Cultures of blood, urine, and other specimens are often appropriate when evaluating patients with vasculitis. Furthermore, patients with established vasculitis are at considerably increased risk of infection when undergoing immunosuppressive therapy, necessitating a low threshold to test for infection in this population. Finally, it is important that some biopsy specimens, especially lung tissue, be sent for culture for both typical and atypical/opportunistic pathogens.

Diagnostic Vascular Imaging

Radiographic assessment of vascular structures has long been an important tool for diagnosing patients with vasculitis. This is especially true when medium and large vessels are involved, because they are much more likely to be visualized by the techniques available.[32] Furthermore, while small- and even medium-sized arteries can often be seen on diagnostic biopsies or surgical specimens, large vessels are not usually amenable to tissue biopsy. Thus diagnostic imaging is crucial to the assessment and management of patients with large vessel vasculitis. The two great challenges inherent in the interpretation of imaging of large vessels are (1) differentiating inflammatory disease from atherosclerotic disease and (2) trying to determine if vascular lesions represent "active" disease. In recent years interest in large vessel vascular imaging has greatly increased, as investigators and clinicians working in vasculitis strive to incorporate properly the advances in various radiologic modalities into practice. Imaging of organs and tissues other than arteries themselves is of obvious benefit for specific syndromes to help understand the extent of disease, facilitate choice of tissue biopsy, and rule out other pathology.

Specialists in vascular medicine need to be aware of the capabilities and limitations of the various modalities described as follows for imaging the vascular system and differentiating atherosclerotic from inflammatory disease. Vascular imaging is much more commonly obtained to evaluate suspected atherosclerotic or structural disease, and thus it is vital that inflammatory disease is recognized even when it is not expected. The increased recognition that atherosclerosis may have an inflammatory component and that vasculitis can result in some changes seen in atherosclerosis makes this differentiation even more challenging. Due to marked differences in treatment and prognosis for these different disorders, continued cooperative work by experts in cardiology, rheumatology, radiology, vascular surgery and other specialties is essential in evaluating patients and interpreting imaging data. The following sections summarize the progress to date in using various imaging modalities for evaluating vascular disease in the inflammatory vasculitides.

Conventional Angiography

Conventional angiography with intravascular injection of radiocontrast dye remains the "gold standard" for detecting stenoses and aneurysms in medium and large arteries and in diagnosing patients with vasculitis, especially Takayasu's arteritis and PAN. It is important to ask radiologists to view the distal runoffs of arteries beyond the trunk, as diagnostic and critical lesions more distally, such as in the axillary artery, may be missed by undue concentration on the proximal vessels. Additional advantages to conventional angiography include the ability to measure intra-arterial blood pressure directly. Such pressure readings are especially important when caring for patients with subclavian or proximal aortic stenoses where peripheral pressure readings may be inaccurate. Finally, conventional angiography is the only current imaging modality that assists catheter-based intervention, including angioplasty and stent placement.

There are several problems with and limitations to conventional angiography for the evaluation of potential vasculitis. The direct toxicities of the contrast dye have the potential for hypersensitivity reactions, renal insufficiency, and volume overload. Catheters can potentially cause vascular injury. The resolution of conventional angiography is limited, and most small vessel disease, such as in the brain or mesentery, is not well imaged by this technique. Additionally, serial studies by conventional angiography, although sometimes necessary, are impractical, incur additive toxicity, and are thus not routinely performed to monitor patients. Finally, conventional angiography does not provide any information about the biologic state of the arterial wall and therefore, except with serial images, cannot determine disease activity.

Magnetic Resonance Imaging (also see Chapter 11)

The use of MRI to help in the diagnosis and management of vasculitis continues to gain acceptance rapidly, although there are few properly done studies on the reliability of MRI for these purposes. MRI and MRA provide detailed information on luminal structures, arterial wall thickness and edema, tissue enhancement (by gadolinium contrast), and blood flow for large and some medium vessels. These structural measures have been proposed as useful in determining vasculitis disease activity. MRI and MRA can be performed repeatedly with little risk to the patient and can thus provide important serial data. The technology for MR continues to improve, and it is anticipated that the reliability and breadth of information it provides in evaluating patients with vasculitis will continue to increase substantially in the next few years, especially for large vessel pathology.

Several problems remain in the use of MR for diagnosing and following patients with vasculitis. First, not all vascular structures are easily imaged, and false-positive scans occur due to problems with imaging artifact and possibly other reasons. Second, neither the protocols for data acquisition nor the methods of image interpretation are standardized, making comparison of research data and studies from different institutions or even different machines problematic. The specificity of MR as a disease activity measure remains controversial. Unlike conventional angiography, MR does not allow for pressure readings or catheter-based interventions. Finally, MR is currently not helpful for small or even most medium vessel disease, although resolution is improving.

Computerized Tomography (also see Chapter 12)

CT is another promising imaging technique for large vessel vasculitis. CT can demonstrate arterial calcification well and, with the newer machines and software, quite precise images are possible. The major drawbacks to CT include the associated toxicities of ionizing radiation and iodinated contrast dye. The best future use of CT may be in combination with other modalities, especially PET (see later).

Ultrasound

Ultrasound has been used to evaluate vascular disease for many years, and well-developed literature is available on this technique. The noninvasive nature, widespread availability, and relatively low cost of ultrasound make it an attractive technique for vascular imaging; however, the work in ultrasound has mostly been on atherosclerotic disease and has focused on specific anatomic areas including the carotid, vertebral, and ophthalmic arterial systems and the abdominal aorta. Recently, investigators have become more interested in the use of ultrasound for inflammatory disease, but the experience and research in this area are still quite limited.

Ultrasound is often the first vascular imaging test obtained for patients with suspected carotid or vertebral arterial disease or aortic aneurysms. The recognition by the examiner that the disease process may be something other than atherosclerosis is vital for proper, early diagnosis. Greater awareness of the differences in foci of disease and in the size and appearances of lesions between atherosclerosis and vasculitis are important to emphasize.

The future use of ultrasound in evaluating inflammatory vascular disease depends on both improved technology that better evaluates arterial wall structures and allows for examination of smaller caliber vessels and demonstration that ultrasound provides insight beyond that obtained from other modalities, such as MR.

Positron Emission Tomography

PET is an exciting and promising new imaging modality for vascular disease. Because PET relies on the uptake of an isotope, it may be able to provide a biologic link to disease activity. Preliminary data are promising on the use of PET in evaluating aortitis, including isolated cases showing resolution of uptake in the aorta following glucocorticoid treatment of active disease. PET holds the promise of providing information on early and clinically unsuspected inflammatory disease; however, the work

TABLE 41-3 TREATMENTS FOR INFLAMMATORY VASCULITIS

Commonly Used Medications/Treatments	Newer and/or Experimental Agents	Surgical/Invasive Treatments
Aspirin	Mycophenolate mofetil	Balloon angioplasty
Glucocorticoids	Leflunomide	Intravascular stents (with or without drug eluting coating)
Cyclophosphamide	Inhibitors of tumor necrosis factor alpha	Vascular bypass or replacement grafts
Azathioprine	Rituximab (anti-CD20)	Reconstructive surgery
Methotrexate	Inhibitors of iInterleukin-1	
Cyclosporine and tacrolimus (FK506)	Many other experimental "biologic" agents	
Antiviral agents		
Plasmapheresis		
Intravenous immunoglobin (IVIG)		

on PET for large vessel vasculitis is still in the early phases, and the lack of standardization, paucity of direct comparisons with MRI, the high cost, and currently limited availability are all important issues delaying the more widespread use of PET for vascular imaging.

Tissue/Biopsy

Given both the need to often exclude infection, malignancy, or other processes, as well as the need for immunosuppressive medications for vasculitis, biopsy evidence is often crucial and empiric therapy is strongly discouraged. With the exception of some cases of large vessel vasculitis and some situations in patients with ANCA-positive disease, tissue biopsy is usually necessary to establish a firm diagnosis of vasculitis.

A temporal artery biopsy is almost always appropriate when GCA is a consideration, even if there are no cranial symptoms. A positive biopsy is such strong evidence for GCA that although a negative temporal artery biopsy does not exclude the diagnosis, a second contralateral biopsy is sometimes advised if the initial specimen is nondiagnostic.

For large vessel diseases other than GCA, a vessel biopsy is almost never obtained, because a medium- to full-thickness biopsy of the aorta or its main branches has obvious morbidity. Obtaining surgical specimens during bypass procedures or biopsies under highly controlled situations such as during aortic valve or graft surgery should, however, be considered when a diagnosis of large vessel disease has not yet been established or when disease activity status is unclear.

For the other vasculitides, it is usually preferred to obtain a biopsy from the most accessible tissue. Skin biopsies are simple, have low risk of morbidity, and can be instrumental in diagnosis. Too often, purpuric lesions are assumed to be vasculitis and biopsies not performed. Additionally, skin biopsies can be examined for evidence of embolic, thrombotic, or infectious diseases.

In the proper settings, biopsies of kidneys or lungs involve moderate risks but can be of high yield, whereas other tissues including sinus mucosa, nerve, and myocardium are lower risks to biopsy but also have lower diagnostic yields. Biopsies of other organs, such as intestine and liver, offer low yields and higher risks but may be appropriate, especially during a surgical procedure, in select circumstances.

TREATMENT OF VASCULITIS

The goals of treatment for inflammatory vasculitis are to stop the active inflammation and prevent permanent damage. Unlike many other systemic inflammatory diseases, true clinical remission is not only possible in many cases of vasculitis but should be the goal of treatment. Thus, protocols are increasingly being referred to as involving either "remission induction" or "remission maintenance" treatments. The mainstays of therapy for vasculitis remain glucocorticoids and various immunosuppressive drugs. Treatment protocols are tailored to the specific type of vasculitis and the extent of disease. Clinical trial data are increasingly available to guide treatment for WG, microscopic polyangiitis, Kawasaki disease, and giant cell arteritis, whereas other diseases rely on either case series for guidance or extrapolated data from studies in related, but not identical, vasculitides. Table 41-3 outlines the treatments used for patients with inflammatory vasculitis.

Ensuring long-term follow-up of patients with inflammatory vasculitis is extremely important. Relapse of vasculitis, even after complete remission, is quite common in many forms, including both large and small vessel diseases. Relapse may occur weeks to years from the time of clinical remission and manifest with different clinical findings, as was seen on initial presentation. For example, aortic aneurysms may be seen in patients with GCA *years* after the patient was believed to be in "remission." Other manifestations may also occur, even in the absence of clinical symptoms, and are more likely be missed when patients are believed to be "cured" of their vasculitis. For example, renal insufficiency in patients with ANCA-associated vasculitis may be undetected due to inadequate surveillance until end-stage renal failure has occurred.

Medical Therapies for Vasculitis

Medical management of patients with vasculitis should only be directed by physicians familiar with both the use of chronic immunosuppressive agents and the clinical presentation and management of vasculitis. The acute and chronic toxicities of these drugs should not be underestimated and can result in significant morbidity. Treatment protocols are beyond the scope of this chapter, but the most commonly used medications for vasculitis are briefly outlined. Many different agents have been used for vasculitis, as outlined in Table 41-3.

Glucocorticoids are used for almost all patients with almost all types of vasculitis during the acute presentation or during flares. They have a rapid onset of action, and high doses often stabilize patients even with severe manifestations such as alveolar hemorrhage or glomerulonephritis. The toxicities of glucocorticoids, especially with prolonged use, are serious and common and include weight gain, osteoporosis, osteonecrosis, glucose intolerance, Cushingoid habitus, adrenal suppression, hypertension, mood disturbances, frank psychosis, cataracts, glaucoma, and many others.

Immunosuppressive drugs are often used in conjunction with glucocorticoids either to provide more effective therapy and induce a remission or to act as "steroid-sparing" drugs allowing for the safe tapering of the glucocorticoids.

Cyclophosphamide is widely considered the most effective agent for inducing and maintaining remission in various types of vasculitis.[12] The introduction of cyclophosphamide-based therapy changed the prognosis of many of these diseases. Although cyclophosphamide is extremely effective, its multiple toxicities are severe and include cytopenias, especially neutropenia with associated infections, gonadal failure, teratogenicity, hemorrhagic cystitis, transitional cell carcinoma of the bladder, myelodysplasia, mucositis, hair loss, and others. Controversy exists about the best route of administration for cyclophosphamide, orally or intravenously.

Multiple alternative agents have been tested and proposed to limit the use of cyclophosphamide. *Methotrexate*, taken orally or intramuscularly weekly, has demonstrated efficacy as both a remission-induction agent and remission-maintenance agent for WG and is used for both purposes for multiple vasculitides.[33] The toxicities of methotrexate include cytopenias, gastrointestinal upset, oral ulcers, teratogenicity, and hepatic disease. *Azathioprine* is another commonly used agent for remission maintenance in vasculitis.[19] Azathioprine can cause cytopenias, infections, nausea, mucositis, hair loss, pancreatitis, and other problems, but like methotrexate, is usually well tolerated even for extended periods. *Mycophenolate mofetil* is increasingly being used for vasculitis despite a relative paucity of efficacy data.[34] Its usefulness in preventing organ transplant allograft rejection and its adoption in protocols to treat SLE have made physicians more comfortable with the drug. It appears to have more rapid onset of action than azathioprine with less toxicity. *Cyclosporine* has long been used in Behçet's disease and occasionally in other vasculitides. Several other immunosuppressive agents have been proposed for use in the vasculitides, although often without data from properly controlled clinical trials to support the recommendations.

Plasmapheresis (plasma exchange) has a central role in treating Goodpasture's syndrome and is used at some centers to treat both alveolar hemorrhage and severe glomerulonephritis in ANCA-associated vasculitis. Pheresis is frequently used to treat acute manifestations of cryoglobulinemic vasculitis and, occasionally, other vasculitides. *Intravenous immunoglobulin (IVIG)* is a mainstay of therapy for Kawasaki disease and has been advocated for several other types of vasculitis, often as a second- or third-line regimen, and based mostly on small case series.

The newest group of drugs to be proposed for use in the inflammatory vasculitides is the so-called *biologics* (see Table 41-1).[18] This rapidly expanding group of agents that inhibit specific targets within the immune system are having a remarkable impact on the care of patients with a wide variety of autoimmune and systemic inflammatory diseases. Inhibitors of TNF-α have shown promise for large vessel vasculitis[35,36] with more definitive trials in progress. Conversely, despite initial enthusiasm,[37] a large trial of etanercept, one of the inhibitors of TNF-α, was found to not be efficacious in the treatment of WG.[38] This experience highlights the need for properly conducted randomized clinical trials in vasculitis. A randomized, double-blinded study of rituximab (anti-CD20 antibody) for the treatment of ANCA-positive vasculitis is under way. Similarly, studies testing the efficacy of inhibitors of interleukin 1 and several other agents listed in Table 41-3 are either currently in process or in the planning stages.

Surgical or Procedural Interventions for Vasculitis

In addition to medical therapies, interventional and surgical treatments for vasculitis remain options for certain types of problems, especially in larger vessels after damage has become permanent. Angioplasty and stent placement have been performed for patients with Takayasu's arteritis and other diseases when severe arterial stenoses occur in large vessels. The results of these interventions are mixed, with restenosis a commonly reported problem. Whether or not the newly introduced drug-eluting stents will offer advantages for the vasculitides remains to be demonstrated.

Surgical bypass or grafts of stenotic vessels, including the aorta and coronary, subclavian, carotid, and renal arteries, are an option for patients with large vessel vasculitides. Several questions are unanswered regarding the proper timing of such surgery in the presence of "active" disease or when patients are on chronic glucocorticoids. Reconstructive surgery also plays a role in the care of patients with vasculitis, especially in patients with WG who suffer deforming damage from nasal collapse or other upper airway and retro-orbital disease.

Miscellaneous Issues in the Treatment of Vasculitis

Pneumocystis carinii Pneumonia Prophylaxis

It is now standard practice to prescribe trimethoprim-sulfamethoxazole or another agent for prophylaxis against *Pneumocystis carinii* pneumonia (PCP) for patients on medium to high doses of glucocorticoids in combination with an immunosuppressive agent.

Gonadal Function and Pregnancy-Related Problems

The treatment of vasculitis often involves drugs that adversely affect patients' gonadal function or are problematic during pregnancy, or both.[39] Cyclophosphamide can cause both male and female sterility and is a highly teratogenic agent. Methotrexate is teratogenic and an abortifacient drug. Glucocorticoids cause significant maternal and some fetal problems. Several of the other treatments in Table 41-3 are either directly contraindicated during pregnancy or their safety during pregnancy has not been established.

It is imperative that patients in their reproductive years be counseled at the time of diagnosis and regularly thereafter regarding issues of fertility, pregnancy, and contraception. Full discussion of these issues often leads to careful planning that may involve freezing sperm, empiric ovarian-preserving medication protocols, and reevaluation of contraceptive choices.

Osteoporosis Prevention

Because patients with inflammatory vasculitis are often treated with repeated courses of high-dose glucocorticoids, it is essential that treating physicians give consideration to preservation of bone mass and assessments of osteoporosis. Almost all patients need to be given calcium and vitamin D supplementation, and many patients may be candidates for bisphosphonates or other treatments for prophylaxis or treatment of glucocorticoid-induced osteoporosis. A baseline bone density scan is often useful for risk stratification.

Accelerated Atherosclerosis

Concern is growing, although there is little firm evidence yet, that patients with inflammatory vasculitis are at increased risk of accelerated atherosclerosis and coronary artery disease as is seen in patients with other chronic inflammatory diseases, such as rheumatoid arthritis and SLE.[40] The etiology of the atherosclerosis is likely multifactorial but includes glucocorticoid usage, lipid disorders associated with disease and treatment regimens, and other treatment-related problems, such as nephrotic syndrome and diabetes mellitus. The impact of chronic inflammation itself, however, may be the most important factor in the development of atherosclerosis. Ongoing research is directed at the interaction between inflammation and atherogenesis. Whether or not chronic therapy with statins or other agents that act via lipid or inflammatory pathways, or both, is appropriate has yet to be proved in clinical studies.

REFERENCES

1. Bloch DA, Michel BA, Hunder GG, et al: The American College of Rheumatology 1990 criteria for the classification of vasculitis. Patients and methods. Arthritis Rheum 33:1068, 1990.
2. Jennette JC, Falk RJ, Andrassy K, et al: Nomenclature of systemic vasculitis, proposal of an international conference. Arthritis Rheum 37:187, 1994.
3. Kissin GY, Merkel PA: Large-vessel vasculitis. In Coffman JD, Eberhardt RT (eds): Peripheral Arterial Disease: Diagnosis and Treatment. Totawa, NJ, Humana Press, 2002, p 319.
4. Weyand CM, Goronzy JJ: Giant-cell arteritis and polymyalgia rheumatica. Ann Intern Med 139:505, 2003.
5. Kerr GS, Hallahan CW, Giordano J, et al: Takayasu arteritis. Ann Intern Med 120:919, 1994.
6. Sakane T, Takeno M, Suzuki N, et al: Behçet's disease. N Engl J Med 341:1284, 1999.
7. Sridharan ST: Relapsing polychondritis. In Hoffman GS, Weyand CM (eds): Inflammatory Diseases of Blood Vessels. New York, Marcel Dekker, 2001, p 675.
8. St Clair EW, McCallum RM: Cogan's syndrome. Curr Opin Rheumatol 11:47, 1999.
9. Rojo-Leyva F, Ratliff NB, Cosgrove DM III, et al: Study of 52 patients with idiopathic aortitis from a cohort of 1,204 surgical cases. Arthritis Rheum 43:901, 2000.
10. Guillevin L: Polyarteritis nodosa and microscopic polyangiitis. In Ball GV, Bridges L (eds): Vasculitis. New York, Oxford University Press, 2002, p 300.
11. Guillevin L, Lhote F, Cohen P, et al: Polyarteritis nodosa related to hepatitis B virus: A prospective study with long-term observation of 41 patients. Medicine 74:238, 1995.
12. Hoffman GS, Kerr GS, Leavitt RY, et al: Wegener granulomatosis: An analysis of 158 patients. Ann Intern Med 116:488, 1992.
13. Hoffman GS, Gross WL: Wegner's granulomatosis: Clinical aspects. In Hoffman GS, Weyand CM (eds): Inflammatory Diseases of Blood Vessels. New York, Marcel Dekker, 2001, p 381.
14. Merkel PA, Lo GH, Holbrook JT, et al: High incidence of venous thrombotic events among patients with Wegener's granulomatosis: The Wegener's Granulomatosis Clinical Occurance of Thrombosis (WeCLOT) Study. Ann Intern Med 142:620, 2005.
15. Walton EW: Giant-cell granuloma of the respiratory tract (Wegener's granulomatosis). Br Med J 2:265, 1958.
16. Reinhold-Keller E, Beuge N, Latza U, et al: An interdisciplinary approach to the care of patients with Wegener's granulomatosis: Long-term outcome in 155 patients. Arthritis Rheum 43:1021, 2000.
17. Langford CA: Treatment of ANCA-associated vasculitis. N Engl J Med 349:3, 2003.
18. Langford CA, Sneller MC: Biologic therapies in the vasculitides. Curr Opin Rheumatol 15:3, 2003.
19. Jayne D, Rasmussen N, Andrassy K, et al: A randomized trial of maintenance therapy for vasculitis associated with antineutrophil cytoplasmic autoantibodies. N Engl J Med 349:36, 2003.
20. Guillevin L, Cohen P, Gayraud M, et al: Churg-Strauss syndrome: Clinical study and long-term follow-up of 96 patients. Medicine 78:26, 1999.
21. Guillevin L, Lhote F, Cohen P: Churg-Strauss syndrome: Clinical aspects. In Hoffman GS, Weyand CM (eds): Inflammatory diseases of blood vessels. New York, Marcel Dekker, 2001, p 399.
22. Barron KS: Kawasaki disease: Etiology, pathogenesis, and treatment. Cleve Clin J Med 69 Suppl 2:SII69, 2002.
23. Saulsbury FT: Henoch-Schönlein purpura. Curr Opin Rheumatol 13:35, 2001.
24. Cacoub P, Costedoat-Chalumeau N, Lidove O, et al: Cryoglobulinemia vasculitis. Curr Opin Rheumatol 14:29, 2002.
25. Calabrese LH, Duna GF, Lie JT: Vasculitis in the central nervous system. Arthritis Rheum 40:1189, 1997.
26. Hajj-Ali RA, Furlan A, Abou-Chebel A, et al: Benign angiopathy of the central nervous system: Cohort of 16 patients with clinical course and long-term followup. Arthritis Rheum 47:662, 2002.
27. Merkel PA: Drug-induced vasculitis. Rheum Dis Clin North Am 27:849, 2001.
28. Merkel PA: Drug-induced vasculitis. In Hoffman GS, Weyand CM (eds): Inflammatory Diseases of Blood Vessels. New York, Marcel Dekker, 2001, p 727.
29. Choi HK, Merkel PA, Walker AM, et al: Drug-associated ANCA-positive vasculitis: Prevalence among patients with high titers of anti-myeloperoxidase antibodies. Arthritis Rheum 43:405, 2000.
30. Niles JL: Antineutrophil cytoplasmic autoantibodies in the classification of vasculitis. Ann Rev Med 47:303, 1996.
31. Merkel PA, Polisson RP, Chang Y, et al: Prevalence of antineutrophil cytoplasmic antibodies in a large inception cohort of patients with connective tissue disease. Ann Intern Med 126:866, 1997.
32. Kissin EY, Merkel PA: Diagnostic imaging in Takayasu arteritis. Curr Opin Rheumatol 16:31, 2004.
33. Langford CA, Sneller MC, Hoffman GS: Methotrexate use in systemic vasculitis. Rheum Dis Clin North Am 23:841, 1997.
34. Langford CA, Talar-Williams C, Sneller MC: Mycophenolate mofetil for remission maintenance in the treatment of Wegener's granulomatosis. Arthritis Rheum 51:278, 2004.

35. Cantini F, Niccoli L, Salvarani C, et al: Treatment of longstanding active giant cell arteritis with infliximab: Report of four cases. Arthritis Rheum 44:2933, 2001.
36. Hoffman GS, Merkel PA, Brasington RD, et al: Anti-tumor necrosis factor therapy in patients with difficult to treat Takayasu arteritis. Arthritis Rheum 50:2296, 2004.
37. Stone JH, Uhlfelder ML, Hellmann DB, et al: Etanercept combined with conventional treatment in Wegener's granulomatosis: A six-month open-label trial to evaluate safety. Arthritis Rheum 44:1149, 2001.
38. WGET Research Group: The Wegener's granulomatosis etanercept trial (WGET): Randomized, double-masked, placebo-controlled trial of etanercept for the induction and maintenance of remission. N Engl J Med 50:3985, 2005.
39. Langford CA, Kerr GS: Pregnancy in vasculitis. Curr Opin Rheumatol 14:36, 2002.
40. Hahn BH: Systemic lupus erythematosus and accelerated atherosclerosis. N Engl J Med 349:2379, 2003.

chapter 42

Takayasu's Arteritis

Kathleen Maksimowicz-McKinnon
Gary S. Hoffman

Takayasu's arteritis (TA) is an idiopathic large-vessel vasculitis that preferentially involves the aorta and its primary branches. Chronic vascular inflammation leads to vessel stenosis and, less commonly, aneurysm formation.

EPIDEMIOLOGY

The peak incidence of TA is in the third decade of life, with women affected about 10 times more frequently than men. TA is a rare disorder, occurring in 2.6 cases/million yearly in Olmstead County, Minnesota, and in 1.2 cases/million yearly in Sweden.[1,2] Autopsy studies in Japan document a higher prevalence, with evidence of TA foundin 1 of every 3000 individuals.[3]

PATHOGENESIS

The etiology of TA is unknown. Although genetic predisposition has been suggested as an important factor in the development of TA, no definite allelic associations have been consistently found and shared by the various affected ethnic groups. Infectious triggers have been extensively studied. Special attention has been directed toward mycobacterial pathogens because of the reported coexistence of TA with previous mycobacterial infection or skin test positivity in a number of ethnic groups. However, this association has only been noted in regions with a high prevalence of mycobacterial disease and not in developed countries such as the United States.

Vessel injury results from the influx and actions of macrophages, cytotoxic T cells, γ-δ T cells, and natural killer cells.[4] Access of leukocytes to the vessel wall is through the vasa vasorum, with subsequent migration to the luminal intima, where various cytokines including perforin, IL-6, RANTES, and tumor necrosis factor-alpha (TNF-α) enhance vascular inflammation.[5] Although the most common response to this process is myointimal proliferation, leading to wall thickening and luminal stenosis, smooth muscle cell and elastic fiber destruction may lead to aneurysm formation, especially in the aortic root and arch (Fig. 42-1).[6]

As lesions progress, all arterial wall layers eventually become involved. Pathologic studies reveal vascular intimal fibrous thickening, destruction of medial smooth muscle cells and elastic layers, and cellular infiltration of the adventitia with resultant thickening.[7] Arterial involvement in TA has been described as affected areas interspersed with regions of normal vessel morphology ("skip lesions"). However, more recent studies suggest that disease progression leads to the secondary, more diffuse vessel involvement with atherosclerotic lesions.[8]

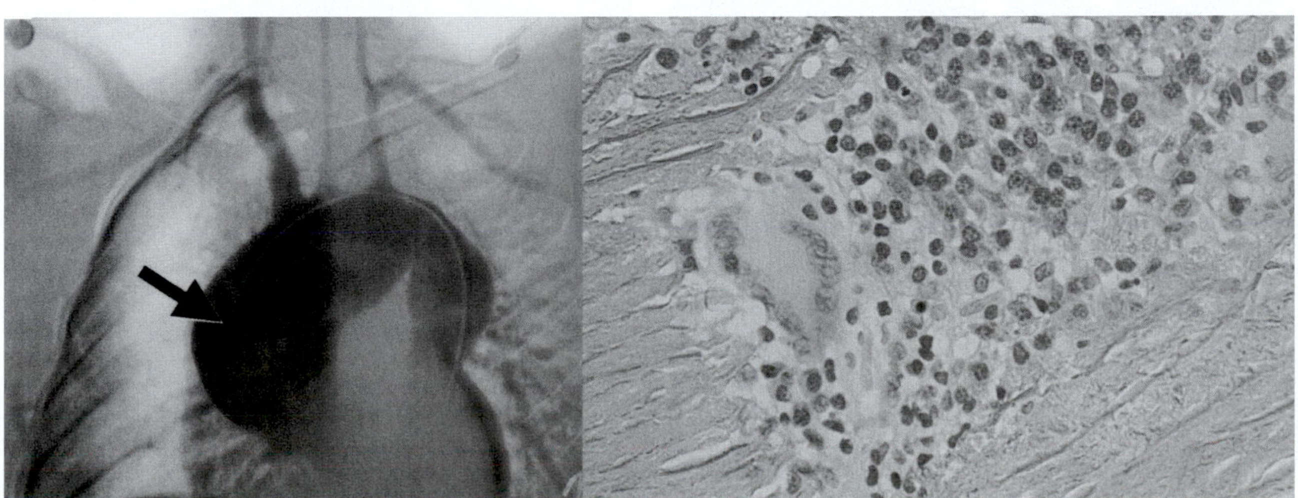

FIGURE 42-1. Granulomatous inflammation leading to destruction of muscle and elastic fibers of the thoracic aorta, with resultant aneurysm formation *(arrow)*.

CLINICAL MANIFESTATIONS

The most common symptom of TA is upper extremity claudication, occurring in more than 60% of patients, reflecting disease predilection for aortic arch vessels (>90% of cases) (Figs. 42-2 through 42-4).[9] The most frequent clinical findings include blood pressure asymmetry in the extremities (96%) and bruits (about 80%), found most often over the carotid, subclavian, and aortic vessels.[10] Aneurysms most often affect the aortic root, resulting in valvular regurgitation in about 20% of patients. Hypertension occurs in at least 40% in U.S. cohorts, and is even more common in Japanese and Indian cohorts. Hypertension is most frequently due to renal artery stenosis, but it may also result from suprarenal aortic stenosis or loss of aortic compliance (Figs. 42-5 through 42-7).[9,11] Coronary arteritis is rare (<5%), with resultant stenoses most often in the ostial regions, but it may occur more distally. Systemic symptoms and signs occur in less than one half of all patients and include fever, weight loss, malaise, and generalized arthralgias and myalgias. Hypertension with vascular bruits or claudication, especially in younger patients, should lead to a suspicion of TA and to further evaluations of all four extremity pulses and blood pressures for asymmetry. Vascular imaging studies should then confirm the diagnosis and delineate the extent of disease and types of lesions.

Classification of TA is based on sites of arterial involvement. One of the most widely accepted schemes separates patients into five types (Fig. 42-8):

1. Type 1: branches of the aortic arch
2. Type 2a: ascending aorta, aortic arch and its branches
3. Type 2b: type 2a plus thoracic descending aorta
4. Type 3: thoracic descending aorta, abdominal aorta, or renal arteries, or a combination
5. Type 4: only abdominal aorta or renal arteries, or both
6. Type 5: segments of the entire aorta and its branches

Type 5 is the most common.

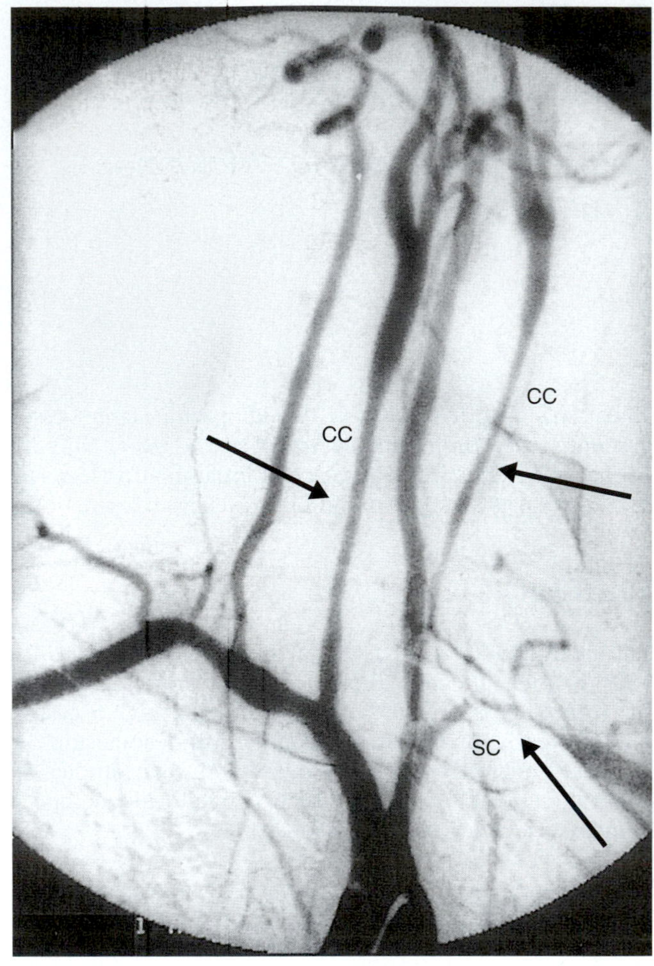

FIGURE 42-3. Smooth-tapering stenoses of the left subclavian *(SC)* and bilateral common carotid *(CC)* arteries (catheter-directed angiography).

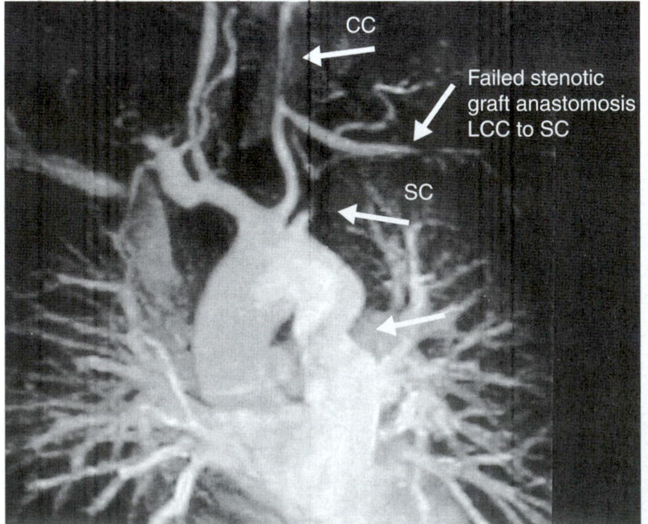

FIGURE 42-2. MRA image of stenotic lesions involving the aorta, left common carotid *(CC)*, and left subclavian *(SC)* arteries. This demonstrates why grafts to and from *CC* to *SC* are ill advised (see text).

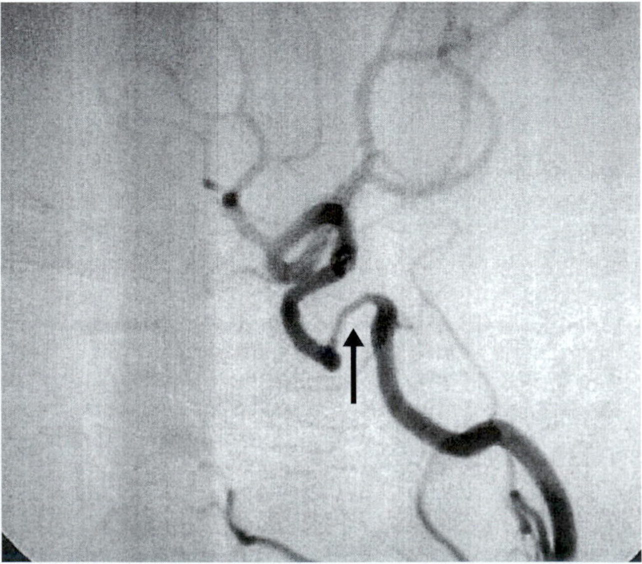

FIGURE 42-4. Arrow indicates stenotic involvement of the distal internal carotid artery (catheter-directed angiography).

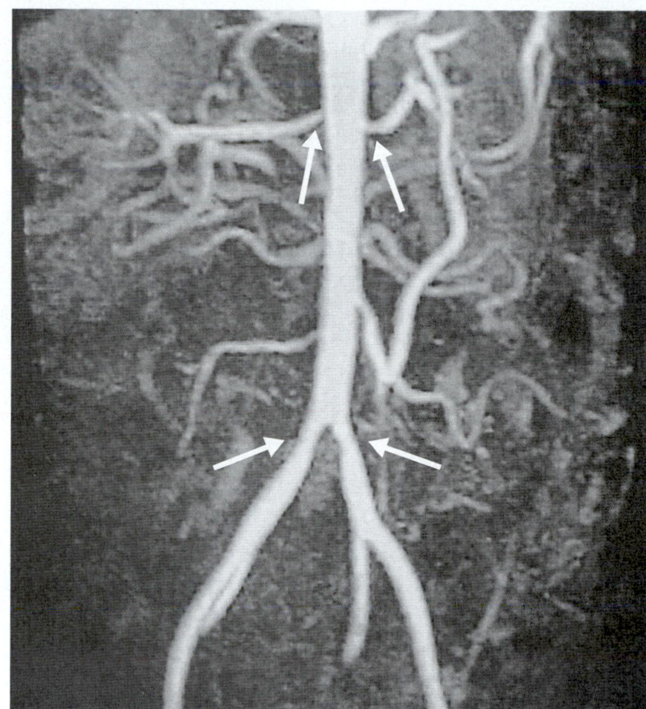

FIGURE 42-5. MRA image of bilateral common iliac and renal arterial stenoses.

Morbidity and mortality in TA result primarily from cardiac, renal, and CNS vascular disease. Undetected and/or untreated hypertension, is a significant cofactor in these disease sequelae (Fig. 42-9). Mortality estimates range from just 3% at 8 years to 35% at 5-years' follow-up.[12,13]

DIFFERENTIAL DIAGNOSIS

A thorough and careful investigation is necessary to distinguish TA from its mimics. Although diseases such as Marfan's syndrome, Ehlers-Danlos syndrome, and other congenital disorders of tissue matrix may present with aortic root and other aneurysms plus valvular insufficiency, they are not generally associated with large vessel stenoses, the hallmark of TA. Additionally, in these genetic disorders, signs and symptoms of systemic inflammation are absent. TA differs from atherosclerotic vascular disease by its prevalence in young females and its predilection for the upper extremities and aortic root (as opposed to vessels of the lower extremities and abdominal aortic involvement in atherosclerosis).

Although other autoimmune disorders such as Cogan's disease, Behçet's disease, systemic lupus erythematosus, and the spondyloarthropathies can be associated with large vessel vasculitis, they are most often distinguished by their other associated disease manifestations and age preferences. Sarcoidosis shares many features with TA.

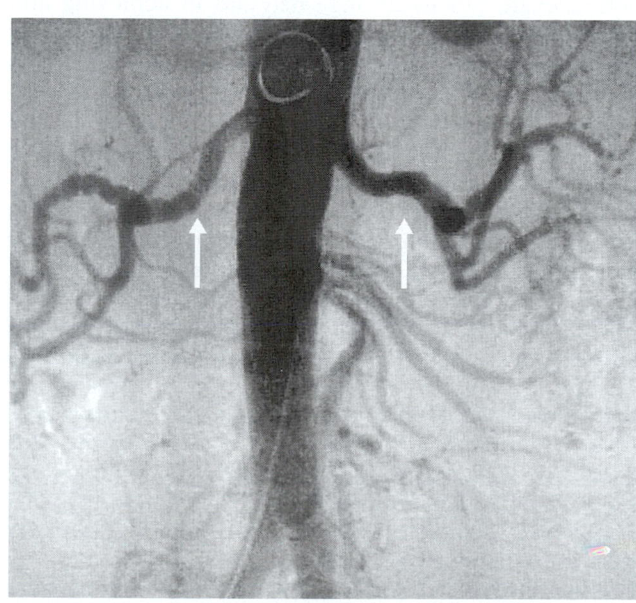

FIGURE 42-6. Bilateral renal artery lesions mimicking fibromuscular dysplasia (catheter-directed angiography).

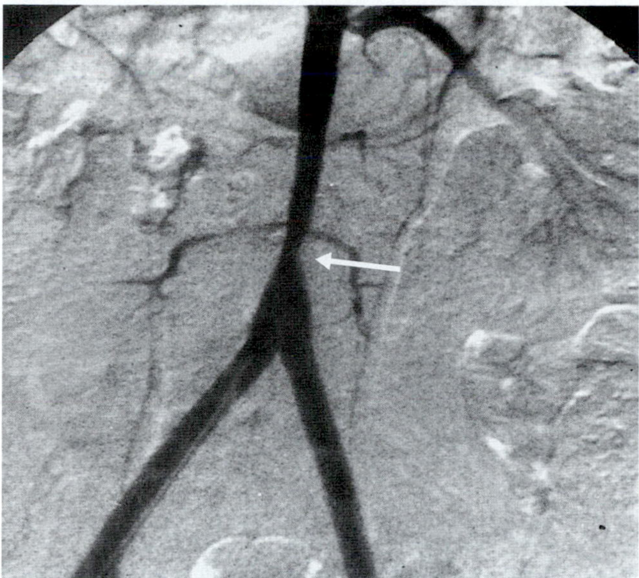

FIGURE 42-7. A tapering stenotic lesion of the abdominal aorta (catheter-directed angiography).

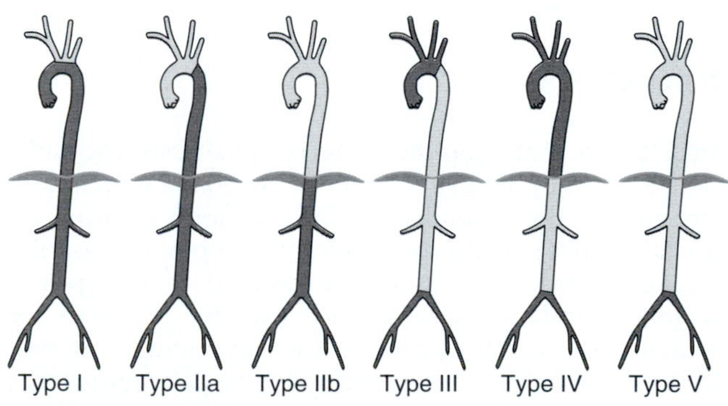

FIGURE 42-8. Classification of Takayasu's arteritis based on vessel involvement according to the International Conference on Takayasu's Arteritis (1994).

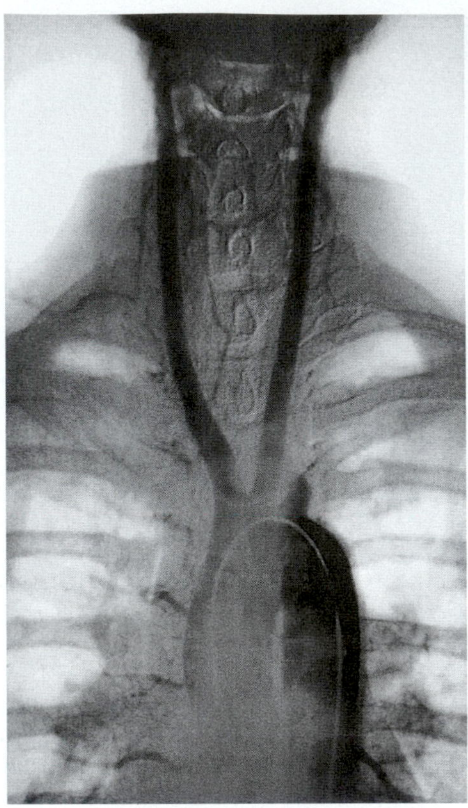

FIGURE 42-9. Bilateral subclavian artery occlusion (catheter-directed angiography). This illustrates the potential difficulty in diagnosis and monitoring of hypertension in Takayasu's arteritis.

The presence of hilar adenopathy, parenchymal lung disease, and synovitis favors sarcoidosis. In some cases, biopsy of involved organs may be required to distinguish among these diseases. A significant and often underappreciated overlap exists between TA and giant cell arteritis, a disease of the elderly (mean age ≈70); however, TA and giant cell arteritis may be indistinguishable in patients who present in middle age (45 to 55 years of age).

Infectious causes of large vessel aneurysms should always be considered, irrespective of age or gender. Previously implicated agents include bacterial, syphilitic, mycobacterial, and mycotic pathogens. Stenosis of arch-branch vessels, however, would be uncommon in the setting of infection.

DIAGNOSIS

There are no radiographic or serological tests with adequate sensitivity and specificity to be considered a gold standard for the diagnosis of TA. Diagnosis is based on clinical findings in the presence of compatible vascular imaging abnormalities. Catheter-directed angiography is the gold standard for diagnostic imaging. It allows for luminal imaging and pressure measurements and provides opportunities for intervention (e.g., angioplasty); however, catheter-directed angiography provides little direct information about the vessel wall per se. New techniques using combined CT and PET or MRA and PET imaging may aid in providing more information about the lumen and the vessel wall, as well as the presence or absence of inflammation within large vessels.

Although systemic signs and symptoms or elevated acute phase reactants may be suggestive of disease activity when present, they are an unreliable means by which to monitor disease status in many patients. Sequential angiographic evaluations have revealed progression of disease, demonstrated by the presence of new vascular abnormalities, in more than 50% of patients with normal erythrocyte sedimentation rates.[12] In addition, histopathologic proof of vascular inflammation has been documented in 44% of bypass specimens from patients with TA who underwent surgery at a time when their disease was believed to be quiescent.

TREATMENT

Essential to ideal therapeutical management is accurate determination of disease activity, a goal that may not always be possible. Kerr and colleagues[9] define active disease as any *two or more* of the following. New or worsening:

1. Signs or symptoms of vascular ischemia or inflammation
2. Increase in sedimentation rate
3. Angiographic features
4. Systemic symptoms not attributable to another disease

Although these features are helpful when present, their absence does not guarantee disease remission. These criteria, combined with sequential imaging, are currently the best, albeit imperfect, means of monitoring disease activity.

Glucocorticoid therapy (e.g., prednisone 1 mg/kg per day) induces improvement in nearly all patients and disease remission in about 50% of patients, with resolution of symptoms and stabilization of radiographic abnormalities. However, in at least 40%, disease relapse occurs with tapering of steroid therapy.[12] In these patients or in patients with steroid-resistant disease, therapy with daily oral cyclophosphamide (1 to 2 mg/kg) or weekly methotrexate (15 to 25/mg) may aid in achieving and maintaining disease remission. Low-dose methotrexate was determined to be efficacious in 13 of 16 patients with glucocorticosteroid-dependent or resistant disease in a National Institutes of Health study.[14] Shelhamer and colleagues[15] demonstrated that cyclophosphamide administered with glucocorticosteroid induced remission in four of six patients with steroid-resistant disease. The authors recommend cyclophosphamide only for patients with severe active disease. In the setting of normal renal function, treatment should be initiated at a dose of 2 mg/kg per day. Patients generally achieve remission and can be tapered to low doses of prednisone (15 mg/day) within 3 to 6 months. At this point cyclophosphamide should be changed to maintenance therapy with weekly methotrexate or azathioprine. This strategy is designed to minimize the risk of long-term cyclophosphamide toxicity. Preliminary studies in a TA cohort have demonstrated efficacy of anti-TNF therapy in 14 of 15 patients with relapsing disease.[16]

About 80% of patients require chronic immunosuppressive therapy over periods that range from 6 months to the remainder of their lives. It has only been over the

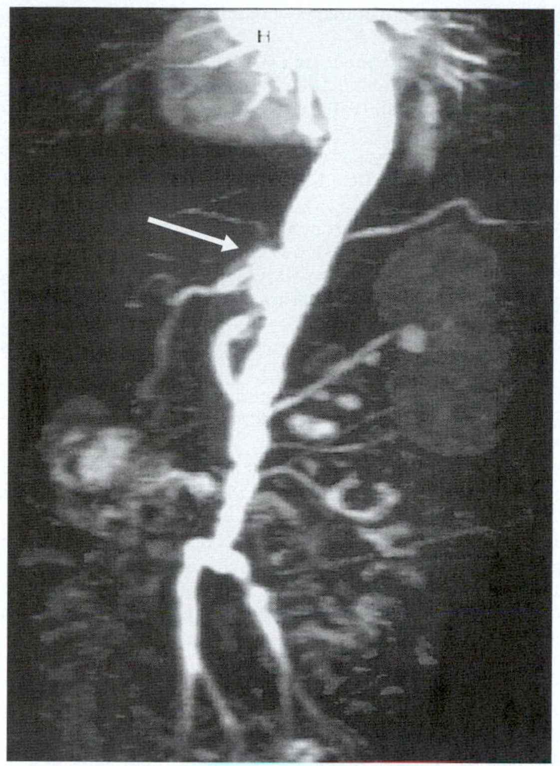

FIGURE 42-10. Diffuse ectasia of the abdominal aorta and bilateral common iliac arteries, with significant stenosis of the left iliac artery (MRA). Also note dilation of the origin of the celiac artery *(arrow)*.

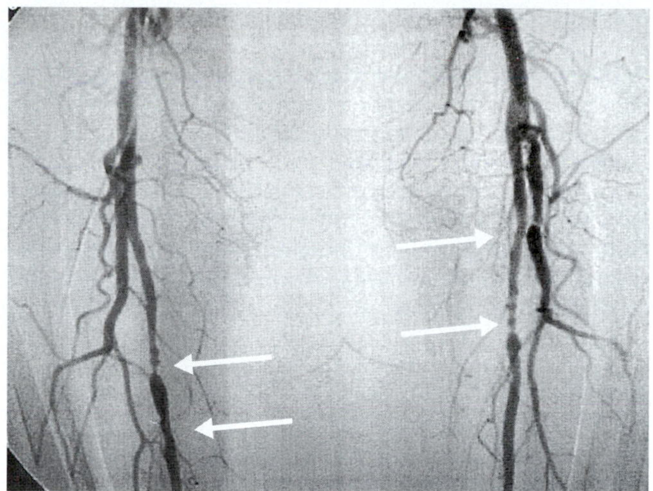

FIGURE 42-11. Multiple stenotic lesions of the deep femoral arteries (catheter-directed angiography).

past 15 years that investigators have recognized the chronic and often treatment-resistant nature of TA. Studies that have incorporated sequential angiography have demonstrated that the majority of patients continue to develop new lesions in new vascular territories, even if patients appear clinically to be in remission.[9,12,14,16] Because clinical symptoms and serology are often unreliable in monitoring disease activity, serial imaging studies (by MRA or CT/PET angiography) have become the gold standard for assessment of disease progression.

Untreated hypertension is a major source of morbidity and mortality in TA. Delay in the diagnosis of hypertension is common because of the high frequency of subclavian and innominate artery involvement, which may result in underestimation of central aortic pressure. Stenotic lesions also may be present in lower extremity vessels, leaving some patients without any extremity capable of providing cuff blood pressure measurements that reliably represent those within the aortic root (Figs. 42-10 and 42-11). This emphasizes the need for complete vascular imaging at the time of diagnosis. Imaging should include the entire aorta and its primary branches. If stenoses are present, especially within upper extremity large vessels, invasive angiography is the preferred study, with inclusion of central aortic pressure measurements and gradient determinations, to establish the accuracy of peripheral blood pressure measurements.

Blood pressure management is crucial but complex in TA. Even with reliable peripheral recordings, determining and attaining a target pressure range in the setting of arterial stenotic lesions affecting major organs (e.g., cerebral or coronary stenoses), without causing compromised perfusion, can be challenging. For this reason, careful monitoring is essential when intervention for blood pressure control is necessary. In addition, angiotensin-converting enzyme inhibitors should be used with caution in the setting of renal artery stenosis, as this therapy blunts the renal autoregulatory response to decreased glomerular pressure. This results in a decrease in the glomerular filtration rate with lowering of blood pressure and may lead to a clinically significant decline in renal function.

All primary branches of the aorta are vulnerable. Arterial stenoses may potentially affect any organ system. Intervention to correct lesions should be considered in the setting of clinically significant symptoms or evidence of significant organ ischemia. Multiple studies demonstrate impressive initial patency of vascular stenoses with percutaneous angioplasty, with success rates of 80% to 100%.[17,18,19] However, even with intravascular stent placement, vascular restenosis occurs frequently, with rates of 20% to 71% reported when followed up to 45 months after the procedure. Drug-eluting stents could potentially increase patency duration but have not yet been studied in TA. Bypass procedures also may be complicated by vessel restenosis, but rates of sustained patency are higher (range 65% to 88%, mean follow-up period 44 to 60 months).[20,21] One postoperative observational study of 29 patients indicates that disease activity at the time of surgery is important in bypass outcomes. In this study, patients with active disease at the time of operative intervention had a 53% bypass graft patency rate at 5 years, whereas patients who were operated on when disease was quiescent had an 88% patency rate over the same period.[21] Thus, when interventions are planned, it is preferred that they occur in the setting of disease remission. Tissue should be obtained from the origin or insertion of grafts, or both. Histopathologic examination may aid in the assessment of disease activity and assist in disease management.

TA patients are generally young, but disease-related complications may increase their surgical risk. A retrospective review of 106 consecutive patients with TA observed 12 perioperative deaths (11.3%) following operative intervention. Most deaths occurred as a result of cardiovascular complications.[22] However, other series document perioperative mortality as low as 0% to 3%.[9,20] Surgical outcomes can be significantly impacted by the experience of the surgical team and medical center in caring for patients with TA.

A multidisciplinary approach to the care of TA patients is optimal. The team should include a rheumatologist; cardiovascular physician; imaging specialist; and, in the setting of critical stenoses or aneurysms, vascular and cardiothoracic surgeons.

REFERENCES

1. Hall S, Barr W, Lie JT, et al: Takayasu arteritis: A study of 32 North American patients. Medicine 64:89, 1985.
2. Waern AU, Anderson P, Hemmingsson A: Takayasu's arteritis: A hospital-region based study on occurrence, treatment, and prognosis. Angiology 34:311, 1983.
3. Nasu T: Takayasu's truncoarteritis in Japan: A statistical observation of 76 autopsy cases. Pathol Microbiol 43:140, 1975.
4. Seko Y, Minota S, Kawasaki A, et al: Perforin-secreting killer cell infiltration and expression of a 65 kD heat shock protein in aortic tissue of patients with Takayasu's arteritis. J Clin Invest 93:750, 1994.
5. Noris M, Daina E, Gamba S, et al: Interleukin-6 and RANTES in Takayasu arteritis: A guide for therapeutic decisions? Circulation 100:55, 1999.
6. Hoffman GS: Large-vessel vasculitis: Unresolved issues. Arthritis Rheum 48:2406, 2003.
7. Numano F: Takayasu's arteritis: Clinical aspects. In Hoffman GS, Weyand CM (eds): Inflammatory Diseases of Blood Vessels. New York, Marcel Dekker, 2002, p 455.
8. Hotchi M: Pathologic studies on Takayasu arteritis. Heart Vessels Suppl 7:11, 1992.
9. Kerr G, Hallahan C, Giordano J, et al: Takayasu arteritis. Ann Intern Med 120:919, 1994.
10. Lupi-Herrara E, Sanchez-Torrez G, Marchushamer J, et al: Takayasu arteritis: Clinical study of 107 cases. Am Heart J 93:94, 1977.
11. Numano F, Kobayashi Y: Takayasu arteritis—beyond pulselessness. Intern Med 38:226, 1999.
12. Hoffman GS: Takayasu arteritis: Lessons from the American National Institutes of Health experience. Int J Cardiol 54(suppl):83, 1996.
13. Morales E, Pineda C, Martinez-Lavin M: Takayasu's arteritis in children. J Rheumatol 18:1081, 1991.
14. Hoffman GS, Leavitt RY, Kerr GS, et al: Treatment of glucocorticoid-resistant or relapsing Takayasu arteritis with methotrexate. Arthritis Rheum 37:578, 1994.
15. Shelhamer JH, Volkman DJ, Parrillo JE, et al: Takayasu's arteritis and its therapy. Ann Intern Med 103:121, 1985.
16. Hoffman GS, Merkel PA, Brassington RD, et al: Anti-tumor necrosis factor therapy in patients with difficult to treat Takayasu arteritis. Arthritis Rheum 50:2296, 2004.
17. Sharma BK, Jain S, Bali HK, et al: A follow-up study of balloon angioplasty and de-novo stenting in Takayasu arteritis. Int J Cardiol 75:S147, 2000.
18. Tyagi S, Gambhir DS, Kaul UA, et al: A decade of subclavian angioplasty: Aortoarteritis versus atherosclerosis. Indian Heart J 48:667, 1996.
19. Bali HK, Bhargava M, Jain AK, et al: De novo stenting of descending thoracic aorta in Takayasu arteritis: Intermediate-term follow-up results. J Invasive Cardiol 12:612, 2000.
20. Liang P, Tan-Ong M, Hoffman GS: Takayasu's arteritis: Vascular interventions and outcomes. J Rheum 31:102, 2004.
21. Pajari R, Hekali P Harjola PT: Treatment of Takayasu's arteritis: An analysis of 29 operated patients. Thorac Cardiovasc Surg 34:176, 1986.
22. Miyata T, Sato O, Koyama H, et al: Long-term survival after surgical treatment of patients with Takayasu's arteritis. Circulation 108:1474, 2003.
23. Lagneau P, Michel JB, Vuong PN: Surgical treatment of Takayasu's disease. Ann Surg 205:157, 1987.

■ ■ ■ chapter 43

Giant Cell Arteritis

Maria C. Cid
Peter A. Merkel

Giant cell (temporal) arteritis (GCA) is a chronic inflammatory arteritis preferentially involving large- and medium-sized arteries. It affects persons after age 50, especially after age 70. Although autopsy studies have shown that the aorta and its major tributaries are almost invariably involved, most of the major clinical manifestations and complications of the disease arise from involvement of the carotid artery branches,[1-3] including headaches, visual loss, and stroke. Aortitis and resulting aneurysms and stenoses, as well as extremity arterial occlusions and claudication, can be seen in GCA, especially in late disease. Histopathologic diagnosis is usually determined from examination of a biopsy of the superficial temporal artery (Figs. 43-1 and 43-2).

Approximately 50% of patients with GCA develop polymyalgia rheumatica (PMR), a clinically defined syndrome consisting of aching and stiffness in the neck, shoulders, or pelvic girdle. PMR can also exist as a distinct entity with no evidence of vascular involvement.[1-3]

This chapter outlines the epidemiology, pathophysiology, clinical manifestations, and treatment options for GCA with particular reference to manifestations likely encountered by vascular medicine specialists.

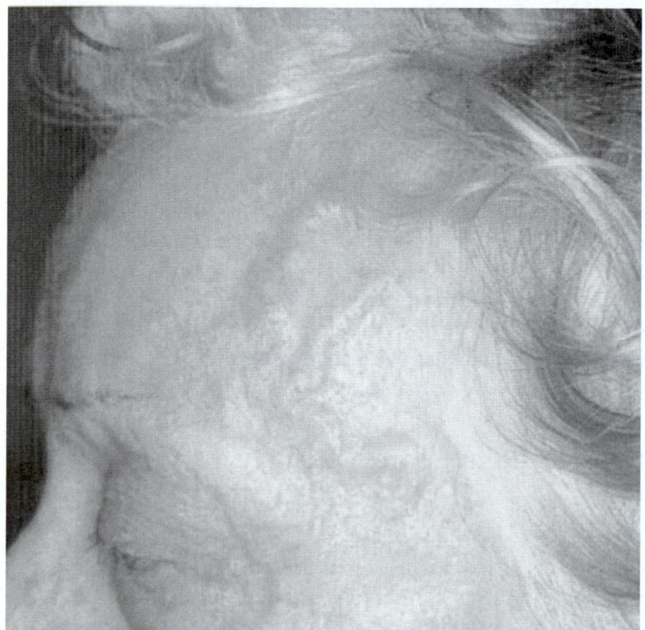

FIGURE 43-1. (See also Color Plate 43-1.) Enlarged, hardened, and pulseless temporal and frontal arteries in a patient with giant cell arteritis.

EPIDEMIOLOGY OF GIANT CELL ARTERITIS

GCA characteristically occurs in people older than 50 years, and its frequency increases with age. The maximal incidence of GCA occurs between 75 and 85 years of age, and it is twice as frequent among women as men. Although there is a markedly increased incidence of GCA among Caucasians in northern Europe and in populations with similar ethnic background,[4,5] the disease can occur in all populations. GCA is not an uncommon disease. Recent studies conducted in northern Europe and North America disclose an annual incidence rate of 19 to 32 cases per 100,000 people older than 50 years,[5-7] and a rate of 49 per 100,000 for individuals in their 80s.[4,7] In Mediterranean countries the annual incidence is lower, about 6 to 10 cases per 100,000.[8,9] Isolated PMR is even more frequent, with an average annual incidence rate of 52 per 100,000 people aged 50 and older.[1,4]

PATHOLOGY OF GIANT CELL ARTERITIS

In the large- and medium-sized arteries involved in GCA, the vessel wall is infiltrated by T lymphocytes and macrophages, frequently producing a granulomatous reaction with the presence of multinucleated giant cells (Fig. 43-3).[10] Scattered polymorphonuclear leukocytes can be occasionally identified; however, B lymphocytes or natural killer cells are virtually absent.[11]

The extent of inflammatory infiltrates is highly variable among patients and even varies in different sections of the same specimen. Inflammatory infiltrates usually extend to the adventitial layer and can span the entire thickness of the vessel. In some patients there is isolated inflammation of vasa vasorum and small vessels surrounding the temporal artery. The internal elastic lamina is usually disrupted, and giant cells often accumulate in its vicinity but are not required for a diagnosis. In well-developed lesions, the lumen is occluded by intimal hyperplasia.

The inflammatory lesions are typically segmental and are preferentially distributed along the carotid and vertebral arteries.[12] Intracranial vessels are usually spared. Small arteries and arterioles in the vicinity of the superficial temporal artery are almost invariably involved.[13] Autopsy studies have demonstrated that inflammatory infiltrates are often detected in the aorta and its major tributaries.[14]

The histopathologic findings in PMR include chronic synovitis and bursitis of proximal joints.[15,16] Synovitis is usually mild, and the inflammatory infiltrates are composed

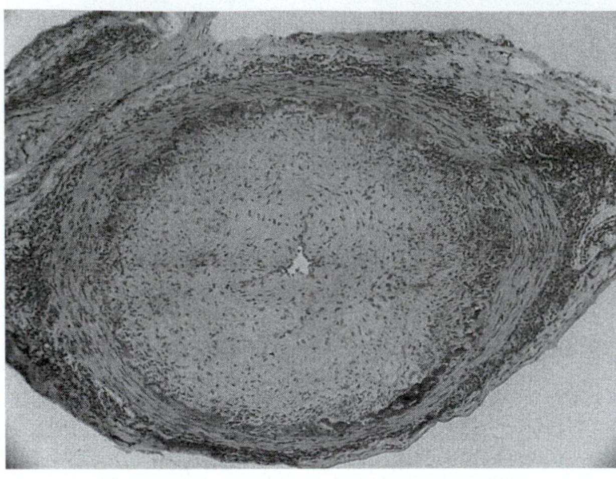

A

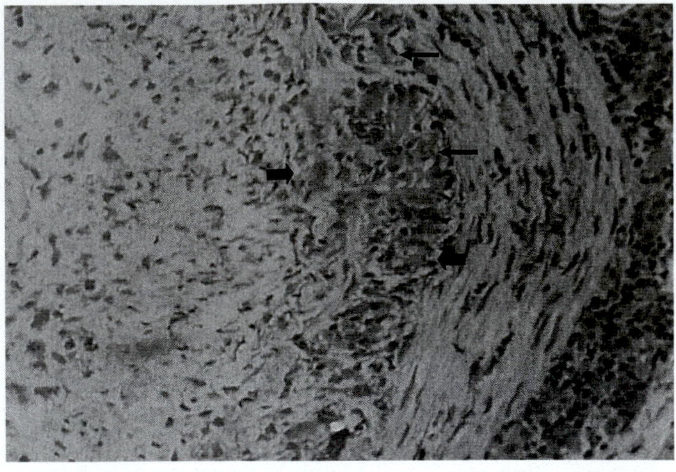

B

FIGURE 43-2. Classic, fully developed lesions in a temporal artery biopsy specimen from a patient with giant cell arteritis. **A,** Inflammatory infiltrates involving the entire arterial wall and predominating at the adventitial layer and at the intima/media junction where a granulomatous reaction with presence of giant cells can be appreciated. A prominent intimal hyperplasia virtually occludes the lumen. **B,** Enlargement of section of intima/media junction from **A**. *Thin arrows* show fragments of the internal elastic lamina. *Thick arrows* indicate multinucleated giant cells.

of CD4 T lymphocytes and macrophages with scarce granulocytes. Muscle biopsies do not disclose specific abnormalities.

PATHOGENESIS OF GIANT CELL ARTERITIS

Genetic Predisposition for Giant Cell Arteritis

The predominance of GCA and PMR among Caucasians, especially in Northern Europe, strongly suggests a genetic component in the pathogenesis of GCA and PMR. A higher prevalence of the HLA class 2 antigen DR4 has been reported among patients with GCA and PMR compared with the general population.[17-19] Certain polymorphisms of genes involved in immune and inflammatory responses, such as tumor necrosis factor-alpha (TNF-α),[20] vascular endothelial growth factor (VEGF),[21] endothelial nitric oxide synthase (NOS),[22] intercellular adhesion molecule-1 (ICAM-1),[23] and mannose-binding lectin[24] appear to be more frequent among patients with GCA than in the general population. The influence of these polymorphisms in the development of GCA remains undefined but is under active investigation.

FIGURE 43-3. Strong tumor necrosis factor-alpha (TNF-α) expression at the granulomatous area in a temporal artery biopsy specimen from a patient with giant cell arteritis. Immunostaining performed with a polyclonal rabbit anti-human TNF-α antibody (Genzyme Corp.) via Avidin-biotin-peroxidase method. (Reproduced with permission from Cid MC, Segarra M, García-Martínez A, Hernández-Rodríguez J: Endothelial cells, anti-neutrophil cytoplasmic antibodies and cytokines in the pathogenesis of systemic vasculitis. Curr Rheum Reports 6:184, 2004.)

Possible Triggering Agents for Giant Cell Arteritis

Several observations suggest that GCA may be caused by a yet undefined environmental triggering agent. Cyclic fluctuations in the incidence of GCA, occurring every 6 to 7 years, have been reported.[7] Additionally, the characteristic granulomatous reaction with multinucleated giant cells has also prompted a search for an infectious agent that may cause a delayed-type hypersensitivity reaction. Attempts to identify specific pathogens, however, including *Chlamydia pneumoniae* and parvovirus B19, have led to conflicting results[25-28]; thus the search for an infectious etiology of GCA continues.[29]

Immunopathogenic Mechanisms in Giant Cell Arteritis

It has been postulated that inflammatory lesions in GCA develop as a consequence of an antigen-specific immune response against epitopes present in the vessel wall. Activated dendritic cells have been detected in inflammatory lesions of GCA,[11,26,30] where they are believed to serve as antigen-presenting cells and provide costimulatory signals for CD4 T cell activation. Immunopathologic studies have demonstrated that inflammatory infiltrates in GCA are mainly composed of macrophages and T lymphocytes, particularly of the CD4 subset,[11] and both cell populations exhibit activation markers such as IL-2 receptors and MHC class 2 antigens. Expansion of IL2R-expressing CD4 T lymphocyte clones derived from different areas of temporal artery biopsy specimens has shown that some of them share identical sequences at the third complementarity-determining region of the T cell receptor,[31] suggesting a specific immune recognition of a disease-relevant antigen. GCA lesions have demonstrated evidence of vigorous production of interferon γ, a key cytokine in macrophage activation and granuloma formation.[32,33] Activated macrophages release various mediators with highly relevant local and systemic consequences.

Mechanisms of Vascular Injury in Giant Cell Arteritis

Multiple processes have been implicated in the vascular injury seen in GCA. Activated macrophages produce oxygen radicals, nitric oxide, and proteolytic enzymes that participate in the disruption of the vessel wall and in tissue destruction.[34,35] Increased levels of lipid peroxidation products,[34] aldose reductase,[34] inducible nitric oxide synthase, nitrotyrosine-containing proteins,[36] and matrix metalloproteases MMP-2 and MMP-9 have been demonstrated in GCA.[37]

Systemic Inflammatory Response in Giant Cell Arteritis

Activated macrophages produce proinflammatory cytokines IL-1, TNF-α, and IL-6, which are the major inducers of the systemic inflammatory response (fever, weight loss, anemia, and hepatic synthesis of acute phase proteins) often prominent in patients with GCA. Expression of these cytokines in the arterial tissue of patients, as well as circulating levels of TNF-α and IL-6, correlate with the intensity of the systemic inflammatory reaction (see Fig. 43-3).[38,39] As discussed later, these cytokines can activate proinflammatory cascades such as chemokine release, adhesion molecule expression, and angiogenesis. Although each of these cascades may amplify and maintain the inflammatory process,[40] some of their effects on vessel wall components might be protective against vascular occlusion.

Vascular Response to Inflammation in Giant Cell Arteritis

Vessel wall components, particularly endothelial cells and smooth muscle cells, actively react to cytokines and growth factors released by infiltrating leukocytes. Vascular response to inflammation leads to amplification and perpetuation of the inflammatory process, as well as vessel occlusion.[40] Inflammation-induced angiogenesis is remarkable in GCA lesions and preferentially occurs at the adventitial layer and within inflammatory infiltrates, particularly in granulomatous areas at the intima/media junction.[41,42]

Neovessels may have a protective role at distal sites where providing new blood supply may prevent organ ischemia.[42] Additionally, neovessels provide a wider endothelial surface and endothelial cells may exert various proinflammatory activities.[41,43] Vascular response to inflammation may eventually lead to vessel occlusion with subsequent ischemia of the tissues supplied by involved vessels.[40] In GCA, vessel occlusion results mostly from intimal hyperplasia.

CLINICAL MANIFESTATIONS OF GIANT CELL ARTERITIS

Patients with GCA may present with a wide variety of clinical features (Table 43-1). Disease-related manifestations may appear rapidly or develop insidiously. A delay of weeks or even months between the beginning of clinical symptoms and diagnosis is common, particularly in patients with predominantly systemic complaints in whom more frequent diseases, such as infections or malignancies, are usually suspected. Ischemic complications tend to accumulate in particular patients and are frequently early events during the course of the disease.[18,44]

Some data suggest that an initial presentation of GCA with signs and symptoms of systemic inflammation (elevated acute phase reactants, fever, anemia, weight loss) is associated with a specific pattern of clinical illness. For unclear reasons, patients with a strong systemic inflammatory response are at lower risk of ischemic events but

TABLE 43-1 CLINICAL FINDINGS IN A SERIES OF 250 PATIENTS WITH GIANT CELL ARTERITIS

General features:	
Age (mean, range)	75 (50-94)
Sex (female/male)	178/72
Weight loss	61%
Fever	47%
Cranial symptoms:	
Headache	77%
Temporal artery abnormality	74%
(swollen, tender, weak/absent pulse)	44%
Jaw claudication	39%
Scalp tenderness	18%
Facial pain	18%
Earache	12%
Odynophagia	8%
Ocular pain	5%
Tongue pain	5%
Carotodynia	5%
Toothache	1%
Trismus	22%
Cerebrovascular accident	2%
Ophthalmic events:	
Blindness (permanent)	14%
Amaurosis fugax	10%
Transient diplopia	4%
Symptomatic large vessel involvement (claudication and/or bruit)	5%
Polymyalgia rheumatica	48%

Modified and reprinted from Cid MS, Hernandez-Rodriquez J, Grau JM: Vascular manifestations in giant-cell arteritis. In Asherson RA, Cervera R (eds): Vascular Manifestations of Systemic Autoimmune Diseases. London, CRC Press, 2001.

are more refractory to therapy[18,38] than patients with a seemingly weaker initial inflammatory response. Similarly, as with cranial ischemic complications, symptomatic stenoses of large vessels have been shown to be negatively associated with prominent inflammatory markers at the time of diagnosis.[45]

Systemic Manifestations of Giant Cell Arteritis

Patients with GCA or PMR frequently experience malaise, anorexia, weight loss, and depression.[1,3,46] Nearly 50% of patients with GCA have fever, and in some patients fever or constitutional symptoms are the most prominent finding. Approximately 10% of patients present with fever of unknown origin with mild or no cranial manifestations.[1,3]

Clinical Manifestations of Cranial Arterial Involvement in Giant Cell Arteritis

Headache is one of the most common and classical symptoms, occurring in about 60% to 98% of cases of GCA.[1,3,47] The intensity and location of headache are highly variable, but headaches frequently predominate at the temporal areas. Scalp tenderness is also common. About 40% of patients experience jaw claudication when eating, a symptom highly specific for GCA but that is occasionally seen in other vascular diseases such as polyarteritis nodosa or systemic amyloidosis. Other manifestations, such as facial swelling, tongue ischemia, or edema, are less frequently seen (see Table 43-1).[1,3,48] Patients may also present with various unusual pains in the craniofacial area, including ocular pain, earache, toothache, odynophagia, odontalgia, and carotidynia. When these symptoms predominate, a substantial delay in diagnosis is common.

Visual impairment is the most feared complication of GCA and occurs in about 15% of cases.[18,49] A wide variety of ophthalmologic problems occur in GCA, but blindness is most commonly due to anterior ischemic optic neuropathy derived from inflammatory involvement of posterior ciliary arteries supplying the optic nerve. Less frequently, central retinal artery thrombosis, retrobulbar neuritis, or cortical blindness can occur. Visual loss can be bilateral or unilateral and either complete or partial; it usually appears suddenly but is often preceded by transient visual loss *(amaurosis fugax)*, diplopia, or blue vision.

Less common ischemic complications include cerebrovascular accidents due to the involvement of carotid or vertebral tributaries and scalp or tongue necrosis. Strokes are more frequent in territories supplied by vertebral arteries. Additional ischemic manifestations include hearing loss and vestibular dysfunction.[50]

Cardiac, Aortic, and Peripheral Vascular Manifestations of Giant Cell Arteritis

Myocardial or mesenteric infarction due to GCA can be infrequently seen. Because GCA occurs in older people, some cases of inflammatory coronary or mesenteric arteritis may be misdiagnosed as due to atherosclerotic disease. Even among patients with GCA, however, atherosclerosis is still a much more common cause of cardiac or mesenteric ischemia than vasculitis. With an increased interest in the role of inflammation in coronary disease and new tools to study the disease process, investigators may now be better able to study the contributions, if any, of inflammatory arteritis to coronary artery disease among patients with GCA and other vasculitides.

Aortitis and inflammatory disease of the main branches of the aorta are more common in GCA than generally appreciated (Figs. 43-4 through 43-7). Autopsy studies and other case series find large vessel vasculitis in many patients with GCA,[12,45,51,52] with the more recent series indicating up to 15% to 27% of patients with large vessel disease. Although fewer patients have clinically significant large vessel disease, this manifestation is almost certainly missed in patients or only diagnosed when a critical event, such as an aneurysmal dissection, occurs. Because aortitis and large vessel occlusions are usually late manifestations of GCA, often occurring years after initial diagnosis, not only are these findings not sought, but when they become clinically significant, they are misdiagnosed as secondary to hypertensive or atherosclerotic disease. Interestingly, unlike noninflammatory aortic disease, there is a markedly increased ratio of thoracic to abdominal aortic aneurysms seen in patients with GCA, and the risk of thoracic disease may be 17-fold higher among patients with a history of GCA.[52]

Patients with GCA should be followed indefinitely for the development of large vessel disease, even when there is no evidence of other active disease. Aortic valvular disease, aortic aneurysms or dissections, and peripheral vascular occlusions should all be considered possibly due to inflammatory disease. The precise methodology and frequency in which to screen such patients is not known, but increased awareness among clinicians of the association between GCA and large vessel disease is a first important step in identifying cases. New vascular bruits, asymmetry in blood pressure readings, weak or absent peripheral pulses, murmurs, and limb claudication or ischemia are all warning signs easily inquired about and examined for in physicians' offices.

Polymyalgia Rheumatica and Other Musculoskeletal Manifestations of Giant Cell Arteritis

Approximately 50% of patients with GCA present with symptoms of PMR, a syndrome clinically defined by the presence of aching and stiffness in the neck, shoulders, or pelvic girdle. Pain is exacerbated with movement. Morning stiffness is a prominent finding and may last for many hours. Proximal muscles are usually tender, but true weakness or myopathy is not seen. Ultrasonography and MRI studies have shown that the underlying abnormalities consist of proximal joint synovitis and inflammation of periarticular structures, characteristically subacromial and subdeltoid bursitis.[46,53] The synovitis of PMR is histologically mild. Macrophages and CD4+ T lymphocytes predominate in inflammatory infiltrates. As in GCA, neutrophils are scarce and B cells are absent.[15,16]

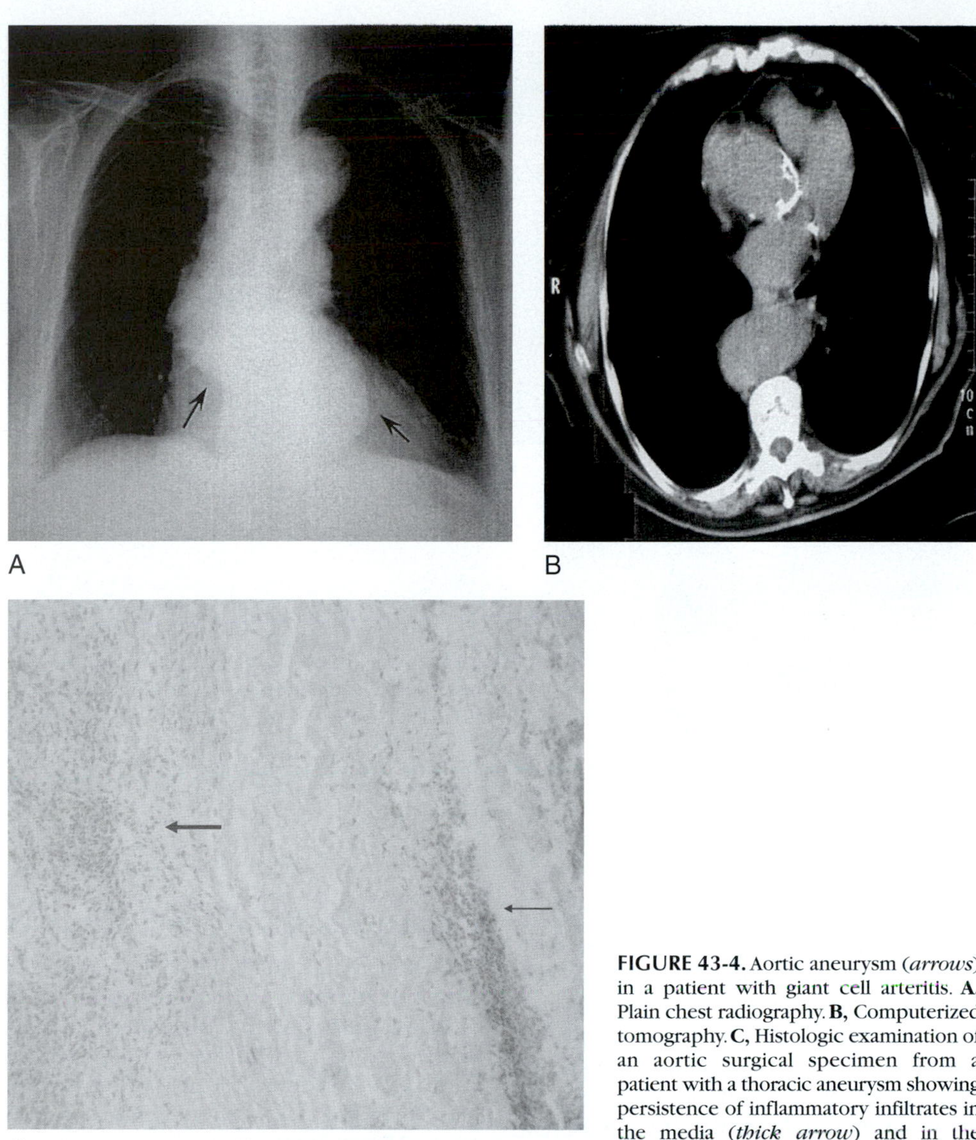

FIGURE 43-4. Aortic aneurysm (*arrows*) in a patient with giant cell arteritis. **A,** Plain chest radiography. **B,** Computerized tomography. **C,** Histologic examination of an aortic surgical specimen from a patient with a thoracic aneurysm showing persistence of inflammatory infiltrates in the media (*thick arrow*) and in the adventitia (*thin arrow*).

Twenty-three percent of patients with GCA develop peripheral synovitis. Knees, wrists, and metacarpophalangeal joints are the most frequently involved joints. Peripheral manifestations usually occur in patients with PMR but may also occasionally appear in patients without proximal symptoms. Other associated manifestations include tenosynovitis, carpal tunnel syndrome, and distal swelling with pitting edema.[46,54-56] Some patients develop a clinical picture indistinguishable from seronegative rheumatoid arthritis.[55]

Relationship Between Polymyalgia Rheumatica and Giant Cell Arteritis

PMR and GCA are closely related, but the nature of their relationship is still unclear. Both conditions have a similar age, sex, and ethnic distribution and share a similar immunogenetic background. Both diseases are characterized by a remarkable acute-phase response, and they both respond remarkably well to glucocorticoid treatment.[57]

PMR can develop simultaneously with cranial symptoms or may emerge months or even years earlier. Some patients with no initial PMR develop PMR symptoms during GCA relapses, and PMR may sometimes be the only clinical manifestation of GCA.

Although PMR can exist as an isolated entity without any evidence of vascular inflammation, temporal artery biopsies disclosing GCA can be demonstrated in about 10% to 20% of patients with apparently isolated PMR. This frequency is much lower, about 1% to 2%, when cranial symptoms are ruled out by a detailed inquiry and abnormalities of the temporal arteries are excluded by careful physical examination.[53,57] Routine temporal artery biopsy is not advised in patients with PMR and no signs or symptoms of cranial disease.

Autopsy studies performed in patients with apparently isolated PMR have revealed inflammatory involvement of the aorta and its branches.[58] More recently, positron emission tomography (PET) studies have demonstrated fluorine-18 (^{18}F)-fluorodeoxyglucose (FDG) uptake in

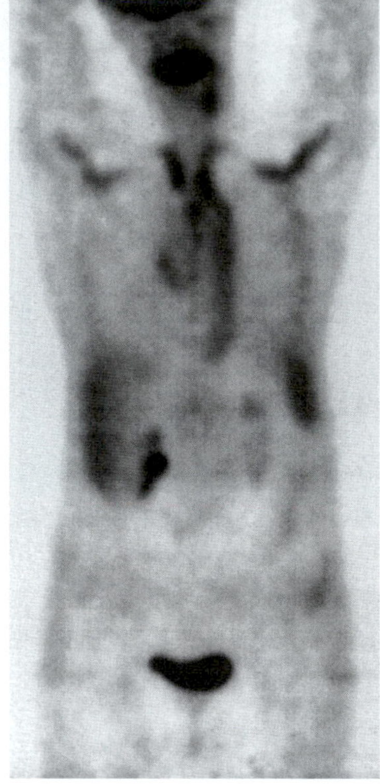

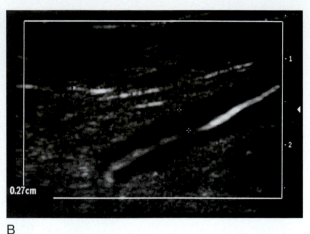

A

B

FIGURE 43-5. Diagnostic images of a patient with giant cell arteritis and a positive temporal artery biopsy. **A,** PET scan demonstrating high uptake in the aorta and the bilateral subclavian and axillary arteries. **B,** A Doppler longitudinal ultrasound scan demonstrating hypoechoic wall thickening around the axillary artery (*indicated by crosses*). (Courtesy of Carlo Salvarani, MD.)

the thoracic aorta or subclavian arteries, or both, in 58% of patients with PMR.[59] However, the number of patients evaluated in this initial series is too small to estimate the real prevalence of aortic involvement in apparently isolated PMR. These data imply that new diagnostic imaging approaches might allow the identification of vascular involvement in a higher proportion of patients with PMR than clinically suspected; however, the prognostic importance and treatment implications of such information have not been established. Nonetheless, it is advised that patients with PMR be followed clinically with the same rigor and frequency as performed with patients with GCA.

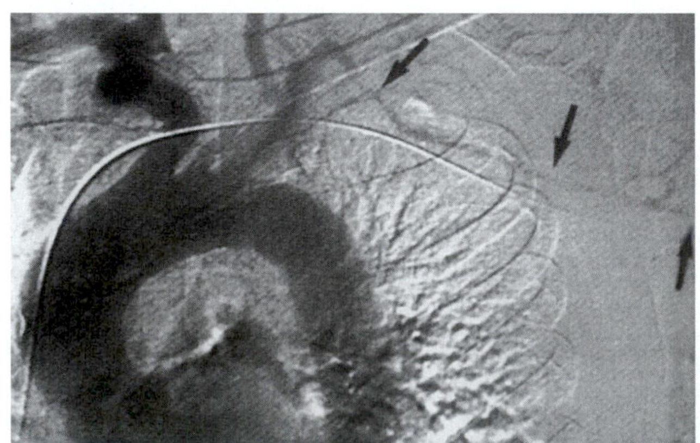

FIGURE 43-6. A conventional digital subtraction angiogram in a patient with giant cell arteritis demonstrating stenosis of the left subclavian artery (*arrows*). (Courtesy of Carlo Salvarani, MD.)

Incidentally Discovered Giant Cell Arteritis

GCA may occasionally be diagnosed only when vascular surgical specimens reveal arteritis, with or without giant cells, and retrospective investigation suggests prior signs or symptoms attributable to GCA. Several retrospective surgical or autopsy series of aortic specimens have demonstrated rates of nonsyphilitic aortitis ranging from 1% to 15%.[60] Most cases of aortitis involved the thoracic aorta, and the majority of cases were in women. Less than 50% of these cases were associated with an identifiable syndrome such as GCA. In a series of 1204 aortic surgical specimens from one institution, 52 (4.3%) demonstrated idiopathic aortitis, and only 12 of the 52 were found to have a non-GCA inflammatory disease.[60] Because a subset of patients with idiopathic aortitis may go on to develop additional clinically important manifestations of GCA, it seems prudent to evaluate and follow such patients as one would cases of more clearly diagnosed GCA.

PHYSICAL EXAMINATION FOR GIANT CELL ARTERITIS

The physical examination is extremely important not only for the initial evaluation of patients with possible GCA but also for following patients after the diagnosis has been established. Blood pressure measurements should be taken in both arms at each visit (and possibly periodically in both legs), with asymmetry of pressures possibly indicating aortic, subclavian, or other peripheral

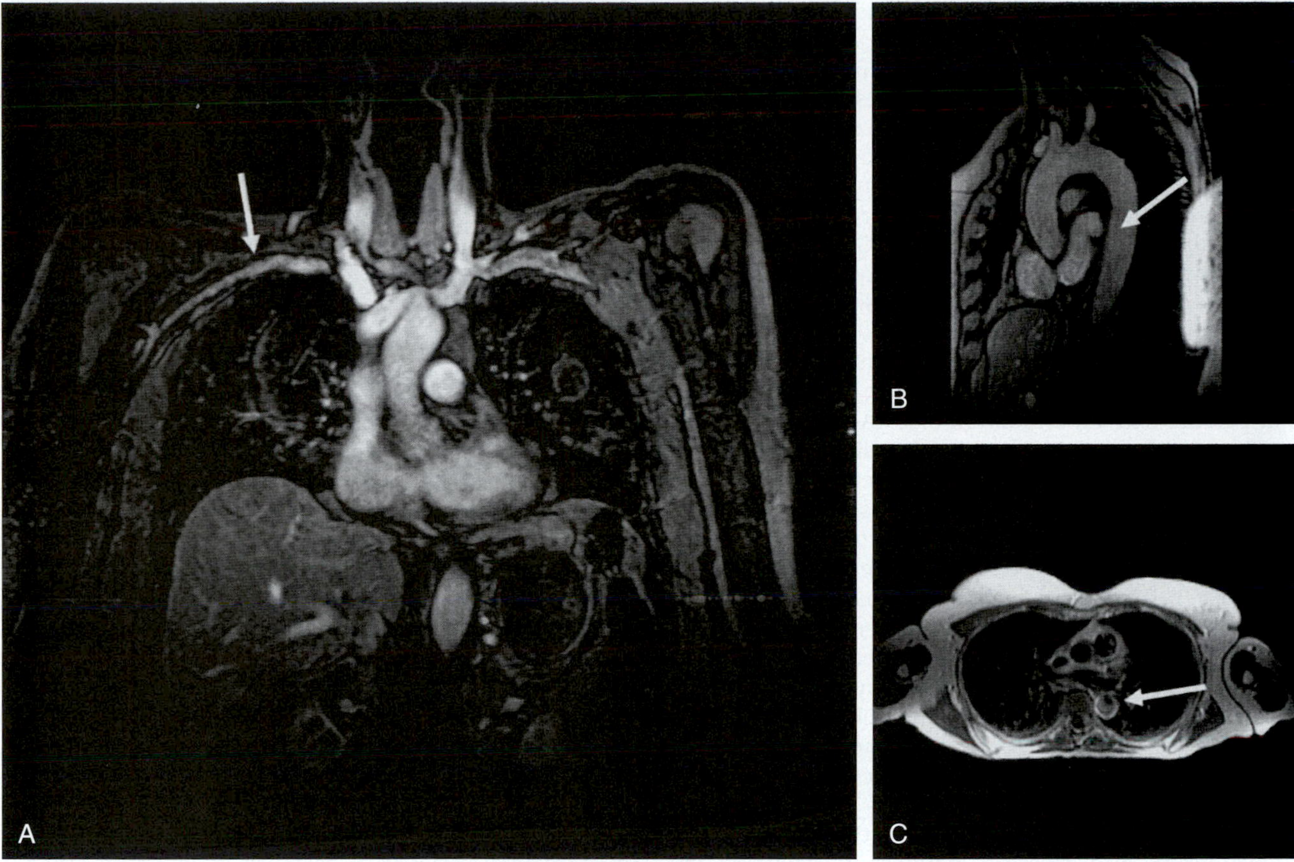

FIGURE 43-7. Magnetic resonance angiogram in giant cell arteritis with irregularities of the subclavian arteries **(A)** and the aortic arch **(B)**. **C,** The aortic wall shows enhancement after application of contrast medium (gadolinium) that is believed to be consistent with inflammation. (Courtesy of Michael Schirmer, MD.)

artery involvement. A careful, comprehensive examination of all pulses is key to the evaluation of GCA. The temporal arteries may be swollen, hard, or pulseless in GCA, although they may also appear normal even in arteries later found to have active arteritis. At times, a slight asymmetry, decrease, or irregularity in the pulse can be detected in temporal or other cranial arteries. Patients should be examined for bruits over carotid, subclavian, axillary, renal, iliac, and other arteries and the aorta. The scalp should be examined for tenderness. Ophthalmologic examination, including funduscopy, visual field, and acuity testing should be performed for evidence of optic ischemia or other abnormalities leading to a diagnosis of GCA or other diseases presenting with visual changes. The rest of a full neurologic examination is important as well. Evidence of synovitis or enthesitis should be sought. A full, general examination is important to help evaluate patients for disorders with overlapping features of GCA.

LABORATORY FINDINGS IN GIANT CELL ARTERITIS

With a few exceptions, both GCA and PMR are characterized by a strong acute-phase reaction. The erythrocyte sedimentation rate (ESR) is usually markedly elevated, frequently around 100 mm/hr (Westergren method). Plasma concentrations of acute phase proteins, such as C-reactive protein, haptoglobin, and fibrinogen, are also elevated. Protein electrophoresis shows an increase in α_2-globulins. Thrombocytosis and anemia of chronic disease are common, and some patients have abnormal liver function tests, particularly increased levels of alkaline phosphatase.[1,3] Hyperbilirubinemia with visible jaundice is rare but may also occur. Symptomatic anemia may occasionally be the first clinical manifestation of GCA. Nonspecific immunologic abnormalities, such as decreased numbers of circulating CD8 lymphocytes and elevated levels of soluble interleukin-2 receptors, are common in GCA and PMR.[1,3]

Several monocyte and endothelial cell activation products can be detected with increased concentrations in plasma from patients with GCA and PMR. These include cytokines such as IL-6 and TNF-α, soluble adhesion molecules such as ICAM-1, and vWF antigen.[1,3,40,61,62] The role these cytokines or cellular markers may play in the diagnosis and management of GCA is an area of active investigation.

DIAGNOSIS OF GIANT CELL ARTERITIS

The diagnosis of GCA is arrived at by a combination of clinical history, physical examination findings, laboratory studies, and arterial biopsy results. No one feature or finding is fully diagnostic by itself, as even "positive" temporal artery biopsies are occasionally seen in other types of arteritis, and many disorders result in systemic features, headaches, or visual changes. Nonetheless, a positive temporal artery biopsy is an extremely strong finding and is almost always diagnostic. Similarly, no feature or finding is absolutely required to make the diagnosis. For example, the ESR may be normal in up to 10% of patients with GCA at presentation. Certain symptoms and findings, however, are notable for establishing a high suspicion of GCA. It is the initial consideration of GCA that is crucial for initiating the diagnostic process and that often leads to empiric treatment even before a diagnosis is fully established.

In parallel with an evaluation of GCA itself, physicians usually need to consider alternative diagnoses such as brain lesions, infections, or malignancies and conduct appropriate evaluations for these disorders. Similarly, even if GCA is established by history and biopsy, other inflammatory vasculitides such as Wegener's granulomatosis or polyarteritis nodosa must at least be considered and sought, because they may rarely present with temporal artery involvement. Finally, although there are differences between patients with GCA and Takayasu's arteritis in terms of the frequency of specific clinical manifestations, responses to therapy, the use of nonglucocorticoid immunosuppressive agents, and outcomes, there are many similar features; thus, all patients with either diagnosis should be screened for manifestations of the other. In evaluating and treating patients with GCA, the best care may require collaborative work among rheumatologists, ophthalmologists, neurologists, and vascular medicine specialists.

Temporal Artery Biopsy

Histopathologic examination of a temporal artery biopsy often provides the definitive diagnosis of GCA (see Figs. 43-1 and 43-2).[10] The area to be excised is carefully selected, guided by physical examination findings and symptoms. At least a 2- to 3-cm fragment should be removed, and multiple histologic sections examined. When the initial biopsy is negative for evidence of GCA, excision of the contralateral artery may increase diagnostic sensitivity. Temporal artery biopsy is highly sensitive for the diagnosis of GCA.[63] Occasionally the temporal artery may be involved in the context of other systemic vasculitides or other disorders, such as systemic amyloidosis.[10,64,65] When involving the temporal artery or its tributaries, systemic necrotizing vasculitis may present with cranial symptoms and complications similar to GCA.[65]

Although the diagnostic yield of a temporal artery biopsy that is performed appropriately is high, a normal temporal artery biopsy does not completely exclude GCA given the segmental distribution of inflammatory infiltrates. In only 10% or less of patients with negative results obtained from a temporal artery biopsy performed and processed under optimal conditions, however, the clinical suspicion is strong enough to indicate long-term glucocorticoid therapy.[63] Due to the frequent existence of overlapping features among vasculitides, criteria sets have been established in order to classify patients with vasculitis into specific categories. The most commonly used classification criteria are those of the American College of Rheumatology, and the set for GCA is outlined in Box 43-1.[66] Although not intended for use diagnostically, these criteria are useful to clinicians when evaluating patients and are adopted for use as inclusion criteria for almost all research studies of GCA. Caution must be used when applying these criteria, however, to ensure patients with nonvasculitic conditions are not mistakenly diagnosed with GCA.

Diagnostic Imaging for Giant Cell Arteritis

Various diagnostic imaging modalities are under investigation for use in the diagnosis and long-term management of GCA.[67] These modalities include ultrasound, MRI, ^{18}F-FDG PET scanning (with or without CT), and conventional contrast angiography (Figs. 43-4 through 43-8). The lack of standardization for these modalities, the wide variation in available equipment, the absence of proper validation studies or long-term data, the need to differentiate findings in GCA from atherosclerotic disease, and the high cost of some studies are all limiting factors to more widespread adoption but are all areas in which progress is anticipated in the next decade. Furthermore, as these imaging techniques continue to be used extensively for evaluation of patients with presumed atherosclerotic disease, additional patients who actually have inflammatory vascular disease are likely to be encountered and diagnosed. Thus, vascular medicine specialists, vascular surgeons, and vascular radiologists need to consider GCA more when reviewing such imaging studies.

Color-duplex ultrasonography has been studied as a diagnostic tool for GCA with conflicting results (see Fig. 43-8).[68-70] It has been proposed that ultrasound may disclose stenosis, occlusion, or a dark hypoechoic halo surrounding the lumen of an affected temporal or

BOX 43-1 American College of Rheumatology Criteria for the Classification of Giant Cell (Temporal) Arteritis*

1. Age at disease onset ≥50 years
2. New onset of headache or new type of localized pain in the head
3. Temporal artery tenderness or decreased pulsation
4. Erythrocyte sedimentation rate ≥50 mm/hr (Westergren)
5. Temporal artery biopsy showing vasculitis with a predominance of mononuclear cells or granulomatous inflammation, usually with multinucleated giant cells.

*A patient is considered to have GCA if at least three of these criteria are present. The presence of any three or more criteria yields a sensitivity of 93.5% and a specificity of 91.2%.

From Hunder GG, Bloch DA, Michel BA, et al: The American College of Rheumatology 1990 criteria for the classification of giant cell arteritis. Arthritis Rheum 33:1122, 1990.

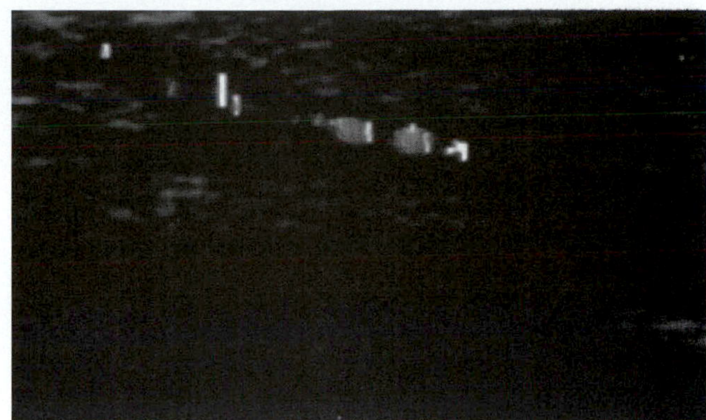

FIGURE 43-8. Patient with giant cell arteritis. A Doppler longitudinal scan shows hypoechoic area around the proximal superficial temporal artery. (Courtesy of Carlo Salvarani, MD.)

branch artery in active GCA and that these combined findings have a high specificity for disease, precluding the need for biopsy.[68] A follow-up study questioned these results, however, finding ultrasound to be of no additional usefulness beyond routine history and physical examination.[70] Thus, at this time, ultrasonography is not powerful enough to be considered as a surrogate diagnostic tool. Its complementary use in the evaluation and follow-up of the extent of disease in terms of involvement of additional vascular territories continues to be assessed.[71] The usefulness of duplex ultrasound for detection of carotid or subclavian artery involvement in GCA is also under investigation.

Conventional angiography may confirm involvement of large vessels in patients with bruits or limb claudication (see Fig. 43-6). Conventional angiography has the additional advantages of being able to measure blood pressure at various locations to evaluate the functional impact of stenoses, as well as provide a means for intervention with angioplasty or stent placement, procedures of some controversy for large vessel disease. The invasive nature and risks of conventional angiography preclude its routine use for screening purposes or for serial examinations.

The use of MRI and angiography is an increasingly used tool for screening and evaluating large vessel disease in GCA (see Fig. 43-7).[67,72,73] Although there are data indicting MRI can detect luminal narrowing, arterial wall thickness, and wall enhancement, corresponding to inflammation, the specificities of these findings as indicators of active vasculitis are unclear, and the tests are certainly not reliable enough to be the sole basis of treatment decisions. Nevertheless, MRI offers a relatively low-risk method to screen and monitor for large vessel disease in GCA and is increasingly part of the standard of care for such patients.

^{18}F-FDG PET scanning is another promising new modality for evaluating patients with suspected GCA (see Fig. 43-5). PET scans have demonstrated FDG uptake in large thoracic arteries in GCA and also in some patients with apparently isolated PMR.[59] As with MRI, the prognostic importance of detecting large arterial changes in asymptomatic patients with GCA is not clear. Furthermore, FDG uptake in the abdominal aorta and lower limbs can also be detected in severe atherosclerosis, and, therefore, specificity is lower in these locations.[74] Although diagnostic sensitivity and specificity need to be tested in larger studies, PET scanning may have a significant role in the evaluation of vascular inflammation in patients with atypical symptoms, fever of unknown origin, and in assessing vascular involvement in patients with an apparently isolated PMR. PET will also likely be combined with scanning by CT as new machines with dual PET-CT function obtain simultaneous images of the same anatomical areas.

Diagnosis of Polymyalgia Rheumatica

The diagnosis of PMR relies, at present, on purely clinical criteria.[46] One of the most widely used criteria sets is outlined in Box 43-2.[75] The diagnosis of PMR requires a careful evaluation to exclude other disorders that may occasionally present with similar symptoms, including rheumatoid arthritis, inflammatory myopathies, other vasculitides, or infections.

MRI and ultrasonography can detect subdeltoid and subacromial bursitis in patients with PMR.[46,76] MRI and ultrasonography may possibly become useful tools in the evaluation of patients with suspected PMR, but their reliabilities need to be evaluated in larger studies.

TREATMENT AND MANAGEMENT OF GIANT CELL ARTERITIS

Glucocorticoid therapy is the treatment of choice for GCA and, in most cases, induces a dramatic amelioration of disease manifestations within a few days. The most widely recommended initial dose is 40 to 60 mg/day of prednisone (or equivalent glucocorticoid). The presence of transient ocular manifestations, such as amaurosis fugax, diplopia, or blue vision, must be considered a medical emergency, and treatment must be started immediately, even before the histologic confirmation of GCA is obtained. Glucocorticoid treatment for several days, and even weeks, does not clear the inflammatory infiltrates and, therefore, does not markedly hinder the histopathologic diagnosis.[77] When visual loss is established,

BOX 43-2 Criteria for the Diagnosis of Polymyalgia Rheumatica*

1. Persistent pain (for at least 1 month) involving two of the following: neck, shoulders, and pelvic girdle
2. Morning stiffness for >1 hour
3. Rapid response to prednisone at ≤20 mg/day
4. Absence of other diseases capable of causing the musculoskeletal symptoms
5. Age older than 50 years
6. Erythrocyte sedimentation rate greater than 40 mm/hr

*The diagnosis of polymyalgia rheumatica is made if all of these criteria are satisfied.

From Healey LA: Long-term follow-up of polymyalgia rheumatica: Evidence for synovitis. Semin Arthritis Rheum 13:322, 1984.

glucocorticoid pulses of 1 gm/day of methylprednisolone (or equivalent glucocorticoid) for 3 days are frequently recommended, although it has not been clearly demonstrated that this dose regimen is more effective than the standard oral treatment.[78,79] Early treatment, within the first 12 to 24 hours, appears to be the major determinant of visual recovery, which can be expected in only 12% of cases.[78-80] Platelet inhibitors are recommended, but their efficacy is not proven.[80] Some patients may lose vision during the first weeks of glucocorticoid treatment, but much of this may be secondary to the already established damage, subsequent scarring with fibrosis, and vessel narrowing, though not necessarily due to ongoing active disease. Visual loss beyond this point or during relapses is rare.

The starting dose of prednisone (or equivalent) is maintained for 2 to 4 weeks, and the daily dose is then progressively tapered by approximately 5 mg per week. Although most patients do well with a daily maintenance dose of 7.5 to 10 mg, some patients may require higher doses. Tapering is guided mainly by clinical evaluation. ESR is a useful parameter in the follow-up of GCA, but therapeutical decisions must not rely solely on ESR values.[1,3] The usual initial dose for patients with isolated PMR is 10 to 20 mg/day of prednisone (or equivalent glucocorticoid). Guidelines for reduction are similar to those recommended for GCA.[1,3,46] Some patients with PMR who have mild symptoms may respond to NSAIDs.[54]

Total duration of therapy may vary, but most patients require 6 months to 2 years. Reductions below the maintenance doses must be made gradually in order to avoid relapses, which are common during the first 2 years after diagnosis. Approximately 25% of patients require low-dose glucocorticoid therapy for several years, some perhaps indefinitely.[81]

In the majority of patients, ESR quickly normalizes after initiation of glucocorticoid therapy; however, other inflammatory markers such as IL-6, C-reactive protein, haptoglobin, and vWFAg are persistently elevated in many patients in apparent clinical remission, possibly indicating a persistent, low-level inflammatory activity.[40,82] The long-term clinical consequences of this residual activity are unknown, and it is not clear whether persistent, low-level inflammatory activity should influence therapeutical decisions.

Complications of glucocorticoid therapy are quite common among patients with GCA and PMR, including osteoporosis, weight gain, mood and sleep disturbances, glucose intolerance, congestive heart failure, cataracts, glaucoma, hypertension, and other problems.[1,3,46,48,81] GCA strikes elderly patients, and this population is particularly susceptible to serious complications of glucocorticoid therapy. Physicians treating GCA should anticipate such complications, screen for them, and, when feasible, prescribe prophylactic treatments such as calcium, vitamin D, and possibly bisphosphonate therapy to prevent osteoporosis.

To help reduce the cumulative toxicity of glucocorticoid therapy, the usefulness of other immunosuppressive drugs as "steroid-sparing agents" has been considered. The most carefully investigated agent for this purpose has been methotrexate, the subject of three randomized, placebo-controlled, double-blind studies.[83-85] These studies yielded conflicting results and, although methotrexate may have some efficacy in sustaining remission, its glucocorticoid-sparing effect is not powerful enough to be recommended for widespread use. Both azathioprine and cyclosporine have been studied in small case series. Based on the current understanding of the pathophysiology of GCA, TNF-α blockade is a reasonable therapeutic approach to study and it has been reported to be effective in a small case series.[86-88] Large, multi-centered efficacy trials of anti-TNF-α agents are currently under way.

Important to note is that patients with both GCA and PMR require long-term follow-up care for many years, if not for life, following apparent disease remission. Disease relapse is common, and the long-term problems of large vessel disease are only now being fully appreciated. Finally, it is imperative that patients and their family members be repeatedly educated and reminded about the warning symptoms of GCA that necessitate urgent medical evaluation.

REFERENCES

1. Hunder G: Giant cell arteritis and polymyalgia rheumatica. Med Clin North Am 81:195, 1997.
2. Cid MC, Coll-Vinent B, Grau JM: Large vessel vasculitides. Curr Opin Rheumatol 10:18, 1998.
3. Salvarani C, Cantini F, Boiardi L, et al: Polymyalgia rheumatica and giant-cell arteritis. N Engl J Med 347:261, 2002.
4. Hunder GG: Epidemiology of giant-cell arteritis. Cleve Clin J Med 69(suppl 2):SII79, 2002.
5. Nordborg E, Nordborg C: Giant cell arteritis: Epidemiological clues to its pathogenesis and an update on its treatment. Rheumatology (Oxford) 42:413, 2003.
6. Baldursson O, Steinsson K, Bjornsson J, et al: Giant cell arteritis in Iceland: An epidemiologic and histopathologic analysis. Arthritis Rheum 37:1007, 1994.
7. Salvarani C, Gabriel SE, O'Fallon WM, et al: The incidence of giant cell arteritis in Olmsted County, Minnesota: Apparent fluctuations in a cyclic pattern. Ann Intern Med 123:192, 1995.
8. González-Gay MA, Alonso MD, Aguero JJ, et al: Temporal arteritis in a northwestern area of Spain: Study of 57 biopsy proven patients. J Rheumatol 19:277, 1992.
9. Sonnenblick M, Nesher G, Friedlander Y, et al: Giant cell arteritis in Jerusalem: A 12-year epidemiological study. Br J Rheumatol 33:938, 1994.
10. Lie J: Histopathologic specificity of systemic vasculitis. Rheum Dis Clin North Am 21:883, 1995.
11. Cid MC, Campo E, Ercilla G, et al: Immunohistochemical analysis of lymphoid and macrophage cell subsets and their immunologic activation markers in temporal arteritis. Influence of corticosteroid treatment. Arthritis Rheum 32:884, 1989.
12. Klein RG, Hunder GG, Stanson AW, et al: Large artery involvement in giant cell (temporal) arteritis. Ann Intern Med 83:806, 1975.
13. Esteban MJ, Font C, Hernández-Rodríguez J, et al: Small-vessel vasculitis surrounding a spared temporal artery: Clinical and pathological findings in a series of twenty-eight patients. Arthritis Rheum 44:1387, 2001.
14. Ostberg G: Temporal arteritis in a large necropsy series. Ann Rheum Dis 30:224, 1971.
15. Meliconi R, Pulsatelli L, Uguccioni M, et al: Leukocyte infiltration in synovial tissue from the shoulder of patients with polymyalgia rheumatica: Quantitative analysis and influence of corticosteroid treatment. Arthritis Rheum 39:1199, 1996.
16. Meliconi R, Pulsatelli L, Melchiorri C, et al: Synovial expression of cell adhesion molecules in polymyalgia rheumatica. Clin Exp Immunol 107:494, 1997.
17. Bignon JD, Barrier J, Soulillou JP, et al: HLA DR4 and giant cell arteritis. Tissue Antigens 24:60, 1984.

18. Cid MC, Font C, Oristrell J, et al: Association between strong inflammatory response and low risk of developing visual loss and other cranial ischemic complications in giant cell (temporal) arteritis. Arthritis Rheum 41:26, 1998.
19. Weyand CM, Hicok KC, Hunder GG, et al: The HLA-DRB1 locus as a genetic component in giant cell arteritis: Mapping of a disease-linked sequence motif to the antigen binding site of the HLA-DR molecule. J Clin Invest 90:2355, 1992.
20. Mattey DL, Hajeer AH, Dababneh A, et al: Association of giant cell arteritis and polymyalgia rheumatica with different tumor necrosis factor microsatellite polymorphisms. Arthritis Rheum 43:1749, 2000.
21. Boiardi L, Casali B, Nicoli D, et al: Vascular endothelial growth factor gene polymorphisms in giant cell arteritis. J Rheumatol 30:2160, 2003.
22. Salvarani C, Casali B, Nicoli D, et al: Endothelial nitric oxide synthase gene polymorphisms in giant cell arteritis. Arthritis Rheum 48:3219, 2003.
23. Salvarani CC, Boiardi B, Ranzi L, et al: Intercellular adhesion molecule 1 gene polymorphisms in polymyalgia rheumatica/giant cell arteritis: Association with disease risk and severity. J Rheumatol 27:1215, 2000.
24. Jacobsen S, Baslund B, Madsen HO, et al: Mannose-binding lectin variant alleles and HLA-DR4 alleles are associated with giant cell arteritis. J Rheumatol 29:2148, 2002.
25. Gabriel SE, Espy M, Erdman DD, et al: The role of parvovirus B19 in the pathogenesis of giant cell arteritis: A preliminary evaluation. Arthritis Rheum 42:1255, 1999.
26. Wagner AD, Gerard HC, Fresemann T, et al: Detection of Chlamydia pneumoniae in giant cell vasculitis and correlation with the topographic arrangement of tissue-infiltrating dendritic cells. Arthritis Rheum 43:1543, 2000.
27. Salvarani C, Farnetti E, Casali B, et al: Detection of parvovirus B19 DNA by polymerase chain reaction in giant cell arteritis: A case-control study. Arthritis Rheum 46:3099, 2002.
28. Regan MJ, Wood BJ, Hsieh YH, et al: Temporal arteritis and Chlamydia pneumoniae: Failure to detect the organism by polymerase chain reaction in ninety cases and ninety controls. Arthritis Rheum 46:1056, 2002.
29. Weck KE, Dal Canto AJ, Gould JD, et al: Murine gamma-herpesvirus 68 causes severe large-vessel arteritis in mice lacking interferon-gamma responsiveness: A new model for virus-induced vascular disease. Nat Med 3:1346, 1997.
30. Krupa WM, Dewan M, Jeon MS, et al: Trapping of misdirected dendritic cells in the granulomatous lesions of giant cell arteritis. Am J Pathol 161:1815, 2002.
31. Weyand CM, Schonberger J, Oppitz U, et al: Distinct vascular lesions in giant cell arteritis share identical T cell clonotypes. J Exp Med 179:951, 1994.
32. Weyand CM, Hicok KC, Hunder GG, et al: Tissue cytokine patterns in patients with polymyalgia rheumatica and giant cell arteritis. Ann Intern Med 121:484, 1994.
33. Weyand CM, Tetzlaff N, Bjornsson J, et al: Disease patterns and tissue cytokine profiles in giant cell arteritis. Arthritis Rheum 40:19, 1997.
34. Rittner HL, Kaiser M, Brack A, et al: Tissue-destructive macrophages in giant cell arteritis. Circ Res 84:1050, 1999.
35. Weyand CM, Goronzy JJ: Medium- and large-vessel vasculitis. N Engl J Med 349:160, 2003.
36. Borkowski A, Younge BR, Szweda L, et al: Reactive nitrogen intermediates in giant cell arteritis: Selective nitration of neocapillaries. Am J Pathol 161:115, 2002.
37. Weyand CM, Goronzy JJ: Arterial wall injury in giant cell arteritis. Arthritis Rheum 42:844, 1999.
38. Hernández-Rodríguez J, Segarra M, Vilardell C, et al: Elevated production of interleukin-6 is associated with a lower incidence of disease-related ischemic events in patients with giant-cell arteritis: Angiogenic activity of interleukin-6 as a potential protective mechanism. Circulation 107:2428, 2003.
39. Hernández-Rodríguez J, Segarra M, Vilardell C, et al: Tissue production of pro-inflammatory cytokines (IL-1beta, TNFalpha and IL-6) correlates with the intensity of the systemic inflammatory response and with corticosteroid requirements in giant-cell arteritis. Rheumatology (Oxford) 43:294, 2004.
40. Cid MC: New developments in the pathogenesis of systemic vasculitis. Curr Opin Rheumatol 8:1, 1996.
41. Cid MC, Cebrián M, Font C, et al: Cell adhesion molecules in the development of inflammatory infiltrates in giant cell arteritis: Inflammation-induced angiogenesis as the preferential site of leukocyte-endothelial cell interactions. Arthritis Rheum 43:184, 2000.
42. Cid MC, Hernández-Rodríguez J, Esteban MJ, et al: Tissue and serum angiogenic activity is associated with low prevalence of ischemic complications in patients with giant-cell arteritis. Circulation 106:1664, 2002.
43. Cid MC: Endothelial cell biology, perivascular inflammation, and vasculitis. Cleve Clin J Med 69(suppl 2):SII45, 2002.
44. Font C, Cid MC, Coll-Vinent B, et al: Clinical features in patients with permanent visual loss due to biopsy-proven giant cell arteritis. Br J Rheumatol 36:251, 1997.
45. Nuenninghoff DM, Hunder GG, Christianson TJ, et al: Incidence and predictors of large-artery complication (aortic aneurysm, aortic dissection, and/or large-artery stenosis) in patients with giant cell arteritis: A population-based study over 50 years. Arthritis Rheum 48:3522, 2003.
46. Salvarani C, Macchioni P, Boiardi L: Polymyalgia rheumatica. Lancet 350:43, 1997.
47. Cid MS, Hernández-Rodríquez J, Grau JM: Vascular manifestations in giant-cell arteritis. In Asherson RA, Cervera R (eds): Vascular Manifestations of Systemic Autoimmune Diseases. London, CRC Press, 2001.
48. Huston KA, Hunder GG, Lie JT, et al: Temporal arteritis: A 25-year epidemiologic, clinical, and pathologic study. Ann Intern Med 88:162, 1978.
49. Hayreh SS, Podhajsky PA, Zimmerman B: Occult giant cell arteritis: Ocular manifestations. Am J Ophthalmol 125:521, 1998.
50. Amor-Dorado JC, Llorca J, García-Porrúa C, et al: Audiovestibular manifestations in giant cell arteritis: A prospective study. Medicine (Baltimore) 82:13, 2003.
51. Ostberg G: Morphological changes in the large arteries in polymyalgia arteritica. Acta Med Scand Suppl 533:135, 1972.
52. Evans JM, O'Fallon WM, Hunder GG: Increased incidence of aortic aneurysm and dissection in giant cell (temporal) arteritis: A population-based study. Ann Intern Med 122:502, 1995.
53. Salvarani C, Cantini F, Boiardi L, et al: Polymyalgia rheumatica. Best Pract Res Clin Rheumatol 18:705, 2004.
54. Chuang TY, Hunder GG, Ilstrup DM, et al: Polymyalgia rheumatica: A 10-year epidemiologic and clinical study. Ann Intern Med 97:672, 1982.
55. Salvarani C, Cantini F, Macchioni P, et al: Distal musculoskeletal manifestations in polymyalgia rheumatica: A prospective followup study. Arthritis Rheum 41:1221, 1998.
56. Salvarani C, Hunder GG: Musculoskeletal manifestations in a population-based cohort of patients with giant cell arteritis. Arthritis Rheum 42:1259, 1999.
57. Cantini F, Niccoli L, Storri L, et al: Are polymyalgia rheumatica and giant cell arteritis the same disease? Semin Arthritis Rheum 33:294, 2004.
58. Hamrin B, Jonsson N, Hellsten S: "Polymyalgia arteritica:" Further clinical and histopathological studies with a report of six autopsy cases. Ann Rheum Dis 27:397, 1968.
59. Blockmans D, Stroobants S, Maes A, et al: Positron emission tomography in giant cell arteritis and polymyalgia rheumatica: Evidence for inflammation of the aortic arch. Am J Med 108:246, 2000.
60. Rojo-Leyva F, Ratliff NB, Cosgrove DM III, et al: Study of 52 patients with idiopathic aortitis from a cohort of 1,204 surgical cases. Arthritis Rheum 43:901, 2000.
61. Roche NE, Fulbright JW, Wagner AD, et al: Correlation of interleukin-6 production and disease activity in polymyalgia rheumatica and giant cell arteritis. Arthritis Rheum 36:1286, 1993.
62. Coll-Vinent B, Vilardell C, Font C, et al: Circulating soluble adhesion molecules in patients with giant cell arteritis: Correlation between soluble intercellular adhesion molecule-1 (sICAM-1) concentrations and disease activity. Ann Rheum Dis 58:189, 1999.
63. Vilaseca J, González A, Cid MC, et al: Clinical usefulness of temporal artery biopsy. Ann Rheum Dis 46:282, 1987.
64. GénéreauT, Lortholary O, Pottier MA, et al: Temporal artery biopsy: A diagnostic tool for systemic necrotizing vasculitis. French Vasculitis Study Group. Arthritis Rheum 42:2674, 1999.
65. Duran E, Merkel PA, Sweet S, et al: ANCA-associated small vessel vasculitis presenting with ischemic optic neuropathy. Neurology 62:152, 2004.

66. Hunder GG, Bloch DA, Michel BA, et al: The American College of Rheumatology 1990 criteria for the classification of giant cell arteritis. Arthritis Rheum 33:1122, 1990.
67. Kissin EY, Merkel PA: Diagnostic imaging in Takayasu arteritis. Curr Opin Rheumatol 16:31, 2004.
68. Schmidt WA, Kraft HE, Vorpahl K, et al: Color duplex ultrasonography in the diagnosis of temporal arteritis. N Engl J Med 337:1336, 1997.
69. Nesher G, Shemesh D, Mates M, et al: The predictive value of the halo sign in color Doppler ultrasonography of the temporal arteries for diagnosing giant cell arteritis. J Rheumatol 29:1224, 2002.
70. Salvarani C, Silingardi M, Ghirarduzzi A, et al: Is duplex ultrasonography useful for the diagnosis of giant-cell arteritis? Ann Intern Med 137:232, 2002.
71. Schmidt WA, Natusch A, Moller DE, et al: Involvement of peripheral arteries in giant cell arteritis: A color Doppler sonography study. Clin Exp Rheumatol 20:309, 2002.
72. Blockmans D: Utility of imaging studies in assessment of vascular inflammation. Cleve Clin J Med 69(suppl 2):SII95, 2002.
73. Tso E, Flamm SD, White RD, et al: Takayasu arteritis: Utility and limitations of magnetic resonance imaging in diagnosis and treatment. Arthritis Rheum 46:1634, 2002.
74. Yun M, Jang S, Cucchiara A, et al: 18F FDG uptake in the large arteries: A correlation study with the atherogenic risk factors. Semin Nucl Med 32:70, 2002.
75. Healey LA: Long-term follow-up of polymyalgia rheumatica: Evidence for synovitis. Semin Arthritis Rheum 13:322, 1984.
76. Cantini F, Salvarani C, Olivieri I, et al: Shoulder ultrasonography in the diagnosis of polymyalgia rheumatica: A case-control study. J Rheumatol 28:1049, 2001.
77. Achkar AA, Lie JT, Hunder GG, et al: How does previous corticosteroid treatment affect the biopsy findings in giant cell (temporal) arteritis? Ann Intern Med 120:987, 1994.
78. Hayreh SS, Zimmerman B, Kardon RH: Visual improvement with corticosteroid therapy in giant cell arteritis: Report of a large study and review of literature. Acta Ophthalmol Scand 80:355, 2002.
79. Foroozan R, Deramo VA, Buono LM, et al: Recovery of visual function in patients with biopsy-proven giant cell arteritis. Ophthalmology 110:539, 2003.
80. González-Gay MA, Blanco R, Rodríguez-Valverde V, et al: Permanent visual loss and cerebrovascular accidents in giant cell arteritis: Predictors and response to treatment. Arthritis Rheum 41:1497, 1998.
81. Proven A, Gabriel SE, Orces C, et al: Glucocorticoid therapy in giant cell arteritis: Duration and adverse outcomes. Arthritis Rheum 49:703, 2003.
82. Weyand CM, Fulbright JW, Hunder GG, et al: Treatment of giant cell arteritis: Interleukin-6 as a biologic marker of disease activity. Arthritis Rheum 43:1041, 2000.
83. Jover JH-G, Morado C; Vargas IC, et al: Combined treatment of giant-cell arteritis with methotrexate and prednisone: A randomized, double-blind, placebo-controlled trial. Ann Intern Med 134:106, 2001.
84. Spiera RF, Mitnick HJ, Kupersmith M, et al: A prospective, double-blind, randomized, placebo controlled trial of methotrexate in the treatment of giant cell arteritis (GCA). Clin Exp Rheumatol 19:495, 2001.
85. Hoffman G, Cid M, Hellmann D, et al: A multicenter placebo-controlled study of methotrexate (MTX) in giant cell artertitis (GCA) [abstract]. Arthritis Rheum 43, 2002.
86. Cantini F, Niccoli L, Salvarani C, et al: Treatment of longstanding active giant cell arteritis with infliximab: Report of four cases. Arthritis Rheum 44:2933, 2001.
87. Airo P, Antonioli CM, Vianelli M, et al: Anti-tumour necrosis factor treatment with infliximab in a case of giant cell arteritis resistant to steroid and immunosuppressive drugs. Rheumatology (Oxford) 41:347, 2002.
88. Tan AL, Holdsworth J, Pease C, et al: Successful treatment of resistant giant cell arteritis with etanercept. Ann Rheum Dis 62:373, 2003.

chapter 44

Thromboangiitis Obliterans (Buerger's Disease)

Jeffrey W. Olin

Thromboangiitis obliterans (TAO) is a nonatherosclerotic segmental inflammatory disease that most commonly affects the small- and medium-sized arteries and veins in both the upper and lower extremities. In the early reports, TAO was exclusively a disease confined to men, however; recently, more women have been diagnosed with Buerger's disease. There is a consistent relationship between tobacco use, usually heavy cigarette smoking, and the occurrence of thromboangiitis obliterans.

In 1879, von Winiwater described a 57-year-old man who complained of pain in his feet for 12 years. The histopathology demonstrated intimal proliferation, thrombosis, and fibrosis. von Winiwater suggested that the endarteritis and endophlebitis that were present in the amputated specimen were distinct from atherosclerosis.[1] This report was the first description of thromboangiitis obliterans, which later became known as Buerger's disease. Twenty-nine years later Leo Buerger stated in his landmark paper, "There is an interesting group of cases characterized by typical symptoms which the Germans have described under the name 'Spontangangran.'"[2] Buerger provided a detailed and accurate description of the pathology of the endarteritis and endophlebitis in 11 amputated limbs.[2] On the basis of his pathologic examination, Buerger called the disease "thromboangiitis obliterans." He made a point to differentiate the clinical and pathologic findings of TAO from atherosclerosis.[3]

Allen and Brown[4] studied 200 cases of TAO seen at the Mayo Clinic from 1922 to 1926. Most of their patients were Jewish males, and all patients smoked large amounts of tobacco. The clinical description of TAO provided by Allen and Brown was quite accurate: "The disease first manifests itself by excessive fatigue in the extremities followed shortly by the pain of claudication ... which is in turn followed by or associated with marked rubor when the extremities are dependent and excessive pallor when they are elevated. Trophic changes occur either in a minor form, such as excessive callosities in the weight bearing areas, or in the major form as gangrenous ulcers of the digits or gangrene involving the toes or the entire foot."[4] The pathologic description in this report was virtually identical to Buerger's original description. Allen and Brown suggested that thromboangiitis obliterans was a disease of infectious origin. This hypothesis has never been proved, and an infectious etiology is not believed to play a major role in the pathogenesis of this disease at the present time.

EPIDEMIOLOGY

Although Buerger's disease has a worldwide distribution, it is more prevalent in the Middle, Near, and Far Eastern regions than in North America and Western Europe.[5,6] The reported number of new patients with Buerger's disease in the United States and Europe has decreased mainly through the adoption of stricter diagnostic criteria. Before the late 1960s, overdiagnosis of Buerger's disease occurred even at Mount Sinai Hospital, where Buerger began his work on TAO: Of the 205 cases diagnosed as Buerger's disease at the hospital from 1933 through 1963, only 33 were later considered to be compatible with the correct diagnosis; the diagnosis was questionable in 28 cases and incorrect in 144 cases.[7]

At the Mayo Clinic, over a 40-year period the annuals patient registration has increased from 166,232 in 1947 to 221,000 in 1986, but the prevalence rate of patients with the diagnosis of Buerger's disease has steadily declined from 104 per 100,000 patient registrations in 1947 to 12.6 per 100,000 patient registrations in 1986.[6,8]

At the International Symposium on Buerger's disease in Bad Gastein, Austria, in 1986, Cachovan[9] reported the following prevalence rate in patients with peripheral arterial occlusive disease in Europe and other countries: 1% to 3% in Switzerland, 0.5% to 5% in West Germany, 1.2% to 5.6% in France, 4% in Belgium, 0.5% in Italy, 0.25% in the United Kingdom, 3.3% in Poland, 6.7% in East Germany, 11.5% in Czechoslovakia, 39% in Yugoslavia, 80% in Israel (Ashkenazim), 45% to 63% in India, and 16% to 66% in Korea and Japan. These rates were calculated from select series of patients treated at specialized institutions rather than from the general population as a whole.

In Asia a much higher proportion of patients with limb ischemia has been attributed to Buerger's disease than that in the United States and Europe. In 1961, McKusick and Harris[10] reported 28 cases of Buerger's disease reviewed at the Presbyterian Medical Center in Chonju, Korea: All patients were male smokers. Of the 28 patients, 23 were farmers or farm laborers, and all 23 were of the lowest socioeconomic status.

In 1973, Hill and colleagues[11] described an analysis of 106 patients with Buerger's disease in Java, Indonesia: All the patients were cigarette smokers, and only one was a woman. In general, the patients were from the lowest socioeconomic sector of the community, and there were no patients who could be judged middle class even by Indonesian standards.

In 1976, the Buerger's Disease Research Committee of the Ministry of Health and Welfare of Japan[12] analyzed 3034 patients (2930 men and 104 women) with the disease from all over Japan and estimated its prevalence to be about 5 per 100,000 population. In 1986, the Epidemiology of Intractable Disease Research Committee of the Ministry of Health and Welfare of Japan[13] estimated that there were 8858 patients with the disease who were treated at various medical institutions in Japan, where the prevalence was about 5 per 100,000 population, and there was no significantly greater prevalence among manual laborers. The number of new patients with Buerger's disease in Japan seems to be decreasing slightly, but the number of the patients under the care of a physician remains almost unchanged due to recurrences.[14]

Buerger's Disease in Women

Buerger's disease was uncommon in women; the reported incidence was 1% to 2% in most published series of cases before 1970. Several series showed a much higher prevalence of women with the disease, beginning with Lie's report,[8] in which 12 (11%) of 109 cases of the disease from 1981 to 1985 in Rochester, Minnesota, were female; 5 (19%) of 26 in 1987 in the Oregon study[15]; 12 (22.6%) of 53 patients in a Swiss study[16]; and 26 (23%) of 112 patients from 1970 to 1987 from the Cleveland study.[17] It is unclear whether the greater number of smokers among young women in recent years is solely responsible for the increased prevalence of Buerger's disease in women or whether the reported prevalence simply varied with the diagnostic criteria adopted. The prevalence of Buerger's disease in Japanese women remains relatively low compared with the increased number of female smokers.[14]

ETIOLOGY AND PATHOGENESIS

The etiology of Buerger's disease is unknown. Pathologically, TAO is a vasculitis.[18] Most vasculitides are immunologically mediated. TAO differs from most forms of vasculitis in that the usual immunologic markers (elevation of acute-phase reactants such as Westergren sedimentation rate and C reactive protein, the presence of circulating immune complexes, and the presence of commonly measured autoantibodies [anti-nuclear antibody, rheumatoid factor, complement levels, etc.]) are usually normal or negative.

Tobacco

An extremely strong association exists between heavy tobacco use and TAO.[17,19] It has been suggested that some patients may be abnormally sensitive or allergic to some component of tobacco and that this sensitivity in some way leads to small vessel occlusive disease.[20,21] The incidence of TAO is higher in countries where the consumption of tobacco is large. In India, many patients who develop TAO are in a low socioeconomic class and smoke bidi (homemade, unrefined tobacco); it has been suggested that this accounts for the higher incidence of TAO in the Indian population.[22,23] A recently published case control study from Bangladesh reported that 35% and 65% of TAO cases were cigarette and bidi smokers, whereas 69.9% and 30.1% of controls were cigarette and bidi smokers, respectively. Using logistic regression analysis, considering cigarette smoking approximately 10 cigarettes per day as a reference, bidi smoking more than 20 cigarettes per day (odds ratio [OR] = 34.76, 95% confidence interval [CI]: 6.11 to 197.67) and 11 to 20 per day (OR = 7.12, 95% CI: 2.35 to 21.63) had greater risk of TAO after adjusting confounding factors.[24]

Kjeldsen and Mozes[25] have demonstrated that patients with TAO had higher tobacco consumption and carboxyhemoglobin levels than patients with atherosclerosis or a control group of patients. There have been reports of TAO in cigar smokers, users of smokeless tobacco, and users of snuff.[26-28]

Whether or not cigarette smoking is causative or contributory to the development of TAO is unknown. What is clearly known is that tobacco use is a major factor in disease progression and continued symptoms associated with TAO.[29] Although passive smoking (secondary smoke) has not been shown to be associated with the onset of TAO, it may be an important factor in the continuation of symptoms in patients during the acute phase of Buerger's disease. Matsuhita, Shionoya, and Matsumoto studied urinary cotinine measurements in patients with Buerger's disease.[30] In their study, cotinine, a major metabolite of nicotine, was used as a marker to determine if patients were actively smoking, being passively exposed to smoke or not smoking at all. A close relationship was found between active smoking and an active course of Buerger's disease. The effect of passive smoking on the disease process was inconclusive in this study.

Lie described one case of pathologically proved Buerger's disease affecting the upper extremities of a 62-year-old man who had "allegedly" discontinued smoking 15 years earlier.[31] However, this report did not contain urinary nicotine measurements, cotinine measurements, or carboxyhemoglobin levels, and thus it is possible that this person was actively smoking.

In summary, most investigators believe that tobacco is an important etiologic factor in patients who develop TAO. As only a small number of smokers worldwide eventually develop TAO, other factors must be involved in the pathogenesis of the disease.

Genetics

Several studies suggest that there may be a genetic predisposition to developing TAO. Considerable differences have been found in the human lymphocyte antigen (HLA) among patients from varied populations. In the United Kingdom, there was a preponderance of HLA-A9 and HLA-B5 antigens, whereas other HLA haplotypes were increased in patients with TAO from Japan, Austria, and Israel.[19,32-34] No consistent pattern exists in HLA haplotypes among patients with Buerger's disease. This may be based on genetic differences in various populations, as well as methodologic differences in each of the studies cited.[35] In the United States, Mills and colleagues performed HLA testing in 11 patients with TAO and found no distinctive pattern identifiable.[15]

Hypercoagulable State

Older reports had failed to identify a specific hypercoagulable state in patients with Buerger's disease.[34] Chaudhury and colleagues[36] showed that the level of urokinase-plasminogen activator was twofold higher and free plasminogen activator inhibitor 1 was 40% lower in patients with TAO compared with healthy volunteers. After venous occlusion, tissue plasminogen activator antigen was increased in both patients with Buerger's disease and healthy volunteers but was much more pronounced in the control group. This suggests that there is some form of endothelial derangement characterized by increased urokinase-plasminogen activator release and decreased plasminogen activator inhibitor 1 release in patients with Buerger's disease. The same group of investigators also showed that there is an increased platelet response to serotonin in patients with Buerger's disease.[37] Carr and colleagues[38] demonstrated that platelet contractile force (PCF) was 82% higher than a normal control in one TAO patient and 340% higher than normal in the second patient. Although elevated PCF has been found in various conditions, such as coronary artery disease and diabetes mellitus, it is unclear whether this plays a role in the pathogenesis of these diseases or simply serves as a marker of enhanced platelet function or endothelial dysfunction, or both.

The Factor V Leiden mutation was demonstrated in 2 of 28 (7.1%) patients with TAO compared with 9 of 262 (3.4%) of controls ($P = .65$) and prothrombin gene mutation 20210A in 1 of 28 (3.6%) of patients with TAO compared with 25 of 262 (9.4%) of controls ($P = .48$).[39] In another case control study, however, the odds ratio for prothrombin 20210A allele compared with G allele was 7.98 (95% CIs 2.45 to 25.93).[40,41]

Two other factors may predispose to abnormal thrombosis in patients with TAO. Elevated plasma homocysteine has been reported in patients with TAO[42,43] and may be related to the high prevalence of heavy cigarette smoking or may in some way be tied into the disease itself. One small series showed that elevated homocysteine levels may be associated with a higher amputation rate compared with those with normal homocysteine levels.[43]

Several reports have shown increased anticardiolipin antibodies in patients with Buerger's disease.[44] A recent study involving patients with TAO ($n = 47$), premature atherosclerosis (pASO) ($n = 48$), and otherwise healthy individuals ($n = 48$) demonstrated that there is a higher prevalence of elevated anticardiolipin antibody titers in patients with TAO (36%) compared with either atherosclerotic (8%; $P = .01$) or healthy individuals (2%; $P < .001$).[45] Patients with TAO and elevated anticardiolipin antibodies had a higher rate of major amputation compared with those without the antibody (100% vs. 17%; $P = .003$). However, several methodologic problems coincided with this study and further research will be necessary to confirm this observation.[46] Another smaller study did not report an increased amputation rate in patients with elevated anticardiolipin antibodies.[43]

Immunology

Numerous studies have examined the immunologic mechanisms in patients with TAO. Adar and colleagues[47] studied 39 patients with Buerger's disease and measured the cell mediated sensitivity for types 1 and 3 collagen by an antigen-sensitive thymidine-incorporation assay. They noted an increased cellular sensitivity to types 1 and 3 collagen (normal constituents of human arteries) in patients with TAO compared with patients with arteriosclerosis obliterans or healthy male controls. In addition, 7 of 39 serum samples from patients with TAO demonstrated a low but significant level of anti-collagen antibody, whereas this antibody was not detected in the control group of patients. Other investigators have found circulating immune complexes in the peripheral arteries of patients with TAO.[48,49]

Additional data from three recent publications suggest that immunologic activation may at least in part be an important pathogenetic factor in TAO.[50-52] The arteries of 9 patients with Buerger's disease were analyzed histologically (33 specimens), including immunophenotyping of the infiltrating cells.[50] Cell infiltration was observed mainly in the thrombus and the intima, whereas the architecture of the vessel wall was well preserved regardless of the stage of disease. Among infiltrating cells, $CD3^+$ T cells greatly outnumbered $CD20^+$ B cells, and $CD68^+$ macrophages or S-100^+ dendritic cells were detected in the intima during acute and subacute stages. Immunoglobulins G, A, and M (IgG, IgA, IgM) and complement factors 3d and 4c were deposited along the internal elastic lamina. These data suggested that Buerger's disease is an endarteritis that is associated with T cell–mediated cellular immunity and by B cell–mediated humoral immunity with associated activation of macro-phages or dendritic cells in the intima.[50]

Immunohistochemical and TUNEL studies were performed in eight patients with TAO for phenotyping of the infiltrating cells with $CD4^+$ (helper T cell), $CD8^+$ (cytotoxic T cell), CD56 (natural killer cell), and CD68 (macrophage); for the identification of cell activation with VCAM-1 and i-NOS; for the presence of cell death with TUNEL analysis; and for inflammatory cytokine detection with RT-PCR.[51]

The T cells were demonstrated in the thrombus, intima, and adventitia. Two interesting observations were noted: (1) among infiltrating cells, CD4+ T cells greatly outnumbered CD8+ cells and (2) VCAM-1 and iNOS were expressed in endothelial cells around the intima in patent segments or vaso vasorum in occluded segments. These findings strongly suggest that T cell–mediated immune inflammation is a significant event in the development of TAO.[51]

Kurata and associates[52] studied the immunohistochemistry in 58 amputated lower extremities with TAO and 5 autopsy controls and showed that TAO has a unique immunophenotype. In patients with definite clinical evidence of TAO, there was a predictable, specific, and highly significant inflammatory response (linear arrangement of macrophages and B- and T-lymphocytes along vascular elastic fibers) to the internal elastic laminae of the affected vessels. This suggests that elastic fibers are an important immunogen in the course of the disease.[52]

Endothelial Dysfunction

Eichhorn and colleagues[53] failed to demonstrate an elevation in various autoantibodies (cANCA, pANCA, ANA, anti-Ro, anticardiolipin antibodies) in 28 patients with TAO. Seven patients with active disease had anti-endothelial cell antibody (AECA) titers of 1857 + 450 arbitrary units (AU) compared with 126 + 15 AU in 30 normal control subjects ($P < .001$) and 461 + 41 AU in 21 patients in clinical remission ($P < .01$). If these findings are confirmed in other studies, assays that measure anti-endothelial cell antibody titers may prove to be useful in following disease activity of patients with Buerger's disease.

It has also been demonstrated that there is impaired endothelium-dependent vasorelaxation in the peripheral vasculature of patients with Buerger's disease.[54] Forearm blood flow (FBF) was measured plethysmographically in the *nondiseased* limb after the infusion of acetylcholine (endothelium-*dependent* vasodilator), sodium nitroprusside (endothelium-*independent* vasodilator) and occlusion-induced reactive hyperemia. After administration of intra-arterial acetylcholine, forearm blood flow was lower in patients with TAO than in healthy controls (14.1 + 2.8 m/min per dl of tissue volume vs. 22.9 + 2.9 ml/min per dL) ($P < .01$). There was no significant difference in FBF response to sodium nitroprusside (13.1 + 4 ml/min per dl vs. 16.3 + 2.5 mL/min per dL) and no significant difference between the two groups after reactive hyperemia. These data indicate that endothelial-dependent vasodilation is impaired even in the nondiseased limb of patients with TAO.

In surgical biopsies obtained from femoral and iliac arteries of patients with TAO, the expressions of ICAM-1, VCAM-1 and E-selectin were increased on the endothelium and inflammatory cells in the thickened intima.[55] Ultrastructural immunohistochemistry revealed contacts between mononuclear blood cells and ICAM-1- and E-selectin-positive endothelial cells. These endothelial cells showed morphologic signs of activation. This study showed that endothelial cells are activated in TAO and that vascular lesions are associated with TNF-α secretion by tissue-infiltrating inflammatory cells, ICAM-1-, VCAM-1- and E-selectin expressions on endothelial cells, and leukocyte adhesion via their ligands. The preferential expression of inducible adhesion molecules in microvessels and mononuclear inflammatory cells suggests that angiogenesis contributes to the persistence of the inflammatory process in TAO.[55]

On the basis of the previous information, there is no single etiologic mechanism present in all patients with TAO. Tobacco seems to play a central role both in the initiation and continuation of the disease. Other contributing factors, such as genetic predisposition, immunologic mechanisms, abnormalities in coagulation, and endothelial dysfunction also play roles in the pathogenesis of the disease.

PATHOLOGY

Buerger's disease is fundamentally an inflammatory thrombosis that affects both arteries and veins, and the histopathology of the involved blood vessels varies according to the chronological age of the disease at which the tissue sample is obtained for examination. The histopathology is most likely to be diagnostic during the acute phase of the disease. It evolves to changes consistent with or suggestive of the disease in the appropriate clinical setting at the immediate stage or subacute phase, and it becomes virtually indeterminate at end-stage or chronic phase when all that remains is organized thrombus and fibrosis of the blood vessels.[2,5,16,56-58]

Dible[58] had acknowledged that the pathologic diagnosis of Buerger's disease was by no means always secure: "There is so much variation from case to case, depending upon the stage of the disease and the characteristic capriciousness of the lesions, that it is difficult to give a succinct account of the histology … " Nevertheless, Dible[58] believed that the histologic distinction between Buerger's disease and atherosclerosis was so clear-cut that a differentiation could be made with a high degree of accuracy by simply examining tissue sections containing digital arteries and veins, the small blood vessels that are not usually affected by arteriosclerosis. An excellent recent review confirms many of the concepts that Dibble described more than 40 years ago.[59]

Acute Phase Lesions

The early, or acute, phase lesion is characterized by acute inflammation involving all coats of the vessel wall, especially of the veins, in association with occlusive thrombosis. Around the periphery of the thrombus are frequently what appear to be collections of polymorphonuclear leukocytes with karyorrhexis, the so-called "microabscesses," in which one or more multinucleated giant cells may be present (Fig. 44-1). This histologic finding in thrombophlebitis is most characteristic of, but may not be specific for, Buerger's disease.[60] This striking inflammatory thrombotic lesion occurs with greater regularity in veins than in arteries and is infrequently seen when organization of the thrombus is well under way.

Whether the vascular lesions of Buerger's disease are primarily thrombotic or primarily inflammatory has never been satisfactorily settled. In either event, the intense inflammatory infiltration and cellular proliferation seen in the acute stage lesions is peculiar and distinctive, especially when the veins are involved. If, by chance, the acute and often tender nodular subcutaneous phlebitic lesion is biopsied at an early stage, one may indeed observe in different segments of the same affected vein several coexisting lesions. These are acute phlebitis without thrombosis, acute phlebitis with thrombosis, and acute phlebitis with thrombus containing microabscess and giant cells.

Intermediate Phase and End-Stage Lesions

The intermediate (or subacute) phase is signified by progressive organization of the occlusive thrombus in the arteries and veins, which is usually accompanied by a prominent inflammatory cell infiltrate within the thrombus and less so in the vessel wall (Fig. 44-2). The chronic phase or end-stage is characterized by complete

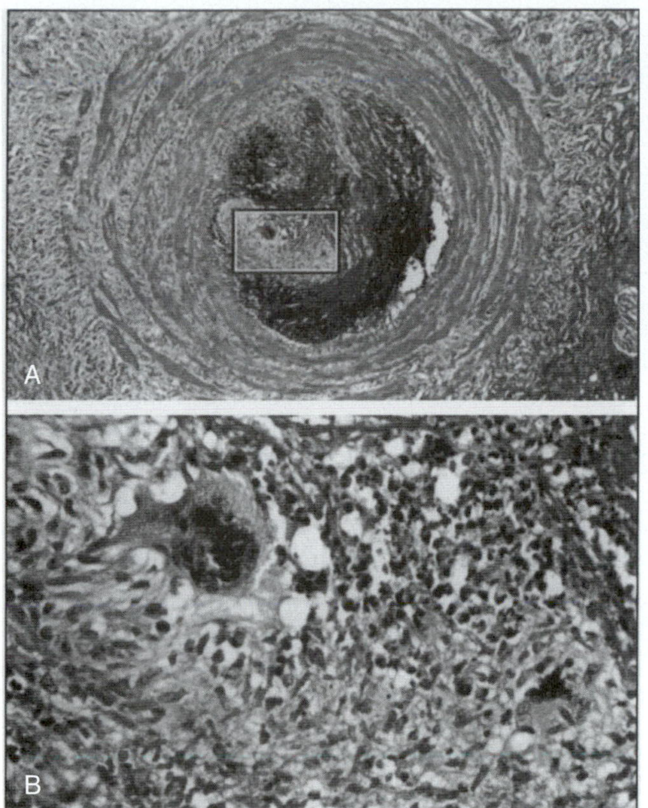

FIGURE 44-1. A, Typical acute histologic lesion of Buerger's disease in a vein with intense thromboangiitis. **B,** Close-up of a boxed area in **A,** showing micro-abscess in the thrombus and two multinucleated giant cells (H&E: **A,** ×64, **B,** ×400). (Reproduced with permission from Lie JT: Pathol Annu 23:257, 1988.)

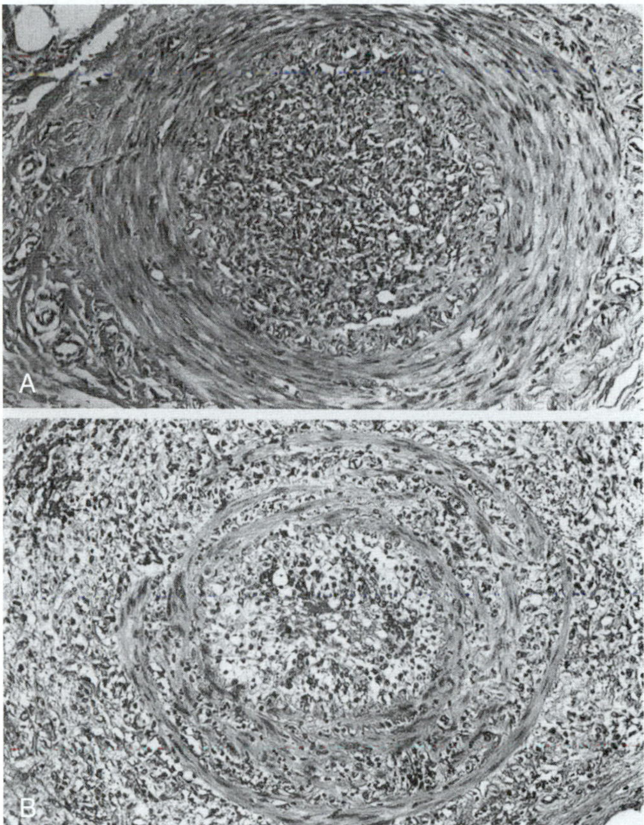

FIGURE 44-2. Digital artery **(A)** and vein **(B)** of the intermediate stage of Buerger's disease. There is a prominent inflammatory infiltrate with early organization of the thrombus (H&E: ×64). (Reproduced with permission from Lie JT: Pathol Annu 23:257, 1988.)

organization of the occlusive thrombus with extensive recanalization, prominent vascularization of the media, and adventitial and perivascular fibrosis (Fig. 44-3). In all three stages, the normal architecture of the vessel wall subjacent to the occlusive thrombus and including the internal elastic lamina remains essentially intact. These findings distinguish thromboangiitis obliterans from arteriosclerosis and from other systemic vasculitides in which there are usually more striking disruptions of the internal elastic lamina and the media, disproportional to those attributable to aging changes.

Buerger's disease is segmental in distribution; "skip" areas of normal vessels between diseased ones are common, and the intensity of the periadventitial reaction may be quite variable in different segments of the same vessel. Bland arterial and venous thrombosis with little or no cellular reaction often intermingle with inflammatory thrombosis in the vascular bed.

Additional Diagnostic Histopathologic Features

Histologic diagnosis of Buerger's disease is usually inconclusive or tentative at best when only the amputated specimens or occluded arteries and veins are examined. The intermediate- and chronic-stage lesions have far fewer characteristic features and are seldom diagnostic. The intermediate lesions coincide with the early phase of organization of the occlusive thrombi in arteries and veins of all sizes. This process is characteristic, if not unique, to Buerger's disease, because of the marked cellular proliferation and inflammatory infiltrate that are rarely seen in the organization of the ordinary, bland arterial and venous thrombi. Lymphohistiocytic cells and, to a much lesser extent, granulocytic leukocytes contribute to the inflammatory infiltrates. Eosinophils may be present, though seldom in excess numbers. The elastic laminae usually remain essentially intact. These changes are frequently observed in small digital blood vessels, which are not normally affected by arteriosclerosis or atherosclerosis.

The end-stage chronic lesions are understandably the least distinctive of the three morphologic stages of Buerger's disease. Occluded arteries and veins characterize the lesions with organized and recanalized thrombi accompanied by fibrosis and neovascularization (see Fig. 44-3). As such, they represent the end products of vascular injury and occlusive thrombosis. The degrees of perivascular fibrosis and lymphoid infiltration observed in the organized thrombi and vessel walls vary throughout the obliterated vascular segments. Focal residual inflammatory reaction of the organized thrombus may still be sufficiently characteristic to suggest Buerger's disease. Overall, these features are consistent with a disease process in which focal or segmental vasculitis, combined with thrombosis and endarteritic changes, affect a variable pattern

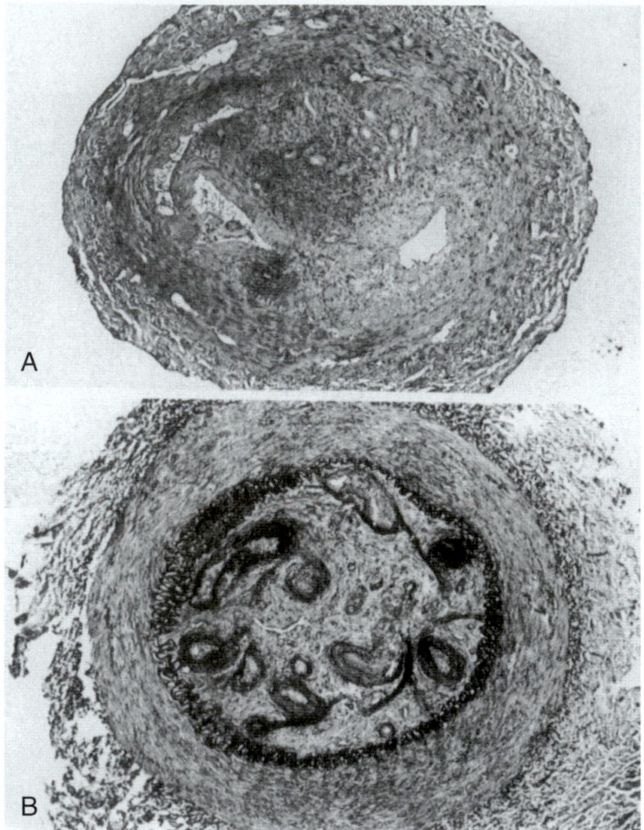

FIGURE 44-3. Chronic phase of Buerger's disease in the radial artery. There is extensive recanalization of the organized thrombus with prominent vascularization of the media. There is an intact internal elastic lamina. (H&E: **A,** ×64, **B,** Elastic Van Gieson stain ×64). (Reproduced with permission from Lie JT: Pathol Annu 23:257, 1988.)

of vascular obliteration that is quite distinct from arteriosclerosis with bland thrombosis. In some patients, especially those older than the age of 40, both Buerger's disease and arteriosclerosis may coexist and thus create further diagnostic uncertainty. Buerger's disease does not confer immunity to atherosclerosis.

Immunochemistry

To date, there have been very few published studies focusing on the cytoskeleton and immunochemistry of the cellular elements in Buerger's disease.[49,61] Soon after the thrombus has occluded the vessel lumen, spindle cells begin to appear in the periphery of the thrombus. They originate in the media and pass through fenestrations along the internal elastic lamella into the intima and from there into the thrombus. These cells express vimentin and α-1-actin (monoclonal marker for smooth muscle actin) and are derived from smooth muscle cells of the media. Capillaries also appear in the marginal zones of the thrombus. The endothelial cells express factor VIII-related antigen and Ulex europaeus agglutinin.

In later stages of thrombus organization, the spindle cells in the thrombus lose their positivity staining for α-1-actin along with their differentiation into fibroblasts. The demonstration of the internal elastic lamella by collagen type 4 markers (Dakopats C 4) confirms that the lamella is intact and that the smooth media muscle cells migrate inward through existing fenestrations to enter the intima. The newly formed capillaries within the thrombus are surrounded by a thin basement membrane mainly composed of type 4 collagen produced by the endothelial cells.

In summary, the process of thrombus organization in TAO is essentially identical to that in ordinary thrombosis but with an added inflammatory component. The invasion of organizing smooth muscle cells from the media of the blood vessel appears more intensified, resulting in a hypercellular thrombus with rapid organization. Prominent inflammatory cell infiltrate and thrombus organization are hallmarks of Buerger's disease. Initial preservation of the internal elastic lamina is another distinguishing feature from arteriosclerosis/atherosclerosis and necrotizing vasculitis.

Buerger's Disease of Blood Vessels in Unusual Locations

Buerger's disease, as already noted, is almost exclusively a disease of the blood vessels in the lower and upper limbs. There have been only occasional reports of involvement of large elastic arteries such as the aorta, the pulmonary arteries,[62] and iliac arteries.[63] Although Buerger[3] had noted that vascular obliteration could affect blood vessels other than those of the limbs, the involvement of the cerebral arteries,[64] coronary arteries,[65,66] renal arteries, mesenteric arteries,[67-73] and internal thoracic arteries[65,74] have been documented in an occasional patient, almost all as single case reports. The most spectacular case of Buerger's disease with combined peripheral and visceral involvement was that of an 18-year-old male cigarette smoker who, in a span of 15 years, underwent bilateral lumbar and dorsal sympathectomies, two bowel resections, and 13 amputations, including bilateral above-elbow and above-knee amputations, before he succumbed at age 33 to another episode of bowel infarction from recurrent Buerger's disease of the mesenteric arteries and veins.[75]

The histopathology of visceral TAO is identical to that observed in blood vessels of the limbs with involvement of both arteries and veins. Verging on being true pathologic curiosities are a unique case of Buerger's disease in a saphenous vein arterial graft[76] and the unusual examples of Buerger's disease in the temporal arteries of young smokers, in some preceded by peripheral ischemia ending in amputations.[77] Also not widely known is the occurrence of Buerger's disease in testicular and spermatic arteries and veins, as was originally described by Buerger.[3]

CLINICAL FEATURES

Classically, Buerger's disease presents in young, male, heavy smokers who often have the onset of symptoms before the age of 45 years. A recent report described a case of Buerger's disease in a 19-year-old female who had only been smoking for 3 years.[78] As noted previously, reports from the United States have suggested an increased incidence of TAO in women.[8,15,17] The predominant clinical presentation is that of ischemia, which begins distally and involves the small- and medium-sized arteries and veins.

Occasionally, large artery involvement has been reported in thromboangiitis obliterans, but this is unusual and rarely occurs in the absence of small vessel occlusive disease.[63] The distribution of arterial involvement in TAO was determined from a nationwide survey carried out in Japan in 1993.[79] There were 749 men and 76 women, with a mean age of 50.8 ± 0.4 years studied. There were 42 patients (5.1%) with upper extremity arterial involvement only, 616 (74.7%) with lower extremity involvement only, and 167 (20.2%) with both. This report was different from previously published reports in that the patients were older and only 25% of the patients had upper extremity involvement[79] compared with other studies showing a much higher prevalence of upper extremity involvement.[17,80]

Initially, patients present with ischemia or claudication of feet, legs, and occasionally the hands. Foot or arch claudication may be the presenting manifestation. Foot claudication is often mistaken for an orthopedic problem and there may be considerable delay before the correct diagnosis is made. Later in the course of the disease, patients may develop ischemic ulcerations in the distal portion of the toes or fingers, or both.

At the Cleveland Clinic Foundation, 112 patients with Buerger's disease were evaluated between 1970 and 1987.[17] The presenting clinical signs and symptoms are demonstrated in Table 44-1. Intermittent claudication occurred in 70 patients (63%). The initial location of claudication was the arch of the foot in many patients. As the disease progresses, claudication often moves proximally to cause typical calf claudication.

Seventy-six percent of patients had ischemic ulcerations at the time of presentation.[17] As stated earlier, however, if there was heightened awareness of the early manifestations of TAO (foot or arch claudication), many patients could be identified and treated before they ever developed ischemic ulcerations (Figs. 44-4 and 44-5).

TABLE 44-1 THROMBOANGIITIS OBLITERANS: DEMOGRAPHIC CHARACTERISTICS, PRESENTING SYMPTOMS AND SIGNS

Variable	Series from 1970-1987*
Patients (*n*)	112
Mean age (yr)	42
Men	86 (77%)
Women	26 (23%)
Intermittent claudication	70 (63%)
Rest pain	91 (81%)
Ischemic ulcers	85 (76%)
Upper extremity	24 (28%)
Lower extremity	39 (46%)
Both	22 (26%)
Thrombophlebitis	43 (38%)
Raynaud's phenomenon	49 (44%)
Sensory findings	77 (69%)
Abnormal Allen test	71 (63%)

*From Olin JW, Young JR, Graor RA, et al: The changing clinical spectrum of thromboangiitis obliterans (Buerger's disease). Circulation 82:IV-3, 1990.

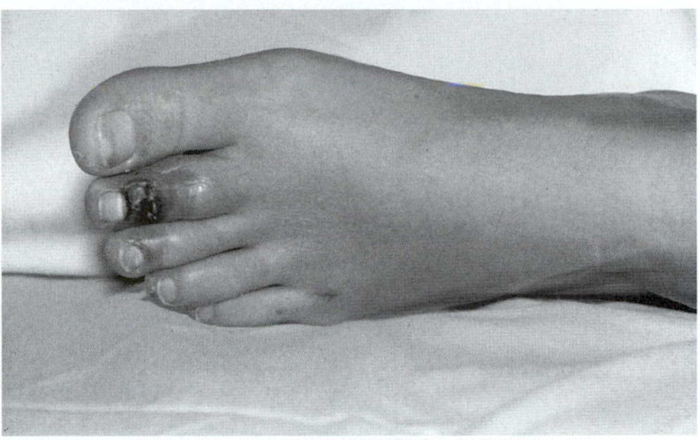

FIGURE 44-4. Ischemic ulcer on the second toe in a young woman with thromboangiitis obliterans.

Two or more limbs are almost always involved in Buerger's disease. Shionoya[81] noted that 2 limbs were affected in 16% of patients, 3 limbs in 41%, and all 4 limbs in 43% of patients.

In patients with lower extremity ulceration in whom Buerger's disease is a consideration, an Allen test should be performed to assess the circulation in the hands and fingers (Fig. 44-6).[82,83] An abnormal Allen test in a young smoker with lower extremity ulcerations is highly suggestive of TAO, because it demonstrates small vessel involvement in both the upper and lower extremities. In the Cleveland Clinic series, 63% of all patients demonstrated an abnormal Allen test. The distal nature of TAO and involvement of the lower and upper extremities help to differentiate TAO from atherosclerosis. Except in patients with end-stage renal disease and diabetes or postrenal transplant, atherosclerosis does not occur in the hand and rarely occurs distal to the subclavian artery.

Superficial thrombophlebitis occurs in approximately 40% of patients with TAO (Fig. 44-7).[17] The thrombophlebitis may be migratory and may parallel disease activity.[19]

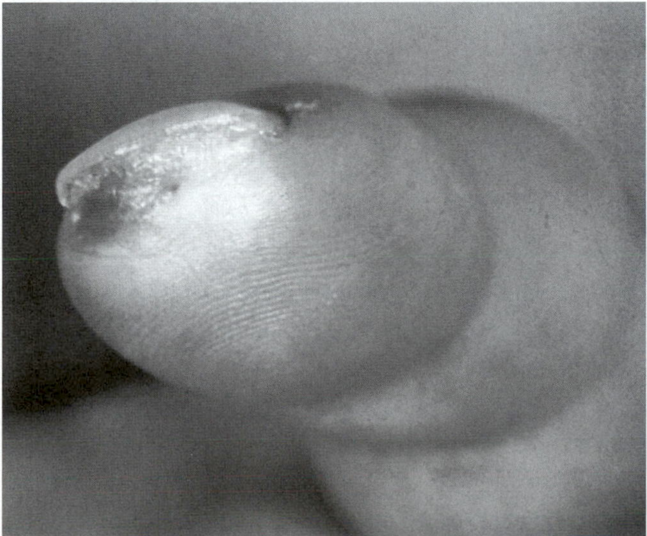

FIGURE 44-5. Ischemic ulcer of the index finger in a patient with Buerger's disease.

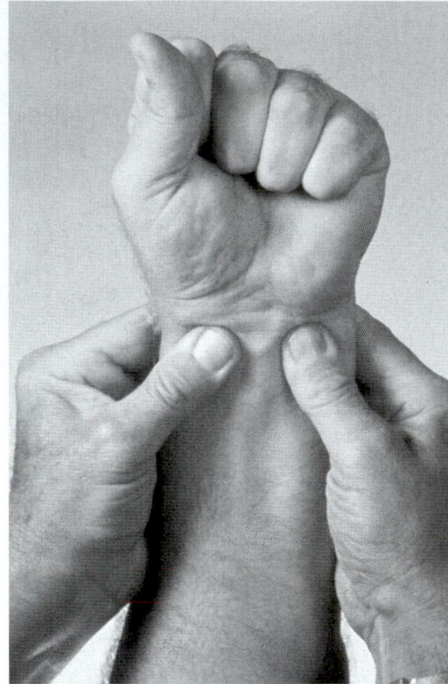

A

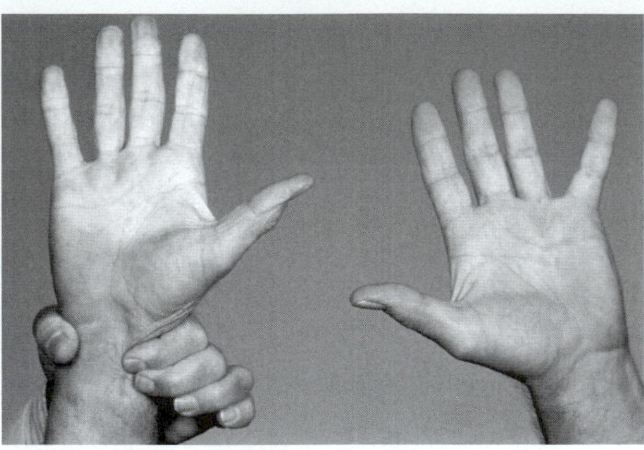

B

FIGURE 44-6. Allen test with occlusion of the radial and ulnar pulse by compression **(A)**. The pressure on the ulnar pulse is released, while the radial is still compressed **(B)**. The hand does not fill with blood, indicating occlusion of the ulnar artery (*right portion of the photograph*). (Reproduced with permission from Olin JW, Lie JT: Current Management of Hypertension and Vascular Disease. In Cooke JP, Frohlich ED (eds): Thromboangiitis Obliterans (Buerger's Disease). St Louis, Mosby-Yearbook, 1992 p 65.)

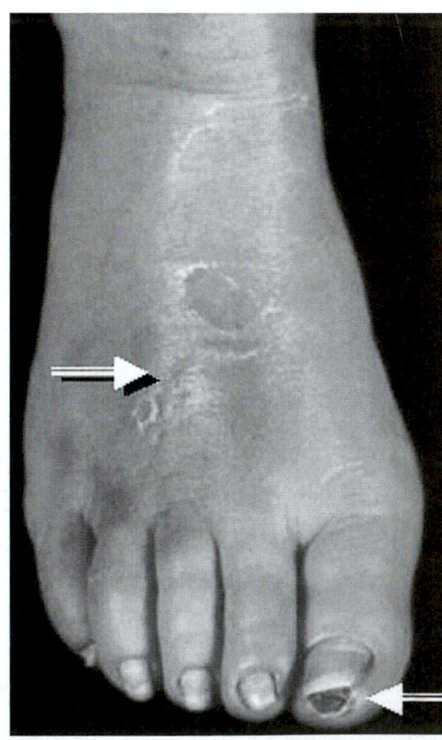

FIGURE 44-7. (See also Color Plate 44-7.) Ischemic ulcer (*arrow*) on the distal great toe in a young man with Buerger's disease. Note the area of superficial thrombophlebitis on the dorsum of the right foot (*arrow*). (Reproduced with permission from Olin JW, Lie JT: Current Management of Hypertension and Vascular Disease. In Cooke JP, Frohlich ED (eds): Thromboangiitis Obliterans (Buerger's Disease). St Louis, Mosby-Yearbook, 1992, p 65.)

Cold sensitivity is common and may be one of the earliest manifestations of TAO. This may be related to ischemia or to markedly increased muscle sympathetic nerve activity, as has been demonstrated in patients with TAO compared with a control group.[84] Typical Raynaud's phenomenon has been reported in approximately 40% of patients. The extremities may be abnormally red or cyanotic. Kimura and colleagues[85] termed this discoloration "Buerger's colour." Using nailfold capillaroscopy, these investigators demonstrated an increase in number and dilatation of capillary loops and correlated this with the cyanotic color change. They suggested that Buerger's color was due to an excessive congestion of venous blood in the subcapillary venous plexus. No other reports have demonstrated similar changes on capillaroscopy.

Sensory findings are common in TAO. They occurred in 69% of cases in the Cleveland Clinic series.[17] Much of these sensory abnormalities are due to ischemic neuropathy, which occurs late in the course of TAO. Some researchers have also suggested that the nerve fibers are encased with the inflammatory or fibrotic material that may occur in Buerger's disease, thus accounting for some of the sensory abnormalities.

Multiple criteria have been proposed for the diagnosis of TAO.[19,26] Shionoya[81] defined a set of criteria that included onset of symptoms before the age of 50, a history of smoking, infrapopliteal arterial occlusions, upper limb involvement or phlebitis migrans, and the absence of atherosclerotic risk factors other than smoking. In addition, an increasing number of individuals fulfill all of the criteria for TAO but have the exclusionary criteria of hypertension or hyperlipidemia. Some of these individuals go on to develop typical atherosclerosis 15 or 20 years after the original diagnosis of TAO. Therefore, if patients meet the criteria of distal extremity involvement,

BOX 44-1 Criteria for the Diagnosis of Thromboangiitis Obliterans[17,29]

Onset before age 45
Current (or recent past) tobacco use
Distal extremity ischemia (infrapopliteal or infrabrachial, or both) such as claudication, rest pain, ischemic ulcers, and gangrene documented with noninvasive testing
Laboratory tests to exclude autoimmune or connective tissue diseases and diabetes mellitus
Exclude a proximal source of emboli with echocardiography and arteriography
Demonstrate consistent arteriographic findings in the involved and clinically noninvolved limbs
A biopsy is rarely necessary to make the diagnosis unless the patient presents with unusual characteristics such as large artery involvement or age older than 45

From Olin JW: Current treatment of thromboangiitis obliterans (Buerger's disease). In Harrison's Online, McGraw-Hill, 2001.

tobacco use, exclusion of a proximal source of emboli or atherosclerosis, in the absence of a definable hypercoagulable state, then hyperlipidemia or hypertension, or both, should not be exclusionary for the diagnosis of TAO (Box 44-1).[17,29]

Laboratory and Arteriographic Findings

No specific laboratory tests aid in the diagnosis of TAO. A complete serologic profile to exclude other diseases that may mimic TAO should be obtained. These include the following: CBC with differential, liver function, renal function, fasting blood sugar, urinalysis, acute-phase reactants (Westergren sedimentation rate and C-reactive protein), anti-nuclear antibody, rheumatoid factor, complement measurements, serologic markers for CREST (calcinosis, Raynaud's phenomenon, esophageal dysmotility, sclerodactyly, telangiectasias) syndrome and scleroderma (anti-centromere antibody and SCL70), and a complete hypercoagulability screen to include antiphospholipid antibodies.

In order to exclude a proximal source of emboli, the patient may need to undergo echocardiography and arteriography. McKusick and colleagues[83,86,87] have described in great detail the arteriographic features present in patients with TAO. Other investigators further defined the arteriographic findings that may occur in patients with TAO.[88] Although the arteriogram may be suggestive of TAO, there are no pathognomonic angiographic findings in TAO. Most patients in these series had clinical or arteriographic evidence of involvement of more than one limb.

Examples of typical arteriographic findings are demonstrated in Figures 44-8 and 44-9. Proximal arteries should be normal, demonstrating no evidence of atherosclerosis, aneurysm, or other source of proximal emboli. Although the disease has been rarely reported in the proximal arteries,[63] in most cases the proximal arteries should be normal. In order to diagnose Buerger's disease with proximal artery involvement, a pathologic specimen

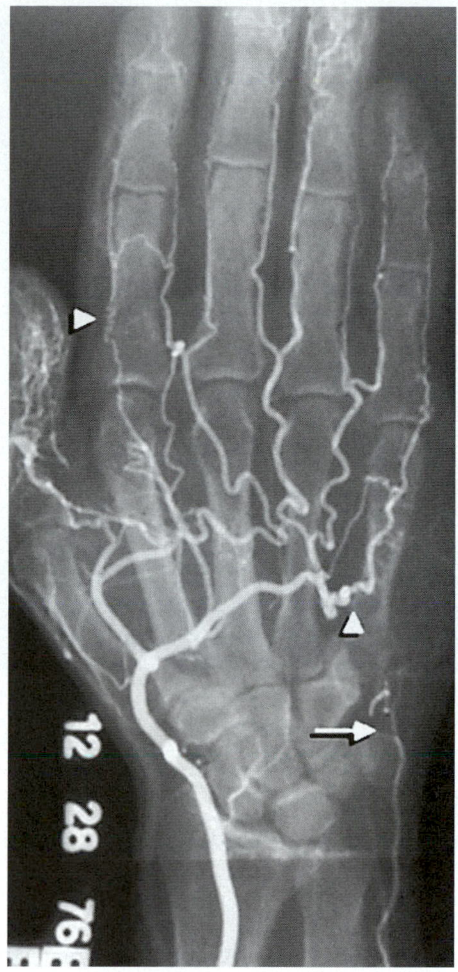

FIGURE 44-8. Arteriogram of the hand demonstrating an extremely small ulnar artery, which eventually occludes distal to the wrist (*arrow*). Note multiple digital artery occlusions and several areas of corkscrew collaterals (*arrow heads*).

is necessary. The disease is confined most often to the distal circulation and is almost always infrapopliteal in the lower extremities and distal to the brachial artery in the upper extremities. There is small- and medium-sized vessel involvement such as the digital arteries in the fingers and toes; the palmar and plantar arteries in the hand and foot; as well as the tibial, peroneal, radial, and ulnar arteries.[86,87] Isolated disease below the popliteal artery virtually never occurs in atherosclerosis. Even the patient with diabetes mellitus often has multisegment disease with some evidence of proximal artery involvement. However, because diabetes is exclusionary for the diagnosis of TAO (in the absence of a pathologic specimen), there should be no confusion between these two diseases.

Arteriographically, TAO is a segmental disorder, demonstrating areas of diseased vessels interspersed with normal blood vessel segments. Evidence of multiple vascular occlusions with collateralization around the obstructions (corkscrew collaterals) is common (see Fig. 44-8). Corkscrew collaterals are not pathognomonic of Buerger's disease, as they may be seen in any small vessel occlusive disease. The arteriographic appearance of Buerger's disease may be identical to that seen in patients with scleroderma

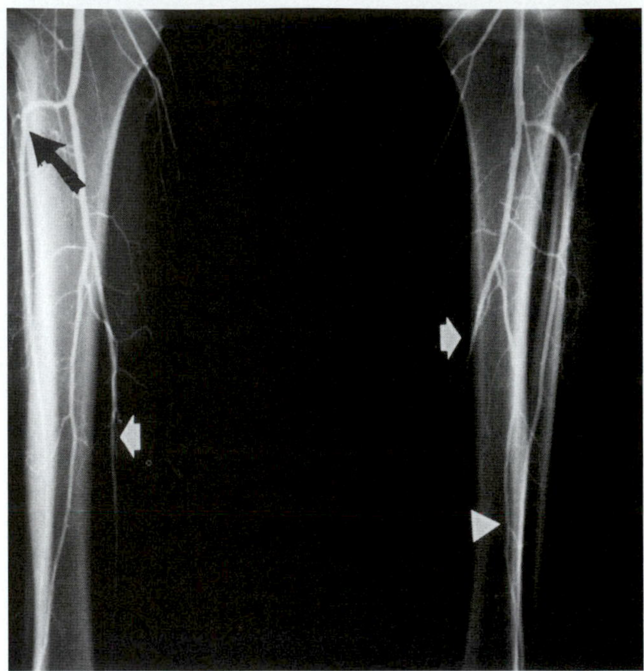

FIGURE 44-9. Severe infrapopliteal disease in a patient with thromboangiitis obliterans. In the right leg the anterior tibial artery (*black arrow*) occludes just distal to its origin. The posterior tibial artery becomes diminutive and then occludes in the midcalf to distal calf (*white arrow*). In the left leg the anterior tibial is patent but the posterior tibial (*white arrow*) is occluded several centimeters from its origin. The peroneal artery (*arrowhead*) becomes diminutive in the midcalf.

or the CREST syndrome. However, the other clinical and serologic manifestations of scleroderma and CREST should help to differentiate these diseases from TAO. Irregularity or calcification of the blood vessel wall should be exclusionary for the diagnosis of Buerger's disease.[19] Figure 44-10 lists the sequential steps in the diagnosis and treatment of TAO.

Differential Diagnosis

The diagnosis of TAO should not be difficult if diseases that mimic TAO are excluded. The most important diseases to exclude are atherosclerosis, emboli and autoimmune diseases such as scleroderma or CREST syndrome. Under most circumstances, with the use of echocardiography and arteriography, atherosclerosis and emboli can be excluded with a high degree of clinical certainty.

The diagnosis in patients who have scleroderma or the CREST syndrome is usually obvious from a clinical examination of the skin, a history of other systemic features that occur in these diseases, and the presence of serological markers such as SCL-70 or anticentromere antibodies. Nailfold capillaroscopy is usually quite distinctive in patients with CREST or scleroderma.

Clinical evidence for features of systemic lupus erythematosus, rheumatoid arthritis, and other types of vasculitides should be sought. Serologic markers often help to eliminate the presence of these conditions. Patients with the antiphospholipid antibody syndrome may present with evidence of both arterial and venous thrombotic events. These patients usually have positive circulating "lupus type" anticoagulants or the presence of high titer anticardiolipin antibodies, or both. Cases of typical Buerger's disease with the presence of elevated anticardiolipin antibodies have been encountered.[43,45,46] A pathologic specimen would clearly differentiate these two entities, as antiphospholipid antibody syndrome is in reality a vasculopathy (the presence of thrombus with no inflammatory components) as opposed to the typical pathological findings in Buerger's disease.

Whereas patients with TAO present with distal extremity ischemia, patients with Takayasu's arteritis or giant cell arteritis present with proximal vascular involvement. The arteriographic features of Takayasu's disease or giant cell arteritis are quite distinctive. Many patients with Takayasu's arteritis have elevations in the acute phase reactants (erythrocyte sedimentation rate and C-reactive protein), but this finding is not invariable and may not correlate with disease activity.[89]

In the presence of lower extremity involvement, the possibility of popliteal artery entrapment syndrome or cystic adventitial disease should be considered, both of which should be readily apparent on arteriography. An aneurysm of the popliteal artery should be easily diagnosed by physical examination.

A careful history should be taken for the possibility of ergotamine abuse, as this may cause severe ischemia in multiple limbs. This, as well as TAO, may cause both lower and upper extremity ischemia. Even if the patient denies a history of migraine headaches or previous ergotamine use, ergotamine blood levels should be obtained to exclude this condition. If there is isolated involvement of the upper extremity, occupational hazards such as vibratory tool use and hypothenar hammer syndrome should be considered.

Cocaine and cannabis ingestion can mimic TAO.[90-93] Marder and Mellinghoff[92] published a detailed case report of heavy cocaine use masquerading as Buerger's disease. The arteriographic findings including the presence of corkscrew collaterals are virtually identical to Buerger's disease. In addition to the other serologic tests recommended previously, blood tests for cocaine, amphetamine, and cannabis may be indicated in the evaluation of some patients. Disdier and colleagues[93] reported on 10 male patients with a mean age of 23.7 years who developed distal ischemia of lower or upper limbs, leading to necrosis in the toes or fingers, or both, and sometimes to distal limb gangrene. Two of the patients also presented with venous thrombosis, and three patients were suffering from Raynaud's phenomenon. Arteriographic evaluation in all cases revealed distal abnormalities in the arteries of feet, legs, forearms, and hands resembling those of Buerger's disease. All patients were moderate tobacco smokers and regular cannabis users. Despite treatment, five amputations were necessary in four patients. It has been shown that δ-8- and δ-9-tetrahydrocanabinols may induce peripheral vasoconstrictor activity. Cannabis arteritis resembles Buerger's disease or may, in fact, be a precipitating factor in addition to tobacco. Therefore, all patients should be questioned about cannabis use. A complete toxicology screen is recommended in patients who present with a clinical picture of TAO, especially if they deny tobacco use.

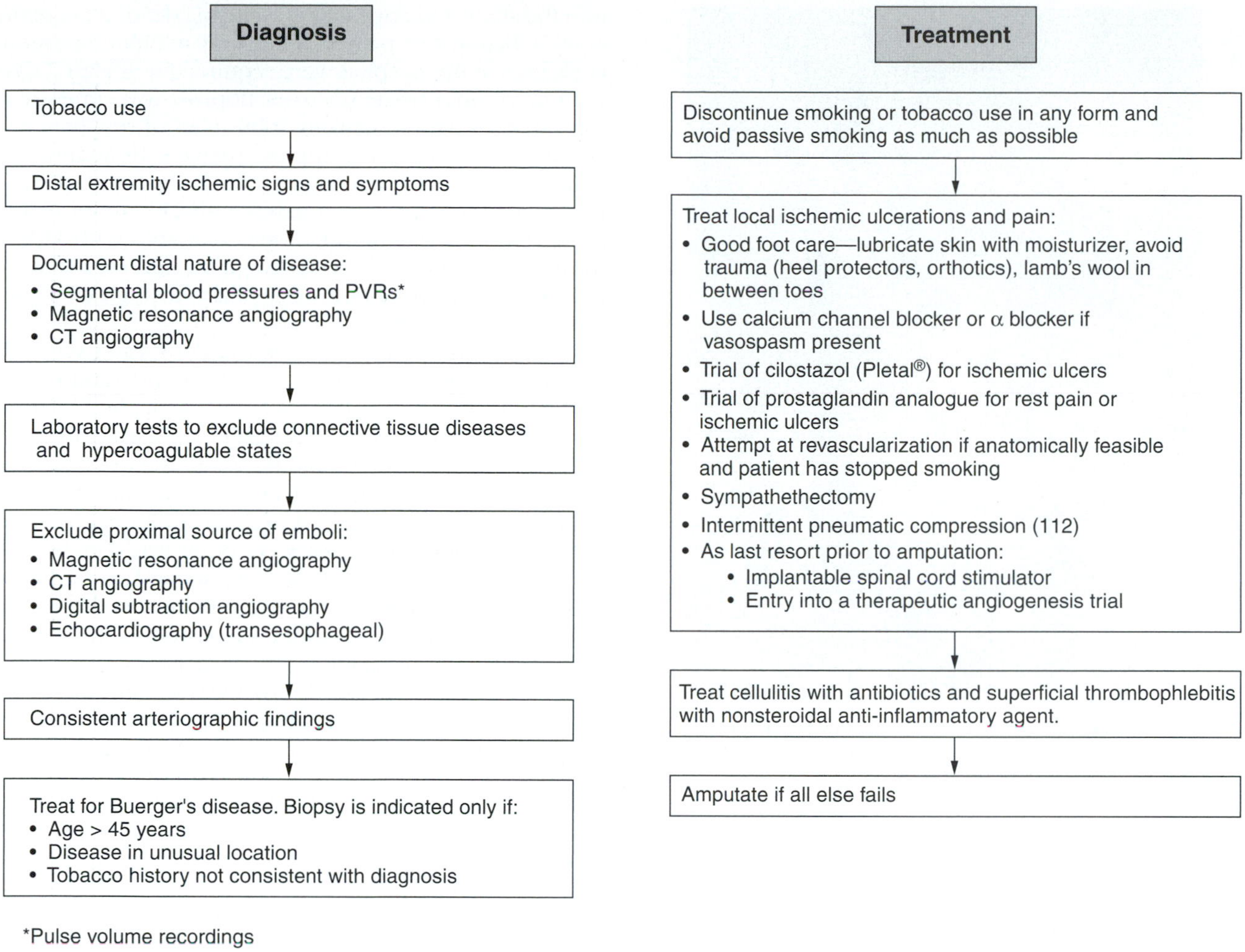

Diagnosis

Tobacco use

↓

Distal extremity ischemic signs and symptoms

↓

Document distal nature of disease:
- Segmental blood pressures and PVRs*
- Magnetic resonance angiography
- CT angiography

↓

Laboratory tests to exclude connective tissue diseases and hypercoagulable states

↓

Exclude proximal source of emboli:
- Magnetic resonance angiography
- CT angiography
- Digital subtraction angiography
- Echocardiography (transesophageal)

↓

Consistent arteriographic findings

↓

Treat for Buerger's disease. Biopsy is indicated only if:
- Age > 45 years
- Disease in unusual location
- Tobacco history not consistent with diagnosis

*Pulse volume recordings

Treatment

Discontinue smoking or tobacco use in any form and avoid passive smoking as much as possible

↓

Treat local ischemic ulcerations and pain:
- Good foot care—lubricate skin with moisturizer, avoid trauma (heel protectors, orthotics), lamb's wool in between toes
- Use calcium channel blocker or α blocker if vasospasm present
- Trial of cilostazol (Pletal®) for ischemic ulcers
- Trial of prostaglandin analogue for rest pain or ischemic ulcers
- Attempt at revascularization if anatomically feasible and patient has stopped smoking
- Sympathethectomy
- Intermittent pneumatic compression (112)
- As last resort prior to amputation:
  - Implantable spinal cord stimulator
  - Entry into a therapeutic angiogenesis trial

↓

Treat cellulitis with antibiotics and superficial thrombophlebitis with nonsteroidal anti-inflammatory agent.

↓

Amputate if all else fails

FIGURE 44-10. Diagnosis and treatment of thromboangiitis obliterans.

THERAPY

Various therapies available for the treatment of TAO are shown in Figure 44-10. The cornerstone of therapy is the complete discontinuation of cigarette smoking or the use of tobacco in any form. It has been demonstrated in many case reports and series that complete abstinence from tobacco is really the only way to halt the progression of Buerger's disease and to avoid future amputations.[17,94,95] Even one or two cigarettes a day are enough to keep the disease active. In patients with documented TAO, smokeless tobacco (chewing tobacco or snuff) has also been reported to cause Buerger's disease and to keep it active once it has already occurred.[27,28] Of 152 patients with Buerger's disease treated at the Cleveland Clinic from 1970 to 1996, long-term follow-up was obtained in 120 patients.[17,43] Fifty-two patients (43%) discontinued cigarette smoking. If gangrene was not present at the time the patient discontinued smoking, amputation did not occur. Forty-nine patients (94%) avoided amputation in the ex-smoking group. In the 68 patients who continued smoking, 29 patients (43%) required one or more amputations.[17,43]

It has often been stated that patients with TAO have a more difficult time stopping smoking than a control group of patients (Figs. 44-11 and 44-12). In reality, patients with Buerger's disease may stop smoking *more frequently* than patients who have atherosclerosis. Olin and associates[17] reported that 42% of the patients with TAO were able to discontinue smoking long term. In the series by Ohta and colleagues,[96] 47 (42.7%) of 110 patients

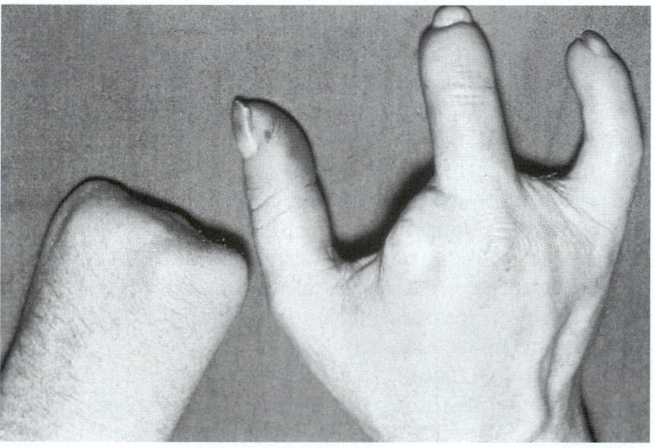

FIGURE 44-11. The result of multiple amputations in a patient with thromboangiitis obliterans who was unable to stop smoking.

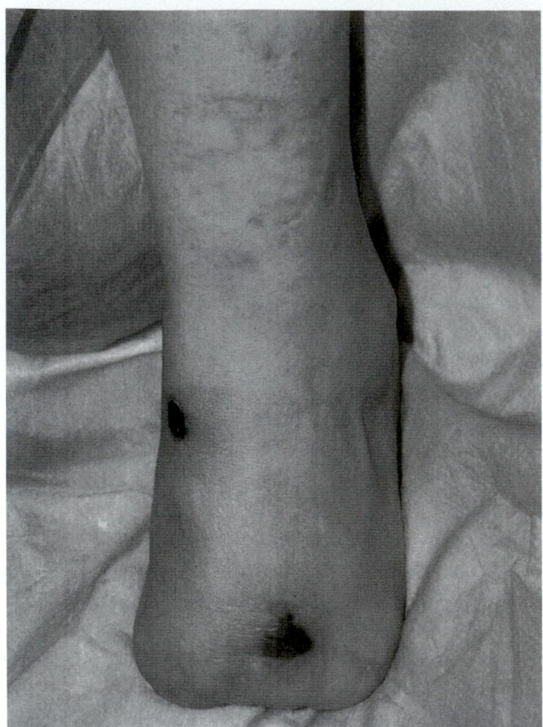

FIGURE 44-12. (See also Color Plate 44-12.) This patient underwent a transmetatarsal amputation in the past. He continued to smoke and has developed several areas of ischemic ulceration on the foot.

underwent either minor or major amputation after onset of disease. Of the patients who stopped smoking, no major limb amputations occurred. Of the 69 patients who continued to smoke, 13 (18.8%) underwent amputation. There was a correlation between continued smoking and limb amputation (P = .007). Matsushita and colleagues[30] used co-nicotine levels to determine whether or not a patient had discontinued cigarette smoking and demonstrated that approximately 50% of their patients had, in fact, stopped. These data illustrate the importance of education and counseling on the part of the physician in trying to get the patients to discontinue tobacco use.

Some investigators have recommended using anecdotes or photographs of patients who had prior amputations or using group meetings with other patients with TAO as a means to get the patient to stop smoking.[28] Education is probably the most important aspect. The patient can be reassured that if he or she is able to discontinue tobacco use, the disease will remit and amputations will not occur as long as critical limb ischemia (gangrene and tissue loss) have not already occurred. If significant arterial segments are occluded, however, the patient may continue to have intermittent claudication or Raynaud's phenomenon, or both.

It is unclear whether involuntary smoking (secondary smoke) can cause TAO. Patients with active TAO should avoid as much involuntary smoking as possible until the disease becomes quiescent.

Other than discontinuation of cigarette smoking, all other forms of therapy are palliative. Fiessinger and Schafer[97] conducted a prospective, randomized, double-blind trial comparing a 6-hour daily infusion of Iloprost (a prostaglandin analog) with aspirin. All patients entered into the study had critical limb ischemia defined as continuous ischemic rest pain in a limb for which continuous analgesics in the hospital were required for at least 7 days with or without tissue necrosis. Iloprost was superior to aspirin at 28 days in causing total relief of rest pain and complete healing of all trophic changes. In addition, at 6 months, 88% of the patients receiving Iloprost responded favorably to therapy as compared with 21% of the aspirin group. Only 6% had amputations compared with 18% in the aspirin group. It has been shown that an oral extended release preparation of Iloprost is pharmacologically equivalent to the IV form.[98]

On the basis of these findings, the European TAO Study Group recently completed a double-blind randomized trial comparing *oral* Iloprost with placebo.[99] Three-hundred and nineteen patients from six European countries were randomized to oral Iloprost (100 or 200 μg) or placebo twice a day for 8 weeks. All patients had rest pain or trophic lesions. There was an additional 6-month follow-up period. The primary endpoint was total healing of the most important lesion. The secondary endpoint was total relief of rest pain without the need for analgesics. The combined endpoint consisted of the patient being alive without major amputation, no lesions, no rest pain, and no analgesic use. Iloprost was significantly more effective than placebo for relief of rest pain without the need for analgesics and for a combined endpoint at 6 months of follow-up, but there was no significant effect on total healing of lesions.[99] It appears that the IV form of Iloprost is more effective than the oral form in ulcer healing.[100] Iloprost may be a useful modality in helping patients with critical limb ischemia get through the early time period when they first discontinue cigarette smoking.

There is no substitute for good general vascular care in the treatment of patients with severe ischemia. A reverse Trendelenburg (vascular) position should be used in patients who have severe ischemic rest pain. Adequate narcotics should be made available during the time period of severe ischemia. Standard anticoagulation has never been demonstrated to be effective in TAO. However, if other options are not available, some clinicians will use anticoagulants in an attempt to buy time and improve collateral flow in a severely ischemic limb. Good foot and hand care should be undertaken. If significant vasospasm is present, calcium channel blocking agents such as nifedipine, nicardipine, or amlodipine should be used.[83] Pentoxifylline has not been formally or adequately studied in patients with TAO. Because this drug increases the RBC membrane flexibility and allows red blood cells to fit through a smaller vascular space, it is not unreasonable to try pentoxifylline in the severely ischemic patient when there are no other good options available. There have been several reports of patients with ischemic ulcerations successfully treated with cilostazol when no other revascularization strategies were possible.[101,102]

Therapeutic angiogenesis has been used to treat the ischemic manifestations of TAO. Seven limbs in six patients (three men, three women; mean age, 33 years; range, 33 to 51 years) who satisfied the criteria for TAO and had signs or symptoms of critical limb ischemia were treated twice, 4 weeks apart, with 2 or 4 mg of vascular endothelial growth factor (phVEGF165), administered by direct IM injection in the ischemic limb.[103] Ulcers that had not healed for more than 1 month before therapy healed completely in three of five limbs after the IM phVEGF165 gene therapy. Nocturnal rest pain was relieved in the remaining two patients, although both continued to have claudication. Evidence of improved perfusion showed on MRI in seven of the seven limbs, and newly visible collateral vessels showed with serial contrast angiography in seven of the seven limbs. The ankle brachial index increased by more than 0.1 in three patients. Transient ankle or calf edema occurred in three of seven limbs. Two patients with advanced distal forefoot gangrene ultimately required below-knee amputation despite the evidence of improved perfusion. This preliminary report suggests that therapeutic angiogenesis with phVEGF165 gene transfer, if instituted before the development of gangrene, may provide an effective therapy for patients with advanced Buerger's disease that is unresponsive to standard medical or surgical treatment methods.[103] A case of upper limb salvage following autologous bone marrow to stimulate blood vessel growth through therapeutic angiogenesis has been reported.[104]

The role of sympathectomy in preventing amputations or in treating pain is unclear. An absence of increased sympathetic nerve activity has been observed in some TAO patients, thus providing further indirect evidence of a local vascular abnormality in TAO.[105,106] In the Cleveland Clinic series, 23 patients underwent sympathectomy and there was no difference in the amputation rate between those undergoing sympathectomy and those not.[17] Occasionally, sympathectomy may help the healing of superficial ischemic ulcerations. Two recent reports have demonstrated that lumbar sympathectomy can be safely and effectively carried out laparoscopically in the lower[107] and upper extremities.[108]

The literature contains a few anecdotal reports on the use of implantable spinal cord stimulators in patients with Buerger's disease. One patient treated with this modality resulted in complete healing of all upper extremity ulcerations.[109] Other reports have demonstrated similar success.[110,111] It may be worthwhile to consider a spinal cord stimulator to help decrease pain and avoid amputation in patients in whom surgical revascularization is not an option and when other forms of therapy are not effective.

In patients without good revascularization options, intermittent compression pump therapy for 6 hours a day may help in wound healing and in relief of rest pain. In the Mayo Clinic series involving 101 patients with extremity ulcers and low TcPO2 levels (<20 mm Hg), healing occurred in 40% of patients and amputation was prevented.[112] This seems to be a particularly useful treatment in patients with small vessel occlusive disease.

There is little information regarding the use of intraarterial thrombolytic therapy as an adjunct for the treatment of Buerger's disease. In one series,[113] selective low-dose intra-arterial streptokinase (10,000 unit bolus followed by 5000 units/hr) was administered to 11 patients with longstanding Buerger's disease who had gangrene or pregangrenous lesions of the toes or feet. Many of these patients had previous lumbar sympathectomies. The investigators report an overall success rate (defined as amputation being avoided or altered) of 58.3%. The efficacy of thrombolytic therapy may not be as successful as reported by Hussain and Dorri.[113] Thrombi in the superficial femoral artery have been successfully lysed, but the severe distal occlusive disease is resistant to thrombolysis (unpublished data). From a pathologic standpoint, a highly inflammatory thrombus quickly becomes encased with connective tissue and fibrous material. Therefore it does not appear logical that thrombolytic therapy would result in substantial improvement in many of these patients. However, if the patient is facing amputation, it is not unreasonable to give a short trial of thrombolytic therapy to see if the circulation can be improved enough to avoid amputation, as long as no contraindications exist.

Surgical revascularization for Buerger's disease is not usually a viable alternative due to the diffuse segmental involvement and extreme distal nature of the disease. There is frequently not a distal blood vessel available for bypass surgery. However, if the patient is severely ischemic and has a distal infrapopliteal blood vessel available as a target, then bypass surgery should be considered with the use of an autogenous vein.[26] Inada and colleagues[114] demonstrated that of 236 patients with Buerger's disease, only 11 (4.6%) patients had lesions that were amenable to surgical revascularization. In the 11 patients who underwent surgical revascularization, the bypass remained patent for 4 months to 7 years with a mean time of 2.8 years. In a series of 216 patients receiving surgical therapy for Buerger's disease, Sayan and associates[115] noted that although the long-term patency of the bypass grafts was not good, the short-term patency was sufficient to allow healing of the ulcerations associated with TAO. Other investigators have agreed with this indication for surgical revascularization.[81]

Dilege and colleagues[116] reported on 27 of 36 (81%) patients with TAO who underwent revascularization procedures. During a 36-month follow-up, the patency rates at 12, 24, and 36 months were 59.2%, 48%, and 33.3%, respectively. However, the limb salvage rate was 92.5%. Although the patency rates do not seem promising, the limb salvation rate was quite satisfactory in this and other series.[116,117]

Another surgical approach in patients with Buerger's disease is that of omental transfer.[118-122] Singh and associates[118] reported on 50 patients with TAO who underwent omental transfer for rest pain or nonhealing ischemic ulcers, or both. All patients showed an improvement in skin temperature, rest pain decreased in 36 patients, and claudication distance increased in 48 patients. The ulcers healed in 32 of 36 patients.

PROGNOSIS

Data on the natural course of life and limb in patients with TAO are scant. In a retrospective study from Japan, Ohta and associates[96] followed 106 men and 4 women (mean age at onset 35 years [range 17 to 49]) for a mean follow-up of 10.6 years. The cumulative survival after initial consultation was 97% at 5 years, 94% at 10 years, 92% at 20 years, and 84% at 25 years. Eleven of 13 (84.6%) patients who underwent amputation lost their jobs ($P < .0001$).

CONCLUSION

TAO is a nonatherosclerotic, segmental, inflammatory disease that affects the small- and medium-sized arteries and veins in the lower and upper extremities. In some way, as yet unexplained, it is causally related to tobacco use. Discontinuation of tobacco is the mainstay of treatment. In those patients who successfully stop smoking, amputation almost never occurs.

REFERENCES

1. von Winiwater F: Ueber eine eigenthumliche form von endarteritis und endophlebitis mit gangran des fusses. Arch Klin Chir 23:202, 1879.
2. Buerger L: Thromboangiitis obliterans: A study of the vascular lesions leading to presenile spontaneous gangrene. Am J Med Sci 136:580, 1908.
3. Buerger L: The circulatory disturbance of the extremities: Including gangrene, vasomotor and trophic disorders. Philadelphia, WB Saunders, 1924.
4. Allen EV, Brown GE: Thrombo-angiitis obliterans: A clinical study of 200 cases. Ann Intern Med 1:535, 1928.
5. Lie JT: Thromboangiitis obliterans (Buerger's disease) revisited. Pathol Annu 23:257, 1988.
6. Lie JT: The rise and fall and resurgence of thromboangiitis obliterans (Buerger's disease). Acta Pathol Jpn 39:153, 1989.
7. Herman BE: Buerger's syndrome. Angiology 26:713, 1975.
8. Lie JT: Thromboangiitis obliterans (Buerger's disease) in women. Medicine (Baltimore) 66:65, 1987.
9. Cachovan M: Epidemiologie und geographisches verteilungsmuster der thromboangiitis obliterans. In Heidrich J (ed): Thromboangiitis Obliterans Morbus Winiwater-Buerger. Stuttgart, New York, George Thieme, 1988, p 31.
10. McKusick VA, Harris WS: The Buerger syndrome in the Orient. Bull Johns Hopkins Hosp 109:241, 1961.
11. Hill GL, Moeliono J, Tumewu F, et al: The Buerger syndrome in Java. A description of the clinical syndrome and some aspects of its aetiology. Br J Surg 60:606, 1973.
12. Annual report of the Buerger's Disease Research Committee of Ministry of Health and Welfare of Japan. Tokyo, 1976, p 3.
13. Nishikimi N, Shionoya S, Mizuno S: Result of national epidemiological study of Buerger's disease. J Jpn Coll Angiol 27:1125, 1987.
14. Shionoya S: Buerger's disease: Diagnosis and management. Cardiovasc Surg 1:207, 1993.
15. Mills JL, Taylor LM Jr, Porter JM: Buerger's disease in the modern era. Am J Surg 154:123, 1987.
16. Leu HJ: Thromboangiitis obliterans Buerger. Pathologisch-anatomische analyse von 53 Fallen. Schweiz Med Wochenschr 115:1080, 1985.
17. Olin JW, Young JR, Graor RA, et al: The changing clinical spectrum of thromboangiitis obliterans (Buerger's disease). Circulation 82:IV3, 1990.
18. Lie JT: Diagnostic histopathology of major systemic and pulmonary vasculitis syndromes. Rheum Dis Clin North Am 16:269, 1990.
19. Papa MZ, Adar R: A critical look at thromboangiitis obliterans (Buerger's disease). Vasc Surg 5:1, 1992.
20. Harkavy J: Tobacco sensitivities in thromboangiitis obliterans, migratory phlebitis, and coronary artery disease. Bull N Y Acad Med 9:318, 1933.
21. Westcott FN, Wright IS: Tobacco allergy and thromboangiitis obliterans. J Allergy 9:555, 1938.
22. Jindal RM, Patel SM: Buerger's disease and cigarette smoking in Bangladesh. Ann R Coll Surg Engl 74:436, 1992.
23. Grove WJ, Stansby GP: Buerger's disease and cigarette smoking in Bangladesh. Ann R Coll Surg Engl 74:115, 1992.
24. Rahman M, Chowdhury AS, Fukui T, et al: Association of thromboangiitis obliterans with cigarette and bidi smoking in Bangladesh: A case-control study. Int J Epidemiol 29:266, 2000.
25. Kjeldsen K, Mozes M: Buerger's disease in Israel: Investigations on carboxyhemoglobin and serum cholesterol levels after smoking. Acta Chir Scand 135:495, 1969.
26. Mills JL, Porter JM: Buerger's disease: A review and update. Semin Vasc Surg 6:14, 1993.
27. Lie JT: Thromboangiitis obliterans (Buerger's disease) and smokeless tobacco. Arthritis Rheum 31:812, 1988.
28. Joyce JW: Buerger's disease (thromboangiitis obliterans). Rheum Dis Clin North Am 16:463, 1990.
29. Olin JW: Thromboangiitis obliterans (Buerger's disease). N Engl J Med 343:864, 2000.
30. Matsushita M, Shionoya S, Matsumoto T: Urinary cotinine measurement in patients with Buerger's disease: Effects of active and passive smoking on the disease process. J Vasc Surg 14:53, 1991.
31. Lie JT: Thromboangiitis obliterans (Buerger's disease) in an elderly man after cessation of cigarette smoking: A case report. Angiology 38:864, 1987.
32. McLoughlin GA, Helsby CR, Evans CC, et al: Association of HLA-A9 and HLA-B5 with Buerger's disease. Br Med J 2:1165, 1976.
33. Otawa T, Jugi T, Kawano N, et al: Letter: HL-A antigens in thromboangiitis obliterans. JAMA 230:1128, 1974.
34. Smolen JS, Youngchaiyud U, Weidinger P, et al: Autoimmunological aspects of thromboangiitis obliterans (Buerger's disease). Clin Immunol Immunopathol 11:168, 1978.
35. Papa M, Bass A, Adar R, et al: Autoimmune mechanisms in thromboangiitis obliterans (Buerger's disease): The role of tobacco antigen and the major histocompatibility complex. Surgery 111:527, 1992.
36. Choudhury NA, Pietraszek MH, Hachiya T, et al: Plasminogen activators and plasminogen activator inhibitor 1 before and after venous occlusion of the upper limb in thromboangiitis obliterans (Buerger's disease). Thromb Res 66:321, 1992.
37. Pietraszek MH, Choudhury NA, Koyano K, et al: Enhanced platelet response to serotonin in Buerger's disease. Thromb Res 60:241, 1990.
38. Carr ME Jr, Hackney MH, Hines SJ, et al: Enhanced platelet force development despite drug-induced inhibition of platelet aggregation in patients with thromboangiitis obliterans: Two case reports. Vasc Endovasc Surg 36:473, 2002.
39. Brodmann M, Renner W, Stark G, et al: Prothrombotic risk factors in patients with thrombangiitis obliterans. Thromb Res 99:483, 2000.
40. Avcu F, Akar E, Demirkilic U, et al: The role of prothrombotic mutations in patients with Buerger's disease. Thromb Res 100:143, 2000.
41. Avcu F, Akar N, Akar E, et al: Prothrombin gene 20210 G→A and Factor V Arg 506 to Gln mutation in a patient with Buerger's disease—a case report. Angiology 51:421, 2000.
42. Caramaschi P, Biasi D, Carletto A, et al: Three cases of Buerger's disease associated with hyperhomocysteinemia. Clin Exp Rheumatol 18:264, 2000.
43. Olin JW, Childs MB, Bartholomew JR, et al: Anticardiolipin antibodies and homocysteine levels in patients with thromboangiitis obliterans. Arthritis Rheum 39:S-47, 1996.
44. Casellas M, Perez A, Cabero L, et al: Buerger's disease and antiphospholipid antibodies in pregnancy. Ann Rheum Dis 52:247, 1993.
45. Maslowski L, McBane R, Alexewicz P, et al: Antiphospholipid antibodies in thromboangiitis obliterans. Vasc Med 7:259, 2002.
46. Olin JW: Are anticardiolipin antibodies really important in thromboangiitis obliterans (Buerger's disease)? Vasc Med 7:257, 2002.
47. Adar R, Papa MZ, Halpern Z, et al: Cellular sensitivity to collagen in thromboangiitis obliterans. N Engl J Med 308:1113, 1983.
48. Gulati SM, Saha K, Kant L, et al: Significance of circulatory immune complexes in thromboangiitis obliterans (Buerger's disease). Angiology 35:276, 1984.
49. Roncon de Albuquerque R, Delgado L, Correia P, et al: Circulating immune complexes in Buerger's disease: Endarteritis obliterans in young men. J Cardiovasc Surg (Torino) 30:821, 1989.
50. Kobayashi M, Ito M, Nakagawa A, et al: Immunohistochemical analysis of arterial wall cellular infiltration in Buerger's disease (endarteritis obliterans). J Vasc Surg 29:451, 1999.
51. Lee T, Seo JW, Sumpio BE, et al: Immunobiologic analysis of arterial tissue in Buerger's disease. Eur J Vasc Endovasc Surg 25:451, 2003.
52. Kurata A, Machinami R, Schulz A, et al: Different immunophenotypes in Buerger's disease. Pathol Int 53:608, 2003.

53. Eichhorn J, Sima D, Lindschau C, et al: Antiendothelial cell antibodies in thromboangiitis obliterans. Am J Med Sci 315:17, 1998.
54. Makita S, Nakamura M, Murakami H, et al: Impaired endothelium-dependent vasorelaxation in peripheral vasculature of patients with thromboangiitis obliterans (Buerger's disease). Circulation 94:II211, 1996.
55. Halacheva K, Gulubova MV, Manolova I, et al: Expression of ICAM-1, VCAM-1, E-selectin and TNF-alpha on the endothelium of femoral and iliac arteries in thromboangiitis obliterans. Acta Histochem 104:177, 2002.
56. Williams G: Recent views on Buerger's disease. J Clin Pathol 22:573, 1969.
57. Leu HJ: Early inflammatory changes in thromboangiitis obliterans. Pathol Microbiol (Basel) 43:151, 1975.
58. Dible JH: The pathology of limb ischemia. Edinburgh, Oliver & Boyd, 1966, p 79.
59. Kurata A, Franke FE, Machinami R, et al: Thromboangiitis obliterans: Classic and new morphological features. Virchows Arch 436:59, 2000.
60. Leu HJ, Bollinger A: Phlebitis saltans sive migrans. Vasa 7:440, 1978.
61. Gulati SM, Madhra K, Thusoo TK, et al: Autoantibodies in thromboangiitis obliterans (Buerger's disease). Angiology 33:642, 1982.
62. Alpaslan M, Akgun G, Doven O, et al: Thrombus in the main pulmonary artery of a patient with thromboangiitis obliterans: Observation by transthoracic echocardiography. Eur J Echocardiogr 2:139, 2001.
63. Shionoya S, Ban I, Nakata Y, et al: Involvement of the iliac artery in Buerger's disease (pathogenesis and arterial reconstruction). J Cardiovasc Surg (Torino) 19:69, 1978.
64. Bozikas VP, Vlaikidis N, Petrikis P, et al: Schizophrenic-like symptoms in a patient with thrombo-angiitis obliterans (Winiwarter-Buerger's disease). Int J Psychiatry Med 31:341, 2001.
65. Donatelli F, Triggiani M, Nascimbene S, et al: Thromboangiitis obliterans of coronary and internal thoracic arteries in a young woman. J Thorac Cardiovasc Surg 113:800, 1997.
66. Becit N, Unlu Y, Kocak H, et al: Involvement of the coronary artery in a patient with thromboangiitis obliterans: A case report. Heart Vessels 16:201, 2002.
67. Deitch EA, Sikkema WW: Intestinal manifestation of Buerger's disease: Case report and literature review. Am Surg 47:326, 1981.
68. Rosen N, Sommer I, Knobel B: Intestinal Buerger's disease. Arch Pathol Lab Med 109:962, 1985.
69. Cho YP, Kwon YM, Kwon TW, et al: Mesenteric Buerger's disease. Ann Vasc Surg 17:221, 2003.
70. Kobayashi M, Kurose K, Kobata T, et al: Ischemic intestinal involvement in a patient with Buerger disease: Case report and literature review. J Vasc Surg 38:170, 2003.
71. Arkkila PE, Kahri A, Farkkila M: Intestinal type of thromboangiitis obliterans (Buerger disease) preceding symptoms of severe peripheral arterial disease. Scand J Gastroenterol 36:669, 2001.
72. Hassoun Z, Lacrosse M, De Ronde T: Intestinal involvement in Buerger's disease. J Clin Gastroenterol 32:85, 2001.
73. Siddiqui MZ, Reis ED, Soundararajan K, et al: Buerger's disease affecting mesenteric arteries: A rare cause of intestinal ischemia—a case report. Vasc Surg 35:235, 2001.
74. Hoppe B, Lu JT, Thistlewaite P, et al: Beyond peripheral arteries in Buerger's disease: Angiographic considerations in thromboangiitis obliterans. Catheter Cardiovasc Interv 57:363, 2002.
75. Cebezas-Moya R, Dragstedt LRI: An extreme example of Buerger's disease. Arch Surg 101:632, 1970.
76. Lie JT: Thromboangiitis obliterans (Buerger's disease) in a saphenous vein arterial graft. Hum Pathol 18:402, 1987.
77. Lie JT, Michet CJ Jr: Thromboangiitis obliterans with eosinophilia (Buerger's disease) of the temporal arteries. Hum Pathol 19:598, 1988.
78. Matsushita M, Kuzuya A, Kobayashi M, et al: Buerger's disease in a 19-year-old woman. J Vasc Surg 38:175, 2003.
79. Sasaki S, Sakuma M, Kunihara T, et al: Distribution of arterial involvement in thromboangiitis obliterans (Buerger's disease): Results of a study conducted by the Intractable Vasculitis Syndromes Research Group in Japan. Surg Today 30:600, 2000.
80. Pokrovskii AV, Kuntsevich GI, Dan VN, et al: Diagnosis of occlusive lesions of upper extremity arteries in patients with thromboangiitis obliterans. Angiol Sosud Khir 9:86, 2003.
81. Shionoya S: Buerger's disease (thromboangiitis obliterans). In Rutherford RB (ed): Vascular Surgery. Philadelphia, WB Saunders, 1989, p 207.
82. Allen EV: Thromboangiitis obliterans: Methods of diagnosis of chronic occlusive arterial lesions distal to the wrist with illustrative cases. Am J Med Sci 178:237, 1929.
83. Olin JW, Lie JT: Thromboangiitis obliterans (Buerger's disease). In Cooke JP, Frohlich ED (eds): Current Management of Hypertension and Vascular Disease. St Louis, Mosby Yearbook, 1992, p 265.
84. Yamamoto K, Iwase S, Mano T, et al: Muscle sympathetic outflow in Buerger's disease. J Auton Nerv Syst 44:67, 1993.
85. Kimura T, Yoshizaki S, Tsushima N, et al: Buerger's colour. Br J Surg 77:1299, 1990.
86. McKusick VA, Harris WS, Ottsen OE: Buerger's disease: A distinct clinical and pathologic entity. JAMA 181:93, 1962.
87. McKusick VA, Harris WS, Ottsen OE, et al: The Buerger's syndrome in the United States: Arteriographic observations with special reference to involvement of the upper extremities and the differentiation from atherosclerosis and embolism. Bull Johns Hopkins Hosp 110:145, 1962.
88. Lambeth JT, Yong NK: Arteriographic findings in thromboangiitis obliterans with emphasis on femoropopliteal involvement. Am J Roentgenol Radium Ther Nucl Med 109:553, 1970.
89. Jaff MR, Olin JW, Young JR: Failure of acute phase reactants to predict disease activity in Takayasu's arteritis. J Vasc Med Biol 4:223, 1994.
90. Noel B: Cocaine and arsenic-induced Raynaud's phenomenon. Clin Rheumatol 21:343, 2002.
91. Noel B: Vascular complications of cocaine use. Stroke 33:1747, 2002.
92. Marder VJ, Mellinghoff IK: Cocaine and Buerger disease: Is there a pathogenetic association? Arch Intern Med 160:2057, 2000.
93. Disdier P, Granel B, Serratrice J, et al: Cannabis arteritis revisited: Ten new case reports. Angiology 52:1, 2001.
94. Corelli F: Buerger's disease: Cigarette smoker disease may always be cured by medical therapy alone: Uselessness of operative treatment. J Cardiovasc Surg (Torino) 14:28, 1973.
95. Gifford RW, Hines EA Jr: Complete clinical remission in thromboangiitis obliterans during abstinence from tobacco: Report of a case. Proc Staff Meetings Mayo Clinic 26:241, 1951.
96. Ohta T, Ishioashi H, Hosaka M, et al: Clinical and social consequences of Buerger disease. J Vasc Surg 39:176, 2004.
97. Fiessinger JN, Schafer M: Trial of iloprost versus aspirin treatment for critical limb ischaemia of thromboangiitis obliterans: The TAO Study. Lancet 335:555, 1990.
98. Hildebrand M: Pharmacokinetics and tolerability of oral iloprost in thromboangiitis obliterans patients. Eur J Clin Pharmacol 53:51, 1997.
99. Oral iloprost in the treatment of thromboangiitis obliterans (Buerger's disease): A double-blind, randomised, placebo-controlled trial. The European TAO Study Group. Eur J Vasc Endovasc Surg 15:300, 1998.
100. Melian EB, Goa KL: Beraprost: A review of its pharmacology and therapeutic efficacy in the treatment of peripheral arterial disease and pulmonary arterial hypertension. Drugs 62:107, 2002.
101. Dean SM, Satiani B: Three cases of digital ischemia successfully treated with cilostazol. Vasc Med 6:245, 2001.
102. Dean SM, Vaccaro PS: Successful pharmacologic treatment of lower extremity ulcerations in 5 patients with chronic critical limb ischemia. J Am Board Fam Pract 15:55, 2002.
103. Isner JM, Baumgartner I, Rauh G, et al: Treatment of thromboangiitis obliterans (Buerger's disease) by intramuscular gene transfer of vascular endothelial growth factor: Preliminary clinical results. J Vasc Surg 28:964, 1998.
104. Taguchi A, Ohtani M, Soma T, et al: Therapeutic angiogenesis by autologous bone-marrow transplantation in a general hospital setting. Eur J Vasc Endovasc Surg 25:276, 2003.
105. Iwase S, Okamoto T, Mano T, et al: Skin sympathetic outflow in Buerger's disease. Auton Neurosci 87:286, 2001.
106. Roncon-Albuquerque R, Serrao P, Vale-Pereira R, et al: Plasma catecholamines in Buerger's disease: Effects of cigarette smoking and surgical sympathectomy. Eur J Vasc Endovasc Surg 24:338, 2002.
107. Watarida S, Shiraishi S, Fujimura M, et al: Laparoscopic lumbar sympathectomy for lower-limb disease. Surg Endosc 16:500, 2002.
108. De Giacomo T, Rendina EA, Venuta F, et al: Thoracoscopic sympathectomy for symptomatic arterial obstruction of the upper extremities. Ann Thorac Surg 74:885, 2002.
109. Swigris JJ, Olin JW, Mekhail NA: Implantable spinal cord stimulator to treat the ischemic manifestations of thromboangiitis obliterans (Buerger's disease). J Vasc Surg 29:928, 1999.

110. Chierichetti F, Mambrini S, Bagliani A, et al: Treatment of Buerger's disease with electrical spinal cord stimulation: Review of three cases. Angiology 53:341, 2002.
111. Pace AV, Saratzis N, Karokis D, et al: Spinal cord stimulation in Buerger's disease. Ann Rheum Dis 61:1114, 2002.
112. Montori VM, Kavros SJ, Walsh EE, et al: Intermittent compression pump for nonhealing wounds in patients with limb ischemia: The Mayo Clinic experience (1998-2000). Int Angiol 21:360, 2002.
113. Hussein EA, el Dorri A: Intra-arterial streptokinase as adjuvant therapy for complicated Buerger's disease: Early trials. Int Surg 78:54,1993.
114. Inada K, Iwashima Y, Okada A, et al: Nonatherosclerotic segmental arterial occlusion of the extremity. Arch Surg 108:663, 1974.
115. Sayin A, Bozkurt AK, Tuzun H, et al: Surgical treatment of Buerger's disease: Experience with 216 patients. Cardiovasc Surg 1:377, 1993.
116. Dilege S, Aksoy M, Kayabali M, et al: Vascular reconstruction in Buerger's disease: Is it feasible? Surg Today 32:1042, 2002.
117. Nishikimi N: Fate of limbs with failed vascular reconstruction in Buerger's disease patients. Int J Cardiol 75(suppl)1:S183, 2000.
118. Singh I, Ramteke VK: The role of omental transfer in Buerger's disease: New Delhi's experience. Aust N Z J Surg 66:372, 1996.
119. Talwar S, Jain S, Porwal R, et al: Free versus pedicled omental grafts for limb salvage in Buerger's disease. Aust N Z J Surg 68:38, 1998.
120. Talwar S, Jain S, Porwal R, et al: Pedicled omental transfer for limb salvage in Buerger's disease. Int J Cardiol 72:127, 2000.
121. Talwar S, Choudhary SK: Omentopexy for limb salvage in Buerger's disease: Indications, technique and results. J Postgrad Med 47:137, 2001.
122. Talwar S, Prasad P: Single-stage lumbar sympathectomy and omentopexy: A new surgical approach towards patients with Buerger's disease. Trop Doct 31:73, 2001.

chapter 45

Kawasaki Disease

David R. Fulton
Jane W. Newburger

Kawasaki disease, initially described by Dr. Tomisaku Kawasaki in 1967,[1] is an acute, systemic vasculitis of uncertain etiology, occurring predominantly in infants and young children. The disease has been described worldwide and affects all racial and ethnic groups. The classic presentation of the illness is marked by at least 5 days of fever, oral mucositis, nonexudative conjunctivitis, erythematous nonvesicular rash, changes in the hands and feet including edema or erythema, and cervical lymphadenopathy (Box 45-1). Coronary artery dilation or aneurysms were identified initially in Japan[2] and affect up to 25% of those who are not treated early in the course of the disease. In some cases, myocardial infarction and death may ensue during the acute phase or months to years later.

EPIDEMIOLOGY

Despite its description in diverse areas of the world, by far the greatest number of cases have been reported in Japan. The most recent statistics from the nationwide survey from 2000 note a total of 168,394 affected children, with higher rates in males and in infants younger than 1 year of age. In the year 2000, the incidence rate was 134.2 per 100,000 children under 5 years.[3] The absence of a mandatory national reporting system in the United States makes statistical analysis difficult, but estimates from regional centers are available. Recent administrative data from hospital discharge abstracts suggested that more than 4000 hospitalizations were associated with Kawasaki disease in the United States in 2000.[4] Current data show that among children under 5 years, the occurrence is greatest in Asians (33.3/100,000), somewhat less in African-Americans (23.4/100,000) and lowest in Caucasians (12.7/100,000).[5] The pattern of involvement is generally endemic, with occasional epidemics primarily among younger children, with a male to female ratio of 1.4:1; however, the illness is being more commonly recognized in older children and adolescents.[6] Outbreaks are more likely in the spring, suggesting an infectious etiology, but a steady background activity of cases is noted throughout the remainder of the year. The disease can recur (approximately 3% in Japan), and person-to-person transmission is unusual.

BOX 45-1 Principal Clinical Findings*

Fever persisting at least 5 days† or more without other source in association with at least 4 principal features:

1. Oral changes that may include erythema or cracking of the lips, strawberry tongue, erythema of the oral mucosa
2. Bilateral, nonexudative conjunctival injection
3. Polymorphous rash, generally truncal involvement, nonvesicular
4. Changes of extremities that may include erythema and edema of the hands or feet; desquamation of fingers and toes 1-3 weeks after onset of illness
5. Cervical lymphadenopathy, often unilateral, with at least 1 node ≥ 1.5 cm

*Patients with fever and fewer than four criteria can be diagnosed with the presence of coronary artery disease by 2-D echocardiography or coronary angiography.

†Many experts believe that in the presence of classic features, the diagnosis of Kawasaki disease can be made by experienced observers before day 5 of fever.

Adapted from Anonymous: Diagnostic guidelines for Kawasaki disease. Circulation 103:335, 2001.

ETIOLOGY

The search for an etiologic agent has been wide-ranging over the course of the past two decades. Features suggesting that the process is infectious include the young age at presentation, the higher frequency of cases in the spring, and clustering of individuals in near proximity albeit without direct interpersonal contact. Prior exposure of index cases to freshly cleaned carpets has been noted for many years by various observers, although no specific organism or toxin has been identified in the rugs. Some investigators favor the theory that an agent triggers a typical immune response resulting in the clinical manifestations of the disease, whereas others believe that the marked immune response is related to exposure of the host to a superantigen.[7] A number of reports have implicated specific superantigens, including TSST-1–secreting strains of *Staphylococcus aureus* and streptococcal pyrogenic exotoxin B- and C-producing streptococci[7-9] in Kawasaki disease, as well as *Lactobacillus casei* inducing coronary arteritis in mice.[10] By contrast, other investigators have found support for a typical antigen immune response by demonstrating oligo-IgA plasma cells and IgA heavy chain genes in vascular tissue of individuals with fatal Kawasaki disease.[11-12]

PATHOGENESIS

Kawasaki disease is accompanied by significant derangements in the immunoregulatory system that lead to coronary inflammation and coronary artery abnormalities (dilatation, aneurysm formation, and giant aneurysms) in some patients. The presence of T-cell activation has been well defined with increased circulating monocytes, activation of helper T cells, and decreased suppressor T cells. B-cell activation has also been shown, with increased secretion of IgG and IgM antibodies.[13-14] These earlier observations have been extended by the fact that a number of investigators have shown stimulation of T cells that bear specific Vβ T-cell receptors capable of interacting with antigen-presenting cells. The markedly skewed expansion of circulating T cells suggests that superantigens may initiate this interaction. Superantigens are known to have specific T-cell receptor Vβ profiles, and the work of some has shown that the Vβ repertoires in Kawasaki disease involving the Vβ2 and Vβ8 are selectively expanded.[9,15-20]

Endothelial cell damage appears to occur as a result of this increased immune activity, although the mechanism is not fully elucidated. Leung and colleagues[21] have reported that IgM antibodies from acute sera can damage cultured human vascular endothelial cells when pretreated with gamma interferon, as have IgG and IgM antibodies when cells are stimulated with interleukin-1 or tumor necrosis factor.[22] It is possible that the cytokines released by stimulated T cells and macrophages incite damage to endothelial cells in the acute phase of the illness. Many investigators have reported on the increased levels of circulating mediators including interleukins,[23-26] soluble selectins,[27] leukotrienes,[28] and tumor necrosis factor.[23] Thus the features of an immune reaction induced by a superantigen are supported by documented Vβ skewing of T lymphocytes, a polyclonal B-lymphocyte activation, and inflammatory cytokine production.[8]

Activation of vascular endothelial growth factor (VEGF) to markedly elevated levels has been identified in the acute phase of Kawasaki disease.[29] This glycoprotein acts on endothelium to increase vascular permeability, an effect that may explain the edema of the distal extremities in the acute phase, as well as the decrease in serum albumin concentration. Microscopic assessment of blood vessels by skin biopsy in the acute phase of the illness shows microvascular dilation and subendothelial edema[30] that could be explained by elevated levels of VEGF. VEGF simulates nitric oxide production in endothelial cells through nitric oxide synthase enzyme expression,[31] and it has been reported that nitric oxide production is greater in those patients with Kawasaki disease who develop coronary aneurysms.[32] Following IV γ-globulin (IVIG) administration, serum VEGF levels have been shown to remain elevated. However, VEGF levels in patients who did not respond to IVIG as manifested by persistent fever were higher than those among patients who were IVIG responders, with serum albumin lower in the IVIG-resistant group.[33] Among the latter, 44% had coronary abnormalities, whereas no coronary abnormalities were evident in IVIG responders. These data may support a contributing role for VEGF in the pathogenesis of coronary artery damage.

Matrix metalloproteinases (MMPs) 2 and 9 degrade extracellular matrix, collagen, and elastin and are in balance with their specific tissue inhibitors (TIMPs). Imbalance between the MMPs and TIMPs has been shown to degrade the tissue matrix in abdominal aortic aneurysms.[34-35] Patients with Kawasaki disease have higher levels of MMPs than afebrile and febrile controls before treatment with IVIG. In addition, Kawasaki disease patients with coronary artery lesions have higher levels of MMPs, as well as higher MMP/TIMP ratios than those without coronary abnormalities,[36] suggesting that these circulating proteins may play an active role in coronary arterial remodeling.

PATHOLOGY

The original pathologic description of Kawasaki disease by Fujiwara and Hamashima was based on autopsy findings of children dying in the acute and subacute phases of Kawasaki disease before available treatment with IVIG.[37] They established four categories of illness on the basis of the time from onset of the disease: stage 1 (0 to 9 days), stage 2 (12 to 25 days), stage 3 (28 to 31 days), and stage 4 (40 days to 4 years). The inflammatory changes in stage I are highlighted by vasculitis of small vessels and microvessels, as well as perivasculitis and endarteritis of the coronary vessels. Pancarditis is present. Pancarditis is seen also in stage II, with panvasculitis of the coronary bed at times with aneurysm formation and coronary thrombosis. By stage 3, the acute inflammation has subsided but myointimal proliferation of the coronary arteries proceeds. In stage 4, stenosis is noted for the first time with scarring. Early in the course of the illness, the authors noted that death was the result of arrhythmia and myocarditis, with increasing trends toward ischemia and infarction as time progressed from the onset of disease. Of note is the concomitant onset of a hypercoagulable state[38] and thrombocytosis in stages 2 and 3, during which intervals the mortality rate is highest.

CLINICAL PRESENTATION

Because no diagnostic test is available for Kawasaki disease, the diagnosis must be made on clinical grounds. Often the illness begins with fever and what appears to be gastroenteritis or otitis media in a child between the ages of 1 and 5 years. The persistence of fever and the onset of the other signs may lead the clinician to consider the diagnosis. First described by Kawasaki on the basis of his observations in Japanese children,[39] the classic criteria have continued to serve as the standard adopted by the American Heart Association (see Box 45-1) for arriving at the diagnosis[40] and include fever for 5 days or more and at least 4 of the 5 following findings: (1) a nonexudative, bilateral conjunctivitis; (2) oral changes with erythematous or dry cracked lips, strawberry tongue, or pharyngitis; (3) a nonvesicular, morbilliform rash involving the trunk, perineum, and extremities, often sparing the face; (4) erythema of the palmar and plantar surfaces, edema of the hands or feet, or periungual desquamation; and (5) anterior cervical lymphadenopathy of 1 cm or greater. Alternatively, the diagnosis can be made with fewer than 4 of 5 criteria in the presence of coronary artery abnormalities on echocardiogram.[41] Not all criteria need to be present simultaneously to make the diagnosis; indeed, it is common for some findings to resolve as others appear, making serial evaluation of the child essential.

Because a sizeable number of children with coronary artery aneurysms never meet the classic criteria, the American Heart Association is currently considering new criteria for IVIG treatment of Kawasaki disease separate from the classic epidemiologic case definition. Other illnesses that may mimic Kawasaki disease include toxin-mediated disease related to staphylococcal or streptococcal diseases, scarlet fever, enterovirus, adenovirus, measles, parvovirus, Epstein-Barr virus, mycoplasma, and rickettsial disease. Infants younger than 6 months old present a particular challenge because they often lack clinical criteria for the diagnosis yet are at greater risk for development of coronary artery abnormalities.[41] The diagnosis should be considered and echocardiography performed in young infants who have fever for more than 5 days without documented source and whose laboratory data are consistent with moderate or severe systemic inflammation.[42-44]

Other supportive signs are present in many children with Kawasaki disease (Box 45-2).The rash when perineal in location often desquamates by the end of the first week of illness.[45] Anterior uveitis can be identified by slit-lamp examination in 83% of patients early in the course.[46] Arthralgia and arthritis of large and small joints may be severe enough that children refuse to walk or perform tasks with their hands, but the arthritis is virtually never chronic.[47] Abdominal signs including vomiting, diarrhea, or hydrops of the gallbladder[48] are common. Other typical findings include sterile pyuria and aseptic meningitis.[49]

BOX 45-2 Other Significant Clinical and Laboratory Findings

Cardiovascular: On auscultation, gallop rhythm or distant heart sounds; ECG changes (arrhythmias; abnormal Q waves; prolonged PR or QT intervals, or both; occasionally low voltage or ST-T wave changes); chest x-ray abnormalities (cardiomegaly); echocardiographic changes (pericardial effusion, coronary aneurysms, or decreased contractility); mitral or aortic valvular insufficiency, or both; and, rarely, aneurysms or peripheral arteries (e.g., axillary), angina pectoris, or myocardial infarction

Gastrointestinal: Diarrhea, vomiting, abdominal pain, hydrops of gallbladder, paralytic ileus, mild jaundice, and mild increase of serum transaminase levels

Blood: Increased erythrocyte sedimentation rate, leukocytosis with left shift, positive C-reactive protein, hypoalbuminemia, and mild anemia in acute phase of illness (thrombocytosis in subacute phase)

Urine: Sterile pyuria of urethral origin and occasional proteinuria

Skin: Perineal rash and desquamation in subacute phase and transverse furrows of fingernails (Beau's lines) during convalescence

Respiratory: Cough, rhinorrhea, and pulmonary infiltrate.

Joint: Arthralgia and arthritis

Neurologic: Mononuclear pleocytosis in CSF fluid; striking irritability; and, rarely, facial palsy

Adapted from Anonymous: Diagnostic guidelines for Kawasaki disease. Circulation 103:335, 2001.

CARDIAC MANIFESTATIONS

Coronary Artery Abnormalities

Kawasaki disease causes coronary artery abnormalities[50] in 15% to 25% of patients who are not treated in the acute phase of the disease with high-dose IVIG.[51] Lesions may be observed by echocardiography as early as 1 week from the onset of fever, with further progression ensuing in the next 3 to 4 weeks. Given the difficulty in reaching diagnostic confirmation of the illness using the classic criteria,[1] identification of those at higher risk for coronary disease and for whom early treatment could reduce extent of involvement has led investigators to focus on predictive factors for coronary artery abnormalities. The Asai score[52] assigned risk by including age younger than 1 year, male gender, fever for more than 14 days, hemoglobin less than 10 g/dl, WBC greater than 30,000 mm^3, erythrocyte sedimentation rate (ESR) greater than 101 mm/hr, and elevation of C-reactive protein (CRP) or ESR beyond 30 days. Other reports have supported the concept of prolonged fever as a marker for ongoing vasculitis.[53-54] In a multicenter prospective trial of IVIG, risk for coronary involvement was increased by male gender, age younger than 1 year, CRP, and higher absolute band count.[55-56] For those treated early with IVIG, a risk assignment methodology has been developed that uses higher baseline neutrophil and band counts, lower hemoglobin concentration, lower platelet count, and fever on the day after IVIG administration.[57] This instrument may provide guidance as to which patients are at risk despite early treatment with IVIG, thereby promoting closer surveillance and early retreatment when indicated. Because of the expense of IVIG in Japan, Harada has proposed a scoring system for identifying those at risk for developing coronary artery abnormalities to determine which patients with Kawasaki disease should be treated.[58]

Myocarditis

In acute Kawasaki disease, myocarditis is a frequent finding at autopsy and by biopsy.[37,59] Gallium-67 citrate scans[60] and technetium 99m-labeled WBC scans[61-62] have also identified inflammatory myocardial changes in 50% to 70% of patients. Congestive heart failure in the acute phase of the illness is generally the result of myocarditis and improves rapidly with IVIG treatment, in many cases within 24 hours from initiation of treatment.[63] Later implications of these early changes is speculative; however, several investigators have evaluated pathology and clinical function late after Kawasaki disease. Myocardial biopsies in patients with long-term follow-up have shown fibrosis, abnormal branching, and hypertrophy of myocytes, unrelated to duration from illness onset.[64] Late noninvasive studies of myocardial function are encouraging, however, with resolution of abnormalities within several years from onset of illness.[65-67]

Valve Regurgitation

Mitral and aortic regurgitations have been associated with Kawasaki disease in both early and chronic phases of the disease. In the acute stage, mitral regurgitation is frequently detected by 2-D echocardiography, related in part to diminished myocardial function, although ischemia and valvulitis are possible etiologies.[68] The frequency of aortic regurgitation has been reported to be as high as 5% in the Japanese population with Kawasaki disease,[69] and there are rare reports of late-onset aortic regurgitation necessitating valve replacement.[70-71] The cause for aortic insufficiency is not known; however, it has been reported that the aortic root enlarges from baseline and remains dilated during the first year after illness onset,[72] raising the possibility that coaptation of the leaflets is disturbed.

LABORATORY FINDINGS

Inflammatory Markers

Kawasaki disease is a systemic vasculitis with laboratory values in the acute phase consistent with systemic inflammation. Acute-phase reactants are markedly increased including ESR, CRP, and α-1 antitrypsin measurements.[73] The WBC count is elevated with a leftward shift, and a normochromic, normocytic anemia[74] is noted within the first week of illness. Thrombocytosis is usually present by the second week of the disease, often peaking at counts greater than 1,000,000 mm^3 in association with hypercoagulability.[38] These parameters often persist over the first month of the illness and gradually decline. Hepatocellular inflammation is accompanied by increases in γ-glutamyltransferase.[75] Sterile pyuria and pleocytosis of CSF,[49] both with mononuclear cells, are found frequently.

Cardiac Testing

Electrocardiographic findings are nonspecific and include sinus tachycardia, prolonged PR interval and diffuse ST-T wave changes. Using 2-D echocardiography, visualization of the proximal coronary arteries in young children is almost always possible and measurements correlate closely with those identified by angiography.[76] In addition to measurements of the proximal left main, anterior descending, circumflex, proximal, and middle right and posterior descending branches, assessment of ventricular function, pericardial fluid, and mitral and aortic regurgitation should be obtained. Coronary artery dilation may be present as early as the end of the first week of illness. Some clinicians believe that "periluminal brightness" may precede dilation, suggesting the presence of inflammatory changes of the endothelium. As a result, echocardiography should be undertaken when the diagnosis is entertained, particularly as an incomplete clinical picture with coronary artery abnormalities is sufficient to make the diagnosis and initiate therapy.[40] Serial studies are obtained at 10 to 14 days from onset of illness to assess for the presence of aneurysm development and at the end of the subacute phase at 6 to 8 weeks from onset.

The definition of normal coronary artery dimensions has been the subject of some controversy. The criteria established by the Japanese Ministry of Health in 1984 defined as abnormal those coronary arteries with lumen diameter greater than 3 mm in children younger than 5 years or greater than 4 mm in those older than age 5; lumen diameter 1.5 times the size of an adjacent segment; or irregular lumen.[52] Others have shown that coronary artery size in normal children correlates linearly with increasing body size.[77] In patients with Kawasaki disease whose coronary arteries are classified as normal by Japanese Ministry of Health criteria, the dimensions are larger than expected when adjusted for body surface area (BSA) in all phases of the disease.[77-79] This observation suggests that the prevalence of coronary artery abnormalities may be underestimated.

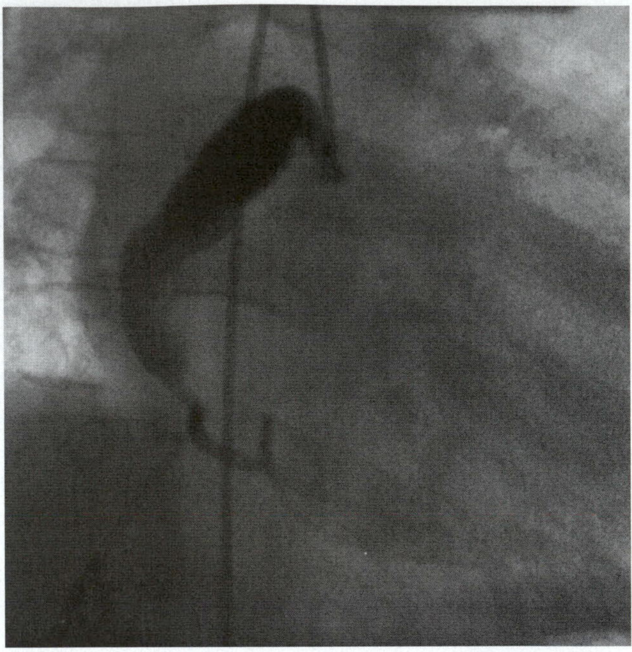

FIGURE 45-1. Isolated giant aneurysm of the left anterior descending coronary artery in a 7-year-old male who received multiple doses of IV γ-globulin and plasmapheresis for persistent fever.

Coronary angiography has been used extensively for diagnostic assessment of coronary abnormalities.[51] With rapid technical improvement in echocardiographic imaging, invasive studies are generally reserved for the child with large aneurysms or those with symptoms suspicious for angina. Aneurysms are described as localized or extensive,[80-81] the former being further subclassified as fusiform or saccular (Fig. 45-1). Extensive aneurysms, those that involve more than one segment, are ectatic (dilated uniformly—Fig. 45-2) or segmented (multiple dilated segments joined by normal or stenotic segments). Aneurysms may also involve other medium- to large-sized extraparenchymal arteries, particularly the subclavian, axillary, femoral, iliac, renal, and mesenteric arteries. Occasionally, aneurysms of the aorta may occur.

MEDICAL TREATMENT

Aspirin has been a mainstay of therapy for Kawasaki disease, both for its anti-inflammatory and antithrombotic effects. Most clinicians use high-dose aspirin, 80 to

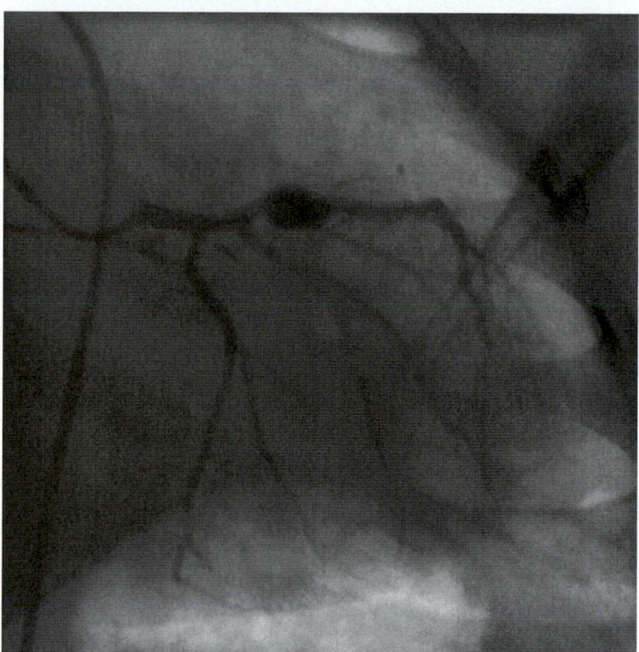

FIGURE 45-2. Ectatic giant aneurysm of the right coronary (maximal diameter 11 mm) from the same subject as in Figure 45-1.

100 mg/kg per day divided into four daily doses, until defervescence, and then reduce the dose to 3 to 5 mg/kg per day, administered once daily until the end of the subacute phase (6 to 8 weeks—Box 45-3), to reduce the likelihood for Reye's syndrome[82] or gastrointestinal bleeding.[83] Meta-analysis has shown that low-dose or high-dose aspirin regimens in conjunction with IVIG have a similar incidence of coronary abnormalities at 30 and 60 days from onset of illness.[84] In patients with aneurysms, low-dose aspirin therapy is continued, sometimes in combination with anticoagulants or other antiplatelet agents.

IVIG was first administered to children with Kawasaki disease in 1984[85] and shown to have beneficial effects in reducing the likelihood of coronary aneurysms and the inflammatory response in the acute phase. Many subsequent studies have confirmed the efficacy of high-dose IVIG.[86-89] The lowest incidence of coronary artery lesions occurs in those patients treated with IVIG, 2 g/kg, administered as a single dose over 8 to 12 hours (Box 45-3).[84,90] The greater efficacy of a single, high-dose infusion of IVIG, compared with multiple doses of lower magnitude, may be related to its higher peak level of serum IgG, which has been reported to be lower among patients who develop coronary abnormalities.[56] The mechanism of action of IVIG remains unknown; clinical studies fail to find significant differences between brands in terms of efficacy,[91-92] although adverse effects vary greatly among different products.[93-94] Of note, although IVIG is generally effective, 8% of patients with Kawasaki disease require additional infusion of IVIG,[92] 5% develop some coronary artery change, and 1% develop giant aneurysms.[95] Children who are acutely ill with Kawasaki disease should be administered IVIG 2g/kg as a single dose no later than the tenth day of illness and ideally within the first 7 days.[96] Patients with fever beyond 10 days of illness should also receive IVIG,[97] as should those with aneurysm formation and evidence for persistent inflammation. Although not tested in a randomized trial, retreatment with IVIG, 2 g/kg, is generally administered to those with recurrent or recrudescent fever more than 36 hours after completion of an initial course of IVIG.

BOX 45-3 Accepted Therapy for Acute Kawasaki Disease

IV γ-globulin 2 g/kg single infusion over 8-12 hours
and:
Aspirin 80-100 mg/kg divided equally 4 times daily until afebrile at least 48 hr
followed by:
Aspirin 3-5 mg/kg as a single daily dose for 6-8 weeks, discontinued if echo is normal at that time

Corticosteroids are widely used in the treatment of other vasculitides but have been generally avoided by most clinicians on the basis of early experience in Japan suggesting that those treated with steroids were more likely to develop aneurysms.[98] It has been hypothesized that such treatment could prevent remodeling of affected vessels[99] or increase hypercoagulability and risk of coronary thrombosis. A retrospective review of children treated with steroids in combination with varying medical regimens indicated shorter duration of fever and decreased prevalence of aneurysm formation.[99] A recent prospective study using IVIG with or without pulse methylprednisolone infusion showed faster resolution of fever, more rapid improvements in markers of inflammation, and shorter length of hospitalization with infrequent adverse effects.[100] No effect on coronary artery dimensions could be demonstrated in this relatively small population of patients. In a randomized trial of patients who failed to respond to an initial dose of IVIG, many of whom already had coronary aneurysms, pulse steroid administration resulted in more rapid resolution of fever and cost reduction but no demonstrable difference on coronary artery outcome.[101] Although it seems likely that steroids are effective in improving the inflammatory response and fever in patients with Kawasaki disease, their effect on coronary outcome remains controversial. Further information is forthcoming from an ongoing NIH-funded, randomized, double-blind clinical trial assessing the impact of corticosteroid therapy on coronary outcome in Kawasaki disease.

Alternative therapies for Kawasaki disease, usually given in combination with IVIG and aspirin, are described in small case series. The initial report of plasmapheresis antedated the use of IVIG[102]; this therapy is technically complex, requiring placement of large-bore catheters and the commitment of the local blood bank to assist in the exchange. As a result, most centers have reserved its use for critically ill patients who fail to respond to IVIG and methylprednisolone. Pentoxifylline is a xanthine derivative used for peripheral arterial disease. A small randomized trial has suggested that high-dose pentoxifylline may have therapeutic benefit in the prevention of coronary aneurysms.[103] Abciximab, a platelet glycoprotein IIb/IIIa receptor inhibitor that prevents platelet aggregation, has been used as an antithrombotic agent in acute Kawasaki disease.[104] Abciximab binds to vitronectin receptors, reducing vascular smooth muscle cell adhesion while inhibiting migration of monocytes at sites of inflammation. It may also play a role in vascular remodeling by promoting apoptosis of smooth muscle cells.[105] A retrospective study reported that patients treated with abciximab had smaller aneurysm size and greater percentage decrease in aneurysm diameter.[106] Though the investigators speculated that abciximab may actively promote vascular remodeling, prospective studies are necessary.

Antithrombotic therapy: The combination of active vasculitis with endothelial damage, thrombocytosis, and hypercoagulable state create the clinical setting for thrombosis of coronary arteries. The peak occurrence for such events is 15 to 45 days from the onset of illness. The current recommendation for therapy is aspirin 3 to 5 mg/k per day for 6 to 8 weeks. If the echocardiogram is normal at that time, the aspirin is discontinued; however, in the presence of dilation or aneurysms, the aspirin is continued until normal vessel lumen size is present. For patients with moderate-sized aneurysms, some clinicians add dipyridamole 3 to 6 mg/k per day in three divided doses[52] or clopidogrel 1 mg/kg per day in a single dose. These antiplatelet agents can be used as a substitute when aspirin is contraindicated. The presence of giant aneurysms places the patient at greater risk for coronary obstruction and subsequent myocardial infarction in the subacute phase.[107-109] Some clinicians have advocated the use of heparin in combination with salicylate therapy in this phase.[52] The long-term options include warfarin, warfarin with aspirin, or the use of two different antiplatelet agents; however, no prospective studies have addressed the appropriate therapeutic approach.

Thrombolytic therapy: On the basis of experience in adult patients with acute coronary thrombosis, thrombolytic therapy has been used in those with acute ischemic events or evolving myocardial infarction following Kawasaki disease. No prospective randomized study has been undertaken to assess the preferred thrombolytic medication because of the limited number of affected patients. Several reports detail the use of such agents in isolated cases.[110-112] Therapy should be instituted as soon as possible; however, even when initiated late, clinical outcomes may be satisfactory. After reperfusion of the affected vessel, anticoagulation is started with the combination of IV heparin and aspirin. This regimen is converted to warfarin in place of heparin for chronic therapy. The optimal therapy in this setting has not yet been determined.[113]

SURGICAL MANAGEMENT

Surgical experience involving revascularization is most extensive in Japan.[114] The decision to undertake coronary artery bypass surgery is generally based on a combination of factors, including evidence of reversible ischemia on stress-imaging tests, viable myocardium in the region of distribution of the affected vessel, and no evidence for severe disease distal to the site of the planned graft. The initial report of bypass grafting in Kawasaki disease involved the use of saphenous veins[115]; however, early failures, particularly among younger children, led to introduction of internal mammary artery grafts.[116] The experience to date has shown increases in the length and diameter of arterial grafts commensurate with somatic growth, as well as improvement in thallium stress testing compared with preoperative assessment. At 90 months following surgery, graft patency was 70% in children operated on when younger than 7 years of age, with 84% patency in those 8 years and older at surgery.

CATHETER INTERVENTION

The widespread experience in adults with the use of percutaneous transluminal coronary angioplasty (PTCA), rotational atherectomy (PTCRA), and stent placement for stenotic coronary lesions makes the applications in Kawasaki disease appealing. There has been limited evaluation of such techniques in children[117,118]; however, the most recent multi-institutional Japanese data show an early success rate for vessel dilation using PTCA to be 86%, PTCRA 96%, and stent placement 90%. At median follow-up (3.6 years, range 4 months to 6 years), restenosis occurred in 29% of arterial segments subjected to PTCA, 28% PTCRA, and 8% following stent implantation. Neoaneurysm formation after PTCA and PTCRA was detected in 6% and 7% of arterial segments, respectively, and believed to be related to the use of high inflation pressures necessary for the stiff arteries found in Kawasaki disease patients.[119]

CLINICAL COURSE

It is widely accepted that the coronary abnormalities in Kawasaki disease tend to regress over time; in one large study of 594 patients, regression occurred in 54% of those with aneurysms over a 13.6-year period, with 90% regressing within two years from the onset of illness.[68] Several investigators have suggested that the potential for aneurysm regression is determined by the initial size of the aneurysm, with smaller abnormalities more likely to improve.[108,121] Other factors related to aneurysm regression are age younger than 1 year at diagnosis, saccular aneurysm morphology, and distal aneurysm location.[81]

Persistent Coronary Artery Abnormalities

Although aneurysm dimension may regress, the prevalence of arterial stenosis increases linearly with time. In one series,[68] among those who eventually developed coronary artery stenoses, 50% had occurred within two years from the onset of illness. Another study reported a similar observation, with progressive stenotic changes over time and highest incidence in arteries with large aneurysms.[121] Giant aneurysms, those with a diameter greater than 8 mm, are at highest risk; stenoses commonly occur at the distal end of these lesions (Fig. 45-3) and, together with sluggish blood flow in the grossly dilated arterial segment, predispose to thrombosis and infarction. Relative to other size aneurysms, giant

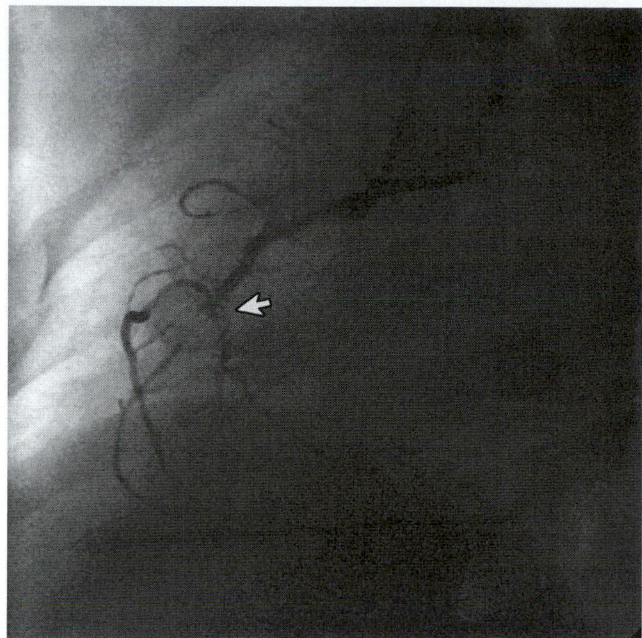

FIGURE 45-3. Calcified thrombotic right coronary artery giant aneurysm in a 10-year-old male diagnosed with Kawasaki disease at 1 year of age. The lesion is stenotic proximally *(arrow)* with recanalized distal vessels.

aneurysms are more frequently associated with late sudden death from infarction.[122-123] The clinical course of giant aneurysms as reported from several Japanese reviews is variable, with some indicating that progression to stenosis occurred in less than 50% of cases.[68,124] At the other extreme, in one series 71% of patients progressed to stenosis or obstruction within 11 months from illness onset, with rare regression.[120] Another series reported 90% occurrence of stenosis in the right or left anterior descending coronary arteries over 15 years from onset[121] and progression to stenosis in all aneurysms 9 mm or greater within 6 months.[125]

Myocardial infarction resulting from Kawasaki disease, though infrequent, is a source of great concern; in the largest series of cases from Japan, many were asymptomatic before their event.[126] Most (73%) had infarction in the initial year following onset of illness, and approximately 50% of infarctions occurred within the first 3 months. Symptoms were more common in those older than 4 years (83%) compared with younger children (17%) and included crying, chest pain, shock, abdominal pain, vomiting, dyspnea, and arrhythmia. Often, infarction occurred during rest or sleep rather than during exercise or play. The first episode was associated with a mortality rate of 22%, most often the result of obstruction of the left main coronary artery or of both the right and left anterior descending coronary arteries. Survivors tended to have involvement of a single artery other than the left main. Mortality rose to 62.5% after a second infarct and to nearly 100% in those with a third infarct. At later follow-up, a sizable proportion (41%) reported no symptoms. Left ventricular ejection fraction has been shown to improve over time in survivors.[127]

The management of patients with persistent aneurysms involves careful serial evaluation of left ventricular function and coronary artery status using both noninvasive and invasive modalities.[128-131] The methods employed for assessment have varied, with one report of normal coronary flow reserve determined by myocardial perfusion imaging in the majority of those with aneurysms.[132] However, other recent reports of noninvasive studies have shown altered myocardial flow reserve using positron emission spectroscopy[133] and abnormal responses to dobutamine infusion using isovolumic contraction, isovolumic relaxation, and ventricular ejection times to derive a systolic/diastolic myocardial performance index.[134] Flow velocity dynamics and coronary flow reserve have been evaluated invasively in patients using intracoronary Doppler flow guidewires, demonstrating flow abnormalities in those with moderate- to large-size aneurysms and in those with stenotic lesions of even mild degree.[135] There appears to be good correlation between invasive measurements of flow reserve in the right or left anterior descending coronary artery and the use of transthoracic Doppler to measure coronary flow velocity reserve in these vessels.[136-137] This technique would appear to have advantages in its application to younger children who are incapable of performing stress testing. More recently, coronary perfusion has been routinely assessed using adenosine stress during cardiac MRI.

Regressed Coronary Aneurysms

Regression of aneurysms occurs as a result of myointimal proliferation,[37,64,138] as identified at postmortem examination and with use of transluminal ultrasound.[139] Histologic examination of regressed aneurysms shows pathologic findings similar to those seen in atherosclerosis,[140] raising the concern that individuals with Kawasaki disease might be predisposed to early onset of coronary disease.[64,81]

Abnormal coronary artery function in regressed aneurysms has been demonstrated in a number of reports. During invasive studies, investigators have identified decreased vascular distensibility,[141] in addition to decreased vasodilator response to IV dipyridamole[142] and nitroglycerine.[143] In a large study of patients with Kawasaki disease receiving isosorbide dinitrate at catheterization, those segments with regressed aneurysms, as well as regions with persistent aneurysms, had diminished reactivity relative to coronary arteries that had never been dilated or to coronary arteries of control patients.[143-145] Furthermore, the decreased reactivity in abnormal areas progressed as duration from illness increased.

No Detectable Lesions

Because children who never have coronary aneurysms comprise the largest subset of patients following Kawasaki disease, data regarding long-term outcome is especially important. Pathologic evaluation is limited. In four children who died early in the acute phase of disease (9 to 22 days), all had inflammatory changes of the coronary arteries without dilation[138]; but it is not possible to determine if these arteries might have dilated had the children survived. In another series, five children who died of incidental causes following Kawasaki disease underwent postmortem examination.[64] Microscopic examination of the coronary arteries revealed intimal thickening and fibrosis indistinguishable from that of atherosclerosis, but correlation with clinical status was not possible.

The diffuse nature of the vasculitis seen in the acute phase of Kawasaki disease has prompted concern about the long-term impact on endothelial function. The absence of plasma 6-keto-prostaglandin F-1α, a metabolite of prostacyclin during the acute and subacute phases of the illness, supports abnormal endothelial cell function.[146] The presence of altered lipid metabolism also implies interference with endothelial cell function.[147] More recently, investigators have found decreased fibrinolytic activity in long-term survivors of Kawasaki disease both with known coronary abnormalities and with normal coronary anatomy.[148]

A study compared children with a history of Kawasaki disease and normal-appearing epicardial arteries to normal controls with regard to myocardial blood flow and flow reserve measured using positron emission tomography. Those with Kawasaki disease had lower myocardial reserve and higher total coronary resistance without regional perfusion abnormalities. The investigators suggest that the abnormal flow reserve and hyperemic blood flow are indicative of damage to the coronary microcirculation.[149] Invasive studies in children with Kawasaki disease and apparently normal epicardial arteries showed abnormal constriction with acetylcholine, an endothelium-dependent vasodilator, whereas response to nitroglycerin, an endothelium-independent vasodilator, was preserved.[150] These findings suggest abnormal endothelial function after Kawasaki disease even in those children in whom coronary dilation was never detected. Resistance coronary artery responses to acetylcholine were well preserved, suggesting normal endothelial and smooth muscle function in these arteries.

High-resolution ultrasound of the brachial artery has shown marked impairment of flow-mediated dilation in Kawasaki disease patients without coronary abnormalities, compared with controls, many years after the onset of disease.[151] Endothelial-independent responses were intact in both groups. These observations were supported by a similar study that showed abnormal hyperemia in brachial artery response among those with Kawasaki disease compared with controls.[152] Interestingly, there was marked improvement in endothelial function following infusion of IV vitamin C in the Kawasaki patients.

Overall, patients who have not had demonstrable coronary artery abnormalities have continued to do well clinically.[68,153] The long-term management of this group should include follow-up assessment every 3 to 5 years after the first year of illness. Particular attention should be paid to minimizing coronary risk factors by maintaining normal blood pressure and healthy dietary habits, assessing lipid profiles every 5 to 10 years, and encouraging routine exercise.

SUMMARY

Kawasaki disease is an acute vasculitis of uncertain etiology in children. Coronary artery aneurysms occur in 2% to 4% of individuals treated in the acute phase of the disease with the optimal regimen of IVIG 2 g/kg and aspirin. Many coronary aneurysms regress to normal lumen diameter by myointimal proliferation, but larger aneurysms may persist and can be associated with progressive stenosis leading to ischemia and myocardial infarction. The latter group needs intensive follow-up with regular stress testing to guide the need for invasive testing and catheter or surgical interventions. Because the long-term outlook for children with Kawasaki disease, both with and without detectable aneurysms, is uncertain, this patient population should be followed at regular intervals appropriate to the severity of their heart disease. Physician awareness is critical for identification and treatment of patients in the acute phase of the illness, as well as for provision of care to the growing population who had Kawasaki disease in childhood.

REFERENCES

1. Kawasaki T: [Acute febrile mucocutaneous syndrome with lymphoid involvement with specific desquamation of the fingers and toes in children]. Arerugi 16:178, 1967.
2. Tanaka N, Sekimoto K, Naoe S: Kawasaki disease: Relationship with infantile periarteritis nodosa. Arch Pathol Lab Med 100:81, 1976.
3. Hayasaka S, Nakamura Y, Yashiro M, et al: Analyses of fatal cases of Kawasaki disease in Japan using vital statistical data over 27 years. J Epidemiol 13:246, 2003.
4. Holman RC, Curns AT, Belay ED, et al: Kawasaki syndrome hospitalizations in the United States, 1997 and 2000. Pediatrics 112:495, 2003.
5. Davis RL, Waller PL, Mueller BA, et al: Kawasaki syndrome in Washington State: Race-specific incidence rates and residential proximity to water. Arch Pediatr Adolesc Med 149:66, 1995.
6. Stockheim JA, Innocentini N, Shulman ST: Kawasaki disease in older children and adolescents. J Pediatr 137:250, 2000.
7. Meissner HC, Leung DY: Superantigens, conventional antigens and etiology of Kawasaki syndrome. Pediatr Infect Dis J 19:91, 2000.
8. Leung DY, Meissner HC, Shulman ST, et al: Prevalence of superantigen-secreting bacteria in patients with Kawasaki disease. J Pediatr 140:742, 2002.
9. Curtis N, Zheng R, Lamb JR, et al: Evidence for a superantigen mediated process in Kawasaki disease. Arch Dis Child 72:308, 1995.
10. Duong TT, Silverman ED, Bissessar MV, et al: Superantigenic activity is responsible for induction of coronary arteritis in mice: An animal model of Kawasaki disease. Int Immunol 15:79, 2003.
11. Rowley AH, Eckerley CA, Jack HM, et al: IgA plasma cells in vascular tissue of patients with Kawasaki syndrome. J Immunol 159:5946, 1997.
12. Rowley AH, Shulman ST, Mask CA, et al: IgA plasma cell infiltration of proximal respiratory tract, pancreas, kidney, coronary artery in acute Kawasaki disease. J Infect Dis 182:1183, 2000.
13. Furukawa S, Matsubara T, Yabuta K: Mononuclear cell subsets and coronary artery lesions in Kawasaki disease. Arch Dis Child 67:706, 1992.
14. Leung DY: Immunologic abnormalities in Kawasaki syndrome. Prog Clin Biol Res 250:159, 1987.
15. Abe J, Kotzin BL, Jujo K, et al: Selective expansion of T cells expressing T-cell receptor variable regions V beta 2 and V beta 8 in Kawasaki disease. Proc Natl Acad Sci U S A 89:4066, 1992.
16. Abe J, Kotzin BL, Meissner C, et al: Characterization of T cell repertoire changes in acute Kawasaki disease. J Exp Med 177:791, 1993.
17. Yamashiro Y, Nagata, Oguchi S, et al: Selective increase of Vβ2+ cells in the small intestional mucosa in Kawasaki disease. Pediatr Res 39:264, 1996.
18. Yoshioka T, Matsutani T, Iwagami S, et al: Polyclonal expansion of TCRβ V2 and TCRβ V6-bearing T cells in patients with Kawasaki disease. Immunology 96:465, 1999.
19. Leung DYM, Giorno R, Kazemi LV, et al: Evidence for superantigen involvement in cardiovascular injury due to Kawasaki syndrome. J Immunol 155:5018, 1995.

20. Brogan PA, Shah V, Klein N, et al: T cell Vβ repertoires in childhood vasculitides. Clin Exp Immunol 131:517, 2003.
21. Leung DY, Collins T, Lapierre LA, et al: Immunoglobulin M antibodies present in the acute phase of Kawasaki syndrome lyse cultured vascular endothelial cells stimulated by gamma interferon. J Clin Invest 77:1428, 1986.
22. Leung DY, Geha RS, Newburger JW, et al: Two monokines, interleukin-1 and tumor necrosis factor, render cultured vascular endothelial cells susceptible to lysis by antibodies circulating during Kawasaki syndrome. J Exp Med 164:1958, 1986.
23. Suzuki H, Uemura S, Tone S, et al: Effects of immunoglobulin and gamma-interferon on the production of tumour necrosis factor-alpha and interleukin-1-β by peripheral blood monocytes in the acute phase of Kawasaki disease. Eur J Pediatr 155:291, 1996.
24. Fujieda M, Oishi N, Kurashige T: Antibodies to endothelial cells in Kawasaki disease lyse endothelial cells without cytokine pretreatment. Clin Exp Immunol 107:120, 1997.
25. Hashimoto H, Igarashi N, Yachie A, et al: The relationship between serum levels of interleukin-6 and thyroid hormone during the follow-up study in children with nonthyroidal illness: Marked inverse correlation in Kawasaki and infectious disease. Endocrine 43:31, 1996.
26. Hirao J, Hibi S, Andoh T, et al: High levels of circulating interleukin-4 and interleukin-10 in Kawasaki disease. Int Arch Allergy Immunol 112:152, 1997.
27. Kim DS, Lee KY: Serum soluble E-selectin levels in Kawasaki disease. Scand J Rheumatol 23:283, 1994.
28. Mayatepek E, Lehmann WD: Increased generation of cysteinyl leukotrienes in Kawasaki disease. Arch Dis Child 72:526, 1995.
29. Terai M, Yasukawa K, Narumoto S, et al: Vascular endothelial growth factor in acute Kawasaki disease. Am J Cardiol 83:337, 1999.
30. Hirose S, Hamashima Y: Morphological observations on the vasculitis in the mucocutaneous lymph node syndrome: A skin biopsy study of 27 patients. Eur J Pediatr 129:215, 1978.
31. Fukumura D, Gohongi T, Kadambi A, et al: Predominant role of endothelial nitric oxide synthase in vascular endothelial growth factor-induced angiogenesis and vascular permeability. Proc Natl Acad Sci U S A 98:2604, 2001.
32. Iizuka T, Oishi K, Sasaki M, et al: Nitric oxide and aneurysm formation in Kawasaki disease. Acta Paediatr 86:470, 1997.
33. Terai M, Honda T, Yasukawa K, et al: Prognostic impact of vascular leakage in acute Kawasaki disease. Circulation 108:325, 2003.
34. Longo GM, Xiong W, Greiner TC, et al: Matrix metalloproteinases 2 and 9 work in concert to produce aortic aneurysms. J Clin Invest 110:625, 2002.
35. Senzaki H, Masutani S, Kobayashi J, et al: Circulating matrix metalloproteinases and their inhibitors in patients with Kawasaki disease. Circulation 104:860, 2001.
36. Gavin PJ, Crawford SE, Shulman ST, et al: Systemic arterial expression of matrix metalloproteinases 2 and 9 in acute Kawasaki disease. Arterioscler Thromb Vasc Biol 23:576, 2003.
37. Fujiwara H, Hamashima Y: Pathology of the heart in Kawasaki disease. Pediatrics 61:100, 1978.
38. Burns JC, Glode MP, Clarke SH, et al: Coagulopathy and platelet activation in Kawasaki syndrome: Identification of patients at high risk for development of artery aneurysms. J Pediatr 105:206, 1984.
39. Kawasaki T, Kosaki F, Okawa S, et al: A new infantile acute febrile mucocutaneous lymph node syndrome (MLNS) prevailing in Japan. Pediatrics 54:271, 1974.
40. Anonymous: Diagnostic guidelines for Kawasaki disease. Circulation 103:335, 2001.
41. Burns JC, Wiggins J, Jr, Toews WH, et al: Clinical spectrum of Kawasaki disease in infants younger than 6 months of age. J Pediatr 109:759, 1986.
42. Schuh S, Laxer RM, Smallhorn JF, et al: Kawasaki disease with atypical presentation. Pediatr Infect Dis 7:201, 1988.
43. Rowley AH, Gonzalez Crussi F, et al: Incomplete Kawasaki disease with coronary artery involvement. J Pediatr 110:409, 1987.
44. Fukushige N, Takahashi N, Ueda K, et al: Incidence and clinical features of incomplete Kawasaki disease. Acta Pediatr 83:1057, 1994.
45. Burns JC, Mason JW, Glode MP, et al: Clinical and epidemiological characteristics of patients referred for evaluation of possible Kawasaki disease. J Pediatr 118:680, 1991.
46. Burns JC, Joffe L, Sargent RA, et al: Anterior uveitis associated with Kawasaki syndrome. Pediatr Infect Dis 4:258, 1985.
47. Rauch AM: Kawasaki syndrome: Critical review of U.S. epidemiology. Prog Clin Biol Res 250:33, 1987.
48. Sty JR, Starshak RJ, Gorenstein L: Gallbladder perforation in a case of Kawasaki disease: Image correlation. J Clin Ultrasound 11:381, 1983.
49. Dengler LD, Capparelli EV, Bastian JF, et al: Cerebrospinal fluid profile in patients with acute Kawasaki disease. J Pediatr Infect Dis 17:478, 1998.
50. Research Committee on Kawasaki Disease: Report of subcommittee on standardization of diagnostic criteria and reporting of coronary artery lesions in Kawasaki disease. Tokyo: Ministry of Health and Welfare, 1984.
51. Kato H, Ichinose E, Yoshioka F, et al: Fate of coronary aneurysms in Kawasaki disease: Serial coronary angiography and long-term follow-up study. Am J Cardiol 49:1758, 1982.
52. Asai T: [Diagnosis and prognosis of coronary artery lesions in Kawasaki disease. Coronary angiography and the conditions for its application (a score chart)]. Nippon Rinsho 41:2080, 1983 (Jpn).
53. Koren G, Lavi S, Rose V, et al: Kawasaki disease: Review of risk factors for coronary aneurysms. J Pediatr 108:388, 1986.
54. Daniels SR, Specker B, Cappanari TE, et al: Correlates of coronary artery aneurysm formation in patients with Kawasaki disease. Am J Dis Child 141:205, 1987.
55. Nakano M: Predictive factors of coronary aneurysm in Kawasaki disease—correlation between coronary arterial lesions and serum albumin, cholinesterase activity, prealbumin, retinal-binding protein and immature neutrophils. Prog Clin Biol Res 250:535, 1987.
56. Newburger JW, Takahashi M, Burns JC, et al: The treatment of Kawasaki syndrome with intravenous gamma globulin. N Engl J Med 315:341, 1986.
57. Beiser AS, Takahashi M, Baker AL, et al: A predictive instrument for coronary artery aneurysms in Kawasaki disease. U.S. Multicenter Kawasaki Disease Study Group. Am J Cardiol 81:1116, 1998.
58. Harada K, Yamaguchi H, Kato H, et al: Indication for intravenous gamma globulin for treatment for Kawasaki disease. In Takahashi M, Taubert K (eds). Proceedings of the Fourth International Symposium on Kawasaki disease. Dallas: American Heart Association, 1993, p 459.
59. Yutani C, Okano K, Kamiya T, et al: Histopathological study on right endomyocardial biopsy of Kawasaki disease. Br Heart J 43:589, 1980.
60. Matsuura H, Ishikita T, Yamamoto S, et al: Gallium-67 myocardial imaging for the detection of myocarditis in the acute phase of Kawasaki disease (mucocutaneous lymph node syndrome): The use of single photon emission computed tomography. Br Heart J 58:385, 1987.
61. Kao CH, Hsieh KS, Wang YL, et al: Tc-99m MHPAO WBC imaging to detect carditis and evaluate the results of high-dose gamma globulin treatment in Kawasaki disease. Clin Nucl Med 17:623, 1992.
62. Kao CH, Hsieh KS, Wang YL, et al: Tc-99m HMPAO labeled WBC scan for the detection of myocarditis in different phases of Kawasaki disease. Clin Nucl Med 17:185, 1992.
63. Moran AM, Newburger JW, Sanders SP, et al: Abnormal myocardial mechanics in Kawasaki disease: Rapid response to gamma-globulin. Am Heart J 139:217, 2000.
64. Tanaka N, Naoe S, Masuda H, et al: Pathological study of sequelae of Kawasaki disease (MCLS): With special reference to the heart and coronary arterial lesions. Acta Pathol Jpn 36:1513, 1986.
65. Hiraishi S, Yahiro K, Oguchi K, et al: Clinical course of cardiovascular involvement in the mucocutaneous lymph node syndrome: Relation between clinical signs of carditis and development of coronary arterial aneurysm. Am J Cardiol 47:323, 1981.
66. Chung KJ, Brandt L, Fulton DR, et al: Cardiac and coronary arterial involvement in infants and children from New England with mucocutaneous lymph node syndrome (Kawasaki disease): Angiographic-echocardiographic correlations. Am J Cardiol 50:136, 1982.
67. Newburger JW, Sanders SP, Burns JC, et al: Left ventricular contractility and function in Kawasaki syndrome: Effect of intravenous gamma globulin. Circulation 79:1237, 1989.
68. Kato H, Sugimura T, Akagi T, et al: Long-term consequences of Kawasaki disease. A 10 to 21 year follow-up study of 594 patients. Circulation 94:1379, 1996.
69. Nakano H, Nojima K, Saito A, et al: High incidence of aortic regurgitation following Kawasaki disease. J Pediatr 107:59, 1985.

70. Gidding SS: Late onset valvular dysfunction in Kawasaki disease. Prog Clin Biol Res 250:305, 1987.
71. Gidding SS, Shulman ST, Ilbawi M, et al: Mucocutaneous lymph node syndrome (Kawasaki disease): Delayed aortic and mitral insufficiency secondary to active valvulitis. J Am Coll Cardiol 7:894, 1986.
72. Ravekes WJ, Colan SD, Gauvreau K, et al: Aortic root dilation in Kawasaki disease. Am J Cardiol 87:919, 2001.
73. Burns JC, Mason WH, Glode MP, et al: Clinical and epidemiologic characteristics of patients referred for evaluation of possible Kawasaki disease. United States Multicenter Kawasaki Disease Study Group. J Pediatr 118:680, 1991.
74. Melish ME: Kawasaki syndrome: A 1986 perspective. Rheum Dis Clin North Am 13:7, 1987.
75. Ting EC, Capparelli EV, Billman GF, et al: Elevated gamma-glutaryltransferase concentrations in patients with acute Kawasaki disease. Pediatr Infect Dis J 17:431, 1998.
76. Capannari TE, Daniels SR, Meyer RA, et al: Sensitivity, specificity and predictive value of two-dimensional echocardiography in detecting coronary artery aneurysms in patients with Kawasaki disease. J Am Coll Cardiol 7:355, 1986.
77. de Zorzi A, Colan SD, Gauvreau K, et al: Coronary dimensions may be misclassified as normal in Kawasaki disease. J Pediatr 133:254, 1998.
78. Arjunan K, Daniels SR, Meyer RA, et al: Coronary artery caliber in normal children and patients with Kawasaki disease but without aneurysm: An echocardiographic and angiographic study. J Am Coll Cardiol 8:1119, 1986.
79. Kurotobi S, Nagai T, Kawakami N, et al: Coronary diameter in normal infants, children and patients with Kawasaki disease. Pediatr Int 44:1, 2002.
80. Suzuki A, Kamiya T, Kuwahara N, et al: Coronary arterial lesions of Kawasaki disease: Cardiac catheterization findings of 1100 cases. Pediatr Cardiol 7:3, 1986.
81. Takahashi M, Mason W, Lewis AB: Regression of coronary aneurysms in patients with Kawasaki syndrome. Circulation 75:387, 1987.
82. Takahashi M, Mason W, Thomas D, et al: Reye syndrome following Kawasaki syndrome confirmed by liver histopathology. In Kato H (ed): Kawasaki disease proceedings of the 5th International Kawasaki Disease Symposium, Fukuoka, Japan, May 22-25, 1995. Amsterdam: Elsevier Science BV, 1995, p 436.
83. Matsubara T, Mason W, Kashani IA, et al: Gastrointestinal hemorrhage complicating aspirin therapy in acute Kawasaki disease. J Pediatr 128:701, 1996.
84. Durongpisitkul K, Gururaj VJ, Park JM, et al: The prevention of coronary artery aneurysm in Kawasaki disease: A meta-analysis on the efficacy of aspirin and immunoglobulin treatment. Pediatrics 96:1057, 1995.
85. Furusho K, Kamiya T, Nakano H, et al: High-dose intravenous gammaglobulin for Kawasaki disease. Lancet ii;1055, 1984.
86. Barron KS, Murphy DJ, Silverman ED, et al: Treatment of Kawasaki syndrome: A comparison of two dosage regimens of intravenously administered immune globulin. J Pediatr 117:638, 1990.
87. Morikawa Y, Ohashi Y, Harada K, et al: A multicenter, randomized, controlled trial of intravenous gamma globulin therapy in children with acute Kawasaki Disease. Acta Paediatr Jpn 36:347,1994.
88. Nagashima M, Matsushima M, Matsuoka H, et al: High-dose gammaglobulin therapy for Kawasaki disease. J Pediatr 110:710,1987.
89. Newburger JW, Takahashi M, Beiser AS, et al: A single intravenous infusion of gamma globulin as compared with four infusions in the treatment of acute Kawasaki syndrome. N Engl J Med 324:1633, 1991.
90. American Academy of Pediatrics. In Pickering LK (ed): Kawasaki Disease. Red Book: Report of the Committee on Infectious Disease, ed 26. Elk Grove Village, IL: American Academy of Pediatrics, 2003, p 394.
91. Burns JC, Glode MP, Caparelli E, et al: Intravenous gammaglobulin treatment in Kawasaki syndrome: Are all brands equal? In Kato H (ed): Kawasaki disease proceedings of the 5th International Kawasaki Disease Symposium, Fukuoka, Japan. Amsterdam: Elsevier Science BV, 1995, p 296.
92. Silverman ED, Huang C, Rose V, et al: IVGG treatment of Kawasaki disease: Are all brands equal? In Kato H (ed): Kawasaki disease proceedings of the 5th International Kawasaki Disease Symposium, Fukuoka, Japan. Amsterdam: Elsevier Science BV, 1995, p 301.
93. Rosenfeld EA, Shulman ST, Corydon KE, et al: Comparative safety and efficacy of two immune globulin products in Kawasaki disease. In Kato H (ed): Kawasaki disease proceedings of the 5th International Kawasaki Disease Symposium, Fukuoka, Japan. Amsterdam: Elsevier Science BV, 1995, p 291.
94. Schneider LC, Geha R, et al: Outbreak of hepatitis C associated with IVGG administration—U.S., October 1993-June 1994. Mor Mortal Wkly Rep CDC Surveill Summ 43:505, 1994.
95. Dajani AS, Taubert KA, Takahashi M, et al: Guidelines for long-term management of patients with Kawasaki disease. Report from the committee on Rheumatic Fever, Endocarditis, and Kawasaki Disease, Council on Cardiovascular Disease in the Young, American Heart Association. Circulation 89:916, 1994.
96. Tse, SML, Silverman ED, McCrindle B, et al: Early treatment with intravenous immunoglobulin in patients with Kawasaki disease. J Pediatr 140:450, 2002.
97. Marasini M, Pongiglione G, Gazzolo D, et al: Late intravenous gamma globulin treatment in infants and children with Kawasaki Disease and coronary artery abnormalities. Am J Cardiol 68:796, 1991.
98. Kato H, Koike S, Yokoyama T: Kawasaki disease: Effect of treatment on coronary artery involvement. Pediatrics 63:175, 1979.
99. Shinohara M, Sone K, Tomomasa T, et al: Corticosteroids in the treatment of the acute phase of Kawasaki disease. J Pediatr 135:465, 1999.
100. Sundel RP, Baker AL, Fulton DR, et al: Corticosteroids in the initial treatment of Kawasaki disease: Report of a randomized trial. J Pediatr 142:611, 2003.
101. Hashino K, Ishii M, Iemura M, et al: Re-treatment for immune globulin-resistant Kawasaki disease: A comparative study of additional immune globulin and steroid pulse therapy. Pediatrics Inter 43:211, 2001.
102. Villain E, Kachaner J, Sidi D, et al: Trial of prevention of coronary aneurysms in Kawasaki's syndrome using plasma exchange of infusion of immunoglobulins [French]. Arch Fr Pediatr 44:79, 1987.
103. Furukawa S, Matsubara T, Umezawa Y, et al: Pentoxifylline and intravenous gamma globulin combination therapy for acute Kawasaki disease. Eur J Pediatr 153:663, 1994.
104. Etheridge S, Tani L, Minich L, et al: Platelet glycoprotein IIb/IIIa receptor blockade therapy for large coronary aneurysms and thrombi in Kawasaki disease. Catheter Cardiovasc Diagn 45:264, 1998.
105. Foster RH, Wiseman LR: Abciximab: An updated review of its use in ischaemic heart disease. Drugs 56:629, 1998.
106. Williams RV, Wilke VM, Tani LY, et al: Does abciximab enhance regression of coronary aneurysms resulting from Kawasaki disease? Pediatrics 109:E4, 2002.
107. Fujiwara R, Fujiwara H, Hamashima Y: Size of coronary aneurysm as a determinant factor of the prognosis in Kawasaki disease: Clinicopathologic study of coronary aneurysms. Prog Clin Biol Res 250:519, 1987.
108. Tatara K, Kusakawa S: Long-term prognosis of giant coronary aneurysm in Kawasaki disease: An angiographic study. J Pediatr 111:705, 1987.
109. Nakano H, Saito A, Ueda K, et al: Clinical characteristics of myocardial infarction following Kawasaki disease: Report of 11 cases. J Pediatr 108:198, 1986.
110. Cheatham JP, Kugler JD, Gumbiner CH, et al: Intracoronary streptokinase in Kawasaki disease: Acute and thrombolysis. Prog Clin Biol Res 250:517, 1987.
111. Levy M, Benson LN, Burrows PE: Tissue plasminogen activator for the treatment of thromboembolism in infants and children. J Pediatr 118:467, 1991.
112. Kato H, Ichinose E, Inoue O, et al: Intracoronary thrombolytic therapy in Kawasaki disease: Treatment and prevention of acute myocardial infarction. Prog Clin Biol Res 250:445, 1987.
113. Terai M, Ogata M, Sugimoto K, et al: Coronary arterial thrombi in Kawasaki disease. J Pediatr 106:76, 1985.
114. Suzuki A, Kamiya T, Ono Y, et al: Indication for of aortocoronary bypass for coronary arterial obstruction due to Kawasaki disease. Heart Vessels 1:94, 1985.
115. Takeuchi Y, Suma K, Shiroma K, et al: Surgical experience with coronary arterial sequelae of Kawasaki disease in children. J Cardiovasc Surg 22:231, 1981.

116. Kitamura S, Kameda Y, Seki T, et al: Long-term outcome of myocardial revascularization in patients with Kawasaki coronary artery disease: A multi-center cooperative study. J Thorac Cardiovasc Surg 107:663, 1994.
117. Ino T, Akimoto K, Ohkubo M, et al: Application of percutaneous transluminal coronary angioplasty to coronary arterial stenosis in Kawasaki disease. Circulation 93:1709, 1996.
118. Sugimura T, Yokoi H, Sato N, et al: Interventional treatment for children with severe coronary artery stenosis with calcification after long-term Kawasaki disease. Circulation 96:3928,1997.
119. Ishii M, Ueno T, Ikeda, et al: Sequential follow-up results of catheter intervention for coronary artery lesions after Kawasaki disease: Quantitative coronary artery angiography and intravascular ultrasound imaging study. Circulation 105:3004, 2002.
120. Nakano H, Ueda K, Saito A, et al: Repeated quantitative angiograms in coronary arterial aneurysm in Kawasaki disease. Am J Cardiol 56:846, 1985.
121. Kamiya T, Suzuki A, Ono Y, et al: Angiographic follow-up study of coronary artery lesions in the cases with a history of Kawasaki disease—with a focus on the follow-up more than ten years after the onset of disease. Kawasaki Disease. In Kato H (ed): Proceedings of the 5th International Kawasaki Disease Symposium, Fukuoka, Japan, May 22-25 1995. Amsterdam: Elsevier Science BV, 1995, p 569.
122. Nakano H, Saito A, Ueda K, et al: Clinical characteristics of myocardial infarction following Kawasaki disease: Report of 11 cases. J Pediatr 108:198, 1986.
123. Fujiwara T, Fujiwara H, Hamashima Y: Frequency and size of coronary arterial aneurysm at necropsy in Kawasaki disease. Am J Cardiol 59:808, 1987.
124. Tatara K, Kusakawa S: Long term prognosis of giant coronary aneurysms in Kawasaki disease. Prog Clin Biol Res 250:579, 1987.
125. Suzuki A, Kamiya T, Arakaki Y, et al: Fate of coronary arterial aneurysms in Kawasaki disease. Am J Cardiol 74:822, 1994.
126. Kato H, Ichinose E, Kawasaki T: Myocardial infarction in Kawasaki disease: Clinical analyses in 195 cases. J Pediatr 108:923, 1986.
127. Suzuki A, Kamiya T, Ono Y, et al: Myocardial ischemia in Kawasaki disease: Follow-up study by cardiac catheterization and coronary angiography. Pediatr Cardiol 9:1, 1988.
128. Fukuda T, Akagi R, Ishibashi M, et al: Noninvasive evaluation of myocardial ischemia in Kawasaki disease: Comparison between dipyridamole stress thallium imaging and exercise stress testing. Am Heart J 135:482, 1998.
129. Kimball TR, Witt SA, Daniels SR: Dobutamine stress echocardiography in the assessment of suspected myocardial ischemia in children and young adults. Am J Cardiol 79:380, 1997.
130. Noto N, Ayusawa M, Karasawa K, et al: Dobutamine stress echocardiography for detection of coronary artery stenosis in children with Kawasaki disease. J Am Coll Cardiol 27:1251, 1996.
131. Pahl E, Sehgal R, Chrystof D, et al: Feasibility of exercise stress echocardiography for follow-up of children with coronary involvement secondary to Kawasaki disease. Circulation 91:122, 1996.
132. Hijazi ZM, Udelson JE, Snapper, et al: Physiologic significance of chronic coronary aneurysms in patients with Kawasaki disease. J Am Coll Cardiol 24:1633, 1994.
133. Furuyama H, Odagawa Y, Katoh C, et al: Altered myocardial flow reserve and endothelial function late after Kawasaki disease. J Pediatr 142:149, 2003.
134. Harada K, Tamura M, Toyono M, et al: Effect of dobutamine on a Doppler echocardiographic index of combined systolic and diastolic performance. Pediatr Cardiol 23:613, 2002.
135. Hamaoka K, Onouchi Z, Kamiya Y, et al: Evaluation of coronary arterial flow-velocity dynamics and flow reserve in patients with Kawasaki disease by means of a Doppler guide wire. J Am Coll Cardiol 31;833, 1998.
136. Hiraishi S, Hirota H, Horiguchi Y, et al: Transthoracic Doppler assessment of coronary flow velocity reserve in children with Kawasaki disease: Comparison with coronary angiography and thallium-201 imaging. J Am Coll Cardiol 40:1816, 2002.
137. Noto N, Karasawa K, Kanamaru H, et al: Non-invasive measurement of coronary flow reserve in children with Kawasaki disease. Br Heart J 87:559, 2002.
138. Fujiwara T, Fujiwara H, Nakano H: Pathological features of coronary arteries in children with Kawasaki disease in which coronary arterial aneurysm was absent at autopsy: Quantitative analysis. Circulation 78:345, 1988.
139. Sugimura T, Kato H, Inoue O, et al: Intravascular ultrasound of coronary arteries in children: Assessment of the wall morphology and the lumen after Kawasaki disease. Circulation 89:258, 1994.
140. Sasaguri Y, Kato H: Regression of aneurysms in Kawasaki disease: A pathological study. J Pediatr 100:225, 1982.
141. Kurisu Y, Azumi T, Sughara T, et al: Variation in coronary artery dimensions (distensible abnormality) after disappearing aneurysm in Kawasaki disease. Am Heart J 114:532, 1987.
142. Matsumura K, Okuda Y, Ito T, et al: Coronary angiography of Kawasaki disease with the coronary vasodilator dipyridamole: Assessment of distensibility of affected coronary arterial wall. Angiology 39:141, 1988.
143. Spevak PJ, Newburger JW, Keane J, et al: Reactivity of coronary arteries in Kawasaki syndrome: An analysis of function [abstract]. Am J Cardiol 60:640, 1987.
144. Sugimura T, Kato H, Inoue O, et al: Vasodilatory response of the coronary arteries after Kawasaki disease: Evaluation by intracoronary injection of isosorbide dintrate. J Pediatr 121:684, 1992.
145. Iemura M, Ishii M, Sugimura T, et al: Long term consequences of regressed coronary aneurysms after Kawasaki disease: Vascular wall morphology and function. Br Heart J 83:307, 2000.
146. Fulton DR, Meissner HC, Peterson MB: Effects of current therapy of Kawasaki disease on eiconsanoid metabolism. Am J Cardiol 61:1323, 1988.
147. Newburger JW, Burns JC, Shen G, et al: Altered lipid metabolism following Kawasaki syndrome. Circulation 76:515, 1987.
148. Albisetti M, Chan A, McCrindle B, et al: Fibrinolytic response to venous occlusion is decreased in patients after Kawasaki disease. Blood Coagul Fibrinolysis 14:181, 2003.
149. Muzik O, Paridon SM, Singh TP, et al: Quantification of myocardial blood flow and flow reserve in children with a history of Kawasaki disease and normal coronary arteries using positron emission tomography. J Am Coll Cardiol 28:757, 1996.
150. Mitani Y, Okuda Y, Shimpo H, et al: Impaired endothelial function in epicardial coronary arteries after Kawasaki disease. Circulation 96:454, 1997.
151. Dhillon R, Clarkson P, Donald A, et al. Endothelial dysfunction late after Kawasaki disease. Circulation 94:2103, 1996.
152. Deng YB, Li TL, Xiang HJ, et al: Impaired endothelial function in the brachial artery after Kawasaki disease and the effects of intravenous administration of vitamin C. Pediatr Infect Dis J 22:34, 2003.
153. Nakamura Y, Yanagawa H, Harada K, et al: Mortality among persons with a history of Kawasaki disease in Japan: The fifth look. Arch Pediatr Adolesc Med 156:162, 2002.

chapter 46

Acute Arterial Occlusion

Kenneth Ouriel

Acute limb ischemia occurs when an extremity is suddenly deprived of adequate blood flow. Symptoms depend on the severity of hypoperfusion. Acute limb ischemia is distinguished from chronic limb ischemia, which is characterized by an insidious onset of symptoms and late presentation of patients after such onset.

In mild cases of limb ischemia, the patient may experience symptoms only with increased muscular demand (e.g., claudication during ambulation). Patients with symptoms of claudication alone are at low risk for amputation, even without treatment. Alternatively, inadequate oxygen delivery occurs even without activity when hypoperfusion is severe. Such patients experience pain at rest and particularly at night, so-called "limb-threatening" symptoms, a situation associated with significant risks of limb loss and even death if the hypoperfusion progresses unchecked (Table 46-1).

The aim of this chapter is to outline the pathophysiology, diagnosis, treatment, and expected clinical outcome of patients with acute limb ischemia—defined for the purposes of discussion as ischemia of 14 days' duration or less.

PATHOPHYSIOLOGY

Acute limb ischemia may occur as the result of embolization or in situ thrombosis (Box 46-1). Emboli originate from the heart in more than 90% of cases and normally lodge at the site of an arterial bifurcation such as the distal common femoral or popliteal arteries.[4,5] The decreasing prevalence of rheumatic heart disease underlies a diminishing proportion of embolic versus thrombotic causes for acute limb ischemia. When embolization occurs, it usually does so in the setting of atrial fibrillation or acute myocardial infarction, when portions of atrial or ventricular mural thrombus detach and embolize to the arterial tree.

Thrombosis as an etiology for acute limb ischemia is a much more diverse category than embolization (Fig. 46-1A-C). With the increased use of peripheral arterial bypass grafts for chronic limb ischemia, and noting the finite patency rate of any bypass graft conduit, it is not surprising that acute graft occlusion is now the most frequent cause of acute lower extremity ischemia in most centers.[1,3,6]

Irrespective of the etiology of ischemia, the end result is the accumulation of toxic byproducts within the ischemic tissue bed. These toxins include the oxygen-derived free radicals, chemically reactive molecules that are responsible for the injury that occurs after ischemia and reperfusion. Ischemia induces leakage of protein and fluid from the capillary bed, resulting in tissue edema.[7] Hydrodynamic pressure in the extravascular space rises to a level that competes with venous outflow, perpetuating a viscous cycle that can eventually impede arterial inflow. At first, this process occurs at a microscopic

TABLE 46-1 OUTCOME OF PATIENTS PRESENTING WITH ACUTE LIMB ISCHEMIA—MORBIDITY AND MORTALITY DEPEND ON SEVERITY OF ISCHEMIA

Study	Year Published	Severity of Ischemia	Amputation Rate	In-Hospital Mortality Rate
Rochester	1994	Class 2B	14%	18%
STILE	1994	Class 1, 2A, 2B	5%	6%
TOPAS	1998	Class 2A, 2B	2%	5%

STILE, Surgery or Thrombolysis for the Ischemic Lower Extremity; TOPAS, Thrombolysis Or Peripheral Arterial Surgery trial.[1-3]

BOX 46-1 Classification of Acute Limb Ischemia

Bypass graft occlusion
- Prosthetic conduit
  - Intimal hyperplasia at the anastomoses (usually distal)
  - Occlusion without a demonstrable lesion
- Autogenous conduit (e.g., saphenous vein graft)
  - Retained valve cusp of an in situ graft
  - Stenosis at the site of a prior venous injury (e.g., superficial phlebitis)

Native arterial occlusion
- Thrombosis at the site of an atherosclerotic stenotic lesion
- Embolism to an arterial bifurcation
- Thrombosis within a near-normal artery, usually as the result of a hypercoagulable state
- Arterial inflammatory diseases such as giant cell arteritis or thromboangiitis obliterans
- Thrombosis of an aneurysm (e.g., popliteal artery aneurysm)
- Rare etiologies (popliteal entrapment syndrome, adventitial cystic disease of the popliteal artery)

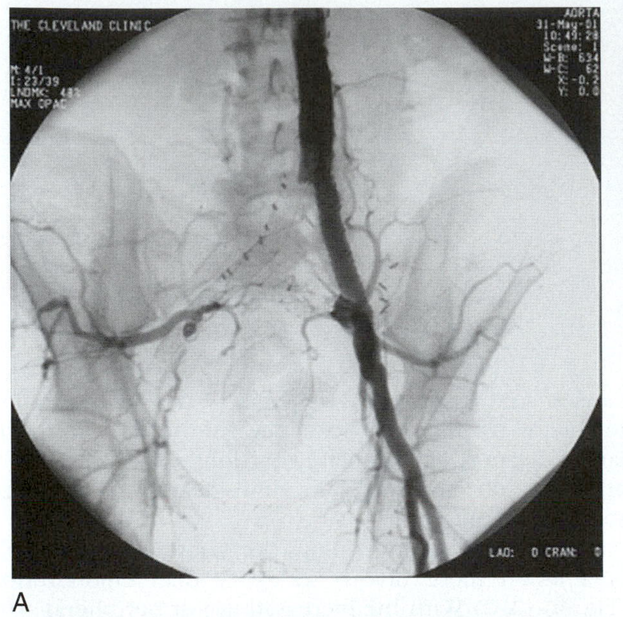

A

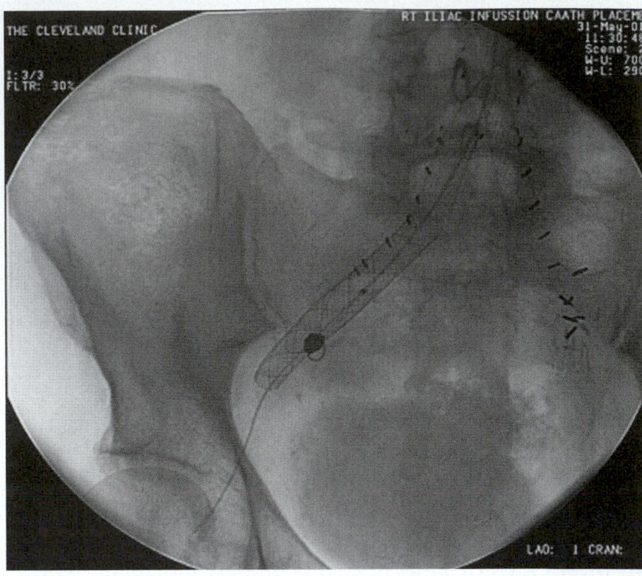

B

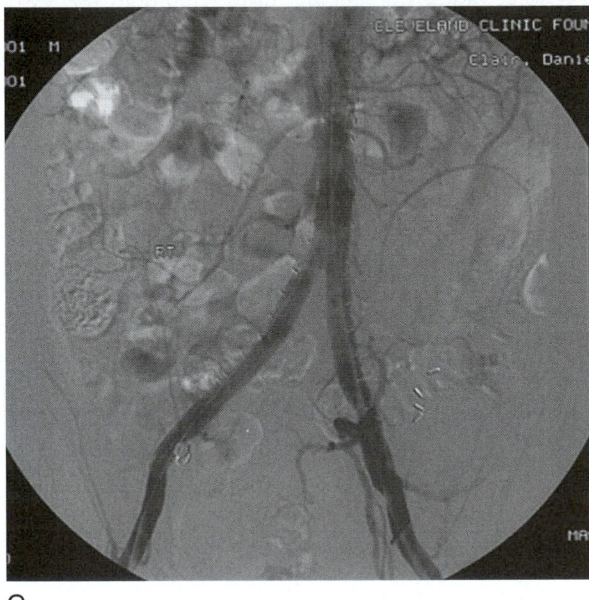

C

FIGURE 46-1. A, Occlusion of the right limb of an aortic endograft. **B,** Placement of a wire and infusion catheter into the occluded right iliac graft limb. **C,** The recanalized right iliac limb, demonstrating a probable stenosis at the origin of the limb.

level, but it may progress to the development of high tissue pressures at a regional level and the clinical entity known as *compartment syndrome.* The development of compartment syndrome is hastened by the abrupt reperfusion of a previously ischemic tissue bed, a phenomenon that explains the relatively frequent need for fasciotomy after intervention for severe limb ischemia (Fig. 46-2).[8,9]

DIAGNOSIS

Acute limb ischemia is a clinical diagnosis. Patients complain of numbness and pain in the extremity, progressing in severe cases to motor loss and muscle rigidity. Examination reveals the absence of palpable pulses, and the location of the pulse deficit allows one to predict the site of arterial occlusion. The "5-Ps" have been used as a mnemonic to remember the presentation of a patient with acute limb ischemia: paresthesia, pain, pallor, pulselessness, and paralysis. In some cases, a sixth "P" is added—"poikilothermia," meaning equilibration of the temperature of the limb to that of the ambient environment (coolness), resulting from a loss of temperature regulation. Inexperienced observers sometimes confuse this process with deep venous thrombosis (DVT). Although DVT may manifest as limb ischemia when severe (phlegmasia cerulea dolens), profound lower extremity edema is uncommon in pure arterial ischemia. Occasionally, a patient with arterial ischemia and pain at rest keeps the extremity in a dependent position and edema may develop; such a scenario is apparent if an adequate history is obtained.

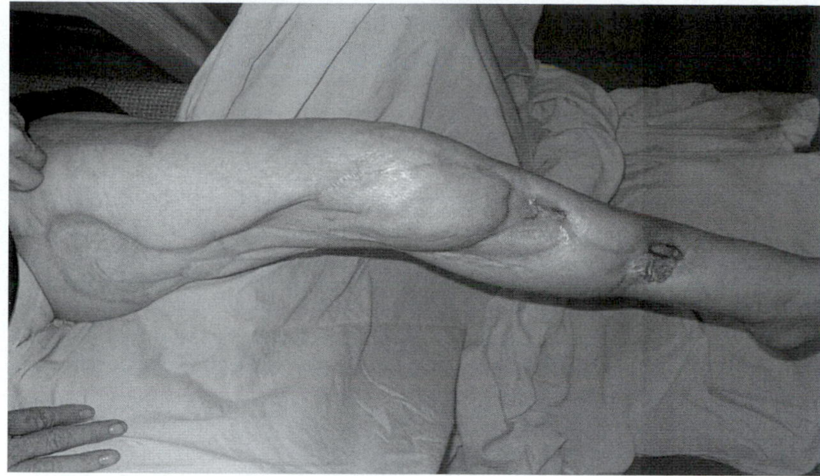

FIGURE 46-2. (See also Color Plate 46-2.) Extensive fasciotomies, skin grafts, and free flaps after successful recanalization of the iliac and femoral arteries with thrombolysis.

In an effort to classify the extent of acute ischemia to standardize reporting of outcome, the Society of Vascular Surgery/International Society of Cardiovascular Surgery (SVS/ISCVS, now SVS) ad hoc committee was established and published what has now come to be known as the "Rutherford criteria," after Dr. Robert Rutherford, the lead author of the article (Table 46-2).[10] Three classes were defined: class 1, in which the limb is viable and remains so even without therapeutic intervention; class 2 for limbs that are threatened and require revascularization for salvage; and class 3 for those limbs that are irreversibly ischemic and infarction has developed such that salvage is not possible. The initial work of the reporting standards committee was revised several years later, dividing the middle category into two subclassifications: 2A for limbs that are not immediately threatened and 2B for limbs that are severely threatened to the point where urgent revascularization is necessary for salvage.

The anatomic level of the arterial stenoses can be predicted from palpation of pulses in the femoral, popliteal, and ankle regions. For example, patients with an acute occlusion of the infrarenal aorta have absent femoral pulses bilaterally. Patients with an acute occlusion of the iliac segment, as may occur with in situ thrombosis over underlying atherosclerotic iliac stenosis, have an absent femoral pulse on the affected side. Patients with common femoral artery emboli may maintain an easily palpable femoral pulse, sometimes even augmented with a "water hammer" characteristic, until such time as the absence of outflow in the external iliac artery causes this vessel to thrombose and the femoral pulse to disappear. When the superficial femoral artery occludes, the femoral pulse is palpable, but no pulses are evident below. For example, a patient with a palpable femoral pulse but absent popliteal pulse is likely to have a superficial femoral artery occlusion. Patients with emboli to the terminus of the popliteal artery, by contrast, usually have a palpable popliteal pulse but no palpable pulses below (dorsalis pedis or posterior tibial). Lastly, a patient with leg ischemia secondary to a popliteal aneurysm usually demonstrates a large and easily palpable popliteal pulse, concurrent with severe calf and foot ischemia. The popliteal pulse is maintained in these patients as a result of the events leading to occlusion—the aneurysm is associated with serial embolic events to the three crural vessels, occluding them one by one until, at the time of the last occlusion, the leg becomes ischemic. The aneurysm itself, however, remains palpable due to the somewhat static column of blood and absent outflow.

TABLE 46-2 SUMMARY OF THE RUTHERFORD CLASSIFICATION OF ACUTE ISCHEMIA[10]

Rutherford Class	Description	Urgency of Revascularization
1	Nonthreatened	Elective or not at all
2A	Threatened	Within days to weeks
2B	Immediately threatened	Within hours
3	Irreversible ischemia	Futile

Even the most astute clinician sometimes has difficulty in discerning his or her own digital pulse from the patient's pedal pulse. For this reason, the use of a Doppler instrument is advantageous to document flow within the smaller arteries and, most importantly, to provide an objective and quantitative assessment of the extent of arterial insufficiency through the calculation of a Doppler-derived ankle-brachial index (ABI) (see also Chapter 10). Normally, the ABI is greater than 1.[11,12] The index is decreased to 0.5 to 0.8 in patients with claudication and to lower levels in patients with pain at rest or tissue loss. The ABI may be normal in some patients with mild arterial narrowing; treadmill exercise has been used in these cases to increase the sensitivity of the test.[13] Patients with diabetes mellitus or renal failure may have calcific lower leg arteries, rendering them incompressible and causing a falsely elevated ABI; in these cases a toe-brachial pressure index can be measured and is more predictive of significant arterial disease.[14] Given the subjective nature of the pulse examination, Doppler segmental pressures are also useful in defining the level of involvement; a drop in pressure of 30 mm Hg or more between two segments predicts arterial occlusion between the two levels.[15] For example, a superficial femoral arterial occlusion would be suggested in a patient with a systolic pressure of 120 mm Hg at the proximal-thigh pressure cuff and 90 mm Hg at the above-knee cuff. Transcutaneous oxygen tension has also been used to assess the severity of peripheral arterial occlusion, as well as to predict the most appropriate level of amputation.[16]

Contrast arteriography remains the gold standard with which all other tests must be compared (see Chapter 13). Even today, standard arteriography is the most accurate test for all but the occasional patient with such slow flow in the tibial or foot vessels that digital subtraction imaging fails to demonstrate a patent artery. Arteriography is, however, a semi-invasive modality and, as such, its use should be confined to those patients for whom a surgical or percutaneous intervention is contemplated. Patients with borderline renal function may experience contrast-induced nephrotoxicity, and in this subgroup the use of alternate contrast agents such as gadolinium or carbon dioxide have been employed.[17,18] Duplex ultrasound has been used in some centers to define the anatomical extent of peripheral artery disease (PAD).[19,20] Although duplex ultrasound has been useful in documenting the patency of a single arterial segment such as a stented superficial femoral artery or a bypass graft, evaluation of the entire lower extremity arterial tree remains imprecise and its adequacy as the sole diagnostic modality for planning a percutaneous or open surgical intervention remains controversial. Magnetic resonance (MR) angiography (see Chapter 11) is being used with greater frequency in patients with PAD.[21,22] Using gadolinium as an MR contrast agent, the specificity and sensitivity of the test exceeds that of duplex ultrasonography and approaches the accuracy of standard arteriography. MR angiography has been effective in demonstrating patent tibial arteries undetected with less sensitive conventional arteriography, identifying potential target vessels for an otherwise unfeasible lower-extremity reconstructive bypass procedure. Today, MR angiography is widely employed in patients with chronic renal insufficiency to limit the dye load. Another noninvasive imaging modality, CT angiography (see Chapter 12), is gaining appeal as a means of delineating anatomy to provide a means of localizing the extent and severity of occlusive disease.[23] With future improvements in hardware and software technology, it is likely that MR and CT angiography will effectively replace conventional diagnostic arteriography, and arterial cannulation will be reserved solely for percutaneous interventional therapies.

TREATMENT

Patients presenting with acute limb ischemia often require revascularization to salvage the leg.[24] In many cases the paucity of preexisting collateral channels renders the limb ischemic after thrombotic or embolic occlusion of the main arterial segment. Symptoms occur with severity and rapidity, forcing the patient to seek treatment almost immediately.

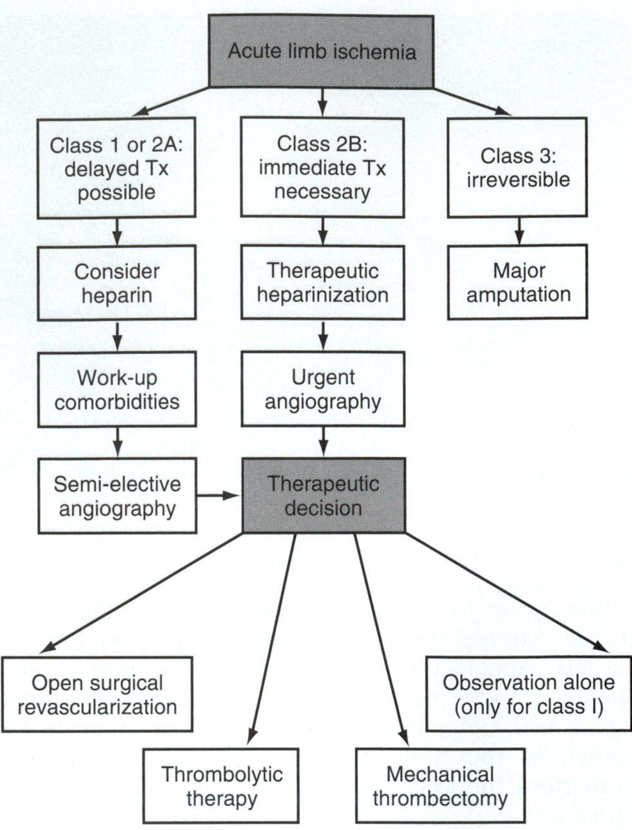

FIGURE 46-3. Paradigm for management of acute limb ischemia.

Once the diagnosis is made, systemic anticoagulation is instituted. A bolus of unfractionated heparin is standard, followed by a continuous infusion to maintain the activated partial thromboplastin time (aPTT) in a therapeutic range. The goal of anticoagulation is twofold: to decrease the risk of thrombus propagation and, in the case of presumed embolic occlusion, to prevent recurrent embolization. Occasionally, if early angiographic evaluation is feasible, heparinization can be withheld, pending the establishment of arterial access. Otherwise, a micropuncture technique (small localizing needle, guidewire, and a 4F sheath) is used to gain access or the anticoagulation is withheld to allow the aPTT to fall within 1.5× control.

Several basic therapeutic options are available for patients with acute limb ischemia (Fig. 46-3):

1. The first option is anticoagulation alone. If the ischemia is nonthreatening (e.g., Rutherford class 1 or 2A), such a nonaggressive course may be appropriate. Angiographic evaluation and elective revascularization may then be undertaken after the patient has been fully prepared and other comorbidities such as concurrent coronary artery disease have been addressed.
2. Patients who present with more severe ischemia (Rutherford class 2B) require some form of intervention to prevent progression to irreversible ischemia

and limb loss. These patients should undergo early angiographic evaluation with adequate imaging of the affected and unaffected extremities. Arterial access is accomplished at a site distant from the ischemic extremity using a contralateral femoral artery or brachial artery approach to avoid the creation of needle entry sites in an artery that might subsequently be infused with a thrombolytic agent.

Early angiographic imaging should be undertaken in all patients, with the sole exception of those patients with common femoral emboli. These individuals can be taken directly to the operating room for embolectomy, but completion angiography is necessary to rule out retained thromboembolic material.[25]

Once adequate diagnostic information has been obtained from the angiogram, the clinician can decide whether to pursue a percutaneous or open surgical option:

A. *Intra-arterial, catheter-directed thrombolytic therapy*. Thrombolytic therapy with the plasminogen activators (urokinase, alteplase, or reteplase) has been demonstrated to lower morbidity and mortality when compared with a traditional approach of immediate operative revascularization.[1-3] These benefits appear to be especially prominent in patients with "hyperacute" ischemia, where revascularization is necessary within just a few hours. The complication rate is high when such patients are taken urgently to open surgical revascularization, a finding that is explained by the frequency and magnitude of comorbid conditions in this frail group of patients.
B. *Percutaneous mechanical thrombectomy*. Removal of intra-arterial thrombus with a mechanical device has gained popularity over the past few years.[26,27] Some devices rely on hydrodynamic, rheolytic forces to extract the thrombus, while others use a rotating basket to fragment the clot. Mechanical thrombectomy devices can be used in conjunction with pharmacological thrombolysis. Although the devices result in clearing much of the occluding thrombus, an infusion of thrombolytic agent is still necessary in many cases to remove smaller amounts of retained mural clot.
C. *Immediate open surgical revascularization*. Early operation has been remarkably effective in restoring adequate blood flow to an ischemic extremity. The relatively simple procedure of balloon catheter thromboembolectomy (e.g., with a Fogarty catheter), however, has fallen into disfavor for all but true embolic occlusions.[28] The underlying lesion responsible for the thrombotic event must be identified and corrected to avoid early reocclusion. For this reason, if an open surgical intervention is elected, patients' acute leg ischemia from occlusion of a bypass graft is best served with the placement of a new bypass graft, if at all possible.[29]

Unfortunately, immediate open surgical interventions have been associated with an unexpectedly high risk of major morbidity and mortality. Blaisdell[30] first reported this finding, noting a 30% perioperative mortality rate in a review of more than 3000 patients in the published works from the 1960s and 1970s. While the results have improved since the publication of Blaisdell's landmark review, mortality rates continue to remain undesirably high.[31] This observation appears to relate to the relatively common occurrence of cardiopulmonary complications developing in these medically compromised patients—patients who are ill prepared to undergo early operative intervention.[32] The severity of ischemia precludes adequate preoperative preparation of the patient, and complications such as perioperative myocardial infarction, cardiac arrhythmia, or pneumonia appear to underlie the unacceptable mortality rate in these patients.

The mortality rate from open surgical treatment of acute limb ischemia has been reconfirmed in numerous studies published after Blaisdell's landmark series. Dale reviewed cases of nontraumatic extremity ischemia and observed an 11% perioperative mortality rate in those with embolism, versus 3% in those with acute thromboses.[33] Several years later, Jivegård and colleagues documented a mortality rate of 20% in patients presenting with acute arterial embolism or thrombosis, a finding that was explained by preexisting cardiac disease in these patients.[34] A study by Edwards and colleagues reported a 1-year mortality rate of 38% in patients undergoing the placement of new autogenous vein grafts for treatment of failed prior grafts in the same leg, with an amputation rate of 6% over the same time frame.[35]

Noting the high morbidity from primary open surgical revascularization in patients suffering from true limb-threatening lower limb ischemia, three randomized, prospective clinical trials were organized to compare thrombolytic therapy and immediate open surgical revascularization. The first study, the Rochester series, compared urokinase to primary operation in a single-center experience of 114 patients presenting with what has subsequently been called "hyperacute ischemia."[2] Patients enrolled in this trial all had severely threatened limbs (Rutherford class 2B) with mean symptom duration of approximately 2 days. After 1 year of follow-up, 84% of patients randomized to urokinase were alive, compared with only 58% of patients randomized to primary operation (Fig. 46-4). By contrast, the rate of limb salvage was identical at 80%. A closer inspection of the raw data revealed that the defining variable for mortality differences was the development of cardiopulmonary complications during the periprocedural period. The rate of long-term mortality was high when such periprocedural complications occurred but relatively low when they did not occur. Only the fact that such complications occurred more commonly in patients taken directly to the operating room explained the greater long-term mortality rate in the operative group.

The second prospective, randomized analysis of thrombolysis versus surgery was the Surgery or Thrombolysis for the Ischemic Lower Extremity (STILE) trial.[3] At its termination, 393 patients were randomized to one of three treatment groups, recombinant tissue plasminogen activator (rt-PA), urokinase, or primary operation. Subsequently, the two thrombolytic groups were combined for purposes of data analysis when the

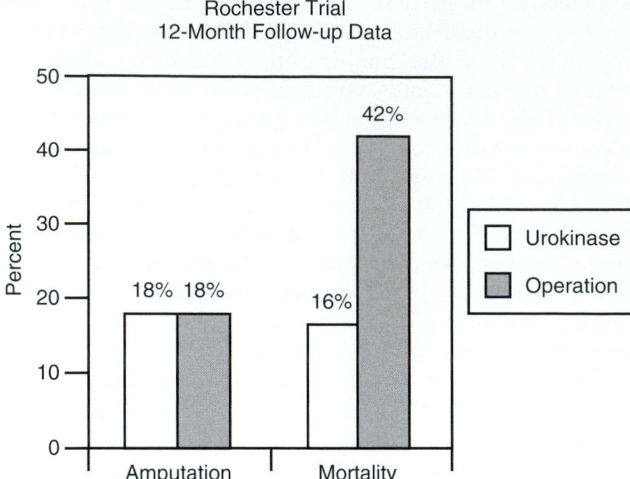

FIGURE 46-4. Frequency of major amputation or death after 1 year in the Rochester trial.

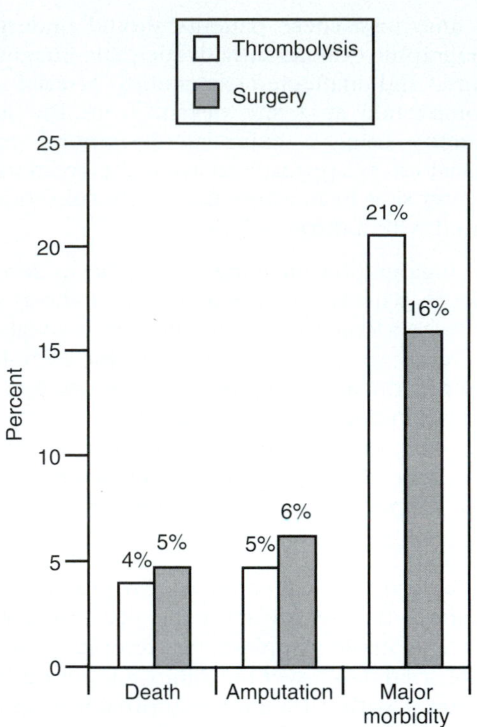

FIGURE 46-5. Frequency of death, amputation, or major morbidity at the time of discharge from the Surgery or Thrombolysis for the Ischemic Lower Extremity trial.

outcome was found to be similar. Although the rate of the composite endpoint of untoward events was higher in the thrombolytic patients, the rates of the more relevant and objective endpoints of amputation and death were equivalent (Fig. 46-5). Articles were written on subgroup analyses of the STILE data, one relating to native artery occlusions[36] and one to bypass graft occlusions.[37] Thrombolysis appeared more effective in patients with graft occlusions. The rate of major amputation was higher in native arterial occlusions treated with thrombolysis (10% thrombolysis vs. 0% surgery at 1 year). By contrast, amputation was lower in patients with acute graft occlusions treated with thrombolysis.

The third and final randomized comparison of thrombolysis and surgery was the Thrombolysis Or Peripheral Arterial Surgery (TOPAS) trial. Following completion of a preliminary dose-ranging trial in 213 patients,[38] 544 patients were randomized to a recombinant form of urokinase or primary operative intervention.[1] After a mean follow-up period of 1 year, the rate of amputation-free survival was identical in the two treatment groups, 68% and 69% in the urokinase and surgical patients, respectively (Fig. 46-6). Although this trial failed to

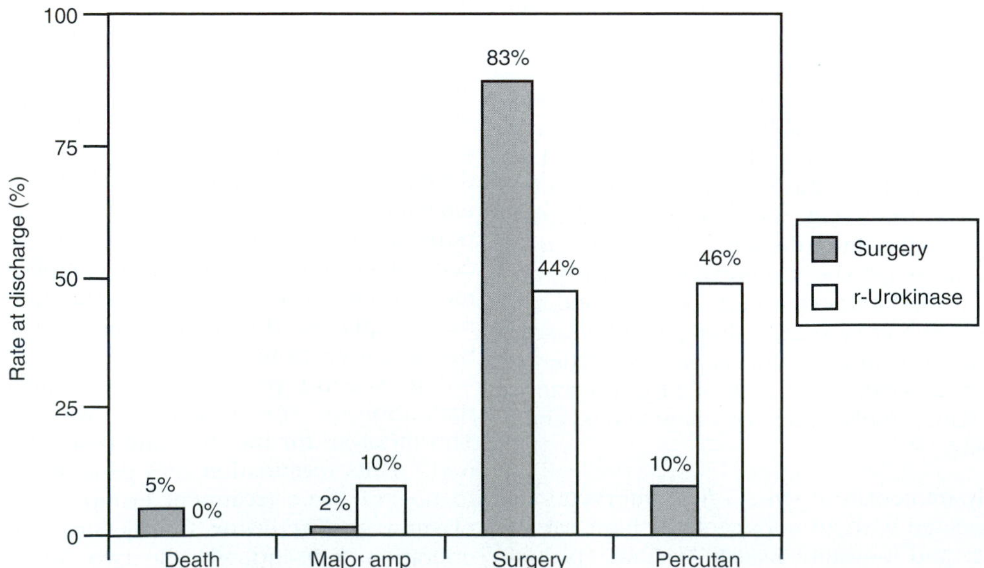

FIGURE 46-6. Frequency of the most severe intervention or event at the time of hospital discharge from the Thrombolysis Or Peripheral Arterial Surgery trial.

document improvement in survival or limb salvage with thrombolysis, after 6 months of follow-up, fully 32% of the thrombolytic patients were alive without amputation and without the need for open surgical revascularization. After 1 year, this number had decreased only slightly, with 26% alive, without amputation and without open surgery. Thus the original goal of the TOPAS trial, to generate data on which regulatory approval of recombinant urokinase would be based, was not achieved. Nevertheless, the findings confirmed that acute limb ischemia could be managed with catheter-directed thrombolysis, achieving similar amputation and mortality rates but avoiding the need for open surgical procedures in a significant percentage of patients.

SUMMARY

Acute limb ischemia develops with the sudden occlusion of a native artery or bypass graft, resulting in hypoperfusion of the distal extremity. When severe, ischemia progresses to infarction and limb loss, the rapidity of which depends on the adequacy of preexisting collateral arterial channels. Treatment is accomplished through the restoration of adequate distal blood flow with open surgical revascularization procedures, pharmacologic thrombolytic therapy, or percutaneous mechanical thrombectomy, or a combination. Morbidity and mortality rates are high, especially in patients with medical comorbidities that render them ill prepared to undergo urgent surgical interventions. The keys to improving outcome lie in rapid diagnosis, effective reperfusion, correction of the culprit lesion that caused the occlusion, and liberal use of antithrombotic therapy. Only through a coordinated approach to care of the patient with acute limb ischemia can reductions in the rate of periprocedural morbidity and mortality be expected.

Acknowledgment

The author would like to thank Lisa Bodzin for her help and support on this chapter.

REFERENCES

1. Ouriel K, Veith FJ, Sasahara AA: A comparison of recombinant urokinase with vascular surgery as initial treatment for acute arterial occlusion of the legs. N Engl J Med 338:1105, 1998.
2. Ouriel K, Shortell CK, DeWeese JA, et al: A comparison of thrombolytic therapy with operative revascularization in the initial treatment of acute peripheral arterial ischemia. J Vasc Surg 19:1021, 1994.
3. Anonymous: Results of a prospective randomized trial evaluating surgery versus thrombolysis for ischemia of the lower extremity. The STILE trial. Ann Surg 220:251, 1994.
4. Raut CP, Cambria RP, LaMuraglia GM, et al: Surgical management of popliteal artery embolism at the turn of the millennium. Ann Vasc Surg 18:79, 2004.
5. Dormandy J, Heeck L, Vig S: Acute limb ischemia. Semin Vasc Surg 12:148, 1999.
6. Davies B, Braithwaite BD, Birch PA, et al: Acute leg ischaemia in Gloucestershire. Br J Surg 84:504, 1997.
7. Bulkley GB: Pathophysiology of free radical-mediated reperfusion injury. J Vasc Surg 5:512, 1987.
8. Heemskerk J, Kitslaar P: Acute compartment syndrome of the lower leg: Retrospective study on prevalence, technique, and outcome of fasciotomies. World J Surg 27:744, 2003.
9. Witz M, Korzets Z, Ellis M, et al: Intraoperative intra-arterial urokinase therapy after failed embolectomy in acute lower limb ischemia. J Cardiovasc Surg (Torino) 43:877, 2002.
10. Rutherford RB, Baker JD, Ernst C, et al: Recommended standards for reports dealing with lower extremity ischemia: Revised version [erratum appears in J Vasc Surg 33:4805, 2001]. J Vasc Surg 26:517, 1997.
11. Ouriel K, Zarins CK: Doppler ankle pressure: An evaluation of three methods of expression. Arch Surg 117:1297, 1982.
12. Smith FB, Lee AJ, Price JF, et al: Changes in ankle brachial index in symptomatic and asymptomatic subjects in the general population. J Vasc Surg 38:1323, 2003.
13. Degischer S, Labs KH, Aschwanden M, et al: Reproducibility of constant-load treadmill testing with various treadmill protocols and predictability of treadmill test results in patients with intermittent claudication. J Vasc Surg 36:83, 2002.
14. de Graaff JC, Ubbink DT, Legemate DA, et al: Evaluation of toe pressure and transcutaneous oxygen measurements in management of chronic critical leg ischemia: A diagnostic randomized clinical trial. J Vasc Surg 38:528, 2003.
15. Moneta GL, Yeager RA, Lee RW, et al: Noninvasive localization of arterial occlusive disease: A comparison of segmental Doppler pressures and arterial duplex mapping. J Vasc Surg 17:578, 1993.
16. Padberg FT, Back TL, Thompson PN, et al: Transcutaneous oxygen ($TcPO_2$) estimates probability of healing in the ischemic extremity. J Surg Res 60:365, 1996.
17. Sam AD, Morasch MD, Collins J, et al: Safety of gadolinium contrast angiography in patients with chronic renal insufficiency. J Vasc Surg 38:313, 2003.
18. Kerns SR, Hawkins IF Jr, Sabatelli FW, et al: Current status of carbon dioxide angiography. Radiol Clin North Am 33:15, 1995.
19. Grassbaugh JA, Nelson PR, Rzucidlo EM, et al: Blinded comparison of preoperative duplex ultrasound scanning and contrast arteriography for planning revascularization at the level of the tibia. J Vasc Surg 37:1186, 2003.
20. Proia RR, Walsh DB, Nelson PR, et al: Early results of infragenicular revascularization based solely on duplex arteriography. J Vasc Surg 33:1165, 2001.
21. Morasch MD, Collins J, Pereles FS, et al: Lower extremity stepping-table magnetic resonance angiography with multilevel contrast timing and segmented contrast infusion. J Vasc Surg 37:62, 2003.
22. Schoenberg SO, Londy FJ, Licato P, et al: Multiphase-multistep gadolinium-enhanced MR angiography of the abdominal aorta and runoff vessels. Invest Radiol 36:283, 2001.
23. Rubin GD, Dake MD, Semba CP: Current status of three-dimensional spiral CT scanning for imaging the vasculature. Radiol Clin North Am 33:51, 1995.
24. Ouriel K: Peripheral arterial disease. Lancet 358:257, 2001.
25. Crolla RM, van de Pavoordt ED, Moll FL: Intraoperative digital subtraction angiography after thromboembolectomy: preliminary experience. J Endovasc Surg 2:168, 1995.
26. Silva JA, Ramee SR, Collins TJ, et al: Rheolytic thrombectomy in the treatment of acute limb-threatening ischemia: Immediate results and six-month follow-up of the multicenter AngioJet registry. Possis Peripheral AngioJet Study AngioJet Investigators. Cathet Cardiovasc Diagn 45:386, 1998.
27. Kasirajan K, Gray B, Beavers FP, et al: Rheolytic thrombectomy in the management of acute and subacute limb-threatening ischemia. J Vasc Interv Radiol 12:413, 2001.
28. AbuRahma AF, Hopkins ES, Wulu JT Jr, et al: Lysis/balloon angioplasty versus thrombectomy/open patch angioplasty of failed femoropopliteal polytetrafluoroethylene bypass grafts. J Vasc Surg 35:307, 2002.
29. Nehler MR, Mueller RJ, McLafferty RB, et al: Outcome of catheter-directed thrombolysis for lower extremity arterial bypass occlusion. J Vasc Surg 37:72, 2003.
30. Blaisdell FW, Steele M, Allen RE: Management of acute lower extremity arterial ischemia due to embolism and thrombosis. Surgery 84:822, 1978.
31. Berridge DC, Kessel D, Robertson I: Surgery versus thrombolysis for acute limb ischaemia: Initial management. Cochrane Database Syst Rev CD002784, 2002.

32. Ouriel K, Veith FJ: Acute lower limb ischemia: Determinants of outcome. Surgery 124:336, 1998.
33. Dale WA: Differential management of acute peripheral arterial ischemia. J Vasc Surg 1:269, 1984.
34. Jivegård L, Holm J, Scherstén T: Acute limb ischemia due to arterial embolism or thrombosis: Influence of limb ischemia versus pre-existing cardiac disease on postoperative mortality rate. J Cardiovasc Surg 29:32, 1988.
35. Edwards JE, Taylor LM Jr, Porter JM: Treatment of failed lower extremity bypass grafts with new autogenous vein bypass grafting. J Vasc Surg 11:136, 1990.
36. Weaver FA, Comerota AJ, Youngblood M, et al: Surgical revascularization versus thrombolysis for nonembolic lower extremity native artery occlusions: Results of a prospective randomized trial. The STILE Investigators. Surgery versus Thrombolysis for Ischemia of the Lower Extremity. J Vasc Surg 24:513, 1996.
37. Comerota AJ, Weaver FA, Hosking JD, et al: Results of a prospective, randomized trial of surgery versus thrombolysis for occluded lower extremity bypass grafts. Am J Surg 172:105, 1996.
38. Ouriel K, Veith FJ, Sasahara AA: Thrombolysis or peripheral arterial surgery: Phase I results. TOPAS Investigators. J Vasc Surg 23:64, 1996.

■ ■ ■ chapter 47

Atheroembolism

Paul A. Tunick
Itzhak Kronzon

ATHEROMA, from the Greek, meaning "crushed grain or porridge"[1]

Atheroembolism is an arterio-arterial embolism emanating from an atheroma, or atherosclerotic plaque. This embolization leads to the occlusion of distal arteries, with resultant organ damage that occurs due to one of two mechanisms—either small- to medium-sized vessel occlusion due to cholesterol crystal embolization or medium- to large-sized vessel occlusion due to thromboembolism. The former, when it affects the digital arteries of the feet, has been recognized for decades as the classic "blue toe syndrome," which is often accompanied by renal failure, livedo reticularis, or intestinal infarction. The latter was recently recognized as being much more frequent than cholesterol crystal embolization, with organ infarction (most often stroke) due to thrombus embolization from unstable plaques in the thoracic aorta. This chapter focuses on these two syndromes, originating primarily from atherosclerotic plaque in the aorta.

EPIDEMIOLOGY

During J. Willis Hurst's cardiology fellowship in the 1940s, he was taught by a historic figure in cardiology, Paul Dudley White, that the risk factors for atherosclerosis were "family history... ; a high-fat, high-cholesterol diet; hypertension; smoking tobacco; lack of exercise; and diabetes mellitus."[2] The importance of these "classic" risk factors for atheroembolism has been borne out in contemporary series of patients, and in addition both older age and male gender have been reported in a majority of those with atheroembolism syndromes.[3] In one study on atheroembolism, the average age of 221 patients with cholesterol crystal embolization was 66 years,[3] and in 111 patients with thromboembolism originating from thoracic aortic plaque, the average age was 76 years and 61% were male.[4]

The "traditional" risk factors of hypertension, age, and smoking positively correlated with severe thoracic aortic atherosclerotic plaque as seen on transesophageal echocardiography in a population-based study.[5] Among those with plaque, the odds of complex atherosclerosis (≥4 mm, ulceration, mobile elements) increased as ambulatory out-of-bed systolic blood pressure increased (odds ratio 1.43 for each 10 mm Hg increase, 95% confidence interval 1.1 to 1.87). Complex aortic plaque was also correlated with hypertension treatment, controlling for age and history of smoking. Other nontraditional risk factors for atherosclerosis have recently been the subject of investigation. In particular, plasma levels of homocysteine have been highly correlated not only with the extent of clinical atherosclerosis[6] but also with the degree of plaque burden in the thoracic aorta, as seen on transesophageal echocardiography.[7] It is thought that endothelial damage due to homocysteine leads to plaque formation.

Perhaps the most intriguing theories currently focus on inflammatory reactions in the pathogenesis of atherosclerosis,[8] and by implication, the atheroemboli syndromes. There is great interest in studying the levels of inflammation markers, such as C-reactive protein (CRP). Considerable evidence exists that CRP levels are, in fact, a risk factor for atherosclerosis and its complications,[9] and there is even evidence that rather than just being a marker for inflammation, CRP could itself help initiate the atherosclerotic process. CRP levels have been found to be associated with the severity of plaque in the thoracic aorta.

CHOLESTEROL CRYSTAL EMBOLIZATION

Cholesterol crystal embolization is a dramatic but uncommon syndrome. It is characterized by diffuse showering of the distal circulation with cholesterol crystals originating from arterial plaque, usually in the aorta (Fig. 47-1). The syndrome may also originate from plaque in the iliac, carotid, and coronary arteries.[10] These crystals lodge

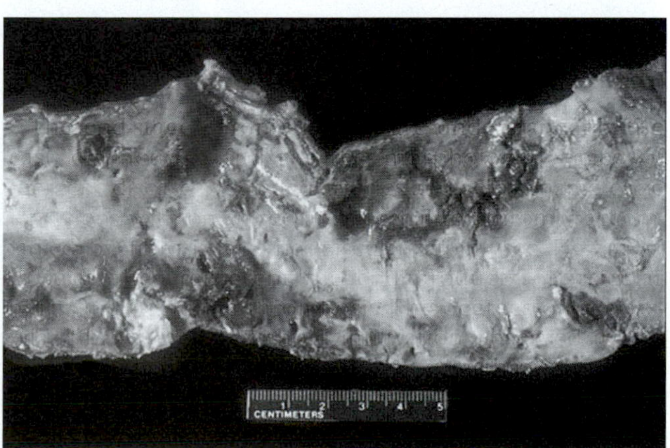

FIGURE 47-1. (See also Color Plate 47-1.) Severely atherosclerotic aorta. Note the ulcerated plaques and superimposed thrombi. (From the University of Utah WebPath and Edward C. Klatt, MD, professor and academic administrator, Florida State University College of Medicine.)

in small- and medium-sized vessels, producing organ damage. This classically occurs in the lower extremities (blue toe syndrome) and also often affects the kidneys. The gastrointestinal tract and upper extremities are less often affected.

The cholesterol crystal embolization syndrome was found in only 5 of 519 patients (1%) with severe thoracic aortic plaque on transesophageal echocardiography, during a mean follow-up time of more than 3 years.[4] Similarly, it occurred in only 1 of 134 warfarin-treated patients (0.7%) with severe aortic plaque in the Stroke Prevention in Atrial Fibrillation III trial.[11]

Clinical Manifestations

The presenting symptoms of cholesterol crystal embolization may be nonspecific, and this may lead to the consideration of many other systemic illnesses. Fever, myalgias, headache, and weight loss are not uncommon.[3] The differential diagnosis of this syndrome is quite broad and includes thrombotic arterial occlusion, vasospastic disorders such as Raynaud's phenomenon or chronic pernio, cyanotic congenital heart disease, secondary syphilis, and pheochromocytoma.[12]

Because of its diverse manifestations, cholesterol crystal embolization may also be included on the list of the "great imitators," along with infections such as syphilis, infectious endocarditis, Whipple's disease, tuberculosis, disseminated mycoses, Lyme disease, and brucellosis; other vascular diseases such as polyarteritis and aortic dissection; and tumors such as cardiac myxoma, lymphoma, and hypernephroma, which are frequent culprits in "fever of unknown origin."[12]

Skin Findings

Although it is often referred to as the blue toe syndrome, blue toes are actually relatively uncommon in this uncommon syndrome (Fig. 47-2).[3] The skin is the most common organ involved. Skin manifestations are most often bilateral and limited to the lower extremities, although some patients have unilateral signs and involvement of the arms, buttocks, scrotum, or torso. Other signs present in the skin are livedo reticularis, gangrene, ulceration, nodules, purpura, and petechiae. Livedo reticularis (Fig. 47-3) is a characteristic reticulated erythema of the skin, which is blanchable. It may be red or blue depending on the degree of blood flow compromise and oxygen desaturation through the affected vessels. The differential diagnosis of livedo reticularis is broad. It may occur due to vasomotor instability (especially in the cold) or Raynaud's phenomenon. It is also seen in patients with vasculitis (polyarteritis nodosa, systemic lupus erythematosus, dermatomyositis, leukocytoclastic angiitis, or rheumatoid vasculitis), infection (syphilis or tuberculosis), cryoglobulinemia, antiphospholipid antibody syndrome, or polycythemia vera. A familial form, Sneddon's syndrome, is associated with cerebrovascular disease.

Although classically the findings in the lower extremities are said to be found in the presence of normal distal pulses, and this is a clinical tip-off to the correct diagnosis, the common concurrence of peripheral arterial disease may produce large-vessel stenosis and occlusion.[3] Cholesterol crystal embolization may be the underlying etiology of leg and foot ulcers, and normal arterial pulsations are often present.[13]

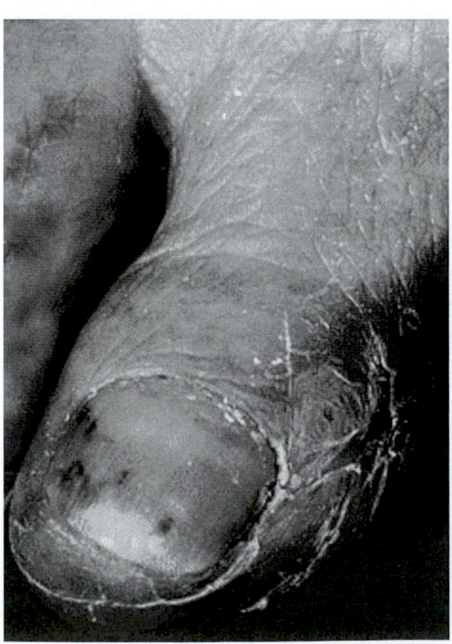
A

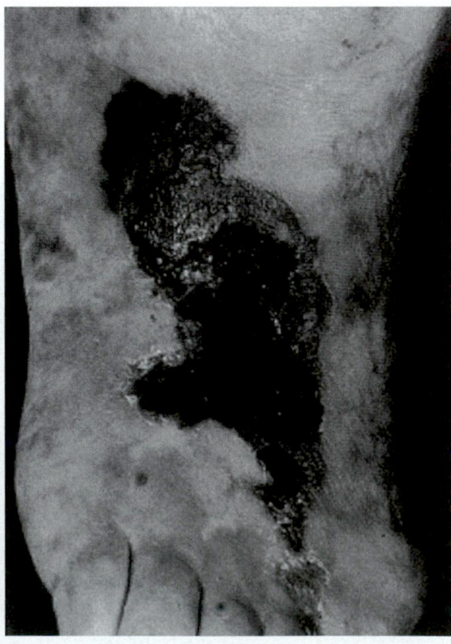
B

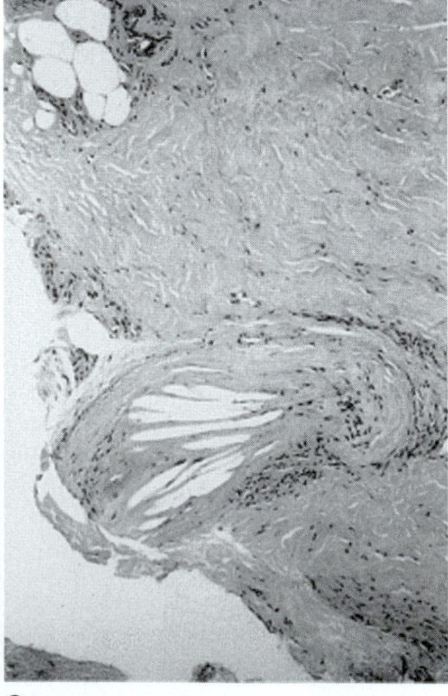
C

FIGURE 47-2. (See also Color Plate 47-2.) Peripheral lesions. **A,** Blue toe. **B,** Necrotic skin ulcer. **C,** Cholesterol clefts in small artery from biopsy of lesion. (From Schanz S, Metzler G, Metzger S, et al: Cholesterol embolism: An often unrecognized cause of leg ulcers. Br J Dermatol 146:1107, 2002.).

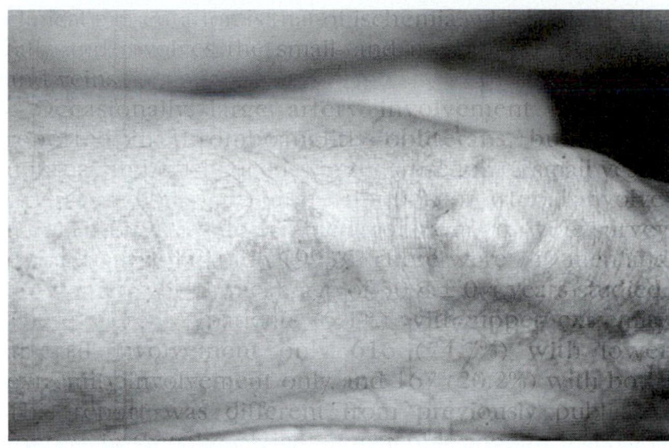

FIGURE 47-3. (See also Color Plate 47-3.) Livedo reticularis. (Copyright-protected material used with permission of the author and the University of Iowa's Virtual Hospital, *www.vh.org*.)

Renal Failure

Acute renal failure may be a life-threatening manifestation of cholesterol crystal embolization. Characteristic cholesterol clefts are found on biopsy specimens (Fig. 47-4).[14] Renal failure most often occurs after invasive vascular procedures (see later discussion on pathophysiology), although it may also occur spontaneously. Renal manifestations are detailed in Table 47-1. The course of renal failure may be steadily downhill (leading to dialysis), it may be relatively benign, or there may be a stuttering course with additional showers of cholesterol embolism. Although loss of renal function following angiography is usually blamed on radiocontrast-induced toxicity, cholesterol crystal embolization should always be considered in patients who are elderly or have other manifestations of atherosclerosis. The course tends to be more protracted when the etiology is cholesterol crystal embolization. Finally, the loss of allograft function following kidney transplantation is not always rejection of the graft—cholesterol crystal embolization may be the culprit (originating from the recipient's aorta or even from the donor).[15]

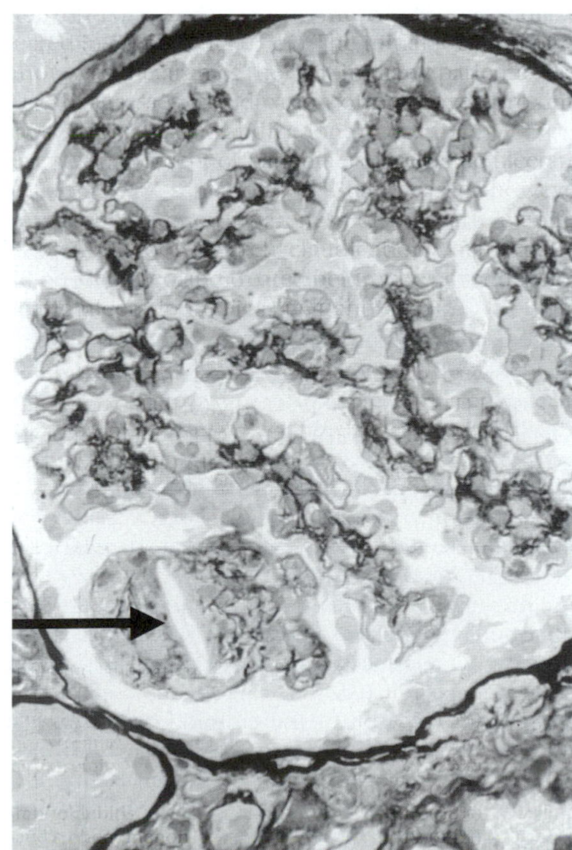

FIGURE 47-4. (See also Color Plate 47-4.) Empty cholesterol cleft (*arrow*) in a glomerulus of a patient with cholesterol crystal embolization. (Courtesy Gloria Gallo, MD, Department of Pathology, New York University School of Medicine.)

TABLE 47-1 RENAL MANIFESTATIONS OF CHOLESTEROL CRYSTAL EMBOLIZATION[3]

Elevated BUN	62/68 (91%)
BUN > 100	17/68 (25%)
Elevated creatinine	43/52 (83%)
Creatinine > 5	13/52 (25%)
Proteinuria	34/63 (54%)
Proteinuria > 2500 mg/24 hr	3/63 (5%)
Hematuria	19/63 (30%)
Pyuria	10/63 (16%)
Casts	25/63 (40%)

BUN, blood urea nitrogen.

Other Signs

In addition to findings in the skin and kidneys, Fine and Kapoor[3] found that gastrointestinal bleeding occurred in 10% of patients and cholesterol crystals occurred in the retina (Hollenhorst plaques, Fig. 47-5) in 6% of patients.

The lesions responsible for blood loss may be present throughout the gastrointestinal tract, from the duodenum

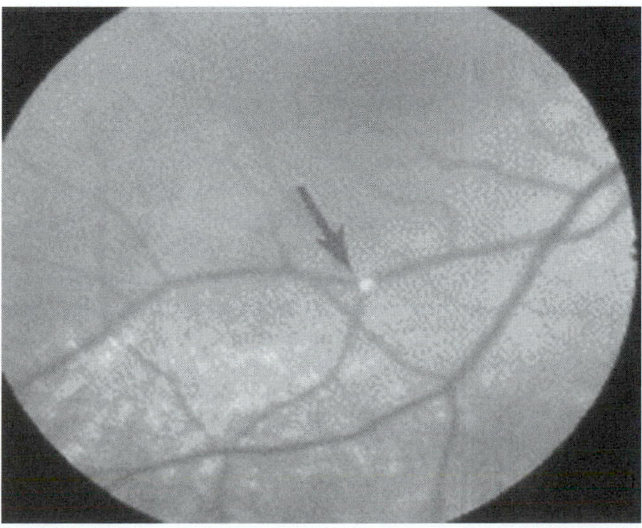

FIGURE 47-5. (See also Color Plate 47-5.) Retina with Hollenhorst plaque (*arrow*). (From the Washington Academy of Eye Physicians and Surgeons, Kory Diement, executive director.)

to the sigmoid colon.[16] Cholesterol crystal embolization may even be a rare cause of bleeding from the stomach, which is usually diagnosed endoscopically as gastritis and only found to be due to cholesterol crystal embolization on surgical pathology or autopsy.[17] The prognosis of intestinal infarction due to cholesterol crystal embolization is poor, with reported mortality rates of 38%[15] to 81%.[3] Rarely, the pancreas, liver, and gallbladder may also be affected by cholesterol crystal embolization.[18]

Although the Hollenhorst plaque[19] may be indicative of diffuse cholesterol crystal embolization elsewhere, the location of the Hollenhorst plaque does not frequently correspond to the location of visual symptoms. Furthermore, the presence of a visible cholesterol crystal does not have strong prognostic importance with respect to stroke or transient ischemic attack: The cerebral hemisphere ipsilateral to asymptomatic Hollenhorst plaques has only a slightly increased risk of a subsequent neurologic event compared with the contralateral side without Hollenhorst plaques.[20] The prevalence of such lesions in the retina of patients with cholesterol crystal embolization to other locations is difficult to assess, as routine careful ophthalmologic examination is not always carried out in patients with other manifestations of the disease. In fact, various reports list the prevalence as 0% to 100%.

Finally, cholesterol crystal embolization probably plays a role in both myocardial and cerebral damage in patients with involvement of the coronary or carotid arteries, but both stroke and myocardial infarction most often occur separately from the typical manifestations of this syndrome.

Pathophysiology

The syndrome of cholesterol crystal embolization may occur spontaneously in approximately half of cases and is precipitated by angiographic or surgical manipulation in the other half. Of the two iatrogenic causes, angiography is more common than vascular surgery; atheroemboli following angiography were recently reported in 85% of iatrogenic cases.[21] The source of the emboli was the abdominal aorta (55%), iliac arteries (24%), and femoropopliteal arteries (21%). Rarely, cholesterol crystal embolization may be precipitated by trauma.[22]

Cardiac catheterization also may precipitate cholesterol crystal embolization.[23] In a prospective study of 1000 consecutive patients undergoing percutaneous coronary interventions, atheromatous material could be retrieved in half of the patients from guiding catheters, which had been passed up the aorta from the femoral artery.[24] However, clinical complications from cholesterol crystal embolization after cardiac catheterization are rare. In a recent study of 1786 patients undergoing catheterization, definite cholesterol crystal embolization was observed in only 0.75%.[25] Of note, the presence of an elevated CRP increased the risk of the syndrome by a factor of 4.6, raising the possibility that an increased inflammatory state (leading to plaque instability) was implicated in the pathogenesis of the complication.

Vascular surgery is a rare precipitating factor of the cholesterol crystal embolization syndrome. Among 1011 patients undergoing surgery involving the infrarenal aorta or the infrainguinal vascular tree over a 90-month period (1986-1993), the syndrome occurred secondary to operative manipulation in only two patients (0.2%) (in an additional 11 patients the syndrome was precipitated by angiography).[21] Although coronary artery bypass surgery rarely results in the syndrome of cholesterol crystal embolization, widespread fatal cholesterol embolization has been reported after this procedure, resulting in diffuse cerebral dysfunction with cutaneous, renal, hepatic, and skin involvement.[26]

There are scattered reports of cholesterol crystal embolization occurring after treatment with medications, especially anticoagulants (heparin or warfarin).[27-29] In fact, anticoagulants are often posited as etiologic (with plaque hemorrhage as the precipitating factor). However, the syndrome occurs uncommonly in patients treated with anticoagulant therapy.[30] In a study of 519 patients treated for severe aortic plaque,[4] it occurred in only 2 patients on warfarin. This was similar to the incidence in the SPAF-3 Trial (0.7% of warfarin-treated patients).[11] Cholesterol crystal embolization may also rarely occur after the use of thrombolytic agents,[31] but a causal relationship has similarly not been established, as there may be several possible etiologic factors in these patients as well.

Pathology

The hallmark of the pathologic diagnosis of cholesterol crystal embolization is the presence of cholesterol crystals seen on the pathologic specimen. These "crystals" are actually empty spaces (clefts) seen when the cholesterol crystals are dissolved by the usual histologic preparation (the birefringent character of cholesterol crystals can be preserved if the specimen is first frozen with liquid nitrogen and then examined with polarized light).[32] The spaces left behind by cholesterol crystals are crescentic (with pointed ends) or elongated ovoid spaces present in small- or medium-sized arteries from affected organs, such as the skin, kidneys, or intestine. They may also be seen in glomeruli. Inflammatory or fibrous intimal proliferation rapidly develops after cholesterol crystal embolization, and this may result in the vascular occlusion that produces organ damage.[33]

The typical lesion seen in the kidney is the occlusion of arcuate and interlobular arteries, as well as the glomerular capillaries, with cholesterol crystals. Although atherosclerotic plaque generally causes stenosis of the main renal arteries and their major branches, cholesterol crystal embolization occludes medium-sized vessels (150 to 200 μm in diameter) and glomerular capillaries. The involvement usually is patchy.[32]

The presence of cholesterol clefts occasionally seen in the pulmonary arteries of patients with the syndrome has not been adequately explained, but as pulmonary arterial atherosclerosis is rare (e.g., in end-stage Eisenmenger's syndrome), the embolic material presumably passes through the systemic capillary bed into the venous system and lungs. Such cholesterol emboli have been seen in 25% of the small pulmonary arteries in a patient with the syndrome.[34]

Diagnosis and Diagnostic Tests

The diagnosis of the cholesterol crystal embolization syndrome often requires a high index of suspicion. If renal failure, abdominal pain, diarrhea (sometimes associated with lactic acidosis indicating bowel infarction), or the typical skin findings occur following cardiac catheterization, angiography, vascular surgery, or blunt trauma to the abdomen, the syndrome should be at or near the top of the list of diagnostic possibilities. This is especially true in a patient with an abdominal aortic aneurysm or in the patient who has diffuse atherosclerotic disease (or one with multiple risk factors). Rarely, the skin findings may be localized distal to a popliteal aneurysm, making the diagnosis more obvious.

Laboratory testing may reveal elevations in the white blood cell count or in the blood urea nitrogen and creatinine (which are often asymptomatic). There may also be abnormalities on urinalysis, as mentioned earlier (sometimes with eosinophiluria), and peripheral eosinophilia may also be present.[35] Eosinophilia has been reported in 14% of cases.[36]

Definitive diagnostic information must come from pathologic examination (biopsy, surgical pathology, or autopsy). However, less invasive testing may be suggestive of the diagnosis. The presence of Hollenhorst plaques, aneurysmal disease on diagnostic ultrasound or other imaging, or the presence of severe thoracic aortic plaque on transesophageal echocardiography may lead to the correct diagnosis. Recently, moving small particulate matter in transit from severe aortic plaque was observed on transesophageal echocardiography in a patient who subsequently died after multisystem involvement from cholesterol embolization (Fig. 47-6).[37]

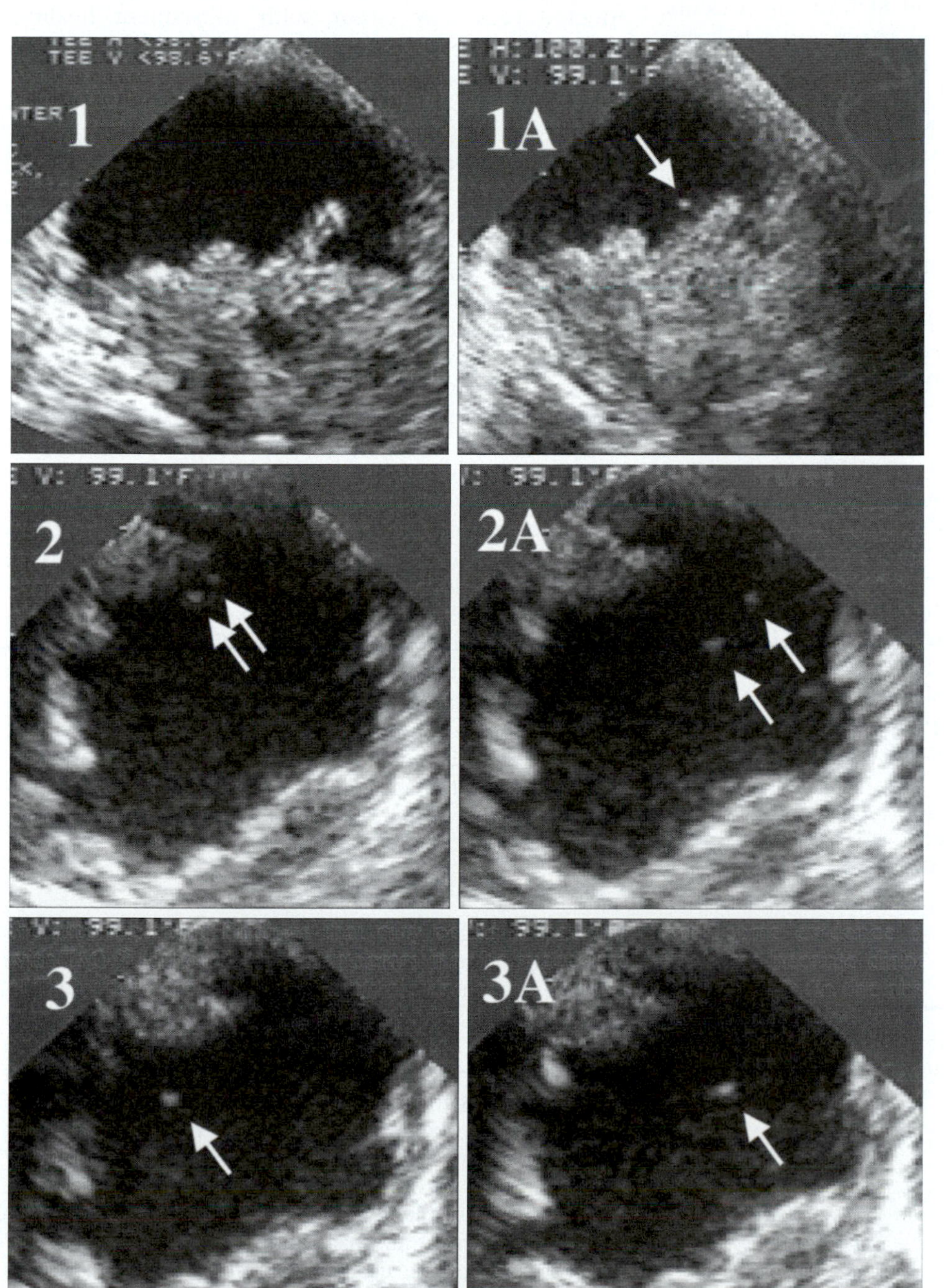

FIGURE 47-6. Emboli in transit. Transesophageal echocardiogram of the descending thoracic aorta in a patient who died of cholesterol crystal embolization syndrome, with intestinal infarction and renal failure. Note the massive atherosclerotic plaque. The pictures on the right **(1A, 2A, 3A)** were taken 1 or 2 seconds after their respective pictures on the left **(1, 2, 3)**. *Arrows* point to small particles of embolic material moving in transit in the aortic lumen. (From Freedberg RS, Tunick PA, Kronzon I: Emboli in transit: The missing link. J Am Soc Echo 11:826, 1998.)

Treatment

Because of the poor prognosis in medically treated patients (with mortality rates as high as 81%),[3] surgical treatment is indicated if a clear embolic source is identified. In a relatively large series, 100 patients underwent surgery (over 12 years) for the cholesterol crystal embolization syndrome.[38] The embolic source was located by a combination of CT scanning, angiography, ultrasound, transesophageal echocardiography, and MRI. Occlusive aortoiliac disease or small aortic aneurysms were the most common sources of emboli. Surgical treatment was aortic bypass or various other vascular procedures. Table 47-2 provides surgery results.[38] In another large surgical series, 62 patients were evaluated at a single institution.[39] Angiography identified the aorta or iliac arteries as the embolic source in 80% of the patients, with the femoral artery, popliteal artery, and subclavian arteries identified in the remaining patients. Surgical bypass grafts were performed in 42 patients (6 extra-anatomic) after exclusion of the native diseased artery. The mortality rate was only 5%. Limb salvage was possible in almost all patients, and there were no recurrent embolic incidents in the involved limbs during a mean follow-up of 20 months.

More recently, covered stents have been surgically implanted in a small number of patients with iliac artery sources of cholesterol crystal embolization,[40] and angioplasty and stenting have also been performed percutaneously in small select groups of patients.[41,42] Currently, definitive recommendations for these procedures cannot be made.

Currently, medical therapy is uncertain in the treatment of patients with the cholesterol crystal embolization syndrome. Small numbers of patients treated with statins, steroids, anticoagulants, and low density lipoprotein apheresis have been reported, but there are no larger trials from which to make evidence-based decisions. The use of statins in larger groups of patients to prevent myocardial infarction, stroke, and atherogenic thromboembolization from aortic plaque (see later) makes these drugs an attractive therapeutic modality. Similarly, the prophylactic use of antiplatelet agents (especially aspirin) seems prudent. Other risk factor modification is also appropriate (blood pressure control, cessation of smoking, aggressive treatment of hyperglycemia). Prospective trials sufficiently powered to evaluate medical treatment are unlikely.

TABLE 47-2 RESULTS OF VASCULAR SURGERY FOR CHOLESTEROL CRYSTAL EMBOLIZATION[38]

Postoperative death	11%
1-yr survival	89%
3-yr survival	83%
5-yr survival	73%
Leg amputation	9%
Toe amputation	10%
Hemodialysis	10%
Recurrent emboli	5%

Wound care is especially important in patients who have developed skin ulceration or gangrene. Systematic assessment of areas with ulceration is essential, with notation of the location, area, and depth of the lesion. The surrounding skin should be frequently evaluated with attention to signs of local infection or gangrene. Deeper infection is possible, despite the lack of systemic signs (fever, leukocytosis). When ulceration is present, surgical débridement with removal of all necrotic tissue may be necessary, along with limitation of weight bearing and systemic antibiotics. Topical antibiotic ointments may also reduce the local bacterial load and provide a barrier to secondary infection. Although soaking and whirlpools should be avoided (as they may aggravate skin breakdown), moist dressings (saline) absorb exudate and aid wound healing.[43] Autoamputation of affected toes may occur, with subsequent healing. Analgesia is essential for the patient with significant discomfort.

ATHEROGENIC THROMBOEMBOLISM

Atherogenic thromboembolism originates from unstable atherosclerotic plaques, which, when they rupture, are the site for clot formation. Organ damage frequently occurs when thrombi detach from the plaques, travel downstream, and lodge in medium-sized or large arteries. Atherogenic thromboembolism can occur anywhere in the arterial system. This section focuses on atherogenic thromboembolism originating from the thoracic aorta. Severe thoracic aortic plaque as an embolic source has been recognized on transesophageal echocardiography since 1990.[44] Perhaps most importantly, the prevalence of severe thoracic aortic plaque in stroke patients (21% to 27%) is on the same order of magnitude as the prevalences of carotid disease (10% to 13%) and atrial fibrillation (18% to 30%) reported in two recent large series of consecutive patients with stroke.[45,46]

Thus atherogenic thromboembolism from the aorta is responsible for a significant percentage of strokes previously labeled as "cryptogenic," much in the way that carotid artery disease became recognized as the etiology of many "cryptogenic" strokes when this entity was described by C. Miller Fisher in the 1950s.

Clinical Manifestations

Severe thoracic aortic plaques are high risk, with strokes occurring at a rate of 12% in one year[47,48] and peripheral emboli in an additional 20% of patients.[46] In the retrospective study mentioned earlier,[4] of 519 patients with severe thoracic aortic plaque on transesophageal echocardiography who were followed for an average of 3 years, there were 111 embolic events (21%). Half of the events were strokes, and the rest were transient ischemic attacks or peripheral emboli.

Atherogenic thromboembolism may involve multiple organs. For example, leg ischemia may occur simultaneously with renal embolization or intestinal infarction. Interestingly, in one case-control study, embolic events more commonly involved the left cerebral hemisphere or the peripheral circulation than the right cerebral hemisphere. This is consistent with the fact that severe plaques more commonly involve the middle or distal aortic arch or descending aorta and are relatively rare in the ascending aorta (and thus less likely to embolize to the innominate artery).[49]

Intraoperative stroke during heart surgery is a particularly devastating clinical manifestation of atherogenic thromboembolism. These strokes in patients with severe aortic arch plaque occur due to cannulation of the aorta for the institution of cardiopulmonary bypass. Such strokes occurred in 12% of 268 patients,[50] which is approximately six times the usual intraoperative stroke risk. Moreover, these intraoperative strokes are particularly severe. The in-hospital mortality for those with intraoperative stroke was 39%, and many survivors were severely disabled. As a result, their recovery room and intensive care unit length of stay was significantly longer, as was their total hospital length of stay. Finally, the in-hospital mortality for the group of 268 patients with severe aortic arch plaque on transesophageal echocardiography was high at 14.9%. Although stroke is the most obvious consequence of cerebral embolization after cannulation of the aorta for heart surgery, it is possible that the cognitive dysfunction that is described in many patients who have undergone cardiopulmonary bypass may also be a manifestation of atherogenic embolism.

Pathophysiology

Atherogenic thromboembolism frequently occurs spontaneously when unstable plaques undergo plaque rupture and thrombosis. The resulting superimposed thrombi are mobile and easily seen in the thoracic aorta on transesophageal echocardiography. Such mobile thrombi are common—they were detected in 127 of 519 patients (24%) with severe thoracic aortic plaque.[4] The instability of these plaques is underscored by the fact that mobile thrombi are often seen in different locations (on different plaques) when transesophageal echocardiography is performed at different times in the same patient.[51] One study measured the size of the lipid pool and the ratio of smooth muscle cells versus macrophages in intact aortic plaques versus plaques with superimposed thrombi.[52] The presence of superimposed thrombus was characteristic of plaques with a high proportion of lipid and with a preponderance of monocyte/macrophages as compared with smooth muscle cells.

Other evidence supports the vulnerable plaque theory. The *absence* of aortic plaque calcification has been found to increase stroke risk.[53] The highest risk was found in patients with noncalcified plaques greater than or equal to 4 mm in thickness. It is likely that these noncalcified plaques may be more lipid laden and therefore more likely to be unstable and responsible for atherogenic thromboembolism. In determining embolic risk, the most important measurable characteristic of aortic plaque is the plaque thickness as seen on transesophageal echocardiography. The French Aortic Plaque in Stroke Group found that the odds ratio for stroke in patients with plaques less than 1 mm was 1 (no increased risk); for 1- to 3.9-mm plaques it was 3.9; and for plaques greater than or equal to 4 mm it was dramatically higher, 13.8.[45] This study also supports causality with respect to arch atheromas and stroke, as the odds ratio for stroke in patients with plaques in the descending aorta (which could not embolize to the head) was only 1.5 for the largest plaques (≥4 mm) vs. 13.8 for those in the arch, upstream from the cerebral circulation.

As mentioned earlier, the physical dislodging of atheroma and thrombus from aortic arch plaques during cannulation for the institution of cardiopulmonary bypass is an important pathophysiologic mechanism as well. Iatrogenic thromboembolism may also infrequently occur during aortic manipulation for angiography and catheterization.

Pathology

Although some of the mobile lesions superimposed on atherosclerotic plaques may be part of the plaque itself ("debris"), early case reports of two patients who underwent aortic arch surgery documented that these mobile components were, in fact, thrombi that were removed from the aortic plaque itself (Fig. 47-7) as well as from

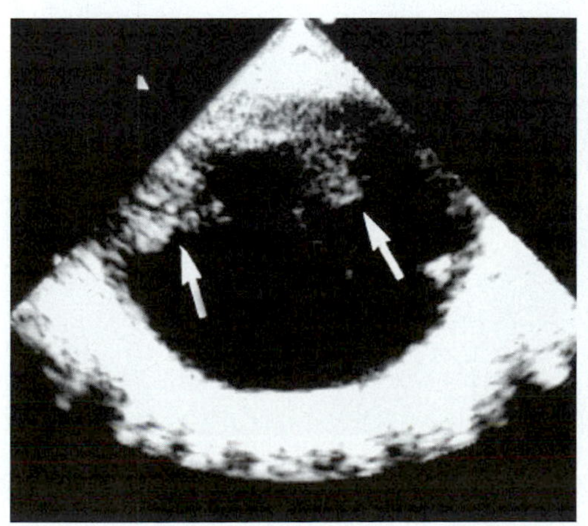

A

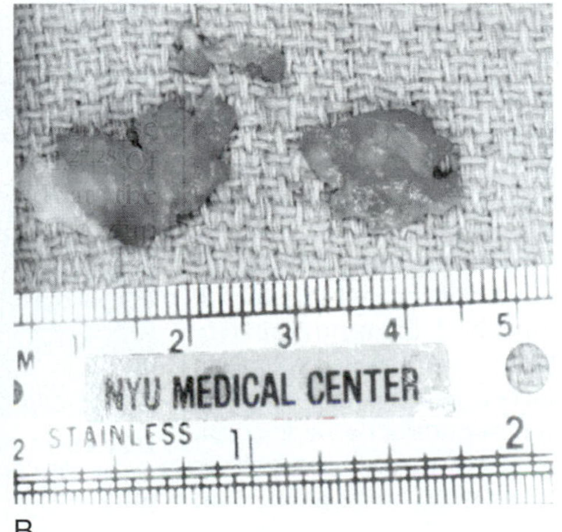

B

FIGURE 47-7. (See also Color Plate 47-7.) **A,** Transesophageal echocardiogram of the distal aortic arch with two mobile clots present *(arrows)*. **B,** Clots removed from the aorta seen in echo on left. (From Tunick PA, Lackner H, Katz ES, et al: Multiple emboli from a large aortic arch thrombus in a patient with thrombotic diathesis. Am Heart J 124:239, 1992.)

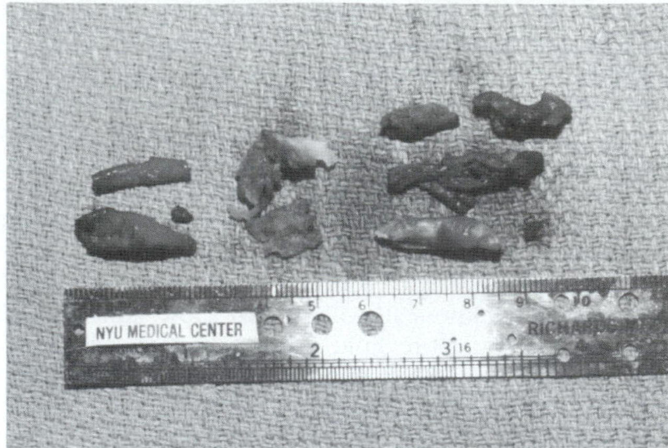

FIGURE 47-8. (See also Color Plate 47-8.) Clots removed from the femoral artery of the same patient seen in the aorta in Figure 47-7.

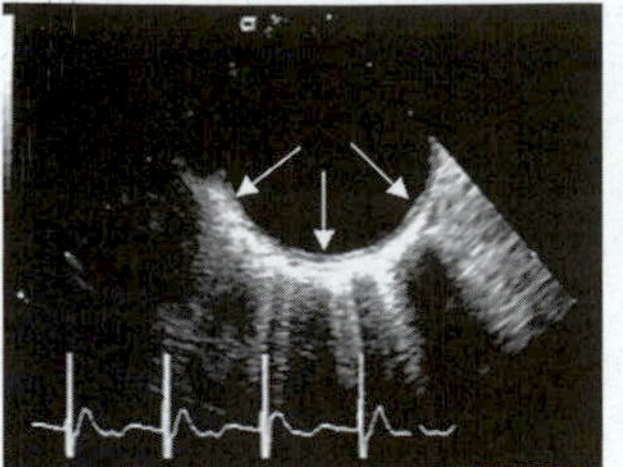

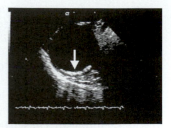

Normal Aorta

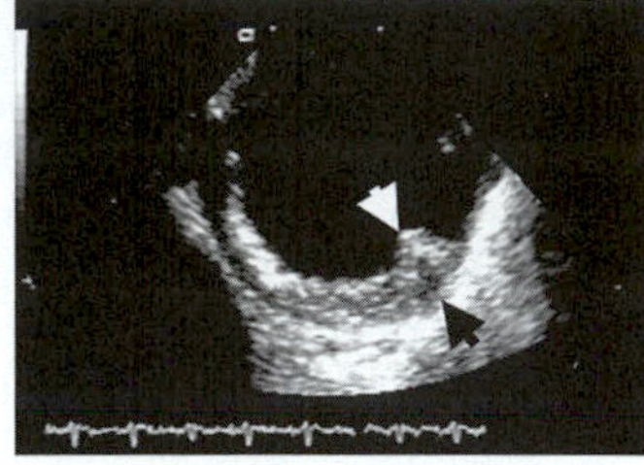

3 mm Plaque

7 mm Plaque

FIGURE 47-9. Three transesophageal echocardiograms of the thoracic aorta. *Upper left,* Normal. *Upper right,* Moderate (3 mm) plaque. *Bottom,* Severe (7 mm) plaque.

the femoral artery (Fig. 47-8) and subclavian artery after embolization.[54,55] This has been corroborated pathologically in additional patients,[56] including one autopsy study that documented aortic thrombi in 17 of 120 consecutive autopsies, as well as a significant association of complex plaque (thrombi, ulceration) with prior emboli.[57] In addition, pathologic examination of mobile lesions in the aorta seen on transesophageal echocardiography was recently reported in six patients with aortic aneurysm or dissection, and thrombi were found at the time of surgery.[58]

Diagnosis and Diagnostic Tests

Transthoracic echocardiography may show severe aortic arch plaque in patients with atherogenic thromboembolism[59]; however, its sensitivity is limited as is its resolution (necessary for measuring the prognostically important plaque thickness and diagnosing mobile thrombi). Ultrasound imaging of the descending thoracic and abdominal aorta is similarly limited. MRI has been used and can identify most severe plaques. However, there are limitations in measuring aortic arch plaque thickness and visualizing mobile thrombi.[60] With the rapid development in computer and MRI technology, this technique is likely to become increasingly valuable. CT is also useful for the detection of aortic plaque.[61] However, this technique subjects the patient to radiation and frequently requires the use of IV contrast.

At this time, transesophageal echocardiography is the procedure of choice for the detection, measurement, and characterization of thoracic aortic plaque (Figs. 47-9 and 47-10). It is relatively noninvasive and has a low complication rate. Although many centers use conscious sedation for patients undergoing transesophageal echocardiography, the procedure may be easily done without sedation in approximately 50% of patients. A full evaluation of the thoracic aorta may be accomplished in approximately 5 minutes, and there is excellent visualization except for a small part of the ascending aorta masked by the tracheal air column. The aortic arch and descending thoracic aorta, critical in patients with atherogenic thromboemboli or cholesterol crystal embolization, may be evaluated in their entirety and with excellent resolution. For patients undergoing cardiac surgery, intraoperative epiaortic ultrasound is useful for the evaluation of the ascending aorta.[62] This technique may complement information about the aortic arch that is obtained with intraoperative transesophageal echocardiography.

Treatment

In contrast with the results obtained from the surgical treatment of cholesterol crystal embolization, surgery has limited applicability in patients with atherogenic thromboembolism. This is because of the high intraoperative stroke rate (35%) that occurs when aortic arch endarterectomy is performed to treat severe arch plaque

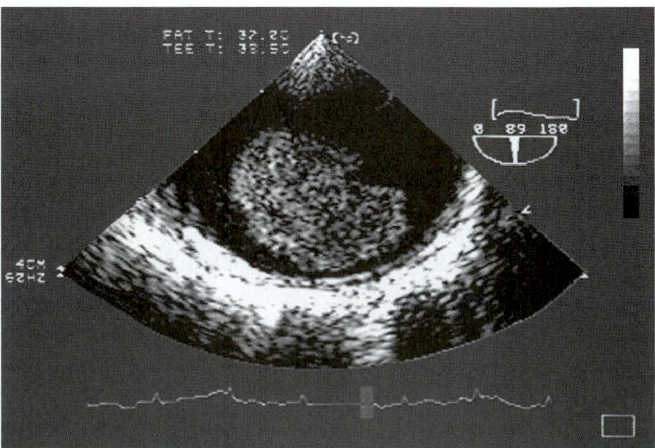

FIGURE 47-10. Transesophageal echocardiogram of the aortic arch, nearly filled by a large, mobile thrombus attached to an atherosclerotic plaque.

before the institution of cardiopulmonary bypass for coronary or valve surgery.[50] In isolated patients who are good operative candidates (especially in the less common younger patient), arch endarterectomy has been performed with good results.[54,55] However, this is a relatively radical approach, requiring hypothermic circulatory arrest. Aortic or carotid filters, which could help prevent complications, are being developed and may theoretically be useful, but they have not been fully evaluated for this purpose.

In contrast, the medical therapy of patients with atherogenic thromboembolism does hold promise. The initial approach to the medical treatment of this condition centered around anticoagulation. Once the pathology (thrombus embolization) became known, warfarin was a logical choice to attempt to prevent embolization. In fact, two studies of the use of warfarin and aspirin in patients with severe aortic plaque reported a potential benefit of warfarin.[63,64] However, both had small numbers of patients and events. The first described 31 patients with mobile thrombi in the aorta on transesophageal echocardiography. There was a higher incidence of events in the patients who were not treated with warfarin than in those who were given warfarin (at the discretion of the referring physicians). Strokes occurred in 3 of 11 patients not treated with warfarin and in none of those on warfarin. The other report was an observational study of 129 patients with previous embolization who were found to have aortic plaque on transesophageal echocardiography. There was a reduction in the number of embolic events in patients with plaques greater than or equal to 4 mm who received oral anticoagulants (0 of 27, vs. 5 events in 23 patients treated with antiplatelet agents).

However, a much larger group of 519 patients, all of whom had severe plaque in the thoracic aorta on transesophageal echocardiography, were evaluated retrospectively.[4] There were a large number of embolic events (111 events, 21%) during an average of 3 years of follow-up. Surprisingly there was no benefit of warfarin or antiplatelet drugs found. However, HMGCoA reductase inhibitors (statins) were independently protective against recurrent events (P = .0001) (Fig. 47-11). The relative risk reduction for embolic events was 59%, and the absolute risk reduction was 17% (yielding a low Number Needed to Treat of only six patients). One of the pleiotropic effects of statin drugs appears to be plaque stabilization, perhaps as a consequence of their anti-inflammatory properties. This may be responsible for the protective effect of statins in patients at risk for atherogenic thromboembolism. There has been no prospective evaluation of the use of statins for this condition (although statins have been shown prospectively to prevent strokes in large numbers of patients with coronary artery disease).

Prospective, randomized data are forthcoming from a recently implemented international trial of warfarin versus aspirin plus clopidogrel (the ARCH Trial), which is overcoming the limitations of the available retrospective data concerning these drugs (although statins are not being randomized). However, it seems possible

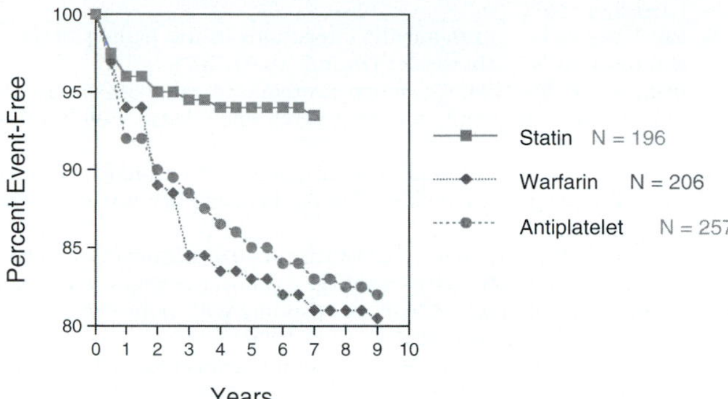

FIGURE 47-11. Event-free survival on statins, warfarin, and antiplatelet drugs. The protective effect of statins was highly significant, with a relative risk reduction of 59%, an absolute risk reduction of 17%, and a Number Needed to Treat of only 6. (From Tunick PA, Nayar AC, Goodkin GM, et al: For the NYU Atheroma Group: Effect of treatment on the incidence of stroke and other emboli in 519 patients with severe thoracic aortic plaque. Am J Cardiol 90:1320, 2002.)

that warfarin does not stabilize plaque and prevent plaque rupture and subsequent thrombosis and embolization.

The use of angiotensin-converting enzyme inhibitors in patients with vascular disease received great interest after the demonstration that ramipril significantly reduces the rates of death, myocardial infarction, and stroke in these patients.[65] Although angiotensin-converting enzyme inhibitors have not been specifically evaluated in patients with severe aortic plaque on transesophageal echocardiography, their use could possibly help prevent embolic events in these patients.

The use of antioxidants is also theoretically attractive for the prevention of atherosclerotic syndromes, but trials to date have been disappointing. The use of B vitamins (folic acid, B_{12}, pyridoxine) does lower plasma homocysteine levels. Information about whether these vitamins may also prevent vascular events is awaited, as are data concerning the efficacy of newer drugs that block cholesterol absorption and affect lipoprotein size and density, or raise HDL.

REFERENCES

1. White PD: Heart Disease, 4th ed. New York, MacMillan, 1951, p 744.
2. Hurst JW: Meaningful quotations from Paul Dudley White. Clin Cardiol 21:617,1998.
3. Fine MJ, Kapoor W, Falanga V: Cholesterol crystal embolization: A review of 221 cases in the English literature. Angiology 38:769,1987.
4. Tunick PA, Nayar AC, Goodkin GM, et al for the NYU Atheroma Group: Effect of treatment on the incidence of stroke and other emboli in 519 patients with severe thoracic aortic plaque. Am J Cardiol 90:1320, 2002.
5. Agmon Y, Khandheria BK, Meissner I, et al: Independent association of high blood pressure and aortic atherosclerosis: A population-based study. Circulation 102:2087, 2000.
6. von Eckardstein A, Malinow MR, Upson B, et al: Effects of age, lipoproteins, and hemostatic parameters on the role of homocyst(e)inemia as a cardiovascular risk factor in men. Arterioscler Thromb 14:460,1994.

7. Konecky N, Malinow MR, Tunick PA, et al: Correlation between plasma homocyst(e)ine and aortic atherosclerosis. Am Heart J 133:534,1997.
8. Fan J, Watanabe T: Inflammatory reactions in the pathogenesis of atherosclerosis. J Atheroscler Thromb 10:63, 2003.
9. Blake GJ, Ridker PM: C-reactive protein and other inflammatory risk markers in acute coronary syndromes. J Am Coll Cardiol 41:S37, 2003.
10. Olin JW: Other peripheral arterial diseases. In Goldman L (ed): Cecil Textbook of Medicine, 21st ed. Philadelphia, WB Saunders, 2000, p 362.
11. The Stroke Prevention in Atrial Fibrillation Investigators Committee on Echocardiography: Transesophageal echocardiography correlates of thromboembolism in high-risk patients with nonvalvular atrial fibrillation. Ann Intern Med 128:639,1998.
12. Abdelmalek MF, Spittell PC: 79-year-old woman with blue toes. Mayo Clin Proc 70:292,1995.
13. Falanga V, Fine MJ, Kapoor WN: The cutaneous manifestations of cholesterol crystal embolization. Arch Dermatol 122:1194,1986.
14. Haas M, Spargo BH, Wit EJ, et al: Etiologies and outcome of acute renal insufficiency in older adults: A renal biopsy study of 259 cases. Am J Kidney Dis 35:433, 2000.
15. Aujla ND, Greenberg A, Banner BF, et al: Atheroembolic involvement of renal allografts. Am J Kidney Dis 13:329,1989.
16. Moolenaar W, Lamers CB: Gastrointestinal blood loss due to cholesterol crystal embolization. J Clin Gastroenterol 21:220,1995.
17. Bourdages R, Prentice RS, Beck IT, et al: Atheromatous embolization to the stomach: An unusual cause of gastrointestinal bleeding. Am J Dig Dis 21:889,1976.
18. Moolenaar W, Lamers CB: Cholesterol crystal embolization to liver, gallbladder, and pancreas. Dig Dis Sci 41:1819,1996.
19. Hollenhorst RW: Significance of bright plaques in the retinal arterioles. JAMA 178:123,1961.
20. Schwarcz TH, Eton D, Ellenby MI, et al: Hollenhorst plaques: Retinal manifestations and the role of carotid endarterectomy. J Vasc Surg 11:635,1990.
21. Sharma PV, Babu SC, Shah PM, et al: Changing patterns of atheroembolism. Cardiovasc Surg 4:573,1996.
22. Baumann DS, McGraw D, Rubin BG, et al: An institutional experience with arterial atheroembolism. Ann Vasc Surg 8:258, 1994.
23. Bashore TM, Gehrig T: Cholesterol emboli after invasive cardiac procedures. J Am Coll Cardiol 42:217, 2003.
24. Keeley EC, Grines CL: Scraping of aortic debris by coronary guiding catheters: A prospective evaluation of 1,000 cases. J Am Coll Cardiol 32:1861,1998.
25. Fukumoto Y, Tsutsui H, Tsuchihashi M, et al, for the Cholesterol Embolism Study (CHEST) investigators: The incidence and risk factors of cholesterol embolization syndrome, a complication of cardiac catheterization: A prospective study. J Am Coll Cardiol 42:211, 2003.
26. Piriou V, Claudel JP, Bastien O, et al: Severe systemic cholesterol embolization after open heart surgery. Br J Anaesth 77:277, 1996.
27. Ribera Pibernat M, Bigata Viscasillas X, et al: [Cholesterol embolism disease: Study of 16 cases]. Rev Clin Esp 200:659, 2000.
28. Nevelsteen A, Kutten M, Lacroix H, et al: Oral anticoagulant therapy: A precipitating factor in the pathogenesis of cholesterol embolization. Acta Chir Belg 92:33,1992.
29. Hyman BT, Landas SK, Ashman RF, et al: Warfarin related purple toe syndrome and cholesterol microembolization. Am J Med 82:1233, 1987.
30. Blackshear JL, Pearce LA, Zabalgoitia M: Low risk of cholesterol crystal embolization (CCE) during warfarin therapy in patients with aortic plaque (AP). Circulation I-101, 1998.
31. Queen M, Biem HJ, Moe GW, et al: Development of cholesterol embolization syndrome after intravenous streptokinase for acute myocardial infarction. Am J Cardiol 65:1042, 1990.
32. Modi KD, Rao VK: Atheroembolic renal disease. J Am Soc Nephrol 12:1781, 2001.
33. Warren BA, Vales O: The ultrastructure of the stages of atheroembolic occlusion of renal arteries. Br J Exp Pathol 54:469, 1973.
34. Case Records of the Massachusetts General Hospital: N Engl J Med 334:973, 1996.
35. Cogan E, Schandene L, Papadopoulos T, et al: Interleukin-5 production by T lymphocytes in atheroembolic disease with hypereosinophilia. J Allergy Clin Immunol 96:427, 1995.
36. Thadhani RI, Camargo CA Jr, Xavier RJ, et al: Atheroembolic renal failure after invasive procedures: Natural history based on 52 histologically proven cases. Medicine (Baltimore) 74:350, 1995.
37. Freedberg RS, Tunick PA, Kronzon I: Emboli in transit: The missing link. J Am Soc Echo 11:826, 1998.
38. Keen RR, McCarthy WJ, Shireman PK, et al: Surgical management of atheroembolization. J Vasc Surg 21:773, 1995.
39. Baumann DS, McGraw D, Rubin BG, et al: An institutional experience with arterial atheroembolism. Ann Vasc Surg 8:258, 1994.
40. Kumins NH, Owens EL, Oglevie SB, et al: Early experience using the Wallgraft in the management of distal microembolism from common iliac artery patholology. Ann Vasc Surg 16:181, 2002.
41. Renshaw A, McCowen T, Waltke EA, et al: Angioplasty with stenting is effective in treating blue toe syndrome. Vasc Endovascular Surg 36:155, 2002.
42. Matchett WJ, McFarland DR, Eidt JF, et al: Blue toe syndrome: Treatment with intra-arterial stents and review of therapies. J Vasc Interv Radiol 11:585, 2000.
43. Sumpio BE: Foot ulcers. N Engl J Med 343:787, 2000.
44. Tunick PA, Kronzon I: Protruding atherosclerotic plaque in the aortic arch of patients with systemic embolization: A new finding seen by transesophageal echocardiography. Am Heart J 120:658, 1990.
45. Amarenco P, Cohen A, Tzourio C, et al: Atherosclerotic disease of the aortic arch and the risk of ischemic stroke. N Engl J Med 331:1474, 1994.
46. Jones EF, Kalman JM, Calafiore P, et al: Proximal aortic atheroma: An independent risk factor for cerebral ischemia. Stroke 26:218, 1995.
47. Tunick PA, Rosenzweig BP, Katz ES, et al: High risk for vascular events in patients with protruding aortic atheromas: A prospective study. J Am Coll Cardiol 23:1085, 1994.
48. Amarenco P, Cohen A for the French Study of Aortic Plaques in Stroke Group: Atherosclerotic disease of the aortic arch as a risk factor for recurrent ischemic stroke. N Engl J Med 334:1216, 1996.
49. Tunick PA, Perez JL, Kronzon I: Protruding atheromas in the thoracic aorta and systemic embolization. Ann Intern Med 115:423, 1991.
50. Stern A, Tunick PA, Culliford AT, et al: Protruding aortic arch atheromas: Risk of stroke during heart surgery with and without aortic arch endarterectomy. Am Heart J 138:746, 1999.
51. Montgomery DH, Ververis JJ, McGorisk G, et al: Natural history of severe atheromatous disease of the thoracic aorta: A transesophageal echocardiographic study. J Am Coll Cardiol 27:95, 1996.
52. Davies MJ, Richardson PD, Woolf N, et al: Risk of thrombosis in human atherosclerotic plaques: Role of extracellular lipid, macrophage, and smooth muscle cell content. Br Heart J 69:377, 1993.
53. Cohen A, Tzourio C, Bertrand B, et al on behalf of the FAPS Investigators: Aortic plaque morphology and vascular events: A follow-up study in patients with ischemic stroke. Circulation 96:3837, 1997.
54. Tunick PA, Lackner H, Katz ES, et al: Multiple emboli from a large aortic arch thrombus in a patient with thrombotic diathesis. Am Heart J 124:239, 1992.
55. Tunick PA, Culliford A, Lamparello P, et al: Atheromatosis of the aortic arch as an occult source of multiple systemic emboli. Ann Intern Med 114:391, 1991.
56. Nihoyannopoulos P, Joshi J, Athanasopoulos G, et al: Detection of atherosclerotic lesions in the aorta by transesophageal echocardiography. Am J Cardiol 71:1208: 1993.
57. Khatibzadeh M, Mitusch R, Stierle U, et al: Aortic atherosclerotic plaque as a source of systemic embolism. J Am Coll Cardiol 27:664, 1996.
58. Vaduganathan P, Ewton A, Nagueh SF, et al: Pathologic correlates of aortic plaques, thrombi and mobile "aortic debris" imaged in vivo with transesophageal echocardiography. J Am Coll Cardiol 30:357, 1997.
59. Weinberger J, Azhar S, Danisi F, et al: A new noninvasive technique for imaging atherosclerotic plaque in the aortic arch of stroke patients by transcutaneous real-time B-mode ultrasonography: An initial report. Stroke 29:673, 1998.

60. Kutz SM, Lee V, Tunick PA, et al: Atheromas of the thoracic aorta: A comparison of transesophageal echocardiography and breath-hold gadolinium-enhanced 3-D magnetic resonance angiography. J Am Soc Echo 12:853, 1999.
61. Tenenbaum A, Garniek A, Shemesh J, et al: Spiral computerized tomography (dual helical mode) as a detector of aortic atheromas in patients with stroke and systemic emboli: Additional benefit of the contrast-enhanced technique. Isr Med Assoc J 2:1, 2000.
62. Wareing TH, Dávila-Román VG, Daily B, et al: Strategy for the reduction of stroke incidence in cardiac surgical patients. Ann Thorac Surg 55:1400, 1993.
63. Dressler FA, Craig WR, Castello R, et al: Mobile aortic atheroma and systemic emboli: Efficacy of anticoagulation and influence of plaque morphology on recurrent stroke. J Am Coll Cardiol 31:134, 1998.
64. Ferrari E, Vidal R, Chevallier T, et al: Atherosclerosis of the thoracic aorta and aortic debris as a marker of poor prognosis: Benefit of oral anticoagulants. J Am Coll Cardiol 33:1317, 1999.
65. The Heart Outcomes Prevention Evaluation Study investigators: Effects of an angiotensin-converting enzyme inhibitor, ramipril, on cardiovascular events in high-risk patients. N Engl J Med 342:145, 2000.

chapter 48

Raynaud's Phenomenon

Mark A. Creager
Jonathan L. Halperin
Jay D. Coffman

"In its simplest form, local syncope is a condition perfectly compatible with health. Persons who are attacked with it are ordinarily females. Under the least stimulus, sometimes without appreciable cause, one or many fingers become pale and cold all at once; in many cases, it is the same finger that is always first attacked; the others become dead successively and in the same order. It is the phenomenon known as 'dead finger.' The attack is indolent, the duration varies from a few minutes to many hours. The determining cause is often the impression of cold; but that which is only commonly produced under the influence of the most severe cold, appears in the subjects of whom I speak on the occasion of the least lowering of temperatures; sometimes even a simple mental emotion is enough … the skin of the affected parts assumes a dead white or sometimes a yellow colour; it appears completely exsanguine. The cutaneous sensibility becomes blunted, then annihilated; the fingers become like foreign bodies to the subject … the slight importance of this local abolition of the circulation is probably due to the fact that it is so transient … the attack is followed by a period of reaction, which is often very painful, and which gives place to a sensation quite analogous to that of being numbed by cold … and in the more pronounced cases, which the patients compared to tingling from cold, or to the stinging of nettles. … Finally, a patch of deep red is formed on the extremities of the fingers. This patch gives place to the normal pink colour, and then the skin is found to have entirely returned to the primitive condition."[1]

Maurice Raynaud

Episodic vasospastic ischemia of the digits was first described by Maurice Raynaud in the quotation above (Fig. 48-1).[1] Raynaud's phenomenon comprises the sequential development of digital blanching, cyanosis, and rubor following cold exposure and subsequent rewarming (Fig. 48-2).[2-4] Emotional stress also precipitates Raynaud's phenomenon. The color changes are usually well demarcated and primarily confined to the fingers or toes. The blanching, or pallor, occurs during the ischemic phase of the phenomenon and is secondary to digital vasospasm. During ischemia, arterioles, capillaries, and venules dilate. Cyanosis results from the deoxygenated blood in these vessels. Cold, numbness, or paresthesias of the digits often accompany the phases of pallor and cyanosis. With rewarming, the digital vasospasm resolves, and blood flow dramatically increases into the dilated arterioles and capillaries. This "reactive hyperemia" imparts a bright red color to the digits. In addition to rubor and warmth, the patients often experience a throbbing sensation during the hyperemic phase. Thereafter, the color of the digits gradually returns to normal. Although the triphasic color response is typical of Raynaud's phenomenon, some patients may develop only pallor and cyanosis. Others may experience only cyanosis.[5]

The classification of Raynaud's phenomenon is broadly separated into two categories: (1) the idiopathic

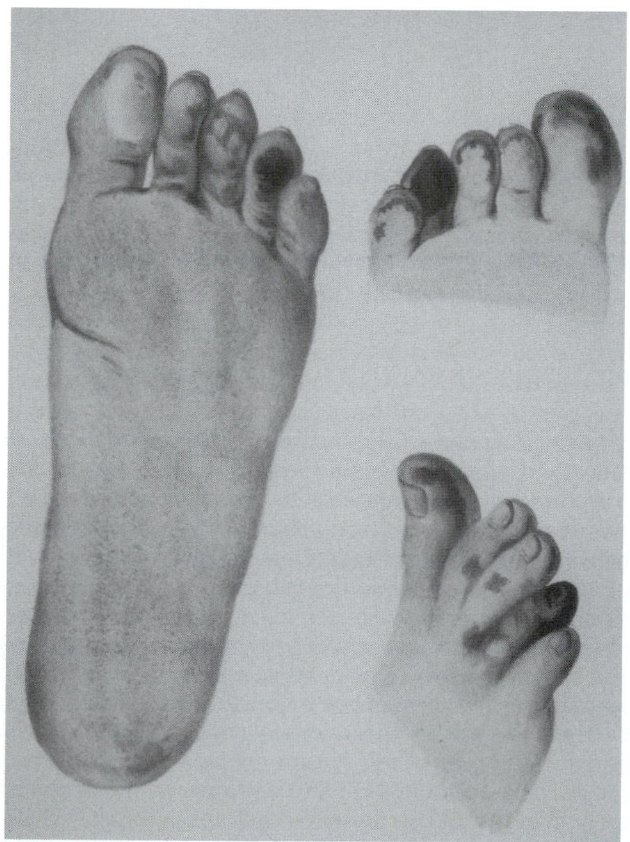

FIGURE 48-1. A patient with Raynaud's phenomenon. (From Raynaud M: Local Asphyxia and Symmetrical Gangrene of the Extremities. London, New Sydenham Society, 1862. Courtesy Boston Medical Library in the Francis A. Countway Library of Medicine.)

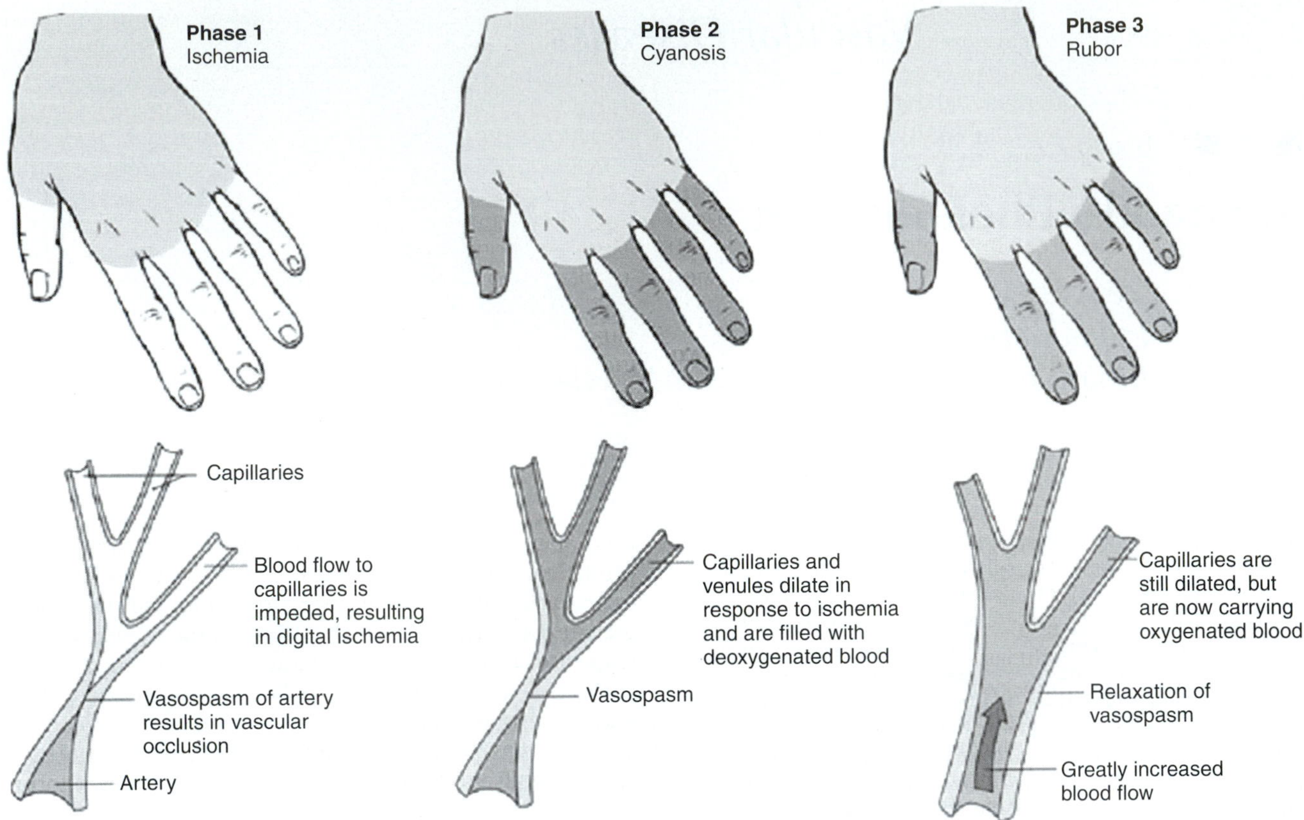
Phase 1
Ischemia
Phase 2
Cyanosis
Phase 3
Rubor
Capillaries
Blood flow to capillaries is impeded, resulting in digital ischemia
Vasospasm of artery results in vascular occlusion
Artery
Capillaries and venules dilate in response to ischemia and are filled with deoxygenated blood
Vasospasm
Capillaries are still dilated, but are now carrying oxygenated blood
Relaxation of vasospasm
Greatly increased blood flow

FIGURE 48-2. (See also Color Plate 48-2.) Raynaud's phenomenon may have three color phases: blanching, cyanosis, and rubor. (From Creager MA: Raynaud's phenomenon. Med Illus 1983;2:84.)

variety, termed *primary Raynaud's phenomenon,* and (2) the secondary variety, which is associated with other disease states or known causes of vasospasm (Box 48-1). The secondary causes of Raynaud's phenomenon include collagen vascular diseases, arterial occlusive disease, thoracic outlet syndrome, several neurologic disorders, blood dyscrasias, trauma, and several drugs.

PRIMARY RAYNAUD'S PHENOMENON

Primary Raynaud's phenomenon, or idiopathic episodic digital vasospasm, is the most common diagnosis of patients who present with Raynaud's phenomenon.[2,3] The diagnosis is based on criteria originally established by Allen and Brown,[6] including (1) intermittent attacks of ischemic discoloration of the extremities; (2) absence of organic arterial occlusions; (3) bilateral distribution; (4) trophic changes—when present, limited to the skin and never consisting of gross gangrene; (5) absence of any symptoms or signs of systemic disease that might account for the occurrence of Raynaud's phenomenon; and (6) duration of the symptoms for 2 years or longer. If a normal sedimentation rate, a normal nailfold capillary examination, and a negative test for antinuclear antibodies are added to these criteria, the diagnosis is more secure.[2,7]

Women are affected approximately five times more frequently than men. In one large study, the average age of onset of Raynaud's phenomenon was 31 years; 78% of the patients were younger than 40 years old when symptoms began.[8] The onset of symptoms in women may occur between menarche and menopause. Raynaud's phenomenon is also known to occur in young children.[9] The prevalence of primary Raynaud's phenomenon varies with climate, with 4.6% of the population affected in warm climates compared with 17% in cooler climates.[10] There is a significant familial aggregation of primary Raynaud's phenomenon. Approximately 26% of patients may know of one or more relatives who have the phenomenon, suggesting a genetic predisposition.[11]

In the vast majority of patients, the fingers are the initial sites of involvement.[2-4] At first blanching or cyanosis may involve only one or two fingers (Fig. 48-3). Later, color changes may develop in additional fingers, and symptoms occur bilaterally. In approximately 40% of patients, Raynaud's phenomenon involves the toes as well as the fingers. Isolated Raynaud's phenomena of the toes occur in only 1% to 2% of patients. Rarely, the ear lobes, tip of the nose, or tongue are affected.

Episodes of Raynaud's phenomenon are usually precipitated by exposure to cool environment or by direct exposure of the extremities to low temperatures. Some patients may experience Raynaud's phenomenon during either cold exposure or emotional stress; infrequently, emotional stress may be the only precipitating factor. The duration, frequency, and severity of Raynaud's phenomenon increase during the cold months.

BOX 48-1 Secondary Causes of Raynaud's Phenomenon

Collagen vascular diseases
- Systemic sclerosis (scleroderma)
- Systemic lupus erythematosus
- Rheumatoid arthritis
- Dermatomyositis and polymyositis
- Mixed connective tissue disease
- Sjögren's syndrome
- Necrotizing vasculitis

Arterial occlusive disease
- Atherosclerosis of the extremities
- Thromboangiitis obliterans (Buerger's disease)
- Thromboembolism

Neurologic disorders
- Carpal tunnel syndrome
- Reflex sympathetic dystrophy
- Stroke
- Intervertebral disk disease
- Syringomyelia
- Poliomyelitis

Thoracic outlet syndrome

Trauma
- Exposure to vibrating tools (vibration white finger)
- Electric shock injury
- Thermal injury
- Percussive injury
- Hypothenar hammer syndrome

Drugs and toxins
- Ergot alkaloids
- Methysergide
- Vinblastine
- Bleomycin
- β-Adrenoceptor antagonists
- Vinyl chloride

Blood dyscrasias
- Hyperviscosity syndrome
- Cold agglutinin disease
- Cryoglobulinemia
- Cryofibrinogenemia
- Myeloproliferative disease

Miscellaneous causes
- Hypothyroidism
- Arteriovenous fistula
- Pulmonary hypertension

Several studies have correlated Raynaud's phenomenon with migraine headaches and variant angina, suggesting a common mechanism for vasospasm.[12-14] An association with vasospasm in the kidney,[15] retina,[16] and pulmonary[17] vessels has also been described. Further evidence is the report of a family with three generations of systemic arterial vasospastic disease involving Raynaud's phenomenon, variant angina, and migraine headaches.[18] Differences in the responses of pharmacologic intervention make the hypothesis of a common mechanism less appealing.[19] Propranolol has been successfully used to prevent migraine headaches.[20] In contrast, β-adrenoceptor blockers are not beneficial in variant angina and may cause Raynaud's phenomenon.[21,22]

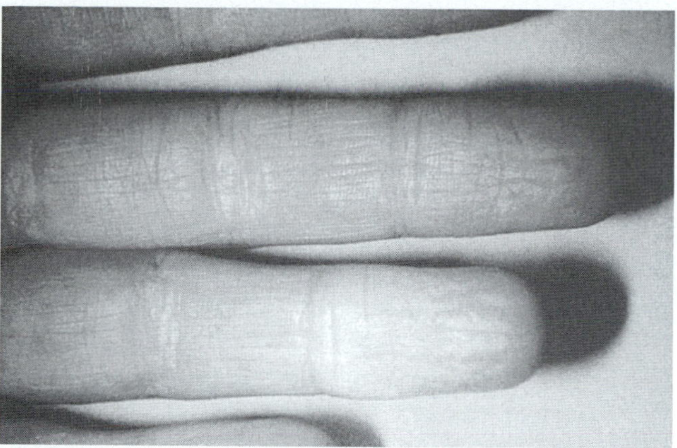

FIGURE 48-3. (See also Color Plate 48-3.) Raynaud's phenomenon presenting as blanching of one finger.

Similarly, nitrates are used for variant angina but are not beneficial in Raynaud's phenomenon and often cause headaches. Ergot alkaloids are effective for treating migraine headaches but can cause coronary and digital vasospasm.[23,24]

The physical examination of patients with primary Raynaud's phenomenon is often entirely normal. Sometimes, the fingers and toes are cool and may perspire excessively. The pulse examination is normal. The radial, ulnar, and pedal pulses should be easily palpable. Trophic changes such as sclerodactyly (thickening and tightening of the digital subcutaneous tissue) have been reported in up to 10% of patients, but these studies preceded nailfold capillaroscopy and antinuclear antibody tests. The physical examination is most important to exclude secondary causes of Raynaud's phenomenon.

Of all the forms of Raynaud's phenomenon, primary Raynaud's phenomenon has the most benign prognosis. In the group of patients identified by Gifford and Hines,[8] followed for a period of 1 to 32 years averaging 12 years, 16% reported worsening of their symptoms, whereas 38%, 36%, and 10% reported no change, improvement, or disappearance of their symptoms, respectively. Sclerodactyly or trophic changes of the digits occurred in approximately 3% of patients during the follow-up, and less than 1% of patients lost part of a digit. In some patients, scleroderma may develop after Raynaud's phenomenon has been present as the only symptom for more than 20 years. Wollersheim and colleagues[25] reported that measuring antinuclear antibodies by immunofluorescence and immunoblotting had a positive predictive value of 65% and 71% and a negative predictive value of 93% and 83%, respectively, for the development of a connective tissue disease in patients with Raynaud's phenomenon.

Pathophysiology

The precise cause of Raynaud's phenomenon has not been clearly identified. It is quite likely that a variety of physiologic and pathologic conditions may contribute to or cause digital vasospasm (Box 48-2) (Fig. 48-4).[2-4,26]

BOX 48-2 Pathophysiology of Raynaud's Phenomenon: Possible Mechanisms

Vasoconstrictive stimuli
- Digital vascular hyperreactivity ("local fault")
- Increased sympathetic nervous system activity
- β-Adrenoceptor blockade
- Circulating vasoactive hormones
  - Angiotensin II
  - Serotonin
  - Thromboxane
  - Endothelin-1
- Exogenous administration of vasoconstrictor agents
  - Ergot alkaloids
  - Sympathomimetic drugs

Decreased intravascular pressure
- Low systemic blood pressure
- Arterial occlusive disorder (e.g., atherosclerosis, thromboangiitis obliterans)
- Digital arterial occlusions (e.g., scleroderma)
- Hyperviscosity

Normally, the regulation of peripheral blood flow depends on several factors including the intrinsic vascular tone; sympathetic nervous system activity; hemorheologic properties such as blood viscosity; and various circulating hormonal substances. In contrast to other regional circulations that are supplied by both vasoconstrictor and vasodilator sympathetic fibers, the cutaneous vessels of the hands and feet are innervated only by sympathetic adrenergic vasoconstrictor fibers. In these vascular beds, neurogenic vasodilation occurs by withdrawal of a sympathetic stimulus. Cooling evokes reflex sympathetic-mediated vasoconstriction in the hands and feet via neurons originating in cutaneous receptors. Environmental cooling, or cooling of specific body parts such as the head, neck, or trunk, normally causes a reduction in digital blood flow. Local digital cooling also induces vasoconstriction; however, digital vasoconstriction caused by local cooling is not mediated by the sympathetic nervous system. Thus digital vasoconstriction may be a physiologic response to local cooling or to reflex activation of the sympathetic nervous system by environmental cold exposure or emotional stress.

Raynaud's phenomenon is not a normal physiologic response but rather an episode of digital artery vasospasm causing cessation of blood flow to the digits. The term *vasospasm* must be distinguished from that of *vasoconstriction*. Vasoconstriction may be defined as the expected reduction in vessel lumen size as a result of endogenous neural, hormonal, or metabolic factors that cause smooth muscle contraction. Vasospasm implies an excessive vasoconstrictor response to stimuli that would normally cause modest smooth muscle contraction but that instead has resulted in obliteration of the vascular lumen. The patency of the digital artery depends on a favorable balance between the contractile forces of the muscular wall of the digital artery and its intraluminal pressure. Thus a situation in which there is excessive vasoconstrictive force or decreased intravascular pressure upsets this balance and results in vasospasm. It is with these rather simple concepts that several theories have been proposed to explain the episodic digital vasospasm that defines Raynaud's phenomenon.

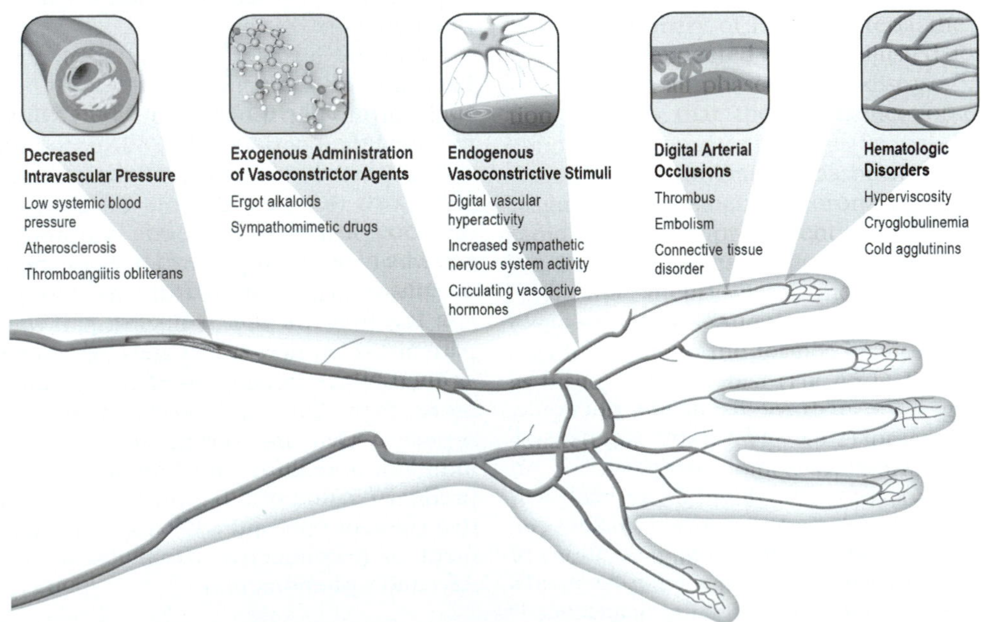

FIGURE 48-4. (See also Color Plate 48-4.) Pathophysiology of digital vasospasm. Digital vasospasm may occur as a consequence of vasoconstrictive stimuli, decreased intravascular pressure, or both. Mechanisms that contribute to exercise vasoconstriction include local vascular hypersensitivity to vasoactive stimuli (e.g., increased α-adrenoceptor sensitivity); sympathetic efferent activity; and local or circulating vasoactive hormones such as angiotensin II, endothelin-1, serotonin, or thromboxane A_2. Low blood pressure, even in a healthy young person, may predispose to Raynaud's phenomenon when the person encounters vasoconstrictive stimuli. Pathologic conditions that may decrease intravascular pressure include arterial occlusion in proximal arteries (e.g., atherosclerosis), digital vascular occlusion (e.g., scleroderma), or hyperviscosity.

Increased Vasoconstrictive Stimuli

Several theories implicate excessive vasoconstrictive stimuli as a cause of Raynaud's phenomenon. Postulated causes include local vascular hyperreactivity; increased sympathetic nervous system activity; elevated levels of vasoconstrictor hormones such as angiotensin II, serotonin, and thromboxane A_2; as well as exogenously administered agents such as ergot alkaloids and sympathomimetic drugs.

Local Vascular Hyperreactivity

The observation that episodic digital vasospasm occurs during cold exposure has led several investigators to consider the possibility that Raynaud's phenomenon occurs as a result of a local vascular hyperreactivity. In 1929 Sir Thomas Lewis observed that following exposure of the finger to cold, vasospasm could be produced even after nerve blockade or sympathectomy.[27] These experiments were repeated and confirmed 60 years later.[28] Therefore the vasospastic response of Raynaud's phenomenon may occur in the absence of efferent digital nerves.

The possibility of local vascular hyperreactivity was examined by Jamieson and coworkers.[29] They compared the magnitude of reflex vasoconstriction in each hand following application of ice to the neck while one hand was kept at 26° C and the other 36° C.[12] At 36° C, the reflex vasoconstrictor response was comparable in normal subjects and patients with primary Raynaud's phenomenon. In the hand cooled to 26° C, however, the reflex vasoconstriction was exaggerated in the patients with Raynaud's phenomenon. This response led these investigators to hypothesize that digital α_1 adrenoceptors were sensitized by cold exposure. A series of studies by Vanhoutte and colleagues[30] have supported the hypothesis that cooling potentiates the vascular response to sympathetic nerve activation. Vasoconstriction, in response to exogenous norepinephrine, also is increased by cooling. Augmentation of adrenergic-mediated vasoconstriction by cooling occurs despite generalized depression of contractile machinery and diminished release of norepinephrine from sympathetic nerve endings in the vessel wall. The most likely hypothesis is that cold causes changes at the level of the adrenoceptor, such as an increase in the affinity for norepinephrine or greater efficacy of the agonist-receptor complex. Vanhoutte and colleagues[30] have reported that α_2 adrenoceptors are more sensitive than α_1 adrenoceptors to change in temperature. Whereas cooling slightly depresses α_1 adrenergic-mediated vasoconstriction, it markedly augments α_2 adrenergic-mediated responses. Conversely, warming augments α_1 adrenergic vasoconstriction and depresses α_2 adrenergic vasoconstriction.[31]

These experimental observations may have important implications regarding the pathophysiology of Raynaud's phenomenon. Flavahan and colleagues[32] examined the distribution of α_1 and α_2 adrenoceptors in arterial tissue from amputated limbs of patients who did not have vascular disease. They reported that α_2 adrenoceptors were more prominent in digital arteries. Chotani and colleagues[33] found that human dermal arterioles selectively expressed α_{2C} adrenoceptors. Jeyaraj and colleagues[34] observed that cooling redistributed α_{2C} adrenoceptors from the Golgi to the plasma membrane in human embryonic kidney cells. It is therefore an intriguing observation by Keenan and Porter that the density of α_2 adrenoceptors is increased in platelets from patients with Raynaud's disease.[35]

In support of these findings, Coffman and Cohen reported that α_2 adrenoceptors were more important than α_1 adrenoceptors in mediating sympathetic nerve-induced vasoconstriction in the fingers.[36] They administered the α_1 antagonist prazosin and the α_2 antagonist yohimbine to patients with Raynaud's phenomenon during reflex sympathetic vasoconstriction caused by body cooling. Whereas prazosin caused no significant change in finger blood flow or finger vascular resistance, yohimbine significantly increased finger blood flow and decreased finger vascular resistance. This study confirmed that postjunctional α_2 adrenoceptors are present in human digits and strongly suggested that these receptors contribute to digital vasoconstriction during environmental cooling in patients with Raynaud's phenomenon. Thereafter Coffman and Cohen demonstrated that patients with Raynaud's phenomenon were hypersensitive to the vasoconstrictor effects of clonidine, an α_2-adrenoceptor agonist, but not to phenylephrine, an α_1-adrenoceptor agonist compared with normal subjects.[37] Cooke and colleagues[38] found that both α_1- and α_2-adrenoceptor antagonists induced digital vasodilation in patients with acute Raynaud's phenomenon yet did not inhibit digital vasoconstriction caused by local digital cooling. Although still speculative, these studies suggest that episodic digital vasospasm may be secondary to a predominance of postjunctional α_2 adrenoceptors in digits of patients with primary Raynaud's phenomenon.

Increased Sympathetic Nervous System Activity

Although appealing as a potential mechanism for digital vasospasm, the concept of exaggerated reflex sympathetic vasoconstrictor responses to cold environment has not been convincingly demonstrated. Increased concentrations of epinephrine and norepinephrine in the peripheral venous blood at the wrist were found higher in patients with primary Raynaud's phenomenon than in normal subjects by one investigator,[39] but others found normal local levels of norepinephrine in brachial arterial and venous blood samples from patients.[40] The latter group of investigators reported that the reflex vasoconstrictor response of the hand to a cold stimulus in the patients is similar to that in a control group of subjects, and there were comparable vasoconstrictor responses to the intraarterial infusion of tyramine, a drug that causes vasoconstriction by releasing norepinephrine from sympathetic nerve terminals. The central thermoregulatory control of skin temperature has also been reported to be comparable in normal individuals and patients with primary Raynaud's phenomenon.[41] Finally, microelectrode recordings of skin sympathetic nerve activity do not demonstrate an abnormality in patients with primary Raynaud's phenomenon.[42] There was no hypersensitivity of the vessels to strong sympathetic stimuli or abnormal increase in sympathetic outflow.

β-Adrenergic Blockade

Raynaud's phenomenon is observed frequently in individuals treated with β-adrenoceptor antagonists.[43-45] It may be inferred from this observation that β-adrenergic vasodilation normally attenuates digital vasoconstrictor tone. Cohen and Coffman[46] examined the effect of isoproterenol and propranolol on fingertip blood flow after vasoconstriction has been induced by a brachial artery infusion of norepinephrine or angiotensin, or reflexly by environmental cooling. Intra-arterial isoproterenol administration increased fingertip blood flow during the infusions of norepinephrine and angiotensin but not during reflex sympathetic vasoconstriction. Conversely, propranolol served to potentiate vasoconstriction caused by intra-arterial norepinephrine but not that caused by reflex sympathetic vasoconstriction. These investigators concluded that a β-adrenergic vasodilator mechanism may be active in human digits but does not modulate sympathetic vasoconstriction. In the absence of pharmacologic blockade of β adrenoceptors, there is no evidence to support the contention that decreased sensitivity or number of β adrenoceptors contributes to the pathophysiology of Raynaud's phenomenon.

Vasoconstriction Caused by Circulating Vascular Smooth Muscle Agonists

Various neurotransmitters, hormones, and platelet release byproducts are capable of constricting vascular smooth muscle and causing digital vasoconstriction. These include angiotensin II, serotonin, thromboxane A_2, and endothelin-1. It would be difficult to attribute all causes of Raynaud's phenomenon to excessive levels of these vasoconstrictor agents, but in some secondary causes of Raynaud's phenomenon, any one of them might contribute to vasoconstriction.

Serotonin (5-hydroxytryptamine [5-HT]) is a neurotransmitter that is synthesized and released by selective neurons and enterochromaffin cells. Serotonin can cause vasoconstriction by directly activating serotoninergic receptors on the smooth muscle cells.[47] Vasoconstriction may also be caused by direct activation of α adrenoceptors on smooth muscle cells or indirectly by facilitating the release of norepinephrine from adrenergic nerve terminal.

Evidence is available that implicates, but does not establish, a role for serotonin in the pathophysiology of Raynaud's phenomenon. The vasoconstrictive effects of serotonin are potentiated at lower temperatures.[48] Cutaneous vessel strips isolated from patients with scleroderma demonstrate hypersensitivity to serotonin.[49] Coffman and Cohen[50] demonstrated that S_2-serotoninergic receptors are present in human fingers and play a role in vasoconstriction of the finger by body cooling. They also found that patients with Raynaud's phenomenon were hypersensitive to the digital vasoconstrictor effects of intra-arterial infusion of 5-HT compared with normal subjects.[36] Halpern and colleagues[51] infused serotonin into the brachial arteries of normal human subjects and patients with Raynaud's phenomenon. Serotonin precipitated digital ischemia and decreased digital temperature in both groups, but the duration of ischemia was more prolonged in the patients. Concurrent administration of a serotonin antagonist attenuated the digital ischemia. The authors hypothesized that serotonin did not initiate Raynaud's phenomenon but rather played a contributing role.

Serotonin antagonists have been used as pharmacologic probes to examine the contribution of serotonin to Raynaud's phenomenon. Ketanserin is a drug that antagonizes serotonergic (5-HT_2) receptors on vascular smooth muscle cells; it also has some α-adrenoceptor blocking properties.[52,53] Ketanserin assists recovery of digital temperature and blood flow following hand immersion in cold water[54] and increases finger blood flow in normal subjects during reflex sympathetic vasoconstriction.[50] Studies examining ketanserin in patients with Raynaud's phenomenon, however, have yielded inconsistent results.[55-58] The contribution of serotonin to digital vasospasm remains speculative.

The possibility that vasoconstrictors released during platelet aggregation may be pertinent to the pathophysiology of Raynaud's phenomenon has been further evaluated by studies that have either measured levels of thromboxane A_2, or administered a thromboxane synthetase inhibitor.[59-63] Coffman and Rasmussen[59] compared the thromboxane synthetase inhibitor dazoxiben to placebo in patients with either primary or secondary Raynaud's phenomenon. Dazoxiben did not affect total fingertip blood flow or fingertip capillary blood flow, whether measured in a warm (28.3° C) or cool (20° C) environment. With chronic treatment, there was a small decrease in the frequency of vasospastic episodes in the patients with primary Raynaud's phenomenon. Studies by other investigators have similarly been unable to establish that dazoxiben improves fingertip blood flow or that it relieves symptomatic digital vasospasm in patients with Raynaud's phenomenon.[60,63] To date, there is insufficient evidence to support a role for thromboxane A_2 in digital vasospasm.

The plasma concentration of the potent vasoconstrictor angiotensin II is rarely elevated in patients with Raynaud's phenomenon. Therefore this hormone is unlikely to contribute to the pathophysiology of digital vasospasm in most patients. The digital vessels in patients with scleroderma are often diseased and potentially hypersensitive to vasoactive stimuli. Thus, in this subgroup of patients, high circulating levels of angiotensin II conceivably could promote intense digital vasoconstriction.

The endothelium-derived substance, endothelin-1, is a powerful and prolonged acting vasoconstrictor agent that has been suggested to play a part in the pathogenesis of Raynaud's phenomenon. It constricts cutaneous blood vessels and rises in response to a cold pressor test in patients.[64] Studies measuring endothelin-1 in primary or secondary Raynaud's phenomenon have been conflicting.[65] It is doubtful that it plays a role in Raynaud's phenomenon.

Decreased Intravascular Pressure

The patency of a blood vessel requires balance between the tension in the arterial wall (favoring closure of the vessel) and the intravascular distending pressure.[66,67]

Landis measured intravascular pressure in patients with Raynaud's phenomenon by introducing a micropipette into a large digital capillary.[68] During cyanosis, capillary pressure fell to approximately 5 mm Hg and flow ceased. These findings suggested that the site of closure was proximal to the capillaries at the arterial level. Interestingly, Thulesius reported that brachial artery blood pressure in patients with primary Raynaud's phenomenon was significantly lower than that in a normal control population.[69] Cohen and Coffman[70] also measured systolic blood pressure at the brachial artery, as well as at the proximal and distal digital arteries, of normal subjects and patients with primary Raynaud's phenomenon. Blood pressure measured at these locations was significantly lower in the patients with Raynaud's disease, averaging 18 mm Hg less than in the normal digits.

A low digital artery pressure may occur in various disorders associated with Raynaud's phenomenon such as large-vessel arterial occlusive disease secondary to atherosclerosis, embolism, or thoracic outlet syndrome. When extrinsic vasoconstrictor force is applied, these vessels may collapse and cause digital ischemia. Distal vascular occlusions secondary to thromboangiitis obliterans (TAO), vasculitis, or vibration injury may also reduce digital arterial pressure distal to the diseased vascular segment.

Hyperviscosity may reduce the velocity of blood flow in the digital vessels, leading to a decrease in intravascular pressure. Indeed, Raynaud's phenomenon occurs in patients with hyperviscosity caused by polycythemia vera or Waldenström's macroglobulinemia.[71,72] In patients with Raynaud's phenomenon secondary to disorders such as cryoglobulinemia and cold agglutinin disease, hyperviscosity caused by cooling may contribute to digital vasospasm.[73-75] Indeed, cooling has been shown to abolish hand blood flow in patients with cold agglutinins, possibly because the vessels become occluded by agglutinated red cells.[75] The data invoking hyperviscosity as a cause of Raynaud's phenomenon in patients who do not have an established blood dyscrasia are less compelling. In multiple studies, it has been impossible to distinguish whole blood or plasma viscosities in patients with Raynaud's phenomenon from those hemorheologic properties in normal individuals, despite cooling the blood to 10°C.[76–78]

SECONDARY CAUSES OF RAYNAUD'S PHENOMENON

The secondary causes of Raynaud's phenomenon include collagen vascular diseases, arterial occlusive disorders, thoracic outlet syndrome, several neurologic disorders, blood dyscrasias, trauma, and several drugs (see Box 48-1).

Collagen Vascular Diseases

Systemic Sclerosis (Scleroderma) Raynaud's phenomenon occurs in 80% to 90% of patients with systemic sclerosis:[2] it may be the presenting symptom in approximately 33% of patients. In some patients scleroderma may develop after Raynaud's phenomenon has been present as the only symptom for many years. The frequency and severity of Raynaud's phenomenon in patients with systemic sclerosis is often worse than that observed in patients with primary Raynaud's phenomenon. The incidence of digital ulceration and gangrene is increased, possibly leading to amputation. The diagnosis of systemic sclerosis is suggested by the appearance of typical sclerotic skin changes. These include tightness, thickening, and nonpitting induration involving the extremities, face, neck, or trunk. When present in the digits, these abnormalities produce changes in the contour of the fingers and toes, referred to as *sclerodactyly*. Other manifestations of systemic sclerosis include pitting scars of the tips of the digits, normal skin pigmentation, and telangiectasia. Visceral manifestations include pulmonary fibrosis, esophageal dysmotility, and colonic sacculation. The kidney and heart may also be involved. As the disease progresses, the skin and subcutaneous tissue of the fingers become stiffer, the joints become immobile, and contractures develop. A variant of systemic sclerosis is the CREST syndrome, a form of limited scleroderma that includes **C**alcinosis, **R**aynaud's phenomenon, **E**sophageal dysmotility, **S**clerodactyly, and **T**elangiectasia in the absence of internal organ involvement.

Several serologic studies are consistent with the diagnosis of scleroderma. The erythrocyte sedimentation rate may be elevated. Antinuclear antibodies are present in the majority of individuals with this disorder; patients may have antibodies to nucleolar antigens, nuclear ribonucleoprotein, and to the centromeric region of metaphase chromosomes. In patients with systemic sclerosis and Raynaud's phenomenon, capillary microscopy often demonstrates enlarged and deformed capillary loops surrounded by relatively avascular areas, particularly in the nailfolds.[80] Angiography frequently demonstrates digital vascular obstruction.

Systemic Lupus Erythematosus Raynaud's phenomenon occurs in approximately 10% to 35% of patients with systemic lupus erythematosus. Persistent digital vasospasm, often due to proliferative endarteritis of the small digital vessels, also occurs and may result in gangrene. Diagnosis of systemic lupus erythematosus is based on the presence of at least four of the following 11 criteria:

1. Malar rash
2. Discoid rash
3. Photosensitivity
4. Oral ulcers
5. Arthritis
6. Serositis including pleuritis or pericarditis
7. Renal disorders, including persistent proteinuria or cellular casts
8. Neurologic disorders, such as seizures and psychosis
9. Hematologic disorders, including hemolytic anemia, leukopenia, lymphopenia, or thrombocytopenia
10. Immunologic disorders
11. Abnormal titers of antinuclear antibody, especially anti-DNA[81]

Rheumatoid Arthritis Raynaud's phenomenon also occurs in patients with rheumatoid arthritis. These patients may have vasculitis of medium-sized vessels, as well as proliferative endarteritis of small vessels. Crops of small brown spots may be observed in the nail beds and digital pulp. Digital blood flow often is reduced in patients with rheumatoid arthritis, and angiography frequently reveals occlusions of one or more digital arteries.[82] The diagnosis is suggested in patients who meet the criteria of the American Rheumatism Association.[83] At least five or six of the following criteria must be present: morning joint stiffness, joint pain or tenderness on motion, joint swelling, subcutaneous nodules, radiological changes typical of rheumatoid arthritis, the presence of rheumatoid factor in the serum, and characteristic histologic changes in the synovium and skin nodules.

Dermatomyositis and Polymyositis Thirty percent of patients with these disorders have associated Raynaud's phenomenon.[2] Muscular manifestations include weakness of the proximal girdle muscles, particularly those involving the lower extremities. Patients may also experience aching in the buttocks, thighs, and calves. Some patients complain of dysphagia or dyspnea. Myocarditis develops in approximately one third of these individuals. The dermatological abnormalities in dermatomyositis include localized or diffuse erythema, a maculopapular rash, and eczematoid dermatitis. A purplish (heliotrope) rash may develop on the upper eyelids, face, chest, limbs, or around the nail beds. Laboratory diagnosis of dermatomyositis and polymyositis is based on elevated serum levels of the skeletal muscle enzymes including creatine kinase, aldolase, serum glutamic oxaloacetic transaminase, and lactic acid dehydrogenase. There may be myoglobinuria, and the erythrocyte sedimentation rate is often elevated. The electromyogram reveals evidence of a myopathy.

Primary Sjögren's Syndrome Sjögren's syndrome is an autoimmune disease that mainly affects exocrine glands leading to dryness of the eyes and mouth but can have extraglandular manifestations. Raynaud's phenomenon has been reported in 13% to 33% of patients and may precede the sicca symptomatology in many.[84] The clinical course is usually milder than in patients with systemic sclerosis. Antinuclear antibody tests are often positive, but the diagnosis is usually made by the clinical picture.

Arterial Occlusive Disease

Occlusive disease of arteries that are proximal to the digital vessels is often associated with Raynaud's phenomenon. Proximal arterial occlusive disease may decrease intravascular pressure and upset the balance between tension in the arterial wall and intravascular distending pressure. This may make the vessel more prone to vasospasm when subjected to sympathetic nervous system stimuli.

Atherosclerosis of the extremities tends to occur most frequently in males older than 50 years and females older than 60 years old. When Raynaud's phenomenon occurs in these individuals, it tends to be unilateral and related to the affected extremity. Usually only one or two digits are involved. The diagnosis is suggested by the clinical history and physical examination. Symptoms of claudication or findings that would suggest atherosclerosis elsewhere, such as in the coronary or cerebral vasculature, often indicate the underlying disorder. Physical findings are noteworthy for decreased or absent pulses in the involved extremity. These abnormalities can be confirmed by noninvasive vascular testing. Severe ischemia may be manifested as persistent digital pallor or cyanosis and must be distinguished from the episodic digital vasospasm of Raynaud's phenomenon.

TAO (Buerger's disease) is an inflammatory occlusive vascular disorder involving small- and medium-sized arteries and veins often accompanied by Raynaud's phenomenon (see Chapter 44). In addition to Raynaud's phenomenon, clinical features of TAO include claudication of the affected extremity and migratory superficial vein thrombosis in a young male.

Thoracic Outlet Syndrome

Compression of the neurovascular bundle as it courses through the neck and shoulder can result in a symptom complex that includes Raynaud's phenomenon, as well as shoulder and arm pain, weakness, paresthesias, and claudication of the affected upper extremity (see Chapter 64). Raynaud's phenomenon may result from the decreased intravascular pressure caused by extrinsic compression of the subclavian artery. Whether compression of the brachial plexus alters sympathetic nervous system activity is unknown.

Neurologic Disorders

Various neurologic conditions, particularly those causing disuse of the limb, may be associated with disorders of circulatory vasomotion. These include stroke, syringomyelia, intervertebral disk disease, spinal cord tumors, and poliomyelitis. The affected limb, including the hand or foot in addition to the digits, may be cool and cyanotic. In contrast to the episodic nature of Raynaud's phenomenon, these changes tend to be persistent.

Raynaud's phenomenon has been reported in approximately 10% of patients with carpal tunnel syndrome.[85] This entrapment neuropathy is caused by compression of the median nerve as it passes through the carpal tunnel. It may result from pregnancy, a localized tenosynovitis, trauma, hypothyroidism, amyloidosis, or activities associated with repeated motion of the wrist. Patients usually experience paresthesias or weakness in the distribution of the median nerve. The diagnosis is suggested when symptoms are reproduced by tapping the volar surface of the wrist (Tinel sign) or by maintaining flexion of the wrist (Phalen maneuver). Nerve conduction tests usually demonstrate abnormalities of the median nerve at the wrist. Supportive treatment includes splints and anti-inflammatory drugs. With severe persistent symptoms, surgical release of the carpal ligament may be beneficial.

Reflex sympathetic dystrophy or causalgia is another neurologic disorder that is associated with cyanotic extremities and involves pain and tenderness of a distal extremity with accompanying vasomotor instability (see Chapter 52).

Blood Dyscrasias

Hyperviscosity syndromes, cold-precipitable plasma proteins, abnormalities of red-cell agglutination, and certain myeloproliferative disorders are associated with Raynaud's phenomenon, as well as with persistent digital ischemia.

Patients with cold agglutinins occasionally develop Raynaud's phenomenon.[2] It is generally thought that Raynaud's phenomenon develops when proteins precipitate on red blood cells and agglutinate within the digital vessel during exposure to cold. Prolonged exposure may cause thrombosis and subsequent digital gangrene. Cold agglutinin disease usually involves IgM antibodies that are reactive with I antigen.[86] The antibody titer is high at 4° C and low at 37° C. These antibodies also may cause cold-induced hemolysis. Agglutination usually does not occur in temperatures above 32° C. Cold agglutinins may arise spontaneously or occur in patients with mycoplasma pneumonia, infectious mononucleosis, or lymphoproliferative disorders. Cold agglutinin disease may be short lived in patients with infectious causes but is often persistent in patients with lymphoproliferative disease.

Cryoglobulins are a group of proteins that precipitate in cold serum and may cause Raynaud's phenomenon.[87] Cryoglobulins are associated with monoclonal and polyclonal gammopathies in disorders such as Waldenström's macroglobulinemia, systemic lupus erythematosus, and rheumatoid arthritis. Cryoglobulinemia has been categorized into three subtypes. Type 1 cryoglobulins include monoclonal immunoglobulins of a single class usually associated with lymphoproliferative disorders, such as multiple myeloma. Type 2 encompasses mixed cryoglobulins containing monoclonal IgM or rheumatoid factor and polyclonal IgG. This may occur in patients with Waldenström's macroglobulinemia or chronic active hepatitis. In patients with Waldenström's macroglobulinemia, about 10% of macroglobulins are cryoglobulins. Type 3 cryoglobulinemia includes polyclonal IgM and IgG immunoglobulins, as may occur in systemic lupus erythematosus. Indeed, approximately 80% of patients with lupus have cold-insoluble precipitates. In these patients, there is a significantly higher level of cryoprecipitating IgM class rheumatoid factors than in other patients.

Cryofibrinogenemia is a rare condition that may be associated with digital vasospasm.[88] The plasma, but not the serum, of patients with cryofibrinogenemia forms a gelatinous precipitate at 4° C. Disorders associated with cryofibrinogenemia include disseminated intravascular coagulation, collagen vascular diseases, thromboembolism, and diabetes mellitus.

Trauma

Various traumatic injuries are associated with Raynaud's phenomenon and have been designated traumatic vasospastic diseases. Causes of traumatic vasospastic disease include electric shock injury, thermal injuries such as frostbite, and mechanical percussive injury associated with piano playing and typing. The most common traumatic cause of Raynaud's phenomenon is repeated exposure to vibrating tools. This has occasionally been referred to as *vibration white finger syndrome*. It has been reported in lumberjacks and other users of chainsaws, stonecutters who use air hammers, operators of pneumatic hand grinders and impact wrenches in the engine manufacturing industry, and road drillers. The prevalence of Raynaud's phenomenon induced by vibration ranges from 33% to 71% among members of populations at risk and increases with exposure time.[89,90] It has been suggested that the combination of vibration and cold exposure in many of these workers is responsible for the development of Raynaud's phenomenon.[91]

Pathophysiologic changes may involve both the vascular and neurologic systems in these individuals and may contribute to digital vasospasm. Intimal thickening of peripheral arteries has been reported in animals exposed to repeated vibration, but pathologic changes of the blood vessels have not consistently been demonstrated.[92] Medial muscular hypertrophy and subintimal fibrosis have been found in biopsy specimens of digital arteries of patients in one study but not in others.[2] Nailbed capillaroscopy has shown a reduction in the number of capillaries. Arteriograms of these patients have shown arterial occlusion of the distal radial and ulnar arteries and frequently of the palmar arch.

Neurophysiologic abnormalities have not been consistently demonstrated in patients with Raynaud's phenomenon secondary to vibration. Although some have found a high instance of abnormal electromyograms, others have found that episodes of Raynaud's phenomena occur independently of electromyographic abnormalities.[93] Peripheral nerve conduction velocities are often abnormal in vibrating tool operators, and pathological changes have also been reported in the nerves of patients with vibration white finger, including axonal degeneration, demyelination, and collagenization of perineurium and endoperineurium.[2] Thus the precise pathophysiology of Raynaud's phenomenon in patients repeatedly exposed to vibratory stimuli is unclear. Some have suggested that overexcitation of the Pacinian corpuscles causes reflex efferent sympathetic nerve activity.[2] Others have suggested that following vibration, cutaneous vessels become more reactive to sympathetic stimuli.

Another trauma-induced cause of Raynaud's phenomenon is the hypothenar hammer syndrome. Patients develop an ulnar artery thrombosis after hammering with the palms of their hands or practicing karate.[2] Raynaud's phenomenon may be unilateral if only one ulnar artery is occluded.

Drugs and Toxins

Various drugs have been implicated in producing Raynaud's phenomenon or digital vasospasm (see Box 48-1).[2] Although some of these drugs act by directly causing vasoconstriction, the mechanism whereby others cause Raynaud's phenomenon is not known.

Ergot derivatives cause vasospasm, primarily by stimulating α adrenoceptors. Ergotamine may stimulate serotonergic receptors as well. Vasospasm usually occurs when excessive doses of these drugs have been administered. Spasm may affect digital vessels, as well as the coronary, carotid, and femoral vessels and the coronary, carotid, femoral, and splanchnic arteries. Bromocriptine mesylate, an ergot derivative with dopamine agonist activity used to treat Parkinson's disease, hyperprolactinemia, and acromegaly, has been associated with Raynaud's phenomenon. Methysergide, used to treat migraine headaches, is another ergot derivative that has been associated with digital ischemia. The tricyclic antidepressant imipramine and the amphetamines also have been reported to cause arterial spasm.

Raynaud's phenomenon has also been associated with the use of two chemotherapeutic agents, vinblastine and bleomycin.[2] Although it is unknown how these compounds cause Raynaud's phenomenon, it has been reported that bleomycin causes pathologic changes in small blood vessels. Vinblastine can induce a peripheral neuropathy and perhaps interfere with the autonomic reflexes.

Industrial exposure to vinyl chloride polymerization processes may cause acro-osteolysis of the distal phalanges of the fingers, changes that are occasionally associated with Raynaud's phenomenon, but one recent study found the phenomenon less frequent among workers than in the population.[94]

β-Adrenoceptor blocking drugs may cause Raynaud's phenomenon.[2] Although the mechanism of action is unknown, possibilities include unopposed stimulation of vascular α adrenoceptors or reflex sympathetic vasoconstriction initiated by the central cardiovascular depressant effect of β-adrenergic blockade. It remains controversial whether cardioselective β-adrenoceptor blocking drugs cause Raynaud's phenomenon less frequently than nonselective drugs, and whether there is less digital vasospasm with drugs that also have α-adrenoceptor blocking properties or intrinsic sympathetic activity. One placebo-controlled study examined both cardioselective and nonselective β-adrenoceptor blockers in patients who already had Raynaud's phenomenon.[95] Compared with placebo, neither metoprolol nor propranolol decreased fingertip blood flow, despite exposure to a cool environment. Furthermore, chronic treatment did not increase the number of vasospastic attacks in patients receiving either drug compared with placebo. One might conclude from these observations that β-adrenoceptor blocking drugs may cause Raynaud's phenomenon in some individuals, but these drugs do not seem to affect the frequency of vasospastic attacks adversely, nor do they decrease finger blood flow in patients with Raynaud's phenomenon.

Miscellaneous Causes

Hypothyroidism may be associated with Raynaud's phenomenon.[96] In these cases, thyroid replacement alleviates the episodes of digital vasospasm. Although the mechanism is unknown, peripheral vasoconstriction may occur in hypothyroid patients to conserve heat. Alternatively, edematous thickening of the vascular wall could predispose to vessel closure during normal sympathetic stimuli.

Patients with arteriovenous fistula may develop Raynaud's phenomenon; it is particularly prevalent in patients undergoing hemodialysis.[97] This may be secondary to decreased blood flow and blood pressure in the digits of the limb with the fistula.

Pulmonary hypertension and Raynaud's phenomenon may occur in the same patients.[2] Some of these may have a connective tissue disorder such as scleroderma.[98] Approximately 30% of patients with pulmonary arterial hypertension have elevated titers of antinuclear antibody.[99,100] Ten percent of women with pulmonary arterial hypertension have Raynaud's phenomenon.[100] This frequency is not different from that which occurs in the general population. Therefore it is not clear whether the association of primary pulmonary hypertension and Raynaud's phenomenon is coincidence or related to a common neurohumoral or immunologic mechanism.

DIAGNOSTIC TESTS

Noninvasive vascular tests may be employed to evaluate patients with Raynaud's phenomenon (see Chapter 10). The effect on finger systolic pressure of local cooling with ischemia is an objective test for Raynaud's phenomenon[101]; however, this is too cumbersome a test for routine use because it involves measuring digital systolic pressure with cooling plus 5 minutes of ischemia at four different temperatures (Fig. 48-5). Patients with Raynaud's phenomenon have a greater reduction or loss of finger systolic pressure with cooling compared with normal subjects who show a gradual decrease.

The pulse volume waveform may distinguish patients with Raynaud's phenomenon who have digital ischemia secondary to vascular occlusive lesions (Fig. 48-6).

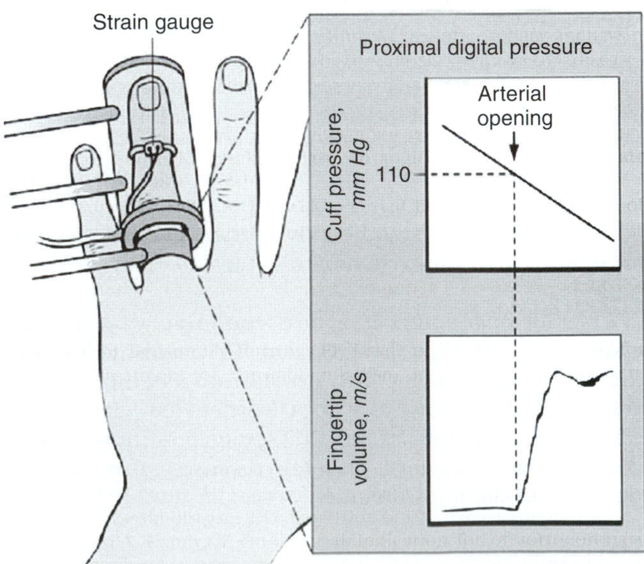

FIGURE 48-5. Measurement of the proximal finger systolic blood pressure using a strain gauge to detect the increase in fingertip volume as the proximal cuff is slowly deflated from suprasystolic pressure. Fingertip pulsations and the volume increase are not detected until the cuff pressure deflates to 110 mm Hg, the point of digital artery opening.

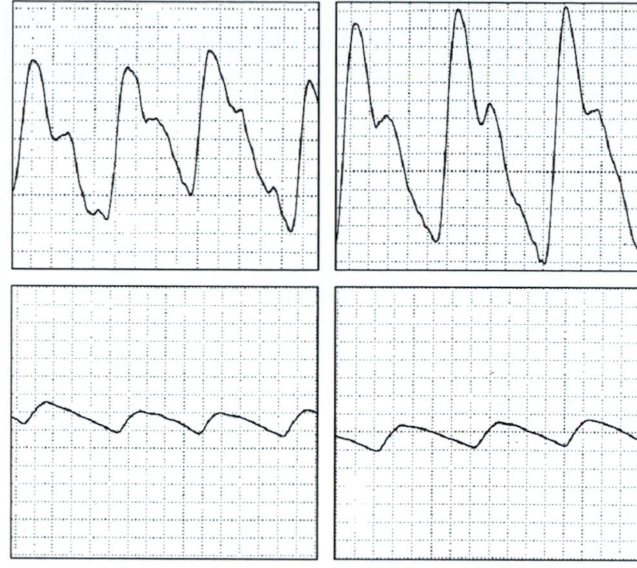

FIGURE 48-6. Digital pulse volume recordings. Digital pulse volume waveforms were recorded during cooling (left; 24° C) and rewarming (right; 44° C). In the healthy subject *(top)*, the pulse volume amplitude increased during warming. In the patient with digital ischemia secondary to vascular occlusion, the pulse volume amplitude is diminished during both cooling and rewarming *(bottom)*.

During local digital warming, the vessel walls become dilated. The pulse waveform is usually normal during warming in patients with Raynaud's phenomenon if obstructive lesions are not present, and may be abnormal if atherosclerosis, TAO, or other fixed obstructive digital vascular pathology impairs digital blood flow.

Various serologic studies such as collagen vascular disorders or blood dyscrasias are useful to screen for secondary causes of Raynaud's phenomenon. These tests include the erythrocyte sedimentation rate; assays for antinuclear antibody, rheumatoid factor, cryoglobulins and cold agglutinins; and serum protein electrophoresis. Indications for these and other serologic studies are usually suggested by the history and physical examination. Nailfold capillary microscopy may be used to detect the deformed capillary loops and avascular areas typical of collagen vascular disorders (Fig. 48-7).[80] Roentgenography of the cervical spine is used to detect cervical ribs.

Angiography is rarely indicated, since Raynaud's phenomenon is a diagnosis based primarily on history. Angiography may be indicated, however, in patients with persistent digital ischemia secondary to atherosclerosis, TAO, or emboli from a subclavian artery aneurysm, in order to plan revascularization procedures (Fig. 48-8).

TREATMENT

Treatment programs must be individualized and designed according to the underlying cause of Raynaud's phenomenon and the severity of the symptoms. Therapy directed specifically at the symptoms of Raynaud's phenomenon can be categorized as follows: (1) conservative measures, (2) pharmacologic intervention, and (3) surgical sympathectomy (Box 48-3). In individuals with well-defined secondary causes of Raynaud's phenomenon, treatment should also be directed specifically at the underlying cause. Thus, for example, if a patient has been taking a vasoactive medication, such as an ergot alkaloid, or has been treated with a β-adrenergic blocking drug for hypertension, removal of the offending agent may reduce or eliminate the Raynaud's phenomenon. Similarly, specific treatment may be directed at other secondary causes such as arterial occlusive disorders, connective tissue diseases, and blood dyscrasias. The following discussion focuses on treatment designed to palliate Raynaud's phenomenon.

Conservative Measures

Patients with primary Raynaud's phenomenon often benefit from reassurance. An explanation describing the

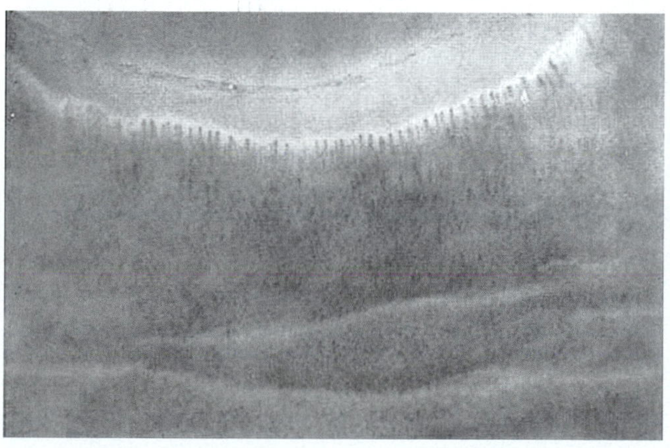

A

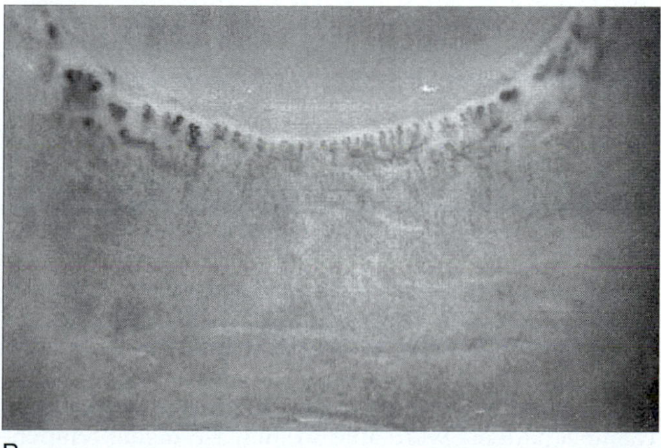

B

FIGURE 48-7. (See also Color Plate 48-7.) Nailfold capillary microscopy is performed using a magnifying glass, ophthalmoscope, or compound microscope (magnification, ×10) to view the clean nailfold covered with immersion oil. Normally **(A)**, the superficial capillaries are regularly spaced hairpin loops. **B,** Results of this test are abnormal in patients with connective tissue disorders. Avascular areas and enlarged and deformed capillary loops are present in the nailfold of this patient with scleroderma. Disorganized nailfold capillaries associated with avascular areas and hemorrhage are present in patients with dermatomyositis and polymyositis (magnification, ×10). (Courtesy H. Maricq, MD.)

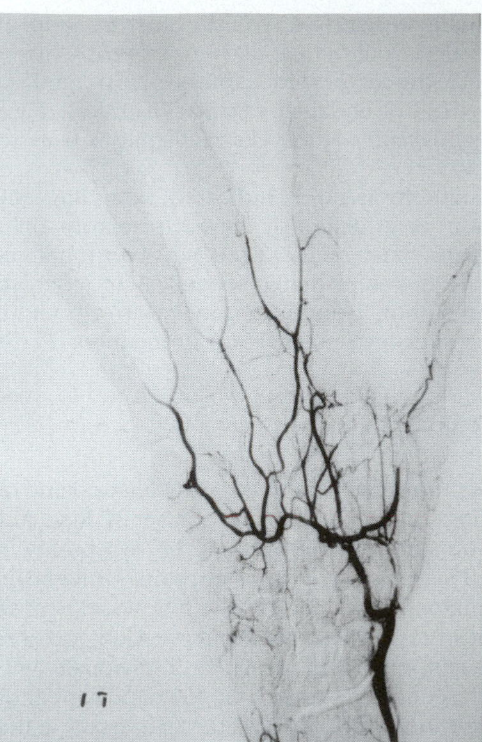

FIGURE 48-8. Angiogram from a young woman with persistent digital ischemia. Multiple areas demonstrate digital vascular occlusion. A blood vessel biopsy was performed to make the diagnosis of necrotizing vasculitis.

frequency of the disease in the general population, its precipitating factors, and its benign prognosis is reassuring and allays fears of amputation. Patients should avoid unnecessary cold exposure and should wear loose and warm clothing. In addition to gloves and adequate foot protection, the trunk and head should be kept warm to avoid reflex vasoconstriction. Moving to a warmer climate is rarely feasible; furthermore, vasospasm may be induced after a move by even small changes in environmental temperature. Patients should use a moisturizing cream on their digits to prevent drying and cracking. Cigarette smoking should be avoided, since nicotine causes cutaneous vasoconstriction.[102]

Because the sympathetic nervous system mediates the vasoconstrictor response to cold and emotional distress, behavioral therapy has been proposed as a means of ameliorating the symptoms of Raynaud's phenomenon. Studies have been reported both supporting and refuting the efficacy of biofeedback training in this disorder.[103-109] The techniques used for biofeedback training in most of these studies were different. Furthermore, objective means of assessing responses varied from determination of digital temperature during cold exposure to queries regarding symptomatic improvement. Several uncontrolled studies indicated that following biofeedback training, patients were able to increase digital temperature and possibly decrease the frequency of vasospastic attacks.[103-107] Patients usually trained to increase their digital temperature during either local or environmental cold exposure. In one controlled study, which compared temperature biofeedback with nifedipine for the treatment of primary Raynaud's phenomenon, biofeedback was not better than control treatment and inferior to the drug.[110] Another form of behavioral therapy, Pavlovian conditioning, has been shown to increase digital temperature during cold exposure.[111] Though behavioral therapy may be effective in some individuals, there are insufficient data to support its routine use for patients with Raynaud's phenomenon.

BOX 48-3 Treatment of Raynaud's Phenomenon

Conservative measures
- Warm clothing
- Avoidance of cold exposure
- Abstinence from nicotine
- Remove offending drug (if present)
- Behavioral therapy

Pharmacologic interventions
- Calcium channel blockers
  - Nifedipine
  - Diltiazem
  - Felodipine
  - Isradipine
  - Amlodipine

Sympathetic nervous system inhibitors
- Prazosin
- Reserpine
- Guanethidine
- Phenoxybenzamine

Classes of drugs with unproven efficacy
- Serotonin antagonists
  - Ketanserin
  - Fluoxetine
- Vasodilator prostaglandins
  - Iloprost
- Thromboxane inhibitors
  - Angiotensin-converting enzyme inhibitors
  - Angiotensin receptor antagonists
  - Organic nitrates

Sympathectomy
- Stellate ganglionectomy
- Lumbar sympathectomy
- Digital sympathectomy

Pharmacologic Intervention

Two classes of drugs are effective for treatment of Raynaud's phenomenon: calcium channel blockers and sympathetic nervous system inhibitors.[3,112,113] Other classes of drugs for which efficacy has not been firmly established include serotonin antagonists, angiotensin-converting enzyme inhibitors, and direct-acting smooth muscle relaxants such as nitrates and vasodilator prostaglandins.

Calcium Channel Blockers

Calcium entry blockers are the most effective drugs for the treatment of Raynaud's phenomenon. Most of the evidence accumulated to date involves nifedipine, which interferes with vascular smooth muscle contraction by antagonizing calcium influx.[114,115] This drug decreases digital vascular resistance in patients with Raynaud's phenomenon during environmental cold exposure and increases digital systolic blood pressure and digital skin temperature during local cold exposure.[116,117] In multiple placebo-controlled trials, nifedipine decreased the frequency and severity of Raynaud's phenomenon.[3,112] It has also been reported to be effective treatment in children.[118] Although nifedipine is not of benefit in all patients, symptoms improve in about two thirds of individuals. Furthermore, patients with primary and secondary Raynaud's phenomenon have shown improvement. Extended-action preparations should be used starting with 30 mg daily and increasing to 60 mg, 90 mg, and 120 mg if necessary.[3,111] Side effects include hypotension, lightheadedness, indigestion, and peripheral edema.

Less information is available about the other calcium channel blocking drugs. Diltiazem, however, has been reported in several studies to improve symptoms of Raynaud's phenomenon.[119,120] One preliminary report also indicated that it was effective in patients with Raynaud's phenomenon secondary to vibration injury.[121] Felodipine, at a dose of 2.5 or 5 mg, may be as effective as nifedipine but has not been as extensively studied.[122,123] Isradipine and amlodipine have been reported to be beneficial in small studies.[3] In contrast, verapamil has not been shown to be effective in patients with Raynaud's phenomenon.[124]

Inhibitors of the Sympathetic Nervous System

The vasoconstrictor response to cold exposure or emotional stress is mediated via the sympathetic nervous system. Sympathetic nervous system inhibitors that have been used to treat Raynaud's phenomenon include prazosin, reserpine, guanethidine, phenoxybenzamine, and methyldopa.

Prazosin hydrochloride is an α_1-adrenoceptor blocker. Since postsynaptic α_1 adrenoceptors are found on digital vessels, clinical improvement following administration of this drug might be anticipated.[3,113] However, one study reported only modest increases in digital blood flow during intra-arterial infusion of prazosin. Uncontrolled observations have suggested that prazosin is effective in approximately 50% of patients with Raynaud's phenomenon. A placebo-controlled double-blind study in a small number of patients suggested that prazosin in doses ranging from 1 to 4 mg twice each day reduced the frequency of Raynaud's phenomenon.[125] Tachyphylaxis may occur with prazosin, often necessitating dosage increments up to 10 mg three times daily. Side effects of prazosin include hypotension, particularly after the first few doses, leading to lightheadedness or syncope. In addition, patients may develop headache, drowsiness, or fatigue. Long acting α_1-adrenoceptor blockers such as doxazosin and terazosin have not been studied in patients with Raynaud's phenomenon but would probably have effects similar to prazosin.

Reserpine is an alkaloid isolated from *Rauwolfia serpentina*. This drug depletes norepinephrine from nerve terminals and may have a brief direct vasodilator action. Reserpine increases fingertip capillary blood flow in patients exposed to a cold environment.[2] Furthermore, the vasoconstrictor responses to the application of ice to the forehead and to intra-arterial tyramine, a drug that releases norepinephrine from adrenergic nerve terminals, are reduced following reserpine.[40] Improvement in Raynaud's phenomenon has been reported following administration of reserpine when given in doses of 0.25 to 0.5 mg. Not all patients achieve long-term benefit from this medication, however, and its use is associated with side effects including nasal congestion, nausea, lethargy, depression, and peptic ulceration. Intra-arterial administration of reserpine has been advocated by some investigators to promote healing of digit ulcerations, but this benefit has not been confirmed by others.[126]

Guanethidine, like reserpine, decreases norepinephrine release from nerve terminals. In one study, guanethidine increased fingertip capillary blood flow in patients with Raynaud's phenomenon secondary to scleroderma.[127] Long-term studies that assess symptomatic responses are lacking. Its utility is significantly limited because of important adverse effects, particularly orthostatic hypotension.

α-Methyldopa is a central adrenergic antagonist that interferes with the formation of dihydroxyphenylethylamine, a precursor of norepinephrine, and inhibits the conversion of 5-hydroxytryptophan to serotonin. Although one group of investigators suggested that this drug was beneficial in Raynaud's phenomenon, no controlled studies attest to its efficacy.[128] Side effects include postural hypotension, lethargy, and impotence. In addition, this drug may cause fever, hemolytic anemia, and hepatic dysfunction.

Phenoxybenzamine is another adrenergic-blocking drug. Several uncontrolled studies have reported favorable results with this drug in patients with Raynaud's phenomenon.[129] The suggested dosage of phenoxybenzamine is 10 to 30 mg once daily. Side effects include postural hypotension, lightheadedness, edema, and ejaculatory dysfunction.

Serotonin Antagonists

Serotonin, as discussed earlier in this chapter, may be pertinent to the pathophysiology of Raynaud's phenomenon. For this reason, ketanserin, a serotonin (5-HT_2) receptor antagonist with some α-adrenoceptor blocking activity, has been evaluated in patients with Raynaud's phenomenon. The results of trials that assess the effect of chronic oral therapy have been conflicting; improvement in symptoms was observed in some but not in others.[55-58] A large placebo-controlled trial involving 222 patients, 50% of whom had primary Raynaud's phenomenon and the rest, Raynaud's phenomenon secondary to connective tissue disorders, was performed.[55] Ketanserin decreased the frequency of digital vasospastic attacks. Digital blood flow measurements were obtained in a subgroup of this study population. Despite symptomatic improvement, there was no evidence that ketanserin improved digital blood flow during exposure to either a warm or cool environment. One small study found that fluoxetine, a selective serotonin uptake inhibitor, reduced the number and severity of vasospastic attacks in 53 patients with primary or secondary Raynaud's phenomenon compared with nifedipine.[130]

Thromboxane Inhibitors

Thromboxane A_2 causes platelet aggregation and vasoconstriction and conceivably could contribute to digital vasospasm in some patients with Raynaud's phenomenon. Dazoxiben is a thromboxane synthetase inhibitor that attenuates the forearm vasoconstrictor response to cold in normal subjects.[60] Dazoxiben decreases thromboxane A_2 levels and improves symptoms in some patients with Raynaud's phenomenon.[113] However, several placebo-controlled trials have failed to show that this drug reduces symptoms.[59,60,63] Furthermore, a combination of a thromboxane-receptor antagonist and a thromboxane synthetase inhibitor did not affect the response of patients with Raynaud's phenomenon to a cold challenge.[131]

Inhibition of the Renin-Angiotensin System

Angiotensin II is unlikely to mediate digital vasospasm in most patients with Raynaud's phenomenon.[132] If this hormone is elevated due to other pathologic conditions, it could conceivably contribute to digital vasospasm in patients already predisposed to Raynaud's phenomenon. One such population is patients with systemic sclerosis and malignant hypertension. One report described two patients with systemic sclerosis, malignant hypertension, renal failure, and digital ischemia who were treated with the angiotensin-converting enzyme inhibitor captopril. Hypertension, renal insufficiency, and digital ischemia all improved following drug administration.[66] However, another study reported that captopril decreased vasospastic attacks in patients with primary Raynaud's phenomenon but not in patients with Raynaud's phenomenon secondary to scleroderma.[133] Other uncontrolled studies have suggested that captopril reduces symptoms in Raynaud's disease.

The angiotensin receptor antagonist losartan has been reported to decrease the frequency and severity of vasospastic attacks in 15 patients with primary Raynaud's phenomenon.[134] More studies of this class of drug are necessary.

Direct Vascular Smooth Muscle Relaxants

The problem with most vasodilators is that they cause a general reduction in vascular resistance and may actually divert blood flow from the affected digits. As a result, patients often experience adverse side effects, including hypotension, without deriving any benefit for Raynaud's phenomenon.

Organic nitrate preparations including nitropaste are often used in patients with Raynaud's phenomenon.[2] One study reported that topical glyceryl trinitrate was an effective therapy for patients with Raynaud's phenomenon but limited in utility because of headache.[135] Nitroprusside has been used in the treatment of severe vasospasm-caused ergotism. No other convincing evidence exists that chronic treatment with nitrate preparations ameliorates Raynaud's phenomenon.[112]

Prostaglandins inhibit platelet aggregation and are vasodilators. Several uncontrolled studies have suggested that IV infusions of prostaglandin E_1 promote healing of digital ulcers in patients with scleroderma.[3,112] In a placebo-controlled, multicenter study, however, IV PGE_1 was no more effective than placebo in reducing symptoms of Raynaud's phenomenon or healing digital ulcers. Several placebo-controlled studies, however, have reported long-term benefit in the treatment of severe Raynaud's phenomenon with IV iloprost, a prostacyclin analogue, for 3 to 5 days, or with prostacyclin for 3 weeks.[3,112] There were significant decreases in the frequency, duration, and severity of vasospastic attacks, or increases in indices of finger blood flow for up to 9 weeks. In one study, comparing intravenous iloprost with oral nifedipine, both drugs were of benefit subjectively while parameters of finger blood flow were only increased with iloprost. Side effects of iloprost depend on dose and include headaches, flushing, nausea, vomiting, and jaw pain. Oral prostacyclin preparations, unfortunately, have not proven of value in the treatment of Raynaud's phenomenon.[3]

Various other direct vasodilators have been proposed as therapeutic agents in patients with Raynaud's phenomenon. These include hydralazine, nicotinic acid, isoxsuprine, cyclandelate, and papaverine. Studies are lacking to prove their benefit.[2]

N-acetylcysteine

N-acetylcysteine, a powerful antioxidant, is postulated to decrease free radical injury of the endothelium. A pilot study of IV drug for 5 days in 22 patients with Raynaud's phenomenon due to systemic sclerosis decreased the vasospastic attack frequency and severity compared with pretreatment values.[136] Controlled studies need to be performed with this interesting compound, which is used safely in other disorders.

Sympathectomy

The success rate of sympathectomy for episodic digital vasospasm of the upper extremity is not as good as might be anticipated. Raynaud's phenomenon recurs in the majority of patients.[2,3,137] Successful relief of digital ischemia is less in patients with secondary forms of Raynaud's phenomenon than in patients with primary Raynaud's phenomenon. In contrast, the majority of patients experience improvement in symptoms in their lower extremities following lumbar sympathectomy. Possibly, lumbar sympathectomy is more complete than thoracodorsal sympathectomy, in which residual sympathetic pathways may develop following surgery.

Digital sympathectomy has been advocated by some surgeons for treatment of digital ischemia, particularly that secondary to severe Raynaud's phenomenon. This technique may improve digital blood flow and allow healing of digital ulcerations.[3,110]

REFERENCES

1. Raynaud M: L'Asphyxie Locale et de la Gangrene Symmetrique des Extremities. Barlow T, trans. London, New Sydenham Society, 1862.
2. Coffman JD: Raynaud Phenomenon. New York, Oxford University Press, 1989.
3. Wigley FM: Raynaud's phenomenon. N Engl J Med 347:1001, 2002.
4. Coffman JD: Raynaud's phenomenon. Curr Opin Cardiol 8:821, 1993.
5. Maricq HR, Weinrich MC, Keil JE, et al: Prevalence of Raynaud's phenomenon in the general population. J Chronic Dis 38:423, 1986.
6. Allen EV, Brown GE: Raynaud's disease: A critical review of minimal requisites for diagnosis. Am J Med Sci 183:187, 1932.
7. LeRoy EC, Medsger TA Jr: Raynaud's phenomenon: A proposal for classification. Clin Exp Rheumatol 10:485, 1991.
8. Gifford RW, Hines EA: Raynaud's disease among women and girls. Circulation 16:1012, 1957.
9. Guntheroth WG, Morgan BC, Harbinson JA, et al: Raynaud's disease in children. Circulation 36: 724, 1967.
10. Maricq HR, Carpentier PH, Weinrich MC, et al: Geographic variation in prevalence of Raynaud's phenomenon. Charleston, SC, USA vs Tarentaise, Savoie France. J Rheumatol 20:70, 1993.
11. Freedman RR, Mayes MD: Familial aggregation of primary Raynaud's disease. Arthritis Rheum 39:1189, 1996.
12. Miller D, Waters DD, Warnica W, et al: Is variant angina the coronary manifestation of a generalized vasospastic disorder? N Engl J Med 304:763, 1981.
13. Zahavi I, Chagnac A, Hering R, et al: Prevalence of Raynaud's phenomenon in patients with migraine. Arch Intern Med 144:742, 1984.
14. O'Keeffe ST, Tsapatsaris NP, Beetham WP Jr: Increased prevalence of migraine and chest pain in patients with primary Raynaud disease. Ann Intern Med 116:985, 1992.
15. Cannon PJ, Hassar M, Case DB, et al: The relationship of hypertension and renal failure in scleroderma (progressive systemic sclerosis) to structural and functional abnormalities of the renal cortical circulation. Medicine 53:1, 1974.
16. Salmenson BD, Reisman J, Sinclair SH, et al: Macular capillary hemodynamic changes associated with Raynaud's phenomenon. Ophthalmology 99:914, 1992.
17. Vergnon J-M, Barthelemy JC, Riffat J, et al: Raynaud's phenomenon of the lung. Chest 101:1312, 1992.
18. Krumholz HM, Goldberger AL: Systemic arterial vasospastic syndrome: Familial occurrence with variant angina. Am J Med 92:344, 1992.
19. Coffman JD, Cohen RA: Vasospasm—ubiquitous? N Engl J Med 304:780, 1981.
20. Tokola R, Hokkanen E: Propranolol for acute migraine. Br Med J 2:1089, 1978.
21. Yasue H, Youyama M, Shimamoto M, et al: Role of autonomic nervous system in the pathogenesis of Prinzmetal's variant form of angina. Circulation 50:534, 1974.
22. Marshal AJ, Roberts CJC, Barritt DW: Raynaud's phenomenon as side effect of β-blockers in hypertension. Br Med J 1:1498, 1976.
23. Schroeder JS, Bolen JL, Quint RA, et al: Provocation of coronary spasm with ergonovine maleate: New test with results in 57 patients undergoing coronary arteriography. Am J Cardiol 40:487, 1977.
24. Curry RC Jr, Pepine CJ, Sabom MB, et al: Effects of ergonovine in patients with and without coronary artery disease. Circulation 56:803, 1977.
25. Wollersheim H, Thien T, Hoet MH, et al: The diagnostic valve of several immunological tests for anti-nuclear antibody in predicting the development of connective tissue disease in patients presenting with Raynaud's phenomenon. Eur J Clin Invest 19:535, 1989.
26. Cohen RA, Coffman JD: Digital vasospasm: The pathophysiology of Raynaud's phenomenon. Int Angiology 3:47, 1984.
27. Lewis T: Experiments relating to the peripheral mechanism involved in spasmodic arrest of the circulation in the fingers, a variety of Raynaud's disease. Heart 15:7, 1929.
28. Freedman RR, Mayes MD, Sabharwal SC: Induction of vasospastic attacks despite digital nerve block in Raynaud's disease and phenomenon. Circulation 80:859, 1989.
29. Jamieson GG, Ludbrook J, Wilson A: Cold hypersensitivity in Raynaud's phenomenon. Circulation 44:254, 1971.
30. Vanhoutte PM, Cooke JP, Lindblad LE, et al: Modulation of postjunctional α-adrenergic responsiveness by local changes in temperature. Clin Sci 68:121s, 1985.
31. Cooke JP, Shepherd JT, Vanhoutte PM: The effect of warming on adrenergic neurotransmission in canine cutaneous vein. Circ Res 54:547, 1984.
32. Flavahan NA, Cooke JP, Shepherd JT, et al: Human postjunctional alpha-1 and alpha-2 adrenoceptors: Differential distribution in arteries of the limbs. J Pharmacol Exp Ther 241:361, 1987.
33. Chotani MA, Mitra S, Su BY, et al: Regulation of α_2-adrenoceptors in human vascular smooth muscle cells. Am J Physiol Heart Circ Physiol 286:H59, 2004.
34. Jeyaraj SC, Chotani MA, Mitra S, et al: Cooling evokes redistribution of α_{2C}-adrenoceptors from Golgi to plasma membrane in transfected human embryonic kidney 293 cells. Mol Pharmacol 60:1195, 2001.
35. Keenan EJ, Porter JM: Alpha-2-adrenergic receptors in platelets from patients with Raynaud's syndrome. Surgery 94:204, 1983.
36. Coffman JD, Cohen RA: Role of alpha-adrenoceptor subtypes mediating sympathetic vasoconstriction in human digits. Eur J Clin Invest 18:309, 1988.
37. Coffman JD, Cohen RA: Alpha-adrenergic and 5-HT_2 receptor hypersensitivity in Raynaud's phenomenon. J Vasc Med Biol 2:100, 1990.
38. Cooke JP, Creager SJ, Scales KM, et al: Role of digital artery adrenoceptors in Raynaud's disease. Vasc Med 2:1, 1997.
39. Peacock JH: Peripheral venous blood concentrations of epinephrine and norepinephrine in primary Raynaud's disease. Circ Res 7:821, 1959.
40. Kontos HA, Wasserman AJ: Effect of reserpine in Raynaud's phenomenon. Circulation 39:259, 1969.
41. Downey JA, Leroy EC, Miller JM III, et al: Thermoregulation and Raynaud's phenomenon. Clin Sci 40:211, 1971.
42. Fagius J, Blumberg H: Sympathetic outflow to the hand in patients with Raynaud's phenomenon. Cardiovasc Res 19:249, 1985.
43. Greenblatt DJ, Koch-Weser J: Adverse reactions to beta-adrenergic receptor blocking drugs. A report from the Boston Collaborative Drug Surveillance Program. Drugs 7:118, 1974.
44. Marshall AJ, Roberts CJC, Barritt DW: Raynaud's phenomenon as side effect of beta-blockers in hypertension. Br Med J 1:1498, 1976.
45. Eliasson K, Lins LE, Sundqvist K: Peripheral vasospasm during beta receptor blockade—a comparison between metoprolol and pindolol. Acta Med Scand Suppl 665:109, 1982.
46. Cohen RA, Coffman JD: Beta-adrenergic vasodilator mechanism in the finger. Circ Res 49:1196, 1981.
47. Vanhoutte PM: 5-Hydroxytryptamine and vascular disease. Fed Proc 42:233, 1983.
48. Vanhoutte PM, Shepherd JT: Effect of temperature on reactivity of isolated cutaneous veins of the dog. Am J Physiol 218:187, 1970.
49. Winkelmann RK, Goldyne ME, Linscheid RL: Hypersensitivity of scleroderma cutaneous vascular smooth muscle to 5-hydroxytryptamine. Br J Dermatol 95:51, 1976.
50. Coffman JD, Cohen RA: Serotonergic vasoconstriction in human fingers during reflex sympathetic response to cooling. Am J Physiol 254:H889, 1988.
51. Halpern A, Kuhn PH, Shaftel HE, et al: Raynaud's disease, Raynaud's phenomenon, and serotonin. Angiology 11:151, 1960.
52. Reimann IW, Frolich JC: Mechanism of antihypertensive action of ketanserin in man. Br Med J 287:381, 1983.
53. Zabludowski JR, Ball SG, Robertson JIS: Ketanserin and $alpha_1$-adrenergic antagonism in humans. J Cardiovasc Pharmacol 7:S123, 1985.
54. Hechtman DH, Jageneau A: Inhibition of cold-induced vasoconstriction with ketanserin. Microvasc Res 30:56, 1985.
55. Coffman JD, Clement DL, Creager MA, et al: International study of ketanserin in Raynaud's phenomenon. Am J Med 87:264, 1989.
56. Seibold JR, Jageneau HM: Treatment of Raynaud's phenomenon with ketanserin, a selective antagonist of the serotonin-2 (5-HT_2) receptor. Arthritis Rheum 27:139, 1984.
57. Stranden E, Roald OK, Krohg K: Treatment of Raynaud's phenomenon with the 5-HT2 receptor antagonist ketanserin. Br Med J 285:1069, 1982.
58. Roald OK, Seem E: Treatment of Raynaud's phenomenon with ketanserin in patients with connective tissue disorders. Br Med J 289:577, 1984.

59. Coffman JD, Rasmussen HM: Effect of thromboxane synthetase inhibition in Raynaud's phenomenon. Clin Pharmacol Ther 36:369, 1984.
60. Ettinger WH, Wise RA, Schaffhauser D, et al: Controlled double-blind trial of dazoxiben and nifedipine in the treatment of Raynaud's phenomenon. Am J Med 77:451, 1984.
61. Jones EW, Hawkey CJ: A thromboxane synthetase inhibitor in Raynaud's phenomenon. Prostaglandins Leukot Med 12:67, 1983.
62. Luderer JR, Nicholas GG, Neumyer MM, et al: Dazoxiben, a thromboxane synthetase inhibitor in Raynaud's phenomenon. Clin Pharmacol Ther 36:105, 1984.
63. Tindall H, Tooke JE, Menys VC, et al: Effect of dazoxiben, a thromboxane synthetase inhibitor on skin blood flow following cold challenge in patients with Raynaud's phenomenon. Eur J Clin Invest 15:20, 1985.
64. Zamora MR, O'Brien RF, Rutherford RB, et al. Serum endothelin-1 concentrations and cold provocation in primary Raynaud's phenomenon. Lancet 336:1144, 1990.
65. Smyth AE, Bell AL, Bruce IN, et al. Digital vascular responses and serum endothelin-1 concentrations in primary and secondary Raynaud's phenomenon. Ann Rheum Dis 59:870, 2000.
66. Burton AC: The physical equilibrium of the small blood vessels. Am J Physiol 164:319, 1951.
67. Krahenbuhl B, Nielsen SL, Lassen NA: Closure of digital arteries in high vascular tone states as demonstrated by measurement of systolic blood pressure in the finger. Scand J Clin Lab Invest 37:71, 1977.
68. Landis EM: Micro-injection studies of capillary blood pressure in Raynaud's disease. Heart 15:247, 1930.
69. Thulesius O: Methods for evaluation of peripheral vascular function in the upper extremities. Acta Chir Scand 465(suppl):53, 1976.
70. Cohen RA, Coffman JD: Reduced fingertip arterial pressure in Raynaud's disease. J Vasc Med Biol 1:21, 1989.
71. Brown GE, Griffin HZ: Peripheral arterial disease in polycythemia vera. Arch Intern Med 46:705, 1930.
72. Imhof JW, Boars H, Verloop MC: Clinical haematologic aspects of macroglobulinaemia Waldenström. Acta Med Scand 163:349, 1959.
73. Marshal RJ, Shepherd JT, Thompson ID: Vascular responses in patients with high serum titres of cold agglutinins. Clin Sci 12:255, 1953.
74. McGrath MA, Penny R: Blood hyperviscosity in cryoglobulinemia: temperature sensitivity and correlation with reduced skin blood flow. Aust J Exp Biol Med Sci 56:127, 1978.
75. Hillestad LK: The peripheral circulation during exposure to cold in normals and in patients with the syndrome of high-titre cold haemagglutination. Acta Med Scand 164:211, 1959.
76. Jahnsen T, Nielsen SL, Skovborg F: Blood viscosity and local response to cold in primary Raynaud's phenomenon. Lancet 2:1001, 1977.
77. Walder DN: Blood viscosity and Raynaud's disease. J R Coll Surg Edinb 18:277, 1973.
78. McGrath MA, Peek R, Penny R: Raynaud's disease: Reduced hand blood flows with normal blood viscosity. Aust N Z J Med 8:126, 1978.
79. Subcommittee for Scleroderma Criteria of the American Rheumatism Association Diagnostic and Therapeutic Criteria Committee: Preliminary criteria for the classification of systemic sclerosis (scleroderma). Arthritis Rheum 23:581, 1980.
80. Maricq HR, LeRoy EC, D'Angelo WA, et al. Diagnostic potential of in vivo capillary microscopy in scleroderma and related disorders. Arthritis Rheum 23:183, 1980.
81. Tan EM, Cohen AS, Fries JF, et al: The 1982 revised criteria for the classification of systemic lupus erythematosus. Arthritis Rheum 25:1271, 1982.
82. Fischer M, Mielke H, Glaefke S, et al: Generalized vasculopathy and finger blood flow abnormalities in rheumatoid arthritis. J Rheum 11:33, 1984.
83. Arnett FC, Edworthy SM, Block DA, et al: The American Rheumatism Association 1987 revised criteria for the classification of rheumatoid arthritis. Arthritis Rheum 31:315, 1988.
84. Garcia-Carrasco M, Siso A, Ramos-Casals M, et al: Raynaud's phenomenon in primary Sjogren's syndrome. Prevalence and clinical characteristics in a series of 320 patients. J Rheumatol 29:726, 2002.
85. Waller DG, Dathan JR: Raynaud's syndrome and carpal tunnel syndrome. Postgrad Med J 61:161, 1985.
86. Cooper RA, Bunn HF: Hemolytic anemia. In E Braunwald et al., eds. Harrison's Principles of Internal Medicine. New York, McGraw-Hill, 1987.
87. Trejo O, Ramos-Casals M, Garcia-Carrasco M, et al: Cryoglobulinemia: Study of etiologic factors and clinical and immunologic features in 443 patients from a single center. Medicine (Baltimore) 80:252, 2001.
88. Jager BV: Cryofibrinogenemia. N Engl J Med 266:579, 1962.
89. Letz R, Cherniack MG, Gerr F, et al: A cross sectional epidemiological survey of shipyard workers exposed to hand-arm vibration. Br J Indust Med 49:53, 1992.
90. Mirbod SM, Yoshida H, Nagata C, et al: Hand-arm vibration syndrome and its prevalence in the present status of private forestry enterprises in Japan. Int Arch Occup Environ Health 64:93, 1992.
91. Davies TAL, Glaser EM, Collins CP: Absence of Raynaud's phenomenon in workers using vibratory tools in warm climate. Lancet 1:1014, 1957.
92. Okada A, Inaba R, Furuno T: Occurrence of intimal thickening of the peripheral arteries in response to local vibration. Br J Ind Med 44:470, 1987.
93. Hisanaga H: Studies of peripheral nerve conduction velocities in vibrating tool operators. Sangyo Igaku 24: 284, 1982.
94. Laplanche A, Clavel-Chapelon F, Contassot JC, et al: Exposure to vinyl chloride monomer: Results of a cohort study after a seven year follow up. The French VCM Group. Br J Ind Med 49:134, 1992.
95. Coffman JD, Rasmussen HM: Effects of beta-adrenoceptor-blocking drugs in patients with Raynaud's phenomenon. Circulation 72:466, 1985.
96. Nielsen SL, Parving H-H, Hansen JEM: Myxoedema and Raynaud's phenomenon. Acta Endocrinol (Copenh) 101:32, 1989.
97. Nielsen SL, Lokkegaard H: Cold hypersensitivity and finger systolic blood pressure in hemodialysis patients. Scand J Urol Nephrol 15:319, 1989.
98. Preston IR, Hill NS: Evaluation and management of pulmonary hypertension in systemic sclerosis. Curr Opin Rheumatol 15:761, 2003.
99. Fuster V, Steele PM, Edwards WD, et al: Primary pulmonary hypertension: Natural history and the importance of thrombosis. Circulation 70:580, 1984.
100. Rich S, Dantzker DR, Ayres SM, et al: Primary pulmonary hypertension. A national prospective study. Ann Intern Med 107:216, 1987.
101. Nielsen SL: Raynaud's phenomena and finger systolic pressure with cooling. Scand J Clin Lab Invest 38:765, 1978.
102. Coffman JD: Effect of propranolol on blood pressure and skin blood flow during cigarette smoking. J Clin Pharmacol 9:39, 1969.
103. Keefe FJ, Surwit RS, Pilon RN: A 1-year follow-up of Raynaud's patients treated with behavioral therapy techniques. J Behav Med 2:385, 1979.
104. Keefe FJ, Surwit RS, Pilon RN: Biofeedback, autogenic training, and progressive relaxation in the treatment of Raynaud's disease: A comparative study. J Appl Behav Anal 13:3, 1980.
105. Rich S, Dantzker DR, Ayres SM, et al: Primary pulmonary hypertension. A national prospective study. Ann Intern Med 107:216, 1987.
106. Yocum DE, Hodes R, Sundstrom WR, et al: Use of biofeedback training in treatment of Raynaud's disease and phenomenon. J Rheumatol 12:90, 1985.
107. Stambrook M, Hamel ER, Carter SA: Training to vasodilate in a cooling environment: A valid treatment for Raynaud's phenomenon? Biofeedback Self-Regul 13:9, 1988.
108. Guglielmi RS, Roberts AH, Patterson R: Skin temperature biofeedback for Raynaud's disease: A double-blind study. Biofeedback Self-Regul 7:99, 1982.
109. Freedman RR, Ianni P, Wenig P: Behavioral treatment of Raynaud's phenomenon in scleroderma. J Behav Med 7:343, 1984.
110. Raynaud's Treatment Study Investigators: Comparison of sustained-release nifedipine and temperature biofeedback for treatment of primary Raynaud's phenomenon. Arch Intern Med 160: 1101, 2000.
111. Jobe JB, Sampson JB, Roberts DE, et al: Induced vasodilation as treatment for Raynaud's disease. Ann Intern Med 97:706, 1982.
112. Coffman JD: Raynaud's phenomenon. Curr Ther Options Cardiovasc Med 2:219, 2000.

113. Belch JJF, Meilen H: Pharmacotherapy of Raynaud's phenomenon. Drugs 52:682, 1996.
114. Antman EM, Stone PH, Muller JE, et al: Calcium channel blocking agents in the treatment of cardiovascular disorders. Part I: Basic and clinical electrophysiologic effects. Ann Intern Med 93:875, 1980.
115. Stone PH, Antman EM, Muller JE, et al: Calcium channel blocking agents in the treatment of cardiovascular disorders. II: Hemodynamic effects and clinical applications. Ann Intern Med 93:886, 1980.
116. Creager MA, Pariser KM, Winston EM, et al: Nifedipine-induced fingertip vasodilation in patients with Raynaud's phenomenon. Am Heart J 108:370, 1984.
117. Nilsson H, Jonason T, Leppert J, et al: The effect of the calcium-entry blocker nifedipine on cold-induced digital vasospasm. A double-blind crossover study versus placebo. Acta Med Scand 221:53, 1987.
118. Matucci Cerinic M, Falcini F, Bartolozzi G, et al: Nifedipine treatment of Raynaud's phenomenon in a paediatric age. Int J Clin Pharm Res 5:67, 1985.
119. Kahan A, Amor B, Menkes CJ: A randomised double-blind trial of diltiazem in the treatment of Raynaud's phenomenon. Ann Rheum Dis 44:30, 1985.
120. Rhedda A, McCans J, Willan AR, et al: A double blind placebo controlled crossover randomized trial of diltiazem in Raynaud's phenomenon. J Rheumatol 12:724, 1985.
121. Matoba T, Chiba M: Effects of diltiazem on occupational Raynaud's syndrome (vibration disease). Angiology 36:850, 1985.
122. Schmidt JF, Valentin N, Nielsen SL: The clinical effect of felodipine and nifedipine in Raynaud's phenomenon. Eur J Clin Pharmacol 37:191, 1989.
123. Kallenberg CGM, Wouda AA, Meems L, et al: Once daily felodipine in patients with primary Raynaud's phenomenon. Eur J Clin Pharmacol 40:313, 1991.
124. Kinney EL, Nicholas GG, Gallo J, et al: The treatment of severe Raynaud's phenomenon with verapamil. J Clin Pharmacol 22:74, 1982.
125. Nielsen SL, Vitting K, Rasmussen K: Prazosin treatment of primary Raynaud's phenomenon. Eur J Clin Pharmacol 24:421, 1983.
126. McFadyen IJ, Housley E, MacPherson AIS: Intraarterial reserpine administration in Raynaud syndrome. Arch Intern Med 132:526, 1973.
127. LeRoy EC, Downey JA, Cannon PJ: Skin capillary blood flow in scleroderma. J Clin Invest 50:930, 1971.
128. Varadi DP, Lawrence AM: Suppression of Raynaud's phenomenon by methyldopa. Arch Intern Med 124:13, 1969.
129. Carter SA: Finger systolic pressures and skin temperatures in severe Raynaud's syndrome: The relationship to healing of skin lesions and the use of oral phenoxybenzamine. Angiology 32:298, 1981.
130. Coleiro B, Marshall SE, Denton CP, et al: Treatment of Raynaud's phenomenon with the selective serotonin reuptake inhibitor fluoxetine. Rheumatology (Oxford) 40:1038, 2001.
131. Gresele P, Volpato R, Migliacci R, et al: Thromboxane does not play a significant role in acute, cold-induced vasoconstriction in Raynaud's phenomenon. Studies with combined thromboxane synthase inhibition and thromboxane receptor antagonism. Thromb Res 66:259, 1992.
132. Challenor VF: Angiotensin converting enzyme inhibitors in Raynaud's phenomenon. Drugs 48:864, 1994.
133. Tosi S, Marchesoni A, Messina K, et al: Treatment of Raynaud's phenomenon with captopril. Drugs Exp Clin Res 13:37, 1987.
134. Dziadzio M, Denton CP, Smith R, et al: Losartan therapy for Raynaud's phenomenon and scleroderma: Clinical and biochemical findings in a fifteen-week, randomized, parallel-group, controlled trial. Arthritis Rheum 42:2646, 1999.
135. Teh LS, Manning J, Moore T, et al: Sustained-release transdermal glyceryl trinitrate patches as a treatment for primary and secondary Raynaud's phenomenon. Br J Rheumatol 34:636, 1995.
136. Sambo P, Amico D, Giacomelli R, et al: Intravenous N-acetylcysteine for treatment of Raynaud's phenomenon secondary to systemic sclerosis: A pilot study. J Rheumatol 28:2257, 2001.
137. de Trafford JC, Lafferty K, Potter CE, et al: An epidemiological survey of Raynaud's phenomenon. Eur J Vasc Surg 2:167, 1988.

chapter 49

Acrocyanosis

Jay D. Coffman

Acrocyanosis was originally described by Crocq in 1896.[1] Classically, patients are young asthenic females whose hands and feet have a bluish discoloration. The cyanosis is reversible when the affected body part is warmed. In contrast to Raynaud's phenomenon, episodic attacks and pallor do not occur. Primary acrocyanosis (of unknown etiology) is benign; pain, ulcers, or gangrene do not occur. Secondary acrocyanosis is due to an underlying condition (e.g., hypoxemia) or disease (e.g., scleroderma) and is usually not benign.

DEMOGRAPHICS

Stern[2] studied patients in a mental institution and found that the sexes were affected equally by primary acrocyanosis. However, many of the inmates did not report spontaneous cyanosis but only had discoloration when their hands were cooled in 20° C water for 15 minutes. Davis[3] reported on 150 patients; the female-to-male ratio was 6:1. Most research studies of small groups of patients involved females, lending strength to the female predominance.[4,5] The age range of patients is usually 20 to 45 years old,[2,3] although primary acrocyanosis has been reported in patients much younger and older. Monticone[6] found that symptoms usually begin at puberty in women and disappear in the fourth decade. Stern[2] reported that 10% of his patients showed a familial pattern occurring in mother and daughter or in siblings. No studies have been conducted on the prevalence, incidence, geographic occurrence, or racial characteristics of patients with primary acrocyanosis. It is believed to occur more frequently in patients with a low body mass index and in cooler climates.

HISTOPATHOLOGY

Cutaneous biopsies of the terminal finger have revealed dilation of the papillary capillaries and, in some patients, the subpapillary capillaries.[7] Biopsies of the dorsal skin of the hands and feet in 12 patients showed that the medial coats of nearly all arterioles from 30 to 150 μm or more in diameter were thickened, although this was considered to be just within the upper limits of normal and more pronounced in the feet.[2] Local edema and skin fibrosis with dilation of the superficial capillaries and new formation of blood vessels sometimes were present. An excess number of arteriovenous anastomoses has been alluded to by only one source.[8]

The nailfold terminal capillaries, as assessed by nailfold microscopy, are dilated at the arterial and venous limbs of the loops from a normal value of 10 to 20 up to 55 μm.[3] Increased numbers of sweat drops are often present.[7] The mean density of capillaries is decreased compared with normal subjects but not as much as in patients with secondary Raynaud's phenomenon.[4,6] The diameter of capillary loops is larger than in normal controls and patients with primary Raynaud's phenomenon.[4] Giant capillaries are rarely seen as in scleroderma.[6] Hemorrhages and pericapillary edema may occur.

PATHOPHYSIOLOGY

Several studies have concerned the pathophysiology of primary acrocyanosis, but the mechanism remains elusive. Abnormalities of arteriolar vasospasm, capillary and venular stasis due to an inability of small vessels to react to stimuli, and altered CNS responses have been postulated. In early studies, it was shown that a structural vascular lesion was unlikely, and a local sensitivity of the blood vessels to cold was proposed.[9-11] Elevation of a cyanotic limb above heart level produced pallor indicating venous obstruction was not present, and pallor induced by pressure on the skin disappeared on release of the pressure. Reactive hyperemia of the fingers was normal. With body heating, the temperature of the fingers reached that of the forehead. Ulnar nerve block relieved the cyanosis of the fifth finger, but the color of the digit did not change until its temperature rose 7°C, which was surmised to mean that the digital arteries opened before "spasm" was relieved in the arterioles.[9]

Vasoconstrictor agents have been shown to produce a normal response in acrocyanotic hands, and body heating combined with sympathetic blocking agents produced vasodilation.[12] The ulnar nerve block would also have blocked sympathetic nerves. Therefore a role for the sympathetic nervous system is suggested. Of interest is a report that the intensely cyanotic hands and forearms of a young girl became warm and red during normal sleep.[13] Her hands responded in the same manner as the rest of the body to heat and cold exposure during phenobarbital-induced sleep. This finding led to the hypothesis that the abnormal vasomotor responses of acrocyanotic patients may be of central origin and not due to a local sensitivity of the blood vessels to cold. Some investigators have implicated red blood cell aggregation and increased blood viscosity as a cause of the cyanosis,[8,14] but others have been unable to find supporting evidence.[4] Most studies have found all blood and noninvasive tests negative. Endothelin-1 levels are elevated before and after exposure of the hands to a 13°C water bath for 5 minutes, and the high levels during cooling persist for at least 90 minutes in patients with acrocyanosis compared with normal control subjects.[15]

The investigators thought that endothelin-1 could contribute by potentiating and prolonging cold-induced vasoconstriction or could be a marker of endothelial damage.

Although several blood flow studies of patients with acrocyanosis have been done, they add little to understanding the underlying mechanism. Normal hand blood flow during local warming to 42° C but low blood flow and skin temperature at 32° C compared with normal controls have been reported.[16,17] Indirect cooling leads to intense vasoconstriction that is not symmetric as in normal subjects and argues against sympathetic nervous system involvement in the pathophysiology.[5] The capillary blood flow in acrocyanotic fingernail folds is not homogeneous. Some capillaries show intermittent flow adjacent to capillaries with continuous flow.[18] Similar variations in blood pressure occur in the capillaries.[19] Delayed or asynchronous arrival of fluorescein sodium in different capillaries occurs.[18] A decrease in red blood cell velocity occurs in the capillaries before and after cold provocation.[4,13] The reason for these abnormalities is unknown.

In summary, the etiology and pathophysiology of primary acrocyanosis remains an enigma, but most evidence points to a local sensitivity of the arterioles to cold, inducing vasospasm with an aggravating sympathetic nervous system component.

CLINICAL PRESENTATION

Patients complain of cold, bluish, discolored hands and feet that intensify with cold exposure or emotional reactions (Fig. 49-1). Sometimes the forearms, ears, lips, nose, or nipples are involved. Typically the patient is a thin, young woman who is not physically active. There is no pain; swelling of the digits and increased perspiration may occur. Patients with the more severe discoloration and moisture may complain that they must avoid social contact. Usually there are no other specific local or systemic complaints.

Examination reveals bluish discoloration of the affected areas and often hyperhidrosis of the same anatomic regions. When the hands are affected, the discoloration may extend proximal to the wrists. The color has also been described as bluish-pink or orange-like tinged with red, but patients may show different hues at various times. Usually cold exposure deepens the color. Pressure on the discolored skin causes pallor, and color returns slowly and irregularly. Fingers may be puffy, but trophic changes do not occur. In primary acrocyanosis, the discoloration affects symmetric parts of the body. A brownish-yellow color on the backs of the hands to the wrists and on the dorsal feet has been described and attributed to exposure to the warmth of the sun, for it is most obvious in the summer.[2]

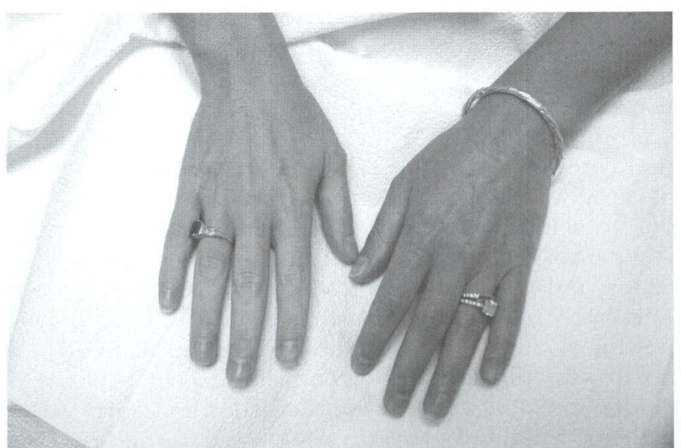

FIGURE 49-1. (See also Color Plate 49-1.) Acrocyanosis of the left hand is evident in this 36-year-old, otherwise healthy woman.

Pulses are normal in the primary syndrome, and there are no abnormal physical findings. Episodes of pallor or redness of the digits do not occur, although patients may have both acrocyanosis and Raynaud's phenomenon. This is especially true in patients with scleroderma or systemic lupus erythematosus as an underlying cause.

DIAGNOSTIC TESTS

No specific tests exist to diagnose primary acrocyanosis. Arterial blood gases help to rule out hypoxemia. Antinuclear antibodies are absent but, if present, may be diagnostic of connective tissue diseases. If the history and physical examination are suggestive, cryoglobulins, antiphospholipid antibodies, cold agglutinins, and antibodies for Epstein-Barr virus should be measured.

Decreased oscillations over the radial artery and decreased digital vessel sounds by Doppler have been described but are nonspecific tests.[8,20] Fingernail capillaroscopy is not diagnostic: It may show capillary dilatation but does not distinguish patients with acrocyanosis from normal subjects or most patients with connective tissue diseases. If megacapillaries and sparse-to-absent areas of capillaries are present, scleroderma or mixed connective tissue is suggested; bushy capillaries implicate systemic lupus erythematosus.

SECONDARY ACROCYANOSIS

Box 49-1 lists the multiple causes of acrocyanosis due to underlying conditions or agents.[21] Most causes are rare. A careful history and physical examination with appropriate laboratory tests are necessary to make these diagnoses. Asymmetric involvement of the extremities, pain, trophic changes of the fingers or toes, and absent pulses suggest a secondary cause. Hypoxemia is probably the most common underlying condition and can be diagnosed by the presence of cyanotic oral mucosa, arterial blood gases, and a search for cardiopulmonary disease. Some cases of pulmonary hypertension[22] and acrocyanosis in infancy are secondary to arterial blood oxygen desaturation.

Recent infection should suggest infectious mononucleosis or cold agglutinins. Auto-anti-M and anti-I antibodies have been found in infectious mononucleosis.[23] Cold agglutinins also occur in lymphoproliferative disorders. Antibiotic treatment of patients with acrocyanosis

BOX 49-1 Causes of Secondary Acrocyanosis

Hypoxemia
Pulmonary hypertension[22]
Acrocyanosis of infancy
Atheromatous embolism
Connective tissue diseases
Rheumatoid arthritis
Anorexia nervosa[26]
Cold agglutinins[23]
Cryoglobulins[25]
Antiphospholipid antibodies[27,28]
Imipramine[29,30]
Interferon α(2a)[31]
Toxicities
  Arsenic[32]
  Blasticidin S[33]
  Butyl nitrite[34]
Heritable diseases
  Ethylmalonic aciduria with muscle cytochrome C deficiency[36]
  Mitochondrial disease (oxidative phosphorylation disorders)[36]
  Palmoplantar keratoderma syndrome[39]
Orthostatic tachycardia syndrome[35]
Spinal cord injury[44]

and cold agglutinins may result in rapid clearing of acrocyanosis.[24] If patients with hepatitis C infection have acrocyanosis, they should be investigated for cryoglobulinemia, although cryoglobulins may also occur in several other diseases.[25]

In one study, 21% of 155 patients with anorexia nervosa had acrocyanosis.[26] It occurred in the more severely ill patients who were emaciated and weighed less than the anorectics without acrocyanosis. They also had pallor of the face and trunk, slow pulse rates, and a higher blood sugar. The hand and calf blood flows were decreased, and vasodilation to a heat stimulus was impaired.

Atheromatous embolism occurs in an older age group than patients with primary acrocyanosis; petechiae and skin lesions with pain are usually present, and patients have other signs of atherosclerosis. Connective tissue diseases and rheumatoid arthritis are entities that may manifest acrocyanosis, but other signs of these diseases are usually present. Patients with scleroderma or systemic lupus erythematosus may have both acrocyanosis and episodic attacks of Raynaud's phenomenon. Antinuclear antibodies or anticardiolipin antibodies may be present with or without connective tissue diseases. The latter were found in 25% of 16 patients with primary acrocyanosis in one study,[27] but the criteria for the diagnosis were not well defined. In the primary antiphospholipid syndrome, 6 of 13 patients compared with 2 of 20 control subjects had acrocyanosis.[28] These antibodies should be determined in patients if there are other cutaneous or vascular lesions.

A child[29] and an adult[30] have been reported developing acrocyanosis while taking imipramine. Tricyclic antidepressants increase norepinephrine levels but also antagonize α adrenoceptors; however, the adult had taken amitriptyline without developing acrocyanosis. One case of acrocyanosis has been reported with interferon α(2a) treatment.[31] Acrocyanosis has been described in 24% of 144 patients with high arsenic levels in the hair and nail clippings compared with 12.5% of control subjects.[32] A fungicide,[33] blasticidin S, and butyl nitrite[34] have also been reported to produce acrocyanosis. Drug and substance toxicity must be ruled out by a careful history.

Adolescents with orthostatic tachycardia syndrome and chronic fatigue syndrome may have acrocyanosis and edema.[35] It was hypothesized that either arteriolar dilation or venodilation due to denervated vessels in the distal extremities caused passive filling of the veins. The heritable diseases with acrocyanosis are easily suspected from their other manifestations. Infants with ethylmalonic aciduria have petechiae, diarrhea, pyramidal signs, and mental retardation.[36] In mitochondrial disease, children may have hair abnormalities, pigmentation disorders, and hypertrichosis[37] or early onset diabetes mellitus, optic atrophy, and deafness (Wolfram's syndrome).[38] Patients with diffuse palmoplantar keratoderma have the characteristic skin lesions; their dusky, well-demarcated acrocyanosis is limited to the lower one third of the arms and legs and disappears with limb elevation.[39]

TREATMENT

Primary acrocyanosis is a benign condition, which means only conservative or nontoxic therapies should be used. Reassurance and the avoidance of cool environments when not dressed warmly often suffice. Some patients are so affected, however, that they avoid social contact. Various drugs have been advocated, but no controlled studies have been performed. Calcium channel blockers, nicotinic acid derivatives, rauwolfia, Cyclospasmol, topical minoxidil, and rutin compounds have been claimed to provide symptomatic improvement.[3,21] Although bromocriptine may induce Raynaud's phenomenon in about one third of patients,[40] it has been reported to relieve acrocyanosis in a few days.[41] Biofeedback training, conditioning of reflexes,[8] and hypnosis may give partial relief. Indoramin, an α-adrenoceptor antagonist given intravenously, increases finger blood flow and decreases vascular resistance in patients with acrocyanosis, but clinical effects have not been described.[42] Cervical sympathectomy has been used but is a radical treatment for a benign disease.[43]

The treatment of secondary acrocyanosis depends on the underlying cause.

REFERENCES

1. Crocq C: De l'acrocyanose. Semin Med 16:297, 1896.
2. Stern ES: The aetiology and pathology of acrocyanosis. Br J Dermatol Syph 49:100, 1937.
3. Davis E: Clinical aspects of acrocyanosis. Adv Microcirc 10:101, 1982.
4. Jacobs MJHM, Breslau PJ, Slaaf DW, et al: A capillary microscopic and hemorheologic study. Surgery 101:136, 1987.
5. Lottenbach K: Vascular response to cold in acrocyanosis. Helvetia Medica Acta 5:437, 1966.

6. Monticone G, Colonna L, Palmeri G, et al: Quantitative nailfold capillary microscopy findings in patients with acrocyanosis compared with patients having systemic sclerosis and normal subjects. J Am Acad Dermatol 42:787, 2000.
7. Sagher F, Davis E, Sheskin J, et al: The small blood vessels of the skin in acrocyanosis. Br J Dermatol 78:586, 1966.
8. Merlen JF: Paradoxes of acrocyanosis. Adv Microcirc 10:95, 1982.
9. Lewis T, Landis EM: Observations upon the vascular mechanism in acrocyanosis. Heart 15:229, 1930.
10. Eliot AH, Evans RD, Stone CS: Acrocyanosis: A study of the circulatory fault. Am Heart J 11:431, 1936.
11. Lambie CG, Morson SM: Acrocyanosis. Med J Aust 2:1070, 1937.
12. Mendlowitz M: The Digital Circulation. New York, Grune & Stratton, 1954.
13. Day R, Klingman WO: The effect of sleep on the skin temperature reactions in a case of acrocyanosis. J Clin Invest 18:271, 1939.
14. Copeman PWM: Acrocyanosis: A blood disease? Proc R Soc Med 66:741, 1973.
15. Mangiafico RA, Malatino LS, Santonocito M, et al: Plasma endothelin-1 concentrations during cold exposure in essential acrocyanosis. Angiology 47:1033, 1996.
16. Peacock JH: Vasodilatation in the human hand: Observations on primary Raynaud's disease and acrocyanosis of the upper extremities. Clin Sci 17:575, 1957.
17. Peacock JH: A comparative study of the digital cutaneous temperatures and hand blood flows in the normal hand, primary Raynaud's disease and primary acrocyanosis. Clin Sci 18:25, 1959.
18. Bollinger A: Function of the precapillary vessels in peripheral vascular disease. J Cardiovasc Pharmacol 7(suppl 3):S147, 1985.
19. Mahler F, Muheim MH, Intaglietta M, et al: Blood pressure fluctuations in human nailfold capillaries. Am J Physiol 236:H888, 1979.
20. Davis E: Oscillometry of radial artery in acrocyanosis and cold sensitivity. J Mal Vasc 17:214, 1992.
21. Nousari HC, Kimyai A, Anhalt GJ: Chronic idiopathic acrocyanosis. J Am Acad Dermatol 45:5207, 2001.
22. Adam A, Patterson DLH: Pulmonary hypertension associated with hepatic cirrhosis and primary acrocyanosis. J R Soc Med 74:689, 1981.
23. Dickerman JD, Howard P, Dopp S, et al: Infectious mononucleosis initially seen as cold-induced acrocyanosis: Association with auto-anti-M and anti-I antibodies. Am J Dis Child 134:159, 1980.
24. Shelley WB, Shelley ED: Acrocyanosis of cold agglutinin disease successfully treated with antibiotics. Cutis 33:556, 1984.
25. Trejo O, Ramos-Casals M, Garcia-Carrasco M, et al: Cryoglobulinemia: Study of etiological factors and clinical and immunologic features in 443 patients from a single center. Medicine 80:252, 2001.
26. Bhanji S, Mattingly D: Acrocyanosis in anorexia nervosa. Postgrad Med J 67:33, 1991.
27. Vayssairat M, Abauf N, Baudot N, et al: Abnormal IgG cardiolipin antibody titers in patients with Raynaud's phenomenon and/or related disorders: Prevalence and clinical significance. J Am Acad Dermatol 38:555, 1998.
28. Naldi L, Locati F, Marchesi L, et al: Cutaneous manifestations associated with antiphospholipid antibodies in patients with suspected primary antiphospholipid syndrome: A case control study. Ann Rheum Dis 52:219, 1993.
29. Anderson RP, Morris BA: Acrocyanosis to imipramine. Arch Dis Child 63:204, 1988.
30. Applelbaum PS, Kapoor W: Imipramine-induced vasospasm: A case report. Am J Psychiatry 140:913, 1983.
31. Campo-Voegeli A, Estrach T, Marti RM, et al: Acrocyanosis induced by interferon alpha (2a). Dermatology 196:361, 1998.
32. Borgono JM, Vincent P, Venturino H, et al: Arsenic in the drinking water of the city of Antofagasta: Epidemiological and clinical study before and after the installation of a treatment plant. Environ Health Perspect 19:103, 1977.
33. Yang CC, Deng JF: Clinical experience in poisonings following exposure to blasticidin S, a curiously strong fungicide. Vet Hum Toxicol 38:1097, 1996.
34. Hoegl L, Thoma-Greber E, Poppinger J, et al: Butyl nitrite-induced acrocyanosis in an HIV infected patient. Arch Dermatol 135:90, 1999.
35. Steward JM, Gewitz MH, Weldon A, et al: Patterns of orthostatic intolerance: The orthostatic tachycardia syndrome and adolescent chronic fatigue. J Pediatr 135:218, 1999.
36. Burlina A, Dionisi-Vici C, Bennett MJ, et al: A new syndrome with ethylmalonic aciduria and normal fatty acid oxidation in fibroblasts. J Pediatr 124:79, 1994.
37. Bodeman C, Rotig A, Rustin P, et al: Hair and skin disorders as signs of mitochondrial diseases. Pediatrics 103:428, 1999.
38. Rotig A, Cormier V, Chatelain P, et al: Deletion of mitochondrial DNA in a case of early-onset diabetes mellitus, optic atrophy, and deafness (Wolfram Syndrome, MM222300). J Clin Invest 91:1095, 1993.
39. Nielsen PG: Diffuse palmoplantar keratoderma associated with acrocyanosis. Acta Derm Venereol (Stockh) 69:156, 1989.
40. Wass JAH, Thorner MO, Basser GM: Digital vasospasm with bromocriptine. Lancet 1:1135, 1976.
41. Morrish DW, Crockford PM: Acrocyanosis treated with bromocriptine. Lancet 2:851, 1976 (letter).
42. Clement DL: Effect of indoramin on finger blood flow in vasospastic patients. Eur J Clin Pharmacol 14:331, 1978.
43. Grima MR: Nursing case study: Bilateral cervical sympathectomy for acrocyanosis. Nurs Times 71:1850, 1975.
44. Twist DJ: Acrocyanosis in a spinal cord injured patient—effects of computer-controlled neuromuscular electrical stimulation: a case report. Phys Ther 70:45, 1990.

■ ■ ■ chapter 50

Erythromelalgia

Mark D.P. Davis
Thom W. Rooke

DEFINITION

Erythromelalgia is a rare condition of the extremities characterized by the triad of redness, warmth, and pain.

HISTORICAL PERSPECTIVE

The symptom complex of intermittent acral warmth, pain, and erythema that defines erythromelalgia has been well documented in the medical literature for more than 150 years. Graves[1] described it as "hot and painful leg" in 1834. The term "erythromelalgia" was coined in 1878 by Mitchell[2] from *erythros* (red), *melos* (extremity), and *algos* (pain). Smith and Allen[3] emphasized another essential component of this syndrome when they renamed it "erythermalgia" in 1938 to denote the heat (*thermé*) in the affected extremity during the periods of redness. Although many authors agree that "erythermalgia" is perhaps more accurate, "erythromelalgia" is the term most commonly used, and it is the term used in this chapter.

The existence of this condition has been debated.[4-6] However, there have been considerable advances in the characterization of this clinical syndrome, with large case series[7-10] and investigations giving some clues as to its pathogenesis. Although the condition is mysterious, it is not as mysterious as was once believed.[9,10]

In previous centuries, symptoms of erythromelalgia may have been ascribed to other recognized diagnostic categories. For example, in William Harvey's day almost every arthropathy was termed gout. Harvey himself had what was termed gout, which he treated with cold water immersion. His choice of therapy raises the possibility that the correct diagnosis was not gout but erythromelalgia.[11]

Much of the current understanding of erythromelalgia derives from the larger case series reported.[7,8,10,12,13]

NOMENCLATURE OF ERYTHROMELALGIA

Considerable confusion exists regarding the nomenclature of erythromelalgia.[14] Many terms have been used, and some authors have proposed that these terms should refer to different forms of erythromelalgia, as detailed later. However, these synonyms are not widely used and most authors now use the term "erythromelalgia," as originally used by Mitchell.

Related names used by some include Weir-Mitchell disease, Mitchell's disease, and acromelalgia. "Erythermalgia," from *thermé* (heat), was suggested in 1938[3] because the term erythromelalgia does not incorporate the cardinal sign of increased skin temperature, which is an integral part of the condition. Michiels and colleagues[15] proposed that the term "erythromelalgia" be restricted to cases due to myeloproliferative disorders responsive to aspirin therapy. They used the term "erythermalgia" to describe idiopathic conditions or conditions due to other diseases that are unresponsive to aspirin therapy. An unwieldy term, "erythermomelalgia," accounts for the four cardinal symptoms and signs of the condition, but it is not in general use.[16] "Erythralgia" has been used.[5,17] "Erythroprosopalgia," derived from *prosopon* (face), is used to describe facial erythromelalgia in the German literature.[5,14,17]

CRITERIA FOR DIAGNOSIS

No objective criteria exist for the diagnosis of erythromelalgia, making it difficult to interpret some of the cases reported in the literature.[14] The diagnosis is most often clinically based, dependent on the medical history and physical findings, because no objective diagnostic or laboratory tests are available[14] and because the physical findings of erythromelalgia may be absent owing to the frequently intermittent nature of the condition.[8]

Different diagnostic criteria have been suggested by different authors. Weir Mitchell[2,8] applied the three inclusion criteria used in the original description of the syndrome: red, hot, and painful extremities. Brown[18] added three additional criteria in 1932: induction and exacerbation of symptoms by warming, relief by cooling, and unresponsiveness to therapy. The criteria were described as follows: (1) during attacks (bilateral or symmetric burning pain in the hands and feet), the affected parts are flushed, congested, and warm; (2) the attacks are initiated or aggravated by standing, exercising, or exposing the extremity to temperatures warmer than 34° C; (3) the symptoms are relieved by elevation of the extremity or exposure of the extremity to cold; and (4) the condition is refractory to treatment. Thompson and colleagues[19] suggested the following five criteria: (1) burning extremity pain, (2) pain aggravated by warming, (3) pain relieved by cooling, (4) erythema of the affected skin, and (5) increased temperature of the affected skin. These five criteria have been used in several publications.[10,14,20-23]

Lazareth and colleagues[24] used three major and two of four minor criteria to satisfy the diagnosis. The major criteria were paroxysmal pain, burning pain, and redness of affected skin. The minor criteria were typical precipitating factors (heat exposure, effort); typical relieving factors (cold, rest); elevated skin temperature in affected skin; and response of symptoms to acetylsalicylic acid. Michiels and colleagues[15] restricted the term "erythromelalgia" to cases due to myeloproliferative disorders responsive to aspirin therapy and used "erythermalgia" for idiopathic cases or conditions due to other diseases unresponsive to aspirin therapy. Drenth and colleagues[25-28] distinguished three types of red, congested, and painful conditions of the extremities that need to be distinguished for effective treatment according to their cause: (1) erythromelalgia in thrombocythemia, (2) primary erythermalgia, and (3) secondary erythermalgia. Kurzrock and Cohen[29] used a classification of early-onset erythromelalgia and late-onset erythromelalgia irrespective of the cause.

Littleford and colleagues[30] used a classification of type 1 erythromelalgia (the typical form) and type 2 erythromelalgia (the abortive form) in which the burning nature of the pain is absent and symptomatic relief is not always provided by cooling or elevation of the limb. Mørk and Kvernebo[14] made the following distinctions: (1) "Syndrome" is used when initial and gradual symptoms localized to the feet and legs appear in childhood or adolescence; a family history of erythromelalgia is seen. "Phenomenon" is used for all other cases. (2) Erythromelalgia is primary when it is idiopathic. It is secondary when symptoms are caused by a primary disease such as a hemorheologic, metabolic, connective tissue, musculoskeletal, or infective disease; induced by drugs; or part of a paraneoplastic phenomenon. (3) "Acute" is used when symptoms reach maximal strength within 1 month after the onset of symptoms. (4) "Borderline erythromelalgia," "erythromelalgia," and "severe erythromelalgia" may be useful.[14]

CLINICAL CONTROVERSIES

Several controversies persist concerning erythromelalgia: the nomenclature, the diagnostic criteria, the scoring systems for clinical severity, and the pathogenesis. Also, the classification of erythromelalgia into primary and secondary types may be controversial because comorbid conditions may be mislabeled as underlying diseases that cause erythromelalgia. The classification of incomplete forms of erythromelalgia is also controversial. For example, some patients report that their feet are blue when symptoms are present. The problem with all definitions is that each criterion depends on clinical subjective judgment. The diagnosis of erythromelalgia is based on history because there are no objective physical findings. This may lead to an erroneous diagnosis.

CLINICAL PRESENTATION

The essential elements of this clinical syndrome, as described by its name, are redness of an acral area (i.e., the extremities or the head and neck area) associated with heat and pain. Common terms used to describe the pain include "piercing," "burning," and "discomfort."[8] The pain and burning sensation can be extremely severe. Patients report that they make major adjustments to their lifestyles to avoid precipitating an event. During an episode, they try to cool their feet in many ways, sometimes resorting to extraordinary measures to alleviate the pain, such as putting their feet in ice or walking barefoot in snow.

Erythromelalgia involves the feet in most circumstances (Fig. 50-1A and B); a minority of these patients have similar symptoms involving the hands.[8] Occasionally, only the hands are involved. Erythromelalgia may extend proximally to the knees in the lower extremities (see Fig. 50-1C) and to the elbows in the upper extremities. Involvement of the extremities is generally symmetric. Rarely, erythromelalgia involves the ears and face. In the largest reported series (168 patients), symptoms predominantly involved feet (148 patients; 88.1%) and hands (43 patients; 25.6%).[8]

In the majority of patients, symptoms are intermittent and the episodes, precipitated by specific triggers, can last from minutes to hours. In a minority of patients, erythromelalgia symptoms are continuous, although they may wax and wane. Patients with continuous symptoms usually report that their symptoms started intermittently and then became more frequent and prolonged until they were continuous. In the series of 168 patients,[8] symptoms were intermittent in 163 patients (97%) and continuous in 5 (3%).

The specific precipitant for erythromelalgia varies from person to person, but the most frequent precipitant is an increase in temperature of the affected acral area. This may be caused by an increase in ambient temperature, and several patients experience increases in severity and frequency of attacks during the summer. Erythromelalgia affecting the feet is often precipitated by an increase in local temperature from aerobic exercise. Symptoms can also be precipitated or intensified by lowering the affected part. Common aggravating factors include warm rooms, floors, or water; placing the extremity near heating appliances; sleeping under bedcovers; and wearing shoes and gloves. Walking, exercise, sitting, dependency of the extremities, and application of skin pressure may intensify the symptoms. However, some patients relate that episodes of erythromelalgia occur spontaneously, without clear precipitating factors.

A decrease in local temperature may decrease the severity of erythromelalgia or even abort an episode. Many patients report that plunging their feet into ice water during an episode relieves their symptoms. Aspirin may dramatically relieve symptoms in a subset of patients with underlying myeloproliferative disease, but otherwise aspirin is rarely effective. Other agents that have been reported to relieve symptoms are presented later in the section on treatment. Patients frequently report that the affected extremities must be exposed to cold surfaces or air-conditioned rooms or be immersed in buckets of cool or ice water to relieve their symptoms. Some patients sleep with their extremities outside the bedcovers, and some engage in unusual behaviors such as sleeping with their feet out a window, putting their feet in a refrigerator, walking barefoot in the snow, or storing shoes in a freezer. Kvernebo[10] described a patient who, for almost 25 years, day and night, lived with a bucket of ice water

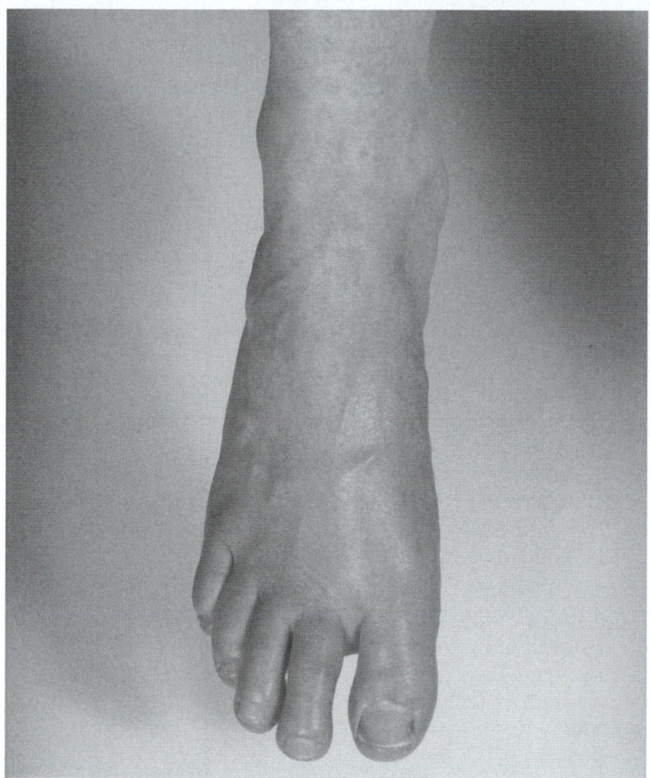

A

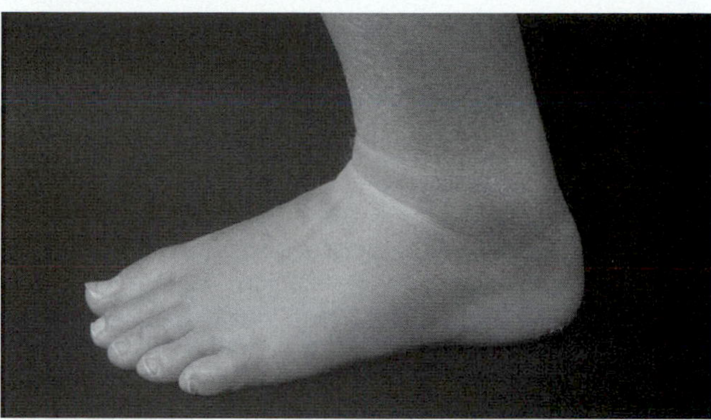

B

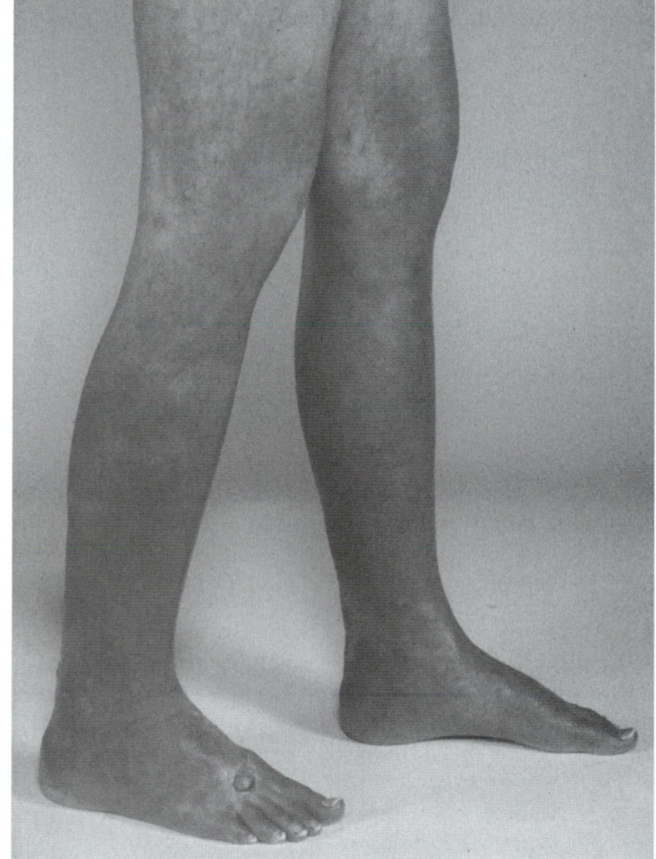

C

FIGURE 50-1. (See also Color Plate 50-1.) Erythromelalgia (red, hot, acral areas) involving the lower extremities may affect the toes only, the distal forefoot (**A**), or the entire foot (**B**), or it may extend up the leg, even beyond the knee (**C**). It is usually bilateral (**C**).

at her side, immersing her feet intermittently for 15 to 30 minutes an hour. Thus, in what superficially appears to be the antithesis of Raynaud's phenomenon, patients seek relief by cooling the affected extremity.

Because symptoms of erythromelalgia are intermittent, the clinical examination findings are usually normal. If the patient is examined during an episode of erythromelalgia, the affected extremity is tender, erythematous, and objectively hot.

The syndrome of erythromelalgia is frequently exacerbated when patients try to relieve their symptoms. For example, patients soak their feet in water and ice, which can lead to a form of immersion foot and irritant contact dermatitis or even frostbite. Allergic contact dermatitis due to substances that have been applied to the affected feet can occur. Other common vascular problems in the lower extremities such as edema, venous insufficiency, and lymphedema can be worsened by erythromelalgia. Patients may have high requirements for pain medications and become addicted to or dependent on narcotic analgesics. Psychiatric problems such as depression and obsessive-compulsive behaviors to avoid episodes of erythromelalgia can occur. The syndrome can be socially disabling if patients avoid exercising, walking, participating in sports, or leaving their homes, which leads to a sense of disablement, isolation, and loneliness. The syndrome frequently affects performance in the workplace (especially with manual work or jobs that entail standing) and at home.

Erythromelalgia predominantly affects people who are white and of any age. In the largest published series,[8] all 168 patients were white, the female-to-male ratio was approximately 3:1, and the mean age was 55.8 years (range, 5 to 91 years). Symptoms had been present since childhood in seven patients (4.2%), and six patients (3.6%) had a first-degree relative with erythromelalgia.

Drenth and colleagues[31] described nine children in whom erythromelalgia was transient (seven girls and two boys; mean age, 11.6 years). The mean duration of each attack was 25 days (range, 6 to 56 days). Intriguingly, seven children were hypertensive, and IV sodium nitroprusside effectively ameliorated the symptoms, with blood pressure decreasing to normal in five patients; pizotifene, labetalol, prostaglandin E_1, and hypnotherapy were effective in each of four separate cases.

DIAGNOSIS OF ERYTHROMELALGIA

Making the diagnosis is often a problem because patients have intermittent symptoms, and objective findings may not be present during the physical examination. Thus the diagnosis may rest on history alone. However, because the differential diagnosis includes many possibilities, it is best to have evidence to support the diagnosis. The following may help:

1. Examine the patient during an episode. Ask the patient to engage in an activity, such as climbing stairs, that will precipitate an episode.
2. If it is not possible to examine a patient during an episode, ask the patient to obtain a photograph of the affected areas during an episode.

CLASSIFICATION

Most authors agree on the fundamentals of the diagnosis of erythromelalgia, but there are many described criteria for diagnosis and many subclassifications of erythromelalgia. Use of these subclassifications may depend on whether one is a "lumper" or "splitter."[26,27,32]

Reported causes of secondary erythromelalgia are presented in Box 50-1. As noted in this box, erythromelalgia has been reported in association with myeloproliferative diseases, blood disorders, drugs, infectious diseases, food ingestion (mushrooms), neoplasms, connective tissue disease, physiologic conditions (pregnancy), and neuropathies. Inheritance in familial, autosomal dominant (29 persons were affected in 5 generations), and X-linked dominant fashions have also been reported. An epidemic in China has been described.[64] The relationship of many underlying disorders to erythromelalgia is sometimes unclear, and the disorder may be a coincidental comorbidity rather than an underlying disease.

Among the reported series, the association with myeloproliferative disease seems most constant.[8,33-35] Evidence of underlying myeloproliferative disease should be sought at diagnosis and subsequently. Erythromelalgia can herald the onset of underlying myeloproliferative disease: erythromelalgia was the presenting symptom of essential thrombocythemia in 26 of 40 patients (65%)[34]; in another series, erythromelalgia was the presenting symptom in 11 of 268 patients with thrombocythemia (4%).[35]

BOX 50-1 Reported Causes of "Secondary Erythromelalgia"

Condition or Agent

Myeloproliferative diseases and blood disorders
- Myeloproliferative disorders[8,33]
- Essential thrombocythemia[34-39]
- Polycythemia rubra vera[40,41]
- Myelodysplastic syndrome[42]
- Pernicious anemia[43]
- Thrombotic thrombocytopenic purpura[44]
- Idiopathic thrombocytopenic purpura[45]

Drugs
- Cyclosporine[46]
- Norephedrine[47]
- Verapamil[48]
- Nicardipine[49,50]
- Nifedipine[51-53]
- Pergolide mesylate[54]
- Bromocriptine[55-57]

Infectious diseases
- Human immunodeficiency virus[58,59]
- Hepatitis B vaccine[60]
- Influenza vaccine[61]
- Infectious mononucleosis[62]
- Pox virus[63]
- Unknown agent[64]

Ingestion
- Mushrooms[22,58]

Neoplastic
- Abdominal cancer[65]
- Paraneoplastic[66]
- Astrocytoma[67]
- Malignant thymoma[68]

Connective tissue disease
- Systemic lupus erythematosus[69-72]
- Vasculitis[73]

Physiologic
- Pregnancy[74]

Neuropathic
- Hereditary sensory neuropathy[75]
- Neuropathy[76]
- Polyneuropathy[77]
- Riley-Day syndrome[78]
- Multiple sclerosis[79]
- Acute diabetic neuropathy[80]
- Neurofibromatosis[81]

Inherited
- X-linked dominant?[82]
- Autosomal dominant[83]
- Unknown[84]
- Familial[85,86]

INCIDENCE

A population-based estimation of the incidence of erythromelalgia does not exist. Incidence and prevalence of the condition are difficult to assess, but as Mørk and Kvernebo[14] have pointed out, erythromelalgia may be more common than previously believed, especially among patients with less severe disease, because they may not present to a physician or the physician may not recognize the condition. The incidence was proposed to be 2.5 to 3.3 per 1 million inhabitants per year in the Norwegian population, with a corresponding annual prevalence of 18 to 20 per 1 million.[10] Cases of borderline erythromelalgia were not included in these figures.[9,10] Davis and colleagues[8] noted that there were 13 cases of erythromelalgia among patients from Olmsted County, Minnesota, between 1970 and 1994. Incidence figures were not reported.

PATHOPHYSIOLOGY

The pathophysiology of erythromelalgia is not clearly understood. Part of the difficulty in understanding erythromelalgia has been the heterogeneity of the affected population.[87] Light has been shed on possible pathophysiologic mechanisms in recent years. Taken together, the underlying pathologic mechanisms are most likely to involve a complex dysregulation of cutaneous blood flow that ultimately results in microvascular ischemia. Determining the nature of this dysfunction has also been challenging because the control of cutaneous blood flow depends on an intricate interplay of systemic and local signals and is not completely understood.[87] A small-fiber neuropathy likely contributes to this dysregulation.[88,89]

The thermoregulatory control of human skin blood flow is vital to the maintenance of normal body temperatures during challenges to thermal homeostasis. Sympathetic neural control of skin blood flow includes the noradrenergic vasoconstrictor system and a sympathetic active vasodilator system, the latter of which is responsible for 80% to 90% of the substantial cutaneous vasodilation that occurs with whole-body heat stress. With body heating, the magnitude of skin vasodilation is striking: skin blood flow can reach 6 to 8 L/min during hyperthermia. Cutaneous sympathetic vasoconstrictor and vasodilator systems also participate in baroreflex control of blood pressure; this is particularly important during heat stress, when such a large percentage of cardiac output is directed to the skin. Local thermal control of cutaneous blood vessels also contributes importantly—local warming of the skin can cause maximal vasodilation in healthy humans and includes roles for both local sensory nerves and nitric oxide. Local cooling of the skin can decrease skin blood flow to minimal levels.[90]

The distribution of the blood flow is largely regulated by two segments of the microvascular bed, the arteriovenous anastomoses and the precapillary sphincters. Arteriovenous anastomoses are most prominent in acral skin, particularly the palms and soles, where blood is shunted away from superficial resistance vessels during vasodilation to increase overall flow and heat dissipation. Located at the end of the terminal arteriole, the precapillary sphincter directly regulates blood flow to capillary beds throughout the circulatory system. In the superficial dermis, the precapillary sphincter controls the flow of blood from the ascending arteriole into the capillaries of the superficial vascular plexus that provide nutrients and oxygen to the papillary dermis and the epidermis.[91] Both these vascular elements respond to multiple systemic stimuli, including core temperature changes, cardiovascular homeostasis, and emotional stress, as well as local stimuli such as pain, inflammation, pressure, and heating or cooling. Vasoconstrictive signals are delivered through the sympathetic nervous system directly to vascular smooth muscle and have the most prominent effects in areas with large concentrations of arteriovenous anastomoses. Local factors such as endothelin 1, which is produced by vascular endothelium, may also mediate vasoconstriction. Vasodilation is mediated by a combination of parasympathetic signals and local production of chemicals with vasomotor activity. Parasympathetic vascular dilation that is acetylcholine mediated depends on production of nitric oxide and prostacyclin, which can also be directly induced by local stimuli.[87]

Erythromelalgia and Raynaud's phenomenon are cutaneous microvascular disorders. Their pathophysiology appears to relate to disorders of local or reflex thermoregulatory control of the skin circulation.[90] Two paradoxic observations concerning blood flow during an episode of erythromelalgia have been made: (1) During symptoms, there is increased blood flow. Sandroni and colleagues,[89] Mørk and colleagues,[9] and Kvernebo[10] confirmed that the observed erythema and warmth are associated with increased blood flow. Using laser Doppler, Sandroni and colleagues measured blood flow during symptoms and demonstrated increased perfusion during attacks. (2) Paradoxically, this increased blood flow is accompanied by local hypoxia. Although there is increased perfusion during attacks, the values for transcutaneous oxygen tension are critically low, low, or unchanged—in other words, during symptoms, the transcutaneous oximetry values decrease or do not change.[9,10,88,89]

To explain this paradox, Mørk and colleagues[23] theorized and demonstrated that the increased blood flow is probably due to shunting through arteriovenous anastomoses, which results in hypoperfusion of the more superficial nutritive capillaries. If available blood is shunted away from normal skin capillaries, the skin will be hypoxic. Mørk and colleagues[23] demonstrated that, despite an increased overall blood flow to the skin, the induction of erythromelalgia symptoms is accompanied by decreased perfusion of the superficial vascular plexus, as evidenced by a decreased density of skin capillaries. Thus their hypothesis is that the dilatation of arteriovenous anastomoses is directly responsible for shunting nutritive blood flow away from the superficial vascular plexus. Furthermore, Mørk and colleagues[21] postulated that erythromelalgia is not a disease but rather a physiologic response to stimuli such as infection, trauma, or tumor and that the symptoms are caused by tissue hypoxia induced by maldistribution of microvascular blood flow in the skin with increased thermoregulatory flow and inadequate perfusion.

Sandroni and colleagues[89] theorized that the effects of diminished perfusion could be exacerbated by increased metabolic demands in response to hyperthermia, ultimately resulting in hypoxic tissue damage and pain. In support of this hypothesis, we have observed in some patients that the temperature of the symptomatic extremity occasionally exceeds core temperature. Pain relief by cooling could be explained by a resultant decrease in the metabolic rate and a corresponding decrease in the need for oxygen.

Littleford and colleagues[30] described an underlying vasoconstrictor tendency in patients with erythromelalgia, which may be related to functional or structural changes in skin microvessels, and noted that basal skin erythrocyte flux and skin temperature were lower in patients with a history of erythromelalgia than in controls. As noted earlier, Raynaud's phenomenon has been described in patients with erythromelalgia.[92,93] Acrocyanosis has also been described.[92] Davis and colleagues[88] have also anecdotally noted that at baseline, the skin may be cool and occasionally cyanotic between episodes.

Several lines of evidence suggest that a neuropathy is associated with erythromelalgia. Erythromelalgia has been described in association with many types of neuropathy (see Box 50-1). In patients with neuropathy (especially autonomic), erythromelalgia may develop.[88] Kazemi and colleagues[94] reported that 72.7% of the patients studied had abnormal sympathetic reflexes, which may result from an abnormality of the sympathetic nerves. A small-fiber neuropathy is common in patients with erythromelalgia—among 57 patients with erythromelalgia who were evaluated with use of an autonomic reflex screen, results for 49 (86%) were abnormal, indicating a small-fiber neuropathy. The commonest abnormalities were sudomotor abnormalities (i.e., absent or reduced sweat production).[88] In an earlier series, findings were similar for 17 of 27 patients (63%); whether the observed neuropathy led to erythromelalgia, or vice versa, is unclear.[89,95] Conversely, in a series of 321 cases of disorders of autonomic neuropathy the majority had erythromelalgia.[96] Orstavik and colleagues[97] used erythromelalgia as a model to study chronic pain and found changes in the conductive properties of C fibers in patients with erythromelalgia, which were indicative of a small-fiber neuropathy. Additionally, an active contribution of mechano-insensitive fibers to chronic pain was postulated. Uno and Parker[98] reported that the density of both acetylcholinesterase-positive and catecholamine-containing nerve terminals in the periarterial and sweat gland plexuses was much less in the skin of the erythermalgic foot than in the unaffected skin of the same patient and much less than in the foot skin of a healthy person. Layzer[99] wrote that it seems plausible to regard erythromelalgia as a problem of polymodal C-fiber receptors in sensitized skin. The threshold of C fibers to activation by heat would decrease to between 32° C and 36° C; activated C fibers would cause vasodilation by axon reflexes, resulting in redness, heat, and swelling. With cooling, the threshold for the nociceptors would increase. Normal sympathetic nerve activity in skin without an associated vasoconstriction response has been found in a patient.[100] Littleford and colleagues[101] also noted findings suggesting that patients with erythromelalgia have diminished sympathetic vasoconstrictor responses to both cold challenge of the contralateral arm and inspiratory gasp. An interplay between neural and vasoactive agents was postulated in the pathophysiology of erythromelalgia.

Thrombin, platelet function, and genetics have also been considered in studies of erythromelalgia. Van Genderen and associates[102] noted that thrombocythemia-associated erythromelalgia may develop despite treatment with oral anticoagulants or heparin, suggesting that the generation of thrombin is not a prerequisite for the development of erythromelalgia. A disordered platelet function affecting the microvasculature has been implicated in thrombocythemia-related erythromelalgia.[103] In a study of five kindreds with multiple cases of primary erythermalgia, there was strong evidence for linkage of the primary erythermalgia locus to markers from 2q31-32.[104]

PATHOPHYSIOLOGIC CONTROVERSIES

Several questions about erythromelalgia remain. Does a neuropathy cause the vasculopathy or does the vasculopathy cause a neuropathy?[88] What causes the neuropathy if it is not caused by the vasculopathy? How does dysfunction of the precapillary sphincter affect this disease? Schechner[87] pointed out that it is unknown whether shunting of blood through arteriovenous anastomoses alone can induce hypoxia severe enough to induce pain, particularly in areas that contain few arteriovenous anastomoses. Potentially inadequate compensatory dilatation, or even inappropriate constriction of the precapillary sphincter, may compound the effects of the relative hypoperfusion. What factors are responsible for vascular dysfunction? Both autonomic neuropathy[21,89] and endothelial injury[105] have been observed in patients with erythromelalgia, but it is not known whether this damage to critical vasoregulatory components is primary or secondary to chronic hypoxia.

DIFFERENTIAL DIAGNOSIS

Any condition causing extremity pain could be mistaken for erythromelalgia. In particular, unwarranted diagnosis of erythromelalgia can result from any clinical situation that includes burning sensations in the limbs.[106] However, the syndrome of erythromelalgia is specific for red, hot extremities. The following conditions are included in the differential diagnosis:

- Neuropathies: peripheral neuropathy, small-fiber neuropathy, reflex sympathetic dystrophy
- Vascular: small-vessel disease, Raynaud's phenomenon, Raynaud's disease, arterial insufficiency, venous insufficiency (which can produce sensations of warm feet, often at bedtime, with edema and an increase in local heat)
- Metabolic: painful crises associated with Fabry's disease (a hereditary sphingolipidosis transmitted on chromosome X that occurs predominantly in men, often starting early in childhood, with a burning sensation in the limbs)
- Skin: dermatitis, immersion foot
- Infectious: erysipelas
- Bone: osteomyelitis
- Exogenous: acrodynia (a rare disease caused by excessive mercury intake and confirmed by high mercury levels in the urine, in which the main sign is vasomotor impairment in the limbs, and the red hands and feet have an intense, paroxysmal, burn-type pain)

INVESTIGATIONS

To investigate the possibility of erythromelalgia, the clinician should take the following steps:

1. Get a detailed history and perform a physical examination with respect to each element of the history outlined earlier.
2. If signs of erythromelalgia are not present during the examination, ask the patient to photograph the affected area when symptoms are apparent.
3. Evaluate the results of a complete blood cell count, including total and differential leukocyte counts.
4. Investigate the possibility of underlying disease as indicated by the patient's age, history, and physical examination.
5. Consider tertiary referral for further investigations as outlined in Box 50-2, especially for small-fiber neuropathy and large-fiber neuropathy, and for noninvasive vascular studies during symptoms and between symptoms, as detailed by Davis and colleagues,[88] to better define the pathophysiology. Results of these tests are useful to confirm the diagnosis and help guide therapy.

BIOPSY FINDINGS

Reports of skin biopsies for erythromelalgia are scant. In the series reported by Davis and colleagues,[8] only 12 of the 168 patients had a biopsy, and the biopsy specimens showed no specific abnormalities.

Three cases of primary erythromelalgia were reported by Drenth and colleagues.[105] The biopsy specimens showed nonspecific changes. A mild perivascular mononuclear infiltrate was described in association with thickened blood vessel basement membranes, abundant perivascular edema, and moderate endothelial swelling. The thickened basal membrane of the blood vessels showed a laminar structure, and abundant perivascular edema and moderate endothelial cell swelling were evident.

The histopathologic changes in cases of erythromelalgia related to thrombocythemia have been characterized by Michiels and associates.[34] Erythromelalgia was the presenting symptom in 26 of 40 patients with thrombocythemia in its primary form or when associated with polycythemia vera. Skin punch biopsy samples from the affected areas showed arteriolar inflammation, fibromuscular intimal proliferation, and thrombotic occlusions. Biopsies were performed 1 to 3 weeks after discontinuation of aspirin therapy, at which time arteriolar changes were present. Specifically, the endothelial cells were often swollen with large nuclei. Narrowing of the lumen resulted from proliferation of smooth muscle cells with vacuolation and swelling of the cytoplasm and deposition of intercellular material. The internal elastic lamina appeared to be split between the proliferated cells, which gave rise to fibromuscular proliferation of the arteriolar intima, and the arterioles were often occluded by thrombi of various ages. Ultimately, the arterioles became completely fibrosed. These vascular changes were restricted to arterioles.[107]

Croue and colleagues[108] reported the histopathologic findings from a case of erythromelalgia related to essential thrombocythemia. Thrombi of various ages occluded small arteries, and intimal proliferation of smooth muscle cells narrowed the lumen. Venules and capillaries were not involved.

Histopathologic findings from punch biopsies from a patient with verapamil-induced erythromelalgia showed a mild perivascular mononuclear infiltrate and moderate perivascular edema.[48] Among patients with erythromelalgia due to bromocriptine, histopathologic examinations of samples from three patients showed a prominent perivascular lymphocytic infiltration and perivascular edema of the dermis without frank vasculitis. This is a reversible, unwanted effect of bromocriptine therapy.[56]

BOX 50-2 Protocol of Investigation for Patients Presenting with Erythromelalgia

- Clinical
  - History
  - Physical examination
- Peripheral vascular laboratory
  - Studies of the following parameters in the affected extremities with and without symptoms:
    - Color change
    - Skin temperature and core temperature
    - Blood flow (laser Doppler flowmetry)
    - Oxygen saturation (transcutaneous oximetry)
    - Ankle-brachial indices
- Neurologic evaluation
  - Electromyography
  - Autonomic nerve studies
    - Quantitative sudomotor axon reflex test (QSART)
    - Heart rate response to deep breathing and Valsalva ratio (cardiovagal functioning)
    - Adrenergic function testing
  - Consultation with neurologist specializing in autonomic nerve studies if results of the above tests are abnormal

From Davis MDP, Sandroni P, Rooke TW, et al: Erythromelalgia: Vasculopathy, neuropathy, or both? A prospective study of vascular and neurophysiologic studies in erythromelalgia. Arch Dermatol 139:1337, 2003.

NATURAL HISTORY AND PROGNOSIS

Prognostic information about erythromelalgia was not published until relatively recently.[8,12] In the study of the natural history of erythromelalgia by Davis and colleagues,[8] at follow-up, 45 of the 168 patients (26.8%) had died. The causes of death included myeloproliferative disease, cardiovascular disease, and cancer. Three with severe symptoms committed suicide. Although the patients represented a heterogeneous population with erythromelalgia, Kaplan-Meier survival curves showed a significant decrease in survival compared with expected survival among people matched for age and sex ($P < .001$). Thus patients with erythromelalgia have significantly increased mortality and morbidity rates compared with the U.S. general population.[8] When 94 patients were questioned about their symptoms after a mean follow-up of 8.7 years (range, 1.3 to 20 years), 30 patients (31.9%) reported that their symptoms had worsened; 25 (26.6%) had not changed; 29 (30.9%) had improved; and 10 (10.6%) had completely resolved.

Different referral patterns may bias reports. For example, patients with erythromelalgia evaluated at a tertiary referral center such as Mayo Clinic probably have more severe symptoms and more comorbid conditions and are seen later in the course of their disease. The outcome is difficult to compare, but a conclusion drawn from these studies is that some patients become worse, some have a stable course, and some get better or even have full resolution of erythromelalgia with time. It is notable that some patients experienced cure.[8]

Kalgaard and colleagues[12] reported that about two thirds of 87 patients had primary cases and about three quarters had some form of chronic condition. Over time, in patients with erythromelalgia, the condition gradually became worse; in patients with primary or secondary acute erythromelalgia, the condition improved; and in patients with primary or secondary chronic erythromelalgia, the condition remained stable.

QUALITY OF LIFE

Although erythromelalgia can have a markedly negative effect on quality of life, only one study has directly measured quality-of-life parameters.[8] The Medical Outcomes Study 36-Item Short Form Health Survey was used, and the results of this questionnaire were compared with the scores obtained from a cohort from the U.S. general population. The questionnaire is a standard survey that measures health-related quality-of-life outcomes and measures each of eight health concepts (or domains) on a five-point Likert scale: physical functioning, role limitations due to physical disease, bodily pain, general health, vitality (energy and fatigue), social functioning, role limitations due to emotional problems, and mental health (psychological stress and psychological well-being). Scores for all but one of the health domains were significantly less in the study population than in the U.S. general population. The lowest scores were in the physical functioning domain.

TREATMENT OF ERYTHROMELALGIA

The management of erythromelalgia is difficult. There are no randomized, controlled studies of treatments for erythromelalgia, and no single treatment is effective in all cases. The literature is replete with case reports and small case series describing a response to one treatment or another; when a larger group of erythromelalgia patients were surveyed, the majority reported that no treatment was very effective (Table 50-1). Various treatments used in the management of erythromelalgia have been reviewed (Box 50-3).[109]

TABLE 50-1 SURVEY OF THE MOST COMMONLY USED THERAPIES AMONG 99 PATIENTS WITH ERYTHROMELALGIA

		RESPONSE, % OF PATIENTS		
Therapy	**Patients, No.**	**Very Useful**	**Somewhat Useful**	**Not Useful**
Aspirin	57	17.5	29.8	52.6
NSAIDs (ibuprofen, indomethacin, nabumetone, naproxen, sulindac)	49	18.4	30.6	51
β Blockers (atenolol, nadolol, propranolol hydrochloride, timolol)	40	22.5	20	57.5
Antihistamines (cyproheptadine hydrochloride, diphenhydramine, phenylpropanolamine, trimeprazine, cimetidine)	28	10.7	14.3	75
Biofeedback, epidural blocks, hypnosis, transcutaneous electrical nerve stimulation	23	17.4	26.1	56.5
Vasodilators (nitroglycerin, nitroprusside, nicotinic acid, nifedipine, diltiazem)	20	10	5	85
Capsaicin	16	12.5	6.3	81.2
Anticonvulsants (carbamazepine, phenytoin)	13	15.4	23.1	61.5
Antidepressants (chlorpromazine, amitriptyline, thioridazine, nortriptyline, fluphenazine, doxepin)	12	16.7	25	58.3
Immunosuppressants (oral corticosteroids, plasma exchange)	12	33.3	8.3	58.4
Antimigraine (ergotamine, methysergide)	10	10	10	80
Pentoxifylline	9	22.2	11.1	66.7
Dipyridamole	7	14.3	14.3	71.4
Sympathetic nerve interruption (surgical or chemical sympathectomy, phenoxybenzamine)	6	0	50	50
Mexiletine hydrochloride	5	0	40	60
Antimitotics (busulfan, hydroxyurea, radioactive phosphorus)	4	75	25	0
Clonidine	4	0	25	75
α Blockers	3	33.3	33.3	33.3
Quinine sulfate	3	0	33.3	66.6
Muscle relaxants (carisoprodol)	2	0	50	50

NSAIDs, nonsteroidal anti-inflammatory drugs.
From Davis MD, O'Fallon WM, Rogers RS III, et al: Natural history of erythromelalgia: Presentation and outcome in 168 patients. Arch Dermatol 136:330, 2000.

BOX 50-3 Approach to Management of Erythromelalgia

1. Educate patient regarding what is known about erythromelalgia, its natural history, and the limitations of studies of treatment options; advise patients regarding availability of support groups.*
2. Teach patient to avoid situations that precipitate erythromelalgia.
3. Teach patient techniques that will cool the affected extremities (such as feet) but do not cause tissue damage.
4. Control pain with the following:
   - Aspirin
   - Nonsteroidal anti-inflammatory agents
   - Systemic narcotics (oral; IV, delivered by pump)
   - Anesthetic agents: local (lidocaine patch), IV (lidocaine), oral (mexiletine), epidural (cervical, lumbar), intrathecal
   - Capsaicin (topical)
   - Drugs acting on the nervous system†
     - Selective serotonin reuptake inhibitors (venlafaxine, sertraline)
     - Tricyclic antidepressants (amitriptyline, imipramine, nortriptyline)
     - Anticonvulsants (gabapentin)
     - Benzodiazepines
     - Ergot alkaloids
   - Sympathectomy; sympathetic nerve block†
   - Nonmedicinal approaches: biofeedback, hypnosis
5. Control secondary factors (leg edema, immersion foot, maceration, dermatitis, addiction to pain medications, psychiatric and psychological complications)
6. Correct underlying disease (e.g., myeloproliferative diseases)
7. Consider disease-modifying drugs and procedures
   - Aspirin
   - Drugs acting on the nervous system
     - Selective serotonin reuptake inhibitors (venlafaxine, sertraline)
     - Tricyclic antidepressants (amitriptyline, imipramine, nortriptyline)
     - Anticonvulsants (gabapentin)
     - Benzodiazepines
     - Ergot alkaloids
   - Drugs acting on the vascular system
     - Calcium antagonists (diltiazem, others)
     - High-dose oral magnesium
     - Sodium nitroprusside infusions
     - Prostaglandin E_1 infusions
   - Antihistamines
   - Surgical procedures: sympathectomy, sympathetic nerve block†

*Example is The Erythromelalgia Association (www.erythromelalgia.org).
†May also improve erythromelalgia.
From Davis MD, Rooke T: Erythromelalgia. Curr Treat Options Cardiovasc Med 4:207, 2002.

Patients learn to avoid behaviors, such as exercise, that precipitate erythromelalgia. During symptoms, they should be advised to avoid applying ice or cold water to the affected areas because those treatments can lead to frostbite or to changes from chronic immersion.

Eradication of erythromelalgia is the ultimate aim of management. Aspirin[3,34,40] has been reported to abolish erythromelalgia, especially in initial reports of the syndrome. It has become increasingly evident that aspirin may be effective in erythromelalgia due to myeloproliferative disease, but it is rarely effective in other forms of erythromelalgia.[8,110]

Increasingly, drugs acting on the nervous system are reported to be useful in inducing remission of disease or in controlling symptoms. Serotonin reuptake inhibitors such as venlafaxine and sertraline,[111,112] tricyclic antidepressants such as amitriptyline,[75] and anticonvulsants such as gabapentin[113] have been reported to be useful. IV lidocaine followed by oral mexiletine[114] has been useful in inducing remission in a patient with longstanding erythromelalgia. Topical capsaicin has been helpful in one report[115] but not in others.[8] Benzodiazepines such as clonazepam have been useful occasionally.[70] Sympathectomy and sympathetic nerve blocks have been reported to both relieve and exacerbate erythromelalgia.[16,116-119] Stereotactic thalamotomy,[120] ankle nerve crushing and neurectomy,[121] and spinal cord stimulation[122] have been reported to be helpful.

Drugs acting on the vascular system (vasoactive drugs) have also been reported to be useful. β blockers such as propranolol[123] and labetalol[31] have been reported to be successful in single cases. Calcium antagonists have been reported to both relieve and exacerbate erythromelalgia.[8,110] Various doses of magnesium have been reported to relieve symptoms.[124] Sodium nitroprusside infusions may be helpful in children with erythromelalgia,[125-128] but one adult experienced worsening of the disease with this medication.[110] Prostaglandin E_1, a potent vasodilator and platelet inhibitor administered intravenously, has successfully induced remission.[10,30,125] Iloprost, a synthetic prostacyclin analog, improved patients' symptoms more than placebo did.[129] The use of ergot alkaloids such as methysergide maleate has been described in isolated case reports.[80,130] Low-molecular-weight heparin has been reported to exacerbate erythromelalgia.[126]

Control of pain is an extremely important factor in erythromelalgia. Anesthetics have been used, including topical lidocaine (lidocaine patch)[131] and epidural infusion of narcotic analgesic medications such as bupivacaine, sometimes in combination with other narcotic drugs.[132-135] Narcotic analgesic drugs may be administered by various routes—oral, IV, IM,[136] epidural,[135] or intrathecal[137] alone or in combination with other drugs. Nonsteroidal anti-inflammatory drugs such as piroxicam[138] may be helpful occasionally.

Pizotyline, a benzocycloheptathiophene derivative used primarily for migraine prophylaxis, has been used for erythromelalgia.[31,139,140] Systemic corticosteroids including prednisone[141] and prednisolone[142] and growth hormone[143] have been useful in single cases. Antihistamines such as cyproheptadine[144] have been reported to help, but many patients find them unhelpful.

A combination of pharmacologic interventions may be of benefit.[61,145] Nonmedicinal therapies such as acupuncture, biofeedback, hypnosis, and magnets have been variably effective.[110,146]

REFERENCES

1. Graves RJ: Clinical Lectures on the Practice of Medicine. Dublin, Fannin, 1834.
2. Mitchell SW: On a rare vaso-motor neurosis of the extremities and on the maladies with which it may be confounded. Am J Med Sci 76:17, 1878.
3. Smith LA, Allen EV: Erythermalgia (erythromelalgia) of the extremities: A syndrome characterized by redness, heat, and pain. Am Heart J 16:175, 1938.
4. Housley E: What is erythromelalgia and how should it be treated? BMJ 293:117, 1986.
5. Lewis T: Clinical observations and experiments relating to burning pain in extremities and to so-called "erythromelalgia" in particular. Clin Sci 1:175, 1933.
6. Snapper I, Kahn AI: Bedside Medicine. 2nd ed. London, William Heinemann Medical Books, 1967, p 106.
7. Babb RR, Alarcon-Segovia D, Fairbairn JF II: Erythermalgia: Review of 51 cases. Circulation 29:136, 1964.
8. Davis MD, O'Fallon WM, Rogers RS III, et al: Natural history of erythromelalgia: Presentation and outcome in 168 patients. Arch Dermatol 136:330, 2000.
9. Mørk C, Kalgaard OM, Kvernebo K: Erythromelalgia: A clinical study of 102 cases (abstract). Australas J Dermatol 38(suppl 2):50, 1997.
10. Kvernebo K: Erythromelalgia: A condition caused by microvascular arteriovenous shunting. VASA J Vasc Dis Suppl 51:1, 1998.
11. Hart FD: William Harvey and his gout. Ann Rheum Dis 43:125, 1984.
12. Kalgaard OM, Seem E, Kvernebo K: Erythromelalgia: A clinical study of 87 cases. J Intern Med 242:191, 1997.
13. Levesque H: Classification of erythermalgia [French]. J Mal Vasc 21:80, 1996.
14. Mørk C, Kvernebo K: Erythromelalgia: A mysterious condition? Arch Dermatol 136:406, 2000.
15. Michiels JJ, Drenth JP, Van Genderen PJ: Classification and diagnosis of erythromelalgia and erythermalgia. Int J Dermatol 34:97, 1995.
16. Zoppi M, Zamponi A, Pagni E, et al: A way to understand erythromelalgia. J Auton Nerv Syst 13:85, 1985.
17. Regli F: Facial neuralgia and vascular facial pain [German]. Praxis 58:210, 1969.
18. Brown GE: Erythromelalgia and other disturbances of the extremities accompanied by vasodilatation and burning. Am J Med Sci 183:468, 1932.
19. Thompson GH, Hahn G, Rang M: Erythromelalgia. Clin Orthop (144):249, 1979.
20. Mørk C, Asker CL, Salerud EG, et al: Microvascular arteriovenous shunting is a probable pathogenetic mechanism in erythromelalgia. J Invest Dermatol 114:643, 2000.
21. Mørk C, Kalgaard OM, Kvernebo K: Impaired neurogenic control of skin perfusion in erythromelalgia. J Invest Dermatol 118:699, 2002.
22. Mørk C, Kalgaard OM, Myrvang B, et al: Erythromelalgia in a patient with AIDS. J Eur Acad Dermatol Venereol 14:498, 2000.
23. Mørk C, Kvernebo K, Asker CL, et al: Reduced skin capillary density during attacks of erythromelalgia implies arteriovenous shunting as pathogenetic mechanism. J Invest Dermatol 119:949, 2002.
24. Lazareth I, Fiessinger JN, Priollet P: Erythermalgia, rare acrosyndrome: 13 cases [French]. Presse Med 17:2235, 1988.
25. Drenth JP, Michiels JJ, van Joost T: Primary and secondary erythermalgia [Dutch]. Ned Tijdschr Geneeskd 138:2231, 1994.
26. Drenth JP, Michiels JJ: Erythromelalgia and erythermalgia: Diagnostic differentiation. Int J Dermatol 33:393, 1994.
27. Drenth JP, Michiels JJ: Erythromelalgia versus primary and secondary erythermalgia. Angiology 45:329, 1994.
28. Drenth JP, van Genderen PJ, Michiels JJ: Thrombocythemic erythromelalgia, primary erythermalgia, and secondary erythermalgia: Three distinct clinicopathologic entities. Angiology 45:451, 1994.
29. Kurzrock R, Cohen PR: Classification and diagnosis of erythromelalgia. Int J Dermatol 34:146, 1995.
30. Littleford RC, Khan F, Belch JJ: Skin perfusion in patients with erythromelalgia. Eur J Clin Invest 29:588, 1999.
31. Drenth JPH, Michiels JJ, Özsoylu S: Erythermlgia Multidisciplinary Study Group: Acute secondary erythermalgia and hypertension in children. Eur J Pediatr 154:882, 1995.
32. Michiels JJ, Drenth JP: Erythromelalgia and erythermalgia: Lumpers and splitters. Int J Dermatol 33:412, 1994.
33. Kurzrock R, Cohen PR: Erythromelalgia and myeloproliferative disorders. Arch Intern Med 149:105, 1989.
34. Michiels JJ, Abels J, Steketee J, et al: Erythromelalgia caused by platelet-mediated arteriolar inflammation and thrombosis in thrombocythemia. Ann Intern Med 102:466, 1985.
35. Itin PH, Winkelmann RK: Cutaneous manifestations in patients with essential thrombocythemia. J Am Acad Dermatol 24:59, 1991.
36. Michiels JJ, ten Kate FJ: Erythromelalgia in thrombocythemia of various myeloproliferative disorders. Am J Hematol 39:131, 1992.
37. McCarthy L, Eichelberger L, Skipworth E, et al: Erythromelalgia due to essential thrombocythemia. Transfusion 42:1245, 2002.
38. Michiels JJ, van Genderen PJ, Lindemans J, et al: Erythromelalgic, thrombotic and hemorrhagic manifestations in 50 cases of thrombocythemia. Leuk Lymphoma 22(suppl 1):47, 1996.
39. Naldi L, Brevi A, Cavalieri d'Oro L, et al: Painful distal erythema and thrombocytosis: Erythromelalgia secondary to thrombocytosis. Arch Dermatol 129:105, 1993.
40. Ongenae K, Janssens A, Noens L, et al: Erythromelalgia: A clue to the diagnosis of polycythemia vera. Dermatology 192:408, 1996.
41. Kudo I, Soejima K, Morimoto S, et al: Polycythemia vera associated with erythromelalgia [Japanese]. Rinsho Ketsueki 29:1055, 1988.
42. Coppa LM, Nehal KS, Young JW, et al: Erythromelalgia precipitated by acral erythema in the setting of thrombocytopenia. J Am Acad Dermatol 48:973, 2003.
43. Mehle AL, Nedorost S, Camisa C: Erythromelalgia. Int J Dermatol 29:567, 1990.
44. Yosipovitch G, Krause I, Blickstein D: Erythromelalgia in a patient with thrombotic thrombocytopenic purpura. J Am Acad Dermatol 26:825, 1992.
45. Rey J, Cretel E, Jean R, et al: Erythromelalgia in a patient with idiopathic thrombocytopenic purpura (letter). Br J Dermatol 148:177, 2003.
46. Thami GP, Bhalla M: Erythromelalgia induced by possible calcium channel blockade by ciclosporin. BMJ 326:910, 2003.
47. Wagner DR, Spengel F, Middeke M: Erythromelalgia unmasked during norephedrine therapy: A case report. Angiology 44:244, 1993.
48. Drenth JP, Michiels JJ, Van Joost T, et al: Verapamil-induced secondary erythermalgia. Br J Dermatol 127:292, 1992.
49. Levesque H, Moore N, Wolfe LM, et al: Erythromelalgia induced by nicardipine (inverse Raynaud's phenomenon?). BMJ 298:1252, 1989.
50. Drenth JP: Erythromelalgia induced by nicardipine (letter). BMJ 298:1582, 1989.
51. Albers GW, Simon LT, Hamik A, et al: Nifedipine versus propranolol for the initial prophylaxis of migraine. Headache 29:215, 1989.
52. Brodmerkel GJ Jr: Nifedipine and erythromelalgia (letter). Ann Intern Med 99:415, 1983.
53. Fisher JR, Padnick MB, Olstein S: Nifedipine and erythromelalgia. Ann Intern Med 98:671, 1983.
54. Monk BE, Parkes JD, Du Vivier A: Erythromelalgia following pergolide administration. Br J Dermatol 111:97, 1984.
55. Dupont E, Illum F, Olivarius BF: Bromocriptine and erythromelalgia-like eruptions (letter). Neurology 33:670, 1983.
56. Eisler T, Hall RP, Kalavar KA, et al: Erythromelalgia-like eruption in parkinsonian patients treated with bromocriptine. Neurology 31:1368, 1981.
57. Calne DB, Plotkin C, Williams AC, et al: Long-term treatment of parkinsonism with bromocriptine. Lancet 1:735, 1978.
58. Dolan CK, Hall MA, Turlansky GW: Secondary erythermalgia in an HIV-1-positive patient. AIDS Read 113:91, 2003.
59. Itin PH, Courvoisier S, Stoll A, et al: Secondary erythermalgia in an HIV-infected patient: Is there a pathogenic relationship? Acta Derm Venereol 76:332, 1996.
60. Rabaud C, Barbaud A, Trechot P: First case of erythermalgia related to hepatitis B vaccination. J Rheumatol 26:233, 1999.
61. Confino I, Passwell JH, Padeh S: Erythromelalgia following influenza vaccine in a child. Clin Exp Rheumatol 15:111, 1997.
62. Clayton C, Faden H: Erythromelalgia in a twenty-year-old with infectious mononucleosis. Pediatr Infect Dis J 12:101, 1993.
63. Zheng ZM, Specter S, Zhang JH, et al: Further characterization of the biological and pathogenic properties of erythromelalgia-related poxviruses. J Gen Virol 73:2011, 1992.
64. Mo YM: An epidemiological study on erythromelalgia [Chinese]. Zhonghua Liu Xing Bing Xue Za Zhi 10:291, 1989.

65. Mørk C, Kalgaard OM, Kvernebo K: Erythromelalgia as a paraneoplastic syndrome in a patient with abdominal cancer (letter). Acta Derm Venereol 79:394, 1999.
66. Kurzrock R, Cohen PR: Paraneoplastic erythromelalgia. Clin Dermatol 11:73, 1993.
67. Levine AM, Gustafson PR: Erythromelalgia: Case report and literature review. Arch Phys Med Rehabil 68:119, 1987.
68. Lantrade P, Didier A, Ille H, et al: Thymome malin et acrosyndromes vasculaires paroxystiques: Une observation. Ann Med Interne (Paris) 131:228, 1980.
69. Cailleux N, Levesque H, Courtois H: Erythermalgia and systemic lupus erythematosus [French]. J Mal Vasc 21:88, 1996.
70. Kraus A: Erythromelalgia in a patient with systemic lupus erythematosus treated with clonazepam. J Rheumatol 17:120, 1990.
71. Michiels JJ: Erythermalgia in SLE. J Rheumatol 18:481, 1991.
72. Alarcon-Segovia D, Diaz-Jouanen E: Case report: Erythermalgia in systemic lupus erythematosus. Am J Med Sci 266:149, 1973.
73. Drenth JP, Michiels JJ, Van Joost T, et al: Erythermalgia secondary to vasculitis. Am J Med 94:549, 1993.
74. Garrett SJ, Robinson JK: Erythromelalgia and pregnancy. Arch Dermatol 126:157, 1990.
75. Herskovitz S, Loh F, Berger AR, et al: Erythromelalgia: Association with hereditary sensory neuropathy and response to amitriptyline. Neurology 43:621, 1993.
76. Staub DB, Munger BL, Uno H, et al: Erythromelalgia as a form of neuropathy. Arch Dermatol 128:1654, 1992.
77. Nagamatsu M, Ueno S, Teramoto J, et al: A case of erythromelalgia with polyneuropathy [Japanese]. Nippon Naika Gakkai Zasshi 78:418, 1989.
78. Tridon P, Vidailhet C, Schweitzer F: The acrodynic form of the Riley-Day syndrome [French]. Pediatrie 44:455, 1989.
79. Cendrowski W: Secondary erythromelalgia in multiple sclerosis [Polish]. Wiad Lek 41:1477, 1988.
80. Vendrell J, Nubiola A, Goday A, et al: Erythromelalgia associated with acute diabetic neuropathy: An unusual condition. Diabetes Res 7:149, 1988.
81. Kikuchi I, Inoue S, Tada S: A unique erythermalgia in a patient with von Recklinghausen neurofibromatosis. J Dermatol 12:436, 1985.
82. van Genderen PJ, Michiels JJ, Drenth JP: Hereditary erythermalgia and acquired erythromelalgia. Am J Med Genet 45:530, 1993.
83. Finley WH, Lindsey JR Jr, Fine JD, et al: Autosomal dominant erythromelalgia. Am J Med Genet 42:310, 1992.
84. Michiels JJ, van Joost T, Vuzevski VD: Idiopathic erythermalgia: A congenital disorder. J Am Acad Dermatol 21:1128, 1989.
85. Cohen IJ, Samorodin CS: Familial erythromelalgia. Arch Dermatol 118:953, 1982.
86. Krebs A, Andres HU: On the clinical features of erythromelalgia: Familial incidence of an idiopathic form in mother and daughter [German]. Schweiz Med Wochenschr 99:344, 1969.
87. Schechner J: Red skin re-read. J Invest Dermatol 119:781, 2002.
88. Davis MDP, Sandroni P, Rooke TW, et al: Erythromelalgia: Vasculopathy, neuropathy, or both? A prospective study of vascular and neurophysiologic studies in erythromelalgia. Arch Dermatol 139:1337, 2003.
89. Sandroni P, Davis MDP, Harper CM Jr, et al: Neurophysiologic and vascular studies in erythromelalgia: A retrospective analysis. J Clin Neuromuscul Dis 1:57, 1999.
90. Charkoudian N: Skin blood flow in adult human thermoregulation: How it works, when it does not, and why. Mayo Clin Proc 78:603, 2003.
91. Braverman IM: The cutaneous microcirculation. J Investig Dermatol Symp Proc 5:3, 2000.
92. Lazareth I, Priollet P: Coexistence of Raynaud's syndrome and erythromelalgia (letter). Lancet 335:1286, 1990.
93. Slutsker GE: Coexistence of Raynaud's syndrome and erythromelalgia (letter). Lancet 335:853, 1990.
94. Kazemi B, Shooshtari SM, Nasab MR, et al: Sympathetic skin response (SSR) in erythromelalgia. Electromyogr Clin Neurophysiol 43:165, 2003.
95. Davis MD, Rooke TW, Sandroni P: Mechanisms other than shunting are likely contributing to the pathophysiology of erythromelalgia. J Invest Dermatol 115:1166, 2000.
96. Liu Y: A study of erythromelalgia in relation to the autonomic nervous system: Report of 321 cases of functional disorders of the autonomic nervous system [Chinese]. Zhonghua Shen Jing Jing Shen Ke Za Zhi 23:47, 1990.
97. Orstavik K, Weidner C, Schmidt R, et al: Pathological C-fibres in patients with a chronic painful condition. Brain 126:567, 2003.
98. Uno H, Parker F: Autonomic innervation of the skin in primary erythermalgia. Arch Dermatol 119:65, 1983.
99. Layzer RB: Hot feet: Erythromelalgia and related disorders. J Child Neurol 16:199, 2001.
100. Sugiyama Y, Hakusui S, Takahashi A, et al: Primary erythromelalgia: The role of skin sympathetic nerve activity. Jpn J Med 30:564, 1991.
101. Littleford RC, Khan F, Belch JJ: Impaired skin vasomotor reflexes in patients with erythromelalgia. Clin Sci (Lond) 96:507, 1999.
102. van Genderen PJ, Lucas IS, van Strik R, et al: Erythromelalgia in essential thrombocythemia is characterized by platelet activation and endothelial cell damage but not by thrombin generation. Thromb Haemost 76:333, 1996.
103. Kurzrock R, Cohen PR: Erythromelalgia: Review of clinical characteristics and pathophysiology. Am J Med 91:416, 1991.
104. Drenth JP, Finley WH, Breedveld GJ, et al: The primary erythermalgia-susceptibility gene is located on chromosome 32. Am J Hum Genet 68:1277, 2001.
105. Drenth JP, Vuzevski V, Van Joost T, et al: Cutaneous pathology in primary erythermalgia. Am J Dermatopathol 18:30, 1996.
106. Lazareth I: False erythermalgia [French]. J Mal Vasc 21:84, 1996.
107. Michiels JJ, ten Kate FW, Vuzevski VD, et al: Histopathology of erythromelalgia in thrombocythaemia. Histopathology 8:669, 1984.
108. Croue A, Gardembas-Pain M, Verret JL, et al: Histopathologic lesions in erythromelalgia during essential thrombocythemia [French]. Ann Pathol 13:128, 1993.
109. Davis MD, Rooke T: Erythromelalgia. Curr Treat Options Cardiovasc Med 4:207, 2002.
110. Cohen JS: Erythromelalgia: New theories and new therapies. J Am Acad Dermatol 43:841, 2000.
111. Rudikoff D, Jaffe IA: Erythromelalgia: Response to serotonin reuptake inhibitors. J Am Acad Dermatol 37:281, 1997.
112. Moiin A, Yashar SS, Sanchez JE, et al: Treatment of erythromelalgia with a serotonin/noradrenaline reuptake inhibitor. Br J Dermatol 146:336, 2002.
113. McGraw T, Kosek P: Erythromelalgia pain managed with gabapentin. Anesthesiology 86:988, 1997.
114. Kuhnert SM, Phillips WJ, Davis MD: Lidocaine and mexiletine therapy for erythromelalgia. Arch Dermatol 135:1447, 1999.
115. Muhiddin KA, Gallen IW, Harries S, et al: The use of capsaicin cream in a case of erythromelalgia. Postgrad Med J 70:841, 1994.
116. Postlethwaite JC: Lumbar sympathectomy: A retrospective study of 142 operations on 100 patients. Br J Surg 60:878, 1973.
117. Shiga T, Sakamoto A, Koizumi K, et al: Endoscopic thoracic sympathectomy for primary erythromelalgia in the upper extremities. Anesth Analg 88:865, 1999.
118. Takeda S, Tomaru T, Higuchi M: A case of primary erythromelalgia (erythermalgia) treated with neural blockade [Japanese]. Masui 38:388, 1989.
119. Seishima M, Kanoh H, Izumi T, et al: A refractory case of secondary erythermalgia successfully treated with lumbar sympathetic ganglion block. Br J Dermatol 143:868, 2000.
120. Kandel EI: Stereotactic surgery of erythromelalgia. Stereotact Funct Neurosurg 54-55:96, 1990.
121. Sadighi PJ, Arbid EJ: Neurectomy for palliation of primary erythermalgia. Ann Vasc Surg 9:197, 1995.
122. Graziotti PJ, Goucke CR: Control of intractable pain in erythromelalgia by using spinal cord stimulation. J Pain Symptom Manage 8:502, 1993.
123. Bada JL: Treatment of erythromelalgia with propranolol. Lancet 2:412, 1977.
124. Cohen JS: High-dose oral magnesium treatment of chronic, intractable erythromelalgia. Ann Pharmacother 36:255, 2002.
125. Kvernebo K, Seem E: Erythromelalgia—pathophysiological and therapeutic aspects: A preliminary report. J Oslo City Hosp 37:9, 1987.
126. Conri CL, Azoulai P, Constans J, et al: Erythromelalgia and low molecular weight heparin [French]. Therapie 49:518, 1994.
127. Ozsoylu S, Coskun T: Sodium nitroprusside treatment in erythromelalgia. Eur J Pediatr 141:185, 1984.
128. Stone JD, Rivey MP, Allington DR: Nitroprusside treatment of erythromelalgia in an adolescent female. Ann Pharmacother 31:590, 1997.

129. Kalgaard OM, Mørk C, Kvernebo K: Prostacyclin reduces symptoms and sympathetic dysfunction in erythromelalgia in a double-blind randomized pilot study. Acta Derm Venereol 83:442, 2003.
130. Pepper H: Primary erythermalgia: Report of a patient treated with methysergide maleate. JAMA 203:1066, 1968.
131. Davis MD, Sandroni P: Lidocaine patch for pain of erythromelalgia. Arch Dermatol 138:17, 2002.
132. Stricker LJ, Green CR: Resolution of refractory symptoms of secondary erythermalgia with intermittent epidural bupivacaine. Reg Anesth Pain Med 26:488, 2001.
133. D'Angelo R, Cohen IT, Brandom BW: Continuous epidural infusion of bupivacaine and fentanyl for erythromelalgia in an adolescent. Anesth Analg 74:142, 1992.
134. Rauck RL, Naveira F, Speight KL, et al: Refractory idiopathic erythromelalgia. Anesth Analg 82:1097, 1996.
135. Mohr M, Schneider K, Grosche M, et al: Cervical epidural infusion of morphine and bupivacaine in severe erythromelalgia [German]. Anasthesiol Intensivmed Notfallmed Schmerzther 29:371, 1994.
136. Trapiella Martinez L, Quiros JF, Caminal Montero L, et al: Treatment of erythromelalgia with buprenorphine (letter) [Spanish]. Rev Clin Esp 197:792, 1997.
137. Macres S, Richeimer S: Successful treatment of erythromelalgia with intrathecal hydromorphone and clonidine. Clin J Pain 16:310, 2000.
138. Calderone DC, Finzi E: Treatment of primary erythromelalgia with piroxicam. J Am Acad Dermatol 24:145, 1991.
139. H'Mila R, Samoud A, Souid M, et al: Erythermalgia: A rare vascular acrosyndrome [French]. Arch Fr Pediatr 48:555, 1991.
140. Guillet MH, Le Noach E, Milochau P, et al: Familial erythermalgia treated with pizotifen [French]. Ann Dermatol Venereol 122:777, 1995.
141. Drenth JP, Michiels JJ: Treatment options in primary erythermalgia? (Letter.) Am J Hematol 43:154, 1993.
142. Kasapcopur O, Akkus S, Erdem A, et al: Erythromelalgia associated with hypertension and leukocytoclastic vasculitis in a child. Clin Exp Rheumatol 16:184, 1998.
143. Cimaz R, Rusconi R, Fossali E, et al: Unexpected healing of cutaneous ulcers in a short child. Lancet 358:211, 2001.
144. Sakakibara R, Fukutake T, Kita K, et al: Treatment of primary erythromelalgia with cyproheptadine. J Auton Nerv Syst 58:121, 1996.
145. Suh DH, Kim SD, Ahn JS, et al: A case of erythromelalgia successfully controlled by systemic steroids and pentazocine: Is it related to a unique subtype of neutrophilic dermatosis? J Dermatol 27:204, 2000.
146. Chakravarty K, Pharoah PD, Scott DG, et al: Erythromelalgia: The role of hypnotherapy. Postgrad Med J 68:44, 1992.

chapter 51

Pernio (Chilblains)

Amjad AlMahameed
Jeffrey W. Olin

Pernio, commonly known as *chilblains*, is a cold-induced, localized, inflammatory condition presenting as skin lesions predominantly on unprotected acral areas. Typically, there is swelling of the dorsa of the proximal phalanges of the fingers and toes (Fig. 51-1). Pernio is a Latin term meaning "frostbite." Chilblains is an Anglo-Saxon term used in older literature meaning "cold sore." The tissue and vascular damage is less severe in pernio than in frostbite, in which the skin is actually frozen. The numerous names used to describe this syndrome created much confusion and misunderstanding of this entity (Box 51-1).[1] In the mid-1800s attempts were made to better classify the disease,[2] and in 1894 Corlett was the first to describe the clinical characteristics of pernio, which he called *dermatitis hiemalis*.[3]

EPIDEMIOLOGY

The first epidemiologic study to explicate the prevalence of chilblains and its impact on productivity in servicewomen was carried out in 1942 by the U.S. Medical Department of the War Office.[4] The study concluded that at least 50% of questionnaire participants had chilblains by age 40 during World War II (1939-1943). Although pernio is most common in young females, it has also been reported in all ages and both sexes.[5-8] The number of reported cases of pernio is higher during times of wet, near-freezing weather and less common in dry, freezing weather or in a bitterly cold climate.[9] Pernio is most commonly encountered in the northern and western parts of the United States, and isolated cases have been reported in warmer climates in times of cooler, damp weather.[5,6,10,11] As shown by a recently reported cross-sectional study conducted by the U.S. Army, the yearly rate of cold weather injuries has declined from 38.2/100,000 in 1985 to 0.2/100,000 in 1999.[12] This and other observations from clinical practice suggest that the disease is becoming less common with higher standards of home and workplace heating and greater use of appropriate clothing during the cold winter months. Also, the study confirmed previous investigations that cold weather injuries in African-American men and women occurred approximately 4 and 2.2 times more often as in their Caucasian counterparts, respectively.

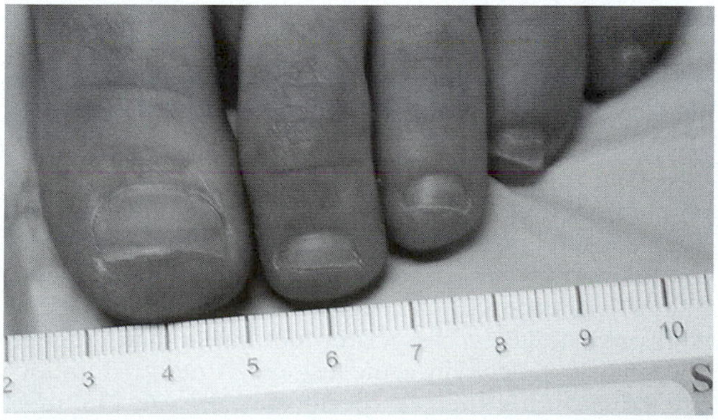

FIGURE 51-1. (See also Color Plate 51-1.) Early manifestation of pernio demonstrating erythema on the dorsum of the phalanges of the toes. At this stage the affected extremities often itch and burn.

PATHOPHYSIOLOGY

The first response to cold exposure is vasoconstriction in the dermis and the subcutaneous tissue. Heat loss is minimized by shutting down the distal capillary beds and diminishing blood supply to the acral portions of the extremities to maintain central body temperature. Stasis and shunting of the blood flow away from the superficial vessels occur secondary to arteriolar constriction, venular relaxation, and the cold-associated increased blood viscosity. The results of these changes are superficial tissue anoxia and ischemia.[7,9,13-15] The arteriolar vasoconstriction described in pernio has been demonstrated in pathologic and radiographic studies.[6,7] The female predominance may be related to an increased responsiveness of the cutaneous circulation to cold. Indeed, there is a higher frequency of vasomotor instability, cold hands and feet, and Raynaud's phenomenon in women.[8,16,17]

BOX 51-1 Names Used in the Literature to Describe Pernio or Pernio-like Conditions

Pernio	Perniosis
Chilblains	Dermatitis hiemalis
Nodular vasculitis	Frostschaeden
Erythrocyanosis	Erythrocyanosis frigida
Erythrocyanose surmalléolair	Erythrocyanosis crurum puellaris
Erythema induratum	Bazin's disease
Lupus pernio	L'engelune
Kibes	Cold panniculitis

TABLE 51-1 CATEGORIES OF DISEASES THAT ARE ASSOCIATED WITH PERNIO

Defective cutaneous vasomotor reactivity	Raynaud's phenomenon
	Acrocyanosis
	Reflex sympathetic dystrophy
	Anterior poliomyelitis
	Syringomyelia
	Livedo reticularis
Underlying chronic limb ischemia	Peripheral arterial disease
	Erythromelalgia (advanced stage)
Hyperviscosity syndrome	Leukemia
	Systemic lupus erythematosus
	Dysproteinemia (cryoproteins)
Abnormal fat distribution	Obese subjects with fat legs
	Inadequate fat pads (anorexia nervosa)

Humidity has an important role in the pathophysiology of pernio, because it enhances air conductivity, thus promoting heat loss from the skin.[5,8] Although most individuals tolerate exposure to nonfreezing damp cold, others may experience pernio, Raynaud's phenomenon, acrocyanosis, or cold urticaria.[8,17] The clinical manifestations of cold injuries are related to the duration, severity, and dampness of cold exposure, as well as the individual's underlying predisposition to cold injury and the stage at which medical attention was sought.[7] The exposed skin of affected subjects remains cool longer and warms slower than that of controls, further highlighting the importance of individual susceptibility for the development of pernio after cold exposure.[6-8,18] The increased incidence of pernio among relatives of affected patients suggests the possibility of genetic predisposition.[4] Several other conditions have been proposed to promote vulnerability to the disease (Table 51-1).

Why one patient exposed to cold develops Raynaud's phenomenon and another pernio is not clear. Raynaud's phenomenon and pernio frequently coexist in the same patient. Thus these diseases may be part of a continuum with Raynaud's phenomenon representing acute and readily reversible vasospasm and pernio representing more prolonged vasospasm with more chronic changes.[8,19]

A number of conditions have been associated with pernio. Weston and Morelli[11] reported the presence of cryoproteins in four of eight children presenting with pernio. Because cryoproteins and cold agglutinins may be detected transiently after viral infections, the researchers hypothesized that exposure to cold, wet weather during the brief cryoproteinemia may lead to exaggerated tissue injury manifesting as pernio. Pernio has been described in women with large amounts of fat in the legs, as well as in women with inadequate fat pads, as seen in anorexia nervosa.[5-7] The possibility that pernio may be a manifestation of a preleukemic state, namely the chronic myelomonocytic type, has been suggested in several case reports in which skin lesions and a clinical course similar to that of pernio were observed.[5,20-22] In some of these cases, leukemia was diagnosed 6 to 36 months after the pernio-like illness.

Viguier and colleagues[19] reported observations over 38 months on a cohort of 33 patients with severe chilblains, defined as duration of lesions longer than 1 month. Two thirds of the patients had clinical or laboratory features, or both, supporting a diagnosis of connective tissue disorders: 12 patients had systemic lupus erythematosus (SLE), and 10 patients presented with at least one of the American College of Rheumatology revised criteria for SLE at the time of the pernio diagnosis. In the latter group, all patients except one had positive ANA titers. These observations led the authors to conclude that, when the lesions persist beyond the cold season, perniotic lesions may be a clue to underlying SLE. Therefore, targeted laboratory investigations to search for conditions listed in Table 51-1, as well as long-term follow-up, are recommended for patients who present with pernio.

HISTOPATHOLOGY OF PERNIO

Although not routinely required to establish the diagnosis, biopsies are occasionally sought by health care providers unfamiliar with the disease.[23] The histopathologic features of perniotic lesions may vary depending on the chronologic stage of the disease and the presence or absence of superimposed secondary pathology such as infection or ulceration.[7,24,25]

The characteristic histopathologic features of pernio are usually seen in the dermis and subcutaneous tissue, but these are not pathognomonic. These consist of edema of the papillodermis, vasculitis characterized by perivascular infiltration of the arterioles and venules of the dermis and subcutaneous fat by mononuclear and lymphocytic cells, thickening and edema of the blood vessel walls, fat necrosis, and chronic inflammatory reaction with giant cell formation.[8] Not all of these changes are necessarily present, and fat necrosis and giant cell formation are frequently absent. The most consistent feature is perivascular lymphocytic or mononuclear infiltrates.[24] Repeated episodes of vasospasm or prolonged vasospasm may cause tissue anoxia, thus causing the identical histopathologic picture that occurs in pernio.[1] The histologic pattern of pernio lesions may mimic that of cutaneous vasculitis but typically lacks the fibrinoid deposition, inflammatory cells in the vessel wall, and thrombosis typical of true vasculitis.[5-7,11,23,25-28] The blood vessels in long-standing pernio resemble those of any chronic occlusive vascular disease. Vascular occlusion and fibrosis in chronic pernio result from long-standing injury. This histopathologic appearance is similar to that seen in other chronic occlusive vascular diseases, usually occurring in subjects with long-standing symptoms.

Review of published case series and case reports support the notion that pernio may display different and loosely related histologic features. Cribier and associates[23] retrospectively compared the biopsies of hand lesions from 17 patients with chilblains with those of 10 patients with proved SLE and associated pernio-like hand lesions. The study included only acute lesions (<1 month duration) occurring during the cold period of the year. The most characteristic finding in chilblains (47% of cases) was the association of edema and reticular dermis infiltrate that showed a perieccrine reinforcement: dermal edema

(70% of chilblains lesions vs. 20% of SLE lesions), superficial (papillary) and deep (reticular) infiltrate (82% vs. 80%), and deep perieccrine reinforcement (76% vs. 0%). The infiltrate was composed of a majority of T cells, predominantly CD3+. Remarkably, 29% of the chilblain lesions in this group showed evidence of microthrombi (compared with 10% in the lupus group), usually a feature seen in vasculitis, and 6% had conspicuous vacuolation (compared with 60% in the lupus group). In another study, Viguier and colleagues[19] prospectively studied 33 patients with severe prolonged chilblains (i.e., lesions persisted >1 month) and attempted to differentiate the histopathologic characteristics of lesions of "idiopathic" pernio from those of pernio-like lesions in patients with connective tissue diseases or lupus pernio. Skin punch biopsies were performed on 5 of 11 patients of the "idiopathic" pernio group, and these showed deep dermal, perisudoral lymphocytic infiltrate (100%), dermal edema (75%), keratinocyte necrosis (62.5%), and keratinocyte vacuolization (50%). In comparison, biopsies from 7 of the 12 patients with the diagnosis of SLE (LE chilblain), demonstrated perisudoral cellular infiltrate in only 2 patients (vs. 8/8 in the "idiopathic" chilblains group, $P = .007$). Biopsy is rarely necessary to make the diagnosis of pernio. However, a biopsy may be helpful in differentiating atheromatous embolization from pernio in an ischemic-looking lesion (Fig. 51-2).

CLINICAL FEATURES

Pernio most commonly affects females in adolescence and early adulthood but may occur at any age and in either gender. The lesions typically affect the acral areas of the toes and the dorsa of the proximal phalanges but may involve the nose, ears, and thighs (Fig. 51-3).[1-4,7,19,29] The location of the lesions seems to depend on the occupation, lifestyle, and clothing habits. The hands and fingers appear more commonly affected in milkers and gardeners; the buttocks have been involved in women

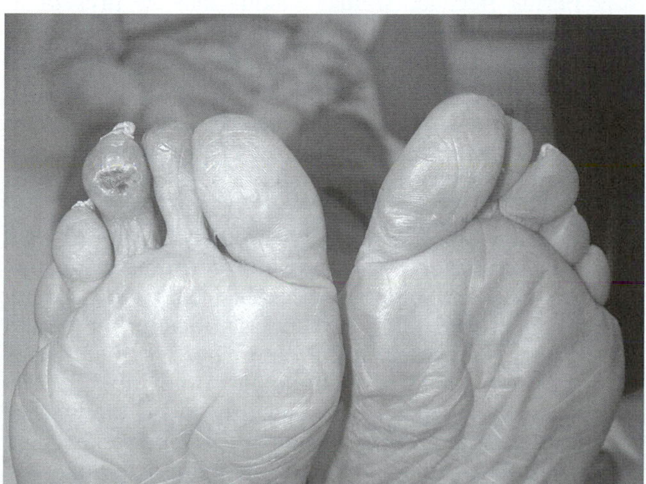

FIGURE 51-2. (See also Color Plate 51-2.) Advanced stage of pernio. The toes are cyanotic, and there is a shallow ulcer on the right third toe. This stage of pernio is often quite painful and may be mistaken for atheromatous embolization in the elderly patient.

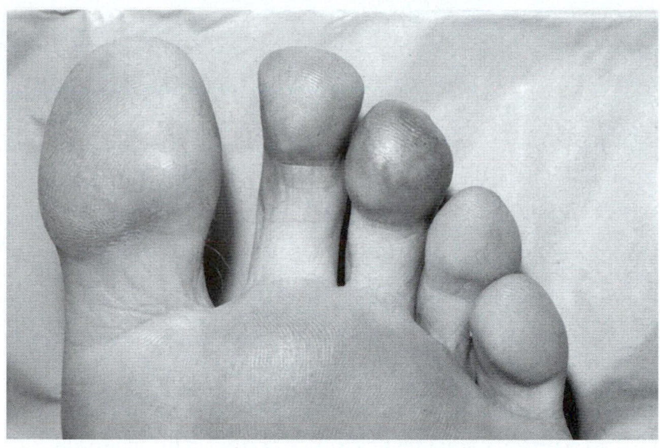

FIGURE 51-3. (See also Color Plate 51-3.) Typical appearance of pernio. Note swelling and brownish yellow appearance of the left third toe. Flaking, itching, burning, and pain are common in pernio.

driving tractors in the winter; and involvement of the lateral thighs has been described in women who wear thin pants and ride horses or motorcycles in the winter.[3,17,30-35] The distal shins and the calves are common sites of involvement in young females who wear short skirts.[36] Facial lesions have been described in infants and rarely in adults.[19,37]

Typically, the initial presentation is one of *acute* pernio, in which the lesions appear during the cold months and disappear when the weather warms up. This may recur for several years and follows a similar seasonal pattern.[7,8] The lesions vary in shape, number, and size and usually are associated with functional symptoms such as itching, burning, or pain. The lesions can be described as brownish, yellow, or cyanotic on a base of doughy subcutaneous swelling or erythema (see Figs. 51-1 and 51-3). They may be cool to touch or cooler than the surrounding skin. The acute lesions may be self-limited and resolve within a few days to few weeks (especially in children) unless cold exposure persists, the lesions become infected, or the skin is broken by iatrogenic causes such as self-treatment with severe heat or vigorous massage. Otherwise, ulceration is not common in acute pernio and, when it happens, the lesions are usually shallow with a hemorrhagic base (see Fig. 51-2).[7,8]

Chronic pernio ensues if repeated and prolonged exposure to cold persists throughout the acute phase or the patient goes through several seasons of acute pernio, or both. The lesions of chronic pernio are similar to those seen in acute pernio but, if they occur over many seasons, may be associated with scarring, atrophy, permanent discoloration, and possibly ulceration (see Fig. 51-2). Initially, pernio may start late in the fall or early winter and resolve in early spring. If left untreated, the lesions of pernio may start earlier in the cold season and resolve later, until eventually all seasonal variation is lost.

Pernio tends to be more severe in adults and may, if left untreated, eventually cause macrovascular occlusive disease.[6,8] Children, on the other hand, tend to have recurrent acute pernio over several seasons. Although most children outgrow the disease, middle-aged individuals presenting with pernio may occasionally recall a history of

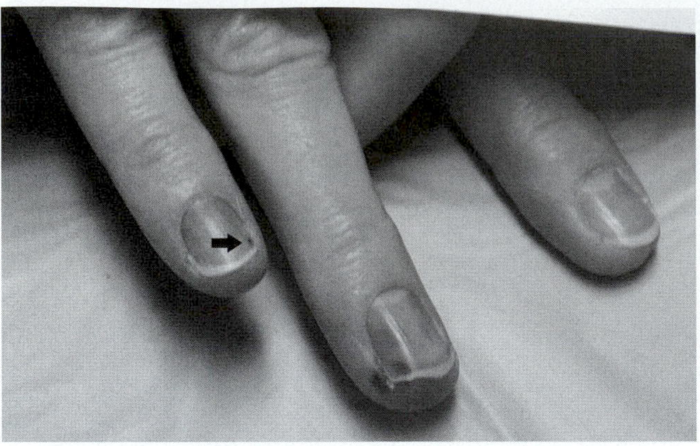

FIGURE 51-4. (See also Color Plate 51-4.) Pernio of the fourth and fifth (*arrow*) fingers of the right hand in a woman exposed to a cold, wet climate. Note the presence of superficial digital infarcts.

acute pernio during childhood. Several different forms of pernio have been described.

Milker's pernio usually affects the hands and can be debilitating enough to force the affected individual to quit milking (Fig. 51-4).[33] *Kibe* is defined as a chapped or inflamed area on the skin, especially on the heel, resulting from exposure to cold or an ulcerated chilblain.[38] This has been described in overweight women who ride horses and wear tight pants, in women who ride motorcycles and wear thin pants, and in men who cross cold rivers with their thighs inadequately clothed.[17,30] The lesions tend to localize on the outer thighs and often cause severe pain and disability. The pain may last up to a week and usually resolves once the lesions heal.[17] A similar form has been described in women who drive tractors in the winter and those who tend to have lesions on the buttocks.[35] *Lupus pernio* applies to papular lesions involving the extremities and is associated with SLE.[39] Whether this is a subtype of pernio or a pernio-like lupus manifestation remains controversial. Although some authors have suggested that most lupus pernio patients have lesions on the hands, this anatomical localization was not a differentiating factor between idiopathic pernio and lupus pernio according to others.[8,19] Features that suggest pernio secondary to SLE include onset of pernio during the third decade, female sex, African origin, and the presence of pernio long after the cold weather has abated. *Erythrocyanosis* affects adolescent girls and young women and typically involves the lower extremities. Some have classified this as the "nodular chronic form" of pernio, and the lesions take on a swollen, dusky red appearance.[8]

DIAGNOSIS

Usually pernio is not difficult to diagnose. A comprehensive history and complete physical examination are the primary means by which the diagnosis of pernio can be correctly established. Chronologic correlation between the onset of typical lesions to nonfreezing cold that improve with the onset of warm weather should strongly suggest the diagnosis.

Within hours of exposure to damp cold, and commonly at the onset of winter, the patient develops violet or yellow blisters, brown plaques, or shallow ulcers on the toes, which often burn, itch, or become painful. These lesions typically disappear when the weather warms up at the beginning of spring. However, in some chronic cases, in which the lesions do not disappear in the warm weather or in which the lesions cause severe pigmentation and disfiguration of the lower part of the leg, the diagnosis may be more difficult.

The main obstacle to establishing the diagnosis of pernio is unfamiliarity of the health care provider with the disease. Because many dermatologic manifestations associated with pernio overlap with other serious diseases, it is not uncommon for pernio patients to be subjected to unnecessary investigations and suffer needless delay in proper treatment.[5,37,40] Characteristically, the peripheral pulses and peripheral blood pressure measurements are normal unless the patient has underlying peripheral arterial disease or the pernio has been of such long duration that chronic occlusive vascular disease has developed.[6] Pulse volume recordings and segmental blood pressures may be abnormal in patients with pernio. This may be due to either vasospasm (the study normalizes with warming of the extremity) or fixed vascular disease due to long-standing pernio.[41]

Because the diagnosis of pernio is a clinical diagnosis, sophisticated laboratory tests are often not necessary. However, it is important to rule out other entities that can mimic pernio. The following tests may be obtained: CBC with differential, antinuclear antibody titer, rheumatoid factor, comprehensive metabolic panel, cryoglobulin, cryofibrinogen, cold agglutinin, and serum viscosity measurements. Arteriography and skin biopsy are not warranted to establish the diagnosis of pernio except in the occasional case when a clear history could not be obtained or a concomitant vascular pathology (such as atheromatous embolization) is suspected.

The differential diagnosis of pernio includes various diseases. Atheromatous emboli (blue toe syndrome) is the most challenging diagnostic entity to differentiate from pernio because similar lesions may be present in each disorder.[42] When the history of cold exposure is uncertain and in patients with established or suspected atherosclerosis, imaging studies often are warranted to demonstrate atheroma in the aorta or iliac vessels. A biopsy of these lesions showing characteristic cholesterol clefts establishes the diagnosis of atheromatous emboli.[42]

The next group of diseases that may be confused with pernio include those with chronic recurrent erythematous, nodular, and ulcerative lesions: erythema induratum, nodular vasculitis, erythema nodosum, and cold panniculitis. Erythema induratum (Bazin's disease) is often, but not always, a cutaneous form of tuberculosis, which usually affects adolescent girls and is manifested by nodular ulcerating lesions of the calves.[7,43] Nontuberculous forms of recurrent painful nodules are called *nodular vasculitis*.[43] Women older than the age of 30 years are usually affected, and no apparent cause is known. Although the nodules of nodular vasculitis are extremely painful, they rarely ulcerate. Erythema nodosum may be differentiated from pernio in that it may be associated with fever, arthralgias, malaise, and an underlying disease. The lesions are painful and generally do not ulcerate. Cold panniculitis, another important entity, is characterized by painful nodules that appear on the skin after cold exposure and can be reproduced by the application of an ice cube. The histology of these lesions reveals fat necrosis.[44] The palpable, purpuric lesion that is sometimes present in pernio must be differentiated from other types of vasculitis, especially leukocytoclastic vasculitis. Lack of the systemic manifestations and laboratory abnormalities that occur in leukocytoclastic vasculitis and the relation of the lesions to cold exposure in pernio serve to separate these two conditions. Rarely, a skin biopsy may be necessary to make a definitive diagnosis.

TREATMENT

Because the primary trigger for the development of pernio is cold exposure, prevention is the mainstay of management. Working in a damp, cold basement or living in a poorly heated apartment may necessitate change of profession or moving to a properly heated residence. Patients do not always volunteer information about the climate of their residence and workplace, and the physician may need to ask specifically about the quality of the heating system and the degree of humidity present. The patient should be instructed on methods of proper dress. Adequate body insulation with gloves, stockings, footwear, and headwear may be necessary. As is the case in treating Raynaud's phenomenon, the entire body must be kept warm.

A dihydropyridine calcium channel blocker such as nifedipine is quite effective in patients with pernio. It also has been shown to be effective in patients with Raynaud's phenomenon.[45] In a double-blinded, placebo-controlled, randomized crossover pilot study, Dowd and colleagues[46] reported that treatment with 20 mg of nifedipine three times daily, when given shortly after the appearance of lesions, led to resolution of the lesions within 7 to 10 days compared with 20 to 28 days with placebo. In addition, the pain disappeared within 5 days in the treated group compared with 20 to 25 days in the group receiving placebo.[46] In a double-blinded, placebo-controlled, randomized trial, Rustin and colleagues[47] have shown that nifedipine, given at a daily dose of 20 to 60 mg, was shown to reduce the severity of symptoms, shorten their duration, enhance resolution of existing lesions, and prevent the development of new lesions. On the basis of these studies and our experience, all patients are prescribed either nifedipine or amlodipine to facilitate the healing of the lesions and prevent their recurrence. When spring and summer approach, the calcium channel blocker is stopped and then restarted the following fall. These pharmacologic therapies should be used in conjunction with other preventive strategies discussed earlier.

Despite speculation that it may enhance the resolution of active lesions and provide subjective improvement, sympathectomy does not prevent recurrence of new lesions and has little effect, if any, on the pigmentation and thickness at the sites of perniotic lesions. Conflicting reports exist about the use of other treatment modalities such as topical vasodilators, topical corticosteroids, calcium, and intramuscular vitamin K. Given the controversy and lack of prospective studies, routine use of these agents is not recommended.[8]

REFERENCES

1. McGovern T, Wright IS, Kruger E: Pernio: A vascular disease. Am Heart J 22:583, 1941.
2. Bazin E: Lecons Theoriques et Cliniques Sur la Scrofule, 2nd ed. Paris: A. Delahue, 1861, p 146.
3. Corlett WT: Cold as an etiological factor in diseases of the skin. Eleventh International Medical Congress in Rome. 1894, p 153.
4. Winner A, Cooper-Willis E: Chilblains in service women. Lancet 1:663, 1946.
5. Goette DK: Chilblains (perniosis). J Am Acad Dermatol 23:257, 1990.
6. Jacob JR, Weisman MH, Rosenblatt SI, et al: Chronic pernio: A historical perspective of cold-induced vascular disease. Arch Intern Med 146:1589, 1986.
7. Lynn RB: Chilblains. Surg Gynecol Obstet 99:720, 1954.
8. Olin JW, Arrabi W: Vascular diseases related to extremes in environmental temperature. In Young JR, Olin JW, Bartholomew JR (eds): Peripheral Vascular Disease, 2nd ed. St Louis, Mosby-Year Book, 1996, pp. 611-613.
9. Purdue GF, Hunt JL: Cold injury: A collective review. J Burn Care Rehabil 7:417, 1986.
10. Wessagowit P, Asawanonda P, Noppakun N: Papular perniosis mimicking erythema multiforme: The first case report in Thailand. Int J Dermatol 39:527, 2000.
11. Weston WL, Morelli JG: Childhood pernio and cryoproteins. Pediatr Dermatol 17:97, 2000.
12. DeGroot DW, Castellani JW, Williams JO, et al: Epidemiology of U.S. Army cold weather injuries, 1980-1999. Aviat Space Environ Med 74:564, 2003.
13. Eubanks RG: Heat and cold injuries. J Ark Med Soc 71:53, 1974.
14. Kulka JP: Vasomotor microcirculatory insufficiency: Observations on nonfreezing cold injury of the mouse ear. Angiology 12:491, 1961.
15. Lewis T: Observations upon the reactions of the vessels of the human skin to cold. Heart 15:177, 1930.
16. Goodfield M: Cold-induced skin disorders. Practitioner 233:1616, 1989.
17. Price RD, Murdoch DR: Perniosis (chilblains) of the thigh: Report of five cases, including four following river crossings. High Alt Med Biol 2:535, 2001.
18. Lewis ST: Observations on some normal and injurious effects of cold upon the skin and underlying tissues: Chilblains and allied conditions. Br Med J 2:837, 1941.
19. Viguier M, Pinquier L, Cavelier-Balloy B, et al: Clinical and histopathologic features and immunologic variables in patients with severe chilblains: A study of the relationship to lupus erythematosus. Medicine (Baltimore) 80:180, 2001.
20. Baker H: Chronic monocytic leukemia with necrosis of pinnae. Br J Dermatol 76:480, 1946.
21. Kelly JW, Dowling JP: Pernio: A possible association with chronic myelomonocytic leukemia. Arch Dermatol 121:1048, 1985.
22. Marks R, Lim CC, Borrie PF: A perniotic syndrome with monocytosis and neutropenia: A possible association with a preleukaemic state. Br J Dermatol 81:327, 1969.
23. Cribier B, Djeridi N, Peltre B, et al: A histologic and immunohistochemical study of chilblains. J Am Acad Dermatol 45:924, 2001.
24. Herman EW, Kezis JS, Silvers DN: A distinctive variant of pernio: Clinical and histopathologic study of nine cases. Arch Dermatol 117:26, 1981.
25. Wall LM, Smith NP: Perniosis: A histopathological review. Clin Exp Dermatol 6:263, 1981.
26. Corbett D, Benson P: Military dermatology. In Zajtchuk R, Bellamy RF (eds): Textbook of Military Medicine. Part III. Diseases of the Environment. Washington, DC, Office of the Surgeon General, 1994.

27. Inoue G, Miura T: Microgeodic disease affecting the hands and feet of children. J Pediatr Orthop 11:59, 1991.
28. Page EH, Shear NH: Temperature-dependent skin disorders. J Am Acad Dermatol 18:1003, 1988.
29. Gourlay RJ: The problem of chilblains: With a note of their treatment with nicotinic acid. Br Med J 1:336, 1948.
30. Winter kibes in horsey women. Lancet 2:1345, 1980.
31. Beacham BE, Cooper PH, Buchanan CS, et al: Equestrian cold panniculitis in women. Arch Dermatol 116:1025, 1980.
32. De Silva BD, McLaren K, Doherty VR: Equestrian perniosis associated with cold agglutinins: A novel finding. Clin Exp Dermatol 25:285, 2000.
33. Duffill MB: Milkers' chilblains. N Z Med J 106:101, 1993.
34. Fisher DA, Everett MA: Violaceous rash of dorsal fingers in a woman. Diagnosis: Chilblain lupus erythematosus (perniosis). Arch Dermatol 132:459, 1996.
35. Thomas EW: Chapping and chilblains. Practitioner 193:755, 1964.
36. Walsh S: More red toes. J Pediatr Health Care 14:193, 2000.
37. Giusti R, Tunnessen WW Jr: Picture of the month: Chilblains (pernio). Arch Pediatr Adolesc Med 151:1055, 1997.
38. The American Heritage Dictionary for the English Language. Boston, New York, Houghton-Mifflin, 2000.
39. Millard LG, Rowell NR: Chilblain lupus erythematosus (Hutchinson): A clinical and laboratory study of 17 patients. Br J Dermatol 98:497, 1978.
40. Parlette EC, Parlette HL III: Erythrocyanotic discoloration of the toes. Cutis 65:223, 2000.
41. Spittell JA Jr, Spittell PC: Chronic pernio: Another cause of blue toes. Int Angiol 11:46, 1992.
42. Rose R, Bartholomew JR, Olin JW: Atheromatous embolization syndrome. In Rutherford RB (ed): Vascular Surgery, 6th ed. Philadelphia, WB Saunders, 2004.
43. Montgomery H, O'Leary PA, Barker NW: Nodular vascular disease of the legs. JAMA 128:335, 1945.
44. Solomon LM, Beerman H: Cold panniculitis. Arch Dermatol 88:897, 1961.
45. Smith CD, McKendry RJ: Controlled trial of nifedipine in the treatment of Raynaud's phenomenon. Lancet 2:1299, 1982.
46. Dowd PM, Rustin MH, Lanigan S: Nifedipine in the treatment of chilblains. Br Med J (Clin Res Ed) 293:923, 1986.
47. Rustin MH, Newton JA, Smith NP, et al: The treatment of chilblains with nifedipine: The results of a pilot study, a double-blind placebo-controlled randomized study and a long-term open trial. Br J Dermatol 120:267, 1989.

chapter 52

Complex Regional Pain Syndrome

Michael Stanton-Hicks

Pain and vasomotor disturbances have been the subjects of a rich and fascinating history. Ever since the 1800s when Claude Bernard implicated pain behavior in animals whose autonomic (sympathetic) control to a region was interrupted, many clinicians including Wolff,[3] Kummell,[4] Sudeck,[5] Fontaine and Herrmann,[6] Livingston,[7] DeTakats,[8] and Homans[9] described pain disorders that were associated with localized vasomotor changes. Undoubtedly, they were all describing what Evans in 1946 ultimately called *reflex sympathetic dystrophy.*[10]

In one of the finest pieces of medical writing, a pupil of Bernard's named Silas Weir Mitchell (1829-1914)[2] described the bizarre inflammatory response of a major nerve in an extremity that suffered a musket shot during the American Civil War. He used the term *causalgia* in contradistinction to the usual neurogenic response seen from such injuries. In a later war, Renee Leriche also noted the peculiarly excessive response in some wounded soldiers and suggested this may be due to what he termed "positive feedback loops" between the central and peripheral nervous systems.[11] Livingston in 1946[7] and Bonica in 1947[12] both observed this response in veterans from World War II, which they attributed to a vicious circle of events that implicated both central and peripheral nervous systems. Sir Sydney Sunderland (1976) spent his life studying the peripheral nervous system and described the same exaggerated response in the few patients who developed causalgia, as previously reported by Mitchell.[2]

Causalgia as a specific entity was officially acknowledged in a British Medical Research Council publication in 1920.[1] It was defined as pain that (1) is spontaneous; (2) is hot and burning in character, intense, diffuse, persistent, and subject to exacerbations; (3) is excited by stimuli that do not necessarily produce a physical effort on the limb; and (4) tends to lead to profound changes in the mental health of the patient. This and other descriptions of causalgic pain associated with a nerve injury are indistinguishable from the clinical characteristics of reflex sympathetic dystrophy that have appeared in the literature (see above).

COMPLEX REGIONAL PAIN SYNDROME

Despite its intended purpose, the *term reflex sympathetic dystrophy* (RSD) in the English speaking world did not satisfy stringent diagnostic criteria and was interpreted variously by different clinicians to the extent that little among consistent clinical reports could be compared because of the differing emphases on clinical signs and symptoms that were applied. For decades the disease entity was viewed with indifference. As a result, many patients received no treatment, their plight being regarded as an exaggerated behavioral aberration to a disease process that was completely misunderstood. Furthermore, its dependency on sympathetic dysfunction, in particular hyperactivity, resulted in making a diagnosis only if analgesia or some relief of pain were obtained by sympathetic block. This had the effect of denying a significant number of patients from receiving appropriate treatment whenever a response to sympathetic blockade was negative. An extension of this premise was the indiscriminate use of surgical sympathectomy for patients suspected of having RSD.

In the 1970s the Committee on Taxonomy of the International Association for the Study of Pain (IASP) attempted to categorize the main features, associated symptoms, signs, and clinical courses of the two conditions, reflex sympathetic dystrophy and causalgia. Much of what appeared in the first edition of the *IASP Classification of Chronic Pain* in 1979 reiterated what Bonica methodically described in his first edition of *The Management of Pain* in 1953[12] (Table 52-1). Reliance on the results of sympathetic blockade as a component of treatment were restated, as well as what was believed to be sympathetic hyperactivity. Gibbons and colleagues[13] introduced a table of signs and symptoms using a weighted score in an attempt to improve the recognition of these syndromes (Box 52-1).

A move to develop reliable diagnostic criteria that could be standardized and conform to those essential features that make up an ideal classification was first attempted in 1993.[14] A group consisting of clinicians and basic scientists gathered for a special Consensus Workshop of the IASP, the specific task of which was to reevaluate the clinical syndromes of causalgia and RSD. Specifically, this group adopted the same principles that form the basis for a classification, along the lines that have been adopted by the International Classification of Diseases, ICD-10, but which essentially would provide a biologic classification in terms of pain. The group agreed that the terms RSD and causalgia should be replaced by terminology that would give no hint to a mechanism but would rather describe the syndromes in clinical terms only. The resultant terms, complex regional pain syndrome type I (CRPS-I) for RSD and complex regional pain syndrome type II (CRPS-II) for causalgia, were proposed and adopted by the Committee on Taxonomy of the IASP.[15] These were published in the second edition of *Classification of Chronic Pain* in 1994.[16] Box 52-1 lists the criteria for the two conditions.

Although causalgia historically preceded a definition and diagnosis of RSD, under the new diagnostic criteria,

TABLE 52-1 INTERNATIONAL ASSOCIATION FOR THE STUDY OF PAIN DIAGNOSTIC CRITERIA FOR COMPLEX REGIONAL PAIN SYNDROME TYPES I AND II[2]

Type I (Reflex Sympathetic Dystrophy)*	Type II (Causalgia)†
1. The presence of an initiating noxious event or a cause of immobilization 2. Continuing pain, allodynia, or hyperalgesia, the pain of which is disproportionate to any inciting event 3. Evidence at some time of edema, changes in skin blood flow, or abnormal sudomotor activity in the region of the pain 4. Diagnosis is excluded by the existence of conditions that would otherwise account for the degrees of pain and dysfunction	1. The presence of continuing pain, allodynia, or hyperalgesia after a nerve injury, not necessarily limited to the distribution of the injured nerve 2. Evidence at some time of edema, changes in skin blood flow, or abnormal sudomotor activity in the region of the pain 3. Diagnosis is excluded by the existence of conditions that would otherwise account for the degrees of pain and dysfunction

*Criteria 2-4 must be satisfied.

†All three criteria must be satisfied.

CRPS-I represents a primary disturbance that usually follows a soft tissue injury (i.e., without a known injury to a nerve). CRPS-II refers to a similar-appearing clinical entity but with a well-defined nerve injury that is necessary for the diagnosis of causalgia to be made. The new taxonomy acknowledges this distinction between the two types of CRPS. Implied with the exception of the injured nerve, however, are similar pathophysiologic events.

The main features of CRPS as defined in the new taxonomy are: pain that is spontaneous; allodynia or hyperalgesia, or both; abnormal vasomotor activity resulting in abnormal regulation of blood flow; sudomotor abnormalities; and edema of the skin and subcutaneous tissues. Clinical changes of the integumentary system and subcutaneous tissues may occur. Although a movement disorder was not considered an absolute criterion for inclusion at the time, it is mentioned in the descriptive terminology and has since been acknowledged by recent research.

The criteria for CRPS-I are as follows:

1. *The presence of an initiating noxious event or cause of immobilization.* This refers to what is usually minor trauma, in some cases with little evidence of bruising, such as a skin lesion, sprain, bone fracture, or surgery. The syndrome may rarely develop after remote visceral trauma such as a stroke or heart attack. CRPS may develop after immobilization following some traumatic event.
2. *Continuing pain, allodynia, or hyperalgesia with which the pain is disproportionate to any inciting event.* The disproportional nature of the symptoms expressed by patients with CRPS distinguishes these patients from those whose symptoms typically are expected after similar injuries. Furthermore, the symptoms are not confined to the territory of an individual nerve or region and, as a corollary, the specific site of the noxious source does not determine the location of symptoms (e.g., CRPS developing in a contralateral extremity after inoculation).
3. *Evidence at some time of edema, changes in skin blood flow (skin color changes, skin temperature changes—more than 1.1° C difference from the homologous body part), or abnormal sudomotor activity in the region of pain.* The patient should be given the benefit of the doubt when acknowledging a history of symptoms that may not be present at the time of his or her clinical visit. The diagnosis is excluded by the existence of conditions that would otherwise account for the degrees of pain and dysfunction. Many clinical conditions share some signs and symptoms of those described in the taxonomy, and it is important to emphasize the need for a careful differential diagnosis of other neuropathic pain syndromes such as peripheral neuropathies in diabetes, infectious or inflammatory disorders, and vasospastic disorders.[17] The criteria for CRPS-II are identical to those of CRPS-I but with the addition of an identifiable nerve lesion.

Perhaps the most significant change in the new diagnostic terminology is removal of the need to make a

BOX 52-1 Diagnostic Criteria for Complex Regional Pain Syndrome

Clinical symptoms and signs

Burning pain
Hyperpathia/allodynia
Temperature/color changes
Edema
Hair/nail growth changes

Laboratory results

Thermometry/thermography
Bone radiograph
Three-phase bone scan
Quantitative sweat test
Response to sympathetic blockade

Interpretation

>6 = Probable complex regional pain syndrome
3-5 = Possible complex regional pain syndrome
< 3 = Unlikely complex regional pain syndrome

From Gibbons JJ, Wilson PR, Lamer TS, Gibson BE: Interscalene blocks for chronic upper extremity pain. Reg Anesth 13:50, 1988.

diagnosis by some form of sympathetic intervention. The concept of sympathetically maintained pain (SMP), originally proposed by Roberts in a hypothesis to explain some of the features of RSD and causalgia, is now defined as *pain that is maintained by sympathetic efferent innervation or by circulating catecholamines*. This is not a clinical diagnosis but rather a clinical phenomenon, the mechanism of which was postulated by Roberts (Fig. 52-1).[18] SMP may be deemed present in a particular disease entity if, following sympatholysis to the painful region, the symptoms are reduced or relieved. The term sympathetically independent pain (SIP), introduced by investigators at Johns Hopkins, can be found in patients who, following a sympatholytic procedure, have no alteration of their symptoms (Fig. 52-2). Interpreting the results of sympathetic blockade may be flawed if less than optimal technical considerations prevail or excessive amounts of local anesthetic agents diffuse to involve not only adjacent somatosensory elements but also the CNS through vascular uptake.[19,20]

The main criticism of the new terminology has been directed toward its relatively low specificity while maintaining a high level of sensitivity.[21,22] As a result, many patients who do not have a diagnosis of CRPS may be included—quite the converse of the previous diagnostic criteria. The other issue is that signs and symptoms including burning pain, atrophy of the skin and nails, dystrophy, and motor abnormalities were not included in the new terminology. On the positive side, however, since its introduction 10 years ago, the new taxonomy has been responsible for a burgeoning literature cataloguing the basic and clinical research of these syndromes. The next section addresses the results of these activities.

EPIDEMIOLOGY

Despite a lack of good prospective epidemiologic studies that address both the incidence and prevalence

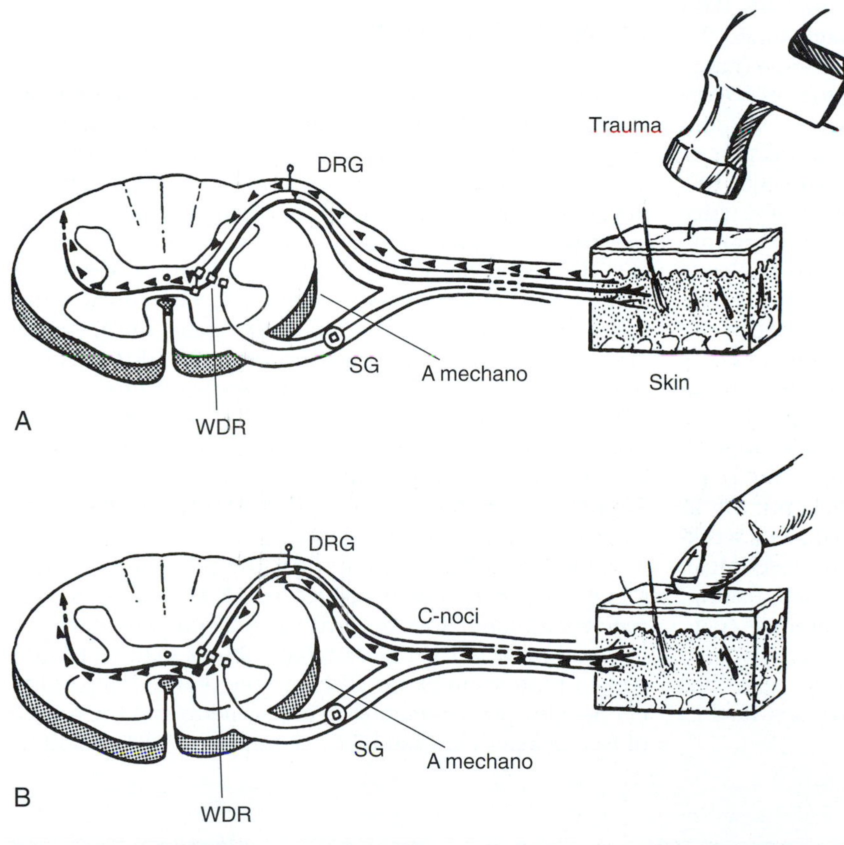

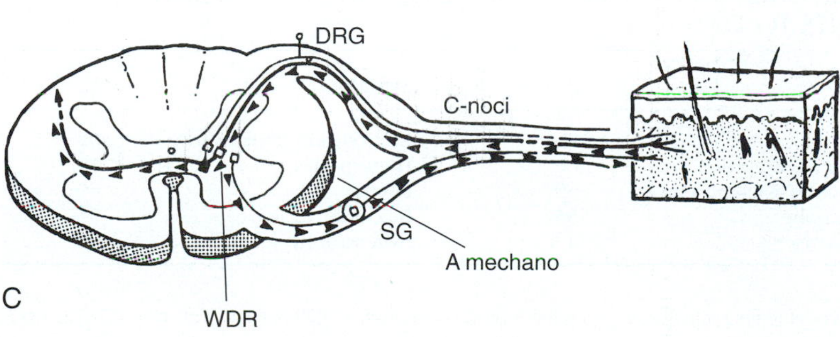

FIGURE 52-1. A schematic representation of Robert's hypothesis on the physiologic basis for causalgia and related pains. **A,** Immediate response to cutaneous trauma. **B,** Sensitization of the wide dynamic-range neurons that respond to the large diameter A mechanoreceptors from light touch. **C,** Allodynia resulting from sensitized wide dynamic-range neurons, the response now being initiated by sympathetic efferent activity. (From WJ Roberts: Practical Management of Pain, 2nd ed. St Louis, Mosby, 1992, p 315.)

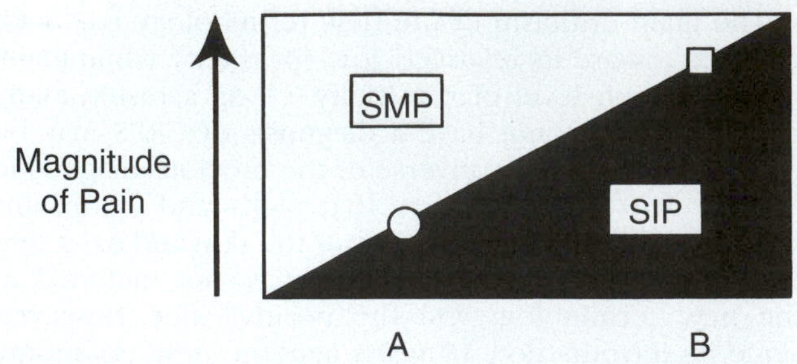

FIGURE 52-2. Demonstrates the relative contribution of sympathetically maintained pain (*SMP*) to total pain. At *A* a patient is predominantly responsive to sympatholysis and therefore has a large component of SMP. At *B* a patient who would barely respond to sympathetic blocks would be regarded as having sympathetically independent pain (*SIP*).

of CRPS, several reports, some quite large, do provide information that was previously only available from anecdotal observations. CRPS was reported in one study to occur in patients with a median age of 41 years (range 4 to 84) and was present for a mean duration of 405 days (Table 52-2); Galer and colleagues[23,24] separately found the prevalence to occur with a median age of 41.8 years (range 18 to 71). Women tend to predominate in a range of 60% to 80%, the mean age of onset varying between 36 and 42 years. Most cases follow an injury such as a fracture or contusion, the incidence of which varies between 10% and 30% of reports. It is well known to occur also after microscopic trauma such as an insect bite or even immunization. In the case of immunization, the disease may present in an extremity that is distant from the site of inoculation. The upper extremity is more frequently affected than the lower in a ratio of 55:45. Bilateral limb involvement occurs in 11% to 16% of patients, (i.e., the disease can be expressed in another extremity with this frequency).

In an excellent review of patients who were injured on the job, 14% occurred in service occupations (e.g., police officers, restaurant workers, and bakers); 8% in clerical and sales professions; 7.4% in manual labor workers (e.g., construction); 5.2% in professional, technical, or managerial occupations; 5.2% in agricultural, fishing, or forestry; 4.4% in bench work occupations (e.g., assembly lines); 2.2% in machine trades (e.g., mechanics); and 4.4% in miscellaneous occupations (e.g., bus drivers and truck drivers). The occupations of a further 5% were not determined.[24]

GENETICS

The fact that patients who develop CRPS may have a genetic predisposition was suggested after a pilot study by Mailis and colleagues.[25] These results are also substantiated by a number of anecdotal reports of siblings and families in which several members have developed the clinical features of CRPS.

PSYCHOLOGICAL FACTORS

Although many attempts have been made to determine whether premorbid psychiatric disease or psychological characteristics might be important for the development of CRPS, an association has not been found. A review by Lynch, who did an exhaustive review of the adult and pediatric literature, found no proof that would be acceptable today or even begin to approach the Cochrane standards in support of premorbid psychological or psychiatric illness in the etiology of CRPS.[26]

PATHOPHYSIOLOGY

The normal (physiologic) inflammatory response to injury includes pain at the site of injury, skin sensitivity, and possibly, depending on its severity, secondary hyperalgesia. This inflammatory response promotes healing and includes a large number of inflammatory mediators—substance P, histamine, calcitonin gene-related peptide (CGRP), bradykinin, leukotrienes, prostaglandins, serotonin, and many other substances. Aδ and C fiber nociceptors mediate this process, and it is postulated that the N-methyl-D-aspartate (NMDA) receptor, substance P, CGRP, and nitric oxide in the CNS are activated in response. Under normal circumstances these inflammatory reactions have a natural history, and the process normally wanes. In CRPS, however, it continues (i.e., an ongoing inflammatory response lasts for months or years). As mentioned already, this aspect was studied by Sudeck in Germany.[5]

Studies by a Dutch group over the past 20 years have focused on what has been described as an exaggerated regional inflammatory response associated with increased microvascular permeability, which allows high-molecular-weight proteins to extravasate into the tissues.[23] Also, high-energy phosphate metabolism impairments and the release of free radicals are claimed to be unique in this condition.

TABLE 52-2 PERCENTAGE IN WHICH SYMPTOMS AND SIGNS ARE EXPRESSED IN THE LARGEST PROSPECTIVE STUDY (829) OF CRPS PATIENTS TO DATE

Symptom	%	Symptom	%	Symptom	%
Paresis	95	Pain	93	Altered skin temperature	92
Skin color changes	92	Limited range of motion	88	Hyperpathia	79
Hyperesthesia	76	Hypoesthesia (stocking/glove)	69	Edema	69
Altered nail or hair growth	60	Muscle atrophy	55	Incoordination	55
Tremor	49	Hyperhidrosis	47	Skin atrophy	40

CRPS, complex regional pain syndrome.
From Veldman PH, Reynen HM, Arnta IE, et al: Signs and symptoms of reflex sympathetic dystrophy: A prospective study of 829 patients. Lancet 342:1012, 1993.

Although for decades it was believed that the sympathetic nervous system was hyperactive, recent investigations have refuted this hypothesis. In fact, plasma catecholamine concentrations drawn from the affected extremity are lower than those taken from other extremities.[27] Laser Doppler and venous occlusion plethysmographic studies of the microcirculation clearly demonstrate a paralysis of vasomotion not only in the symptomatic limb but also in other extremities.[28] Although a paucity of histochemical studies have been undertaken, those in the literature report no atypical fibers in the hyperalgesic skin of CRPS patients. Also, no increase in the catecholamine receptor population is found in skin biopsies.[29] No correlation between skin temperature and vasomotor activity has been found. Lastly, a significantly large number of patients meeting criteria for CRPS do not respond positively with pain relief to sympathetic blocking.

In fact, ample evidence favors an upregulation of adrenergic receptor activity, particularly with progression of this syndrome. Similar findings have also been identified in patients with post-herpetic neuralgia.

SENSORY ABNORMALITIES

The commonest pain of which CRPS patients complain is a deep-seated, spontaneous, burning pain. This pain is out of proportion in intensity to the inciting event. Movement causes a deeply felt pain (somatic allodynia). These findings have been reported by clinicians for years. In fact, it is the basis for a particular form of exercise therapy termed "stress loading," which uses isometric exercises as one of its components to avoid pain that arises from joint movement.[30] Both central and peripheral sensitization are postulated to explain the allodynia or hyperalgesia, or both, that occur in the affected extremity.

A comparatively recent observation is that hemicorporeal hypoesthesia and hypoalgesia can be demonstrated ipsilateral to the disease process.[31] In fact, quantitative sensory testing (QST) demonstrates the decreased thresholds to noxious stimuli from mechanical, cold, and heat sources. There appears to be a direct correlation with duration of the illness and these responses. Because of the precise anatomical distribution of these sensory abnormalities, the source must involve processing in the CNS, most likely involving the midbrain thalamus and cortex. Recent PET studies have correlated changes in the thalamus with progression of the disease.[32] Similarly, electromyogram (EMG) studies have also demonstrated a reduction in the representations of finger and thumb in the S1 cortex of the painful side.[33] The foregoing sensory changes are irreversible and are well described by patients, even after resolution of their main clinical signs, suggesting irreversible neuroplastic changes have occurred in the CNS.[34]

Butler has postulated a "neglect-like" syndrome.[35] In a manner like patients after a stroke, patients with CRPS often regard the affected limb as "not being a part of them." In fact, it can be quite difficult and may take some time before a patient can initiate movement in the affected extremity. The same author also suggested that the "neglect-like" syndrome results from neuroplastic changes in the brain, particularly that part involving autonomic control. This explanation is in contradistinction to the previously held view that guarding the affected extremity results from a patient's fear of movement-induced pain. Although similar changes are seen following prolonged casting of an extremity, patients without CRPS rapidly reverse these changes with exercise.

SYMPATHETICALLY MAINTAINED PAIN

Recent studies in humans have provided some insight to this phenomenon.[36,37] In patients with CRPS of an extremity, the cutaneous sympathetic vasoconstrictor outflow was activated by whole body cooling. The ipsilateral extremity, however, was clamped to 35° C to obviate any thermal effects on nociceptors. The intensity of spontaneous pain and mechanical hyperalgesia (both static and dynamic) significantly increased in patients who had previously been classified as having SMP after a positive result from sympathetic blockade. Patients classified as having SIP had no increase in symptoms.[38] The investigators noted that the sympathetic challenge only influenced cutaneous sympathetic vasoconstrictor fibers without affecting the sympathetic supply innervating deep somatic structures (muscle vasoconstrictor neurons).[39,40] The authors suggested that interaction of the sympathetic terminals and afferent nociceptors is most likely located in the skin, as has been demonstrated by the injection of intracutaneous norepinephrine, which elicits an increase in symptoms of patients who have CRPS-II. The relief of both spontaneous and evoked pain was much more evident after sympathetic blockade than any changes that might be elicited through experimental activation of the sympathetic nervous system.[39] The results also suggest that the *extreme* joint pain experienced by some patients with CRPS may be due to the sympathetic-afferent interaction, particularly in deep somatic tissues such as bone, muscle, and joint.[39,40]

The underlying mechanisms of SMP postulated are a coupling between the noradrenergic sympathetic efferent neurons and the primary afferent (PA) fibers in the periphery.[41] Although several well-established animal models have been used to study this effect after nerve lesions, there are no suitable animal models to study SMP in CRPS. For this reason it is impossible to infer that the SMP phenomenon can be explained simply by a similar mechanism. Many animal experiments, however, have explored the possibility of sympathetic afferent coupling in animals, which do not involve efferent activity in sympathetic fibers. Certainly, the potentiation of the inflammatory response from substances such as nerve growth factor (NGF), bradykinin, and others may be extremely important to the genesis of pain that is experienced in CRPS. Also, coupling of sympathetic activity to nociceptive neurons by adrenomedullary release of epinephrine can lead to the sensitization of nociceptors in this model. Of what importance this association may be to humans with CRPS is unknown.

Finally, in what manner sympatholysis can provide prolonged relief of pain in patients with CRPS and therefore be categorized as having SMP remains an enigma. In some cases, the effect of this block can be permanent.

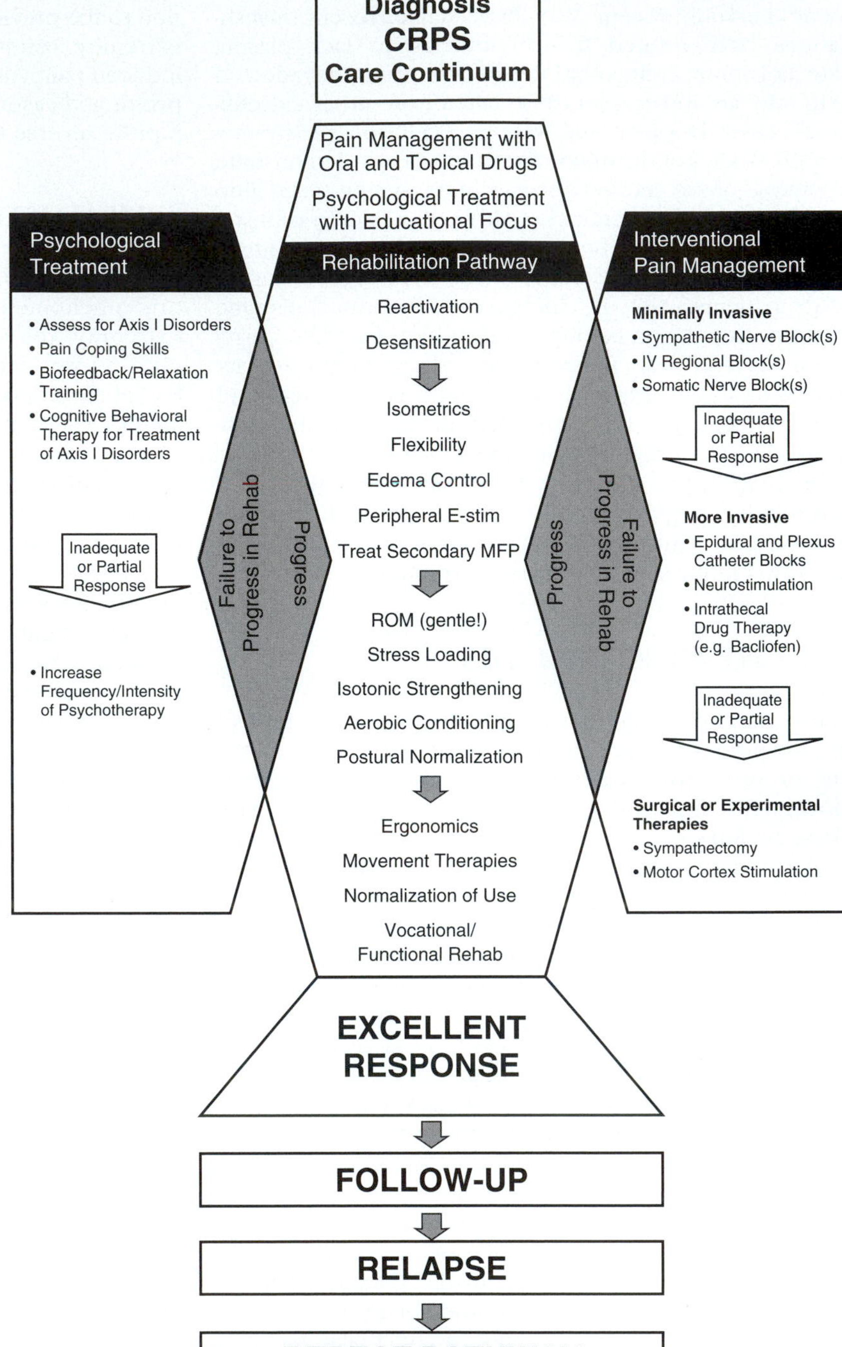

FIGURE 52-3. Postulated relationship of sympathetically maintained pain to other medical conditions and a proposed association in patients with autonomic signs.

This question has been asked by Baron and colleagues[37] who suggest that the activity in sympathetic neurons, of central origin, may maintain a positive feedback circuit via the primary afferent neurons. Although no animal models have demonstrated this effect, these authors suggested that a central state of hyperexcitability of central neurons—in the dorsal horn—are stimulated by the intense nociceptive input. They suggested that this central hyperexcitability is temporarily relieved by sympathetic block lasting at least the pharmacologic duration of the local anesthetic used and then remains quiescent in some cases. Perhaps the sympathetic distribution to deep somatic tissues is more important for a hypothetic positive feedback, a hypothesis that requires experimental exploration. The reader is reminded that SMP can be demonstrated in numerous medical conditions (Fig. 52-3).

SYMPATHETIC DYSREGULATION

A typical clinical sign in early CRPS-I is warm, frequently hyperhidrotic skin. In later CRPS-I many patients (79%) have hypohidrotic skin.[42] The resting sweat output (RSO) and axon reflex sweating (stimulated) is increased in patients with CRPS-I. The increase in sweat production can only be explained by a central mechanism. In a number of studies by Wasner and colleagues,[43] sympathetic effector organ function was studied by measuring bilateral changes in temperature and blood flow by laser Doppler flowmetry. Normally, sympathetic reflexes do not show side-to-side differences. These investigators found three distinct patterns:

1. In a **warm regulation type** (duration of CRPS <6 months) the affected limb was warm and skin perfusion values higher than the contralateral extremity throughout the entire spectrum of sympathetic activity. Of note is that total body cooling and respiratory stimuli failed to demonstrate any activity in the sympathetic vasoconstrictor neurons. Noradrenaline levels from the affected region were reduced in the ipsilateral extremity.
2. In the **intermediate type**, the temperature and perfusion were either higher or lower depending on the degree of sympathetic activity.
3. In the **cold type** (CRPS >6 months), both temperature and perfusion were lower on the affected side throughout the entire thermoregulatory cycle. Norepinephrine levels, however, were lower on the affected side.

To summarize the foregoing results, those alterations of cutaneous vasoconstrictor and respiration-related reflex activities that occur in acute CRPS-I patients are most likely to result from central changes in the cutaneous vasoconstrictor system rather than changes of neurovascular transmission (development of super sensitivity in vascular smooth muscle). With successful treatment of CRPS, these are reversible.

Secondary changes of neurovascular transmission that have been observed and related to the supersensitivity of vascular smooth muscle (resulting from chronically decreased vasoconstrictor neuronal activity) could explain the severe vasoconstriction and cold skin that are hallmarks of chronic CRPS-I. Radioisotope labeling shows an increase in α-adrenoceptors from skin biopsies of patients with CRPS-I.

MYOFASCIAL DYSFUNCTION

Motor dysfunction is observed in more than 70% of all patients with CRPS.[44,45] Specifically, fine movements are impaired, but conduction and electromyographic studies are normal other than in patients who have advanced disease. One half of the patients have a postural or action tremor and 10% of the patients demonstrate dystonia of the affected hand or foot.

Recent experiments strongly suggest that the somatomotor changes are of a central nature due to a changed activity in the α-motor neurons, possibly due to a change in spinal reflex circuitry.[45] Why the motor abnormalities immediately disappear after sympathetic block is unknown.

Kinematic analysis of "target reaching" and grip force analysis have been used to assess motor deficits in CRPS patients. Abnormal central programming and processing of motor tasks may have at their bases a pathologic sensory motor integration in the parietal cortex. Interestingly, some contralateral impairment was also observed in these experiments. Magnet encephalography (MEG) analysis suggested that the 20-Hz motor cortex interoscillation to tactile stimulation in CRPS patients was altered, implying a sustained inhibition of the motor cortex.[45]

INFLAMMATION

One of the commonest signs in acute CRPS is persistent edema that extends well beyond the territory of the inciting trauma.[46] This edema responds clinically to aggravating stimuli such as loud noise, emotion, movement of the part, and mechanical- or thermal-induced stimulation. The dramatic reduction in edema—within 2 hours—after sympathetic blockade suggests its dependence on activity in postganglionic sympathetic neurons. Although the mechanism is unknown, it has been suggested that there is incongruence between the vasoconstrictor activity of precapillary and postcapillary blood vessels. In fact, venous occlusion plethysmography has demonstrated that a higher hydrostatic pressure is necessary to achieve capillary filtration on the affected side of patients with CRPS.[28]

Scintigraphic studies using radiolabeled immunoglobulins demonstrate extensive plasma extravasation in patients with acute CRPS-I. Skin microdialysis in CRPS patients demonstrates increased serum levels of calcitonin gene–related peptide (CGRP) and neurogenic inflammatory activation of peptidergic afferents. Increased levels of IL-6 and tumor necrosis factor-alpha are noted in artificially produced skin blisters ipsilateral to the disease. Although these findings certainly demonstrate an unusual form of inflammatory response, it cannot be stated clearly whether they are a consequence of neuroprocesses or whether they are the primary event. What is clear, however, is that in some way the sympathetic nervous system effects the intensity of inflammation that occurs in CRPS.

PSYCHOLOGICAL FACTORS

As stated earlier, no recent extensive review of the psychological literature has identified premorbid psychological factors. Ochoa and colleagues,[47] who have written extensively on this subject, suggest that the clinical features of CRPS are primarily of a psychogenic nature. They postulate that because they cannot demonstrate by neurophysiologic testing any definable abnormality and because many patients demonstrate a placebo response to various interventions, the clinical entity must be of a psychogenic nature. To substantiate this hypothesis, electrodiagnostic testing should be normal in cases of CRPS-I. Additionally, however, testing by neurophysiologic means does not have the specificity to unravel the pathophysiology associated with CRPS in humans. No tests of altered CNS processing, peripheral altered receptor affinity, or the observance of aberrant synapse formation are available to evaluate at this time.[48] All of the reported placebo responses were derived from single-blinded placebo trials, suggesting bias, and therefore render the responses invalid.

SYMPTOMATOLOGY

Without specific mechanistic-based laboratory tests to corroborate a diagnosis of CRPS, the clinician is left with the presenting symptoms and signs to make a diagnosis. In the absence of evidence-based criteria, validation studies have been used to support a clinical diagnosis. Typical examples of diagnostic criteria are those for migraine by the International Headache Society and those for depression, which appear in the *Diagnostic and Statistical Manual*.[49,50] Three recent studies are reported to assess the validity of self-reported symptoms in the diagnosis of CRPS.[22,51,52] The pattern of frequencies across signs and symptoms is important to its diagnosis. As described in the new taxonomy, however, objective signs are useful, acknowledging the fact that, as in many medical conditions, these signs may vary over time.[21,23,53]

SITE/INCIDENCE OF SPREAD AND RECURRENCE

The commonest site for the expression of CRPS is the distal portion of a limb. CRPS is also reported to occur in the face, breast, and genitalia. CRPS may also spread to other body regions with an incidence of 10%. This spread has been divided into three categories: (1) contiguous, (2) contralateral, and (3) distant.[54] After remission, the syndrome may recur in the same or other limb.[75]

Common to this condition is a proximal myofascial disturbance that is manifested by burning dysesthesia, muscle irritability, and spasm similar to those experienced in the primary site. As the disease progresses, both shoulder and pelvic girdles, respectively, become symptomatic and reflect progression of the disease. In the upper extremity it is common for the ipsilateral side of the face and neck to become involved.

Vasomotor changes are manifested by side-to-side temperature differences that are variable during the acute stage but later become cold.[46] These are associated with changes in skin color that may vary from mottled purple and pale to bright red. Changes vary with ambient temperature and also with time. Color changes correlate with the skin temperature. Some patients develop rashes and, in particular, punctate skin lesions that are of an ischemic nature, initially vesicular and later ulcerating. The regional skin typically becomes dry and scaly, with loss of turgor.

Edema may be mild to pitting, and sometimes patients complain of a feeling of swelling without there being any clinical evidence of edema. Sweat abnormalities include hyperhidrosis, generally early in the disease, and reduced sweating later or in chronic cases. The latter dysfunction is typically manifested by dry and scaly skin.[46]

Although the motor abnormalities have not been accorded the distinction of a specific movement disorder, changes in muscle activity have been clinically described for decades. Most patients admit to weakness and an inability to hold objects. Also, with CRPS of the lower extremities, patients typically report that they stumble or trip on uneven surfaces. This degree of muscle dysfunction has been overlooked by clinicians despite early observations by Evans and Livingstone, the latter of whom described muscle spasms as being a key to his postulated vicious cycle.[7,10]

Trophic changes, classically of the integument, are much less common than previously believed. These include altered hair growth, slow or rapid nail growth, brittle nails, tendon shortening, capsular swelling, and muscular atrophy. Although such changes tend to occur more frequently in chronic cases, they are not included in the new taxonomy because of the comparatively small numbers of patients exhibiting such obvious features.

LABORATORY TESTS

Although the CRPS criteria do not call for supplemental laboratory tests, four tests are cited repeatedly in the literature as being helpful to substantiate a clinical diagnosis.

Autonomic Testing The quantitative sudomotor axon reflex test (QSART) is a test of the axon reflex that induces sweating.[55] The QSART test depends on activity in peripheral sudomotor units and is responsible for increased sudomotor activity early in the course of the disease. Later, however, it tends to be decreased (i.e., in patients with long-standing CRPS). In a recent prospective evaluation, the originators of this study have validated their data.[51,52,56] Results suggest a concordance of approximately 78% in patients with a clinical diagnosis of CRPS.

Thermographic Imaging This has undergone rigorous testing, the results of which suggest its validity as a diagnostic tool in CRPS when there are temperature side-to-side differences of at least 0.6° C.[53] The method of temperature measurement has optimal sensitivity and specificity. If this test is performed in conjunction with the cold pressor test, delay in any cooling or rewarming of ipsilateral and contralateral extremities is strongly suggestive of autonomic dysfunction, which, with good clinical criteria, support the diagnosis. The latter results have not been validated however.

Electrodiagnostic Studies As indicated earlier in this account, electromyography and nerve conduction testing may indicate large fiber injury consistent with a diagnosis of CRPS-II. However, quantitative sensory testing can provide information regarding axonal function in small and large fibers. In particular, the function in fibers subserving thermal, cold, and vibration modalities reflect axonal loss consistent with conditions like CRPS. This is a sensitive test.[57]

Bone Scan Bone scintigraphy (three-phase bone scan) has been proposed as a useful diagnostic tool in support of a clinical diagnosis of CRPS since 1981.[58] Originally, a sensitivity of 67% and specificity of 86% were claimed; however, several subsequent studies have questioned its veracity.[59] Most recently, fourth and fifth phases have been added to the testing sequence. These results have not been validated by prospective studies.

TREATMENT

Of all the treatments and remedies that have been introduced over the years, none can be said to effect a cure for CRPS. Treatment approaches have tended to reflect the particular resources of each medical discipline or treating clinician and, in most cases, have been monotherapies that do not acknowledge the varying clinical presentations and pathophysiologies of these syndromes. Excellent and extensive reviews of the literature have been published by Kingery and Tanelian.[60,61] The published literature demonstrates a few prospective, controlled clinical trials, although more recently some prospective studies of monotherapies have reported symptomatic benefit for CRPS.[62-64] Most significant, however, is a lack of published trials that affirm any long-term improvement of function. It should also be stressed that although classic teaching has supported the use of sympathetic nerve blockade, no data exist to suggest any *long-term* efficacy with this treatment.

What is now clear, however, is that management of CRPS, rather than its treatment to effect a remission, requires a multidisciplinary approach. The aim of treatment is to support the patient psychologically and medically to reduce the impact of symptoms on the disease course and to promote active functional restoration. The physician's role is crucial in this respect. Irrespective of the clinical background, his or her purpose is to coordinate a treatment team that can identify and manage any comorbid behavioral features such as anxiety, post-traumatic stress disorder, and depression that would, if untreated, hinder a successful outcome. The role of exercise therapy, both physical and occupational, is the crux of treatment. In the absence of a known mechanism that would otherwise be the target for medical treatment, all interventions, whether pharmacologic, regional anesthetic, surgical, or behavioral, must be fully integrated if the management of these patients is to be successful.

In 1998 clinical guidelines were published to assist clinicians in building a treatment plan around a pathway of functional restoration.[64] Monotherapy, by itself, is unlikely to be successful in the management of CRPS-I and CRPS-II. These guidelines emphasize certain principles that include motivation, desensitization, and mobilization, the last of which is assisted by the relief of pain. Although it was felt that the proposed therapeutic pathway would be more useful than the previously isolated monotherapeutic measures that have been the hallmarks of traditional therapy, the initial algorithm did not allow for the fact that these syndromes have varying temporal rates of progression. In fact, CRPS may represent a multitude of patient subgroups with different pathophysiologic mechanisms and etiologic factors that are influenced by multiple factors. Thus, while describing this syndrome as a single disease entity, one must respond to these multiple presentations. Most recently, an "updated" clinical pathway (guideline) has been published (Fig. 52-4).[65]

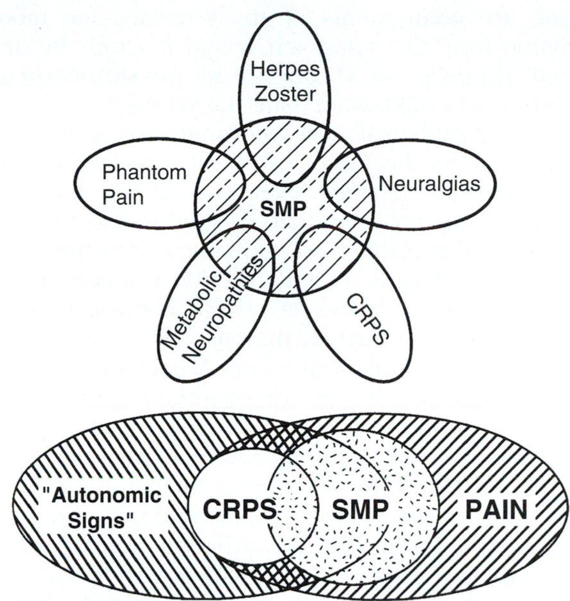

FIGURE 52-4. Physiotherapeutic pathway and algorithm for complex regional pain syndrome. Different therapeutic options are shown on either side of the rehabilitation pathway. There are no constraints as to when any modality may be employed. Rather, the failure to progress is sufficient reason to use whatever means is considered appropriate at the time.[66] (From Stanton-Hicks M, Burton AW, Bruehl SP, et al: An updated interdisciplinary clinical pathway for CRPS: Report of an expert panel. Pain Pract 2:1, 2002.)

This guideline also comprises the same three domains, namely rehabilitation, pain management, and psychological treatment. It likewise emphasizes the interdisciplinary, time-contingent guidance that is the foundation of the previous guideline, but it differs in an important aspect by allowing access to any therapeutic modality at any time during the course of functional restoration, rather than the concept of only using more invasive modalities when other simpler methods have been exhausted. Clinical experience with this disease process clearly underscores the need to respond rapidly to any deterioration or failure in the response to current therapy. In fact, time may not be an ally of the treating physician because of the biologic neuroplastic changes to chronic pain that have been demonstrated in laboratory animals. These changes are irreversible.

REHABILITATION

Functional restoration is the primary treatment, and for CRPS-I and CRPS-II it is quite different from the type of exercise therapy used for other injuries. Patients must be assessed by the therapist to determine the degree of motivation and set goals, but most importantly, to evaluate the patient's compliance in relation to his symptoms. The concept of "stress loading" introduced by Watson and Carlson in 1987 acknowledges the change in mechanoreceptor function that has been demonstrated in animals.[30] With good education, adequate analgesia, and encouragement, the physical modalities of desensitization, isometric exercises, and gentle resisted range of motion are components of the stress-loading model. Deviation from this approach would not only be detrimental to progress through the physiotherapeutic algorithm but could exacerbate the syndrome.

The associated myofascial syndrome must be addressed concurrently by the use of electrical stimulation, trigger point injections, postural exercises, and, if the lower extremities are involved, gait correction. Validated evidence is now available to support these measures in the management of patients with CRPS.[64] Concurrent with these physical modalities is edema control. This may require elevation; retrograde massage; the use of compression stockings; pumps; sympathetic blocks; diuretics; and, in the presence of SMP, the use of adrenoceptor-blocking agents such as terazosin, prazosin, or phenoxybenzamine.

To maintain progress along the functional restoration pathway, stress-loading techniques including scrubbing, distraction, and general aerobic conditioning are incorporated. Should pain or an exacerbation of the syndrome prevent further progress, immediate attention should be focused on the treatments at this juncture and whatever intervention is felt appropriate at the time should be instituted. Behavioral management of patients with CRPS should focus on quality of life; cognitive behavioral psychotherapy where indicated; and, most importantly, helping the patient to develop coping skills. Most patients confronted with their diagnosis are apprehensive, not only because of the degree of their disability but because of the misinformation they have received through contemporary means, particularly the Internet. As a result, patients may have an extremely negative view of their future and therefore require strong psychological support, which should be a major component of education. Education should include the importance for reactivation of their affected extremity and all measures that will be used to achieve this purpose.

Obviously, psychological factors play increasing parts as the disease progresses. Any comorbid Axis I (meaning clinical psychiatric diagnosis) psychiatric disorders require identification and treatment. Relaxation training is used for pain control and as an integral part of cognitive behavioral psychotherapy. The use of surface EMG biofeedback or other biofeedback modalities can be helpful. A particular advantage of EMG biofeedback is its ability to anticipate possible secondary myofascial pain that accompanies CRPS. Family members should be recruited in the overall program of functional restoration. Although well meaning, they can also interfere with the patient's progress, such as when they have unrealistic concerns regarding pain and tissue damage. An intimate collaboration among the psychologist, physical and occupational therapists, and physician is critical to a successful outcome.

PAIN MANAGEMENT

As this is the cardinal feature of CRPS syndromes, any treatment program that omits the control of pain is doomed to failure. Management of pain control must be flexible and dynamic in response to temporal change of the disease. Although less invasive strategies form the basis of management, the use of regional anesthetic techniques or more surgically invasive techniques must be considered whenever these are no longer effective or if the patient's condition markedly deteriorates.

Pharmacologic management should be symptomatic and include drugs that have been found useful in the treatment of neuropathic pain, such as tricyclic antidepressants (e.g., amitriptyline), antiepileptics (gabapentin, in particular), and the antiarrhythmic, mexiletine. Steroids during the onset of the condition are efficacious for treating the inflammatory component and in some cases do affect a remission. The use of anti-inflammatory agents, either the COX-1 or COX-2 inhibiting nonsteroidal anti-inflammatory drugs, may help with the deep-seated musculoskeletal symptoms. Biphosphonates such as pamidronate have a demonstrated efficacy in early CRPS. The α_2-adrenoceptor agonist clonidine has undergone significant investigation and may be used either transdermally or by epidural administration. Off-label experience with N-methyl-D-aspartate antagonists such as ketamine has demonstrated some efficacy, although the results of long-term outcome following treatment is wanting and no prospective clinical studies have been developed. Preclinical studies have, however, demonstrated promising results.

REGIONAL ANESTHETIC PROCEDURES

Local anesthetic blocks, particularly sympathetic, should be considered as adjuncts to rehabilitation rather than primary therapeutic modalities, notwithstanding that in a small number of cases the response may be salutary. Most sympathetic blocks—stellate ganglion or lumbar sympathetic for the upper and lower extremities, respectively—are useful diagnostic procedures that may reveal the presence of SMP. In such cases a trial of oral α-adrenoceptor blocking agents such as terazosin, phenoxybenzamine, or prazosin may prove useful in the ongoing management of this type of pain. A continuous somatosensory block by epidural infusion can be used to provide prolonged analgesia over a period of weeks or months. This technique can be used to assist rehabilitation. The advantages of the epidural route allow a number of agents, including local anesthetics, opiates, and α_2-adrenergic agonists to be used. In the largest randomized-blinded trial of epidural analgesia, Rauck and colleagues demonstrated significantly reduced pain scores compared with placebo in patients who receive epidural clonidine.[67] In the past, IV regional anesthesia was used widely for upper extremity pain. Recent data suggest that this relief is only of a comparatively short duration. For this reason, the technique requires a much larger, randomized, controlled trial to determine its place as a therapeutic adjunct.

NEUROSTIMULATION

Until recently there was only anecdotal evidence to support the use of neurostimulation, particularly spinal cord stimulation for pain management in CRPS patients.

A randomized, prospective, controlled trial by Kemler and colleagues[61] has highlighted the usefulness of spinal cord stimulation. Two other studies have demonstrated a significant improvement in not only pain but also a reduction in the motor dysfunction of patients with CRPS.[68,69] The Kemler study demonstrated a significantly reduced pain intensity and higher global perceived effect (GPE).

Peripheral nerve stimulation has also been used successfully to manage CRPS-II pain. In a prospective trial of 32 consecutive patients with CRPS, Hassenbusch and colleagues[70] reported favorable results. The long-term response rate was rated as good to fair relief in 63%. Twenty percent of these patients returned to work. Both allodynia and spontaneous pain were significantly reduced in all responders.

INTRATHECAL DRUG DELIVERY

In a prospective, randomized, controlled crossover study, Van Hilten and colleagues[63] reported that 50% of patients who suffered from severe dystonia of the upper extremities receiving continuous intrathecal baclofen regained normal hand function, and a further 33% who had complete impairment of lower extremity function regained their ability to walk. Side effects were said to be mild to moderate.

SYMPATHECTOMY

Evidence in support of sympathectomy is limited. Although it is more common now to use radiofrequency neurolysis at the sympathetic chain in patients who have been determined to suffer from SMP, no prospective, large, controlled trials have been undertaken. Data concerning surgical sympathectomy in CRPS patients are all taken from retrospective studies. The purported successful outcomes range from 70% to 85%. In one study, Schwartzman and colleagues[71] found that of 29 patients, those who had a significantly long duration of symptoms before their surgery did poorly in comparison with those with shorter histories. However, a number of reports indicate that patients who had surgical sympathectomy were distinctly worse in terms of their symptoms and general function.[72]

MOTOR CORTEX AND DEEP BRAIN STIMULATION

Although no specific study on deep brain stimulation for the management of CRPS has been conducted, improvement in approximately 30% to 40% of patients with intractable neuropathic pain has been reported.[73] Epidural motor cortex stimulation, which has been proposed for the treatment of some central pain states, has been successful in reducing the dysesthetic pain, particularly heat hyperalgesia in a small number of CRPS patients.[74] These patients have failed all other previous pharmacologic and nonpharmacologic invasive techniques.

CONCLUSION

Although the key to managing CRPS is early diagnosis, management of the clinical entity should follow a multidisciplinary approach, the goal of which is functional restoration. This requires the coordination of medical specialists, exercise therapists, and behavioral treatment to motivate and encourage the patient along a physiotherapeutic pathway. Although pain relief is fundamental to any success, the outcome is less predictable and likely to fail if therapeutical measures do not include stress management, supportive psychotherapy, and the treatment of any comorbid psychological aspects. At best, a complete remission of the syndrome is possible in a high percentage of cases. Early diagnosis, however, is paramount if the foregoing measures are to prove successful. Importantly, more invasive management should not be withheld in the event that a failure to progress or worse, a decrement in progress, should occur. No treatment that is without significant improvement over a period of 10 to 12 weeks should continue before alternative measures or more interventional management is implemented. Until such time as treatment can be based on a mechanism, the foregoing measures can be successful in achieving a remission and more favorable outcomes than have been reported in the past.

REFERENCES

1. Medical Research Council: The diagnosis and treatment of peripheral nerve injuries. Med Res Counc Spec Rep 54:1, 1920.
2. Mitchell SW: On the diseases of nerves, resulting from injuries. In Flint A (ed): Contributions relating to the causation and prevention of disease, and to camp diseases. New York, U.S. Sanitary Commission Memoirs, 1867.
3. Wolff J, Uebereine N: Fall von Ellenogengelenks-Reaktion: Arch Klin Chir 20:771, 1877.
4. Kummell H: Ueber die traumatischen Erkrankungen der Wirbelsäule. Deutsch Med Wchnschr 21:18, 1895.
5. Südeck P: Ueber die akute enzündliche Knochenatrophie. Arch Klin Chir 62:147, 1900.
6. Fontaine R, Herrmann LG: Post-traumatic painful osteoporosis. Ann Surg 97:26, 1933.
7. Livingston WK: Post-traumatic pain syndromes. West J Surg Obstet Gynecol 46:341, 1938.
8. DeTakats G: Reflex sympathetic dystrophy of extremities. Arch Surg 34:939, 1937.
9. Homans J: Minor causalgia. N Engl J Med, 222:870, 1940.
10. Evans JA: Reflex sympathetic dystrophy. Surg Gynecol Obstet 82:36, 1946.
11. Leriche R: Da La causalgie envisageé comme une nevrite du sympathique et des son traitement par la dénudation et l'exision des plexus nerveux periartériels. Presse Med 17:8, 1916.
12. Bonica JJ: The management of pain. Philadelphia, Lea & Febiger, 1953.
13. Gibbons JJ, Wilson PR, Lamer TS, Gibson BE: Interscalene blocks for chronic upper extremity pain. Reg Anesth 13:50, 1988.
14. Stanton-Hicks M, Jänig W, Hassenbusch S, et al: Reflex sympathetic dystrophy: Changing concepts and taxonomy. Pain 63:127, 1995.
15. Stanton-Hicks M, Jänig W, Hassenbusch S, et al: Reflex sympathetic dystrophy: Changing concepts and taxonomy. Pain 63:127, 1998.
16. Merskey H, Bogduk N: Classification of chronic pain: Descriptions of chronic pain syndromes and definition of pain terms, 2nd ed. Seattle, IASP Press, 1994.
17. Boas RA: Complex regional pain syndrome: Symptoms, signs and differential diagnosis. In Jänig W, Stanton-Hicks M (eds): Reflex sympathetic dystrophy: A reappraisal. Progress in pain research and management, vol 6. Seattle, IASP Press, 1996, pp 79-92.

18. Roberts WJ: A hypothesis on the physiologic basis for causalgia and related pains. Pain 24:297, 1986.
19. Backonja N, Gombar K: Serum lidocaine levels following stellate ganglion sympathetic blocks and intravenous lidocaine injection. J Pain Symptom Manage 7:2, 1992.
20. Wulf H, Glein M, Schele HA: Plasma concentrations of bupivacaine after lumbar sympathetic block. Anesth Analg 79:918, 1994.
21. Galer BS, Bruehl S, Harden RN: IASP diagnostic criteria for complex regional pain syndrome: A preliminary empirical validation study. Clin J Pain 14:48, 1998.
22. Harden RN, Bruehl S, Galer BS, et al: Complex regional pain syndrome: Are the IASP diagnostic criteria valid and sufficiently comprehensive? Pain 83:211, 1999.
23. Veldman PH, Reynen HM, Arntz IE, et al: Signs and symptoms of reflex sympathetic dystrophy: A prospective study of 829 patients. Lancet 342:1012, 1993.
24. Allen G, Galer BS, Schwartz L: Epidemiological review of 134 patients with complex regional pain syndrome assessed in a chronic pain clinic. Pain 80:539, 1999.
25. Mailis A, Wade J: Profile of Caucasian women with possible genetic predisposition to reflex sympathetic dystrophy: A pilot study. Clin J Pain 10:210, 1994.
26. Lynch ME: Psychological aspects of reflex sympathetic dystrophy: A review of the adult and pediatric literature. Pain 49:337, 1992.
27. Harden RN, Duc TA, Windress TR, et al: Norepinephrine and epinephrine levels in affected versus unaffected limbs in sympathetically maintained pain. Clin J Pain 10:324, 1994.
28. Schurmann M, Zaspel J, Gradl G, et al: Assessment of the peripheral microcirculation using computer-assisted venous occlusion plethysmography in post-traumatic complex regional pain syndrome type I. J Vasc Res 38:453, 2001.
29. Drummond PD, Skipworth S, Finch PN: Alpha-1 adrenoceptors in normal and hyperalgesic human skin. Clin Sci (Colch) 91:737, 1996.
30. Watson Hk, Carlson L: Treatment of reflex sympathetic dystrophy of the hand with an active "stress loading" program. J Hand Surg [Am] 12:729, 1987.
31. Rommel O, Gehling M, Dertwinkel R, et al: Hemisensory impairment in patients with complex regional pain syndrome. Pain 80:95, 1999.
32. Iadorola MJ, Max MB, Berman KF, et al: Unilateral decrease in thalamic activity observed with positron emission tomography in patients with chronic neuropathic pain. Pain 63:55, 1995.
33. Gelnar PA, Krauss BR, Sheehe PR, et al: A comparative fMRI study of cortical representations for thermal painful, vibrotactile and motor performance tasks. Neuroimage 10:460, 1999.
34. Woolf CJ, Mannion RJ: Neuropathic pain: Etiology, symptoms, mechanisms and magnagement. Lancet 353:1859, 1999.
35. Galer BS, Butler S, Jensen M: Case reports and hypothesis: A neglect-like syndrome may be responsible for the motor disturbance in reflex sympathetic dystrophy. J Pain Symptom Manage 10:385, 1995.
36. Baron R, Maier C: Reflex sympathetic dystrophy: Skin blood flow, sympathetic vasoconstrictor reflexes in pain before and after surgical sympathectomy. Pain 67:317, 1996.
37. Baron R, Schattschnider J, Binder A, et al: Relation between sympathetic vasoconstrictor activity in pain and hyperalgesia in complex regional pain syndromes: A case control study. Lancet 359:1655, 2002.
38. Raja SN, Treede R-D, Davis KD, Campbell JN: Systemic alpha-adrenergic blockade with phentolamine: A diagnostic test of sympathetically maintained pain. Anesthesiology 74:691, 1991.
39. Janig W, McLachlan EM: Neurobiology of the autonomic nervous system. In Mathias CJ, Bannister R (eds): Autonomic failure, 4th ed. Oxford, Oxford University Press, 1999, pp 3-15.
40. Jänig W, Habler HJ: Sympathetic nervous system: Contribution to chronic pain. Prog Brain Res 129:451, 2000.
41. Jänig W, Levin JD, Michaelis N: Interactions of the sympathetic and primary afferent neurons following nerve injury and tissue trauma. Prog Brain Res 113:161, 1996.
42. Birklein F, Sittle R, Spitzer A, et al: Sudomotor function in sympathetic reflex dystrophy. Pain 69:49, 1997.
43. Wasner G, Schattschneider J, Heckmann K, et al: Vascular abnormalities in reflex sympathetic dystrophy (CRPS I): Mechanisms and diagnostic value. Brain 124:587, 2001.
44. Schwartzman RJ, Kerrigan J: The movement disorder of reflex sympathetic dystrophy. Neurology 40:57, 1990.
45. Rashiq S, Galer BS: Proximal myofascial dysfunction in complex regional pain syndrome: A retrospective prevalence study. Clin J Pain 15:151, 1999.
46. Blumberg H, Hoffman U, Mohadjer M, Scheremet R: Clinical phenomenology and mechanisms of reflex sympathetic dystrophy: Emphasis on edema. In Gephardt GF, Hammond DL, Jensen TS (eds): Proceedings of the 7th World Congress on Pain. Seattle, IASP Press, 1994, pp 455-481.
47. Ochoa JL, Verdugo RJ, Campero M: Pathophysiological spectrum of organic and psychogenic disorders in neuropathic pain patients fitting the description of causalgia and reflex sympathetic dystrophy. In Jänig W, Stanton-Hicks M (eds): Proceedings of the 7th World Congress on Pain. Progress in Pain Research and Management, vol 2. Seattle, IASP Press, 1994, pp 483-494.
48. Juottonen K, Gockel M, Silen T, et al: Altered central sensorimotor processing in patients with complex regional pain syndrome. Pain 98:315, 2002.
49. American Psychiatric Association: Diagnostic and statistical manual of mental disorders (DSM-IV), 4th ed, Washington DC, 1994.
50. Oleson J: International Headache Society classification and diagnostic criteria for headache disorders, cranial neuralgias and facial pain. Cephalgia 8:57, 1988.
51. Bruehl S, Harden RN, Galer BS, et al: External validations of IASP diagnostic criteria for complex regional pain syndrome and proposed research diagnostic criteria. Pain 81:47, 1999.
52. Bruehl S, Harden RN, Galer B, Backonja M: Factor, analysis of signs and symptoms of complex regional pain syndrome: A partial validation of IASP diagnostic criteria and suggestions for change. Neurology 50(suppl 4):A254, 1998.
53. Bruehl S, Lubenow TR, Nath H, Ivankovich O: Validation of thermography in the diagnosis of reflex sympathetic dystrophy. Clin J Pain 12:316, 1996.
54. Maleki J, LeBela A, Bennett JG, Schwartzman RJ: Patterns of spread in complex regional pain syndrome type I (reflex sympathetic dystrophy). Pain 88:259, 2000.
55. Low PA, Caskey PE, Tuck RR, et al: Quantitative sudomotor axon reflex test in normal neuropathic subjects. Ann Neurol 14:573, 1983.
56. Sandroni P, Low PA, Ferrer T, et al: Complex regional pain syndrome (CRPS I): Prospective study and laboratory evaluation. Clin J Pain 14:282, 1998.
57. Dellemijn HL, Fields RR, Allen WR, et al: The interpretation of pain relief and sensory changes following sympathetic blockade. Brain 117:309, 1994.
58. Kozin F, Soin JS, Ryan LM, et al: The reflex sympathetic dystrophy syndrome. Radiology 38:437, 1981.
59. Mailis A, Meindok H, Papagapiou M, Pham D: Alterations of the three-phase bone scan after sympathectomy. Clin J Pain 10:146, 1994.
60. Kingery WS: A critical review of controlled clinical trials for peripheral neuropathic pain and complex regional pain syndromes. Pain 73:123, 1997.
61. Tanelian DT: Reflex sympathetic dystrophy: A re-evaluation of the literature. Pain Forum 5:247, 1996.
62. Kemler MA, Berendse GA, van Kleef M, et al: Spinal cord stimulation in patients with complex regional pain syndrome. N Engl J Med 343:618, 2000.
63. van Hilten BJ, van der Beek WJ, Hoff JL, et al: Intrathecal baclofen for the treatment of dystonia in patients with reflex sympathetic dystrophy. N Engl J Med 343:625, 2000.
64. Oerlemans H, Oostenderp RA, de Boo T, et al: Adjuvant physical therapy versus occupational therapy in patients with reflex sympathetic dystrophy/complex regional pain syndrome type I. Arch Phys Med Rehabil 81:49, 2000.
65. Stanton-Hicks M, Baron R, Boas R, et al: Complex regional pain syndromes: Guidelines for therapy. Clin J Pain 14:155, 1998.
66. Stanton-Hicks M, Burton AW, Bruehl SP, et al: An updated interdisciplinary clinical pathway for CRPS: Report of an expert panel. Pain Pract 2:1, 2002.
67. Rauck RL, Eisenach JC, Jackson K, et al: Epidural clonidine treatment for refractory reflex sympathetic dystrophy. Anesthesiology 79:1163, 1993.

68. Oakley JC, Weiner RL: Spinal cord stimulation for complex regional pain syndrome: A prospective study of 19 patients at 2 centers. Neuromodulation 2:47, 1999.
69. Bennett DS, Alo KM, Oakley JJ, Feler CA: Spinal cord stimulation for complex regional pain syndrome I (RSD): A retrospective multicenter experience from 1995 to 1998 of 101 patients. Neuromodulation 2:202, 1999.
70. Hassenbusch SJ, Stanton-Hicks M, Schoppa D, et al: Long-term results of peripheral nerve stimulation for reflex sympathetic dystrophy. J Neurosurg 84:415, 1996.
71. Schwartzman RJ, Liu JE, Smullens SN, et al: Long-term outcome following sympathectomy for complex regional pain syndrome type I (RSD). J Neurol Sci 150:149, 1997.
72. Furlan AD, Mailis A, Papagapio U: Are we paying too high a price for surgical sympathectomy? A systematic literature review of later complications. J Pain 1:245, 2000.
73. Rezai AR, Lozano AM: Deep brain stimulation (DBS) for pain. In Burchiel KJ (ed): Surgical Management of Pain. New York, Thieme Medical Publishers, 2002, pp 565-576.
74. Nguyen JP, Lefaucheur JP, Decq P, et al: Chronic motor cortex stimulation in the treatment of central and neuropathic pain: Correlations between electrophysiological and anatomical data. Pain 82:245, 1999.

chapter 53

Venous Thrombosis

Jack E. Ansell

In the past decade, tremendous advances have been made with respect to the diagnosis and treatment of venous thrombosis and thromboembolism. The use of invasive techniques to diagnose venous thromboembolism (VTE) is being rapidly replaced with accurate yet noninvasive, diagnostic modalities. The therapy of VTE is undergoing exciting changes with the development of targeted antithrombotics with greater therapeutic efficacy and safety, as well as considerably greater ease of use. This chapter focuses on the clinical entity of deep venous thrombosis (DVT) with an emphasis on diagnostic evaluation and management.

EPIDEMIOLOGY OF VENOUS THROMBOEMBOLISM

In its broadest context, arterial and venous thrombosis is the most common cause of death in the United States. VTE occurs in approximately 1 per 1000 individuals,[1] with 40% representing DVT and 60%, pulmonary embolism (PE). The rate increases with increasing age (Fig. 53-1).[2] Of interest is an apparent reduction in the rate of PE over the past 15 years whereas the rate of DVT has remained constant.[1] Other analyses concur that the rate of fatal PE has decreased by two thirds during this time[3] but also show that the rate of postoperative DVT has decreased by approximately 50%, whereas non-postoperative DVT has remained constant. These changes may represent improved prophylactic measures and their greater use in surgical patients, although surveys in the 1990s also indicated that there is considerable room for improvement.[4,5] In another trend analysis of VTE in patients discharged from a hospital between 1979 and 1999, similar trends were seen initially, but somewhat different findings were noted from 1989-1999, with significant increases in the diagnoses of DVT and PE in the latter 10 years, possibly related to the greater use and availability of noninvasive diagnostic testing.[6]

ETIOLOGY AND PATHOGENESIS

Venous thrombi are intravascular deposits consisting of varying degrees of fibrin, red blood cells, and platelets. Arterial thrombi tend to have a greater proportion of platelets relative to red blood cells and thus a paler appearance (i.e., white thrombi) compared with the darker, jelly-like appearance of pure venous thrombi. Thrombi tend to occur in areas of low flow, such as valve cusp pockets in the veins of the lower extremity.[7] They may also occur at sites of vascular trauma, as happens during surgery, or from intravascular foreign devices (i.e., central venous catheters).

Significant advances have been made in recent years in the understanding of the etiology of venous thrombosis. Virchow's triad continues to serve as the unifying concept in the pathogenesis of VTE, but what has become apparent is the significance of the interplay between the elements of Virchow's triad and environmental or acquired risk factors.[8] Box 53-1 identifies commonly recognized acquired risk factors for VTE.[9] Tremendous strides have also been made in recent years in understanding the inherited risk factors for VTE.[10]

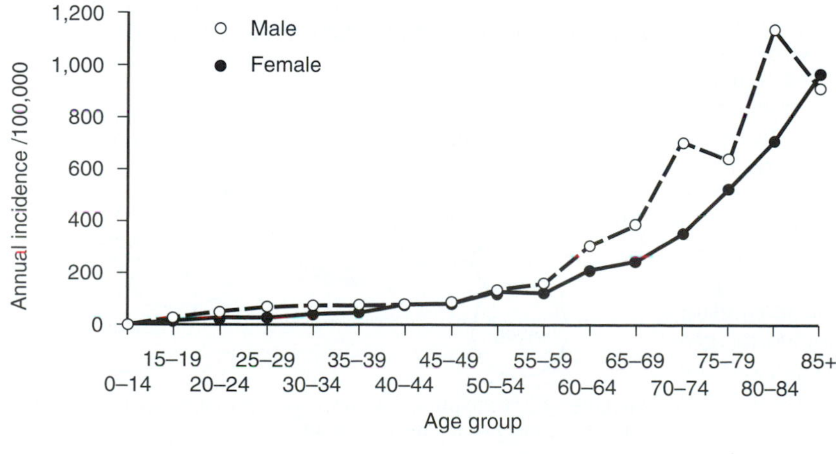

FIGURE 53-1. Annual incidence of venous thromboembolism among Olmsted County, Minn., residents, 1966-1990, by age and gender. (From Silverstein M, Heit JA, Mohr D, et al: Trends in the incidence of deep vein thrombosis and pulmonary embolism: A 25 year population based study. Arch Intern Med 158:585, 1998.)

BOX 53-1 Risk Factors Associated with the Development of Deep Venous Thrombosis

Strong risk factors (odds ratio >10)
- Fracture (hip or leg)
- Hip or knee replacement
- Major general surgery
- Major trauma
- Spinal cord injury

Moderate risk factors (odds ratio 2-9)
- Arthroscopic knee surgery
- Central venous lines
- Chemotherapy
- Congestive heart or respiratory failure
- Hormone replacement therapy
- Malignancy
- Oral contraceptive therapy
- Paralytic stroke
- Pregnancy, postpartum
- Previous venous thromboembolism
- Thrombophilia

Weak risk factors (odds ratio <2)
- Bed rest >3 days
- Immobility due to sitting (e.g., prolonged car or air travel)
- Increasing age
- Laparoscopic surgery
- Obesity
- Pregnancy, antepartum
- Varicose veins

From Anderson FA Jr, Spencer FA: Risk factors for venous thromboembolism. Circulation 107:I-9, 2003.

BOX 53-2 Inherited Changes Intrinsic to the Blood That Influence the Risk of Deep Venous Thrombosis

Common
- G1691A mutation in the factor V gene (factor V_{Leiden})
- G20210A mutation in the prothrombin gene
- Homozygous C677T mutation in the methylenetetrahydrofolate reductase gene

Rare
- Antithrombin deficiency
- Protein C deficiency
- Protein S deficiency

Very rare
- Dysfibrinogenemia
- Homozygous homocystinuria

Probably inherited
- Increased levels of factor VIII, factor IX, factor XI, or fibrinogen

Modified from Seligsohn U, Lubetsky A: Genetic susceptibility to venous thrombosis. N Engl J Med 344:1222, 2001.

To a large extent these represent changes in the blood (Box 53-2) leading to a hypercoagulable state. It is now believed that the risk of thrombosis is greatest when there is interaction between acquired risk factors and elements of Virchow's triad. Thus Virchow's triad is best expressed as a Venn diagram with overlapping areas representing varying levels of risk for a clinical event (Fig. 53-2).

The pathogenesis of venous thrombosis usually represents an imbalance between prothrombotic and antithrombotic forces in the blood.[11] The prothrombotic forces are those encompassed by Virchow's triad and include factors such as stasis of blood flow, vascular damage, or changes intrinsic to the blood. The latter forces include not only inherited prothrombotic factors (e.g., factor V_{Leiden}) but the generation of cytokines that can lead to endothelial cell activation (e.g., tumor necrosis factor [TNF]) and expression of tissue factor or the direct activation of the coagulation cascade by bacteria (e.g., endotoxin).[12] The antithrombotic forces include a range of natural anticoagulant properties including the natural anticoagulant proteins such as antithrombin, protein C, protein S, and tissue factor pathway inhibitor; the proteins of the fibrinolytic system; the natural anticoagulant properties of vascular endothelial cells including glycosaminoglycans, prostacyclin, and nitric oxide; and the compartmentalization of coagulation interactions and the diluting force of blood flow.[13]

Venous thrombosis confined to the superficial veins is often the result of an inflammatory condition of a superficial vein (e.g., infection or indwelling catheter), with thrombosis being a secondary event.[14] However, superficial vein thrombosis is also associated with many of the same factors as DVT such as cancer[14] and acquired and inherited thrombophilias.[15,16] Superficial venous thrombosis may be characterized by distinct clinical syndromes such as Mondor's disease,[17] a thrombophlebitis of a superficial vein segment of the anterolateral chest wall, and thrombophlebitis migrans,[14] or recurrent episodes of thrombophlebitis involving short segments of superficial veins in various parts of the body, often associated with an underlying malignancy.

NATURAL HISTORY OF VENOUS THROMBOSIS

Venous thrombosis can occur in any venous segment, but the clinical syndromes typically involve the deep veins of the lower or upper extremity with or without embolization to the lungs. Superficial thrombosis in veins

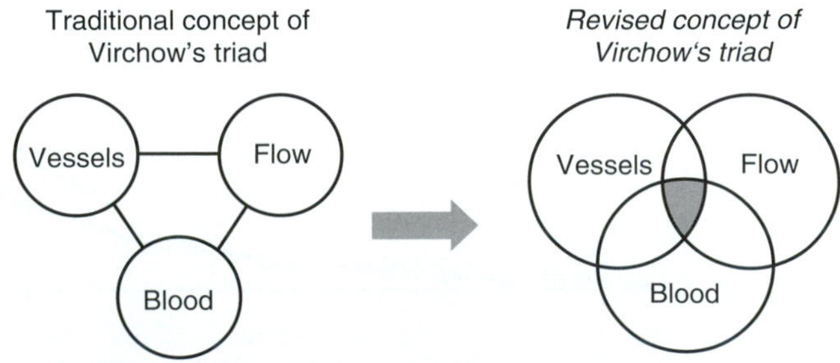

FIGURE 53-2. Pathophysiology of venous thromboembolism based on changing concepts of Virchow's triad.

of the lower extremity often occurs in varicosities or superficial veins that have become inflamed or infected; it may be associated with DVT in calf or proximal leg veins.[18] This is particularly true when the greater saphenous or lesser saphenous vein is involved.[19] DVT is clinically more important because of the potential for embolization.[7] DVT frequently originates in the calf veins, where it is more likely to be asymptomatic and less likely to produce pulmonary embolization. Left untreated, calf vein thrombosis has the potential to extend more proximally in approximately 25% of cases, although studies indicate a wide range of extension risk (5% to 30%).[7,20] Symptomatic PE as a result of isolated calf vein thrombosis is uncommon (<5%), although asymptomatic PE may occur in up to 20% to 30% of such patients. Proximal DVT results in pulmonary emboli in up to 50% of cases if carefully sought, although most of these cases are asymptomatic.[21] Fatal PE, however, is most likely to occur in the setting of proximal vein DVT.

Venous thrombosis of the upper extremities is not uncommon, representing about 4% of patients with VTE[22] and about 0.2% of all admissions to a community hospital.[23] It is seen more frequently today because of the common use of central venous catheters.[24] Upper extremity thrombosis most commonly occurs as a result of trauma, repetitive venous injury, or anatomical conditions that impinge on the venous system in the area of the shoulder.[25] Approximately 25% may be idiopathic, and these may be associated with an underlying thrombophilic condition.[26] Cancer is often an underlying associated condition, even in those without an indwelling central line.[23] The rate of recurrence is more likely to occur in those with an underlying thrombophilic condition.[25] A surprisingly high incidence of pulmonary embolization occurs in untreated upper extremity venous thrombosis, as much as 16% in one study of catheter-related DVT,[27] although the clinical sequelae may be less severe than those from the lower extremities.[28]

Once established, thrombi may lyse spontaneously, become organized, persist as an obstruction, recanalize partially, or extend more proximally.[7] Spontaneous lysis occurs in about one third of cases. The remaining thrombi become organized and develop varying degrees of recanalization. A consequence of DVT, especially of the proximal system, is the postphlebitic syndrome, manifested by varying degrees of pain, swelling, increased pigmentation, and ulcer formation.[29] The frequency of these findings ranges from 25% to 90% of patients depending on the study population.[7]

CLINICAL FEATURES AND DIFFERENTIAL DIAGNOSIS

The clinical features of DVT are nonspecific. Signs and symptoms can reflect other conditions that affect the lower extremities such as cellulitis, congestive heart failure (CHF), or ruptured Baker's cyst.[30] Thus one cannot simply rely on clinical findings to establish a diagnosis.[31,32] Pain, redness, and warmth are common symptoms reported by patients, and swelling, tenderness to palpation, and erythema are common signs of a DVT.[33] Venous distention and the presence of a palpable cord may be seen with a superficial venous thrombosis. Homans' sign, or pain in the calf on active dorsiflexion of the foot, is often not present, in contrast to earlier reports. Studies measuring the sensitivity and specificity of the most reliable signs or symptoms have been inconsistent,[34,35] and in one study, if reliance on clinical findings alone were the basis for diagnosis, 42% of patients in the cohort without DVT as determined by objective testing would have received anticoagulant treatment.[35] Table 53-1 summarizes the findings from one study of confirmed alternative diagnoses in patients who were suspected of having a DVT but found to have negative venograms.[30] The clinical findings and the context in which the symptoms develop, however, are helpful in establishing one's a priori suspicion of DVT, and, together with other parameters, are helpful in directing a diagnostic evaluation.[31]

TABLE 53-1 ALTERNATIVE DIAGNOSES IN 87 CONSECUTIVE PATIENTS WITH CLINICALLY SUSPECTED VENOUS THROMBOSIS AND NEGATIVE VENOGRAMS

Diagnosis	Patients (%)
Muscle strain	4
Direct twisting injury to leg	10
Leg swelling in paralyzed limb	9
Lymphangitis, lymphatic obstruction	7
Venous reflux	6
Muscle tear	5
Baker's cyst	3
Cellulitis	2
Internal abnormality of knee	1
Unknown	26

From Hull RD, Hirsch J, Sackett DL, et al: Clinical validity of a negative venogram in patients with clinically suspected venous thrombosis. Circulation 64:622, 1981.

The diagnosis of superficial venous thrombosis is often made on the basis of clinical findings; objective diagnostic tests are less well studied. Signs and symptoms include swelling, pain, erythema, and tenderness along a segment of the involved vein.[14] Compression ultrasonography, when used, shows a noncompressible venous lumen with echogenic material within. The clinical picture may often mimic cellulitis. Other differential considerations include lymphangitis, erythema nodosum, polyarteritis nodosa, sarcoid granuloma, and Kaposi's sarcoma.[36]

Clinical Prediction Rules

In recent years a number of investigators have studied patient populations with DVT in an effort to construct formal rules or indices for the diagnosis of DVT.[31,37-39] The construct is often based first on an evaluation of a cohort of patients with established disease, followed by applying it prospectively to another cohort. The best-known predictive model is that of Wells and colleagues.[38,39] By integrating the results of the clinical index with the results of an ultrasound examination, one could enhance the predictive accuracies of a positive ultrasound to 100%, 96%, and 63% in high, moderate, and low

TABLE 53-2 CLINICAL PREDICTION INDEX OF WELLS AND COLLEAGUES[40]

Clinical Feature	Score
Active cancer	1
Paralysis, recent plaster cast	1
Recent immobilization or major surgery	1
Tenderness along deep veins	1
Swelling of entire leg	1
>3 cm difference in calf circumference compared with other leg	1
Pitting edema	1
Collateral superficial veins	1
Alternative diagnosis likely	−2

A score of ≥3 represents high probability, 1-2 represents moderate probability, and ≤0 correlates with low probability for a pretest probability of deep venous thrombosis.

probability groups, respectively, and the negative predictive accuracies of a normal ultrasound to 98%, 84%, and 68% in low, moderate, and high probability groups, respectively.[38] Table 53-2 illustrates a revised model of Wells' prediction index that establishes a simplified scoring system.[40] When tested prospectively in a cohort of 593 patients with suspected DVT, it correctly established a diagnosis in 74.6%, 16.6%, and 3% of patients assigned to high, moderate, and low pretest probability groups, respectively.[38]

DIAGNOSTIC EVALUATION OF VENOUS THROMBOEMBOLISM

Objective diagnostic testing for acute DVT has changed considerably over the past two decades.[6] The gold standard, ascending venography, was used extensively through the early 1980s but experienced a rapid decline thereafter in association with a surge in venous ultrasound, including B-mode ultrasound, duplex, and color flow ultrasound studies.[6] Impedance plethysmography (IPG) was also popular in the early 1980s but has since fallen out of favor. Continuing changes are likely in diagnostic modalities with the combined use of clinical prediction models, D-dimer assays, and objective imaging studies, as well as with new techniques such as magnetic resonance direct thrombus imaging.

Ultrasonography

Real-time, B-mode compression ultrasonography is currently the diagnostic method of choice for identifying DVT in patients who are symptomatic, although the sensitivity varies according to which venous segment is involved (see Chapter 10).[41] In some asymptomatic patients venous ultrasonography is insensitive,[42,43] especially in postoperative patients, and venography is the test of choice. Absence of vein compressibility is the most important criterion indicating proximal venous thrombosis.[44,45] With venography as the standard, studies confirm a sensitivity between 93% and 97% and a specificity between 96% and 99%[46] for symptomatic proximal venous thrombosis. Other parameters, such as echogenicity or change in venous diameter during a Valsalva maneuver, are less reliable. Duplex ultrasonography involves both B-mode imaging (compressibility) and blood flow imaging using the pulsed Doppler signal. Absence of phasic blood flow and failure to augment blood flow by manual compression, leg elevation, or Valsalva indicate obstruction. Studies support a sensitivity of 95% and specificity of 93% in symptomatic outpatients.[46] Color-coded duplex ultrasonography appears to provide even greater accuracy with a sensitivity and specificity of 97% each.[46]

In the past, ultrasonography has shown insufficient sensitivity or specificity for the diagnosis of DVT isolated to the calf veins[47,48] in symptomatic patients. As calf vein thrombosis extends to the proximal veins in approximately 25% of patients[7,20] and proximal DVT is most likely to lead to PE, investigators have studied the usefulness of repeated venous ultrasound examinations in suspected DVT of the calf veins looking for extension before initiating treatment. Using this rationale, a repeat negative venous ultrasound 5 to 7 days after the initial ultrasound examination provides sufficient assurance that a DVT does not exist or that proximal extension will not occur.[43,49] A pooled analysis of studies of serial venous ultrasound testing found an incidence of 0.8% (17/2073) in the 3 months following the initial presentation with negative serial ultrasound examinations.[46]

More recently ultrasound imaging of calf veins has improved, and investigators have assessed the usefulness of a single comprehensive duplex ultrasound of the entire leg.[50-52] Using compressibility as the sole criterion, Stevens and colleagues[53] withheld anticoagulation in 385 patients with suspected DVT and a negative test, and over a 3-month follow-up, only 3 patients (0.8%) developed symptomatic venous thrombosis. This is still a relatively new capability, and more studies are necessary to confirm its sensitivity and specificity.

Impedance Plethysmography

IPG employs the principle that electrical impedance between two electrodes placed on the calf is inversely proportional to the volume of blood in the calf, which can be manipulated by inflation of a pneumatic cuff around the thigh.[33,54,55] With obstruction of blood flow out of the calf, the rate of change in impedance can identify such obstruction. IPG was a popular noninvasive diagnostic alternative to venography in the 1980s before the refinement of the Doppler and duplex ultrasound, but it has since been largely replaced by ultrasonography. Numerous studies established the diagnostic accuracy of IPG in symptomatic patients using venography as the comparator, yielding sensitivity rates of 86% to 90% and specificity rates of 94% to 96%, with the predictive value of an abnormal test being 89%.[56] Early studies of IPG tended to provide higher sensitivity and specificity rates than those achieved later. Analyses of these studies[57] identified a number of potential biases in multiple studies that may have accounted for such variability. IPG is relatively insensitive to calf vein thrombosis, as well as being variably sensitive to nonobstructing proximal vein thrombosis.[33,56,58] IPG is also influenced by external venous outflow obstruction due to such factors as compression with pregnancy or tumors, or even poor flow found in severe CHF. Finally, IPG has insufficient sensitivity or specificity to be used as a screening tool for patients with asymptomatic DVT.[43] As with compression ultrasound, serial IPGs have been employed to identify those who can be followed safely without treatment. Pooled results from a number of studies of serial, negative IPGs found an incidence of DVT of 1.5% (21/1395) over a 3-month follow-up. During the serial testing, four symptomatic PEs occurred (0.3%) for a total incidence of 1.8%.[46]

Venography

Venography remains the gold standard for the diagnosis of DVT, but its use has diminished considerably with the development of reliable noninvasive techniques,[6] especially for proximal DVT. Venography is of particular value in the diagnosis of asymptomatic DVT, in which ultrasonography is less reliable. It is used extensively in clinical trials of DVT prophylaxis when asymptomatic DVT is typically a major clinical endpoint. Venography is a complex, invasive procedure and requires considerable expertise.[33] With contrast venography, one can visualize the entire deep venous system of the leg, with similar sensitivity and specificity for both calf vein and proximal DVT. Most other techniques are insufficiently sensitive to detect calf vein thrombosis. A venogram must be technically adequate, and the interpreter should follow strict diagnostic criteria to provide reliable results with minimal interinterpreter differences.[59] The most reliable abnormality is the presence of an intraluminal filling defect that is constant and seen in at least two views.[33] Other criteria include a sharp cutoff of contrast dye in a venous segment or nonfilling of a venous segment.

Contrast venography does, however, have drawbacks, including the need for extensive resources and expertise, venous access that may be difficult if not impossible in some patients, and the inability to do repetitive examinations. Side effects include pain and discomfort at the site of injection or in the calf; the risk of allergic reactions to the contrast dye; and a postvenography syndrome of pain and induced venous thrombosis, which may be superficial or deep.[60,61] One must carefully weigh the value of contrast venography in patients with renal failure or who are at risk of renal failure, because both nonionic and high-ionic contrast dyes may cause or aggravate such problems.[62]

Magnetic Resonance Imaging

Magnetic resonance (MR) venography is a sensitive means of detecting proximal venous thrombi but is not useful for distal (below-knee) disease. The MR signal can discern stationary thrombus from flowing blood by differential signals.[63] These and other noninvasive studies indicate thrombi by filling defects or by other indirect means (e.g., IPG, D-dimer). Most recently, promising results have been found with a technique called MR direct thrombus imaging (MRDTI), in which thrombi are visualized against a suppressed background (positive image) and IV contrast is not necessary.[64] For lower extremity DVT, this technique can identify both proximal and calf vein thrombi, although its sensitivity is greater in the larger veins. It also allows imaging of the lower extremities and the chest in one sitting. In a comparative study against venography in 101 patients, two independent readers had sensitivities of 94% and 96% and specificities of 90% and 92%.[65] The sensitivities were in the range of 80% to 90% for isolated calf vein thrombosis, 97% for femoropopliteal DVT, and 100% for iliofemoral DVT. Although still early in development, this technique offers another promising noninvasive modality for the diagnosis of VTE.

Plasma D-dimers

Although much attention has focused on changes in the blood to understand the pathophysiology of DVT, blood tests are of little help in the identification or confirmation of a DVT but may be helpful in the exclusion of one. In the process of fibrin formation and the simultaneous activation of the fibrinolytic system, the lysis of fibrin results in the generation of fibrin breakdown or degradation products. One such fragment of crosslinked fibrin is known as a D-dimer (Fig. 53-3).[66] Immunologic D-dimer assays are particularly sensitive for the presence of intravascular thrombosis, but they have low specificity for DVT.[67,68] Thus a negative assay may be helpful in the exclusion of an acute thrombotic process.[69-71] Sensitive enzyme-linked immunosorbent assays (ELISAs) have been studied for their predictive negative values in excluding a DVT, and D-dimer assays have been included as part of diagnostic algorithms to help physicians diagnose DVT with a minimum of invasive testing. One must be careful, however, in understanding the type of D-dimer assay used in this process because standard latex agglutination assays have a much lower sensitivity compared with ELISA assays (Table 53-3).[72,73] Evidence from prospective studies indicates that a negative D-dimer (sensitive assay) in the setting of a low clinical suspicion is sufficient to exclude the presence of a DVT.

On the basis of the likelihood of a DVT being present at baseline and the results of a sensitive D-dimer assay and objective testing, a number of investigators have developed algorithms for the diagnostic approach to confirming a DVT with the ultimate goal of avoiding invasive testing (i.e., venogram). Figure 53-4 illustrates an approach recommended by Bates and colleagues[70] using such an algorithm.

The Diagnostic Evaluation of Thrombophilia in Patients with a Deep Vein Thrombosis

When a patient is diagnosed with a DVT, the physician tries to determine its cause. This is particularly important in guiding antithrombotic therapy, especially the duration of therapy. As discussed previously, the pathophysiology of VTE should be considered in the context of Virchow's triad with an attempt to understand what factors have disturbed blood flow (e.g., immobility), vascular endothelium (e.g., trauma), or the hemostatic process (e.g., defective inhibition of coagulation factors). Some inciting factors are obvious, such as postoperative DVT, whereas others are more obscure (e.g., idiopathic DVT). Furthermore, it is the combination of risk factors that

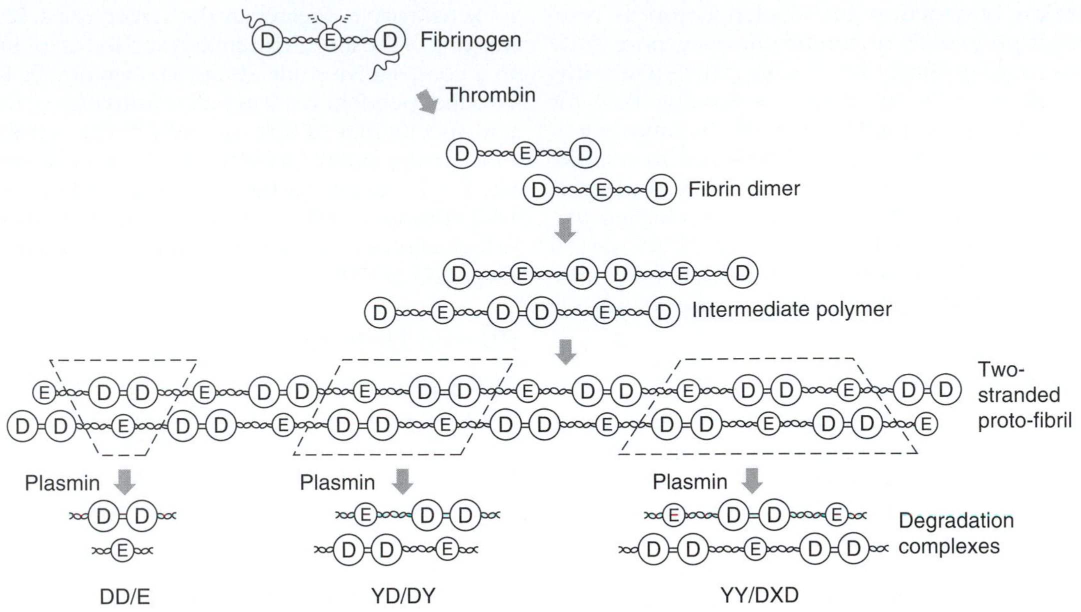

FIGURE 53-3. Schematic representation of D-dimer fragment as a plasmin digest of polymerized fibrin. The D-dimer fragment is pictured in the lower left portion of the figure. (From Francis CW, Marder VJ: Mechanisms of fibrinolysis. In Williams WJ, Beutler E, Erslev AJ, Lichtman MA [eds]: Hematology, 4th ed. New York, McGraw-Hill, 1990, pp 1313-1321.)

seems to put the patient at highest risk. A challenging aspect of this evaluation is to know when to test, and what to test for, when considering a thrombophilic condition. Bauer[74] has addressed this question and recommends categorizing patients into strongly or weakly thrombophilic groups and stratifying testing accordingly. Thus age, a history of recurrent thrombosis, and a positive family history may help in guiding a thrombophilic evaluation (Table 53-4).

PREVENTION OF VENOUS THROMBOEMBOLISM

The prevention of postoperative DVT and PE has been the subject of extensive study over the past 40 years. Without prophylaxis, the incidence of postoperative VTE may be as high as 70% in orthopedic surgery, the surgical procedure with the highest risk of VTE. The development of ^{125}I iodinated fibrinogen scans to identify prospectively the nascent development of DVT was immensely helpful in establishing baseline rates of DVT.[20] Early studies identified PE as the most preventable cause of hospital death.[75] Some 25 years ago it was estimated that more than 600,000 symptomatic PEs occur annually in the United States and that as many as 200,000 individuals die of such events.[76] Many of these individuals die suddenly without any warning. Thus not only can appropriate prophylaxis improve this situation, but many of the benefits of increased prophylaxis have already been achieved.[1] Despite these advances, there is still substantial evidence that prophylaxis is not uniformly employed by many physicians.[4,5]

The rationale for VTE prophylaxis is based not only on its high prevalence in select conditions but also on the silent nature of the disease. The clinical diagnosis of VTE is unreliable and requires objective documentation.[31,32] One can either perform prospective testing in patients at risk or employ a pharmacologic or physical method to prevent its development. Unfortunately, noninvasive testing is not sufficiently sensitive as a screening tool in asymptomatic patients and as the first manifestation of disease may be a fatal PE, it makes most sense to prevent its occurrence.

Sevitt and Gallagher[77] were among the first to clearly show in a small randomized study that a vitamin K antagonist could prevent PE in injured patients. It was not until the 1970s that a simple and reliable method of prophylaxis, low-dose heparin, was shown to be effective.[78] Twenty years later, low-molecular weight heparin (LMWH) became the agent of choice for many conditions. Today, newer agents such as fondaparinux have been shown to be as effective, and perhaps better, for some conditions. One important advance in the past 15 years was the recognition that not only surgical patients are at

TABLE 53-3 ACCURACY OF D-DIMER ASSAYS FOR DETECTING VENOUS THROMBOSIS

Assay	Sensitivity (%)	Specificity (%)
ELISA	95-99	32-46
Latex agglutination	78-96	48-72
RBC agglutination (SimpliRED)	77-100	54-75
Rapid ELISA (Vidas DD)	92-100	29-62

ELISA, enzyme-linked immunosorbent assay; RBC, red blood count.
From Frost SD, Brotman DJ, Michota FA: Rational use of D-dimer measurement to exclude acute venous thromboembolic disease. Mayo Clin Proc 78:1385, 2003 and Bounameaux H, de Moerloose P, Perrier A, et al: D-dimer testing in suspected venous thromboembolism: An update. QJM 90:437, 1997.

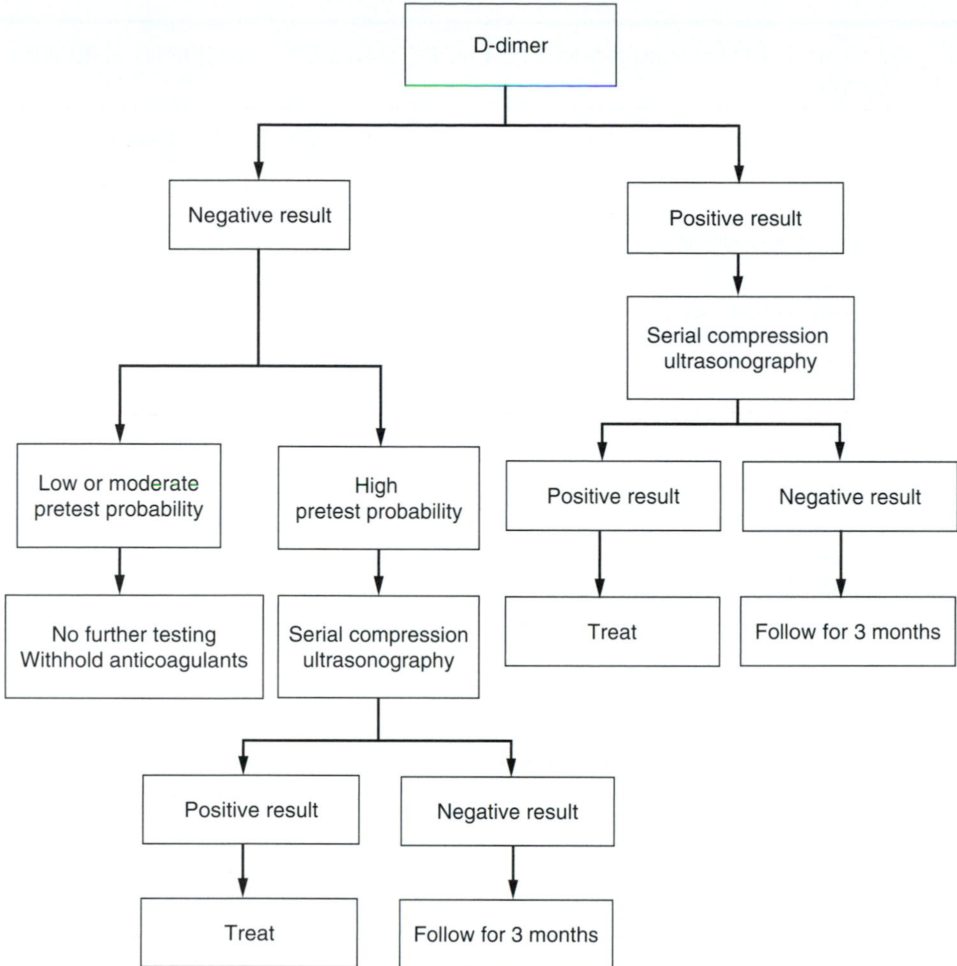

FIGURE 53-4. Systematic approach to the diagnosis of deep venous thrombosis using clinical suspicion, D-dimer, and ultrasound. (From Bates SM, Kearon C, Crowther M, et al: A diagnostic strategy involving a quantitative latex D-dimer assay reliably excludes deep venous thrombosis. Ann Intern Med 138:787, 2003.)

TABLE 53-4 CHARACTERIZATION OF PATIENTS WITH VENOUS THROMBOEMBOLISM

Clinical History	Weakly Thrombophilic	Strongly Thrombophilic
Age at onset <50 yr	Negative	Positive
Recurrent thrombosis	Negative	Positive
Family history	Negative	Positive
Screening assays for thrombophilic patients		
Activated protein C resistance (screening assay)		
Confirm positive results of APCR assay by factor V_{Leiden} genetic assay		
Prothrombin^{G20210A} genetic assay		
Antithrombin functional assay		
Protein C functional assay		
Protein S functional assay and immunologic assays of total and free protein S		
Lupus anticoagulant clotting assay and immunologic antiphospholipid antibody assay		
Fasting total plasma homocysteine assay		

APCR, activated protein C resistance.
Modified from Bauer KA: The thrombophilias: Well-defined risk factors with uncertain therapeutic implications. Ann Intern Med 135;367, 2001.

risk of VTE but that hospitalized medical patients have a substantial risk, and the same strategies employed in postoperative patients have now been studied in medical patients.[79]

The key to sensible prophylaxis is risk stratification among different surgical procedures, medical illnesses, and underlying patient factors. Table 53-5 summarizes the risk in surgical patients without prophylaxis, categorizing patients by intensity of surgery and associated other risk factors. The following discussion focuses on a number of these specific conditions and the outcomes achieved with different modalities of prophylaxis.

Specific Surgical and Medical Conditions

Orthopedic Surgery Compared with other surgical settings, total hip replacement (THR), total knee replacement (TKR), and hip fracture surgery have the highest rate of postoperative DVT, up to 70% for total VTE and 30% for proximal VTE occurring 7 to 14 days after surgery.[80,81] PE may occur in up to 10% of untreated patients. It is now well documented that the risk continues postoperatively for up to at least 30 days after THR, although the majority

TABLE 53-5 RISK OF VENOUS THROMBOEMBOLISM IN PATIENTS UNDERGOING SURGERY AND NOT RECEIVING PROPHYLAXIS

Level of Risk *(Examples)*	**Calf** *DVT %*	**Proximal** *DVT %*	**Clinical** *PE %*	**Fatal** *PE %*
Low risk Minor surgery in patients <40 yr with no additional risk factors	2	0.4	0.2	0.002
Moderate risk Minor surgery in patients with additional risk factors; nonmajor surgery in patients aged 40-60 yr with no additional risk factors; major surgery in patients <40 yr with no additional risk factors	10-20	2-4	1-2	0.1-0.4
High risk Nonmajor surgery in patients >60 yr or with additional risk factors; major surgery in patients >0 yr or with additional risk factors	20-40	4-8	2-4	0.4-1
Highest risk Major surgery in patients >40 yr plus prior VTE, cancer, or molecular hypercoagulable state; hip or knee arthroplasty; hip fracture surgery; major trauma; spinal cord injury	40-80	10-20	4-10	0.2-5

DVT, deep venous thrombosis; PE, pulmonary embolism; VTE, venous thromboembolism.
Data from references 75-77.

of these are asymptomatic.[82-84] Physical measures such as elastic stockings or intermittent pneumatic compression boots are not sufficiently effective in reducing postoperative VTE compared with other modalities, especially for proximal DVT prevention.[80]

Among the pharmacologic approaches, neither aspirin nor low-dose heparin is sufficiently effective. Warfarin, which is commonly used in the United States, is effective prophylaxis when started preoperatively or soon after surgery and dosed to achieve an international normalized ratio (INR) of between 2 and 3.[80,85-88] Warfarin also has the convenience to be continued in the weeks following surgery. LMWH has been studied in numerous trials and, compared with warfarin, achieves an equivalent outcome in hip replacement surgery.[80,85-89] Table 53-6 summarizes the results of various prophylactic modalities in patients undergoing either THR or TKR surgery. Hull and colleagues[90,91] have recently shown that the timing of perioperative dosing is key to achieving optimal efficacy but also influences the rates of bleeding. Thus LMWH given approximately 6 hours after surgery can achieve even better results than warfarin but at a price of more bleeding.

Recent studies with fondaparinux, an indirect factor Xa inhibitor, suggest that this agent may provide even greater protection than LMWH (enoxaparin).[92] Two randomized controlled trials in more than 4500 patients undergoing THR surgery showed a 25% to 56% relative risk reduction in the occurrence of total VTE over enoxaparin.[93,94] Fondaparinux was dosed approximately 6 hours after surgery in each trial compared with 12 hours preoperatively in one trial and 12 hours postoperatively in the other for enoxaparin. Major bleeding was not significantly increased in the fondaparinux group.

TABLE 53-6 POOLED OUTCOME RESULTS OF DVT IN PATIENTS UNDERGOING THR OR TKR SURGERY WITH VARIOUS PROPHYLACTIC AGENTS

	TOTAL HIP REPLACEMENT		**TOTAL KNEE REPLACEMENT**	
Regimen	*Total DVT*	*Proximal DVT*	*Total DVT*	*Proximal DVT*
	expressed as % prevalence and (relative risk reduction)			
Placebo/control	54.2 (–)	26.6 (–)	64.3 (–)	15.3 (–)
Elastic stockings	41.7 (23)	25.5 (4)	60.7 (6)	16.6 (–)
Aspirin	40.2 (26)	11.4 (57)	56 (13)	8.9 (42)
Low-dose heparin	30.1 (45)	19.3 (27)	43.2 (33)	11.4 (25)
Warfarin	22.1 (59)	5.2 (80)	46.8 (27)	10 (35)
LMWH	16.1 (70)	5.9 (78)	30.6 (52)	5.6 (63)
Adjusted-dose heparin	14 (74)	10.2 (62)	–	–

DVT, deep venous thrombosis; LMWH, low-molecular weight heparin; THR, total hip replacement; TKR, total knee replacement.
Modified from Geerts WH, Heit JA, Clagett GP, et al: Prevention of venous thromboembolism. Chest 119(suppl):132S, 2001.

In hip fracture surgery both LMWH and warfarin provide important reductions in VTE, although no studies have compared the two agents.[80] Recently, a randomized controlled trial of fondaparinux versus enoxaparin showed a significant reduction in total VTE favoring fondaparinux (8.3% vs. 19.1%) in more than 1600 patients randomized.[95] There was also a decrease in proximal DVT (0.9% vs. 4.3%), whereas there was no difference in major bleeding.

The rates of thrombosis and outcomes with different prophylactic regimens in TKR differ somewhat from those in total hip replacement surgery, mainly in that TKR is associated with higher rates of VTE in the short term,[82] and the benefits of LMWH over warfarin are even more substantial.[80,87,89] The pooled results from several randomized trials of LMWH versus warfarin clearly demonstrate the superiority of LMWH (see Table 53-6).[80]

Fondaparinux has also been studied in knee replacement surgery. One trial of 1000 patients randomized to fondaparinux versus enoxaparin showed a greater than 50% relative risk reduction for total VTE in the fondaparinux group (12.5% vs. 27.8%) and an almost significant reduction in proximal DVT.[96] The fondaparinux patients did experience a significant increase in major bleeding with the fondaparinux dosing at approximately 6 hours postoperatively, whereas the enoxaparin was given 12 hours after surgery.

The ideal duration of postoperative prophylaxis in orthopedic surgery is not known, but recent studies clearly indicate a continuing risk for at least up to 30 days. In a meta-analysis of four clinical studies of short-term prophylaxis only, Douketis and coworkers[82] found a post-prophylaxis rate of symptomatic nonfatal VTE of 2.2%, with a 3-month fatal PE rate of 0.05%. The rate of VTE was higher following hip surgery (2.5%) versus knee surgery (1.4%). Several studies have shown the value of extended therapy for up to 4 to 6 weeks. Thus, patients (THR) treated with warfarin experienced fewer symptomatic events (2.3%) compared with those given no treatment (3.3%) up to 6 weeks after surgery,[97] whereas those treated with LMWH also had fewer symptomatic events (0.5%) compared with those given no treatment (5.1%) up to 4 weeks after THR.[98] Similar results were noted with fondaparinux (0.3%) compared with untreated controls (2.7%) up to 4 weeks after hip fracture surgery.[84] In the latter study, the rate of venogram-documented DVT between the two groups was 1.4% and 35%, respectively. There was a trend toward increased major bleeding in the fondaparinux group (2.4% vs. 0.6%). In a pooled analysis of six studies, Hull and colleagues[99] found that 22% of untreated patients had a positive venogram versus 8% of those who had extended treatment. Symptomatic DVT was significantly lower at 4.2% and 1.4%, respectively.

Nonorthopedic Surgery Gynecologic surgery is associated with a 15% to 20% incidence of DVT in untreated patients.[80] Those patients with cancer are at the higher end of this spectrum. Of the various prophylactic modalities, low-dose unfractionated heparin (LDUH) has been studied most extensively. Pooled analyses of studies indicate a risk of documented DVT of approximately 7% with LDUH.[80] LMWH has not been well studied in this condition, although one case-controlled series with symptomatic DVT as an endpoint reported an incidence of only 0.3% in more than 2000 patients.[100]

Although general surgery is associated with a 20% to 30% incidence of objectively documented DVT in untreated patients,[80] general surgeons still suffer from a complacency toward the use of prophylaxis. On the basis of a review of physician practices in Oklahoma hospitals in 1995, Bratzler and coworkers[5] found that only 38% of select Medicare general surgery patients received prophylaxis with no variation in use on the basis of their risk of VTE. A higher rate of use was found by Stratton and colleagues,[101] 75% for major abdominal surgery in a review of records from 10 teaching and community hospitals between 1996 and 1997. LDUH given twice daily has been extensively tested in general surgery and shown to yield a greater than 60% reduction in DVT[80] and reduce proximal DVT, PE, and fatal PE. LMWH has not been shown to be substantially better,[80,102] although it does have the advantages of once-daily dosing and a lower incidence of heparin-induced thrombocytopenia. As noted earlier for orthopedic surgery, timing of LMWH dosing also influences outcomes.

Medical Illnesses Major medical illnesses include patients with many of the risk factors discussed earlier including advanced age; immobility or paralysis; stroke; myocardial infarction; cancer; need for intensive care; CHF; and varying degrees of respiratory disease, infection, or failure.[79,80] The incidence of DVT in such patients, when untreated, ranges from 10% to 20%.[80] LDUH, 5000 units twice daily or three times daily, when compared with placebo, effectively reduces the rate of DVT,[80,103] but dosing three times daily may be more effective. One study found an 80% reduction in DVT compared with placebo without an increase in major bleeding when low-dose heparin was dosed three times daily.[104] When LMWH was compared with placebo,[105] 20 mg/day was ineffective, but 40 mg/day significantly reduced the incidence of total and proximal DVT (15% to 5.5% and 5% to 1.7%, respectively). Treatment was for 6 to 14 days, and the outcomes remained unchanged when the patients were followed up at 3 months. The incidence of PE was not significantly lower in the treated group, nor was the incidence of major or minor bleeding. When LMWH at a dose of 20 mg daily (enoxaparin) is compared with LDUH (5000 units twice daily), no differences in outcome are seen (thrombosis or hemorrhage).[106]

Leizorovicz and colleagues[107] randomized 3700 patients with heart failure, respiratory failure, infection, and other disorders between dalteparin and placebo. Overall reductions in VTE of at least 30% were achieved with the LMWH (2.8% vs. 5%, respectively) in proximal DVT (1.8% vs. 3.7%, respectively) and symptomatic DVT (0.3% vs. 0.6% respectively). The PRIME trial[108] randomized 885 patients between enoxaparin, 40 mg daily versus UFH 5000 units three times daily for 7 days. The major diagnoses were heart failure, respiratory failure, and cancer. There was no significant difference in VTE between the two groups or in major bleeding. A similar result occurred in the PRINCE trial,[109] with 665 patients randomized between enoxaparin 40 mg daily and UFH 5000 units three times daily (8.4% and 10.4%, respectively). In the subgroup of patients with CHF, there was a significant reduction in VTE (9.7% for LMWH vs. 16.1% for UFH; $P = .014$). The enoxaparin group also experienced fewer adverse events, bleeding, and deaths.

Spinal cord injury (SCI) has the highest risk of VTE of the nonsurgical conditions with rates approaching 100%,[80] mostly in the acute postinjury period (3 months). No large, well-controlled studies of various agents in this condition have been conducted, but smaller studies have shown that LDUH is inadequate when given in a fixed dose of 5000 units twice a day when compared with the outcomes with LMWH[110] or adjusted-dose heparin (ADH).[111] Green and coworkers[111] showed superiority of ADH over LDUH with rates of DVT of 7% versus 31%, respectively, and in another study[110] of LMWH over LDUH with rates of DVT of 0% versus 26%, respectively. The optimal duration of therapy in these patients is uncertain. Patients with complete motor paralysis but no other risk factors should receive prophylaxis for approximately 8 weeks.[112] Those with high cervical spine lesions and paralyses of the upper and lower extremities should receive at least 12 weeks of prophylaxis. Associated injuries and other medical problems may influence the actual duration of therapy. Ongoing therapy is generally not required because the risk of VTE markedly decreases over the long term in association with regression of the deep venous system and an increase in fibrinolytic activity. If therapy is required, warfarin with an INR target of 2.5 is recommended.[80]

TREATMENT OF VENOUS THROMBOSIS

Unfractionated heparin followed by warfarin therapy has been traditional treatment for acute venous thrombosis. Both agents have undergone tremendous refinements in management over the past four decades, but they continue to have major pharmacologic, as well as practical, limitations. The introduction of low-molecular weight fractions of heparin in the 1980s provided a major improvement in therapy and was responsible for allowing management of DVT outside the hospital. Major additional changes are likely in the near future with the development of new targeted and direct-acting coagulation factor inhibitors that may significantly change the long-term management of VTE.

Acute Treatment

Unfractionated heparin (UFH) is a glycosaminoglycan composed of long chains of repeating saccharide units (iduronic acid and glucosamine) (average chain length 45 units).[113] Its anticoagulant activity is dependent on binding to the serine protease inhibitor, antithrombin (AT), via a unique pentasaccharide sequence, and potentiating its activity. For neutralization of thrombin (IIa), UFH must bind to antithrombin and to a heparin-binding domain on thrombin. This additional binding is not required for neutralization of its other major target, Xa. UFH also catalyses the inactivation of thrombin through another cofactor, heparin cofactor II, that is independent of antithrombin. The UFH-antithrombin complex also catalyses the inactivation of other serine proteases including factors IXa, XIa, and XIIa. After an IV bolus of approximately 5000 units, UFH has an effective half-life of about 1 hour.[114] Its half-life increases with increasing doses. Although it is eliminated through the kidney, modification of dosing is generally not required with impaired renal function. At therapeutic doses, heparin is largely bound to endothelial cells and macrophages where it is depolymerized. Most importantly following injection, a variable amount of heparin is bound to plasma proteins and is unavailable for binding to antithrombin.[115] This fraction varies among individuals, making the effective therapeutic dose unpredictable[116] and thus requiring an assay to monitor its anticoagulant effect. This assay is the activated partial thromboplastin time (aPTT).[117] Binding to plasma proteins can occasionally lead to relative degrees of heparin resistance.

The response of the aPTT to UFH also depends on the reagent and instrument used in the assay. There is no methodology for equilibrating results across laboratories as there is with the prothrombin time (e.g., the INR). Thus it is recommended that each laboratory perform a heparin titration curve with the particular reagent/instrument in use to determine how the aPTT correlates with therapeutic heparin levels that, by protamine sulfate titration, are 0.2 to 0.4 IU/ml, or by anti-Xa assay 0.3 to 0.7 U/ml.[118]

A major problem with heparin therapy is failure to promptly achieve and remain in a targeted therapeutic range on the basis of traditional dosing schemes.[119,120] Several randomized studies have confirmed the necessity of achieving an aPTT ratio of at least 1.5. Hull and coworkers[121] compared continuous IV dosing with intermittent subcutaneous dosing of IV UFH in patients with proximal DVT and found a high incidence of recurrent VTE in patients who failed to promptly reach a therapeutic aPTT. Thus 24.5% of patients with an aPTT response below the lower limit for 24 hours or more had recurrent VTE, compared with only 1.6% who achieved a therapeutic level. Most failures occurred in the intermittent dosing group. Similar results occurred when oral anticoagulants alone were compared with UFH for the initial treatment of patients with proximal DVT.[122] Recurrent VTE occurred in 20% of patients treated only with oral anticoagulants over the first 3 months compared with 6.7% in those initially treated with UFH and then oral anticoagulants.

In the past decade, a number of heparin-dosing algorithms have been tested to gauge their ability to achieve therapeutic levels more promptly. The most popular algorithm is that of Rashke and colleagues (Table 53-7).[123] In a study by the Rashke group,[123] recurrent VTE was more frequent in the standard dosing group (5000 unit bolus followed by 1000 units/hr infusion) compared with those treated according to the nomogram (80 units/kg bolus followed by 18 units/kg/hr infusion). The key advantage to such algorithms, besides standardization of dosing increments, is to force physicians to use higher amounts of UFH both for the bolus dose and continuous infusion, thus achieving effective aPTT levels more

TABLE 53-7 HEPARIN DOSING NOMOGRAM

Check baseline aPTT, INR, CBC/platelet count
Give heparin bolus, 80 units/kg IV
Begin IV heparin infusion, 18 units/kg/h
Target aPTT for institution-specific therapeutic range*

aPTT	Dose Adjustment
<35 sec*	80 units/kg bolus; increase drip by 4 units/kg/hr
35-50 sec*	40 units/kg bolus; increase drip by 2 units/kg/hr
51-70 sec*	No change
71-90 sec*	Reduce drip by 2 units/kg/hr
>90 sec*	Hold heparin for 1 hr; reduce drip by 3 units/kg/hr

*Each laboratory must perform its own in vitro heparin titration curve to establish the therapeutic range for the specific aPTT reagent in use, which is equivalent to a heparin concentration of 0.3-0.7 anti Xa U/ml (by anti Xa assay) or 0.2-0.4 U/ml (by protamine titration assay). The therapeutic range varies depending on the aPTT reagent in use.
aPTT, activated partial thromboplastin time; CBC, complete blood count; INR, international normalized ratio
Modified from Raschke RA, Reilly BM, Guidry JR, et al: The weight-based heparin dosing nomogram compared with a "standard care" nomogram. A randomized controlled trial. Ann Intern Med 119:874, 1993.

promptly. The problem of underdosing of heparin has been confirmed by others.[119,124-126] In one audit of three university affiliated hospitals, Wheeler and colleagues[125] found that 60% of patients failed to achieve a therapeutic aPTT (ratio of ≥1.5) during the initial 24 hours and that up to 40% of patients remained subtherapeutic over the next 3 to 4 days.

In another study, Raschke and colleagues[127] audited 15 randomized controlled trials comparing UFH with LMWH and found that only 20% of trials used a validated aPTT therapeutic range. Hylek and coworkers[128] found a similar inadequacy of heparin therapy during the initial treatment of various thrombotic conditions including different magnitudes of initial heparin boluses, the frequency of monitoring, and the time to achieve a therapeutic range. Only 20% of patients met the recommended 4 days or more of heparin and warfarin overlap until the INR was in a therapeutic range for 2 consecutive days.

Although subtherapeutic heparin levels early in therapy are associated with a higher incidence of recurrent disease, the evidence to suggest that bleeding is a consequence of overanticoagulation, as measured by the aPTT, is unclear. The risk of bleeding with UFH does correlate with dose,[114] but other factors are also important. Hull and colleagues[129] showed that the risk of bleeding with supertherapeutic aPTTs was related not so much to the elevation of the aPTT but to the underlying risk of bleeding per individual patient. Bleeding complications occurred in 8 of 93 (8.6%) patients with supertherapeutic aPTTs compared with 13 of 106 patients (12.3%) without supertherapeutic aPTTs, and major bleeding occurred in 3.2% and 9.4%, respectively. Patients who were considered at low risk for bleeding had a low frequency of major bleeding, even if they had the higher heparin dose, whereas those considered at high risk for bleeding had more bleeding even though they received a lower dosage of heparin. From an analysis of many studies, the overall risk of major bleeding with heparin ranges from 0% to 7%,[130] with fatal bleeding in 0% to 2% of cases.

Low-Molecular Weight Heparin and Fondaparinux

After the discovery in 1976[131,132] that low-molecular weight fractions of UFH had antithrombotic properties, a number of products were developed on the basis of different fractionation processes, each having slightly different pharmacokinetic profiles. LMWHs are produced by chemical or enzymatic depolymerization of unfractionated heparin.[133] Various preparations are available, most with an average molecular weight of between 4000 and 6500 Da. They contain the essential pentasaccharide for AT binding, enabling the AT-LMWH complex to neutralize factor Xa, but they lack a substantial number of the larger monosaccharide chains (18 or more) required for binding to thrombin. Thus the ratio of the relative neutralizing potency for Xa:IIa, which for unfractionated heparin is 1:1, is approximately 3:1 for LMWH. Although varying degrees of anti-Xa:anti-IIa neutralizing capacities have been suggested to confer favorable attributes of one LMWH preparation over another, little solid evidence backs this up.

LMWHs have qualities that make them better anticoagulants than unfractionated heparin. These pharmacologic attributes are mostly related to their reduced ability to bind to plasma proteins, endothelial cells, and blood cells, making them more available for binding to AT and producing an anticoagulant effect. Consequently, they have a greater bioavailability and predictability of response and do not require monitoring. They are also more uniformly absorbed from subcutaneous depots and have a longer plasma half-life, in the range of 3 to 5 hours. LMWHs are excreted predominantly from kidneys. Alteration of dosing is required in renal failure, in which it is recommended that full-dose therapy be instituted only with the aid of anti-X_a monitoring.

These agents have undergone extensive testing in a wide range of thromboembolic conditions in which they have proved not only safe and effective but decidedly simpler to use. LMWHs have been shown to be effective and safe in the treatment of DVT and PE.[114] Because different LMWH products differ in molecular weight, half-life, ratio of anti-Xa:anti-IIa activity, and other characteristics, products are tested and approved by licensing agencies individually for prophylaxis and for treatment. Several meta-analyses of the effectiveness of LMWHs have been conducted.[134-136] A recent analysis by Dolovich and colleagues[136] compared several LMWHs and various aspects of their effectiveness in the treatment of VTE (Figs. 53-5 through 53-8). Perhaps the greatest impact that LMWH has had on the treatment of VTE is allowing for treatment to move out of the hospital and into the home. Levine and others[137] and Koopman and coworkers[138] showed that LMWH was both as effective and safe as standard unfractionated heparin treatment in patients with DVT treated at home versus in the hospital (Table 53-8). Although most analyses indicate that LMWH is as effective as standard treatment, some investigators have found evidence for improved outcomes with LMWH. Thus Breddin[139] showed both improved thrombus

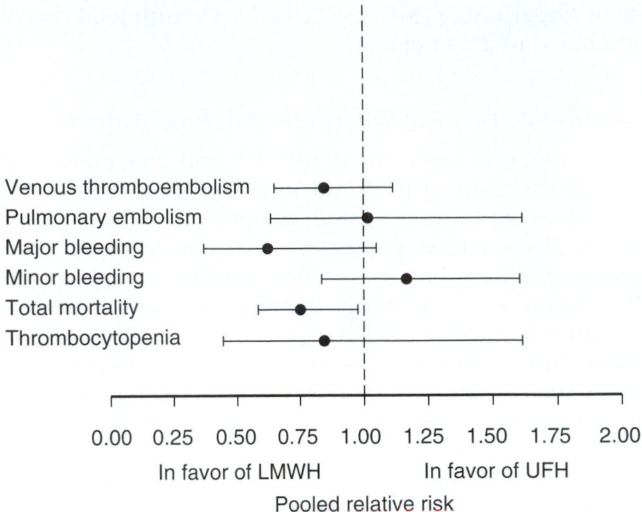

FIGURE 53-5. The effects of low-molecular weight heparin (LMWH) versus unfractionated heparin (UFH) in the acute treatment of venous thromboembolism. (From Dolovich LR, Ginsberg JS, Douketis JD, et al: A meta-analysis comparing low molecular weight heparins with unfractionated heparin in the treatment of venous thromboembolism: Examining some unanswered questions regarding location of treatment, product type, and dosing efficiency. Arch Intern Med 160:181, 2000.)

regression on repeat venogram and decreased VTE recurrence with LMWH given twice daily for one week versus unfractionated heparin. Although studies comparing LMWH with UFH have been criticized because of the poor dose management of UFH and the inability to achieve a therapeutic range, it is just this attribute of LMWH that makes it such a more favorable anticoagulant over UFH.[140]

Another controversial area where the benefits of LMWH have been debated is its use in the treatment of DVT in patients with cancer and the impact on survival in patients with cancer and VTE. Cancer is a known risk factor for the development of VTE,[7] and patients with cancer and VTE have poorer survival rates than those with cancer but without DVT.[135] There also appears to be a higher failure rate (i.e., recurrence of DVT) in patients treated with warfarin despite being in therapeutic range when recurrence occurs.[141-143] Two recent studies indicate the potential benefit of LMWH over warfarin in cancer-related DVT. Meyer and colleagues,[144] in a randomized open-label study of more than 130 patients, found that those who received warfarin experienced a higher rate of failure (recurrent DVT or major bleeding) (21.1%) compared with enoxaparin (10.5%) (*P* = .09%) with fewer deaths and hemorrhagic deaths in the LMWH group. In an open-label study by Lee and colleagues,[145] there was a significant difference in recurrent DVT between those randomized to 3 months of dalteparin (27/336) versus dalteparin followed by warfarin (53/336) in patients with VTE and cancer. No significant difference in major bleeding or death occurred in these two groups.

A recent further refinement on the heparin molecule is fondaparinux, a synthetic form of the pentasaccharide sequence of UFH that binds to antithrombin.[146] Because fondarparinux lacks longer saccharide chains than in UFH or even LMWH, it lacks ability to bind to thrombin and thus has no antithrombin effect. It is a specific inhibitor of activated factor X via its binding to antithrombin. Whether this conveys an antithrombotic advantage is unknown and can only be tested through comparative clinical trials. Fondaparinux is almost 100% bioavailable when administered by subcutaneous injection. It has little protein binding. It has a predictable antithrombotic effect and requires no coagulation monitoring. Fondaparinux has good absorption from subcutaneous depots, reaches peak concentrations in 1 to 3 hours, and has an effective half-life of approximately 17 hours. Fondaparinux does not induce heparin-induced thrombocytopenia. It is excreted entirely by the kidneys and is not recommended in patients with renal impairment (creatinine clearance of <30 ml/min).

Fondaparinux underwent initial studies in prophylaxis of VTE in patients undergoing elective orthopedic joint replacement or in hip fracture surgery[93-96] (see previous discussion) and has recently undergone studies in the treatment of acute DVT and PE.[147,148] In a double-blinded

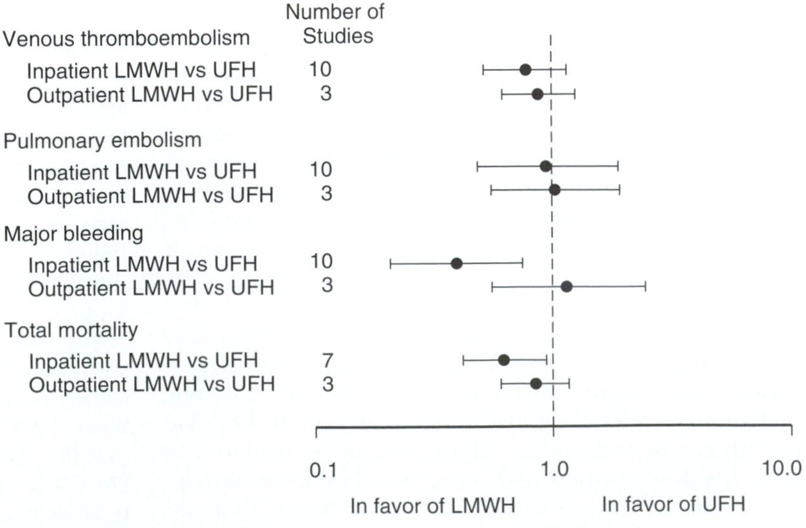

FIGURE 53-6. A comparison of inpatient versus outpatient treatment with low-molecular weight heparin (LMWH) versus unfractionated heparin (UFH). (From Dolovich LR, Ginsberg JS, Douketis JD, et al: A meta-analysis comparing low molecular weight heparins with unfractionated heparin in the treatment of venous thromboembolism: Examining some unanswered questions regarding location of treatment, product type, and dosing efficiency. Arch Intern Med 160:181, 2000.)

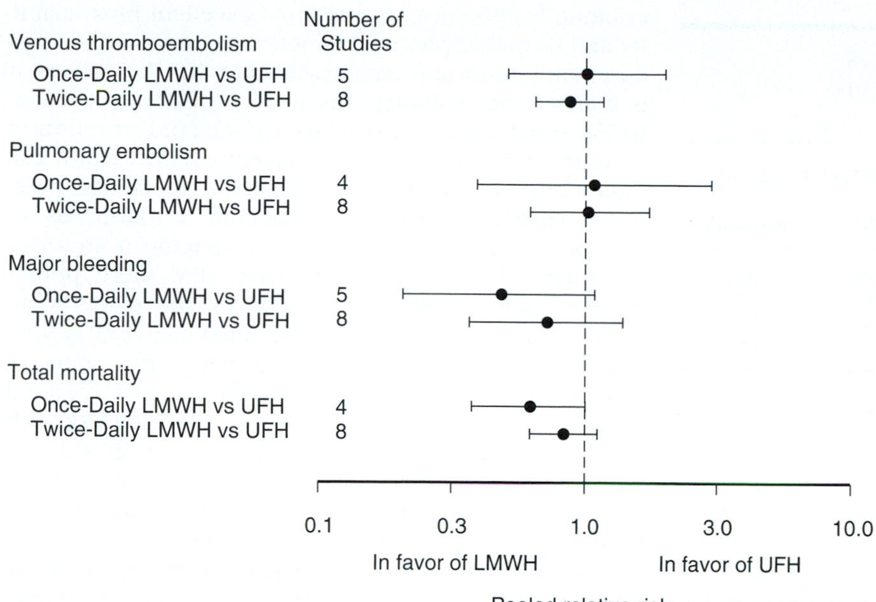

FIGURE 53-7. A comparison of once-daily or twice-daily low-molecular weight heparin (LMWH) versus unfractionated heparin (UFH). (From Dolovich LR, Ginsberg JS, Douketis JD, et al: A meta-analysis comparing low molecular weight heparins with unfractionated heparin in the treatment of venous thromboembolism: Examining some unanswered questions regarding location of treatment, product type, and dosing efficiency. Arch Intern Med 160:181, 2000.)

study of more than 2000 patients with acute DVT randomized between fondaparinux and enoxaparin for the initial 7- to 10-day treatment followed by warfarin for 3 months, there was no significant difference in recurrence of VTE (3.9% and 4.1%, respectively) or major bleeding (1.1% and 1.2%, respectively).[147] In an open-label study of fondaparinux versus UFH for the first 7 to 10 days followed by warfarin in more than 2000 patients with PE, the outcomes were similar: recurrent DVT/PE 2.4% versus 3.6%, respectively, and major bleeding 1.3% versus 1.1%, respectively.[148]

The treatment for upper extremity DVT has undergone changes in recent years. Traditionally, supportive care including elevation, warm compresses, and anti-inflammatory

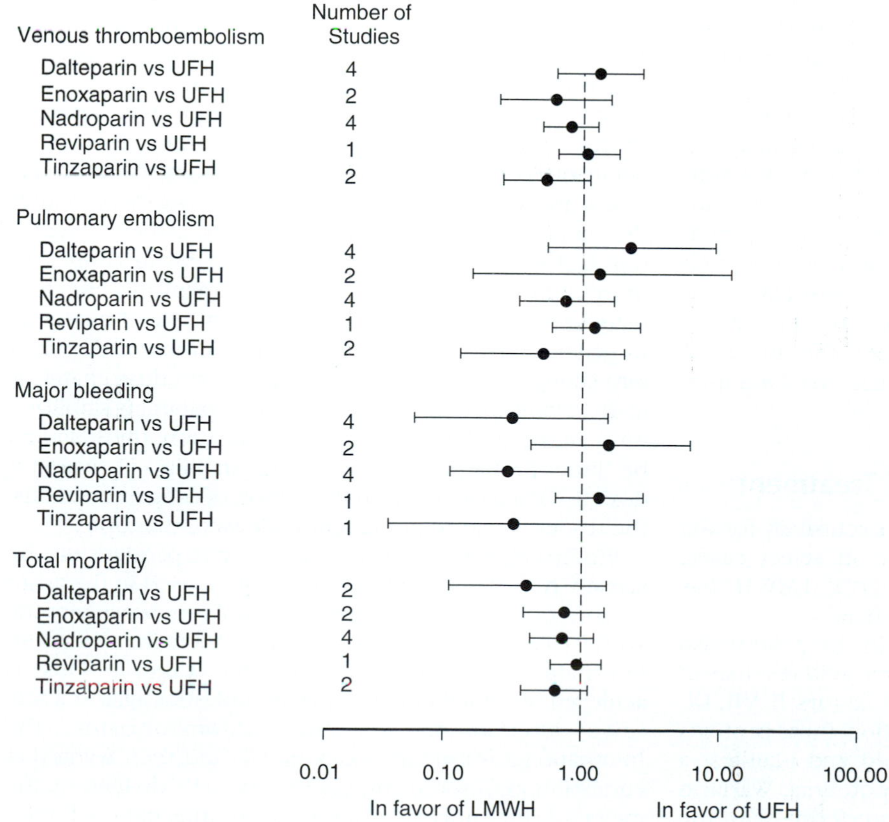

FIGURE 53-8. A comparison of different low-molecular weight heparin (LMWH) products versus unfractionated heparin (UFH). (From Dolovich LR, Ginsberg JS, Douketis JD, et al: A meta-analysis comparing low molecular weight heparins with unfractionated heparin in the treatment of venous thromboembolism: Examining some unanswered questions regarding location of treatment, product type, and dosing efficiency. Arch Intern Med 160:181, 2000.)

TABLE 53-8 INPATIENT (UFH) VERSUS PREDOMINANTLY OUTPATIENT (LMWH) TREATMENT OF DVT

	LEVINE ET AL[137]		KOOPMAN ET AL[138]	
Regimen	**UFH**	**Enoxaparin**	**UFH**	**Nadroparin**
Patients	253	247	198	202
Rec Thromb	6.7 %*	5.3%	8.6%	6.9%
Bleeding	1%	2%†	2%	0.5%
Hospital stay (days)	6.5	1.1‡	8.1	2.7§

Rec Thromb; recurrent thrombosis
*2 fatal pulmonary embolisms
†2 fatal bleeds
‡48% never hospitalized
§36% never hospitalized
DVT, deep venous thrombosis; LMWH, low-molecular weight heparin; UFH, unfractionated heparin

analgesics was the standard. With both a greater recognition of PE as a complication and to prevent post-thrombotic symptoms, anticoagulant therapy with UFH or LMWH followed by warfarin is now often used, but there is little information to guide the physician as to how long to treat.[149] Three months are usually provided depending on how the patient responds. Other options for treatment include local thrombolysis,[150] surgical thrombectomy, stenting, and superior vena caval filters when anticoagulation is contraindicated or unsuccessful.[151]

The optimal treatment for superficial venous thrombosis is less well characterized than that for lower extremity DVT. Often a conservative approach is used, withholding anticoagulants while administering anti-inflammatory agents. Compression stockings are often applied. UFH, when used, is given subcutaneously; larger doses may be more beneficial than lower prophylactic doses.[152] LMWH, in either a low dose (40 mg daily) or high dose (1.5 mg/kg daily) is also effective,[153] as is warfarin. Patients with superficial venous thrombosis are often referred for ligation surgery or venous stripping, but there is currently no standard of care for such patients. Because superficial vein thrombosis may occur in the setting of DVT in as many as 10% to 12% of patients,[18] it is important to consider the presence of DVT before instituting less intense therapy for superficial venous thrombosis.

Chronic Treatment/Duration of Treatment

Vitamin K antagonists are used almost exclusively for the long-term treatment of DVT, although in select cases, such as patients with cancer and DVT, LMWH has recently been shown to be more beneficial.

Vitamin K_1 is an essential cofactor in the posttranslational γ-carboxylation of several glutamic acid residues in the vitamin K–dependent coagulation factors II, VII, IX, and X.[154] In the absence of γ-carboxylation, these proteins cannot bind calcium and phospholipid and manifest a reduced coagulant (i.e., enzymatic) potential. Warfarin produces its anticoagulant effect by interfering with the cyclic interconversion of vitamin K and its 2,3 epoxide (vitamin K epoxide). Owing to its excellent bioavailability and favorable pharmacokinetics, warfarin is the most commonly used oral anticoagulant in North America. It is highly water soluble, rapidly absorbed from the gastrointestinal tract, and reaches a peak concentration in 60 to 90 minutes. Warfarin is a racemic mixture of R and S stereoisomers, each with distinctive metabolic pathways, half-lives, and potency. Racemic warfarin has an average half-life of 36 to 42 hours, ranging from 15 to 60 hours. The S form of warfarin (the more potent isomer) is metabolized primarily by the cytochrome P450 system, specifically the enzyme CYP2C9.[155] Genetic polymorphisms in this enzyme affect rates of drug metabolism and influence both the dose required to achieve a therapeutic level and the bleeding risk with warfarin therapy.[156,157] Specifically, the CYP2C9*2 and CYP2C9*3 alleles are associated with lower dose requirements and higher bleeding complication rates compared with the wild type enzyme CYP2C9*1.

Drug interactions with warfarin commonly occur by affecting its pharmacokinetic or pharmacodynamic behavior.[158] Drug interactions may also interfere with gastrointestinal absorption of warfarin, resulting in a reduction in plasma levels, or interfere with the metabolism of warfarin, leading to a reduction or increase in clearance and consequently higher or lower plasma warfarin levels. The latter effects may be stereospecific in that only one of the stereoisomers is affected, or they may be nonspecific in that both isomers are affected. Interference in the metabolism of the S isomer, usually by affecting the P450 cytochrome system (CYP2C9), is more common and has greater potential for enhancing the intensity of anticoagulation because the S isomer is several times more potent than the R isomer. Drugs may also decrease plasma warfarin levels by enhancing the metabolic clearance of racemic warfarin.

The pharmacodynamics of warfarin may also be altered when drugs interfere with other aspects of hemostasis or vitamin K_1 homeostasis. Some drugs or disease states (e.g., liver disease, hyperthyroidism) can alter the metabolism of coagulation factors, inhibit coagulation factor interactions by other mechanisms (heparin), or inhibit other aspects of hemostasis (aspirin's effect on platelet function) and lead to a greater risk of bleeding. In general, such interactions are most problematic when interacting drugs are added or deleted (or a dose change is made) from a patient's regimen. Once a patient is stabilized on warfarin and an interacting medication, there should be little problem in maintaining stability of warfarin dosing. For a more detailed discussion of drug interactions, the reader is referred to recent reviews of the topic.[159]

Prothrombin time results are highly dependent on the sensitivity of the thromboplastin reagent used in the assay. To correct for differences in thromboplastin sensitivity, the World Health Organization recommended the use of an international standard prothrombin time.[160] This is achieved by equilibrating all thromboplastins against a sensitive international reference thromboplastin (the International Sensitivity Index or ISI) and then using that equilibration factor to convert PT ratios (PT divided by the mean of the normal range) to an international ratio (the INR). The INR is essentially the PT ratio one would obtain if the international reference thromboplastin had been used to measure the PT. By converting all PT ratios to INRs one can interpret a patient's PT result regardless of where it is performed. Use of the INR does not eliminate all discrepancies in prothrombin time reporting,[161,162] but it significantly improves on the reporting of PT results using raw seconds or the PT ratio when monitoring patients on warfarin.

Therapy with warfarin is properly initiated using an average maintenance dose (5 mg) for the first 2 or 3 days,[163] although starting with a single 10-mg dose has also been shown to be safe and effective.[164] Additionally, lower than 5 mg starting doses might be appropriate in the elderly, in patients with impaired nutrition or liver disease, and in patients at high risk of bleeding.The dose required to maintain a therapeutic range for patients older than the age of 60 years has been shown to decrease with increasing age,[165] and older patients are more likely to have other factors that might influence INR stability or might influence the risk of bleeding such as a greater number of other medical conditions or concurrent drug use. Heparin should be given concurrently with warfarin, and both drugs overlap for a period of 4 to 5 days. Heparin is discontinued when the INR has been in the therapeutic range on two measurements at least 24 hours apart. Estimation of the maintenance dose is based on observations of the INR response following a fixed dose of warfarin over a few days' interval. Prothrombin time monitoring is performed frequently until the therapeutic range has been achieved and then less frequently as stability is maintained.

Patients receiving long-term warfarin therapy often have unexpected fluctuations in dose response that require careful management. A nontherapeutic (e.g., elevated) INR can be managed by discontinuing warfarin, administering vitamin K_1, or infusing fresh frozen plasma or prothrombin concentrate.[166] Recombinant factor VII_a has also been shown to correct an elevated INR due to warfarin.[167] Recent studies confirm earlier reports that oral administration of vitamin K is predictably effective and has the advantages of safety and convenience over parenteral routes.[168] Table 53-9 summarizes the latest American College of Chest Physicians (ACCP) guidelines for management of nontherapeutic INRs.

Clinicians are often confronted with the challenge of managing anticoagulation in individuals requiring noncardiac surgery or other invasive procedures, especially in individuals with prosthetic heart valves.[169] There is a paucity of critical studies examining the alternative choices for anticoagulation in this setting. Physicians must assess the risk of bleeding from a procedure if anticoagulation is continued versus the risk of thrombosis if anticoagulation is discontinued, as well as the cost of alternative anticoagulation options. LMWH offers a less complex alternative to UFH in that it requires no monitoring and can be given at home.[170-172]

Once treatment is initiated, a number of factors determine the appropriate duration of therapy. Principal among these is the likelihood of a recurrent event if anticoagulation is discontinued versus the risk of major bleeding with continued oral anticoagulation.The risk of bleeding on continued oral anticoagulation depends on a number of risk factors,[173,174] especially the quality of dose management.[175] A recent meta-analysis by Linkins and colleagues[176] of bleeding events from nine randomized studies of patients who received extended therapy (>3 months) found a rate of major bleeding of 2.74% with a rate of fatal bleeding of 0.63%.The case-fatality for major bleeding was 9.1%.

TABLE 53-9 RECOMMENDATIONS FOR MANAGING ELEVATED INRs OR BLEEDING IN PATIENTS RECEIVING VITAMIN K ANTAGONISTS

INR above therapeutic but <5 No significant bleeding	Lower or omit dose, monitor more frequently, and resume at lower dose when INR is therapeutic; if only minimally above therapeutic range, no dose reduction may be required **(grade 2C).**
INR >5 but <9 No significant bleeding	Omit next one or two doses, monitor more frequently, and resume at lower dose when INR is therapeutic. Alternatively, omit dose and give vitamin K_1 (≤5 mg) orally, particularly if patient is at increased risk of bleeding. If faster reversal is required because the patient requires urgent surgery, vitamin K_1 (2 to 4 mg) orally can be given with the expectation that a reduction of the INR will occur in 24 hr. If the INR is still high, additional vitamin K_1 (1 to 2 mg) orally can be given **(grade 2C).**
INR >9 No significant bleeding	Hold warfarin and give higher dose of vitamin K_1 (5-10 mg) orally with the expectation that the INR will be reduced substantially in 24-48 hrs. Monitor more frequently and use additional vitamin K_1 if necessary. Resume therapy at lower dose when INR is therapeutic **(grade 2C).**
Serious bleeding at any elevation of INR	Hold warfarin and give vitamin K_1 (10 mg) by slow IV infusion and supplemented with fresh plasma or prothrombin complex concentrate depending on the urgency of the situation; recombinant factor VIIa may be considered as alternative to prothrombin complex concentrate. Vitamin K_1 can be repeated every 12 hr **(grade 1C).**
Life-threatening bleeding	Hold warfarin and give prothrombin complex concentrate supplemented with vitamin K_1, 10 mg by slow IV infusion; recombinant factor VIIa may be considered as alternative to prothrombin complex concentrate; repeat if necessary depending on INR **(grade 1C).**

Note: If continuing warfarin therapy is indicated after high doses of vitamin K_1, then heparin or LMWH can be given until the effects of vitamin K_1 have been reversed and the patient becomes responsive to warfarin therapy. INR values >4.5 are less reliable than values in or near the therapeutic range. Thus these guidelines represent an approximate guide for high INRs.

INR, international normalized ratio

From Ansell J, Hirsh J, Poller P, et al: The pharmacology and management of the vitamin K antagonists. Chest 126(3 suppl): 204S, 2004.

Historically, patients have been routinely treated for 3 to 6 months with little consideration of factors that might require a shorter or longer duration of treatment. Recent studies have identified criteria, however, that are used to stratify patients into risk categories of those who have a low risk of recurrence and require a short duration of treatment and those with a high risk of recurrence and require a longer duration.[177-180] Patients who develop an initial DVT in the setting of a major, transient, reversible risk factor as the precipitating cause are recommended for 3 months of therapy. A British study of 712 patients found a trend toward lower recurrence in patients treated for 12 weeks (4%) compared with 6 weeks (7.8%)[181]; however, no difference was noted in those with postoperative DVT where the recurrence rate was low in both groups (≈2.6%), suggesting that a short duration of treatment was appropriate for this group. Levine and coworkers[182] found similar outcomes for patients with reversible transient risk factors who received 3 months of therapy (0% recurrence after 11 months of follow-up) versus those with risk factors (12.3% recurrence). Prandoni and colleagues[183] confirmed the low risk of recurrence in a long-term, 8-year, follow-up study of patients with transient risk factors (hazard ratio 0.36; confidence interval 0.21 to 0.62) compared with those with ongoing risk factors (hazard ratio 1.72 for cancer and 1.44 for impaired coagulation inhibition).

Of greater concern are those patients who have ongoing risk factors such as cancer or patients with idiopathic DVT. Kearon and coworkers[184] showed that 10 months of therapy were significantly better than 3 months (1.3% per patient year recurrence vs. 27.4% per patient year). However, Agnelli and coworkers[185] showed that even after 1 year of continued treatment, the recurrence rate was the same but occurred later, compared with those having only 3 months of treatment (15.7% recurrence at 3 years vs. 15.8% recurrence). The rate of recurrence was the same for both groups but was simply delayed in those who continued treatment longer.

Most recently, two groups have assessed the value of longer-term therapy in patients with idiopathic or unprovoked DVT. In an effort to balance the risks of bleeding against the benefit of DVT prevention, Ridker and colleagues[186] randomized 508 patients after approximately 6 months of standard therapy to either low-dose warfarin (INR 1.5 to 2) or placebo. After a mean of 2.1 years of follow-up, recurrent VTE occurred in 37 placebo patients (7.2 per 100 patient years) versus 14 low-dose warfarin patients (2.6 per 100 patient years) ($P < .001$). There was no difference in major bleeding. Once stable, the warfarin group was monitored about every 2 months. In contrast, Kearon and colleagues[187] assessed the value of low-dose warfarin (INR 1.5 to 1.9) versus full-dose warfarin (INR 2 to 3) in a similar group of 738 patients who were randomized after 3 or more months of therapy and followed for a mean of 2.4 years. Recurrence of VTE was seen in 16 patients in the low-dose group (1.9 per 100 patient years) versus 6 in the conventional-dose group (0.7 per 100 patient years) ($P = .03$). Of note, there was no difference in major bleeding between the two groups (1.1 vs. 0.9 per 100 patient years). Table 53-10 compares these results with a new oral anticoagulant, ximelagatran, discussed later, as prevention of recurrent VTE after a course of standard duration treatment.

TABLE 53-10 COMPARISON OF THREE TRIALS OF EXTENDED, LONG-TERM PROPHYLAXIS FOR DVT RECURRENCE AFTER A STANDARD COURSE OF TREATMENT

	PREVENT	ELATE	THRIVE
No. of patients	508	738	1223
Mean follow-up	2.1 yr	2.3 yr	1.5 yr
VTE recurrence*			
Treatment†	2.6 (LD warfarin)	0.7 (FD warfarin)	1.9 (Ximelag)
Comparator†	7.2 (PLC)	1.9 (LD warfarin)	8.4 (PLC)
Major bleed*			
Treatment†	0.9	0.9	0.7
Comparator†	0.4	1.1	0.9

*No. per 100 patient yr
†Results expressed as %
DVT, deep venous thrombosis; FD, full dose; LD, low dose; PLC, placebo; VTE, venous thromboembolism
Data from PREVENT trial[186]; ELATE trial[187]; Thrive trial.[196]

These data provide strong evidence that the rate of VTE recurrence is high (≈8% to 10% per year) after 6 months of anticoagulation treatment in patients with idiopathic or unprovoked DVT or with ongoing risk factors. Continued treatment with either low-dose warfarin (INR 1.5 to 2) or full-dose warfarin (INR 2 to 3) is effective, although full-dose warfarin is more effective, as one might expect. The risk of bleeding was low in all groups studied and not statistically different. This lack of a difference in bleeding might be due to the fact that the studies were not sized to detect such a difference, that patients were already 3 to 6 months out from initiation of therapy and those who bled early were not enrolled, or that anticoagulation control was optimized under study conditions. The safety of full-intensity therapy in a non-study environment may not be as ideal, and thus either low-dose or full-dose long-term therapy is a reasonable approach depending on patient characteristics and the availability of high-quality dose management.

Recently, investigators have identified markers that may serve as risk factors for recurrent disease in patients treated for 6 months, thus enabling further stratification of those who should or should not receive continuing therapy. These include elevated D-dimer levels or residual vein thrombus on ultrasound detected after a course of anticoagulation is completed.[188,189] In 610 patients studied, Eichinger and colleagues[188] found that the cumulative probability of recurrent VTE at 2 years was 3.7% for patients with D-dimer levels below 250 ng/ml compared with 11.5% for patients with higher levels. Cosmi and coworkers[189] found a recurrence rate of 13.3% versus 5.7% in patients with and without residual vein thrombosis after a standard course of therapy, and 8.3% versus 3.4% for patients with an elevated D-dimer versus those without. The rate was 16.5% for those with both a positive D-dimer and residual vein thrombosis.

NEW ANTICOAGULANT AGENTS

A number of new anticoagulants are undergoing study to determine their efficacy and safety compared with standard therapy in the treatment of VTE.[190] Several of these agents are unique in that they are small-molecule, direct inhibitors of specific coagulation factors as opposed to indirect inhibitors such as heparin, LMWH, or fondaparinux[191-193]; they are orally available without many of the drawbacks of the vitamin K antagonists; and they have pharmacokinetic characteristics that make them more attractive for long-term outpatient use.[194] One agent of particular interest is the oral, direct thrombin inhibitor ximelagatran. Although not currently approved for clinical use in the United States, ximelagatran has undergone extensive phase 3 testing for VTE prophylaxis and treatment, as well as for stroke prevention in patients with atrial fibrillation.[195-198] In approximately 2500 patients with acute DVT randomized to receive ximelagatran or enoxaparin followed by warfarin for 6 months, ximelagatran was found to be noninferior to standard therapy (2.1% recurrence vs. 2%, respectively), with no difference in major bleeding.[195]

In a study of 1200 patients with DVT treated for 6 months with standard therapy and then randomized to treatment with ximelagatran versus placebo for the next 18 months, ximelagatran was significantly better, resulting in a 78% relative risk reduction in recurrent VTE (2.8% vs. 12.6%, respectively) with no difference in major bleeding.[196] This compares favorably with studies by Ridker and colleagues[186] and Kearon and coworkers[187] using full-dose or low-dose warfarin (see Table 53-10), although direct comparison of ximelagatran with full-dose or low-dose warfarin over an 18-month period after the initial 6 months of therapy has yet to be performed.

Ximelagatran has also been studied extensively in hip and knee replacement surgery and, depending on the dose or timing of administration, or both, has proved to be equivalent or better than prophylaxis with warfarin or enoxaparin.[199,200] Other oral direct coagulation factor inhibitors are being studied, and one of interest is razaxaban, a direct, oral Xa inhibitor showing favorable results in a phase 2 study against LMWH for prophylaxis in TKR surgery.[193] Lastly, agents such as idraparinux, an indirect Xa inhibitor variant of fondaparinux with a prolonged half-life that allows for once weekly subcutaneous dosing, has undergone phase 2 trials in acute DVT[194] and is currently undergoing a phase 3 trial in acute and chronic treatments of DVT and PE, as well as preliminary trials in stroke prevention in atrial fibrillation.

VENOUS THROMBOEMBOLISM IN PREGNANCY

VTE is a particular problem in pregnancy.[201,202] PE remains an important cause of maternal mortality; the underlying risk factors for VTE can predispose to complications of pregnancy other than VTE including miscarriage, intrauterine growth retardation, eclampsia, placental problems, and fetal death; the treatment or prevention of these problems with the usual agents is fraught with its own set of problems; and finally, the need for effective treatment is increasing as more women at risk are identified. Women with thrombophilia (e.g., factor V_{Leiden} or prothrombin^{G20210A} gene variant) are at increased risk of fetal loss.[203-205] This is an even greater problem and often a marker of disease for those with the antiphospholipid syndrome.[206]

The use of anticoagulants to prevent these complications of pregnancy or to prevent VTE in patients who have not had a previous event is controversial, especially in North America, whereas in several European countries, treatment is more likely to be instituted. Of particular concern are the complications experienced with the use of anticoagulants. Vitamin K antagonists can induce an embryopathy if used during the first trimester of pregnancy, although the actual occurrence is rather low.[202] Unfractionated heparin, given by subcutaneous injection in adjusted doses, is the usual alternative, although a pooled analysis of multiple reports indicates that UFH may lead to fetal complications (e.g., miscarriage, congenital fetal anomalies, fetal wastage) in 20% to 40% of pregnancies.[202] LMWH has not been systematically studied in randomized trials of pregnant women, but in a number of cohort studies, outcomes have been as effective as those reported with UFH,[211-213] and LMWH is less difficult to manage. Women who have mechanical prosthetic heart valves and become pregnant are at great risk for valve thrombosis or systemic embolism. The alternative treatment of choice in this setting has been less clear because of the concern that LMWH is inadequate to prevent valve thrombosis.[214,215] A systematic review of case reports or series of pregnant patients treated with LMWH who have mechanical valves indicates that LMWH is effective in this setting and may be better than UFH when used appropriately.[216]

REFERENCES

1. Silverstein M, Heit JA, Mohr D, et al: Trends in the incidence of deep vein thrombosis and pulmonary embolism: A 25 year population based study. Arch Intern Med 158:585, 1998.
2. Heit JA: Venous thromboembolism epidemiology: Implications for prevention and management. Semin Thromb Hemost 28(suppl 2): 3, 2001.
3. Cohen AT: Discoveries in thrombosis care for medical patients. Semin Thromb Hemost 28(suppl 2):13, 2002.
4. Anderson FA Jr, Wheeler HB, Goldberg RJ, et al: Physician practices in the prevention of venous thromboembolism. Ann Intern Med 115:591, 1991.
5. Bratzler DW, Raskob GE, Murray CK, et al: Under use of venous thromboembolism prophylaxis for general surgery patients: Physician practices in the community hospital setting. Arch Intern Med 158:1909, 1998.
6. Stein PD, Hull RD, Chali WA, et al: Tracking the uptake of evidence: Two decades of hospital practice trends for diagnosing deep vein thrombosis and pulmonary embolism. Arch Intern Med 163:1213, 2003.
7. Leclerc JR: Natural history of venous thromboembolism. In Leclerc JR (ed): Venous Thromboembolic Disorders. Malvern, PA, Lea & Febiger, 1991, pp 166-175.
8. Phillips MD: Interrelated risk factors for venous thromboembolism. Circulation 95:1749, 1997.
9. Anderson FA Jr, Spencer FA: Risk factors for venous thromboembolism. Circulation 107:I-9, 2003.

10. Seligsohn U, Lubetsky A: Genetic susceptibility to venous thrombosis. N Engl J Med 344:1222, 2001.
11. Rosenberg RD, Aird WC: Vascular-bed-specific hemostasis and hypercoagulable states. N Engl J Med 340:1555, 1999.
12. Thomas RH: Hypercoagulability syndromes. Arch Intern Med 161:2433, 2001.
13. Coleman RW, Hirsh J, Marder VJ, et al: Overview of coagulation, fibrinolysis and their regulation. In Colman RW, Hirsh J, Marder VJ, et al (eds): Hemostasis and Thrombosis, Philadelphia, Lippincott Williams & Wilkins, 2001, pp 17-20.
14. Grondin L, Raymond-Martimbeau P: Superficial venous system disorders. In Leclerc JR (ed): Venous Thromboembolic Disorders. Malvern, PA, Lea & Febiger, 1991, pp 412-429.
15. Schonauer V, Kyrle PA, Weltermann A, et al: Superficial thrombophlebitis and risk for recurrent venous thromboembolism. J Vasc Surg 37:834, 2003.
16. de Godoy JM, Batigalia F, Braile DM: Superficial thrombophlebitis and anticardiolipin antibodies-report of association. Angiology 52:127, 2001.
17. de Godoy JM, Godoy MA, Batigalia F, et al: The association of Mondor's disease with protein S deficiency: Case report and review of literature. J Thromb Thrombolys 13:187, 2002.
18. Skillman JJ, Kent KC, Porter, et al: Simultaneous occurrence of superficial and deep thrombophlebitis in the lower extremity. J Vasc Surg 11:818, 1990.
19. Ascher E, Hanson JN, Salles-Cunha S, et al: Lesser saphenous vein thrombophlebitis: Its natural history and implications for management. Vasc Endovasc Surg 37:421, 2003.
20. Kakkar VV, Howe CT, Flanc C, et al: Natural history of post-operative deep vein thrombosis. Lancet 2:230, 1969.
21. Meignan M, Rosso J, Gauthier H, et al: Systematic lung scans reveal a high frequency of silent pulmonary embolism in patients with proximal deep venous thrombosis. Arch Intern Med 160:159, 2000.
22. Bolgiano EB, Foxwell MM, Browne BJ, et al: Deep venous thrombosis of the upper extremity: Diagnosis and treatment. J Emerg Med 8:85, 1990.
23. Mustafa S, Stein P, Kalpesh P, et al: Upper extremity deep venous thrombosis. Chest 123:1953, 2003.
24. Horattas MC, Wright DJ, Fenton AH, et al: Changing concepts of deep venous thrombosis of the upper extremity: Report of a series and review of the literature. Surgery 104:561, 1988.
25. Martinelli I, Cattaneo M, Panzeri D, et al: Risk factors for deep venous thrombosis of the upper extremities. Ann Intern Med 126:707, 1997.
26. Heron E, Lozinguez O, Alhenc-Gelas M, et al: Hypercoagulable states in primary upper-extremity deep vein thrombosis. Arch Intern Med 160:382, 2000.
27. Monreal M, Raventos A, Lerma R, et al: Pulmonary embolism in patients with upper extremity DVT associated to venous central lines: A prospective study. Thromb Haemost 72:548, 1994.
28. Heron E, Lozinguez O, Emmerich J, et al: Long-term sequelae of spontaneous axillary-subclavian venous thrombosis. Ann Intern Med 131:510, 1999.
29. Mulder DS: Chronic venous insufficiency syndrome: Etiology, pathogenesis and treatment. In Leclerc JR (ed): Venous Thromboembolic Disorders. Malvern, PA, Lea & Febiger, 1991, pp 74-83.
30. Hull RD, Hirsh J, Sackett DL, et al: Clinical validity of a negative venogram in patients with clinically suspected venous thrombosis. Circulation 64:622, 1981.
31. Kahn SR: The clinical diagnosis of deep venous thrombosis: Integrating incidence, risk factors, and symptoms and signs. Arch Intern Med 158:2315, 1998.
32. Anand SS, Wells PS, Hunt D, et al: Does this patient have deep vein thrombosis? JAMA 279:1094, 1998.
33. Leclerc JR, Illescas F, Jarzem P: Diagnosis of deep vein thrombosis. In Leclerc JR (ed): Venous Thromboembolic Disorders. Malvern, PA, Lea & Febiger, 1991, pp 176-228.
34. Haeger K: Problems of acute deep venous thrombosis. I. The interpretation of signs and symptoms. Angiology 20:219, 1969.
35. Sandler DA, Martin JF, Duncan JS, et al: Diagnosis of deep vein thrombosis: Comparison of clinical evaluation, ultrasound, plethysmography, and venoscan with X-ray venogram. Lancet 2:716, 1984.
36. Samlaska CP, James WD: Superficial thrombophlebitis. II. Secondary hypercoagulable states. J Am Acad Dermatol 23:1, 1990.
37. Landefeld CS, McGuire E, Cohen AM: Clinical findings associated with acute proximal deep vein thrombosis: A basis for quantifying clinical judgement. Am J Med 88:382, 1990.
38. Wells PS, Hirsh J, Anderson DR, et al: Accuracy of clinical assessment of deep vein thrombosis. Lancet 345:1326, 1995.
39. Wells PS, Anderson DR, Bormanis J, et al: Value of assessment of the pretest probability of deep vein thrombosis in clinical management. Lancet 350:1795, 1997.
40. Wells PS, Anderson DR, Bormanis J, et al: Application of a diagnostic clinical model for the management of hospitalized patients with suspected deep vein thrombosis. Thromb Haemost 81:493, 1999.
41. Birdwell BG, Raskob GE, Whitsett TL, et al: Predictive value of compression ultrasonography for deep vein thrombosis in symptomatic outpatients: Clinical implications of the site of vein noncompressibility. Arch Intern Med 160:309, 2000.
42. Wells PS, Lensing AW, Davidson BL, et al: Accuracy of ultrasound for the diagnosis of deep venous thrombosis in asymptomatic patients after orthopedic surgery: A meta-analysis. Ann Intern Med 122:47, 1995.
43. Kearon C, Julian JA, Newman TE, et al: Noninvasive diagnosis of deep venous thrombosis. McMaster Diagnostic Imaging Practice Guidelines Initiative. Ann Intern Med 128:663, 1998.
44. Lensing AW, Prandoni P, Brandjes D, et al: Detection of deep-vein thrombosis by real-time B-mode ultrasonography. N Engl J Med 320:342, 1989.
45. White RH, McGahan JP, Daschbach MM, et al: Diagnosis of deep vein thrombosis using duplex ultrasound. Ann Intern Med 111:297, 1989.
46. Kraaijenhagen RA, Lensing AW, Wallis JW, et al: Diagnostic management of venous thromboembolism. In Pineo GF, Hull RD (eds): Bailliere's Clinical Haematology, Prevention, Diagnosis and Management of Venous Thromboembolic Disease. London, Bailliere Tindall, 1998, pp 541-586.
47. Mitchell DC, Grasty MS, Stebbings WS, et al: Comparison of duplex ultrasonography and venography in the diagnosis of deep venous thrombosis. Br J Surg 78:611, 1991.
48. Simons GR, Skibo LK, Polak JF, et al: Utility of leg ultrasonography in suspected symptomatic isolated calf deep venous thrombosis. Am J Med 99:43, 1995.
49. Birdwell BG, Raskob GE, Whitsett TL, et al: The clinical validity of normal compression ultrasonography in outpatients suspected of having deep venous thrombosis. Ann Intern Med 128:1, 1998.
50. Wolf B, Nichols DM, Duncan JL: Safety of a single duplex scan to exclude deep venous thrombosis. Br J Surg 87:1525, 2000.
51. Schellong SM, Schwarz T, Halbritter K, et al: Complete compression ultrasonography of the leg veins as a single test for the diagnosis of deep vein thrombosis. Thromb Haemost 89:228, 2003.
52. Elias A, Mallard L, Elias M, et al: A single complete ultrasound investigation of the venous network for the diagnostic management of patients with a clinically suspected first episode of deep venous thrombosis of the lower limbs. Thromb Haemost 89:221, 2003.
53. Stevens SM, Elliott CG, Chan KJ, et al: Withholding anticoagulation after a negative result on duplex ultrasonography for suspected symptomatic deep venous thrombosis. Ann Intern Med 140:985, 2004.
54. Wheeler HB: Diagnosis of deep vein thrombosis: Review of clinical evaluation and impedance plethysmography. Am J Surg 150:7, 1985.
55. Hull R, Taylor DW, Hirsh J, et al: Impedance plethysmography: The relationship between venous filling and sensitivity and specificity for proximal vein thrombosis. Circulation 58:898, 1978.
56. Hull RD, Hirsh J, Sackett DL, et al: Combined use of leg scanning and impedance plethysmography in suspected venous thrombosis: An alternative to venography. N Engl J Med 296:1497, 1977.
57. Kearon C, Hirsh J: Factors influencing the reported sensitivity and specificity of impedance plethysmography for proximal deep vein thrombosis. Thromb Haemost 72:652, 1994.
58. Prandoni P, Lensing AW, Huisman MV, et al: A new computerized impedance plethysmography: accuracy in the detection of proximal deep vein thrombosis in symptomatic outpatients. Thromb Haemost 65:229, 1991.
59. McLachlan MS, Thomson JG, Taylor DW, et al: Observer variation in the interpretation of lower limb venograms. AJR Am J Roentgenol 132:227, 1979.
60. Bettman MA, Paulin S: Leg phlebography: The incidence, nature and modification of undesirable side effects. Radiology 122:101, 1977.

61. Cohan RH, Dunnick NR: Intravascular contrast media: Adverse reactions. AJR Am J Roentgenol 149:665, 1987.
62. Bettman MA, Robbins A, Braun SD, et al: Contrast venography of the leg: Diagnostic efficacy, tolerance, and complication rates with ionic and nonionic contrast media. Radiology 165:113, 1987.
63. Evans AJ, Sostman HD, Knelson MH, et al: Detection of deep venous thrombosis: Prospective comparison of MR imaging with contrast venography. AJR Am J Roentgenol 161:131, 1993.
64. Kelly J, Hunt BJ, Moody A: Magnetic resonance direct thrombus imaging: A novel technique for imaging venous thromboemboli. Thromb Haemost 89:773, 2003.
65. Fraser DGW, Moody AR, Morgan PS, et al: Diagnosis of lower-limb deep venous thrombosis: A prospective blinded study of magnetic resonance direct thrombus imaging. Ann Intern Med 136:89, 2002.
66. Bockenstedt P: D-dimer in venous thromboembolism. N Engl J Med 349:1203, 2003.
67. Freyburger G, Trillaud H, Labrouche S, et al: D-dimer strategy in thrombosis exclusion: A gold standard study in 100 patients suspected of deep venous thrombosis or pulmonary embolism: 8 DD methods compared. Thromb Haemost 79:32, 1998.
68. van der Graaf F, van den Borne H, van der Kolk M, et al: Exclusion of deep venous thrombosis with D-dimer testing: Comparison of 13 D-dimer methods in 99 outpatients suspect of deep venous thrombosis using venography as reference standard. Thromb Haemost 83:191, 2000.
69. Kearon C, Ginsberg JS, Douketis J, et al: Management of suspected deep venous thrombosis in outpatients by using clinical assessment and D-dimer testing. Ann Intern Med 135:108, 2001.
70. Bates SM, Kearon C, Crowther M, et al: A diagnostic strategy involving a quantitative latex D-dimer assay reliably excludes deep venous thrombosis. Ann Intern Med 138:787, 2003.
71. Wells PS, Anderson DR, Rodger M, et al: Evaluation of D-dimer in the diagnosis of suspected deep-vein thrombosis. N Engl J Med 349:1227, 2003.
72. Frost SD, Brotman DJ, Michota FA: Rational use of D-dimer measurement to exclude acute venous thromboembolic disease. Mayo Clin Proc 78:1385, 2003.
73. Bounameaux H, de Moerloose P, Perrier A, et al: D-dimer testing in suspected venous thromboembolism: An update. QJM 90:437, 1997.
74. Bauer KA: The thrombophilias: Well-defined risk factors with uncertain therapeutic implications. Ann Intern Med 135:367, 2001.
75. Dismuke SE, Wagner EH: Pulmonary embolism as a cause of death: The changing mortality in hospitalized patients. JAMA 255:2039, 1986.
76. Dalen JE, Alpert JS: Natural history of pulmonary embolism. Prog Cardiovasc Dis 17:259, 1975.
77. Sevitt S, Gallagher NG: Prevention of venous thrombosis and pulmonary embolism in injured patients: A trial of anticoagulant prophylaxis with phenindione in middle-aged and elderly patients with necks of femur. Lancet 2:981, 1959.
78. Kakkar VV, Field ES, Nicolaides AN, et al: Low doses of heparin in prevention of deep vein thrombosis. Lancet 2:669, 1971.
79. Lederle FA: Heparin prophylaxis for medical patients? Ann Intern Med 128:768, 1998.
80. Geerts WH, Heit JA, Clagett GP, et al: Prevention of venous thromboembolism. Chest 119(suppl):132S, 2001.
81. Nicolaides AN, Bergqvist D, Hull R, et al: Prevention of VTE: International consensus statement. Int Angiol 16:3, 1997.
82. Douketis JD, Eikelboom JW, Quinlan DJ, et al: Short-duration prophylaxis against venous thromboembolism after total hip or knee replacement. Arch Intern Med 162:1465, 2002.
83. O'Donnell M, Linkins LA, Kearon C, et al: Reduction of out-of-hospital symptomatic venous thromboembolism by extended thromboprophylaxis with low molecular weight heparin following elective hip arthroplasty. Arch Intern Med 163:1362, 2003.
84. Eriksson BI, Lassen MR, et al: Duration of prophylaxis against venous thromboembolism with fondaparinux after hip fracture surgery. Arch Intern Med 163:1337, 2003.
85. Hull R, Raskob G, Pineo G, et al: A comparison of subcutaneous low molecular weight heparin with warfarin sodium for prophylaxis against deep vein thrombosis after hip or knee implantation. N Engl J Med 329:1370, 1993.
86. Hamulyak K, Lensing AWA, van der Meer J, et al: Subcutaneous low molecular weight heparin or oral anticoagulants for the prevention of deep vein thrombosis in elective hip and knee replacement? Thromb Haemost 74:1428, 1995.
87. Leclerc JR, Geerts W, Desjardin L, et al: Prevention of venous thromboembolism after knee arthroplasty: A randomized, double-blind trial comparing enoxaparin with warfarin. Ann Intern Med 124:619, 1996.
88. The RD Heparin Arthroplasty Group: RD heparin compared with warfarin for the prevention of venous thromboembolic disease following total hip or knee arthroplasty. J Bone Joint Surg Am 76:1174, 1994.
89. Zimlich RH, Fulbright BM, Friedman RJ: Current status of anticoagulation therapy after total hip and total knee arthroplasty. J Am Acad Orthop Surg 4:54, 1996.
90. Hull RD, Pineo GF, Stein PD, et al: Timing of initial administration of low molecular weight heparin prophylaxis against deep vein thrombosis in patients following elective hip arthroplasty: A systematic review. Arch Intern Med 161:1952, 2001.
91. Hull RD, Pineo GF, Bharadia V, et al: Timing of initial administration of prophylaxis against deep vein thrombosis in patients following hip surgery. Chest 122(suppl):212, 2002.
92. Turpie AG, Gallus AS, Hoek JA, for the Pentasaccharide Investigators: A synthetic pentasaccharide for the prevention of deep vein thrombosis after total hip replacement. N Engl J Med 344:619, 2001.
93. Turpie AG, Bauer KA, Eriksson BI, et al: Postoperative fondaparinux versus postoperative enoxaparin for prevention of venous thromboembolism after elective hip replacement surgery: A randomized double-blind trial. Lancet 359:1721, 2002.
94. Lassen MR, Bauer KA, Eriksson BI, et al: Postoperative fondaparinux versus preoperative enoxaparin for prevention of venous thromboembolism in elective hip replacement surgery: A randomized double-blind comparison. Lancet 359:1715, 2002.
95. Eriksson BI, Bauer KA, Lassen MR, et al: Fondaparinux compared with enoxaparin for the prevention of venous thromboembolism after hip fracture surgery. N Engl J Med 345:1298, 2001.
96. Bauer KA, Eriksson BI, Lassen MR, et al: Fondaparinux compared with enoxaparin for the prevention of venous thromboembolism after elective major knee surgery. N Engl J Med 345:1305, 2001.
97. Samama CM, Vray M, Barre J, et al. Extended venous thromboembolism prophylaxis after total hip replacement: A comparison of low-molecular-weight heparin with oral anticoagulants. Arch Intern Med 162:2191, 2002.
98. Prandoni P, Bruchi O, Sabbion P, et al: Prolonged thromboprophylaxis with oral anticoagulants after total hip arthroplasty: A prospective controlled randomized study. Arch Intern Med 162:1966, 2002.
99. Hull RD, Pineo GF, Stein PD, et al: Extended out-of-hospital low-molecular-weight heparin prophylaxis against deep venous thrombosis in patients after elective hip arthroplasty: A systematic review. Ann Intern Med 135:858, 2001.
100. Haas S, Flosbach CW: Antithromboembolic efficacy and safety of enoxaparin in general surgery: German Multicentre Trial. Eur J Surg 571(suppl):37, 1994.
101. Stratton MA, Anderson FA, Bussey HI, et al: Prevention of venous thromboembolism. Adherence to the 1995 American College of Chest Physicians Consensus Guidelines for Surgical Patients. Arch Intern Med 160:334, 2000.
102. Nurmohamed MT, Rosendaal FR, Buller HR, et al: Low molecular weight heparin versus standard heparin in general and orthopaedic surgery: A meta-analysis. Lancet 340:152, 1992.
103. Mismetti P, Laporte-Simitsidis S, Tardy B, et al: Prevention of venous thromboembolism in internal medicine with unfractionated or low molecular weight heparins: A meta-analysis of randomized clinical trials. Thromb Haemost 83:14, 2000.
104. Belch JJ, Lowe GD, Ward AG, et al: Prevention of deep vein thrombosis in medical patients by low-dose heparin. Scott Med J 26:115, 1981.
105. Samama MM, Cohen AT, Darmon JY, et al: A comparison of enoxaparin with placebo for the prevention of venous thromboembolism in acutely ill medical patients. Prophylaxis in Medical Patients with Enoxaparin Study Group. N Engl J Med 341:793, 1999.
106. Bergmann JF, Neuhart E: A multicenter randomized double-blind study of enoxaparin compared with unfractionated heparin in the prevention of venous thromboembolic disease in elderly in patients bedridden for an acute medical illness. Thromb Haemost 76:529, 1996.

107. Leizorovicz A, Goldhaber SZ: New Developments in Cutting Edge Therapeutics. Presented at the 32nd Annual Critical Care Congress of the Society of Critical Care Medicine; January 31, 2003; San Antonio, TX.
108. Lechler E, Schramm W, Flosbach CW: The venous thrombotic risk in non-surgical patients: Epidemiological data and efficacy/safety profile of low molecular weight heparin (enoxaparin). The Prime Study Group. Haemostasis 26(suppl 2):49, 1996.
109. Kleber FX, Witt C, Vogel G, et al: Randomized comparison of enoxaparin with unfractionated heparin for the prevention of venous thromboembolism in medical patients with heart failure or severe respiratory disease. Am Heart J 145:614, 2003.
110. Green D, Lee MY, Lim AC, et al: Prevention of thromboembolism after spinal cord injury using low molecular weight heparin. Ann Intern Med 113:571, 1990.
111. Green D, Lee MY, Ito VY, et al: Fixed vs adjusted dose heparin in the prophylaxis of thromboembolism in spinal cord injury. JAMA 260:1255, 1988.
112. Green D: Prevention and treatment of venous thromboembolism in neurologic and neurosurgical patients. In Kitchens C, Alving B, Kessler G (eds): Consultative Hemostasis and Thrombosis. Philadelphia, WB Saunders, 2002, pp 549-556.
113. Hirsh J: Heparin. N Engl J Med 324:1565, 1991.
114. Hirsh J, Warkentin TE, Shaughnessy SG, et al: Heparin and low molecular weight heparin: Mechanisms of action, pharmacokinetics, dosing, monitoring, efficacy, and safety. Chest 119(suppl): 64S, 2001.
115. Young E, Prins MH, Levine MN, et al: Heparin binding to plasma proteins: An important mechanism for heparin resistance. Thromb Haemost 67:639, 1992.
116. Hirsh J, van Aken WG, Gallus AS, et al: Heparin kinetics in venous thrombosis and pulmonary embolism. Circulation 53:691, 1976.
117. Basu D, Gallus AS, Hirsh J, et al: A prospective study of value of monitoring heparin treatment with the activated partial thromboplastin time. N Engl J Med 287:324, 1972.
118. Brill-Edwards P, Ginsberg JS, Johnston M, et al: Establishing a therapeutic range for heparin therapy. Ann Intern Med 119:104, 1993.
119. Fennerty AG, Thomas P, Backhouse G, et al: Audit of control of heparin treatment. Br Med J 290:27, 1985.
120. Reilly B, Raschke R, Sandhya S, et al: Intravenous heparin dosing; Patterns and variations in internist's practices. J Gen Intern Med 8:536, 1993.
121. Hull RD, Raskob GE, Hirsh J, et al: Continuous intravenous heparin compared with intermittent subcutaneous heparin in the initial treatment of proximal vein thrombosis. N Engl J Med 315:1109, 1986.
122. Brandjes DP, Heijboer H, Buller HR, et al: Acenocoumarol and heparin compared with acenocoumarol alone in the initial treatment of proximal vein thrombosis. N Engl J Med 327:1485, 1992.
123. Raschke RA, Reilly BM, Guidry JR, et al: The weight-based heparin dosing nomogram compared with a "standard care" nomogram: A randomized controlled trial. Ann Intern Med 119:874, 1993.
124. Cruickshank MK, Levine MN, Hirsh H, et al: A standard nomogram for the management of heparin therapy. Arch Intern Med 151:333, 1991.
125. Wheeler AP, Jaquiss RD, Newman JH: Physician practices in the treatment of pulmonary embolism and deep venous thrombosis. Arch Intern Med 148:1321, 1988.
126. Elliott GC, Hiltunen SJ, Suchyta M, et al: Physician guided treatment compared with a heparin protocol for deep vein thrombosis. Arch Intern Med 154:999, 1994.
127. Raschke R, Hirsh J, Guidry JR: Suboptimal monitoring and dosing of unfractionated heparin in comparative studies with low molecular weight heparin. Ann Intern Med 138:720, 2003.
128. Hylek EM, Regan S, Henault LE, et al: Challenges to the effective use of unfractionated heparin in the hospitalized management of acute thrombosis. Arch Intern Med 163:621, 2003.
129. Hull RD, Raskob GE, Rosenbloom D, et al: Optimal therapeutic level of heparin therapy in patients with venous thrombosis. Arch Intern Med 152:1589, 1992.
130. Levine MN, Raskob G, Landefeld S, et al: Hemorrhagic complications of anticoagulant treatment. Chest 119(suppl 1):108S, 2001.
131. Johnson EA, Kirkwood TB, Stirling Y, et al: Four heparin preparations: Anti-Xa potentiating effect of heparin after subcutaneous injection. Thromb Haemost 35:586, 1976.
132. Andersson LO, Barrowcliffe TW, Holmer E, et al: Anticoagulant properties of heparin fractionated by affinity chromatography on matrix-bound antithrombin III and by gel filtration. Thromb Res 9:575, 1976.
133. Weitz JI: Low molecular weight heparin. N Engl J Med 337:688, 1997.
134. Hettiarachchi RJ, Prins MH, Lensing AW, et al: Low molecular weight heparin versus unfractionated heparin in the initial treatment of venous thromboembolism. Curr Opin Pulm Med 4:220, 1998.
135. Gould MK, Dembitzer AD, Doyle RL, et al: Low molecular weight heparin compared with unfractionated heparin for treatment of acute deep venous thrombosis. Ann Intern Med 130:800, 1999.
136. Dolovich LR, Ginsberg JS, Douketis JD, et al: A meta-analysis comparing low molecular weight heparins with unfractionated heparin in the treatment of venous thromboembolism: Examining some unanswered questions regarding location of treatment, product type, and dosing efficiency. Arch Intern Med 160:181, 2000.
137. Levine M, Gent M, Hirsh J, et al: A comparison of low molecular weight heparin administered primarily at home with unfractionated heparin administered in the hospital for proximal deep-vein thrombosis. N Engl J Med 334:677, 1996.
138. Koopman MM, Prandoni P, Piovella F, et al: Treatment of venous thrombosis with intravenous unfractionated heparin administered in the hospital as compared with subcutaneous low molecular weight heparin administered at home. The Tasman Study Group. N Engl J Med 334:682, 1996.
139. Breddin HK, Hach-Wunderle V, Nakov R, et al for the CORTES Investigators: Effects of a low molecular weight heparin on thrombus regression and recurrent thromboembolism in patients with deep vein thrombosis. N Engl J Med 344:626, 2001.
140. Montalescot G, Polle V, Collet JP, et al: Low molecular weight heparin after mechanical heart valve replacement. Circulation 101:1083, 2000.
141. Sorensen HT, Mellemkjaer L, Olsen JH, et al: Prognosis of cancers associated with venous thromboembolism. N Engl J Med 343:1846, 2000.
142. Hutten BA, Prins MH, Gent M, et al: Incidence of recurrent thromboembolic and bleeding complications among patients with venous thromboembolism in relation to both malignancy and achieved international normalized ratio: A retrospective analysis. J Clin Oncol 18:3078, 2000.
143. Prandoni P, Lensing AW, Piccioli A, et al: Recurrent venous thromboembolism and bleeding complications during anticoagulant treatment in patients with cancer and venous thrombosis. Blood 100:3484, 2002.
144. Meyer G, Marjanovic Z, Valcke J, et al: Comparison of low molecular weight heparin and warfarin for the secondary prevention of venous thromboembolism in patients with cancer. Arch Intern Med 162:1729, 2002.
145. Lee AY, Levine MN, Baker RI, et al: Low molecular weight heparin versus a coumarin for the prevention of recurrent venous thromboembolism in patients with cancer. N Engl J Med 349:146, 2003.
146. Turpie AG: Pentasaccharides. Semin Hematol 39:158, 2002.
147. Buller HR, Davidson BL, Decousus H, et al: Fondaparinux or enoxaparin for the initial treatment of symptomatic deep venous thrombosis. Ann Intern Med 140:867, 2004.
148. The Matisse Investigators: Subcutaneous fondaparinux versus intravenous unfractionated heparin in the initial treatment of pulmonary embolism. N Engl J Med 349:1695, 2003.
149. Shah MK, Black-Schaffer RM: Treatment of upper limb deep vein thrombosis with low molecular weight heparin. Am J Phys Med Rehabil 82:415, 2003.
150. Druy E, Trout H, Giordano J, et al: Lytic therapy in the treatment of axillary and subclavian vein thrombosis. J Vasc Surg 2:821, 1985.
151. Spence LD, Gironta MG, Malde HM, et al: Acute upper extremity deep venous thrombosis: Safety and effectiveness of superior vena caval filters. Radiology 210:53, 1999.
152. Marchiori A, Verlato F, Sabbion P, et al: High versus low doses of unfractionated heparin for the treatment of superficial thrombophlebitis of the leg: A prospective, controlled, randomized study. Haematologica 87:523, 2002.
153. The Superficial Thrombophlebitis Treated by Enoxaparin Study Group: A pilot randomized double-blind comparison of a low-molecular-weight heparin, a nonsteroidal anti-inflammatory agent,

and placebo in the treatment of superficial vein thrombosis. Arch Intern Med 163:1657, 2003.

154. Hirsh J, Dalen JE, Anderson DR, et al: Oral anticoagulants: Mechanism of action, clinical effectiveness, and optimal therapeutic range. Chest 119(suppl):8S, 2001.
155. Miners JO, Birkett DJ: Cytochrome P4502C9: An enzyme of major importance in human drug metabolism. Br J Clin Pharmacol 45:525, 1998.
156. Aithal GP, Day CP, Kesteven PJ, et al: Association of polymorp hisms in the cytochrome P450 CYP2C9 with warfarin dose requirement and risk of bleeding complications. Lancet 353:717, 1999.
157. Higashi M, Veenstra DL, Kondo LM, et al: Influence of CYP2C9 genetic variants and anticoagulation-related outcomes during warfarin therapy. JAMA 287:1690, 2002.
158. Hirsh J: Oral anticoagulant drugs. N Engl J Med 324:1865, 1991.
159. Hansten P, Wittkowsky AK: Warfarin drug interactions. In Ansell JE, Oertel LB, Wittkowsky AK (eds): Managing Patients on Oral Anticoagulants: Clinical and Operational Guidelines, Gaithersburg, MD, Aspen Publishers, 1997, pp 7:1-7:11.
160. Kirkwood TBL: Calibration of reference thromboplastins and standardization of the prothrombin time ratio. Thromb Haemost 49:238, 1983.
161. Hirsh J, Poller L: The International Normalized Ratio: A guide to understanding and correcting its problems. Arch Intern Med 154:282, 1994.
162. Poller L: International normalized ratios (INR): The first 20 years. J Thromb Haemost 2:849, 2004.
163. Harrison L, Johnston M, Massicotte MP, et al: Comparison of 5 mg and 10 mg loading doses in initiation of warfarin therapy. Ann Intern Med 126:133, 1997.
164. Kovacs MJ, Rodger M, Anderson DR, et al: Comparison of 10 mg and 5 mg warfarin initiation nomograms together with low molecular weight heparin for outpatient treatment of acute venous thromboembolism: A randomized, double-blind, controlled trial. Ann Intern Med 138:714, 2003.
165. Gurwitz JH, Avorn J, Ross-Degnan D, et al: Aging and the anticoagulant response to warfarin therapy. Ann Intern Med 116:901, 1992.
166. Ansell J, Hirsh J, Dalen J, et al: Managing oral anticoagulant therapy. Chest 119:22S, 2001.
167. Berntorp E, Stigendal L, Lethagen S, et al: NovoSeven in warfarin-treated patients. Blood Coag Fibrinolys 11(suppl 1):S113, 2000.
168. Crowther MA, Donovan D, Harrison L, et al: Low dose oral vitamin K reliably reverses over anticoagulation due to warfarin. Thromb Hemost 79:1116, 1998.
169. Kearon C, Hirsh J: Management of anticoagulation before and after elective surgery. N Engl J Med 336:1506, 1997.
170. Johnson J, Turpie AG: Temporary discontinuation of oral anticoagulants: Role of low molecular weight heparin. Thromb Hemost Supplement:62, 1999.
171. Tinmouth A, Kovacs MJ, Cruickshank M, et al: Outpatient perioperative and peri-procedure treatment with dalteparin for chronically anticoagulated patients at high risk for thromboembolic complications. Thromb Hemost Supplement:662, 1999.
172. Spandorfer JM, Lynch S, Weitz HH, et al: Use of enoxaparin for the chronically anticoagulated patient before and after procedures. Am J Cardiol 84:478, 1999.
173. Landefeld CS, Goldman L: Major bleeding in outpatients treated with warfarin: Incidence and prediction by factors known at the start of outpatient therapy. Am J Med 87:144, 1989.
174. Beyth RJ, Quinn LM, Landefeld S: Prospective evaluation of an index for predicting the risk of major bleeding in outpatients treated with warfarin. Am J Med 105:91, 1998.
175. Ansell JE: Anticoagulation management as a risk factor for adverse events: Grounds for improvement. J Thromb Thrombolys 5(suppl 1):S13, 1998.
176. Linkins LA, Choi PT, Douketis JD: Clinical impact of bleeding in patients taking oral anticoagulant therapy for venous thromboembolism: A meta-analysis. Ann Intern Med 139:893, 2003.
177. Heit JA, Mohr DN, Silverstein MD, et al: Predictors of recurrence after deep vein thrombosis and pulmonary embolism. Arch Intern Med 160:761, 2000.
178. Douketis JD, Foster GA, Crowther MA, et al: Clinical risk factors and timing of recurrent venous thromboembolism during the initial 3 months of anticoagulant therapy. Arch Inter Med 160:3431, 2000.
179. Hansson PO, Sorbo J, Eriksson H: Recurrent venous thromboembolism after deep vein thrombosis: Incidence and risk factors. Arch Intern Med 160:769, 2000.
180. Baglin T, Luddington R, Brown K, et al: Incidence of recurrent venous thromboembolism in relation to clinical and thrombophilic risk factors: Prospective cohort study. Lancet 362:523, 2003.
181. Research Committee of the British Thoracic Society: Optimum duration of anticoagulation for deep vein thrombosis and pulmonary embolism. Lancet 340:873, 1992.
182. Levine MN, Hirsh J, Gent M, et al: Optimal duration of oral anticoagulant therapy: A randomized trial comparing four weeks with three months of warfarin in patients with proximal deep vein thrombosis. Thromb Haemost 74:606, 1995.
183. Prandoni P, Lensing AW, Cogo A, et al: The long-term clinical course of acute deep venous thrombosis. Ann Intern Med 125:1, 1996.
184. Kearon C, Gent M, Hirsh J: A comparison of three months of anticoagulation with extended anticoagulation for a first episode of idiopathic venous thromboembolism. N Engl J Med 340:901, 1999.
185. Agnelli G, Prandoni P, Santamaria MG, et al: Three months versus one year of oral anticoagulant therapy for idiopathic deep venous thrombosis. N Engl J Med 345:165, 2001.
186. Ridker PM, Goldhaber SZ, Danielson E, et al: Long-term, low-intensity warfarin therapy for the prevention of recurrent venous thromboembolism. N Engl J Med 348:1425, 2003.
187. Kearon C, Ginsberg JS, Kovacs MJ, et al: Comparison of low-intensity warfarin therapy with conventional-intensity warfarin therapy for long-term prevention of recurrent venous thromboembolism. N Engl J Med 349:631, 2003.
188. Eichinger S, Minar E, Bialonczyk C, et al: D-dimer levels and risk of recurrent venous thromboembolism. JAMA 290:1071, 2003.
189. Cosmi B, Leganani C, Cini M, et al: D-dimer and residual vein thrombosis assessed at 3 months after anticoagulation withdrawal are independent risk factors for recurrent venous thromboembolism. Thromb Haemost 89:(electronic abstract), 2003.
190. Weitz JI, Hirsh J: New anticoagulant drugs. Chest 119(suppl 1):95S, 2001.
191. Gustafsson D, Nystrom J-E, Carlsson S, et al: The direct thrombin inhibitor melagatran and its oral prodrug H376/95: Intestinal absorption properties, biochemical and pharmacodynamic effects. Thromb Res 101:171, 2001.
192. Eriksson UG, Bredberg U, Gislen K, et al: Pharmacokinetics and pharmacodynamics of ximelagatran, a novel oral direct thrombin inhibitor, in young healthy male subjects. Eur J Clin Pharmacol 59:35, 2003.
193. Lassen MR, Davidson BL, Gallus A, et al: A phase II randomized, double-blind, five-arm, parallel-group, dose-response study of a new oral directly acting factor Xa inhibitor, razaxaban, for the prevention of deep vein thrombosis in knee replacement surgery. Blood 102:15a, 2003.
194. The PERSIST investigators: A novel long-acting synthetic factor Xa inhibitor (SanOrg34006) to replace warfarin for secondary prevention in deep vein thrombosis: A phase 22 evaluation. J Thromb Haemost 2:47, 2003.
195. Francis CW, Ginsberg JS, Berkowitz SD, et al: Efficacy and safety of the oral direct thrombin inhibitor ximelagatran compared with standard therapy for acute symptomatic deep vein thrombosis, with or without pulmonary embolism: The THRIVE treatment study. Blood 102:6a, 2003.
196. Schulman S, Wahlander K, Lundstron T, et al: Secondary prevention of venous thromboembolism with the oral direct thrombin inhibitor ximelagatran. N Engl J Med 349:1713, 2003.
197. SPORTIF III Investigators. Stroke prevention with the oral direct thrombin inhibitor ximelagatran compared with warfarin in patients with non-valvular atrial fibrillation: Randomized controlled trial. Lancet 362:1691, 2003.
198. Halperin J, on behalf of the SPORTIFV investigators: Efficacy and safety study of oral direct thrombin inhibitor ximelagatran compared with dose-adjusted warfarin in the prevention of stroke and systemic embolic events in patients with atrial fibrillation.

Presented at the American Heart Association Annual Scientific Meeting, Orlando, Fla, November 9-12, 2003.

199. Eriksson BI, Agnelli G, Cohen AT, et al: The direct thrombin inhibitor melagatran followed by oral ximelagatran compared with enoxaparin for the prevention of venous thromboembolism after total hip or knee replacement. J Thromb Haemost 1:2490, 2003.

200. Mismetti P: Prevention of venous thromboembolism after major orthopedic surgery: New clinical trials for new antithrombotic agents. J Thromb Haemost;1:2474, 2003.

201. Toglia MR, Weg JG: Venous thromboembolism during pregnancy. N Engl J Med 335:108, 1996.

202. Ginsberg JS, Greer I, Hirsh J: Use of antithrombotic agents during pregnancy. Chest 119:122S, 2001.

203. Brenner B, Sarig G, Weiner Z, et al: Thrombophilic polymorphisms are common in women with fetal loss without apparent cause. Thromb Haemost 82:6, 1999.

204. Ridker PM, Miletich JP, Buring JE, et al: Factor V_{Leiden} mutation as a risk factor for recurrent pregnancy loss. Ann Intern Med 128:1000, 1998.

205. Kupferminc MJ, Eldor A, Steinman N, et al: Increased frequency of genetic thrombophilia in women with complications of pregnancy. N Engl J Med 340:9, 1999.

206. Eldor A: Management of thrombophilia and antiphospholipid syndrome during pregnancy. In Kitchens C, Alving B, Kessler C (eds): Consultative Hemostasis and Thrombosis, Philadelphia, WB Saunders, 2002, pp 449-458.

207. Brill-Edwards P, Ginsberg JS, Gent M, et al: Safety of withholding heparin in pregnant women with a history of venous thromboembolism. N Engl J Med 343:1439, 2000.

208. Zotz RB, Gerehardt A, Scharf RE: Antithrombotic prophylaxis for women with thrombophilia and pregnancy complications. J Thromb Haemost 2:1182, 2004.

209. Paidas M, Ku DH, Triche E, et al: Does heparin therapy improve pregnancy outcome in patients with thrombophilias? J Thromb Haemost 2:1194, 2004.

210. Middeldorp S: Antithrombotic prophylaxis for women with thrombophilia and pregnancy complications—No. J Thromb Haemost 1:2072, 2003.

211. Dulitzki M, Pauzner R, Langevitz P, et al: Low molecular weight heparin during pregnancy and delivery: Preliminary experience with 41 pregnancies. Obstet Gynecol 87:380, 1996.

212. Hunt BJ, Doughty HA, Majumdar G, et al: Thromboprophylaxis with low molecular weight heparin (Fragmin) in high risk pregnancies. Thromb Haemost 77:39, 1997.

213. Nelson-Piercy C, Letsky EA, de Swiet M: Low molecular weight heparin for obstetric thromboprophylaxis: Experience of 69 pregnancies in 61 women at high risk. Am J Obstet Gynecol 176:1062, 1997.

214. Chan WS, Anand S, Ginsberg JS: Anticoagulation of pregnant women with mechanical heart valves: A systematic review of the literature. Arch Intern Med 160:191, 2000.

215. Ginsberg JS, Chan WS, Bates SM, et al: Anticoagulation of pregnant women with mechanical heart valves. Arch Intern Med 163:694, 2003.

216. Oran B, Ansell J: Low molecular weight heparin for the prophylaxis of thromboembolism in women with prosthetic mechanical heart valves during pregnancy. Thromb Haemost 92:747, 2004.

chapter 54

Pulmonary Embolism

Nils Kucher
Samuel Z. Goldhaber

Pulmonary embolism (PE) and deep venous thrombosis (DVT) comprise venous thromboembolism (VTE), a complex illness that warrants primary management or consultation by vascular medicine specialists. In Western countries, the annual incidence of VTE in adults is about 1 in 1000.[1] The incidence of VTE increases with age; it is especially common in older, institutionalized patients.[2,3] The death rate among consecutive patients exceeds 15% within 3 months of diagnosis.[4]

RISK FACTORS FOR VENOUS THROMBOEMBOLISM

VTE is often associated with acquired (Box 54-1) or inherited (Box 54-2) risk factors. Prior VTE increases the risk of recurrence.

In the prospective DVT FREE registry of 5451 patients, the most common acquired comorbidities were hypertension (50%), surgery within 3 months (38%), immobility within 30 days (34%), cancer (32%), and obesity (27%).[5] Cancer augments the risk of VTE[6] through numerous mechanisms including intrinsic tumor procoagulant activity and extrinsic factors such as chemotherapeutic agents and indwelling central venous catheters. Pancreatic, lung, gastric, genitourinary tract, and breast malignancies are associated with a particularly high risk of DVT and PE. The most common laboratory manifestations of hypercoagulability include elevation of clotting factor levels (fibrinogen, factors V, VIII, IX, and XI); fibrin degradation products; or platelets. Chemotherapy further increases levels of coagulation factors, suppresses anticoagulant and fibrinolytic activity, and directly damages the endothelium.

Fatal PE associated with long-haul air travel has captivated the attention of the lay public. Although rare, the risk of massive PE increases progressively when the flight distance exceeds 5000 kilometers.[7]

VTE can adversely affect women's health. Oral contraceptives,[8] pregnancy,[9] and postmenopausal hormone replacement therapy[10] increase the risk of PE and DVT. Most oral contraceptives are "second-generation" agents that double or triple the VTE risk.[8] Newer, "third-generation" agents have desogestrel or gestodene as the progestogen component and cause less acne and hirsutism; however, they appear to cause acquired resistance to activated protein C, with an incremental doubling or tripling of the VTE risk compared with "second-generation" contraceptives.[8]

The antiphospholipid antibody syndrome is the most ominous acquired risk factor and is associated with arterial and venous thromboembolism, as well as recurrent pregnancy loss. Autoantibodies bind to endothelial receptors to promote the release of tissue factor and suppress cell surface plasminogen activation.[11]

Thrombophilia is often inherited.[11] A family history of VTE should be sought in all patients with DVT or PE. Whether laboratory testing should routinely be undertaken for patients with PE is highly controversial. The factor V Leiden mutation, a single-base mutation (substitution of A for G at position 506), is a common genetic polymorphism associated with activated protein C resistance (Fig. 54-1).[5] This genetic mutation is also a risk factor for recurrent pregnancy loss, probably due to placental vein thrombosis. The use of oral contraceptives in patients with factor V Leiden is associated with about

BOX 54-1 Common Acquired Risk Factors for Venous Thromboembolism

Immobilization/trauma/surgery
Cancer
Prior venous thromboembolism
Medical comorbidities, including obesity
Increasing age
Pregnancy/postpartum
Oral contraceptives/hormonal replacement therapy
Indwelling central venous catheter
Lupus anticoagulant/antiphospholipid antibody syndrome
Hyperhomocysteinemia due to folic acid deficiency
Long-distance airplane travel

BOX 54-2 Inherited Hypercoagulable States Associated with Venous Thromboembolism

Factor V Leiden
Prothrombin G20210 mutation
Protein C deficiency
Protein S deficiency
Antithrombin III deficiency
Dysfibrinogenemia
Disorders of plasminogen

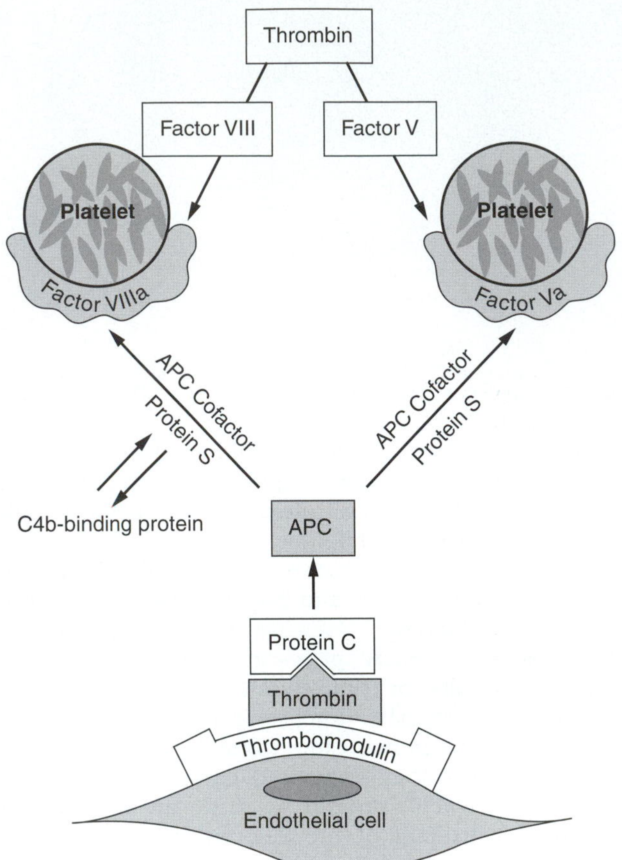

FIGURE 54-1. Thrombin converts factors VIII and V to their activated forms, factors VIIIa and Va. A complex of thrombin with the endothelial cell receptor thrombomodulin activates protein C. APC inactivates factors VIIIa and Va on the platelet surface. This reaction is accelerated by APC cofactor, which is thought to be inactivated factor V, as well as by free protein S. (From Bauer KA: Hypercoagulability—A new cofactor in the protein C anticoagulant pathway. N Engl J Med 330:566, 1994.)

a 10-fold higher risk of VTE.[8] The prothrombin gene mutation is a less common thrombophilic mutation identified in the 3′ untranslated region of the prothrombin gene (substitution of A for G at position 20210). This mutation causes an increased prothrombin concentration and is associated with about a threefold increase in the risk of VTE.[11] This chapter focuses on the clinical presentation and treatment of PE; Chapter 57 focuses on venous thrombosis.

PATHOPHYSIOLOGY

PE can manifest the following pathophysiologic effects:[12] (1) **increased pulmonary vascular resistance** due to vascular obstruction, neurohumoral agents, pulmonary artery baroreceptors, or increased pulmonary artery pressure; (2) **impaired gas exchange** due to increased alveolar dead space from vascular obstruction and hypoxemia from alveolar hypoventilation, low ventilation perfusion units, and right-to-left shunting, as well as impaired carbon monoxide transfer owing to loss of gas exchange surface; (3) **alveolar hyperventilation** from reflex stimulation of irritant receptors; (4) **increased airway resistance** as a result of bronchoconstriction; and (5) **decreased pulmonary compliance** because of lung edema, lung hemorrhage, and loss of surfactant.

Arterial hypoxia and an increase in the alveolar-arterial oxygen tension gradient are the most common gas exchange abnormalities. Mismatching of ventilation and perfusion is the most common cause of impaired pulmonary oxygen transfer. PE causes redistribution of blood flow so that some lung gas exchange units have low ratios of ventilation to perfusion, whereas other lung units have excessively high ratios of ventilation to perfusion. A right-to-left shunt further contributes to arterial hypoxia as venous blood enters the systemic arterial system without passing through ventilated gas exchange units of the lung. Low cardiac output due to right ventricular dysfunction leads to increased extraction of oxygen in the tissues, thereby further decreasing the partial pressure of oxygen in venous blood.

Hemodynamic alterations are common in patients with acute PE. Increased pulmonary vascular resistance and pulmonary artery pressure cause right ventricular shear stress and microinfarction. Although increased myocardial shear stress can be quantified with brain natriuretic peptide levels,[13] elevated troponin levels indicate myocardial ischemia and microinfarction.[14] Myocardial ischemia and microinfarction are probably caused by two mechanisms: (1) increased oxygen demand of the failing right ventricle and (2) reduced coronary perfusion as a consequence of a decreased systemic cardiac output.

As the extent of embolic occlusion of the pulmonary vascular bed increases, right ventricular and pulmonary artery pressure rises to abnormally high levels. As right ventricular dilatation and dysfunction evolve, reduced right ventricular output impairs left ventricular filling. Left ventricular distensibility may be further compromised due to a shift of the interventricular septum toward the left ventricle.

PREVENTION

PE is easier and less expensive to prevent than to diagnose or treat. Virtually all patients hospitalized for more than a day should receive prophylactic measures against VTE. Detailed guidelines for prevention of VTE with various mechanical measures and pharmacologic agents are available from American[15] and European[16] consensus conferences. The type of prophylaxis strategy that is selected should match the level of risk for developing venous thrombosis (Table 54-1).

Despite the availability of effective measures to prevent VTE, prophylaxis continues to be underused, even among high-risk hospitalized patients. In the DVT FREE registry of 5451 patients with ultrasound-confirmed DVT, only 42% of the inpatients had received prophylaxis within 30 days before diagnosis.[6] At our institution, most deaths among patients initially hospitalized for reasons other than PE occurred in the setting of inadequate rather than omitted prophylaxis.[17] Prevention programs should be implemented to establish and enforce protocols that are streamlined and standardized. Computer-generated prompting can increase the usage of prophylactic measures.[18]

TABLE 54-1 POSSIBLE PROPHYLAXIS STRATEGIES

Condition	Prophylaxis Strategy
General surgery	Enoxaparin 40 mg qd Dalteparin 2500 or 5000 U qd Unfractionated heparin 5000 U bid/tid
Total hip replacement	Enoxaparin 40 mg qd Fondaparinux 2.5 mg qd Warfarin
Total knee replacement	Enoxaparin 40 mg qd Fondaparinux 2.5 mg qd
Hip fracture surgery	Enoxaparin 40 mg qd Fondaparinux 2.5 mg qd
Neurosurgery	Graduated compression stockings and intermittent pneumatic compression PLUS unfractionated heparin 5000 U bid or enoxaparin 40 mg qd, PLUS predischarge venous ultrasound in patients with brain tumor
Trauma (not brain)	Enoxaparin 40 mg qd
Thoracic surgery	Graduated compression stockings, intermittent pneumatic compression, and unfractionated heparin 5000 U tid
Medical patients	Unfractionated heparin 5000 U SC tid Graduated compression stockings or intermittent pneumatic compression Enoxaparin 40 mg qd Dalteparin 5000 U qd

qd, once daily; bid, twice daily; SC, subcutaneous; tid, three times daily.

Mechanical prophylaxis measures use graduated compression stockings (GCSs) and intermittent pneumatic compression (IPC). GCSs increase venous blood flow and prevent perioperative venodilation of the legs. They are inexpensive, simple, and free of serious complications such as hemorrhage. In randomized trials evaluating GCSs for prevention of venous thrombosis after nonorthopedic surgery (general surgery, gynecologic surgery, or neurosurgery), there was an overall reduction of 72% in DVT.[19] IPC devices compress the veins more forcefully than GCSs and also stimulate the endogenous fibrinolytic system.[20]

Subcutaneous administration of unfractionated or low molecular weight heparins (LMWHs) helps prevent perioperative VTE. Collins and colleagues[21] pooled data from 78 randomized controlled unfractionated heparin trials with 15,598 patients undergoing surgery. There was a 40% reduction in nonfatal PE and 64% reduction in fatal PE among patients treated prophylactically with heparin. Patients assigned to heparin had about one third as many DVTs as control patients, regardless of whether they had undergone general, urologic, elective orthopedic, or trauma surgery.

LMWHs have several advantages over unfractionated heparin. They exhibit less binding to plasma proteins and to endothelial cells than unfractionated heparin. Consequently, they tend to have a more predictable dose-response, a more dose-independent mechanism of clearance, and a longer plasma half-life than unfractionated heparin. Furthermore, osteoporosis and heparin-induced thrombocytopenia appear to be less common with LMWHs than with unfractionated heparin. In most prevention trials, LMWHs are administered as once or twice daily subcutaneous injections in fixed or weight-adjusted doses, without laboratory monitoring or dose adjustment.

Fondaparinux, a pentasaccharide, is effective in preventing VTE after orthopedic surgery in a fixed low dose of 2.5 mg daily.[22,23] Ximelagatran, an oral direct thrombin inhibitor, does not require dose adjustment or serial blood testing, and may be at least as effective and safe as enoxaparin or warfarin in a dose of 24 mg twice daily.[24,25]

DIAGNOSIS

Clinical Suspicion of Pulmonary Embolism

PE is difficult to diagnose despite the availability of contemporary imaging techniques such as spiral chest CT and MRI. Thus appreciating the clinical setting and maintaining a high degree of clinical suspicion for possible PE are of paramount importance. The most common symptoms and signs are nonspecific: dyspnea, tachypnea, chest pain, and tachycardia. Usually, patients who present with chest pain or with hemoptysis have an anatomically small PE near the periphery of the lung, where nerve innervation is greatest and where pulmonary infarction is most likely to occur owing to poor collateral circulation. Ironically, patients with life-threatening PEs often have a painless presentation characterized by dyspnea, syncope, or cyanosis.

Assessment of the clinical pretest probability may improve the diagnostic accuracy in patients with suspected PE. Wells and coworkers[26] have tested a bedside assessment score to estimate the clinical pretest probability for PE. The following clinical variables are required to calculate the score: signs or symptoms of DVT (3 points), no alternative diagnosis (3 points), a heart rate greater than 100 beats/min (1.5 points), immobilization or surgery within 4 weeks (1.5 points), a history of VTE (1.5 points), hemoptysis (1 point), and cancer (1 point). In this study, more than one third of the patients had a Wells score less than or equal to 2. PE was confirmed in only 2% of these patients. In contrast, one half of the patients with a Wells score greater than 6 had PE diagnosed on further testing.

PE should be suspected in hypotensive patients when (1) there is evidence of, or there are predisposing factors for, venous thrombosis and (2) there is clinical evidence of acute cor pulmonale (acute right ventricular failure) such as distended neck veins, an S3 gallop, a right ventricular heave, tachycardia, or tachypnea, especially if there is electrocardiographic evidence of acute cor pulmonale manifested by a new S1 Q3 T3 pattern, new incomplete right bundle branch block, T wave inversion in V1 through V3, or a Qr pattern in V1 (Box 54-3).[27]

TESTS FOR PULMONARY EMBOLISM

Chest Radiography Enlargement of a central pulmonary artery, especially with progressive enlargement on serial radiographs, is a cardinal radiographic sign of PE. The chest radiograph can also help exclude diseases such as lobar pneumonia or pneumothorax that have similar clinical presentations; however, these latter patients can also have concomitant PE.

BOX 54-3 Electrocardiographic Findings in Pulmonary Embolism

Sinus tachycardia
Incomplete or complete right bundle branch block
S1 Q3 T3
QRS transition zone shift to V5
QRS axis > 90 degrees or indeterminate axis
Qr in V1
T wave inversion in leads V1-V3
Low limb lead voltage

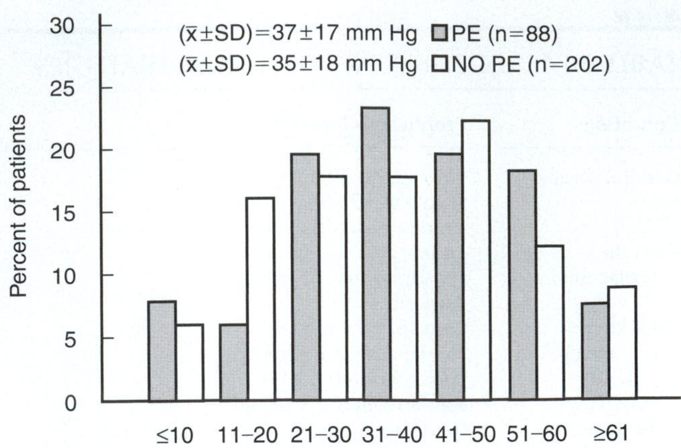

FIGURE 54-3. Distribution of alveolar-arterial oxygen gradient among 88 patients with angiographically proven pulmonary embolism (PE) and no preexisting cardiac or pulmonary disease and 202 patients in whom PE was excluded with normal pulmonary angiograms. (From Stein PD, Terrin ML, Hales CA, et al: Clinical, laboratory, roentgenographic, and electrocardiographic findings in patients with acute pulmonary embolism and no pre-existing cardiac or pulmonary disease. Chest 100:598, 1991.)

Arterial Blood Gas Analysis Neither room air arterial blood gases (Fig. 54-2) nor calculation of the alveolar-arterial oxygen gradient (Fig. 54-3) helps to differentiate patients with a confirmed PE at angiography from those with a normal pulmonary angiogram.[28] Therefore arterial blood gases should not be obtained as a screening test in patients suspected of PE.

D-Dimer D-dimer is a specific proteolytic degradation product released into the circulation by endogenous fibrinolysis of a cross-linked fibrin clot. An abnormally elevated level of plasma D-dimer (>500 ng/ml), performed with a quantitative ELISA (Fig. 54-4), has a greater than 90% sensitivity for angiographically proven PE.[29] In a meta-analysis, the ELISA D-dimer test had a sensitivity of 94% and a specificity of 45% for the diagnosis of PE.[30]

The role of D-dimer as a "rule-out" test can be extended to diagnose PE as a "rule-in" test. The specificity of the ELISA D-dimer to predict PE may be increased by using the D-dimer/fibrinogen (D/F) ratio.[31] Functional fibrinogen, measured by the Clauss method (g/l), is increased in most conditions that mimic PE symptoms and signs; however, in PE, the fibrinogen level decreases with increasing pulmonary arterial occlusion. In one study all patients with a D/F ratio greater than 1000 had PE confirmed on further testing.[31]

Ventilation Perfusion Scanning Lung scanning has been the principal noninvasive diagnostic test for suspected PE for many years; however, an increasing number of hospitals restrict lung scanning to patients with allergy to radiographic contrast agents, severe renal insufficiency, or pregnancy. Ventilation perfusion scanning is nondiagnostic

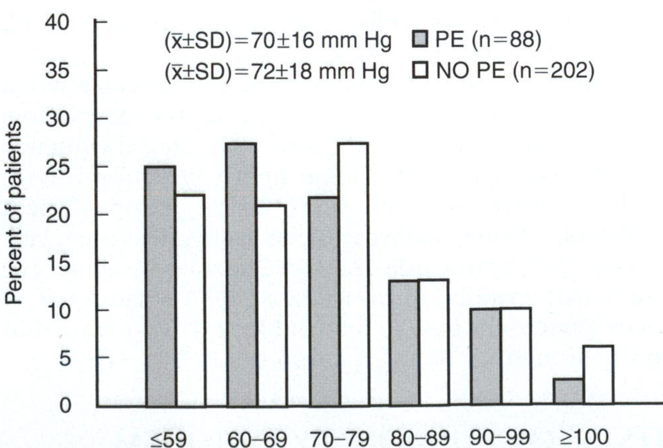

FIGURE 54-2. Distribution of partial pressure of oxygen in arterial blood (PO_2), while breathing room air, among 88 patients with angiographically proven PE and no preexisting cardiac or pulmonary disease and 202 patients in whom PE was excluded with normal pulmonary angiograms. (From Stein PD, Terrin ML, Hales CA, et al: Clinical, laboratory, roentgenographic, and electrocardiographic findings in patients with acute pulmonary embolism and no pre-existing cardiac or pulmonary disease. Chest 100:598, 1991.)

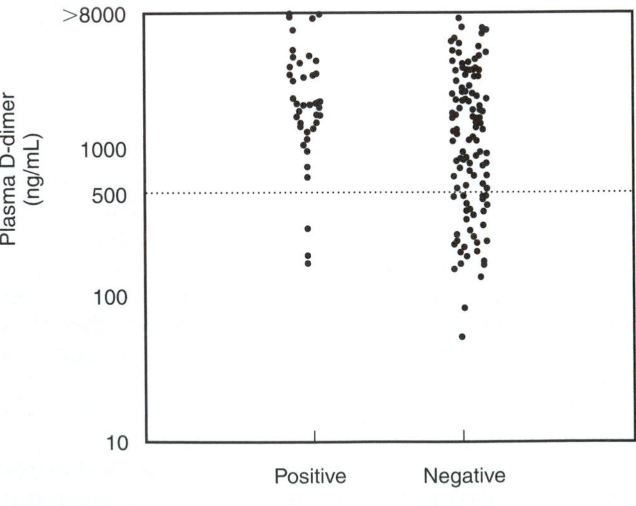

FIGURE 54-4. Distribution of plasma D-dimer ELISA levels, sorted according to angiographic findings, among 173 patients with suspected acute pulmonary embolism. (From Goldhaber SZ, Simons GR, Elliott CG, et al: Quantitative plasma D-dimer levels among patients undergoing pulmonary angiography for suspected pulmonary embolism. JAMA 270:2819, 1993.)

TABLE 54-2 PIOPED: PULMONARY EMBOLISM STATUS

	CLINICAL PROBABILITY (%)			
	80-100	**20-79**	**0-19**	**0-100**
Lung Scan Category	*n/n (%)*	*n/n (%)*	*n/n (%)*	*n/n (%)*
High	28/29(96)	70/80(88)	5/9(56)	103/118(87)
Intermediate	27/41(66)	66/236(28)	11/68(16)	104/345(30)
Low	6/16(40)	30/191(16)	4/90(4)	40/296(14)
Very low	0/5(0)	4/62(6)	1/61(2)	5/128(4)
Total	61/90(68)	170/569(30)	21/228(9)	252/887(28)

Modified from the PIOPED Investigators: Value of the ventilation/perfusion scan in acute pulmonary embolism. JAMA 263:2757, 1990.

(low or intermediate probability scans) in the majority of patients with suspected PE. The diagnostic accuracy of lung scanning may be improved when scans are interpreted in conjunction with clinical pretest probability (Table 54-2).[32]

Contrast-Enhanced Chest Computed Tomography Chest CT has become the most useful imaging test in patients with clinically suspected acute PE. Newer generation scanners involve continuous movement of the patient through the scanner with concurrent scanning by a constantly rotating gantry and detector system. Rapid, continuous volume acquisitions can be obtained during a single breath, thereby facilitating imaging in critically ill patients. The latest generation of multidetector CT scanners (Fig. 54-5) permits image acquisition of the entire chest with 1-mm or submillimeter resolution and a breath-hold of less than 10 seconds. They reveal emboli in the main, lobar, or (sub)segmental pulmonary arteries with greater than 90% sensitivity and specificity.[33] Spiral chest CT is also useful in detecting alternative diagnoses such as aortic dissection, pneumonia, or pericardial tamponade.

Pulmonary Angiography Classic invasive contrast pulmonary arteriography is the established "gold standard" imaging test for the diagnosis of PE. Currently, pulmonary angiography is rarely performed because multiplanar chest CT scanning, incorporated into a noninvasive diagnostic strategy, seems to be equally accurate.

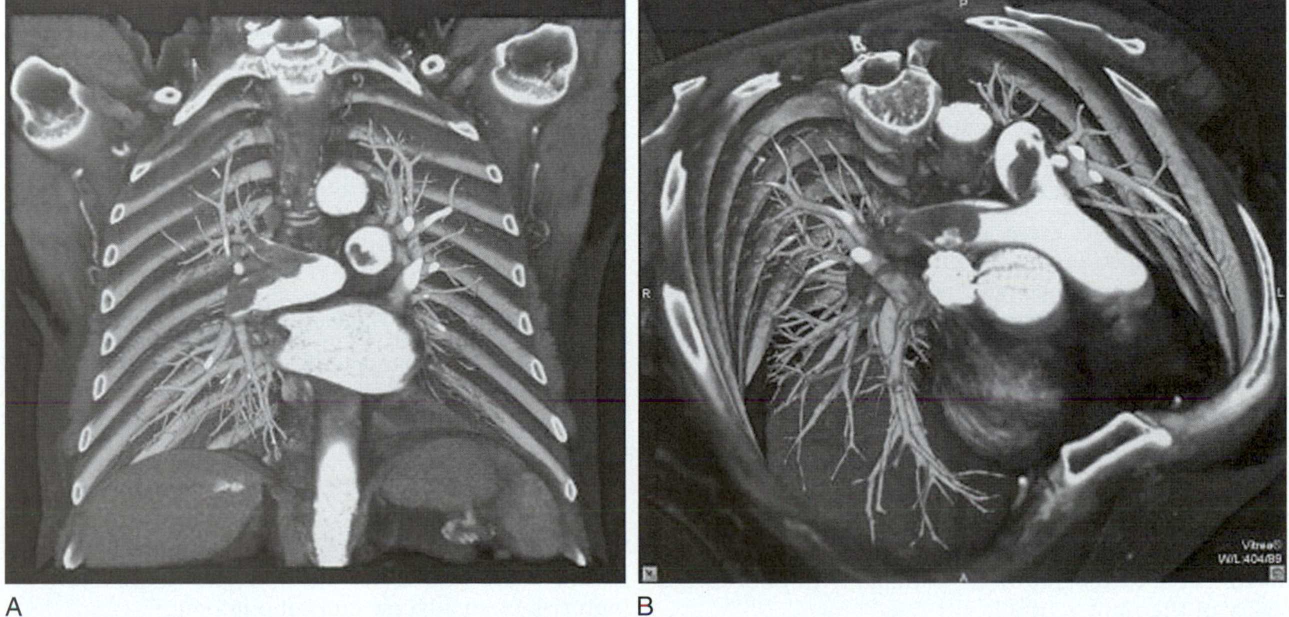

FIGURE 54-5. (See also Color Plate 54-5.) Contrast-enhanced multislice CT in a 72-year-old man with acute central pulmonary embolism showing a "saddle embolus." Colored volume rendering technique seen from an anterior-cranial **(A)** and anterior **(B)** perspective allows intuitive visualization of location and extent of embolism. (Figures kindly provided by Joseph Schoepf, MD, Department of Radiology, Brigham and Women's Hospital, Boston.)

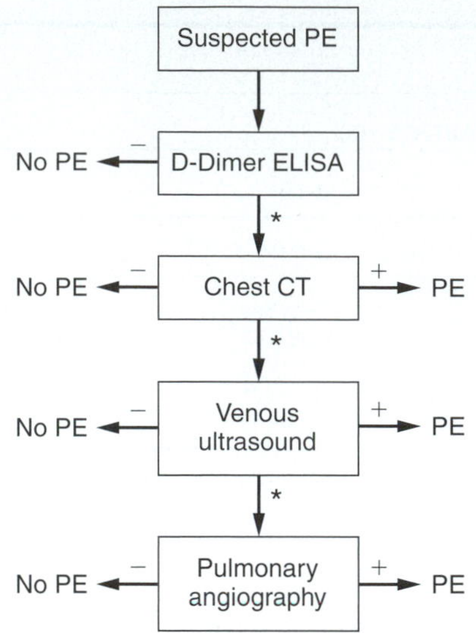

FIGURE 54-6. Suggested diagnostic strategy for patients with suspected pulmonary embolism (PE) without cardiogenic shock. In this strategy, chest CT is used as the principal imaging test.
*Further testing should be considered if the test is inconclusive or negative with a persistent suspicion of PE.

Gadolinium-Enhanced Magnetic Resonance Angiography MRI avoids ionizing radiation or iodinated contrast agents. MRI also allows assessment of left and right ventricular function and size, potentially important for risk stratification of PE patients. When MRI is performed under optimal conditions, it appears to be almost as sensitive and specific for PE as pulmonary angiography.[34]

Venous Ultrasonography Ultrasonography of the deep veins is noninvasive, cost effective, and accurate in diagnosing proximal leg DVT in symptomatic patients. Ultrasound is considered diagnostic for PE if it confirms DVT in patients with PE symptoms; however, one third to one half of PE patients have no ultrasound or venogram evidence of leg DVT, probably because the thrombus has already embolized to the lungs. Therefore, if clinical suspicion of PE is high, patients without clinical or imaging evidence of DVT should still be worked up for PE.

Echocardiography Echocardiography is not useful routinely to diagnose PE because it is normal in about half of consecutive patients with suspected PE[35]; however, transthoracic echocardiography assists evaluation of hemodynamically unstable patients with clinically suspected PE. Potentially life-saving therapy including thrombolysis, catheter fragmentation, or surgical embolectomy can be rapidly initiated on the basis of echocardiographic evidence of severe right ventricular dysfunction without necessarily obtaining time-consuming PE imaging tests.[36] Transesophageal echocardiography helps visualize centrally located thrombi and is an alternative to transthoracic echocardiography for patients with poor image quality of the right ventricle.[37]

Overall Diagnostic Strategy The initial assessment includes a history, physical examination, ECG, and chest radiograph. A plasma D-dimer ELISA should be obtained in all outpatient or emergency department patients. If the D-dimer is below the assay-specific cut-off level, PE is essentially excluded. If D-dimer levels are elevated, we recommend obtaining a spiral chest CT (Fig. 54-6). In all patients with significant impairment of renal function, pregnancy, or allergy to contrast agents, ventilation perfusion scanning may be performed as the primary imaging test. When the diagnosis remains uncertain, a venous ultrasound study is the next step. If a high clinical suspicion for PE persists despite a negative ultrasound study, we recommend pulmonary angiography. This strategy is safe and requires pulmonary angiography in less than 10% of patients.[38]

MANAGEMENT

Risk Stratification

PE spans a wide spectrum of morbidity and mortality. With therapeutic levels of anticoagulation, most patients have a benign clinical course. Unfortunately, some PE patients suffer rapid clinical deterioration, including death from right ventricular failure or the need for escalation of therapy such as cardiopulmonary resuscitation, mechanical ventilation, administration of pressor agents, rescue thrombolysis, or surgical embolectomy. Early risk assessment is paramount in selecting the appropriate management strategy. Previously, risk assessment deemed patients at high risk only when the systemic arterial pressure declined to less than 90 mm Hg and was unresponsive to pressor agents. Contemporary risk stratification focuses on rapid detection of right ventricular dysfunction even while the systemic arterial pressure remains normal. Right ventricular dysfunction is an independent predictor of early death.[39]

Clinical Evaluation Severe dyspnea, cyanosis, and syncope usually indicate life-threatening PE. The clinical examination may show signs of acute right ventricular dysfunction including tachycardia, a low arterial blood pressure, distended neck veins, an accentuated pulmonic component of the second heart sound, or a tricuspid regurgitation murmur. The Geneva Prognostic Index predicts clinical outcome.[40] This scoring system has a maximum of 8 score-points: systolic blood pressure less than 100 mm Hg (+2), history of cancer (+2), congestive heart failure (+1), deep venous thrombosis (+1), hypoxemia (+1), or evidence of DVT by ultrasound (+1). As the score increases, prognosis worsens. In contrast, carefully selected patients with a Geneva Prognostic Index less than or equal to 2 can safely be treated on an entirely outpatient basis.

Electrocardiography T wave inversion in V1 through V3 and a pseudoinfarction pattern (Qr) in V1 indicate severe right ventricular dilation and dysfunction and high risk of an adverse clinical outcome.[27]

Echocardiography Transthoracic echocardiography has emerged as the most important tool for risk assessment and treatment guidance in patients with acute PE.

Echocardiography is also the principal imaging test to diagnose a patent foramen ovale in patients with suspected paradoxic embolism and directly visualize thrombi in the main pulmonary artery, right heart chambers, or vena cava. Echocardiography is also useful to detect conditions that mimic PE, such as myocardial infarction, aortic dissection, or pericardial tamponade.

Right ventricular systolic function is usually assessed qualitatively. Patients with acute PE may show a specific regional wall motion abnormality of the right ventricle known as the *McConnell sign:* hypokinesis of the right ventricular free wall combined with preserved systolic contraction of the right ventricular apex.[41] Right ventricular dilatation is an indirect sign of right ventricular pressure overload. A right ventricular-to-left ventricular size ratio of greater than or equal to 1 in the apical four-chamber view indicates right ventricular dilation. Right ventricular pressure overload may cause a paradoxic (systolic) septal motion toward the left ventricle. In the parasternal short axis view, the interventricular septum may flatten and cause a "D-shaped" left ventricle (Fig. 54-7). Other indirect signs of right ventricular dysfunction include increased tricuspid regurgitant velocity greater than 2.6 m/sec and reduced inspiratory collapse of a dilated inferior vena cava.

Cardiac Biomarkers Cardiac troponins I and T, as well as N-terminal pro brain natriuretic peptide (proBNP) and brain natriuretic peptide (BNP), have emerged as promising tools for risk stratification in PE.

Cardiac troponins are the most sensitive and specific markers of myocardial cell damage. Elevations of troponin levels in PE patients are mild and of short duration compared with patients with acute coronary syndromes. In acute PE, troponin levels correlate well with the presence of right ventricular dysfunction.[14,42] Myocardial ischemia due to alterations in oxygen supply and demand of the failing right ventricle probably plays a major role in the pathogenesis of troponin release. This is supported by finding elevated troponin levels in PE patients without angiographic coronary artery disease.[14]

The natriuretic peptides are useful diagnostic and prognostic markers for patients with congestive heart failure. The stimulus for BNP synthesis and secretion is cardiomyocyte stretch. ProBNP in normal ventricular myocytes is not stored in a significant amount. Thus it takes several hours for the plasma natriuretic peptide levels to increase significantly after the onset of acute cardiomyocyte stretch. This includes myocardial BNP messenger ribonucleic acid (mRNA) synthesis, proBNP synthesis, and proBNP release into the circulation. An initially normal BNP level in a newly symptomatic PE patient should be interpreted with caution. Elevations in BNP and proBNP are associated with the presence of right ventricular dysfunction in acute PE.[13,43,44]

Troponins and natriuretic peptides are similarly accurate in identifying low-risk PE patients. The negative predictive value for in-hospital death ranges from 97% to 100% for these assays (Table 54-3). The cut-off levels for troponins are the lower detection limits for myocardial ischemia reported by the manufacturer. The cut-off level for the BNP Triage assay to predict a benign clinical outcome in PE patients is lower (<50 pg/ml) than the "congestive heart failure" cut-off level of 90 pg/ml.

Cardiac biomarker test results should be interpreted in context with other risk stratification tools. In hemodynamically stable PE patients with increased troponin

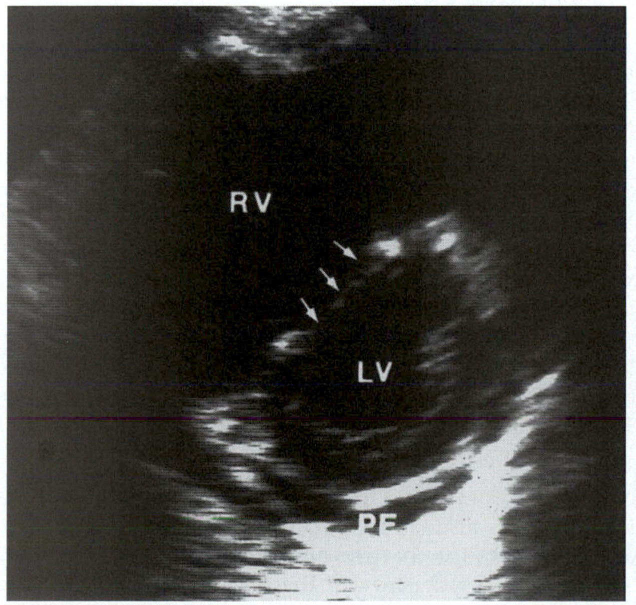

A

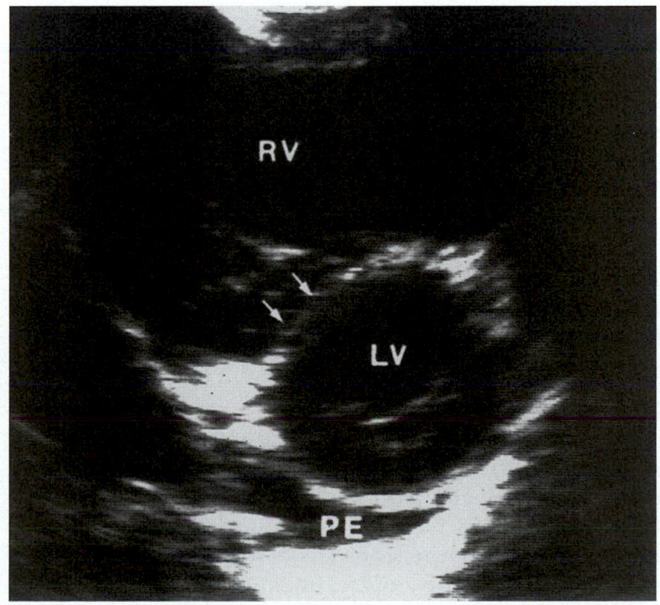

B

FIGURE 54-7. Parasternal short axis views of the right ventricle (*RV*) and left ventricle (*LV*) in diastole **(A)** and systole **(B)**. There is diastolic and systolic bowing of the interventricular septum (*arrows*) into the left ventricle compatible with right ventricular volume and pressure overloads, respectively. The right ventricle is appreciably dilated and markedly hypokinetic, with little change in apparent right ventricular area from diastole to systole. PE, small pericardial effusion. (From Come PC: Echocardiographic evaluation of pulmonary embolism and its response to therapeutic interventions. Chest 101:151S, 1992.)

TABLE 54-3 CARDIAC BIOMARKERS FOR THE PREDICTION OF IN-HOSPITAL DEATH IN PATIENTS WITH PULMONARY EMBOLISM

Biomarker	Assay	Cut-off Level	NPV %	PPV %
TnI[42]	Centaur, Bayer	0.07 ng/ml	98	14
TnT[42]	Elecsys, Roche	0.04 ng/ml	97	12
TnT[14]	TropT, Roche	0.10 ng/ml	97	44
TnT[45]	Elecsys, Roche	0.09 ng/ml	99	34
TnT[46]	Elecsys, Roche	0.01 ng/ml	100	25
BNP[44]	Shionoria, CIS	21.7 pmol/l	99	17
BNP[13]	Triage, Biosite	50 pg/ml	100	12
ProBNP[43]	Elecsys, Roche	500 pg/ml	100	12

BNP, brain natriuretic peptide; NPV, negative predictive value; PPV, positive predictive value; ProBNP, N terminal pro brain natriuretic peptide; TnI, troponin I; TnT, troponin T.

or BNP levels, further risk stratification with echocardiography should be undertaken due to the low specificity of the assays for PE-related right ventricular dysfunction. However, in patients with biomarker levels below the assay-specific cut-off, echocardiography generally shows normal right ventricular function and does not provide incremental prognostic information.

Anticoagulation

When DVT or PE is diagnosed or strongly suspected, anticoagulation therapy should be initiated immediately unless a major contraindication exists.

Unfractionated Heparin as a "Bridge" to Warfarin

A bolus of IV unfractionated heparin (80 U/kg) followed by 18 U/kg per hour is an effective and safe approach to initiate anticoagulation.[47] The activated partial thromboplastin time (aPTT) should be followed at 6-hour intervals until it remains consistently in the therapeutic range of 1.5 to 2.5 times the upper limit of the normal range. Oral anticoagulation with warfarin can be started as soon as the aPTT is within the therapeutic range. Patients should receive at least 5 days of heparin while an adequate level of oral anticoagulation is established. The prothrombin time, used to adjust the dose of oral anticoagulation, should be reported according to the International Normalized Ratio (INR), not the prothrombin time ratio or the prothrombin time expressed in seconds.

Low Molecular Weight Heparin Two trials have shown that therapy with LMWH is as safe and effective as therapy with unfractionated heparin in hemodynamically stable patients with acute PE.[48,49] In Geneva, carefully selected low-risk patients were treated with LMWH on a completely outpatient basis.[50] The FDA has approved enoxaparin for outpatient treatment of symptomatic DVT, with or without PE, as a bridge to warfarin. Two dosing regimens exist: 1 mg/kg subcutaneously every 12 hours for both outpatients and inpatients and 1.5 mg/kg subcutaneously once daily for inpatients. Extended 3-month therapy with enoxaparin as monotherapy without warfarin for symptomatic acute PE is feasible and shortens the duration of hospitalization compared with patients receiving standard treatment.[51]

Cancer patients are at particularly high risk for both recurrent VTE and major bleeding while receiving warfarin. A recent randomized, controlled trial of 672 cancer patients compared dalteparin monotherapy without warfarin versus dalteparin as a "bridge" to warfarin.[52] Patients randomized to dalteparin 200 U/kg once daily for 6 months had a 50% lower VTE recurrence rate (8.8%) compared with standard therapy patients (17.4%), without an increase in major bleeding.

Anti-Xa levels may be used to monitor LMWH dosing in the presence of obesity, renal dysfunction, or pregnancy. A peak therapeutic anticoagulant level, taken 3 to 6 hours after LMWH administration, is in the approximate range of 0.5 to 1 units/ml using the HEPRN pack (Dupont) assay.

Warfarin The vitamin K antagonist warfarin sodium inhibits γ-carboxylation activation of coagulation factors II, VII, IX, and X and proteins C and S. The full anticoagulant effect of warfarin requires about 5 days of therapy, even if the INR is in the intended therapeutic range. Warfarin is a difficult drug to dose and monitor, with multiple drug-drug and drug-food interactions.[53] Excessive warfarin anticoagulation may cause major bleeding events, including intracranial hemorrhage, and may contribute to in-hospital death and other adverse clinical outcomes.[53] In one study of hospitalized patients, there was a trend toward increasing warfarin-related hemorrhage from 1995 to 2002.[54]

New Anticoagulant Drugs Pentasaccharides such as idraparinux and fondaparinux are promising new anti-Xa agents for the prevention and treatment of VTE. The PERSIST study showed that monotherapy with idraparinux (2.5 mg subcutaneously once weekly) was as safe and effective in the treatment of acute DVT as enoxaparin twice daily.[55] The MATISSE studies found that fondaparinux 7.5 mg subcutaneously once daily was at least as safe and effective as unfractionated heparin or LMWH.[56]

Ximelagatran, an oral direct thrombin inhibitor, is promising for the treatment of acute VTE. In a randomized trial of 2489 patients with acute DVT, ximelagatran monotherapy was as effective and safe as enoxaparin "bridged" to warfarin.[57]

Optimal Duration and Intensity of Anticoagulation

The optimal intensity and duration of anticoagulation in patients with idiopathic VTE is controversial (Table 54-4). In PREVENT,[58] a double-blind, randomized, controlled trial of idiopathic VTE patients who had completed an average of 6 months of full-intensity warfarin, low-intensity warfarin (target INR of 1.5 to 2) for an average of 2 years reduced the recurrence rate by two thirds. Patients required INR testing only once every 8 weeks. The strategy of long-term, low-intensity warfarin was highly effective in preventing recurrence in all subgroups, even in those with factor V Leiden or the prothrombin gene mutation.

In the THRIVE III trial of 1233 patients who had completed 6 months of full-intensity anticoagulation with warfarin, an additional 18 months of anticoagulation with ximelagatran (24 mg twice daily) reduced the composite endpoint of death and recurrent VTE by 77% compared with placebo.[59] In the ELATE study of 739 patients with idiopathic VTE,[60] indefinite-duration, full-intensity warfarin (target INR 2 to 3) was more effective and as safe as indefinite-duration, low-intensity warfarin therapy (target INR 1.5 to 1.9).

Certain patients at particularly high risk for recurrent VTE (e.g., patients with antiphospholipid antibodies or combined thrombophilias) may require indefinite-duration, full-intensity anticoagulation. Serial D-dimer measurements may identify patients at increased risk for recurrent VTE events after discontinuation of anticoagulation. Normal D-dimer levels measured 1 month after withdrawal of anticoagulation have a high negative predictive value for recurrence.[61]

Thrombolytic Therapy

Systemic thrombolysis is lifesaving and considered standard therapy in patients with massive PE and cardiogenic shock. Thrombolysis rapidly reverses severe right ventricular dysfunction by dissolution of pulmonary arterial thrombi that might otherwise lead to chronic pulmonary hypertension. Thrombolysis may also dissolve much of the source of the residual thrombus in the deep veins, thereby minimizing the likelihood of recurrent PE. In patients with acute PE, thrombolysis is effective up to 2 weeks after the onset of symptoms. The only contemporary FDA-approved thrombolytic regimen is a continuous IV infusion of 100 mg alteplase/2 hr.

In the largest thrombolysis study (MAPPET-3) of patients with submassive PE, heparin plus alteplase as a continuous infusion over 2 hours was compared with heparin alone.[66] Compared with heparin alone, thrombolysis markedly reduced adverse clinical outcomes from 25% to 11%, defined as the need for cardiopulmonary resuscitation, mechanical ventilation, administration of pressors, secondary "rescue" thrombolysis, or surgical embolectomy. No significant increase in major bleeding occurred, and there was no intracranial bleeding with alteplase among these carefully selected PE patients.

In the absence of PE-related cardiogenic shock, administration of systemic thrombolysis remains controversial because a significant mortality benefit in favor of thrombolysis has not yet been shown. There are only 10 randomized PE trials of thrombolysis versus heparin alone, with a total of 717 patients. In an overview, there is a trend toward mortality reduction (relative risk 0.63, 95% confidence interval 0.32 to 1.23) and a twofold increase in the hazard of major hemorrhage with thrombolysis compared with heparin alone (relative risk 1.76, 95% confidence interval 1.04 to 2.98).[67] Therefore low-risk PE patients with preserved systemic arterial pressure and normal/near normal right ventricular function should not be treated with thrombolysis because the risk of bleeding exceeds the expected benefits.

TABLE 54-4 OPTIMAL DURATION AND INTENSITY OF ANTICOAGULATION IN PATIENTS WITH IDIOPATHIC PULMONARY EMBOLISM OR DEEP VENOUS THROMBOSIS

Trial	Regimens Tested	Findings
DURAC[62]	Warfarin for 6 wk vs. warfarin for 6 mo	Recurrence rate was halved in 6-mo group
Kearon[63]	Warfarin, INR 2-3, vs. placebo, after initial 3 mo anticoagulation	Warfarin group had 95% reduction in recurrence, but borderline statistically increased major bleeding
WODIT-DVT[64]	Warfarin for 3 mo vs. warfarin for 12 mo	The initial decreased recurrence rate in the 12-mo group is not maintained after warfarin is discontinued
WODIT-PE[65]	Warfarin for 3 mo vs. warfarin for 12 mo	The initial decreased recurrence rate in the 12-mo group is not maintained after warfarin is discontinued
ELATE[60]	Warfarin, INR 1.5-2, vs. warfarin, INR 2-3	Warfarin, INR 2-3, had fewer recurrences and no increased bleeding compared with warfarin, INR 1.5-2
THRIVE III[59]	Ximelagatran 24 mg twice daily for 18 mo vs. placebo, after initial 6 mo of anticoagulation	Ximelagatran group had 85% fewer recurrences, without increased major bleeding
PREVENT[58]	Warfarin, INR 1.5-2 vs. placebo, after initial average 6-mo anticoagulation	Warfarin more than halved recurrence without increased major bleeding

INR, international normalized ratio.

TABLE 54-5 INTERVENTIONAL DEVICES FOR THE THERAPY OF MASSIVE PULMONARY EMBOLISM

Device	Mechanism
Greenfield catheter	Suction embolectomy
Pigtail catheter	Fragmentation without embolectomy
Amplatz device	Clot maceration via high-speed impeller rotation without embolectomy ("clot buster")
AngioJet	Embolectomy via high-pressure saline injection (Venturi effect)
Hydrolyser	Embolectomy via rheolytic effect

Catheter Intervention

Interventional thrombus fragmentation with or without embolectomy is an alternative to systemic thrombolysis or surgical embolectomy in patients with massive PE. Catheter fragmentation can be combined with local or systemic thrombolysis. An ideal interventional catheter for PE has not yet been developed (Table 54-5).

Surgical Embolectomy

Emergency pulmonary embolectomy should be considered in patients with life-threatening PE in the setting of (1) a high bleeding risk from thrombolysis; (2) failed thrombolysis; or (3) the presence of right atrial and ventricular thrombi. The operation involves a median sternotomy incision, institution of cardiopulmonary bypass, and deep hypothermia with circulatory arrest periods. In a cohort study of 29 patients presenting with massive PE within a 2-year period, the survival rate after emergency embolectomy was 89%.[68]

Vena Cava Interruption

The two principal indications for vena caval filter placement are major contraindications to anticoagulation and recurrent embolism despite adequate therapy. There was an extraordinarily high rate (24%) of vena caval filter use for secondary prevention in patients with PE in the DVT FREE registry.[6] Only half of these patients had clear indications for a vena caval filter, including failure of anticoagulation, contraindication to anticoagulation, or major bleeding. This is a disturbing finding because patients with filters are more than twice as likely as nonfilter patients to require rehospitalization for DVT due to formation of thrombus proximal to the filter or on the proximal tip of the filter.[69] Rare complications of inferior vena cava (IVC) filter failure include filter migration or improper filter positioning, allowing thrombi to bypass the filter. Occasionally, IVC obstruction due to complete filter thrombosis may occur. Temporary filters have been placed in individuals deemed at extremely high risk for DVT yet unable to receive anticoagulant prophylaxis, such as certain trauma patients.[70] Retrievable filters can be removed within 2 weeks after placement or can remain permanently, if necessary, because of a trapped thrombus or a persistent contraindication to anticoagulation.

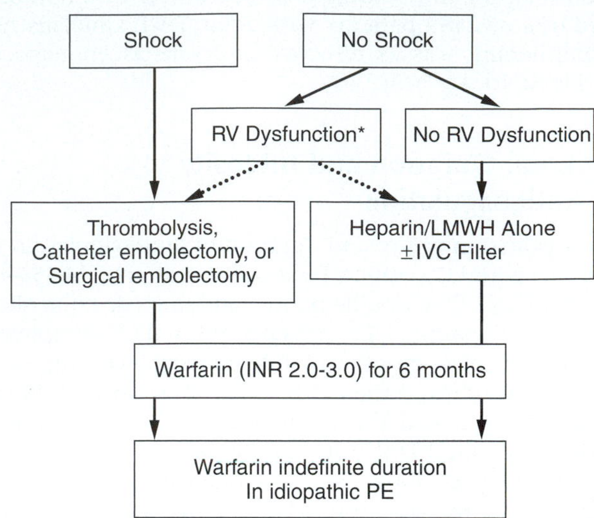

FIGURE 54-8. Suggested management strategy for pulmonary embolism. *Patients with right ventricular dysfunction and a preserved arterial blood pressure are candidates for thrombolysis in the absence of contraindications.

Overall Management Strategy

Treatment decisions in acute PE are primarily based on the hemodynamic presentation of the patient (Fig. 54-8). Although patients with massive PEs and cardiogenic shock should be rapidly treated with a reperfusion regimen (thrombolysis, catheter embolectomy, or surgical embolectomy), the decision on how to treat a patient with preserved systemic arterial pressure remains controversial but depends mostly on the presence of moderate or severe right ventricular dysfunction. Future studies will show whether cardiac biomarkers are useful to guide treatment decisions. Abnormally elevated proBNP, BNP, or troponin levels may help select patients who benefit from further confirmation of right ventricular dysfunction by echocardiography. Normal proBNP or BNP levels might help identify low-risk patients who benefit from anticoagulation alone.

PE patients should be treated with full-dose anticoagulation for at least 6 months. Anticoagulation is usually discontinued after 6 months in patients with transient VTE risk factors, such as surgery or trauma within 90 days. Indefinite-duration, low-intensity anticoagulation with warfarin (INR 1.5 to 2) is effective and safe for most patients with idiopathic PE or DVT. Some patients at particular high risk for recurrent VTE may require indefinite-duration, full-dose anticoagulation with warfarin. Cancer patients may benefit from long-term anticoagulation with dalteparin rather than warfarin.

EMOTIONAL SUPPORT

Although PE can be as devastating emotionally as myocardial infarction, the psychological burden for PE patients may be greater because the general public does not have as good an understanding of PE, particularly regarding the possibility of long-term disability and incomplete recovery. Young patients with PE repeatedly voice a common theme. Although they appear healthy, they often have difficulty expressing their fears and feelings about this potentially life-threatening illness to close family and friends.

Discussion of the implications of VTE with the patient and family may help to reduce the emotional burden. One example is a PE support group led by a nurse-physician team. Although these sessions have an educational component, the major emphasis is peer support to alleviate the anxieties that occur in the aftermath of PE.

REFERENCES

1. White RH: The epidemiology of venous thromboembolism. Circulation 107:4, 2003.
2. Heit JA, Silverstein MD, Mohr DN, et al: Risk factors for deep vein thrombosis and pulmonary embolism: A population-based case-control study. Arch Intern Med 160:809, 2000.
3. Kearon C: Natural history of venous thromboembolism. Circulation 107:22, 2003.
4. Goldhaber SZ, Visani L, De Rosa M: Acute pulmonary embolism: Clinical outcomes in the International Cooperative Pulmonary Embolism Registry (ICOPER). Lancet 353:1386, 1999.
5. Goldhaber SZ, Tapson VF, for the DVT FREE Steering Committee: DVT FREE: A prospective registry of 5451 patients with confirmed deep vein thrombosis. Am J Cardiol 93:259, 2004.
6. Lee AY, Levine MN: Venous thromboembolism and cancer: Risks and outcomes. Circulation 107:17, 2003.
7. Lapostolle F, Surget V, Borron SW, et al: Severe pulmonary embolism associated with air travel. N Engl J Med 345:779, 2001.
8. Vandenbroucke JP, Rosing J, Bloemenkamp KW, et al: Oral contraceptives and the risk of venous thrombosis. N Engl J Med 344: 1527, 2001.
9. Greer LA: Prevention and management of venous thromboembolism in pregnancy. Clin Chest Med 24:123, 2003.
10. Rossouw JE, Anderson GL, Prentice RL, et al: Risks and benefits of estrogen plus progestin in healthy postmenopausal women: Principal results from the Women's Health Initiative randomized controlled trial. JAMA 288:321, 2002.
11. Joffe HV, Goldhaber SZ: Laboratory thrombophilias and venous thromboembolism. Vasc Med 7:93, 2002.
12. Goldhaber SZ, Elliot CG: Acute pulmonary embolism: Part I: Epidemiology, pathophysiology, and diagnosis. Circulation 108: 2726, 2004.
13. Kucher N, Printzen G, Goldhaber SZ: Prognostic role of brain natriuretic peptide in acute pulmonary embolism. Circulation 107:2545, 2003.
14. Giannitsis E, Muller-Bardorff M, Kurowski V, et al: Independent prognostic value of cardiac troponin T in patients with confirmed pulmonary embolism. Circulation 102:211, 2000.
15. Geerts WH, Heit JA, Clagett GP, et al: Prevention of venous thromboembolism. Chest 119:132S, 2001.
16. Prevention of venous thromboembolism: International Consensus Statement Guidelines compiled in accordance with the scientific evidence. Int Angiol 20:1, 2001.
17. Goldhaber SZ, Dunn K, MacDougall RC: New onset of venous thromboembolism among hospitalized patients at Brigham and Women's Hospital is caused more often by prophylaxis failure than by withholding treatment. Chest 118:1680, 2000.
18. Durieux P, Nizard R, Ravaud P, et al: A clinical decision support system for prevention of venous thromboembolism: Effect on physician behavior. JAMA 283:2816, 2000.
19. Wells PS, Lensing AW, Hirsh J: Graduated compression stockings in the prevention of postoperative venous thromboembolism. A meta-analysis. Arch Intern Med 154:67, 1994.
20. Kessler CM, Hirsch DR, Jacobs H, et al: Intermittent pneumatic compression in chronic venous insufficiency favorably affects fibrinolytic potential and platelet activation. Blood Coagul Fibrinolysis 7:437, 1996.
21. Collins R, Scrimgeour A, Yusuf S, et al: Reduction in fatal pulmonary embolism and venous thrombosis by perioperative administration of subcutaneous heparin. Overview of results of randomized trials in general, orthopedic, and urologic surgery. N Engl J Med 318: 1162, 1988.
22. Lassen MR, Bauer KA, Eriksson BI, et al: Postoperative fondaparinux versus preoperative enoxaparin for prevention of venous thromboembolism in elective hip-replacement surgery: A randomised double-blind comparison. Lancet 359:1715, 2002.
23. Bounameoux H, Perneger T: Fondaparinux: A new synthetic pentasaccharide for thrombosis prevention. Lancet 359:1710, 2002.
24. Francis CW, Davidson BL, Berkowitz SD, et al: Ximelagatran versus warfarin for the prevention of venous thromboembolism after total knee arthroplasty. A randomized, double- blind trial. Ann Intern Med 137:648, 2002.
25. Eriksson BI, Agnelli G, Cohen AT, et al: Direct thrombin inhibitor melagatran followed by oral ximelagatran in comparison with enoxaparin for prevention of venous thromboembolism after total hip or knee replacement. Thromb Haemost 89:288, 2003.
26. Wells PS, Anderson DR, Rodger M, et al: Derivation of a simple clinical model to categorize patients' probability of pulmonary embolism: Increasing the models utility with the SimpliRED D-dimer. Thromb Haemost 83:416, 2000.
27. Kucher N, Walpoth N, Wustmann K, et al: QR in V1—an ECG sign associated with right ventricular dysfunction and adverse clinical outcome in pulmonary embolism. Eur Heart J 24:1113, 2003.
28. Stein PD, Terrin ML, Hales CA, et al: Clinical, laboratory, roentgenographic, and electrocardiographic findings in patients with acute pulmonary embolism and no pre-existing cardiac or pulmonary disease. Chest 100:598, 1991.
29. Goldhaber SZ, Simons GR, Elliott CG, et al: Quantitative plasma D-dimer levels among patients undergoing pulmonary angiography for suspected pulmonary embolism. JAMA 270:2819, 1993.
30. Brown MD, Rowe BH, Reeves MJ, et al: The accuracy of the enzyme-linked immunosorbent assay D-dimer test in the diagnosis of pulmonary embolism: A meta-analysis. Ann Emerg Med 40:133, 2002.
31. Kucher N, Kohler HP, Doernhoefer T, et al: Accuracy of D-dimer/fibrinogen ratio to predict pulmonary embolism: A prospective diagnostic study. J Thromb Haemost 1:708, 2003.
32. PIOPED Investigators: Value of the ventilation/perfusion scan in acute pulmonary embolism. Results of the Prospective Investigation of Pulmonary Embolism Diagnosis (PIOPED). JAMA 263:2753, 1990.
33. Schoepf UJ, Holzknecht N, Helmberger TK, et al: Subsegmental pulmonary emboli: Improved detection with thin-collimation multi-detector row spiral CT. Radiology 222:483, 2002.
34. Oudkerk M, van Beek EJ, Wielopolski P, et al: Comparison of contrast-enhanced magnetic resonance angiography and conventional pulmonary angiography for the diagnosis of pulmonary embolism: A prospective study. Lancet 359:1643, 2002.
35. Goldhaber SZ: Echocardiography in the management of pulmonary embolism. Ann Intern Med 136:691, 2002.
36. Kucher N, Luder CM, Dornhofer T, et al: Novel management strategy for patients with suspected pulmonary embolism. Eur Heart J 24:366, 2003.
37. Pruszczyk P, Torbicki A, Kuch-Wocial A, et al: Diagnostic value of transesophageal echocardiography in suspected haemodynamically significant pulmonary embolism. Heart 85:628, 2001.
38. Musset D, Parent F, Meyer G, et al: Diagnostic strategy for patients with suspected pulmonary embolism: A prospective multicentre outcome study. Lancet 360:1914, 2002.
39. Grifoni S, Olivotto I, Cecchini P, et al: Short-term clinical outcome of patients with acute pulmonary embolism, normal blood pressure, and echocardiographic right ventricular dysfunction. Circulation 101:2817, 2000.
40. Wicki J, Perrier A, Perneger TV, et al: Predicting adverse outcome in patients with acute pulmonary embolism: A risk score. Thromb Haemost 84:548, 2000.
41. McConnell MV, Solomon SD, Rayan ME, et al: Regional right ventricular dysfunction detected by echocardiography in acute pulmonary embolism. Am J Cardiol 78:469, 1996.
42. Konstantinides S, Geibel A, Olschewski M, et al: Importance of cardiac troponins I and T in risk stratification of patients with acute pulmonary embolism. Circulation 106:1263, 2002.

43. Kucher N, Printzen G, Doernhoefer T, et al: Low pro-brain natriuretic peptide levels predict benign clinical outcome in acute pulmonary embolism. Circulation 107:1576, 2003.
44. ten Wolde M, Tulevski II, Mulder JW, et al: Brain natriuretic peptide as a predictor of adverse outcome in patients with pulmonary embolism. Circulation 107:2082, 2003.
45. Pruszczyk P, Bochowicz A, Torbicki A, et al: Cardiac troponin T monitoring identifies high-risk group of normotensive patients with acute pulmonary embolism. Chest 123:1947, 2003.
46. Janata K, Holzer M, Laggner AN, et al: Cardiac troponin T in the severity assessment of patients with pulmonary embolism: Cohort study. BMJ 326:312, 2003.
47. Raschke RA, Reilly BM, Guidry JR, et al: The weight-based heparin dosing nomogram compared with a "standard care" nomogram. A randomized controlled trial. Ann Intern Med 119:874, 1993.
48. Simonneau G, Sors H, Charbonnier B, et al: A comparison of low-molecular-weight heparin with unfractionated heparin for acute pulmonary embolism. N Engl J Med 337:663, 1997.
49. The Columbus Investigators: Low-molecular-weight heparin in the treatment of patients with venous thromboembolism. N Engl J Med 337:657,1997.
50. Beer HJ, Burger M, Gretener S, et al: Outpatient treatment of pulmonary embolism is feasible and safe in a substantial proportion of patients. J Thromb Haemost 1:186, 2003.
51. Beckman JA, Dunn K, Sasahara AA, et al: Enoxaparin monotherapy without oral anticoagulation to treat acute symptomatic pulmonary embolism. Thromb Haemost 89:953, 2003.
52. Lee AY, Levine MN, Baker RI, et al: Low-molecular-weight heparin versus a coumarin for the prevention of recurrent venous thromboembolism in patients with cancer. N Engl J Med 349:146, 2003.
53. Koo S, Kucher N, Nguyen P, et al: Excessive anticoagulation increases mortality and morbidity in hospitalized patients with anticoagulation-related hemorrhage. Arch Intern Med 164:1557, 2004.
54. Kucher N, Castellanos L, Quiroz R, et al: Time-trends in warfarin-related hemorrhage. Am J Cardiol 94:403, 2004.
55. The PERSIST Investigators: A novel long-acting synthetic factor Xa inhibitor (idraparinux sodium) to replace warfarin for secondary prevention in deep vein thrombosis. The 44th Annual Meeting of the American Society of Hematology [abstract 301], 2002. Available at http://www.hematology.org/meeting/abstracts.cfm
56. Buller HR, Davidson BL, Decousus H, et al: Subcutaneous fondaparinux versus intravenous unfractionated heparin in the initial treatment of pulmonary embolism. N Engl J Med 349:1695, 2003.
57. Huisman MV for the THRIVE Investigators: Efficacy and safety of the oral direct thrombin inhibitor ximelagatran compared with current standard therapy for acute symptomatic deep vein thrombosis, with or without pulmonary embolism: A randomized, double-blind, multinational study [abstract OC003]. International Society on Thrombosis and Hemostasis, 2003.
58. Ridker PM, Goldhaber SZ, Danielson E, et al: Long-term, low-intensity warfarin therapy for the prevention of recurrent venous thromboembolism. N Engl J Med 348:1425, 2003.
59. Schulman S, Wahlander K, Lundstrom T, et al: Secondary prevention of venous thromboembolism with the oral direct thrombin inhibitor ximelagatran. N Engl J Med 30;349:1713, 2003.
60. Kearon C, Ginsberg JS, Kovacs MJ, et al: Comparison of low-intensity warfarin therapy with conventional-intensity warfarin therapy for long-term prevention of recurrent venous thromboembolism. N Engl J Med 349:631, 2003.
61. Palareti G, Legnani C, Cosmi B, et al: Predictive value of D-Dimer test for recurrent venous thromboembolism after anticoagulation withdrawal in subjects with a previous idiopathic event and in carriers of congenital thrombophilia. Circulation 108:313, 2003.
62. Schulman S, Rhedin AS, Lindmarker P, et al: A comparison of six weeks with six months of oral anticoagulant therapy after a first episode of venous thromboembolism. Duration of Anticoagulation Trial Study Group. N Engl J Med 332:1661, 1995.
63. Kearon C, Gent M, Hirsh J, et al: A comparison of three months of anticoagulation with extended anticoagulation for a first episode of idiopathic venous thromboembolism. N Engl J Med 340:901, 1999.
64. Agnelli G, Prandoni P, Santamaria MG, et al: Three months versus one year of oral anticoagulant therapy for idiopathic deep venous thrombosis. Warfarin Optimal Duration Italian Trial Investigators. N Engl J Med 345:165, 2001.
65. Agnelli G, Prandoni P, Becattini C, et al: Extended oral anticoagulant therapy after a first episode of pulmonary embolism. Ann Intern Med 139:19, 2003.
66. Konstantinides S, Geibel A, Heusel G, et al: Heparin plus alteplase compared with heparin alone in patients with submassive pulmonary embolism. N Engl J Med 347:1143, 2002.
67. Thabut G, Thabut D, Myers RP, et al: Thrombolytic therapy of pulmonary embolism: A meta-analysis. J Am Coll Cardiol 40:1660, 2002.
68. Aklog L, Williams CS, Byrne JG, et al: Acute pulmonary embolectomy: A contemporary approach. Circulation 105:1416, 2002.
69. White RH, Zhou H, Kim J, et al: A population-based study of the effectiveness of inferior vena cava filter use among patients with venous thromboembolism. Arch Intern Med 160:2033, 2000.
70. Offner PJ, Hawkes A, Madayag R, et al: The role of temporary inferior vena cava filters in critically ill surgical patients. Arch Surg 138:591, 2003.

chapter 55

Varicose Veins

Edwin C. Gravereaux
Magruder C. Donaldson

Varicose veins are pathologically enlarged subcutaneous venous channels. In the lower extremity, varicose veins involve the superficial, extrafascial greater and lesser saphenous veins and their tributaries. Estimates indicate that more than 10% of the adult population harbors significant varicose veins for which symptomatic relief might be sought at one time or another. If asymptomatic or mildly symptomatic veins are considered as well, the prevalence of varicose veins is substantially higher, up to 40%, and if small reticular malformations are included, the prevalence may be as high as 80%.[1] Though females more commonly present for therapy, there is evidence that prevalence of varicose veins may be at least as great if not greater among men.[1]

In *primary* varicose veins, the problem originates within the superficial system, with no involvement of the deep subfascial veins (Figs. 55-1 and 55-2). In the case of *secondary* varicose veins, superficial veins become enlarged as a result of disease originating in the deep venous system by way of communicating veins that connect the deep and superficial systems (Figs. 55-3 and 55-4). Among a large number of patients presenting for therapy at the Mayo Clinic, 72% were thought to have primary varicose veins and 28% to have secondary veins. The greater saphenous system was involved five to six times more often than the lesser saphenous.[2]

PATHOGENESIS AND PATHOPHYSIOLOGY

Patients seeking therapy for varicose veins are most commonly beyond their third decade of life, with advancing age clearly associated with increasing incidence and severity of varicose veins.[1,2] Suggested mechanisms of pathogenesis of primary varicose veins include defective structure and function of valves in the saphenous vein, intrinsic weakness of the vein walls, and the presence of tiny arteriovenous connections that gradually lead to venous engorgement.[3] More than 50% of people with primary varicose veins have a family history,[2] suggesting that there is an inherited defect in vein structure or function that predisposes to varicosity. In one study, saphenofemoral reflux detected by Doppler ultrasound was twice as common in children of parents with varicose veins as in children of parents without varicosities.[4] Some observers have noted attenuation and disorganization of connective tissue and smooth muscle components in varicose veins and postulated that a cellular synthetic

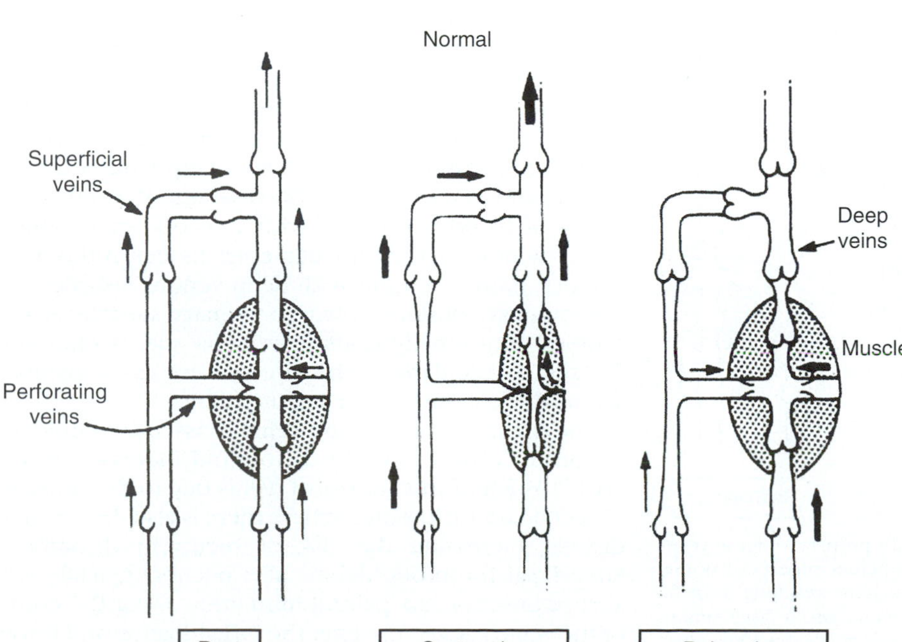

FIGURE 55-1. Normal action of the "muscle pump." Blood flows up the deep veins with systolic muscle contraction against competent distal and perforator valves. Flow through the open distal valves into the empty pump occurs during diastole. (From Sumner DS: Venous dynamics—varicosities. Clin Obstet Gynecol 24:743, 1981).

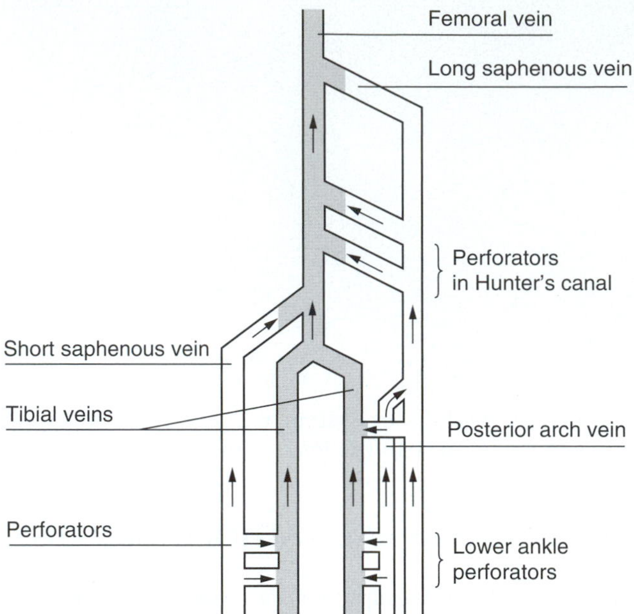

FIGURE 55-2. Diagrammatic representation of flow from superficial veins (*clear*) through perforators into the deep system (*shaded*). (From Haeger K: The anatomy of the veins of the leg. In JT Hobbs [ed]: The Treatment of Venous Disorders. Philadelphia, Lippincott, 1977, p 19).

defect may predispose toward varicosity, perhaps on a familial basis.[3] Events during pregnancy include increased intravascular volume, elevated pressure on the intra-abdominal and pelvic veins, and perhaps softening of vein walls along with many other connective tissue elements, which helps to explain the 2:1 female-to-male prevalence ratio of significant varicose veins.[5,6]

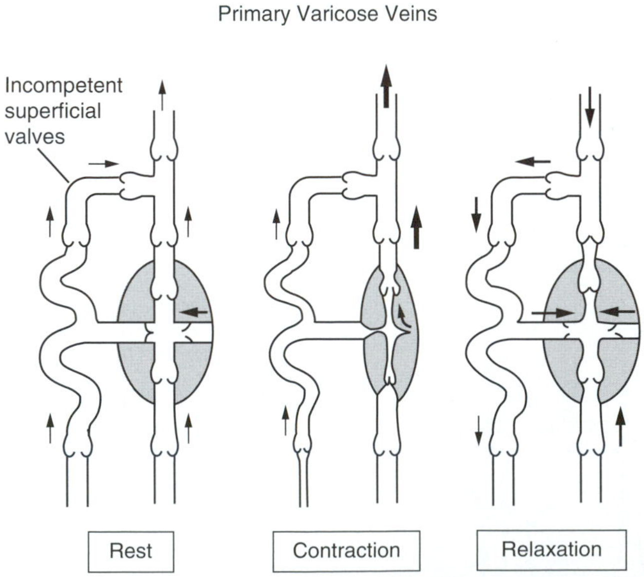

Primary Varicose Veins

Incompetent superficial valves

Rest | Contraction | Relaxation

FIGURE 55-3. Abnormal "muscle pump" with primary varicose veins. Significant reflux of blood down the incompetent superficial system occurs, with filling of pump from proximal veins, resulting in inefficient circular flow of blood and impaired reduction in distal venous pressure. (From Sumner DS: Venous dynamics—varicosities. Clin Obstet Gynecol 24:743, 1981).

Anatomic study[7,8] and careful survey using Doppler ultrasound[9] have found evidence of minute arteriovenous fistulas connecting to the varicose system. It is unclear whether these fistulas are causative or arise at a later stage of development of the lesions, and the contribution of these connections to typical varicose veins remains controversial. Fistulas do not occur in the Klippel-Trenaunay syndrome, where large superficial varicosities occur on a congenital basis, associated with cutaneous nevi and bone and soft-tissue hypertrophy.[10-12]

By definition, secondary varicose veins arise as a result of disease of the deep veins. Most often, deep vein thrombosis (DVT) is the inciting factor, with deep valvular incompetence leading to communicator incompetence or deep vein occlusion causing enlargement of superficial veins as collateral channels. In a minority of patients, primary valvular reflux in the deep veins or communicating veins gives rise to secondary varicosities without prior DVT.[13]

Greater saphenous vein enlargement is a common early abnormality in the great majority of patients with primary varicose veins. It has become clear, however, that proximal sources of reflux other than the greater saphenous exist in about 10% of patients, including the pelvic veins via vulvar tributaries, muscular veins presenting on the back or sides of the thigh, or veins accompanying the sciatic nerve.[14] Regardless of the source, reflux distally enhances further venous enlargement with distraction of valve leaflets and further valvular incompetence and reflux into sections of adjacent distal vein. With time, this process propagates into peripheral branches and also into communicating veins when they become exposed to blood below an incompetent valve in the main channel. As the segment of engorged vein becomes longer, the hydrostatic pressure exerted by the uninterrupted column of blood increases. Furthermore, with exercise, pressures fail to decrease normally because effective valves are absent. When communicator incompetence is present, activation of the muscle pump forcefully ejects blood outward into the superficial system, greatly increasing pressures on the subcutaneous tissues. With return to the deep system through adjacent competent communicators, ineffective circuitous motion of venous blood occurs with each muscle contraction. With high pressures and inefficient emptying of the leg, edema and microscopic extravasation of cellular elements of blood can occur, with a secondary inflammatory reaction in the subcutaneous tissues. Although it is much more common with deep venous insufficiency, this process confined solely to primary superficial varicosities occasionally leads to eczema and ulceration of the skin, particularly in the more severe cases involving secondary communicator incompetency.[15]

The presence of varicose veins is associated epidemiologically with a twofold to fourfold increased risk of DVT.[16] Much of this statistical risk is due to the presence of secondary varicosities, where there is also deep venous disease, increasing the risk of recurrent thrombosis. Superficial thrombophlebitis also occurs, typically with abrupt onset of red, painful induration along the course of the vein. In some patients, the inflammation and thrombosis is triggered by blunt trauma such as contusion to

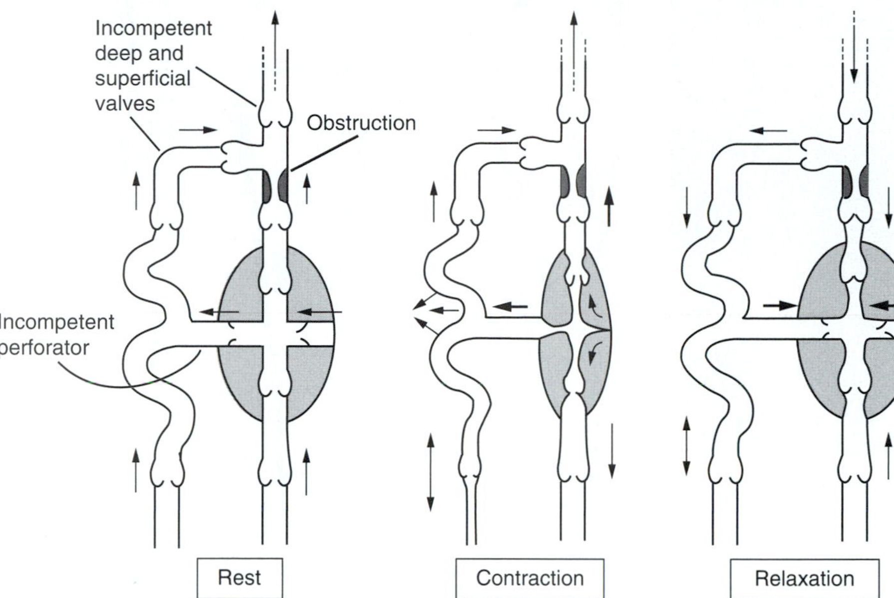

FIGURE 55-4. Abnormal "muscle pump" with deep venous insufficiency and secondary varicose veins. Muscle contraction with some proximal obstruction and incompetent deep, communicating, and superficial veins causes retrograde flow in all veins, resulting in high pressures in distal leg. (From Sumner DS: Venous dynamics—varicosities. Clin Obstet Gynecol 24:743, 1981).

the varicosity. In uncommon instances, the process tracks down a communicating vein goes into the saphenofemoral junction to reach the deep system.[17,18] Thrombophlebitis of the superficial veins alone presents no significant threat of postphlebitic syndrome or pulmonary embolism. Patients with repetitive attacks of superficial thrombophlebitis may be harboring a malignancy.

CLINICAL MANIFESTATIONS

History

The most common complaint of patients with varicose veins concerns the cosmetic appearance of their legs.[19] Often a relatively small cluster of veins becomes visible in a young woman with a family history, and there is concern about arresting the process before it becomes unmanageable. Many patients are also concerned about the possibility of developing dangerous blood clots in the veins. In addition, however, most patients with involvement of a long segment of vein that extends across the knee or ankle joint have some discomfort. The typical syndrome involves a dull ache, heaviness, or pressure sensation in the area of the vein, particularly after a period of standing, with relief on elevation of the leg. In women, these complaints are usually more noticeable just before the menses and become dramatically worse during pregnancy. Superficial thrombophlebitis occurs episodically in some patients. A small percentage of patients with extensive primary varicose veins develop eczema and ulceration at the ankle level.[15,20] Finally, some extremely superficial varicose veins may be subject to rupture with a startling amount of bleeding, which can be dangerous because it is painless and therefore can go unheeded.

Physical Findings

Simple examination of the legs demonstrates most varicosities, which are more easily seen over the calf and ankle than over the thigh. The dependent position with oblique lighting enhances visibility (Figs. 55-5 and 55-6). If the subcutaneous tissue is thick, veins are not as evident, in which case palpation is helpful. Enlarged veins can generally be balloted, particularly with the leg dependent. Percussion ("tap test") of a distal portion of a vein transmits a fluid wave proximally, proving continuity. When valvular competence is in question, percussion of a vein proximally transmits a fluid wave distally when the valves are not functional. The wave force is dampened by a competent valve. Similar abnormal retrograde pulse transmission can be elicited by coughing when all proximal valves are incompetent. In some patients, the saphenous bulb in the groin may protrude dramatically with coughing or the Valsalva maneuver. Varicosities should be sought in both greater and lesser saphenous vein distributions.

Primary and secondary varicosities can often be differentiated by the Brodie-Trendelenburg test (Fig. 55-7).[21] The leg is raised to empty the veins, and a tourniquet is placed above the knee to obstruct flow of blood through the superficial veins. The leg is then lowered to a dependent position while the examiner watches for filling of distal varicosities over the calf and ankle. Prompt filling of the varicosities with the thigh tourniquet in place indicates reflux of blood through incompetent communicators from an incompetent deep venous system, which makes the varicose veins *secondary*. On the other hand, if filling of the varicosities with a thigh tourniquet in place takes more than 20 seconds, with rapid filling only after removal of the tourniquet, the source of reflux is the superficial system, indicating that the varicose veins

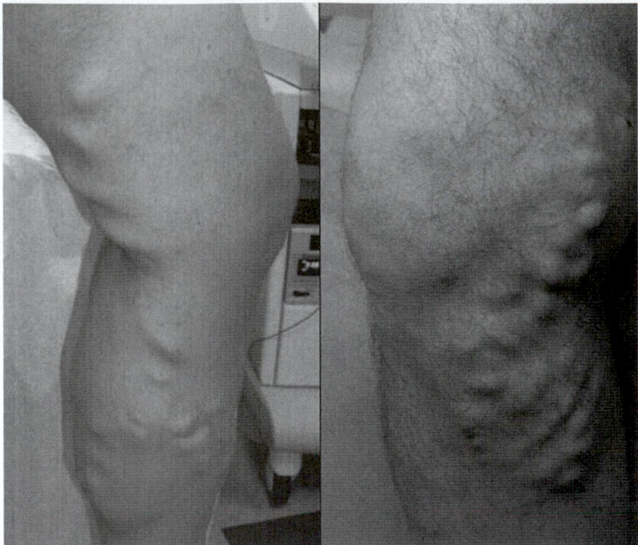

FIGURE 55-5. Primary varicose veins involving the greater saphenous vein and calf tributaries.

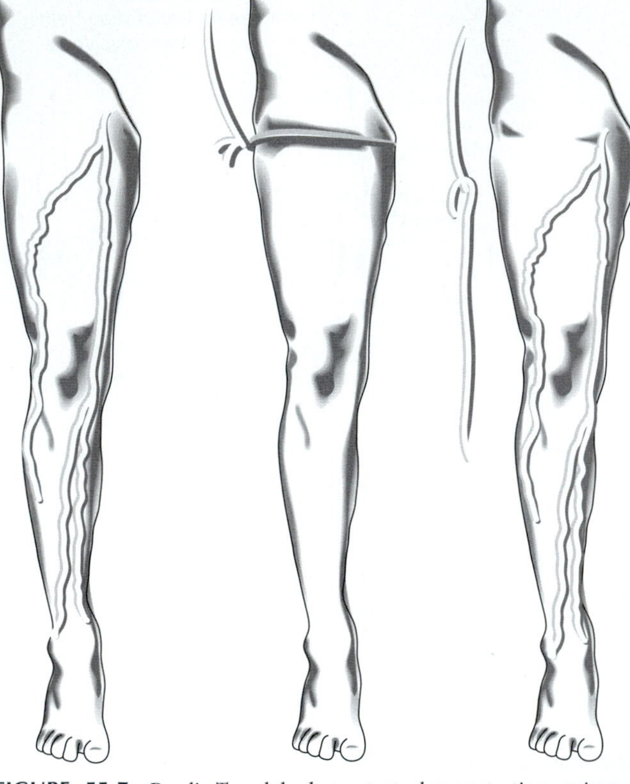

FIGURE 55-7. Brodie-Trendelenburg test demonstrating primary varicosity of the greater saphenous vein. Vein fills with leg dependency and no tourniquet (*left*). After elevation to empty the vein, tourniquet is applied to obstruct abnormal retrograde filling of varicosity with dependency (*center*). Release of the tourniquet allows prompt reflux to fill the varicose system (*right*). (From Dodd H, Cockett FB: The Pathology and Surgery of the Veins of the Lower Limb. Edinburgh, Livingstone, 1976, p 82.)

are *primary*. In some patients both deep-communicator and superficial incompetence are identified by the Brodie-Trendelenburg test.

Other findings of significance associated with varicose veins in some patients are thickened cords over chronically occluded superficial veins and changes such as induration and hyperpigmentation in the skin and subcutaneous tissue of the ankle and distal calf, indicating the presence of chronic venous hypertension. Superficial thrombophlebitis produces a linear indurated cord with erythema, swelling, and tenderness and is frequently mistaken for abscess. Edema may be present in patients with severe primary varicosities or with deep venous disease and secondary varicosities. Small-branched veins, "spider" veins, and telangiectasias are common in many patients, particularly after middle age, with or without trunk varicosities related to saphenous incompetence. Physical findings associated with Klippel-Trenaunay syndrome include enlargement of the involved extremity, cutaneous nevi, and an unusually extensive pattern of superficial varicosities.

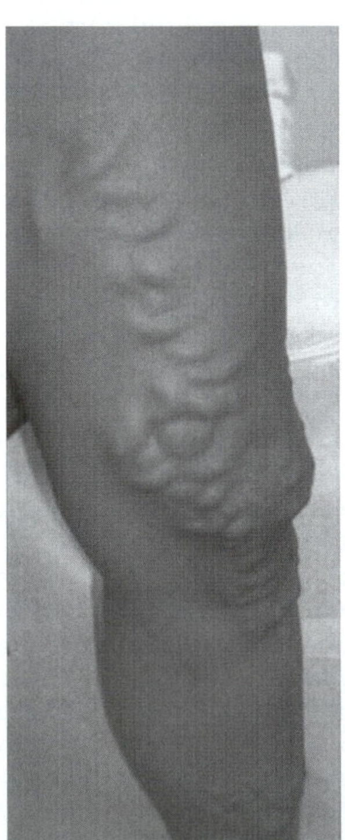

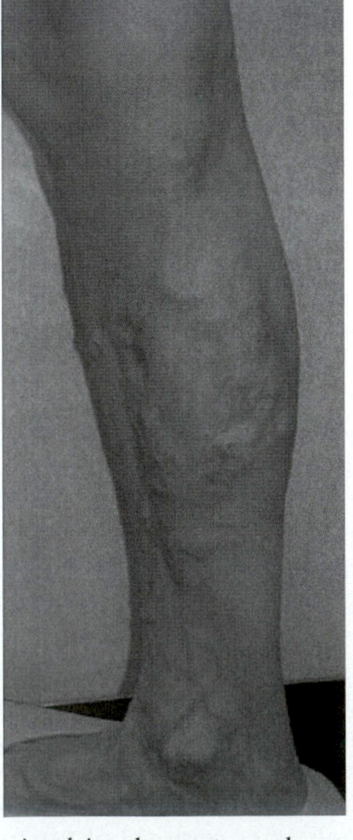

FIGURE 55-6. Primary varicose veins involving the greater saphenous vein and calf tributaries.

Laboratory

Laboratory study of varicose veins should be used selectively, usually only if ablation is being considered. Nonetheless, certain laboratory techniques may be helpful to supplement the physical examination, particularly when there is question about the status of the deep venous system. Using continuous wave Doppler ultrasound to detect flow, the percussion tests can be performed with greater precision, and reflux and vein continuity thus assessed. In recent years, duplex ultrasound has become the most popular method for mapping the anatomy and filling patterns of varicose systems, with relatively easy detection of valvular reflux and occlusions in superficial and deep veins, as well as location of communicating veins.[22,23] Routine use of duplex ultrasound in all cases has been advocated by some, but most would emphasize selective use for patients with recurrent varicose veins, a history of DVT, clinical evidence of deep venous insufficiency, venous ulcer, and unclear sources of reflux, particularly when involving the popliteal fossa and lesser saphenous system.[14,24] Duplex ultrasound is helpful when the cause of phlebitis appears unrelated to preexisting varicose veins, in which case a systemic hypercoagulable state may create associated DVT. If the phlebitic segment of vein is adjacent to the saphenofemoral or saphenopopliteal junction, duplex ultrasound is the best way to exclude involvement of adjacent deep veins by contiguity.

In some laboratories, a variant of the Brodie-Trendelenburg test can be performed using the photoplethysmograph, which detects blood volume in the subcutaneous capillary bed.[25] After a baseline reading is obtained at the ankle level, ankle flexion several times in succession normally decreases blood volume in the veins, reducing the baseline tracing dramatically. Refilling of the veins after exercise normally takes more than 20 seconds. In the presence of valvular reflux, emptying with ankle flexion is less efficient and venous refill time after exercise occurs in less than 20 seconds. Placement of a tourniquet just below the knee normalizes refilling time if reflux is via the superficial veins (*primary* varicosities). If refilling time remains shortened with such a tourniquet in place, reflux must be occurring via incompetent communicating veins from a diseased deep system (*secondary* varicosities).

Ascending venography is a precise means of defining venous anatomy.[26] It is rarely indicated in evaluating varicose veins but may be used occasionally as an adjunct in some clinics employing catheter-based ablation techniques for saphenous trunk reflux. Radiographic dye is introduced into a foot or other peripheral superficial vein and, with a tourniquet placed at the ankle level, the dye is forced to flow into the deep system outlining the deep veins. If incompetent communicators are present, reflux back into the superficial system is detected. With no ankle tourniquet, dye introduced at the foot level remains largely superficial, outlining the saphenous vein and associated varicosities. Venography by direct puncture of a varicosity may be useful to outline unusual vein patterns.

MANAGEMENT

Conservative Measures

An important aspect of management of varicose veins is patient education about their natural history, emphasizing the small potential for major impact on health. It is particularly helpful to differentiate between venous disease and the more ominous course of arterial disease, and between superficial and deep venous disease, especially with regard to potential for thrombosis and pulmonary embolism. Understanding of the pathophysiology of varicose veins encourages compliance with conservative measures to reduce symptoms and retard progression of vein enlargement.

Among these measures, elastic support is most useful and should allow pursuit of normal occupational and recreational activities.[27,28] Numerous brands of pantyhose or styled stocking are commercially available for both men and women. To be effective, stockings must fit firmly with diminishing compression as the garment ascends the leg, avoiding a proximal constricting band.[29] Graduated external compression should provide a counterbalance to the graduated hydrostatic pressure change within the superficial veins. The most precise physiologic control is afforded by prescription stockings measured to fit properly and available either off the shelf or by custom tailoring. These prescription stockings can be designed to provide compression pressures at the ankle ranging from 20 to 60 mm Hg. Compression at the ankle of 20 to 30 mm Hg is sufficient for most patients with primary varicose veins. Knee-length hose are quite satisfactory, though thigh-length or pantyhose-style hose with sufficient elasticity may be preferred by women. Special maternity brands with an expandable lower abdominal panel are advisable during the last trimester of pregnancy. Trial and error of various types may be necessary to balance efficacy against comfort, cost, and appearance. Stockings lose their elasticity with wear and washing, and patients should be aware that new garments will be needed every few months.

Skin hygiene and moisturizing cream are helpful in avoiding dermatitis and eczema in patients with extensive varicosities to the ankle level. Topical steroid cream may help control early inflammation in these patients. Startling bleeding caused by cracking or injury of skin over superficial varicose branches is easily controlled acutely by steep leg elevation and pressure using an elastic bandage. Local branch ligation or sclerotherapy may be necessary to avoid recurrences. Acute episodes of superficial thrombophlebitis are best managed by a short course of a nonsteroidal anti-inflammatory medication. Systemic anticoagulation may be warranted in patients who fail to respond to anti-inflammatory therapy or who have associated or contiguous DVT. In a few patients with extensive or recurrent superficial thrombophlebitis, ablative surgery may be indicated.

Ablative Measures

If symptoms persist despite use of support, a number of options are available for ablation of varicose veins with minimal morbidity. Sclerotherapy has been used extensively in Europe and is regaining popularity in North America with the introduction of new sclerosant agents. In properly selected patients, it has the major advantage of avoiding hospital costs since it is easily performed in the office setting. The principle of therapy is to inject a material into the varicosities that induces inflammation and scarring sufficient to seal the lumen. The U.S. Food and Drug Administration has approved sodium tetradecyl sulfate, sodium morrhuate, and ethanolamine oleate for treatment of varicose veins and cutaneous telangiectasias. Sclerotherapy is most effective when application is limited to superficial "spider" veins and telangiectasias, small (1 to 3 mm) diameter varicose branches without associated saphenous reflux, or residual or early recurrent varicosities after saphenous ablation.[30]

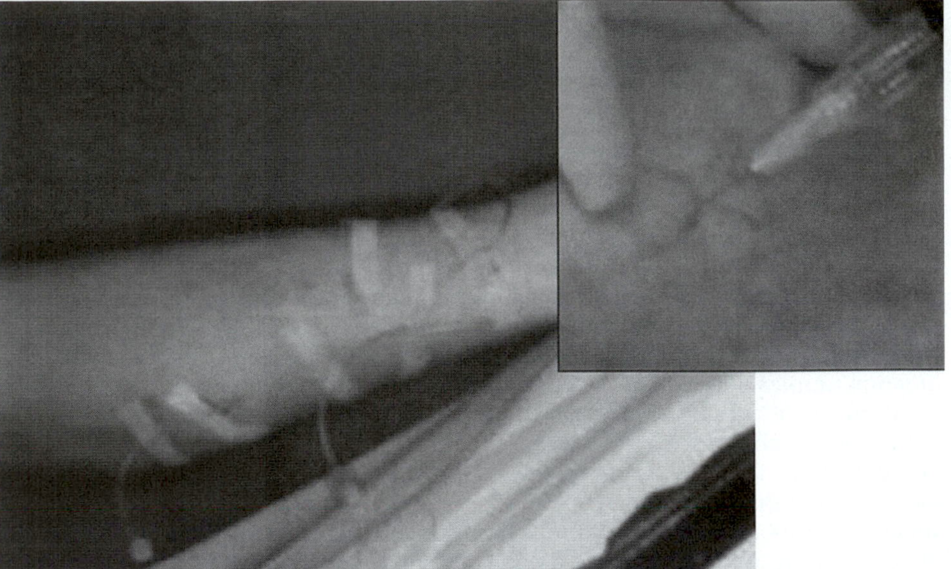

FIGURE 55-8. Technique of varicose vein sclerotherapy, multiple simultaneous venous cannulations in an elevated calf, and single injection (*inset*).

In general, the technique involves insertion of a small-gauge needle on a syringe containing the sclerosant into the target vein while the leg is dependent. The syringe is taped to the leg while two or three other varicosities are punctured. The leg is then elevated to empty the veins, and a small volume of the sclerosant is slowly injected into the vein at each site (Fig. 55-8). Compression with a gauze pad and tape is provided over the vein as the needle is withdrawn. At the completion of the injections, with the leg still elevated, a firm elastic bandage is wrapped carefully from the foot to 6 inches above the most proximal injection site. Patients are instructed to maintain their usual activities, to avoid prolonged sitting or standing, and to leave the bandage in place for several days. Depending on the agent used, the size and number of veins injected, and the practitioner's experience, various regimens of compression and postinjection activity are recommended to optimize efficacy and minimize morbidity.[30]

Allergic reactions to sclerosing agents have been estimated to occur in 0.01% to 3% of patients depending on the agent, with rare episodes of fatal anaphylaxis.[31] Mild local reactions such as edema, ecchymosis, and matting or induration occur in up to 20% of patients, and extravasation of sclerosant at the injection site may cause occasional skin necrosis. Hyperpigmentation over the course of the injected vein occurs in 10% to 30% of patients but almost invariably resolves over 6 to 12 months. Results or sclerotherapy are generally excellent when the method is applied selectively, as indicated earlier. Results are poor, however, when sclerotherapy is applied to patients with saphenous trunk incompetence, with up to 80% recurrence rate at 5 years in some studies.[32,33]

Control of proximal superficial vein reflux is an important prerequisite to long-term control of associated calf varicosities. Two minimally invasive techniques have been introduced to allow percutaneous endovascular ablation of incompetent proximal saphenous veins. Heating of the venous wall by radiofrequency microwave[34-38] or laser[39,40] energy delivered endoluminally by catheter under ultrasound guidance results in closure of the vein in up to 90% of patients (Fig. 55-9). In carefully selected patients, the procedure can be performed on an ambulatory basis with local anesthesia without incurring hospital expenses. Recovery is prompt, with return to work and other activities after a day or two of minimal discomfort. Occasional hematomas from vein perforation or skin injury or neuropathy from heat have been reported.

The procedure is best applied to patients with early symptoms based on saphenous reflux, with small or moderate-sized calf branches that are potentially amenable to simultaneous or subsequent ambulatory ligation or sclerotherapy. In general patients with large, extensive symptomatic calf branches require a more definitive approach involving surgical branch ligation or ablation with a powered phlebectomy device[41] under regional or general anesthesia. Under these circumstances, the potential cost and comfort advantages of minimally invasive, ambulatory ablation are less compelling and a comprehensive surgical approach to both trunks and branches in one setting is more appropriate.

Surgical therapy is directed at control of the source of reflux via the incompetent saphenous system and removal of significant varicose branches to prevent persistent filling by capillary inflow and collateral routes. Ligation of the saphenous origin without stripping of the trunk has been shown to provide only temporary relief in most cases because of such collaterals. Removal of the saphenous trunk by stripping or other methods provides the best long-term control.[42,43] Despite this evidence, it is reasonable in some cases to use selective use of surgery directed at specific segments and branches of the main veins when it appears important to try to preserve the main saphenous trunk vein as a potential conduit for arterial bypass.

The procedure requires a spinal, epidural, or general anesthetic but can usually be performed without

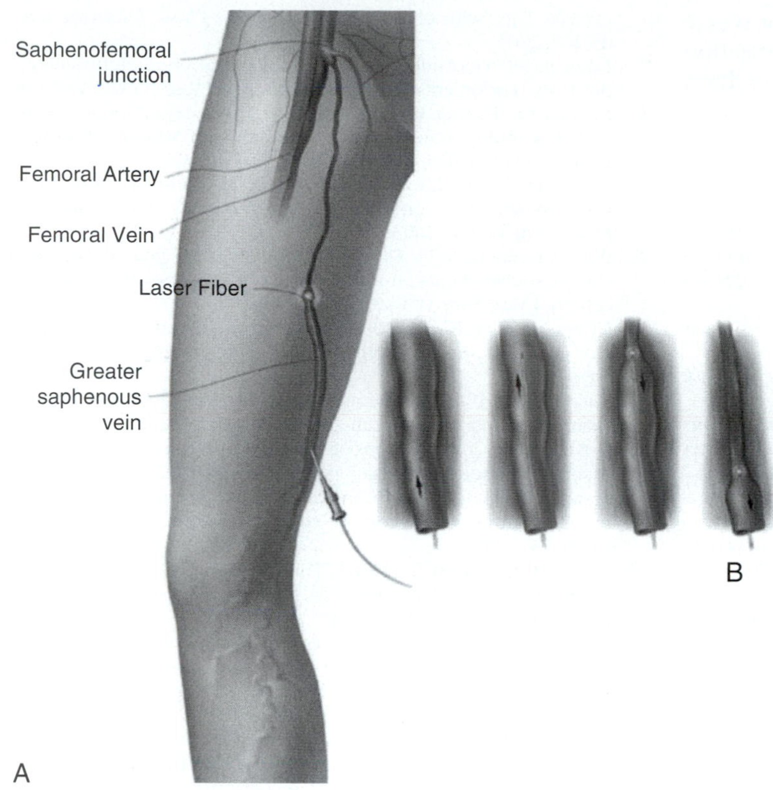

FIGURE 55-9. Endovenous laser ablation of the greater saphenous vein (GSV): Through a venous sheath placed into the GSV at the knee (**A**), the laser is withdrawn from just distal to the saphenofemoral junction down the length of the vein, obliterating the lumen behind the probe (**B**).

overnight hospitalization. Typically, the vein pattern is marked with the patient standing immediately preoperatively. A small incision is placed at the distal end of the involved vein, near the medial malleolus at the ankle in the case of the greater saphenous. An internal vein stripper is advanced proximally up the greater saphenous trunk, a counterincision is made over the saphenofemoral junction, and the stripper secured. The ends of the vein are ligated, leaving the proximal saphenous vein flush with the common femoral vein. The stripper is then used to pull the vein out in a downward direction toward the foot, which reduces the likelihood of traumatic saphenous neuropathy compared with pulling the vein upward.[44,45] Side branches and communicating veins are avulsed during this process. Any significant residual branches can be removed separately with an internal or external stripper or simply ligated through a series of several stab incisions. An alternative method uses a series of small punctures placed over the course of branches of the varicose system, employing a small hook to pull the veins out for ligation or removal and enabling preservation of much of the main saphenous trunk.[46-49]

Postoperatively, the leg is wrapped with an elastic bandage and ambulation held to a minimum for 12 hours. There is receding postoperative pain for a few days, as well as ecchymosis and edema over the track of the vein, which resolve within 3 weeks. Return to many activities is possible within a week, using compression for comfort. Occasional hemorrhage, infection, and local neuropathy occur, but DVT and other significant morbidity and mortality are rare.[48]

With a thorough surgical approach to the saphenous trunk and its main varicose tributaries, about 85% of patients remain free of recurrence at 5 years.[48,50] Hobbs, in a controlled trial comparing surgery and sclerotherapy, found a 12% incidence of recurrence at 5 years among patients treated surgically for large saphenous system veins.[51] On the other hand, the 5-year recurrence rate of lower-limb communicating veins and superficial small veins treated surgically was about 56%, suggesting that these smaller veins may be best treated by primary sclerotherapy. Optimal ablative therapy of varicose veins combines either endovascular intervention or surgery and sclerotherapy, depending on the presenting pathology.[48,49]

SPIDER VEINS

Clusters of small cutaneous veins occur frequently, particularly in women after childbirth and as middle age approaches. These lesions often appear to arise from a single feeding vein with a caput medusa pattern of serpiginous branches. This arrangement has led to the names *venous telangiectasia, spider hemangioma,* and *spider vein*. Alternatively, the veins may take a linear pattern. Their distribution varies from a few isolated locations in the thigh or calf to diffuse involvement throughout the legs, most heavily around the ankles and feet. Self-consciousness about appearance of the legs is the usual complaint.

Therapy emphasizes education about the veins and their natural history. Hose and makeup are effective ways of covering the veins in many instances. Alternatively, sclerotherapy using a 30-gauge needle, magnification, and a suitable sclerosant solution is possible.

Patients should be warned that a blemish as bad or worse than the vein could result should there be extravasation at the site of injection. Lasers and electrocautery have also been used to obliterate spider veins.[48]

REFERENCES

1. Evans CJ, Fowkes FG, Ruckley CV, et al: Prevalence of varicose veins and chronic venous insufficiency in men and women in the general population: Edinburgh Vein Study. J Epidemiol Community Health 53:149, 1999.
2. Lofgren EP: Treatment of long saphenous varicosities and their recurrence: A long-term follow-up. Surg Veins 285, 1985.
3. Rose SS, Ahmed A: Some thoughts on the aetiology of varicose veins. J Cardiovasc Surg 27:534, 1986.
4. Reagan B, Folse R: Lower limb venous dynamics in normal persons and children of patients with varicose veins. Surg Gynecol Obstet 132:15, 1971.
5. Bergan JJ: Causes of venous varicosities and telangiectasias: Implications for treatment. J Vasc Biol Med 85:1101, 1995.
6. Clarke GH, Vasdekis SN, Hobbs JT, et al: Venous wall function in the pathogenesis of varicose veins: Role of venous elasticity in the development of varicose veins. Surgery 111:402, 1992.
7. Schalin S: Arteriovenous communications localised by thermography and identified by operative microscopy. Acta Chir Scand 147:409, 1981.
8. Piulachs P, Vidal-Barraquer F: Pathogenic study of varicose veins. Angiology 4:59, 1953.
9. Haimovici H: Role of precapillary arteriovenous shunting in the pathogenesis of varicose veins and its therapeutic implications. (erratum appears in Surgery 102:54, 1987). Surgery 101:515, 1987.
10. Gloviczki P, Stanson AW, Stickler AW, et al: Klippel-Trenaunay syndrome: The risks and benefits of vascular interventions. Surgery 110:469, 1991.
11. Baskerville PA, Ackroyd JS, Browse NL: The etiology of the Klippel-Trenaunay syndrome. Ann Surg 202:624, 1985.
12. Noel AA, Gloviczki P, Cherry KJ Jr, et al: Surgical treatment of venous malformations in Klippel-Trenaunay syndrome. J Vasc Surg 32:840, 2000.
13. Almgren B, Eriksson I, Bylund H, et al: Phlebographic evaluation of nonthrombotic deep venous incompetence: New anatomic and functional aspects: Primary deep venous incompetence in limbs with varicose veins. J Vasc Surg 11:389, 1990.
14. Labropoulos N, Tiongson J, Pryor L, et al: Nonsaphenous superficial vein reflux. J Vasc Surg 34:872, 2001.
15. Hoare MC, Nicolaides AN, Miles CR, et al: The role of primary varicose veins in venous ulceration. Surgery 92:450, 1982.
16. Nicolaides AN, Irving D: Clinical factors and the risk of deep venous thrombosis. In Nicolaides AN (ed): Thromboembolism, Baltimore, University Park Press, 1975, p 193.
17. Skillman JJ, Kent KC, Porter DH, et al: Simultaneous occurrence of superficial and deep thrombophlebitis in the lower extremity. J Vasc Surg 11:818, 1990.
18. Lerche A, Jorgensen M, Urhammer S, et al: The incidence of deep venous thrombosis in patients with superficial thrombophlebitis of the lower limbs. J Intern Med 234:457, 1993.
19. Bradbury A, Evans C, Allan P, et al: What are the symptoms of varicose veins? Edinburgh vein study cross sectional population survey. Br Med J 318:353, 1999.
20. Sethia KK, Darke SG: Long saphenous incompetence as a cause of venous ulceration. Br J Surg 71:754, 1984.
21. Bradbury A, Ruckley CV: Clinical assessment of patients with venous disease. Handbook of Venous Disorders, London, Chapman and Hall Medical, 2001, pp 80-97.
22. Mattos MA, Sumner DS: Direct noninvasive tests (duplex scan) for the evaluation of chronic venous obstruction and valvular incompetence. Handbook of Venous Disorders, London, Chapman and Hall Medical, 2001, p 120.
23. Nicolaides AN, Szendro G, Irvine AT, et al: Duplex scanning in the assessment of deep venous incompetence. J Vasc Surg 5:148, 1987.
24. Wong JKF, Duncan JL, Nichols DM: Whole leg duplex mapping for varicose veins: Observations on patterns of reflux in recurrent and primary legs, with clinical correlation. Eur J Vasc Endovasc Surg 25:267, 2003.
25. Papadakis K, Nicolaides AN, Al-Kutoubi A, et al: Photoplethysmography in the assessment of venous insufficiency. J Vasc Surg 7:215, 1988.
26. Kamida CB, Kistner RL, Eklof B, et al: Lower extremity ascending and descending phlebography. Handbook of Venous Disorders, London, Chapman and Hall Medical, 2001, p 132.
27. Ibegbuna V, Delis KT, Nicolaides AN, et al: Effect of elastic compression stockings on venous hemodynamics during walking. J Vasc Surg 37:420, 2003.
28. Buhs CL, Bendick PJ, Glover JL: The effect of graded compression elastic stockings on the lower leg venous system during daily activity. J Vasc Surg 30:830, 1999.
29. Godin MS, Rice JC, Kerstein MD: Effect of commercially available pantyhose on venous return in the lower extremity. J Vasc Surg 5:844, 1987.
30. Villavicencio JL: Sclerotherapy guidelines. Handbook of Venous Disorders, London, Chapman and Hall Medical, 2001, p 253.
31. Goldman MP: Complications of sclerotherapy. Handbook of Venous Disorders, London, Chapman and Hall Medical, 2001, p 279.
32. Freiman DB, Gatenby R, Hobbs CL, et al: Surgery and sclerotherapy in the treatment of varicose veins: A random trial. Arch Surg 116:1377, 1981.
33. Neglen P, Einarsson E, Eklof B: The functional long-term value of different types of treatment for saphenous vein incompetence. J Cardiovasc Surg 34:295, 1993.
34. Lurie F, Creton D, Eklof B, et al: Prospective randomized study of endovenous radiofrequency obliteration (Closure procedure) versus ligation and stripping in a selected patient population (EVOLVEeS Study). J Vasc Surg 38:207, 2003.
35. Sybrandy JE, Wittens CH: Initial experiences in endovenous treatment of saphenous vein reflux. J Vasc Surg 36:1207, 2002.
36. Chandler JG, Pichot O, Sessa C, et al: Treatment of primary venous insufficiency by endovenous saphenous vein obliteration. J Vasc Surg 34:201, 2000.
37. Manfrini S, Gasbarro V, Danielsson G, et al: Endovenous management of saphenous vein reflux. Endovenous Reflux Management Study Group. J Vasc Surg 32:330, 2000.
38. Rautio T, Ohinmaa A, Perala J, et al: Endovenous obliteration versus conventional stripping operation in the treatment of primary varicose veins: A randomized controlled trial with comparison of the costs. J Vasc Surg 35:958, 2002.
39. Proebstle TM, Lehr HA, Kargl A, et al: Endovenous treatment of the greater saphenous vein with a 940-nm diode laser: Thrombotic occlusion after endoluminal thermal damage by laser-generated steam bubbles. J Vasc Surg 35:729, 2002.
40. Min RJ, Zimmet SE, Isaacs MN, et al: Endovenous laser treatment of the incompetent greater saphenous vein. J Vasc Intervent Radiol 12:1167, 2001.
41. Cheshire N, Elias SM, Keagy B, et al: Powered phlebectomy (TriVex) in treatment of varicose veins. Ann Vasc Surg 16:488, 2002.
42. Winterborn RJ, Foy C, Earnshaw JJ: Causes of varicose vein recurrence: Late results of a randomized controlled trial of stripping the long saphenous vein. J Vasc Surg 40:634, 2004.
43. Sarin S, Scurr JH, Coleridge Smith PD: Stripping of the long saphenous vein in the treatment of primary varicose veins. Br J Surg 81:1455, 1994.
44. Cox SJ, Wellwood JM, Martin A: Saphenous nerve injury caused by stripping of the long saphenous vein. Br Med J 1:415, 1974.
45. Morrison C, Dalsing MC: Signs and symptoms of saphenous nerve injury after greater saphenous vein stripping: Prevalence, severity, and relevance for modern practice. J Vasc Surg 38:886, 2003.
46. Large J: Surgical treatment of saphenous varices, with preservation of the main saphenous trunk. J Vasc Surg 2:886, 1985.
47. Samson RH, Yunis JP, Showalter DP: Is thigh saphenectomy a necessary adjunct to high ligation and stab avulsion phlebectomy? Am J Surg 176:168, 1998.
48. Bergan JJ, Goldman MP: Varicose Veins and Telangiectasias: Diagnosis and Management. St. Louis, Quality Medical Publishing, 1993.
49. Teruya TH, Ballard JL: New approaches for the treatment of varicose veins. Surg Clin North Am 84:1397, 2004.
50. Darke SG: The morphology of recurrent varicose veins. Eur J Vasc Surg 6:512, 1992.
51. Hobbs JT: Surgery and sclerotherapy with the treatment of varicose veins: A random trial. Arch Surg 109:793, 1974.

chapter 56

Venous Insufficiency

Edwin C. Gravereaux
Magruder C. Donaldson

The general term *venous insufficiency* refers to the physiologic consequence of either deep vein obstruction, valvular incompetence, or a combination of both lesions. The terms *postphlebitic* and *post-thrombotic* are commonly used to describe the pathologic and clinical features of venous insufficiency arising from deep vein thrombosis (DVT), the most common etiology of deep venous disorders. Modern prospective analysis has demonstrated that within 5 years after DVT, up to 80% of patients have signs, symptoms, or laboratory findings of venous insufficiency.[1-5] From an epidemiologic standpoint, cutaneous manifestations of deep venous insufficiency of the lower extremities were found in about 20% of employees in one study, with severe changes in 9%, and a history of ulceration in 1.3%.[6] The prevalence of venous insufficiency in America and Europe has been estimated at 0.5% to 3% of the adult population.[7]

PATHOGENESIS AND PATHOPHYSIOLOGY

Valvular Incompetence

The most important cause of chronic venous insufficiency in the lower extremities is valvular incompetence of the deep veins.[8] In most instances this arises after DVT, when most veins eventually become partially or totally recanalized.[1,3] In the process of phlebitic inflammation, the extremely delicate valve leaflets become thickened, shortened, or embedded into the scarred vein wall, rendering them incapable of promoting antegrade flow and of halting retrograde flow of blood. Rather than a fine, reactive unidirectional channel, the vein becomes a rigid, thick-walled tube with remnants of ineffectual valves and fibrous synechiae strung across its lumen. Secondary valvular incompetence arises in areas distal to either chronic obstruction or significant reflux, where high pressures distend the vein, causing the leaflets to elongate, separate, and leak. Though not yet proven, there is hope that rapid clearance of acute DVT with fibrinolytic agents may protect valve leaflets from damage sufficiently to diminish the impact of postphlebitic sequelae.[9,10]

Floppy valves with redundant leaky cusps may occur as a primary disorder without previous DVT; they have been studied in some detail.[11,12] Valvular reflux occurs in normal asymptomatic subjects[13]; therefore pathologic incompetence may simply be an accentuation of a physiologic phenomenon. More severe degrees of primary reflux can lead to symptoms and secondary communicator involvement with varicose veins. Reduced numbers of valves and rare congenital absence[14,15] of venous valves have been recognized.

Valvular reflux to the popliteal and tibial levels is more damaging than is isolated reflux at more proximal levels.[16,17] In the presence of valvular incompetence, efficient directional flow of blood and emptying of the deep veins cannot occur (see Fig. 55-4). With activation of the muscle pump, blood is driven partially in retrograde directions determined by the pattern of valve damage. Pressure in the distal venous tree and deep tissues fails to decrease normally during muscle activity.[18,19] Secondary communicating vein and superficial system engorgement and valvular failure occur, subjecting the subcutaneous tissues to high pressures, particularly during muscle contraction.[20,21]

Muscle biopsies from patients with valvular incompetence reveal atrophic changes and enlargement and fibrosis of the interstitial space.[22] There is an increase in the number of capillaries in the subcutaneous tissue, with abnormally high levels of fibrinogen and fibrin in the interstitial space.[23] Macrophages and other inflammatory cells appear, leading to pericapillary fibrosis manifested as subcutaneous thickening and induration. Hemosiderin deposits result from erythrocyte lysis, causing brown pigmentation. Recurring episodes of barotrauma and persistent venous capillary hypertension, interstitial edema, and inflammation cause local hypoxia and malnutrition. Fat necrosis and liposclerosis occur, followed by loss of skin integrity with consequent eczema and ulceration. At this stage, secondary bacterial colonization and invasion can occur, with cellulitis greatly aggravating the process. Secondary lymphatic insufficiency occurs with progressive sclerosis of lymph channels in the face of increased demands for clearance of interstitial fluid.[24] With chronicity, tissue fibrosis causes relative fixation of the ankle joint, with subsequent disuse atrophy of the involved muscular apparatus. In a small number of long-standing chronic ulcers, malignant degeneration occurs to form a Marjolin ulcer.

Obstruction

In the lower extremity, DVT accounts for the bulk of chronically occluded veins. Though the majority of veins recanalize to some extent after thrombosis, large proximal veins are more likely to remain occluded than distal ones.[25] Other rare causes of intrinsic obstruction are recognized, including venous aplastic lesions, webs in the vena cava[26] or iliac veins, and primary venous tumors, seen most frequently in the vena cava.[27] The May-Thurner syndrome is produced by extrinsic obstruction of the left common iliac vein by the right common iliac artery crossing anterior to the vein.[28,29] Other examples of extrinsic compression include fibrous bands across the iliac vein, tumor masses, and aneurysms arising in arteries such as the femoral or popliteal, which are adjacent to major veins. Important veins are occasionally ligated or removed by surgery or become obstructed in association with trauma or radiation. For years, vena cava and femoral vein ligations were carried out to prevent pulmonary embolism. Modern nonocclusive caval filtering devices led to caval occlusion in 4% to 5% of patients.

Isolated obstructions in smaller veins of the lower extremity, such as those below the knee, produce little hemodynamic impact on the limb as a whole. Obstruction at levels at or above the popliteal vein may produce significant compromise in venous flow, depending on the availability of collaterals. The effects of obstruction are most marked immediately after an abrupt occlusion of a major vein. In acute experiments on dogs,[30] ligation of the common femoral vein causes an abrupt decrease in femoral artery flow to 50% of baseline values, with a slow recovery to 80% of baseline after a few hours. The clinical parallel to this experiment would be acute iliofemoral thrombosis, producing phlegmasia alba dolens with arterial spasm and insufficiency, followed within a short time by phlegmasia cerulea dolens with plethora and venous congestion from virtual cessation of venous flow in the entire limb.

As acute obstruction becomes chronic, increased distal venous pressure causes increased flow through all available collateral channels. Increased flow gradually enlarges these preexisting channels, starting within moments of occlusion and continuing over a period of weeks. With sufficient enlargement of vein caliber to produce valvular insufficiency, communicating veins become incompetent, resulting in secondary varicosities in the superficial veins. Chronic communicator incompetence below an obstruction promotes stasis changes in the overlying subcutaneous tissues.

Even in the presence of extensive collaterals, venous volume and pressure may remain elevated when measured in resting recumbency.[31,32] With exercise, arterial flow into the limb dramatically increases, with a consequent increased demand on the venous system to return blood to the vena cava. In the face of significant obstruction and fixed resistance of the collateral bed, distal venous volume and pressure increase (Fig. 56-1).[31] A combination of increased deep compartment pressure, which causes stretching of fascial envelopes, decreased capillary inflow of nutrients, and clearance of metabolic byproducts, results in pain termed *venous claudication*. With cessation of exercise the severe physiologic aberrations recede, and pain is relieved.

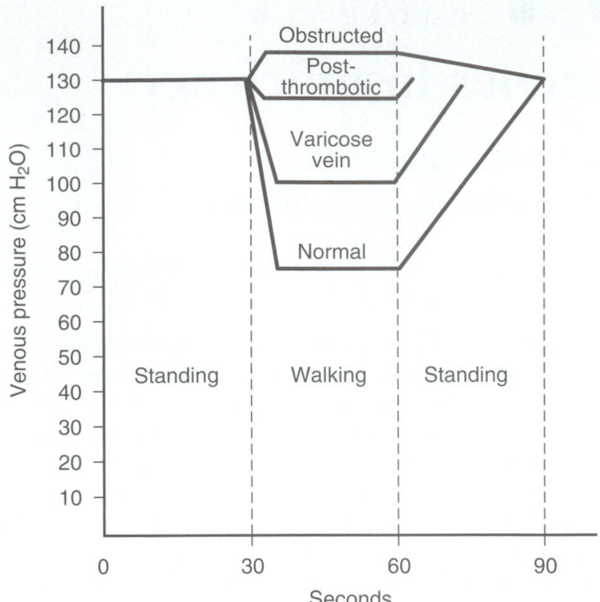

FIGURE 56-1. Ambulatory pedal pressure curves (diagrammatic). Pressure is greatly reduced in the normal system with a gradual return to baseline after exercise. The presence of varicose veins decreases the efficiency of the muscle pump, with more impairment in the presence of deep vein incompetence, causing less pressure reduction and a prompt return to baseline due to passive reflux. Obstructed proximal veins may actually cause pressure to increase. (From DeWeese JA: Venous and lymphatic disease. In Schwartz SI [ed]: Principles of Surgery, 4th ed. New York, McGraw-Hill, 1983, p 975.)

CLINICAL MANIFESTATIONS

History

Though venous insufficiency is most frequently the result of DVT, there may be no supporting history, since DVT may have been asymptomatic or undiagnosed because of nonspecific symptoms. If past DVT is known to have occurred, it is helpful to obtain documentation, particularly noninvasive vascular or radiologic evidence of the location and extent of involvement. A detailed history of previous surgery or trauma is important. Other historic clues may reveal the presence of a pelvic malignancy or other cause for extrinsic compression of a major vein.

As mentioned earlier, valvular incompetence and obstruction are often present simultaneously.[33] When *valvular incompetence* predominates, early symptoms consist of heaviness and dull, bursting pressure in the lower leg with dependency. Edema of the foot and ankle may occur if dependency is prolonged. These symptoms are relieved with elevation. Later in the course, secondary superficial varicosities may become evident, usually over the medial aspect of the leg and ankle where communicating veins emerge from the deep system. Foci of hyperpigmentation gradually appear in the subcutaneous tissues. Pain, itching, and eczema may arise spontaneously, followed by overt skin ulceration. More diffuse subcutaneous inflammation may develop with varying degrees of cellulitis.

If significant *venous obstruction* predominates, its contribution to symptoms may be relatively mild at rest when collateral channels more easily decompress the lower limb. Exercise elicits the most important symptoms of obstruction including deep, intense pressure in the distal leg that is relieved by rest. This pattern of venous claudication is generally stereotyped in each patient. Though cutaneous manifestations are not prominent in cases of pure obstruction, skin breakdown and ulceration may occur in conjunction with secondary incompetence of communicating veins.

Physical Findings

Examination may reveal evidence of hemodynamic compromise, with increased leg circumference, peripheral edema, tightness of muscle compartments, and cyanosis and plethora of the feet with dependency. Secondary varicose veins are generally present, and in cases of predominant obstruction, the location of visible superficial collaterals over the leg or lower abdomen indicates the site of obstruction. Brawny induration is obvious under healed skin lesions and surrounding other sites of old minor trauma or inflammation (Fig. 56-2). Most of these lesions are distributed medially over the ankle and lower leg, with the highest frequency just above the medial malleolus. Untreated ulcerations are usually punched out and necrotic, with copious drainage from the open bed. Frequently there are signs of surrounding cellulitis, occasionally ascending up the leg with lymphangitic involvement. Chronicity usually results in stiffening of the ankle joint and loss of proximal muscle bulk and strength.

Laboratory

The noninvasive vascular laboratory provides an objective baseline for following the natural history of the disease and for later reference when symptoms of recurrent acute DVT overlap those of the postphlebitic syndrome. In addition, noninvasive screening is an important means of detecting candidates for more specific approaches to treatment. Magnetic resonance venography (MRV) or computed tomographic angiography (CTA) are appropriately used for diagnosis and therapeutic planning in some instances. Contrast venography is only rarely necessary for diagnosis but is increasingly employed in concert with catheter-based endovascular interventions.

Duplex ultrasound is the single most useful modality for routine documentation of venous anatomy, obstruction, and valvular incompetence (see also Chapter 10).[34-36] Except in cases of obstruction in the pelvis or abdomen, ultrasound can directly visualize the site of venous obstruction and often map collateral patterns, typically involving the saphenous system in the case of superficial femoral vein occlusion and cross-pudendal routes in the case of iliac vein occlusion. Valvular dysfunction can be characterized by ultrasound, ranging from total reflux through a valve that is all but invisible, to minimal reflux evident only during the Valsalva maneuver through a leaflet that may be slightly scarred or redundant. Incompetent communicating veins may be mapped.

Physiologic tests are less widely available but useful in selected circumstances. Plethysmography by one of the available techniques can document in most instances the hemodynamic abnormality caused by proximal vein obstruction, though this test can be normal at rest in the presence of large collaterals. Exercise testing using foot vein pressure monitoring or photoplethysmography can demonstrate poor emptying of the distal veins and hypertension in the presence of venous insufficiency, with abnormal recovery patterns after cessation of exercise.[37-39]

Anatomic study by MRV, CT, or contrast venography is valuable mainly to confirm patterns of obstruction, particularly if extrinsic venous compression is suspected. Though still regarded by some as the "gold standard," dynamic diagnostic ascending and descending venography is only occasionally used in some centers to characterize patterns of obstruction and reflux (Fig. 56-3).[40,41]

A recent study provided evidence that venous hypertension may result in markers detected outside the vascular system. Hemosiderin was present in the urine of patients with chronic venous insufficiency, and the amount of hemosiderin correlated with the severity of disease.[42]

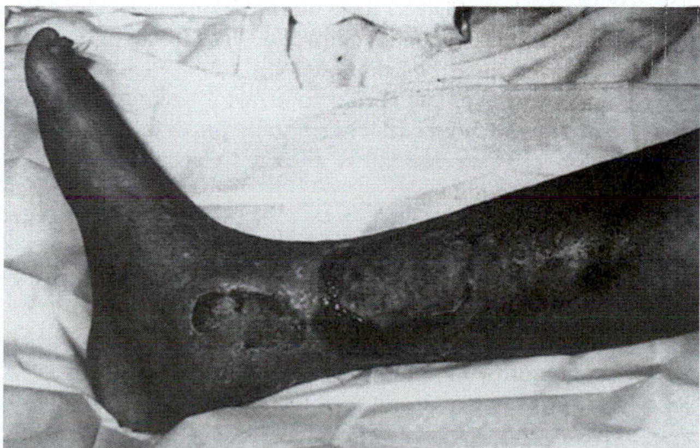

FIGURE 56-2. Chronic venous stasis changes in the leg. Note the hyperpigmentation of skin, ulcers above the malleolus, and muscular atrophy.

MANAGEMENT

Conservative Measures

Therapy of venous insufficiency, whether caused by obstruction, valvular reflux, or the common combination of both lesions, is directed at countering the damaging effects of peripheral venous hypertension. Thorough education of the patient about the underlying problem and the pathophysiology involved is essential, with counseling about beneficial changes in lifestyle. Prolonged standing or sitting promotes stasis and sustained hypertension in the lower leg. Prescription graduated compression stockings with 30 to 40 mm Hg pressure at the ankle should be obtained and worn during the day, as they help control edema and may tend to reduce valvular reflux.[43-45] Exercise and usual ambulatory activities are recommended to enlarge and maintain venous collaterals, provided adequate stocking support is employed. Jogging or other exercise that involves cyclic-dependent thrusting of the legs should be replaced by gentler sports such as rowing or swimming. Moderate tipping of the bed into a head-down position promotes mobilization of edema and relief of muscle compartment tension at night. All of these measures help to protect patent veins from recurrent DVT. A regular schedule of noninvasive laboratory evaluations should be maintained to detect possible repeat episodes of thrombosis and further deterioration.

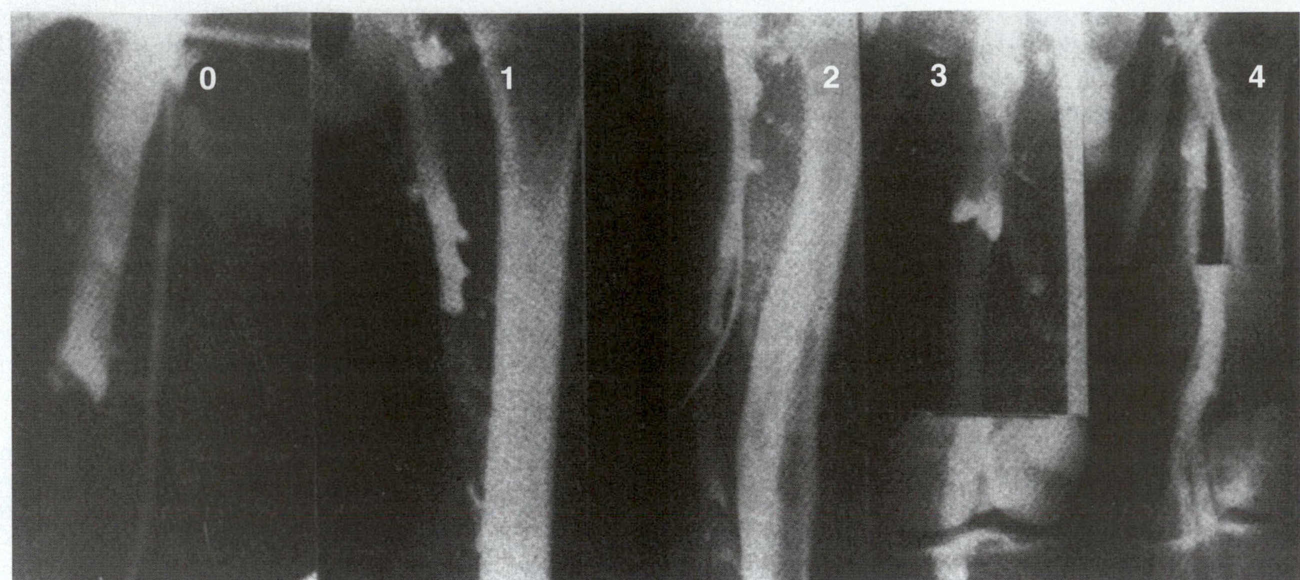

FIGURE 56-3. Descending venography, demonstrating degrees of valvular incompetence in the leg ranging from none (*0*) to minimal (*1*) in the presence of healthy valves, to free retrograde flow (*4*) to calf level with gross valvular damage. (From Kistner RL, Ferris EB, Randhawa G, et al: A method of performing descending venography. J Vasc Surg 4:464, 1986.)

When eczema and skin ulceration supervene, a few days of recumbency combined with careful hygiene and protective dressings usually provide early control. If bacterial cellulitis or lymphangitis is suspected, antibiotics should be directed initially against staphylococcal and streptococcal skin colonizers, modified later as cultures dictate. Open ulcers should be treated initially with a gentle debriding regimen of dressing changes two to four times a day using wet-to-dry normal saline on coarse mesh gauze. Once the ulcer is clean and cellulitis appears controlled, less frequent dressing changes must be combined with continued firm compression over the region to achieve healing. Use of several hours of intermittent pneumatic compression daily has been shown to accelerate healing.[46,47] A practical and effective method is Unna's paste boot,[48] which combines support to combat venous hypertension and edema with a mixture of zinc oxide, calamine, and gelatin to gently medicate the open ulcer. The patient can maintain most normal activities, and essentially no care is required between changes of the boot every 1 to 3 weeks. Closed compression bandage treatment should only be employed on relatively clean ulcers, since cellulitis may be exacerbated under the dressing if the ulcer is infected. If the ulcer is large or persistent, split-thickness skin grafts can be applied to ulcers after sufficient preparation.

Surgical Measures

Previous ulceration or a prolonged history of venous insufficiency makes durable success with conservative measures less likely. In these instances of severe disease, interventions directed at the underlying causes of venous hypertension may be indicated.

Interruption of incompetent communicating veins reduces barotrauma to the subcutaneous tissues. Optimally, any ulcer should be healed or small and free of cellulitis before surgery, and preoperative imaging should confirm communicator anatomy and incompetence. In selected instances, direct exposure of communicators adjacent to the ulcer site may be helpful. Because many ulcers do not have communicating veins at their base[49] and collateral channels connected to adjacent communicators from a severely diseased deep system may predispose to recurrent postoperative ulceration, a more general approach to elimination of all communicating veins in the region of the ulcer is probably optimal.

With improved anatomic mapping and less invasive surgical techniques, it is not necessary to perform the procedure advocated by Linton,[50] which involved an incision from the ankle to the proximal calf with subfascial ligation of all communicating veins. Subfascial endoscopic perforator surgery (SEPS) allows minimally invasive access to the subfascial plane of the leg and fiberoptic visualization and interruption of the communicating veins as they perforate the fascial envelope.[51-53] SEPS has dramatically reduced operative wound morbidity compared with open subfascial ligation techniques. Ulcer healing rates are comparable to open techniques, but there appears to be a lower recurrent ulceration rate, with about 12% recurrence after SEPS compared with 22% after open ligation.[54,55] Results appear to be best for patients with primary deep valvular incompetence compared with those with post-thrombotic insufficiency and when long-term postoperative use is made of support stockings.

In addition to subfascial ligation of communicating veins in patients with extensive valvular dysfunction, methods have been developed to directly correct deep vein valve reflux.[56,57] Kistner and colleagues[56] developed a valvuloplasty operation that can be applied to patients with primary valvular reflux due to redundancy and laxity of the valve leaflets. After careful documentation of

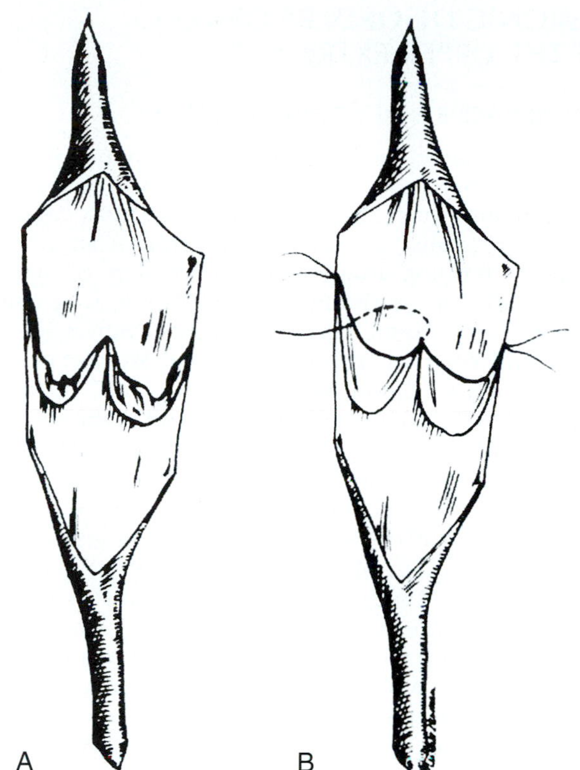

FIGURE 56-4. Valvuloplasty to repair floppy valve allowing reflux. **A,** Vein opened through valve commissure during surgery, showing redundant, leaky valve leaflets. **B,** Fine sutures placed at valve corners to correct redundancy by reefing leaflets. (From Kistner RL: Transvenous repair of the incompetent femoral vein valve. In Bergan JJ, Yao JST: Venous Problems. Chicago, Year Book, 1978, p 503.)

reflux and valve anatomy by descending venography, the valve is exposed and opened between the valve leaflets. Fine sutures are used to reef the lax leaflets, restoring competency (Fig. 56-4).

When valves are too damaged to be reparable, a new competent valve may be juxtaposed into the incompetent system. If the superficial femoral vein is involved and the saphenous vein is normal, end-to-end transposition of the competent proximal saphenous vein into the distal femoral vein introduces a valve into the system (Fig. 56-5). Alternatively, the profunda femoris vein can be transposed into the superficial femoral vein. When no normal valve is available nearby, a segment of the axillary vein containing a competent valve may be transplanted into the femoral or popliteal vein.[58] Cryopreserved venous allografts have even been used for this purpose in highly selected patients, with reasonable midterm results reported.[59]

All of these valvular reconstructive procedures are applicable only to a relatively small number of patients who have been found by careful evaluation to have appropriate pathophysiology and a favorable anatomic situation. Apparently there is a cumulative 60% ulcer-free rate by life-table analysis after autogenous vein valve transplant in selected patients, with segmental venous occlusion in less than 10% when postoperative anticoagulation is used.[55,60] Interestingly, it has sometimes been difficult to demonstrate dramatic improvement in objective measures of venous physiology commensurate with apparent clinical improvement.

Interventional recanalization of veins occluded by thrombus is only practicable in the acute phase. Surgical thrombectomy or fibrinolytic therapy has been used with inconsistent success.[61-63] With chronic thrombotic occlusion, veins become fibrotic, and attempts to open them are usually unsuccessful. On the other hand, if external compression or a discrete intraluminal web is present, efforts to relieve the obstruction may occasionally be helpful. In rare instances of iliac vein compression by the crossing iliac artery, a bridge-like prosthesis has actually been devised to lift the iliac artery off the caval bifurcation.[64]

Surgical bypass of venous occlusions has been employed in selected instances for some 30 years. Palma and Esperon[65] and then Dale and Harris[66] described a procedure in which the contralateral saphenous vein is mobilized and tunneled across the pubis to the femoral vein to direct flow from the leg away from an obstructed iliac system (Fig. 56-6). This procedure has been used successfully in palliating disabling symptoms in patients with pelvic malignancy. Another operation makes use of the ipsilateral saphenous vein connected to the popliteal vein to provide a collateral channel around obstruction or incompetence limited to the superficial femoral and proximal popliteal veins.[67]

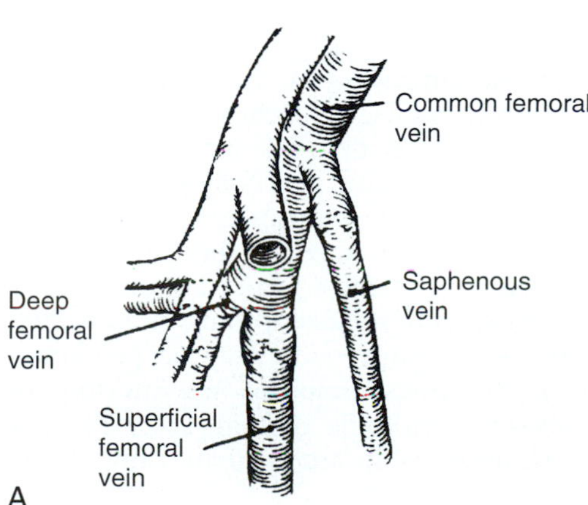

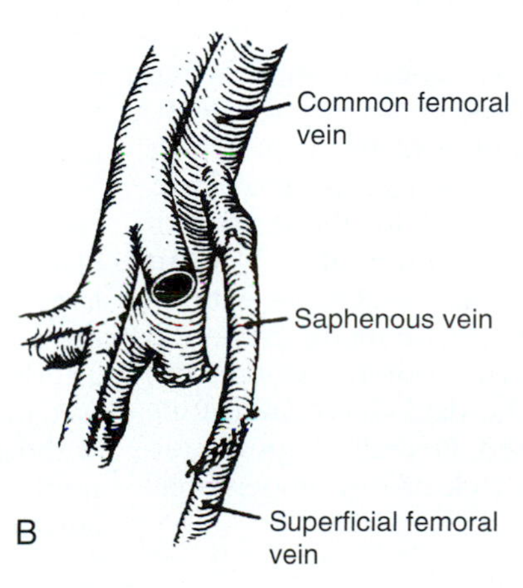

FIGURE 56-5. Vein transposition. **A,** Anatomy of proximal femoral region, with incompetent valves in superficial femoral vein. **B,** Restoration of superficial femoral vein competence by transposition below normal valve in saphenous vein. (From Queral LA, Whitehouse WM Jr, Flinn WR, et al: Surgical correction of chronic deep venous insufficiency by valvular transposition. Surgery 87:688, 1980).

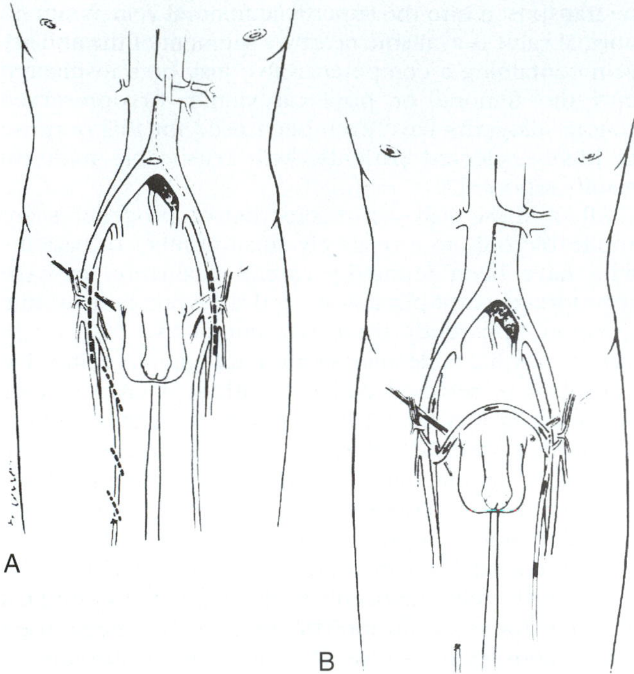

FIGURE 56-6. Palma-Dale cross-pubic bypass, using mobilized saphenous vein (**A**) to drain contralateral femoral system through a subcutaneous tunnel to relieve symptoms from iliac vein obstruction (**B**). (From Bergan JJ, Yao JS, Flinn WR, et al: Surgical treatment of venous obstruction and insufficiency. J Vasc Surg 3:174, 1986.)

Prosthetic grafts have been used from time to time in the femoral, cross-femoral, and iliocaval positions.[68] Experimental work suggests that externally supported polytetrafluoroethylene is the preferred prosthetic among those currently available, as it appears to be least thrombogenic and resists collapse under pressure from surrounding tissues.[69] Endothelial seeding of such grafts appears to improve patency only slightly in the canine experimental model.[70] A complementary temporary arteriovenous fistula (AVF) probably improves long-term patency of venous bypass grafts, particularly prosthetics. An AVF increases flow velocity, reduces platelet deposition on the graft surface,[71] and augments the capacity of autogenous collateral channels. It has been suggested that a primary, temporary AVF might be a reasonable means of enlarging collaterals, with improvement in venous hemodynamics after closure of the fistula.[72]

Surgical reconstructions have good results when assessed by symptom relief, physiologic improvement, or bypass patency. In a compilation of the largest published series of procedures designed to relieve obstruction, clinical improvement occurred in about 80% of patients at varied postoperative intervals.[73,74] Graft patency does not appear to be as durable as symptomatic relief.[75] Some surgeons recommend a period of anticoagulation with warfarin sodium (Coumadin) after surgery, though there are no data clearly indicating that bypass patency is improved. Overall surgical morbidity is low, with a surprising lack of thromboembolic complications.

CHRONIC DISORDERS OF VEINS OF THE UPPER EXTREMITY

Pathogenesis and Pathophysiology

Valvular incompetence is of no consequence in veins of the upper extremity, but chronic proximal obstruction can be an important clinical problem. The most common cause of proximal occlusion of the subclavian veins is thrombus forming around the wide variety of central-access catheters currently in use[76,77] and, to a much smaller extent, around pacemaker wires. Primary spontaneous axillary or subclavian vein thrombosis also occurs, usually in association with fibrous bands, muscular hypertrophy, or bony compression found in the thoracic outlet syndrome. Intermittent subclavian vein occlusion has been detected rarely as a precursor to thrombosis and has been reported in 1.5% to 3.5% of patients with thoracic outlet syndrome.[78,79] Vigorous arm activity can precipitate so-called *effort thrombosis* (Paget–von Schroetter syndrome), seen most commonly in athletes such as swimmers or baseball pitchers in whom extreme abduction and extension of the shoulder apparently traumatizes the axillary and subclavian veins.[76] Finally, extrinsic compression by mediastinal fibrosis or malignancy can cause obstruction of the superior vena cava, with compromised venous drainage of the brachiocephalic regions.

Acute axillary or subclavian vein thrombosis may be quite dramatic but is rarely severe enough to threaten the arm[80]; it is associated with clinically important pulmonary embolism in 4% to 12% of patients.[78] Recanalization of proximal arm thrombosis probably occurs in a majority of cases, particularly those caused by intravascular catheters that have been removed. If the cause of thrombosis persists, as in the thoracic outlet syndrome, restoration of an adequate venous channel is less likely. With residual chronic obstruction, a rich collateral network develops around the shoulder and upper chest, but hemodynamic impairment is sufficient to produce long-term symptoms in 40% to 85% of patients.[76,78] In one series, 39% of subjects were forced to change their occupation to accommodate arm disability.[81]

CLINICAL MANIFESTATIONS

History

Symptoms are most impressive in the acute stage of thrombosis, with sudden onset of tightness and bursting pain, which is worse with dependency and exercise. As the course becomes chronic and collaterals develop, resting symptoms become less prominent than venous claudication induced by exercise, or the limb may be largely asymptomatic. If thoracic outlet compression is the cause of venous occlusion, symptoms of associated arterial or neurologic compression may be prominent (see Chapter 64).[79] If venous compression is intermittent, without thrombosis, symptoms of temporary obstruction of the subclavian vein are evident only during certain arm activities.

Physical Findings

Physical findings are absent or subtle in many patients with proximal segmental occlusions located in the axillary or subclavian veins. Large subcutaneous collateral veins around the shoulder are usually evident on inspection. In more severe cases, increased arm circumference, tightness of muscle compartments, cyanosis, and venous engorgement are evident. In the presence of thoracic outlet syndrome, there may be tenderness over the brachial plexus, findings of ulnar neuropathy, or aggravation of symptoms and loss of the radial pulse with hyperextension and abduction of the arm.

Laboratory

The noninvasive vascular laboratory can be used to gather confirmatory evidence of venous occlusion (see Chapter 10).[82] Ultrasound is capable of detecting occlusion in the arm and interference with normal flow dynamics caused by more proximal occlusion. Resting venous pressure measured in a forearm vein is elevated compared with the contralateral normal arm. With intermittent subclavian vein compression, pressure gradients can be measured across the point of impingement at the thoracic outlet.[83] Though experience with noninvasive techniques is evolving, particularly the use of MRV to evaluate central venous anatomy and disease, venography remains the most accurate diagnostic method. Provocative positioning (arm abduction) during venography can elicit evidence of venous compression through the thoracic outlet.

Management

Thrombosis around central venous catheters responds well in most instances to removal of the catheter and a short course of anticoagulation, when possible. Spontaneous thrombosis is more difficult to manage, with a higher likelihood of long-term sequelae.[76,78] Surgical thrombectomy has a role if used within a few days of thrombosis, but there is a substantial incidence of recurrent clotting.[79] Systemic or local fibrinolytic therapy is often applicable and has gained popularity as a means of opening veins acutely, with satisfactory long-term patency, provided that extrinsic causes of thrombosis are also promptly addressed.[84,85] This often means decompression of the thoracic outlet by first-rib resection[86] or scalenectomy followed by anticoagulation for several months.[78] More recent treatments have used balloon angioplasty of the affected subclavian vein following operative thoracic outlet decompression with first-rib resection, with excellent results.[87,88] Adjuvant subclavian vein stenting has not shown wide success.[89]

In the chronic situation, therapy is almost exclusively conservative because there are few good alternatives. Careful patient education is critical, with counseling about possible changes in occupation to decrease stress on the involved arm. Gentle exercise should be encouraged to enlarge and maintain collaterals. Compression sleeves may be necessary in some instances to control symptoms and swelling. If venous obstruction is intermittent, thoracic outlet decompression should be performed to prevent thrombosis. Experience with direct surgical approaches to chronically occluded veins is limited. In selected patients with segmental proximal subclavian obstruction, the ipsilateral jugular vein can be used to provide a bypass around the obstruction.[90] Superior vena cava reconstruction is possible using autogenous spiral vein grafts or prosthetic substitutes.[68]

REFERENCES

1. Johnson BF, Manzo RA, Bergelin RO, et al: Relationship between changes in the deep venous system and the development of the postthrombotic syndrome after an acute episode of lower limb deep vein thrombosis: A one- to six-year follow-up. J Vasc Surg 21:307, 1995.
2. Johnson BF, Manzo RA, Bergelin RO, et al: The site of residual abnormalities in the leg veins in long-term follow-up after deep vein thrombosis and their relationship to the development of the post-thrombotic syndrome. N Engl J Med 335:670, 1996.
3. Lindner DJ, Edwards JM, Phinney ES, et al: Long-term hemodynamic and clinical sequelae of lower extremity deep vein thrombosis. J Vasc Surg 4:436, 1986.
4. Meissner MH, Caps MT, Bergelin RO, et al: Propagation, rethrombosis and new thrombus formation after acute deep venous thrombosis. J Vasc Surg 22:558, 1995.
5. Meissner MH, Caps MT, Zierler BK, et al: Determinants of chronic venous disease after acute deep venous thrombosis. J Vasc Surg 28:826, 1998.
6. Widmer LK, Zemp E , Maggs M: Varicose veins and chronic venous insufficiency—a disorder or disease? A critical epidemiological review. Vasa 15:126, 1986.
7. Biland L, Widmer LK: Varicose veins (VV) and chronic venous insufficiency (CVI). Medical and socio-economic aspects, Basle study. Acta Chir Scand Suppl 544:9, 1988.
8. Markel A, Manzo RA, Bergelin RO, et al: Incidence and time of occurrence of valvular incompetence following deep vein thrombosis. Wien Med Wochenschr 144:216, 1994.
9. Comerota AJ, Throm RC, Mathias SD, et al: Catheter-directed thrombolysis for iliofemoral deep venous thrombosis improves health-related quality of life. J Vasc Surg 32:130, 2000.
10. Mewissen MW, Seabrook GR, Meissner MH, et al: Catheter-directed thrombolysis for lower extremity deep venous thrombosis: Report of a national multicenter registry. Radiology 211:39, 1999.
11. Kistner RL: Proceedings: Post-phlebitic syndrome: Cure by surgical repair of the incompetent femoral value. J Cardiovasc Surg 17:85, 1976.
12. Almgren B, Eriksson I, Bylund H, et al: Phlebographic evaluation of nonthrombotic deep venous incompetence: New anatomic and functional aspects. J Vasc Surg 11:389, 1990.
13. Bishara RA, Sigel B, Rocco K, et al: Deterioration of venous function in normal lower extremities during daily activity. J Vasc Surg 3:700, 1986.
14. Friedman EI, Taylor LM Jr, Porter JM: Congenital venous valvular aplasia of the lower extremities. Surgery 104:465, 1988.
15. Sales CM, Rosenthal D, Petrillo KA, et al: The valvular apparatus in venous insufficiency: A problem of quantity? Ann Vasc Surg 12:153, 1998.
16. Moore DJ, Himmel PD, Sumner DS: Distribution of venous valvular incompetence in patients with the postphlebitic syndrome. J Vasc Surg 3:49, 1986.
17. Gooley NA, Sumner DS: Relationship of venous reflux to the site of venous valvular incompetence: Implications for venous reconstructive surgery. J Vasc Surg 7:50, 1988.
18. Fukuoka M, Sugimoto T, Okita Y: Prospective evaluation of chronic venous insufficiency based on foot venous pressure measurements and air plethysmography findings. J Vasc Surg 38:804, 2003.
19. Arnoldi CC: On the conditions for the venous return from the lower leg in healthy subjects and in patients with chronic venous insufficiency. Angiology 17:153, 1966.

20. Christopoulos D, Nicolaides AN, Cook A, et al: Pathogenesis of venous ulceration in relation to the calf muscle pump function. Surgery 106:829, 1989.
21. Delis KT, Husmann M, Kalodiki E, et al: In situ hemodynamics of perforating veins in chronic venous insufficiency. J Vasc Surg 33:773, 2001.
22. Taheri SA, Heffner R, Williams J, et al: Muscle changes in venous insufficiency. Arch Surg 119:929, 1984.
23. Burnand KG, Whimster I, Naidoo A, et al: Pericapillary fibrin in the ulcer bearing skin of the leg. Br Med J 285:1071, 1982.
24. Eliska O, Eliskova M: Morphology of lymphatics in human venous crural ulcers with lipodermatosclerosis. Lymphology 34:111, 2001.
25. Killewich LA, Bedford GR, Beach KW, et al: Spontaneous lysis of deep venous thrombi: Rate and outcome. J Vasc Surg 9:89, 1989.
26. Ono J, Sakoda K, Kawada T: Membranous obstruction of the inferior vena cava. Ann Surg 197:454, 1983.
27. Fischer MG, Gelb AM, Nussbaum M, et al: Primary smooth muscle tumors of venous origin. Ann Surg 196:720, 1982.
28. Ferris EJ, Lim WN, Smith PL, et al: May-Thurner syndrome. Radiology 147:29, 1983.
29. Kibbe MR, Ujiki M, Goodwin AL, et al: Iliac vein compression in an asymptomatic patient population. J Vasc Surg 39:937, 2004.
30. Hobson RW II, Howard EW, Wright CB, et al: Hemodynamics of canine femoral venous ligation: Significance in combined arterial and venous injuries. Surgery 74:824, 1973.
31. Killewich LA, Martin R, Cramer M, et al: Pathophysiology of venous claudication. J Vasc Surg 1:507, 1984.
32. Delis KT, Bountouroglou D, Mansfield AO: Venous claudication in iliofemoral thrombosis: Long-term effects on venous hemodynamics, clinical status, and quality of life. Ann Surg 239:118, 2004.
33. Neglen P, Thrasher TL, Raju S: Venous outflow obstruction: An underestimated contributor to chronic venous disease. J Vasc Surg 38:879, 2003.
34. Baker SR, Burnand KG, Sommerville KM, et al: Comparison of venous reflux assessed by duplex scanning and descending phlebography in chronic venous disease. Lancet 342:400, 1993.
35. Mattos MA, Sumner DS: Direct noninvasive tests (duplex scan) for the evaluation of chronic venous obstruction and valvular incompetence. In Gloviczki P, Yao JST (eds): Handbook of Venous Disorders. London, Arnold, 2001, p 120.
36. Neglen P, Raju S: A comparison between descending phlebography and duplex Doppler investigation in the evaluation of reflux in chronic venous insufficiency: A challenge to phlebography as the "gold standard." J Vasc Surg 16:687, 1992.
37. Padberg FT Jr, Johnston MV, Sisto SA: Structured exercise improves calf muscle pump function in chronic venous insufficiency: A randomized trial. J Vasc Surg 39:79, 2004.
38. Haenen JH, Janssen MC, van Langen H, et al: The postthrombotic syndrome in relation to venous hemodynamics, as measured by means of duplex scanning and strain-gauge plethysmography. J Vasc Surg 29:1071, 1999.
39. Pearce WH, Ricco JB, Queral LA, et al: Hemodynamic assessment of venous problems. Surgery 93:715, 1983.
40. Kistner RL, Ferris EB, Randhawa G, et al: A method of performing descending venography. J Vasc Surg 4:464, 1986.
41. Masuda EM, Kistner RL: Prospective comparison of duplex scanning and descending venography in the assessment of venous insufficiency. Am J Surg 164:254, 1992.
42. Zamboni P, Izzo M, Fogato L, et al: Urine hemosiderin: A novel marker to assess the severity of chronic venous disease. J Vasc Surg 37:132, 2003.
43. Buhs CL, Bendick PJ, Glover JL: The effect of graded compression elastic stockings on the lower leg venous system during daily activity. J Vasc Surg 30:830, 1999.
44. Ibegbuna V, Delis KT, Nicolaides AN, et al: Effect of elastic compression stockings on venous hemodynamics during walking. J Vasc Surg 37:420, 2003.
45. Mayberry JC, Moneta GL, DeFrang RD, et al: The influence of elastic compression stockings on deep venous hemodynamics. J Vasc Surg 13:91, 1991.
46. Smith PC, Sarin S, Hasty J, et al: Sequential gradient pneumatic compression enhances venous ulcer healing: A randomized trial. Surgery 108:871, 1990.
47. Coleridge-Smith PC, Sarin S, Hasty J, et al: Sequential gradient pneumatic compression enhances venous ulcer healing: A randomized trial. Surgery 108:871, 1990.
48. Kitka MJ, Schuler JJ, Meyer JP, et al: A prospective, randomized trial of Unna's boots versus hydroactive dressing in the treatment of venous stasis ulcers. J Vasc Surg 7:478, 1988.
49. Hanrahan LM, Araki CT, Rodriguez AA, et al: Distribution of valvular incompetence in patients with venous stasis ulcers. J Vasc Surg 13:805, 1991.
50. Linton RR: The post-thrombotic ulceration of the lower extremity: Its etiology and surgical therapy. Ann Surg 138:415, 1953.
51. Bergan JJ, Murray J, Greason K: Subfascial endoscopic perforator vein surgery: A preliminary report. Ann Vasc Surg 10:211, 1996.
52. Gloviczki P, Bergan JJ, Menawat SS, et al: Safety, feasibility, and early efficacy of subfascial endoscopic perforator surgery: A preliminary report from the North American registry. J Vasc Surg 25:94, 1997.
53. Sybrandy JE, van Gent WB, Pierik EG, et al: Endoscopic versus open subfascial division of incompetent perforating veins in the treatment of venous leg ulceration: Long-term follow-up. J Vasc Surg 33:1028, 2001.
54. Gloviczki P, Bergan JJ, Rhodes JM, et al: Mid-term results of endoscopic perforator vein interruption for chronic venous insufficiency: Lessons learned from the North American subfascial endoscopic perforator surgery registry. The North American Study Group. J Vasc Surg 29:489, 1999.
55. Gloviczki P, Yao JST: Handbook of Venous Disorders: Guidelines of the American Venous Forum. London, Arnold, 2001.
56. Kistner RL, Eklof B, Masuda EM: Deep venous valve reconstruction. Cardiovasc Surg 3:129, 1995.
57. Raju S, Berry MA, Neglen P: Transcommissural valvuloplasty: Technique and results. J Vasc Surg 32:969, 2000.
58. Raju S, Neglen P, Doolittle J, et al: Axillary vein transfer in trabeculated postthrombotic veins. J Vasc Surg 29:1050, 1999.
59. Dalsing MC, Raju S, Wakefield TW, et al: A multicenter, phase I evaluation of cryopreserved venous valve allografts for the treatment of chronic deep venous insufficiency. J Vasc Surg 30:854, 1999.
60. Raju S, Fredericks RK, Neglen PN, et al: Durability of venous valve reconstruction techniques for "primary" and postthrombotic reflux. J Vasc Surg 23:357, 1996.
61. Raju S, Owen S Jr, Neglen P: The clinical impact of iliac venous stents in the management of chronic venous insufficiency. J Vasc Surg 35:8, 2002.
62. Arnesen H, Hoiseth A, Ly B: Streptokinase of heparin in the treatment of deep vein thrombosis. Follow-up results of a prospective study. Acta Med Scand 211:65, 1982.
63. Kakkar VV, Lawrence D: Hemodynamic and clinical assessment after therapy for acute deep vein thrombosis: A prospective study. Am J Surg 150:54, 1985.
64. Trimble C, Bernstein EF, Pomerantz M, et al: A prosthetic bridging device to relieve iliac venous compression. Surg Forum 23:249, 1972.
65. Palma EC, Esperon R: Vein transplants and grafts in the surgical treatment of the postphlebitic syndrome. J Cardiovasc Surg (Torino) 1:94, 1960.
66. Dale WA, Harris J: Cross-over vein grafts for iliac and femoral venous occlusion. J Cardiovasc Surg (Torino) 10:458, 1969.
67. Husni EA: In situ saphenopopliteal bypass graft for incompetence of the femoral and popliteal veins. Surg Gynecol Obstet 130:279, 1970.
68. Gloviczki P, Pairolero PC, Cherry KJ, et al: Reconstruction of the vena cava and of its primary tributaries: A preliminary report. J Vasc Surg 11:373, 1990.
69. Robison RJ, Peigh PS, Fiore AC, et al: Venous prostheses: Improved patency with external stents. J Surg Res 36:306, 1984.
70. Herring M, Gardner A, Peigh P, et al: Patency in canine inferior vena cava grafting: Effects of graft material, size, and endothelial seeding. J Vasc Surg 1:877, 1984.
71. Plate G, Hollier LH, Gloviczki P, et al: Overcoming failure of venous vascular prostheses. Surgery 96:503, 1984.
72. Sawchuk AP, Dalsing MC, Emerick SC, et al: A temporary distal arteriovenous fistula improves venous hemodynamics in a model of venous occlusion. Surgery 102:256, 1987.
73. Dale WA: Reconstructive venous surgery. Arch Surg 114:1312, 1979.

74. O'Donnell TF Jr, Mackey WC, Shepard AD, et al: Clinical, hemodynamic, and anatomic follow-up of direct venous reconstruction. Arch Surg 122:474, 1987.
75. Halliday P, Harris J, May J: Femoro-femoral crossover grafts (Palma operation): A long term follow-up study. In Bergan JJ, Yao JS (eds): Surgery of the Veins. New York, Grune & Stratton, 1985, p 241.
76. Hill SL, Berry RE: Subclavian vein thrombosis: A continuing challenge. Surgery 108:1, 1990.
77. Gonsalves CF, Eschelman DJ, Sullivan KL, et al: Incidence of central vein stenosis and occlusion following upper extremity PICC and port placement. Cardiovasc Intervent Radiol 26:123, 2003.
78. Gloviczki P, Kazmier FJ, Hollier LH: Axillary-subclavian venous occlusion: The morbidity of a nonlethal disease. J Vasc Surg 4:333, 1986.
79. Rutherford R, Piotrowski J: Axillary-subclavian vein thrombosis. Vasc Surg 3:883, 1989.
80. Smith BM, Shield GW, Riddell DH, et al: Venous gangrene of the upper extremity. Ann Surg 201:511, 1985.
81. Tilney N, Griffiths H, Edwards E: Natural history of major venous thrombosis of the upper extremity. Arch Surg 101:792, 1970.
82. Sullivan ED, Reece CI, Cranley JJ: Phleborheography of the upper extremity. Arch Surg 118:1134, 1983.
83. Schubart PJ, Haeberlin JR, Porter JM: Intermittent subclavian venous obstruction: Utility of venous pressure gradients. Surgery 99:365, 1986.
84. Arko FR, Cipriano P, Lee E, et al: Treatment of axillosubclavian vein thrombosis: A novel technique for rapid removal of clot using low-dose thrombolysis. J Endovasc Ther 10:733, 2003.
85. Sabeti S, Schillinger M, Mlekusch W, et al: Treatment of subclavian-axillary vein thrombosis: Long-term outcome of anticoagulation versus systemic thrombolysis. Thromb Res 108:279, 2002.
86. Taylor LM Jr, McAllister WR, Dennis DL, et al: Thrombolytic therapy followed by first rib resection for spontaneous ("effort") subclavian vein thrombosis. Am J Surg 149:644, 1985.
87. Schneider DB, Dimuzio PJ, Martin ND, et al: Combination treatment of venous thoracic outlet syndrome: Open surgical decompression and intraoperative angioplasty. J Vasc Surg 40:599, 2004.
88. Lee MC, Grassi CJ, Belkin M, et al: Early operative intervention after thrombolytic therapy for primary subclavian vein thrombosis: An effective treatment approach. J Vasc Surg 27:1101, 1998.
89. Urschel HC Jr, Patel AN: Paget-Schroetter syndrome therapy: Failure of intravenous stents. Ann Thorac Surg 75:1693, 2003.
90. Jacobson JH, Haimov M: Venous revascularization of the arm: Report of three cases. Surgery 81:599, 1977.

chapter 57

Pulmonary Arterial Hypertension

Laura B. Kane
Joseph Loscalzo

NORMAL PULMONARY CIRCULATION

The normal pulmonary arterial circulation is a highly distensible, high-flow, low-pressure system with minimal resting vascular tone that functions to carry deoxygenated blood into the alveolar capillaries, where gas exchange occurs. The low-pressure nature of this system is reflected in its thin, sparsely muscularized vessel walls and the thin-walled, crescentic right ventricle (RV). The architecture of the pulmonary vascular tree is crucial to its low resting tone. The main pulmonary artery arises from the RV and divides into the left and right pulmonary arteries, and sequentially into small muscular arteries, arterioles, and alveolar capillaries that create the gas exchange surface. The progressive branching of vessels increases the cross-sectional area at each level, decreasing blood flow velocity and allowing for optimal gas exchange at the smallest branches.

Like other elastic arteries, pulmonary arteries (PAs) are composed of three layers:

1. Intima: a single layer of endothelial cells (ECs) with underlying elastic lamina and connective tissue
2. Media: smooth muscle cells (SMCs) and fine elastic fibers, although normally much less muscularized than systemic vessels
3. Adventitia: a poorly defined layer of connective tissue and fibroblasts

Each layer also contains extracellular matrix (ECM) components including collagen, elastin, glycosaminoglycans, and fibronectin, which help maintain vessel elasticity and assist cell migration and proliferation.

In normal adults the PA lumen is wide and the media is thin, comprising less than 10% of the PA cross-sectional area. As the diameter of the arterial lumen decreases, the elastic laminae become less prominent and are replaced by smooth muscle. Beyond the terminal bronchioles, muscularization of the arteries decreases with size until there is no smooth muscle found in the smaller intra-acinar arteries. The major sites of pulmonary vascular resistance (PVR) are the small muscular arteries (100 to 1000 μm) and the precapillary arterioles (<100 μm). Even small changes in vascular tone or lumen size at this level increase resistance and, consequently, pulmonary artery pressure (PAP) significantly.[1]

Pulmonary Vascular Resistance

Pulmonary vessels are highly distensible. Even when blood flow increases substantially (as with increased cardiac output [CO] during exercise), minimal increases in PAP occur. This effect is due to distension of perfused vessels and recruitment of normally unused vessels, which result in a functional increase in the cross-sectional area of the pulmonary vascular bed and a substantial decrease in PVR. Pulmonary hypertension (PH) may occur with a loss of vascular compliance or increase in PVR due to a loss of vascular surface area. Several conditions may cause this decreased surface area, such as obstruction or loss of pulmonary arteries (PAs) (e.g., pulmonary embolus, PA stenosis, decreased number of PAs in congenital PH); occlusion of PAs by remodeling in pulmonary arterial hypertension (PAH); hypoxia-induced vasoconstriction; or chronic obstructive lung disease.

Resistance is the measure of a vessel's hindrance to blood flow. It is calculated as the drop in pressure across the pulmonary circulation divided by the rate of flow across it, analogous to Ohm's law of electrical resistance:

$$\text{PVR} = (\text{mean PAP} - \text{PVP})/\text{CO},$$
where PVP = pulmonary venous pressure

Left atrial pressure or pulmonary artery wedge pressure is used to estimate pulmonary venous pressure. When pressures are measured in mm Hg and CO in L/min, normal PVR is less than 1 Wood unit, but it is usually expressed in dyne/sec-cm^{-5} by multiplying by the conversion factor of 80, in which normal PVR is approximately 100.

Vasomotor Mechanisms That Regulate Pulmonary Blood Flow

Hypoxia

Unlike the systemic circulation, hypoxia induces vasoconstriction in the pulmonary vasculature. Hypoxia causes adaptive shifting of blood away from poorly ventilated areas to improve ventilation-perfusion matching and gas exchange. This adaptive mechanism preserves arterial oxygenation when localized to an isolated, underventilated lung segment, as is the case when flow is reduced to an area of lung with pneumonia. Chronic, sustained hypoxia causes sustained hypoxic pulmonary vasoconstriction with vascular remodeling, PH, and, ultimately, right heart failure and death.[2]

Biochemical Mediators

Vasodilator prostaglandins help maintain the low resting tone of the pulmonary circulation and oppose the effects of thromboxane A_2. Pulmonary ECs express prostacyclin synthetase, whereas platelets express thromboxane synthase, both of which convert cyclic endoperoxide precursors into active eicosanoids. Prostacyclin (prostaglandin I_2) is a potent, short-lived vasodilator that inhibits platelet activation and aggregation through activation of adenylyl cyclase; it is also antiproliferative and antithrombotic. Thromboxane A_2 is a potent vasoconstrictor, mitogen, and agonist of platelet aggregation. Other important vasoactive substances include the vasoconstrictors and mitogens endothelin, serotonin, and angiotensin II and the vasodilating, antithrombotic, and antiproliferative agent, nitric oxide (NO). Leukotrienes have also been shown to cause pulmonary vasoconstriction.[1]

Nitric oxide has effects similar to prostacyclin. Like prostacyclin, NO is produced by normal ECs and is an important regulator of basal vascular tone. It is synthesized from the amino acid L-arginine by NO synthases. Nitric oxide diffuses from ECs to SMCs, where it induces smooth muscle relaxation by activating guanylyl cyclase, as well as altering cation transport. Release of NO occurs in response to bradykinin, thrombin, and shear stress. Nitric oxide also inhibits platelet activation and aggregation, as well as migration and growth of vascular SMCs. Unlike prostacyclin, NO also impairs platelet adhesion.[3] Production of NO by pulmonary ECs may be protective in that it may limit the vasoconstrictive response to biochemical and mechanical stimuli. Absence of NO impairs relaxation and induces excessive pulmonary vasoconstriction in response to contractile stimuli.[4]

Neural Input

In an unstressed state, the autonomic nervous system is not a major contributor to pulmonary vascular tone. Vagal stimulation dilates and sympathetic stimulation constricts pulmonary vessels. There are α- and β-adrenergic receptors on pulmonary vascular smooth muscle, predominantly in the larger vessels. Norepinephrine, a potent α-agonist, causes pulmonary vasoconstriction, and the β-agonist isoproterenol induces vasodilation.[1]

DEFINITION AND CLASSIFICATION

PH is an elevation of PAP that can result from a wide range of conditions. PAH is a rare, progressive disorder usually defined as a mean PAP of greater than or equal to 25 mm Hg at rest or greater than or equal to 30 mm Hg during exercise, with a normal pulmonary artery wedge pressure, in the absence of any known cause. It is accompanied by pathologic changes in precapillary pulmonary arteries. Until improved therapeutic options became available during the past decade, PAH was a rapidly progressive, devastating condition that led to death from right heart failure by a median of 2.8 years from the time of diagnosis.[5]

PAH gained attention in the late 1960s when an epidemic occurred in Europe following the introduction of the over-the-counter appetite suppressant aminorex. The increased attention to this disorder led to a multicenter registry of patients with PAH organized by the National Institutes of Health (NIH) in an effort to describe epidemiologic and clinical characteristics of the disease. A symposium on PAH sponsored by the World Health Organization (WHO) in Evian, France, in 1998 led to a reclassification of pulmonary hypertensive disorders.[6] The 2003 Third World Symposium on Pulmonary Arterial Hypertension held in Venice addressed the usefulness of, and introduced modifications to, the Evian classification (Box 57-1).[7]

The WHO classification of PH presented in 1998 introduced the category of PAH. Previously PH was classified

BOX 57-1 Clinical Classification of Pulmonary Hypertension (Venice 2003)*

1. **Pulmonary arterial hypertension (PAH)**
   - a. Idiopathic (IPAH)
   - b. Familial (FPAH)
   - c. Associated with:
     - Collagen vascular disease
     - Congenital systematic-to-pulmonary shunts
     - Portal hypertension
     - HIV infection
     - Drugs and toxins
     - Other (thyroid disorders, glycogen storage disease, Gaucher's disease, hereditary hemorrhagic telangiectasia, hemoglobinopathies, myeloproliferative disorders, splenectomy)
   - d. Associated with significant venous or capillary involvement
     - Pulmonary veno-occlusive disease
     - Pulmonary capillary hemangiomatosis
   - e. Persistent pulmonary hypertension of the newborn
2. **Pulmonary hypertension with left heart disease**
   - Left atrial or left ventricular heart disease
   - Left-sided valvular heart disease
3. **Pulmonary hypertension associated with lung diseases or hypoxemia, or both**
   - Chronic obstructive pulmonary disease
   - Interstitial lung disease
   - Sleep-disordered breathing
   - Alveolar hypoventilation disorders
   - Chronic exposure to high altitude
   - Developmental abnormalities
4. **Pulmonary hypertension due to chronic thrombotic or embolic disease, or both**
   - Thromboembolic obstruction of proximal pulmonary arteries
   - Thromboembolic obstruction of distal pulmonary arteries
   - Nonthrombotic pulmonary embolism (tumor, parasites, foreign material)
   - Sickle-cell disease
5. **Miscellaneous**
   - Sarcoidosis, histiocytosis X, lymphangiomatosis, compression of pulmonary vessels (adenopathy, tumor, fibrosing mediastinitis)

Modified from Simonneau G, Galie N, Rubin JL, et al: Clinical classification of pulmonary hypertension. J Am Coll Cardiol 43:5S, 2004.

as either primary (idiopathic or unexplained) or secondary. The term "primary PH" was replaced with "idiopathic pulmonary arterial hypertension" at the Venice meeting in 2003. The classification of PAH recognized the clinical, histopathologic, and therapeutic similarities between idiopathic PAH and PAH associated with other conditions. The disorders encompassed by the term PAH share distinctive vascular changes in the precapillary arteries. The term PAH now includes idiopathic PAH (IPAH); familial PAH (FPAH); PAH related to collagen vascular diseases, HIV infection, portal hypertension, toxin or drug exposure (including appetite suppressants), congenital systemic-to-pulmonary shunts; and PAH related to rarer diseases such as hereditary hemorrhagic telangiectasia, thyroid disorders, splenectomy, chronic myeloproliferative disorders, and metabolic diseases. This classification distinguishes these intrinsic causes of PH from pulmonary venous hypertension (characterized by elevated pulmonary venous pressure and caused by left-sided heart disease) and PH associated with respiratory diseases or hypoxemia, chronic thromboembolic diseases, or diseases that directly impair the pulmonary vasculature. These broad categories are generally grouped according to shared treatment modalities.[6]

The PVR equation incorporates the pressure drop across the pulmonary circulation. This pressure drop is also called the transpulmonary pressure gradient (TPG):

TPG = PADP − mean PAWP,
where *PADP* is PA diastolic pressure and *PAWP* is PA wedge pressure

This gradient is useful in distinguishing "postcapillary" PH (pulmonary venous hypertension) from "precapillary" PH, or PAH. In postcapillary PH the rise in PVR is passive and due to elevated pulmonary venous pressure (≥15 mm Hg) with normal TPG. A TPG greater than 10 mm Hg has been used as another defining characteristic of PAH.

EPIDEMIOLOGY

Epidemiologic data were obtained from the NIH Registry for the characterization of IPAH, which included 187 patients, between 1981 and 1985. The registry excluded patients with other conditions in the PAH category except for those with exposure to appetite suppressant drugs.[8] The incidence of IPAH is estimated at one to two cases per million people in the general population, although the actual frequency of the disease may be higher. The disease affects women more frequently than men (1.7:1). This female predominance is exaggerated in the black population (4.3:1), although the overall racial distribution of patients reflects that in the general population. Primary PH presents most commonly in the fourth decade of life; ages range from 1 to 81 with 9% of the patients older than 60 years of age.[8] Some sources cite a similar gender ratio among children diagnosed with the disease, whereas others note an equal distribution between male and female children.[9] Primary PH is difficult to diagnose because it is rare and presents with nonspecific symptoms. The average time from the onset of symptoms to diagnosis was 2 years in the NIH Registry.[8]

PATHOLOGY OF PULMONARY ARTERIAL HYPERTENSION

In humans the natural history of PAH lesions is unknown, as patients usually present when the disease is advanced. The pathologic appearance of severe PH is similar regardless of the cause and reflects the end stage of a common response to pulmonary vascular injury. The histopathology of PAH shows a heterogeneous occlusive pulmonary arteriopathy with a wide range of abnormalities in ECs, SMCs, and ECM.

The major characteristics of PAH histology are medial smooth muscle hypertrophy, concentric and eccentric intimal proliferation (onionskin lesions), fibrosis leading to obliteration of small pulmonary arteries, *in situ* thrombosis with recanalized thrombi, and plexiform lesions (Fig. 57-1). There is thickening of muscular arteries of all sizes, most pronounced in the intimal layer, and appearance

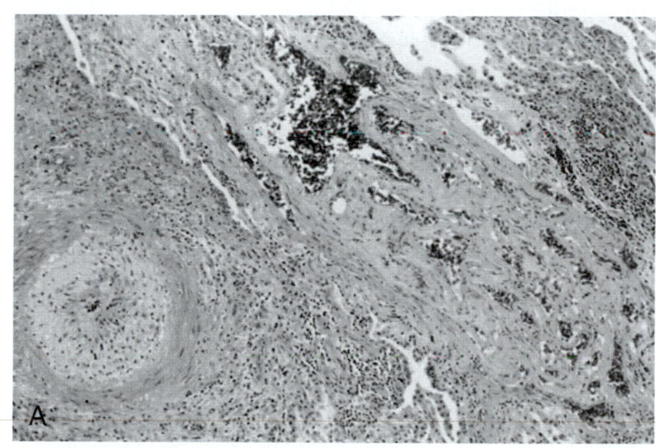

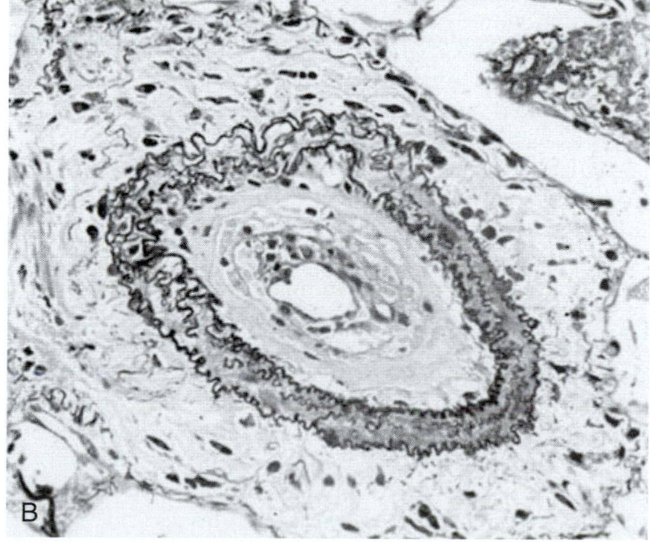

FIGURE 57-1. Pathology of pulmonary arterial hypertension. **A,** Hematoxylin and eosin stain of a histologic section of the lungs of an idiopathic pulmonary arterial hypertension (IPAH) patient demonstrates characteristic vascular lesions: a completely occluded vessel with severe concentric intimal fibrosis and medial thickening (*left*) and a plexiform lesion with multiple lumina (*right*). **B,** Elastin von Gieson stain of internal and external elastic laminae demonstrates the medial hypertrophy and neointimal formation in a small muscular pulmonary artery in a patient with IPAH. (Courtesy JL Faul, MD, Stanford University.)

of muscle in normally nonmuscular intra-acinar arteries, resulting in a reduction in peripheral arterial volume. The mechanism of this muscularization is unknown but may involve recruitment of interstitial fibroblasts from the surrounding lung parenchyma and their transdifferentiation into smooth muscle-like cells. In more proximal muscular arteries there are hypertrophy and hyperplasia of the medial smooth muscle layer, causing a fixed narrowing of the lumen. There is also dissolution of the elastic laminas, deposition of elastin and collagen, and proliferation of fibroblasts.[2]

Plexiform lesions are present in approximately 40% to 80% of lungs examined *post-mortem*. A plexiform lesion is a dilatation of a small pulmonary artery filled with a disorganized mesh of vessels lined with proliferating ECs, resembling a glomerulus. Plexiform lesions are not specific for IPAH, as they are found in severe PAH of any cause. Because the lesions occur in a patchy distribution, they may be missed on examination of biopsy specimens. Some sources suggest that plexiform lesions may originate from the medial and adventitial layers in addition to the endothelial layer.[10]

There is controversy as to the cell types and mechanisms responsible for the development of plexiform lesions and other remodeling changes. Some propose SMC transformation into myofibroblasts, whereas others believe ECs are the source—proliferating in response to cytokines, growth factors, and vascular injury. The usual location of a plexiform lesion near a bifurcation of a small artery suggests a role for the blood flow pattern in its development.[11] The discovery of monoclonal ECs in plexiform lesions in IPAH, in contrast with polyclonal cells in secondary forms of PH, supports the hypothesis of Tuder and colleagues[12] that plexiform lesions represent an abnormal form of angiogenesis with neoplasia-like dysregulated EC growth. Their studies use the plexiform lesion to demonstrate the key role of endothelial dysfunction in the pathogenesis of IPAH. Using markers specific for ECs (including vascular EC growth factor [VEGF] and its receptor VEGFR-2) and for SMCs, they demonstrated that plexiform and concentric lesions in IPAH, as well as in scleroderma and HIV, are formed by ECs, and that SMCs are not present in plexiform lesions.[12] Concentric lesions are located proximal to plexiform lesions. It is not known whether these lesions evolve or regress as plexiform lesions develop, nor whether the lesions are associated in some way with plexiform lesion formation.[13]

Plexogenic and thrombotic arteriopathies were originally considered distinct manifestations of unique diseases. Studies of lung specimens from family members with FPAH, however, demonstrated that the two lesions coexist in families of patients with FPAH and even in patients. Thus these arteriopathic processes are probably different manifestations of the same disease.[14]

The most commonly used histologic grading classification of PAH was described by Heath and Edwards.[15] The summary from the WHO symposium on PAH published in 1998, however, recommended that their pathologic classification of pulmonary vascular disease be abandoned because it is too restrictive, does not correlate with clinical findings, and does not enhance understanding of disease pathogenesis.[6] The one potential indication for obtaining a specimen for pathological analysis is in the subgroup of patients with PAH caused by congenital systemic-to-pulmonary shunts in which the information is used to guide decisions on surgical repair.

GENETICS

Background

PAH, initially labeled *primary PH,* was first described by Dresdale and colleagues in 1951, who also described the presence of this disease among family members in 1954.[16] The true incidence of FPAH is unknown. It is widely accepted that at least 6% to 10% of cases show an autosomal dominant pattern of inheritance, on the basis of the NIH Registry for IPAH in which 12 of the 187 IPAH patients (6.4%) reported a first-degree relative with the disease.[8] This is likely an underestimate because the low penetrance and variable expression of the disease lead to "skipped generations" in FPAH and the frequent misdiagnosis of sporadic disease. Multiple cases of sporadic PAH have been reported in which a remote, common ancestry was later discovered or in which inheritance of a mutated gene from an unaffected parent was found.[17,18]

Idiopathic Pulmonary Arterial Hypertension: Familial versus Sporadic

Sporadic IPAH and FPAH are identical histologically and clinically and in their response to therapy. Patients in the NIH Registry with FPAH had no distinguishing demographic or clinical characteristics and had a similar gender ratio, age of onset, and natural disease course.[8]

Familial Pulmonary Arterial Hypertension: Pattern of Inheritance

Transmission studies of families who were collected through the national FPAH registry revealed vertical transmission in up to five generations in one family, strongly suggesting a single dominant gene.[15] Other characteristics of FPAH transmission include genetic anticipation, varying age of onset, incomplete penetrance, and female predominance. It has also been observed that there are fewer males born in PAH families (female-to-male ratio of offspring is 1.3:1), suggesting that the PAH gene might influence fertilization or cause male fetal demise.[17]

Genetic Anticipation

Genetic anticipation is defined as an increase in the severity of a disease in subsequent generations. This pattern has been demonstrated in FPAH, with an earlier age of death in successive generations.[19] The only known mechanism described to cause genetic anticipation is the expansion of microsatellite repeat sequences, which is the mechanism of Huntington's disease and several other neurologic diseases. Approximately 10% of the human genome is composed of sequences of DNA repeats, which are stable in offspring. Certain trinucleotide repeats may become unstable and prone to expansion, which affects the expression of neighboring genes. Such instability can lead to different lengths of repeats in members of the same family and a variation in the clinical severity of disease.[20] Analysis of the coding sequence of the PAH gene (bone morphogenetic protein receptor type 2 [BMPR2], see later) in 50 families did not reveal any triplet-repeat sequences or expansion of repeats. Other possible mechanisms to explain genetic anticipation in PAH may be expansion of an intronic triplet repeat in the PAH gene or in a modifying gene; alternatively, genetic anticipation in PAH may be caused by a previously undescribed mechanism.[21]

Identifying the Gene for Pulmonary Arterial Hypertension: PPH1

Recognition of PAH in families led to gene localization using linkage analysis studies. In 1997 two independent groups performed a whole genome screen using polymorphic microsatellite markers. Linkage was established between PAH and the long arm of chromosome 2 (2q31-32), designated PPH1.[22,23] The initial candidate interval was 27cM, which was subsequently reduced by identifying recombinant events within families to 5cM. A positional candidate transcript map of genes within the locus was created, which enabled the description of genes spanning the PPH1 region.[24]

The PPH1 gene was discovered in 2000. Sequencing of positional candidate genes revealed heterozygous mutations in the gene encoding BMPR2, which is a member of the transforming growth factor beta (TGF-β) superfamily.[25,26]

Bone Morphogenetic Protein Receptor Type 2 Mutations

Mutations in the gene for BMPR2 have been detected in 40 (55%) of 73 families with PAH. Forty-six unique BMPR2 mutations have been identified. All mutations have been shown to segregate with disease in families, and each mutation is transmitted in a given family.[18,21,25,26] No BMPR2 mutations have been found in more than 350 controls analyzed in the literature.[27,28] Despite the close correlation between BMPR2 mutations and FPAH, 45% of families with PAH do not appear to exhibit a mutation in this gene. One explanation may be that the direct-sequencing methods used may not detect all heterozygous mutations. Alternatively, there may be mutations in portions of the gene that have not been sequenced, such as promoter, intronic, regulatory, or untranslated regions[21]; or there may be a separate genetic defect, possibly for another component of the TGF-β signaling pathway.

What is Bone Morphogenetic Protein Receptor Type 2?

The BMPR2 gene was considered a likely candidate for the PPH1 locus because the receptor, BMPR-II, is a member of the TGF-β superfamily of receptors. The TGF-β superfamily is critical in endothelial and SMC growth, differentiation, matrix production, and angiogenesis, as well as in maintaining the function and integrity of the normal vasculature.[29] BMPR-II is ubiquitously expressed. The principal ligands for BMPR2, bone morphogenetic proteins (BMPs), were initially identified as cellular products in normal bone that regulate growth and differentiation of bone and cartilage but were later discovered to be multifunctional cytokines that regulate growth, differentiation, and apoptosis of multiple cell types. BMPs are members of the TGF-β superfamily of circulating proteins that regulate growth and tissue repair (there are more than 30 members of the BMP subfamily). The other protein subfamilies in the TGF-β superfamily include the three TGF-β isoforms (TGF-β 1,2,3), the activins, and the inhibins. The effect of BMP and TGF-β signaling is cell specific and can cause proliferation or growth inhibition. Generally TGF-β and BMPs inhibit the proliferation and migration of vascular SMCs and ECs.[30,31]

Transforming Growth Factor β Superfamily Signaling

TBG-β receptors are of three classes: types 1, 2, and 3. The receptors are transmembrane signaling molecules with serine-threonine kinase activity. The current paradigm for TGF-β signaling is that ligand binds the type 2 receptor, which recruits and phosphorylates the type 1 receptor to activate one of a class of intracellular signaling molecules, the Smads, by phosphorylation. There are at least nine Smad proteins, which ultimately dictate the cellular response to specific TGF-β superfamily proteins by moving to the nucleus and interacting with specific transcription factors. There is considerable plasticity to this signaling system. Depending on the specific ligand-receptor combination, receptor expression, cell type, Smad intermediate, and transcriptional response, the signal can either promote or inhibit proliferation of the cell. BMPs bind to the complex formed by the heterodimerization of BMPR-II and a type 1 receptor (BMPR-1a, BMPR-1b, or activin receptor-1), leading to phosphorylation of Smads 1, 5, or 8, which associate with Smad 4 to modulate transcription of factors that regulate cell growth.[32] The BMPR2 mutation in FPAH may lead to a loss of the inhibitory action of BMP on the growth of pulmonary vascular SMCs, thereby triggering a proliferative response.[16]

Bone Morphogenetic Protein Receptor Type 2 and Disease

How BMPR2 mutations lead to the disease phenotype is unknown. Direct sequence analysis of the protein-encoding portion of the BMPR2 gene has revealed germline heterozygous missense, nonsense, and frameshift mutations. The mutations are predicted to lead to premature truncation or defective protein, which may interrupt BMP-mediated signaling, allowing transmission of a proliferative rather than apoptotic signal in the cell.[21] Possible mechanisms include simple haploid insufficiency from decreased protein expression, haploid insufficiency in combination with a second somatic mutation or regulatory event affecting the wild type allele, or a dominant-negative effect of the mutant BMPR2 receptor. The heterogeneity of the BMPR2 mutations and variability of clinical patterns make haploid insufficiency with additional epigenetic factors a plausible explanation.[33] This explanation supports the hypothesis that the BMPR2 signaling pathway is essential for the maintenance of the normal pulmonary vascular phenotype, and that target cells are sensitive to a reduced level of the BMPR2 gene or its transcription.[21,28]

BMPR2 Mutations in Nonfamilial Pulmonary Arterial Hypertension

BMPR2 Mutations in Sporadic Idiopathic Pulmonary Arterial Hypertension

BMPR2 mutations have also been found in one study of patients with sporadic PAH. Thomson and colleagues[34] sequenced the coding regions and intron/exon boundaries of the BMPR2 gene in 50 unrelated patients with acquired PAH and found that the "sporadic" form of the disease is associated with germline mutations of the BMPR2 gene in 13 (26%) cases. None of the patients had a family history of the disease, but genetic testing indicated three patients had inherited the mutated gene from a parent and two patients did not have parental samples for testing.[35] More recent studies of sporadic IPAH have demonstrated a BMPR2 mutation in only 11% of cases.[36]

BMPR2 Mutations in PAH Associated with Appetite Suppressants

BMPR2 mutations have also been detected in patients with PAH who have been exposed to the appetite suppressants fenfluramine and dexfenfluramine. Humbert and colleagues[27] screened the BMPR2 gene in 35 patients who had taken fenfluramine or dexfenfluramine, or both, and developed PAH and found that 9% of patients had BMPR2 mutations. The disease was identical in patients with and without BMPR2 mutations, but the patients with BMPR2 mutations had a significantly shorter duration of exposure to fenfluramines than patients in whom BMPR2 mutations were not detected (median use 1 month vs. 4 months).[27] Further study is needed to confirm that fenfluramine exposure behaves as an environmental factor that augments expression of a mutated gene. The study did not evaluate family members of patients with BMPR2 mutations; thus it is not possible to conclude that exposure to fenfluramines increases disease penetrance.

PPH2—Possible Second Locus

The possibility of locus heterogeneity was investigated by one group, and a second PAH locus was found proximal to the PPH1 region in a large kindred without germline mutation in BMPR2. The investigators used stress Doppler echo to identify gene carriers (family members with abnormal PAP response to exercise), as well as patients with established PAH, and found a second PAH gene that mapped to 2q31-32. This gene has not yet been identified.[37]

Hereditary Hemorrhagic Telangiectasia

The argument that TGF-β superfamily signaling features strongly in the pathogenesis of PAH is buttressed by the finding that a mutation in another TGFβ receptor may result in a disease phenotypically identical to IPAH. Hereditary hemorrhagic telangiectasia (HHT), or Osler-Weber-Rendu syndrome, is a rare, autosomal dominant disorder characterized by the occurrence of vascular dysplastic lesions including vascular dilatations and arteriovenous malformations in many organs. A small percentage of these patients also develop the occlusive arteriopathy and elevated pulmonary vascular resistance found in PAH. HHT is associated with mutations in two genes, endoglin and activin receptor-like kinase-1 (Alk1), which encode different components of the TGF-β receptor complex. Endoglin is a TGF-β type 3 receptor that assists the association of receptor types 1 and 2. Alk1 is an activin type 1 receptor, the function of which is unclear, but that appears to be abundant in the pulmonary vasculature, particularly in ECs. Trembath and colleagues[38] identified mutations in the gene for Alk1 in members of families with HHT who also had PH. One patient with HHT, PAH, and a mutation in the endoglin gene has recently been reported.[39] Alk1 signaling, like BMP signaling in ECs, is mediated by phosphorylation of Smads 1,5, or 8, which may explain why IPAH and HHT share some vascular abnormalities. These two receptors have not been shown to interact directly, but they may have a similar effect on another component of the signaling pathway.[32]

Epigenetic and Environmental Factors

How does a genetic defect, present since birth, cause a disease limited to the pulmonary vasculature, affect only a small percentage of individuals with the mutation, and manifest late in life? BMPR2 is known to be essential for development, because mice homozygous for the mutation die *in utero*. The mere presence of a mutation is not sufficient to cause disease, as only 20% of patients with BMPR2 mutations develop PAH (and heterozygous mice are phenotypically normal and have normal pulmonary pressures). The clinical variability among family members with the identical genetic mutation, including nonpenetrance of disease, further indicates the requirement for additional environmental or genetic factors in disease pathogenesis. The female predominance of patients argues that there may be a hormonal factor involved, although this has not been demonstrated in epidemiologic studies.[21] TGF-β behaves as a tumor suppressor gene, and numerous components of the TGF-β signaling pathway are mutated in various cancers. Perhaps there is a second insult or somatic mutation in the TGF-β signaling pathway that results in the disease phenotype.[40]

PATHOGENESIS OF PULMONARY ARTERIAL HYPERTENSION

The pathogenesis of PAH is a complex, poorly understood process involving a genetic predisposition and environmental triggers. The sustained elevation in PVR is caused by a combination of pulmonary vascular remodeling, vasoconstriction, and thrombosis *in situ*. The remodeling seen in PAH results from pulmonary vascular injury of myriad causes. The diseases that are categorized under the rubric of PAH were grouped for their similarities in histopathology, disease course, and response to therapy. It is unknown whether they share a common pathogenic mechanism, but the end results are indistinguishable. It seems likely that the initial injury in these diseases varies, and that they subsequently evolve along a common pathway of remodeling. Pulmonary vascular remodeling probably involves a combination of endothelial injury, dysregulation of cell growth, activation of matrix production, and stimulation by growth factors and vasoactive mediators. It also remains enigmatic as to how myriad, diverse stimuli trigger the same cellular abnormalities—the inflammation associated with collagen vascular diseases, the mechanical forces associated with congenital heart diseases, exposure to serotonin analogs such as dexfenfluramine, viral infection, and BMPR2 or Alk1 mutations. The pathogenic commonalities remain unexplained, but severe PH seems to represent the end stage of a diverse group of diseases that initially induce pulmonary endothelial dysfunction and damage.

It is impossible to study the earliest changes in human PAH vessels, as the disease is not diagnosed until it is advanced, and obtaining a biopsy for diagnosis is rarely indicated. Consequently, research on PAH relies on studying advanced disease in humans or animal models, which are limited representations of the human disease.

In broad summary, it seems clear that any severe type of PH begins with genetic susceptibility in association with epigenetic factors, either disease-modifying genes or environmental determinants of disease expression. In this setting, injury to the pulmonary vasculature triggers a wide range of cellular and molecular responses to create an environment that is mitogenic, vasoconstricting, and thrombotic. Historically, the elevated PVR in PAH was attributed to an imbalance between mediators of vasoconstriction and vasodilation. More recently it has become clear that the vasoactive view of PAH pathogenesis is limited. The vasoconstrictor, or mechanical, explanation of the pathogenesis of PH does not address the crucial role of a dysfunctional endothelium in triggering the disease process, nor does it incorporate the importance of genetic mutations. The range of mechanisms proposed as contributing to remodeling and abnormally high resistance is wide (Fig. 57-2). Each of these pathobiologic mechanisms is discussed later, in turn.

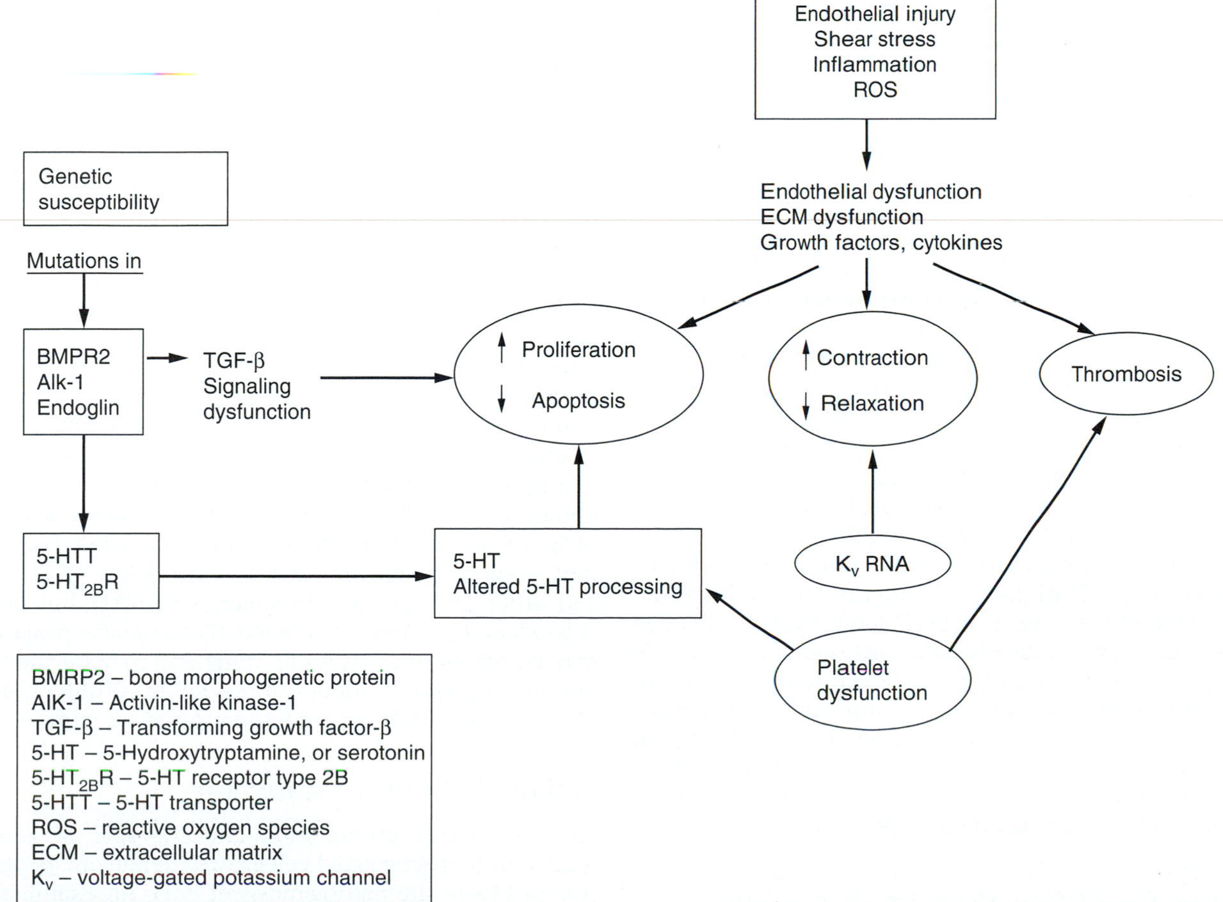

FIGURE 57-2. Schematic of possible pulmonary arterial hypertension (PAH) pathogenesis. PAH probably requires genetic susceptibility followed by endothelial injury, leading to changes in endothelial cells, smooth muscle cells, platelets, and extracellular matrix favoring proliferation, vasoconstriction, and thrombosis.

TGF-β and BMPR2 Mutations

Direct causal evidence implicating BMPR2 mutations in PAH has not been shown. However, recent observations support a role for BMPR2 mutations in the pathogenesis of PAH. Morrell and colleagues[29] demonstrated an abnormal propensity for growth in IPAH cells in a study showing that TGF-β1 and BMPs suppressed proliferation of pulmonary artery smooth muscle cells (PASMCs) from patients with secondary forms of PH and control patients, but PASMCs from patients with IPAH were resistant to those antiproliferative effects. Failure of BMP-induced growth suppression, then, may contribute to the abnormal proliferation of vascular smooth muscle cells and adverse vascular remodeling in PAH. Interestingly, cells from all PAH patients in the study behaved similarly, regardless of the presence of a mutation in BMPR2, suggesting that there may be another abnormality in the TGF-β superfamily contributing to abnormal growth not explained by interruptions in BMPR2 signaling. This idea is strengthened by the finding that the cells had a heightened growth response to TGF-β1, which is not a known ligand for BMPR2.[29]

Atkinson and colleagues[41] studied the cellular localization of BMPR2 in FPAH, sporadic IPAH, secondary PH, and normal control patients. In the normal circulation, BMPR2 was located in the endothelium. Pulmonary vascular BMPR2 expression was reduced in all patients with severe PH, including PAH without a BMPR2 mutation and in secondary forms of PH, although expression was lowest in patients with an underlying BMPR2 mutation. This observation suggests that reduced BMPR2 signaling may have a role in the pathogenesis of PH even in patients without germline mutations in BMPR2, possibly even in secondary PH.[41] However, reduced expression of BMPR2 has not been clearly demonstrated to induce dysfunctional pulmonary vascular cell growth.

Du and colleagues[42] addressed the question of whether there exists a common molecular mechanism for pulmonary vascular remodeling in PH caused by diverse etiologies. In their study of 42 patients with various types of PH, they found that BMPR1a, a type 1 receptor that forms a complex with BMPR2 in the presence of a BMP ligand, was downregulated in patients with PAH, as well as four different acquired forms of PH. Furthermore, they found increased expression of angiopoietin-1, an angiogenic factor produced by SMCs, in PH from all causes. Phosphorylation of the angiopoietin-1 receptor, TIE2, was minimal in control patients and correlated with clinical severity of PH in diseased patients. The study further demonstrated that angiopoietin-1 downregulates BMPR1a mRNA and protein levels, and that elevated levels of angiopoietin-1 are a cause, not a consequence of PH. This study links FPAH and other causes of PH by demonstrating that dose-dependent inactivation of the BMPR complex—either by BMPR2 mutations or by downregulation of BMPR1a transcription through increased angiopoietin-1—is a hallmark of the disease.[42]

Dysfunctional Endothelial Cell Growth

Historically, pulmonary vascular changes and plexiform lesions were considered the result of progressive scarring of pulmonary arteries, a pathologic finding late in the disease course, and not pathogenically significant.[41] The recent observations implicating abnormal signaling in pulmonary vascular cells, as well as analysis of plexiform lesions, have shed new light on the importance of endothelial and SMC proliferation in the development of disease. These studies lend support to the idea that changes in vascular cell growth may be the primary event, rather than a consequence of elevated pulmonary arterial pressures.

Tuder and colleagues[12] argue that EC injury causes apoptosis, accompanied by the selective growth of an apoptosis-resistant EC clone. This cell line is then prone to proliferate due to an acquired somatic mutation in a growth regulatory gene, causing monoclonal, neoplasia-like growth. Proliferation continues due to the increased presence of angiogenesis-inducing molecules, including VEGF, VEGFR2, and hypoxia-inducible factor-1.[12] VEGF stimulates EC growth via platelet-derived growth factor (PDGF) and TGF-β. There is prominent VEGF expression in plexiform lesions, and VEGFR-2 inhibition was shown to exacerbate hypoxic PH in rats by causing EC proliferation. This observation suggests a protective role of VEGF in endothelial function and also supports the role of apoptosis because the proliferation and PH were blocked by the addition of an agent that prevents apoptosis.[43]

Further support for the role of abnormal EC growth came from Lee and colleagues,[44] who studied EC proliferation in plexiform lesions and demonstrated that 77% of these lesions in patients with IPAH (and PAH associated with appetite suppressants) were monoclonal. By contrast, in secondary types of PH (including scleroderma or congenital systemic-to-pulmonary shunts), all of the lesions demonstrated polyclonality. Because a monoclonal cell population originates from a single cell that develops a somatic mutation, the presence of monoclonal EC proliferation in IPAH supports the concept that an acquired somatic mutation may be involved in the pathogenesis of the disease, similar to the early pathogenesis of neoplasms. Polyclonal EC proliferation in plexiform lesions of secondary PH suggests that the cells proliferate in response to another primary stimulus, such as high shear stress associated with increased blood flow or inflammation.[44] Yeager and colleagues[45] hypothesized that genomic instability may lead to spontaneous somatic mutations in PH. They performed microdissection studies of ECs from plexiform lesions and found microsatellite mutations and reduced protein expression of TGF-βR2 and other growth regulatory genes in IPAH, but not in secondary PH. They concluded that somatic mutations may be acquired in sporadic IPAH and may be the "second hit" required to induce abnormal EC proliferation in FPAH, acting much like a tumor suppressor gene.[45]

Endothelial Cell Dysfunction

Endothelial cell proliferation and the role of genetic mutations in dysregulated cell growth define one potential role of ECs in the pathogenesis of PAH. An examination of EC function and how it is altered in PAH demonstrates the importance of ECs in regulating blood flow and PVR. ECs provide a semipermeable, antithrombotic barrier that suppresses the migration and growth of the underlying SMC population. ECs produce substances that regulate the tone of the underlying smooth muscle, control cell migration and proliferation, and maintain the antithrombotic milieu. Biochemical and mechanical stimuli that modulate these phenotypic properties include increased shear stress, hypoxia, oxidant damage, acidosis, inflammation, and exposure to toxins. Following vascular injury, regenerated ECs are dysfunctional, with altered morphological appearance and impaired relaxation.[46]

Imbalance of Vasoactive Mediators

PH has historically been considered a disease caused by an imbalance in vasoconstricting and vasodilating mediators. Although this may not prove to be the instigating event in the disease, there is considerable evidence to suggest that this imbalance plays a key role in disease progression, and it is the pathway that has been targeted most effectively in treatment. EC injury, crucial to the proliferative aspect of the disease, also underlies some of the abnormalities in vasoactive mediators. The complexity of interactions among these mediators makes it impossible to identify a single culprit mechanism in disease pathogenesis.

As discussed earlier, the normally low resting tone of the pulmonary vascular bed is regulated by the balance between the endothelium-derived vasodilators prostacyclin and NO and the vasoconstrictors serotonin, endothelin, and thromboxane A_2. Patients with IPAH have increased release of thromboxane A_2, a platelet activator in addition to vasoconstrictor, and decreased prostacyclin synthesis compared with controls. Pulmonary artery ECs in IPAH were found to have reduced expression of prostacyclin synthase and endothelial nitric oxide synthase, and increased expression of endothelin-1 and endothelin synthase.[47] It was later demonstrated that NO production in the lung is preserved or increased, as is urinary excretion of cGMP, suggesting that the normal response of the pulmonary circulation is to increase these effectors in an effort to restore normal vascular tone. The decrease in exhaled NO is probably due to increased oxidation of NO to NO_2^-/ NO_3^- or $OONO^-$.[48]

Endothelin-1

The endothelins comprise a family of highly potent vasoconstrictor peptides, including endothelin (ET)-1,2, and 3. ET-1 is both a potent vasoconstrictor and comitogen/proliferation factor for vascular smooth muscle. The main source of ET-1 is ECs, but it is also produced by SMCs, in which it may have autocrine proliferative effects.[49] Plasma levels and lung expression of ET-1 are elevated in both PAH and secondary PH, and plasma levels correlate with disease severity in PAH.[50] ET-1 levels in the pulmonary circulation have been shown to correlate with PVR.[51]

Endothelin has also been shown to have vasodilating properties. Two subtypes of the ET receptor have been cloned and sequenced. The ETA receptor is selective for ET-1 and mediates vasoconstriction. The ETB receptor is nonselective and mediates vasodilation when present on the vascular endothelium or contraction when present on vascular SMCs. Occupancy of endothelial ETB receptors by ET-1 permits NO and prostacyclin release, promoting vasodilation, and also removes ET-1 from the circulation. It is theorized that ETB downregulation or desensitization may promote PH by reducing its vasodilating effects. Support for this theory comes from the finding that transgenic ETB receptor-deficient rats had higher plasma ET-1 levels, lower levels of NO and prostacyclin metabolites, and exaggerated hypoxic PH responses.[52] ET receptor antagonists are effective in decreasing PAP in patients with PH.

Angiotensin II

Angiotensin II plays an important role in systemic hypertensive vascular remodeling. It has been shown to stimulate the growth of human PASMCs. Endothelial angiotensin-converting enzyme (ACE) expression is increased in peripheral pulmonary arteries of patients with IPAH and secondary PH. ACE inhibitors have been shown to block the development of PH in hypoxic rats. Increased angiotensin II generated by ACE in small precapillary pulmonary arteries may contribute to increasing PVR. In small case studies, long-term administration of ACE inhibitors reduced pulmonary vascular resistance[53]; however, the response to ACE inhibitor therapy in PAH patients has not been significant.

Serotonin (5-Hydroxytryptamine)

Serotonin (5-hydroxtryptamine [5-HT]) is a potent pulmonary vasoconstrictor and growth factor for vascular SMCs. It is secreted by enterochromaffin cells in the intestine, stored mainly in platelets in dense (delta) granules, and released on platelet activation. Free serotonin in plasma is rapidly metabolized by the endothelial monoamine oxidase enzymatic system in the liver and lungs. Normally the pulmonary vascular bed is only minimally exposed to serotonin owing to hepatic metabolism and the large serotonin storage capacity of platelets.

Several findings implicate serotonin in the pathogenesis of PAH. In 1990 there was a reported case of a patient with a rare platelet delta storage pool disease who was found to have PAH. The platelet delta storage pool defect impairs the platelet's ability to store serotonin and leads to elevated plasma serotonin levels. This association compelled investigators to consider serotonin in the pathogenesis of PAH. The importance of serotonin in PAH was reemphasized when the disease was found to occur in patients who took appetite suppressants that interfere with serotonin transport. Patients with PAH have significantly reduced platelet serotonin levels and elevated plasma serotonin levels compared with controls. Following normalization of pulmonary pressures through heart-lung transplantation, platelet serotonin storage remains impaired and serotonin levels remain elevated. Serotonin levels are not elevated in patients with secondary forms of PH. These findings suggest that the platelet serotonin abnormality is not secondary to elevated pulmonary pressures, and that it may play a role in the pathogenesis of PAH.[54]

The vasoconstricting action of 5-HT is mediated mainly through the serotonin receptors. The mitogenic effect depends on internalization of 5-HT by the 5-HT transporter (5-HTT). The exact mechanism of 5-HTT involvement in PAH is not clear. Eddahibi[56] showed that PASMCs from patients with IPAH grow faster than comparable cells from control patients when stimulated by serotonin, which was associated with increased expression of 5-HTT. 5-HTT expression is also increased in platelets and lungs of patients with IPAH. Drugs that block 5-HTT also inhibit the mitogenic effects of 5-HT on SMCs.[55] Support for the role of 5-HTT in PH has been provided in animal models of hypoxic PH: 5-HTT transcription and 5HTT levels are increased in hypoxic rats, increased plasma 5-HT augments PH in hypoxic rats (an effect that is prevented by treatment with 5-HTT inhibitors), and mice with disruption of the 5-HTT gene develop less hypoxic PH than controls.[55]

A 5-HTT gene promoter polymorphism is associated with 5-HTT overexpression and increased SMC growth. The promoter may contain either a 44 kb insertion (long, or L allele) or deletion (short, or S allele). The L allele is associated with a twofold to threefold higher level of 5-HTT expression, and the LL genotype was considerably more common in IPAH patients than in controls (70% to 80% compared with 20% to 30%), which implies that this polymorphism may confer susceptibility to PAH.[56] As fenfluramine is a 5-HTT ligand, one group proposed that patients who develop PH after fenfluramine exposure might have a higher frequency of this gene polymorphism; however, this population has the same proportion of this polymorphism, as do other PH patients. It is not clear why patients without the polymorphism can also have an abnormal proliferative response to 5-HT. One possibility is that under normal conditions, the mitogenic effects of 5-HT may balance the antiproliferative effects of BMPR2. Dysfunctional BMPR2 signaling may leave the proliferative effects of 5-HTT unopposed. This imbalance, in conjunction with 5-HTT overexpression from the gene promoter polymorphism, may lead to the proliferative phenotype.[57]

One type of 5-HT receptor, 5-HT_{2B} (5-HT_{2B}R), has been particularly implicated in the development of PH. Pulmonary arterial ECs and SMCs express mRNAs for multiple 5-HT receptors. Dexfenfluramine binds weakly to the 5-HT receptors, but its active metabolite, N-de-ethylated dexfenfluramine (norDF), is a high-affinity ligand for 5-HT_{2B}R, where it acts as a potent agonist. Activation by norDF at the 5-HT_{2B}R raises intracellular calcium levels and mediates the mitogenic actions of 5-HT. Expression of 5-HT_{2B}R is increased in patients with PH. Launay and colleagues[58] completely prevented the development of hypoxia-induced PH in mice by inactivation of 5-HT_{2B}Rs, demonstrating that activation of the 5-HT_{2B}R is a limiting step in the development of PH. In the mouse, this effect is not at the level of acute vasoconstrictive responses but rather at the level of hypoxia-induced signaling mechanisms important in remodeling, including TGF-β. The authors propose that, in humans, the level of 5-HT_{2B}R expression may delineate susceptibility to PH.[58]

Recognition of the role of serotonin in PAH led investigators to consider whether other diseases involving platelet dysfunction or abnormal 5-HT availability might be associated with PAH. A deficiency of dense granules in platelets might result in a diminished capacity to take up circulating 5-HT and an increase in blood concentration of 5-HT. PAH has been reported in patients with abnormal platelet serotonin storage. Type 1a glycogen storage disease is an autosomal recessive disorder caused by a deficiency of glucose-6-phosphatase (von Gierke's disease) with an estimated incidence of 1 per 100,000 people. Since its initial description in 1980, seven cases of severe PH in patients with type 1a glycogen storage disease have been described, and the lungs of these patients were described pathologically as having pulmonary hypertensive arteriopathy, like the lesions seen in PAH.[59] To test the hypothesis that PAH in type 1a glycogen-storage disease could be due to abnormal levels of 5-HT, Humbert and colleagues[60] measured the plasma serotonin concentrations in patients with this disease, patients with severe PAH, one patient with both, and healthy controls. They found elevated 5-HT concentrations in patients with either severe PAH or type 1a glycogen storage disease and an extremely high concentration in the patient with both conditions, compared with controls. Most patients with glycogen storage disease do not develop PAH, again demonstrating the requirement for individual susceptibility determinants or other genetic or environmental factors. The patient in this study had no sequence variants in BMPR2 or Alk1 exons or 5-HTT polymorphisms.[60] The genetic mutation leading to type 1a glycogen-storage disease has been cloned, and several mutations have been detected, demonstrating the genetic heterogeneity of this condition. It is unknown whether a possible gene mutation predisposing to PH is present in the same region of the chromosome (17q21).[60]

Thrombosis

Whether hypercoagulability occurs in response to PAH or plays a role in its initiation is unclear, but thrombosis *in situ* is a prominent histopathologic finding in peripheral pulmonary arteries and leads to occlusion of vessels. There is also evidence of increased platelet activity in patients with PAH. PAH patients have diminished fibrinolysis and elevated plasminogen activator inhibitor type 1.[61] As discussed later, anticoagulant therapy improves survival in PAH. The decreased elaborations of prostacyclin, NO, and thrombomodulin also contribute to the loss of the antithrombotic function of ECs. Furthermore, shear stress may also generate a thrombogenic surface. PAH is also associated with certain prothrombotic conditions such as splenectomy (in which PAH occurs in the setting of postsplenectomy thrombocytosis), hemoglobinopathies, thrombotic thrombocytopenic purpura (TTP), and chronic myeloproliferative disorders. These conditions may predispose to PAH due to activation of platelets rather than simply to thrombosis.[62]

K Channels

Voltage-gated potassium (Kv) channels are transmembrane proteins with a K^+-selective pore. They are tonically active in vascular SMCs, which allows a slow efflux of K^+ along the concentration gradient (145/5 mmol/L, intracellular/extracellular). Kv channels are one of many types of potassium channels. Decreased activity of these channels causes accumulation of K^+ inside the cell, making the membrane potential more positive. This depolarization activates the voltage-gated L-type calcium channel, allowing calcium influx, prompting contraction. Acute hypoxic vasoconstriction occurs by inhibiting PASMC Kv channels.[48] In PASMCs of patients with PAH, there is reduced mRNA for certain types of Kv channels and an abnormally low channel current. Calcium concentrations in SMCs from PAH patients are significantly higher than in SMCs from patients with secondary PH or from controls. The downregulation or dysfunction of Kv channels and elevation in cytoplasmic calcium within SMCs in PAH are similar to the changes observed in response to chronic hypoxia, demonstrating a common pathway resulting in vasoconstriction and remodeling in these two conditions.[48,63]

Interestingly, reduced expression of Kv channels has been found in PASMCs after the addition of fenfluramine, illustrating that control of Kv channel gene regulation may be a possible mechanism of PH triggered by exposure to anorexigens.[64] Further evidence for the role of Kv channel deficiency in PH comes from a model of chronic hypoxic PH in rats in which aerosolized gene transfer was used to administer voltage-gated K^+ channel type 1.5 into the pulmonary circulation. The animals with the Kv gene transfer had transiently reduced PVR and regression of medial hypertrophy and RVH compared with control animals.[65]

Shear Stress

Few studies have implicated shear stress in remodeling, but it is a major contributor to PAH in patients with congenital systemic-to-pulmonic shunts and is probably a factor in other types as well. Shear stress can alter the expression of genes important in regulating endothelial and SMC growth. The endothelium is the interface between hemodynamic forces and the vascular wall. Shear stresses are mechanically transmitted from the cytoskeleton to focal adhesion molecules, which tether the cell to underlying matrix proteins. Cells then transduce those mechanical stimuli into secondary signals, which are not well understood. The EC responds to those signals with various changes, including calcium fluxes, Kv channel activation, NO and prostacyclin release, cell shape, and an increased rate of cell proliferation.[2]

Botney[66] proposes that neointimal formation occurs in the presence of both endothelial injury and changes in pulmonary artery hemodynamics. Systemic vessels develop neointimal lesions after injury. By contrast, pulmonary vessels are usually spared from developing neointimal disease, possibly owing to a protective effect of the substantially lower pressures in pulmonary arteries. The argument for the etiologic role of shear stress is supported by the fact that animal models only develop significant neointimal lesions when the endothelial injury is compounded by increased shear stress by limiting circulation to one lung (with pneumonectomy).[66]

Extracellular Matrix

Pulmonary vascular remodeling in PAH involves increased production of ECM, including collagen, elastin, fibronectin, and tenascin, a matrix glycoprotein that amplifies the proliferative response of SMCs to growth factors. The internal elastic lamina, which separates the endothelium from SMCs in muscular arteries, is fragmented in PAH. Rabinovitch[67] speculates that endothelial injury causes a loss of its barrier function and allows leakage of a serum factor into the normally isolated subendothelium. This serum factor could induce activity of endogenous vascular elastase or matrix metalloproteinases with release of matrix-bound SMC mitogens. The result is smooth muscle hypertrophy and proliferation and increased synthesis of connective tissue proteins and tenascin. Tenascin then contributes to the differentiation of precursor cells into the SMCs that appear in the normally nonmuscular, small peripheral PAs, and causes hypertrophy in muscularized arteries. *In vitro* administration of elastase and matrix metalloproteinase inhibitors to pulmonary arteries from pulmonary hypertensive animals lowered tenascin levels, induced apoptosis of SMCs, and reversed PH-associated remodeling with a reduction in ECM components.[67] In a rat model, an elastase inhibitor was also shown to reverse pulmonary vascular disease completely, with normalization of pulmonary artery pressure, apoptosis, and resorption of the ECM with regression of the hypertrophied vessel wall.[68]

Inflammation

Inflammation seems to play an important role in the initiation or progression of PH. A large proportion of patients with PAH show evidence of autoimmunity or active inflammation, including circulating antinuclear antibodies and elevated levels of proinflammatory cytokines, including IL-1 and IL-6. These cytokines are mitogens and are also known to promote thrombosis, leading to the hypothesis that inflammation may contribute to remodeling and *in situ* thrombosis.[69] Inflammatory cells are present around remodeled vascular lesions, particularly mast cells, macrophages, and T and B lymphocytes. In addition to cytokines, inflammatory cells release growth factors and reactive oxygen species. Expression of 5-lipoxygenase (5-LO) and the membrane-bound 5-LO activating protein (FLAP) are increased in lungs from patients with PAH, and *in vitro* studies show that 5-LO inhibitors block the growth of human pulmonary artery ECs.[70,71]

Numerous inflammatory mediators appear to be likely contributors to PAH. Leukocytes can secrete angiogenic factors such as VEGF, PDGF, interleukins, and TGF-β1. Mast cells and macrophages also release vasoactive and angiogenic factors. Anti-inflammatory drugs, such as leukotriene inhibitors and HMG-CoA reductase inhibitors, have induced resolution of animal models of PH, further suggesting that inflammation contributes to abnormal hemodynamics and remodeling.[72,73]

Reactive Oxygen Species

Oxidative stress likely also plays an important role in pulmonary vascular remodeling. Reactive oxygen species enhance the proliferation of pulmonary vascular cells. Superoxide has been shown to mediate the proliferation of PASMC and fibroblasts stimulated by 5-HT, ET-1, PDGF, FGF, and dexfenfluramine.[2]

PULMONARY ARTERIAL HYPERTENSION RISK FACTORS AND ASSOCIATED CONDITIONS

The WHO PAH symposium in 1998 led to a description of conditions associated with the development of PAH (Table 57-1). The rarity of PAH makes definitive statements of causality or association with risk factors difficult. Associations are based on epidemiologic or controlled studies, case series, registries, or observations. "Factors not associated" are postulated risk factors that have not been found to have any association with PAH from controlled epidemiologic studies. Risk factors may include demographic characteristics, diseases, drugs, or toxic exposures.[6] Even the confirmed risk factors only cause PAH in an extremely small percentage of patients exposed, indicating the requirement for individual susceptibility for the disease.

Demographic and Comorbid Conditions

There is a greater risk for PAH in women, although in childhood the gender distribution is equal in males and females. PAH can occur at any age but is more common in young adults, with a mean age at diagnosis of 40 years and a peak of incidence in the third and fourth decades. There is no documented geographic or racial predominance, although in the NIH Registry there was a greater incidence in black females. There are reports of PAH onset during pregnancy, but it is unknown whether this is caused by the increased pulmonary blood flow in pregnancy or by hormonal changes.[74] There seems to be a trend toward higher systolic blood pressure in patients with PAH, but there have not been enough patients studied to confirm this finding. Obesity has not been an observed independent risk factor. Splenectomy has been noted as a possible risk factor for PAH, most likely due to loss of the platelet-buffering function and associated thrombocytosis. More than 5% of patients referred to one center for severe PH had a prior splenectomy. Asplenia is associated both with PAH and with chronic thromboembolic PH.[74]

Drugs and Toxins

Appetite Suppressants

The most firmly established risk factor for developing PH is exposure to appetite-suppressant drugs. These drugs are amphetamine-like agents that enhance serotonin release and inhibit serotonin reuptake in the brain, causing appetite suppression. An epidemic of PAH was

TABLE 57-1 PAH RISK FACTORS AND ASSOCIATED CONDITIONS

Factors Associated with the Development of PAH	Factors Not Associated with the Development of PAH
Drugs and Toxins	*Drugs and Toxins*
Aminorex	Antidepressants
Fenfluramine	Oral contraceptives
Dexfenfluramine	Estrogen therapy
Toxic rapeseed oil	Cigarette smoking
Amphetamines	
L-tryptophan	
Meta-amphetamines	
Cocaine	
Chemotherapeutic agent	
Crotalaria plant species	
Demographic and Medical Conditions	*Demographic and Medical Conditions*
Female sex	Obesity
Pregnancy	
Systemic hypertension	
Splenectomy	
Diseases	
HIV infection	
Congenital systemic-to-pulmonary cardiac shunts	
Portal hypertension	
Collagen vascular diseases	
Hereditary hemorrhagic telangiectasia (Osler-Weber-Rendu disease)	
Type 1a glycogen storage disease (von Gierke's disease)	
Lipid storage disorders (Gaucher's disease)	
Hemoglobinopathies (sickle-cell disease, thalassemia, spherocytosis)	
Chronic myeloproliferative disorders	
Thyroid disorders	

PAH, pulmonary arterial hypertension.

attributed to aminorex fumarate use in the late 1960s. More than 60% of the 582 patients with PAH at that time had taken aminorex, but only 0.1% of people who took aminorex developed the disease. A similar outbreak occurred in the 1990s associated with the widespread use of fenfluramine and dexfenfluramine. (In the United States fenfluramine was commonly coprescribed with phentermine, and marketed as "fen/phen.") Aminorex and fenfluramine were withdrawn from the U.S. and European markets.[48] The relative risk of PAH following exposure to fenfluramines is 6, but the risk increases significantly with duration of use, to a 23-fold increase in risk if exposed for greater than 3 months. Some patients, however, developed severe disease even with a short duration of use.[75]

The mechanism by which appetite suppressants cause PAH is unknown. Attempts to reproduce the disease with these agents in laboratory animals have been unsuccessful. Fenfluramine interacts with the serotonin transporter, causes release of serotonin from platelets, and inhibits its reuptake, raising free serotonin concentrations in plasma.[76] As described earlier, activation of the 5-HT receptor type 2B by the dexfenfluramine metabolite may be crucial to the development of PH by this agent.[58] Fenfluramine and aminorex inhibit voltage-gated potassium channels in pulmonary vascular smooth muscle, promoting vasoconstriction. These agents also lower the threshold for platelet activation.

Amphetamines

It is not clear whether isolated exposure to amphetamines can cause PAH. A small number of cases of PAH were reported in association with the sympathomimetic appetite suppressant Amfepramone (diethylpropion) in Belgium between 1995 and 2000.[77] There have been no reported cases of PAH associated with Amfepramone in the United States.[78]

L-Tryptophan

L-tryptophan is a food supplement that has been used to treat a wide range of conditions and has been etiologically associated with eosinophilia-myalgia syndrome. Eosinophilia-myalgia syndrome can develop into a progressive, severe, multisystemic disorder. Descriptions of pulmonary involvement include eosinophilic pneumonitis, vasculitis, interstitial lung disease, and a few cases of PH. Neither the multisystemic presentation nor corresponding biopsy information has demonstrated a strong etiological link to PAH.[74]

Toxic Rapeseed Oil

In 1981 a major epidemic of PAH occurred after rapeseed oil contaminated with aniline dye, intended for industrial use, was sold illegally in Spain. More than 20,000 people developed a multisystemic disease with pneumonitis, myalgias, and eosinophilia, and 20% developed PAH. In most cases the PAH regressed spontaneously, but 2% developed a progressive form that was histologically indistinguishable from IPAH. The toxic rapeseed oil syndrome is also characterized by endothelial damage. The pathogenic products in the aniline dye included fatty acid oleyl anilides and the monoester and diester of 3-phenylamino-1,2-propanediol. There was a higher incidence of progressive PAH among females who consumed the contaminated product.[48]

Other Toxins

PH has been reported in association with inhaled exposure to toluene (glue), methamphetamine, and propylhexedrine, as well as with smoking crack cocaine. A proposed mechanism involves a background of genetic susceptibility to sympathomimetic exposure, with subsequent toxic and hypoxic endothelial injury, vasospasm, vasculitis, and dysregulation of mediators of vascular tone.[79] Cocaine causes stimulation of α-adrenergic receptors on vascular SMCs, inducing increased mRNA and protein synthesis of ET-1, PDGF, and VEGF. This process results in proliferation of SMC and fibroblasts, hypertrophy, and vasoconstriction. It can be difficult to distinguish PAH due to toxin exposure via IV drugs from the other causes of PH associated with IV drug use, particularly emboli, HIV infection, or portal hypertension in the setting of hepatitis C virus.[80] There have been no reported cases of PAH associated with the use of marijuana. Cigarette smoking is the major cause of the most prevalent diseases causing secondary PH, but it is not an independent risk factor for PAH.

Monocrotaline is a pyrrolizidine alkaloid found in *Crotalaria* plants. It is commonly used to induce an inflammatory model of PH in laboratory rats. Jamaican bush tea is made with the seeds and leaves of this plant and has been reported to be associated with a few cases of PAH.[74]

Oral Contraceptives and Estrogen Therapy

An association between estrogen and PAH has been postulated because of the increased prevalence of the disease among women, but epidemiologic data have not confirmed a link with the use of oral contraceptives or hormone replacement therapy.

Antidepressants

Selective serotonin reuptake inhibitors (SSRIs) such as fluoxetine have an effect on serotonin reuptake similar to that of fenfluramine; however, no case of PAH has been reported in association with these widely prescribed drugs. This difference in response suggests that the increase in serotonin availability is not alone sufficient to explain the increased risk of PAH associated with serotonin-modulating appetite suppressants. Another possible explanation may be that, unlike appetite suppressants, SSRIs do not interact with the serotonin transporter.[74]

Diseases

Human Immunodeficiency Virus

First described in 1987, HIV-associated PAH is now a widely recognized, although rare, complication of the infection. Although IV drug use is the primary risk factor, PAH is seen in patients with all routes of HIV infection.

There is no observed correlation between PAH and the degree of immunosuppression or presence of opportunistic infections. HIV-associated PAH is more aggressive and fatal than IPAH, with a 1-year survival rate, if untreated, of 51% compared with 68% in IPAH.[80]

Only an estimated 0.5% of HIV-infected individuals develop PAH, again demonstrating the requirement for individual susceptibility to this disease. Mutations in the BMPR2 gene have not been found in HIV-associated PAH. The histopathology of HIV-associated PAH is similar to other forms of PAH. Pulmonary veno-occlusive disease is also seen in some HIV-infected individuals. PAH has been diagnosed in patients with HIV in the absence of other risk factors; thus it seems likely that the pulmonary arteriopathy is due to the HIV infection itself. The mechanism of PAH in HIV infection is unknown. HIV does not directly infect the endothelium. It probably acts indirectly through mediator release and through the production of cytokines. HIV may also alter the metabolism of vasoactive mediators in the lung, favoring a vasoconstrictive phenotype. Small studies have suggested a possible genetic polymorphism expressed in specific human leukocyte antigen class II alleles in HIV-associated PAH compared with HIV-infected controls.[80] A recent retrospective study concluded that the most important prognostic factors for survival in HIV-associated PAH are a CD4 lymphocyte count of more than 212 cells/mm^3, the use of combined antiretroviral therapy, and treatment with epoprostenol.[81]

Persistent Pulmonary Hypertension of the Newborn

Fetal circulation is characterized by a high PVR. Because fetal lungs do not supply oxygen, the circulation shunts blood away from the lungs by intense vasoconstriction of small pulmonary arteries. Normally with the first breath, expansion of the lungs and increased PO_2 cause an abrupt drop in PVR. Pulmonary artery pressure drops to 50% of systemic pressures by 24 hours of life and approaches normal adult values (<15% of systemic pressures) by 4 weeks. Persistent PH of the newborn is characterized by persistent elevation of PVR, right-to-left shunting, and severe hypoxemia. It can occur with pulmonary parenchymal diseases including sepsis, meconium aspiration, pneumonia, maladaptation of the pulmonary vascular bed, or without an apparent cause. Persistent PH in newborns may lead to death during the neonatal period, or it may be transient, leading to spontaneous and complete recovery.[9]

Inadequate production of NO may be an important contributor to persistent PH in infants. NO is critical in the transition to a pulmonary circulation at birth and in subsequent regulation of PVR. Endothelial cells generate NO from its precursor L-arginine, and Pearson and colleagues[82] demonstrated lower plasma concentrations of arginine and NO metabolites in neonates with PH compared with controls.

Congenital Systemic-to-Pulmonary Shunts (Eisenmenger's Syndrome)

Congenital heart defects with systemic-to-pulmonary shunts and high pulmonary blood flow at high pressure induce progressive PAH with impaired growth of pulmonary arteries and a loss of surface area in the pulmonary arteriolar bed. Pulmonary vascular disease caused by a congenital heart defect with communication between the pulmonary and systemic circulations is called Eisenmenger's syndrome. It develops after a hyperkinetic period with increased pulmonary blood flow but normal PVR. Increased pulmonary blood flow will cause an initial decrease in PVR to maintain PAP at normal levels; however, if pulmonary blood flow is increased beyond the capacity of the pulmonary vascular bed to compensate, PAP will rise. Eisenmenger's syndrome is usually caused by atrial or ventricular septal defects or a patent ductus arteriosus. The risk of developing Eisenmenger's syndrome depends on the size and location of the intracardiac defect, the magnitude of the shunt, and individual susceptibility factors. PAH develops in 50% of patients with a large (>1.5-cm diameter) ventricular septal defect or patent ductus arteriosus and in 10% of those with an atrial septal defect.[81]

The prognosis in Eisenmenger's syndrome is substantially better than in other forms of PAH. Median survival reported at one center with 109 patients was 53 years of age.[83] The progression of pulmonary vascular remodeling may be slower in this disease, allowing time for the RV to adapt to increasing vascular resistance. Another explanation for better survival is preservation of right ventricular wall thickness in congenital heart disease in contrast to the normal loss of muscularization in the adult RV. The shunt itself also plays a protective role; it unloads right ventricular strain and preserves left ventricular CO by maintaining left ventricular (LV) filling, preventing the hypertrophied RV from obstructing LV outflow.[83]

Approximately one third of patients with uncorrected congenital heart disease die from PAH. The decision to repair a defect surgically is difficult, because it is challenging to identify those patients who will have persistent disease following surgery, and surgical risk may be prohibitive. Therefore it is crucial to determine the degree of reversibility of vascular disease before surgical correction. Congenital heart disease is one of the few conditions in which information gained from tissue examination is likely to alter clinical decision-making, and biopsies are commonly used for this indication. Reversibility can usually be predicted if the remodeling changes are limited to early medial hypertrophy and vasoconstriction; irreversibility of PAH is associated with arteritis and plexiform lesions. The timing of surgical repair also influences the outcome. If the shunt is repaired within the first 8 months of life, patients tend to have normal pulmonary pressures regardless of pathologic findings; by contrast, patients operated on after age 2 tend to have persistent PAH. As an alternative to surgical biopsy, pulmonary arteriograms can be used to estimate structural changes: wedge angiography can demonstrate the rate of tapering of arteries and predict the severity of structural disease and the probability of postoperative improvement in pulmonary pressures. Importantly, when PVR equals or exceeds systemic vascular resistance, surgical correction of a shunt will increase the load on an already overburdened RV, worsen the clinical condition of the patient, and not reverse PAH.[84]

The development of PAH in congenital heart disease is multifactorial. Pathologic studies have indicated that PAH may be present from birth, or it may develop later in some patients. Shear stress due to increased pulmonary blood flow seems to play a greater role in congenital heart disease–related PAH than in other types of PAH. However, in some children, PAH-like lesions have been seen in patients without a significant left-to-right shunt, suggesting an idiopathic type of PAH. Pathologic findings also vary according to the age of the child. In younger children, there is a failure of the neonatal vasculature to open and a reduction in arterial number. Older children tend to demonstrate intimal hyperplasia and occlusive changes in arterioles, as well as plexiform lesions, which are notably absent in infants.

Hereditary Hemorrhagic Telangiectasia

Please see earlier discussion.

Portal Hypertension

Portal hypertension is an important cause of PAH. Approximately 9% of patients with severe PAH are reported to have portal hypertension. Portopulmonary hypertension is defined as PAH associated with portal hypertension (portal pressure > 10 mm Hg), with or without hepatic disease. Because patients with nonhepatic causes of portal hypertension have been reported with this entity, it appears that it is the portal hypertension and not cirrhosis that triggers the development of PH. The mechanism of portopulmonary hypertension is unknown. Patients with portal hypertension may develop PH from an inability of the liver to metabolize serotonin and other vasoactive substances. The shear stress from increased pulmonary blood flow may result in endothelial injury, triggering a cascade of events that result in the characteristic adverse remodeling as described earlier.[85]

PH affects 4% to 6% of patients referred for liver transplantation. Liver transplantation perioperative mortality is significantly increased in patients with a mean PAP greater than 35 mm Hg.[86] The diagnosis of PH is usually made 4 to 7 years after the diagnosis of portal hypertension, but it has occasionally been reported to precede the onset of portal hypertension. The risk of PH increases with duration of disease. The correlation between the severity of portal hypertension and development of PH is debated. The female predominance of IPAH is not seen in portopulmonary hypertension. Survival is much worse than in PAH of other causes, with a median survival of 6 months.[85]

Collagen Vascular Diseases

PAH has been reported in association with every type of collagen vascular disease, most commonly with scleroderma. PAH is clinically apparent in up to 10% of patients with collagen vascular disease, and histopathologic changes consistent with PAH are present at autopsy in up to 80% of individuals.[87] PAH and coincident collagen vascular disease has a much worse prognosis than either diagnosis alone. Scleroderma is a progressive, multisystem disease variably involving the vasculature and connective tissue of the skin, gastrointestinal tract, kidney, heart, and lung. Pulmonary manifestations include interstitial fibrosis, constriction of the chest wall, chronic aspiration due to esophageal dysmotility, and PAH.

PH can result from severe interstitial fibrosis-induced vascular obliteration, renal crisis, or cardiomyopathy with diastolic dysfunction. In the diffuse form of systemic scleroderma, these secondary causes of PH predominate. PAH is more common in the limited cutaneous form of systemic sclerosis, also described as CREST (Calcinosis, Raynaud's phenomenon, Esophageal dysmotility, Sclerodactyly, Telangiectasias), than in frank scleroderma (systemic sclerosis). In this context PAH does not occur with interstitial fibrosis and is pathologically similar to IPAH.[87] After ACE inhibitor therapy was shown to improve survival from renal crisis in scleroderma, PAH became the leading cause of death in CREST patients.[88] PAH has been reported in approximately 10% to 30% of patients with mixed connective tissue disease, 5% to 10% of patients with systemic lupus erythematosus, and more rarely in the settings of rheumatoid arthritis, dermatomyositis, and polymyositis. Sjögren's syndrome may rarely be complicated by rapidly progressive PAH. It is particularly important to distinguish between PAH and thromboembolic PH in patients with systemic lupus erythematosus and antiphospholipid syndrome.[89]

Thyroid Disease

PAH has been associated with hyperthyroidism, hypothyroidism, and the presence of antithyroglobulin antibodies on the basis of case reports and retrospective studies. Chu and colleagues[90] hypothesized that autoimmune thyroid disease and PAH may have a shared immunogenetic cause and demonstrated the presence of autoimmune thyroid disease in approximately one half of their patients with PAH, on the basis of a prospective observational study of 63 adults. Nearly 30% of the patients were newly diagnosed. There was an equal distribution of hyperthyroid, hypothyroid, and euthyroid patients.[90]

Platelet Storage Pool Diseases

As discussed earlier, PAH has been reported in patients with abnormal platelet serotonin storage including type 1a glycogen storage (von Gierke's disease) and platelet delta storage pool disease.

Chronic Myeloproliferative Disorders

Several studies have demonstrated an association between the chronic myeloproliferative disorders (CMPD) (polycythemia vera, essential thrombocythemia, and myelofibrosis with myeloid metaplasia) and the development of PAH. A cohort study of patients with CMPD from the Mayo Clinic revealed that the annual incidence of PAH in this population is approximately 1 to 8 cases per 100,000, which is much greater than the 0.2 cases per 100,000 population observed for idiopathic PAH, suggesting an etiologic link.

Platelets appear to be central to the pathogenesis of PH related to CMPD. Most cases are associated with thrombocytosis; moreover, treatment to reduce platelet counts resulted in improvements in PAP in some patients. Platelets stimulate smooth muscle hyperplasia via the release of factors such as serotonin and PDGF, and by this mechanism may contribute to medial hypertrophy of the pulmonary arterioles. Additionally, patients with CMPD are hypercoagulable with a known increased propensity for both arterial and venous thromboses. Microthrombi in the pulmonary vasculature likely occurs in these patients with a resultant increase in PAP. Additionally, in one study, there was evidence of direct obstruction of pulmonary arterioles by circulating megakaryocytes in these patients. The relatively high incidence of portal hypertension in patients with myelofibrosis with myeloid metaplasia (up to 17% in one series) suggests that PH may result from mechanisms similar to those causing portopulmonary hypertension.[91]

Overall, the prognosis for patients with PH related to CMPD is poor, with a median survival time of 18 months. Death is caused by PH and right heart failure in approximately 50%. Although some patients have improved PAP with treatment of thrombocytosis, many do not, suggesting that once it develops, the course of PH is independent of the underlying CMPD.[91] Further study of this disease entity is necessary to clarify the pathogenesis of PH related to CMPD and investigate possible treatment options for these patients.

PATHOPHYSIOLOGY

The pulmonary vascular bed has a remarkable capacity to dilate and recruit unperfused vessels, adapting easily to large increases in blood flow. In PAH these properties are lost. Right ventricular function is highly afterload dependent and works less efficiently with increases in PVR. With increased afterload, the RV hypertrophies and dilates. In the early stages of PAH, resting PAP remains normal and cardiac output is maintained, but with exercise PAP becomes abnormally high and the RV is unable to increase CO. With progressive PH there may eventually be a decrease in the measured PAP due to a decrease in CO, while the PVR remains elevated. Cardiac function is characterized by RV systolic and diastolic overload from tricuspid regurgitation. The left ventricle is not directly affected by pulmonary vascular disease, but when PAP rises to the extent that the RV changes from its normal crescentic shape to expand into the left ventricle, it can impair LV filling, increase LV end diastolic pressure, and decrease CO, a phenomenon described as the "reverse Bernheim effect."

The two most frequent causes of death in PAH are progressive RV failure and sudden death. RV failure may be exacerbated by pneumonia, because alveolar hypoxia can cause further vasoconstriction and greater impairment of CO. Sudden death may be caused by arrhythmias that arise in the setting of hypoxemia and acidosis, acute pulmonary emboli, massive pulmonary hemorrhage, and sudden subendocardial RV ischemia.[9]

DIAGNOSTIC EVALUATION

Initial Approach

There is no pathognomonic finding in PAH; thus the diagnosis is one of exclusion. A thorough evaluation must be performed to reveal potentially contributing factors, including causes of secondary forms of PH that require a different treatment approach. It is important to probe for a family history of PH, early unexplained deaths, congenital heart disease, and collagen vascular disease. A thorough history should also include all associated risk factors of PH to uncover a possible explanation for the onset of PAH and exclude secondary causes of PH. A functional assessment should be made on the basis of the New York Heart Association (NYHA/WHO) functional classification of heart failure, which was adopted for PAH at the WHO-sponsored symposium.[6] In addition to a comprehensive history, the diagnostic evaluation should include physical examination, exercise capacity testing (e.g., 6-minute walk), chest radiograph, electrocardiography, pulmonary function tests, arterial blood gas and other blood tests, noninvasive cardiac and pulmonary imaging, and cardiac catheterization with measurement of response to vasodilator administration (Fig. 57-3).

Symptoms

PAH has no early symptoms or signs. By the time patients develop symptoms, PAH is usually advanced and CO is reduced. The nonspecific nature of presenting symptoms causes a long delay in diagnosis in most patients. The mean interval from the onset of symptoms to diagnosis was 2 years in the NIH Registry.[8] The most common presenting symptom is dyspnea on exertion, which affects nearly 100% of patients as the disease progresses. Other presenting symptoms include fatigue, syncope or near syncope, chest pain, lower extremity edema, or palpitations.[8] Dyspnea is caused by impaired oxygen delivery during exercise due to the inability to increase CO with increased oxygen demand. Syncope occurs when CO is severely limited and inadequate cerebral blood flow with exertion ensues. Chest pain in PAH is caused by subendocardial RV ischemia.

Physical Findings

Clinical findings in PAH are initially subtle. The first signs of disease may be a right ventricular heave, a loud pulmonic second heart sound, and a right-sided fourth heart sound. Eventually a right-sided third heart sound and a left parasternal systolic murmur of tricuspid regurgitation may be audible. The findings of jugular venous distension, ascites, and peripheral edema indicate overt right heart failure. Physical examination must include evaluation for signs associated with specific diseases associated with PAH, including collagen vascular disease, liver disease, HIV, HHT, thyroid disease, and all secondary causes of PH.

Laboratory Studies

Secondary causes of PAH should be sought with serology for HIV and collagen vascular diseases, liver function

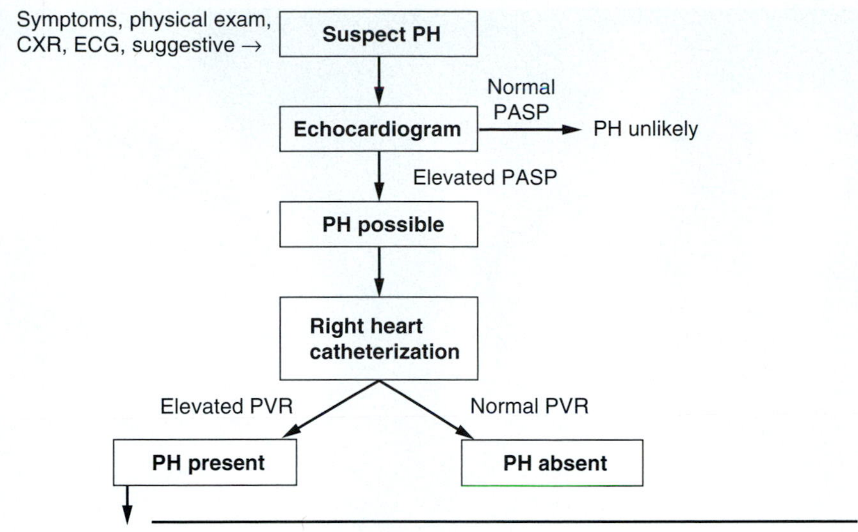

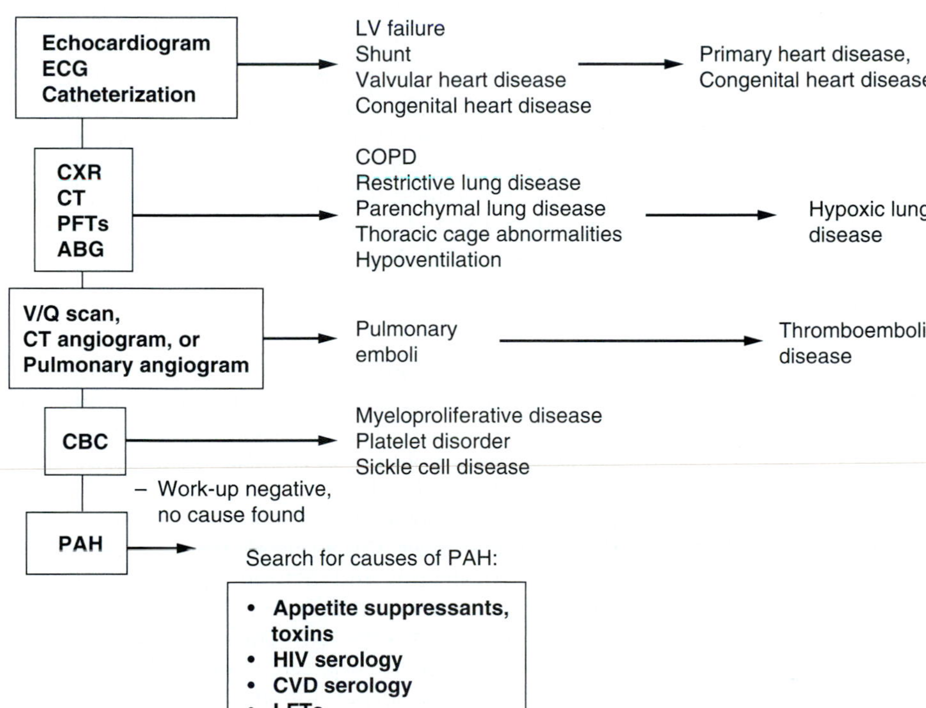

FIGURE 57-3. Diagnostic evaluation for suspected pulmonary arterial hypertension. Please refer to Chapter 58 for a discussion of secondary causes of pulmonary hypertension. ABG, arterial blood gas; CBC, complete blood count; COPD, chronic obstructive pulmonary disease; CPET, cardiopulmonary exercise test; CT, computed tomography scan; CVD, collagen vascular disease; LFTs, liver function tests; LV, left ventricle; PASP, pulmonary arterial systolic pressure; PFTs, pulmonary function tests; PVR, pulmonary vascular resistance; V/Q scan, ventilation and perfusion nucleotide scan.

tests (LFTs), and toxic exposures. Thyroid function should be evaluated. Thrombocytopenia may be present in severe PAH and has multiple contributing causes, including platelet activation and aggregation, pulmonary vascular sequestration, hepatosplenomegaly with splenic sequestration, as well as an autoimmune-mediated syndrome similar to idiopathic thrombocytopenic purpura.[92] Thrombocytopenia may accompany microangiopathic hemolysis when blood flows through fibrin deposits in plexiform lesions with subsequent shearing of red blood cells and platelets. Prostacyclin may also induce thrombocytopenia.[62] Thrombocytosis may be present in patients following splenectomy.

In patients with PH, high levels of atrial natriuretic peptide (ANP) and brain natriuretic peptide (BNP) parallel decreased RV function. Levels of both peptides decrease with prostacyclin treatment and ensuing hemodynamic improvement. A subsequent increase in plasma BNP has been demonstrated to be an independent predictor of mortality.[93]

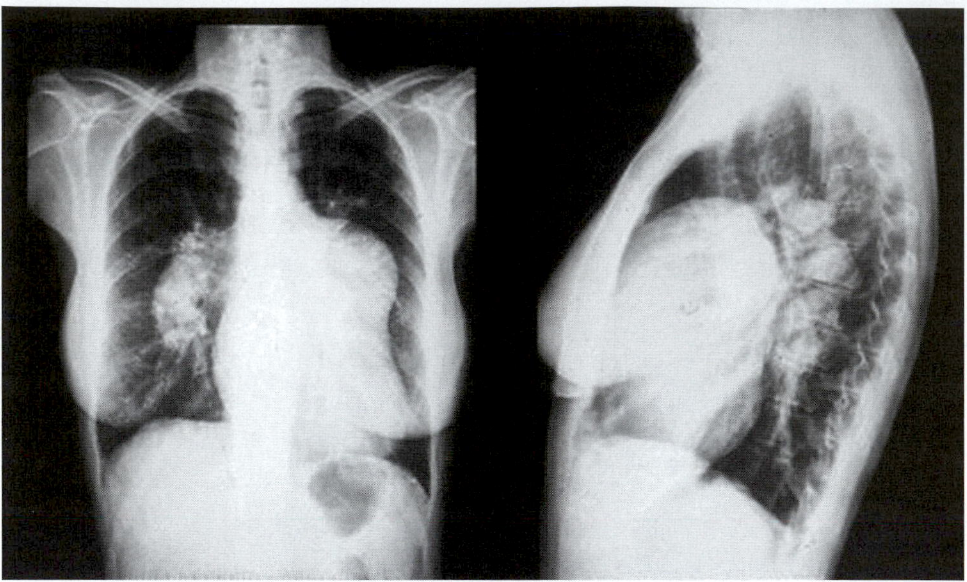

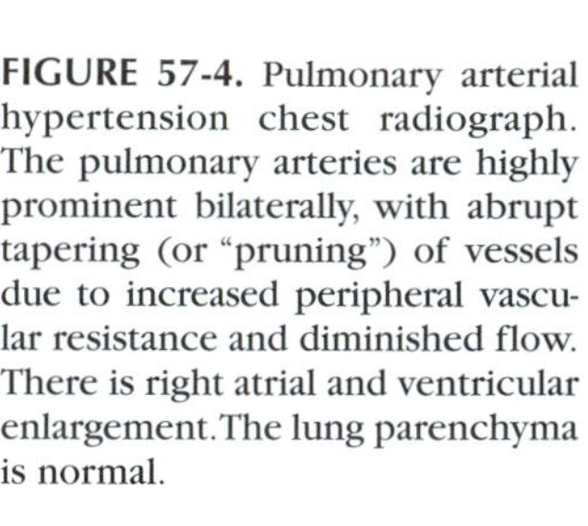

FIGURE 57-4. Pulmonary arterial hypertension chest radiograph. The pulmonary arteries are highly prominent bilaterally, with abrupt tapering (or "pruning") of vessels due to increased peripheral vascular resistance and diminished flow. There is right atrial and ventricular enlargement. The lung parenchyma is normal.

Radiographic Studies

Chest radiographs in PH usually show an enlarged pulmonary trunk and hilar pulmonary arteries, pruning of peripheral vessels, and obliteration of the retrosternal clear space by the enlarged RV (Fig. 57-4). Occasionally the chest radiograph may appear normal.[8] High-resolution CT is used to evaluate the lung parenchyma for interstitial lung disease. Helical CT is used to evaluate the central pulmonary arteries for the presence of thrombi. Ventilation/perfusion scans are used to search for chronic pulmonary thromboemboli (see Fig. 57-4). In patients with PAH these scans are normal or show only patchy defects. If inconclusive, a pulmonary angiogram, which will show pruning of peripheral vessels in PAH, must be performed to definitively exclude thromboembolic disease. The use of pulmonary MRA has not been widely reported but has recently been shown to identify patients with PAH with high sensitivity and negative predictive values.[93]

Electrocardiogram

The ECG may provide hints to the presence of PAH, but it is not a sensitive or specific screening tool. In advanced disease the ECG usually shows signs of right heart strain and enlargement, including right axis deviation and evidence of right ventricular hypertrophy. The presence of a conduction abnormality is not typical of PAH. Electrocardiographic evidence of right heart strain has been associated with decreased survival.[5]

Pulmonary Function Tests

Pulmonary function tests (PFTs) are important in excluding secondary causes of PH, particularly chronic obstructive airways disease. Airway obstruction is not typical of PAH, although cases of bronchial obstruction due to enlarged pulmonary arteries have been reported. PAH patients typically demonstrate borderline restrictive physiology, a reduced diffusing capacity for carbon monoxide (DLCO), and hypoxemia with hypocapnea.[8] The reduction in DLCO results from the reduced blood volume in the alveolar capillaries. A recent study of pulmonary function in 79 patients presenting with PAH demonstrated a significantly reduced DLCO (mean 68% of predicted values) in 75% of patients and mild restrictive physiology in 50%.[94]

Echocardiography

Transthoracic echocardiography is a crucial diagnostic tool in evaluating patients for PH. It can determine the presence of left-sided heart disease, valvular disease, and intracardiac shunts, and it allows the noninvasive measurement of elevated PAP. A finding of an abnormal PAP must be further evaluated with pulmonary artery catheterization. Echocardiography of PAH patients frequently shows RV hypertrophy and dilation, right atrial enlargement, and a decrease in the size of the LV cavity due to bowing of the interventricular septum in advanced disease. The inferior vena cava, too, is distended and does not collapse during inspiration in advanced disease.[95] Systolic PAP can be estimated using Doppler measurement of the tricuspid regurgitant flow velocity. The upper limit of normal systolic PAP is generally considered 40 to 50 mm Hg at rest, corresponding to a tricuspid regurgitant velocity of 3 to 3.5 m/s (although this value varies with age, body mass index, and right atrial pressure). Limitations to Doppler measurement of PAP do exist, however. Studies have documented false-negative examinations in patients with poor-quality views or moderate elevations in PAP. Although interobserver variability has been reported to be less than 5%, Doppler estimates of pressures are operator dependent. Studies comparing Doppler-derived PAP values with pressures determined by catheterization yield varying results, with some reporting underestimation of systolic PAP by Doppler.[93] Echocardiography is probably best employed for its negative predictive value. In high-risk patients, echocardiography should be performed annually.

Exercise echocardiography is a more sensitive test for the presence of early PAH, which is particularly valuable in pediatric cases in which it may influence decisions regarding surgery. Exercise echocardiography has been studied as a screening tool to identify asymptomatic carriers of a mutated BMPR2 in PAH families. In two German families with PAH, all family members with a pathologic rise in PAP during exercise were carriers of the mutated gene. In that study, exercise echocardiography had a sensitivity of 87.5% and a specificity of 100%.[96]

A resting echocardiogram or cardiac catheterization demonstrating normal PA pressure usually excludes a diagnosis of PH. However, when PAS is strongly suspected, or a patient has unexplained dyspnea, exercise echocardiography or catheterization performed during exercise may reveal exercise-induced PAH.

Cardiac Catheterization

Cardiac catheterization remains the "gold standard" for establishing the diagnosis and type of PH. This procedure can directly measure right heart and PA pressures, as well as pulmonary capillary wedge pressure and CO. It can also be used to assess the vasodilation reserve (see explanation later in the section on vasodilator therapy) and is the major determinant in prognosis of PH. Cardiac catheterization can also be performed with exercise to assess the possibility of exercise-induced PH, in which the resting PAP is normal but PAP during exercise is abnormally high.

Exercise Testing

Exercise testing is not required for a diagnosis of PH, but it may provide valuable information regarding prognosis. The most widely used exercise test, and the most reproducible, is the 6-minute walk test. This test is usually done after the diagnosis is confirmed by cardiac catheterization and at regular intervals to monitor functional status. The distance walked in 6 minutes has been shown to decrease in proportion to the NYHA functional class and is a strong, independent predictor of mortality. Patients with PAH who walked 300 or more meters and decreased arterial oxygen saturation by 10% at maximal distance had a significantly increased mortality.[93] Maximal exercise testing must be avoided, as syncope and sudden death have been reported. Cardiopulmonary exercise testing has been used in research studies but is not routinely used in practice.

Screening

It is unknown whether early treatment of PAH changes progression of disease. It seems plausible that treating patients during a period of reversible pathogenic events would reverse or stabilize the disease and prevent or slow the onset of RV failure, although this has not been proved. Whatever its cause, PH tends to become self-perpetuating because increased resistance in vessels will compound the initial injury with further increases in shear stress. Screening should be performed in asymptomatic patients at high risk for PAH, although the exact population recommended for screening is controversial because the prevalence of disease is low even in categories of patients at increased risk. Screening asymptomatic or minimally symptomatic patients should begin with a thorough history and physical examination to elicit symptoms or signs consistent with PH, followed by diagnostic testing if inconclusive. The transthoracic echocardiogram is the best noninvasive test used for screening patients.

The WHO PAH symposium recommended echocardiographic screening for patients with scleroderma or with any decline in respiratory status annually. Annual screening is also recommended for all patients with portal hypertension who are being evaluated for liver transplantation. As discussed earlier, perioperative mortality is significantly increased in patients with portal hypertension and PH. Echocardiography is accurate in excluding the diagnosis. If echocardiographic findings are positive, right heart catheterization is required to confirm the presence of PH, because patients with portal hypertension due to cirrhosis are predisposed to elevated right-sided pressures from a hyperdynamic circulation and increased intravascular volume. Patients with portopulmonary hypertension are frequently asymptomatic from a pulmonary perspective.[86]

Families of patients with IPAH should undergo echocardiography at the time of the diagnosis and subsequently every 3 to 5 years or whenever symptoms arise. Patients with PAH and their families should be evaluated for the presence of HHT, and families with mutations in Alk1 and endoglin should undergo screening for PAH as recommended for FPAH. The optimal screening method for asymptomatic family members is uncertain. As described earlier, exercise echocardiography is a more sensitive test than resting echocardiography for revealing carriers of a mutated BMPR2 gene and it may prove to be a sufficient screening modality. The following groups of patients should be evaluated for PAH only if they present with symptoms suggestive of the disease: those with collagen vascular disease other than scleroderma, HIV, IV drug users, patients exposed to appetite-suppressant drugs, and patients with portal hypertension who are not being considered for transplantation.[6]

Genetic Testing

The risk for disease in first-degree relatives of a patient with PAH is low, which has led to uncertainty in screening their family members. Before the identification of BMPR2 mutations, the risk of asymptomatic family members was estimated to be 5% to 10%. If DNA of the patient is available, analysis of BMPR2 can be used to determine the risk to relatives. Genetic testing requires DNA sequencing of the proband, because mutations of BMPR2 are unique to each family. If no BMPR2 mutation is found, the patient is diagnosed with sporadic PAH and the risk to other family members is only marginally increased over that in the general population. If a BMPR2 mutation is found, relatives can be tested for the presence of a mutation. If available, this information should probably be offered to family members of patients with PAH until other screening methods are more extensively studied. Importantly, the results of genetic testing might lead to confusion. If family members have not inherited the mutation, their risk is low. If they have inherited the mutation, there is still an approximately 80% chance that they will not develop the disease phenotype, given the low penetrance of disease. Genetic testing may result in detrimental psychological, employment, and insurance effects and must be supported by appropriate genetic counseling.

Screening asymptomatic individuals enhances our knowledge of the prevalence of FPAH and may shed light on whether early treatment influences the pathogenesis of disease. Screening also allows at-risk individuals to be aware of known risks that theoretically may augment penetrance of the disease.[59]

Disease Course

The NIH Registry reflects the natural course of untreated disease because it was completed before the widespread use of vasodilator therapy. It reported a median survival of 2.8 years, with single-year survival rates of 68% at 1 year, 48% at 3 years, and 34% at 5 years.[5] Prognosis is related to RV function. Worse prognosis correlated with NYHA functional classification, the distance walked during the 6-minute walk test, the mean right atrial pressure, cardiac index, and systemic arterial and mixed oxygen saturation.[93] Other markers of earlier mortality in the NIH Registry included lower DLCO and the presence of Raynaud's phenomenon.[5] Echocardiographic predictors of adverse outcomes in PAH include pericardial effusion (which is more common in NYHA class IV), right atrial enlargement, septal displacement, and poor RV function.[93]

TREATMENT

There is no known cure for PAH. Until the development of vasodilating agents over the past 15 years, a diagnosis of PAH was invariably fatal. Current therapeutic options have dramatically changed the survival and quality of life for patients with PAH. The approach to treatment is based on what is known about the physiology and pathobiology of the disease (Fig. 57-5). The mainstays of treatment include anticoagulation and vasodilating drugs. Oxygen should be administered if hypoxemia is present. It is not clear whether PAH patients in functional class II benefit from vasodilating therapy rather than witholding treatment and monitoring for disease progression.

General Measures

Avoiding circumstances and substances that exacerbate the disease is important. Any behavior that increases oxygen demand or CO can worsen PH and RV failure.

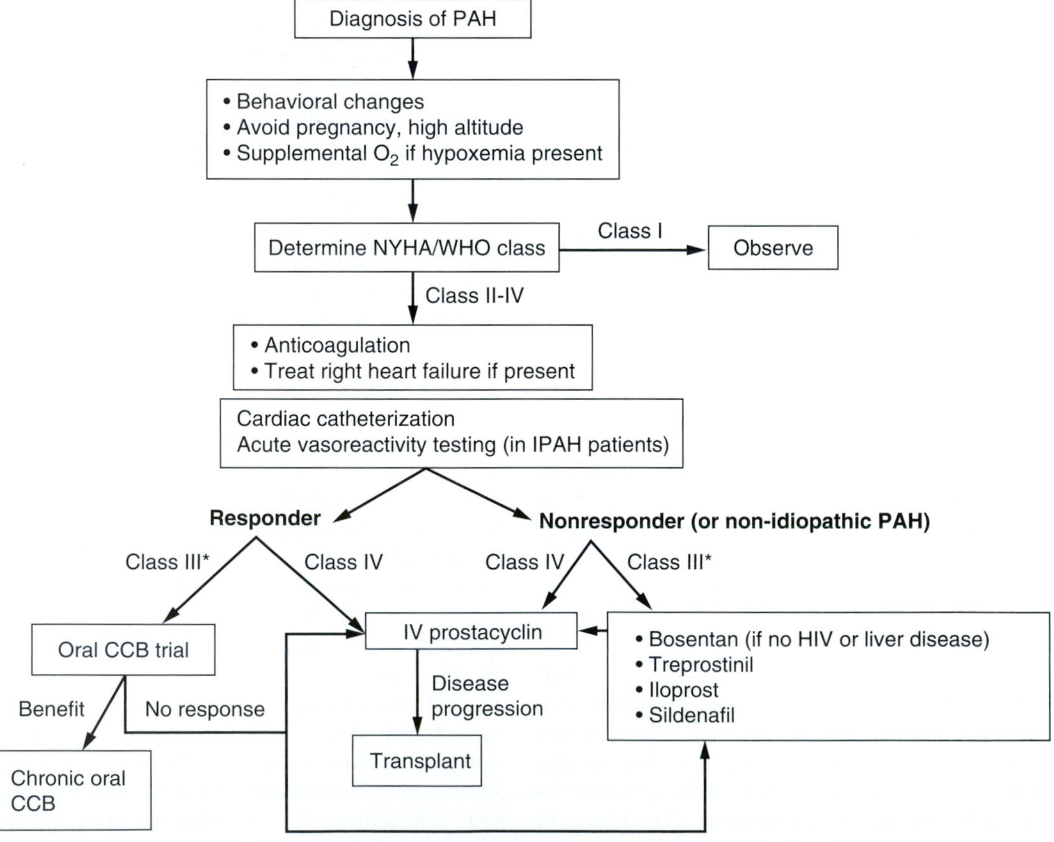

FIGURE 57-5. Algorithm for treatment of pulmonary arterial hypertension. CCB, calcium-channel blockers. *PAH patients in functional class II may be included. The natural course of disease in patients diagnosed at this early stage is unknown. Therefore, it is unclear whether these patients benefit from early vasodilating therapy rather than monitoring for disease progression.

Heavy physical exertion should be avoided. High altitude and nonpressurized airplane cabins can induce hypoxia and hypoxia-induced PH. Supplemental oxygen should be used if it is necessary for the patient to be exposed to high altitude. PAH is one of the true contraindications to pregnancy, because it may precipitate fatal right heart failure. Oral contraceptives are theoretically contraindicated due to the increased risk of hypercoagulability causing thromboembolic PH, although they are often used in nonsmoking women with PAH without a history of thromboembolic disease.

Anticoagulation

Anticoagulation has been incorporated into the treatment of PAH on the basis of the presence of thrombosis in small PAs, the risk of compounding PAH with a thromboembolic component, and the increased risk of deep venous thrombosis in the setting of a low CO. There is no controlled trial of anticoagulation in PAH, but it is used on the basis of the improved survival of patients who received warfarin in three small studies, two retrospective[97,98] and one prospective.[99] The optimal dose of warfarin was not determined in these studies. The usual recommended range is an international normalized ratio of 2 to 2.5. Although prostacyclin inhibits platelet aggregation, additional anticoagulation is usually used in the absence of a contraindication. Because patients with congenital systemic-to-pulmonary shunts are at greater risk for hemoptysis, some practitioners do not recommend anticoagulation in those cases.[62]

Oxygen Therapy

Use of supplemental oxygen therapy should be considered in patients with hypoxemia at rest (PaO2 < 55 mm Hg or SaO_2 < 88%). Shunt-induced hypoxemia in patients with patent foramen ovale or intracardiac shunt is refractory to supplemental oxygen therapy. A controlled trial has not been performed, but oxygen therapy can improve the quality of life by improving dyspnea and exercise capacity, although oxygen equipment can limit mobility. Supplemental oxygen treatment should be decided on a case-by-case basis.

Treatment of Right Heart Failure

Diuretics are used to reduce intravascular volume and hepatic congestion. Cautious use of loop and thiazide diuretics may be required for adequate management. Overdiuresis must be avoided, however, as it can impair CO by decreasing RV preload. Digoxin is generally not used in PAH except for rate control of arrhythmias.[100] IV dobutamine and dopamine may acutely improve symptoms of right heart failure, although they are not feasible as chronic agents and the long-term effects are unknown.

Vasodilator Therapy

The scientific rationale for vasodilator therapy was based on the finding of abnormal vasoactive mediators in patients with PAH. Patients who are likely to respond are identified by their acute response to vasodilating drugs. The most widely used drugs for acute vasoreactivity testing include inhaled NO and IV prostacyclin (epoprostenol), adenosine, and iloprost, a prostacyclin analog with less effect on the systemic vasculature. NO has several advantages, including kinetic specificity for the pulmonary vasculature, early peak effect at 5 to 10 minutes, easier mode of delivery, and lower cost. The recommended dose is 10 parts per million. Because inhaled NO has no systemic effects, the acute drop in PVR reflects the pulmonary vasodilatory capacity. A significant response to vasodilator testing is generally accepted as a drop in PVR by greater than 25%.

Other parameters used include a greater than 20% decrease in systolic PAP, a greater than 10-mm Hg drop in mean PAP, or an increase in cardiac index by greater than or equal to 30%. Testing more than one drug offers no advantage. Vasodilator challenge must be performed with care as drug-induced systemic hypotension (such as with prostacyclin) may reduce RV coronary blood flow and cause RV ischemia. Most studies on PAH report the proportion of responders to vasodilators as between 12% and 25%. There is no particular clinical or disease characteristic that reliably predicts vasodilator response. The lack of response to acute vasodilators predicts the response to oral vasodilator therapy (i.e., nonresponders to inhaled NO do not respond to oral calcium-channel blockers). Response to acute vasodilators, however, does *not* predict a response to prostacyclin. A trial of long-term calcium-channel blocker therapy is usually recommended in PAH patients who respond to vasodilator challenge with a decrease in PVR of greater than or equal to 50%.[93]

Calcium-Channel Blockers

Calcium-channel blockers are the oral drugs of choice for treating patients who have a significant response to acute vasodilators. These agents have been shown to improve hemodynamics, RV function, and survival in a small minority (<25%) of patients with PAH.[99,101,102] Both nifedipine and diltiazem are effective. The choice between these two drugs is guided by resting heart rate; if the heart rate is greater than 80 beats/min, diltiazem is usually used for initial therapy. The doses of these drugs required to lower PVR are much higher than those used for other indications (up to 240 mg/day of nifedipine or 960 mg/day of diltiazem), which makes systemic side effects a significant problem, particularly systemic hypotension and lower extremity edema. Verapamil is not used because of its greater negative inotropic effects. Acute administration of amlodipine causes pulmonary vasodilation, but its long-term efficacy has not been studied.[100]

Prostacyclin and Prostacyclin Analogs

Epoprostenol

Prostacyclin is a prostaglandin (prostaglandin I_2) produced from arachidonic acid in vascular endothelial and SMCs. It causes vasodilation and inhibits platelet aggregation. It also has antiproliferative and weak fibrinolytic activities. Prostacyclin acts by increasing intracellular cyclic adenosine monophosphate (AMP) levels through activation of adenylyl cyclase. IV prostacyclin (epoprostenol or Flolan) was first used to treat PAH in the early 1980s. Since then, multiple trials of epoprostenol have demonstrated improved survival, exercise capacity, and hemodynamics in patients with PAH compared with conventional treatment.[5,103,104] Epoprostenol was approved for use in PAH by the United States Food and Drug Administration (FDA) in 1995 and is now considered the treatment of choice in patients with NYHA/WHO class IV PAH and is an alternative to lung transplantation. McLaughlin and colleagues[105] treated 162 PAH patients with epoprostenol and reported improved survival rates at 1, 2, and 3 years of 88%, 76%, and 63%, respectively, compared with the expected survival rates of 59%, 46%, and 35% based on historical controls. A remodeling effect of epoprostenol has been suggested by several findings: Patients who have no acute response may demonstrate a delayed hemodynamic improvement, hemodynamic improvement increases in patients who show an initial response, and RV dysfunction improves after long-term therapy.[95]

Epoprostenol has an extremely short half-life (approximately 3 to 6 minutes) and must be administered through a central venous catheter. The patient must reconstitute the medication from powder form, and it must be kept cold, requiring use of a cold pack with a pump. Long-term dose requirements are highly variable among patients. Selecting the appropriate dose requires striking a balance between hemodynamic and symptomatic improvements on the one hand and side effects of the drug on the other. Common side effects include jaw pain, headache, diarrhea, flushing, leg pain, nausea, and vomiting. Epoprostenol is started in the hospital, employing a PA catheter, with continuous monitoring. Initiation of epoprostenol can lead to increased CO with LV strain, or isolated pulmonary edema, with rapid clinical deterioration. Dose initiation is variable, but one method is a starting dose of 2 ng/kg/min increasing by 2 ng/kg/min every 15 minutes, depending on patient tolerance, until 10 ng/kg/min is reached. Some clinicians continue the dose escalation until limited by side effects or until there is a plateau in the hemodynamic response. The patient is then discharged from the hospital, and further dose increases are made on an outpatient setting on the basis of clinical symptoms, exercise testing, and hemodynamic measurements. The major limitations to use of epoprostenol include the need for permanent central venous access with the associated small risk of catheter-related infection or air embolism, the capacity to handle the catheter and pump, and the extremely high cost of the drug (approximately $125,000 per patient per year). Patients also tend to develop tachyphylaxis to epoprostenol over time.[100]

Prostacyclin Analogs: Treprostinil, Iloprost, and Beraprost

The complexities of epoprostenol administration have led investigators to search for alternative agents. Prostacyclin analogs, treprostinil, iloprost, and beraprost were tested in 12-week placebo-controlled trials. All of these agents showed significant improvements in mean exercise capacity. Treprostinil (Remodulin, UT-15) has a longer half-life (approximately 4 hours) than epoprostenol and can be delivered intravenously or subcutaneously with a pump system similar to that used with subcutaneous insulin. Treprostinil does not require reconstitution nor cold temperature. Pain at the site of subcutaneous infusion is a frequent problem that requires cessation of the drug in 8% to 12% of patients. Iloprost is another chemically stable analog that can be given intravenously and by inhaled routes. Iloprost can be used in a nebulized form that must be inhaled 6 to 9 times daily for a continuous effect.[106] Beraprost is an analog that can be taken orally four times daily. A 12-month double-blinded, randomized, placebo-controlled trial demonstrated that early, mild improvement in exercise capacity in beraprost-treated patients was transient.[106a] Treprostinil and iloprost are FDA approved for PAH and may be considered for PAH patients in NYHA/WHO class III.

Endothelin-1 Receptor Antagonists

Bosentan

Endothelin (ET-1) is an endogenous protein with vasoconstrictor, mitogenic, and profibrotic effects. PAH is associated with elevated plasma levels of ET-1. Bosentan (Tracleer) is an antagonist to both endothelin receptor subtypes A and B. Two double-blinded, placebo-controlled trials of patients in NYHA classes III and IV with IPAH or PAH associated with collagen vascular disease showed improvements in exercise capacity, NYHA functional class, and hemodynamics. Because bosentan is administered orally twice daily, this treatment provides an excellent combination of easy administration and efficacy. The most frequent side effect is a dose-dependent increase in liver transaminases, which necessitated discontinuation in 2% and dose adjustment in 8% to 12% of patients. The recommended starting dose is 62.5 mg twice daily, which is increased to 125 mg twice daily if there is no evidence of toxicity.[107] The major drawbacks of this medication are hepatic toxicity and delayed hemodynamic benefit compared with the immediate effect of epoprostenol. Bosentan is indicated for patients with stable functional class III PAH. Bosentan is not recommended for patients with HIV who are taking antiretroviral drugs, due to drug interactions.

Sitaxsentan and Ambrisentan

Sitaxsentan is a specific antagonist of ET receptor A. Specific inhibition of ETA receptors may provide more benefit by decreasing the vasoconstrictor effects of ETA while allowing the vasodilator and ET-1 clearance functions of ETB receptors. A small pilot 12-week trial of patients with NYHA classes II, III, and IV who received once-daily oral sitaxsentan demonstrated improvements in exercise capacity and hemodynamics, but there were two cases of acute hepatitis, one of which was fatal.[108] Sitaxsentan use also has been complicated by supertherapeutic anticoagulation. A 1-year open-label extension of this trial, with eleven patients treated with sitaxsentan 100 mg once daily showed significant improvements in exercise capacity, functional class, and hemodynamics. One patient worsened at 7 months. There were no serious adverse events, hepatotoxicity, or bleeding events.[108a] A third endothelin antagonist, ambrisentan, is currently in phase III clinical trials.

Phosphodiesterase Inhibitors

Sildenafil

NO exerts its vasodilatory effects through the second messenger cyclic guanosine monophosphate (cGMP). Sildenafil selectively inhibits the cGMP-specific enzyme phosphodiesterase type 5, enabling endogenous NO to exert a more sustained effect. This phosphodiesterase is highly abundant in the pulmonary vasculature compared with systemic vessels, making sildenafil a relatively selective pulmonary vasodilator. (Sildenafil has been used extensively to treat erectile dysfunction because this enzyme is also present in the corpus cavernosa). Initial data on the effect of sildenafil come only from short-term use in small case series. In patients with lung fibrosis and PAH, acute administration of sildenafil surpassed the vasodilating effect of NO. The effect was similar to IV epoprostenol except sildenafil showed more selectivity for better-ventilated areas of the lung, resulting in improved gas exchange.[109] Clinical and hemodynamic improvements have also been reported with use of sildenafil in patients with IPAH and PAH associated with congenital shunts, SLE,[110] and HIV.[11,111] In three patients being treated with IV epoprostenol, the addition of sildenafil improved hemodynamic measurements and the 6-minute walking distance after 5 months of treatment.[112] A 3-month, multicenter, double-blinded, randomized, placebo-controlled study of sildenafil treatment for PAH demonstrated significant improvements in exercise ability and quality of life. A long-term open-label extension study is currently ongoing. Sildenafil is FDA-approved for the treatment of PAH.[112a,112b]

Surgical Treatment

Atrial Septostomy

Survival in PAH is based largely on right ventricular function. Any method of relieving stress on the RV could theoretically improve PAH. The rationale for creating an interatrial orifice is based on clinical and laboratory observations. Among PAH patients, those with a patent foramen ovale or with Eisenmenger's syndrome have better cardiac function and survival than patients without intracardiac defects. Animal studies showed improved systemic blood flow after interatrial septostomy. With this background, it was proposed that creating an atrial septal defect would allow right-to-left shunting, unload a strained RV, improve systemic output, and improve oxygen transport, despite a drop in systemic arterial oxygen saturation. The first blade balloon atrial septostomy (AS) was performed in 1983.

A review of 64 cases reported in the literature found improved clinical status in 47 of 50 patients. Procedure-related mortality for the 64 cases reported worldwide was 16%. Ten patients died perioperatively; all had been considered terminally ill. Patients had overall improvements in functional class and exercise tolerance though the hemodynamic changes were mild or moderate. Long-term clinical outcome reflected hemodynamic response immediately following the procedure. Compared with treatments available before epoprostenol, AS seemed to improve survival in patients with severe PAH. The median survival of the 54 patients who survived the procedure was 19.5 months (range 2 to 96 months). AS should be considered a palliative procedure, because the underlying pulmonary vascular disease will eventually progress. One potential complication involves creating too great a shunt, in which case severe RV failure would be replaced by refractory hypoxemia. The procedure can be performed in patients with severe PAH and should be considered as a treatment option in the setting of recurrent syncope or RV failure despite maximal medical therapy or as a bridge to transplantation, and it should only be attempted in centers with experience in the procedure.[113]

Lung Transplantation

Before the introduction of epoprostenol, transplantation was the treatment of choice for severe PAH. It is still the last option in treating PAH and the only available cure. Heart-lung and single- and double-lung transplantations have been successfully performed in patients with PAH. The best choice for patients with PAH is uncertain. Single-lung transplantation is desirable considering the scarcity of donor organs. However, there may be less functional recovery and higher graft-related complications with single-lung transplant. The allograft receives nearly the entire CO because of the markedly elevated PVR in the native lung, but ventilation is evenly divided. This marked ventilation-perfusion mismatching makes any complication in the transplanted lung a risk for a severe gas exchange disturbance. However, overall mortalities in single- and double-lung transplantations for PAH are similar. Lung transplantation has demonstrated that severe RV dysfunction is reversible, indicating that heart transplantation is not necessary unless the patient has cardiac disease unrelated to PH.[100] The outcome in patients with PAH is similar to that of general transplantation patients. Survival rates at 1, 3, and 5 years after transplantation are 65%, 55%, and 44%, respectively.[114] PAH has not been reported to recur after transplantation.[100] Transplantation should be reserved for patients who are unable to tolerate medical therapy or who have progressive RV failure despite maximal medical management.

Previously, patients with collagen vascular disease were precluded from transplantation, but they have recently demonstrated survival rates similar to those of other patient groups. Transplantation should be considered an option for collagen vascular disease patients in whom extrapulmonary manifestations are not severe.[89] Because of the high intraoperative and perioperative risks, liver transplantation has generally not been offered to patients with portopulmonary hypertension. Pulmonary hemodynamics have been reported to improve with liver transplantation, however, and the risk of mortality at surgery is minimal if the mean PAP is less than 35 mm Hg. If the PAP is greater than 35 mm Hg, pretransplantation management with epoprostenol may decrease the mortality risk, and it is used as a bridge to transplantation.[85]

Hemodynamic responses to a 3-month epoprostenol infusion may help identify a subset of PAH patients who might benefit from being considered earlier for lung transplantation. A recent study demonstrated poor survival in patients with NYHA functional classes III and IV who remained in that class or failed to achieve a 30% decrease in PVR after 3 months on continuous IV epoprostenol.[115]

Treatment of Pulmonary Arterial Hypertension Associated with Specific Diseases

There are numerous reports on the efficacy of IV epoprostenol in patients with collagen vascular diseases and PAH. Skin lesions in patients with scleroderma may also improve substantially with this treatment.[89] As in IPAH, baseline hemodynamic data do not predict a response to epoprostenol in PAH associated with scleroderma. The acute vasodilator response is present in an even smaller proportion of patients with collagen vascular diseases than with IPAH. Accordingly, calcium-channel blockers are not beneficial in this group of patients.[87] As mentioned earlier, patients with CREST/scleroderma were included in the efficacious bosentan trial. There have also been case reports of successful epoprostenol treatment of PAH in patients with SLE[116]; however, treatment in this group has been complicated by severe thrombocytopenia.[92] There are a few case reports of regression of PH with immunosuppressive therapy in patients with various forms of collagen vascular diseases, though there have been no clinical trials to follow up these observations.[89] IV epoprostenol has recently been shown to improve functional capacity, oxygen saturation, and hemodynamics in a small group of adults with Eisenmenger's syndrome, and NYHA classes III and IV.[117] Epoprostenol has also been used successfully in patients with PAH and HIV infection.

Epoprostenol and its analogs have been used successfully in patients with portopulmonary hypertension. There are reports of improvement in this condition with the use of β-blockers and nitrates, which may also decrease the incidence of variceal bleeding. Anticoagulation in these patients is controversial because of the risk of hemorrhage. The liver toxicity associated with bosentan and sitaxsentan make these unacceptable choices for patients with hepatic disease.[85]

Experimental Therapies

Vasoactive intestinal peptide (VIP) is a neuropeptide with potent systemic and pulmonary vasodilating effects. A deficiency of VIP has been demonstrated in serum and lung tissue of patients with IPAH. Administration of aerosolized VIP to eight patients with NYHA functional class III or IV IPAH acutely improved hemodynamics. After 3 months of aerosolized VIP four times daily, there were significant improvements in mean PAP, CO, mixed venous oxygen saturation, 6-minute walk distance, and degree of dyspnea.[118]

The antiproliferative properties of prostacyclin have extended the search for therapeutic agents that may act on cell proliferation. Simvastatin, a cholesterol-lowering drug that is a 3-hydroxymethyl-3-methylglutaryl-coenzyme A (HMG CoA)-reductase inhibitor, or statin, has been shown to attenuate vascular injury and remodeling in a rat model of PAH induced by the combined insults of the toxin, monocrotaline, and shear stress induced by pneumonectomy. The cholesterol-independent effects of the statins may include anti-inflammatory and antiproliferative effects on the vascular wall.[119] There are no reports of statin use in patients with IPAH.

Gene Replacement Therapy

The recent advances in our understanding of the genetics and pathogenesis of PAH have raised the prospect of gene replacement therapy. Possible therapeutic targets include replacing a mutated BMPR2 gene or inducing overexpression of vasodilator genes including endothelial NO synthase or prostacyclin synthetase.[9]

REFERENCES

1. Fishman AP: Pulmonary circulation. In Geiger SR (ed): Handbook of Physiology: The Respiratory System. Baltimore: Williams & Wilkins, 1985, p 93.
2. Jeffery TK, Morrell NW: Molecular and cellular basis of pulmonary vascular remodeling in pulmonary hypertension. Prog Cardiovasc Dis 45:173, 2002.
3. Loscalzo J: Nitric oxide and vascular disease. N Engl J Med 333:251, 1995.
4. Stamler JS, Loh E, Roddy MA, et al: Nitric oxide regulates basal systemic and pulmonary vascular resistance in healthy humans. Circulation 89:2035, 1994.
5. D'Alonzo GE, Barst RJ, Ayres SM, et al: Survival in patients with primary pulmonary hypertension: Results from a national prospective registry. Ann Intern Med 115:343, 1991.
6. Rich S: Executive Summary from the World Symposium on Primary Pulmonary Hypertension. www.who.int/en1-29, 1998. 6-27-03. Ref type: Electronic citation.
7. Simonneau G, Galie N, Rubin JL, et al: Clinical classification of pulmonary hypertension. J Am Coll Cardiol 43:5S, 2004.
8. Rich S, Dantzker DR, Ayres SM, et al: Primary pulmonary hypertension: A national prospective study. Ann Intern Med 107:216, 1987.
9. Widlitz A, Barst RJ: Pulmonary arterial hypertension in children. Eur Respir J 21:155, 2003.
10. Meyrick B: The pathology of pulmonary artery hypertension. Clin Chest Med 22:393, 2001.
11. Runo JR, Loyd JE: Primary pulmonary hypertension. Lancet 361: 1533, 2003.
12. Tuder RM, Cool CD, Yeager M, et al: The pathobiology of pulmonary hypertension. Endothelium. Clin Chest Med 22:405, 2001.
13. Cool CD, Kennedy D, Voelkel NF, et al: Pathogenesis and evolution of plexiform lesions in pulmonary hypertension associated with scleroderma and human immunodeficiency virus infection. Hum Pathol 28:434, 1997.
14. Loyd JE, Atkinson JB, Pietra GG, et al: Heterogeneity of pathologic lesions in familial primary pulmonary hypertension. Am Rev Respir Dis 138:952, 1988.
15. Wagenvoort CA, Heath D, Edwards JE: The pathology of the pulmonary vasculature. In Thomas C (ed): Springfield, IL: 1964, p 224.
16. Loscalzo J: Genetic clues to the cause of primary pulmonary hypertension. N Engl J Med 345:367, 2001.
17. Loyd JE, Butler MG, Foroud TM, et al: Genetic anticipation and abnormal gender ratio at birth in familial primary pulmonary hypertension. Am J Respir Crit Care Med 152:93, 1995.
18. Newman JH, Wheeler L, Lane KB, et al: Mutation in the gene for bone morphogenetic protein receptor II as a cause of primary

pulmonary hypertension in a large kindred. N Engl J Med 345:319, 2001.
19. Loyd JE, Slovis B, Phillips JA, III, et al: The presence of genetic anticipation suggests that the molecular basis of familial primary pulmonary hypertension may be trinucleotide repeat expansion. Chest 111:82S, 1997.
20. Thomson JR, Trembath RC: Primary pulmonary hypertension: The pressure rises for a gene. J Clin Pathol 53:899, 2000.
21. Machado RD, Pauciulo MW, Thomson JR, et al: BMPR2 haploinsufficiency as the inherited molecular mechanism for primary pulmonary hypertension. Am J Hum Genet 68:92, 2001.
22. Morse JH, Jones AC, Barst RJ, et al: Mapping of familial primary pulmonary hypertension locus PPH1 to chromosome 2q31-q32. Circulation 95:2603,1997.
23. Nichols WC, Koller DL, Slovis B, et al: Localization of the gene for familial primary pulmonary hypertension to chromosome 2q31-32. Nat Genet 15:277, 1997.
24. Deng Z, Haghighi F, Helleby L, et al: Fine mapping of PPH1, a gene for familial primary pulmonary hypertension, to a 3-cM region on chromosome 2q33. Am J Respir Crit Care Med 161:1055, 2001.
25. Deng Z, Morse JH, Slager SL, et al: Familial primary pulmonary hypertension gene PPH1 is caused by mutations in the bone morphogenetic protein receptor-II gene. Am J Hum Genet 67:737, 2000.
26. Lane KB, Machado RD, Pauciulo MW, et al: Heterozygous germline mutations in BMPR2, encoding a TGF-beta receptor, cause familial primary pulmonary hypertension. The International PPH Consortium. Nat Genet 26:81, 2000.
27. Humbert M, Deng Z, Simonneau G, et al: BMPR2 germline mutations in pulmonary hypertension associated with fenfluramine derivatives. Eur Respir J 20:518, 2000.
28. Loyd JE: Genetics and pulmonary hypertension. Chest 122:284S, 2002.
29. Morrell NW, Yang X, Upton PD, et al: Altered growth responses of pulmonary artery smooth muscle cells from patients with primary pulmonary hypertension to transforming growth factor-beta1 and bone morphogenetic proteins. Circulation 104:790, 2001.
30. Massague J, Blain SW, Lo RS: TGF beta signaling in growth control, cancer, and heritable disorders. Cell 103:295, 2000.
31. Blobe GC, Schiemann WP, Lodish HF: Role of transforming growth factor beta in human disease. N Engl J Med 342:1350, 2000.
32. van den Driesche S, Mummery CL, Westermann CJ: Hereditary hemorrhagic telangiectasia: An update on transforming growth factor beta signaling in vasculogenesis and angiogenesis. Cardiovasc Res 58:20, 2003.
33. De Caestecker M, Meyrick B: Bone morphogenetic proteins, genetics and the pathophysiology of primary pulmonary hypertension. Respir Res 2:193, 2001.
34. Thomson JR, Machado RD, Pauciulo MW, et al: Sporadic primary pulmonary hypertension is associated with germline mutations of the gene encoding BMPR-II, a receptor member of the TGF-beta family. J Med Genet 37:741, 2000.
35. Tuder RM, Yeager ME, Geraci M, et al: Severe pulmonary hypertension after the discovery of the familial primary pulmonary hypertension gene. Eur Respir J 17:1065, 2001.
36. Newman JH, Trembath RC, Morse JA, et al: Genetic basis of pulmonary arterial hypertension: Current understanding and future directions. J Am Coll Cardiol 43:33S, 2004.
37. Janssen B, Rindermann M, Barth U, et al: Linkage analysis in a large family with primary pulmonary hypertension: Genetic heterogeneity and a second primary pulmonary hypertension locus on 2q31-32. Chest 121:54S, 2002.
38. Trembath RC, Thomson JR, Machado RD, et al: Clinical and molecular genetic features of pulmonary hypertension in patients with hereditary hemorrhagic telangiectasia. N Engl J Med 345:325, 2001.
39. Chaouat A, Coulet F, Favre C, et al: Endoglin germline mutation in a patient with hereditary haemorrhagic telangiectasia and dexfenfluramine associated pulmonary arterial hypertension. Thorax 59:446, 2004.
40. Attisano L, Wrana JL: Signal transduction by the TGF-beta superfamily. Science 296:1646, 2002.
41. Atkinson C, Stewart S, Upton PD, et al: Primary pulmonary hypertension is associated with reduced pulmonary vascular expression of type II bone morphogenetic protein receptor. Circulation 105: 1672, 2002.
42. Du L, Sullivan CC, Chu D, et al: Signaling molecules in nonfamilial pulmonary hypertension. N Engl J Med 348:500, 2003.
43. Taraseviciene-Stewart L, Kasahara Y, Alger L, et al: Inhibition of the VEGF receptor 2 combined with chronic hypoxia causes cell death-dependent pulmonary endothelial cell proliferation and severe pulmonary hypertension. FASEB J 15:427, 2001.
44. Lee SD, Shroyer KR, Markham NE, et al: Monoclonal endothelial cell proliferation is present in primary but not secondary pulmonary hypertension. J Clin Invest 101:927, 1998.
45. Yeager ME, Halley GR, Golpon HA, et al: Microsatellite instability of endothelial cell growth and apoptosis genes within plexiform lesions in primary pulmonary hypertension. Circ Res 88:E2, 2001.
46. Weidinger FF, McLenachan JM, Cybulsky MI, et al: Persistent dysfunction of regenerated endothelium after balloon angioplasty of rabbit iliac artery. Circulation 81:1667, 1990.
47. Christman BW, McPherson CD, Newman JH, et al: An imbalance between the excretion of thromboxane and prostacyclin metabolites in pulmonary hypertension. N Engl J Med 327:70, 1992.
48. Archer S, Rich S: Primary pulmonary hypertension: A vascular biology and translational research "Work in progress." Circulation 102: 2781, 2000.
49. Wort SJ, Woods M, Warner TD, et al: Endogenously released endothelin-1 from human pulmonary artery smooth muscle promotes cellular proliferation: relevance to pathogenesis of pulmonary hypertension and vascular remodeling. Am J Respir Cell Mol Biol 25:104, 2001.
50. Rubens C, Ewert R, Halank M, et al: Big endothelin-1 and endothelin-1 plasma levels are correlated with the severity of primary pulmonary hypertension. Chest 120:1562, 2001.
51. MacLean MR: Endothelin-1 and serotonin: Mediators of primary and secondary pulmonary hypertension? J Lab Clin Med 134:105, 1999.
52. Ivy DD, Yanagisawa M, Gariepy CE, et al: Exaggerated hypoxic pulmonary hypertension in endothelin B receptor-deficient rats. Am J Physiol Lung Cell Mol Physiol 282:L703, 2002.
53. Orte C, Polak JM, Haworth SG, et al: Expression of pulmonary vascular angiotensin-converting enzyme in primary and secondary plexiform pulmonary hypertension. J Pathol 192:379, 2000.
54. Herve P, Launay JM, Scrobohaci ML, et al: Increased plasma serotonin in primary pulmonary hypertension. Am J Med 99:249, 1995.
55. Eddahibi S, Raffestin B, Hamon M, et al: Is the serotonin transporter involved in the pathogenesis of pulmonary hypertension? J Lab Clin Med 139:194, 2002.
56. Eddahibi S, Humbert M, Fadel E, et al: Serotonin transporter overexpression is responsible for pulmonary artery smooth muscle hyperplasia in primary pulmonary hypertension. J Clin Invest 108:1141, 2001.
57. Rabinovitch M: Linking a serotonin transporter polymorphism to vascular smooth muscle proliferation in patients with primary pulmonary hypertension. J Clin Invest 108:1109, 2001.
58. Launay JM, Herve P, Peoc'h K, et al: Function of the serotonin 5-hydroxytryptamine 2B receptor in pulmonary hypertension. Nat Med 8:1129, 2002.
59. Humbert M, Trembath RC: Genetics of pulmonary hypertension: From bench to bedside. Eur Respir J 20:741, 2002.
60. Humbert M, Labrune P, Sitbon O, et al: Pulmonary arterial hypertension and type-I glycogen-storage disease: The serotonin hypothesis. Eur Respir J 20:59, 2002.
61. Farber HW, Loscalzo J: Prothrombotic mechanisms in primary pulmonary hypertension. J Lab Clin Med 134:561, 1999.
62. Herve P, Humbert M, Sitbon O, et al: Pathobiology of pulmonary hypertension: The role of platelets and thrombosis. Clin Chest Med 22:451, 2001.
63. Yuan JX, Aldinger AM, Juhaszova M, et al: Dysfunctional voltage-gated K+ channels in pulmonary artery smooth muscle cells of patients with primary pulmonary hypertension. Circulation 98: 1400, 1998.
64. Wang J, Juhaszova M, Conte JV Jr, et al: Action of fenfluramine on voltage-gated K+ channels in human pulmonary-artery smooth-muscle cells. Lancet 352:290, 1998.
65. Pozeg ZI, Michelakis ED, McMurtry MS, et al: In vivo gene transfer of the O2-sensitive potassium channel Kv1.5 reduces pulmonary hypertension and restores hypoxic pulmonary vasoconstriction in chronically hypoxic rats. Circulation 107:2037, 2003.
66. Botney MD: Role of hemodynamics in pulmonary vascular remodeling: Implications for primary pulmonary hypertension. Am J Respir Crit Care Med 159:361, 1999.

67. Cowan KN, Jones PL, Rabinovitch M: Elastase and matrix metalloproteinase inhibitors induce regression, and tenascin-C antisense prevents progression, of vascular disease. J Clin Invest 105:21, 2000.
68. Cowan KN, Heilbut A, Humpl T, et al: Complete reversal of fatal pulmonary hypertension in rats by a serine elastase inhibitor. Nat Med 6:698, 2000.
69. Eddahibi S, Morrell N, d'Ortho MP, et al: Pathobiology of pulmonary arterial hypertension. Eur Respir J 20:1559, 2002.
70. Walker JL, Loscalzo J, Zhang YY: 5-Lipoxygenase and human pulmonary artery endothelial cell proliferation. Am J Physiol Heart Circ Physiol 282:H585, 2002.
71. Tuder RM, Lee SD, Cool CC: Histopathology of pulmonary hypertension. Chest 114:1S, 1998.
72. Tuder RM, Voelkel NF: Pulmonary hypertension and inflammation. J Lab Clin Med 132:16, 1998.
73. Carmeliet P: Angiogenesis in health and disease. Nat Med 9:653, 2003.
74. Humbert M, Nunes H, Sitbon O, et al: Risk factors for pulmonary arterial hypertension. Clin Chest Med 22:459, 2001.
75. Abenhaim L, Moride Y, Brenot F, et al: Appetite-suppressant drugs and the risk of primary pulmonary hypertension: International Primary Pulmonary Hypertension Study Group. N Engl J Med 335:609, 1996.
76. Egermayer P, Town GI, Peacock AJ: Role of serotonin in the pathogenesis of acute and chronic pulmonary hypertension. Thorax 54: 161, 1999.
77. Amfepramone; New cases of primary pulmonary hypertension reported. Available at http://www.who.int/medicines/library/pnewslet/npn0101.html. 2001.
78. WHO Questionnaire for Review of Dependence-Producing Psychoactive Substances by the Thirty-third Expert Committee on Drug Dependence. Available at http://www.fda.gov/ohrms/dockets/dailys/02/Jul02/070202/02n-0101-let0002-vol1.pdf, 2-5. 2002.
79. Schaiberger PH, Kennedy TC, Miller FC, et al: Pulmonary hypertension associated with long-term inhalation of "crank" methamphetamine. Chest 104:614, 1993.
80. Klings ES, Farber HW: The pathogenesis of HIV-associated pulmonary hypertension. In Barbaro G (ed): HIV Infection and the Cardiovascular System. Basel, Switzerland: Karger, 2003, p 71.
81. Nunes H, Humbert M, Sitbon O, et al: Prognostic factors for survival in human immunodeficiency virus-associated pulmonary arterial hypertension. Am J Respir Crit Care Med 167:1433, 2003.
82. Pearson DL, Dawling S, Walsh WF, et al: Neonatal pulmonary hypertension: Urea-cycle intermediates, nitric oxide production, and carbamoyl-phosphate synthetase function. N Engl J Med 344:1832, 2001.
83. Granton JT, Rabinovitch M: Pulmonary arterial hypertension in congenital heart disease. Cardiol Clin 20:441, 2002.
84. Rabinovitch M: Pulmonary hypertension: Pathophysiology as a basis for clinical decision making. J Heart Lung Transplant 18:1041, 1999.
85. Budhiraja R, Hassoun PM: Portopulmonary hypertension: A tale of two circulations. Chest 123:562, 2003.
86. Fallon MB: Portopulmonary hypertension: New clinical insights and more questions on pathogenesis. Hepatology 37:253, 2003.
87. Klings ES, Hill NS, Ieong MH, et al: Systemic sclerosis-associated pulmonary hypertension: short- and long-term effects of epoprostenol prostacyclin. Arthritis Rheum 42:2638, 1999.
88. Steen V, Medsger TA Jr: Predictors of isolated pulmonary hypertension in patients with systemic sclerosis and limited cutaneous involvement. Arthritis Rheum 48:516, 2003.
89. Hoeper MM: Pulmonary hypertension in collagen vascular disease. Eur Respir J 19:571, 2002.
90. Chu JW, Kao PN, Faul JL, et al: High prevalence of autoimmune thyroid disease in pulmonary arterial hypertension. Chest 122:1668, 2002.
91. Dingli D, Utz JP, Krowka MJ, et al: Unexplained pulmonary hypertension in chronic myeloproliferative disorders. Chest 120:801, 2001.
92. Horn EM, Barst RJ, Poon M: Epoprostenol for treatment of pulmonary hypertension in patients with systemic lupus erythematosus. Chest 118:1229, 2000.
93. Chemla D, Castelain V, Herve P, et al: Haemodynamic evaluation of pulmonary hypertension. Eur Respir J 20:1314, 2002.
94. Sun XG, Hansen JE, Oudiz RJ, et al: Pulmonary function in primary pulmonary hypertension. J Am Coll Cardiol 41:1028, 2003.
95. Klings ES, Farber HW: Current management of primary pulmonary hypertension. Drugs 61:1945, 2001.
96. Grunig E, Janssen B, Mereles D, et al: Abnormal pulmonary artery pressure response in asymptomatic carriers of primary pulmonary hypertension gene. Circulation 102:1145, 2000.
97. Fuster V, Steele PM, Edwards WD, et al: Primary pulmonary hypertension: Natural history and the importance of thrombosis. Circulation 70:580, 1984.
98. Frank H, Mlczoch J, Huber K, et al: The effect of anticoagulant therapy in primary and anorectic drug-induced pulmonary hypertension. Chest 112:714, 1997.
99. Rich S, Kaufmann E, Levy PS: The effect of high doses of calcium channel blockers on survival in primary pulmonary hypertension. N Engl J Med 327:76, 1992.
100. Sitbon O, Humbert M, Simonneau G: Primary pulmonary hypertension: Current therapy. Prog Cardiovasc Dis 45:115, 2002.
101. Rubin LJ: Calcium channel blockers in primary pulmonary hypertension. Chest 88(suppl 4):257S, 1985.
102. Rich S, Brundage BH: High-dose calcium channel-blocking therapy for primary pulmonary hypertension: Evidence of long-term reduction in pulmonary arterial pressure and regression of right ventricular hypertrophy. Circulation 76:135, 1987.
103. Higenbottam T, Wheeldon D, Wells F, et al: Long-term treatment of primary pulmonary hypertension with continuous intravenous epoprostenol prostacyclin. Lancet 8385:1046, 1984.
104. Shapiro SM, Oudiz RJ, Cao T, et al: Primary pulmonary hypertension: Improved long-term effects and survival with continuous intravenous epoprostenol infusion. J Am Coll Cardiol 30:343, 1997.
105. McLaughlin VV, Shillington A, Rich S: Survival in primary pulmonary hypertension: The impact of epoprostenol therapy. Circulation 106:1477, 2002.
106. Galie N, Manes A, Branzi A: The new clinical trials on pharmacological treatment in pulmonary arterial hypertension. Eur Respir J 20;1037, 2002.
106a. Barst RJ, McGoon M, McLaughlin V, et al: Beraprost therapy for pulmonary arterial hypertension. J Am Coll Cardiol 41:2119, 2003.
107. Rubin LJ, Badesch DB, Barst RJ, et al: Bosentan therapy for pulmonary arterial hypertension. N Engl J Med 346:896, 2002.
108. Barst RJ, Rich S, Widlitz A, et al: Clinical efficacy of sitaxsentan, an endothelin-A receptor antagonist, in patients with pulmonary arterial hypertension: Open-label pilot study. Chest 121:1860, 2002.
108a. Langleben D, Hirsch AM, Shalit E, et al: Sustained symptomatic, functional and hemodynamic benefit with the selective endothelin-A receptor antagonist, sitaxsentan, in patients with pulmonary arterial hypertension: A 1-year follow-up study. Chest 126:1377, 2004.
109. Ghofrani HA, Wiedemann R, Rose F, et al: Sildenafil for treatment of lung fibrosis and pulmonary hypertension: A randomised controlled trial. Lancet 360:895, 2002.
110. Molina J, Lucero E, Luluaga S, et al: Systemic lupus erythematosus-associated pulmonary hypertension: Good outcome following sildenafil therapy. Lupus 12:321, 2003.
111. Bharani A, Mathew V, Sahu A, et al: The efficacy and tolerability of sildenafil in patients with moderate-to-severe pulmonary hypertension. Indian Heart J 55:55, 2003.
112. Stiebellehner L, Petkov V, Vonbank K, et al: Long-term treatment with oral sildenafil in addition to continuous IV epoprostenol in patients with pulmonary arterial hypertension. Chest 123:1293, 2003.
112a. Badesch D, Burgess G, Parpia T et al: Sildenafil citrate in patients with pulmonary arterial hypertension (PAH): Results of a multicenter, multinational, randomized, double-blind, placebo-controlled trial by WHO functional class (FC). Proc Am Thorac Soc 2: A206, 2005.
112b. Pepke-Zaba J, Brown MCJ, Parpia T, et al: The impact of sildenafil citrate on health-related quality of life in patients with pulmonary arterial hypertension (PAH): Results of a multicenter, multinational, randomized, double-blind, placebo-controlled trial. Proc Am Thorac Soc 2:A299, 2005.

113. Sandoval J, Rothman A, Pulido T: Atrial septostomy for pulmonary hypertension. Clin Chest Med 22:547, 2001.
114. Trulock EP: Lung transplantation for primary pulmonary hypertension. Clin Chest Med 22:583, 2001.
115. Sitbon O, Humbert M, Nunes H, et al: Long-term intravenous epoprostenol infusion in primary pulmonary hypertension: Prognostic factors and survival. J Am Coll Cardiol 40:780, 2002.
116. Robbins IM, Gaine SP, Schilz R, et al: Epoprostenol for treatment of pulmonary hypertension in patients with systemic lupus erythematosus. Chest 117:14, 2000.
117. Fernandes SM, Newburger JW, Lang P, et al: Usefulness of epoprostenol therapy in the severely ill adolescent/adult with Eisenmenger physiology. Am J Cardiol 91:632, 2003.
118. Petkov V, Mosgoeller W, Ziesche R, et al: Vasoactive intestinal peptide as a new drug for treatment of primary pulmonary hypertension. J Clin Invest 111:1339, 2003.
119. Nishimura T, Faul JL, Berry GJ, et al: Simvastatin attenuates smooth muscle neointimal proliferation and pulmonary hypertension in rats. Am J Respir Crit Care Med 166:1403, 2002.

chapter 58

Secondary Pulmonary Hypertension

Elizabeth S. Klings
Joseph Loscalzo

Secondary pulmonary hypertension was originally defined as pulmonary hypertension (PH) occurring in the setting of another cardiopulmonary disease. Recently, secondary PH has been further subclassified into diseases associated with (a) pulmonary venous hypertension; (b) chronic hypoxemia; (c) thrombotic or embolic diseases; and (d) direct involvement of the pulmonary vasculature (see Chapter 57, Table 57-1).[1] This chapter serves as an overview of the disorders associated with secondary forms of PH and a guide to their management.

PULMONARY VENOUS HYPERTENSION

Left-Sided Congestive Heart Failure

PH occurs in the setting of left-sided congestive heart failure (CHF) as a result of a passive increase in pulmonary venous pressure. Acutely, a reversible dysregulation of vascular smooth muscle tone occurs. Over the long term, however, there is structural remodeling of the pulmonary vasculature, which is irreversible.

Pathogenesis

The endothelium is the primary mediator of vascular tone in the pulmonary circulation. In the setting of left ventricular (LV) dysfunction, cytokines and neurohormones are released. These mediators, in combination with elevated shear stress, produce phenotypic changes within the endothelium. There is increased endothelial production of the vasoconstrictor endothelin-1 (ET-1) in PH related to left-sided CHF, and plasma levels of ET-1 correlate with pulmonary artery pressure (PAP) and pulmonary vascular resistance.[2,3] Additionally, there appears to be deficient production of the vasodilator nitric oxide (NO) and a decrease in endothelium-dependent vasodilation.[2] The overall effect of these changes is an increased propensity to vasoconstriction and smooth muscle proliferation, leading to remodeling within the pulmonary vasculature.

Diagnosis and Treatment

Symptomatically, these patients develop dyspnea, orthopnea, paroxysmal nocturnal dyspnea, and lower extremity edema due to the presence of left- and right-sided CHF. PH may confer an independent risk factor for impaired exercise tolerance and increased mortality in patients with left-sided CHF.[4] Echocardiography is the key diagnostic study in these patients, elucidating the presence of LV dysfunction or left-sided valvular disease. In some cases, right heart catheterization is necessary for confirmation of the diagnosis. Treatment for these patients is primarily limited to conventional treatment of heart failure. ACE inhibitors, β-blockers, digoxin and most vasodilators reduce PVR.[2] IV epoprostenol, which is clinically useful in the treatment of pulmonary arterial hypertension (PAH), results in increased mortality when used in this population.[5] The endothelin receptor antagonists, bosentan and sitaxsentan, have only been studied in small case series but appear to have potential therapeutic benefit. Cardiac transplantation is the only curative therapy available for PH related to left-sided CHF; elevated PAP resolve quickly post-transplantation.[2]

Fibrosing Mediastinitis

Fibrosing and granulomatous mediastinitis can manifest across a clinical spectrum from benign disease with minor symptomatology to severe PH and death.[6] Although PH is a rare complication of this condition, occurring in less than 15% of patients, it is the most common cause of morbidity and mortality.[6] PH occurs in the setting of fibrosing mediastinitis secondary to direct obstruction of pulmonary arteries, veins, or both by large, often calcified masses.[6]

Pathogenesis

Fibrosing mediastinitis is an uncommon complication of granulomatous disease, particularly histoplasmosis, the etiology of which is unclear and likely multifactorial. Fibrosis of the mediastinal structures is believed to occur via an immunologic response to caseous nodes, resulting in an intense fibrotic response. The rarity of this presentation suggests an alteration in the host response with an overproduction of collagen in response to immunological stimuli.[6] The development of fibrosing mediastinitis appears to be a late consequence of infection, as organisms are rarely isolated from the lesions.[6]

Pulmonary Veno-Occlusive Disease (also see Chapter 59)

Pulmonary veno-occlusive disease (PVOD) is a rare clinicopathologic condition that accounts for a small number of cases of pulmonary hypertension annually. PVOD is a histopathologic diagnosis, leading to an underestimation of its true incidence as an etiology of PH. Pooling of patients from seven case series of PH (465 patients) found that PVOD accounted for approximately 10% of cases of PH. This frequency suggests an overall incidence of 0.1 to 0.2 cases per million in the general population. PVOD affects patients of all ages with a male-to-female ratio of approximately 1:1. PVOD portends a poor prognosis for patients—most die within 2 years of diagnosis.[7]

Pathophysiology

It is hypothesized that PVOD represents a common pathological response to various possible insults. Characteristic of PVOD is the extensive and diffuse occlusion of pulmonary veins by fibrous tissue.[7] This fibrous tissue may be edematous early in the course of the disease but generally becomes more sclerotic over time. Although this is primarily a disease of the pulmonary veins, arterioles exhibit moderate to severe medial hypertrophy in approximately one half of cases. Notably, plexiform lesions and arteritis are generally absent.[8] Histologically, the most common parenchymal change observed is interstitial edema, particularly in the lobular septa (Fig. 58-1). This pathology can be differentiated from interstitial edema due to left-sided CHF in later stages by the presence of collagen deposition and progression to fibrosis. Other pathologic findings include hemosiderosis, type 2 pneumocyte hyperplasia, focal lymphocytic infiltrates, dilated pulmonary lymphatics, and engorged alveolar capillaries.[7]

Various risk factors have been identified for the development of PVOD, mainly via case reports and small case series. They include infection, genetic factors, toxic exposures, thrombosis, and the presence of autoimmune disorders. These proposed risk factors have not been substantiated by case-control or cohort studies specifically addressing potential etiologies of PVOD, and thus a unifying theory concerning predisposing factors for this condition has not been well established.

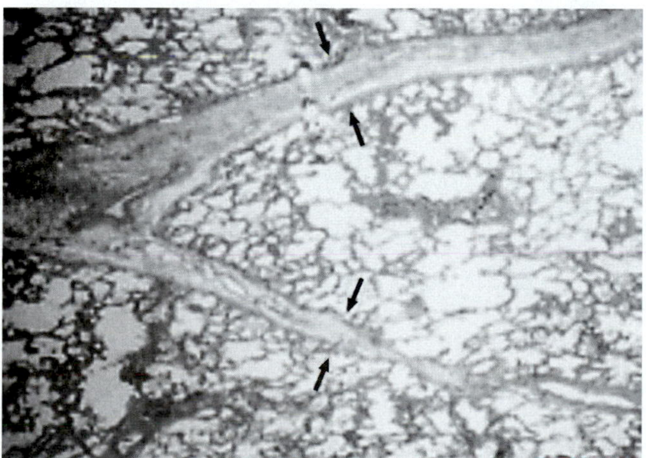

FIGURE 58-1. (See also Color Plate 58-1.) Histopathology of pulmonary veno-occlusive disease. Longitudinal section of lobular septa (*arrows*), which are widened by interstitial edema and fibrosis (hematoxylin & eosin, ×4).[7]

Diagnosis and Treatment

Clinically, patients with PVOD present with primarily progressive dyspnea, similarly to how they present with other forms of PH. Patients often present after a nonresolving respiratory infection[7] or with symptoms of orthopnea, both of which are rare in PAH. Physical examination findings are similar to those observed in other forms of PH and right-sided congestive heart failure. Additionally, specific to PVOD is the presence of auscultatory crackles in patients with prominent pulmonary infiltrates.[7]

Chest radiography in PVOD frequently demonstrates pleural effusions and Kerley B lines resulting from postcapillary obstruction, which leads to elevated pulmonary capillary and visceral pleural capillary hydrostatic pressures.[7] Additionally, there may be engorgement of the central pulmonary vessels. CT scans may reveal diffuse or mosaic ground glass opacities or septal thickening[7] of unclear pathologic significance (Fig. 58-2). Ventilation-perfusion scanning reveals normal ventilation with areas of hypoperfusion (mismatched defects) similar to those observed in chronic thromboembolic pulmonary hypertension.[7] Pulmonary function tests usually reveal a decreased single-breath diffusing capacity for carbon monoxide (D_LCO) and may demonstrate restrictive physiology.[7] Although not necessary diagnostically, bronchoscopy may reveal intense hyperemia and vascular engorgement of the lobar and segmental bronchi.[9]

Right heart catheterization generally reveals elevated pulmonary arterial (PA) pressures with a normal pulmonary artery occlusion pressure (PAOP). It is often difficult to obtain a PAOP because when the distal port of the PA catheter is flushed while in the wedge position, the infused saline may become trapped between the catheter tip and the narrowed pulmonary veins. Clinically, the diagnosis of PVOD is suggested by the triad of severe PAH, a normal PAOP, and radiographic evidence

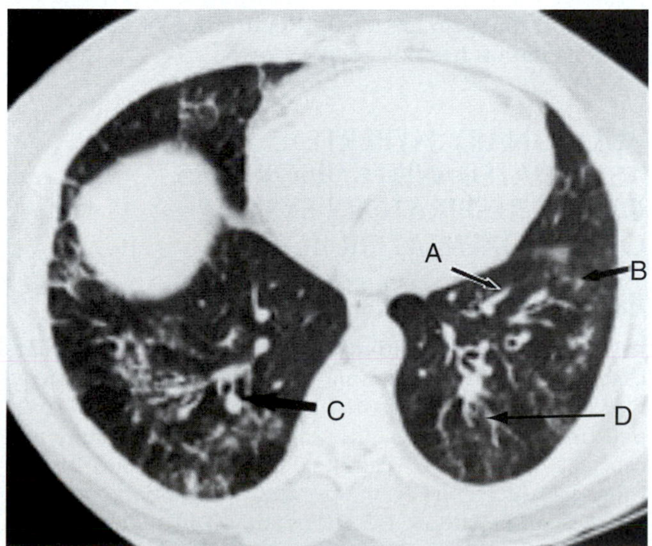

FIGURE 58-2. (See also Color Plate 58-2.) CT scan of a patient with pulmonary veno-occlusive disease demonstrating numerous thickened septal lines (**D**) and patchy foci of ground glass attenuation (**B**). The arteries are enlarged (**C**), whereas the pulmonary veins appear of normal caliber (**A**).[7]

of pulmonary edema. Because many patients do not have this triad, however, open lung biopsy is recommended for definitive diagnosis.[7]

Treatment

The prognosis for PVOD is poor, with a survival rate of less than 2 years after diagnosis. On the basis of literature generated in the PAH population, long-term anticoagulation and oxygen therapy to correct hypoxemia are recommended for all patients with PVOD without contraindications to these therapies.[7] Unlike PAH, vasodilators have not been helpful in treating PVOD and can be life threatening due to the development of acute pulmonary edema. It is believed that this adverse effect is due to dilation of the pulmonary arterioles and increased hydrostatic pressure on the fixed-resistance, narrowed pulmonary venules. A limited number of patients experience therapeutic benefit from epoprostenol with associated dilation of the pulmonary venules. Because of this possibility, a cautious trial of a short-acting vasodilator such as inhaled NO, adenosine, or epoprostenol may be performed. Patients who develop a therapeutic hemodynamic response to these medications without the development of pulmonary edema may be candidates for long-term epoprostenol, but it is unclear what effect, if any, this treatment has on survival. Immunosuppressive medications, such as glucocorticoids and antimetabolites, have been used in patients with PVOD and extensive interstitial lung disease without a standardization of treatment regimens across institutions, making conclusions regarding efficacy difficult to ascertain.[7]

The only therapy for PVOD associated with improved survival is single- or double-lung transplantation, and it is recommended to refer patients for transplants at the time of diagnosis. Even so, as the average waiting time for lung transplants in the United States is longer than most patients' life expectancies, this definitive therapy is not an option for many patients.[7] Recurrence of PVOD after transplantation has not been reported.

PULMONARY HYPERTENSION ASSOCIATED WITH DISORDERS OF THE RESPIRATORY SYSTEM OR HYPOXEMIA, OR BOTH

Pathophysiology

PH is a common complication of chronic lung diseases associated with hypoxemia including chronic obstructive lung disease, interstitial lung disease, cystic fibrosis, and bronchiectasis, resulting in increased morbidity and mortality (Box 58-1).[10] Pathologically, PH related to chronic lung disease results from sustained pulmonary vasoconstriction and response to various stimuli, including chronic alveolar hypoxia, inflammation, and shear stress.[11] This pathobiology results in a vasculopathy characterized by remodeling of the pulmonary resistance vessels and reductions in the number of blood vessels and vascular density of the lung.[12] Remodeling of the pulmonary resistance vessels occurs via hypertrophy and hyperplasia of vascular smooth muscle cells, leading to medial thickening and encroachment on the vessel lumen (Fig. 58-3). The mechanisms responsible for vascular remodeling include chronic hypoxia, inflammation, shear stress, and endothelial dysfunction (see Chapter 57 for more details).[13-15]

BOX 58-1 Clinical Conditions Associated with Hypoxia-Induced Pulmonary Hypertension

Chronic obstructive pulmonary disease
Interstitial lung disease
Bronchiectasis
Sleep-disordered breathing
Alveolar hypoventilation disorders
Cystic fibrosis
Chronic exposure to high altitude

CLINICAL CONDITIONS ASSOCIATED WITH CHRONIC HYPOXEMIA AND PULMONARY HYPERTENSION

Chronic Obstructive Pulmonary Disease

Chronic obstructive pulmonary disease (COPD) is the most common cause of hypoxemia-induced PH and right-sided CHF or cor pulmonale, accounting for more than 80% of cases. PH associated with chronic lung disease is

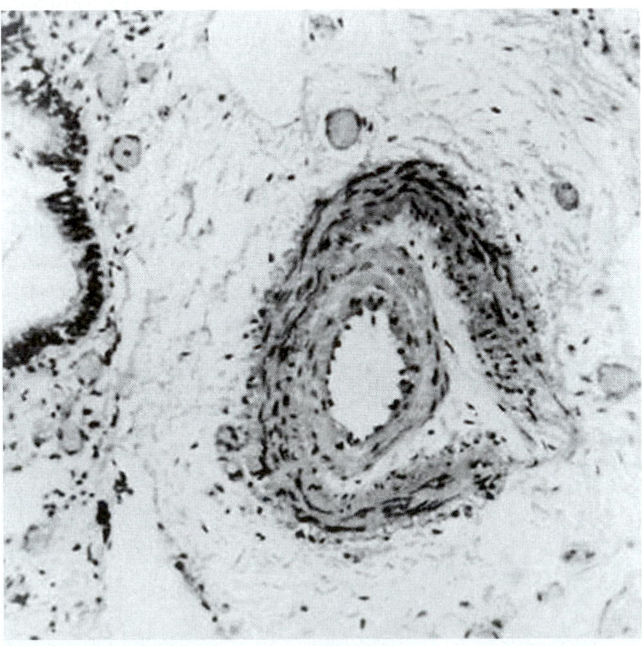

FIGURE 58-3. Histopathology of hypoxia-induced pulmonary hypertension. Slightly oblique section of a muscular pulmonary artery from a patient with pulmonary fibrosis and hypoxia-induced pulmonary hypertension demonstrating hypertrophy of the vascular media (hematoxylin & eosin, ×175).

defined as a mean PAP of greater than 20 mm Hg at rest, slightly lower than the definition of PAH. Patients with PH related to chronic hypoxemia, particularly those with COPD, exhibit only modest elevations in PA pressure, usually with a mean PAP of less than 40 mm Hg.[16] The progression of PH in these patients is also less rapid than that observed in PAH, with an average change in mean PAP of 0.5 mm Hg/year.[16] In COPD, increases in PAP occur in association with worsening hypoxemia, such as observed during exercise, sleep, and acute exacerbations of their disease process. The presence of PH appears to be an independent risk factor for death in COPD patients; a mean PAP of 20 to 35 mm Hg is associated with a 5-year survival of 50%, regardless of FEV_1.[16]

Diagnosis

Assessing patients for PH related to COPD often presents a challenge for the physician. Clinical signs of PH and cor pulmonale are often obscured in COPD patients due to the hyperinflation of their chests. As a result, it is often difficult to determine jugular venous distension or to auscultate a loud pulmonic component of the second heart sound. Similarly, the detection of right ventricular hypertrophy by chest radiography or electrocardiography is poorly sensitive.[16] The noninvasive diagnosis of PH related to COPD is presently being determined by echocardiography. This allows for an estimation of the right ventricular systolic pressure (which should be identical to the PA systolic pressure) by calculation of the transtricuspid pressure gradient from the peak velocity of the tricuspid regurgitant jet and application of the Bernoulli equation.[16] Recent studies have suggested that this estimation may not be as sensitive a measure of detection as originally believed,[17] suggesting that other, more sensitive studies may need to be developed to detect PH in these patients.

Interstitial Lung Disease

PH is a recognized complication of long-standing interstitial lung disease. In addition to chronic hypoxia, the increase in pulmonary vascular resistance observed results, in part, from anatomic compression of arterioles and capillaries by the fibrosing process. One study that can aid in the determination of PH in this patient group is a measurement of the main pulmonary artery diameter (MPAD) by CT scan; a MPAD greater than or equal to 29 mm was 84% sensitive and 75% specific for PH related to interstitial lung disease.[18]

Obstructive Sleep Apnea

In patients with obstructive sleep apnea (OSA), pulmonary hemodynamic alterations can be observed transiently during apnea-associated periods of hypoxia.[19] Additionally, daytime PH may occur as a result of long-term effects of hypoxic pulmonary vasoconstriction, resulting in endothelial dysfunction and vascular remodeling.[20] Unlike other forms of hypoxia-induced PH, there may be a reversible component observed in OSA patients. Treatment of OSA with continuous positive pressure airway pressure (CPAP) to reverse nocturnal hypoxemia was associated with a decrease in PA pressure after 4 months of treatment.[20]

PULMONARY HYPERTENSION SECONDARY TO CHRONIC THROMBOTIC OR EMBOLIC DISEASE, OR BOTH

Chronic Thromboembolic Pulmonary Hypertension

PH is a long-term complication of thromboembolic disease, occurring in 0.1% to 0.5% of those who survive an acute pulmonary embolism (PE).[21] In many patients there is not a clear antecedent history of thromboembolic disease due to either an asymptomatic initial presentation or inadequate diagnostic evaluation at the time of presentation.[22] This, and the fact that patients with chronic thromboembolic PH (CTEPH) remain asymptomatic for years before clinical presentation, make the early natural history of this disorder unclear. The extent of pulmonary vascular obstruction appears to be a key determinant for the development of CTEPH, requiring generally more than 40% obstruction of the pulmonary vascular bed.[22] Without intervention, the rate of survival relates directly to the degree of PH; mean pulmonary artery pressures above 30 to 40 mm Hg appear to be markers for poor prognosis—30% of patients have 5-year survival rates.[22]

Pathophysiology

The etiology of CTEPH is unclear and likely multifactorial. Obstruction of the pulmonary vasculature may occur via several mechanisms: incomplete resolution of one or more acute PEs; recurrent thromboembolism; and in situ thrombosis. Incomplete resolution of thrombus occurs more commonly than originally believed and is associated with the presence of an anticardiolipin antibody in 10% of patients.[22] In situ thrombosis is believed to occur as a result of increased stasis and resultant hypercoagulability in the pulmonary vasculature. Although thrombosis of the pulmonary arteries plays an important role in the pathogenesis of CTEPH, many patients exhibit evidence of pulmonary vascular remodeling and development of an arteriopathy similar to that observed in other forms of PH. This hypothesis is supported clinically by the poor correlation between the level of central vascular obstruction and the degree of PH and the progression of symptoms and hemodynamic derangements observed without documented evidence of recurrent thromboembolism or in situ thrombosis.[22] Histologically, pulmonary hypertensive arteriopathy is present in vessels that are distinct from the site of thrombus, suggesting that the presence of thrombus triggers a more diffuse injury to the pulmonary vasculature. The mechanism by which this process occurs is unclear.

Diagnosis and Treatment

Clinically, patients with CTEPH present similarly to those with other forms of PH, with progressive exertional dyspnea being the primary symptom. Late in the course of

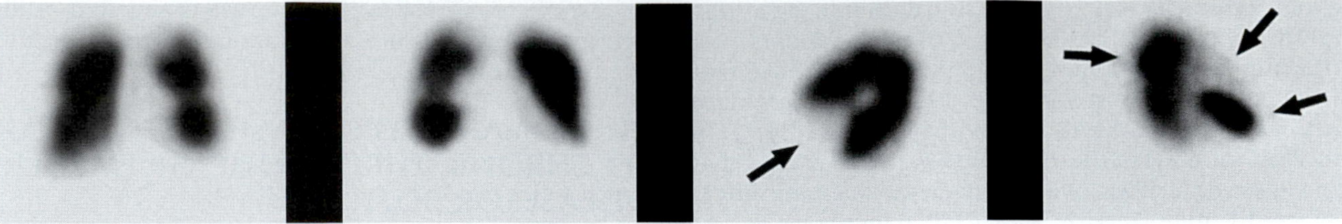

FIGURE 58-4. Perfusion scan of a patient with chronic thromboembolic pulmonary hypertension.The ventilation scan was normal. The perfusion scan demonstrates multiple defects (*arrows*).[27]

their disease, signs and symptoms of decreased right-sided cardiac output, such as exertional chest pain, increased abdominal girth and lower extremity edema, and syncope/near-syncope can occur. Physical examination findings are mainly similar to those of other forms of PH. One differentiating feature of CTEPH is the presence of a bruit auscultated over the lung fields, which may be present in up to 30% of patients[22] and likely results from turbulent flow through a partially occluded pulmonary vessel.

Clinically, it is important to differentiate patients with CTEPH from those with other forms of PH as it greatly affects their long-term treatment. Several diagnostic modalities are extremely useful for this purpose. Duplex ultrasound scanning of the lower extremities reveals evidence of prior deep vein thrombosis in up to 45% of patients with CTEPH.[22] Ventilation perfusion (V/Q) scanning has traditionally been the best study to evaluate patients for the presence of CTEPH. Patients with CTEPH invariably demonstrate one or more mismatched, segmental, or larger defects (Fig. 58-4). In contrast, those with primary PH typically have either normal scans or small subsegmental defects present on the perfusion scans.[22] CT scans of the chest may provide additional information about the presence of thrombus in the central vessels but appear to be most useful in evaluating patients who have unilateral perfusion defects on V/Q scans to rule out other disorders such as fibrosing mediastinitis, adenopathy, and tumors of the pulmonary artery, all of which can mimic CTEPH in their presentation (Table 58-1).

Pulmonary angiography should be performed in all patients being considered for surgical intervention to determine the extent and proximal extension of thromboemboli and thereby their surgical accessibility.[22] Angiographically, chronic thromboembolic disease is characterized by complex patterns of recanalization and partially occluding thrombi, which differ greatly from the well-defined intraluminal filling defects observed with acute PE.[22] Pulmonary angioscopy, a diagnostic fiberoptic device, was developed for preoperative assessment of patients with CTEPH. Approximately 60% of patients have this procedure performed as part of their work-up. Vessels that are afflicted by chronic emboli exhibit pitted masses of chronic embolic material within the lumen, roughening or pitting of the intimal surface, and evidence of partial recanalization. The main use for this diagnostic procedure is to assess operability in patients who would not meet surgical criteria by angiographic findings alone.[22]

The treatment of choice for CTEPH is pulmonary thromboendarterectomy, which results in improved symptoms, hemodynamics, and mortality in patients with symptomatic disease at rest or with exertion.[22-24] The key factor determining operability in these patients is the location and hemodynamic significance of the proximal thromboembolic obstruction.[22] The best candidates for surgery are those who have significant hemodynamic compromise from thrombus originating in main, lobar, or proximal segmental arteries.[22] Thrombotic material originating more distal than the proximal segmental arteries is generally not surgically accessible. As such, if distal thrombus or small vessel arteriopathy appears to be the major component of hemodynamic impairment, it is unlikely that thromboendarterectomy will improve PH postoperatively. The only absolute contraindication to this surgery is the presence of severe obstructive or restrictive lung disease.[22]

TABLE 58-1 CLINICAL FEATURES OF TAKAYASU'S ARTERITIS, PAS, AND CTEPH

	Takayasu Arteritis	PAS	CTEPH
Symptoms			
Dyspnea	+	+	+
Chest pain	+	+	+
Hemoptysis	+	+	+
Symptoms of arterial insufficiency	+	—	—
Systemic symptoms	+	+	—
Physical examination			
Pulmonary artery bruits	+	+	+
Systemic artery bruits	+	—	—
Hypertension	+	—	—
Diminished or absent pulses	+	—	—
Laboratory data			
Anemia	+	+	—
Elevated ESR	+	+	—
Radiography			
Abnormal pulmonary artery contour	+	+	+
Abnormal aortic contour/aortic aneurysm	+	—	—
Areas of decreased perfusion on V/Q scan	+	+	+

CTEPH, chronic thromboembolic pulmonary hypertension; ESR, erythrocyte sedimentation rate; PAS, pulmonary artery sarcoma; V/Q, ventilation-perfusion. From Kerr KM, Auger WR, Fedullo PR, et al: Large vessel pulmonary arteritis mimicking chronic thromboembolic disease. Am J Resp Crit Care Med 152:367, 1995.

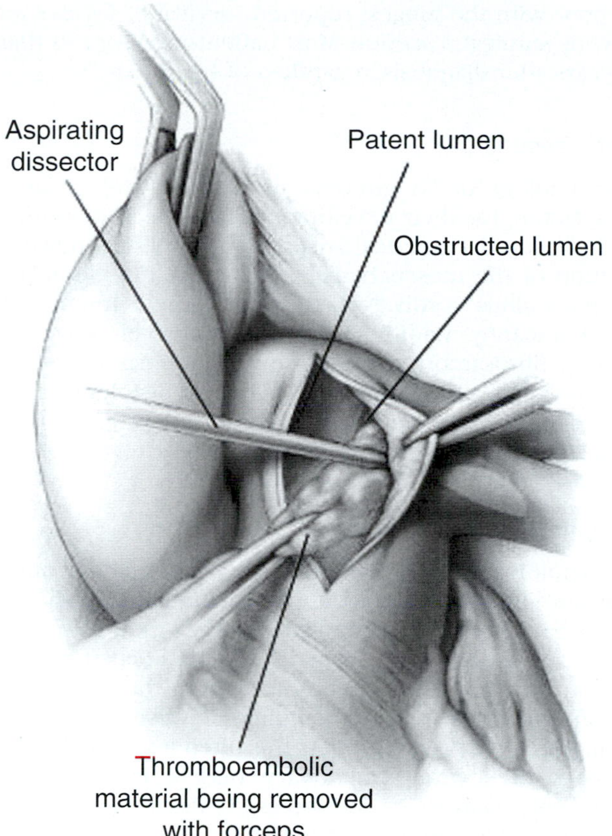

FIGURE 58-5. (See also Color Plate 58-5.) Intraluminal view of the pulmonary artery during thromboendarterectomy. The thromboembolic material is grasped with a forceps and circumferentially dissected from the vessel wall by an aspirating dissector. The process is repeated until all the material has been removed and the patency of the vessel restored.[27]

Surgically, the procedure performed is an endarterectomy because often the thromboembolic material is fibrotic and adherent to the vessel wall (Fig. 58-5). Right and left thromboarterectomies are performed sequentially through a median sternotomy after hypothermic circulatory arrest and cardiopulmonary bypass. An incision is made in the right PA where it passes the aorta to the division of the lower lobe branches. On the left, the incision extends from the main PA to the origin of the left upper lobe branch.[22] An endarterectomy plane is created in each vessel between the intima and the embolic material, and the obstructing material is grasped with a forceps and dissected off the vessel wall.[22] More than 2000 thromboendarterectomies have been performed worldwide; more than two thirds of these were done at a single center. Since 1996 case series have reported mortality rates of 5% to 24%, with the best results observed at the most experienced centers.[23,24]

In addition to the risk of major cardiothoracic surgery, the main risks for death postoperatively are reperfusion lung injury—a neutrophil-mediated form of high permeability pulmonary edema—and right ventricular failure secondary to residual PH. Therapy for each of these conditions is primarily supportive including ventilatory support and use of inotropic agents and inhaled NO to improve gas exchange. For most patients, the outcome from surgery is favorable with a mean reduction in PVR of approximately 65%[22] with associated improvement in New York Heart Association functional class.[24]

Lifelong anticoagulation is recommended for all patients, irrespective of whether or not they undergo thromboendarterectomy. Vasodilators are considered as second-line therapy for those patients who are inoperable and have only been studied in small trials in CTEPH. In patients with CTEPH, inhaled NO and aerosolized iloprost result in acute pulmonary vasodilation; iloprost may also produce long-term improvements in symptoms, hemodynamics, and survival. In select patients, there may be benefit from long-term treatment with epoprostenol or sildefanil.[22,25] Additionally, lung transplantation may be an option for those with inoperable disease or an incomplete response to thromboendarterectomy.[22]

Sickle Cell Disease

PH is becoming an increasingly recognized complication of sickle cell disease (SCD), occurring in 30% to 40% of patients.[26,27] PH in SCD has emerged as an important cause of morbidity and mortality over the past decade with the emergence of life-prolonging treatments such as transfusion therapy, antibiotic prophylaxis, and hydroxyurea. The presence of PH in SCD appears to be an independent risk factor for increased mortality in these patients, with 2-year mortality rates approaching 50%.[27] Additionally, evidence of pulmonary arteriopathy is found in a high percentage of autopsy studies performed on SCD patients who experience sudden cardiac death.[28]

Pathogenesis

The etiology of PH related to SCD is likely multifactorial. Although PH was traditionally believed to occur as a result of multiple episodes of acute chest syndrome, recent evidence supports the notion that patients with SCD experience a spectrum of vaso-occlusive processes over their lifetime and that subclinical pulmonary vasoocclusion may play a role in the development of sickle cell chronic lung disease.[26] Placing these patients at particular risk for the development of PH is the occurrence of increased cytokine production, shear stress, and localized hypoxia during pulmonary vasoocclusion, each of which has been implicated in the pathogenesis of primary PH. Additionally, the presence of PH in other hemolytic disorders such as thalassemia, hereditary spherocytosis, and paroxysmal nocturnal hemoglobinuria suggests a role for cell-free hemoglobin in this process.[29-31] One potential mechanism by which free hemoglobin can play a role in the development of PH is via its role as a scavenger of NO.[32] Additionally, the sickle RBC is a source of reactive oxygen species such as superoxide (O_2^-) and hydrogen peroxide (H_2O_2), which, on lysis, can be released into the bloodstream and react with NO to form nitrosative metabolites, thereby decreasing NO bioavailability[33,34] and promoting pulmonary vasoconstriction.

Autopsy studies of SCD patients have demonstrated that evidence of pulmonary arteriopathy is much more widespread than expected by clinical presentation.

Of 20 SCD patients who underwent autopsies after dying from various causes in one study, all had evidence of pulmonary vascular disease. Approximately 50% of patients had evidence of the irreversible plexiform lesions in their lungs, although many had more reversible lesions of PH, such as medial hypertrophy, intimal fibroelastosis, and cellular intimal hyperplasia present.[28] These data suggest that the incidence of PH in the SCD population is likely grossly underestimated by current antemortem clinical testing and that this represents an important area of future investigative work.

Diagnosis and Treatment

Limited data are available regarding the diagnosis and treatment of PH secondary to SCD. Although patients with end-stage disease present similarly to those with other forms of PH with progressive dyspnea, screening echocardiograms and autopsy studies suggest that many with PH related to SCD are asymptomatic. In general, these patients are older than SCD patients without PH, with a mean age of approximately 37 years.[27] Although patients with hemoglobin SS disease generally have more symptomatic vaso-occlusive events and more evidence of end-organ disease, interestingly, this may not be the case for PH related to SCD, which in some studies occurs in equal frequency in those without SS disease. A recent large-scale study evaluating 175 patients with SCD found PH in approximately 33%,[26] confirming the results observed in the older smaller studies. Right-heart catheterization of 20 patients with PH related to SCD demonstrated mean PA pressures that are moderately elevated (≈36 mm Hg), but in contrast to other forms of PH, there was a persistently high cardiac output observed (≈8.6 L/min).[26] This high output cardiac failure likely relates to the anemic states of these patients.

Studies evaluating the treatment of PH related to SCD have been quite limited. In two small studies, containing four and eight patients respectively, IV epoprostenol had acute therapeutic hemodynamic effects in approximately 75% of the patients.[26] As the median survival of patients who underwent right-heart catheterization evidence of PH was 25.6 months, it appears to be essential that larger scale trials of vasodilators such as epoprostenol be conducted in this population.

PULMONARY HYPERTENSION SECONDARY TO DISORDERS DIRECTLY AFFECTING THE PULMONARY VASCULATURE

Pulmonary Artery Sarcoma

Neoplasms of the pulmonary artery (PA) are uncommon, with several hundred cases reported in the medical literature. PA sarcoma, first described at autopsy by Mandelstam in 1923, represents the most common of these disorders.[35] These tumors are frequently misdiagnosed as CTEPH and historically were only diagnosed postmortem. Recent advances in diagnostic modalities and heightened clinical suspicion have led to earlier diagnosis in the past decade. Overall, the prognosis of PA sarcoma is poor with the longest reported survival of 5 years following surgical resection. Most patients survive less than 2 years after diagnosis, regardless of treatment.[35]

Pathogenesis

The etiology of PA sarcomas is obscure, and no clear risk factors for their development have been identified. It is believed that they arise from neoplastic transformation of the mesenchymal cells of the muscle anlage of the bulbus cordis.[36] Histologically, these tumors are predominantly undifferentiated spindle cell sarcomas (34%), fibrosarcomas or fibromyxosarcomas (21%), or leiomyosarcomas (20%). Regardless of histologic type, the clinical presentation and long-term prognosis are similar among all cases of PA sarcoma.[37]

Diagnosis and Treatment

Epidemiologically, PA sarcomas affect men and women equally, with an average age at presentation of 55 (although cases have been reported to affect all age groups).[37] Most of these tumors arise from the dorsal area of the PA trunk, although they can originate from the distal right or left pulmonary artery, the pulmonic valve, or the right ventricular outflow tract.[35] As this often leads to obstruction of the central pulmonary vessels, PH and right ventricular failure can develop as the disease progresses.

Usually, this tumor results in a fixed obstruction of the pulmonary vasculature. However, if the tumor grows on a stalk, the obstruction and symptomatology can be more intermittent.[37] The presentation is similar to CTEPH with dyspnea, chest pain, cough, and hemoptysis being the predominant symptoms (see Table 58-1). In contrast to those with CTEPH, all patients have evidence of systemic disease, typically characterized by weight loss, anemia, and fever. Eighty percent of patients in one series had an elevated erythrocyte sedimentation rate.[37] Most commonly, chest radiography reveals an abnormal hilar mass, although an elevated hemidiaphragm, pleural effusion, or a pulmonary nodule with or without cavitation can be observed. The presence of pulmonary nodules in this disease results from embolic metastatic spread of the disease, which, in some cases, can lead to pulmonary infarction.[37]

Surgery remains the treatment of choice for PA sarcomas, although in most cases, the disease is uniformly fatal in less than 2 years. Surgical resection of the tumor followed by pneumonectomy has resulted in a 5-year survival in one patient[35]; before that report, the longest survival reported was 3.5 years.[35,37] The responses of these tumors to chemotherapy and radiation therapy have not been extensively studied.[37]

Malignant Fibrous Histiocytoma

This tumor, first characterized by O'Brien and Stout, is the most common soft tissue sarcoma of adults.[38] Although most of these tumors involve the extremities, retroperitoneum, and intra-abdominal cavity, 21 cases of malignant fibrous histiocytoma involving the pulmonary parenchyma have been described in the literature[38]; in only one did the tumor arise from the pulmonary artery.[38]

In these cases PH resulted from obstruction of the main pulmonary arteries. These tumors, which originate from tissue histiocytes, are also often misdiagnosed as CTEPH as their clinical presentations are similar. The presence of fever and weight loss can help to distinguish patients with malignant fibrous histiocytoma from those with CTEPH.[38] Ultimately, the diagnosis is made histopathologically. Surgery is the treatment of choice for malignant fibrous histiocytoma with long-term survival of up to 10 years being reported in one case.[38] Most patients, however, survive less than 2 years. The roles of chemotherapy and radiation therapy in treatment are not well established.

Sarcoidosis

PH commonly affects patients with pulmonary sarcoidosis, occurring in up to 28% of these patients.[39] It appears to be more common in those with advanced disease; 50% of patients with stage 3 sarcoidosis have evidence of PH at rest, and all have elevated PAPs with exercise.[39]

Pathophysiology

The etiology of PH associated with sarcoidosis is unclear and likely multifactorial. Initially, it was believed to result from fibrosis of the pulmonary vasculature occurring in the setting of extensive parenchymal disease; however, a growing body of literature supports a role for direct invasion of the intima and media of the pulmonary arteries with noncaseating granulomas, thereby resulting in encroachment of vascular flow.[39] In addition to histopathologic evidence of pulmonary vascular granulomatous disease, the favorable clinical response observed in these patients treated with vasodilators suggests that this is an important contributor to the disease process. This correlates with the observation, in some patients, that the severity of PH is worse than the extent of parenchymal disease.[39]

Treatment

In a number of small clinical studies, PH secondary to sarcoidosis has been responsive to vasodilators. Two studies demonstrated an acute hemodynamic response to epoprostenol in a small number of patients with PH related to sarcoidosis. Preston and colleagues[39] demonstrated an acute hemodynamic response in seven of eight patients to inhaled NO, four of six patients to epoprostenol, and two of five patients to calcium-channel blockers. Long-term inhaled NO resulted in improved symptoms and hemodynamics after 1 year of treatment.[39]

Pulmonary Capillary Hemangiomatosis

First described by Wagenvoort and colleagues in 1978,[40] this disorder, characterized by uncontrolled proliferation of capillaries infiltrating vascular, bronchial, and interstitial pulmonary structures, has been associated with PH in 37 cases reported in the literature (Fig. 58-6). Clinically, this disorder is indistinguishable from pulmonary veno-occlusive disease. Dyspnea is the most common presenting symptom; fever, hemoptysis, cyanosis, and chest pain can occur as well. Signs of postcapillary PH including elevated pulmonary capillary wedge pressure, Kerley B lines consistent with interstitial edema, and pleural effusions on chest radiographs can be present in up to 50%, particularly those with later-stage disease. Pleural effusions, seen in approximately one third of patients, are usually transudative but can be hemorrhagic.[40]

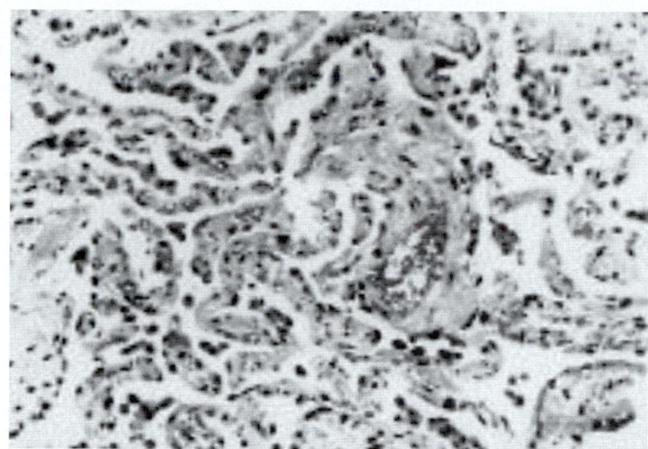

FIGURE 58-6. Histopathology of a case of pulmonary capillary hemangiomatosis. Interalveolar septae thickened with irregular fibrosis and proliferation of numerous dilated capillaries (hematoxylin & eosin, ×200).[42]

Pathogenesis

The etiology of PH related to pulmonary capillary hemangiomatosis is unclear, but it is believed to relate to vascular obstruction secondary to in situ thrombosis or vascular narrowing from the proliferation of intravascular capillaries. Another possible hypothesis includes the local production of vasoconstrictors as a result of endothelial injury.[40]

Diagnosis and Treatment

The diagnosis of pulmonary capillary hemangiomatosis is difficult secondary to the patchy nature of the disease. As such, multiple sites of biopsy are often required. Making this diagnosis histologically in patients suspected of having this disease is important because it greatly alters the treatment regimen. Most patients with PH secondary to pulmonary capillary hemangiomatosis are treated supportively for CHF with diuretics, angiotensin-converting enzyme (ACE) inhibitors, oxygen, and warfarin. These treatments, although beneficial symptomatically, have no impact on the progression of disease.[40] Because this disease is a postcapillary form of PH, it responds poorly to prostaglandins with a high incidence of worsening hypoxemia, pulmonary edema, and death. Due to these adverse effects, their use is contraindicated in PH related to pulmonary capillary hemangiomatosis. Steroids have been determined to have no clinical value in this disease entity.[40] Interferon α-2a ($IFN_{\alpha 2a}$) represents a new, promising treatment option for these patients; three patients treated with this medication in open-labeled studies demonstrated clinical improvements. The mechanism of action of $IFN_{\alpha 2a}$ is unclear, but in vitro studies have demonstrated that it is effective in inhibiting EC proliferation and migration, suggesting that it may have antiangiogenic properties.[40]

Takayasu's Arteritis (see Chapter 42)

This large vessel vasculitis, originally described in Japan, has a worldwide distribution and classically affects young women with an average age of onset of 30 years. PA involvement is a relatively common complication of this disorder, occurring in 14% to 86% of patients in different case series.[41] Usually, disease of the pulmonary arteries occurs in conjunction with systemic arterial disease. In rare instances patients can present with PA manifestations of Takayasu's arteritis alone, although on further examination, evidence of more widespread systemic disease is always present.[41]

Pathogenesis

Histologically, this disease is characterized by a progressive giant cell arteritis. Early lesions demonstrate a lymphoplasmacytic infiltration of the media associated with adventitial fibrosis and intimal proliferation. Later in the disease, the vessels appear more sclerotic with little or no inflammatory infiltrate. There appear to be three vascular lesions specific to the pulmonary arteries in this disease: stenosis/recanalization lesion, in which a new muscular artery derived from the vasa vasorum develops in the vessel wall; angiomatoid dilatation of small vessels; and cellular arteritis in small muscular arteries.[41]

Diagnosis and Treatment

Clinically, PH complicating Takayasu's arteritis manifests similarly to CTEPH (see Table 58-1). Although dyspnea, chest pain, and hemoptysis are the primary manifesting symptoms of both disorders, systemic symptoms such as fever, malaise, and weight loss and symptoms of arterial insufficiency such as headache, claudication, and vision loss are seen only in PH secondary to Takayasu's arteritis.[41] Chest radiographs in both disorders reveal irregularly contoured pulmonary arteries with areas of enlargement and narrowing. Additionally, ventilation/perfusion scans demonstrate decreased perfusion to multiple segments of the lungs. Evidence of aortic arteritis by aortography is diagnostic of Takayasu's arteritis and obviates the need for an open lung biopsy.[41]

Steroids are the treatment of choice for Takayasu's arteritis, although their efficacy has not been proved in prospective, long-term controlled trials. Use of daily prednisone in 29 patients with Takayasu's arteritis resulted in a decrease in systemic inflammatory symptoms and erythrocyte sedimentation rate within several weeks. Shelhamer and colleagues[41] determined that, in those patients who do not respond to steroids, cyclophosphamide is a useful treatment adjunct. The Systemic Vascular Disorders Research Committee of Health and Welfare of Japan established a standardized treatment policy for treatment of Takayasu's arteritis. Patients with evidence of active arteritis characterized by fever, pain, increased erythrocyte sedimentation rate, and increased C-reactive protein should be treated with 30 mg prednisone daily or its equivalent.[42] The use of platelet inhibitors and anticoagulation should be strongly considered in those with evidence of ischemic changes or infarction of major organs. Additionally, there have been several cases reported in the literature of successful surgical correction of stenosis of the main pulmonary arteries secondary to Takayasu's arteritis.[41]

REFERENCES

1. Rich S (ed): Primary Pulmonary Hypertension: Executive Summary from the World Symposium. World Health Organization, 1998.
2. Moraes DL, Colucci WS, Givertz MM: Secondary pulmonary hypertension in chronic heart failure: The role of the endothelium in pathophysiology and management. Circulation 102:1718, 2000.
3. Cody RJ, Haas GJ, Binkley PF, et al: Plasma endothelin correlates with the extent of pulmonary hypertension in patients with chronic congestive heart failure. Circulation 85:504, 1992.
4. Abramson SV, Burke JF, Kelly JJ Jr, et al: Pulmonary hypertension predicts mortality and morbidity in patients with dilated cardiomyopathy. Ann Intern Med 116:888, 1992.
5. Califf RM, Adams KF, McKenna WJ, et al: A randomized controlled trial of epoprostenol therapy for severe congestive heart failure: The Flolan International Randomized Survival Trial (FIRST). Am Heart J 134:44, 1997.
6. Berry DF, Buccigrossi D, Peabody J, et al: Pulmonary vascular occlusion and fibrosing mediastinitis. Chest 89:296, 1986.
7. Mandel J, Mark EJ, Hales CA: Pulmonary veno-occlusive disease. Am J Resp Crit Care Med 162:1964, 2000.
8. Wagenvoort CA, Wagenvoort N, Takahashi T: Pulmonary veno-occlusive disease: Involvement of the pulmonary arteries and review of the literature. Hum Pathol 16:1033, 1985.
9. Matthews AW, Buchanan R: A case of pulmonary veno-occlusive disease and a new bronchoscopic sign. Respir Med 84:503, 1990.
10. Hopkins N, McLoughlin P: The structural basis of pulmonary hypertension in chronic lung disease: Remodeling, rarefaction or angiogenesis. J Anat 201:335, 2002.
11. Voelkel NF, Tuder RM: Cellular and molecular mechanisms in the pathogenesis of severe pulmonary hypertension. Eur Respir J 8:2129, 1995.
12. Peinado VI, Barbera JA, Ramirez J, et al: Endothelial dysfunction in pulmonary arteries of patients with mild COPD. Am J Physiol 274:L908, 1998.
13. Okada K, Tanaka Y, Bernstein M, et al: Pulmonary hemodynamics modify the rat pulmonary artery response to injury: A neointimal model of pulmonary hypertension. Am J Pathol 151:1019, 1997.
14. MacLean MR: Endothelin-1 and serotonin: Mediators of primary and secondary pulmonary hypertension? J Lab Clin Med 134:105, 1999.
15. Fagan KA, Fouty BW, Tyler RC, et al: The pulmonary circulation of homozygous or heterozygous eNOS-null mice is hyperresponsive to mild hypoxia. J Clin Invest 103:291, 1999.
16. Weitzenblum E: Chronic cor pulmonale. Heart 89:225, 2003.
17. Arcasoy SM, Christie JD, Ferrari VA, et al: Echocardiographic assessment of pulmonary hypertension in patients with advanced lung disease. Am J Respir Crit Care Med 167:735, 2003.
18. Tan RT, Kuzo R, Goodman LR, et al: Utility of CT scan evaluation for predicting pulmonary hypertension in patients with parenchymal lung disease. Chest 113:1250, 1998.
19. Marrone O, Bonsignore MR: Pulmonary haemodynamics in obstructive sleep apnoea. Sleep Med Rev 6:175, 2002.
20. Sajkov D, Wang T, Saunders NA, et al: Continuous positive airway pressure treatment improves pulmonary hemodynamics in patients with obstructive sleep apnea. Am J Respir Crit Care Med 65:152, 2002.
21. Moser KM, Auger WR, Fedullo PF: Chronic major-vessel thromboembolic pulmonary hypertension. Circulation 81:1735, 1990.
22. Fedullo PF, Auger WR, Kerr KM, et al: Current concepts: Chronic thromboembolic pulmonary hypertension. N Engl J Med 345:1465, 2001.

23. Jamieson SW, Kapelanski DP: Pulmonary endarterectomy. Curr Probl Surg 37:165, 2000.
24. Archibald CJ, Auger WR, Fedullo PF, et al: Long-term outcome after pulmonary thromboendarterectomy. Am J Resp Crit Care Med 160:523, 1999.
25. Ghofrani HA, Schermuly RT, Rose F, et al: Sildenafil for long-term treatment of nonoperable chronic thromboembolic pulmonary hypertension. Am J Resp Crit Care Med 167:1139, 2003.
26. Gladwin MT, Sachdev V, Jison ML, et al: Pulmonary hypertension as a risk factor for death in patients with sickle cell disease. N Engl J Med 350:880, 2004.
27. Castro O, Hoque M, Brown BD: Pulmonary hypertension in sickle cell disease: Cardiac catheterization results and survival. Blood 101:1257, 2003.
28. Haque AK, Gokhale S, Rampy BA, et al: Pulmonary hypertension in sickle cell hemoglobinopathy: A clinicopathologic study of 20 cases. Hum Pathol 33:1037, 2002.
29. Aessopos A, Farmakis D, Karagiorga M, et al: Cardiac involvement in thallassemia intermedia: A multicenter study. Blood 97:3411, 2001.
30. Hayag-Barin JE, Smith RE, Tucker FC Jr: Hereditary spherocytosis, thrombocytosis, and chronic pulmonary emboli: A case report and review of the literature. Am J Hematol 57:82, 1998.
31. Heller PG, Grinberg AR, Lencioni M, et al: Pulmonary hypertension in paroxysmal nocturnal hemoglobinuria. Chest 102:642, 1992.
32. Reiter CD, Wang X, Tanus-Santos JE, et al: Cell-free hemoglobin limits nitric oxide bioavailability in sickle cell disease. Nat Med 8:1383, 2002.
33. Schachter L, Warth JA, Gordon EM, et al: Altered amount and activity of superoxide dismutase in sickle cell disease. FASEB J 2:237, 1998.
34. Hebbel RP, Eaton JW, Balasingam M, et al: Spontaneous oxygen radical generation by sickle erythrocytes. J Clin Invest 70:1253, 1982.
35. Mattoo A, Fedullo PF, Kapelanski D, et al: Pulmonary artery sarcoma: A case report of surgical cure and 5-year follow-up. Chest 122:745, 2002.
36. Baker PB, Goodwin RA: Pulmonary artery sarcoma. Arch Pathol Lab Med 109:35, 1985.
37. Parish JM, Rosenow EC, Swensen SJ, et al: Pulmonary artery sarcoma: Clinical features. Chest 110:1480, 1996.
38. Carlin BW, Moser KM: Pulmonary artery obstruction related to malignant fibrous histiocytoma. Chest 92:173, 1987.
39. Preston IR, Klinger JR, Landzberg MJ, et al: Vasoresponsiveness of sarcoidosis-associated pulmonary hypertension. Chest 120:866, 2001.
40. Almagro P, Julia J, Sanjaume M, et al: Pulmonary capillary hemangiomatosis associated with primary pulmonary hypertension: Report of 2 new cases and review of 35 cases from the literature. Medicine 81:417, 2002.
41. Kerr KM, Auger WR, Fedullo PR, et al: Large vessel pulmonary arteritis mimicking chronic thromboembolic disease. Am J Resp Crit Care Med 152:367, 1995.
42. Ito I: Medical treatment of Takayasu arteritis. Heart Vessels Suppl 7:133, 1992.

chapter 59

Pulmonary Veno-occlusive Disease

Jess Mandel

Pulmonary veno-occlusive disease (PVOD) is among the most lethal and most poorly understood pulmonary vascular disorders.[1,2] In contrast to major breakthroughs in the understanding and therapy that idiopathic pulmonary arterial hypertension (IPAH) and related conditions have undergone in the past two decades, knowledge of PVOD remains primitive and therapy is largely unsatisfactory.

The clinicopathologic syndrome of PVOD was first described in 1934 by Julius Höra at the University of Munich.[3] The index patient was a 48-year-old previously healthy baker, who died in the year after presenting with progressive dyspnea, edema, and cyanosis. Before his death, the patient was assumed to be suffering from mitral stenosis, but at autopsy, diffuse obstruction of the pulmonary venules with loose fibrous tissue was noted in the absence of mitral valve disease or other causes of left atrial hypertension. Höra hypothesized an infectious explanation for the pathologic findings, although no organisms could be demonstrated by stains or cultures.

The condition was referred to as "isolated pulmonary venous sclerosis," "obstructive disease of the pulmonary veins," or "the venous form of primary pulmonary hypertension" for the next several decades, until the term "pulmonary veno-occlusive disease" was popularized in the mid-1960s.[4-7] PVOD does not encompass and should be differentiated from stenosis of one or more of the four main pulmonary veins, which may occur as a congenital anomaly or become acquired as a complication of cardiothoracic surgery or radiofrequency ablation procedures for atrial fibrillation.[8-10]

EPIDEMIOLOGY

The true incidence and prevalence of PVOD are difficult to estimate precisely because less severe cases may not come to medical attention, and many cases are probably misclassified as IPAH because of the difficulty in distinguishing the two syndromes without tissue biopsy. An imprecise estimate of the annual incidence of PVOD can be extracted from analysis of IPAH series in which the fractions of patients fulfilling criteria for PVOD were reported. Pooling of seven such series published between 1970 and 1991 and comprising a total of 465 patients suggests that the incidence of PVOD is approximately 10% that of true IPAH .[11-18] If one accepts an annual incidence of IPAH of 1 to 2 cases per million persons in the general population, this suggests an annual incidence of PVOD of around 0.1 to 0.2 cases per million persons in the general population.[19,20] However, this may represent an underestimate of the true incidence of PVOD, because a number of cases are probably alternatively misclassified as interstitial lung disease or heart failure, but no studies have thoroughly examined the magnitude of this phenomenon.

Unlike IPAH, which appears to be more common in women, there does not appear to be a clear gender imbalance among patients with PVOD.[2,21,22] The age at diagnosis has ranged from within 9 days of birth to the seventh decade of life.

PATHOLOGY

The most prominent pathologic feature of PVOD is the extensive and diffuse obliteration of small pulmonary veins or venules by fibrous tissue, which may be either loose and edematous or dense and sclerotic (Fig. 59-1A and B).[2,11,23,24] Venous lesions tend to be eccentric or trabeculated, similar to changes seen in arterial structures that have undergone recanalization following thrombotic occlusion.[25] The media of the venules may undergo arterialization with an increase in elastic fibers, which become calcified in some cases.

Pulmonary arteriolar changes frequently accompany venous changes, although it is not clear if they develop concomitantly with them or as a consequence of them. In approximately 50% of patients with PVOD, pulmonary arterioles demonstrate marked medial hypertrophy. Capillaries become engorged and tortuous, occasionally leading to a misdiagnosis of pulmonary capillary hemangiomatosis.[26] Plexiform lesions are less commonly encountered than in IPAH, and arteritis or venulitis is distinctly uncommon.[27,28] Lymphatics, both in the pleura and in the lung, can become markedly dilated, presumably because of increased movement of fluid from capillaries to the interstitial space as a result of elevated capillary hydrostatic pressure.[29]

In contrast to many other causes of pulmonary hypertension (PH), pulmonary parenchymal abnormalities are common in PVOD. Interstitial edema is commonly observed and is particularly distinct in lobular septae (Fig. 59-2). Collagen deposition in these areas, and occasionally also involving alveolar walls, can appear similar to changes observed in longstanding mitral stenosis.[30] Lymphocytes and monocytes are commonly seen in the interstitium and may be sufficiently numerous to lead to the misdiagnosis of an idiopathic interstitial pneumonitis.[24]

Areas of microscopic pulmonary hemorrhage or hemosiderosis are frequently observed and presumably reflect the extravasation of erythrocytes as a consequence of

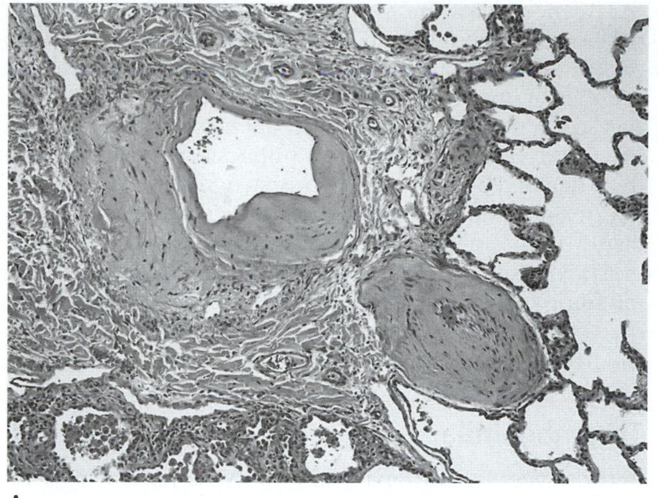
A

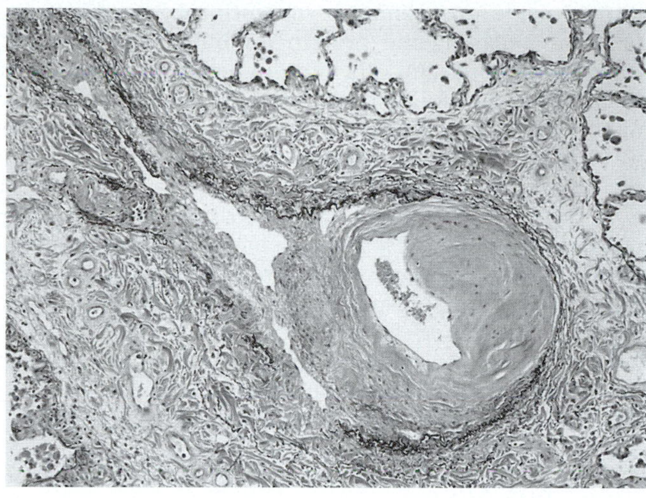
B

FIGURE 59-1. (See also Color Plate 59-1.) High magnification (original magnification ×100) photomicrograph showing venous sclerosis and occlusion in pulmonary veno-occlusive disease. **A,** hematoxylin & eosin stain. **B,** Verhoeff Van Gieson stain. There is marked luminal narrowing resulting from sclerosis of the intima. (Courtesy Jeffrey L. Myers, MD.)

pulmonary capillary hypertension. Determining whether observed areas of pulmonary hemorrhage are due to PVOD or reflect tissue disruption by biopsy procedures can be problematic. Patients with PVOD commonly demonstrate hemosiderin in alveolar macrophages or the interstitium, and in some cases this feature is of such prominence that the diagnosis of idiopathic pulmonary hemosiderosis or a vasculitis (e.g., Wegener's granulomatosis) is considered.[2,31]

ETIOLOGY

The etiology of PVOD remains speculative. No case-control or cohort studies have been performed specifically to explore the potential causes of this condition.

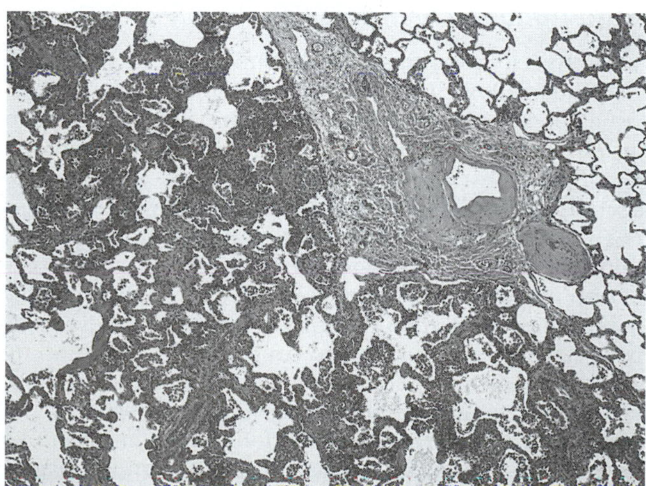

FIGURE 59-2. Low magnification (hematoxylin & eosin stain, original magnification ×40) photomicrograph illustrating venous sclerosis and associated alveolar septal congestion in pulmonary veno-occlusive disease. (Courtesy Jeffrey L. Myers, MD.)

The situation is further complicated by the fact that PVOD likely represents a final common clinicopathologic pathway that may be triggered in a susceptible host by a number of discrete causes. Nonetheless, various risk factors have been proposed on the basis of case reports and small case series.

Genetic Factors

Reports of PVOD developing in siblings have fueled suspicions that a genetic predisposition may underlie development of the disease. Most such cases have developed before the third decade of life. Unaffected siblings have also been detailed in a number of these families.[7,17,24,32,33] No definite genetic abnormality has been demonstrated in these sibling pairs, and the development of disease in these cases could also reflect common exposures to environmental or infectious agents.

Since the identification of mutations of the bone morphogenic protein receptor type 2 (BMPR2) gene as a major cause of familial pulmonary arterial hypertension in 2000, there has been speculation that abnormalities at this site may also be involved in the pathogenesis of PVOD.[34-36] In 2003 a BMPR2 mutation (deletion of a cytosine residue 44 bases from the translation start site in exon 1, resulting in production of a truncated, nonfunctional protein) was described in a patient who developed PVOD at age 36.[37] The patient's mother had died of PH several decades earlier, but lung tissue had not been examined to determine if she suffered from IPAH or PVOD. The authors reported that at the time of manuscript submission, the index patient had been stable for 5 years while receiving continuous IV epoprostenol, a clinical course that is somewhat atypical in PVOD.

The finding of a BMPR2 mutation in PVOD suggests the possibility that IPAH and PVOD may share a common genetic basis and the pathologic phenotype that develops may be due to modifier genes or differing environmental exposures. Presumably, the loss of a functional

BMPR2 allele may diminish the antiproliferative effects of bone morphogenic protein on pulmonary vascular endothelial and smooth muscle cells and result in unchecked proliferation in response to other ligands of the transforming growth factor-β family. The genetic mechanism may be by haploinsufficiency or may be due to a dominant-negative effect.[38]

A common BMPR2 defect would also help explain the development of scattered venous lesions in some patients with predominantly precapillary disease and the presence of precapillary lesions and abnormal precapillary resistance in many patients with PVOD.[39-41] Over the next several years, more extensive genotyping of patients with PVOD should help clarify the role of BMPR2 mutations in the development of this condition.

Infectious Agents

Since the initial description of PVOD, speculation has abounded that it was related to an infectious cause.[42] Höra believed that streptococcal infection played a role in his patient's illness, but in the decades that followed, nonbacterial agents have been more frequently hypothesized to play a role.[3] Recent influenza-like illness and serological evidence of recent infection with agents such as measles or *Toxoplasma gondii* have been documented at the time of PVOD diagnosis, and some patients have had manifestations of Epstein-Barr virus or cytomegalovirus infection such as lymphadenopathy, fever, and erythrophagocytosis.[4,5,43-45] Several cases have been reported in association with human immunodeficiency virus (HIV) infection.[46-48]

In contrast to HIV or other lentivirus infections, it is difficult to reconcile the time courses of acute infectious illnesses and PVOD, given that it requires months to years to develop severe right ventricular hypertrophy and the symptom complex with which PVOD patients commonly present. More likely, the significance of an acute illness near the time of PVOD diagnosis is that it may bring an undiagnosed patient to medical attention and stimulate a diagnostic evaluation that ultimately demonstrates the presence of PVOD.

Toxic Exposures

An association between certain drugs or chemicals and the development of PVOD has been postulated. As an example, the disease developed in a 14-year-old boy with a two-year history of ingesting and sniffing a powdered cleaning product containing silica, soda ash, dodecyl benzyl sulfonate, and trichloro-s-triazinetriome.[49]

As awareness developed that patients could develop hepatic veno-occlusive disease (HVOD) following antineoplastic chemotherapy, reports began to emerge linking PVOD to these agents as well. Many of these patients received radiation and various different antineoplastic drugs over several years, making identification of a specific culprit agent difficult, but the most commonly implicated compounds are bleomycin, mitomycin, carmustine (BCNU), and gemcitabine.[50-56] Anecdotal reports suggest that PVOD may be more common following either allogeneic or autologous bone marrow transplantation than routine cytoreductive chemotherapy.[57-62]

The mechanism by which certain drugs might produce pulmonary venous remodeling is unknown. Because endothelial cells in the pulmonary circulation perform a number of important metabolical functions, it is possible that certain chemotherapeutic agents may be metabolized to toxic intermediates in pulmonary capillaries and then damage pulmonary venous structures.

Cocaine, amphetamines, and anorectic agents are associated with pulmonary arterial hypertension but have not been linked to PVOD.[19,20] Similarly, "bush teas" containing pyrrolizidine alkaloids have been responsible for case clusters of HVOD but have not been associated with the development of PVOD.[63,64]

Thrombophilia

Because venules and small veins in PVOD have an appearance similar to recanalized, thrombotically occluded arteries, and lung specimens occasionally have evidence of fresh thrombi in affected vessels, a number of researchers have suspected that thrombophilia may play a role in the pathogenesis of PVOD. Coagulation and rheologic parameters have not been assessed in PVOD patients by state-of-the-art techniques, but several reports from the 1960s described increased platelet adhesiveness in patients with the disorder, in one case to a degree four standard deviations above the mean for normals.[4,65] A number of cases of PVOD have occurred in patients with risk factors for hypercoagulability such as pregnancy or oral contraceptive use.[66,67]

However, although cases of PVOD have occurred in the setting of documented thrombophilia, such comorbidities have been unusual.[68] The thrombophilia hypothesis also fails to explain the fact that extrapulmonary venous or arterial thrombi, which would be expected to develop commonly in hypercoagulable states, are infrequent in patients with PVOD. Finally, examination of lung specimens from the majority of patients with PVOD fails to demonstrate acute pulmonary venous thrombi.[29]

Autoimmune Disorders

Venulitis, either primary or secondary to an infectious vasculitis, followed by thrombosis, remodeling, or both, could presumably explain the pathologic changes seen in PVOD, but it is not a typical feature of the disorder. Granulomatous venulitis rarely has been described to accompany sarcoidosis, and a similar vascular lesion has been described in a 21-year-old marijuana-smoking man with the clinical syndrome of PVOD.[28,69]

Although most patients with PVOD do not display manifestations of autoimmunity, a number of individuals have developed PVOD in the context of positive antinuclear antibodies, alopecia, myopathy, rheumatoid arthritis, Felty's syndrome, systemic lupus erythematosus, or the scleroderma spectrum of conditions (including features such as calcinosis, Raynaud's phenomenon, esophageal dysmotility, sclerodactyly, and telangiectasias).[70-78] However, the fact that only a minority of cases display associated autoimmune findings argues against autoimmunity playing a fundamental role in PVOD.

CLINICAL MANIFESTATIONS

The majority of patients with PVOD present with nonspecific symptoms of PH such as dyspnea on exertion and fatigue.[22] Patients may develop a chronic cough (either productive or nonproductive), and many patients are initially diagnosed with an acute respiratory infection; PVOD is subsequently found after they fail to improve significantly after treatment with antimicrobial agents.[5,45,79] As PH progresses, patients may develop right upper quadrant pain (secondary to hepatic congestion), pedal edema, or exertional syncope. Orthopnea reportedly is more common and severe in patients with PVOD than in those with IPAH or other causes of pulmonary arterial hypertension.[31] Unusual clinical presentations of PVOD include symptomatic diffuse alveolar hemorrhage or sudden cardiac death.[80-82] Chronic subacute alveolar hemorrhage appears common on the basis of lung histopathologic findings; if hemoptysis is present clinically, it is rarely massive and life threatening.[80]

Physical examination also tends to reveal nonspecific findings of PH, with or without overt right ventricular failure, such as increased intensity of the pulmonic component of the second heart sound or a right ventricular heave/lift, or both. Murmurs of tricuspid regurgitation and, less commonly, pulmonic insufficiency, may be appreciated, and a right-sided fourth heart sound, elevated jugular venous pressure, hepatomegaly, and edema may also be apparent. Any murmurs or gallops present generally are augmented with inspiration, consistent with their right-sided location.[83] Digital clubbing is sometimes present, and basilar rales are appreciated in some cases.[45]

Pleural effusions are relatively common in patients with PVOD, in contrast to their infrequent association with IPAH and related precapillary causes of PH.[84,85] The most likely explanation for this observation is that PVOD and other postcapillary causes of PH produce elevated pulmonary capillary and visceral pleural hydrostatic pressures, leading to transudation of fluid into the pleural space. In contrast, the high-resistance areas of the pulmonary circulation are precapillary in IPAH, and thus pleural effusions do not generally accumulate until elevated hydrostatic pressure develops in the central systemic veins, leading to elevations in hydrostatic pressure in the parietal pleural capillaries.

Radiographic Findings

Chronic pulmonary capillary hypertension can result in transudation of fluid into the pulmonary interstitium, resulting in engorgement of pulmonary lymphatics, appearing radiographically as Kerley B lines on plain chest films (Fig. 59-3A and B). Central pulmonary arteries generally are visibly enlarged, peribronchial cuffing can be seen, and scattered parenchymal opacities may be present.[4,86] However, the absence of any or all of these findings does not eliminate the possibility of PVOD.[22,76,87,88]

CT images may display smooth thickening of the septae; diffuse or mosaic ground glass opacities; multiple well or poorly defined, small, noncalcified nodules; pleural effusions; or areas of alveolar consolidation that may be gravitationally dependent (Fig. 59-4).[84,89-92] The pathologic correlate of ground glass attenuation seen in these patients is not entirely clear; alveolar hemorrhage, nonspecific interstitial inflammation, or alveolar septal thickening with associated epithelial hyperplasia have each been proposed to explain the finding. The central pulmonary veins and the left atrium are not enlarged, in contrast to patients with mitral stenosis, cor triatriatum, or left atrial myxoma. Prominent mediastinal lymphadenopathy has been reported in several cases.[1,92-94]

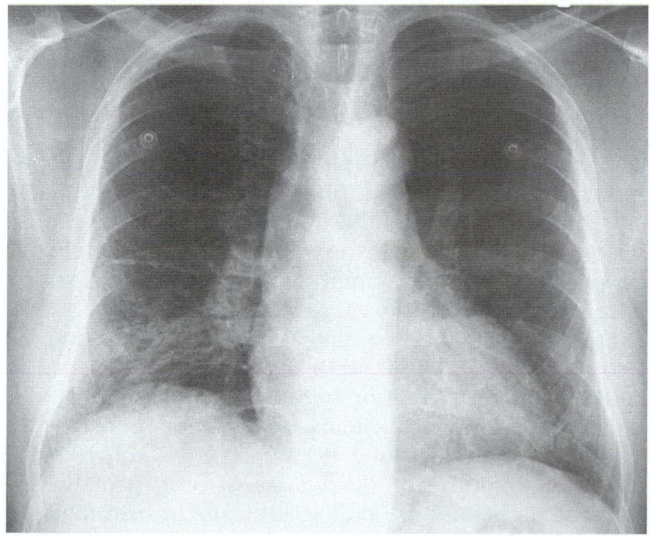
A

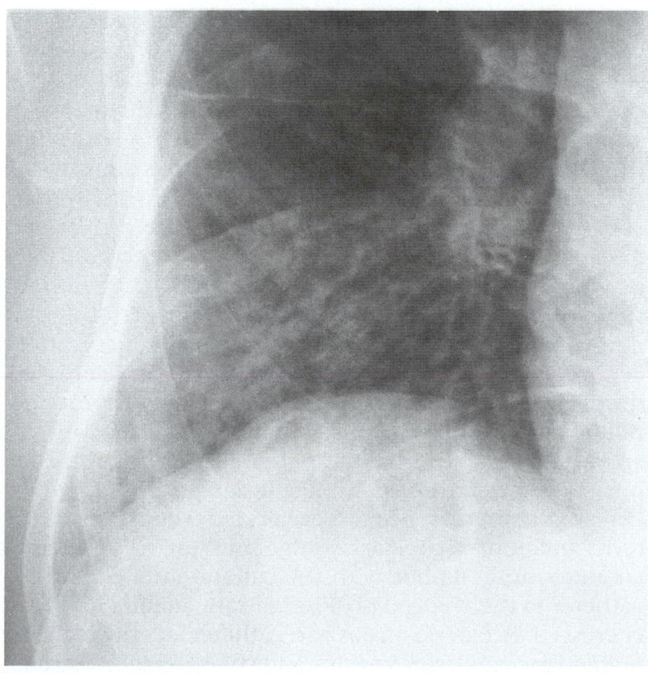
B

FIGURE 59-3. Posteroanterior chest radiograph (**A**) showing enlarged hila, a normal-sized cardiac silhouette, fluid in the minor fissure, and thickened septal lines (Kerley B lines) in the lower lobes, which are better appreciated on the magnified view of the right lower lobe (**B**).

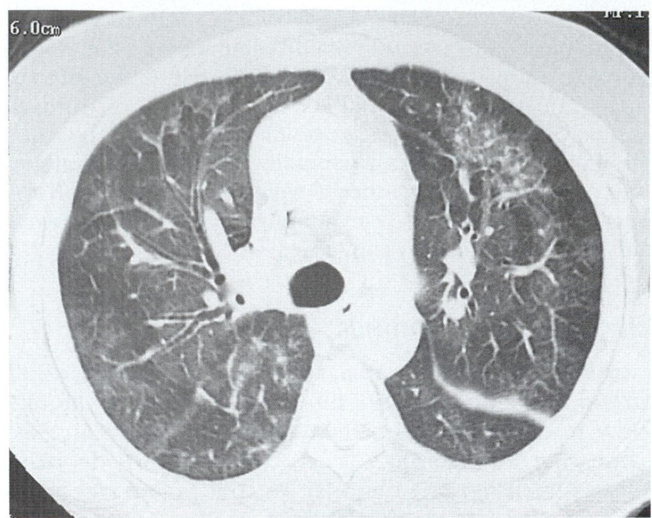

FIGURE 59-4. CT image showing thickened septal lines at the periphery, patchy foci of ground glass attenuation, and enlargement of arteries relative to associated bronchi.

Radionuclide ventilation-perfusion images display normal ventilation but commonly reveal multiple focal areas of hypoperfusion, sometimes in a segmental pattern.[95] This finding may be misinterpreted as supporting the diagnosis of chronic thromboembolic PH.[22,31,79,80,88,89,96-99]

Cardiac Catheterization

It is frequently difficult to obtain a satisfactory pulmonary artery occlusion (wedge) pressure in patients with PVOD. When the distal port of the catheter is flushed while the balloon is inflated (i.e., in the wedged position), there is often a disproportionate rise in recorded pressure, which then falls extremely slowly to baseline; these phenomena reflect impaired runoff of infused saline because of the diminished cross-sectional area of the pulmonary venules and small veins.[4,80,100] To document successful catheter wedging in this situation, it may be necessary to demonstrate that blood gas analysis of a sample slowly drawn from the distal catheter port while the balloon is inflated demonstrates values similar to a specimen drawn simultaneously from an arterial source.

If a pulmonary artery occlusion pressure can be successfully measured, it is recommended to record values in several different locations to ensure that spurious values have not been obtained because of local phenomena. In patients with PVOD, the pulmonary artery occlusion pressure is generally normal or decreased, despite the fact that postcapillary obstruction produces pulmonary capillary hypertension.[45] The cause of this apparent paradox is that the pulmonary artery occlusion pressure is determined by left atrial pressures, not by hydrostatic pressures in the pulmonary capillaries, as the term "pulmonary capillary wedge pressure" is sometimes taken to imply. Rather, with the balloon inflated and the catheter in the wedged position, a static column of blood is created. It extends from the catheter tip through the pulmonary capillaries, venules, and veins to the left atrium, the latter of which determines the recorded pressure, and is generally normal in PVOD. Extensive stenosis of the small pulmonary veins in PVOD tends to dampen this pressure tracing to some degree but does not fundamentally alter the fact that structures distal to the pulmonary venules determine the pulmonary artery occlusion pressure, and these structures are unaffected in this condition.[101,102]

Short-acting pulmonary arterial vasodilators are frequently administered to patients with PH at the time of cardiac catheterization to determine if pulmonary vasoreactivity is present.[20] However, in patients with PVOD, such medications may produce acute life-threatening pulmonary edema, and the development of this complication strongly suggests that PVOD is present.[45,94] Presumably, pulmonary edema develops in this circumstance because of pulmonary arterial vasodilation without concomitant pulmonary venodilation, causing a rapid increase in transcapillary hydrostatic forces and transudation of fluid into the pulmonary interstitium and alveoli.

Other Studies

Patients with PVOD generally display normal spirometry. The single-breath diffusing capacity for carbon monoxide ($D_{L_{CO}}$) is usually reduced, and a mild to moderate restrictive ventilatory defect is seen in some cases.[45,88,89] Laboratory parameters are generally unremarkable, although isolated cases have displayed otherwise unexplained features such as microangiopathic hemolytic anemia,[54] heavy proteinuria,[5] or elevated IgG or IgM concentrations.[72]

The finding on bronchoscopy of intense hyperemia and longitudinal vascular engorgement of the lobar and segmental bronchi has been reported in PVOD.[97] As these abnormalities were not seen in the trachea and main bronchi, where systemic bronchial veins are well developed, they likely result from engorgement of the bronchial arterial system, which in segmental and more distal bronchi normally drains into the impaired pulmonary circulation characteristic of PVOD.

Diagnosis

The triad of severe PH, radiographic evidence of pulmonary edema, and a normal pulmonary artery occlusion pressure is frequently sufficient to warrant a clinical diagnosis of PVOD.[102] However, many patients with PVOD do not have all three components of this triad. Thus its absence cannot reliably exclude the diagnosis.

Delays in diagnosis are almost universally encountered by patients with PVOD, with many patients believed to suffer from heart failure because of radiographic evidence of pulmonary edema and pleural effusions or chronic thromboembolic PH because of nonresolving radionuclide perfusion defects. In cases of PVOD where interstitial changes are radiographically or histologically prominent, alternative diagnoses of diffuse parenchymal lung diseases such as sarcoidosis, pneumoconioses, cystic fibrosis, or idiopathic interstitial pneumonias may be considered.[103]

Definitive diagnosis is possible only by surgical lung biopsy, and this procedure should be considered to confirm the clinical suspicion of PVOD. Although the need for lung biopsy has been questioned because therapy for PVOD is so unsatisfactory, establishing the diagnosis has significant implications for prognosis, medical therapy, and timing of lung transplantation and therefore should be considered in patients in whom the diagnosis is suspected and surgical risk is not prohibitive.

The demonstration of occult pulmonary hemorrhage by bronchoalveolar lavage in the proper clinical setting may support the diagnosis if lung tissue has not been obtained.[104] Transbronchial biopsy almost never yields enough tissue for a firm pathologic diagnosis and carries significant risks when performed in the setting of PH.

PROGNOSIS AND TREATMENT

The prognosis of PVOD is poor, with most patients dying within 2 years of diagnosis. Nonetheless, cases have been reported where individuals have survived in excess of 5 years, generally when therapy with oral calcium channel antagonists or IV epoprostenol therapy has been well tolerated.[37,105,106]

Because PVOD is a rare disease, large treatment trials cannot be easily performed, and the degree to which any of the current therapies influence survival and quality of life is unclear.[107] With the possible exceptions of lung transplantation and IV epoprostenol (if tolerated), the impact of current therapies does not seem profound.

Calcium Channel Antagonists and Epoprostenol

A minority of patients with IPAH display acute pulmonary vasoreactivity (defined as a 20% decrease in mean pulmonary artery pressure and pulmonary vascular resistance) in response to vasodilator medications such as adenosine, epoprostenol, inhaled nitric oxide, or calcium channel antagonists.[108,109] Such patients tend to have an excellent prognosis when treated with calcium channel antagonists. In IPAH patients without an acute hemodynamic response and who cannot be treated with calcium channel antagonists, therapy with continuous IV epoprostenol has been associated with improved survival.[110,111]

The generalizability of such data to PVOD is unclear. Theoretically, a reduction in pulmonary arterial resistance without a concomitant reduction in pulmonary venous resistance could cause pulmonary edema, whereas a parallel decrease in both arterial and venous resistance should be well tolerated and advantageous.

The clinical experience with vasodilator medications in patients with PVOD has been mixed. Modest improvements in hemodynamics and exercise tolerance have been reported in a small number of patients with nifedipine, hydralazine, and prazosin, but in general these benefits have not been well maintained over time.[106,112] Epoprostenol has been reported to have salutary effects on pulmonary hemodynamics and to decrease vasomotor tone in pulmonary venules in some patients, but it has produced fulminant pulmonary edema and death in others.[37,45,94,105,113,114] There is limited experience with inhaled nitric oxide or iloprost in this condition, although some descriptions of the use of these agents in this context have suggested that improvement in cardiac output resulted without the development of pulmonary edema.[115]

Because the therapeutic options in PVOD are so limited, a cautious trial of epoprostenol is generally indicated. If tolerated, patients are generally initiated on epoprostenol at a dose of 2 to 4 ng/kg/min, then uptitrated by 1 to 2 ng/kg/min every 2-4 weeks as permitted by side effects.

Lung Transplantation

Either single-lung or double-lung transplantation can be performed to treat PVOD.[116] Heart-lung transplantation is rarely required, as impaired right ventricular function almost always improves with the transplantation of normal lungs.[116,117] Recurrence of PVOD after transplantation appears unusual, although the precise risk is not known, because the number of transplantations performed for this diagnosis has been relatively small.[90,118,119,119a]

Given the poor prognosis of PVOD, patients generally should be evaluated for possible lung transplantation at the time of diagnosis. Unfortunately, the usefulness of lung transplantation is diminished by limited organ availability and prolonged waiting times. Furthermore, median survival following lung transplantation is only approximately 4 years, an outcome that hardly permits the procedure to be considered curative. Bronchiolitis obliterans syndrome and infection remain the major causes of mortality among successfully transplanted individuals.[120]

Conventional Supportive Therapy

Patients with PVOD should receive conventional supportive therapy similar to that prescribed for patients with IPAH unless contraindications are present.[109] Of note, none of these therapies has been documented in high-quality randomized trials to be efficacious in patients with PH of *any* cause; these therapies are employed because of theoretic consideration and case reports or case series that have suggested possible benefit.

Warfarin generally is titrated to an international normalized ratio of approximately 2 on the basis of the suggestion of several nonrandomized studies in PPH that survival may be modestly improved.[108,121] Episodic small-volume hemoptysis generally does not require discontinuation of anticoagulation, but the medication is usually stopped if more than 50 ml of blood are expectorated over a 24-hour period, significant extrapulmonary hemorrhage occurs, or syncope or other risk factors for head trauma develop.

Long-term oxygen therapy should be initiated if an oxygen saturation of 89% or an arterial pO_2 of 59 mm Hg or less is documented. These recommendations are based on clinical trials of oxygen therapy in patients with chronic obstructive pulmonary disease rather than primary pulmonary vascular disease, and not all patients with PH show improvement in pulmonary hemodynamics after oxygen therapy is begun.[122-124]

Transtracheal oxygen therapy permits delivery of oxygen at higher flow rates than via nasal cannulae and may be considered when epistaxis is problematic, although local bleeding complications at the insertion site can occur.[125]

Diuretics should be used as necessary to maintain euvolemia. Both dehydration and hypervolemia can be hazardous, and patients should monitor their weight daily. On the basis of the improvement in cardiac output described in patients with IPAH treated with digoxin, the drug is generally prescribed to patients with PVOD unless contraindications are present.[126]

Immunosuppressive Agents

Immunosuppressive medications such as glucocorticoids and azathioprine occasionally have been employed in the treatment of PVOD, although protocols have been neither standardized nor randomized, making unequivocal conclusions about their effectiveness difficult to draw. Nonetheless, only rare responses to therapy have been reported and only a minority of these cases have shown sustained improvements.[58,72,127] Most patients do not have prominent autoimmune features or biochemical indices suggestive of an inflammatory process.[2,103]

Generally immunosuppressive agents do not have a role in the treatment of PVOD, although a 4-week trial of 0.75 to 1 mg/kg of prednisone may be undertaken in patients with associated nonspecific interstitial pulmonary inflammation or autoimmune features such as arthritis, alopecia, or an elevated erythrocyte sedimentation rate. If improvements are seen in symptoms, radiographs, diffusing capacity, or alveolar-arterial oxygen gradient, the dose is slowly tapered to 20 to 40 mg per day.

Experimental Therapies

Although endothelin-1 receptor antagonists such as bosentan, and phosphodiesterase-5 inhibitors such as sildenafil are finding roles in the treatment of pulmonary arterial hypertension, there is no published experience with these medications in the treatment of PVOD.[128-131] Both classes of medications could either prove beneficial or deleterious in PVOD for similar reasons as vasodilators, and at present their use is not recommended.

A number of experimental therapies have been investigated for HVOD such as defibrotide, recombinant tissue plasminogen activator (rtPA), or antithrombin-III concentrate.[132,133] No data are available regarding the potential usefulness of these treatments in PVOD, and given the likely differences in pathogenesis of the two conditions, none of these agents is recommended to treat patients with PVOD pending specific data supporting their efficacy.

CONCLUSION

PVOD remains a highly lethal and poorly understood syndrome, with basic and critical questions about its etiology and optimal treatment remaining unanswered despite the seven decades since its initial description. Its diagnosis requires a high degree of clinical suspicion and frequently necessitates surgical lung biopsy, but the prognosis and management of PVOD are sufficiently different from other causes of PH that such efforts are generally justified. In particular, the approach to timing of lung transplantation and medical therapy with prostanoids or endothelin-1 receptor antagonists are different than in IPAH, and significant harm or death may occur if PVOD goes unrecognized. Additional research is required to more precisely delineate risk factors for the syndrome and to define optimal therapy for it.

REFERENCES

1. Veeraraghavan S, Koss M, Sharma O: Pulmonary veno-occlusive disease. Curr Opin Pulm Med 5:310, 1999.
2. Mandel J, Mark E, Hales C: Pulmonary veno-occlusive disease. Am J Respir Crit Care Med 162:1964, 2000.
3. Höra J: Zur histologie der klinischen "primaren Pulmonalsklerose." Frankfurt Z Pathol 47:100, 1934.
4. Brown C, Harrison C: Pulmonary veno-occlusive disease. Lancet 2:61, 1966.
5. Heath D, Segel N, Bishop J: Pulmonary veno-occlusive disease. Circulation 34:242, 1966.
6. Weisser K, Wyler F, Gloor F: Pulmonary veno-occlusive disease. Arch Dis Child 42:322, 1967.
7. Rosenthal A, Vawter G, Wagenvoort C: Intrapulmonary veno-occlusive disease. Am J Cardiol 31:78, 1973.
8. Robbins I, Colvin E, Doyle T, et al: Pulmonary vein stenosis after catheter ablation of atrial fibrillation. Circulation 98:1769, 1998.
9. Arentz T, Jander N, von Rosenthal J, et al: Incidence of pulmonary vein stenosis 2 years after radiofrequency catheter ablation of refractory atrial fibrillation. Eur Heart J 24:963, 2003.
10. Spray T, Bridges N: Surgical management of congenital and acquired pulmonary vein stenosis. Semin Thorac Cardiovasc Surg Pediatr Card Surg Annu 2:177, 1999.
11. Pietra G, Edwards W, Kay J, et al: Histopathology of primary pulmonary hypertension: A qualitative and quantitative study of pulmonary blood vessels from 58 patients in the National Heart, Lung, and Blood Institute Primary Pulmonary Hypertension Registry. Circulation 80:1198, 1989.
12. Palevsky H, Schloo B, Pietra G, et al: Primary pulmonary hypertension: Vascular structure, morphometry, and responsiveness to vasodilator agents. Circulation 80:1207, 1989.
13. Wagenvoort C: Lung biopsy specimens in the evaluation of pulmonary vascular disease. Chest 77:614, 1980.
14. Kinare S, Deshpande J: Primary pulmonary hypertension in India (autopsy study of 26 cases). Indian Heart J 39:9, 1987.
15. Burke A, Farb A, Virmani R: The pathology of primary pulmonary hypertension. Mod Pathol 4:269, 1991.
16. Pietra G: The pathology of primary pulmonary hypertension. In Rubin L, Rich S (eds): Primary Pulmonary Hypertension. New York, Marcel Dekker, 1997.
17. Bjornsson J, Edwards W: Primary pulmonary hypertension: A histopathologic study of 80 cases. Mayo Clin Proc 60:16, 1985.
18. Wagenvoort C, Wagenvoort N: Primary pulmonary hypertension: A pathologic study of the lung vessels in 156 clinically diagnosed cases. Circulation 42:1163, 1970.
19. Abenhaim L, Moride Y, Brenot F, et al: Appetite-suppressant drugs and the risk of primary pulmonary hypertension. N Engl J Med 335:609, 1996.
20. Rubin L: Primary pulmonary hypertension. N Engl J Med 336:111, 1997.
21. Wagenvoort C: Pulmonary veno-occlusive disease: Entity or syndrome? Chest 69:82, 1976.
22. Thadani U, Burrow C, Whitaker W, Heath D: Pulmonary veno-occlusive disease. Q J Med 64:133, 1975.
23. Rubin E, Farber J: The respiratory system. In Rubin E, Farber J (eds): Pathology. Philadelphia, JB Lippincott, 1994, p 557.

24. Wagenvoort C, Wagenvoort N: The pathology of pulmonary veno-occlusive disease. Virchows Arch A Pathol Anat Histol 364:69, 1974.
25. Chazova I, Robbins I, Loyd J, et al: Venous and arterial changes in pulmonary veno-occlusive disease, mitral stenosis and fibrosing mediastinitis. Eur Respir J 15:116, 2000.
26. Schraufnagel D, Sekosan M, McGee T, Thakkar M: Human alveolar capillaries undergo angiogenesis in pulmonary veno-occlusive disease. Eur Respir J 9:346, 1996.
27. Wagenvoort C, Wagenvoort N, Takahashi T: Pulmonary veno-occlusive disease: Involvement of pulmonary arteries and review of the literature. Hum Pathol 16:1033, 1985.
28. Crissman J, Koss M, Carson R: Pulmonary veno-occlusive disease secondary to granulomatous venulitis. Am J Surg Pathol 4:93, 1980.
29. Carrington C, Liebow A: Pulmonary veno-occlusive disease. Hum Pathol 1:322, 1970.
30. Cortese D: Pulmonary function in mitral stenosis. Mayo Clin Proc 53:321, 1978.
31. Glassroth J, Woodford D, Carrington C, Gaensler E: Pulmonary veno-occlusive disease in the middle-aged. Respiration 47:309, 1985.
32. Davies P, Reid L: Pulmonary veno-occlusive disease in siblings: Case reports and morphometric study. Hum Pathol 13:911, 1982.
33. Voordes C, Kuipers J, Elema J: Familial pulmonary veno-occlusive disease: A case report. Thorax 32:763, 1977.
34. Deng Z, Morse J, Slager S, et al: Familial primary pulmonary hypertension (gene PPH1) is caused by mutations in the bone morphogenetic protein receptor-II gene. Am J Hum Genet 67:737, 2000.
35. Thomas A, Carneal J, Markin C, et al: Specific bone morphogenic protein receptor II mutations found in primary pulmonary hypertension cause different biochemical phenotypes in vitro. Chest 121:83S, 2002.
36. Lane K, Machado R, Pauciulo M, et al: Heterozygous germline mutations in BMPR2, encoding a TGF-beta receptor, cause familial primary pulmonary hypertension: The International PPH Consortium. Nat Genet 26:81, 2000.
37. Runo J, Vnencak-Jones C, Prince M, et al: Pulmonary veno-occlusive disease caused by an inherited mutation in bone morphogenetic protein receptor II. Am J Respir Crit Care Med 167:889, 2003.
38. Machado R, Pauciulo M, Thomson J, et al: BMPR2 haploinsufficiency as the inherited molecular mechanism for primary pulmonary hypertension. Am J Hum Genet 68:92, 2001.
39. Chazova I, Loyd J, Zhdanov V, et al: Pulmonary artery adventitial changes and venous involvement in primary pulmonary hypertension. Am J Pathol 146:389, 1995.
40. Dorfmuller P, Humbert M, Sanchez O, et al: Significant occlusive lesions of pulmonary veins are common in patients with pulmonary hypertension associated to connective tissue diseases [abstract]. Presented at the American Thoracic Society 99th International Conference, Seattle, 2003.
41. Fesler P, Pagnamenta A, Vachiery J, et al: Single arterial occlusion to locate resistance in patients with pulmonary hypertension. Eur Respir J 21:31, 2003.
42. Pulmonary veno-occlusive disease. Br Med J 3:369, 1972.
43. Stovin P, Mitchinson M: Pulmonary hypertension due to obstruction of the intrapulmonary veins. Thorax 20:106, 1965.
44. McDonnell P, Summer W, Hutchins G: Pulmonary veno-occlusive disease: Morphological changes suggesting a viral cause. JAMA 246:667, 1981.
45. Holcomb BJ, Loyd J, Ely E, et al: Pulmonary veno-occlusive disease: A case series and new observations. Chest 118:1671, 2000.
46. Ruchelli E, Nojadera G, Rutstein R, Rudy B: Pulmonary veno-occlusive disease: Another vascular disorder associated with human immunodeficiency virus infection? Arch Pathol Lab Med 118:664, 1994.
47. Escamilla R, Hermant C, Berjaud J, et al: Pulmonary veno-occlusive disease in an HIV-infected intravenous drug abuser. Eur Respir 8:1982, 1995.
48. Hourseau M, Capron F, Nunes H, et al: Pulmonary veno-occlusive disease in a patient with HIV infection: A case report with autopsy findings. Ann Pathol 22:472, 2002.
49. Liu L, Sackler J: A case of pulmonary veno-occlusive disease: Etiological and therapeutic appraisal. Angiology 23:299, 1973.
50. Doll D, Yarbro J: Vascular toxicity associated with chemotherapy and hormonotherapy. Curr Opin Oncol 6:345, 1994.
51. Joselson R, Warnock M: Pulmonary veno-occlusive disease after chemotherapy. Hum Pathol 14:88, 1983.
52. Knight B, Rose AG: Pulmonary veno-occlusive disease after chemotherapy. Thorax 40:874, 1985.
53. Swift G, Gibbs A, Campbell I, et al: Pulmonary veno-occlusive disease and Hodgkin's lymphoma. Eur Respir J 6:596, 1993.
54. Waldhorn R, Tsou E, Smith F, Kerwin D: Pulmonary veno-occlusive disease associated with microangiopathic hemolytic anemia and chemotherapy of gastric adenocarcinoma. Med Pediatr Oncol 12: 394, 1984.
55. Gagnadoux F, Capron F, Lebeau B: Pulmonary veno-occlusive disease after neoadjuvant mitomycin chemotherapy and surgery for lung carcinoma. Lung Cancer 36:213, 2002.
56. Vansteenkiste JF, Bomans P, Verbeken EK, et al: Fatal pulmonary veno-occlusive disease possibly related to gemcitabine. Lung Cancer 31:83, 2001.
57. Williams L, Fussell S, Veith R, et al: Pulmonary veno-occlusive disease in an adult following bone marrow transplantation: Case report and review of the literature. Chest 109:1388, 1996.
58. Hackman R, Madtes D, Petersen F, Clark J: Pulmonary venoocclusive disease following bone marrow transplantation. Transplantation 47:989, 1989.
59. Kuga T, Kohda K, Hirayama Y, et al: Pulmonary veno-occlusive disease accompanied by microangiopathic hemolytic anemia 1 year after a second bone marrow transplantation for acute lymphoblastic leukemia. Int J Hematol 64:143, 1996.
60. Salzman D, Adkins D, Craig F, et al: Malignancy-associated pulmonary veno-occlusive disease: Report of a case following autologous bone marrow transplantation and review. Bone Marrow Transplant 18:755, 1996.
61. Trobaugh-Lotrario A, Geffe B, Deterding R, et al: Pulmonary veno-occlusive disease after autologous bone marrow transplant in a child with stage IV neuroblastoma: Case report and literature review. J Pediatr Hematol Oncol 25:405, 2003.
62. Seguchi M, Hirabayashi N, Fujii Y, et al: Pulmonary hypertension associated with pulmonary occlusive vasculopathy after allogenic bone marrow transplantation. Transplantation 69:177, 2000.
63. Kumana C, Ng M, Lin H, et al: Herbal tea induced hepatic veno-occlusive disease: Quantification of toxic alkaloid exposure in adults. Gut 26:101, 1985.
64. Tandon B, Tandon H, Tandon R, et al: An epidemic of veno-occlusive disease of the liver in central India. Lancet 2:271, 1976.
65. Clinicopathological conference: A case of veno-occlusive disease. Demonstrated at the Royal Postgraduate Medical School. Br Med J 1:818, 1968.
66. Tsou E, Waldhorn R, Kerwin D, et al: Pulmonary venoocclusive disease in pregnancy. Obstet Gynecol 64:281, 1984.
67. Townend J, Roberts D, Jones E, Davies M: Fatal pulmonary veno-occlusive disease after use of oral contraceptives. Am Heart J 124:1643, 1992.
68. Hussein A, Trowitzsch E, Brockmann M: Pulmonary veno-occlusive disease, antiphospholipid antibody and pulmonary hypertension in an adolescent. Klin Padiatr 211:92, 1999.
69. Hoffstein V, Ranganathan N, Mullen J: Sarcoidosis simulating pulmonary veno-occlusive disease. Am Rev Respir Dis 134:809, 1986.
70. Scully R, Mark E, McNeely B: Case records of the Massachusetts General Hospital: Weekly clinicopathologic exercises. Case 14—1983: A 67-year-old woman with pulmonary hypertension. N Engl J Med 308:823, 1983.
71. Scully R, Mark E, McNeely W, McNeely B: Case records of the Massachusetts General Hospital: Weekly clinicopathologic exercises, Case 37—1992: A 68-year-old woman with rheumatoid arthritis and pulmonary hypertension. N Engl J Med 327:873, 1992.
72. Sanderson J, Spiro S, Hendry A, Turner-Warwick M: A case of pulmonary veno-occlusive disease responding to treatment with azathioprine. Thorax 32:140, 1977.
73. Morassut P, Walley V, Smith C: Pulmonary veno-occlusive disease and the CREST variant of scleroderma. Can J Cardiol 8:1055, 1992.
74. Kishida Y, Kanai Y, Kuramochi S, Hosoda Y: Pulmonary venoocclusive disease in a patient with systemic lupus erythematosus. J Rheumatol 20:2161, 1993.
75. Katz D, Scalzetti E, Katzenstein A, Kohman L: Pulmonary veno-occlusive disease presenting with thrombosis of pulmonary arteries. Thorax 50:699, 1995.

76. Leinonen H, Pohjola-Sintonen S, Krogerus L: Pulmonary veno-occlusive disease. Acta Med Scand 221:307, 1987.
77. Liang M, Stern S, Fortinn P, et al: Fatal pulmonary venoocclusive disease secondary to a generalized venopathy: A new syndrome presenting with facial swelling and pericardial tamponade. Arthritis Rheum 34:228, 1991.
78. Devereux G, Evans M, Kerr K, Legge J: Pulmonary veno-occlusive disease complicating Felty's syndrome. Respir Med 92:1089, 1998.
79. Calderon M, Burdine J: Pulmonary veno-occlusive disease. J Nucl Med 15:455, 1974.
80. Chawla S, Kittle C, Faber L, Jensik RJ: Pulmonary venoocclusive disease. Ann Thorac Surg 22:249, 1976.
81. Bolster M, Hogan J, Bredin C: Pulmonary vascular occlusive disease presenting as sudden death. Med Sci Law 30:26, 1990.
82. Cagle P, Langston C: Pulmonary veno-occlusive disease as a cause of sudden infant death. Arch Pathol Lab Med 108:338, 1984.
83. Wiedemann H: Cor pulmonale. In Rose B (ed): UpToDate, vol 11.1. Wellesley, Mass. UpToDate, 2003.
84. Swensen S, Tashjian J, Myers J, et al: Pulmonary venoocclusive disease: CT findings in eight patients. AJR Am J Roentgenol 167:937, 1996.
85. Weiner-Kronish J, Goldstein R, Matthay R, et al: Lack of association of pleural effusion with chronic pulmonary arterial and right atrial hypertension. Chest 92:967, 1987.
86. Gluecker T, Capasso P, Schnyder P, et al: Clinical and radiographic features of pulmonary edema. Radiographics 19:1507, 1999.
87. Scheibel R, Dedeker K, Gleason D, et al: Radiographic and angiographic characteristics of pulmonary veno-occlusive disease. Radiology 103:47, 1972.
88. Elliott C, Colby T, Hill T, Crapo R: Pulmonary veno-occlusive disease associated with severe reduction of single-breath carbon monoxide diffusing capacity. Respiration 53:262, 1988.
89. Maltby J, Gouverne M: CT findings in pulmonary venoocclusive disease. J Comput Assist Tomogr 8:758, 1984.
90. Cassart M, Gevenois P, Kramer M, et al: Pulmonary venoocclusive disease: CT findings before and after single-lung transplantation. AJR Am J Roentgenol 160:759, 1993.
91. Worthy S, Müller N, Hartman T, et al: Mosaic attenuation pattern on thin section CT scans of the lung: Differentiation among infiltrative lung, airway, and vascular diseases as a cause. Radiology 205:465, 1997.
92. Resten A, Maitre S, Humbert M, et al: Pulmonary arterial hypertension: Thin section CT predictors of epoprostenol therapy failure. Radiology 222:782, 2002.
93. Scully R, Mark E, McNeely W, McNeely B: Case records of the Massachusetts General Hospital: Weekly clinicopathologic exercises, Case 48-1993: A 27-year-old woman with mediastinal lymphadenopathy and relentless cor pulmonale. N Engl J Med 329:1720, 1993.
94. Dufour B, Maitre S, Humbert M, et al: High-resolution CT of the chest in four patients with pulmonary capillary hemangiomatosis or pulmonary venoocclusive disease. AJR Am J Roentgenol 171:1321, 1998.
95. Bailey C, Channick R, Auger W, et al: "High probability" perfusion lung scans in pulmonary venoocclusive disease. Chest 162:1974, 2000.
96. Rich S, Pietra G, Kieras K, et al: Primary pulmonary hypertension: Radiographic and scintigraphic patterns of histologic subtypes. Ann Intern Med 105:499, 1986.
97. Matthews A, Buchanan R: A case of pulmonary veno-occlusive disease and a new bronchoscopic sign. Respir Med 84:503, 1990.
98. Nawaz S, Dobersen M, Blount SJ, et al: Florid pulmonary veno-occlusive disease. Chest 98:1037, 1990.
99. Shackelford G, Sacks E, Mullins J: Pulmonary venoocclusive disease: Case report and review of the literature. AJR Am J Roentgenol 128:643, 1977.
100. Rapidly progressive dyspnea in a teenage boy. Clinical pathological conference. JAMA 223:1243, 1973.
101. Weed H: Pulmonary "capillary" wedge pressure not the pressure in the pulmonary capillaries. Chest 100:1138, 1991.
102. Rambihar V, Fallen E, Cairns J: Pulmonary veno-occlusive disease: Antemortem diagnosis from roentgenographic and hemodynamic findings. Can Med Assoc J 120:1519, 1979.
103. De Vries T, Weening J, Roorda R: Pulmonary veno-occlusive disease: A case report and a review of therapeutic possibilities. Eur Respir J 4:1029, 1991.
104. Rabiller A, Humbert M, Sitbon O, et al: Bronchoalveolar lavage (BAL) as a diagnostic tool in pulmonary hypertension: Occult alveolar haemorrhage is a common feature of pulmonary veno-occlusive disease (PVOD). Presented at the American Thoracic Society 99th International Conference, Seattle, 2003.
105. Okumura H, Nagaya N, Kyotani S, et al: Effects of continuous IV prostacyclin in a patient with pulmonary veno-occlusive disease. Chest 122:1096, 2002.
106. Salzman G, Rosa U: Prolonged survival in pulmonary veno-occlusive disease treated with nifedipine. Chest 95:1154, 1989.
107. Lagakos S: Clinical trials and rare diseases. N Engl J Med 348:2455, 2003.
108. Rich S, Kaufmann E, Levy P: The effect of high doses of calcium-channel blockers on survival in primary pulmonary hypertension. N Engl J Med 327:76, 1992.
109. Runo J, Loyd J: Primary pulmonary hypertension. Lancet 361: 1533, 2003.
110. Barst R, Rubin L, Long W, et al: A comparison of continuous intravenous epoprostenol (prostacyclin) with conventional therapy for primary pulmonary hypertension: The Primary Pulmonary Hypertension Study Group. N Engl J Med 334:296, 1996.
111. McLaughlin V, Shillington A, Rich S: Survival in primary pulmonary hypertension: The impact of epoprostenol therapy. Circulation 106:1477, 2002.
112. Palevsky H, Pietra G, Fishman A: Pulmonary veno-occlusive disease and its response to vasodilator agents. Am Rev Respir Dis 142:426, 1990.
113. Davis L, deBoisblanc B, Glynn C, et al: Effect of prostacyclin on microvascular pressures in a patient with pulmonary veno-occlusive disease. Chest 108:1754, 1995.
114. Palmer S, Robinson L, Wang A, et al: Massive pulmonary edema and death after prostacyclin infusion in a patient with pulmonary veno-occlusive disease. Chest 113:237, 1998.
115. Hoeper M, Eschenbruch C, Zink-Wohlfart C, et al: Effects of inhaled nitric oxide and aerosolized iloprost in pulmonary veno-occlusive disease. Respir Med 93:62, 1999.
116. Gammie J, Keenan R, Pham S, et al: Single- versus double-lung transplantation for pulmonary hypertension. J Thorac Cardiovasc Surg 115:397, 1998.
117. Bando K, Armitage J, Paradis I, et al: Indications for and results of single, bilateral, and heart-lung transplantation for pulmonary hypertension. J Thorac Cardiovasc Surg 108:1056, 1994.
118. Kramer M, Estenne M, Berkman N, et al: Radiation-induced pulmonary veno-occlusive disease. Chest 104:1282, 1993.
119. Stewart S, McNeil K, Nashef S, et al: Audit of referral and explant diagnoses in lung transplantation: A pathologic study of lungs removed for parenchymal disease. J Heart Lung Transplant 14:1173, 1995.
119a. Izbicki G, Shitrit D, Schechtman I, et al: Recurrence of pulmonary veno-occlusive disease after heart-lung transplantation. J Heart Lung Transplant 24:635,2005.
120. Hertz M, Taylor DO, Trulock EP. et al: The registry of the international society for heart and lung transplantation: Nineteenth official report—2002. J Heart Lung Transplant 21:950, 2002.
121. Frank H, Mlczoch J, Huber K, et al: The effect of anticoagulant therapy in primary and anorectic drug-induced pulmonary hypertension. Chest 112:714, 1997.
122. Continuous or nocturnal oxygen therapy in hypoxemic chronic obstructive lung disease: A clinical trial. Nocturnal Oxygen Therapy Trial Group. Ann Intern Med 93:391, 1980.
123. Long term domiciliary oxygen therapy in chronic hypoxic cor pulmonale complicating chronic bronchitis and emphysema: Report of the Medical Research Council Working Party. Lancet 1:681, 1981.
124. Morgan J, Griffiths M, du Bois R, Evans T: Hypoxic pulmonary vasoconstriction in systemic sclerosis and primary pulmonary hypertension. Chest 99:551, 1991.
125. Eckmann D: Transtracheal oxygen delivery. Crit Care Clin 16:463, 2000.

126. Rich S, Seidlitz M, Dodin E, et al: The short-term effects of digoxin in patients with right ventricular dysfunction from pulmonary hypertension. Chest 114:787, 1998.
127. Gilroy RJ, Teague M, Loyd J: Pulmonary veno-occlusive disease: Fatal progression of pulmonary hypertension despite steroid-induced remission of interstitial pneumonitis. Am Rev Respir Dis 143:1130, 1991.
128. Rubin L, Badesch D, Barst R, et al: Bosentan therapy for pulmonary arterial hypertension. N Engl J Med 346:896, 2002.
129. Cheng J: Bosentan. Heart Dis 5:161, 2003.
130. Kothari S, Duggal B: Chronic oral sildenafil therapy in severe pulmonary artery hypertension. Indian Heart J 54:404, 2002.
131. Prasad S, Wilkinson J, Gatzoulis M: Sildenafil in primary pulmonary hypertension [letter]. N Engl J Med 343:1342, 2000.
132. Richardson P, Murakami C, Jin Z, et al: Multi-institutional use of defibrotide in 88 patients after stem cell transplantation with severe veno-occlusive disease and multisystem organ failure: Response without significant toxicity in a high-risk population and factors predictive of outcome. Blood 100:4337, 2002.
133. Willner I: Veno-occlusive disease. Curr Treat Options Gastroenterol 5:465, 2002.

chapter 60

Diseases of the Lymphatic Circulation

Stanley G. Rockson
John P. Cooke

Diseases of the lymphatic circulation may be developmental or acquired. Developmental disorders may be due to hypoplasia or maldevelopment of the lymphatic circulatory structures, with accompanying disorders of lymph transit. Secondary lymphatic disease is most often due to disruption of lymphatic channels, typically in the setting of trauma, infection, neoplasia, or surgical interventions.

Without regard to the cause, when regional lymphatic flow is insufficient to maintain tissue homeostasis, interstitial fluid accumulates and swelling ensues. When lymph stasis is chronic, variable degrees of cutaneous and subcutaneous fibrosis may ensue, often accompanied by the deposition of substantial adipose tissue within the subcutaneous compartment. Collectively, these pathological alterations characterize the lymphatic disorder known clinically as lymphedema. Lymphedema may also accompany proliferative disorders of the lymphatic microvasculature that, in turn, lead to a functionally incompetent vasculature. Lymphatic insufficiency of the viscera can also lead to profound metabolic disturbances. Regional and systemic immune function is compromised by lymphatic disease.

Historically, the rather limited therapeutic options for lymphatic disease have reflected an incomplete understanding of the pathophysiology of lymphedema; nevertheless, recent advances in imaging and therapeutics, as well as insights gained from vascular biology, hold promise of more definitive therapy.

ANATOMY OF THE LYMPHATIC CIRCULATION

Recognition of the lymphatic system and comprehension of its importance came relatively late to the medical and scientific communities. Although a number of early anatomists and physicians made oblique references to various aspects of the lymphatic circulation, it was not until the seventeenth century that Gasparo Aselli recognized the lymphatics as a distinct anatomic entity.[1] The gifted professor of anatomy and surgery from Milan was frequently asked by friends and colleagues to perform his elegant vivisections, and on July 23, 1622, he intended to demonstrate to them the action and innervation of the canine diaphragm.

"While I was attempting this, and for that purpose had opened the abdomen and was pulling down with my hand the intestines and stomach ... I suddenly beheld a great number of cords, as it were, exceedingly thin and beautifully white, scattered over the whole of the mesentery and the intestine, and starting from almost innumerable beginnings.... I noticed that the nerves belonging to the intestine were distinct from these cords, and wholly unlike them, and besides, were distributed quite separately from them. Wherefore struck by the novelty of the thing, I stood for some time silent. ... When I gathered my wits together for the sake of the experiment, having laid hold of a very sharp scalpel, I pricked one of these cords and indeed one of the largest of them. I had hardly touched it, when I saw a white liquid like milk or cream forthwith gush out. Seeing this, I could hardly restrain my delight."[1]

The chylous return from the intestine of the recently fed animal allowed Aselli to recognize the lymphatics; when he repeated the demonstration several days later, no vessels were to be seen. Aselli eventually realized the relation between feedings and the visibility of the mesenteric lymphatics and duplicated the work in several species (Fig. 60-1). Over the following half century, Aselli's work was extended by Pecquet, Bartholinus, and Rudbeck, who defined the gross anatomy of the lymphatic system in toto.[1] By the eighteenth century, smaller lymphatic channels were visualized by Anton Nuck using mercury injections. Using those techniques, Sappey observed and recorded the human lymphatic system in exquisite detail (Fig. 60-2). Even greater resolution of the anatomy was provided by von Recklinghausen in 1862 with his discovery that the lymphatic endothelium stained darkly with silver nitrate. Using that technique, von Recklinghausen differentiated the lymphatic capillaries from the blood vessel capillaries. Most recently, substantial advances in the techniques of immunohistochemistry and transmission electron microscopy have enabled the certain identification of the lymphatic microcirculation and its distinction from the blood vasculature.[2,3]

We now know that lymphatic capillaries are blind-ended tubes formed by a single layer of endothelial cells. The endothelial cells of lymphatic capillaries closely resemble those of blood vessels and have a common embryonic origin.[4] Like vascular endothelium, lymphatic

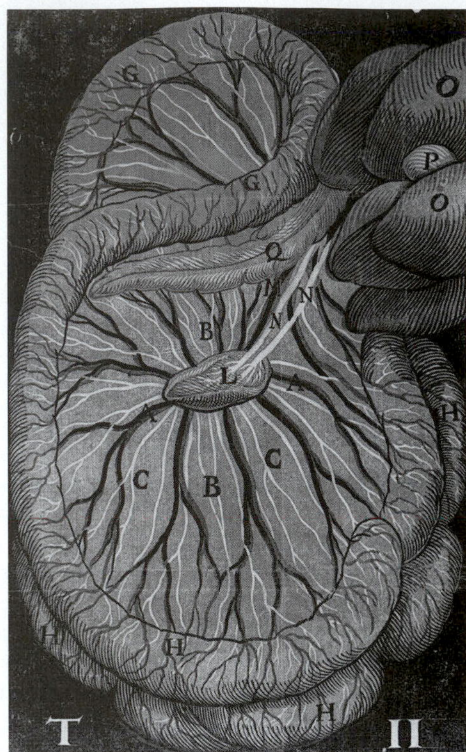

FIGURE 60-1. The original anatomic illustration of the visceral lymphatics by Gasparo Aselli. (From the monograph *De Lactibus Sive Lacteis Venis,* courtesy Harvard Medical Library, Francis A. Countway Library of Medicine.)

endothelial cells in culture form confluent "cobblestone" monolayers, which "sprout" to form tubules and which demonstrate identical histologic markers (von Willebrand factor, F-actin, fibronectin, and Weibel-Palade bodies). Unlike systemic capillaries, the basement membrane of lymphatic capillaries is absent or widely fenestrated, allowing greater access to interstitial proteins and particles.

The capillaries join to form larger vessels (100 to 200 μm), which are invested with smooth muscle and capable of vasomotion. Those vessels in turn merge to form larger conduits composed of three distinct layers: intima, media, and adventitia. Those conduits possess intraluminal valves that are usually tricuspid, are located a few millimeters to centimeters apart, and ensure that the flow of interstitial fluid (now called *lymph*) is directed centrally.[5,6]

In the lower limbs, the larger conduits form a system of lymphatic return that is divided into superficial and deep components. The superficial component comprises medial and lateral channels. The medial channel originates on the dorsum of the foot and along the course of the saphenous vein. The lateral channel begins on the lateral aspect of the foot and ascends to the midleg, where the tributaries cross anteriorly to the medial side to follow the course of the medial lymphatics up to the inguinal nodes. Deep lymphatics do not usually communicate with the superficial system except through the popliteal and inguinal lymph nodes. Those vessels originate

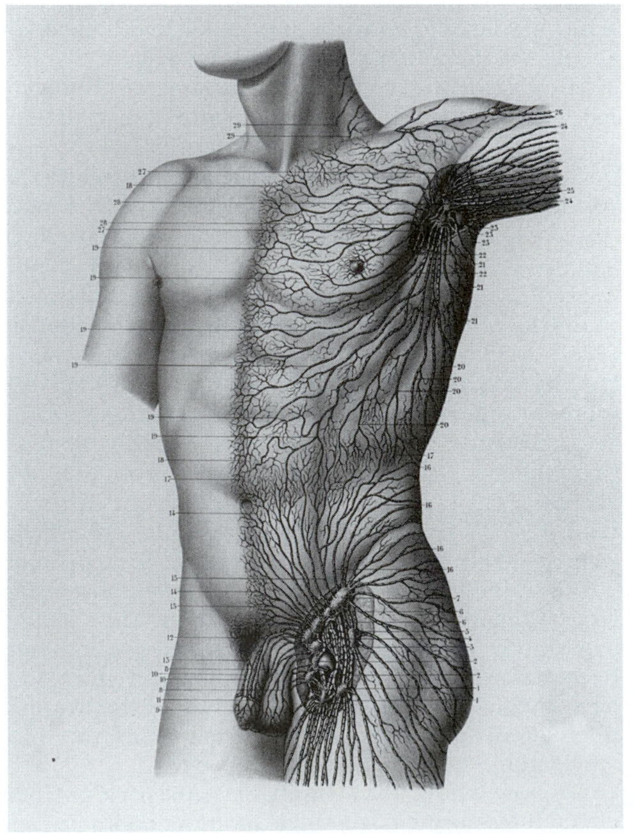

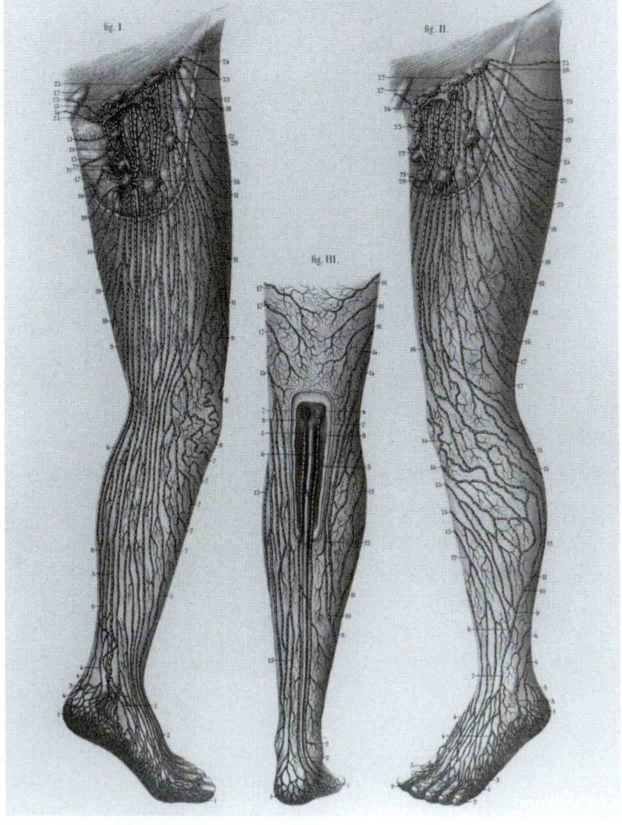

FIGURE 60-2. Nineteenth-century anatomic delineation of the cutaneous lymphatics. (From the text *Anatomi, Physiologie, Pathologie des Vaisseaux Lymphatiques*, by PC Sappey [1874], courtesy Harvard Medical Library, Francis A. Countway Library of Medicine.)

subcutaneously, follow the course of the deep blood vessels, and eventually pass through the inguinal nodes.

Small- and medium-sized lymphatic vessels empty into main channels, of which the thoracic duct is the largest. That vessel, roughly 2 mm wide and 45 cm long, ascends from the abdomen through the lower chest just to the right of and anterior to the vertebral column. At approximately the level of the fifth thoracic vertebra, it crosses to the left of the spine, where it continues to ascend through the superior mediastinum to the base of the neck and eventually empties into the left brachiocephalic vein. Other large right- and left-sided lymphatic ducts may exist, although their arrangement, size, and course are highly variable. Those vessels join with the main thoracic duct or empty directly into great veins; they provide important collateral conduits should the thoracic duct become obstructed.

PHYSIOLOGY OF THE LYMPHATIC CIRCULATION

In 1786 William Hunter and two of his pupils, William Cruikshank and William Hewson, published the results of their work, laying a foundation for the physiology of the lymphatic system.[1] They correctly inferred from clinical observation that the lymphatics were involved in the response to infection, as well as in the absorption of interstitial fluid. A century later, their theories received experimental support from the physiologic studies of Karl Ludwig and Ernest Starling. Ludwig cannulated lymph vessels, collected and analyzed the lymph, and proposed that it was a filtrate of plasma. Starling elucidated the forces governing fluid transfer from the blood capillaries to the interstitial space and offered evidence that the same forces apply to the lymphatic capillaries. He proposed that an imbalance in those forces could give rise to edema formation:

"In health, therefore, the two processes, lymph production and absorption are exactly proportional. Dropsy depends on a loss of balance between these two processes—on an excess of lymph-production over lymph-absorption. A scientific investigation of the causation of dropsy will therefore involve, in the first place, an examination of the factors which determine the extent of these two processes and, so far as is possible, the manner in which these processes are carried out."[7]

As first enunciated by Starling, interstitial fluid is largely an ultrafiltrate of blood. Its rate of production reflects the balance between factors that favor filtration out of capillaries (capillary hydrostatic pressure and tissue oncotic pressure) and those that favor reabsorption (interstitial hydrostatic pressure and capillary oncotic pressure).[8] Under normal conditions, filtration exceeds reabsorption at a rate sufficient to create 2 to 4 L of interstitial fluid per day. There is a net filtration of protein (primarily albumin) from the vasculature into the interstitium; approximately 100 g of circulating protein may escape into the interstitial space daily. The interstitial fluid also receives the waste products of cellular metabolism, as well as foreign matter or microbes that enter through breaks in the skin or by hematogenous routes.

The volume and the composition of the interstitial fluid are kept in balance by the lymphatic system. The functions of that system include (1) transport of excess fluid, protein, and waste products from the interstitial space to the blood stream; (2) distribution of immune cells and substances from the lymphoid tissues to the systemic circulation; (3) filtration and removal of foreign material from the interstitial fluid; and (4) in the viscera, to promote the absorption of lipids from the intestinal lumen.

Several forces drive fluid through the lymphatic system. The lymphatic vessels in skeletal muscle are compressed by extrinsic muscular contractions that propel the fluid centrally through the unidirectional valves. In other tissues, such as the splanchnic and cutaneous systems, it is primarily contractions of lymphatic smooth muscle that generate the driving force.[9,10] These contractions are increased in frequency and amplitude by elevated filling pressure, sympathetic nerve activity, and shock, and they may be modulated by circulating hormones and prostanoids.[11-15] Considerable force can be generated by those contractions; experimentally induced obstruction of the popliteal lymphatic system augments the strength and frequency of contraction, generating pressures of up to 50 mm Hg.[16] Other factors that may contribute to lymphatic flow include intermittent compression from arterial pulsations and gastrointestinal peristalsis. In addition, it has most recently been proposed that the initial lymphatics (the small lymphatic capillaries that begin blindly in the tissues) most likely possess a two-valve system.[17,18] In addition to the classically described, secondary intralymphatic valves, the initial lymphatics are thought to possess a primary valve system at the level of the endothelium to ensure unidirectional flow at this level. Once lymph enters the thorax, negative intrathoracic pressure generated during inspiration aspirates fluid into the thoracic duct (the "respiratory pump").[16]

LYMPHATIC INSUFFICIENCY (LYMPHEDEMA)

Pathogenesis of Edema

Edema develops when the production of interstitial fluid (lymph) exceeds its transport through the lymphatic system. Thus an overproduction of lymph (enhanced lymphatic load) or a decreased ability to remove fluid (defective transport) from the interstitium may result in edema. Conditions associated with overproduction of lymph include elevated venous pressures, increased capillary permeability, and hypoproteinemia. Elevated hydrostatic pressure in the veins results in increased filtration of plasma from venules and blood capillaries (as seen in right-sided congestive heart failure, tricuspid regurgitation, and deep vein thrombosis). Conversely, local inflammation increases capillary permeability, accelerating the loss of protein and fluid to the interstitium despite a normal capillary hydrostatic pressure. This increases lymph production by 10- to 20-fold, exceeding lymphatic transport and resulting in marked edema.[19] Hypoproteinemia also may lead to marked edema, in which case hydrostatic pressure and capillary permeability are normal, but capillary oncotic pressure is reduced, favoring osmotic flow to the interstitium. The edema that ensues in these conditions can, strictly speaking, be called lymphedema only when there is objective evidence of impaired lymphatic clearance or evidence of the pathognomonic lymphedematous changes in the skin or subcutaneous tissues.

Pathogenesis of Lymphedema

Lymphedema occurs whenever lymphatic vessels are absent, underdeveloped, or obstructed. Impedance to lymphatic flow may be due to an inborn defect (primary lymphedema) or an acquired loss of lymphatic patency (secondary lymphedema).

Primary Lymphedema

Prevalence estimates for the heritable causes of lymphedema are difficult to ascertain and vary substantially. Primary lymphedema is thought to occur in approximately 1 of every 6 to 10,000 live births. Females are affected 2- to 10-fold more commonly than males.[20-22] Primary lymphedema represents a heterogeneous group of disorders, and therefore its classification schemata are numerous. Affected individuals can be classified by age of onset, by functional anatomic attributes, or by clinical setting.

Age of Onset

When distinguished by age of clinical onset, primary lymphedema can typically be divided into the following categories:[23]

1. Congenital lymphedema, clinically apparent at or near birth
2. Lymphedema praecox, with onset after birth and before age 35; lymphedema praecox, a term used by Allen in 1934,[27] most typically appears in the peripubertal years
3. Lymphedema tarda appears after the age of 35

Anatomic Patterns

An alternative classification scheme relies on an anatomic description of the lymphatic vasculature.[24-26]

1. Aplasia: no collecting vessels identified
2. Hypoplasia: a diminished number of vessels are seen
3. Numeric hyperplasia (as defined by Kinmonth): an increased number of vessels are seen
4. Hyperplasia: in addition to an increase in number, the vessels have valvular incompetence and display tortuosity and dilation (megalymphatics)

Approximately one third of all cases are secondary to agenesis, hypoplasia, or obstruction of the distal lymphatic vessels, with relatively normal proximal vessels.[26,27] In those cases the swelling is usually bilateral and mild and affects females much more frequently than males. The prognosis in such cases is good. Generally, after the first year of symptoms, there is little extension in the same limb or to uninvolved extremities. Although the extent of involvement is established early in the disease in about 40% of patients, the girth of the limb continues to increase.

In more than half of all cases, the defect primarily involves obstruction of the proximal lymphatics or nodes, with initial lack of involvement of distal lymphatic vessels. Pathologic studies reveal intranodal fibrosis.[18] In those cases, the swelling tends to be unilateral and severe; there may be a slight predominance of females in this group.[26,27] In patients with proximal involvement, the extent and degree of the abnormality is more likely to progress and require surgical intervention. Initially uninvolved distal lymphatic vessels may become obliterated with time.

A minority of patients have a pattern of bilateral hyperplasia of the lymphatic channels or tortuous dilated megalymphatics. In these less common forms of primary lymphedema, there is a slight male predominance. Megalymphatics are associated with a greater extent of involvement and a worse prognosis.

Clinical Characteristics

As a third alternative, the primary lymphedemas can often be characterized by associated clinical anomalies or abnormal phenotype.[28] Although sporadic instances of primary lymphedema are more common,[29] the tendency for congenital lymphedema to cluster in families is significant. The syndrome of a familial predisposition to congenital lymphedema, ultimately determined to ensue from an autosomal dominant form of inheritance with variable penetrance, was first described by Milroy in 1892.[30] He reported "hereditary edema" affecting 22 individuals of one family over six generations.[30] Although Milroy ultimately came to consider not only congenital lymphedema, but also praecox and tarda forms, as variants of the syndrome that bears his name,[31] the praecox form of primary lymphedema more often carries the eponym of Meige's disease.[32]

In fact, a long list of disorders are associated with heritable forms of lymphedema. Increasingly these disorders have yielded to chromosomal mapping techniques. Lymphedema-cholestasis, or Aagenaes syndrome, has been mapped to chromosome 15q.[33] In several family cohorts of Milroy's disease, it has been determined that the disorder reflects missense inactivating mutations in the tyrosine kinase domain of vascular endothelial growth factor receptor 3 (VEGFR3),[34,35] thus underscoring the likelihood that the pathogenesis of this condition likely reflects an inherited defect in lymphatic vasculogenesis. Several additional lymphedema syndromes have recently lent themselves to successful genetic mapping.[28] Lymphedema-distichiasis, an autosomal dominant, dysmorphic syndrome in which the lymphedema presents in association with a supplementary row of eyelashes arising from the meibomian glands, has been linked to truncating mutations in the forkhead-related transcription factor FOXC2[36]; mutations in FOXC2 have subsequently been associated with a broad variety of primary lymphedema presentations.[37] Similarly, a more unusual form of congenital lymphedema, hypotrichosis-lymphedema-telangiectasia, has been ascribed to both recessive and dominant forms

BOX 60-1 Hereditary Conditions Associated with Lymphedema

Chromosomal aneuploidy
- Trisomy 13
- Trisomy 18
- Trisomy 21
- Triploidy
- Klinefelter's syndrome
- Turner's syndrome

Dysmorphogenic-genetic disturbances
- Noonan's syndrome
- Noone-Milroy hereditary lymphedema
- Meige's lymphedema (lymphedema praecox)
- Lymphedema-distichiasis
- Cholestasis-lymphedema syndrome (Aagenaes syndrome)[10]
- Lymphedema-microcephaly-chorioretinopathy[19]
- Neurofibromatosis type I (von Recklinghausen)
- Lymphedema-hypoparathyroidism syndrome
- Klippel-Trénaunay-Weber syndrome

From Rockson SG: Syndromic lymphedema: Keys to the kingdom of lymphatic structure and function? Lymph Res Biol 1:181, 2003.

of inheritance of mutations in the transcription factor gene SOX18.[38] It is altogether plausible that further elucidation of the molecular pathogenesis of these diseases linked to FOXC2 and SOX18 mutations will lead to enhanced insights into mechanisms of normal and abnormal lymphatic development.

In general, autosomal or sex-linked recessive forms of congenital lymphedema occur less commonly than the dominant forms of inheritance.[26,39,40] Nevertheless, the list of heritable lymphedema-associated syndromes is long and growing (Box 60-1). Primary lymphedema has been described in association with various forms of chromosomal aneuploidy, such as Turner's and Klinefelter's syndromes, with various dysmorphogenic-genetic anomalies such as Noonan's syndrome and neurofibromatosis, and with various as yet unrelated disorders such as yellow nail syndrome, intestinal lymphangiectasia, lymphangiomyomatosis, and arteriovenous malformation.[41-46] The association of lymphedema with vascular anomalies belies the common anlage of the lymph and blood vessels.

Secondary Lymphedema

Secondary lymphedema is an acquired condition that ensues after loss or obstruction of previously adequate lymphatic channels. A wide variety of pathologic processes may lead to such lymphatic obliteration.

Infection

Recurrent episodes of bacterial lymphangitis lead to thrombosis and fibrosis of the lymphatic channels and are one of the most common causes of lymphedema.[47] The responsible bacteria are almost always streptococci, which tend to enter through breaks in the skin or fissures induced by trichophytosis. Recurrent bacterial lymphangitis is also a frequent complicating factor of lymphedema from any cause.

Filariasis, a nematode infection endemic to regions of Asia and Africa, is the most common cause of secondary lymphedema in the world. The World Health Organization estimates that 90 million people may be affected by filarial infections; in India alone there are up to 14 million symptomatic cases.[48,49] Common tropical filaria include *Wuchereria bancrofti* and *Brugia malayi* or *timori*.[50,51] Other Brugia species are found in North America and occasionally cause lymphatic obstruction.[52-54]

The microfilaria are transmitted by a mosquito vector and induce recurrent lymphangitis and eventual fibrosis of lymph nodes.[55] It is unclear whether filaria themselves produce the lymphangitis or simply predispose those afflicted to recurrent episodes of bacterial lymphangitis. The filaria also can be identified in blood specimens of tissue obtained by fine-needle biopsy of the affected areas, and eosinophilia is a common local and systemic feature.[38] Diethylcarbamazine remains the most popular drug for treating filariasis; although side effects are frequent,[51,56] it is extremely efficacious.[57] Ivermectin is a new antifilarial agent that may replace diethylcarbamazine; it is less toxic, and a single oral dose (25 μg/kg) appears to be as efficacious as a 2-week course of diethylcarbamazine.[58]

Lymphatic Trauma

Within this category, by far the most common mechanism of lymphedema relates to the surgical excision of lymph nodes.[59] This occurs most commonly in the setting of cancer therapeutics. Breast cancer–associated lymphedema is the most common form of this condition in the United States. Both axillary lymph node dissection and adjuvant radiation therapy, particularly of the axilla itself, predispose to the development of secondary lymphedema of the upper extremity.[60] Recent observations suggest that, after periods of up to 13 years of follow-up, a late incidence of postmastectomy lymphedema of 14% can be expected in surgically treated patients with adjuvant postoperative irradiation.[61] Even less radical surgery (e.g., lumpectomy) can occasionally be complicated by lymphedema. Despite improvements in surgical and radiotherapeutic techniques, lymphedema remains a potential complication.[62,63] Similarly, edema of the leg may occur after surgery for pelvic or genital cancer, particularly when there has been inguinal and pelvic lymph node dissection or irradiation.[64] Its reported frequency varies between 1% and 47%.[65,66] Pelvic irradiation increases the frequency of leg lymphedema after cancer surgery[67] for such conditions as malignant melanoma, prostate cancer, and gynecologic malignancies.

Lymphedema can also ensue from other mechanisms of lymphatic trauma, among them burns, large or circumferential wounds of the extremity, or other iatrogenic causes.

Malignant Diseases

In addition to cancer therapeutics, various malignancies may induce secondary lymphedema. Tumor cells may obstruct lymphatic vessels, inducing lymphedema directly or by predisposing the patient to bacterial lymphangitis. In males the most common neoplastic etiology is prostate cancer; in females it is lymphoma.[6]

Other Causes

Other conditions leading to or associated with obstruction of lymphatic channels include tuberculosis, contact dermatitis, rheumatoid arthritis, and pregnancy.[46,67-69] Autoimmune destruction of the lymphatics remains an interesting but unproven etiology.[70] Factitious lymphedema (oedema bleu) also occurs; that condition usually affects the hand or arm, or both; is unilateral; and is induced by applications of tourniquets, self-inflicted cellulitis, or maintenance of the limb in an immobile and dependent state.[71] Chronic subcutaneous injections of drugs (most notably, pentazocine hydrochloride) also may lead to lymphatic sclerosis and obstruction.

Pathology of Lymphedema

Early in the natural history of lymphedema, there is variable thickening of the epidermis: the skin becomes rough, with hyperkeratosis and accentuation of the skin folds. Organization and fibrosis may lead to the development of papillomatosis. Early on, substantial edema of the dermis may occur. On cut section of gross specimens, the dermis is firm and gray, as is the deep fascia.[72] Usually later in the course, but sometimes quite early, there may be expansion of the subcutaneous adipose tissue, often septated by prominent fibrous strands. In some specimens compression causes lymph to exude from the dermis and subcutaneous tissue, although this is not a prominent feature. Microscopic examination reveals hyperkeratosis with prominent dermal fibrosis, as well as variable degrees of dermal edema (Fig. 60-3).[72] Abundant subcutaneous fat with prominent fibrous septa is apparent in all cases. Often, perivascular inflammatory cells (lymphocytes, plasma cells, and occasionally eosinophils) can be seen. The lymphatic vessels often are difficult to visualize and may be obliterated or thrombosed by previous inflammatory episodes or may be congenitally absent or hypoplastic. Dilatation of the lymphatics may be seen.

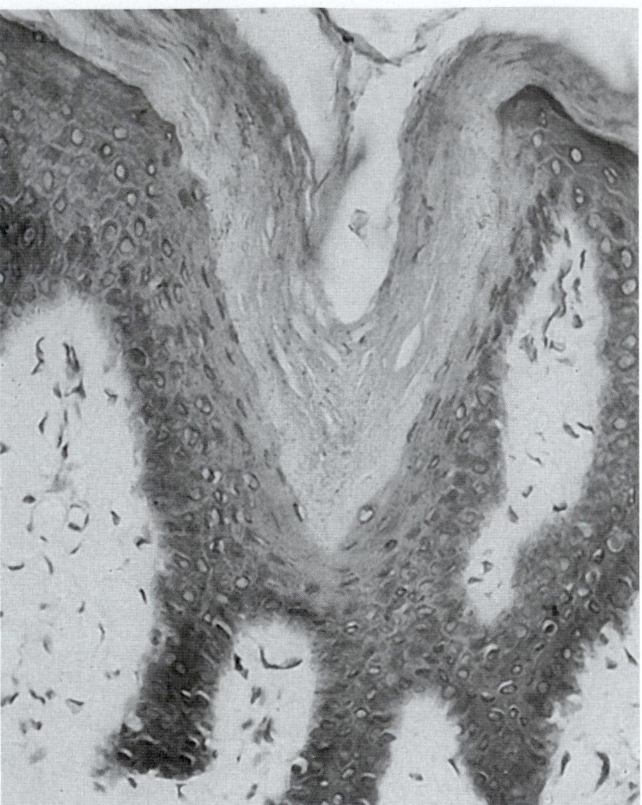

FIGURE 60-3. Skin biopsy in chronic lymphedema discloses characteristic hyperkeratosis and hypercellularity.

Clinical Presentation

The clinical signs of lymphedema largely depend on the duration and severity of the disease. Initially, the interstitial space is expanded by an excess accumulation of relatively protein-rich fluid volume. The swelling produced by that fluid collection typically is soft, is easily displaced with pressure ("pitting edema"), and may substantially decrease with elevation of the limb. In the lower extremities, the edema typically extends to the distal aspects of the feet, resulting in the characteristic "square toes" seen in this condition. Over a period of years, the limb may take on a woody texture as the surrounding tissue becomes indurated and fibrotic (Fig. 60-4). In these later stages, pitting edema is no longer a major component and limb elevation or external compression is much less successful at reducing the girth of the extremity.

Proliferation of subcutaneous connective and adipose tissue leads to thickening of the skin and loss of flexibility; the affected limb is grossly enlarged, and a mossy or cobblestone skin texture may develop. Correlates of these changes that can be sought on physical examination include the peau d'orange that reflects cutaneous and subcutaneous fibrosis, and the so-called *Stemmer sign* (inability to tent the skin at the base of the toes), which is considered to be pathognomonic of lymphedema when present in a swollen limb.[73] In many cases of long-standing lymphedema, the deposition of substantial amounts of subcutaneous adipose tissue has been described,[74] hypothetically ascribable to abnormalities of adipogenesis or lipid accumulation that accompany chronic stagnation of lymph.[75] However, the mechanisms of this component of chronic lymphatic circulatory insufficiency have not yet been delineated.

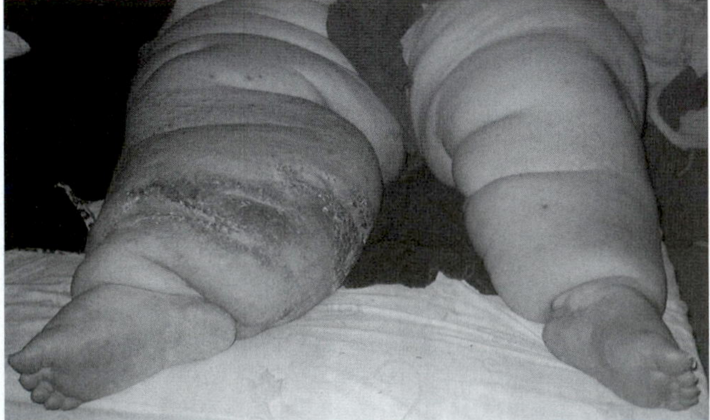

FIGURE 60-4. (See also Color Plate 60-4.) Profound cutaneous and subdermal changes in chronic lower extremity lymphedema.

Natural History and Differential Diagnosis

The natural history of lymphedema is quite variable and often may encompass a substantial interval of subclinical, asymptomatic disease. For example, even 3 years following modified radical mastectomy and axillary lymph node dissection, more than 20% of women remain free of any overt clinical evidence of lymphatic impairment, despite the extensive iatrogenic destruction of the lymphatic architecture in these patients.[76,77] Similarly, in many forms of primary lymphedema, there may be a protracted phase of apparently adequate lymphatic function, despite the inherited anatomic or functional pathology. The precipitating factors for the appearance of overt lymphedema are unknown. At the onset of clinical lymphedema, swelling of the involved extremity is typically described as puffy, and, at times, the edematous changes may even be intermittent. With chronicity, the involved structures develop the characteristic features of induration and fibrosis.[78] In many of these patients, the maximal volume increase of the involved limb is determined within the first year after clinical onset unless there are supervening complications like recurrent cellulitis. The propensity to recurrent soft-tissue infection is one of the most troublesome aspects of long-standing lymphedema. In addition to the proinfectious features of accumulated fluid and proteins, the lymphatic dysfunction also impairs local immune responses.[79,80] With recurrent infections, there is progressive damage of lymphatic capillaries.

In rare cases long-standing, chronic lymphedema may be complicated by the local development of malignant tumors. Although it is unnecessary to burden the patient about the possibility of malignancy, the patient should be alerted to report any changes in the appearance of the limb. Neoplastic transformation of the blood or lymph vessels can develop in long-standing lymphedema of any cause, including primary or secondary lymphedema.[6,81-83] Angiosarcomas or lymphangiosarcomas are potentially devastating but fortunately uncommon complications of long-standing lymphedema, occurring in less than 1% of cases.[84,85] Lymphangiosarcomas can be either sclerotic plaques or multicentric lesions with blue-tinged nodules or bullous changes. Early detection and amputation can be lifesaving, but recognition of the condition is often delayed by a lack of awareness on the part of the patient and the physician. Other malignancies including lymphoma, Kaposi's sarcoma, squamous cell cancer, and malignant melanoma have been reported in association with chronic lymphedema.[86,89]

The hypertrophied limb with thickened skin seen in chronic lymphedema has little similarity to the edematous limb of deep venous insufficiency. In the latter case, a soft pitting edema is prominent and seen in association with stasis dermatitis, hemosiderin deposition, and superficial venous varicosities. The history and examination easily differentiate chronic lymphedema from venous disorders and other causes of limb swelling (see Fig. 60-4). Earlier in the presentation, however, it may be more difficult to distinguish lymphedema from venous disease, reflex sympathetic dystrophy, or other causes of limb swelling.

Myxedema can be characterized by lower extremity edema that superficially resembles lymphedema. In hypothyroidism, edema arises when abnormal mucinous deposits accumulate in the skin. Hyaluronic acid–rich protein deposition in the dermis produces edema with resulting abnormal structural integrity and reduced skin elasticity. In thyrotoxicosis, this process is localized to the pretibial region. Myxedema is characterized by roughening of the skin of the palms, soles, elbows, and knees; brittle, uneven nails; dull, thinning hair; yellow-orange discoloration of the skin; and reduced sweat production.

Lipedema is a condition that affects women almost exclusively, although it can be seen in men with a feminizing disorder. The edema is caused by accumulation of subcutaneous adipose tissue in the leg, with sparing of the feet. Although the pathophysiology of lipedema is uncertain, it does involve an increase of subcutaneous adipocytes with structural alterations in the small vascular structures within the skin. Indeed, regional abnormalities of the circulation may cause the initial accumulation of fat in the affected regions. The characteristic distribution, with sparing of the feet, should suggest the correct diagnosis. The absence of a Stemmer sign is an additional clue. Most often, lipedema arises within 1 to 2 years after the onset of puberty. In addition to the near lifelong history of heavy thighs and hips, affected patients often complain of painful swelling. In addition, these individuals are commonly predisposed to easy bruising, perhaps a result of increased fragility of capillaries within the adipose tissue.

Diagnostic Modalities

Sometimes it is necessary to obtain more information about the nature and degree of lymphatic involvement when (1) the etiology of a swollen limb remains uncertain, (2) the diagnosis is evident but the etiology is unclear, or (3) a surgical drainage procedure is being considered.

Lymphangiography

Human lymphatics were first visualized in vivo by Hudack and McMaster at the Rockefeller Institute in 1933.[1] They used one another as subjects to demonstrate superficial lymphatic plexuses along the forearm and inner thigh, using subcutaneous injection of vital dyes. In 1948 Glenn cannulated a lymphatic vessel in the dog hind limb and injected contrast media to produce a lymphangiogram in the canine leg and groin.[1] Subsequently, Servelle and Deysson visualized the lymphatics in patients with elephantiasis using retrograde injection.[1] Visualization of the dilated lymph channels, however, depended on partial or complete valvular incompetence. Lymphangiography as such was developed by Kinmonth and coworkers[90] in 1952. The technique involves identification of a distal vessel made visible by an intradermal injection of a vital dye into the metatarsal web spaces. The vessel is isolated and cannulated, and iodinated contrast material is injected. Following the injection, the contrast material is visualized radiographically as it progresses proximally through lymphatic channels.

There are several drawbacks to the procedure, including frequent requirements for surgical exposure in the edematous limb, microsurgical techniques to achieve direct cannulation, and, occasionally, the need for general anesthesia.[27] Of greater importance is the fact that the irritation caused by the contrast agent results in lymphangitis in one third of the studies and potentially can worsen the lymphedema.[91] For these reasons, the use of lymphangiography as a diagnostic modality for the edematous limb has largely been abandoned and is contraindicated in patients with lymphedema.

Lymphoscintigraphy

Lymphoscintigraphy involves the injection of technetium containing colloids into the subcutaneous tissue of the distal aspect of the affected extremity (e.g., the dorsum of the foot). The progress of the radionuclide through the lymphatic system is followed by a radioscintigraphic camera. In primary lymphedema, channels are obliterated or absent; in a small percentage of cases, they are ectatic and incompetent. In secondary lymphedema, often with dilatation of the vascular channels, the level of obstruction can often be determined.[92] In lymphedema of any cause, the proximal progression of the radionuclide is delayed and its accumulation distally in the dilated channels of the dermis is manifested as a "dermal backflow" pattern (Fig. 60-5).

Lymphoscintigraphy is easier to perform than lymphangiography and is not reported to cause lymphangitis. It lacks the spatial resolution of lymphangiography; resolution is maximized by reducing the swelling of the extremity as much as possible before the study (reducing dilution of the radionuclide in stagnant lymph). Effective use of lymphoscintigraphy to plan therapeutic interventions requires an understanding of the pathophysiology of lymphedema and the influence of technical factors such as selection of the radiopharmaceutic, imaging times after injection, and patient activity after injection on the images.[93]

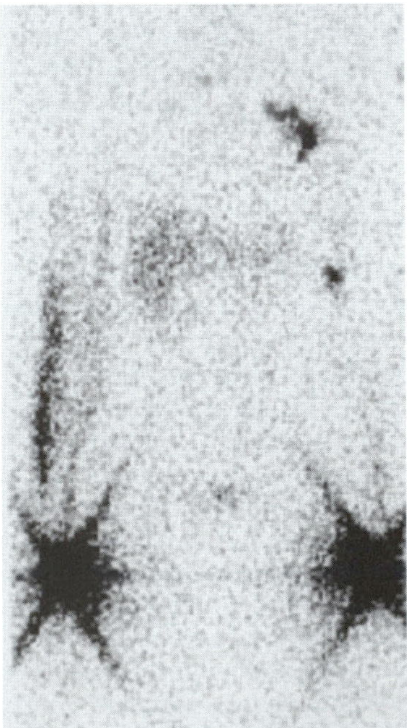

FIGURE 60-5. Bilateral upper extremity lymphoscintigraphy is accomplished by subcutaneous, interdigital injection of radiolabeled sulfur colloid. The study illustrates the absence of nodal uptake in the right axilla, along with prominent "dermal backflow" in the right forearm. These findings confirm the diagnosis of unilateral lymphedema.

Computed Tomography

CT scans of a lymphedematous limb are characterized by a honeycomb pattern in the affected area.[94] CT cannot localize the level of obstruction.[95] This technique can, however, provide insight into volume changes within various compartments visualized on cross-sectional images of the affected limb.[96] The greatest utility of CT is its ability to distinguish some of the causes of secondary lymphedema (e.g., lymphoma, pelvic tumor). Certainly, the typical honeycomb pattern of lymphedema can be sought. In addition, elements of the differential diagnosis (venous obstruction, obesity, hematoma, ruptured popliteal cyst) can be further delineated through the CT images.

Magnetic Resonance Imaging

MRI is an alternative, and most likely superior, technique to image the soft tissues in edema.[97] Among the discernible attributes by MRI are: cutaneous thickening with a honeycomb pattern in the subdermis, dilated lymphatic channels (when present as a consequence of lymphangioma or lymph reflux), and dermal accumulation of free fluid with surrounding fibrosis. This technique has particular virtue in differentiating lymphedema from lipedema.

Treatment

Medical Therapy

Successful treatment of lymphedema requires close collaboration between the patient and the physician. To that end, the physician should (1) carefully instruct the patient in the details of the medical program and (2) attend to the psychological impact of the disease. Associated emotional problems are not uncommon and are often neglected by physicians.[32] The need to address the psychological aspects of long-term disfigurement, especially with adolescent patients, cannot be overemphasized. In discussing these issues with the patient, the physician should be realistic about the possibility of progression but should emphasize the patient's ability to modulate the course of the disease by careful attention to the details of the medical program.

The physiotherapeutic approach to lymphedema has been termed *decongestive lymphatic therapy.* Meticulous attention to control of edema may reduce the likelihood of disease progression and limit the incidence of soft-tissue infections.[98] The elements of this therapeutic approach have been designed to accomplish the initial reduction in edematous limb volume, to maintain these therapeutic gains, and to ensure optimal health and functional integrity of the skin.[99-102] In addition to the acute reduction in limb volume that ensues from treatment, well-maintained therapy has been demonstrated to accelerate lymph transport and to enhance the dispersal of accumulated protein.[102] Decongestive lymphatic therapy integrates elements of meticulous skin care, massage, bandaging, exercise, and the use of compressive elastic garments.

To hydrate and soothe the skin, water soluble emollients should be applied in a consistent and diligent manner. For excessive hyperkeratosis, these emollients can be supplemented with application of salicylic acid ointments. Where skin cracking is prominent, meticulous attention to hygiene can be coupled with topical antiseptic agents.

The specialized massage technique for these patients (so-called *manual lymphatic drainage* or *therapy*) is an empirically derived technique. Its goal is to enhance lymphatic contractility and to augment and redirect lymph flow through the unobstructed cutaneous lymphatics. Manual lymphatic drainage should not be confused with other forms of therapeutic massage that do not share this ability to augment lymphatic contractility and may, in fact, be detrimental to lymphatic function (e.g., athletic massages). The mild tissue compression during manual lymphatic drainage results in enhanced filling of the initial lymphatics and improves transport capacity, through the cutaneous lymphatic dilatation and the development of accessory lymph collectors.[103] Typically, 8 to 15 consecutive daily sessions of manual lymphatic drainage are required to achieve optimal reduction of limb volume in a previously untreated patient.

During this acute approach to volume reduction, nonelastic, compressive bandages should be applied in multiple layers after each session of manual lymphatic drainage (Fig. 60-6). These are worn during muscular exertion (which is encouraged) to prevent reaccumulation of fluid and to promote lymph flow during exertion. Multilayer bandaging can also help to reverse skin changes, soften the subcutaneous tissues, and reduce the degree of lymphorrhea, when present. In the maintenance phase of lymphedema care, the use of multilayer bandages is most often supplanted by the daily use of compressive elastic garments.

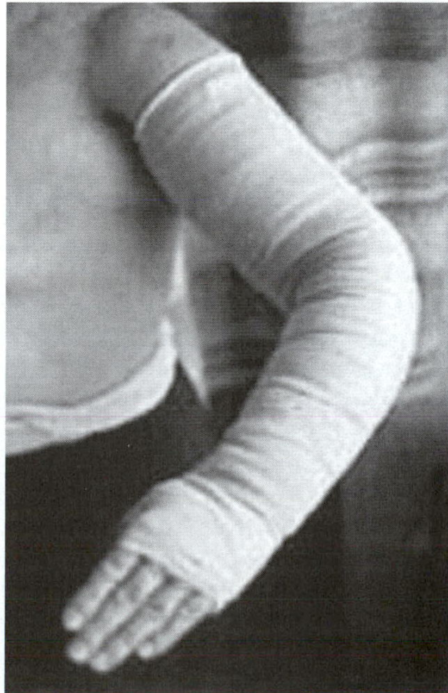

FIGURE 60-6. Short-stretch multilayer compression bandaging in secondary lymphedema of the upper extremity.

Elastic support hose should be fitted to the patient's limb after the edema in the extremity has been maximally reduced by compression and elevation.[47,104] This is an important detail. The stocking or sleeve does not reduce the size of the limb but maintains the circumference to which it is fitted. However, if the limb is fitted for a stocking while in a swollen state, the limb will be maintained by the stocking in a swollen state. The prescription of compressive garments is a necessary adjunct to all other forms of maintenance lymphedema therapy. Relatively inelastic sleeves, stockings, and underwear that transmit high-grade compression (40 to 80 mm Hg) will prevent reaccumulation of fluid after successful decongestive treatments.[105-107] Garments must be fitted properly and replaced when they lose their elasticity (every 3 to 6 months). In addition to the standard, fitted garments for upper and lower extremities, various additional appliances are now available. They provide the capacity to maintain limb volume during sleep, when the sleeve or stocking is removed, and during various forms of activity.

Without guidance from the physician, some patients become sedentary in response to uncomfortable or heavy sensations in the affected limb. Reduced physical activity at work and at home leads to apathy and malaise; that consequence can be averted by encouraging physical activity with proper support hose. Regular exercise appears to reduce lymphedema as long as elastic support (or hydrostatic pressure) is applied.[104] Swimming is a particularly good physical activity for these patients because the hydrostatic pressure of the surrounding water negates the need for compressive support.

Although the elements of decongestive lymphatic therapy were initially derived empirically, the efficacy of these interventions has now been demonstrated in numerous prospective observations.[108-110] Long-term efficacy is particularly enhanced when there is attention to focused patient instruction in maintenance self-care.[109]

Various adjunctive treatment approaches have been investigated. Of these, perhaps the most useful is intermittent pneumatic compression (IPC). Multichamber pneumatic devices are available that intermittently compress the limb; techniques that employ sequential graduated compression (in which the cuffs are inflated sequentially from distal to proximal sites with a pressure gradient from the most distal cuff to the most proximal) are the most efficacious.[111,112] Pneumatic compression techniques cannot, however, clear edema fluid from adjacent noncompressed sections of the limb. Consequently, as fluid shifts occur during pneumatic compression, the root of the limb must be decompressed with the aforementioned manual techniques.

The incorporation of IPC into a multidisciplinary, therapeutic approach long has been advocated empirically by some physiotherapeutic schools.[113,114] Individual reports of complications and lack of efficacy have reduced enthusiasm for the use of pneumatic compression as stand-alone therapy.[111,115,116] More recently, it has been demonstrated that when IPC is used adjunctively with the other, established elements of decongestive lymphatic therapy, it enhances the therapeutic response, both in the initial and maintenance approaches to the patient. Pneumatic compression is well tolerated and remarkably free of complications.[117] However, it must be stressed that any form of compressive therapy requires a sufficient arterial blood supply to the limb. In cases where severe peripheral arterial disease is coexisting, any form of sustained compression can further compromise arterial blood flow.

Other physical forms of therapy are under investigation. Low-level laser therapy may be effective in postmastectomy lymphedema: in one small series, subjective improvement accompanied an objective documentation of improved bioimpedance and reduced extracellular and intracellular fluid accumulation.[118] In other hands, such techniques as local hyperthermia[119] or the intra-arterial injection of autologous lymphocytes[120] have independently produced favorable results. In the latter approach, it is postulated that regression of edema is linked to the expression of L-selectin, a lymphocyte-specific adhesion molecule.[120] The observations in these pilot studies must be confirmed in larger controlled trials.

Additional, standard treatment approaches are directed toward prevention and control of infection. Recurrent cellulitis and local infections pose a constant threat of exacerbation. Skin hygiene is essential. In addition to the application of emollients to the skin, trauma must be avoided (when ambulatory, the feet should be covered by slippers or shoes; a podiatrist should attend to nail care as needed). Fungal infections should be aggressively treated with topical antifungal agents. The patient should be instructed to take antibiotics at the earliest sign of cellulitis and should be given a prescription for a course of an oral semisynthetic penicillin or (for penicillin-sensitive patients) erythromycin. In lymphedema, acute inflammatory episodes may not elicit typical, clearly demarcated erythematous skin responses or associated systemic evidence of infection. Nevertheless, these more subtle presentations should be treated aggressively with antibiotics. After a course of therapy, the edema once again responds to compressive therapy and the tenderness resolves. Various broad-spectrum oral antibiotics can be used to good effect, particularly with attention to the spectrum of activity against streptococcal and staphylococcal species.

Other than antibiotic therapy, where needed, pharmacotherapy has little role in the management of lymphedema. Diuretics, although widely prescribed for this chronic, edematous condition, are rarely useful and may in fact be deleterious. On the other hand, in edema of mixed origin, these agents may have a beneficial effect through their ability to reduce circulating blood volume and thereby reduce capillary filtration. An understanding of the mechanisms inducing the proliferation of subcutaneous connective tissue and lymphedema may lead to more definitive treatment. Agents might then be designed to alter the relationship between the deposition and lysis of collagen fibers such that lysis is favored, thereby reducing fibrosis.[5,121] Benzopyrones (coumarin, hydroxyethylrutin) represent a class of agents that have been reported to reduce volume in affected limbs, purportedly by stimulating tissue macrophages, which in turn increase interstitial proteolysis. Although initial trials appeared favorable,[122,123] subsequent evaluation suggests that the therapeutic gains are small[124,125]; furthermore, the utility of coumarin is significantly hampered by the risk of drug-related hepatotoxicity.[126] An important question left unanswered is whether coumarin is additive in its effects to the usual compressive measures. The agent is not yet approved by the FDA for use in the United States. Another experimental therapy is intralymphatic injections of steroids, which may help by inhibiting the proliferation of connective tissue.[127] The development of angiogenic steroids that have some tissue specificity could make this a feasible approach. Alternatively, flavonoids such as hesperidin and diosmin have been employed to beneficial effect. Their use is supported by preclinical, experimental investigations that suggest the agents have the capacity to improve microvascular permeability and augment lymphatic contractile activity.[128,129] Extract of horse chestnut seed containing escin, a bioflavonoid, has been shown to reduce venular capillary permeability and edema of lymphatic or venous etiology.

Surgical Treatment

Surgery is a last resort, and only for selected cases. It should not be considered lightly. When the lymphatic obstruction is of a proximal type and the lymphatic channels distal to the obstruction are of adequate diameter, a *drainage procedure* is occasionally feasible under certain well-defined circumstances, and only by skilled operators. Even then, successful drainage is gained in only about 50% of cases and is often temporary.

Flaps of tissue rich in lymphatics have been implanted into the edematous region.[130] In theory, if the lymphatic vessels in the flap remain functional, they eventually may anastomose with the surrounding lymphatics and provide an alternative pathway for drainage from the edematous area. The myocutaneous flap (using latissimus dorsi) has been reported to be useful for the upper extremity, and the intestinal flap (enteromesenteric bridge) may improve drainage in the lower extremity.[131,132]

Direct microsurgical anastomotic procedures also have been used. Lymphovenous anastomoses can be made between lymphatic vessels distal to an obstruction in nearby small veins; these allow lymph from the obstructed region to flow directly into the venous system.[131] Anastomoses also can be made from the lymph nodes to the adjacent vein. One of the latest techniques involves harvesting normal autogenous lymphatic vessels for use as bypass grafts around a lymphatic obstruction. All of these microsurgical techniques require the presence of dilated lymphatic vessels distal to the obstruction.[130,133] These operations obviously are of no value when the lymphatic obstruction is at the level of the smaller distal vessels. The argument has been made, however, that lymphatic bypass operations should be performed as soon as possible after the onset of obstruction to avoid the cutaneous changes of chronic lymphedema, as well as the gradual destruction of the distal lymphatic channels.[134] An appropriate candidate for such surgery would be an individual with a recent onset of lymphedema secondary to trauma and with an otherwise normal lymphatic system proximal and distal to the area of obstruction. In a recently published, large series of such appropriately selected patients, microsurgical lymphatic-venous anastomosis accomplished objective reduction of limb volume in 85% of the cases.[135]

Reduction procedures have been employed generally for limbs that have become so bulky or unsightly that they constitute a significant impairment to daily living. Such procedures are generally considered a patient's last resort and, by themselves, result in a limb that is scarred and disfigured, albeit more mobile. The procedures involve resection of a portion of the skin and subcutaneous tissue and subsequent closure of the wound to reduce the limb diameter. Acute complications include wound infection or necrosis of the skin flaps; late complications include recurrent cellulitis or verrucous hyperplasia of the skin grafts. Swelling of the extremity is more likely to progress if recurrent bouts of cellulitis are not adequately controlled, or if adequate compressive support is not provided postoperatively (the procedure does not correct the obstruction to lymph efflux). These limbs require lifelong compressive support and, because of their vulnerability to infection, fastidious attention to hygiene. Some of the most challenging patients cared for by a lymphedema center are those who have had aggressive reduction surgery, producing a painful mutilated limb that is immunocompromised and ravaged by recurrent fungal and bacterial infections.

Currently, medical therapy is directed at preventing complications and retarding progression of the disorder, whereas surgery is palliative. Of interest are recent reports of therapeutic success of liposuction in advanced, stable lymphedema. Surgical liposuction of chronic postmastectomy lymphedema has been reported to produce excellent results, with sustained reduction of excess volume. In one series, an average long-term reduction of edema volume of 106% was observed in 28 patients with an average edema volume of 1845 ml.[74] Liposuction combined with long-term decongestive compression therapy reduces edema volume more successfully than does compression therapy alone. However, the volume reduction is unsuccessful unless compression therapy is maintained after the surgical intervention.[136]

Prospects for Molecular Therapy

Although many therapeutic strategies for lymphedema effectively reduce excess volume, minimize complications, and optimize function, the disease currently lacks a cure. For these reasons, there has been emphasis on the possible application of effective molecular therapies. Among these, the most exciting to date is therapeutic lymphangiogenesis, which is based on insights into the developmental biology of the lymphatics.

Among the mitogenic substances that initiate and regulate the growth of vascular structures, those in the VEGF family play a central role.[137,138] VEGF-C and VEGF-D direct the development and growth of the lymphatic vasculature in embryonic and postnatal life through binding to VEGFR-3 receptors on lymphatic endothelia.[139-142] Exogenous administration of VEGF-C upregulates the VEGFR-3 receptor, leading to a lymphangiogenic response[143] and, in transgenic mice that overexpress VEGF-C, the lymphatic vessels demonstrate a hyperplastic, proliferative response, with secondary cutaneous changes.[141]

These molecular observations have shed light on the mechanisms that contribute to disease expression in the most common heritable form of lymphedema, the autosomal dominant condition known as Milroy's disease. This disease has been linked to the FLT4 locus, encoding vascular VEGFR-3.[34] Disease-associated alleles contain missense mutations that produce an inactive tyrosine kinase, thereby preventing downstream gene activation. It is believed that the mutant form of the receptor is excessively stable, as well as inactive, so that the normal signaling mechanism is blunted, leading to hypoplastic development of the lymphatic vessels.[144]

The prospects for therapeutic lymphangiogenesis in human lymphedema have been underscored by the recent description of a mouse model of inherited limb edema based on mutations in the VEGFR-3 signaling mechanism and pathology that resembles human disease.[145] In this model, therapeutic overexpression of VEGF-C using a viral vector induces the generation of new, functional lymphatics and the amelioration of lymphedema. Similarly, in a rodent model of acquired, postsurgical lymphatic insufficiency (i.e., resembling postmastecomy lymphedema), the exogenous administration of human recombinant VEGF-C restores lymphatic flow (as assessed by lymphoscintigraphy),[146] increases lymphatic vascularity, and reverses the hypercellularity that characterizes the untreated lymphedematous condition (Fig. 60-7).

Intensive future investigation is necessary to verify the therapeutic potential of such approaches, as well as to establish dose-response relationships and durability of the therapeutic response. As with other forms of angiogenic therapy, the relative virtues of growth factor therapy versus gene therapy must be established.

DISEASES OF THE LYMPHATIC VASCULATURE

Complex Vascular Pathology with Lymphatic Anomalies (also see Chapter 66)

There is a broad constellation of developmental anomalies of the arteriovenous circulation that concurrently distort lymphatic anatomy or function, or both. These mixed vascular deformities are best characterized by the dominant vascular anomaly, whether angiomatous, venous, or arteriovenous.[25]

Klippel-Trénaunay Syndrome

Klippel-Trénaunay syndrome is the most common congenital venous anomaly to affect the entire limb. It is a

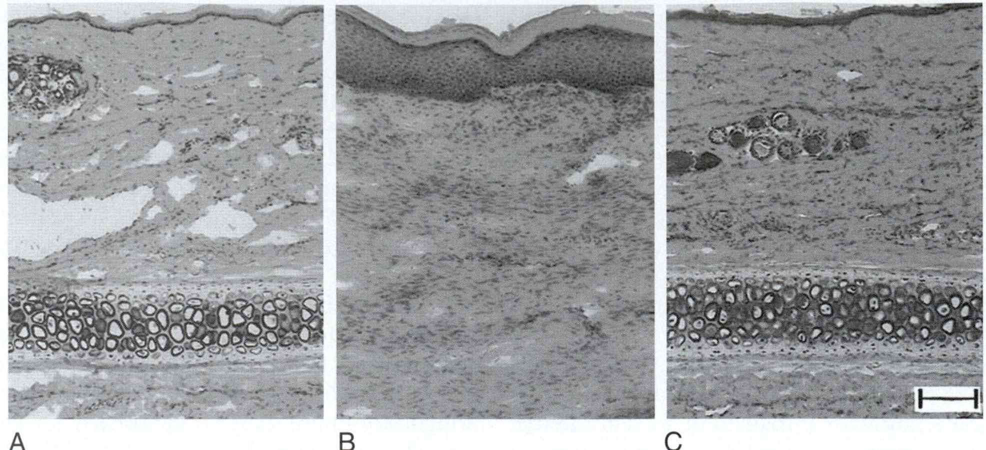

FIGURE 60-7. (See also Color Plate 60-7.) Postmortem histology (H&E stained frozen sections) of rabbit skin after recombinant human VEGF-C therapy (**A**) and in untreated lymphedema (saline control) (**B**). Histology of a normal skin specimen (**C**) is provided for comparison. The thickening of the dermal and epidermal structures in untreated lymphedema is so profound that, in contrast to both normal and VEGF-C–treated specimens, visualization of the subdermal cartilage within the microscopic field is rendered impossible. All three panels were photographed at the same magnification (scale = 100 μm). (From Szuba A, Skobe M, Karkkainen MJ, et al: Therapeutic lymphangiogenesis with human recombinant VEGF-C. FASEB J 16:1985, 2002.)

congenital disorder in which varicose veins, cutaneous nevi, and limb hypertrophy are observed.[147] Lymphedema is reported in 5% of these patients.[148] It has been suggested that this syndrome reflects a generalized disturbance of mesodermal development, thereby engendering the commonly associated anomalies: bony overgrowth, soft tissue hypertrophy, syndactyly, hypospadias, and lymphatic hypoplasia.[149] Treatment is generally restricted to meticulous skin care (i.e., hydration, protection from trauma); compressive therapy for the associated lymphedema and venous insufficiency; prevention of superficial bleeding from the varicose veins; and prophylaxis against deep venous thrombosis.

Maffucci's Syndrome

The Maffucci syndrome is described as severe dyschondroplasia in association with multiple lymphangiomata (see later). In this condition, lymphatic vasculature and nodes are typically hypoplastic.[25]

Parkes Weber Syndrome

This syndrome is characterized by the presence of multiple arteriovenous fistulae with associated enlargement of the girth of a single limb. The condition can be ascribed, at least in part, to the concomitant dilated, tortuous lymphatics and consequent lymphedema.[150] The pathophysiology of this disorder likely reflects the enormous increase in blood flow consequent to the multiple arteriovenous fistulae; this increase in capillary filtration would then lead to an increase in lymphatic load, producing first vascular dilatation and, ultimately, insufficiency. The lymph reflux in the limb may lead to the appearance of lymph vesicles in the skin, which should be treated conservatively. We have had some initial success with percutaneous and intravascular, catheter-based embolization of associated arteriovenous fistulae (unreported observations).

Proliferative Growth of Lymphatic Vascular Structures and Neoplasm

(also see Chapter 66)

Lymphangioma

This developmental malformation is first detectable in infants. These are not, despite their name, strictly speaking, tumors. Rather, these lesions are composed of profuse numbers of dilated, thin-walled lymphatic vascular structures. They can occur throughout the body but are seen most commonly on the proximal extremities and at the limb girdle. Small, clear vesicles are observed in the skin, sometimes with associated cutaneous bleeding. When these lesions are encountered in the setting of dyschondroplasia, the designation of Maffucci's syndrome is applied.[151]

Cavernous Lymphangioma and Cystic Hygroma

These hamartomatous lesions appear within the first years of life, if not present at birth. Like lymphangiomata, these lesions contain dilated lymphatic vascular structures. The cavernous lesions are typically found in the mouth, in the mesentery, and on the extremities; cystic hygromas present in the neck, axilla, and groin. These lesions are often surgically resected to prevent complications.

Lymphangiomatosis

This is a rare developmental condition in which proliferation of lymphatic vascular structures involves dermis, soft tissue, bone, and parenchyma in a diffuse manner. The organs most typically affected are liver, spleen, lung, and pleura.[152] Associated lymphangiectasia can be observed in numerous additional organs including liver, kidney, testes, lymph nodes, adrenals, and intestines. Involvement of the viscera typically confers a poor prognosis. When chylothorax is present, repeated thoracentesis and pleurodesis is often required. In one small series, all patients died within 6 to 33 months of clinical presentation.[153]

Lymphangiosarcoma

Lymphangiosarcomas, malignant angiosarcomas that develop in association with lymphedema, develop as multicentric lesions that have a high propensity for systemic metastasis.[151,152] The vast majority of such lesions have been observed in lymphedema patients that are breast cancer survivors with chronic, significant edema. It is seen only rarely in other forms of lymphedema.[154,155] Whatever the clinical substrate, the prognosis for survival is poor, even following radical amputation.

Visceral Lymphatic Disorders

Chylous Reflux, Chylothorax, Chylous Ascites

When the lymphatics are incompetent, obstructed, or hypoplastic, fluid has the capacity to reflux. In visceral disease, this fluid can be lymph or chylous lymph. The presence of chylous lymph denotes incompetence of lymphatic flow that extends to the level of the lacteals, at the point where they join the preaortic lymphatics and the cisterna chyli. The anatomical substrate of this problem can be either primary or secondary. In the former case, hypoplastic or dilated incompetent lymphatics reflect the inherited defect of lymphatic development; in secondary forms, thoracic duct obstruction occurs through surgical mishap, trauma, malignancy, or the damage created by filariasis.

Lymph or chyle reflux can occur directly into the lower limbs. The abnormal fluid drains directly from vesicles on the surface of the leg or on the genitalia. Variants of this same presentation can produce chylothorax, chylous ascites, chylous arthritis, and chyluria. In general, if chyle is present in the refluxing body fluid, the therapeutic approach should include a fat-restricted diet with supplementation of medium chain triglycerides; if the response is not satisfactory, complete elimination of chyle from the fluid can be accomplished, at least temporarily, with total parenteral nutrition.

The prognosis for such presentations is not favorable. The natural history of reflux reflects the tendency for the condition to worsen with the passage of time. In some patients, there may be an episodic pattern of leakage with sudden exacerbations; others experience a steady, increasing tendency to lymphorrhea and reflux. In patients with the secondary form, an assiduous search for predisposing malignancy or extrinsic lymphatic obstruction should always be undertaken. In patients with the various forms of visceral involvement, complex surgical interventions are sometimes required to mitigate the functional and symptomatic consequences of reflux into the serous cavities.

Protein-Losing Enteropathy

The presence of visceral lymphatic vascular disease can predispose to a life-threatening form of metabolic insufficiency called *protein-losing enteropathy.* When chyle refluxes back into the villi as a consequence of the effective blockade of its passage into the central lymphatics, this condition engenders weight loss, diarrhea, and steatorrhea as protein, fat, calcium, and fat-soluble vitamins are malabsorbed. In addition to the secondary forms of lymphatic obstruction (usually malignant), the primary hypoplastic and lymphangiectatic disorders can also predispose to enteropathy; in these cases lymphedema of an extremity often precedes or accompanies the appearance of the enteropathy. As with other forms of reflux, the initial therapeutic strategy should entail medium chain triglyceride supplementation with restriction of total dietary fat intake.[157,158] Where the response to conservative therapy is insufficient, it has been suggested that systemic treatment with octreotide may help to alleviate the severity of the disorder, although the mechanism of benefit is not entirely understood.[158,159]

REFERENCES

1. Kanter MA: The lymphatic system: An historical perspective. Plast Reconstr Surg 79:131, 1987.
2. Rockson SG: Preclinical models of lymphatic disease: The potential for growth factor and gene therapy. Ann N Y Acad Sci 979:64, 2002.
3. Shin WS, Szuba A, Rockson SG: Animal models for the study of lymphatic insufficiency. Lymph Res Biol 1:159, 2003.
4. Oliver G: Lymphatic vasculature development. Nat Rev Immunol 4:35, 2004.
5. Baldwin M, Stacker S, Achen M: Molecular control of lymphangiogenesis. Bioessays 24:1030, 2002.
6. Gashev A: Physiologic aspects of lymphatic contractile function: Current perspectives. Ann N Y Acad Sci 979:178, 2002.
7. Starling EH: Classics in lymphology. Lymphology 17:83, 1984.
8. Sparks HV, Rooke TW: Essentials of Cardiovascular Physiology. Minneapolis, University of Minnesota Press, 1987.
9. Cotton KD, Hollywood MA, McHale NG, Thornbury KD: Outward currents in smooth muscle cells isolated from sheep mesenteric lymphatics. J Physiol 503(pt 1):1, 1997.
10. von der Weid PY, Zawieja DC: Lymphatic smooth muscle: The motor unit of lymph drainage. Int J Biochem Cell Biol 36:1147, 2004.
11. Gashev AA, Zawieja DC: Physiology of human lymphatic contractility: A historical perspective. Lymphology 34:124, 2001.
12. Muthuchamy M, Gashev A, Boswell N, et al: Molecular and functional analyses of the contractile apparatus in lymphatic muscle. FASEB J 17:920, 2003.
13. Thornbury KD, Harty HR, McGeown JG, McHale NG: Mesenteric lymph flow responses to splanchnic nerve stimulation in sheep. Am J Physiol 264:H604, 1993.
14. Harty HR, Thornbury KD, McHale NG: Neurotransmission in isolated sheep mesenteric lymphatics. Microvasc Res 46:310, 1993.
15. McHale NG, Thornbury KD, Hollywood MA: 5-HT inhibits spontaneous contractility of isolated sheep mesenteric lymphatics via activation of 5-HT(4) receptors. Microvasc Res 60:261, 2000.
16. Hall JL, Morris B, Wooley L: Intrinsic rhythmic propulsion of lymph in anesthetized sheep. J Physiol 180:336, 1965.
17. Trzewik J, Mallipattu SK, Artmann GM, et al: Evidence for a second valve system in lymphatics: Endothelial microvalves. FASEB J 15:1711, 2001.
18. Mendoza E, Schmid-Schonbein GW: A model for mechanics of primary lymphatic valves. J Biomech Eng 125:407, 2003.
19. Samuels LD: Lymphoscintigraphy. Lymphology 20:4, 1987.
20. Browse NL: The diagnosis and management of primary lymphedema. Vasc Surg 3:181, 1986.
21. Rockson SG: Primary lymphedema. In Ernst CB, Stanley JC (eds): Current Therapy in Vascular Surgery, 4th ed. Philadelphia, Mosby, 2000.
22. Rockson SG: Lymphedema. Am J Med 110:288, 2001.
23. Szuba A, Rockson SG: Lymphedema: Classification, diagnosis and therapy. Vasc Med 3:145, 1998.

24. Kinmonth JB: Primary lymphoedema: Classification and other studies based on oleo-lymphography and clinical features. J Cardiovasc Surg (Torino). Special number for the XVII Congress of the European Society of Cardiovascular Surgeons 1969;65.
25. Kinmonth JB: The Lymphatics, 2nd ed. London, Arnold, 1982.
26. Wolfe JHN: The prognosis and possible cause of severe primary lymphoedema. Ann R Coll Surg Engl 66:251, 1984.
27. Allen EV: Lymphedema of the extremities: Classification, etiology and differential diagnosis: A study of three hundred cases. Arch Intern Med 54:606, 1934.
28. Rockson SG: Syndromic lymphedema: Keys to the kingdom of lymphatic structure and function? Lymph Res Biol 1:181, 2003.
29. Wolfe JHN, Kinmonth JB: The prognosis of primary lymphedema of the lower limbs. Arch Surg 116:1157, 1981.
30. Milroy WF: An undescribed variety of hereditary edema. N Y Med J 56:505, 1892.
31. Milroy WF: Chronic hereditary edema: Milroy's disease. JAMA 91:1172, 1928.
32. Smeltzer DM, Stickler GB, Schirger A: Primary lymphedema in children and adolescents: A followup study and review. Pediatrics 76:206, 1985.
33. Bull LN, Roche E, Song EJ, et al: Mapping of the locus for cholestasis-lymphedema syndrome (Aagenaes syndrome) to a 6.6-cM interval on chromosome 15q. Am J Hum Genet 67:994, 2000.
34. Karkkainen MJ, Ferrell RE, Lawrence EC, et al: Missense mutations interfere with VEGFR-3 signalling in primary lymphoedema. Nat Genet 25:153, 2000.
35. Irrthum A, Karkkainen MJ, Devriendt K, et al: Congenital hereditary lymphedema caused by a mutation that inactivates VEGFR3 tyrosine kinase. Am J Hum Genet 67:295, 2000.
36. Fang J, Dagenais SL, Erickson RP, et al: Mutations in FOXC2 (MFH-1), a forkhead family transcription factor, are responsible for the hereditary lymphedema distichiasis syndrome. Am J Hum Genet 67:1382, 2000.
37. Finegold DN, Kimak MA, Lawrence EC, et al: Truncating mutations in FOXC2 cause multiple lymphedema syndromes. Hum Mol Genet 10:1185, 2001.
38. Irrthum A, Devriendt K, Chitayat D, et al: Mutations in the transcription factor gene SOX18 underlie recessive and dominant forms of hypotrichosis-lymphedema-telangiectasia. Am J Hum Genet 72:1470, 2003.
39. Lewis JM, Wald ER: Lymphedema praecox. J Pediatr 104:641, 1984.
40. Dahlberg PJ, Borer WZ, Newcomer KL, Yutuc WR: Autosomal or X-linked recessive syndrome of congenital lymphedema, hypoparathyroidism, nephropathy, prolapsing mitral valve, and brachytelephalangy. Am J Med Genet 16:99, 1983.
41. Mucke J, Hoepffner W, Scheerschmidt G, et al: Early onset lymphoedema, recessive form—a new form of genetic lymphoedema syndrome. Eur J Pediatr 145:195, 1986.
42. Henriksen HM: Turner's syndrome associated with lymphoedema, diagnosed in the newborns. Z Geburtshilfe Perinatol 184:313, 1980.
43. White SW: Lymphedema in Noonan's syndrome. Int J Dermatol 23:656, 1984.
44. Venencie PY, Dicken CH: Yellow nail syndrome: Report of five cases. J Am Acad Dermatol 10:187, 1984.
45. Wheeler ES, Chan V, Wassman R, et al: Familial lymphedema praecox: Meige's disease. Plast Reconstr Surg 67:362, 1981.
46. Abe R, Kimura M, Airosaki A: Retroperitioneal lymphangiomyomatosis with lymphedema of the legs. Lymphology 13:62, 1980.
47. Schirger A: Lymphedema. Cardiovasc Clin 13:293, 1983.
48. Lymphatic filariasis—tropical medicine's origin will not go away. Lancet (Editorial) 1:1409, 1987.
49. Dandapat MC, Mahapatro SK, Dash DM: Management of chronic manifestations of filariasis. J Indian Med Assoc 84:219, 1986.
50. Tan TJ, Kosin E, Tan TH: Lymphographic abnormalities in patients with Brugia malayi filariasis and "idiopathic tropical eosinophilia." Lymphology 18:169, 1985.
51. Ottesen EA: Efficacy of diethylcarbamazine in eradicating infection with lymphatic-dwelling filariae in humans. Rev Infect Dis 7:341, 1985.
52. Baird JK, Alpert LI, Friedman R, et al: North American brugian filariasis: Report of nine infections of humans. Am J Trop Med Hyg 35:1205, 1986.
53. Clark WR, Lieber MM: Genital filariasis in Minnesota. Urology 28:518, 1986.
54. Leonard JC, Humphrey GB, Basmadjian G: Lymphedema secondary to filariasis. Clin Nucl Med 10:203, 1985.
55. Jayaram G: Microfilariae in fine needle aspirates from epididymal lesions. Acta Cytol 31:59, 1987.
56. Partono F: Treatment of elephantiasis in a community with timorian filariasis. Trans R Soc Trop Med Hyg 79:44, 1985.
57. Bockarie M, Tisch D, Kastens W, et al: Mass treatment to eliminate filariasis in Papua New Guinea. N Engl J Med 347:1841, 2002.
58. Kumaraswami V, Ottesen EA, Vijayasekaran V, et al: Ivermectin for the treatment of *Wuchereria bancrofti* filariasis: Efficacy and adverse reactions. JAMA 259:3150, 1988.
59. Szuba A, Rockson S: Lymphedema: A review of diagnostic techniques and therapeutic options. Vasc Med 3:145, 1998.
60. Rockson SG: Precipitating factors in lymphedema: Myths and realities. Cancer 83:2814, 1998.
61. Hojris I, Andersen J, Overgaard M, Overgaard J: Late treatment-related morbidity in breast cancer patients randomized to postmastectomy radiotherapy and systemic treatment versus systemic treatment alone. Acta Oncol 39:355, 2000.
62. Tengrup I, Tennval-Nittby L, Christiansson I, Laurin M: Arm morbidity after breast-conserving therapy for breast cancer. Acta Oncol 39:393, 2000.
63. Petrek JA, Heelan MC: Incidence of breast carcinoma-related lymphedema. Cancer 83(suppl 12):2776, 1998.
64. Fiorica JV, Roberts WS, Greenberg H, et al: Morbidity and survival patterns in patients after radical hysterectomy and postoperative adjuvant pelvic radiotherapy. Gynecol Oncol 36:343, 1990.
65. Werngren-Elgstrom M, Lidman D: Lymphoedema of the lower extremities after surgery and radiotherapy for cancer of the cervix. Scand J Plast Reconstr Surg Hand Surg 28:289, 1994.
66. Soisson AP, Soper JT, Clarke-Pearson DL, et al: Adjuvant radiotherapy following radical hysterectomy for patients with stage IB and IIA cervical cancer. Gynecol Oncol 37:390, 1990.
67. Lynde CW, Mitchell IC: Unusual complication of allergic contact dermatitis of the hands-recurrent lymphangitis and persistent lymphoedema. Contact Dermatitis 8:279, 1982.
68. Kyle VM, DeSilva M, Hurst G: Rheumatoid lymphoedema. Clin Rheumatol 1:126, 1982.
69. Reed BR, Burke S, Bozeman M, et al: Lymphedema of the lower abdominal wall in pregnancy. J Am Acad Dermatol 12:930, 1985.
70. Majeski I: Lymphedema tarda. Cutis 38:105, 1985.
71. Brunning I, Gibson AG, Perry M: Oedema bleu: A reappraisal. Lancet 1:810, 1980.
72. Sakulsky SB: Lymphedema: Results of surgical treatment in 64 patients (1936-1984). Lymphology 10:15, 1977.
73. Stemmer R: Ein klinisches Zeichen zur fruh-und differential-Diagnose des Lymphodems. (A clinical symptom for the early and differential diagnosis of lymphedema). Vasa 5:261, 1976.
74. Brorson H, Svensson H: Complete reduction of lymphoedema of the arm by liposuction after breast cancer. Scand J Plast Reconstr Surg Hand Surg 31:137, 1997.
75. Rosen E: The molecular control of adipogenesis, with special reference to lymphatic pathology. Ann N Y Acad Sci 979:143, 2002.
76. Gregl A, Poppe H, Pohls H, et al: Häufigkeit, Pathogenese und klinische Symptomatic des Armodems beim Mammakarzmom. (Occurrence, pathogenesis and clinical symptoms of arm edema in breast carcinoma). Strahlentherapie 133:499, 1967.
77. Clodius L: Secondary arm lymphedema. In Clodius L (ed): Lymphedema. Stuttgart, Georg Thieme, 1977, p 147.
78. Schirger A, Harrison EG, Janes JM: Idiopathic lymphedema: Review of 131 cases. JAMA 182:124, 1962.
79. Mallon E, Powell S, Mortimer P, Ryan TJ: Evidence for altered cell-mediated immunity in postmastectomy lymphoedema. Br J Dermatol 137:928, 1997.
80. Beilhack A, Rockson SG: Immune traffic: A functional overview. Lymph Res Biol 1:219, 2003.
81. Muller R, Hajdu SI, Brennan MF: Lymphangiosarcoma associated with chronic filarial lymphedema. Cancer 59:179, 1987.
82. Alessi E, Sala F, Berti E: Angiosarcoma in lymphedematous limbs. Am J Dermatopathol 8:371, 1986.
83. Benda JA, Al Jurf AS, Benson AB III: Angiosarcoma of the breast following segmental mastectomy complicated by lymphedema. Am J Clin Pathol 87:651, 1987.

84. Servelle M: Surgical treatment of lymphedema: A report on 652 cases. Surgery 101:485, 1987.
85. Schmitz-Rixen T, Horsch S, Arnold G, et al: Angiosarcoma in primary lymphedema of the lower extremity—Stewart-Treves syndrome. Lymphology 17:50, 1984.
86. Tatnall PM, Mann BS: Non-Hodgkin's lymphoma of kin associated with chronic limb lymphoedema. Br J Dermatol 113:75, 1985.
87. Ruocco V, Astarita C, Guerrera V, et al: Kaposi's sarcoma on a lymphedematous immunocompromised limb. Int J Dermatol 23:56, 1984.
88. Epstein JI, Mendelsohn G: Squamous carcinoma of the foot arising in association with long-standing verrucous hyperplasia in a patient with congenital lymphedema. Cancer 54:943, 1984.
89. Bart AH, Pinsky CM: Malignant melanoma appearing in a postmastectomy lymphedematous arm: A novel association of double primary tumors. J Surg Oncol 30:316, 1985.
90. Kinmonth JB, Taylor GW, Harper RK: Lymphangiography: A technique for its clinical use in the lower limb. Br Med J 1:940, 1955.
91. O'Brien BM, et al: Effect of lymphangiography on lymphedema. Plast Reconstr Surg 68:922, 1981.
92. Vaqueiro M, et al: Lymphoscintigraphy in lymphedema: An aid to microsurgery. J Nucl Med 27:1125, 1986.
93. Szuba A, Shin WS, Strauss HW, Rockson S: Lymphoscintigraphy in the evaluation of lymphedema. J Nucl Med 44:43, 2003.
94. Hadjis NS, Carr DH, Banks L, Pflug JJ: The role of CT in the diagnosis of primary lymphedema of the lower limb. AJR Am J Roentgenol 144:361, 1985.
95. Gamba JL, Silverman PM, Ling D, et al: Primary lower extremity lymphedema: CT diagnosis. Radiology 149:218, 1983.
96. Vaughan BF: CT of swollen legs. Clin Radiol 41:24, 1990.
97. Liu NF, Wang CG: The role of magnetic resonance imaging in the diagnosis of peripheral lymphatic disorders. Lymphology 31:319, 1998.
98. Gniadecka M: Localization of dermal edema in lipodermatosclerosis, lymphedema, and cardiac insufficiency: High-frequency ultrasound examination of intradermal echogenicity. J Am Acad Dermatol 35:37, 1996.
99. Rockson SG, Miller LT, Senie R, et al: American Cancer Society Lymphedema Workshop. Workgroup III: Diagnosis and management of lymphedema. Cancer 83:2882, 1998.
100. Morgan RG, Casley-Smith JR, Mason MR, Casley-Smith JR: Complex physical therapy for the lymphoedematous arm. J Hand Surg [Br] 17:437, 1992.
101. Foeldi M: Treatment of lymphedema. Lymphology 27:1, 1994.
102. Foeldi E, Foeldi M, Weissleder H: Conservative treatment of lymphedema of the limbs. Angiology 36:1711, 1985.
103. Kubik S: The role of the lateral upper arm bundle and the lymphatic watersheds in the formation of collateral pathways in lymphedema. Acta Biologica Academiae Scientiarum Hungaricae 31:191, 1980.
104. Schirger A, Peterson LFA: Lymphedema. In Jergens JL, Spittell JA, Fairbairn JF II (eds): Peripheral Vascular Diseases. Philadelphia, Saunders, 1980, p 823.
105. Zeissler RH, Rose GB, Nelson PA: Postmastectomy lymphoedema: Late results of treatment in 385 patients. Arch Phys Med Rehabil 53:159, 1972.
106. Swedborg I: Effects of treatment with an elastic sleeve and intermittent pneumatic compression in post-mastectomy patients with lymphoedema of the arm. Scand J Rehabil Med 16:35, 1984.
107. Bertelli G, Venturini M, Forno G, et al: An analysis of prognostic factors in response to conservative treatment of postmastectomy lymphedema. Surg Gynecol Obstet 175:455, 1992.
108. Ko DS, Lerner R, Klose G, Cosimi AB: Effective treatment of lymphedema of the extremities. Arch Surg 133:452, 1998.
109. Szuba A, Cooke JP, Yousuf S, Rockson SG: Decongestive lymphatic therapy for patients with cancer-related or primary lymphedema. Am J Med 109:296, 2000.
110. Badger CM, Peacock JL, Mortimer PS: A randomized, controlled, parallel-group clinical trial comparing multilayer bandaging followed by hosiery versus hosiery alone in the treatment of patients with lymphedema of the limb. Cancer 88:2832, 2000.
111. Zanolla R, Monzeglio C, Balzarini A, et al: Evaluation of the results of three different methods of postmastectomy lymphedema treatment. J Surg Oncol 26:210, 1984.
112. Compression for lymphoedema. Lancet (Editorial) 1:896, 1986.
113. Leduc O, Leduc A, Bourgeois P, Belgrado JP: The physical treatment of upper limb edema. Cancer 83:2835, 1998.
114. Brennan MJ, Miller LT: Overview of treatment options and review of the current role and use of compression garments, intermittent pumps, and exercise in the management of lymphedema. Cancer 83:2821, 1998.
115. Richmand DM, O'Donnell TF Jr, Zelikovski A: Sequential pneumatic compression for lymphedema: A controlled trial. Arch Surg 120:1116, 1985.
116. Kim-Sing C, Basco VE: Postmastectomy lymphedema treated with the Wright linear pump. Can J Surg 30:368, 1987.
117. Szuba A, Achalu R, Rockson SG: Decongestive lymphatic therapy for patients with breast carcinoma-associated lymphedema: A randomized, prospective study of a role for adjunctive intermittent pneumatic compression. Cancer 95:2260, 2002.
118. Piller NB, Thelander A: Treatment of chronic postmastectomy lymphedema with low level laser therapy: A 2.5 year follow-up. Lymphology 31:74, 1998.
119. Casley-Smith J, Casley-Smith J: Other physical therapy for lymphedema: Pumps, heating, etc. In Casley-Smith J, Casley-Smith J (eds): Lymphedema. Adelaide, Australia: Lymphedema Association of Australia, 1991, p 155.
120. Ogawa Y, Yoshizumi M, Kitagawa T, et al: Investigation of the mechanism of lymphocyte injection therapy in treatment of lymphedema with special emphasis on cell adhesion molecule (L-selectin). Lymphology 32:151, 1999.
121. Piller NB: Lymphoedema, macrophages and benzopyrones. Lymphology 13:109, 1980.
122. Casley-Smith JR, Morgan RG, Piller NB: Treatment of lymphedema of the arms and legs with 5,6-benzo-(alpha)-pyrone. N Engl J Med 329:1158, 1993.
123. Casley-Smith JR, Wang CT, Zi-hai C: Treatment of filarial lymphoedema and elephantiasis with 5,6-benzo-alpha-pyrone (coumarin). Brit Med J 307:1037, 1993.
124. Taylor HM, Rose KE, Twycross RG: A double-blind clinical trial of hydroxyethylrutosides in obstructive arm lymphoedema. Phlebology 8(suppl 1):22, 1993.
125. Mortimer PS, Badger C, Clarke I, et al: A double-blind, randomized parallel-group, placebo-controlled trial of o-(b-hydroxyethyl)-rutosides in chronic arm oedema resulting from breast cancer treatment. Phlebology 10:51, 1995.
126. Loprinzi CL, Kugler JW, Sloan JA, et al: Lack of effect of coumarin in women with lymphedema after treatment for breast cancer. N Engl J Med 340:346, 1999.
127. Fyfe NC, Rutt DL, Edwards JM, Kinmonth JB: Intralymphatic steroid therapy for lymphoedema: Preliminary studies. Lymphology 15:23, 1982.
128. Zelikovski A, Haddad M, Reiss R: Non-operative therapy combined with limited surgery in management of peripheral lymphedema. Lymphology 19:106, 1986.
129. Miller TA: Surgical approach to lymphedema of the arm after mastectomy. Am J Surg 148:152, 1984.
130. Savage RC: The surgical management of lymphedema. Surg Gynecol Obstet 160:283, 1984.
131. Medgyesi S: A successful operation for lymphoedema using myocutaneous flap as a "wick." Br J Plast Surg 36:64, 1983.
132. Hurst PA, Stewart G, Kinmonth JB, Browse NL: Long term results of the enteromesenteric bridge operation in the treatment of primary lymphoedema. Br J Surg 72:272, 1985.
133. Ho LCY, Lai MF, Kennedy PJ: Micro-lymphatic bypass in the treatment of obstructive lymphoedema of the arm: Case report of a new technique. Br J Plast Surg 36:350, 1983.
134. Fyfe NC, Wolfe JH, Kinmonth JB: "Die-back" in primary lymphedema-lymphographic and clinical correlations. Lymphology 15:66, 1982.
135. Campisi C, Boccardo F: Microsurgical techniques for lymphedema treatment: Derivative lymphatic-venous microsurgery. World J Surg 28:609, 2004.
136. Brorson H: Liposuction in arm lymphedema treatment. Scand J Surg 92:287, 2003.
137. Olofsson B, Jeltsch M, Eriksson U, et al: Current biology of VEGF-B and VEGF-C. Curr Opin Biotechnol 10:528, 1999.
138. Veikkola T, Karkkainen M, Claesson-Welsh L, et al: Regulation of angiogenesis via vascular endothelial growth factor receptors. Cancer Res 60:203, 2000.

139. Joukov V, Pajusola K, Kaipainen A, et al: A novel vascular endothelial growth factor, VEGF-C, is a ligand for the Flt4 (VEGFR-3) and KDR (VEGFR-2) receptor tyrosine kinases. EMBO J 15:1751, 1996.
140. Kaipainen A, Korhonen J, Mustonen T, et al: Expression of the fms-like tyrosine kinase 4 gene becomes restricted to lymphatic endothelium during development. Proc Natl Acad Sci U S A 92:3566, 1995.
141. Jeltsch M., Kaipainen A, Joukov V, et al: Hyperplasia of lymphatic vessels in VEGF-C transgenic mice. Science 276:1423, 1997.
142. Oh SJ, Jeltsch MM, Birkenhager R, et al: VEGF and VEGF-C: Specific induction of angiogenesis and lymphangiogenesis in the differentiated avian chorioallantoic membrane. Dev Biol 188:96, 1997.
143. Enholm B, Karpanen T, Jeltsch M, et al: Adenoviral expression of vascular endothelial growth factor-C induces lymphangiogenesis in the skin. Circ Res 88:623; 2001.
144. Karkkainen MJ, Petrova TV: Vascular endothelial growth factor receptors in the regulation of angiogenesis and lymphangiogenesis. Oncogene 19:5598, 2000.
145. Karkkainen MJ, Saaristo A, Jussila L, et al: A model for gene therapy of human hereditary lymphedema. Proc Natl Acad Sci U S A 98:12677, 2001.
146. Szuba A, Skobe M, Karkkainen MJ, et al: Therapeutic lymphangiogenesis with human recombinant VEGF-C. FASEB J 16:1985, 2002.
147. Klippel M, Trénaunay P: Du noevus variqueux osteo-hypertrophiques. Archives Générale Médicale (Paris) 185:641, 1900.
148. Baskerville PA, Ackroyd JS, Lea Thomas M, Browse NL: The Klippel-Trénaunay syndrome: Clinical, radiological and haemodynamic features and management. Br J Surg 72:232, 1985.
149. Baskerville PA, Ackroyd JS, Browse NL: The etiology of the Klippel-Trénaunay syndrome. Ann Surg 202:624, 1985.
150. Robertson DJ: Congenital arteriovenous fistulae of the extremities. Ann R Coll Surg Engl 18:73, 1956.
151. Suringa DW, Ackerman AB: Cutaneous lymphangiomas with dyschondroplasia (Maffucci's syndrome): A unique variant of an unusual syndrome. Arch Dermatol 101:472, 1970.
152. Ramani P, Shah A: Lymphangiomatosis: Histologic and immunohistochemical analysis of four cases. Am J Surg Pathol 17:329, 1993.
153. Sordillo PP, Chapman R, Hajdu SI, et al: Lymphangiosarcoma. Cancer 48:1674, 1981.
154. Stewart NJ, Pritchard DJ, Nascimento AG, Kang YK: Lymphangiosarcoma following mastectomy. Clin Orthop 135, 1995.
155. Alessi E, Sala F, Berti E: Angiosarcomas in lymphedematous limbs. Am J Dermatopathol 8:371, 1986.
156. Andersson HC, Parry DM, Mulvihill JJ: Lymphangiosarcoma in late-onset hereditary lymphedema: Case report and nosological implications. Am J Med Genet 56:72, 1995.
157. Jeffries GH, Chapman A, Sleisenger M: Low-fat diet in intestinal lymphangiectasis. N Engl J Med 270:761, 1964.
158. Ballinger AB, Farthing MJ: Octreotide in the treatment of intestinal lymphangiectasia. Eur J Gastroenterol Hepatol 10:699, 1998.
159. Kuroiwa G, Takayama T, Sato Y, et al: Primary intestinal lymphangiectasia successfully treated with octreotide. J Gastroenterol 36:129, 2001.

chapter 61

Vascular Infection

M. Burress Welborn
R. James Valentine

Vascular infection is a rare but serious problem associated with potentially disastrous complications. Considering the numerous episodes of bacteremia that humans experience in a lifetime, it is somewhat surprising that vascular infection is so uncommon in the general population. Resistance to infection is attributable to a number of teleologic mechanisms, many of which can be conveniently grouped into immune, architectural, and anatomic themes. The reticuloendothelial and immune systems rapidly clear organisms from the circulation, providing excellent first-line protection against blood-borne invasion. The continuous endothelial cell lining of the arterial tree represents an important barrier to organism invasion. The tough adventitial outer lining and the deep anatomical location of most arteries make external penetration unlikely. Many other resistance mechanisms are related to arterial wall function that are considered elsewhere in this text. Overall, resistance to vascular infection is comprehensive, redundant, and efficient.

The presence of arterial infection implies profound homeostatic failure. Risk factors include arterial injury, underlying arterial pathology, endothelial cell dysfunction, immune deficiency, and the presence of a foreign body such as prosthetic graft material. Prosthetic graft infections are far more common than primary arterial infections, and there are important differences in presentation, treatment, and outcome between the two. This chapter describes current concepts of vascular infection, considering primary arterial infections and prosthetic graft infec-tions separately. Primary venous infections are considered in a third section. The continuously evolving experience in all three areas promises better understanding of prevention and treatment of these difficult problems.

PRIMARY ARTERIAL INFECTIONS

The first published experience with primary arterial infection is generally credited to Koch,[1] who reported a patient with a ruptured superior mesenteric artery aneurysm in 1851. Arterial infections were not appreciated before this time because the basic tenets of bacteriology and infection had not been developed. Breakthroughs in human bacteriologic research by Pasteur and others in the mid-19th century set the stage for a basic understanding of the pathophysiology and classification of vascular infections.

Classification and Etiology Nearly all primary arterial infections result in the formation of aneurysms or pseudoaneurysms. Osler coined the term "mycotic aneurysm" in 1885 to describe infected aortic arch aneurysms containing "fresh fungal vegetation" in a patient who had concomitant aortic valve vegetations.[2] Although "mycotic" aneurysms apply only to the subset of individuals with infected aneurysms caused by septic emboli, the term has been loosely applied to include all infected aneurysms, regardless of etiology. This practice is confusing and prevents meaningful comparison of the numerous small series of infected aneurysms reported in the modern literature.

The most widely accepted classification of arterial infections was introduced by Wilson and colleagues[3] in 1978. Typical features are shown in Table 61-1. In keeping with

TABLE 61-1 CLASSIFICATION OF PRIMARY ARTERIAL INFECTIONS

	Mycotic Aneurysm	Infected Aneurysm	Microbial Arteritis	Traumatic Infected Aneurysm	Contiguous Arterial Infection
Status of preinfected artery	Normal	Preexisting aneurysm	Normal or atherosclerotic	Normal	Normal
Etiology	Endocarditis	Bacteremia	Bacteremia	Bacteremia	Direct spread
Sites of predilection	Visceral, intracranial, and peripheral arteries	Distal aorta	Aortoiliac segment, superficial femoral arteries	Femoral, carotid, and sites of injection	Aorta, superior mesenteric artery

Modified from Wilson SE, van Wagenen P, Passaro E Jr: Arterial infection. Curr Prob Surg 15:1, 1978.

the traditional definition introduced by Osler, the authors classified a *mycotic aneurysm* as one that occurred in an otherwise normal, nonaneurysmal artery as a result of septic emboli of endocardial origin. A pre-established aneurysm that became infected as a result of bacteremia is classified as an *infected aneurysm. Microbial arteritis* refers to infection of a normal or atherosclerotic (i.e., nonaneurysmal) artery that has become infected as a result of bacteremia. This most often results in rupture, with formation of a pseudoaneurysm. *Traumatic infected aneurysms* include infected aneurysms due to trauma or iatrogenic injury (e.g., complications of arteriography). *Contiguous arterial infection* is due to direct extension of an adjacent infection into the wall of the artery, such as infected aortitis associated with vertebral osteomyelitis. The specific classification based on etiology is acknowledged wherever appropriate in this chapter. However, for purposes of clarity and simplification, the generic term "infected aneurysm" is applied to include all arterial infections discussed later.

The etiology of infected aneurysms has changed in the past 150 years. In the preantibiotic era, 86% of patients with arterial infections had evidence of endocarditis.[4] Following widespread use of antibiotics, the incidence of infective endocarditis has relegated the true mycotic aneurysm to a rare entity. In 1984, Brown and associates[5] reported a collective series of infected aneurysms on the basis of a search of the English literature. The etiology could be determined in 75% of the 180 subjects, as shown in Table 61-2. The authors separated the reported experience into cases occurring before 1965 and those occurring since that time. The accuracy of the results suffers due to important differences in diagnosis and reporting frequency between the two periods. Nevertheless, this collective experience remains the largest comparative analysis of infected aneurysms to date. In the earlier part of the series, endocarditis was still the leading cause of infected aneurysms, but arterial trauma of all types became the leading cause after 1965. The authors attributed this etiologic shift to a substantial change in the pattern of antibiotic usage for the treatment of sepsis and trauma.[5] Other explanations include an increased prevalence of IV drug abuse and the widespread application of transarterial interventional procedures. The increase in interventional procedures was particularly notable after the pioneering work of Grunzig and others in the 1970s. The enthusiasm for endovascular technology seen in recent years suggests that arterial trauma may soon become an even more important cause of arterial infection.

TABLE 61-2 ETIOLOGY OF INFECTED ANEURYSMS BASED ON A COLLECTED SERIES OF 243 ANEURYSMS IN 180 PATIENTS

	Before 1965	After 1965	Total
Arterial trauma	4 (10%)	71 (51%)	75 (42%)
• Iatrogenic			
• Traumatic			
• IV drug abuse			
Endocarditis	15 (37%)	14 (10%)	29 (16%)
Local infection	3 (7%)	6 (4%)	9 (5%)
Bacteremia	—	9 (6%)	9 (5%)
Retroperitoneal abscess	2 (5%)	2 (1%)	4 (2%)
Gastrointestinal source	1 (2%)	3 (2%)	4 (2%)
Oropharynx	—	3 (2%)	3 (2%)
Pneumonia	1 (2%)	—	1 (<1%)
Carcinoma	—	1 (1%)	1 (<1%)
Unknown	15 (36%)	30 (22%)	45 (25%)
TOTAL	41	139	180

Modified from Brown SL, Busuttil RW, Baker JD, et al: Bacteriologic and surgical determinants of survival in patients with mycotic aneurysms. J Vasc Surg 1:541, 1984.

Pathogenesis of Infected Aneurysms The basic mechanisms leading to the formation of infected aneurysms have been studied most extensively in the abdominal aorta. Chronic, uninfected abdominal aortic aneurysms (AAAs) are thought to form as a result of both elastin and collagen degradation. Elastolytic matrix metalloproteinases (MMPs) play a central role, leading to initial aortic dilation.[6] However, it is collagen failure that eventually leads to gross enlargement and eventual rupture of the AAA.[7]

A number of important differences have been noted between infected and uninfected aneurysms of the abdominal aorta. In contrast to chronic AAAs, infected AAAs follow a more rapid course, have a predilection for the suprarenal aorta, and may be isolated to a small segment of an otherwise normal aorta. Recent studies have revealed a number of interesting findings related to etiology of infected AAAs. First, Buckmaster and associates[8] have shown that elastolytic activity is derived from host leukocytes, not from the infectious organisms. However, infectious organisms play a central role in collagen degradation. Many bacterial isolates produce collagenases,[6] and bacteria are capable of activating the collagenase promoter in macrophage-like cells.[9] Furthermore, various bacterial proteases activate MMP-1, -8, and -9.[6] Therefore, infected AAAs appear be the consequence of bacterial proteases causing rapid collagen breakdown in a previously normal aorta.[6] The collagenase activity may be relatively localized, leading to formation of a saccular AAA or pseudoaneurysm in an otherwise normal-appearing vessel. Collagenase activity may also be intensive, which may explain the rapid course associated with infected AAAs. The reason that infected AAAs are predisposed to the suprarenal aorta has not been elucidated.

Anatomic Location In their 1984 study, Brown and associates[5] documented 243 infected aneurysms in 180 patients in the following distribution: 38% femoral artery, 31% abdominal aorta, 8% superior mesenteric artery, 7% brachial artery, 6% iliac artery, 5% carotid artery, 3% ulnar/radial arteries, 1% hepatic artery, <1% subclavian artery, and <1% popliteal artery. Notably, there were no cases involving the suprarenal or thoracoabdominal aorta in this series. More recent reports have documented a much higher prevalence of infected aortic aneurysms involving the segments proximal to the renal arteries,[10-12] suggesting that the aorta is the most frequent site of involvement.

Bacteriology Approximately 75% of clinically infected aneurysms are associated with positive culture results.[5] There have been significant shifts in the bacteriologic patterns of infected aneurysms that have paralleled the changes in etiology. Before 1960, gram-positive organisms predominated, particularly *Streptococcus pneumoniae, Streptococcus pyogenes,* and *Staphylococcus aureus.*[3] More recent series have reported a higher prevalence of gram-negative organisms, paralleling the increasing number of arterial infections due to bacteremia, particularly *Salmonella* species.[11,13] Gram-negative sepsis in elderly patients is a frequent clinical scenario in these circumstances.[14] Apparently the bacteriologic pattern is continuing to evolve. At least two reports within the past 5 years have identified *S. pneumoniae* as an increasingly frequent cause of infected aortic aneurysms.[12,15] The prevalence of organisms associated with opportunistic infections such as fungus and *Mycobacteria* species may also be on the rise due to the increasing prevalence of chronic diseases associated with impaired immunity.

Salmonella infections deserve special emphasis. For uncertain reasons, *Salmonella* organisms tend to infect the abdominal aorta. Up to 36% of all infected aneurysms of the aorta are due to *Salmonella* species; conversely, 65% of *Salmonella* vascular infections are localized to the aorta.[16] Humans become infected by ingestion of contaminated food or water. Of the patients who develop *Salmonella* gastroenteritis, a small proportion develop bacteremia that may result in extraintestinal seeding and infection. The interval between the onset of gastrointestinal (GI) symptoms and development of aortic infection may be several weeks.[16] *Salmonella* aortitis is an extremely morbid condition associated with mortality rates of 50% and a high rate of reinfection after revascularization.[16] Diagnosis can be difficult because the signs and symptoms are nonspecific: More than one half of patients have ruptured aneurysms before the diagnosis is made.[16] Common isolates from aortic wall specimens have included *Salmonella choleraesuis, Salmonella typhimurium,* and *Salmonella enteritides.*

Infected Aortic Aneurysms

The definition of aortic aneurysm infection has been confounded by the fact that 10% to 15% of patients with uninfected, chronic AAA have positive culture results from intraluminal thrombus removed at the time of aneurysm repair. Fortunately, positive culture results are not associated with an increased risk of late graft infection.[17,18] However, this underscores the fact that the definition of infected AAA relies on other criteria such as operative findings (inflammation and purulence); clinical symptoms (fever, pain, leukocytosis); aneurysm architecture (saccular or localized); and positive aneurysm wall culture.[11]

Modern series of infected aortic aneurysms reveal that the majority of affected patients have comorbid conditions associated with immunosuppression such as diabetes, chronic renal failure, chronic steroid use, human immunodeficiency virus, or cancer.[11,19] Nearly 50% of patients have had a recent documented infection such as pneumonia or urinary tract infection,[11] while several reports have documented direct extension of vertebral osteomyelitis.[12,20,21]

Features Infected aneurysms of the aorta may involve any segment from the ascending arch to the distal infrarenal area. In a series of 43 patients with infected aortic aneurysms treated at the Mayo Clinic over a 25-year period, Oderich and colleagues[11] documented a wide distribution of lesions. No segment of the aorta was spared. As indicated in Figure 61-1, 40% of infected aneurysms were localized to the infrarenal aorta, while the remaining lesions were almost evenly distributed in the juxta/-pararenal, paravisceral, thoracoabdominal, and descending thoracic segments. A similar distribution has been observed by others.[12,22]

The majority of aortic infections can be classified as bacterial aortitis. Most lesions are saccular and well localized in an otherwise normal-appearing aorta (Fig. 61-2). This appearance is highly suggestive of a ruptured aortic pseudoaneurysm, which is pathognomonic for aortic infection. In a minority of cases, infection of a pre-existing aortic aneurysm may make diagnosis difficult. In these circumstances, suspicion of infection is completely reliant on clinical information.

Diagnosis The majority of patients with infected aortic aneurysms are symptomatic. In the series by Oderich and colleagues,[11] 93% of patients had symptoms, the most common of which were fever, back pain, and leukocytosis (Table 61-3). Blood cultures are positive in approximately 75% of cases.[11] The degree of symptomatology

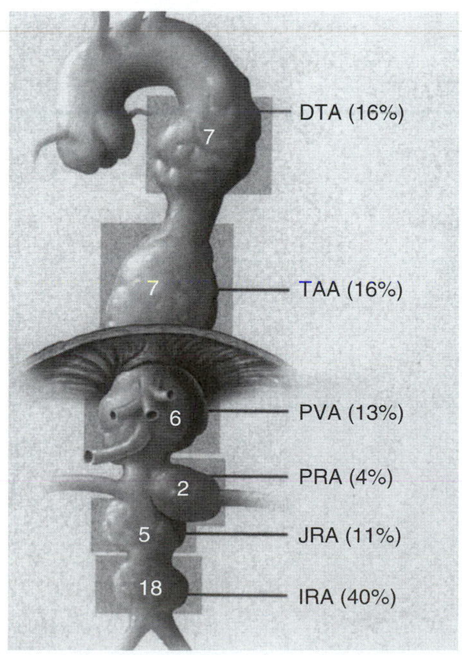

FIGURE 61-1. Distribution of infected aortic aneurysms in a series of 43 patients treated at the Mayo Clinic. (From Oderich GS, Panneton JM, Bower TC, et al: Infected aortic aneurysms: Aggressive presentation, complicated early outcome, but durable results. J Vasc Surg 34:900, 2001, with permission from the Society for Vascular Surgery and the American Association for Vascular Surgery.)

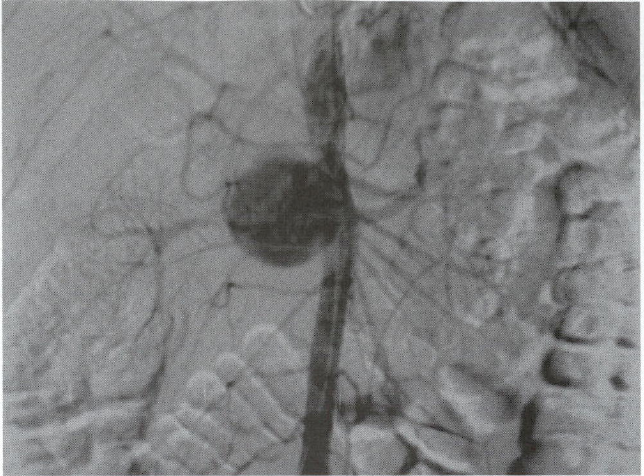

FIGURE 61-2. Arteriogram of an infected aneurysm in the suprarenal abdominal aorta. Note the saccular shape and normal appearance of the aorta above and below the lesion. (From Fillmore AJ, Valentine RJ: Surgical mortality in patients with infected aortic aneurysms. J Am Coll Surg 196:435, 2003, with permission from the American College of Surgeons.)

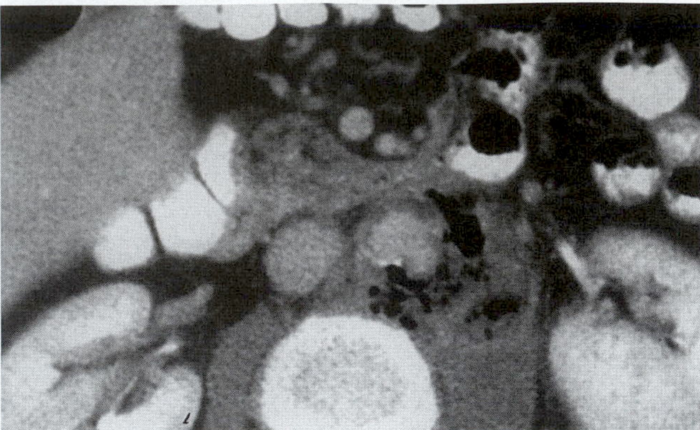

FIGURE 61-3. Enhanced CT scan demonstrating gas bubbles and periaortic fat stranding suggestive of an infected aortic aneurysm. (From Oderich GS, Panneton JM, Bower TC, et al: Infected aortic aneurysms: Aggressive presentation, complicated early outcome, but durable results. J Vasc Surg 34:900, 2001, with permission from the Society for Vascular Surgery and the American Association for Vascular Surgery.)

may be an important indicator of prognosis. Recent data suggest that the systemic inflammatory response syndrome (SIRS), a marker for sepsis, is associated with increased morbidity and mortality in patients with infected aortic aneurysms.[12,23] Diagnostic criteria for SIRS include the presence of two or more of the following: body temperature higher than 38°C or lower than 36°C; heart rate higher than 90 beats/min; respiratory rate greater than 20 breaths/min or $PaCO_2$ less than 32 torr; and WBC greater than 12,000 cells/mm^3, less than 4000 cells/mm^3, or 10% immature (band) forms.[23]

Diagnosis of infected aortic aneurysms relies on a number of imaging techniques. The presence of a saccular aneurysm in a patient with typical symptoms is pathognomonic, and the diagnosis is confirmed if blood cultures are positive. Gas bubbles and periaortic fat stranding on MRI or enhanced CT scans are also diagnostic for infection (Fig. 61-3) but are not universally present. More subtle signs include periaortic stranding, proximity to abnormal fluid collections or nearby infections such as vertebral osteomyelitis, and rapid aneurysm expansion over several days. Indium-111-labeled white blood cell scans have been used in some patients, but the 80% sensitivity and specificity of this test suggest that it has limited usefulness. Angiography has been recommended to localize the infection and to plan appropriate operative treatment in all patients. As an alternative, newer imaging techniques such as CT angiography can be used to assess periaortic tissues, localize the infectious process, and evaluate vascular anatomy. This technique has the advantage of being minimally invasive compared to standard angiography, and it essentially combines two tests into one.

TABLE 61-3 CLINICAL PRESENTATION AND LABORATORY FINDINGS IN 43 PATIENTS TREATED AT THE MAYO CLINIC FOR INFECTED AORTIC ANEURYSMS

	No. Patients (%)
Symptomatic	40 (93)
Fever	33 (77)
Pain (abdominal or back)	28 (65)
Leukocyte count > 12,000/mm^3	23 (54)
Chills	22 (51)
Sweats	12 (28)
Enlarging aneurysm	12 (28)
Nausea/vomiting or diarrhea	10 (25)
Pulsatile mass	7 (16)
Hemodynamic instability	3 (7)

Modified from Oderich GS, Panneton JM, Bower TC, et al: Infected aortic aneurysms: Aggressive presentation, complicated early outcome, but durable results. J Vasc Surg 34:900, 2001.

Clinical Course The natural history of infected aortic aneurysms depends on the classification. The more common bacterial aortitis is associated with inexorable expansion of the pseudoaneurysm and eventual rupture. Rapid expansion over 2 to 3 days has been documented; in more than half of cases, the pseudoaneurysm has already ruptured at the time of diagnosis. Contiguous and traumatic infections of the aorta, also associated with pseudoaneurysms, have a similar natural history. Urgent repair of these lesions is always indicated. Infections involving preexisting aortic aneurysms are relatively rare, and the natural history is unknown. However, due to the potential for rapid expansion and rupture, as well as recurrent bacteremia, urgent repair is indicated for these lesions as well. Patients with true mycotic aneurysms have two problems: the aortic aneurysm and the primary cardiac valvular lesion. Treatment may require extensive preoperative stabilization before the aneurysm is repaired.

Treatment Treatment of infected aortic aneurysms is surgical. The urgent nature of infected aortic aneurysms cannot be overstated due to the potential for rupture with exsanguination. Once the diagnosis is confirmed with appropriate imaging tests, preoperative preparation should be completed as rapidly as possible—usually within 2 or 3 hours. Patients with hemodynamic instability should be transported immediately to the operating room. Stable patients should be admitted to an ICU for rapid fluid repletion, institution of broad-spectrum IV antibiotics, and placement of appropriate monitoring devices. Blood should be typed and crossmatched, and at least four units of packed RBCs should be available in the operating room.

Surgical treatment of infected aortic aneurysms depends on the location and extent of the infection. The most common operation is ligation and débridement of the infected arterial segment, with revascularization of the lower extremities using grafts brought through uninfected tissues remote from the infected site ("extra-anatomic bypass").[22,24] For example, infected aneurysms of the infrarenal aorta can be treated with ligation of the abdominal aorta distal to the renal arteries and revascularization of the lower extremities using axillofemoral bypass grafts. However, proximal aortic aneurysms involving the renal arteries, visceral aorta, or descending thoracic aorta are much more complicated. These aortic segments require direct revascularization to preserve blood flow to the kidneys, intra-abdominal organs, and the spinal cord. In these cases, aortic débridement with direct revascularization of the affected segment within the infected bed ("in situ reconstruction") is appropriate. In situ reconstruction has been performed with prosthetic graft, but the reinfection rate of up to 20% makes this option unattractive except in patients who are unstable at the time of operation.[25,26]

Prolonged administration of antibiotics is generally recommended in these patients.[27] As an alternative, a rifampin-bonded, gelatin-impregnated Dacron graft has been recommended in patients with arterial infections caused by susceptible organisms such as *S. aureus*[28]; however, these grafts are not effective against methicillin-resistant *S. aureus* or *E. coli* infections.[29] Additional alternatives include human allografts and autogenous vein grafts. In 1993 Kieffer and colleagues[30] reported their experience with in situ replacement using preserved allografts in 43 patients with infected aortic aneurysms. During a mean follow-up of 14 months, there was only one recurrent infection. However, 26% of surviving patients had pathologic changes in the allografts, and one third of these individuals required repeat operations. The experience with autogenous superficial femoral-popliteal vein (SFPV) grafts has been more encouraging. Several small series attest to the negligible reinfection rates and excellent durability associated with in situ SFPV reconstruction.[12,31] The early enthusiasm for this option is buoyed by the excellent experience using the SFPV to replace infected prosthetic grafts of the aorta (see later).

Infected Femoral Artery Aneurysms

The superficial location of the femoral artery makes it an excellent choice for access to the central arterial circulation, but it also provides a convenient route of access for drug abusers. Femoral artery infections tend to be extensive and are often associated with virulent organisms or those that are resistant to standard antibiotics. Proper treatment requires radical débridement and careful consideration of the options for revascularization. Errors in surgical decision often result in recurrent femoral artery infections, with disastrous complications.

Femoral Artery Infections Associated with Invasive Procedures Compared with alternative approaches involving direct puncture of the axillary artery or the abdominal aorta, the transfemoral approach is associated with the lowest risk of complications. Modern results indicate that the overall arterial complication rate of transfemoral catheterizations is less than 1%; the risk of femoral artery infection is exceedingly rare.[32,33] However, the increasing popularity of transcatheter techniques suggests that the absolute number of patients with catheter-related complications is likely to rise.

In an effort to reduce the incidence of pseudoaneurysms, many interventionalists use percutaneous closure devices to mechanically seal the arterial puncture site. Compared with manual compression, these devices have resulted in earlier mobilization and discharge of patients after arterial catheterization. However, these devices have been associated with a slightly higher risk of femoral artery infection. Recent series estimate the overall risk to be 0.3% to 0.7% of patients who receive the devices.[34,35] Use of a percutaneous closure device is not the only risk factor for femoral artery infection: Hollis and colleagues[34] also noted a higher prevalence of diabetes mellitus and obesity in their patients who developed femoral artery infections after percutaneous catheterization.

Primary femoral artery infections present as pseudoaneurysms. Common findings include pain at the puncture site, fever with chills, and a pulsatile groin mass. The onset of symptoms may be delayed up to several weeks after the original puncture. Gram-positive organisms predominate, especially *S. aureus*, but gram-negative bacteria are common isolates. Treatment involves institution of broad-spectrum antibiotics, débridement of the infected arterial segment, removal of all closure device material, and excision of grossly infected adjacent tissues. Direct revascularization with autogenous saphenous vein or SFPV has been associated with a high risk of reinfection and vein graft blowout.[34] Simple ligation of the common femoral artery may be preferable if the femoral bifurcation is uninvolved.[36] If revascularization is necessary, the bypass should be routed through extra-anatomic tissues to avoid infected areas. A transobturator bypass is ideally suited to this situation.[37]

Femoral Artery Infections in Intravenous Drug Abusers These complex lesions are extremely difficult to treat. In addition to the acute infection-related problems, many affected patients have serious comorbidities such as seropositivity for HIV and hepatitis B. These individuals are notoriously unreliable due to psychiatric disorders associated with chronic addiction, and most do not return for follow-up after hospital discharge. Therefore most authorities recommend conservative treatment approaches that emphasize avoidance of reinfection and late complications.

Approximately three fourths of all admissions for accidental IV drug injections involve the lower extremity, and the femoral artery is the most common site of involvement.[38] Most patients present with a painful, pulsatile groin mass, often associated with overlying cellulitis. The most commonly cultured organism is *S. aureus*. Appropriate treatment involves ligation of the affected arterial segment to reduce the risk of hemorrhage and débridement of all grossly contaminated tissue to remove the septic focus. The advisability of subsequent revascularization remains controversial.

Many authors recommend ligation without revascularization, even if this leads to amputation. Repeated use of superficial veins for drug injection eliminates available autogenous conduits, necessitating the use of prosthetic material in many cases. The incidence of reinfection is extremely high in these circumstances, risking graft disruption and life-threatening hemorrhage.

Avoidance of revascularization rarely leads to amputation. Earlier reports documented an 11% amputation rate when one artery was ligated and a 33% amputation rate after triple-vessel ligation.[39] More recent reports suggest that the incidence of amputation is much lower. Ting and colleagues[40] performed routine ligation in 34 infected femoral pseudoaneurysms, including 24 that involved the femoral bifurcation. The mean postoperative ankle-brachial index was .43 after triple ligation and .52 with single-vessel ligation. Although 88% of patients had some degree of intermittent claudication after discharge, there were no instances of delayed limb loss. Cheng and colleagues[41] reported a similar rate of claudication after single- or triple-vessel ligation, but one patient (5%) required above-knee amputation.

The consensus of modern opinion is that infected femoral aneurysms in drug addicts are best treated with ligation alone. Most patients will suffer some degree of claudication, but the risk of early and late amputation is low. Immediate revascularization should be limited to cases in which no Doppler signal is detected at the ankle after femoral artery ligation.[42] In the vast majority, staged revascularization should be considered in patients with limiting claudication after the infection has been completely cleared. The known propensity for prosthetic graft infection from remote injection site suggests that autogenous tissue is preferable in these circumstances. In the absence of a usable saphenous vein, the superficial femoral-popliteal vein represents an excellent alternative.

Infected Aneurysms of the Superior Mesenteric Artery

The superior mesenteric artery (SMA) is the third most common site of visceral aneurysms from all causes, but it is the most common site for infected aneurysms in the splanchnic circulation.[43,44] Original studies from more than 20 years ago reported that approximately 60% of SMA aneurysms had an infectious etiology,[45] but this proportion appears to be decreasing. More recent series have reported an infectious etiology in 5% to 33% of reported cases.[43,44,46] Infected SMA aneurysms usually occur secondary to subacute bacterial endocarditis, and the most commonly isolated organism is nonhemolytic *Streptococcus*.[43,47]

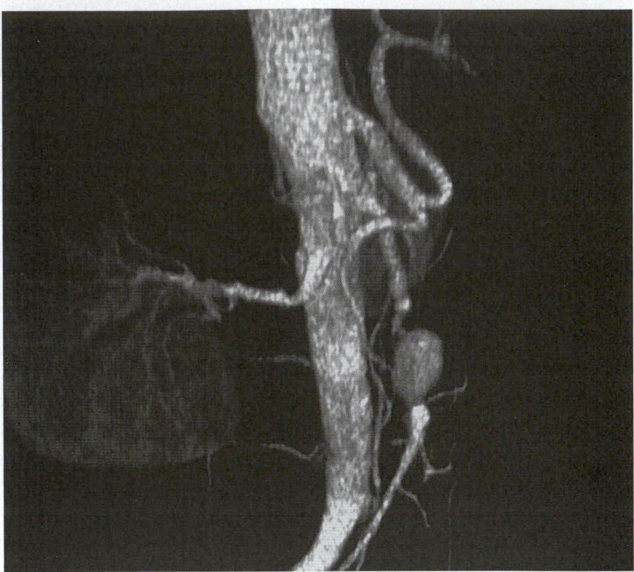

FIGURE 61-4. Computerized tomographic arteriogram demonstrating an infected superior mesenteric aneurysm in a 32-year-old female with endocarditis.

Most infected SMA aneurysms occur in patients younger than 50 years; men and women are equally affected.[43,45] Only 10% of patients are completely asymptomatic.[43] Some degree of abdominal discomfort is present in two thirds, and up to half have a tender, mobile, pulsatile mass.[45] Fever, nausea, vomiting, GI hemorrhage, and jaundice may also be present.

SMA aneurysms tend to occur within 5 cm of the SMA origin, but any segment may be affected. Aneurysms may be suspected when vascular calcifications are seen on plain radiographs of the abdomen. Diagnosis should be confirmed with appropriate imaging studies that also localize the extent of the aneurysm, such as standard mesenteric angiography or CT angiography (Fig. 61-4). Most infected SMA aneurysms are single, with variable involvement of visceral branches.

The natural history of infected SMA aneurysms is one of progression and eventual rupture; in fact, rupture has occurred at the time of presentation in 38% to 50% of patients.[43] The reported mortality rate after rupture approaches 30%.[46] Treatment includes transabdominal exploration and ligation of the arterial segments proximal and distal to the aneurysm. Complete excision is hazardous due to the proximity of the superior mesenteric vein and pancreas; therefore débridement should be limited to exposed portions of the aneurysm wall and to the aneurysm sac contents. In the vast majority of cases, extensive mesenteric collateralization preserves bowel viability after SMA ligation. Therefore ligation with resection of short segments of nonviable intestine is almost always appropriate. Direct revascularization is necessary in approximately 15% of cases. Bypass should be performed with autogenous tissue; the superficial femoral-popliteal vein is an excellent alternative, with superior patency compared with the saphenous vein.[48]

Infected Carotid Artery Aneurysms

Infected aneurysms are rare in the extracranial carotid circulation. In a series of 67 carotid artery aneurysms treated over a 35-year period at the Texas Heart Institute, only one was infected.[49] Most patients present with fever and a tender, pulsatile neck mass. Medial deviation of the pseudoaneurysm may lead to clinical findings suggestive of a parapharyngeal mass. Before the antibiotic era, most carotid artery infections were the consequence of direct spread from pharyngeal infections. Most lesions are currently due to septicemia from bacterial endocarditis.

Gram-positive organisms, especially *S. aureus* and *S. pyogenes*, are common isolates from infected carotid aneurysms, but *Salmonella* infections have also been reported.[50,51] Treatment involves ligation of all infected segments, even if this requires ligation of the internal and external carotid branches. Due to the potential for graft disruption and exsanguinating hemorrhage, revascularization is rarely indicated. To prevent propagation of the internal carotid thrombus into the middle cerebral artery circulation, systemic anticoagulation with warfarin is recommended. Anticoagulation should theoretically be continued until the thrombus becomes stable, a period not longer than 6 weeks. Although most patients can be expected to tolerate internal carotid ligation without sequelae, temporary occlusion with a balloon catheter should be performed in the preoperative period. Patients who develop neurologic deficits during balloon occlusion should be considered for prophylactic extracranial-intracranial bypass through remote, uninfected tissues. As an alternative, some patients may benefit from hypertensive therapy combined with hypervolemia and hemodilution.[51]

Other Infected Aneurysms

Primary arterial infections of the upper extremity are rare and generally the consequence of arterial trauma. Infected aneurysms of the axillary, brachial, radial, and ulnar arteries have been reported most frequently in IV drug abusers, but these lesions are also seen after percutaneous catheterization for diagnostic procedures. Infected radial artery aneurysms are frequently associated with indwelling catheters used for arterial monitoring. The most common isolates are gram-positive organisms, usually *S. aureus*. Patients may present with a tender mass and overlying cellulitis, but digital embolization has been the first manifestation in many cases. Treatment involves ligation of the arteries proximal and distal to the aneurysm, followed by excision of infected tissues. Following excision, single involvement of the radial or ulnar artery does not usually require revascularization due to adequate collateral flow in the hand. However, revascularization may be required in rare cases of incomplete hand circulation. More proximal arteries should be revascularized using autogenous tissue such as saphenous veins.

Aside from femoral artery aneurysms, infected aneurysms of the lower extremity are exceedingly rare. The vast majority of infected popliteal artery aneurysms are a consequence of septic embolization from infective endocarditis.[52] Mycotic aneurysms of the tibioperoneal trunk and tibial vessels have also been reported. Most infections involve gram-positive organisms such as *Streptococcus*, but *Salmonella* species have been recovered in a significant number of recently reported cases. The most common presentation is rupture, although thrombosis with foot ischemia has also been described. Treatment involves excision of the infected arterial segment and revascularization using autogenous bypass grafts.

PROSTHETIC GRAFT INFECTIONS

Development of a prosthetic graft infection remains a daunting complication. Despite improvements in diagnosis and management, modern morbidity and mortality rates remain prohibitively high. Even after successful treatment, the recovery from operative therapy is often prolonged and many patients require extensive rehabilitation. Clinical diagnosis remains challenging, as many graft infections follow an insidious course. In fact, most patients present with complications of latent graft infections such as graft occlusions or pseudoaneurysms months to years after implantation. Despite the improvements in imaging modalities, radiologic diagnosis remains exceedingly difficult. A high index of suspicion is required to diagnose graft infections before otherwise inevitable catastrophic complications. Once the diagnosis is made, careful operative planning is required to minimize the risk of loss of life and limb and to assure that recurrent infection does not occur. The advent of new endovascular approaches to the management of arterial disease has not eliminated the problem of graft infections; rather, these devices have created a new set of diagnostic and management challenges for surgeons and internists alike.

Risk Factors and Pathogenesis

The pathogenesis of graft infections is multifactorial and partly related to the site of implantation. Contamination before implantation due to failed sterilization techniques or breaks in packaging is thought to occur infrequently. Likewise, gross breaks in sterile technique are rare. Most graft infections occur as a result of unrecognized bacterial contamination at the time of implantation. Exposure of the graft material to surrounding skin is a likely source, as viable bacteria remain in the dermis of the skin despite antiseptic preparation.[53] Graft contamination can also occur from remote infections such as cellulitis or pyelonephritis. Wet gangrene of a toe can increase the risk of infection in a prosthetic femoropopliteal bypass graft. Similarly, concurrent intra-abdominal procedures such as cholecystectomy or appendectomy can expose an aortic graft to the patient's enteric flora, thereby increasing the risk of graft infection.

A number of specific risk factors have been associated with aortic graft infections. Colonic ischemia following the repair of ruptured and nonruptured aortic aneurysms is associated with a high risk of graft infection due either to direct contamination or to hematogenous seeding from bacterial translocation.[54] It is well recognized that graft infections are more common after emergency repair of ruptured aortic aneurysms compared with elective operations.[55] The emergent nature of ruptured AAA repair likely leads to inadvertent breaks in sterile techniques as the surgical team rushes to gain vascular control. In addition, patients presenting with either acute occlusion of the aorta or rupture of an aortic aneurysm are at high risk to develop a postoperative systemic inflammatory response syndrome (SIRS). This SIRS response leads to an initial production of a proinflammatory cytokine response followed by a compensatory anti-inflammatory cytokine response. This response renders the patient immunocompromised and at risk for nosocomial infections. Theoretically, this immunocompromised state may contribute to the increased risk of graft infection by hematogenous seeding during episodes of bacteremia.

Aortic grafts are uniquely prone to primary bacterial colonization at the time of aortic aneurysm repair. As noted earlier, many studies have demonstrated that the mural thrombus found in aneurysms is frequently colonized with bacteria. Macbeth and colleagues[56] found that up to 43% of arterial walls were culture positive for bacteria at the time of surgery. In this series, all of the aortic graft infections (0.9%) occurred exclusively in patients with positive aortic wall cultures. The most common isolate was *Staphylococcus epidermidis* (71%) followed by *Streptococcus* species (13%) and other isolates (16%).[56] Similarly, Buckels and colleagues[57] in 1985 found that graft infection occurred more frequently in patients with positive cultures of aortic contents compared with those with negative cultures. More contemporary studies have failed to confirm an absolute association between positive aortic cultures and subsequent graft infections. Farkas and colleagues[18] reported positive cultures in 37% of 500 aortic aneurysms. However, only one patient with a positive culture developed a graft infection. In contrast, 6 of 296 patients with negative cultures developed aortic graft infections during follow-up.[18] On the basis of these observations, it is clear that colonization of the mural thrombus by bacteria plays, at most, a minor role in the pathogenesis of aortic graft infection. The results from more contemporary experiences may be due to the consistent use of perioperative antibiotic therapy.

Local and regional factors may also play a role in the development of graft infections. The use of groin incisions (e.g., aortobifemoral bypass) can more than double the risk of graft infection compared with aortic grafts that remain completely intra-abdominal (e.g., aortobiiliac bypass or aortic tube graft repairs). This may be related to the local environment of the groin, an area associated with one of the highest concentrations of *Staphylococcus* species found on the body.[53] In addition, dissection in the groin disrupts abundant femoral lymphatics, leading to risk of lymph leak, groin wound breakdown, and direct graft contamination. Furthermore, the lymphatic system transports bacteria from distal sites of infection to the groin lymph nodes; opening these channels exposes the graft to potential contamination. Translocated bacteria have been demonstrated in animals and humans. In patients presenting with complex foot infections, positive lymphatic cultures at the time of amputation have been demonstrated in up to 20% of patients.[58] Cultures of groin lymph nodes at the time of vascular reconstruction have revealed bacteria in 11%. However, these cultures do not correlate with subsequent groin wound infections.[59]

Recurrent operations in the same location, particularly the groin, represent a significant risk for graft infection. Repeated catheter access also increases the overall risk. Aortofemoral bypass grafts placed for treatment of occlusive disease, while durable, do thrombose and are frequently revised by either lysis or thrombectomy. Procedures used to reestablish flow through occluded grafts, whether surgical or endovascular, expose the graft to potential contamination. It is common to find that patients with late graft infections have had multiple procedures to reestablish arterial flow through such grafts.

Graft material also plays a role in the pathogenesis of graft infections. The immune system responds to the foreign body by walling off the offending agent. The initial response is an acute inflammation, with influx of neutrophils followed by macrophages. These inflammatory cells produce cytokines and release proteases in an attempt to eliminate the foreign body. This initial response has a negative effect on bacterial survival; however, if the inoculum is large, some bacteria may survive. The graft interstices may offer a safe haven for bacteria and allow them to survive the initial inflammatory phase. After the acute inflammatory response, a reparative phase begins. This stage is characterized by fibroblasts depositing collagen in response to locally secreted cytokines. A resulting connective tissue barrier shields bacterium from detection and obliteration by immune-competent cells. This results in a closed space for the bacteria to thrive and grow on exudative proteins existing in an acidic and ischemic environment. In the absence of infection, the reparative phase culminates in tissue ingrowth and incorporation of the graft. However, if bacterial colonization is present, the graft fails to incorporate and chronic inflammation continues. Failure to incorporate may be due to fibroblast inhibition by the bacterial components found in the perigraft fluid.[60] This results in the failure to obliterate the closed space around the graft and failure of incorporation. The bacteria are left to thrive in this closed space, eventually becoming an abscess. This can manifest as perigraft fluid that may express through incisions with sinus tract formation. In addition, the artery may be degraded at suture lines, resulting in pseudoaneurysm formation.

Clearly, multiple factors play a role in the establishment of graft infections following the vascular reconstructions. Despite this, the incidence of graft infection remains low, at less than 5% for all reconstructions. Vascular graft infections can be categorized into two general groups: aortic graft infections and graft infections following infrainguinal arterial reconstruction. These two broad groups can be further subdivided into prosthetic and autogenous graft infections. Virtually all graft infections following aortic reconstructions are prosthetic graft infections, but infection following infrainguinal reconstructions can occur in both autogenous and synthetic grafts. The anatomic configuration of the graft and the material that comprises the graft alter both the diagnostic and therapeutic modalities. Diagnosis and management of aortic and infrainguinal graft infections are considered separately in the following sections.

Aortic Graft Infection

Over the past two decades, refinements in the diagnosis and operative management of aortic graft infections have resulted in improved mortality and morbidity. Mortality during the early experience of aortic graft infection approached 50%, and limb loss rates were as high as 75%. With refinement in technique, the respective mortality and limb loss rates have decreased to 20% or less in many series.[61]

Incidence

The exact incidence of graft infection following aortic reconstruction is not precisely known because most series are retrospective and suffer from lack of inclusive follow-up. The best estimates suggest that the incidence of graft infection following aortic reconstructions ranges from 1% to 5%.[62,63] More contemporary data can be abstracted from the UK Small Aneurysm Trial, a randomized study of AAA repair in patients with small aneurysms. Although this study did not directly report the incidence of aortic graft infection, a number of graft-related complications were documented. Three patients in the UK Small Aneurysm Trial had late aortic rupture following AAA repair, and four patients died following the development of aortoenteric fistula. Most of these complications can be assumed to represent complications from aortic graft infection and represent 2% of the total patients.[64] Although the true incidence of aortic graft infection remains inadequately described, most authorities agree the incidence is quite low and certainly less than 2% in the contemporary experience.

Classification

To better understand the pathogenesis and natural history of graft infections, classification systems have been developed. Wound complications following vascular reconstruction were first classified by Szilagyi and colleagues[65] in 1972. The authors characterized wound complications following prosthetic graft placement in terms of anatomical involvement. *Grade I* lesions involved only the dermis. *Grade II* lesions extended into the subcutaneous tissue without involvement of the graft, while *grade III* lesions involved the graft by direct extension.[65] Grade III lesions can be considered technical problems associated with wound closure. Certainly, local factors such as ischemic tissue play a significant role in wound infections, but they may be avoidable. This grading scheme is important only for early graft infections, which comprise less than 1% of all graft infections.[66] It does not take into account graft infections that present during late follow-up after aortic reconstruction. This grading scheme is more relevant to infections that follow infrainguinal arterial reconstructions, which result most frequently from complications of wound infections.

More relevant to the understanding of aortic graft infection is the scheme developed by Bandyk, who categorized aortic graft infections in terms of the time of presentation after graft implantation.[66] This classification scheme offers better insight into the origin of graft infections and is a better predictor of the type of bacteria that is found infecting the graft. Bandyk defined an *early* graft infection as one that occurred less than 4 months after implantation, while *late* graft infections manifested after 4 months. Graft infections are subcategorized in terms of presentation: perigraft infection, graft-enteric erosion, and graft-enteric fistula (Table 61-4). Most early perigraft infections represent the sequela of Szilagyi grade III wound infection (i.e., extension of local wound infections to involve the graft). Remote sites of infection (e.g., wet gangrene) or immunosuppression play a minor role in early graft infections.[66] The diagnosis of these early perigraft infections is usually obvious. Most patients present with purulent drainage from the wound, signs of sepsis with bacteremia, pseudoaneurysm formation, or anastomotic disruption with hemorrhage. These infections can be expected to contain any one of various organisms including gram-positive and gram-negative organisms. Early infections are manifest almost exclusively in wounds located at or below the femoral level. In contrast, late perigraft infections tend to occur months to years following implantation. Most will present more than 1 year following implantation, and the majority result from *S. epidermidis* infection with biofilm production.

TABLE 61-4 CLASSIFICATION OF AORTIC GRAFT INFECTIONS BY TIME AND TYPE OF PRESENTATION

Clinical Presentation	Time Interval After Implantation	Pathogens
Perigraft infection	Early*	*Staphylococcus aureus* *Streptococcus* *Escherichia coli* *Klebsiella* *Pseudomonas*
	Late†	*Staphylococcus epidermidis*
Graft enteric erosion	Late	*E. coli* *Enterococcus* *Bacteroides*
Graft enteric fistula	Early	*E. coli* *S. aureus*
	Late	*E. coli* *Klebsiella* *S. epidermidis*

*Early graft infection is defined as infection within 4 mo of implantation.
†Infection occurring more than 4 mo after implantation.
Modified from Bandyk DF: Aortic graft infection. Semin Vasc Surg 3:122, 1990.

Bandyk further subdivided graft enteric fistulas into graft enteric erosions and graft enteric fistulas. Graft enteric *erosions* appear late and are thought to result from erosion of the graft into a contiguous loop of bowel by mechanical forces. Most graft enteric erosions occur in the body of the graft, but some may extend to involve the anastomosis. Bacterial cultures from these graft infections will yield predominantly gram-negative pathogens. Graft enteric erosions are attributed to inadequate retroperitoneal closure over the prosthetic graft at the time of aortic reconstruction. However, graft enteric erosions may be a manifestation of unrecognized perigraft infection. The infective process involves the overlying retroperitoneum with extension to the bowel and eventual graft enteric erosion. Mechanical forces and inadequate coverage of the graft likely contribute, but in our opinion, most erosions are the result of latent perigraft infections.

Unlike graft enteric erosions, graft enteric *fistulas* are the result of a perigraft infection. These fistulas rarely occur in the early postoperative period. Perigraft infection leads to anastomotic breakdown and pseudoaneurysm formation. The pseudoaneurysm then erodes into the overlying bowel, leading to fistula formation. Like erosions, culture of graft enteric fistulas yields predominantly gram-negative enteric pathogens.

These classification systems are not all-encompassing. All aortic graft infections will not fall into a single category, but such systems serve as a useful guide and allow one to anticipate the pathogens likely to be encountered.

Etiology

Most aortic graft infections are thought to occur by direct contamination or extension of adjacent infections. No good evidence exists confirming that bacteremia contributes to aortic graft infection in humans. However, there is ample evidence from animal studies that bacteremia can result in prosthetic graft infections.[67,68] Antibiotic therapy during bacteremia in dog models prevents prosthetic graft infections.[68] All of these models consist of bacteremia immediately following graft implantation. In humans, bacteremia frequently occurs after aortic surgery, yet the rate of acute graft infection is low. Bacteremia likely plays only a minor role in acute aortic graft infections. The role of bacteremia in late-occurring graft infection is unknown, but it is likely an uncommon cause of late graft infection. In contrast to patients with prosthetic cardiac valves, patients with prosthetic vascular grafts are rarely given prophylactic antibiotics before dental procedures. Late-occurring graft infections are caused only rarely by organisms found in the mouth flora.[69] Graft incorporation may act as a barrier to bacteremia and prevent late graft infections.

Clinical Presentation

The signs of aortic graft infection can vary widely, from obvious to subtle. Early graft infections can be easy to identify, as they represent complications of wound infections. Affected patients usually present with one or more of the following: induration and cellulitis at the wound, purulent wound drainage, or wound dehiscence with exposed graft. In patients with aortic reconstructions confined to the abdomen, presenting symptoms tend to manifest without wound involvement. Patients can present with failure to thrive, ileus, fever, elevated white blood cell (WBC) count, or frank sepsis. Similarly, malaise, weight loss, and vague constitutional symptoms may be the only manifestations of graft infection. Graft infections can be difficult to diagnose in these patients, and the diagnosis is made fortuitously during work-up of more common sources. Alternatively, the patient may present with pseudoaneurysm formation or catastrophic aortic anastomotic rupture.

Any patient with a wound infection overlying a prosthetic graft requires careful wound exploration. These wounds should be examined in the operating room unless the infection is clearly confined to the subcutaneous tissue or is manifest solely as cellulitis. Cellulitis with drainage requires exploration for an underlying abscess. In the operating room, the wound is explored and opened to the deepest depth of involvement. If the deep tissues are unaffected, most grafts are not contaminated. Operative exploration is mandatory because the exterior wound can be deceptive; only direct exploration can reveal that the infective process involves the body of the graft.

The clinical presentation of late graft infection can be subtle. Latent graft infections can present as chronic femoral pseudoaneurysms. At repair, the graft will be poorly incorporated with surrounding perigraft fluid. These findings are considered to be diagnostic for graft infection and have been associated with positive cultures in 71% of cases.[70] Lack of graft incorporation is more sensitive for graft infection: Padberg and colleagues[70] found that 97% of incorporated grafts were not infected. Infection may be a primary process for the formation of anastomotic femoral pseudoaneurysm. Up to 60% of clinically uninfected femoral pseudoaneurysms will be culture positive at repair.[71] The presence of a latent graft infection should be considered in all cases of femoral pseudoaneurysms. Another subtle sign of latent graft infection is graft thrombosis. This is particularly true if the graft has failed in the past, requiring revision either surgically or by thrombolysis. All patients with graft limb thrombosis or femoral pseudoaneurysms should have CT scan imaging of the graft to rule out infection before repair or revision. Hydronephrosis may also herald a latent graft infection.[72] All patients with prior aortic surgery should have a CT to evaluate for latent graft infection when hydronephrosis is encountered.

Less subtle presentations of latent graft infections include draining sinuses from groin wounds and a history of bleeding from a groin pseudoaneurysm. Bleeding from the groin in the presence of a pseudoaneurysm is a surgical emergency and must be addressed immediately. Such bleeding episodes are herald bleeds and result in life-threatening hemorrhage if not dealt with expeditiously. Graft infection may also present as GI bleeding in a patient with prior aortic surgery. All such patients should be considered to have an aortoenteric fistula until proven otherwise. Rupture of a previously repaired aneurysm or pseudoaneurysm at the proximal anastomosis should be considered the sequelae of graft infection. A summary of the clinical manifestations of aortic graft infections in the University of Texas Southwestern experience is found in Table 61-5.[62] This experience is similar to other published series.[69,73]

Diagnosis

Numerous modalities have been used to diagnose aortic graft infection, including CT, MRI, tagged WBC scans, ultrasonography, sinography, percutaneous aspiration,

TABLE 61-5 CLINICAL MANIFESTATIONS OF GRAFT INFECTIONS IN 31 PATIENTS—THE UNIVERSITY OF TEXAS SOUTHWESTERN MEDICAL CENTER EXPERIENCE*

Clinical Manifestation	No. Patients (%)
Groin sinus or abscess	12 (39)
Graft thrombosis	8 (26)
Femoral artery pseudoaneurysm	
Stable	7 (23)
Acute rupture	5 (16)
Sepsis	4 (13)
Gastrointestinal hemorrhage	3 (10)
Postoperative femoral wound infection	1 (3)

*10 patients had more than one sign.
Modified from Valentine RJ: Diagnosis and management of aortic graft infections. Semin Vasc Surg 14:292, 2001.

arteriography, and operative exploration. Each method has its strengths and weaknesses, and often several are used in concert to assure accurate diagnosis.

Computed Tomography Scan The CT scan remains the gold standard for diagnosis of aortic graft infections. Findings on CT that are suggestive of graft infections include loss of continuity of the aortic wrap (i.e., the residual native aortic wall closed over the graft at the time of repair), pseudoaneurysms, perigraft fluid, perigraft inflammation with loss of tissue plains, perigraft air, and focal bowel wall thickening (Fig. 61-5). The relative frequency of these findings in cases of confirmed graft infection is demonstrated in Table 61-6. The presence of any of these findings is highly suggestive of aortic graft infection. The reported sensitivity and specificity of CT scans to diagnose all graft infections are 95% and 85%, respectively.[74] The sensitivity and specificity approach are 100% when findings of perigraft fluid, perigraft inflammation,

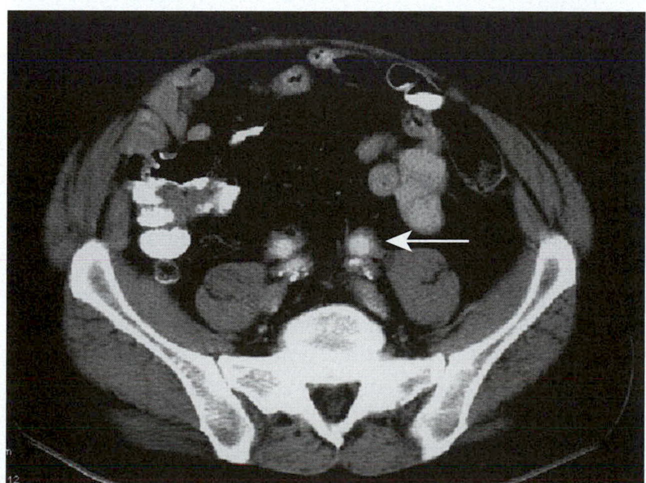

FIGURE 61-5. CT scan of a patient with an infected aortobifemoral bypass demonstrating the presence of perigraft fluid. The *arrow* points to the perigraft fluid.

TABLE 61-6 CT SCAN FINDINGS IN PATIENTS WITH LATE AORTIC GRAFT INFECTION

CT Finding	Percent
Increased perigraft soft tissue	90
Loss of continuity of aortic wrap	53
Increased tissue between wrap and graft	50
Focal bowel wall thickening	37
Ectopic gas	34
Perigraft fluid	28
Pseudoaneurysm	20

Modified from Low RN, Wall SD, Jeffrey RB Jr, et al: Aortoenteric fistula and perigraft infection: Evaluation with CT. Radiology 175:157, 1990.

or ectopic gas are present.[72,74] However, CT scanning may not be able to accurately diagnose subtle graft infections manifest solely by the presence of perigraft fluid. While CT imaging of low-grade aortic graft infection has a specificity of 100%, the sensitivity is only 55%.[72] The other disadvantage of CT scanning is the requirement for contrast. This may be contraindicated in patients with chronic renal insufficiency or radiocontrast allergies. However, the CT modality is readily available, safe, inexpensive, and familiar to clinicians; it remains the imaging modality of choice for initial evaluation.

Magnetic Resonance Imaging The major advantage of MRI, in comparison to CT scanning, is the ability to diagnose small fluid collections and differentiate inflammatory changes from chronic hematomas. Perigraft fluid has low to medium signal intensity on T1-weighted images and high intensity on T2-weighted images (Fig. 61-6). Uninfected aortic grafts have perigraft fibrosis without the characteristic bright fluid "halo" seen surrounding infected grafts on heavily weighted T2 images. Tissue surrounding infected aortic grafts frequently exhibits heterogeneous increased signal intensity that is not seen in association with sterile grafts.[75] Aufferman and colleagues[76] found the sensitivity and specificity of MRI for the diagnosis of graft infections to be 85% and 100%, respectively. The ability of MRI to detect small fluid collections on T2-weighted images gives this modality a distinct advantage over CT scanning to diagnose low-grade *S. epidermidis* graft infections. CT scans should be considered as the initial imaging modality, and MRI used to find latent graft infections not detected by CT.

Radionuclide Scanning Radionuclide scanning relies on labeled WBCs to localize areas of infection and inflammation. Various scanning techniques have been developed to aid in diagnosis. The major pitfall of such imaging techniques is false-positive results. Initially, gallium[67] and indium[111] were used without WBC labeling. The sensitivities and specificities of imaging with gallium and indium were quite high. However, these tracers have been largely abandoned due to uptake by the GI tract and kidneys that obscures the aorta and makes analysis difficult. More recently, WBC labeling techniques have become the norm. Indium[111] oxine-labeled WBC

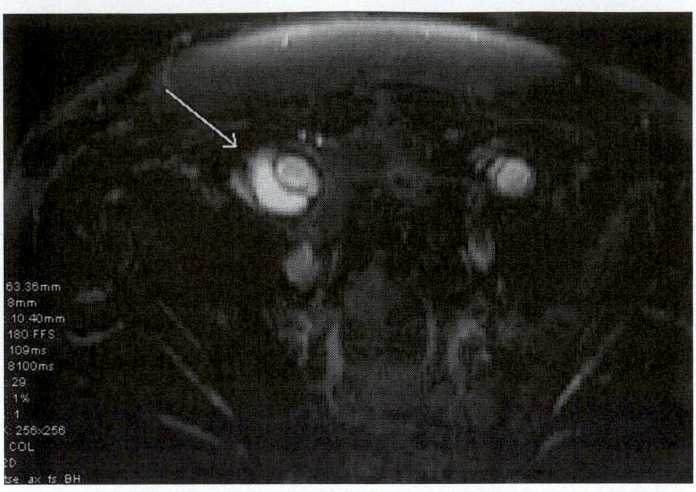

FIGURE 61-6. MRI with heavily weighted T2 imaging of a patient with an infected aortobifemoral bypass. The perigraft fluid is seen as a bright (*white*) signal surrounding the graft (*arrow*). Note the bright fluid "halo" surrounding the infected graft.

scans have been found to be sensitive (82% to 100%) but have a lower specificity (80% to 83%).[77-79] The low specificity of this technique is due to colabeling of platelets that can deposit on uninfected graft surfaces, resulting in an unacceptably high false-positive rate.

Other techniques have been employed in an attempt to increase the sensitivity of radionuclide scanning. These include labeling WBC with technetium-99m-hexametazime or technetium-99m-d,l-hexamethylpropylene amine oxide (Tc-99HMPAO). These techniques are less expensive and do not suffer from the colabeling problems seen with indium. Liberatore and colleagues[80] reported a sensitivity for Tc-HMPAO of 100% and a specificity of 92%. Other techniques included indium^{111}-labeled IgG and avidin/indium^{111}-labeled biotin scintigraphy.[75] Both of these techniques appear to have increased specificity compared with indium-labeled WBCs, but the published experience has been limited. The role of radionuclide scanning is not entirely clear; some centers use radionuclide scanning as the primary mode of imaging for graft infections. Like all nuclear medicine imaging technique, the results depend on the skill and experience of the interpreting radiologist. The most rational approach is to use such scanning techniques as an adjunct to both CT scanning and MRI.

Ultrasound Ultrasonography has limited applicability in the diagnosis of aortic graft infection. Although ultrasound can accurately diagnose the presence of perigraft fluid, the intra-abdominal portion of grafts is not readily imaged. The primary utility of US is to diagnose femoral pseudoaneurysms and perigraft fluid around infrainguinal grafts or aortic grafts that extend to the groin.

Sinography Injection of draining sinuses associated with aortic grafts has been reported. A positive study demonstrates contrast tracking from the sinus to fill a perigraft fluid collection around an unincorporated graft. The utility of such studies is not known, and it is doubtful that such studies add any new information from what can be gleaned from CT or MRI. In addition, injection of contrast into an infected perigraft fluid collection could result in bacteremia or bleeding. Almost all draining sinuses after vascular prosthetic grafting represent external expression of an infection, and thus sinography is unlikely to yield any information not already known to the clinician.

Percutaneous Aspiration Some authors have advocated percutaneous aspiration to confirm the diagnosis of a suspected graft infection.[81,82] In the routine diagnosis of graft infection, this modality offers little additional information beyond conventional noninvasive imaging techniques, and percutaneous aspiration can lead to introduction of bacteria into an otherwise sterile fluid collection. Percutaneous aspiration may offer some assistance in the high-risk patient to confirm the diagnosis before embarking on surgical repair. Concurrent placement of an external drainage catheter can be used as a therapeutic measure. Belair and colleagues[81] reported a series of 11 patients treated with percutaneous drainage and antibiotic therapy. In this retrospective series, four patients were successfully treated. The remaining patients required adjunctive procedures (two surgical drainage, four graft excision), and one patient died as a complication of hemorrhage following drainage.[81] Percutaneous drainage with lifelong antibiotic therapy may be an option for the high-risk patient who is not anticipated to survive graft excision.

Arteriography Arteriography has little role in the diagnosis of aortic graft infection. Unsuspected pseudoaneurysm may be uncovered on arteriography, but the images obtained give little insight to potential infectious etiologies. However, arteriography is vital for preoperative planning and should be obtained before any planned surgical therapy for infected grafts.

Operative Exploration In rare circumstances, there may be a high index of suspicion for graft infection with no supporting evidence on imaging of graft infection. In such situations, operative exploration may be the only way to determine the presence of a latent graft infection. As noted earlier, the finding of a nonincorporated graft is not necessarily diagnostic for graft infection, but the finding of a well-incorporated graft does rule out the diagnosis of infection. Operative exploration may be most helpful in determining the extent of graft infection. If preservation of a portion of a graft is entertained, operative exploration is often the only mechanism to determine if a graft infection is isolated to a segment of the graft or whether the entire graft is infected. Careful preoperative planning is required before such operative explorations to ensure that noninvolved graft is not inadvertently contaminated.

Diagnostic Pitfalls with Early Graft Infection Although most early graft infections are obvious, normal findings in the immediate postoperative period may be misconstrued as signs of graft infection. There is no good diagnostic solution in such cases. Fluid and air surrounding the graft are common findings in the early postoperative period and are not necessarily indicative of infection. The finding of air around the graft is seen routinely until 1 week following implantation; air is not considered to be pathognomonic for infection until 4 to 7 weeks have elapsed.[83,84] Likewise, fluid around the graft is a common finding. Virtually all patients have some degree of hematoma around the graft in the early postoperative period. However, fluid persisting past 3 months is abnormal and highly suspicious for graft infection.[72] MRI evaluation for early graft infection suffers from the same pitfalls as CT scanning. MRI cannot distinguish between air and calcium in the aortic wall remnant, and thus suspicion for infection depends on the finding of perigraft fluid. Labeling of WBCs for scintigraphy is also unreliable in the early postoperative period. Ramo and colleagues[85] found that 29% of Tc-99m-HMPAO–labeled WBC scans were positive in 24 patients examined 2 weeks following surgery. At 3 months, 4 of 24 studies continued to be positive. Only one patient was ultimately found to have an infected graft.[85]

Sedwitz and colleagues[86] found a similar lack of specificity for the diagnosis of early graft infection (<3 months) using indium-labeled WBC scintigraphy. Direct aspiration of perigraft fluid is not helpful in diagnosis of early graft infection and is not recommended in the early postoperative period. As noted earlier, such procedures may introduce bacteria into an otherwise sterile fluid collection.[75] Any of these imaging modalities may be helpful in the early postoperative period if they are negative. A negative study leads the clinician to entertain other diagnoses to explain the clinical findings that have raised the suspicion of an early graft infection. However, a positive study is not useful; the clinician must rely on judgment, and operative exploration may be the only solution to this vexing clinical dilemma.

Diagnosis of Aortoenteric Fistula The diagnosis of aortoenteric fistula can be as challenging as diagnosing and early graft infection. Any patient presenting with GI hemorrhage and a history of aortic reconstruction should be considered to have an aortoenteric fistula until proven otherwise. Both MRI and CT can fail to diagnose graft enteric fistulas. MRI can fail to clearly demonstrate ectopic air that may be misinterpreted as aortic wall calcifications. CT scanning may fail to diagnose the fistulas due to limited inflammation or fluid around the graft, resulting in misinterpretation.[75] If the patient is stable, then either MRI or CT should be obtained. Concerning findings are the absence of a soft tissue plane between adjacent bowel and the graft, as well as ectopic air or perigraft fluid. Extravasation of contrast into the bowel is virtually never seen. All stable patients should undergo upper endoscopy to include the fourth portion of the duodenum. Endoscopy rarely demonstrates visible graft, but endoscopy should be performed to rule out other causes of upper GI hemorrhage. In unstable patients or patients in whom no other source of bleeding is found, operative exploration is necessary to rule out a graft-enteric fistula. During exploration, the entire duodenum and any other adherent bowel must be dissected entirely free to rule out a fistula.

Bacteriology

A wide variety of bacterial pathogens can be cultured from infected grafts. The type of pathogen that will be isolated can be anticipated from the timing of presentation (see Table 61-4). The culture results from Yeager's experience treating 60 infected grafts are typical and presented in Table 61-7.[87] In late-occurring graft infections, staphylococcal species are predominant, with *S. epidermidis* found most frequently. Bandyk reported that 60% of late-occurring graft infections were culture positive for *S. epidermidis.*[88] The most commonly cultured organism responsible for early graft infection is *S. aureus.*[66] Early graft infections have a higher frequency of gram-negative rods and atypical organisms such as anaerobes and yeast. Aortoenteric fistulas and graft erosions are characterized by gram-negative rod infections. Pseudomonal infections are notorious for their virulent course. Graft and arterial disruption are common. This is related to the production of elastase and alkaline proteases by *Pseudomonas*, leading to arterial degradation

TABLE 61-7 AORTIC PROSTHETIC GRAFT CULTURE RESULTS IN 32 PATIENTS

Organism	No. Cases (%)
Staphylococcus aureus	14 (44)
Staphylococcus epidermidis	14 (44)
Bacteroides	3 (9)
Escherichia coli	2 (6)
Streptococcus	2 (6)
Klebsiella	1 (3)
Pseudomonas	1 (3)
Enterococcus	1 (3)
Clostridium	1 (3)
Serratia	1 (3)
Candida	1 (3)
Corynebacterium	1 (3)
Propionibacterium	1 (3)
No growth	2 (6)
Multiple organisms	10 (31)

Modified from Yeager RA, Taylor LM, Moneta GL: Improved results with conventional management of infrarenal aortic infection. J Vasc Surg 30:900, 1999.

and eventual disruption.[53] The time of presentation of the graft infection and the pathogens found at the time of therapy guide antibiotic therapy.

The optimal length of treatment with antibiotics after graft excision is not known. Some authorities have recommended a 6-week course of parenteral antibiotics, followed by 6 months of suppressive therapy to treat concurrent arterial wall infection.[56] Macbeth and colleagues[56] described sending pathologic specimens and aortic biopsies for culture at the time of infected graft excision. Patients with positive arterial wall cultures who were treated with only minimal débridement and short-term antibiotics all suffered aortic stump disruption or other arterial wall disruption.[56] Consequent to these findings, the authors advocated 6 weeks of parenteral antibiotics, followed by 6 months of oral suppressive therapy in patients with positive arterial wall cultures.[56]

Treatment of Aortic Graft Infection

The basic tenet of management of infected arterial grafts is excision of the infected graft and revascularization through uninvolved tissue planes (extra-anatomic bypass). The traditional management of infected aortic grafts has been axillary to femoral bypass, followed by graft excision and ligation of the aortic stump. This technique is plagued by the poor graft durability, the risk of bypass infection, and aortic stump blowout. More recent innovations have included in-line reconstruction with antibiotic-impregnated grafts, arterial homografts, and reconstruction with autogenous superficial femoral/popliteal veins. Each approach has its advantages and disadvantages, and operative therapy must be tailored to suit the individual patient.

Antibiotic Therapy Limited treatment using lifelong antibiotic therapy or percutaneous drainage and antibiotic therapy are options for the most high-risk patient with a limited life expectancy. Little data support such treatment regimens. Roy and Grove[89] reported a series of high-risk patients treated with antibiotic therapy alone for proven or suspected graft infections. Only two of the patients had proven infections of preexisting grafts. All patient were alive at the median follow-up of 36 months without systemic symptoms of infection.[89] Only latent graft infections by *S. epidermidis* should be considered for management in this fashion. This therapy should be condemned in all but the most high-risk patients. Infection by more virulent bacteria has a grave prognosis, and antibiotic therapy alone has little impact on the natural history of the infection.

Total Graft Excision without Revascularization In the early experience of management of aortic graft infections, graft excision without arterial reconstruction was commonly used. The infected graft would be excised, and a wait-and-see strategy would be used to determine if the limbs required revascularization. This approach led to unacceptably high rates of amputation and death. Graft excision alone can be considered in patients with occluded grafts who do not have severe ischemia. Most patients tolerate excision of thrombosed, infected grafts without worsening of their preexisting ischemia; however, the risk of interrupting important collaterals during graft excision should be borne in mind. Patients who undergo aortic grafting for claudication may tolerate graft excision without revascularization. Such patients can be expected to return to their preoperative degree of ischemia after graft removal. This technique should be reserved for patients who have had end-to-side aortic grafting for aortoiliac occlusive disease. Preoperative arteriography must be obtained to determine if the native circulation remains intact. Thrombosis of the native aorta is common following end-to-side aortobifemoral bypass grafting and must be ruled out before graft excision. In most patients, and virtually all patients operated on for aortic aneurysmal disease, graft excision without revascularization can be expected to result in lower extremity amputation.

Total Graft Excision and Extra-anatomic Revascularization Total graft excision with extra-anatomic bypass is the traditional treatment for infected aortic graft. This treatment strategy consists of extra-anatomical bypass by axillary-femoral-femoral bypass, or bilateral axillary to femoral bypasses with total graft excision. Axillary-femoral-femoral bypasses are employed for treatment of infected grafts that do not involve the femoral arteries, while bilateral axillary to femoral bypasses are used to treat infected aortobifemoral bypass grafts. The approach for infected aortobifemoral bypass requires careful planning and inventive tunneling. To prevent cross-contamination of the new graft, the femoral vessels are approached through uninvolved tissue planes, typically lateral to the sartorius muscle. Bypasses are performed from the axillary artery to the profunda femoris artery or to the superficial femoral artery, if it is disease free. Axillary to popliteal artery bypasses have poor patency and have largely been abandoned.

After completing the extra-anatomic bypass, the infected graft is removed. The timing of the two stages is controversial. The extra-anatomic bypass can be performed just before removal of the infected graft during the same operative procedure, or the procedures can be staged with extra-anatomic bypass performed several days before removal of the infected graft. Staging procedures gives the patient time to recover from the initial bypass and avoids a long procedure. Proponents of the staged procedure report a lower operative mortality and increased limb salvage than the single-stage operative strategy.[90,91]

There are several disadvantages to extra-anatomic bypass with total graft excision. The most worrisome complication is infection of the new bypass graft. Reinfection rates can be as high as 20%, but most series report a low reinfection rate of less than 10%.[62,91] Durability of the extra-anatomic bypass is also a concern. The highest reported primary patency rate for axillary-femoral-femoral bypass is higher than 75%, but the primary patency rate of unilateral axillary-femoral bypasses is approximately 60% at 3.5 years.[90,92] The most devastating complication of this procedure is disruption of the oversewn aortic stump (aortic stump blowout). Fortunately, this lethal complication is rare.

Because of these disadvantages, many other options for graft excision and revascularization have been introduced.

Total Graft Excision with In Situ Replacement Using Prosthetic Graft In situ replacement of an infected graft with a new prosthetic graft is technically the simplest method of revascularization and avoids the potential for aortic stump blowout. However, replacing an infected prosthetic graft with a new prosthesis poses the real potential for recurrent graft infection. In situ prosthetic replacement may be best used as a salvage operation for unstable patients with either aortoenteric fistula or ruptured proximal pseudoaneurysms. The reported rate of clinically apparent reinfection following in situ replacement for aortoenteric fistula is surprisingly low (<15%).[93,94] Replacement with new graft may be appropriate for localized graft infections such as those found in the setting of an aortoenteric fistula. Recurrent infection in the setting of gross graft infection has been disappointing. The authors use in situ replacement with prostheses as a bridge to definitive therapy, with autogenous replacement at a later operation.

The advent of antibiotic-bonded Dacron grafts appeared to offer improved results for in situ prosthetic replacement. This modality seems to be most appropriate for the treatment of graft infections with the biofilm producing *S. epidermidis* or *S. aureus*. Young and colleagues[94] reported a series of nine patients treated with rifampin-soaked grafts and found that the reinfection rate was 11%. Bandyk and Hayes[95,96] both concluded that rifampin-bonded grafts are acceptable for treatment of low-grade biofilm graft infections by *S. epidermidis* and *S. aureus*. Bandyk[95] found that recurrent infection occurred in less than 10% of patients. Hayes[96] only reported reinfection in patients with methicillin-resistant *S. aureus* (MRSA) infections. Apparently antibiotic-bonded grafts may offer improved results but only in selected patients with low-grade *S. epidermidis* and, possibly, *S. aureus* infections. They are usually not appropriate in cases involving more virulent organisms.

Total Graft Excision with In Situ Replacement Using Arterial Allograft An alternative to in situ replacement with prosthetic graft is replacement with arterial allograft. Animal studies have demonstrated that the allograft is relatively resistant to infection when antibiotic loaded.[97] The experience in humans has confirmed this finding. Leseche and colleagues[98] reported of a series of 28 patients treated with allografts for graft infection or infected aortic aneurysms. They reported no recurrent infection. In a series of 49 patients, Vogt and colleagues[99] reported 2 patients with recurrent infections that resulted in death. However, in this series there were four deaths related to allograft technical complications. In three patients, allograft side branch rupture resulted in three aortoenteric fistulas that were uniformly fatal. A fourth patient died intraoperatively from rupture of a friable allograft.[99] Less favorable results have been reported by the U.S. Cryopreserved Aortic Allograft Registry. Of the 53 patients entered into the registry, 9% developed recurrent infection with bleeding complications. Other complications include limb occlusion (9%) and pseudoaneurysm (2%).[11] Reoperation for degenerative changes in such grafts is common (9% to 17%), and pathologic changes are seen in up to 26% of patients.[30,98] Allograft replacement for infected aortic grafts appears to yield better results than in situ replacement with prosthetic grafts, but reinfection is common and late degenerative changes in the grafts are problematic. In situ allograft and prosthetic graft replacement may be best used as a temporizing technique until more definitive therapy can be undertaken.

Total Graft Excision with In Situ Replacement Using Autogenous Veins Perhaps the best solution for management of prosthetic graft infection is in situ reconstruction with a superficial femoral/popliteal vein (SFPV). This conduit has proven to be the most resistant conduit to infection, has unchallenged patency rates, avoids the risk of aortic stump blowout, and rarely degenerates. Operative mortality following aortic reconstruction with SFPV has been reported as less than 10%.[100-102] Reinfection is rare. In the UT Southwestern experience, only one patient suffered infection of an SFPV graft, and the offending organism was *Candida*. Franke and Voit[103] noted two cases of SFPV infection that occurred in the face of overwhelming *Pseudomonas* infection. In the UT Southwestern experience, all patients with pseudomonal infections were treated successfully; however, none of the patients presented with overwhelming sepsis. Patients with overwhelming sepsis may be better served by extra-anatomic bypass and graft excision. SFPV is durable, with primary patency rates of greater than 80% and less than 5% of grafts requiring revision.[100,102] Venous morbidity is minimal.

Most patients are suitable for aortic reconstruction with SFPV regardless of the bacterial pathogen. The only downside to this management strategy is the length of the operative procedure. Harvest of the SFPV requires two teams, and mean operative time is 8 hours. Due to the length of time required, SFPV aortic reconstruction is not appropriate for unstable patients, particularly patients with bleeding aortoenteric fistulas. However, such patients can be treated with in situ prosthetic replacement with delayed conversion to SFPV after a period of stabilization and recovery. Extra-anatomic bypass with graft excision has been the standard for treatment of aortic graft infection, but autogenous replacement with SFPV has earned a place as the new gold standard for management of such patients.

Partial Graft Excision With improvement in imaging techniques, some authors have advocated partial graft excision if the aortic graft infection can be localized to the femoral portion on preoperative imaging. Reconstruction can be carried out by extra-anatomic bypass or in situ grafting. This technique is most appropriate for patients with late *S. epidermidis* infections. It is not appropriate for patients with early graft infections because the entire graft is almost invariably involved. Towne and colleagues[104] described treating 14 patients with confirmed

S. epidermidis or *S. aureus* infection using partial graft excision, wide local débridement, and in situ replacement with PTFE graft. Only 2 of the 14 patients ultimately developed infection in the remaining graft, but the new PTFE grafts remained uninfected.[104]

Calligaro and colleagues[105] demonstrated that graft patch remnants on infrainguinal vessels can be safely left in situ at the time of graft excision in more than 92% of patients. Reilly and colleagues[61] have described good results with partial graft excision and extra-anatomic bypass; in the authors' most recent experience, only 63% of patients require total graft excision. In our experience, subtotal graft excision can be attempted if the body of the graft is found to be incorporated at the time of surgical exploration. In these situations, planned reconstruction with SFPV has a real advantage. The body of the graft can be explored before violating the clearly infected portion. If the entire graft is infected, total graft excision and reconstruction with SFPV can be undertaken. If the body of the graft is not infected, the graft can be divided and sewn to the SFPV. The wound is closed, the infected portion of the graft is removed, and the reconstruction completed. Subtotal graft excision should only be considered in high-risk patients with late-occurring graft infections. Such patients should be followed closely, and infection of the residual graft should be anticipated.

Graft Infection Following Endovascular Repair The incidence of graft infection following stent graft repair of aneurysm is unknown, as only case reports have surfaced in the literature. As of 2002, there have been 10 reports of infected aortic stent grafts and 8 reports of aortoenteric fistulas.[106] As with traditional aortic surgery, aortoenteric fistula should be considered in any patient experienc-ing GI hemorrhage who has been treated with aortic stent grafting. The presentation of patients with infected aortic stent grafts is anticipated to be atypical. We had one patient who developed an infected aortic stent graft following urosepsis. The typical clinical presentation and radiographic finding associated with stent graft infections are not well described and await a more mature experience with these endovascular techniques.

PERIPHERAL GRAFT INFECTIONS

The incidence of graft infection following infrainguinal peripheral arterial reconstruction ranges from 2% to 5%.[107] Most peripheral graft infections occur after extension of local wound infections. Late infections of autogenous grafts are rare and most frequently occur in thrombosed grafts. Late infections occur more commonly in prosthetic grafts. As most infections result from extension of a local wound infections (Szilagyi grade III), the microbiology can be varied, with gram-negative rods playing a prominent role. In a series of 68 patients with infected infrainguinal autogenous grafts, Treiman and colleagues[108] found *S. aureus* and *S. epidermidis* most commonly, followed closely by *Pseudomonas.*

Peripheral graft infections can present as drainage of pus from the wound, graft occlusion, or graft disruption with hemorrhage. A patient presenting with bleeding from the site of an infrainguinal arterial reconstruction should be considered to have a graft infection, and operative exploration is mandatory. In less obvious cases, the diagnosis of such infections is similar to that of aortic graft infections. CT scanning is most helpful and demonstrates perigraft fluid collections and inflammation. MRI can successfully diagnose infected prosthetic grafts that have surrounding perigraft fluid. Ultrasound may also be helpful in such cases. The grafts are easily accessible, and ultrasound is particularly good at identifying perigraft fluid.

The mainstay of therapy is arterial reconstruction through uninfected fields and graft removal. In patients with occluded grafts who do not have limb-threatening ischemia, the graft can be excised without arterial reconstruction. However, patients operated on for limb-threatening ischemia who undergo graft excision can anticipate needing revascularization or they will face inevitable amputation.

In patients who require concurrent revascularization at the time of infected graft excision, the management options are different for prosthetic grafts versus autogenous graft. In virtually all cases of prosthetic graft infection, the entire graft is involved in the infectious process. This requires total graft excision with revascularization through uninfected tissues. Revascularization is performed first with autogenous conduit, if possible. Careful planning and inventive tunneling are required if cross contamination is to be avoided. If the graft originates from the femoral artery, the profunda femoris artery, approached lateral to the sartorius muscle, can be used as the donor artery. If the profunda femoris artery is diseased, the iliac artery can be used for inflow and the graft can be tunneled through the obturator foramen into the thigh. The recipient artery or runoff artery must be one level below the infective process. If the above-the-knee popliteal artery is involved in the infective process, then the new runoff vessel must be the below-the-knee popliteal artery or the tibial vessels. More distal reconstruction to uninvolved tibial vessels is required if the infected graft terminates at the below-the-knee popliteal vessel or a tibial vessel. Often the graft needs to be tunneled through the lateral thigh to avoid the previously violated medial thigh. The below-the-knee popliteal artery, peroneal artery, and the anterior tibial artery can all be approached through lateral leg incisions. After reestablishing flow and closing the wounds, the prosthetic graft is excised. If possible, the entire graft should be excised with autogenous patching of the donor and recipient arteries to avoid late complications from infected graft remnants. Well-incorporated remnants of prosthetic grafts can be left in place with successful healing and few late complications, but these patients require close observation.[105]

Virtually all autogenous graft infections occur at the site of a wound infection. An autogenous graft infection is often localized to the segment of the graft located directly beneath the infected wound. In these cases, the uninvolved portion of the graft can be left in place and a new autogenous graft can originate from these uninvolved portions. As with prosthetic graft infections, the best option is revascularization through uninfected tissue planes. However, new autogenous grafts can be placed in the infected tissue planes with concurrent coverage by well-vascularized muscle flaps. In patients with infected grafts but without graft disruption, graft preservation may be attempted. The graft may be left in situ, covered with muscle flaps, and treated with IV antibiotics.

Calligaro and colleagues,[109] in a series of 16 patients with autogenous graft infections without disruption, successfully salvaged 11 grafts. Of these patients, six were treated with muscle flap coverage, with only one failure and no graft-associated mortality. Patients treated with operative débridement and antibiotic-soaked dressing changes had more complications and a higher mortality from graft complications. Limb salvage was obtained in 6 of 10 patients. In this series, the overall operative mortality was 19% and the amputation rate was 8%.[109] Tukiainen and colleagues[110] reported improved results with graft preservation, aggressive débridement, and muscle flap coverage. In a series of 14 patients with autogenous graft infections, 30-day graft preservation and limb salvage were obtained in 13 patients with aggressive débridement with muscle flap coverage. One patient required a late amputation due to ongoing graft infection, and four patients had late graft occlusions. All four patients with late graft occlusions had in situ replacement with new grafts for graft disruption and hemorrhage. There were no graft-related mortalities and no graft disruptions from recurrent infection.[110] Treiman and colleagues[108] identified graft disruption with bleeding, elevated WBCs, fever, and renal insufficiency as the only predictors for graft failure and limb loss following selective graft preservation.

In our experience, wound infections that involve autogenous grafts without graft disruption represent graft contamination rather than graft infections. Such grafts can be treated by graft preservation and muscle flap coverage. It is imperative that well-vascularized muscle be used to cover such grafts. If the graft is not covered by muscle, continued wound sepsis with progression to frank graft infection and disruption can be anticipated. True graft infections manifest as graft degradation and hemorrhage. Invariably, pathologic examination of such grafts reveals pathogens in the wall of the graft. Such grafts should be treated by graft ligation with revascularization through uninfected tissue planes; uninfected portions of the graft may be left place. In situ reconstruction with new autogenous graft with muscle flap coverage should be reserved only for patients with limited autogenous conduit; close observation with prolonged antibiotic therapy is necessary. Such patients should be observed in the ICU setting until wound healing and absence of recurrent graft infection is assured. Graft ligation with or without primary amputation may be the safest course in such patients.

SUPPURATIVE THROMBOPHLEBITIS

Due to the widespread use of IV therapy in hospital patients, primary venous infections are more common than their arterial counterparts. The term "suppurative thrombophlebitis" implies a localized infection of the vein wall associated with intraluminal thrombosis, which should be differentiated from catheter-related sepsis. Although the two may be temporally related in the same patient, they can usually be distinguished by the following characteristics: (1) catheter sepsis is not usually associated with vein wall suppuration, and (2) in catheter sepsis, the intraluminal thrombus is adherent to the catheter, not the vein wall. The following discussion focuses on diagnosis and management of suppurative thrombophlebitis; more complete information on catheter sepsis is available elsewhere.[111]

Suppurative thrombophlebitis can be classified into five areas: superficial, central/pelvic, portal (pylephlebitis), cavernous sinus, and jugular (Lemierre's syndrome).

Peripheral Vein Suppurative Thrombophlebitis

Thrombophlebitis is the most common complication of peripheral vein infusion, occurring in up to one fourth of hospitalized patients receiving IV therapy via veins of the forearm or hand.[112] The pathogenesis has been related to irritation of the vein from the catheter material, infusate, or bacteria. Thrombosis occurs as a result of localized stasis and prostaglandin-mediated activation of the coagulation cascade.[113] *Suppurative superficial thrombophlebitis* results from infection of the thrombus, which is estimated to occur in 0.2% to 2% of peripheral vein catheter insertions.[114] The onset of infection is a serious development, resulting in significant morbidity and prolonged hospital stay. Development of life-threatening infections such as osteomyelitis or endocarditis may occur after a single episode of superficial suppurative thrombophlebitis. This complication is more common with plastic catheters than with steel ("scalp vein") cannulas and is related to duration of IV catheterization.[115] Prolonged catheterization is the most important predictor of peripheral vein infusion thrombophlebitis; this has led to the recommendation by the Centers for Disease Control and Prevention that short peripheral IV catheters should be changed every 72 hours.

Although there is a higher risk of suppurative superficial thrombophlebitis from catheters inserted in the lower extremity, upper extremity involvement is the more common presentation. Affected patients have signs of local inflammation including tenderness, erythema, induration, and warmth over the involved superficial vein. Differentiation between uninfected and suppurative thrombophlebitis may be difficult. Systemic signs of infection such as fever, tachycardia, and leukocytosis are not universally present. Bacteremia occurs in the majority of patients, and gross pus within the vein lumen may be found in up to half the cases.[115] Diagnosis often relies on a positive culture of the indwelling catheter tip. *S. aureus* is the most common isolate, but gram-negative organisms are becoming more frequent. Antibiotic resistance is common.

Treatment of superficial suppurative thrombophlebitis involves removal of the IV catheter, institution of broad-spectrum antibiotics, and excision of the involved vein. The involved vein should be explored proximal to the highest anticipated site of involvement—usually several centimeters above the inflamed area. The infected vein segment and its tributaries should be completely excised using a patent, noninflamed vein segment as the endpoint. Incisions should be left open to heal by secondary intention. Postoperatively, antibiotics should be continued for an undetermined period of time. Empiric recommendations suggest continuation of culture-directed antibiotics for at least 2 to 3 weeks.

Central Vein Suppurative Thrombophlebitis

Two classic scenarios have been described for suppurative thrombophlebitis of central veins: (1) residual central thrombosis following central line sepsis and (2) pelvic suppurative thrombophlebitis associated with gynecologic complications. Suppurative thrombophlebitis of thoracic veins occurs in the chronic setting, whereas suppurative pelvic thrombophlebitis occurs more acutely.

Central Suppurative Thrombophlebitis Following Intravenous Line Sepsis Suppurative thrombophlebitis often follows prolonged IV therapy in immunocompromised patients. The condition is most common in patients receiving total parenteral nutrition, in critically ill patients receiving IV therapy through central venous catheters, and in those with long-term cannulation devices such as Hickman or Broviac catheters. Central suppurative thrombophlebitis may also be the consequence of IV drug abuse (see earlier discussion). Catheter infections are usually due to microorganisms that migrate from the skin entry site, but hematogenous seeding and contaminated fluids have also been implicated.[111] Suppurative thrombophlebitis occurs subsequent to infection of the thrombus that typically develops around the IV device. The thrombus becomes attached to the central vein wall and causes localized inflammation.

Central suppurative thrombophlebitis should be suspected in any patient who fails to improve after removal of an infected central venous catheter. Systemic signs of infection are more common than venous obstructive symptoms such as arm edema. Diagnosis can be made by demonstrating a deep vein thrombosis (by duplex ultrasonography, venography, or MRI) in a septic patient with positive blood cultures who does not have other sources of primary infection.[116] CT scans may be useful to demonstrate a vein thrombosis, especially if gas is detected in the vein lumen.[115]

Treatment of central suppurative thrombophlebitis involves removal of central catheters, use of broad-spectrum antibiotics, and anticoagulation with heparin. In some cases, fibrinolytic therapy[117] or surgical thrombectomy[118] may be required. Long-term anticoagulation with warfarin is recommended to reduce the risk of embolization and recurrent thrombosis. A 2- to 3-week course of culture-directed antibiotics is usually appropriate.

Pelvic Suppurative Thrombophlebitis Infection of the deep pelvic veins usually develops 2 to 3 weeks postpartum or after gynecologic complications such as criminal abortions or other severe pelvic infections. Diagnosis of pelvic suppurative thrombophlebitis should be suspected in a postpartum woman with high fevers, chills, and abdominal pain. Large veins may cause ureteral obstruction, resulting in severe flank pain.[115] Nearly 80% of cases are on the right side due to compression of the right ovarian vein at the pelvic brim by the gravid uterus.[115] Although a tender vein can be palpated on pelvic examination in up to 30% of women, the physical examination may be normal.[115] CT scanning and MRI have both been useful to confirm deep pelvic vein thrombosis; a positive test in the clinical setting of sepsis confirms the diagnosis. Pelvic suppurative thrombophlebitis usually responds to broad-spectrum IV antibiotics. It remains controversial whether patients benefit from anticoagulation with heparin. Occasionally, patients do not respond to conservative treatment and drainage of a pelvic abscess or ligation of the affected vein is required.

Suppurative Thrombophlebitis of the Portal Vein (Pylephlebitis)

Suppurative thrombophlebitis of the portal vein usually follows infection of an organ drained by the portal vein or a contiguous structure. Historically, pylephlebitis was most commonly due to appendicitis.[119] The condition is now rare due to widespread use of antibiotics, as well as early diagnosis and intervention for abdominal infections. Most modern cases occur as a complication of abdominal infections such as perforated appendicitis or diverticulitis.[119] However, some are due to secondary infection of portal vein thrombosis associated with a hypercoagulable disorder such as cirrhosis or malignancy.[120]

The clinical presentation of patients with pylephlebitis is nonspecific: Most have fevers of unknown origin with variable signs of systemic toxicity. Ultrasound may be helpful to detect thrombus within the lumen of the portal vein, but CT is the more common test to confirm the diagnosis. MRI may be able to discern acute from chronic thrombus.[120] Many patients have other intra-abdominal processes such as abscesses or common bile duct stones. Small intrahepatic liver abscesses may also be present.

Treatment of pylephlebitis involves use of broad-spectrum IV antibiotics and eradication of the underlying infection. Early treatment is critical to reduce the risk of ischemic bowel infarction from mesenteric vein thrombosis. Although systemic administration of broad-spectrum antibiotics is usually adequate, catheter infusion of antibiotics directly into the portal vein may result in more prompt improvement.[121] Intra-abdominal infections should be treated promptly by percutaneous drainage or surgical intervention. Although controversial, anticoagulation may be useful in patients with hypercoagulable states who have persistent infection unresponsive to antibiotics.[120] Fortunately, development of acute portal hypertension with variceal hemorrhage is uncommon.

Septic Thrombosis of the Cavernous Sinuses

Widespread use of antibiotics has dramatically reduced the incidence of cavernous sinus thrombophlebitis, but it is still occasionally seen in patients with severe head and neck infections. Infection of the ethmoid and sphenoid sinuses is the most common primary source that leads to cavernous sinus thrombophlebitis.[122] *S. aureus* is isolated in approximately 60% to 70% of cases, followed by *S. pneumoniae*, gram-negative bacilli, and anaerobes.[122] Early diagnosis and treatment are extremely important, as mortality rates of 20% to 30% are still reported in the modern era.[123]

Patients with cavernous sinus thrombophlebitis typically present with fever, ptosis, proptosis, chemosis, and external ophthalmoplegia.[122] The ocular signs are due to damage of nerves that traverse the cavernous sinus. Headache, papilledema, and periorbital swelling are present in more than half of affected patients. Diagnosis may be established by high-resolution CT scans or by MRI. Management includes treatment of the underlying infection (sinusitis, dental abscess, tonsillitis) and use of broad-spectrum antibiotics. Cavernous sinus drainage is almost never performed.[122] At least one study[124] suggests that anticoagulation with heparin may reduce the mortality rate in survivors. Severe sequelae have been reported in most survivors including lung, brain, and orbital abscesses and prolonged cranial nerve dysfunction. Early diagnosis and treatment remain the keys to reducing potential disasters in these patients.

Septic Thrombophlebitis of the Internal Jugular Vein

This disorder was first described in 1936 by Lemierre, who reported a 90% mortality rate in his patients.[125] Widespread use of antibiotics has reduced the prevalence and mortality of septic thrombophlebitis of the internal jugular vein (also known as postanginal septicemia or Lemierre's syndrome), but the rarity of the syndrome also means that it is often overlooked. Several stages have been described.[126] Septic thrombophlebitis of the internal jugular vein usually follows an acute oropharyngeal infection; a sore throat is the most common presentation. In the second stage, local invasion of the parapharyngeal space leads to septic thrombophlebitis of the internal jugular vein. This most commonly presents as swelling and tenderness of the neck, which should be considered a serious development in a patient with pharyngitis. Metastatic infections occur in the third stage, most commonly the lungs and joints.

Diagnosis of Lemierre's syndrome should be considered in any patient with current or recent pharyngitis who presents with tenderness in the anterior cervical triangle. Clinical signs during the course of disease include fever, abdominal pain, and hyperbilirubinemia.[126] Most patients have already developed metastatic infections at the time of diagnosis. A triad of pharyngitis, tender/swollen neck, and noncavitating pulmonary infiltrates has been described.[126] The most common isolate is *Fusobacterium necrophorum*, an anaerobic gram-negative rod that is a normal inhabitant of the oral cavity.[126] Diagnostic tests such as ultrasonography, CT, or MRI should be used to confirm the presence of internal jugular vein thrombosis. CT or MRI may be helpful to delineate the presence of neck abscesses that require drainage; these tests are also useful to follow the local anatomy once treatment has been instituted. Treatment involves a 3- to 6-week course of IV antibiotics; surgical excision of the internal jugular vein is only necessary in patients with uncontrolled sepsis or recurrent septic emboli despite appropriate antibiotic therapy (<10% of cases).

CONCLUSION

Primary arterial infections, graft infections, and suppurative thrombophlebitis remain daunting problems for clinicians. A high index of suspicion and modern imaging techniques are required to make the diagnosis of arterial infection, whether primary or following arterial reconstruction. Suppurative thrombophlebitis should be suspected in any patient who does not improve after removal of an infected venous catheter or in any patient with a fever of unknown origin. With the advent of inventive management strategies, the mortality and morbidity associated with arterial infections has steadily improved. SFPV is the conduit of choice for reconstruction of large arteries with primary infections such as the carotid and mesenteric vessels. Aortic reconstruction with SFPV is the optimal management strategy for most patients with primary aortic infections or prosthetic aortic graft infections. Long-term administration of antibiotics represents the mainstay of treatment for primary venous infections; surgical excision is reserved for infections involving superficial veins and for deep veins in patients who do not improve on appropriate antibiotic therapy.

REFERENCES

1. Koch R: Ueber aneurysma der arteria mesenterica superior Inaug Dural-Abhandlung. Barfus'schen Universitaetes Buchdruckerei, 1851.
2. Osler W: The Gulstonian lectures on malignant endocarditis. Br Med J 1: 467, 1885.
3. Wilson SE, Van Wagenen P, Passaro E Jr: Arterial infection. Curr Probl Surg 15:1, 1978.
4. Stengel A, Wolferth CC: Mycotic (bacterial) aneurysms of intravascular origin. Arch Intern Med 31:527, 1923.
5. Brown SL, Busuttil RW, Baker JD, et al: Bacteriologic and surgical determinants of survival in patients with mycotic aneurysms. J Vasc Surg 1:541, 1984.
6. Tilson MD: Pathogenesis of mycotic aneurysms. Cardiovasc Surg 7:1, 1999.
7. Dobrin PB, Mrkvicka R: Failure of elastin or collagen as possible critical connective tissue alterations underlying aneurysmal dilatation. Cardiovasc Surg 2:484, 1994.
8. Buckmaster MJ, Curci JA, Murray PR, et al: Source of elastin-degrading enzymes in mycotic aortic aneurysms: Bacteria or host inflammatory response? Cardiovasc Surg 7:16, 1999.
9. Pierce RA, Sandefur S, Doyle GA, et al: Monocytic cell type-specific transcriptional induction of collagenase. J Clin Invest 97:1890, 1996.
10. Gomes MN, Choyke PL, Wallace RB: Infected aortic aneurysms. A changing entity. Ann Surg 215:435, 1992.
11. Oderich GS, Panneton JM, Bower TC, et al: Infected aortic aneurysms: Aggressive presentation, complicated early outcome, but durable results. J Vasc Surg 34:900, 2001.
12. Fillmore AJ, Valentine RJ: Surgical mortality in patients with infected aortic aneurysms. J Am Coll Surg 196:435, 2003.
13. Oz MC, Brener BJ, Buda JA, et al: A ten-year experience with bacterial aortitis. J Vasc Surg 10:439, 1989.
14. McNamara MF, Roberts AB, Bakshi KR: Gram-negative bacterial infection of aortic aneurysms. J Cardiovasc Surg (Torino) 28:453, 1987.
15. Brouwer RE, van Bockel JH, van Dissel JT: *Streptococcus pneumoniae*, an emerging pathogen in mycotic aneurysms? Neth J Med 52:16, 1998.
16. Katz SG, Andros G, Kohl RD: Salmonella infections of the abdominal aorta. Surg Gynecol Obstet 175:102, 1992.

17. van der Vliet JA, Kouwenberg PP, Muytjens HL, et al: Relevance of bacterial cultures of abdominal aortic aneurysm contents. Surgery 119:129, 1996.
18. Farkas JC, Fichelle JM, Laurian C, et al: Long-term follow-up of positive cultures in 500 abdominal aortic aneurysms. Arch Surg 128:284, 1993.
19. Gouny P, Valverde A, Vincent D, et al: Human immunodeficiency virus and infected aneurysm of the abdominal aorta: Report of three cases. Ann Vasc Surg 6:239, 1992.
20. McHenry MC, Rehm SJ, Krajewski LP, et al: Vertebral osteomyelitis and aortic lesions: Case report and review. Rev Infect Dis 13:1184, 1991.
21. Hagino RT, Clagett GP, Valentine RJ: A case of Potts' disease of the spine eroding into the suprarenal aorta. J Vasc Surg 24:482, 1996.
22. Muller BT, Wegener OR, Grabitz K, et al: Mycotic aneurysms of the thoracic and abdominal aorta and iliac arteries: experience with anatomic and extra-anatomic repair in 33 cases. J Vasc Surg 33:106, 2001.
23. Ihaya A, Chiba Y, Kimura T, et al: Surgical outcome of infectious aneurysm of the abdominal aorta with or without SIRS. Cardiovasc Surg 9:436, 2001.
24. Pasic M, Carrel T, Tonz M, et al: Mycotic aneurysm of the abdominal aorta: Extra-anatomic versus *in situ* reconstruction. Cardiovasc Surg 1:48, 1993.
25. Robinson JA, Johansen K: Aortic sepsis: Is there a role for *in situ* graft reconstruction? J Vasc Surg 13:677, 1991.
26. Hollier LH, Money SR, Creely B, et al: Direct replacement of mycotic thoracoabdominal aneurysms. J Vasc Surg 18:477, 1993.
27. Fichelle JM, Tabet G, Cormier P, et al: Infected infrarenal aortic aneurysms: When is *in situ* reconstruction safe? J Vasc Surg 17:635, 1993.
28. Gupta AK, Bandyk DF, Johnson BL: *In situ* repair of mycotic abdominal aortic aneurysms with rifampin-bonded gelatin-impregnated Dacron grafts: A preliminary case report. J Vasc Surg 24:472, 1996.
29. Koshiko S, Sasajima T, Muraki S, et al: Limitations in the use of rifampicin-gelatin grafts against virulent organisms. J Vasc Surg 35:779, 2002.
30. Kieffer E, Bahnini A, Koskas F, et al: *In situ* allograft replacement of infected infrarenal aortic prosthetic grafts: Results in forty-three patients. J Vasc Surg 17:349, 1993.
31. Benjamin ME, Cohn EJ Jr, Purtill WA, et al: Arterial reconstruction with deep leg veins for the treatment of mycotic aneurysms. J Vasc Surg 30:1004, 1999.
32. Oweida SW, Roubin GS, Smith RB III, et al: Postcatheterization vascular complications associated with percutaneous transluminal coronary angioplasty. J Vasc Surg 12:310, 1990.
33. McCann RL, Schwartz LB, Pieper KS: Vascular complications of cardiac catheterization. J Vasc Surg 14:375, 1991.
34. Whitton HH Jr, Rehring TF: Femoral endarteritis associated with percutaneous suture closure: New technology, challenging complications. J Vasc Surg 38:83, 2003.
35. Cherr GS, Travis JA, Ligush J Jr, et al: Infection is an unusual but serious complication of a femoral artery catheterization site closure device. Ann Vasc Surg 15:567, 2001.
36. Arora S, Weber MA, Fox CJ, et al: Common femoral artery ligation and local debridement: A safe treatment for infected femoral artery pseudoaneurysms. J Vasc Surg 33:990, 2001.
37. Patel A, Taylor SM, Langan EM III, et al: Obturator bypass: A classic approach for the treatment of contemporary groin infection. Am Surg 68:653, 2002.
38. Buerger R, Benitez P: Surgical emergencies from intravascular injection of drugs. In Bergan JJ, Yao JST (eds): Vascular Surgical Emergencies. Orlando, Fla, Grune & Stratton, 1987, p 309.
39. Reddy DJ, Smith RF, Elliott JP Jr, et al: Infected femoral artery false aneurysms in drug addicts: Evolution of selective vascular reconstruction. J Vasc Surg 3:718, 1986.
40. Ting AC, Cheng SW: Femoral pseudoaneurysms in drug addicts. World J Surg 21:783, 1997.
41. Cheng SW, Fok M, Wong J: Infected femoral pseudoaneurysm in intravenous drug abusers. Br J Surg 79:510, 1992.
42. Padberg F Jr, Hobson R, Lee B, et al: Femoral pseudoaneurysm from drugs of abuse: Ligation or reconstruction? J Vasc Surg 15:642, 1992.
43. Lorelli DR, Cambria RA, Seabrook GR, et al: Diagnosis and management of aneurysms involving the superior mesenteric artery and its branches—a report of four cases. Vasc Endovascular Surg 37:59, 2003.
44. Stone WM, Abbas M, Cherry KJ, et al: Superior mesenteric artery aneurysms: Is presence an indication for intervention? J Vasc Surg 36:234, 2002.
45. Stanley JC, Wakefield TW, Graham LM, et al: Clinical importance and management of splanchnic artery aneurysms. J Vasc Surg 3:836, 1986.
46. Messina LM, Shanley CJ: Visceral artery aneurysms. Surg Clin North Am 77:425, 1997.
47. Zimmerman-Klima PM, Wixon CL, Bogey WM Jr, et al: Considerations in the management of aneurysms of the superior mesenteric artery. Ann Vasc Surg 14:410, 2000.
48. Modrall JG, Sadjadi J, Joiner DR, et al: Comparison of superficial femoral vein and saphenous vein as conduits for mesenteric arterial bypass. J Vasc Surg 37:362, 2003.
49. El Sabrout R, Cooley DA: Extracranial carotid artery aneurysms: Texas Heart Institute experience. J Vasc Surg 31:702, 2000.
50. Grossi RJ, Onofrey D, Tvetenstrand C, et al: Mycotic carotid aneurysm. J Vasc Surg 6:81, 1987.
51. Nader R, Mohr G, Sheiner NM, et al: Mycotic aneurysm of the carotid bifurcation in the neck: Case report and review of the literature. Neurosurgery 48:1152, 2001.
52. Safar HA, Cina CS: Ruptured mycotic aneurysm of the popliteal artery. A case report and review of the literature. J Cardiovasc Surg (Torino) 42:237, 2001.
53. Seabrook GR. Pathobiology of graft infections. Semin Vasc Surg 3:81, 1990.
54. Woodcock NP, el Barghouti N, Perry EP, et al: Is bacterial translocation a cause of aortic graft sepsis? Eur J Vasc Endovasc Surg 19:433, 2000.
55. Reilly LM, Altman H, Lusby RJ, et al: Late results following surgical management of vascular graft infection. J Vasc Surg 1:36, 1984.
56. Macbeth GA, Rubin JR, McIntyre KE Jr, et al: The relevance of arterial wall microbiology to the treatment of prosthetic graft infections: Graft infection vs. arterial infection. J Vasc Surg 1:750, 1984.
57. Buckels JA, Fielding JW, Black J, et al: Significance of positive bacterial cultures from aortic aneurysm contents. Br J Surg 72:440, 1985.
58. Fisher DF Jr, Clagett GP, Fry RE, et al: One-stage versus two-stage amputation for wet gangrene of the lower extremity: A randomized study. J Vasc Surg 8:428, 1988.
59. Josephs LG, Cordts PR, DiEdwardo CL, et al: Do infected inguinal lymph nodes increase the incidence of postoperative groin wound infection? J Vasc Surg 17:1077, 1993.
60. Henke PK, Bergamini TM, Watson AL, et al: Bacterial products primarily mediate fibroblast inhibition in biomaterial infection. J Surg Res 74:17, 1998.
61. Reilly L: Aortic graft infection: Evolution in management. Cardiovasc Surg 10:372, 2002.
62. Valentine RJ: Diagnosis and management of aortic graft infection. Semin Vasc Surg 14:292, 2001.
63. Hallett JW Jr, Marshall DM, Petterson TM, et al: Graft-related complications after abdominal aortic aneurysm repair: Reassurance from a 36-year population-based experience. J Vasc Surg 25:277, 1997.
64. Long-term outcomes of immediate repair compared with surveillance of small abdominal aortic aneurysms. N Engl J Med 346:1445, 2002.
65. Szilagyi DE, Smith RF, Elliott JP, Vrandecic MP: Infection in arterial reconstruction with synthetic grafts. Ann Surg 176:321, 1972.
66. Bandyk DF: Aortic graft infection. Semin Vasc Surg 3:122, 1990.
67. White JV, Freda J, Kozar R, et al: Does bacteremia pose a direct threat to synthetic vascular grafts? Surgery 102:402, 1987.
68. Goeau-Brissonniere O, Leport C, Lebrault C, et al: Antibiotic prophylaxis of late bacteremic vascular graft infection in a dog model. Ann Vasc Surg 4:528, 1990.
69. Jones L, Braithwaite BD, Davies B, et al: Mechanism of late prosthetic vascular graft infection. Cardiovasc Surg 5:486, 1997.
70. Padberg FT Jr, Smith SM, Eng RH: Accuracy of disincorporation for identification of vascular graft infection. Arch Surg 130:183, 1995.
71. Seabrook GR, Schmitt DD, Bandyk DF, et al: Anastomotic femoral pseudoaneurysm: an investigation of occult infection as an etiologic factor. J Vasc Surg 11:629, 1990.
72. Orton DF, LeVeen RF, Saigh JA, et al: Aortic prosthetic graft infections: Radiologic manifestations and implications for management. Radiographics 20:977, 2000.

73. Sharp WJ, Hoballah JJ, Mohan CR, et al: The management of the infected aortic prosthesis: a current decade of experience. J Vasc Surg 19:844, 1994.
74. Low RN, Wall SD, Jeffrey RB Jr, et al: Aortoenteric fistula and perigraft infection: Evaluation with CT. Radiology 175:157, 1990.
75. Modrall JG, Clagett GP: The role of imaging techniques in evaluating possible graft infections. Semin Vasc Surg 12:339, 1999.
76. Olofsson PA, Auffermann W, Higgins CB, et al: Diagnosis of prosthetic aortic graft infection by magnetic resonance imaging. J Vasc Surg 8:99, 1988.
77. Brunner MC, Mitchell RS, Baldwin JC, et al: Prosthetic graft infection: Limitations of indium white blood cell scanning. J Vasc Surg 3:42, 1986.
78. Reilly DT, Grigg MJ, Cunningham DA, et al: Vascular graft infection: The role of indium scanning. Eur J Vasc Surg 3:393, 1989.
79. Lawrence PF, Dries DJ, Alazraki N, et al: Indium 111-labeled leukocyte scanning for detection of prosthetic vascular graft infection. J Vasc Surg 2:165, 1985.
80. Liberatore M, Iurilli AP, Ponzo F, et al: Clinical usefulness of technetium-99m-HMPAO-labeled leukocyte scan in prosthetic vascular graft infection. J Nucl Med 39:875, 1998.
81. Belair M, Soulez G, Oliva VL, et al: Aortic graft infection: The value of percutaneous drainage. AJR Am J Roentgenol 171:119, 1998.
82. Harris KA, Kozak R, Carroll SE, et al: Confirmation of infection of an aortic graft. J Cardiovasc Surg (Torino) 30:230, 1989.
83. Qvarfordt PG, Reilly LM, Mark AS, et al: Computerized tomographic assessment of graft incorporation after aortic reconstruction. Am J Surg 150:227, 1985.
84. O'Hara PJ, Borkowski GP, Hertzer NR, et al: Natural history of periprosthetic air on computerized axial tomographic examination of the abdomen following abdominal aortic aneurysm repair. J Vasc Surg 1:429, 1984.
85. Ramo OJ, Vorne M, Lantto E, et al: Postoperative graft incorporation after aortic reconstruction—comparison between computerised tomography and Tc-99m-HMPAO labelled leucocyte imaging. Eur J Vasc Surg 7:122, 1993.
86. Sedwitz MM, Davies RJ, Pretorius HT, et al: Indium 111-labeled white blood cell scans after vascular prosthetic reconstruction. J Vasc Surg 6:476, 1987.
87. Yeager RA, Taylor LM Jr, Moneta GL, et al: Improved results with conventional management of infrarenal aortic infection. J Vasc Surg 30:76, 1999.
88. Bandyk DF, Berni GA, Thiele BL, et al: Aortofemoral graft infection due to *Staphylococcus epidermidis*. Arch Surg 119:102, 1984.
89. Roy D, Grove DI: Efficacy of long-term antibiotic suppressive therapy in proven or suspected infected abdominal aortic grafts. J Infect 40:184, 2000.
90. Seeger JM, Pretus HA, Welborn MB, et al: Long-term outcome after treatment of aortic graft infection with staged extra-anatomic bypass grafting and aortic graft removal. J Vasc Surg 32:451, 2000.
91. Reilly LM, Stoney RJ, Goldstone J, et al: Improved management of aortic graft infection: The influence of operation sequence and staging. J Vasc Surg 5:421, 1987.
92. Yeager RA, Moneta GL, Taylor LM Jr, et al: Improving survival and limb salvage in patients with aortic graft infection. Am J Surg 159:466, 1990.
93. Walker WE, Cooley DA, Duncan JM, et al: The management of aortoduodenal fistula by *in situ* replacement of the infected abdominal aortic graft. Ann Surg 205:727, 1987.
94. Young RM, Cherry KJ Jr, Davis PM, et al: The results of *in situ* prosthetic replacement for infected aortic grafts. Am J Surg 178:136, 1999.
95. Bandyk DF, Novotney ML, Back MR, et al: Expanded application of *in situ* replacement for prosthetic graft infection. J Vasc Surg 34:411, 2001.
96. Hayes PD, Nasim A, London NJ, et al: *In situ* replacement of infected aortic grafts with rifampicin-bonded prostheses: The Leicester experience (1992 to 1998). J Vasc Surg 30:92, 1999.
97. Knosalla C, Goeau-Brissonniere O, Leflon V, et al: Treatment of vascular graft infection by *in situ* replacement with cryopreserved aortic allografts: An experimental study. J Vasc Surg 27:689, 1998.
98. Leseche G, Castier Y, Petit MD, et al: Long-term results of cryopreserved arterial allograft reconstruction in infected prosthetic grafts and mycotic aneurysms of the abdominal aorta. J Vasc Surg 34:616, 2001.
99. Vogt PR, Brunner-LaRocca HP, Lachat M, et al: Technical details with the use of cryopreserved arterial allografts for aortic infection: Influence on early and midterm mortality. J Vasc Surg 35:80, 2002.
100. Valentine RJ, Clagett GP: Aortic graft infections: Replacement with autogenous vein. Cardiovasc Surg 9:419, 2001.
101. Cardozo MA, Frankini AD, Bonamigo TP: Use of superficial femoral vein in the treatment of infected aortoiliofemoral prosthetic grafts. Cardiovasc Surg 10:304, 2002.
102. Daenens K, Fourneau I, Nevelsteen A: Ten-year experience in autogenous reconstruction with the femoral vein in the treatment of aortofemoral prosthetic infection. Eur J Vasc Endovasc Surg 25:240, 2003.
103. Franke S, Voit R: The superficial femoral vein as arterial substitute in infections of the aortoiliac region. Ann Vasc Surg 11:406, 1997.
104. Towne JB, Seabrook GR, Bandyk D, et al: *In situ* replacement of arterial prosthesis infected by bacterial biofilms: Long-term follow-up. J Vasc Surg 19:226, 1994.
105. Calligaro KD, Veith FJ, Valladares JA, et al: Prosthetic patch remnants to treat infected arterial grafts. J Vasc Surg 31:245, 2000.
106. Jackson MR, Joiner DR, Clagett GP: Excision and autogenous revascularization of an infected aortic stent graft resulting from a urinary tract infection. J Vasc Surg 36:622, 2002.
107. Chang JK, Calligaro KD, Ryan S, et al: Risk factors associated with infection of lower extremity revascularization: Analysis of 365 procedures performed at a teaching hospital. Ann Vasc Surg 17:91, 2003.
108. Treiman GS, Copland S, Yellin AE, et al: Wound infections involving infrainguinal autogenous vein grafts: A current evaluation of factors determining successful graft preservation. J Vasc Surg 33:948, 2001.
109. Calligaro KD, Veith FJ, Schwartz ML, et al: Management of infected lower extremity autologous vein grafts by selective graft preservation. Am J Surg 164:291, 1992.
110. Tukiainen E, Biancari F, Lepantalo M: Deep infection of infrapopliteal autogenous vein grafts—immediate use of muscle flaps in leg salvage. J Vasc Surg 28:611, 1998.
111. Sitges-Serra A, Girvent M: Catheter-related bloodstream infections. World J Surg 3:589 1999.
112. Tagalakis V, Kahn SR, Libman M, Blostein M: The epidemiology of peripheral vein infusion thrombophlebitis: A critical review. Am J Med 113:146, 2002.
113. Lewis GBH, Hecker JF: Infusion thrombophlebitis. Br J Anaesth 57:220, 1985.
114. Stratton CW: Infection related to intravenous infusions. Heart Lung 11:123, 1982.
115. Bayer AS, Scheld WM: Endocarditis and intravascular infections. In Mandell GL, Bennett JE, Dolen R (eds): Principles and Practice of Infectious Diseases, 5th ed. New York, Churchill Livingstone, 2000, p 857.
116. Miceli M, Atoui R, Thertulien R, et al: Deep septic thrombophlebitis: An unrecognized cause of relapsing bacteremia in patients with cancer. J Clin Oncol 22:1529, 2004.
117. Andes DR, Urban AW, Archer CW, et al: Septic thrombosis of the basilic, axillary, and subclavian veins caused by a peripherally inserted central venous catheter. Am J Med 105:446, 1998.
118. Kuiemeyer HW, Grabitz K, Buhl R, et al: Surgical treatment of septic deep venous thrombosis. Surgery 118:49, 1995.
119. Plemmons RM, Dooley DP, Longfield RN: Septic thrombophlebitis of the protal vein (pylephlebitis): Diagnosis and management in the modern era. Clin Inf Dis 2:1114, 1995.
120. Singh P, Yadav N, Visvalingam V, et al: Pylephlebitis—diagnosis and management. A J Gastroenterol 96:1312, 2001.
121. Pelsang RE, Johlin F, Dhada R, et al: Management of suppurative pylephlibitis by percutaneous drainage: Placing a drainage catheter into the portal vein. A J Gastroenterol 96:3192, 2001.
122. Ebright JR, Pace MT, Niazi AF: Septic thrombosis of the cavernous sinuses. Arch Intern Med 161:2671, 2001.
123. Yarington CT: Cavernous sinus thrombosis revisited. Proc R Soc Med 70:456, 1977.
124. Levine SR, Twyman RE, Gilman S: The role of anticoagulation in cavernous sinus thrombosis. Neurology 28:517, 1988.
125. Lemierre A: On certain septicemias due to anaerobic organisms. Lancet 1:701, 1936.
126. Chirinos JA, Lichtstein DM, Garcia J, et al: The evolution of Lemierre syndrome: Report of two cases and review of the literature. Medicine 81:458, 2002.

chapter 62

Lower Extremity Ulceration

Bauer E. Sumpio
Jacek Paszkowiak
John Aruny
Peter Blume

Chronic ulceration of the lower extremity is a relatively common condition that causes significant discomfort and disability. An ulcer is a disruption of the skin with erosion of the underlying subcutaneous tissue.[1] This breach may extend further to the contiguous muscle and bone. Minor trauma, often footwear related, is a frequent inciting event. A chronic ulcer is a full thickness skin defect with no significant re-epithelialization for more than 4 weeks.

Common causes of leg ulcerations are responsible for almost 95% of leg ulcers; about 40% to 80% of ulcers are a result of underlying venous disease, 10% to 20% are caused by arterial insufficiency, 15% to 25% are a consequence of diabetes mellitus, and in 10% to 15% of patients a combination of two or more causes exists. Prolonged pressure and local infection are common causes of leg ulcers with minimal vascular compromise. Rare causes are responsible for less than 5% of all leg ulcers (Box 62-1).[2] The disease entities that usually underlie leg ulceration, such as venous insufficiency, peripheral arterial disease, and diabetes mellitus, are associated with significant patient morbidity and mortality. A detailed knowledge of the clinical picture, pathogenesis, relevant diagnostic tests, treatment modalities, and differential diagnosis of leg ulcerations is essential in planning the optimal treatment strategy (Table 62-1). An incorrect or delayed initial diagnosis may harm the patient and increase the risk of serious complications, including permanent disability and amputations.

The exact prevalence of lower extremity ulcers in the United States is unknown. The prevalence of leg ulceration in the general population of Western nations has been reported to be from 1% to 3.5%, with the prevalence increasing to 5% in the geriatric population.[3-6] The data from these studies most likely underestimate the true prevalence because they do not include patients with leg ulcers who are not known to the health care system.

The cost of treating leg ulceration is staggering. Epidemiologic studies from Sweden estimated annual costs of treatment of lower extremity ulcers at $25 million. In England, the estimated cost of care for patients with leg ulcers in a population of 250,000 was about $130,000 annually per patient.[7] Items factored into the equation include physician visits, hospital admissions, home health care, wound care supplies, rehabilitation, time lost from work, and jobs lost. Adding to the cost is the chronic nature of these wounds, the high rate of recurrence, and the propensity to become infected. It is also evident that a true accounting of the cost is difficult because of the unknown prevalence of disease.

The social cost of leg ulcers also becomes a factor as the disease affects a patient's lifestyle and attitude. The ability to work may be temporarily or permanently affected by the condition.[8] Reduction in working capacity adds to the total cost. An estimated 10 million workdays are lost in the United States annually from lower extremity ulcers, and this figure may be low.[9,10] A report in 1994 focused on the financial, social, and psychological implications of lower extremity lesions in 73 patients.[11] Among the study patients, 68% reported feelings of fear, social isolation, anger, depression, and negative self-image because of the ulcers. In addition, 81% of the patients felt that their mobility was adversely affected. Within the younger population that was still actively working, there was a correlation between lower extremity ulceration and adverse effect on finances, time lost from work, and job loss. In addition, there was a strong correlation between time spent on ulcer care and feelings of anger and resentment. These factors combined to have a negative emotional impact on their lives.

BIOMECHANICS OF WALKING AND ULCER FORMATION

An appreciation of the biomechanics required for walking is essential in understanding the etiology of foot ulcers. The foot is a complicated biologic structure containing 26 bones, numerous joints, and a network of ligaments, muscles, and blood vessels. Gait is a complex set of events that requires triplanar foot motion and control of multiple axes for complete bipedal ambulation (Fig. 62-1A).[12] When the heel hits the ground, its outer edge touches first. The foot is in a supinated position, which makes it firm and rigid. The soft tissue structures (muscles, tendons, and ligaments) then relax, allowing the foot to pronate. The foot becomes less rigid and is able to flatten, absorb the shock of touchdown, and adapt to uneven surfaces. During midstance, the heel lies below the ankle joint complex, the front and back of the foot are aligned, and the foot easily bears weight. Toward the end of midstance, the soft tissue structures begin to tighten; the foot resupinates and regains its arch. The foot is again firm, acting as a rigid lever for propulsion.

BOX 62-1 Causes of Lower Extremity Ulcers

Vascular
Common:
- Venous disease and insufficiency
- Peripheral atherosclerotic disease

Rare:
- Vasculitis
- Autoimmune disease (scleroderma)
- Hypertension (Martrell ulcer)
- Thromboangiitis obliterans (Buerger's disease)
- Lymphedema
- Hematologic disorders (sickle cell anemia)
- Clotting disorders (antiphospholipid syndrome)

Neurotrophic
Diabetes mellitus
Uremia
AIDS
Nutritional deficiencies

Biomechanical
Charcot foot
Rheumatoid arthritis (Felty's syndrome)
Fracture, dislocations

Others
Infectious diseases
Physical or chemical injury (trauma, pressure ulcers, burns, frostbite)
Metabolic diseases (porphyria, calciphylaxis)
Neoplastic (melanoma, basal cell carcinoma, squamous cell carcinoma, sarcomas)
Drug reactions or side effects (steroids, Coumadin)
Ulcerating skin diseases (pyoderma gangrenosum)

The heel lifts off the ground, it swings slightly to the inside, and the toes push weight off the ground.

Sensory input from the visual and vestibular systems, as well as proprioceptive information from the lower extremities, is necessary to modify learned motor patterns and muscular output to execute the desired action. Various external and internal forces[13] affect foot function. The combination of body weight pushing down and ground reactive force pushing up creates friction and compressive forces. Shear results from the bones of the foot sliding parallel to their plane of contact during pronation and supination. Foot deformities or ill-fitting footwear enhance pressure points because they focus the forces on a smaller area. When the foot flattens too much or overpronates, the ankle and heel do not align during midstance and some bones are forced to support more weight. The foot strains under the body's weight, causing the muscles to pull harder on these areas, making it more difficult for tendons and ligaments to hold bones and joints in proper alignment. Over time, swelling and pain on the bottom of the foot or near the heel may occur. Bunions can form at the great toe joint, and hammertoe deformities can form at the lesser toes. Abnormal foot biomechanics resulting from limited joint mobility and foot deformities magnify shearing forces, resulting in increased plantar pressure on the foot during ambulation (see Fig. 62-1B and C). This can represent critical causes for tissue breakdown.

PATHOPHYSIOLOGY OF ULCER FORMATION

Venous Disorders

Venous leg ulcers are the most frequently occurring chronic lower extremity wounds (Fig. 62-2A) (also see Chapter 56). The prevalence of lower extremity ulceration secondary to chronic venous disease in European and Western populations is estimated to be 0.5% to 1%. In the United States, it is estimated that between 600,000 and 2.5 million patients have venous ulcerations. Treatment costs in the United States are estimated to be between $2.5 and $3 billion dollars with a corresponding loss of 2 million workdays per year.[14] The estimated annual cost of treatment for venous ulcer patients is almost $40,000 per patient.[15]

The pathophysiology of venous ulceration is straightforward. Blood returns from the lower extremities against gravity to the inferior vena cava, through the deep and superficial venous systems. The deep veins are located within the muscles and deep fascia of the legs. The superficial system consists of the greater saphenous vein and the lesser saphenous vein and is located within the subcutaneous fat. Valves are present within all three systems and prevent retrograde flow of the blood. A portion of blood from the superficial system is directed to the deep system through the communicating perforators. While standing, about 22% of the total blood volume is localized to the lower extremities and hydrostatic pressure in the foot veins can reach 80 mm Hg. In healthy

TABLE 62-1 LOWER EXTREMITY ULCERS CHARACTERIZED BY ETIOLOGY

	Site	Skin Appearance	Ulcer Characteristics	Other Findings
Venous	Lower third of leg; malleolar area	Edema, hemosiderin, dermatitis, eczema	"Weeping," irregular borders, painful	Varicose veins, "bottle" leg, ABI normal
Arterial	Most distal areas, toes	Thin, atrophic, dry, "shiny," hair loss	Round, regular borders, no bleeding, dry base, very painful	Weak/absent pulse, poor capillary refill, ABI < 0.8
Neurotrophic (diabetes mellitus)	Pressure sites; heel and metatarsal heads	Cellulitis	Round, deep, purulent discharge, painless	Sensory deficit; ABI often > 1.3 due to vascular calcification

ABI, ankle brachial index.

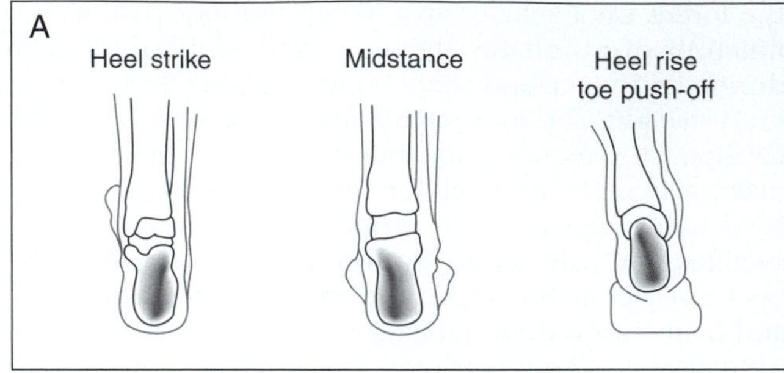

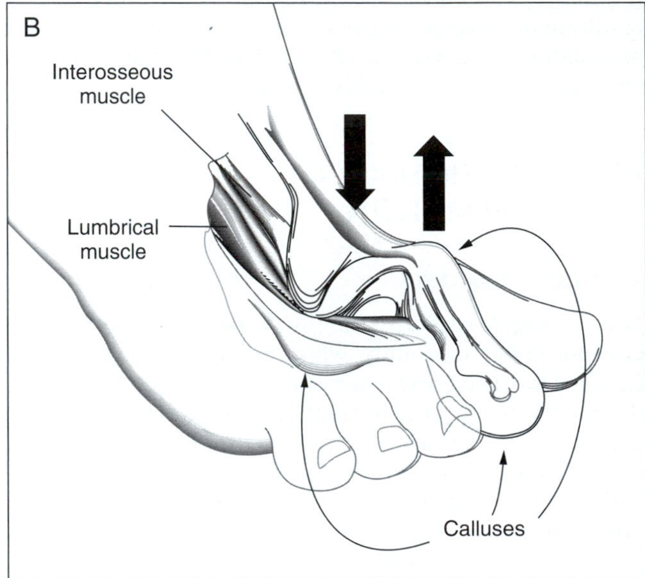

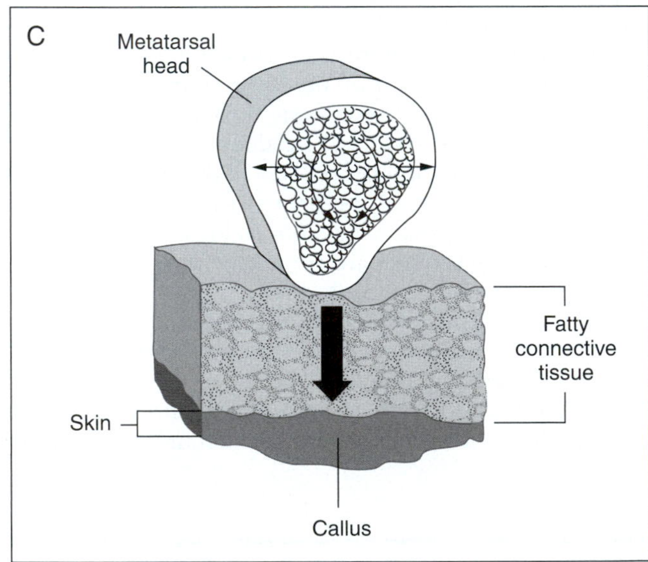

FIGURE 62-1. Biomechanics of ulceration.

individuals with competent venous valves, the efficient calf muscle pump can reduce venous pressure by two thirds during exercise. Venous insufficiency occurs when any of these elements do not function adequately. The pressure in the venous system increases and, most importantly, the ambulatory venous pressure rises during leg exercise. The primary cause of venous hypertension is insufficiency of the valves of the deep venous system and the perforating veins of the lower leg.

The exact mechanism by which ulcerations develop in patients with venous insufficiency is not clear. One theory is that ulceration results as a consequence of increased intraluminal pressure within the capillary system of the leg. The capillaries become dilated and elongated. Blood flow is sluggish, resulting in microthrombi formation and frequently leading to occlusion of the capillaries. Fibrin, albumin, and various macromolecules leak into the dermis, where they bind to and trap growth factors, making them unavailable for the tissue repair process.[16] Leakage of fibrinogen through capillary walls results in deposition of pericapillary fibrin cuffs,[17] which has been suggested as a physical barrier impeding the passage of oxygen.[18] Iron deposition, white blood cell accumulation, decreased fibrinolytic activity, and a myriad of inflammatory responses to the vascular damage are all postulated to be the final pathways leading to venous ulcerations, but it is still not clear whether they represent causative factors.

Tissue hypoxia appears to be the major underlying factor in developing venous ulceration. Unlike ulcers associated with arterial insufficiency, this hypoxic state is not caused by decreased blood flow to the legs; patients with venous insufficiency usually have adequate blood flow to their lower extremities. Direct measurements of transcutaneous oxygen levels on the lower leg have demonstrated that exercise produces a marked rise in skin oxygen tension in normal legs but not in those affected by venous insufficiency. Exercise reduces venous pressure in patients with competent valves, thus removing the stimulus for reflex vasoconstriction. In patients with compromised valves, the venous pressure remains high during exercise and reflex vasoconstriction persists.[19]

On the basis of these findings, it is clear that management of lower extremity ulcers caused by venous insufficiency must include measures that improve the abnormal venous blood return from the affected extremity. Leg elevation, compression therapy, local wound care, and surgical correction of selected underlying pathology are all important components of the treatment plan.

Arterial Disease

The incidence of lower extremity ulcers (see Fig. 62-2B) caused by peripheral arterial disease is increasing in Western nations.[6] The general "aging" of the population and better diagnostic techniques may provide possible explanations for this observation. Risk factors for the development of atherosclerotic lesions causing leg ischemia include diabetes mellitus, smoking, hyperlipidemia, hypertension, obesity, and age. Lack of perfusion decreases tissue resilience, leads to rapid death of tissue, and impedes wound healing (see Chapter 16). Wound healing and tissue regeneration depend on an adequate blood supply to the region. Ischemia due to vascular disease impedes healing by reducing the supply of oxygen, nutrients, and soluble mediators that are involved in the repair process.[20]

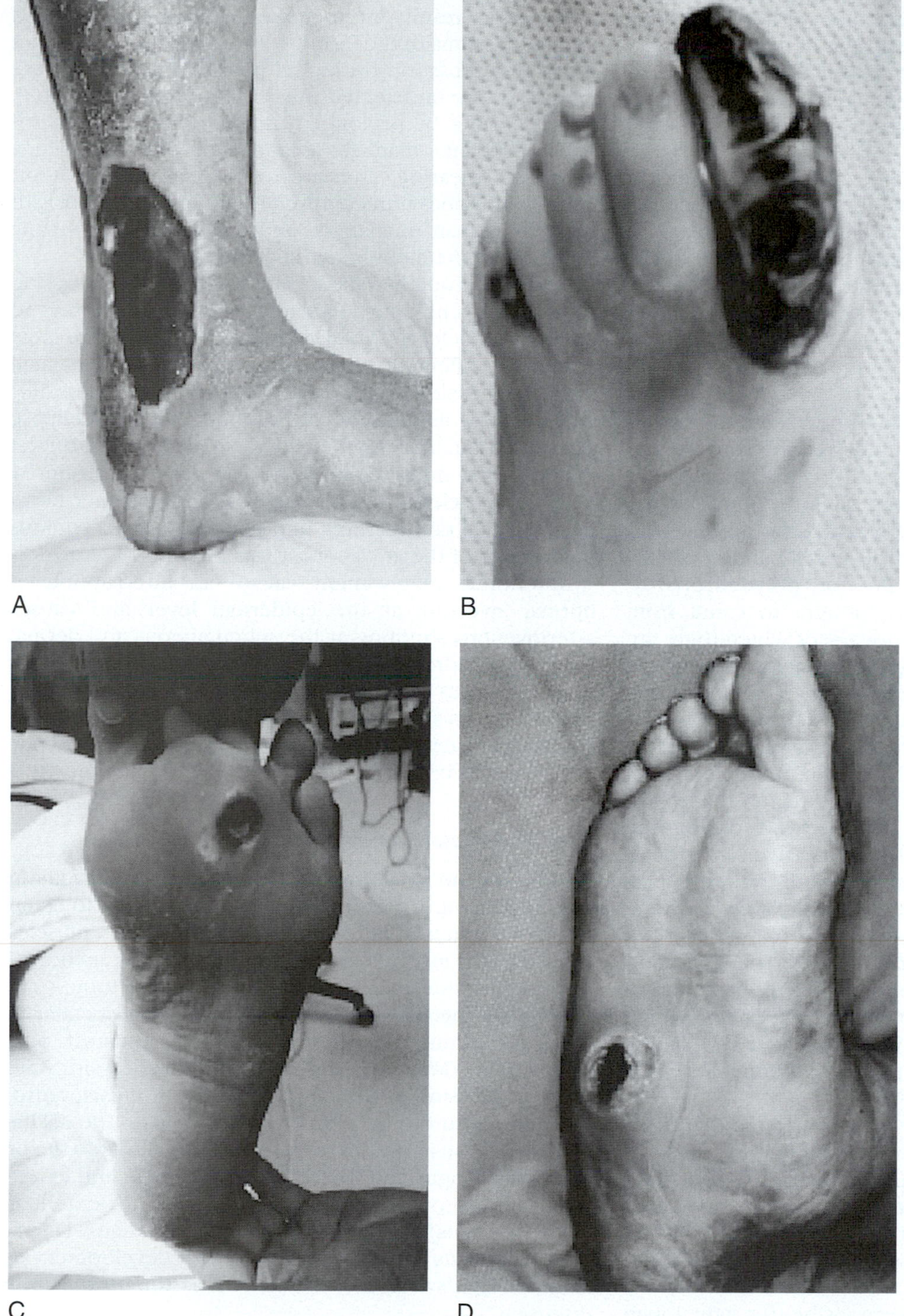

FIGURE 62-2. Various foot ulcers. **A,** Venous stasis. **B,** Ischemic. **C,** Neurotrophic. **D,** Charcot's foot.

The Diabetic Foot

Persons with diabetes mellitus are particularly prone to foot ulcers. The American Diabetes Association consensus group found that among persons with diabetes, the risk of foot ulceration was increased among men, patients who had had diabetes for more than 10 years, and patients with poor glucose control or cardiovascular, retinal, or renal complications.[21] It is estimated that 15% of U.S. patients with diabetes will develop manifestations of diabetic foot disease in their lifetime.[22,23] In this population, the prevalence of lower extremity ulcers ranges from 4% to 10% with an annual incidence of 2% to 3%.[24] Although representing only 6% of the population, patients with diabetes account for 46% of the 162,000 hospital admissions for foot ulcers annually. Diabetic foot ulcers and their sequelae, amputations, are the major cause of disability, morbidity, mortality, and costs for these patients.[23] Ulceration and infection of lower extremities are also the leading causes of hospitalization in patients with diabetes.[25] Treatment of pedal soft-tissue deficits in the diabetic patient population continues to be a medical and surgical challenge, thereby extending the length of their disability and significantly increasing the cost of medical care.

Development of diabetic foot disease can be attributed to several primary risk factors including neuropathy, ischemia, infection, and immune impairment.[23,26] Four foot-related risk factors have been identified in the genesis of pedal ulceration: altered biomechanics, limited joint mobility, bony deformity, and severe nail pathology.[21]

Neuropathy

Neuropathy is the most common underlying etiology of foot ulceration and frequently involves the somatic and autonomic fibers. Although there are many causes of peripheral neuropathy, diabetes mellitus is by far the most common (see Box 62-1). Neuropathy is present in 42% of diabetic patients after 20 years[27] and is usually a distal symmetric sensorimotor polyneuropathy. The peripheral neuropathy is thought to result from abnormalities in metabolic pathways, of which there are several hypotheses including deficiencies in sorbitol metabolism via the polyol pathway.[26,28] Neurotrophic ulcers typically form on the plantar aspect of the foot at areas of excessive focal pressures, which are most commonly encountered over the bony prominences of the metatarsal heads and the forefoot region due to the requirements of midstance and heel off during the gait cycle (see Fig. 62-2C). Loss of protective sensation in the foot can rapidly lead to ulceration if patient education and preventive measures are not taken. Diabetic patients are especially prone to development of a neuro-osteoarthropathy, Charcot's foot.[29] This condition is thought to involve autonomic-nerve dysfunction resulting in abnormal perfusion to foot bones, which leads to bony fragmentation and collapse (see Fig. 62-2D). The resulting "rocker-bottom foot" is prone to tissue breakdown and ulceration.[23,29]

Several investigators[30,31] have demonstrated that there is an increase in both static and dynamic foot pressures when evaluating the neuropathic foot. To date, high pressures alone have not been shown to cause foot ulceration. Rheumatoid patients with high plantar foot pressures but no sensitivity deficit have almost no evidence of foot ulceration.[32]

Type-A sensory fibers are responsible for light touch sensation, vibratory sensation, pressure, proprioception, and motor innervation to the intrinsic muscles of the foot. Type-C sensory fibers detect painful stimuli, noxious stimuli, and temperature. When these fibers are affected, protective sensation is lost. This manifests as a distal, symmetric loss of sensation described in a "stocking" distribution and proves to be the primary factor predisposing patients to ulcers and infection.[33] Patients are unable to detect increased loads, repeated trauma, or pain from shearing forces. Injuries such as fractures, ulceration, and foot deformities therefore go unrecognized. Repeat stress to high-pressure areas or bone prominences, which would be interpreted as pain in the non-neuropathic patient, also go unrecognized. Sensory dysfunction results in increased shearing forces and repeated trauma to the foot.[30,34] Patients have inadequate protective sensation during all phases of gait; therefore high loads are undetected due to loss of pain threshold, which results in prolonged and increased forces.[30,31] These problems manifest as abnormal pressure points, increased shearing, and greater friction to the foot. Because this goes unrecognized in the insensate foot, gait patterns remain unchanged and the stresses eventually cause tissue breakdown and ulceration.

Motor neuropathy is associated with demyelinization and motor end-plate damage, which contribute to conduction defects. The distal motor nerves are the most commonly affected, resulting in atrophy of the small intrinsic muscles of the foot. Wasting of the lumbrical and interosseous muscles of the foot results in collapse of the arch and loss of stability of the metatarsal-phalangeal joints during mid-stance of the gait. Overpowering by extrinsic muscles can lead to depression of the metatarsal heads, digital contractures, and cocked-up toes; equinus deformities of the ankle; or a varus hindfoot.[35]

Autonomic involvement causes an interruption of normal sweating at the epidermal level, and causes arteriovenous shunting at the subcutaneous and dermal level. Hypohidrosis leads to a noncompliant epidermis that increases the risk of cracking and fissuring. Arteriovenous shunting diminishes the delivery of nutrients and oxygen to tissue regions, and skin and subcutaneous tissues become more susceptible to breakdown.[36]

Musculoskeletal Deformities

Atrophy of the small muscles within the foot results in nonfunctioning intrinsic foot muscles referred to as an "intrinsic minus foot" (see Fig. 62-1B).[37] The muscles showing early involvement are the flexor digitorum brevis, lumbricales, and interosseous muscles. These groups act to stabilize the proximal phalanx against the metatarsal head preventing dorsiflexion at the metatarsal phalangeal joint (MTPJ) during midstance in the gait cycle. With progression of the neuropathy, these muscles atrophy and fail to function properly. This causes the MTPJs to become unstable, allowing the long flexors (flexor digitorum longus and flexor hallucis longus) and extensors (extensor digitorum longus and extensor hallucis longus) to act unchecked on the digits. Dorsal contractures develop at the MTPJs with development of hammer digit syndrome, also known as *intrinsic minus disease.*

The deformity acts to plantarflex the metatarsals, making the heads more prominent and increasing the plantar pressure created beneath them (see Fig. 62-1B). It also acts to decrease the amount of toe weight bearing during the gait cycle, which also increases pressure on the metatarsal heads. Normal anatomy consists of a metatarsal fat pad located plantar to the MTPJs. This structure helps to dissipate pressures on the metatarsal heads from the ground. When the hammer digit deformity occurs, the fat pad migrates distally and becomes nonfunctional. This results in elevated plantar pressures that increase the risk of skin breakdown and ulceration due to shearing forces.[1]

Overpowering by the extrinsic foot muscles also leads to an equinus deformity at the ankle, and a varus hindfoot. A cavovarus foot type can develop, leading to decreased range of motion of the pedal joints, an inability to adapt to terrain, and low tolerance to shock. In essence, a mobile adapter is converted to a rigid lever. Pressure is equal to body weight divided by surface area, thus decreasing surface area below a metatarsal head with concomitant rigid deformities and leading to increased forces or pressure to the sole of the foot. When neuropathic foot disease is associated with congenital foot deformities such as long or short metatarsals, a plantarflexed metatarsal, abnormalities in the metatarsal parabola, or a Charcot's foot (see Fig. 62-2D), there is a higher propensity toward breakdown as a result of increased and abnormal plantar foot pressures.

Increasing body weight and decreasing the surface area of contact of the foot components with the ground increases pressure. A low pressure but constant insult over an extended period can have the same ulcerogenic effect as high pressure over a shorter period. This is typical of the effect of tight-fitting shoes. If the magnitude of these forces in a given area is large enough, either skin loss or hypertrophy of the stratum corneum (callus) occurs (see Fig. 62-1C). The presence of callus in patients with neuropathy should raise a red flag because the risk of ulceration in a callused area is increased by two orders of magnitude.

Arterial Disease

One of the major factors affecting diabetic foot disease is the development of lower extremity arterial disease. Peripheral arterial disease is estimated to be 2 to 4 times more common in persons with diabetes than in others (see Chapter 14).[23,38] Atherosclerosis occurs at a younger age in persons with diabetes than in others, and its hallmark is the involvement of the tibioperoneal vessels with sparing of the pedal vessels. In addition to being more prevalent in diabetics, atherosclerosis is more accelerated and results in a higher rate of amputations.[39-41] Lesions in persons with diabetes tend to localize to the infracrural region. The relative sparing of the pedal vessels often assists pedal bypass. Occlusive lesions affecting the foot and precluding revascularization are not common in diabetic patients.[23]

Purely ischemic diabetic foot ulcers are uncommon, representing only 10% to 15% of ulcers in patients with diabetes. More commonly, ulcers have a mixed ischemic and neuropathic origin, representing 33% of diabetic foot ulcers.[23] The initiation of an ischemic ulcer usually requires a precipitating factor such as mechanical stress. Ulcers often develop on the dorsum of the foot, over the first and fifth metatarsal heads. A heel ulcer can develop from constant pressure applied while the heel is in a dependent position or during prolonged immobilization and bed rest. Once formed, the blood supply necessary to allow healing of an ulcer is greater than that needed to maintain intact skin. This leads to chronic ulcer development unless the blood supply is improved.

Infection

Patients with diabetes appear to be more prone to various infections than their nondiabetic counterparts. Several factors increase the risk of development of diabetic foot infections including diabetic neuropathy, peripheral arterial disease, and immunologic impairment. Several defects in immunologic response relate to increased infection risk in diabetics. Diabetic patients demonstrate a decrease in function of polymorphonuclear leukocytes that can manifest as a decrease in migration, phagocytosis, and decreased intracellular activity. Evidence suggests impaired cellular immune response, as well as abnormalities in complement function.[42,43] Some of the defects appear to improve with control of hyperglycemia.[44]

Undiagnosed clean neuropathic foot ulcers often convert to acute infections with abscess and/or cellulites.[45] Diabetic foot infections can be classified into those that are nonthreatening and those that are life or limb threatening. Non-limb-threatening diabetic foot infections arc often mild infections associated with a superficial ulcer. They often have less than 2 cm of surrounding cellulitis and demonstrate no signs of systemic toxicity. These infections have on average 2.1 organisms (Table 62-2).[45] Aerobic gram-positive cocci are the sole pathogens in 42% of these cases, with the most notable

TABLE 62-2 PERCENT FREQUENCY OF BACTERIAL ISOLATES FROM DIABETIC FOOT INFECTION

Organism	Louie (20)	Sapico (32)	Gibbons (100)	Wheat (54)	Calhoun (850)	Scher (65)	Grayson (96)	Leichter (55)
Staphylococcus aureus	35	25	54	37	45.9	35.4	56	27.3
Coagulase-negative staphylococci	30	9.3	32	32	22.6	27.7	12.5	40
Enterococcus	45	40.6	32	27	28.7	N/A	29	29
Proteus mirabilis	55	28.1	22	17	26.1	55.8	7.3	12.4
Pseudomonas aeruginosa	20	15.6	14	7	15.9	23.1	7.3	9.1
Bacteroides sp.	85	67	67	33	15.6	84.6	31	9.1

Modified from Caballero E, Frykberg R: Diabetic foot infections. J Foot Ankle Surg 37:248, 1998.

organisms being *Staphylococcus aureus*, coagulase-negative *S. aureus*, and streptococci. These less-severe infections can often be managed with local wound care, rest, elevation, and oral antibiotics on an outpatient basis. A foot infection in a diabetic patient can present with a more severe, life- or limb-threatening picture. In these patients, there is usually a deeper ulceration or an undrained abscess, gangrene, or necrotizing fasciitis. They tend to have greater than 2 cm of surrounding cellulitis, as well as lymphangitis and edema of the affected limb. These more severe cases generally present with fever, leukocytosis, and hyperglycemia.

In contrast to nondiabetic individuals, complex foot infections in diabetic patients usually involve multiple organisms. Studies report an average of five to eight different species per specimen.[46-49] These included a combination of gram-positive and -negative, as well as aerobic and anaerobic organisms. The most prevalent organisms identified were *S. aureus*, coagulase-negative *Staphylococcus*, group B *Streptococcus, Proteus, Escherichia coli, Pseudomonas*, and *Bacteroides*. Recently, methicillin-resistant *S. aureus* (MRSA) infection has become more common in diabetic foot ulcers and is associated with previous antibiotic treatment and prolonged time to healing.[50-52] Anaerobic infections with *Clostridium* are also not uncommon. These patients require immediate hospitalization, broad-spectrum IV antibiotics, and aggressive surgical débridement. Superficial wound cultures are often unreliable, as they may demonstrate organisms responsible for colonization that do not affect the associated infection. Deep wound or bone cultures are the best way to accurately assess the microbiology in a diabetic foot infection and to assess for osteomyelitis.

ASSESSMENT OF THE PATIENT WITH A LOWER EXTREMITY ULCER

Accurate diagnosis of the underlying cause of lower extremity ulceration is essential for successful treatment. The etiology of most leg ulcers can be ascertained quite accurately by careful, problem-focused history taking and physical examination. Diagnostic and laboratory studies are occasionally necessary to establish the diagnosis but are more often performed to guide treatment strategy.

History

Patients with ulcers due to venous insufficiency usually complain of aching and swelling of the legs. They may recount a history of recurrent cellulitis, previous deep vein thrombosis, or previous superficial venous surgery. Symptoms are often worse at the end of the day, exacerbated when the leg is dependent, and relieved by leg elevation.

Arterial insufficiency is suggested by a history of underlying cardiac or cerebrovascular disease, complaints of leg claudication or impotence, or pain in the distal foot when supine (rest pain) (see Chapter 17). Symptoms of arterial insufficiency occur because of inadequate perfusion to the lower extremity relative to its metabolism. Tissue hypoxia and the subsequent increase in concentration of lactic acid produce pain. Patients may complain of pain in the buttocks or calves brought on with activity and relieved with rest (intermittent claudication) or pain in the forefoot aggravated by elevation and relieved by dependency (rest pain). The presence of an extremity ulcer is an easily recognized but late sign of peripheral vascular insufficiency. Patients with lower extremity ulcers resulting from atherosclerotic disease usually have a risk-factor profile that includes: older age, male sex, smoking, diabetes mellitus, hypertension, hypercholesterolemia, and obesity.[23,53] Patients with leg ulcers and multiple atherosclerotic risk factors often have atherosclerosis in other arterial beds.[54]

Up to one third of patients with diabetes mellitus can have significant atherosclerotic disease, without specific symptoms. Most common complaints are those of neuropathic disease, which include history of numbness, paresthesias, and burning pain in the lower extremities. Patients often report previous episodes of foot ulcers and chronic skin infections.

Physical Examination

A complete examination can only be performed with the patient supine in an examination gown. The patient's vital signs are recorded and abnormalities noted. The patient's temperature, respiratory rate, heart rate, and blood pressure in both upper extremities should be obtained. Fever may indicate the presence of an infected ulcer, and the presence of tachycardia and tachypnea may support the diagnosis of a septic foot.

A classic look, listen, and feel examination includes inspection of the skin of the extremities, palpation of all peripheral pulses, measurement of ankle-brachial indices, assessment of extremity temperature, auscultation for bruits, and a thorough neurologic examination.

Visual inspection coupled with an accurate history can determine the presence of a chronic vascular condition (Fig. 62-3A). The color of the skin is conferred by the blood in the subpapillary layer and varies with the position of the extremity, temperature of the skin, and degree of blood oxygenation (reduced hemoglobin → blue). Also in chronic arterial insufficiency, the arterioles are maximally dilated as a compensatory response to the chronic ischemia intensifying color changes. In acute arterial occlusion the venules empty, leading to a chalky white appearance regardless of extremity position. Partial but inadequate perfusion either from an incomplete acute or chronic occlusion allows for pooling of blood in the venules, which may be red in the cold or blue at higher temperatures.

When the extremity is at the level of the heart, the pooled blood masks the color imparted by the arterial flow. Elevation of the extremity above the level of the central venous pressure (rarely >25 cm) allows the pooled venous blood to drain, enabling an accurate assessment of the degree of arterial flow. The normal extremity remains pink, whereas that with arterial insufficiency becomes pallid. Conversely, allowing the extremity to become dependent causes an intense rubor

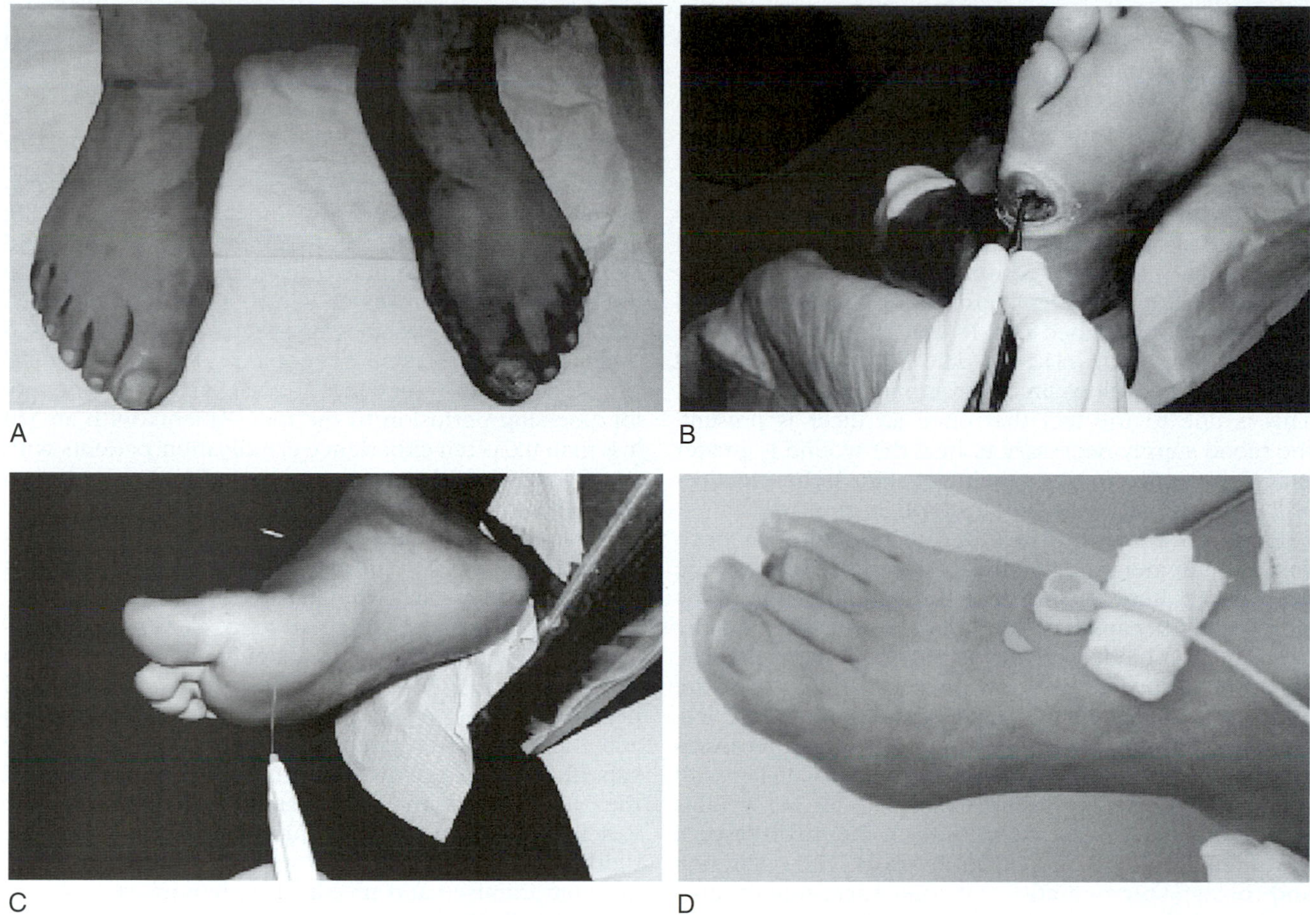

FIGURE 62-3. Examination of the foot. **A,** Visual. **B,** Probing the wound. **C,** Using Semmes-Weinstein monofilament. **D,** Transcutaneous oximetry.

or cyanosis. The time of return of blood to the dependent extremity is a useful marker of the severity of the deficit (normally <20 seconds). With a diminished nutritional supply to the skin, there is thinning and functional loss of the dermal appendages, evident as dry, shiny, and hairless skin. The nails may become brittle and ridged. Comparison of color and trophic changes between extremities gives a good indication of the severity of the process unless a bilateral deficit is present, in which case the experience of the examiner is required to make an accurate diagnosis.

Skin temperature is a reliable indicator of the blood flow rate in the dermal vessels, though flow is governed primarily by constriction or dilation of the arterioles to maintain a constant core temperature. Nevertheless, the temperature of the skin as a marker of perfusion is useful and can be assessed by lightly palpating the skin with the back of the hand and comparing similar sites from one extremity to the other. An ischemic limb is cool, and demarcation of temperature gives a rough indication of the level of the occlusion. Again, assessment of temperature differences is confounded when both extremities are affected.

In limbs of patients with venous insufficiency there is evidence of chronic edema. Venous hypertension causes transudation of serous fluid and RBCs into the subcutaneous tissue. Hemoglobin from the RBCs breaks down to produce the pigment hemosiderin, leading to hyperpigmentation, especially in the medial paramalleolar areas. Patients with venous insufficiency commonly develop stasis dermatitis. This eczematic process may spread from the area of the medial malleolus and involve the leg circumferentially. The recurrent cellulitis can cause contraction of the subcutaneous tissue in the lower third of the leg, below the knee, and together with the chronic edema can produce a "bottle leg" appearance.

Ulcer Evaluation

A thorough evaluation of ulcers of the lower extremity is critical in ascertaining the etiology and to institute an appropriate treatment strategy. Specific characteristics of the ulcer such as location, size, depth, and appearance should be recorded during the initial evaluation and with each subsequent follow-up visit to record progress and evaluate the treatment regimen. Ulcers of the foot should be gently examined with a cotton-tipped probe to establish the presence of a sinus tract. The margins of the ulcer should be undermined to evaluate the extent of tissue destruction. Ulcer extension to tendon, bone, or joint should be sought. A positive probe-to-bone finding (see Fig. 62-3B) has a high predictive value for osteomyelitis and is an extremely sensitive and cost-effective screen.[55]

Extremity ulcerations have a characteristic appearance depending on their origin. Ulcerations caused by ischemia are typically located on the tips of the toes (Fig. 62-2B) and between the digits. The lesions often appear punched out and are painful but exhibit little bleeding. Ischemic ulcers are characterized by absence of bleeding, pain, and a precipitating trauma or underlying foot deformity. They also often develop on the dorsum of the foot and over the first and fifth metatarsal heads. Ischemic ulcers are uncommon on the plantar surface as the pressure is usually less sustained and the perfusion better. A heel ulcer can develop from constant pressure applied while the heel is in a dependent position or during prolonged immobilization and bed rest. It should not be a surprise that a patient with relatively mild symptoms of arterial insufficiency develops limb-threatening extremity ulcers. This is due to the fact that once an ulcer is present, the blood supply necessary to heal the wound is greater than that needed to maintain intact skin. A chronic ulcer will develop unless the blood supply is improved.

Elevated venous pressure due to perforator or deep vein incompetency or venous thrombosis reduces the pressure gradient for perfusion. Inadequate tissue perfusion results because elevated venous pressure and the venous stasis hinder clearance of breakdown products. However, venous ulcers rarely present in the foot and are commonly located in the "gaiter" distribution of the leg, around the medial malleolus, where the venous pressures are highest. These are associated with a swollen leg with a distinctive skin appearance (see Fig. 62-2A). Venous ulcerations occur most commonly on the medial aspect of the ankle and are surrounded by areas with induration and brown pigmentation of the surrounding area (brawny induration) and scaling skin. These ulcers are often exquisitely tender and weep copious serous fluid.

The appearance of the extremity in venous insufficiency is distinctive and rarely poses a problem distinguishing between it and arterial insufficiency. It is important to differentiate the rubor associated with vascular insufficiency and cellulitis accompanying an infective process. Cellulitic color changes will persist despite extremity elevation. With isolated venous insufficiency, the extremity is warm and variably swollen with the characteristic skin changes described earlier. Acute or chronic arterial vascular insufficiency may be superimposed on the changes of chronic venous insufficiency, impairing the healing of the venous ulcer. In these situations, lower extremity revascularization may be required to assist in healing a venous ulceration that is not responding appropriately to compression therapy. Furthermore, the presence of significant lower extremity swelling or skin changes can complicate arterial reconstructions by altering the surgical approach to distal arterial target sites.

Neuropathic ulcerations typically occur at the heel or over the metatarsal heads on the plantar surface at pressure points (mal perforans ulcer) (see Fig. 62-2C) but may also occur in less characteristic locations secondary to trauma. They usually are painless. The sensory neuropathy in the diabetic patient may allow the destructive process to go unchecked, with extension into the deep plantar space and minimal appreciation by the patient.

In addition to ulcers, patients may present with varying degrees of tissue loss or frankly gangrenous digits, forefoot, or hindfoot. The presence of dry gangrene is a relatively stable process allowing for a complete vascular evaluation; however, any progression to an infected wet gangrene requires immediate surgical débridement.

Vascular Examination

A careful physical examination should be performed in patients with leg ulcers to elucidate the underlying cause of leg ulcers (see Chapter 9). The handheld Doppler ultrasound should be used in case of inability to easily palpate a given vessel. These can be supplemented with noninvasive vascular tests (see Chapter 10) and other diagnostic tests as necessary for each clinical situation. An ankle-brachial index is an important tool for assessing perfusion to the foot. Patients with an ABI less than 0.6 often experience claudication; patients with an ABI less than 0.3 may complain of rest pain; and in patients with tissue loss, the ABI is often less than 0.5.[56] In patients with diabetes and renal failure due to calcification of the vessel, ABI may be falsely elevated and is not reliable to evaluate the level of ischemia.

If the physical examination suggests venous insufficiency, a Trendelenburg test should be performed to assess valve function of the deep venous system and perforators. The patient is placed in a supine position and the legs are elevated. After decompression of the superficial veins occurs, a tourniquet is placed around the patient's thigh and the patient is asked to stand. If the varicose veins do not fill within 60 seconds below the tourniquet, the valves in deep system and perforators are not compromised and proximal saphenous vein incompetence is likely.

Neurologic Examination

The lower extremity neurologic examination is essential and should include testing for motor strength; deep-tendon reflexes; and vibratory, proprioceptive, and protective sensation. Chronic ischemia can cause varying patterns of sensory loss that is usually within the affected arterial distribution. Neuropathy occurs in 42% of patients with diabetes within 20 years after diagnosis of the disease.[27] The neuropathy alters motor, sensory, and autonomic function, which directly affect the dynamic function of the foot during gait. The gait of the patient should be observed to detect any gross asymmetry or unsteadiness.

Motor neuropathy is associated with demyelinization and motor end-plate damage, which contribute to conduction defects. Atrophy of the small intrinsic muscles of the foot occurs secondary to the distal motor nerve damage. Wasting of the lumbric and interosseous muscles of the foot results in collapse of the arch and loss of stability of metatarsal-phalangeal joints during midstance of the gait.[1] Overpowering by extrinsic muscles can lead to depression of the metatarsal heads, digital contractures, and cocked-up toes. These changes result in abnormal pressure points, increased shearing, and ulcer formation.

Diabetic sensory neuropathy is typically a glove-and-stocking distribution and is associated with a decrement in vibration and two-point discrimination. Loss of protective sensation due to peripheral neuropathy is the most common cause of ulceration in the diabetic population.

The use of monofilament gauges (Semmes-Weinstein) is a good objective way of assessing diabetic neuropathy (see Fig. 62-3C). Patients with normal foot sensation usually can feel a 4.17 monofilament (equivalent to 1 g of linear pressure). Patients who cannot detect a 5.07 monofilament when it buckles (equivalent to 10 g of linear pressure) are considered to have lost protective sensation.[57,59] Several cross-sectional studies have indicated that foot ulceration is strongly associated with elevated cutaneous pressure perception thresholds. Magnitudes of association, however, were provided in a case-control study,[60] where an unadjusted sevenfold risk of ulceration was observed in those patients (97% male) with insensitivity to the 5.07 monofilament.

The presence of neuropathy mandates attention to the biomechanics of the foot. The role of the podiatrist or foot surgeon in the evaluation of these patients cannot be underscored enough. Use of a computerized gait analysis system to assess abnormally high pressure areas has led to greater use of orthotic devices in the prevention of skin breakdown. For example, an F scan system uses an ultrathin Tekscan sensor consisting of 960 sensor cells (5 mm^2 each). The sensor is used in a floor mat system designed to measure barefoot or stocking-foot dynamic plantar pressures, indicating those subjects with pressures greater than or equal to 6 kg/cm^2. Abnormal mechanical forces that can result in ulcerations should be addressed with the use of offloading devices or other modalities in order to assist in wound healing.

Particular attention should be paid to documenting a complete neurologic examination on patients who have suffered from a previous stroke, as much of the rationale for extremity salvage hinges on the potential for rehabilitation. The remainder of the physical examination should be undertaken with attention to the presence of comorbidities, which may influence the decision-making process.

Tests and Imaging Techniques

The use of non-diagnostic imaging techniques by Duplex ultrasound has been covered in depth (see Chapter 10). Other noninvasive imaging methods useful in the assessment of patients with leg ulcers include plain radiography, MRI, and angiography (MRA) (see Chapter 11). Imaging techniques can be used to diagnose osteomyelitis and confirm the presence of bony deformities. Plain film radiography is used primarily to exclude bony lesions as a cause of a patient's pain complaints, assess the presence of osteomyelitis beneath a ulcerated foot lesion, and assess the degree of vascular wall calcification (usually in concert with standard IV contrast angiography). Plain films of the foot are relatively inexpensive and can show soft-tissue swelling, disruption of bone cortex, and periosteal elevation. MRI can provide details of pathologic anatomic features and has a high sensitivity for assessment of deep space infection and the presence of osteomyelitis in the diabetic foot.

The assessment of a patient with foot ulcers stemming from peripheral vascular disease encompasses a thorough history and physical examination with the adjunctive use of the noninvasive vascular laboratory to confirm, localize, and grade lesions.[56] While multiple noninvasive and invasive methods are available to assess the peripheral vasculature, it should be obvious that not every patient requires an exhaustive battery of tests in order to evaluate his or her vascular status. In general, only those tests likely to provide information that alters the course of action should be performed. Differing clinical syndromes mandate the extent of peripheral vascular testing. It is imperative that flow-limiting arterial lesions are evaluated and reconstructed or bypassed if ischemic foot ulcers are to heal.

MANAGEMENT OF ULCERS

General

Aggressive mechanical débridement, systemic antibiotic therapy, and strict non–weight bearing are the cornerstones for effective wound care.[61] Sharp débridement in the operating room or at the bedside, when applicable, allows for thorough removal of all necrotic material and optimizes the wound environment. All necrotic bone, plus a small portion of the uninvolved bone, soft tissue, and devascularized structures, should be excised, and the degree of penetration of the infection should be established. Curettage of any exposed or remaining cartilage is important to prevent this avascular structure from becoming a nidus of infection. Foot soaks, whirlpool therapy, or enzymatic débridement have a use but are rarely effective and may lead to further skin maceration or wound breakdown. No prospective randomized studies have demonstrated the superiority of dressing products compared with standard saline wet to dry sterile gauze in establishing a granulation bed. Use of moist dressings in clean, granulating wounds is recommended to enhance the wound environment.[20,62] An "ideal" dressing not only provides protection against further bacterial contamination but also maintains moisture balance, optimizes the wound pH, absorbs fibrinous fluids, and reduces local pain. Various dressings are currently available to target specific characteristics of the wound[63]; however, moist normal-saline dressings are probably sufficient for most wounds. These inexpensive dressings are highly absorptive of exudative drainage and maintain the moist environment.

In the presence of infection and cellulitis, oral antimicrobial therapy should be instituted on the basis of the suspected pathogen and clinical findings. Severe infections should be treated with broad-spectrum IV antibiotics.[64] After bacterial contamination has been controlled, small ulcers can usually be excised and closed immediately. Large open wounds, however, are treated with a staged approach, with frequent débridement and establishment of a granulation base. The clean wounds can then be closed with healthy tissue, with the use of local or free-flap coverage and soft-tissue repair. Meticulous surgical reconstruction of these wounds can help avert the production of inelastic scar tissue over weight-bearing surfaces. Any remaining extrinsic or intrinsic pressures can be reduced with the postoperative use of orthoses.

Surgical correction of biomechanical defects, plastic and soft-tissue reconstruction, and appropriate measures to minimize foot pressure are all essential to enable the patient to walk effectively again. In cases of gross wound infections and rampant cellulitis, use of a silver-containing medication such as Silvadene may be necessary in the initial setting to reduce the bacterial load. Oral antimicrobial therapy should be instituted on the basis of the suspected pathogen and clinical findings. IV antimicrobials should be administered for severe infections. Future advances such as use of bioactive drugs (e.g., Recombinant PDGF, Regranex) or skin substitutes (e.g., Apligraf, Dermagraft) are showing promising results and have proven useful under specific circumstances. A clinical practice algorithm for foot ulcers is seen in Figure 62-4.[65]

Off-loading strategies such as total contact casting or removable walkers has resulted in significant decreases in healing times. The stresses placed on the foot can be intrinsic, as was previously described with respect to

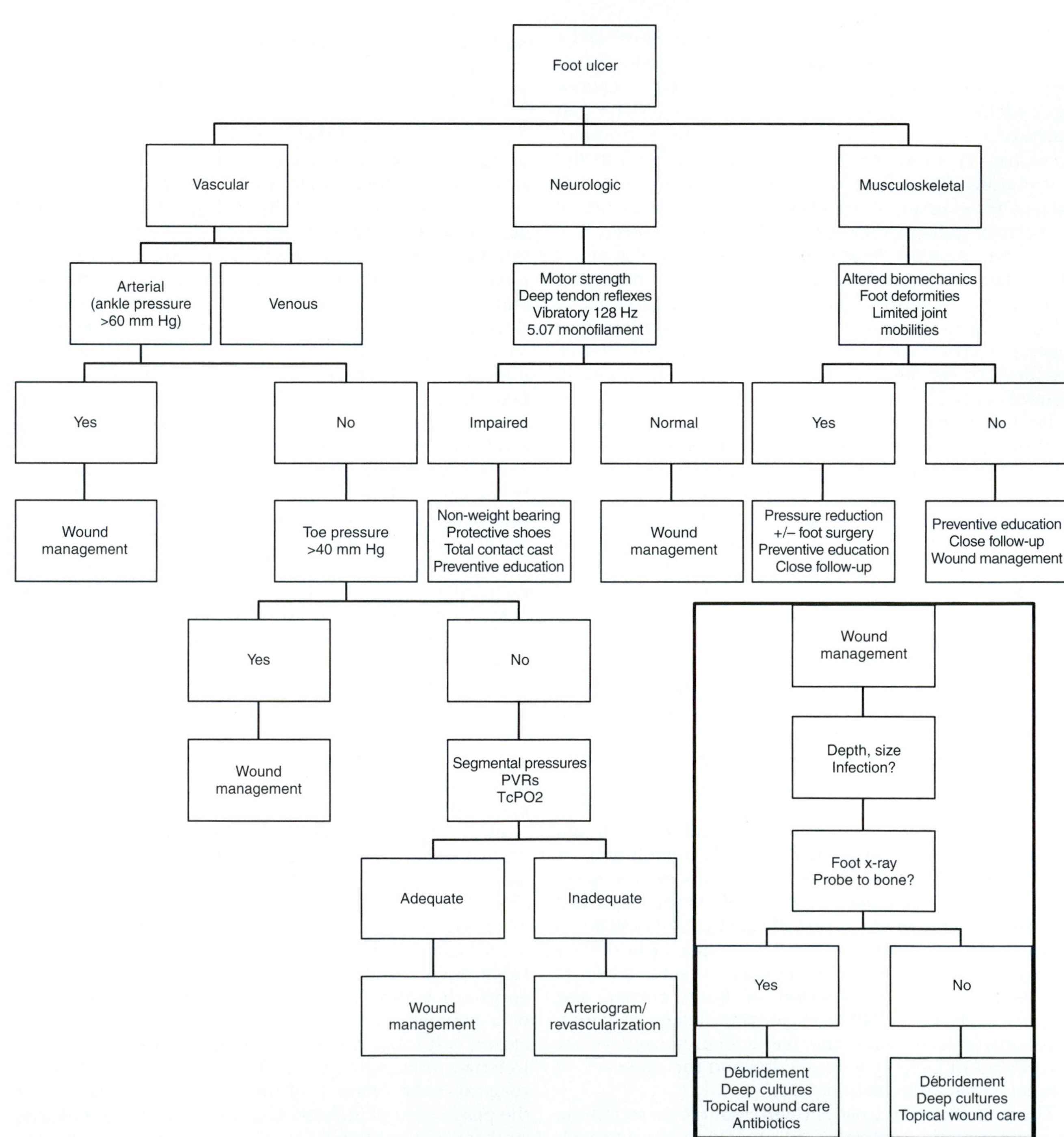

FIGURE 62-4. Algorithm for evaluation and management of foot ulcers.

digital contractures, or extrinsic in nature. These external forces can result from inappropriate footwear, traumatic injury, or foreign bodies. Shoes that are too tight or too shallow are a frequent yet preventable component to the development of neuropathic ulcers. Various shoe modifications such as the rocker-sole design and different types of insoles have made it possible to reduce plantar foot pressures, thus decreasing the risks of ulceration.[66,67]

Venous Ulcers

Elevation of the leg is a simple maneuver that can effectively but temporarily eliminate venous hypertension. All patients should be encouraged to elevate the affected leg above the level of the heart for 2 to 3 hours during the day and when lying in bed at night. Compression therapy is also effective in controlling edema and accelerates healing of ulcerations. However, before compression is applied to the limb, significant occlusive arterial disease should be excluded. Compression therapy is generally contraindicated in patients with an ABI less than 0.7 or with other signs and symptoms of compromised blood supply to the leg. Many different types of compression devices are available, including elastic and nonelastic bandages, graduated compression stockings, and compression pumps. The most effective way of delivering compression must be decided on an individual basis. Compression should be applied just before arising from bed and removed at bedtime.

Treatment of stasis dermatitis minimizes further trauma to the skin from scratching. Pruritus can be controlled by topically applied corticosteroids or orally administered antihistamines, or both. The goal of local wound care in patients with venous ulcers is to minimize stasis; decrease bacterial contamination of the ulcer; and provide a healthy, moist wound environment that promotes healing. Heavily contaminated venous ulcers with surrounding cellulitis may require systemic antibiotic therapy in addition to local wound control. The predominant organisms cultured from chronic ulcers are gram-positive pathogens like *S. aureus* and *Streptococcus pyogenes*. The most common gram-negative bacteria are *Pseudomonas aeruginosa*, especially in the diabetic population. Various moisture-retentive dressings can be used in conjunction with compression therapy to relieve pain, debride necrotic tissue, and promote granulation tissue formation.

The goal of surgical treatment in venous insufficiency is to correct underlying pathology. Surgical intervention can result in healing up to 90% of ulcers and modest long-term results if the diagnostic studies can adequately characterize and localize the incompetent superficial or perforating system valves.[68] Ulcer recurrence is significantly less after superficial venous surgery and use of compression stockings when compared with compression therapy alone.[69,70] If reflux exists in the deep venous system, ligation and stripping of the superficial veins has a poor result and high ulcer recurrence rate. For patients who are young and understand the importance of long-term compression therapy and adjunctive antiplatelet or anticoagulant therapy, reconstruction of vein valves can be recommended.[71,72]

Ischemic Ulcers

Management of ischemic ulcers follows some basic guiding principles. It is imperative that flow-limiting arterial lesions be evaluated and reconstructed or bypassed. In general, the optimal strategy is to perform revascularization, if indicated, as soon as possible. Closure of the ulcer by primary healing or secondary reconstructive surgery will then be expedited. If revascularization of an ischemic ulcer is not possible for medical or technical reasons, amputation of the foot or limb will most likely result. Contraindications to revascularization include nonambulatory patients and a foot phlegmon with sepsis or excessive foot gangrene, precluding a functional foot despite adjunctive plastic surgical procedures such as skin grafts and free flaps.

Nonoperative management of patients with lower extremity ischemia consists of general wound care measures. As a rule, however, severe ischemia of the lower limb generally requires an interventional approach. The method of revascularization of the affected limb depends on several factors, among the most important being the indications for surgery, the patient's operative risk, arteriographic findings, and available graft material. Chapter 20 reviewed these important issues.

Diabetic Ulcers

The role of a multidisciplinary group of consultants in the management of diabetic ulcers cannot be overemphasized. Successful management of foot ulcers involves recognition and correction of the underlying etiology, as well as appropriate wound care and prevention of recurrence. Assessment of the ulcer consists of determining the size and depth of the wound and inspection of the surrounding area for local signs of infection or gangrene. Several classification systems have been devised for descriptive purposes and act as prognostic indicators.[73]

The absence of systemic manifestations such as fever, chills, or leukocytosis is an unreliable indicator of underlying infection, especially in the diabetic immunocompromised population. The use of plain films to rule out osteomyelitis or deep culture of the wound is frequently necessary.

Neuropathic and Musculoskeletal Management

Reconstructive foot surgery may often become the conservative treatment in order to avoid major amputations in these chronic neuropathic wounds. The endpoint for chronic diabetic foot wounds should include reduction in the number of major amputations, prevention of infection, decreased probability of ulceration, maintenance of skin integrity, and improvement of function. Successful outcomes for diabetic foot reconstruction should result in less intrinsic pressures via minor amputations, arthroplasties, osteotomies, condylectomies, exostosectomies, tendon procedures, and joint arthrodesis. Open wounds can be treated in one stage and are primarily closed with premorbid tissue using local flap reconstruction and soft tissue repair.[74] Plastic surgical repair of these wounds can help avoid the production of inelastic scar tissue over weight-bearing surfaces. Extrinsic and intrinsic pressures can be further neutralized with postoperative accommodative shoe gear. Prophylactic diabetic foot surgery is an increasingly used option to prevent recurrent ulceration and reduce the risk of major amputations.[75,76] Surgical biomechanics, plastic and soft tissue reconstruction, and appropriate offloading are all essential to creating a stable platform from which to keep these difficult patients free from tissue breakdown and as functional as possible.

Treatment of these pedal soft tissue deficits in the diabetic patient population continues to be a medical and surgical challenge, which extends the length of the patient's disability and significantly increases the cost of medical care. Simple closure of these wounds is often difficult because of preexisting bone deformity, tissue inelasticity, location of the defect, and superimposed osteomyelitis. Clinical pathways related to diabetic foot ulcers frequently involve persistent sharp débridement, expensive wound care products, long-term IV antibiotics, total contact casting, total contact casting with tendo-Achilles lengthening, use of skin equivalents, electrical stimulation, multiple offloading orthopedic devices, and even amputation.

Wounds are often allowed to granulate, contract, and heal by secondary intention. When these wounds occur on the plantar aspect of the foot, they frequently recur since the resulting scar has decreased extensibility and mobility. Attempted primary wound closure of diabetic pedal defects is frequently unsuccessful and may be a sequela of inadequate wound assessment, lack of proper evaluation of comorbidities, and an inadequate treatment plan. Reconstructive surgery has traditionally been performed on select patients with severe deformities that cannot be accommodated by custom footwear. Recently, some authors have stressed the importance of addressing the underlying bony pathology in treating diabetic foot problems and have dispelled the unfounded fear of performing surgery on diabetic feet.[74-76]

Reconstructive surgery can range from simple metatarsal head resections to subtotal calcanectomies. Local flaps that are often difficult to elevate and inset are more easily mobilized and incised when concomitant bone resection is achieved at the time of flap creation. In addition, a local flap results in greater exposure and direct visualization of the underlying osseous structures compared with a single linear or semielliptical incision. The implementation of local random flaps can eliminate the need for additional incisions often deemed necessary to gain access to a forefoot, midfoot, or rearfoot bony defect.

SUMMARY

Chronic leg ulcers are frequently encountered in clinical practice. The cost of chronic nonhealing wounds is enormous. Considerable morbidity and mortality are associated with ulcerations of the lower limbs in diabetic and nondiabetic patients. The role of the primary care physician in the evaluation, diagnosis, and management of lower extremities wounds is critical. Careful assessment of vascular disease, evaluation and management of biomechanical and metabolic abnormalities, and aggressive treatment of any infections are required. The multidisciplinary approach provides a comprehensive treatment protocol and significantly increases the chances of successfully healing the ulcer and preventing recurrence.

Acknowledgment

Bauer E. Sumpio is supported by grants from the National Institute of Health (R01-HL47345) and the Veterans Administration (Merit Review). This work was supported in part from an unrestricted grant from the North American Foundation for Limb Preservation.

REFERENCES

1. Sumpio B: Foot ulcers. N Engl J Med 343:787, 2000.
2. Mekkes J, Loots M, Van Der Wal A, et al: Causes, investigation and treatment of leg ulceration. Br J Dermatol 148:388, 2003.
3. Clement D: Venous ulcer reappraisal: Insights from an international task force. Veins International Task Force. J Vasc Res 36:42, 1999.
4. Beauregard S: A survey of skin problems and skin care regimens in the elderly. Arch Dermatol 1:1638, 1987.
5. De Wolfe V: The prevention and management of chronic venous insufficiency. Prac Cardiol 1187:202, 1980.
6. Phillips T: Chronic cutaneous ulcers: Etiology and epidemiology. J Invest Dermatol 102:38S, 1994.
7. Ellison D, Hayes L, Lane C, et al: Evaluating the cost and efficacy of leg ulcer care provided in two large UK health authorities. J Wound Care 11:47, 2002.
8. Phillips T, Dover J: Leg ulcers. J Am Acad Dermatol 25:965, 1991.
9. Browse N, Burnand K: The postphlebitic syndrome: A new look. In Bergan J, Yao J (eds): Venous Problems. Chicago, Year Book, 1978, p 395.
10. Goldman M, Fronek A: The Alexander House Group: Consensus paper on venous leg ulcers. J Dermatol Surg Oncol 18:592, 1992.
11. Phillips T, Stanton B, Provan A: A study of the impact of leg ulcers on quality of life: Financial, social, and psychological implications. J Am Acad Dermatol 31:49, 1994.
12. Hutton W, Stokes I: The mechanics of the foot. In Klenerman L (ed): The Foot and Its Disorders. Oxford, Blackwell Scientific Publications, 1991, p 11.
13. Murray H, Boulton A: The pathophysiology of diabetic foot ulceration. Clin Podiatric Med Surg 12:1, 1995.
14. Phillips T: Leg ulcer management. Dermatol Nurs 8:333, 1996.
15. O'Donnell T, Browse N, Burnand K, et al: The socioeconomic effects of an iliofemoral venous thrombosis. J Surg Res 22:483, 1977.
16. Falanga V, Eaglstein W: The "trap" hypothesis of venous ulceration. Lancet 341:1006, 1993.
17. Burnand K, Clemenson G, Whimpster I, et al: Extravascular fibrin deposition in response to venous hypertension—the cause of venous ulcers. Br J Surg 63:660, 1976.
18. Browse NL: The etiology of venous ulceration. World J Surg 10:938, 1986.
19. Dodd H, Gaylarde P, Sarkany I: Skin oxygen tension in venous insufficiency of the lower leg. J R Soc Med 78:373, 1985.
20. Singer A, Clark R: Cutaneous wound healing. N Engl J Med 341: 738, 1999.
21. American Diabetes Association: Preventive foot care in people with diabetes [position statement]. Diabetes Care 26:S78, 2003.
22. Reiber G, Lipsky B, Gibbons G: The burden of diabetic foot ulcers. Am J Surg 176:5S, 1998.
23. Knox R, Dutch W, Blume P, et al: Diabetic foot disease. Int J Angiol 1:1, 2000.
24. Reiber GE, Boyko EJ, Smith DG: Lower extremity foot ulcers and amputations. In Harris M. (eds): Diabetes in America. Bethesda, Md, National Institutes of Health Publication, 1995, p 409.
25. Boulton A: The diabetic foot: A global view. Diabetes Metab Res Rev 16:S2, 2000.

26. Kamal K, Powell RJ, Sumpio BE: The pathobiology of diabetes mellitus: Implications for surgeons. J Am Coll Surg 183:271, 1996.
27. O'Brien I, Corrall R: Epidemiology of diabetes and its complications. N Engl J Med 318:1619, 1988.
28. Laing P: The development and complications of diabetic foot ulcers. Am J Surg 176:11S, 1998.
29. Lee L, Blume P, Sumpio B: Charcot joint disease in diabetes mellitus. Ann Vasc Surg 17:571, 2003.
30. Boulton A, Hardisty C, Betts R, et al: Dynamic foot pressure and other studies as diagnostic and management aids in diabetic neuropathy. Diabetes Care 6:26, 1983.
31. Veves A, Fernando D, Walewski P, et al: A study of plantar pressures in a diabetic clinic population. Foot 2:89, 1991.
32. Masson E, Hay E, Stockley I, et al: Abnormal foot pressures alone may not cause ulceration. Diabet Med 6:426, 1989.
33. Levin M: Diabetes and peripheral neuropathy. Diabetes Care 21: 1, 1998.
34. Fernando D, Masson E, Veves A, et al: Relationship of limited joint mobility to abnormal foot pressures and diabetic foot ulceration. Diabetes Care 14:8, 1991.
35. Morag E, Pammer S, Boulton A, et al: Structural and functional aspects of the diabetic foot. Clin Biomech 12:S9, 1997.
36. Saltzman C, Pedowitz W: Diabetic foot infection. AAOS Instructional Course Lectures 48:317, 1999.
37. Habershaw G, Chzran J: Biomechanical considerations of the diabetic foot. In Hutton W, Stokes I (eds): Management of Diabetic Foot Problems. Philadelphia, WB Saunders, 1995, p 53.
38. Bullock G, Stavosky J: Surgical wound management of the diabetic foot. Surg Technol Int 301, 2001.
39. Bild D, Selby J, Sinnock P, et al: Lower-extremity amputation in people with diabetes. Epidemiology and prevention. Diabetes Care 12:24, 1989.
40. Melton L, Macken K, Palumbo P, et al: Incidence and prevalence of clinical peripheral vascular disease in a population-based cohort of diabetic patients. Diabetes Care 3:650, 1980.
41. Kannel W, McGee D: Diabetes and cardiovascular disease. The Framingham study. JAMA 241:2035, 1979.
42. Hostetter M: Handicaps to host defense. Effects of hyperglycemia on C3 and *Candida albicans*. Diabetes Care 39:271, 1990.
43. Hostetter M, Krueger R, Schmeling D: The biochemistry of opsonization: Central role of the reactive thioester of the third component of complement. J Infect Dis 150:653, 1984.
44. MacRury S, Gemmell C, Paterson K, et al: Changes in phagocytic function with glycemic control in diabetic patients. J Clin Pathol 42:1143, 1989.
45. Caballero E, Frykberg R: Diabetic foot infections. J Foot Ankle Surg 37:248, 1998.
46. Louie T, Bartlett J, Tally F, et al: Aerobic and anaerobic bacteria in diabetic foot ulcers. Ann Intern Med 85:461, 1976.
47. Sapico F, Canawati H, Witte J, et al: Quantitative aerobic and anaerobic bacteriology of infected diabetic feet. J Clin Microbiol 12:413, 1980.
48. Sapico F, Witte J, Canawati H, et al: The infected foot of the diabetic patient: Quantitative microbiology and analysis of clinical features. Rev Infect Dis 6:S171, 1984.
49. Wheat L, Allen S, Henry M: Diabetic foot infections. Bacteriologic analysis. Arch Intern Med 146:1935, 1986.
50. Tentolouris N, Jude E, Smirnof I, et al: Methicillin-resistant *Staphylococcus aureus*: An increasing problem in a diabetic foot clinic. Diabet Med 16:767, 1999.
51. Dang C, Prasad Y, Boulton A, et al: Methicillin-resistant *Staphylococcus aureus* in the diabetic foot clinic: A worsening problem. Diabet Med 20:159, 2003.
52. Day M, Armstrong D: Factors associated with methicillin resistance in diabetic foot infections. J Foot Ankle Surg 36:322, 1997.
53. Sumpio B, Pradhan S: Artherosclerosis: Biological and surgical considerations. In Ascher E, Hollier L, Strandness D (eds): Haimovici's Vascular Surgery. Malden, Mass, Blackwell Science 2004, p 137.
54. Weitz J, Bynre J, Clagett P: Diagnosis and treatment of chronic arterial insufficiency of the lower extremities: A critical review. Circulation 94:3026, 1996.
55. Grayson M, Gibbons G, Balogh K, et al: Probing to bone in infected pedal ulcers: A clinical sign of underlying osteomyelitis in diabetic patients. JAMA 273:721, 1995.
56. Collins KA, Sumpio BE: Vascular assessment. Clin Podiatr Med Surg 17:171, 2000.
57. Armstrong D, Lavery L: Diabetic foot ulcers: Prevention, diagnosis and classification. Am Fam Physician 57:1325, 1998.
58. Kumar S, Fernando D, Veves A, et al: Semmes-Weinstein monofilaments: A simple, effective and inexpensive screening device for identifying diabetic patients at risk of foot ulceration. Diabetes Res Clin Pract 13:63, 1991.
59. Birke J, Sims D: Plantar sensory threshold in the ulcerative foot. Leprosy Rev 57:261, 1986.
60. McNeely M, Boyko E, Ahroni J, et al: The independent contributions of diabetic neuropathy and vasculopathy in foot ulceration: How great are the risks? Diabetes Care 18:216, 1995.
61. Steed D, Donohoe D, Webster M, et al: Effect of extensive debridement and treatment on the healing of diabetic foot ulcers. J Am Coll Surg 183:61, 1996.
62. Bergstrom N, Cuddigan J: Treating pressure ulcers, vol 1. Guideline Technical Report Number 15. Clinical Practice Guideline, National Center for Health Services Research 1-525, 1994.
63. Bello Y, Phillips T: Recent advances in wound healing. JAMA 283:716, 2000.
64. Joshi N, Caputo G, Weitekamp M, et al: Infections in patients with diabetes mellitus. N Engl J Med 341:1906, 1999.
65. Frykberg R, Armstrong D, Giurini J: Diabetic foot disorders. A clinical practice guideline. For the American College of Foot and Ankle Surgeons and the American College of Foot and Ankle Orthopedics and Medicine. J Foot Ankle Surg 1:1, 2000.
66. Barrow J, Hughes J, Clark P, et al: A study of the effect of wear on the pressure-relieving properties of foot orthosis. Foot 1:195, 1992.
67. Nawoczenski D, Birke J, Coleman W: Effect of rocker sole design on plantar forefoot pressures. J Am Podiatr Med Assoc 78:455, 1988.
68. Bello M, Scriven M, Hartshorne T, et al: Role of superficial venous surgery in the treatment of venous ulceration. Br J Surg 86:755, 1999.
69. Barwell J, Taylor M, Deacon J: Surgical correction of isolated superficial venous reflux reduces long-term recurrence rate in chronic venous leg ulcers. Eur J Vasc Endovasc Surg 20:363, 2000.
70. Ghauri A, Nyamekye I, Grabs A, et al: Influence of a specialised leg ulcer service and venous surgery on the outcome of venous leg ulcers. Eur J Vasc Endovasc Surg 16:238, 1998.
71. Plagnol P, Ciostek P, Grimaud J, et al: Autogenous valve reconstruction technique for post-thrombotic reflux. Ann Vasc Surg 13:339, 1999.
72. Eriksson I: Reconstruction of deep venous valves of the lower extremity. Surg Annu 24:211, 1992.
73. Frangos S, Kilaru S, Blume P, et al: Classification of diabetic foot ulcers: Improving communication. Int J Angiol 11:158, 2002.
74. Blume PA, Paragas LK, Sumpio BE, et al: Single-stage surgical treatment of noninfected diabetic foot ulcers. Plast Reconstr Surg 109:601, 2002.
75. Armstrong D, Lavery L, Stern S, et al: Is prophylactic diabetic foot surgery dangerous? J Foot Ankle Surg 35:585, 1996.
76. Catanzariti A, Blitch E, Karlock L: Elective foot and ankle surgery in the diabetic patient. J Foot Ankle Surg 34:23, 1995.

chapter 63

Vascular Trauma

James O. Menzoian
Joseph D. Raffetto
Christopher H. Gram
Melinda Aquino

The management of patients with vascular injuries has been enhanced by the pioneering studies of DeBakey and Simeone reporting on their experience in World War II,[1] Hughes reporting on the experience from the Korean Conflict,[2] and Rich and Hughes reporting on the experience from the Vietnam Conflict.[3,4] Although the severity and complications of military injuries are usually greater than those incurred from civilian trauma, management principles gleaned from these experiences have greatly benefited our treatment of these complex injuries. Rapid triage, adequate resuscitation, control of bleeding, management of fractures and soft tissue, and principles of surgical repair used in the management of civilian vascular injuries are based on lessons learned from extensive military experience. The following pages detail the epidemiology, pathophysiology, evaluation, and treatment of patients with vascular injuries incurred from blunt, penetrating, and iatrogenic trauma.

EPIDEMIOLOGY OF CIVILIAN VASCULAR TRAUMA

Etiology and Incidence

The etiology of civilian vascular trauma is either blunt or penetrating injury. Most series report a 10% to 15% incidence of blunt injuries, mostly from motor vehicle accidents.[5] The remaining injuries are penetrating, with about 50% firearm injury and 30% to 40% from sharp instruments such as knives or glass. Arterial injuries are most common, and isolated venous injuries are least common.[5] A venous injury is more likely to occur in combination with arterial injury. Traumatic vascular injuries are most common in the extremities, which account for 75% of vascular injury. Of these injuries, lower extremity injuries are slightly more common than upper extremity injuries. Other common sites of arterial trauma (in decreasing order) are cervical, visceral, and aortic injuries. Most series report young males to be the most frequent vascular trauma victims. Therefore the majority have few, if any, other significant health problems. In the elderly patient, the preexistence of atherosclerotic disease, particularly peripheral arterial disease, is important in the assessment of the magnitude of injury and consideration for repair.

Data obtained from the American College of Surgeons National Trauma Data Bank Report of 2002 reveal a change in pattern of trauma in the United States. Penetrating injuries occur predominantly in males, with a peak frequency between ages 18 and 21 and a second peak between ages 36 and 37. Curiously, of all the injuries in this large database, 11% are injuries due to violence (gunshots, shotguns, and fights). Gunshot wounds had the highest mortality with more than 16% of these patients dying from their injuries.

Pathophysiology of Vascular Trauma

Thorough knowledge of the mechanism of injury is essential in the initial patient assessment. With penetrating injuries, it is helpful to know the type of weapon, angle of entry, and depth of penetration, but this information is often unknown. Vascular injuries caused by blunt trauma are increasing as traffic and roadways increase and the size of vehicles increases. The vector of the blunt force may directly traumatize a vascular structure (Fig. 63-1). Another type of blunt injury is caused by the shearing force of rapid deceleration on a fixed point in a blood vessel. This most commonly occurs in the thoracic aorta distal to the left subclavian artery at the attachment of the ligamentum arteriosum. Vehicular accidents often cause multiple injuries, and frequently an

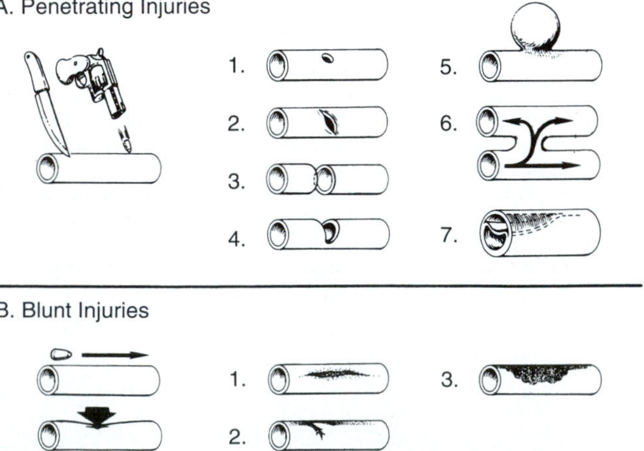

FIGURE 63-1. Mechanisms of vascular injury. **A,** Penetrating injury: (1) puncture, (2) laceration, (3) complete transection, (4) partial transection, (5) aneurysm, (6) arteriovenous fistula, and (7) dissection. **B,** Nonpenetrating injury (external compression or blast effect): (1) intimal contusion, (2) intimal flap, and (3) intimal injury with thrombosis.

associated fracture or dislocation causes vascular damage. The popliteal artery and vein, for example, are likely to be traumatized by a posterior dislocation of the knee.

With penetrating wounds from sharp instruments and low-velocity bullets, the damage is usually limited to the wound tract (see Fig. 63-1). The energy carried in higher-velocity missiles is transmitted to the surrounding tissues, outside the wound tract. This "blast effect" can cause vessel damage, even if the bullet itself does not strike the vascular structures. Severe concomitant soft-tissue injury can occur with high-velocity missiles, as well as with close-range but lower-velocity gunshot wounds.

Iatrogenic vascular injuries resulting from diagnostic and therapeutic intervention, as well as those from IV drug abuse, are increasingly common. Penetrating injuries result in punctures, lacerations, and transections of blood vessels. Indirect bullet injury may cause an intimal disruption, although the outer layers of the arterial wall remain intact. Similar intimal injury may also result from blunt trauma, which may crack the intima, raising a flap that protrudes into the lumen, or denude the endothelial surface, providing a nidus for thrombosis (Fig. 63-2).

The puncture site of an artery may form a false aneurysm, which may be detected at the time of puncture or at a later date. False aneurysms are prone to infection or rupture. A fistula between an artery and vein may result from injury to both structures. These may develop at the time of the initial injury or at a later date. Embolization of arterial wall or missile fragments from the entry site to a distant location is a rare but reported occurrence. A dissection of the arterial wall, forming a false lumen, may occasionally result from blunt or penetrating trauma. It is most often seen, however, in iatrogenic catheter injury.

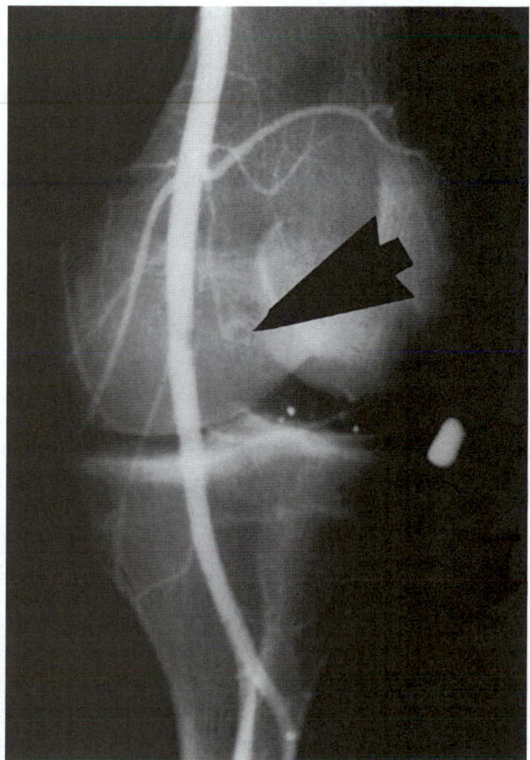

FIGURE 63-2. Gunshot wound of the popliteal fossa. Patient had intact pedal pulses. An angiogram was performed and showed an intimal disruption (*arrowhead*). At surgery the popliteal artery had thrombosed.

The multilayer wall structure of the artery and vein influence the outcome of vascular injury. The more muscular medial layer of the artery permits an injured artery to contract and thrombose more readily than the thin-walled vein. The intact intima of the artery and vein has numerous mechanisms to prevent thrombosis, whereas the underlying medial and adventitial layers are actually thrombogenic. Therefore endothelial injury promotes intravascular thrombosis.

The anatomic proximity of nerves to arteries and veins is important in the recognition of vascular injury. A neurologic deficit may alert the astute physician to the possibility of an arterial or venous injury that may not otherwise be readily apparent. In one report, compression neuropathies of the brachial plexus were the first sign of traumatic pseudoaneurysms of the axillary artery.[6]

A compartment syndrome may result from vascular injury, or it may cause extrinsic vascular compression and thrombosis. This syndrome occurs when increased pressure in the noncompliant fascia of extremities compromises circulation and neuromuscular function in that anatomic space. Major soft-tissue injury, arterial or venous bleeding, prolonged ischemia, or intra-arterial injection of drugs are the more common causes of compartment syndrome. Increased pressure within the compartment further compromises circulation, leading to muscle edema, higher compartment pressures, and a progressively worsening ischemic limb. If left untreated, this syndrome causes permanent destruction of the neurovascular structures in the compartment. Systemic manifestations of advanced compartment syndrome are also seen. The toxic effects of severe ischemic muscle catabolism lead to systemic acidosis, hyperkalemia, and hypovolemia, which may result in multisystem failure and death.

Initial Clinical Assessment and Management

Initial assessment of the trauma victim should begin with the primary survey, including the establishment of a definitive airway if needed, and assurance of adequate ventilation. In a hemodynamically unstable patient, control of the airway precedes any further evaluation.

Assessment of the hemodynamic status of a patient is next. Initially, this includes measurement of the pulse and blood pressure. The presence of a peripheral pulse correlates with a systolic blood pressure of at least 90 mm Hg, and the absence of a peripheral pulse with a present carotid pulse usually correlates with a systolic pressure of about 60 mm Hg. Tachycardia is an early but nonspecific sign of hypovolemia and possibly hemorrhagic shock. However, most healthy trauma victims can maintain a near-normal blood pressure with tachycardia and peripheral vasoconstriction until their blood losses exceed 30%. Therefore a "normal" blood pressure in a trauma patient should not be interpreted as assurance of a stable patient. The Advanced Cardiac Life Support study has categorized hemorrhagic shock into four stages (Table 63-1).

TABLE 63-1 CLASSIFICATION OF HEMORRHAGIC SHOCK (ACLS,* 1993)

	Class I	Class II	Class III	Class IV
Blood loss (ml)	<750 ml	750-1500 ml	1500-2000 ml	>2000 ml
Blood loss (%)	<15%	15-30%	30-40%	>40%
Heart rate	<100	100-120	120-140	>140
Respiratory rate	14-20	20-30	30-35	>35
Urinary output	>30	20-30	5-15	None
Level of consciousness	Anxious	Agitated	Confused	Lethargic
Blood pressure	Normal	Normal	Decreased	Decreased

*ACLS, Advanced Cardiac Life Support.

The initial evaluation should proceed with assessment of the major injuries, including those to the neck, chest, mediastinum, abdomen, and pelvis, and obvious extremity deformities. Large-bore IV access is established, and a Foley catheter is placed if there is no sign of pelvic trauma. In the case of vascular injuries with hemorrhagic shock, control of bleeding is a priority before aggressive fluid resuscitation. Sudden increases in blood pressure should be avoided. Hemodynamically unstable patients should have a radiologic assessment of their cervical spine, chest, and pelvis (usually with portable radiographs) and either a focused abdominal sonogram in trauma (FAST) ultrasound or diagnostic peritoneal lavage (DPL) to quickly assess the source of bleeding before operative management.

In a hemodynamically stable patient with possible vascular injury, a careful history is essential. The mechanism of injury should be obtained from the patient, emergency personnel, and witnesses. For example, the size, type, and trajectory of the weapon are critical in determining the likelihood of injury.

The clinical signs of vascular trauma are divided into "hard" and "soft" signs (Table 63-2). These signs should be carefully elicited through the history and physical examination because the presence or absence of these signs stratify patients into high, moderate, and low likelihoods of sustaining vascular injury. Patients with one or more hard signs have a high likelihood of having sustained an arterial injury. In one study, the presence of a bruit or thrill had a 100% correlation with arterial injury, absent pulses had a 90% correlation, and active hemorrhage correlated with arterial injury in 82% of patients.[5] In any suspected injury, an arterial pressure index (API) should be determined. This is the measurement of systolic pressure in the injured limb divided by that in the uninjured limb. In one study, an API of less than 0.9 had 95% sensitivity and 97% specificity for identifying occult arterial injury. Soft signs should alert the physician to the possibility of vascular injury that may not have been otherwise diagnosed. Therefore a large blood loss or pulsatile bleeding witnessed at the scene indicate possible arterial injury, even if there is no obvious bleeding at the time of the examination. This underscores the importance of a careful history.

TABLE 63-2 HARD AND SOFT SIGNS OF ARTERIAL INJURY

Hard Signs	Soft Signs
Pulsatile arterial bleeding from the wound	Neurologic injury in proximity to a major vessel
Ischemia	Unexplained hypotension
• Pulselessness	History of pulsatile blood loss at the scene
• Paresthesias	Nonexpanding hematoma
• Pallor	Unexplained hypotension
• Poikilothermy	
Bruit or thrill	
Rapidly expanding hematoma	
Arterial pressure index <.9	

Any history of preexisting vascular disease such as intermittent claudication or rest pain is helpful in evaluating patients with suspected vascular injury. This is especially true in elderly patients, where absent pulses could be related to long-standing atherosclerosis and not to vascular trauma.

The physical assessment for vascular injuries should proceed in a systematic fashion. The injury should be evaluated first for hard signs of vascular injury, including the presence or absence of pulses, skin temperature, sensory and motor deficits, or the presence of a hematoma or thrill. If these hard signs are absent, the wound should be assessed for its proximity to major vessels. If injury is suspected, the API should be obtained. The presence of a deformity or fracture is important, since certain orthopedic injuries have a high correlation with vascular injuries (e.g., posterior knee dislocation, popliteal artery injury, distal humerus fracture, brachial artery injury). However, in patients who do not have these signs but rather have an injury that is simply in proximity to a major vessel, only 20% were found to have positive findings on exploration. Therefore angiography is used for patients with an injury in proximity to a major vessel, if there are diminished or unequal pulses, or if the API is less than 0.9.[7]

Noninvasive Evaluation

Doppler assessment of an injured extremity is especially helpful in patients with absent distal pulses. The quality of the Doppler sound, as well as a Doppler ankle-brachial index (ABI) (see Chapter 10) determination, is helpful in diagnosing an arterial injury, as well as providing a baseline that can be followed during the course of therapy. A decreased ABI and abnormal arterial waveform analysis should raise suspicion of a significant arterial injury. Noninvasive evaluation using Doppler assessment can reliably exclude major occult arterial damage in injured extremities. Screening for such injuries using the ABI and reserving arteriography for those extremities in which the ABI is less than 0.9 is safe, accurate, and cost effective.[8]

Duplex ultrasonography has been advocated in diagnosing arterial injuries.[9-11] Its advantages are that it is noninvasive, can be promptly obtained even in the emergency department setting, and can eliminate the risks of invasive arteriography. Studies have reported excellent sensitivity and specificity when comparing the results of duplex scanning with arteriography in the management of vascular trauma. It may be that in centers where this modality is available on a 24-hour basis, duplex imaging could replace conventional angiography. As usual with any modality, it is suggested that each center assess the sensitivity and specificity of duplex ultrasonography compared with conventional angiography or surgical exploration, or both. In a clinical study comparing duplex ultrasonography with arteriography, duplex ultrasonography was able to reproduce the results of arteriography in diagnosing vascular injuries of the limbs and neck.[12] In patients with proximity-penetrating extremity trauma, duplex ultrasound was helpful in the detection of occult venous injuries.[13]

Radiography

Plain films of the injured area should be obtained to confirm obvious bone injuries. Additionally, the chest radiograph may demonstrate mediastinal widening or capping of the apical pleura in patients with significant mediastinal vascular or thoracic outlet injuries. Abdominal films may demonstrate obliteration of the psoas muscle margin, suggesting retroperitoneal hematoma.

Arteriography

The liberal yet judicious use of arteriography has been extremely helpful in evaluating patients with possible vascular injuries.[14,15] In extremity injuries, if time permits and the patient is hemodynamically stable, angiography can specifically localize the injury (Fig. 63-3). On the other hand, immediate surgical exploration is warranted if the patient or the extremity is at risk due to active bleeding or severe ischemia. In this case, an intraoperative angiogram can be performed if needed.

In patients with injuries in proximity to major vessels, arteriography may be useful, since about 12% of these patients show a significant finding on angiography that was not clinically suspected (Fig. 63-4).[5,16,17] Recent data, however, have suggested that this approach may be less fruitful than expected and that proximity angiography may not be indicated in all instances.[18-21]

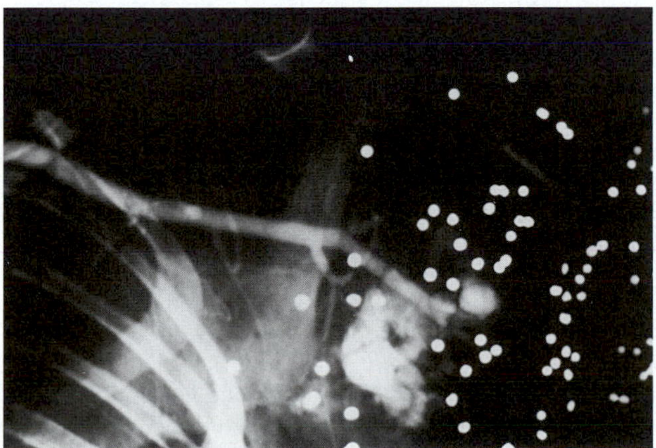

FIGURE 63-3. This angiogram was obtained to localize the clinically evident arterial injury. The axillary artery is thrombosed, and evidence of a pseudoaneurysm (contrast extravasation) exists. The massive amount of soft tissue injury precluded clinical localization of the arterial injury, making arteriography invaluable for localization and operative planning.

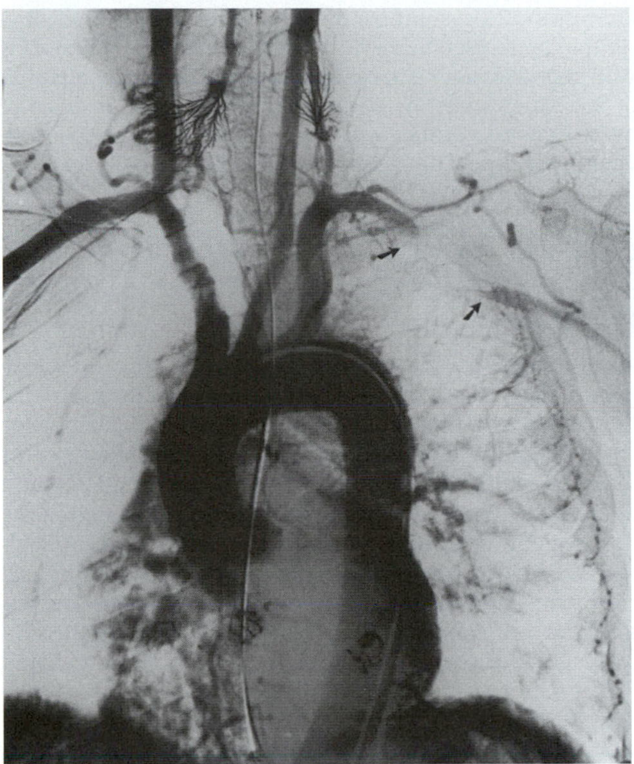

FIGURE 63-4. Patient with a fractured left clavicle from blunt trauma that had a diminished radial artery pulse. Angiogram reveals a thrombosed axillary artery (*arrows*) secondary to direct trauma with arterial contusion and thrombosis.

Arteriography is essential in patients with a widened mediastinum or first-rib fractures with the possibility of thoracic outlet injury. Patients with hematuria and suspected renal artery injuries, large retroperitoneal hematomas, and pelvic fractures with significant blood loss should also undergo arteriography, although each patient must be evaluated individually.

The use of MRA can also be helpful in certain types of injuries. This has been especially rewarding in injuries to the carotid and vertebral vessels. It can also be helpful in extremity trauma. However, in order to achieve a high-quality examination, a cooperative, stable patient is a requirement, and this is often not the case in trauma victims.[22,23]

CT angiography has been of increasing value in trauma victims. It has the advantage of being an extremely fast study with good resolution.[24] A cooperative patient is also necessary, but because the time required to complete the test is shorter, the study has a relative advantage over MRA.[23]

Associated Injuries

In the complete evaluation of a traumatically injured patient, an awareness of associated injuries is essential in evaluating the possibility of a significant vascular injury. The association of vascular injuries with pelvic fractures, knee dislocation, supracondylar fractures of the femur, first-rib fractures, distal humerus fractures, and tibial fractures is well known. If any of these injuries exist, further evaluation of the patient must be undertaken, even in the absence of overt signs of significant vascular injury. The use of arteriography is especially helpful in these instances.

GENERAL ASPECTS OF TREATMENT

Priorities

As discussed earlier, the first objective is the establishment of the airway, breathing, and assessment of circulation. After this, the patient can be further evaluated for the possibility of a vascular injury. In the presence of active bleeding, direct pressure is the preferred method of control. Exploration of wounds in the emergency department for control of bleeding vessels is not recommended because it is impossible to get adequate vessel exposure, and the possibility of further injuring the vessels and associated nerves is high. A firm compression bandage over the site of bleeding should be attempted first, or alternatively, a blood pressure cuff placed above the site of injury should be inflated to greater than the systolic pressure. If this is unsuccessful, direct digital pressure is achieved by inserting a gloved finger in the wound. Manual pressure should not be released until the patient is in the operating room, where the surgeon can gain proximal and distal control of the injured vessel. This often requires prepping the patient while maintaining vascular control in the operative field. The use of a tourniquet to control hemorrhage is generally contraindicated, since it can cause significant soft-tissue ischemia. In select circumstances, however, it may be useful to achieve temporary control of active bleeding from an injured extremity until the time of surgical exploration.

In patients with significant chest trauma and the potential of superior vena cava, inferior vena cava, or subclavian vein injury, IV lines should not be placed in the injured extremity because the resuscitative fluids could be infused into the thoracic cavity. In cases of abdominal and pelvic trauma with hemodynamic instability, the use of an abdominal-pelvic towel wrap or C-clamp for external pelvic reduction can be helpful in tamponading active bleeding. Obvious fractures should be stabilized in the emergency department because, in many instances, this controls bleeding and enhances perfusion of the injured extremity.

In patients with active bleeding, direct transfer to the operating room is essential. Here, further resuscitative measures can be undertaken and prompt surgical exploration for the control of bleeding can be completed. Patients who have obvious vascular injury to an organ or limb that is not life threatening can undergo further stabilization and evaluation in the emergency department, but urgent surgical exploration should follow.

Preoperative Preparation

In patients requiring urgent surgery, preoperative preparation should include chest radiograph, electrocardiogram, baseline blood chemistries, evaluation of hemoglobin and hematocrit, a coagulation profile, and a blood bank sample. Baseline blood gases also are helpful. A Foley catheter should be placed to assess adequate fluid resuscitation. In penetrating injuries, a dose of preoperative antibiotics is also given (usually a first-generation cephalosporin) because repair of the vascular injury may require the placement of a prosthetic graft.[25] These should be continued for a total of no more than 24 hours.

Preoperative anticoagulants are generally contraindicated in patients with vascular injuries due to the high risk of hemorrhage. Limited exceptions exist, however. In patients with acute arterial occlusion, such as with a posterior dislocation of the knee and subsequent contusion and thrombosis of the popliteal artery, the judicious use of heparin can prevent clot propagation (away from the area of injury) that might occlude collateral blood supply to the injured extremity. These patients, however, require vigilant observation for the possibility of hemorrhage into the injured soft tissue.

Anesthesia

The type of anesthesia used for operative intervention in these patients should depend on the preference and expertise of the anesthesiologist. For many patients, regional anesthesia such as axillary or interscalene block for the upper extremity or spinal/epidural anesthesia for abdominal, pelvic, and lower-extremity injuries is safe and effective. However, general inhalation anesthesia can be administered more promptly and is usually the technique of choice. In patients in whom a significant blood loss is anticipated, the placement of a central venous or pulmonary artery (Swan-Ganz) catheter is helpful in monitoring hemodynamics and cardiac function. Intraoperatively, close monitoring of cardiac output, blood pressure, and urine production is critical. Significant blood loss should be replaced with blood, fresh frozen plasma, platelets, and calcium after multiple transfusions. Additionally, autotransfusion (cell-saver) systems are useful if there is no gross contamination in the operative field.

Arterial, Venous, and Orthopedic Injuries

In extremity trauma with combined vascular and orthopedic injuries, traditional teaching advocates orthopedic stabilization followed by vascular repair. In the case of a nonperfused limb, however, where prompt reperfusion is critical to limb salvage, the vascular repair must take priority.[26] In this case, fasciotomy usually is performed first, followed by repair of arterial and venous injuries, and finally by orthopedic stabilization. A critical amount of time can be lost if orthopedic stabilization is attempted first. An awareness of the need for fasciotomy is critical, since tissue perfusion suffers if a compartment syndrome exists. Once fasciotomy and vascular repair have been completed, close observation of the repaired vessels is necessary to ensure that there is no tension on the repair or injury to the graft during the period of orthopedic stabilization.

In patients with extensive soft-tissue trauma in association with vascular and orthopedic injuries, external fixation of the fracture is preferred. This allows for adequate postoperative monitoring of the soft-tissue injury, as well as arterial flow and neurologic function without obstruction from a cast. The external fixation device can then be removed and replaced with internal fixation once the soft tissue is healed or skin grafting is performed.

In the presence of an arterial injury, temporary indwelling synthetic shunts can be used to bridge the gap in the injured vessel and provide perfusion while other injuries are attended to.[27] Initial temporary vascular shunting in selected patients with combined skeletal soft tissue and vascular injury of the extremity may reduce the complications resulting from prolonged ischemia and also allow time for attention to other injuries.[28]

Numerous methods of repairing arterial injuries exist, including simple suturing of lacerations, end-to-end anastomosis of transected vessels, and interposition bypass grafts when the extent of the arterial defect precludes end-to-end repair. An autogenous vein is the preferred conduit, preferably the saphenous vein from the noninjured extremity. Vein grafts in young trauma victims have been demonstrated to have excellent long-term results.[29] If a saphenous vein is not available, a cephalic or basilic vein from the upper extremity can be used. When none of these is available, a synthetic material must be used. However, this is usually suboptimal, since these materials have greater potential for graft thrombosis and infection. Polytetrafluoroethylene (PTFE) has been shown to be far superior to Dacron in traumatic vascular repair.

Once the arterial repair is complete, angiography should be performed. Angiography delineates any technical problems, as well as any distal thrombosis that may not be clinically evident. This should be done in the operating room, with fluoroscopy if available. Once identified, any problems can be corrected, avoiding the possibility of a return to the operating room and minimizing the risk of subsequent graft thrombosis.

Significant venous injuries should be repaired if the patient's general condition allows. In some instances, venous ligation is necessary due to other multiple complex injuries.[30] When injured veins are repaired, there is less resultant soft-tissue edema and improved limb perfusion.[31] This is especially true when there are combined arterial and venous injuries.[32,33] Major veins can be repaired by lateral suture techniques; end-to-end anastomosis; and, in some instances, interposition vein grafts. An analysis of 191 major venous injuries by Sharma and colleagues[34] offered a treatment algorithm dictating which major venous injuries should be repaired or ligated. Considerations included hemodynamic stability, extent and location of injury, and clinical measurement of venous hypertension. In hemodynamically stable patients, major venous injuries were repaired. If the patient was hemodynamically unstable, an assessment of venous pressure either by direct stump pressure measurement or by clinical assessment was undertaken. If markedly engorged veins were present (suggesting venous hypertension), venous repair was performed.

One criticism of the repair of venous injuries has been the high rate of thrombosis following repair. Some evidence suggests that patients who undergo a venous repair with subsequent venous thrombosis can have recanalization of this thrombosed segment and thus have improved venous drainage of the extremity.[35]

In the case of soft tissue injury, devitalized tissue should be debrided aggressively. In patients with a large tissue defect or a fasciotomy, every effort should be made to cover the area of vascular repair with living tissue. The subcutaneous layer can be left open and subsequently repaired by delayed primary closure or by split-thickness skin grafting.

Postoperative Management

Following vascular repair, the patient must be monitored closely for signs of continued bleeding, failure of the arterial repair, progressive ischemia, and compartment syndrome. Anticoagulation is not routinely used following the repair of vascular injuries. In fact, anticoagulation is contraindicated in the face of significant concomitant soft-tissue and orthopedic injuries. The rare exception is those patients with isolated vascular injury undergoing venous repair who receive heparin to prevent local venous thrombosis. In this case, heparin is continued for a limited time in the postoperative period. Long-term anticoagulation is not recommended. In addition to this short course of heparin, external pneumatic compression devices are used to minimize edema, augment venous flow, and diminish the incidence of venous thrombosis.[36] Prophylactic antibiotic therapy is continued for a total of 24 hours in the perioperative period in patients with a penetrating injury and in those with a prosthetic vascular graft. If an autogenous vein is used for vascular repair in the absence of a penetrating injury, postoperative antibiotics are not necessary.

Reperfusion edema can occur following repair of an extremity vascular injury. This is manifest by pitting edema that develops rather precipitously and is likely related to a loss of capillary integrity during the ischemic period. If significant edema develops, an ultrasound evaluation of the extremity should be performed to assess for deep vein thrombosis. Reperfusion edema is usually short lived and disappears within a week to 10 days. Postoperative deep vein thrombosis is well known following vascular injury and is probably related to immobility and venous stasis in the injured extremity. In some patients, however, debilitating edema can persist. In these cases, compression-gradient elastic stockings should be used. If there is evidence of deep vein thrombosis, anticoagulant therapy should be initiated with IV heparin followed by oral warfarin sodium for at least 6 months.

Postoperative physical therapy is essential for patients with injured extremities and should be pursued as aggressively as possible given an individual patient's capabilities and injuries. Physical therapy has been shown to increase blood flow, decrease venous stasis and edema, and result in enhanced earlier mobility.

COMPLICATIONS OF VASCULAR TRAUMA

Complications of vascular trauma may be broadly divided into perioperative and late groups. Although these complications are similar to those encountered in vascular surgery in general, several problems characteristically occur in the setting of trauma.

Perioperative Complications

In the early postoperative period after vascular trauma, patients must be monitored closely. This requires serial vascular examinations. Two of the more commonly encountered early complications are thrombosis of the repaired vessel and hemorrhage. Numerous factors contribute to these early problems. Perioperative use of heparin and systemic coagulopathies in transfused patients, as well as those with severe multisystem injury, can contribute to hemorrhage. Most often, however, a discrete bleeding point is encountered.

The coexistence of extensive soft-tissue injury, as well as long-bone fractures, may contribute to early occlusion. These same factors may promote vascular spasm. This spasm may be particularly severe in the young trauma patient with otherwise normal vessels. Although this problem is frequently encountered, in general, ischemia in the early postoperative period should not be attributed to spasm without an arteriogram that demonstrates vascular patency.

Reperfusion injury is a perioperative complication that encompasses a wide range of pathologic effects. These can be classified either as local effects or systemic effects (Fig. 63-5). The pathologic endpoints of reperfusion injury may include limb loss or death, or both. The goal for anyone taking care of a patient who manifests the signs and symptoms of reperfusion syndrome should be to minimize the damage by anticipating its development and promptly treating it.

Local Effects of Reperfusion Injury: Compartment Syndrome

One of the most serious and preventable local complications of reperfusion injury is acute compartment syndrome. Of all the tissue present in the extremity compartments, nerve and skeletal muscle are the most vulnerable to ischemia. Ischemic tissue releases inflammatory cytokines that cause vasodilatation and increased capillary permeability. After 3 hours of muscle ischemia, one can anticipate that significant edema will develop after restoration of perfusion. This edema quickly becomes threatening to the affected extremity as the noncompliant fascial compartments resist expansion and intracompartment pressure quickly rises above capillary perfusion pressure.

Once this occurs, the patient has between 4 and 6 hours before permanent debilitating muscle loss occurs. This is a surgical emergency that requires immediate fasciotomy to prevent gangrene and limb loss. Although compartment syndrome can occur in numerous areas of the upper and lower extremity, the calf with its four compartments is at greatest risk. Furthermore, the anterior compartment of the calf, which contains the deep peroneal nerve, is almost always involved when compartment syndrome affects the leg.

The most important factor in preventing morbidity from compartment syndrome is early diagnosis and treatment. Early diagnosis depends on a high index of suspicion and careful examination. Compartment syndrome should be anticipated in the setting of delayed vascular repair (>6 hours), combined arterial and venous injuries, and associated soft-tissue injuries.

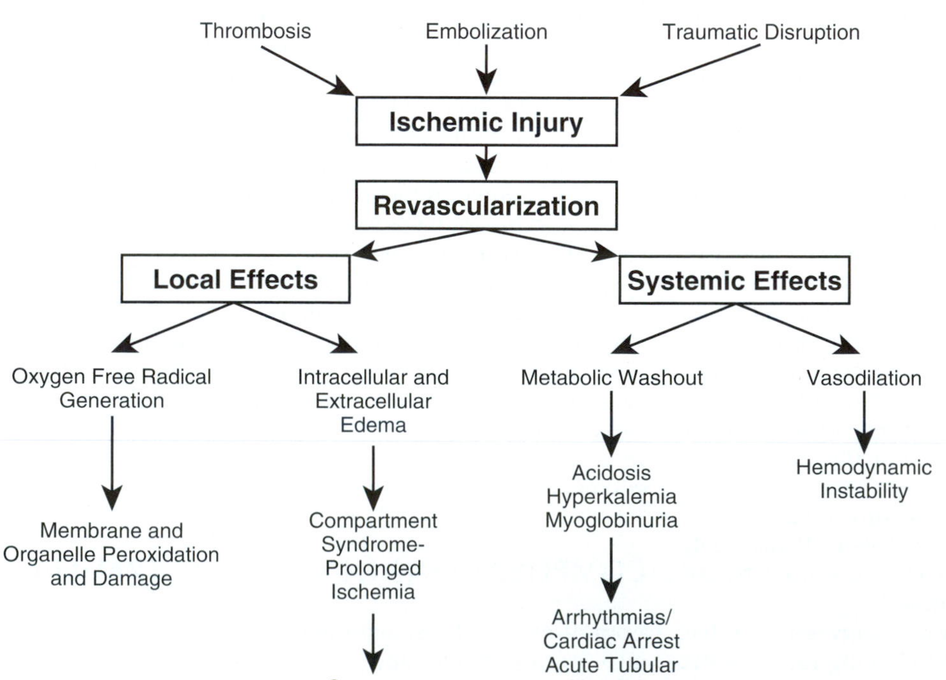

FIGURE 63-5. Ischemia-reperfusion syndrome. Combined local and systemic effects of reperfusion of ischemic muscle. See text for explanation.

Signs and symptoms of increasing compartment pressures include numbness and paresthesia in the extremity, pain over the compartments, firm compartments on examination, and decreased Doppler perfusion pressure. The presence of palpable arterial pulses is of no value in ruling out compartment syndrome, as pulses may persist long after capillary pressure is exceeded and nutrient flow has stopped. If a compartment syndrome is suspected, pressure measurements can be obtained using a Stryker solid-state transducer needle. Compartmental pressures are normally below 10 mm Hg. Pressures above 20 mm Hg are abnormal, and those above 40 mm Hg require surgical decompression.

The standard treatment of compartment syndrome is fasciotomy. Although multiple published techniques exist, a direct and simple method is described here. A medial longitudinal skin incision is made parallel and 2 cm posterior to the tibia, through which the superficial and deep posterior compartments are decompressed by incising the fascia overlying each compartment. An anterolateral incision between the tibia and fibula is then made, and the anterior and lateral compartments are decompressed in a similar fashion. When compartment syndrome is anticipated, prophylactic fasciotomies can be done at the time of the initial vascular repair.

A second mechanism for local tissue injury is the inflammatory cascade that occurs following restoration of perfusion. An ischemic limb usually has zones of varying degrees of ischemia, and it is in the marginal zone between reversibly and irreversibly damaged tissue that the mediators of inflammation have their greatest effect.[37] This reperfusion injury is mediated by oxygen-derived free radicals, which are generated by cellular enzymes when oxygen is reintroduced. The resultant superoxide, peroxide, and hydroxyl radicals lead to damage of the cell membranes through peroxidation of phospholipids. Membrane-bound organelles, such as lysosomes and mitochondria, are also disrupted. The potential therapeutic benefits of free radical scavengers, including superoxide dismutase and mannitol, have been demonstrated in various tissues including skeletal muscle.[38]

Activation of the clotting cascade causes further microvascular thrombosis and muscle damage, creating a vicious circle of worsening injury in the marginal zone. One method to arrest this process is the institution of systemic anticoagulation, usually with heparin. Heparin has been shown to have multiple beneficial effects in this situation. It acts primarily to prevent ongoing thrombosis, but it has also been found to decrease capillary leak in the involved tissue and so reduce the amount of interstitial edema.[39] Heparin also acts to inhibit the local inflammatory response when given in sufficient doses to completely stop clot propagation. To achieve an appropriate level of heparin in the affected tissue, larger-than-usual doses of the drug may be used, at least initially, until the inflammation-mediated vasospasm has abated. Heparin's beneficial effects, however, must be weighed against the potential for bleeding in the multiple-injured patient. Hence each patient needs individual assessment before instituting systemic heparin.

Systemic Effects of Reperfusion Injury

Reperfusion of a traumatized ischemic limb may have a profound systemic impact leading to a cascade of complications that may ultimately threaten the patient's life. Previously, renal failure was thought to be the predominant morbidity following reperfusion. With improvements in resuscitation and hemodynamic monitoring, pulmonary injury has replaced renal failure as the primary morbidity in these patients.

When perfusion is restored to the limb that has suffered ischemic myonecrosis, large amounts of acidic metabolites and potassium enter into the systemic circulation, resulting in acute acidosis and hyperkalemia, which can then cause vasomotor shock and cardiac arrhythmias or arrest. The magnitude of the systemic effect is proportional to the muscle mass of the involved limb and the duration of ischemia. Distal extremity trauma is expected to manifest predominantly local effects, while more proximal injuries have a greater chance of causing life-threatening systemic effects. The myonecrosis results in the release of myoglobin, which enters the circulation. Within a few hours the myoglobin appears in the urine, where acidic conditions lead to precipitation in the renal tubules. Oliguria with progression to acute tubular necrosis may result if prompt recognition does not occur and therapy is not employed.

Recognition is based on observation of the characteristic cherry-red urine discoloration, as well as urine chemistries detecting myoglobin. Treatment consists of alkalinization of the urine and the maintenance of a brisk osmotic diuresis with mannitol. Aggressive fluid replacement to maintain intravascular volume is essential. When prolonged ischemia (>6 hours) in the traumatized limb has resulted in a large necrotic muscle mass, the risk of morbid systemic effects in the face of a negligible chance of limb salvage may necessitate primary amputation. Currently the mainstays of treatment for systemic manifestation of reperfusion injury include aggressive fluid resuscitation, careful electrolyte management, and diuresis.

Late Complications of Vascular Trauma

The vast majority of late complications of vascular trauma are directly related to circumstances surrounding the vascular repair or injuries that were missed or underestimated at the time of injury. A wide variety of late complications have been reported. The most common and troublesome include graft infections, false aneurysm formation, arteriovenous fistulas, and post-traumatic pain syndrome (causalgia, reflex sympathetic dystrophy), which is known now as *complex regional pain syndrome (CRPS).*

Graft Infections (also see Chapter 61)

Infection of prosthetic vascular grafts is one of the most dreaded complications in vascular surgery. Under the ideal circumstances of clean, elective vascular procedures with appropriate prophylactic antibiotics, graft infection rates from 1.34% to 6% have been reported.[40] Infection generally presents months to years after the original surgery and can be a significant source of morbidity and mortality. Infection is usually related to direct contamination at the time of surgery. The incidence is increased in grafts involving groin anastomoses, contaminated wounds, and prolonged or emergent procedures. The infection may result in thrombosis or in infected false aneurysms when an anastomosis is involved or simply persistent sepsis when the graft is involved away from an anastomosis. Successful management of an infected graft is one of the greatest challenges in vascular surgery and depends on prompt recognition. The principles of treatment include removal of the infected graft, débridement of the infected tissue, effective antibiotic coverage, and revascularization through uninfected tissue planes.

The superior patency and resistance to infection of autogenous graft (such as saphenous vein) has led to its preferential use. This has been especially true in the setting of vascular trauma, where the emergent nature of the surgery and contaminated wounds are thought to predispose to infection of prosthetic graft material. Feliciano and associates[41] have reported on the use of 236 PTFE grafts in vascular wounds. Although long-term follow-up is limited, they found an acceptable patency (5.8% early arterial occlusion) and no graft infections in the absence of exposure of the graft or osteomyelitis. Advantages of PTFE grafts cited by these authors include immediate availability in various sizes and maintenance of structural integrity in the setting of infection (where autogenous vein grafts may weaken and rupture).

Regardless of the conduit ultimately chosen for vascular repair, successful avoidance of infection depends on adhering to several basic principles. These include the use of perioperative antibiotics, extensive débridement of devitalized and contaminated tissue, copious local irrigation with local antibiotic solution, and prompt revascularization of the ischemic tissue.

Traumatic Aneurysms

Chronic traumatic aneurysms generally arise from missed arterial injuries. In most instances, localized arterial disruption leads to a perivascular hematoma, which goes on to form a pseudoaneurysm. In other cases, blunt arterial injury leads to arterial wall weakening and true aneurysm formation. Traumatic aneurysms generally present as painless expanding pulsatile masses in patients with a previous history of trauma. Distal ischemia may occur in the setting of secondary thrombosis, and symptoms of neural compression may also occur. Abdominal and thoracic aneurysms are usually asymptomatic and often go unrecognized until a complication develops. Diagnostic work-up is based on complete angiographic evaluation. In some cases, ultrasound and CT scanning may be useful. Operative management is recommended because of the possibility of rupture, thrombosis, compression syndromes, and other problems.

The size of the aneurysm dictates the most appropriate treatment. Small distal aneurysms may be managed by simple ligation. Larger, more proximal aneurysms require more formal repair. After obtaining proximal and distal control, the aneurysm may be directly entered and the vessel repaired from within. In other cases where the artery is significantly damaged or distorted, resection of the aneurysm with repair by an interposition graft may be necessary. The results of these repairs are usually excellent.

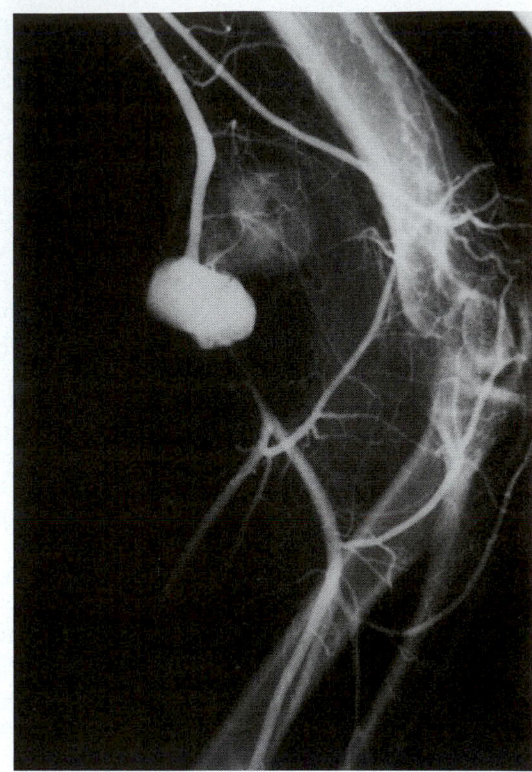

FIGURE 63-6. Brachial artery mycotic pseudoaneurysm secondary to IV drug abuse.

Another approach that is less invasive and increasingly common is the endovascular approach. This is especially useful in high-risk patients or in patients where the aneurysm is in an anatomically challenging area such as the subclavian artery (see later section on endovascular repair).

An increasingly common and difficult problem is mycotic pseudoaneurysm formation in drug abusers. These occur at various sites, but the femoral and brachial arteries are most commonly involved (Fig. 63-6). They usually result from direct arterial injury from contaminated needles, although secondary bacterial seeding from endocarditis is not unusual. *Staphylococcus aureus* accounts for the majority of these infections.[42] These patients often present late, after secondary complications have developed. Management generally involves wide excision, débridement, and aggressive antibiotic coverage. Vascular reconstruction is best reserved for cases demonstrating limb-threatening ischemia. These reconstructions usually require more complicated extra-anatomic bypass to avoid infection.

Chronic Traumatic Arteriovenous Fistulas

Traumatic arteriovenous (AV) fistulas generally result from penetrating injuries to contiguous arteries and veins. This allows the higher pressure arterial blood to flow directly into the lower pressure vein, which maintains the patency of the connection in the form of a fistula.

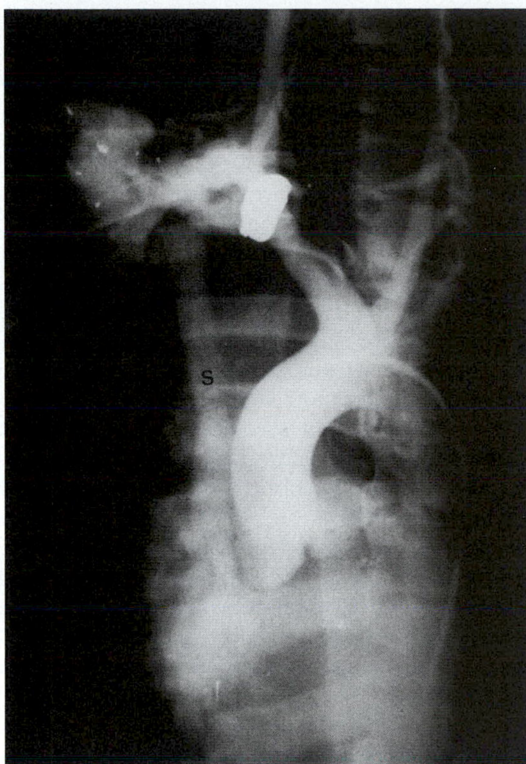

FIGURE 63-7. A traumatic arteriovenous fistula of the right subclavian artery and vein caused by a gunshot wound. Note the prompt filling of the superior vena cava (S).

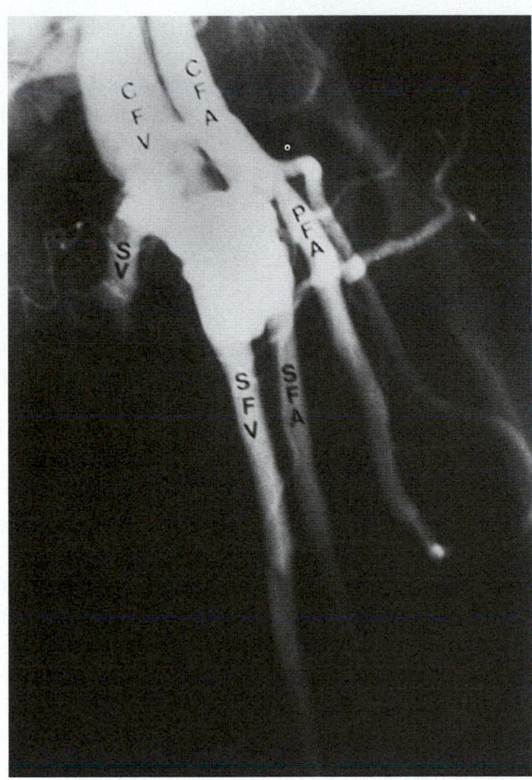

FIGURE 63-8. Combined injury with arteriovenous fistula and pseudoaneurysm secondary to a stab wound to the left groin. Note the early venous filling of the common femoral vein. CFA, common femoral artery; CFV, common femoral vein; PFA, profunda femoris artery; SFA, superficial femoral artery; SFV, superficial femoral vein; SV, saphenous vein.

These fistulas are rare and may be associated with traumatic aneurysms when they occur in the extremities (Figs. 63-7 and 63-8). Unlike traumatic aneurysms, however, AV fistulas may appear anywhere in the body. The presenting symptoms depend on the size of the fistula. The patient may note a pulsating mass or a thrill in the region of previous penetrating trauma. Large extremity fistulas may have the warmth of overlying skin, which contrasts with distal coolness. There may be signs of venous hypertension, including varicosities, and chronic venous insufficiency. Large fistulas may impose significant hemodynamic stresses including high-output cardiac failure.

The natural history of traumatic arteriovenous fistulas is one of gradual enlargement with increasingly severe hemodynamic changes. Operative repair is therefore recommended in low-risk patients. Preoperative evaluation should include complete angiographic studies to assess the size and location of the fistula. In some cases angiographic embolization may be sufficient to obliterate smaller distal fistulas. As with traumatic aneurysms, the type of repair depends on the location and size of the fistula. Small distal fistulas may be treated effectively by simple ligation of the involved artery and vein proximal and distal to the fistula. However, the repair of larger fistulas must restore continuity of both the arterial and venous conduits.

Well-established fistulas may be repaired by separating the artery and vein and suturing each primarily. Preferentially, however, a portion of the artery and vein is resected along with the fistula. The vessels can then be mobilized and repaired end to end, or an interposition vein graft can be used to restore continuity to both vessels. Successful repair generally leads to prompt hemodynamic and peripheral vascular improvement. As with traumatic aneurysms, endovascular treatment is becoming increasingly popular in the treatment of traumatic arteriovenous fistulas (see later section on endovascular repair).

Posttraumatic Pain Syndromes

Complex regional pain syndrome (CRPS) is a heterogeneous group of disorders involving neuropathic pain and multiple etiologies (see Chapter 52). The neuropathic symptoms may be due to abnormalities in any or all of the segments of the nervous system. The precise pathophysiology and appropriate treatment of this disease remain elusive. Many interventions to relieve pain have been tried in an effort to alleviate the symptoms. Most success has been achieved through a multidisciplinary approach with an understanding that relief may be a gradual process.[43,44] CRPS has been classified as either type I or type II.

In CRPS I (formerly known as reflex sympathetic dystrophy), there is no nerve lesion. Burning, deep, spontaneous pain is the characteristic complaint. One also sees disturbances of the skin circulation, abnormal sweating, and trophic disturbances of the joints and bones. The sympathetic dysfunction may lead to either vasodilatation or vasoconstriction. Surgical sympathectomy can be an effective treatment, but many patients will have residual symptoms requiring further therapy.

CRPS II (formerly known as causalgia) develops following a peripheral nerve injury. The symptoms are identical to CRPS I. Treatment can also include sympathectomy if other methods are unsuccessful.[45]

Although poorly understood, the posttraumatic syndrome of causalgia is a well-recognized and difficult problem. Causalgia occurs in both the upper and lower extremities following trauma. This trauma may or may not involve peripheral nerves. Although manifestations vary, the salient features include severe pain, sympathetic dysfunction, hyperhidrosis, delayed functional recovery, and trophic changes. Burning pain occurs in the distal extremity and may be accompanied by a severe cutaneous dysesthesia. The sympathetic dysfunction may lead to either vasodilatation or vasoconstriction. Surgical sympathectomy is the most effective treatment of this disabling pain syndrome. Although most patients are relieved of their pain, many have some residual symptoms. A sympathetic nerve block may be useful in confirming the diagnosis and in predicting the response to surgical sympathectomy. Chemical sympathectomy following sympathetic nerve block may be an alternative form of sympathetic ablation in some cases.

SPECIFIC ASPECTS OF DIAGNOSIS AND TREATMENT

Heart Injuries

Trauma to the heart may cause injury to the pericardium, free cardiac wall, cardiac septum, valves, or coronary arteries. The right ventricle is the most frequently injured chamber because of its anterior presentation, followed by the left ventricle, the right atrium, and the left atrium. Penetrating wounds of the heart can be caused by missiles, knives, ribs, or sternal bone fragments. They are frequently seen with precordial injury but may also be associated with injury to the neck, lateral thorax, back, or abdomen. The clinical course and presentation following penetrating heart injuries depend on the size of the hole in the heart, the associated coronary and intracardiac injury, and whether the pericardium remains open or fills with blood. The various signs and symptoms that may accompany penetrating cardiac injury include hemothorax, hemoperitoneum, hemorrhage, or cardiac tamponade. The physical signs of cardiac tamponade may include hypotension, paradoxic pulse (pulsus paradoxus is defined as a 10 mm Hg drop in systolic pressure during inspiration), narrow pulse pressure, a hypodynamic and rapid pulse, distant heart tones, or elevated central venous pressure (CVP). If cardiac tamponade is suspected, an immediate thoracotomy should be performed. In the stable patient who is suspected of having a hemopericardium, an echocardiogram can be helpful. All precordial penetrating injuries occurring between the nipple lines laterally, the clavicles superiorly, and the epigastrium inferiorly should be assumed to involve the heart until ruled out. Furthermore, all gunshot injuries with an entrance and exit wound that cross the mediastinum should be assumed to involve the heart until proven otherwise. If hemothorax is present, a thoracostomy tube should be placed, and the collected blood can be autotransfused.

If anesthesia is required, the patient should be prepped and draped before induction of anesthesia. A median sternotomy incision is made. The pericardium is opened parallel to the phrenic nerves, and all intrapericardial blood is quickly evacuated. Bleeding from the heart, if present, is controlled digitally, and the heart is inspected for other injuries and to assess its performance. The cardiac wound is then repaired primarily, if possible. Rarely, an injury to the free wall cannot be repaired primarily or an associated intracardiac injury might require cardiopulmonary bypass, with repair carried out with or without the use of prosthetic or bioprosthetic material.

Most intracardiac wounds are of such a magnitude that the patient does not survive the preoperative preparation and resuscitative stage. If a patient does make it to the operating room with an intracardiac injury, it is usually small enough to be managed surgically at a later date, following repair of the free cardiac wall injury and subsequent cardiac catheterization. Wounds of small, terminal branches of the coronary arteries are ligated, whereas all other wounds of the coronaries should be repaired by saphenous vein bypass graft.

Neck Injuries

The neck is anatomically divided into three zones. Zone I is the area from the thoracic outlet (the level of the clavicle) to the cricoid cartilage, zone II is between the cricoid cartilage and the angle of the mandible, and zone III is above the angle of the mandible to the base of the skull. These zones are important because of the relationship of the major neurovascular structures to the thoracic outlet, mandible, cervical spine, and skull base, along with the proximal aerodigestive tract.

The zone of injury and clinical presentation of the patient dictates the diagnostic tests and therapy required. In general, hemodynamically unstable patients with vascular neck injuries regardless of the zone are brought emergently to the operating room for exploration.

In stable patients, the management of zone II injuries of the neck is the source of some debate among trauma centers. Previously, all zone II injuries were explored because of the relative ease of exposure, coupled with the many vital structures passing through this region. More recently, the trend has been selective exploration of those with a proven injury after further diagnostic evaluation. Usually, this evaluation includes serial physical examinations, esophagoscopy and bronchoscopy, and angiography or duplex scanning when vascular injury is suspected.[46-49] Centers that have evaluated penetrating neck injuries in hemodynamically stable patients using angiography have found only 13% to 17% of these patients have major vascular (carotid and vertebral) injuries requiring repair.[48,49] Because of this, some have begun to advocate angiography only in cases of suspected vascular injury and report very few missed injuries with this approach. More recent studies have also advocated CT scanning as an adjunct to the physical examination in zone II neck injuries.

In zones I and III, hemodynamically and neurologically stable patients usually undergo angiography to diagnose or define the presence and location of injury in these anatomically complex areas. Zone III vascular injuries are frequently amenable to coil embolization. Zone III injuries usually require evaluation of the nasopharynx and upper aerodigestive tract. Zone I injuries similarly require laryngoscopy, bronchoscopy, and rigid esophagoscopy to diagnose occult injuries.

Surgical exposure of the neck differs markedly depending on the zone of injury. Exposure of zone II injuries is usually best done through a standard incision along the anterior border of the sternocleidomastoid. Injuries in zone I, on the other hand, generally require a median sternotomy for adequate exposure, and often with an extension of the incision obliquely into the neck, similar to the incision used for zone II. Zone III injuries are best approached by lateral mandibulotomy,[50] subluxation of the temporomandibular joint followed by the application of arch bars and intermaxillary wires, or the simple application of a towel clip in the mandible to use as a retractor to maintain this position.

Trauma to the Carotid Artery

The most common cause of carotid arterial injury is penetrating trauma, which may manifest with pulsatile hematomas, pulsatile bleeding, or carotid artery thrombosis. Occasionally, blunt trauma to the head may result in carotid-jugular arteriovenous fistula. Depending on the details of the injury, various neurologic deficits may result from these injuries.

Blunt trauma to the internal carotid artery often results in intimal tears in the distal internal carotid artery. The dissection and thrombosis that eventually occur are especially difficult to treat because of the distal location. Blunt injury to the carotid artery can have devastating consequences because of the lack of specific symptoms, delay in neurologic symptoms well after the onset of injury has even been diagnosed, and initial presentation with other concomitant injuries and closed head injuries that mask a suspected blunt carotid injury. It is imperative that carotid injury be suspected in patients presenting with blunt trauma to the head and neck, skull base, and chest who have normal or abnormal neurologic status at presentation.

Expedited diagnostics with duplex ultrasonography and angiography are essential to avoid catastrophic and irreversible neurologic events. The accepted treatment for blunt carotid injury is anticoagulation, and occasionally direct surgical and endovascular repair is used for patients who have failed anticoagulation or have a pseudoaneurysm of the artery, or both.[51-53] Patients with major head trauma may also present with carotid cavernous fistulas, which are best treated by balloon occlusion of the fistula. Under ideal conditions, a balloon can be placed such that it occludes the fistula and still maintains patency of the internal carotid artery.[54]

Carotid Artery Ligation

The major clinical dilemma involving patients with injuries to the common or internal carotid artery is whether to ligate or repair the vessels of those who have developed a major stroke or frank coma early after their injury. The classic argument against revascularization is that acute reperfusion of the ischemic brain converts an ischemic infarct into a hemorrhagic infarct. Little evidence supports this theory, however. Autopsy studies of patients dying after acute reperfusion have demonstrated that cerebral edema and herniation (not hemorrhagic infarct) was the most common cause of death.[55] In general, the carotid artery should be repaired if prograde flow is present or if the internal carotid artery is thrombosed at the time of operative exploration and if the neurologic deficit is of short duration (<3 hours). When the neurologic deficit has been present for a long time (as is common after blunt trauma), the neurologic outcome is likely to be unsatisfactory (Glasgow Coma Scale <8), and the patient's carotid artery is thrombosed with no prograde flow, revascularization is probably of no benefit and the carotid artery should be ligated to control bleeding and prevent embolization.[47,56] Others have also recommended that patients with penetrating carotid injury who have a neurologic deficit should undergo repair rather than ligation of the carotid artery.[47,57] Patients with a thrombosed internal carotid artery who are neurologically intact can be treated with anticoagulation. From the data available, it appears that if patients present with neurologic deficits and a carotid injury that is repaired promptly, the majority have improvement in their neurologic status and improved outcomes versus those having ligation. Most injuries of the intracranial internal carotid artery can be treated nonoperatively, but all such injuries should be evaluated on an individual patient basis by a vascular surgeon, neurosurgeon, and neurologist.[54] Rarely, extracranial-intracranial (EC-IC) bypass may be beneficial after an injury to the distal carotid artery has required ligation and a neurologic deficit develops shortly thereafter.[58]

Vertebral Artery Injury

Vertebral artery injuries are being seen with increasing frequency in recent years, probably because of the widespread availability of safe cervical cranial angiography. The first portion of the vertebral artery can be easily exposed through a supraclavicular incision. Exposure of the second portion (in the bony canal of the transverse vertebral processes) or the third portion (posterior to the atlas) is a difficult operative procedure. If the contralateral vertebral artery is normal and if no major branches to the spinal cord arise from the injured vertebral artery, then ligation of the vertebral artery or placement of an occlusive balloon catheter at the site of injury is appropriate treatment. Certain patients who are at extremely high risk and who would otherwise present challenging exposure of the injured vessel should have endovascular consideration for definitive treatment. This has been advocated by a number of centers with experience in the placement of low-profile, endovascular-covered stents; however, further improvements and long-term results are necessary before endovascular grafts are considered the therapy of choice in injuries to the vertebral artery.[59]

Jugular Vein

Lateral venorrhaphy is preferred for repair of an uncomplicated, injured jugular vein, but ligation is usually performed if a unilateral injury is extensive. A single internal jugular vein may be ligated with impunity, but if bilateral ligation is required, transient cerebral edema and airway problems may result. The internal jugular vein is exposed by a standard oblique cervical incision, and control may be at the site of injury or may require mobilization for proximal and distal control.

Thorax and Thoracic Outlet

Penetrating Injury

Penetrating wounds to the thoracic aorta are rarely seen clinically, as most patients exsanguinate before arrival to the hospital emergency department. If a precordial wound is present and the patient is in shock or cardiac arrest, and if any report from witnesses at the scene or from the emergency personnel suggest that the patient had vital signs or signs of life (spontaneous breathing, eye opening, supraventricular rhythm) at the time of injury before arrival to the emergency department, then a left or bilateral anterolateral thoracotomy just below the nipple in the male or the retracted breasts in a female should be performed immediately to gain control of the thoracic aorta and quickly identify the thoracic injury for temporizing and resuscitation. Wounds of the ascending or descending thoracic aorta can often be controlled with the application of partially occluding clamps in young trauma victims, but wounds of the transverse arch must be controlled with finger pressure while primary repair is undertaken.

Occasionally, the patient with a penetrating wound to the thorax may present hemodynamically stable with a hematoma or with a "proximity" injury alone. In the patient with an expanding hematoma and hypotension, however, with or without an associated hemothorax, immediate thoracotomy is necessary. With an anterior stab wound, the ascending or transverse aortic arch is likely to be injured, and a median sternotomy can be considered if clamping of the descending thoracic aorta will not be necessary. For this reason, gunshot wounds, which may create posterior, descending thoracic perforations, are best approached through a bilateral anterolateral thoracotomy incision. In a stable patient with a small, nonexpanding hematoma or a proximity wound, retrograde arch aortography or CT angiography is indicated if it can be obtained expeditiously.

Blunt Injury: Traumatic Aortic Disruption

Blunt trauma to the thoracic aorta is a classic traumatic injury that usually occurs following deceleration injury in motor vehicle accidents and falls. This injury is seen characteristically just distal to the fixed ligamentum arteriosum in the descending thoracic aorta (Fig. 63-9). In 85% of these cases, the tear is large enough that exsanguinating hemorrhage ensues at the scene. In those who survive transport, however, this injury may present asymptomatically or with dramatic hemodynamic instability. This is because the aortic injury may be an intimal disruption, a full thickness tear with hematoma, or a near full-thickness disruption, with only a layer of adventitia in place.

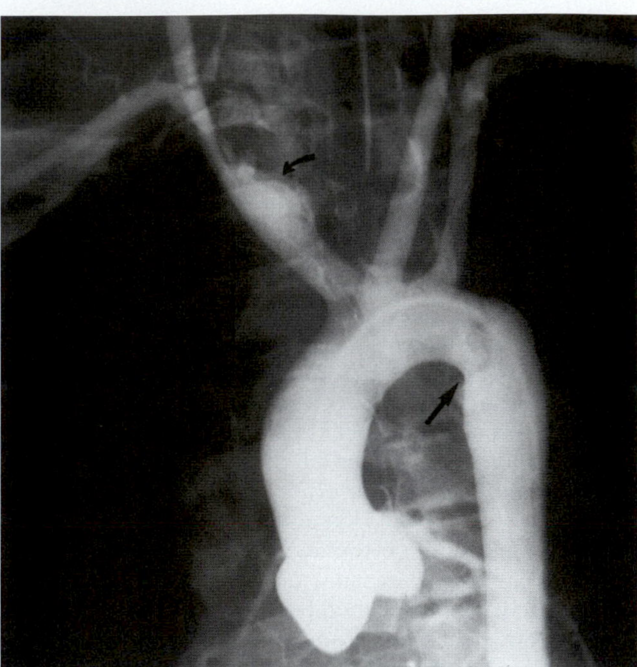

FIGURE 63-9. An example of blunt chest trauma and rapid deceleration causing a shearing force injury in the thoracic aorta just distal to the left subclavian artery, where the aorta is fixed by the attachment of the ligamentum arteriosum (*long arrow*). Note a similar injury to the innominate artery (*curved arrow*).

Once in the hospital, however, the mortality of untreated patients is approximately 1%/hr, and therefore early diagnosis and treatment is mandatory.[60] In unconscious patients, the mechanism of injury coupled with the appearance of precordial contusions (especially the classic imprint of the hub of the steering wheel) warrants further emergent studies. In stable patients without vertebral or spinal cord injury, an anteroposterior chest radiograph is obtained while the patient is sitting up and leaning forward approximately 115 degrees (Ayella maneuver). For aortic injuries, this is the initial test of choice. Widening of the superior mediastinum more than 8 cm or obliteration of the aortic knob on this film confirms the need for immediate aortography or CT angiography. Other radiographic findings on the chest radiograph suggesting the need for further studies include fractures of the first or multiple ribs, sternum, scapula, or fracture-dislocation of the thoracic vertebrae. Occasionally, findings such as a left apical cap, depression of the left main stem bronchus, and an associated left hemothorax or deviation of the nasogastric tube, endotracheal tube, or trachea to the right may help indicate the need for further evaluation. In hypotensive patients with marked widening of the superior mediastinum and obliteration of the aortic knob, no further evaluation is necessary. Instead, these patients require emergent operative intervention.

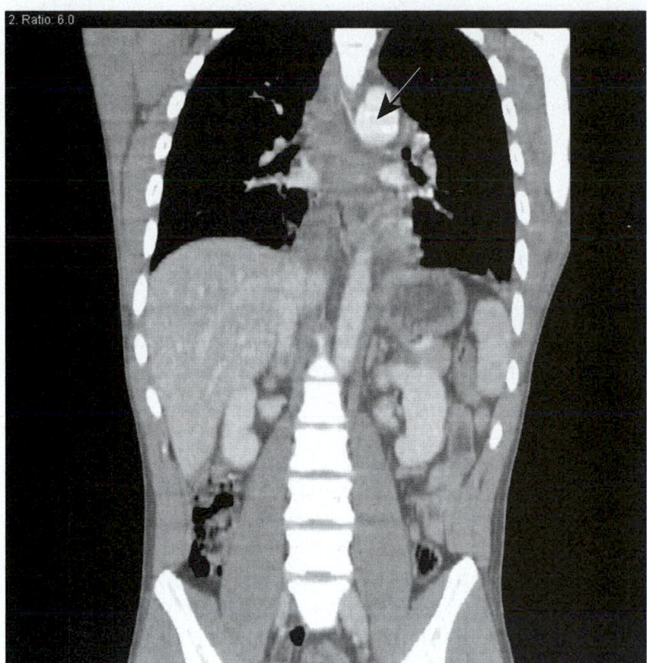

FIGURE 63-10. Spiral CT imaging showing a traumatic thoracic aortic disruption, with surrounding hematoma. *Arrow* points to the aortic dissection.

Several modalities are used to further diagnose traumatic aortic disruption. Aortography still remains the gold standard for evaluating the thoracic aorta and can definitively localize the injury. However, other diagnostic studies are emerging that approach the sensitivity and specificity of aortography. Spiral CT scans, which are less prone to motion artifact and much faster than their predecessors, are proving to be effective in imaging the aorta.[61-63] One recent study showed 100% sensitivity and 99.7% specificity of spiral CT for diagnosing aortic disruption (Fig. 63-10).[64] Transesophageal echocardiography is another sensitive and valuable imaging study for aortic trauma. Its accuracy varies according to the expertise of the institution and examiner, but it has the distinct advantage of being available in the operating room and is especially useful in the patient who becomes unstable in the operating room without having had previous aortic imaging. Transesophageal echocardiography has a sensitivity and specificity of 91% and 100% for diagnosing traumatic aortic injuries.[65]

The classic tear in the proximal descending thoracic aorta is approached through a left posterolateral thoracotomy at the fourth intercostal space after the insertion of a double-lumen endobronchial tube. Techniques of repair include (1) simple cross-clamping of the aorta ("clamp/repair") without shunt or bypass; (2) left-sided heart or aortic bypass using heparin-bonded shunts or external pumps and systemic heparinization; and (3) partial or complete cardiopulmonary bypass using an oxygenator and systemic heparinization. A recent cohort study and systematic review identifying 20 studies involving a total of 618 patients found that regardless of the surgical technique, the mortality rates were similar (ranging from 8% to 17%), but that paraplegia was highest for the clamp and repair without a shunt/bypass during aortic cross-clamping (7%; range from 0% to 7%).[66] Other studies have also emphasized the importance of distal aortic perfusion during aortic clamping to reduce the risk of paraplegia.[67]

Patient positioning is usually in a modified right lateral decubitus position. The femoral arteries should remain accessible in case femoral-femoral bypass is necessary. The arterial line should be placed on the right side because the left subclavian is usually clamped during the repair. Once proximal and distal control of the thoracic aorta has been obtained, the aortic hematoma is opened. Repair is usually by insertion of a woven Dacron tube graft, although primary repair is occasionally possible. Mortality with clamp/repair or shunt techniques is between 10% and 15%, and postoperative paraplegia rates range from 8% to 10%.

Innominate, Common Carotid, and Subclavian Arteries

Patients with penetrating wounds to the innominate, common carotid, and subclavian arteries present similarly to that described from penetrating wounds to the thoracic aorta; that is, they are either profoundly hypotensive and may require thoracotomy in the emergency department, or they are stable enough to be transported to the operating room or to an angiographic suite. In patients with exsanguinating hemorrhage into the ipsilateral pleural cavity from an injury to the subclavian artery, a high anterolateral thoracotomy with transpleural apical packing on the right or clamping of the intrapleural proximal left subclavian artery may be lifesaving.

Penetrating injuries to the distal common carotid artery occur more frequently than those proximally. However, injuries to the subclavian and innominate artery are rare. These injuries have a significant morbidity and mortality if not recognized and treated expeditiously. The majority of patients are either in extremis or have clinical signs of subclavian artery injury requiring immediate surgical exploration and repair. Approximately one third of patients are hemodynamically stable and can undergo angiography for diagnostics and localization of the injury in helping with the surgical planning. With rapid diagnosis and treatment of patients with penetrating injuries to the subclavian artery, the limb salvage rates are 100% and mortality less than 5%.[68,69] Associated penetrating injuries of the subclavian artery include subclavian vein (44%) and brachial plexus (31%), the latter accounting for significant morbidity in the long term.[70]

Blunt trauma to the subclavian and common carotid arteries is rare, but blunt disruption of the innominate artery at the origin of the aortic arch is not rare in trauma centers where victims of deceleration injury are commonly seen. Many of these individuals have a peculiar "pointed" appearance to the right side of the widened superior mediastinum.

Operative Management

In the operating room, a median sternotomy followed by mobilization of the left innominate vein allows for adequate exposure of the proximal innominate artery and left common carotid artery, as well as the superior vena cava. A right cervical or supraclavicular extension with or without resection of the clavicle allows for proximal exposure of the right common carotid and right subclavian arteries, respectively. The same extensions on the left allow for distal exposure of the left common carotid artery and the second and third portions of the left subclavian artery, respectively. The intrapleural proximal left subclavian artery, which is rarely injured, is approached through a left anterolateral thoracotomy in the third or fourth intercostal space.

Various techniques including cardiopulmonary bypass, moderate or profound hypothermia, and shunts for perfusion of the right common carotid artery have been used for repair of injuries to the innominate artery. In the absence of profound intraoperative hypotension or the need to simultaneously occlude the left common carotid artery and the innominate artery, none of these adjuncts is necessary in the young trauma patient. When these conditions are present, however, an internal shunt for carotid perfusion should be considered. In the patient with a blunt tear to the innominate artery at its origin, an 8 to 12 mm prosthetic graft is generally sewn to the side of the ascending aorta before entering the hematoma. Once proximal and distal control of the injured vessel is obtained, the injured segment is resected, the origin of the innominate artery is oversewn and the prosthetic graft is sewn to the distal innominate artery proximal to its bifurcation.

Exposure for injuries to the second and third nonmediastinal portion of either subclavian artery is enhanced by resection of the clavicle through the supraclavicular incision.[71] Resection or division may be performed in a subperiosteal plane if time is available, or the clavicle may simply be divided completely. If one chooses the latter approach, great care must be taken to avoid injury to the underlying and adherent subclavian vein. No morbidity results from resection of the clavicle. If division only is used, the clavicle can be approximated using either a dynamic compression plate or Kirschner wires.

Results

In series in which penetrating wounds predominate, a survival rate of 85% to 95% can be expected with wounds to the innominate or subclavian arteries when the patient has not suffered a cardiac arrest either in the field or shortly after arrival in the emergency department.[72]

Upper Extremity Injuries

Axillary Artery Injuries

Axillary artery injuries are frequently associated with benign-appearing wounds when evaluated clinically. Associated brachial or subclavian vessel injuries, or both (34%), and concomitant brachial plexus injuries (35%) have been noted in civilian series.[73] The latter accounts for the majority of the long-term morbidity. Progressive signs of brachial plexus injury by an adjacent hematoma is the most common indication for exploration of axillary artery injuries in stable patients who do not have rapidly expanding hematomas. Preservation of collateral vessels is essential in operative exposure and repair. The approach to the axillary artery is made via an infraclavicular incision that can easily be extended down the medial aspect of the arm if exposure of the brachial artery is necessary. The axillary artery is then exposed by separation of the pectoralis major muscle fibers and lateral retraction of the pectoralis minor tendon. Interposition bypass grafting with 6 or 8 mm expanded PTFE is the most commonly used means of repair. However, the details of the type of injury, its location, associated findings, and the general condition of the patient might suggest another type of treatment including ligation.

Brachial Artery Injuries

As in axillary injuries, the major morbidity of brachial artery injuries arises primarily from associated nerve and soft-tissue injury. Almost half of patients who present with major nerve injury will have neurologically dysfunctional limbs after long-term follow-up. Associated fractures in the arm are usually repaired before vascular repair. Brachial artery injuries can be successfully repaired by primary repair if the injury is localized and adequate mobilization of uninjured artery offers a tension-free anastomosis. Otherwise, interposition grafting with either autogenous vein or prosthetic is used in cases with extensive loss of arterial tissue. Ligation of the brachial artery may lead to amputation in approximately 35% of the cases; therefore every attempt should be made to repair this artery.

Radial and Ulnar Artery Injuries

Although there is general agreement that all major brachial artery injuries should be repaired, reconstruction of minor arteries (brachial profunda, radial, and ulnar) is thought by some investigators to be warranted only in cases of complete or near-complete severance of the upper extremity, when signs of severe ischemia are present, or when both the radial and ulnar arteries are injured. Johnson and associates[74] reported that the patency following repair of radial and ulnar arteries was approximately 50%. Delayed hand symptoms, if they developed, were related to nerve or tendon damage and not to arterial patency. Their recommendation was that in the absence of acute hand ischemia, ligation of the radial or ulnar artery was appropriate. Smith and coworkers demonstrated that no postoperative functional deficit occurred after ligation of most upper extremity injuries, including brachial arteries. Nevertheless, given the current state of the art, it seems reasonable to attempt repair of injured forearm and arm vessels to obtain the best possible result, as long as the patient's general condition permits.

Abdominal and Pelvic Vascular Injuries

Patients with penetrating abdominal vascular injuries often present with exsanguinating hemorrhage or contained hematomas.[75] The sequence of vascular repair versus repair of the bowel is determined by the presentation. All intra-abdominal hematomas from penetrating injury should be explored. This includes supramesocolic, inframesocolic, perirenal, pelvic, portal, and mesenteric hematomas. Gunshot wounds are responsible for 70% to 78% of abdominal vascular injuries, and the arteries most commonly injured are the aorta, inferior vena cava, and external iliac. The overall mortality rate for penetrating abdominal vascular injuries is 45%, but injuries to the abdominal aorta, hepatic veins and retrohepatic vena cava, and portal vein carry a mortality rate of up to 90%.[47,76] Rapid control of bleeding and preventing profound hypothermia are paramount factors in improving survival.

Abdominal vascular injuries can also result from blunt trauma, usually from avulsed mesenteric vessels, partial avulsion of the renal veins, or other pelvic vessels associated with adjacent fractures. Direct injury to the abdominal aorta from blunt trauma is reported but is rare, occurring in 0.04% of all nonpenetrating abdominal trauma.[77] The most common abdominal vascular injury is to the mesenteric vessels, which is a shearing deceleration injury often accompanied by bowel injury. If this injury is missed, it can present in a delayed fashion with bowel perforation from resultant ischemia.[78] Mesenteric vascular injury is treated with bowel resection rather than arterial or venous repair.

As with penetrating injury, midline supramesocolic and inframesocolic, portal, and mesenteric hematomas should be routinely explored. However, in the presence of a normal preoperative CT of the kidney, lateral perirenal retroperitoneal hematomas are not ordinarily opened in the case of blunt trauma. Similarly, pelvic hematomas that are not expanding are not routinely opened and explored, since this bleeding is usually secondary to venous injury.

Supramesocolic Hematomas

A midline supramesocolic hematoma or active hemorrhage from this area is generally best approached laterally unless the site of hemorrhage can be easily visualized in the lesser sac. If hemorrhage is rapid, an aortic compression device or an assistant's hand may be used to occlude the aorta at the diaphragmatic hiatus before formal dissection and clamping. Furthermore, if the supramesocolic injury is close to the abdominal aortic hiatus, the left chest should be also prepped and draped for possible thoracic aortic clamping through a left anterolateral thoracotomy. Injuries to the supramesocolic area include suprarenal aorta, celiac axis, proximal superior mesenteric artery, or renal artery. The left colon, left kidney, spleen, tail of the pancreas, and gastric fundus are then rapidly mobilized past the midline by a combination of sharp and blunt dissection. Occasionally, a partial left radial phrenotomy (division of the left hemidiaphragm) further improves the exposure. Once the aorta is palpated and exposed, a long DeBakey aortic clamp is used to occlude it. Dissection then proceeds distally so that the actual bleeding site in the aorta or one of the visceral branches is exposed and distal vascular control obtained.

Inframesocolic Hematomas

An inframesocolic hematoma or hemorrhage is approached directly in the midline just below the mesocolon, similar to the exposure of the aorta in an aneurysm repair. Hematomas to the inframesocolic region are associated with infrarenal aorta or vena cava injuries. Stab wounds or small-caliber gunshot wounds of the abdominal aorta can be repaired with a running suture of 4-0 or 5-0 polypropylene. If excessive narrowing results, a patch aortoplasty using expanded PTFE or Dacron may then be performed to improve blood flow. When the aorta suffers extensive destruction, as can occur in seatbelt-associated blunt abdominal aortic trauma,[79] a prosthetic interposition graft is inserted. Extensive experience with aortic prosthesis in the face of enteric or fecal contamination from penetrating wounds has clearly demonstrated that this is a surprisingly safe approach.[80]

If the celiac artery is injured, it can be ligated with impunity in a young trauma patient. Surprisingly, little morbidity results from this maneuver due to a generous collateral circulation via the superior mesenteric artery.

Conversely, injuries to the superior mesenteric artery are treacherous and often present a challenging problem. Wounds requiring ligation of this artery at its origin lead to ischemia of the entire midgut. Plus, the origin of this artery is precariously close to the pancreas and presents commonly with associated pancreatic injury. The potential for a pancreatic leak near the arterial anastomosis may prevent direct repair of this vessel in the setting of pancreatic injury. Retrograde bypass grafting with saphenous vein or PTFE from the distal infrarenal abdominal aorta to the superior mesenteric artery avoids anastomotic dehiscence and prevents the development of an ischemic midgut.[16]

Renal Artery Injury

When life-threatening hemorrhage necessitates ligation of the renal artery, a nephrectomy should be performed. On rare occasions in stable patients with penetrating renal artery injury, bypass grafting from the infrarenal abdominal aorta to the distal renal artery may be justified. When renal artery thrombosis secondary to an intimal contusion from blunt trauma is recognized soon after it occurs, resection of the renal artery with an end-to-end anastomosis is preferred.[81] As soon as the abdomen is entered, the affected kidney is packed in ice and flushed with cold Collins solution. If the warm ischemia time is longer than 6 hours, nephrectomy is recommended. A recent retrospective multicenter study determined that renal injuries from blunt trauma had a worse salvage rate than those from penetrating trauma, and renal injuries requiring arterial reconstruction (vs. only venous reconstruction) also had a poor prognosis. The study concluded that patients with blunt renal vascular injuries who also sustained significant parenchymal disruption should have an immediate nephrectomy, in the presence of a functioning contralateral kidney.[82]

Vena Cava Injuries

Injuries to the vena cava are rare and are usually the result of penetrating injury. They are also highly lethal, however, with only 50% surviving to present to the emergency department. Among those who present with signs of life, mortality has been estimated to be as high as 60%.[83,84] Determinant of survival is based on the severity of patient presentation, anatomic location of the caval injury, and associated aortic injury.

Exposure of the infrahepatic inferior vena cava and both renal veins is done by mobilizing the right colon and hepatic flexure past the midline and performing an extended Kocher maneuver. The retrohepatic vena cava is exposed by dividing the triangular and anterior and posterior coronary ligaments of the hepatic lobe and mobilizing this lobe to the midline. Vascular control of the infrarenal vena cava is initially obtained by applying sponge sticks proximally and distally to the injury. Because of extensive paired lumbar veins merging with the vena cava at this level, control of a large portion of this vessel can be challenging. With injuries at the level of the renal veins, both renal veins should be encircled with vessel loops and clamped, and the vena cava should be controlled at the infrarenal level and at the suprarenal infrahepatic level as it passes beneath the liver. In the case of worsening hemodynamic status, coagulopathy, or multiple associated injuries, the infrarenal vena cava can be quickly ligated with no change in outcome.[85] Ligation above the renal arteries, however, is associated with a high rate of renal congestion and failure.

Injury to the retrohepatic vena cava presents one of the most challenging exposures and repair in trauma surgery. This segment of the vena cava is about 7 cm in length and is located between the right adrenal vein inferiorly and the phrenic vein superiorly. It lies in a groove posterior to the liver and just posterior to the portal vein. Immediately distal to the diaphragm, the retrohepatic vena cava is joined by two or three major hepatic veins and several smaller hepatic vein tributaries. These short veins tether the vena cava to the liver at this location and make circumferential control treacherous. Furthermore, hepatic suspensory ligaments attach the liver to the diaphragm here. In most instances, these suspensory ligaments serve to contain retrohepatic bleeding from the vena cava unless the liver itself or one of the ligaments is disrupted.[86]

In the hemodynamically stable patient, simultaneous cross-clamping of the portal triad, suprahepatic (intraabdominal) vena cava, and suprarenal vena cava (below the liver) occasionally slows bleeding enough to allow for the placement of sutures. If this maneuver fails, or if the patient is unstable, a sternotomy incision is added to the celiotomy incision and an atriocaval shunt is placed. Umbilical tape tourniquets around the vena cava are pulled tightly on the shunt, thus excluding the area of injury and allowing direct repair. Patients requiring an atriocaval shunt for a retrohepatic caval injury have a mortality rate of between 50% and 90%. Occasionally, in the patient with an extensive hepatic injury, a deep hepatotomy without the aid of a shunt may be used to approach the perforation directly.[87]

The vena cava is repaired preferably in a transverse fashion using a running suture of 4-0 or 5-0 polypropylene. Primary venorrhaphy has been demonstrated to be effective, especially for anterior cava perforations, and has low thrombotic and embolic complications.[88] Extensive suprarenal injuries below the liver should be treated by patch venoplasty or the insertion of an externally supported polytetrafluoroethylene conduit of appropriate size. The right renal vein and left renal vein near the left kidney are repaired by lateral venorrhaphy, and the left renal vein at the midline may be ligated.

Exposure and Control of Iliac Vessels

Injuries to the iliac arteries and veins present with lateral pelvic hemorrhage or hematomas. Proximal vascular control is obtained by exposing the infrarenal abdominal aorta and vena cava in the midline. Distal control is obtained by dividing the peritoneum over the external iliac vessels just proximal to the inguinal ligament as the vessels come out of the pelvis. Full exposure of the right iliac vessels usually necessitates mobilization of the cecum and right colon. On the left, the sigmoid colon must be mobilized for complete exposure. The confluence of the common iliac veins is difficult to expose and may necessitate temporary transection of the right common iliac artery with mobilization to the left of midline, and following repair of the venous injury a primary end-to-end reanastomosis of the artery.

Destructive injuries to the common or external iliac arteries in the presence of extensive enteric or fecal contamination are best treated by ligation rather than insertion of a vascular conduit, as infection and blowout may occur. In such a patient, a fasciotomy in the ipsilateral leg is probably necessary. The extremity may develop significant ischemia, requiring an extra-anatomic femorofemoral or axillofemoral bypass graft. Extensive injuries to the internal iliac vessels or iliac veins should be ligated. Appropriate precautions such as extremity elevation and wrapping must be taken in the postoperative period.[89]

Lower Extremity Injuries

Techniques of exposure, clinical examination, diagnostic tests, indications for surgery, and basic principles of repair have been described previously in this chapter. Careful handling of small vessels; use of small vascular clamps, bulldog clamps, or vascular loops; and an open anastomosis technique are keys to the successful completion of an end-to-end anastomosis or insertion of a vascular conduit in an extremity.[7] Distal thrombus should always be removed with an embolectomy catheter once vascular control has been achieved. Regional heparin should then be injected to prevent thrombosis of distal collateral vessels during the period of vascular occlusion. Completion arteriography is mandatory. Postoperative care includes the use of IV antibiotics, monitoring of arterial pulses, wound assessment, and elevation and wrapping for all major venous ligations. In certain patients with clinically occult vascular injuries from penetrating extremity trauma, it appears safe to treat them nonoperatively solely on the basis of clinical examination and if follow-up is available. In one study, a group of patients was followed for a mean of 9.1 years. Only 9% required surgical treatment of the injured extremity artery within 1 month of the injury.[90]

Common Femoral and Profunda Femoris Arteries

Common femoral and profunda femoris arterial injuries can often be repaired primarily, although interposition bypass grafting or patch angioplasty with autogenous or prosthetic material is also frequently employed. Ligation of the common femoral artery injuries during World War II carried an 81% amputation rate[1]; therefore, all common femoral artery injuries are repaired unless operative repair seems to jeopardize the patient's life. Ligation of distal branches of the profunda femoris artery can be performed safely. The approach to the common and proximal profunda femoris artery is made via a standard vertical groin incision, exactly like that used for elective femoral popliteal reconstructive procedures. The incision can easily be extended proximally for retroperitoneal exposure of the iliac vessels, if vascular control at a more proximal level is necessary.

Superficial Femoral Artery

The proximal superficial femoral artery can be exposed through the vertical groin incision described in the previous section. For injuries in the more distal aspects of the femoral artery, an appropriately positioned incision can be placed on the medial aspect of the thigh, reflecting the sartorius muscle laterally. Associated femoral venous trauma should be repaired if the patient is stable. The seminal work by Rich and associates[4] from the Vietnam Vascular Registry, and the clinical[17] and experimental[91] observations of Hobson and colleagues have made repair of concomitant venous injuries the standard of good surgical care.

Popliteal Artery

Injury to the popliteal artery has the highest amputation rate of all arterial injuries to the lower extremity. Some recent civilian series have reported amputation rates as high as 42%.[92] Blunt injury to the knee with resultant popliteal artery injury is an especially difficult problem to manage. Blunt injury sufficient enough to disrupt the stabilization of the knee often causes direct injury to the popliteal artery with resultant thrombosis. This vessel also does not have the collateral supply of the tibial vessels and is functionally an isolated arterial conduit to the lower leg. Diagnosis and management of these injuries is difficult and may have a high amputation rate if unrecognized and left untreated for more than 6 to 8 hours.[93,94] The presence of pedal pulses in the presence of a posterior knee dislocation followed by reduction does not guarantee freedom from a popliteal injury. Because of the severe morbidity and limb loss of a missed popliteal arterial injury, a high index of suspicion is mandatory and a low threshold for angiography or ultrasonography, or both, is warranted to diagnose and expeditiously repair the popliteal artery.[94,95]

The approach to the popliteal artery can be through a standard incision in the medial aspect of the knee or through a posterior approach, making a horizontal S-shaped incision through the popliteal space, with the horizontal portion of the incision parallel to the skin crease in the knee. If the injury is isolated to the popliteal artery (as it often is), a pneumatic tourniquet placed around the midthigh can be lifesaving because it allows immediate proximal control during the prepping, draping, and surgical exposure of the artery.

Associated venous injury is common in popliteal artery injury, and on occasion, an isolated popliteal venous injury is encountered during exploration of the injured knee for other reasons. As with femoral venous injuries, all popliteal venous injuries are repaired for the reason outlined earlier. The postoperative patency of repaired veins in the extremities can be improved with the use of intermittent pneumatic compression devices applied distally, because these devices increase the rate of blood flow across the venous repair site and prevent stasis, with its attendant thrombosis.[36]

Tibial and Peroneal Artery

Injuries to the tibial or peroneal arteries (collectively referred to as the *tibial arteries*) present a special problem because, in most cases, they do not cause severe ischemia unless two of the three vessels are interrupted. Arteriographic survey of these patients is essential to determine if indeed there is a significant problem. This is especially true in a patient who has multiple wounds as the result of a shotgun blast. In a patient who has penetrating trauma to the lower leg resulting in occlusion of one tibial artery without bleeding or open fracture, the injury can be accepted without arterial repair. Such patients should be observed with clinical examination and pulse assessment rather than direct operation. Surgical exploration of a single tibial artery injury is customarily performed only if it is bleeding or if an arteriovenous fistula or false aneurysm is seen on the arteriogram. In contrast, patients with injuries of two tibial arteries should have one of these vessels repaired to ensure adequate function of the extremity.[96-98] A study by Neville and colleagues[99] reported that ischemic symptoms were worse in blunt tibial injuries when compared with penetrating tibial injuries. In patients with a single arterial injury, a plan of observation or ligation resulted in no amputations. Some patients with two tibial vessels injured did not have ischemic complications unless the single remaining tibial vessel was the peroneal artery. Their recommendation based on experience is that if the only remaining tibial vessel is the peroneal artery, then one of the other tibial vessels should be revascularized.

Iatrogenic Vascular Injuries

As diagnostic and therapeutic techniques have become more advanced and invasive, the incidence of iatrogenic complications has increased. The nature of these invasive procedures places the vascular system at high risk for iatrogenic injury. The injuries sustained in this setting are often less dramatic than those suffered in penetrating or blunt injuries and are therefore underemphasized in the surgical literature. Many early reports of the vascular trauma experience from large centers fail to even mention iatrogenic injuries. Unfortunately, the compromised health of patients undergoing diagnostic or therapeutic invasive procedures makes them ill suited to contend with hemorrhagic, thrombotic, and embolic iatrogenic complications.

Operations for iatrogenic vascular complications comprise 10% to 29% of all surgery for civilian vascular trauma.[100] Ninety percent of these operations are for arterial trauma, whereas 10% are for venous injuries.[101] The experience with surgery for iatrogenic vascular injuries at the Walter Reed Army Medical Center has been extensively reviewed.[102] Approximately 30% of these injuries were related to cardiac catheterization, 30% to angiography including percutaneous transluminal angioplasty, 30% to various surgical complications including injuries secondary to intra-aortic balloon counterpulsation, and 10% to miscellaneous procedures (central venous, arterial, and pulmonary arterial catheter complications). Since many of the vascular complications of these miscellaneous procedures do not require surgical intervention, their incidence is underestimated.

The most common iatrogenically injured artery is the femoral artery (42%), followed by the brachial (17%), axillary (14%), iliac arteries (11%), and aorta (4%). Most injuries can be repaired by vascular suture or simple thrombectomy, but approximately 20% require complex vascular reconstruction.[102]

The most important factor in limiting mortality and morbidity of iatrogenic vascular injuries is prompt recognition and treatment. In one series, a delay in repair of an iatrogenic vascular injury was an important factor in six of eight permanent functional disabilities and three of four amputations.[103] Other important factors include attention to details of technique, judicious management of anticoagulants, a sound knowledge of anatomy, and recognition of when the risks of continued intervention outweigh the benefits.

The following sections discuss the most common types of iatrogenic vascular injuries.

Vascular Complications of Angiography

Angiography has become a standard diagnostic modality that is available in nearly every general and tertiary care hospital. Its broad application has resulted in a significant amount of iatrogenic vascular injury. Hessel and associates[104] conducted a national survey of hospitals to determine the incidence of angiography-related complications. They found that the incidence of complications, including vascular injuries, was highly dependent on the site of cannulation. The more common transfemoral approach had a 1.73% incidence of complications, whereas the translumbar and transaxillary routes had a 2.89% and 3.29% incidence, respectively. There were 30 deaths out of 118,591 examinations. At least 10 of these were related to vascular injuries, including aortic dissection or aneurysm rupture (eight cases), aortic occlusion (one case), and bowel infarction (one case). An inverse relationship was found between the complication rate and annual number of arteriograms performed.

The major types of arterial injuries are related to vessel cannulation and guidewire manipulation. These injuries include (in descending order) vessel perforation and hemorrhage, thrombosis, embolism, pseudoaneurysm formation, arterial dissection, and arteriovenous fistula. Special problems with the axillary approach are well recognized and are related to the location, small size, constraints of the axillary sheath, and relative mobility of this artery. These factors make hemostasis difficult and predispose to brachial plexus compression injuries, as well as cerebral emboli.[6,105] Catheter-induced vessel thrombosis is influenced by the relationship of catheter size to the vessel being cannulated. This factor explains the relatively high incidence of thrombosis in the axillary artery and in children who are subjected to angiography.[106]

The risks of cerebral angiography warrant special consideration. The risk of neurologic deficits is approximately 1% with the transfemoral approach.[104,107] The majority of these deficits are transient, however, with the incidence of completed stroke being somewhat lower. Cerebral emboli account for the majority of neurologic events. Neurotoxic effects of contrast agents, however, may play a role in some cases.

Iatrogenic complications of coronary angiography can be a source of significant morbidity and mortality. As with peripheral angiography, the rate of these complications seems to vary with the cannulation site. The reported incidence of myocardial infarction, cerebrovascular accidents, and death varies, with some studies showing the superiority of the transfemoral route and others demonstrating the superiority of the transbrachial route. As with peripheral angiography, however, the incidence of peripheral vascular complications is higher when the transbrachial route is employed.[108] In the Coronary Artery Surgery Study, the complications of 7551 coronary angiograms were reviewed.[109] The rates of arterial embolization, thrombosis, and dissection were each higher for the transbrachial route, and the overall vascular complication rate was 2.85%, versus 0.45% for the transfemoral route.

The brachial artery route has been found to be especially dangerous in women undergoing coronary angiography. One study demonstrated a relative risk of a vascular complication of 11.6 for females compared with males with the brachial approach.[110] Patients undergoing coronary angiography are often highly compromised. Fortunately, the brachial artery often has excellent collateral flow and observation may be warranted after brachial artery thrombosis when the hand is not compromised.[111] In patients with hand ischemia, and occasionally forearm ischemia, heparin should be instituted immediately. In patients who respond to anticoagulation with return of hand perfusion, clinical observation is acceptable. In patients with persistent ischemia, however, immediate surgical exploration with thrombectomy or bypass, or both, is mandatory to avoid digital necrosis and functional impairment.

Vascular complications appear to occur more frequently when coronary angioplasty is performed.[112] The most frequent complications of diagnostic angiography are the development of false aneurysms and arteriovenous fistulas. The management of these two specific injuries is the subject of some debate. It may be that small arteriovenous fistulas and small pseudoaneurysms may resolve on their own. The questions of which can be observed and which require repair are unresolved.

Apparently, a number of these types of vascular injuries resolve.[113-116] Most asymptomatic arteriovenous fistulas are observed. In the event that a high-flow arteriovenous fistula causes symptoms including heart failure, limb ischemia, or extremity edema, recommendations are to repair. Management of false aneurysms and some arteriovenous fistulas can be treated with ultrasound-guided compression.

Ultrasonography is used to identify the neck of the false aneurysm or the arteriovenous fistula, and then a downward compression is applied with the transducer until flow in the false aneurysm or fistula is eliminated. Potential problems of this approach involve discomfort associated with the compression and the possibility of thrombosis of the compressed vessel. The utilization of this modality has been reported by various authors and with variable success rates.[115,117,118] Recently, the use of duplex ultrasound-guided thrombin injection of pseudoaneurysms has been demonstrated to be effective and the treatment of choice in obliterating arterial pseudoaneurysms.[119-121] The procedure is performed under ultrasound guidance to identify the pseudoaneurysm sac, while a needle is placed into the sac, thrombin is injected, and thrombosis of the sac is monitored. A study comparing ultrasound-guided thrombin injection to ultrasound compression found that the thrombosis of the pseudoaneurysm was accomplished in 96% of cases with thrombin injection compared with only 75% with ultrasound-guided compression.[120] The benefits of duplex ultrasound-guided thrombin injection of pseudoaneurysms are patient comfort (avoiding pain related to forceful compression), effectiveness of the therapy, and few repeat interventions with thrombin injections. Potential complications of intra-arterial thrombin injection, with arterial thrombosis or embolization and pseudoaneurysm rupture, occur in 4% of patients and require surgical intervention.[120]

Ultrasound-guided thrombin injection of pseudoaneurysms has also been reported to be effective in anatomically difficult and high-risk patients. These have been described by single institutions as case reports involving the treatment of pseudoaneurysms of the inferior epigastric artery following a rectus sheath hematoma,[122] hepatic artery following liver transplantation,[123] and in a pancreatitis-induced arterial pseudoaneurysm.[124]

Percutaneous Transluminal Balloon Angioplasty

Percutaneous transluminal angioplasty of the iliac, femoral, and popliteal arteries has gained widespread acceptance. This may be attributed to several factors, including an acceptable safety record, cost effectiveness, and initial results comparable with those of reconstructive surgery. Nonetheless, overall complication rates ranging between 2% and 25% have been reported, with many of these representing vascular injuries. Weibull and associates[125] collectively reviewed the literature to determine the complication rate of percutaneous transluminal angioplasty. In 2043 percutaneous angioplasties, there was an 8.6% overall complication rate. Vascular complications requiring surgical intervention included distal embolization (2%), vessel thrombosis (1.8%), groin hematoma (0.25%), retroperitoneal hemorrhage (0.1%), pseudoaneurysm (0.1%), and intimal injury (0.1%). Other complications that did not require surgery included groin hematoma (2%), subintimal dissection (0.75%), guidewire perforation of the vessel (0.25%), and arteriovenous fistula (0.25%). The incidence of complications was inversely related to the angiographer's experience.

A report of 4988 coronary percutaneous transluminal angioplasty procedures revealed a complication rate of 1%. Pseudoaneurysm was the most frequent complication, followed by arteriovenous fistula and hemorrhage at the puncture site. Age, female gender, thrombolytic therapy, and anticoagulation correlated with the risk of complications.[126]

Vascular Complications of Surgical Procedures

Complications of surgical procedures constitute approximately 30% of iatrogenic vascular injuries. Because of the wide variety of surgical operations, these injuries have involved nearly every artery in every imaginable location. This wide range of potential injuries has been reflected in numerous case reports, as well as in large surgical series of iatrogenic vascular injuries.[127] Furthermore, these complications have occurred in nearly every surgical discipline including general surgery, orthopedics, urology, neurosurgery, obstetrics, and gynecology. A series by Youkey and associates[102] found that 4 of 6 gynecologic complications, 10 of 11 urologic complications, and the single general-surgery vascular complication all occurred during difficult dissections for retroperitoneal tumor. The complex nature of these operations, the proximity of major vessels, and the disruption of normal anatomic planes by tumor all contributed to these injuries. Other well-described vascular injuries include iliac artery and vein injury during lumbar disc surgery, vascular injury during trocar insertion for laparoscopy, inadvertent arterial injury during venous stripping, iliofemoral injuries related to cardiac bypass, and femoral artery and vein injuries during inguinal hernia repair.[102,107,127]

Various vascular injuries have been reported with orthopedic surgical procedures. These include direct vascular trauma related to open reduction and internal fixation, total joint arthroplasty, and acute compartment syndromes induced by constricting casts. Prompt recognition of the ischemic limb and treatment is mandatory and may require angiographic diagnosis for planning revascularization and removal of the constricting cast and possible fasciotomy to relieve the compartment syndrome.

Complications of Intra-aortic Balloon Counterpulsation

The insertion and operation of intra-aortic balloon pumps (IABPs) are a major source of surgically induced iatrogenic vascular injury. These injuries accounted for 15% of all iatrogenic vascular injuries in one series, and complication rates as high as 36% have been reported.[100]

The 8.8% vascular complication rate noted by Perler and associates[128] in their series is more typical. These complications included ischemic injuries (4.5%), arterial injury (2.5%), and hemorrhagic complications (0.9%), as well as septic complications. The limb ischemia was due to either thromboembolism or arterial obstruction by the large intraluminal balloon catheter and sheath. This usually necessitated removal of an IABP to the contralateral leg, embolectomy of the femoral vessel, or both. In a series of 1454 patients treated with intra-aortic balloon counterpulsation, Friedell and associates[129] reported the use of femorofemoral crossover grafting to treat limb-threatening ischemia in 80 (5%) of patients. The arterial injuries included both local injuries at the insertion site and dissection of the iliac arteries and aorta. The local injuries were easily managed with simple repair. Complications of the arterial dissections were devastating, however, with five of six patients dying from bowel infarction or aortic occlusion. Complications appear to correlate with a history of peripheral vascular disease, diabetes, and female gender.[130] A study by Barnett and colleagues[131] on vascular complications in 72 patients demonstrated that a history of peripheral vascular disease, female gender, history of cigarette smoking, and postoperative insertion were independent predictors of vascular complications. However, the risk for most vascular complications could not be explained by these factors alone.

Several factors are important in the prevention of IABP complications. Most important is careful selection of the insertion site based on physical examination and, if necessary, preinsertion angiography. Selection of the appropriate size of balloon catheter, careful insertion, and movement to the contralateral side when the balloon does not pass easily are other important factors. Although the overall incidence of vascular complications related to IABP has not changed, the severity of these complications has decreased due to careful patient selection and early recognition and treatment of the limb in jeopardy.[131]

Vascular Complications of Invasive Monitoring

Sophisticated hemodynamic monitoring techniques have had a significant impact on complementing the clinician's ability to care for critically ill patients. Unfortunately, the invasive nature of these monitoring devices has resulted in various complications including iatrogenic vascular injuries.

One of the more common invasive procedures performed is central vein cannulation. In addition to hemodynamic monitoring, this technique is useful for various purposes including fluid resuscitation, parenteral nutrition, and hemodialysis access. A wide variety of complications have been reported with both the subclavian and internal jugular approach. The major vascular complication is arterial puncture of the carotid or subclavian vessels, which occurs in 3.3% to 6.7% of cases depending on the experience of the physician and the condition of the patient.[132] These injuries may result in significant hematomas, as well as hemithoraces. Hemorrhage from the subclavian artery is particularly troublesome, as it cannot be directly tamponaded because of the anatomic location and surrounding clavicle. Other complications of central venous lines include catheter-induced venous thrombosis and catheter embolization. Venous thrombosis has been reported in 6% of central venous cannulations and may result in pulmonary emboli.[133] This, however, is an underestimate, since not all patients with central catheter access have confirmatory studies.

Flow-directed pulmonary artery catheterization is subject to the same complications as central venous cannulation, as well as several additional vascular injuries. One of the most serious of these is catheter-induced pulmonary artery perforation, which occurred in 4 of 6245 cases in one large series.[134] Barash and associates[135] reviewed six such cases and identified pulmonary hypertension, anticoagulation, and hypothermia as significant risk factors. The major causes identified included catheter-tip erosion through the pulmonary artery, eccentric balloon inflation, and balloon overinflation. The authors stress several factors in preventing those complications: avoidance of overinsertion of the catheter, avoidance of overinflating the balloon, and a reliance on pulmonary artery diastolic pressures whenever possible.

Another important vascular complication of pulmonary artery catheterization is pulmonary infarction, resulting when the balloon remains inflated or the catheter migrates into the wedged position. Other more unusual complications include cardiac valve and wall damage and intravascular knotting of the catheter.

Indwelling arterial catheters allow continuous blood pressure monitoring and assist frequent blood sampling. In most instances the radial artery is the site of choice. The major risk associated with radial artery cannulation is radial artery thrombosis with secondary vascular insufficiency of the hand and digits. Fortunately, although radial artery thrombosis is common, ischemic damage is rather unusual. In a series of 1699 consecutive short-term percutaneous radial artery cannulations, Slogoff and colleagues[136] found that the radial artery was occluded or partially occluded in 25% of cases. Despite that finding, no ischemic damage or hand disability occurred in any patient. It is generally held that documentation of collateral flow from the ulnar artery with an Allen test is an important factor in preventing ischemic complications.

These authors, however, did not find the Allen test to be a useful predictor of ischemia, with 16 patients having an uncomplicated radial artery cannulation despite a positive test. When percutaneous insertion is not possible and radial artery cutdown is necessary, the incidence of complications increases to 50%.[137] In this situation it may be prudent to switch to a percutaneous femoral approach rather than a radial cutdown. Two prospective studies have compared percutaneous radial and femoral artery cannulation and found that the complication rates are similar and that the femoral catheters are more durable.[137,138] Due to the relative size of the catheter and vessel, arterial occlusion is unusual in the femoral artery. When there is preexisting peripheral vascular disease, however, the complication rate of femoral artery cannulation increases significantly, and this route should be avoided, if possible.[137]

Pediatric Vascular Trauma

Principles of evaluation and treatment of vascular injuries in the pediatric population are similar to those in adults. However, important differences must be considered. Spasm of blood vessels is a major factor in pediatric vascular injuries both in iatrogenic injuries and in traumatic injuries. Because of the small size of a child's vessels, vasospasm can result in thrombosis and permanent occlusion. In pediatric patients, in whom spasm is thought to be the cause of the arterial insufficiency, anticoagulation with IV heparin is indicated with a defined period of observation before deciding to surgically intervene. Depending on the condition of the injured extremity, the period of observation can be as short as 6 hours, as suggested by Flanigan and associates,[139] or as long as 48 hours, as suggested by Klein and associates,[140] before taking the patient to the operating room.

Another major consideration in the pediatric population that is different than in adults is the consequence of altered limb growth. It is well documented that in the pediatric population with vascular injuries there is a retardation of limb growth, which can occur if blood flow is interrupted for any significant period of time. The infant population is extremely vulnerable to retardation of limb growth when the vascular occlusion is not recognized. Attenuated limb growth can also occur if the vascular injury is not promptly recognized and the patient has a significant delay in repair of the vascular injury. Awareness of the possibility of a vascular injury is essential because of the risk of stunted limb growth.[141]

Signs of vascular insufficiency may not be as clear as they would be in an adult; thus the likelihood of a missed vascular injury is much greater in this population. All authors of pediatric vascular trauma publications clearly point out the need for thorough evaluation of the injured extremity, a heightened awareness of the possibility of vascular injury, prompt recognition and diagnosis of vascular injury with a thorough physical examination including Doppler ultrasound examination and arteriography, and the immediate institution of appropriate therapy to repair the injury.[142-144]

Principles of repair in the pediatric population are generally similar to those in adults. Some recommendations, however, indicate that more liberal use of gentle vessel dilatation with heparinized papaverine solutions may be important.[145] Other technical considerations, including long spatulation of the anastomoses using interrupted sutures for the repair to allow the anastomosis to grow with the child, may be important. In addition, there have been some suggestions of the possibility of using absorbable sutures[145,146]; however, most surgeons in practice favor fine (6-0 or 7-0) nonabsorbable monofilament sutures for the anastomoses. The choice of conduit in the pediatric population is probably similar to adults, with saphenous vein being the preferable conduit because of the matched size and because it contains endothelium with the potential to lengthen as the child grows.

Issues of aneurysmal dilatation in the pediatric population have been raised, since the autogenous graft must last for the entire life of the young patient. Because the venous conduit may become aneurysmal, some authors have suggested the use of autografts using the hypogastric artery. This is only appropriate when a relatively short graft is available, but it also has the disadvantage of requiring an abdominal incision. General use of the hypogastric artery is appropriate in a limited number of circumstances.[145] Postoperative management of such patients has special considerations due to the relatively small size of the repaired vessel. Many authors believe that continued use of heparin and low molecular weight dextran in the postoperative period, if possible, may be appropriate to prevent thrombosis.[146]

In a review by Harris and associates,[147] the authors retrospectively evaluated 19 children who underwent upper or lower extremity revascularization due to both penetrating and blunt trauma. The mean age was 13.9 years, and 79% of the patients had associated nonvascular injuries. There were no deaths, and 95% of the limbs were salvaged. Although only nine patients were available for late follow-up, the authors found that 75% of patients resumed normal activity at a mean of 1.5 months, and the remaining 25% of patients with deficits in function had originally concomitant orthopedic injuries.

Cardneau and associates[148] investigated limb-length discrepancy in 14 children who underwent 16 lower extremity revascularizations with greater saphenous vein. The main objective was to evaluate vein graft durability and efficacy of the revascularizations. Patient extremity bypasses were assessed with ABI, ultrasonography, and limb length with a mean follow-up of 5.7 years. Of the grafts evaluated at follow-up, 36% remained unchanged, 50% developed nonaneurysmal dilation, and 14% had aneurysmal expansion. When evaluating all grafts, 11.2% developed aneurysmal expansion at an average time of 10.7 years. The authors also found that limb-length discrepancies were reduced in 70% of children and concluded that saphenous vein graft reconstructions of the lower extremity are durable in children.

Other venous conduits including the basilic vein have been used. In a study by Lewis and associates,[149] eight 3- to 10-year olds had supracondylar humeral fracture with brachial arterial injuries. The basilic vein from the ipsilateral arm was used in a reverse fashion for revascularization. There were no postoperative thromboses, and at a minimum of 1 year follow-up, all patients had patent vein grafts.

As in adults, pediatric patients with knee dislocations pose special problems because of the high likelihood of direct injury to the popliteal artery. In a series of 37 knee dislocations in 35 patients reported by Kendall and associates,[150] all patients with a popliteal artery injury had a pulse deficit, signs of peripheral ischemia, or both. Angiography was only used in selected cases. Basic principles of popliteal artery repair follow those of adults.

Endovascular Repair of Vascular Injuries

With the advancements of endovascular technology (EVT) and the benefit of less invasive therapy, a number of institutions have applied endovascular repair of vascular injuries routinely involving arteriovenous fistulas and pseudoaneurysms in both central and peripheral located vessels.[59,151,152] Advantages to repairing traumatic vascular injuries by EVT include: remote access from the injured vessel; ability to repair vessels in anatomically challenging locations; avoidance of major incisions for vascular control; less invasion; and decreased blood loss. It is also ideal for critically ill patients with coexisting injuries or medical comorbidities. Disadvantages and limitations of EVT in traumatic vessel injuries include: difficulty with disrupted and thrombosed vessels; contrast load that may be nephrotoxic in the hypovolemic hypotensive patient; accessibility to the angiographic suite in an emergent setting; institutional experience and resources; necessity for continued surveillance; and lack of long-term follow-up in an evolving new technology.

Reports of EVT in both acute and chronic traumatic rupture of the thoracic aorta have been described with initial feasibility and success.[153,154] A study by Marty-Ane[153] of nine patients undergoing EVT repair of the thoracic aorta, with a follow-up ranging from 4 to 20 months, demonstrated no perioperative deaths, renal failure, or neurologic complications. Only one patient required a second stent graft for a proximal endoleak.

A favorable application of EVT is in patients presenting with injuries to the innominate, subclavian, and axillary arteries. Case reports of EVT repair of the rare injury involving blunt trauma of the innominate artery have had good technical success and follow-up to 18 months.[155,156] Similarly, several institutions have reported treating penetrating injuries of the subclavian and axillary arteries by EVT. Du Toit and associates[157] evaluated stable patients with thoracic outlet arterial injuries and found that 66% of the patients considered were candidates for stent graft repair (seven subclavian arteries, one axillary artery, two carotid arteries). EVT was successful in all, with no complications at the 7-month follow-up. The proximal (zone I) and distal (zone III) carotid artery injuries due to penetrating, blunt, or iatrogenic causes can present difficult surgical management. In a study by Bush and associates,[158] pseudoaneurysms of the carotid artery in five symptomatic patients were treated by endoluminal stent graft, followed by coil embolization of the pseudoaneurysm. At a mean of 8.5 months, all patients were symptom free and in three patients angiograms confirmed carotid patency at a mean of 11.7 months. In another case report by McNeil and associates,[159] a penetrating injury of the internal carotid artery in zone III was treated successfully by EVT.

EVT treatment of vascular injuries of the upper extremity,[160] lower extremity arteriovenous fistula,[161] and dissection of the renal artery following blunt trauma[162] has been described. It is difficult to assess how successful these techniques will be, but early limited experience seems to suggest that EVT may become a valuable and increasingly popular tool for management of vascular injuries in the future.[161] Further studies and long-term follow-up are necessary to determine if EVT treatment of specific traumatic vascular injuries will replace open surgical approaches.

To Repair or Not To Repair?

A trend toward adopting a less aggressive approach to vascular injuries is growing. At one time, all penetrating extremity injuries were surgically explored due to the possibility of finding a significant vascular injury. This approach was subsequently modified so that physical findings, noninvasive evaluations, and arteriography could be used to assess the need for surgical exploration. This was further modified to the point where it was thought that in the absence of any hard findings on physical examination or Doppler evaluation, no further evaluation was necessary. Simultaneously, some authors reported that minor vascular injuries such as small pseudoaneurysms and arteriovenous fistulas, as well as certain intimal defects, need not undergo surgical repair because they were insignificant injuries and did not result in permanent injury to the patient. A publication by Perry[163] cautions us about the morbidity of missed arterial injuries and suggests that further analyses are necessary before we continue in this relatively conservative approach to vascular injuries. Furthermore, the natural history of iatrogenic injuries occurring under controlled circumstances may be different from injuries resulting from blunt and penetrating trauma.

REFERENCES

1. DeBakey ME: Battle injuries of arteries in World War I: An analysis of 2,471 cases. Ann Surg 123:534, 1946.
2. Hughes CW: Arterial repair during the Korean war. Ann Surg 147:555, 1958.
3. Rich NM, Hughes CW: Vietnam vascular registry: A preliminary report. Surgery 65:218, 1969.
4. Rich NM, Baugh JH, Hughes CW: Significance of complications associated with vascular repairs performed in Vietnam. Arch Surg 100:646, 1970.
5. Chobanian AV, Menzoian JO, Shipman J, et al: Effects of endothelial denudation and cholesterol feeding on in vivo transport of albumin, glucose, and water across rabbit carotid artery. Circ Res 53:805, 1983.
6. Gallen J, Wiss DA, Cantelmo N, et al: Traumatic pseudoaneurysm of the axillary artery: Report of three cases and literature review. J Trauma 24:350, 1984.
7. LaMorte WW, Menzoian JO, Sidawy A, et al: A new method for the prediction of peripheral vascular resistance from the preoperative angiogram. J Vasc Surg 2:703, 1985.
8. Johansen K, Lynch K, Paun M, et al: Non-invasive vascular tests reliably exclude occult arterial trauma in injured extremities. J Trauma 31:515, 1991.
9. Bergstein JM, Blair JF, Edwards J, et al: Pitfalls in the use of color-flow duplex ultrasound for screening of suspected arterial injuries in penetrated extremities. J Trauma 33:395, 1992.
10. Fry WR, Smith RS, Sayers DV, et al: The success of duplex ultrasonographic scanning in diagnosis of extremity vascular proximity trauma. Arch Surg 128:1368, 1993.
11. Fry WR, Dort JA, Smith RS, et al: Duplex scanning replaces arteriography and operative exploration in the diagnosis of potential cervical vascular injury. Am J Surg 168:693, 1994.
12. Kuzniec S, Kauffman P, Molnar LJ, et al: Diagnosis of limbs and neck arterial trauma using duplex ultrasonography. Cardiovasc Surg 6:358, 1998.
13. Gagne PJ, Cone JB, McFarland D, et al: Proximity penetrating extremity trauma: The role of duplex ultrasound in the detection of occult venous injuries. J Trauma 39:1157, 1995.
14. Hood DB, Weaver FA, Yellin AE: Changing perspectives in the diagnosis of peripheral vascular trauma. Semin Vasc Surg 11:255, 1998.
15. Keen JD, Keen RR: The cost-effectiveness of exclusion arteriography in extremity trauma. Cardiovasc Surg 9:441, 2001.
16. Accola KD, Feliciano DV, Mattox KL, et al: Management of injuries to the suprarenal aorta. Am J Surg 154:613, 1987.
17. Geuder JW, Hobson RW II, Padberg FT Jr, et al: The role of contrast arteriography in suspected arterial injuries of the extremities. Am Surg 51:89, 1985.

18. Weaver FA, Yellin AE, Bauer M, et al: Is arterial proximity a valid indication for arteriography in penetrating extremity trauma? A prospective analysis. Arch Surg 125:1256, 1990.
19. Kaufman JA, Parker JE, Gillespie DL, et al: Arteriography for proximity of injury in penetrating extremity trauma. J Vasc Interv Radiol 3:719, 1992.
20. Gardner GP, Cordts PR, Gillespie DL, et al: Can air plethysmography accurately identify upper extremity deep venous thrombosis? J Vasc Surg 18:808, 1993.
21. Schwartz MR, Weaver FA, Bauer M, et al: Refining the indications for arteriography in penetrating extremity trauma: A prospective analysis. J Vasc Surg 17:116, 1993.
22. Bok AP, Peter JC: Carotid and vertebral artery occlusion after blunt cervical injury: The role of MR angiography in early diagnosis. J Trauma 40:968, 1996.
23. James CA: Magnetic resonance angiography in trauma. Clin Neurosci 4:137, 1997.
24. Ofer A, Nitecki SS, Braun J, et al: CT angiography of the carotid arteries in trauma to the neck. Eur J Vasc Endovasc Surg 21:401, 2001.
25. Kaiser AB, Clayson KR, Mulherin JL Jr, et al: Antibiotic prophylaxis in vascular surgery. Ann Surg 188:283, 1978.
26. Modrall JG, Weaver FA, Yellin AE: Vascular considerations in extremity trauma. Orthop Clin North Am 24:557, 1993.
27. Nichols JG, Svoboda JA, Parks SN: Use of temporary intraluminal shunts in selected peripheral arterial injuries. J Trauma 26:1094, 1986.
28. Sriussadaporn S, Pak-art R: Temporary intravascular shunt in complex extremity vascular injuries. J Trauma 52:1129, 2002.
29. Dorweiler B, Neufang A, Schmiedt W, et al: Limb trauma with arterial injury: Long-term performance of venous interposition grafts. Thorac Cardiovasc Surg 51:67, 2003.
30. Timberlake GA, Kerstein MD: Venous injury: to repair or ligate, the dilemma revisited. Am Surg 61:139, 1995.
31. Borman KR, Jones GH, Snyder WH III: A decade of lower extremity venous trauma: Patency and outcome. Am J Surg 154:608, 1987.
32. Ierardi RP, Rich N, Kerstein MD: Peripheral venous injuries: A collective review. J Am Coll Surg 183:531, 1996.
33. Pappas PJ, Haser PB, Teehan EP, et al: Outcome of complex venous reconstructions in patients with trauma. J Vasc Surg 25:398, 1997.
34. Sharma PV, Ivatury RR, Simon RJ, et al: Central and regional hemodynamics determine optimal management of major venous injuries. J Vasc Surg 16:887, 1992.
35. Nypaver TJ, Schuler JJ, McDonnell P, et al: Long-term results of venous reconstruction after vascular trauma in civilian practice. J Vasc Surg 16:762, 1992.
36. Hobson RW II, Lee BC, Lynch TG, et al: Use of intermittent pneumatic compression of the calf in femoral venous reconstruction. Surg Gynecol Obstet 159:284, 1984.
37. Blaisdell FW: The pathophysiology of skeletal muscle ischemia and the reperfusion syndrome: A review. Cardiovasc Surg 10:620, 2002.
38. Walker PM, Lindsay TF, Labbe R, et al: Salvage of skeletal muscle with free radical scavengers. J Vasc Surg 5:68, 1987.
39. Wright JG, Kerr JC, Valeri CR, et al: Heparin decreases ischemia-reperfusion injury in isolated canine gracilis model. Arch Surg 123:470, 1988.
40. Fry WJ, Lindenauer SM: Infection complicating the use of plastic arterial implants. Arch Surg 94:600, 1967.
41. Feliciano DV, Mattox KL, Graham JM, et al: Five-year experience with PTFE grafts in vascular wounds. J Trauma 25:71, 1985.
42. Johnson JR, Ledgerwood AM, Lucas CE: Mycotic aneurysm. New concepts in therapy. Arch Surg 118:577, 1983.
43. Yung Chung O, Bruehl SP: Complex regional pain syndrome. Curr Treat Options Neurol 5:499, 2003.
44. Rho RH, Brewer RP, Lamer TJ, et al: Complex regional pain syndrome. Mayo Clin Proc 77:174, 2002.
45. Baron R, Binder A, Ulrich W, et al: [Complex regional pain syndrome. Sympathetic reflex dystrophy and causalgia]. Schmerz 17:213, 2003.
46. McIntyre WB, Ballard JL: Cervicothoracic vascular injuries. Semin Vasc Surg 11:232, 1998.
47. Davis TP, Feliciano DV, Rozycki GS, et al: Results with abdominal vascular trauma in the modern era. Am Surg 67:565, 2001.
48. Mittal VK, Paulson TJ, Colaiuta E, et al: Carotid artery injuries and their management. J Cardiovasc Surg (Torino) 41:423, 2000.
49. van As AB, van Deurzen DF, Verleisdonk EJ: Gunshots to the neck: Selective angiography as part of conservative management. Injury 33:453, 2002.
50. Dichtel WJ, Miller RH, Feliciano DV, et al: Lateral mandibulotomy: A technique of exposure for penetrating injuries of the internal carotid artery at the base of the skull. Laryngoscope 94:1140, 1984.
51. Carrillo EH, Osborne DL, Spain DA, et al: Blunt carotid artery injuries: Difficulties with the diagnosis prior to neurologic event. J Trauma 46:1120, 1999.
52. Kraus RR, Bergstein JM, DeBord JR. Diagnosis, treatment, and outcome of blunt carotid arterial injuries. Am J Surg 178:190, 1999.
53. Cogbill TH, Moore EE, Meissner M, et al: The spectrum of blunt injury to the carotid artery: A multicenter perspective. J Trauma 37:473, 1994.
54. Welling RE, Saul TG, Tew JM Jr, et al: Management of blunt injury to the internal carotid artery. J Trauma 27:1221, 1987.
55. Ledgerwood AM, Mullins RJ, Lucas CE: Primary repair vs ligation for carotid artery injuries. Arch Surg 115:488, 1980.
56. Chandler WF: Penetrating injuries of the carotid artery. Chandler WF (ed): Carotid Artery Injuries. New York, Futura, 1982, p 77.
57. Kuehne JP, Weaver FA, Papanicolaou G, et al: Penetrating trauma of the internal carotid artery. Arch Surg 131:942, 1996.
58. Gewertz BL, Samson DS, Ditmore QM, et al: Management of penetrating injuries of the internal carotid artery at the base of the skull utilizing extracranial-intracranial bypass. J Trauma 20:365, 1980.
59. Sanchez LA, Veith FJ, Ohki T, et al: Early experience with the Corvita endoluminal graft for treatment of arterial injuries. Ann Vasc Surg 13:151, 1999.
60. Hudson HM II, Woodson J, Hirsch E: The management of traumatic aortic tear in the multiply-injured patient. Ann Vasc Surg 5:445, 1991.
61. Melton SK, McGiffin D, McGwin G, Rue LW: The evolution of chest computed tomography for the definitive diagnosis of blunt aortic injury: A single-center experience. J Trauma Inj Infect Crit Care 56:243, 2004.
62. Fabian TR, Croce MA, Smith JS, et al: Prospective study of blunt aortic injury: Multicenter Trial of the American Association for the Surgery of Trauma. J Trauma Inj Infect Crit Care 42:374, 1997.
63. Gavant MM, Fabian T, Flick PA, et al: Blunt traumatic aortic rupture: Detection with helical CT of the chest. Radiology 197:125, 1995.
64. Mirvis SSKBJRA: Use of spiral computed tomography for the assessment of blunt trauma patients with potential aortic injury. J Trauma Inj Infect Crit Care 45:922, 1998.
65. Vignon PG, Vedrinne JM, Lagrange P, Lang RM: Role of transesophageal echocardiography in the diagnosis and management of traumatic aortic disruption. Circulation 92:2959, 1995.
66. Jahromi AS, Kazemi K, Safar HA, et al: Traumatic rupture of the thoracic aorta: Cohort study and systematic review. J Vasc Surg 34:1029, 2001.
67. Langanay T, Verhoye JP, Corbineau H, et al: Surgical treatment of acute traumatic rupture of the thoracic aorta a timing reappraisal? Eur J Cardiothorac Surg 21:282, 2002.
68. Kalakuntla V, Patel V, Tagoe A, et al: Six-year experience with management of subclavian artery injuries. Am Surg 66:927, 2000.
69. Demetriades D, Asensio JA: Subclavian and axillary vascular injuries. Surg Clin North Am 81:1357, 2001.
70. Heise M, Kruger U, Ruckert R, et al: Correlation between angiographic runoff and intraoperative hydraulic impedance with regard to graft patency. Ann Vasc Surg 17:509, 2003.
71. Elkin DC, Cooper FW. resection of the clavicle in vascular injuries. J Trauma 20:537, 1980.
72. Johnston RH Jr, Wall MJ Jr, Mattox KL: Innominate artery trauma: A thirty-year experience. J Vasc Surg 17:134, 1993.
73. Brown MF, Graham JM, Feliciano DV, et al: Carotid artery injuries. Am J Surg 144:748, 1982.
74. Johnson M, Ford M, Johansen K: Radial or ulnar artery laceration. Repair or ligate? Arch Surg 128:971, 1993.
75. Jackson MR, Olson DW, Beckett WC Jr, et al: Abdominal vascular trauma: A review of 106 injuries. Am Surg 58:622, 1992.
76. Tyburski JG, Wilson RF, Dente C, et al: Factors affecting mortality rates in patients with abdominal vascular injuries. J Trauma 50:1020, 2001.
77. Pisters PW, Heslin MJ, Riles TS: Abdominal aortic pseudoaneurysm after blunt trauma. J Vasc Surg 18:307, 1993.
78. Yasuhara H, Naka S, Kuroda T, et al: Blunt thoracic and abdominal vascular trauma and organ injury caused by road traffic accident. Eur J Vasc Endovasc Surg 20:517, 2000.
79. Randhawa MP Jr, Menzoian JO: Seat belt aorta. Ann Vasc Surg 4: 370, 1990.

80. Buchness MP, LoGerfo FW, Mason GR: Gunshot wounds of the suprarenal abdominal aorta. Am Surg 42:1, 1976.
81. Spirnak JP, Resnick MI: Revascularization of traumatic thrombosis of the renal artery. Surg Gynecol Obstet 164:22, 1987.
82. Knudson MM, Harrison PB, Hoyt DB, et al: Outcome after major renovascular injuries: A Western Trauma Association Multicenter Report. J Trauma 49:1116, 2000.
83. Kuehne J, Frankhouse J, Modrall G, et al: Determinants of survival after inferior vena cava trauma. Am Surg 65:976, 1999.
84. Asensio JA, Chahwan S, Hanpeter D, et al: Operative management and outcome of 302 abdominal vascular injuries. Am J Surg 180:528, 2000.
85. Burch JM, Feliciano DV, Mattox KL, et al: Injuries of the inferior vena cava. Am J Surg 156:548, 1988.
86. Buckman RF Jr, Badellino MM, Mauro LH, et al: Penetrating cardiac wounds: Prospective study of factors influencing initial resuscitation. J Trauma 34:717, 1993.
87. Pachter HL, Spencer FC, Hofstetter SR, et al: The management of juxtahepatic venous injuries without an atriocaval shunt: Preliminary clinical observations. Surgery 99:569, 1986.
88. Carr JA, Kralovich KA, Patton JH, et al: Primary venorrhaphy for traumatic inferior vena cava injuries. Am Surg 67:207, 2001.
89. Mullins RJ, Lucas CE, Ledgerwood AM: The injuries of the axilla. Ann Surg 195:232, 1982.
90. Dennis JW, Frykberg ER, Veldenz HC, et al: Validation of nonoperative management of occult vascular injuries and accuracy of physical examination alone in penetrating extremity trauma: 5- to 10-year follow-up. J Trauma 44:243, 1998.
91. Hobson RW II, Howard EW, Wright CB, et al: Hemodynamics of canine femoral venous ligation: Significance in combined arterial and venous injuries. Surgery 74:824, 1973.
92. Orcutt MB, Levine BA, Root HD, et al: The continuing challenge of popliteal vascular injuries. Am J Surg 146:758, 1983.
93. Van Wijingaarden M: Management of blunt vascular trauma to the extremities. Surg Gynecol Obstet 771:41, 1993.
94. Kirby L, Abbas J, Brophy C: Recanalization of an occluded popliteal artery following posterior knee dislocation. Ann Vasc Surg 13:622, 1999.
95. Gable DR, Allen JW, Richardson JD: Blunt popliteal artery injury: Is physical examination alone enough for evaluation? J Trauma 43:541, 1997.
96. Lange RH, Bach AW, Hansen ST Jr, et al: Open tibial fractures with associated vascular injuries: prognosis for limb salvage. J Trauma 25:203, 1985.
97. Segal D, Brenner M, Gorczyca J: Tibial fractures with infrapopliteal arterial injuries. J Orthop Trauma 1:160, 1987.
98. Shah DM, Corson JD, Karmody AM, et al: Optimal management of tibial arterial trauma. J Trauma 28:228, 1988.
99. Neville RF, Padberg FT Jr, DeFouw D, et al: The arterial wall response to intimal injury in an experimental model. Ann Vasc Surg 6:50, 1992.
100. Orcutt MB, Levine BA, Gaskill HV III, et al: Iatrogenic vascular injury. A reducible problem. Arch Surg 120:384, 1985.
101. Rich NM, Hobson RW II, Fedde CW: Vascular trauma secondary to diagnostic and therapeutic procedures. Am J Surg 128:715, 1974.
102. Youkey JR, Clagett GP, Rich NM, et al: Vascular trauma secondary to diagnostic and therapeutic procedures: 1974 through 1982. A comparative review. Am J Surg 146:788, 1983.
103. Mills JL, Wiedeman JE, Robison JG, et al: Minimizing mortality and morbidity from iatrogenic arterial injuries: The need for early recognition and prompt repair. J Vasc Surg 4:22, 1986.
104. Hessel SJ, Adams DF, Abrams HL: Complications of angiography. Radiology 138:273, 1981.
105. Molnar W, Paul DJ: Complications of axillary arteriotomies. An analysis of 1,762 consecutive studies. Radiology 104:269, 1972.
106. Franken EA Jr, Girod D, Sequeira FW, et al: Femoral artery spasm in children: Catheter size is the principal cause. AJR Am J Roentgenol 138:295, 1982.
107. Mani RL, Eisenberg RL, McDonald EJ Jr, et al: Complications of catheter cerebral arteriography: Analysis of 5,000 procedures. I. Criteria and incidence. AJR Am J Roentgenol 131:861, 1978.
108. McCollum CH, Mavor E: Brachial artery injury after cardiac catheterization. J Vasc Surg 4:355, 1986.
109. Davis K, Kennedy JW, Kemp HG Jr, et al: Complications of coronary arteriography from the Collaborative Study of Coronary Artery Surgery (CASS). Circulation 59:1105, 1979.
110. Harris JM Jr: Coronary angiography and its complications. The search for risk factors. Arch Intern Med 144:337, 1984.
111. Corson JD, Johnson WC, LoGerfo FW, et al: Doppler ankle systolic blood pressure. Prognostic value in vein bypass grafts of the lower extremity. Arch Surg 113:932, 1978.
112. Ricci MA, Trevisani GT, Pilcher DB: Vascular complications of cardiac catheterization. Am J Surg 167:375, 1994.
113. Rivers SP, Lee ES, Lyon RT, et al: Successful conservative management of iatrogenic femoral arterial trauma. Ann Vasc Surg 6:45, 1992.
114. Kent KC, McArdle CR, Kennedy B, et al: A prospective study of the clinical outcome of femoral pseudoaneurysms and arteriovenous fistulas induced by arterial puncture. J Vasc Surg 17:125, 1993.
115. McCann RL, Schwartz LB, Pieper KS: Vascular complications of cardiac catheterization. J Vasc Surg 14:375, 1991.
116. Kotval PS, Khoury A, Shah PM, et al: Doppler sonographic demonstration of the progressive spontaneous thrombosis of pseudoaneurysms. J Ultrasound Med 9:185, 1990.
117. Fellmeth BD, Roberts AC, Bookstein JJ, et al: Postangiographic femoral artery injuries: Nonsurgical repair with US-guided compression. Radiology 178:671, 1991.
118. Dorfman GS, Cronan JJ: Postcatheterization femoral artery injuries: Is there a role for nonsurgical treatment? Radiology 178:629, 1991.
119. Sultan S, Nicholls S, Madhavan P, et al: Ultrasound guided human thrombin injection. A new modality in the management of femoral artery pseudo-aneurysms. Eur J Vasc Endovasc Surg 22:542, 2001.
120. Khoury M, Rebecca A, Greene K, et al: Duplex scanning-guided thrombin injection for the treatment of iatrogenic pseudoaneurysms. J Vasc Surg 35:517, 2002.
121. Olsen DM, Rodriguez JA, Vranic M, et al: A prospective study of ultrasound scan-guided thrombin injection of femoral pseudoaneurysm: A trend toward minimal medication. J Vasc Surg 36:779, 2002.
122. Shabani AG, Baxter GM: Inferior epigastric artery pseudoaneurysm: Ultrasound diagnosis and treatment with percutaneous thrombin. Br J Radiol 75:689, 2002.
123. Patel JV, Weston MJ, Kessel DO, et al: Hepatic artery pseudoaneurysm after liver transplantation: Treatment with percutaneous thrombin injection. Transplantation 75:1755, 2003.
124. Manazer JR, Monzon JR, Dietz PA, et al: Treatment of pancreatic pseudoaneurysm with percutaneous transabdominal thrombin injection. J Vasc Surg 38:600, 2003.
125. Weibull H, Bergqvist D, Jonsson K, et al: Complications after percutaneous transluminal angioplasty in the iliac, femoral, and popliteal arteries. J Vasc Surg 5:681, 1987.
126. Oweida SW, Roubin GS, Smith RB III, et al: Postcatheterization vascular complications associated with percutaneous transluminal coronary angioplasty. J Vasc Surg 12:310, 1990.
127. Natali J, Benhamou AC: Iatrogenic vascular injuries. A review of 125 cases (excluding angiographic injuries). J Cardiovasc Surg (Torino) 20:169, 1979.
128. Perler BA, McCabe CJ, Abbott WM, et al: Vascular complications of intra-aortic balloon counterpulsation. Arch Surg 118:957, 1983.
129. Friedell ML, Alpert J, Parsonnet V, et al: Femorofemoral grafts for lower limb ischemia caused by intra-aortic balloon pump. J Vasc Surg 5:180, 1987.
130. Kantrowitz A, Wasfie T, Freed PS, et al: Intraaortic balloon pumping 1967 through 1982: Analysis of complications in 733 patients. Am J Cardiol 57:976, 1986.
131. Barnett MG, Swartz MT, Peterson GJ, et al: Vascular complications from intraaortic balloons: Risk analysis. J Vasc Surg 19:81, 1994.
132. Sznajder JI, Zveibil FR, Bitterman H, et al: Central vein catheterization. Failure and complication rates by three percutaneous approaches. Arch Intern Med 146:259, 1986.
133. Borow M, Crowley JG: Prevention of thrombosis of central venous catheters. J Cardiovasc Surg (Torino) 27:571, 1986.
134. Karmody AM, Leather RP, Shah DM, et al: Peroneal artery bypass: A reappraisal of its value in limb salvage. J Vasc Surg 1:809, 1984.
135. Barash PG, Nardi D, Hammond G, et al: Catheter-induced pulmonary artery perforation. Mechanisms, management, and modifications. J Thorac Cardiovasc Surg 82:5, 1981.
136. Slogoff S, Keats AS, Arlund C: On the safety of radial artery cannulation. Anesthesiology 59:42, 1983.
137. Russell JA, Joel M, Hudson RJ, et al: Prospective evaluation of radial and femoral artery catheterization sites in critically ill adults. Crit Care Med 11:936, 1983.

138. Soderstrom CA, Wasserman DH, Dunham CM, et al: Superiority of the femoral artery of monitoring. A prospective study. Am J Surg 144:309, 1982.
139. Flanigan DP, Keifer TJ, Schuler JJ, et al: Experience with iatrogenic pediatric vascular injuries. Incidence, etiology, management, and results. Ann Surg 198:430, 1983.
140. Klein MD, Coran AG, Whitehouse WM Jr, et al: Management of iatrogenic arterial injuries in infants and children. J Pediatr Surg 17:933, 1982.
141. Schnitzer JJ, Fitzgerald D: Peripheral vascular injuries from plastic bullets in children. Surg Gynecol Obstet 176:172, 1993.
142. Evans WE, King DR, Hayes JP: Arterial trauma in children: Diagnosis and management. Ann Vasc Surg 2:268, 1988.
143. Navarre JR, Cardillo PJ, Gorman JF, et al: Vascular trauma in children and adolescents. Am J Surg 143:229, 1982.
144. Meagher DP Jr, Defore WW, Mattox KL, et al: Vascular trauma in infants and children. J Trauma 19:532, 1979.
145. McNeil JW, Thomas WO III, Luterman A, et al: Penetrating thermal vascular injury in a child: A case report. J Vasc Surg 18:1060, 1993.
146. Shaker IJ, White JJ, Signer RD, et al: Special problems of vascular injuries in children. J Trauma 16:863, 1976.
147. Harris LM, Hordines J: Major vascular injuries in the pediatric population. Ann Vasc Surg 17:266, 2003.
148. Cardneau JD, Henke PK, Upchurch GR Jr, et al: Efficacy and durability of autogenous saphenous vein conduits for lower extremity arterial reconstructions in preadolescent children. J Vasc Surg 34:34, 2001.
149. Lewis HG, Morrison CM, Kennedy PT, et al: Arterial reconstruction using the basilic vein from the zone of injury in pediatric supracondylar humeral fractures: A clinical and radiological series. Plast Reconstr Surg 111:1159, 2003.
150. Kendall RW, Taylor DC, Salvian AJ, et al: The role of arteriography in assessing vascular injuries associated with dislocations of the knee. J Trauma 35:875, 1993.
151. Ohki T, Veith FJ, Marin ML, et al: Endovascular approaches for traumatic arterial lesions. Semin Vasc Surg 10:272, 1997.
152. Risberg B, Lonn L: Management of vascular injuries using endovascular techniques. Eur J Surg 166:196, 2000.
153. Marty-Ane CH, Berthet JP, Branchereau P, et al: Endovascular repair for acute traumatic rupture of the thoracic aorta. Ann Thorac Surg 75:1803, 2003.
154. Gawenda M, Landwehr P, Brunkwall J: Stent-graft replacement of chronic traumatic aneurysm of the thoracic aorta after blunt chest trauma. J Cardiovasc Surg (Torino) 43:705, 2002.
155. Axisa BM, Loftus IM, Fishwick G, et al: Endovascular repair of an innominate artery false aneurysm following blunt trauma. J Endovasc Ther 7:245, 2000.
156. Miles EJ, Blake A, Thompson W, et al: Endovascular repair of acute innominate artery injury due to blunt trauma. Am Surg 69:155, 2003.
157. du Toit DF, Strauss DC, Blaszczyk M, et al: Endovascular treatment of penetrating thoracic outlet arterial injuries. Eur J Vasc Endovasc Surg 19:489, 2000.
158. Bush RL, Lin PH, Dodson TF, et al: Endoluminal stent placement and coil embolization for the management of carotid artery pseudoaneurysms. J Endovasc Ther 8:53, 2001.
159. McNeil JD, Chiou AC, Gunlock MG, et al: Successful endovascular therapy of a penetrating zone III internal carotid injury. J Vasc Surg 36:187, 2002.
160. Ohki T, Veith FJ, Kraas C, et al: Endovascular therapy for upper extremity injury. Semin Vasc Surg 11:106, 1998.
161. Marin ML, Veith FJ, Panetta TF, et al: Percutaneous transfemoral insertion of a stented graft to repair a traumatic femoral arteriovenous fistula. J Vasc Surg 18:299, 1993.
162. Lee JT, White RA: Endovascular management of blunt traumatic renal artery dissection. J Endovasc Ther 9:354, 2002.
163. Perry MO: Complications of missed arterial injuries. J Vasc Surg 17:399, 1993.

■ ■ ■ chapter 64

Vascular Compression Syndromes

David A. Rigberg
Julie A. Freischlag
Herbert I. Machleder

Arterial and venous structures can be compressed by adjacent tissues in several areas in the body. Although not common, there are clinical sequelae to these situations. The anatomic regions most associated with compression syndromes are the thoracic outlet, the popliteal fossa, and the proximal portion of the celiac artery as it passes the arcuate ligament. The basic pathophysiology of these lesions is occasionally seen elsewhere in unusual diseases such as the nutcracker syndrome (compression of the left renal vein between the aorta and superior mesenteric artery), adductor canal compression syndrome (abnormal bands from the adductor magnus compressing the superficial femoral artery), or compression of the distal external iliac artery in bicyclists just proximal to the inguinal ligament. This chapter focuses on the more commonly encountered syndromes.

THORACIC OUTLET SYNDROME

The thoracic outlet syndrome (TOS) describes a spectrum of symptoms and signs all related to the passage of key anatomical structures through a narrow aperture on their way to the upper extremity. This syndrome is manifest in three main forms on the basis of the tissues damaged: neurogenic, venous, and arterial. Considerable controversy surrounds the diagnosis and, some would even argue, the existence of the neurogenic form.

The major shift in the modern conception of TOS occurred in 1956 with Peet and colleagues' coining of the term *thoracic outlet syndrome* and their description of a therapeutic exercise program, essentially the first physical therapy program for TOS.[1] This also coincided with the therapeutic focus shifting to the first rib. In 1962 Clagett described high thoracoplasty for first rib resection, an operation requiring the division of the trapezius and rhomboid muscles.[2] In 1966 Roos described what has become for many the modern treatment of choice for TOS, the transaxillary first rib resection.[3] This operation was fashioned after the transaxillary sympathectomy. First rib resection by this route offered reasonable exposure and minimal morbidity, especially when compared with previously employed techniques.

Anatomy of the Thoracic Outlet

The limited space and large number of important structures that must traverse the neck and chest areas on their way to the upper arm make the thoracic outlet an area like no other in the body. Although any number of anatomic anomalies predispose or directly cause compression to the neural, venous, or arterial structures within its confines, the normal anatomy itself does not leave much room for stress positioning.

Definitions may vary from author to author, but it is generally accepted that the thoracic outlet is the area from the edge of the first rib extending medially to the upper mediastinum and superiorly to the fifth cervical nerve. The clavicle and subclavius muscles can be pictured as forming a roof, while the superior surface of the first rib forms the floor. Machleder's description of the thoracic outlet as a triangle with its apex pointed toward the manubrium is helpful in visualizing the three-dimensional orientation of the structures, as well as the dynamic changes that can lead to injury.[4] In this model, the clavicle and its underlying subclavius muscle and tendon form the superior limb, while the base is the first thoracic rib. The point at which these two structures "overlap" medially can be pictured as the fulcrum of a pair of scissors that opens and closes as the arm moves, potentially causing compression of the thoracic outlet contents (Fig. 64-1).

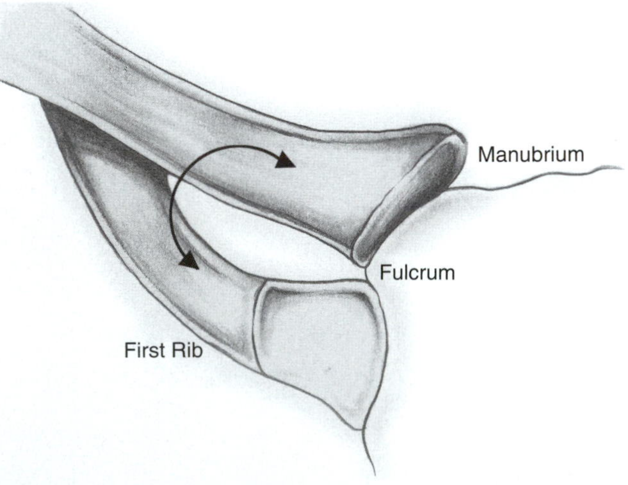

FIGURE 64-1. A useful schematic for visualizing the thoracic outlet, which demonstrates the "scissoring" effect between the clavicle and first rib. Although this is a simplification, it does suggest how removal of either the clavicle or the first rib can decompress the region.

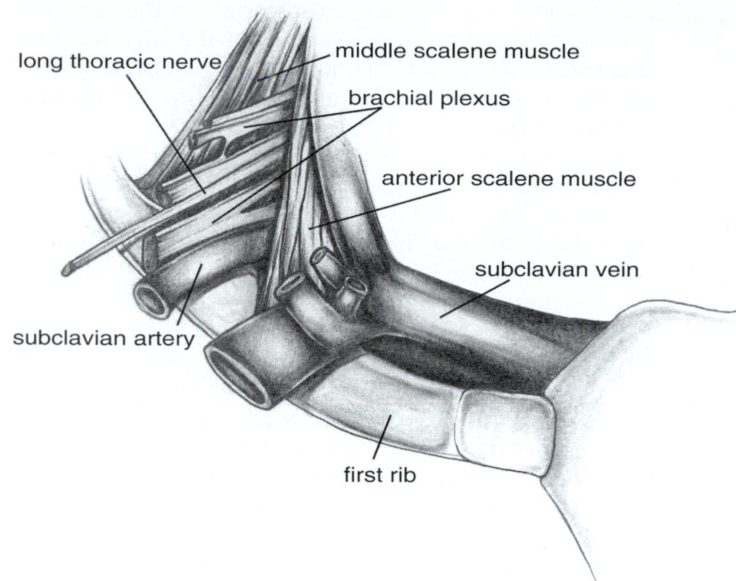

FIGURE 64-2. This diagram shows the complex anatomic relationships within the thoracic outlet, including the broad-based attachment of the middle scalene muscle. The clavicle has been removed for exposure.

Although most TOS symptoms are related to nerve compression, almost any structure that travels through the thoracic outlet can be involved. Moving from medial to lateral, one first encounters the exiting of the subclavian vein, usually positioned adjacent to the region where the first rib and clavicular head fuse to form a fibrocartilaginous joint with the manubrium. Immediately lateral to the vein is the anterior scalene muscle, which inserts onto a prominence on the first rib. Lateral to this site is the subclavian artery, so that the anterior scalene muscle lies between the subclavian artery and vein, with the artery deep, lateral, and somewhat cephalad. The brachial plexus is the next structure encountered. The C4-C6 roots are superiorly oriented, and the C7-T1 roots inferior. Posterior and lateral to the plexus, there is a generally rather broad attachment of the middle scalene muscle to the first rib (Fig. 64-2).

Other structures encountered in the thoracic outlet include the phrenic and dorsal scapular nerves, the stellate ganglion, the thoracic duct, and the cupola of the lung. The thoracic duct may be encountered if a left supraclavicular approach is undertaken, and care must be taken not to injure it or to ligate it if injury occurs. Finally, one must watch for pleural injury in any approach to TOS and be prepared to evacuate pneumothoraces when indicated.

Pathophysiology of Thoracic Outlet Syndrome

The cervical rib is the most obvious bony abnormality contributing to TOS, and autopsy studies indicate that roughly 0.5% of the general population has this structure (Fig. 64-3).[5] Series from the United States generally report cervical ribs in 10% of TOS patients, although others have reported these are present in up to 65% of TOS patients.[5] The European literature reports that cervical ribs are present in approximately 25% of TOS patients.[6] The reason for this discrepancy is not known. Cervical ribs can be completely formed or rudimentary. In the latter case, there is almost always a compressive band of tissue extending to the first thoracic rib. As they project from transverse processes, cervical ribs displace the involved structures forward. The subclavian artery is particularly vulnerable to damage in this configuration, and some surgeons feel that arterial changes secondary to TOS rarely occur in the absence of a cervical rib.

A number of other bony abnormalities are found in association with TOS. Post-traumatic changes following clavicular or first rib fractures are commonly reported, with callous formation at the clavicle and pseudoarthroses of the first rib. Elongated C7 transverse processes also are seen occasionally. These changes frequently can be appreciated radiographically.

The majority of TOS cases are associated with some form of soft tissue anomaly. Work by Juvonen, Raymond, and others led to appreciation of the multiple forms of TOS.[7] However, the classification system of Roos is the

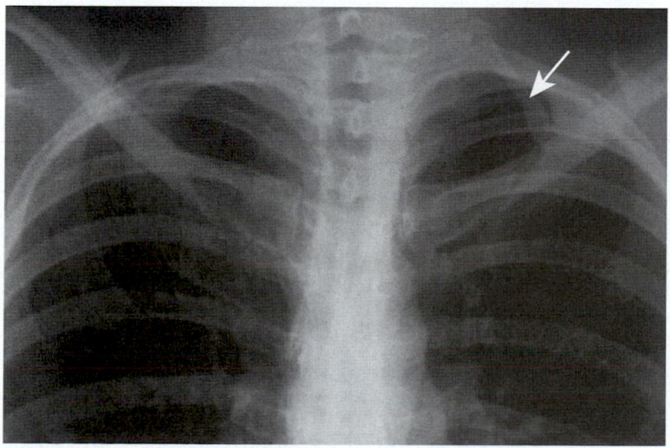

FIGURE 64-3. Chest radiogram demonstrating a left cervical rib (*arrow*).

TABLE 64-1 ROOS CLASSIFICATION SYSTEM FOR THORACIC OUTLET SYNDROME ANATOMY

I	Incomplete cervical rib with fibrous band connected to rib
II	Abortive cervical rib (band only)
III	Accessory muscle between neck and tubercle of first rib
IV	Enlarged middle scalene muscle compressing T1 nerve root
V	Scalenus minimus muscle
VI	Scalenus minimus muscle with a band to the endothoracic fascia
VII	Band from the middle scalene to the sternum or costal cartilages
VIII	Similar to type VII, but band passes beneath the subclavian vein
IX	Web filling the inner surface of the first rib
X	Double band from cervical rib to first rib, with a limb to the sternum

most thorough, with 10 distinct anomalies with several subtypes observed intraoperatively (Table 64-1).[8]

In addition to these anatomic arrangements, hypertrophy of the normal musculature or tendons has been implicated in TOS. For example, some surgeons see a link between Paget-Schroetter syndrome and subclavius tendon hypertrophy, particularly in the presence of an enlarged insertion tubercle. Others have implicated a role for the pectoralis minor muscle.[9] Another association occurs with weight lifting, frequently in a young man, with hypertrophied scalene musculature. Anatomic studies have documented the compression of the subclavian vein into the costoclavicular notch by this muscle.[10] This has clear implications for axillo-subclavian vein thrombosis.

Trauma in general is implicated in the pathogenesis of TOS, particularly when the trauma is localized to the neck and shoulder. Hyperextension, or whiplash injury, occurs in this patient population with some frequency. This can also be seen with repetitive motion-type injuries. In a review of operative TOS patients by Sanders and Hammond,[11] 86% had a history of trauma. This prevalence of trauma is considerably higher than in many other reports but stresses the role that trauma can play in the disorder.[11]

Presentation of Thoracic Outlet Syndrome

Neurogenic

Patients can present with the symptoms of neurogenic TOS at any age, although the usual case is a young to middle-aged adult with no other major health issues. When confronted by the pediatric or younger teenage patient with purely neurogenic symptoms, clinical practice is usually to recommend a period of waiting to see if growth allows the symptoms to abate. The neurogenic symptoms can range in severity from nuisance to severely debilitating pain. Motor effects are seen, and although gross dysfunction of the upper extremity is unusual, a degree of weakness is not. This occasionally manifests as a decrease in grip strength. Gilliat's description of classic neurogenic TOS with muscle wasting in the hand is not common.[12]

The pain may originate anywhere in the upper extremity, but the most common site is the back of the shoulder. The supracapsular portion of the trapezius may be involved. From the shoulder, pain can spread up the ipsilateral extremity, along the back and neck or even up the face. This situation can lead to hemicranial headaches that can be labeled migraines.

Pain involving the arm can be focused to a particular nerve distribution or generalized. When localized, ulnar symptoms tend to be the most common, leading to difficulties with the ring and small fingers. Many authors report that these "lower plexus" (C8-T1) symptoms are more common than "upper" (C5-C7) manifestations.

Patients may report pain at rest that is not relieved by positioning. However, the typical patient reports that stress positioning exacerbates symptoms. This is particularly the case with work-related situations. People who must perform tasks with elevated arms or hold their arms in other awkward positions note they are no longer able to perform these tasks. Examples include waitresses, mechanics, and truck drivers. With prolonged stress positioning, patients may report finger discoloration, coolness of the extremity, or even swelling. Driving an automobile can be difficult with the concomitant numbness and tingling in the fingers that can occur.

Patients often report that their symptom complex started following a traumatic event. These can be chronic, repetitive-type injuries such as seen with pitchers and other athletes. Direct injury to the chest wall or shoulder can also precipitate symptoms, particularly if associated with a clavicular fracture or an acromioclavicular joint dislocation. Whiplash-type injuries are also associated with TOS. Even a relatively minor injury can "unmask" the syndrome in a previously completely asymptomatic individual.

Paget-Schroetter Syndrome

Paget-Schroetter syndrome (axillosubclavian vein thrombosis or "effort" thrombosis) usually presents suddenly in a previously healthy patient with no symptoms of neurogenic TOS. Typically, the patient is a young athlete or worker with a component to their sport or job that requires prolonged or repetitive stressful positioning of the arm. Examples include baseball players, swimmers, weight lifters, volleyball players, and mechanics. This presentation is dramatic compared to neurogenic TOS, and patients usually seek medical attention immediately.

The involved extremity is swollen and often has a degree of discoloration, from rubor to cyanosis. The redness may be confused with the erythema of an infection, leading to a delay in diagnosis. Physical examination may reveal the presence of dilated collateral veins around the shoulder and upper arm. The remainder of the physical examination is usually normal.

If the condition is left untreated, the swelling resolves over the course of days or weeks. The patient typically does not have symptoms at rest but cannot use the arm for any period of time, particularly in a stressed (abducted, externally rotated) position. The collateral channels that develop and allow the swelling to abate are almost never adequate to accommodate the increased venous return that occurs with activity.

An alternate presentation is associated with an acute traumatic injury. Typically, the patient has an injury to the shoulder area. After a few days pass, some degree of ipsilateral arm swelling occurs. The natural history of this variant of Paget-Schroetter syndrome is the same, reflecting the fact that the injury most likely contributed to compression in the thoracic outlet so that the thrombosis associated with injury is really the same insult seen in "spontaneous" thrombosis.

Symptoms of neurogenic TOS are not usually associated with Paget-Schroetter syndrome. Although not common, ipsilateral sympathetic hyperactivity is not rare in this setting.

Arterial Complications of Thoracic Outlet Syndrome

Subclavian artery compression can lead to a number of injuries, and its presentation is the most varied of all forms of TOS. Damage to the subclavian artery itself can result in arterial pathology ranging from a small stenosis to aneurysm formation or complete occlusion. Each of these occurrences then can have its own sequelae secondary to embolization or thrombosis or the extremely rare rupture of a subclavian aneurysm.

Patients not infrequently are misdiagnosed with collagen vascular disease because of cold sensitivity, Raynaud's phenomena, and other symptoms. These patients may develop frank ischemic conditions of the hands, with parenchymal ulcers or fingertip gangrene. If the subclavian artery is completely occluded, patients may present with early fatigue of the involved side. This may be described as "crampy" pain with exercise and has led to the term "arm claudication."

Diagnosis of Thoracic Outlet Syndrome

It is important to point out that there is no generally accepted battery of tests that must be performed to confirm the presence of TOS. Most surgeons routinely dealing with the disorder require at a minimum a physical examination consistent with the symptoms, cervical films to rule out disc disease, and a chest radiograph to visualize any bony abnormalities one may encounter. Various other tests may be applied in different clinical situations or when the diagnosis is not clear. Different specialists also can have differing approaches to the diagnosis, and the need for invasive or expensive tests is an area of considerable debate.

History and Physical Examination

An extensive history should be taken from the patient including any injuries, as well as the patient's occupation. Activities that worsen and improve the discomfort or other symptoms should be ascertained. In conjunction with a good history, most cases of TOS are diagnosed on the basis of physical examination. In addition, the physical examination plays an important role in ruling out other causes of a patient's symptoms. A thorough examination should focus not only on the site of complaints, but also on other areas commonly involved in neurologic conditions. This includes the general appearance of the patient and other signs of symptom impact. Note should be made of symmetry of the muscle groups of the shoulders and upper extremities.

Serratus anterior atrophy is occasionally present with TOS, as demonstrated by a winged scapula. Although cervical symptoms are common with TOS, limited cervical range of motion is not and there should not be excessive tenderness over the vertebral bodies. The presence of either of these suggests an alternate diagnosis. Deep-tendon reflexes, grip strength, and pulses should be routinely assessed. Palmar hyperhidrosis should be noted, if present. Machleder points out that even in neurogenic TOS, changes in pulses can sometimes be readily detected.[13] Specific provocative neurologic maneuvers, such as downward compression of the head to rule out cervical disc disease, can be used when necessary. After this general neurologic assessment, tests more specific for the presence of thoracic outlet compression can be undertaken.

Patients with TOS generally do not have obvious muscle atrophy and, in fact, have nearly normal gross baseline sensory and motor examinations. However, useful information can still be obtained if one uses an organized approach. Initial palpation of the structures of the chest wall, cervical area, and shoulder can be useful before undertaking provocative testing. The region overlying the anterior scalene muscle is frequently exquisitely tender in the face of brachial plexus entrapment or irritation. In addition, percussion of the clavicle can reproduce pains and paresthesias in TOS patients. These simple maneuvers should be performed before more complex maneuvering of the patient, which may cloud later findings.

The most used of the TOS tests is probably the elevated arm stress test (EAST), which was originally described by Roos in 1966 as a means for eliciting upper extremity claudication and neurologic symptoms.[14] In the test, the patient is asked to completely elevate the shoulders and arms ("hold-up position") and then to repeatedly clench and unclench his or her hands. This positioning is designed to constrict the costoclavicular space, and by many reports will bring on weakness and paresthesias in the ulnar and median nerve distributions in patients with TOS within 3 minutes. Its proponents argue that it is specific for TOS and that the time of onset of symptoms correlates with the severity of TOS. In addition, it is thought by many that the test is good for reproducing the symptoms that patients suffer while using their upper extremities at work. Attention should also be made to the color of the hands during the EAST, as one may become pale and ischemic if arterial compromise is involved.

This test is not without its detractors. Although anecdotally reported to have excellent specificity, a study from 1985 found a positive test in more than 80% of patients with carpal tunnel syndrome. An earlier study by this same group found a positive EAST in almost all healthy patients, although they did note that the positive tests occurred earlier in patients with TOS.[15] Additionally, some question the anatomic basis for the test, particularly how clenching and unclenching of the hand can lead to stress of the brachial plexus.[16]

Closely related to the EAST is the abduction and external rotation (AER) test. The arm is abducted and rotated and held in that position. This test works by a similar mechanism and likewise produces the weakness and numbness seen with EAST in a similar distribution, namely the C8 to T1 fibers supplying the median and ulnar nerves. In addition, one can sometimes detect a bruit below the lateral portion of the clavicle that is attributable to partial compression of the axillary artery. Both of these tests appear particularly suited to work-related and repetitive motion–associated TOS.[17]

Additional information can be gained by adding pulse examination to the previously mentioned tests. The original Adson test consisted of assessment of the radial pulse following rotation of the neck to the contralateral side and deep inspiration. "Adson sign" is the subsequent loss of the radial pulse. This test is notoriously nonsensitive and has been reported to be positive in less than 3% of TOS patients.[18] In 1945 Wright described the hyperabduction position, which is also of little clinical utility given its positive result in most healthy individuals. However, measurements that quantify blood pressure are more sensitive, and a drop of 20 mm Hg after movement from neutral position, or the same pressure difference from one extremity to the other, is frequently present in TOS. Using the Doppler probe assists these tests. None of these aforementioned tests is pathognomonic, but the presence of one or more of them can help to support the diagnosis of TOS. Combined with the proper history, other disorders can be effectively ruled out and other tests avoided.

Objective Testing

The cervical spine film and chest radiograph are the most important objective studies needed in making the diagnosis of TOS. Clearly, cervical disease must be excluded as a cause of neurologic symptoms, and the bony abnormalities of TOS (cervical ribs, elongated C7 transverse processes, fractures with exostosis, or callus formation) can be appreciated on plain chest films. The use of MRI and CT is advocated by some, but the utility of these studies has yet to be proved. Ongoing studies are addressing this issue.

The use of objective neurodiagnostic tests for TOS has met with some success, although it continues to be an area of considerable controversy. Perhaps the main criticism of these tests is that they only tend to be positive in patients with advanced disease, in whom history and physical examination should be sufficient. Thus no less an authority than Dr. David Roos suggests they offer "little definitive diagnostic information" and that one "still must rely on careful history and physical..."[15] All of this reflects the fact that most electrophysiologic tests evaluate larger myelinated nerve fibers, not the smaller fibers whose injury mediates the pain associated with TOS. A recent study by Franklin and coauthors found that of 158 TOS patients, only 7.6% had abnormalities in their electrodiagnostic tests.[19] Nonetheless, these tests can aid in making the diagnosis of TOS and in excluding other conditions.

Neurophysiologic testing came to the forefront in the early 1960s, but the anatomic constraints of attempting to measure changes across the brachial plexus have always made its application in this position difficult. Nerve conduction studies can offer limited information in the work-up of TOS and can show evidence of carpal tunnel syndrome, either alone or in conjunction with the double-crush syndrome. Conduction studies do not offer definitive diagnostic information as specifically related to TOS. To measure velocities usefully, the nerve must be stimulated proximal to the potential point of injury. For compression at the thoracic outlet, this could mean stimulation at the roots, a site not conducive to easy testing.

Several authors have described their experience using ulnar conduction velocity from Erb's point (above the clavicle and lateral to the insertion of the sternocleidomastoid muscle) to the elbow to assess TOS, but this technique has been criticized.[13] However, if there is severe disease with concomitant axonal damage, changes in ulnar action potentials can be demonstrated. A reasonable approach to conduction studies includes sensory testing of the median and ulnar nerves at the wrist to screen for carpel tunnel syndrome and TOS, respectively. The addition of motor nerve conduction velocities can be considered if additional information is necessary to rule out carpel tunnel syndrome or ulnar entrapment neuropathy. However, no specific motor pathways for demonstrating TOS have been determined.

Electromyography is also capable of showing objective data supporting the diagnosis of TOS, although this is again in a setting of advanced disease. This study can demonstrate spontaneous firing of acutely denervated muscle fibers (positive sharp waves, fibrillation potentials), but this is not the usual clinical situation for TOS. Rather, after reinnervation, prolonged and irregular potentials are seen. Because this is a reflection of previous denervation injury, many of these patients have atrophy of the involved muscle groups and the electromyogram (EMG) can confirm that the lower trunk of the brachial plexus was injured. However, in patients without evidence of atrophy, this test is not likely to reveal these findings. This fact is supported by studies showing that standard EMG tests are negative in 62% of TOS patients.[20] However, these tests can be used to examine the paraspinal muscles, which can be important in ruling out radiculopathy as the cause of the patient's symptoms.

EMG has an additional role that bears mentioning, that of an adjunct to needle placement for scalene block. This test has utility as a predictor of surgical outcome for neurogenic TOS, with relaxation of the anterior scalene muscle approximating the decompression achieved with first rib resection/scalenectomy. Inadvertent needle placement can confuse the results of this test or cause injury, particularly to the brachial plexus itself or even the sympathetic ganglia at that level. Patients are given a series of injections of either lidocaine or saline, and then pain with provocative maneuvers is assessed (generally the EAST). Jordan and Machleder[21] reported on 122 patients in whom this technique was used and found a 90% positive predictive value for correlation with the clinical diagnosis of TOS. In addition, for patients undergoing first rib resection for TOS, those with a positive scalene block had a much greater chance of a good outcome

(94%) than those with a negative preoperative scalene block (50%). This test can be positive with other disorders, particularly radiculopathies, yet is another useful adjunct not only for the diagnosis of TOS, but also to predict the likelihood of surgical benefit.

F-wave studies are an attractive concept for evaluating TOS because they allow for propagation of the stimulus back to the spinal cord, thus crossing the brachial plexus and obviating the need for proximal nerve access. In this technique, nerve stimulation at the wrist leads to not only an immediate action potential in the affected muscle groups, but also to this proximal propagation with a concomitant reflection from the cord leading to a secondary action potential. This returning potential is the F-wave. Generally, multiple trials are recorded and the shortest period between percutaneous stimulus and the secondary response is taken as the latency. This period is delayed if the nerve fibers are damaged, as can be seen with TOS. These tests tend to be poorly tolerated by many patients, and it is prudent to avoid their use unless other tests have proved unrewarding and further diagnostic information is required.

Somatosensory evoked potentials (SSEPs) can play a role in the work-up of TOS. Currently, assessment of the ulnar and median nerves can be used for evidence of their compression at the thoracic outlet. These studies, when abnormal, tend to show lower plexus injury (ulnar) with normal median function. This is seen primarily as a blunting of the Erb point peak. Machleder and colleagues[22] showed that 74% of their patients carrying a clinical diagnosis of TOS had abnormal evoked responses. Furthermore, when these patients were studied following operative decompression of their thoracic outlets, more than 90% had correlation between improved symptoms and normalization of their SSEPs.[22] Increases of the sensitivity of these tests can be achieved with provocative maneuvers, such as arm positioning, although these maneuvers can also cause SE changes in patients with no clinical evidence of TOS.

Diagnosis of Paget-Schroetter Syndrome

In the TOS patient who presents with upper extremity swelling, the diagnosis of axillo-subclavian vein thrombosis is suggested by the history and physical examination described earlier. Assessment of the venous system is usually initiated with noninvasive duplex ultrasonography and dynamic phlebography. Provocative positioning, such as external rotation and abduction, can increase the sensitivity of these tests. Other authors describe a two-position technique, with the arms fully adducted and then 90 degrees abducted. It is not clear at this time how useful magnetic resonance venography is for axillosubclavian evaluation. It appears to have anatomic limitations similar to duplex ultrasonography, with poor quality of images in the retroclavicular space.

Most patients undergo a diagnostic venogram, which is the gold standard for thrombosis in this situation (Fig. 64-4). Although this test confirms the diagnosis of thrombosis, the occasional patient needs further clarification as to its cause. Neurogenic symptoms are usually not present, and one must often rely on the exclusion of causes of venous thrombosis other than TOS in this situation.

Diagnosis of Arterial Disease in Thoracic Outlet Syndrome

As discussed in a previous section, a number of symptoms and signs are a consequence of arterial involvement in TOS. Thus the diagnostic algorithm is not straightforward. Physical examination may be helpful, with the presence of subclavian bruits, pulse changes with provocative positioning, and blood pressure differentials between the extremities. The stress positions described previously can be used. Patients may initially be evaluated with digital plethysmography or upper extremity arterial duplex ultrasonography. These may be abnormal depending on the lesion, and arteriography is almost always

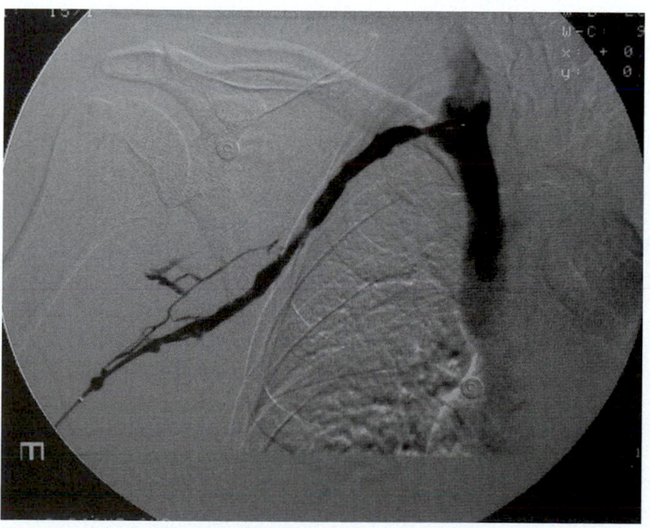

A

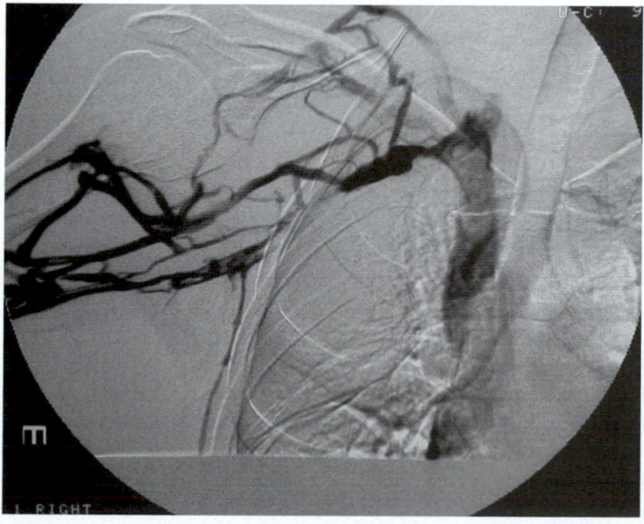

B

FIGURE 64-4. These two images clearly display compression of the axillo-subclavian vein when the arm is placed in the neutral position (**A**) and stressed, abducted position (**B**). The images must be obtained with and without stress positioning to confirm the diagnosis.

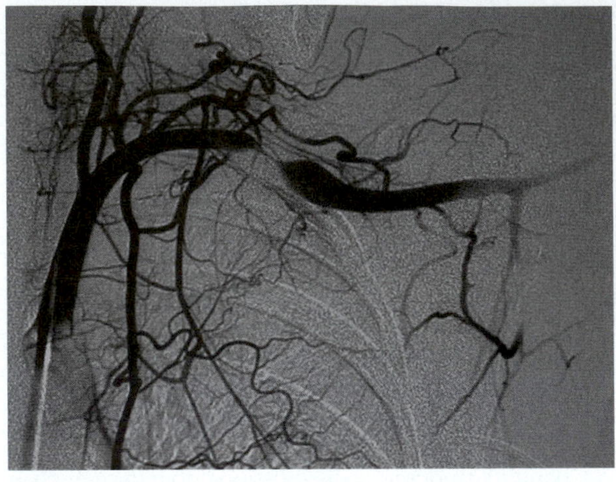

A

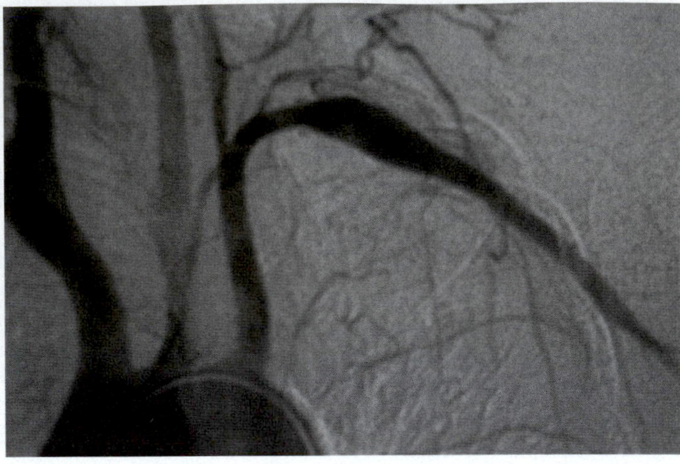

B

FIGURE 64-5. Angiogram demonstrating occlusion of the subclavian artery when the arm is abducted (**A**), with resumption of flow when the arm is returned to the neutral position (**B**). Note the presence of poststenotic dilatation when the arm is fully adducted.

required in this setting. When arterial compression is suspected, attention should first be toward an arch study to include the subclavian and axillary arteries more distally.

Frequently, arterial compression can be better visualized if the arm is abducted 90 degrees, and most studies are obtained with the arms in these two positions (Fig. 64-5). When distal embolization is suggested, the angiography should encompass the target sites, often requiring studies of the hand on the affected side. As experience has been gained with MRA, this technique has also been applied to TOS. Again, provocative positioning (abduction) is frequently useful in this setting.

Treatment of Thoracic Outlet Syndrome

The vast majority of patients with neurogenic TOS, in all likelihood, go undiagnosed and thus receive no therapy. This reflects the range of severity inherent in the spectrum of symptoms associated with TOS. For those seeking medical intervention, it is clear that most have substantial improvement without operation. Although the numbers are controversial and dependent on the modalities used to make the diagnosis, more than 95% of patients avoid operation. Currently, considerable debate surrounds neurogenic TOS surgery, with several groups reporting no long-term benefit from operation versus physical therapy. Nonetheless, most surgeons with considerable experience with neurogenic TOS report good surgical results with properly selected patients.

For many TOS surgeons, referral patterns are such that patients have already undertaken unsuccessful conservative therapy before seeking further consultation. It is important for surgeons to be aware of this selection bias. It is also important to have an algorithm for conservative treatment so that the correct patients are selected for operation. A minimum of 6 weeks of physical therapy is required before its effects can be evaluated. It is also key that the correct program is used, as it has been recognized that inappropriate physical therapy can worsen TOS symptoms. In general, these programs are designed to relax muscle groups that tighten the thoracic outlet while conditioning those that open it. Aligne and Barral thus described a program in which the trapezius, levator scapulae, and sternocleidomastoid muscles are strengthened and the middle scalene, subclavius, and pectoralis muscles relaxed.[23]

Other nonsurgical interventions are available. Following the concept of diagnostic scalene blocks, attempts have been made at therapeutic blockade of the scalene muscles. Steroid injection has not been successful, and early attempts at using botulinum toxin were complicated by dysphagia in up to 20% of attempts. However, recent work by Jordan and coauthors[24] demonstrated that electrophysiologic and fluoroscopic guidance of needle placement decreased the incidence of dysphagia and relieved symptoms for a mean duration of 88 days. This technique may prove to be a useful tool either in relieving symptoms in the preoperative period or in allowing the patient to tolerate an extended period of physical therapy or other adjustments, such as in their ergonomics at work.

Surgical Treatment

When a symptomatic patient who has sought treatment fails to improve with physical therapy, surgical intervention is warranted. First, rib resection can be performed via either the transaxillary or supraclavicular approach. The patient is placed in the lateral decubitus position, with the head neutral. No paralytic agents are used. Various devices are available for elevation of the arm on the operative side, all of which should permit easy lowering of the extremity intermittently throughout the procedure to allow periods of increased arterial inflow and decreased tension on stretched nerves (Fig. 64-6). The incision is placed between the pectoralis major and the latissimus dorsi in the lower aspect of the axilla. Dissection is carried out, with care taken to identify intercostal brachial cutaneous nerves. These structures should be avoided and preserved when possible, but it is

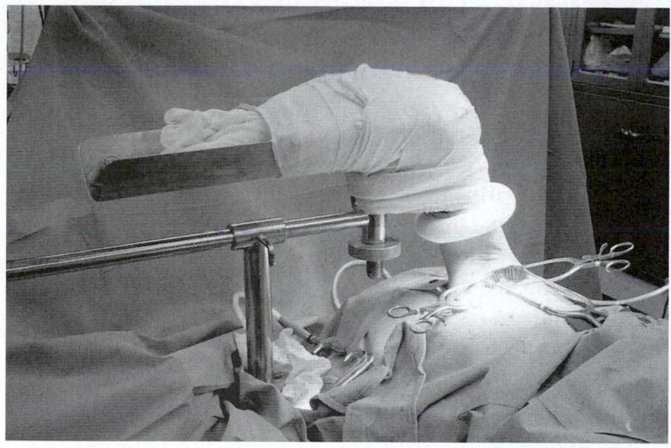

FIGURE 64-6. Proper positioning of the patient for transaxillary first rib resection is shown. Although it is possible to perform the procedure using an assistant to support the ipsilateral upper extremity, customized retractor systems are the preferred method. There should be a mechanism for convenient intermittent lowering of the arm to allow perfusion in a less stressed position during the course of the operation.

preferable to sacrifice them rather than to leave them injured, thereby subjecting the patient to possible causalgic pain. Care must be taken in the region of the posterior scalene muscle to identify the long thoracic nerve, as injury with resulting winged scapula has been reported when this structure aberrantly passes close to the midaxillary line.

After the connective tissue over the thoracic outlet is opened using blunt techniques, the subclavian vein and artery, anterior scalene muscle, and lower trunk of the brachial plexus can be identified and cleared. The anterior scalene muscle is now carefully separated from the subclavian vessels, and its attachment to the first rib can be divided. The subclavius tendon is also divided. Before the rib can be removed, further attachments between it and the middle scalene and first intercostal muscle must be released, with particular care taken not to injure the T1 nerve. A right-angled rib shear is next positioned posteriorly over the first rib so that it approaches the transverse process of T1. Anteriorly, the rib is divided almost at the level of the costal cartilage. Considerable care must be taken following removal of the rib to smooth the posterior stump to prevent any subsequent T1 injury. At this point, any further encountered anomalies (fibromuscular bands, scalenus minimus muscles) should be resected. Cervical ribs are resected in a similar fashion to the first rib, requiring division of their attachments to the middle scalene and intercostal muscles.

Before closure, irrigation is placed into the wound and inspection is made for a pleural leak. In the presence of a leak, a small chest tube can be used for pleural drainage. This can usually be removed the following day. A postoperative chest radiograph is obtained. Most patients are discharged to home on postoperative day 1 or 2. Careful follow-up and physical therapy are also employed in the early postoperative period.

Scalenectomy is considered for TOS in three situations. The first is when the patient's symptoms are particularly suggestive of upper brachial plexus involvement (as opposed to the more common lower plexus). As described by Roos,[35] it is reasonable to use an approach in which these nerves can be more directly decompressed. The second situation is that in patients who have undergone transaxillary operation but now have upper plexus symptoms. The third situation is one in which some surgeons believe that the supraclavicular approach is as effective as the transaxillary operation and safer; thus they use this approach routinely. The first rib can also be resected as a component of this procedure, although some argue that it cannot be done with the same margins as the transaxillary approach.

As with the transaxillary approach, no paralytics are used so that nerve function can be assessed intraoperatively. The patient is placed in the semi-Fowler position, with the head turned away from the operative side. An incision is placed two fingerbreadths above the clavicle, extending from the external jugular vein to the sternocleidomastoid muscle. This muscle is subsequently mobilized medially, while the omohyoid muscle must usually be transected. The scalene fat pad is carefully divided, taking care to avoid the underlying phrenic nerve. This structure must be protected throughout the course of the operation. Underlying the nerve is the anterior scalene muscle. This is divided inferiorly at its insertion on the first rib. There are usually adhesions between the muscle and the subclavian artery and brachial plexus components that also must be freed, and the origin end of the muscle is divided medially to expose the C5-C7 roots. The area between the C7 root and the subclavian artery is next cleaned, including the division of a subclavius minimus muscle if present. At this point, the five roots should be completely cleaned and tested using a nerve stimulator, although many surgeons have noted that it is often difficult to assess the T1 nerve root in this manner.

If the operation is to include first rib resection, the middle scalene muscle must be divided. The rib is divided posteriorly and a finger used to dissect it from the pleura while elevating the divided end. The subclavian artery must be freed from the anterior portion of the rib before it is divided. It can then be carefully extracted.

Irrigation is placed in the wound to assess for pleural leak. If present, the soft closed suction drain can be positioned so that the tip drains the pleural space. Otherwise, the drain can be placed to drain the wound. Postoperative chest radiograph is obtained, and the patient is usually discharged home within 1 or 2 days.

A brief mention should be made here of thoracoscopic first rib resection. This procedure has not gained widespread acceptance, as some question the benefits versus the transaxillary approach. Nonetheless, it is offered at several centers, and it remains to be seen what place this operation will play in the treatment of TOS.[25]

Treatment of Venous Thrombosis

Venous occlusion at the thoracic outlet should be treated expeditiously. Although this disease was once treated with anticoagulation and arm elevation, therapeutic protocols now stress the importance of dissolving the clot, maintaining patency of the axillo-subclavian veins, and correcting any anatomic abnormalities contributing to the thrombosis. Once the diagnosis has been established, the patient should be taken for catheter-directed fibrinolysis of the clot. Streptokinase, urokinase, and tPA have all been used successfully. In addition to the clot-directed therapy, patients should receive heparin and then warfarin (Coumadin). Work by Machleder and Kunkle[26] demonstrated that a period of 1 to 3 months of anticoagulation allowed for intimal healing of the damaged vein before the patient was taken for definitive surgery with first rib resection. Following surgery, the vein is again assessed. If residual stricture exists, the patient undergoes further catheter-based treatment.

In attempts to decrease the period of disability between the initial lysis and the definitive operation, some authors have advocated first rib resection during the initial hospitalization. Angle and authors[27] recently reported a series of patients treated in this fashion and noted no increased morbidity compared with patients with delayed operation. In particular, none of the theoretical concerns for bleeding following thrombolytic instillation were realized, nor were there particular technical problems secondary to the inflammation associated with the venous thrombosis. It is likely that a policy of early surgical intervention will be employed by many vascular specialists, even though no randomized prospective trial has yet to compare these two protocols.

Angioplasty for residual stricture appears to work quite well following correction of the anatomical problems.[27] Stenting, however, has not been particularly useful.[28] In some cases the vein is so severely damaged that the only operative repair possible is a jugular-subclavian bypass, although this is rarely undertaken.

Thrombus that resists thrombolysis suggests a component of chronic disease. Machleder and colleagues[22] observed that these patients may have intermittent periods of clot propagation for which their collaterals are not adequate to compensate. It is during these times that there is "acute" swelling. It is unclear what the ideal treatment is in this situation. If the patient has resolution of the acute symptoms, anticoagulation is a reasonable option. For symptomatic patients, either surgical or endovascular treatment tailored to the particular problem is warranted. A first rib resection may be helpful in improving symptoms in patients with a completely occluded vein that resists attempts at recanalization. This is particularly true in the case of long-segment axillo-subclavian occlusions.

Treatment of Arterial Complications of Thoracic Outlet Syndrome

As previously discussed, a number of arterial problems can arise from thoracic outlet obstruction, although they are not common. The area of arterial involvement is usually the retroscalene subclavian artery to the prepectoral region of the axillary artery. The urgency of intervention depends on the severity of the problem, with ischemia requiring an expeditious approach. Transaxillary first rib resection followed by arterial repair is the treatment of choice in most cases. If treating a patient with emboli, catheter-based thrombolysis is usually necessary before addressing the source of embolism.

Aneurysms secondary to TOS usually are treated with resection and graft reconstruction, as is done with aneurysms caused by atherosclerosis. This is also the treatment for axillosubclavian poststenotic dilatation and obstruction. Standard approaches are used, with a high anterior thoracotomy for proximal lesions on the left and a median sternotomy for proximal lesions on the right. For more distal lesions, various supra- and infra-clavicular incisions may be used. Graft material is a matter of surgeon's preference, but synthetic material, vein grafts and arterial grafts all have been used with success in this position. Postoperative anticoagulation usually is not indicated, and patients tend to do well if the thoracic outlet is adequately decompressed and the vessel is no longer subjected to trauma.

An additional consideration in these patients is the presence of reflex sympathetic dystrophy, causalgia, or other autonomic dysfunction (see Chapter 52). Cervicodorsal or cervicothoracic sympathectomy may be helpful in these patients and can often be performed at the time of the arterial repair by standard approaches.

Prognosis of Thoracic Outlet Syndrome

For the majority of patients diagnosed with TOS, the prognosis is excellent, with improvement in symptoms following physical therapy or other adjustments in their working postures or activities. However, for the patients with more debilitating symptoms who require surgical intervention, the long-term prognosis is not clear. In addition, it is difficult to study objectively the outcomes following surgery for neurogenic TOS. Various endpoints have been examined, but no prospective outcome-based study has been published evaluating operation for TOS. Nonetheless, many results have been reported.

Several series have had recurrence rates between 15% and 20% following first rib resection by either the transaxillary or supraclavicular route. Sanders and colleagues[29] reported a similar range and noted that the vast majority of these occur within 2 years of the initial operation. In this same study, it was reported that the subjectively determined immediate postoperative success rate of 84% decreased to 59% at 2 years, 69% at 5 years, and to as low as 41% at the 10- to 15-year interval using life-table analysis. Reoperation for these patients resulted in improvement so that at the 5- to 10-year interval, 86% of patients still were reporting subjective benefits from their procedures. Patients with symptoms that were persistent, rather than recurrent, also tended to be worse following reoperation.

A study by Sharp and coauthors[30] focused on patients' ability to return to work following TOS surgery, noting that 80% of the patients in their study were able to do so and that 85% of the patients subjectively described their outcomes as good to excellent. Employment and disability issues complicate outcomes in TOS. In Franklin and colleagues'[16] Washington state workers' compensation study, 40% of postoperative TOS patients were still not working 2 years after their operations; this percentage was actually worse at 5 years (44%). Interestingly, the conservatively treated patients in this study did better in this regard, although this was a retrospective study where the cohorts were not particularly well matched. Numerous other studies have shown worse outcomes when the patients have work-related or legal issues related to their TOS.[31]

Other factors predicting outcome following TOS surgery have been studied. Trauma as the event precipitating TOS is associated with poor outcomes in several series, but not in others.[32,33] In addition, preoperative depression has been linked to worse outcome as well. In a report by Axelrod and colleagues,[34] those patients with preoperative depression were more likely to have continued functional and vocational disability following operation. This study combined preoperative and postoperative interviews, psychological evaluations, and patient examinations, with an overall 67% subjectively reported "good or average" outcome. At an average of 47 months' follow-up, 64% of patients were satisfied with their outcomes and 69% reported they would undergo operation again if faced with the same symptoms. Eighteen percent of the patients considered themselves disabled.

In one of the largest series of TOS patients, Roos reported that in 1844 transaxillary first rib resections, 90% of patients were able to return to performing tasks they had been unable to perform preoperatively. In addition, 97% said that they would recommend rib resection to other patients with symptoms from TOS. There was a 5% recurrence, which was better than the 19% seen with scalenectomy (although this was without rib resection).[35] Green and colleagues[36] also reported higher recurrence following anterior approach, although other authors have reported that the two approaches yielded equivalent recurrence rates.[37]

The prognosis for untreated axillo-subclavian venous thrombosis had been one of progressive disability. Even after the institution of immobilization and anticoagulation, a study in 1970 revealed that 75% of patients had poor outcomes.[38] Following modern treatment protocols, most patients can resume normal activities. This is of particular importance in this group of predominantly young and otherwise healthy patients. The most important factor is the time to treatment following thrombosis, with most treatment failures occurring if treatment is delayed. Feugier and colleagues[39] reported that all treated patients were asymptomatic after an average follow-up of 45 months. Long-term sequelae are not common if patients are treated expeditiously and if complete recanalization of the vein is achieved and the compressive rib is removed. If this cannot be accomplished, repeated venous problems occur, and these can lead to debilitating outcomes.

The prognosis for patients with arterial involvement in TOS is highly variable and depends on the pattern of disease. If the compressive element of the process is removed, the principal issue affecting prognosis is the result of the arterial repair. The outcomes of subclavian artery repairs generally mirror those of repairs done for other disease processes and are generally good.

POPLITEAL ARTERY ENTRAPMENT SYNDROME

Popliteal entrapment syndrome is a rare disorder that most often presents as claudication in otherwise healthy young patients. It is usually caused by one of five anatomical variations in the configuration of the popliteal fossa, with the medial head of the gastrocnemius usually contributing significantly to compression of the popliteal artery (Table 64-2). The syndrome has been recognized since the late nineteenth century, when Stuart described in some detail both the aberrant course of the artery and the associated aneurysmal degeneration.[40] The syndrome received its name from Love and Whelan in 1965.[41] Diagnostic modalities and treatment have evolved so that the disorder should be diagnosed and treatable by the vascular specialist.

TABLE 64-2 TYPES OF POPLITEAL ENTRAPMENT

Type 1	Popliteal artery deviates medial to medial head of normally configured gastrocnemius
Type 2	Abnormally lateral insertion of medial head of gastrocnemius displacing popliteal artery medially
Type 3	Normal popliteal artery is compressed by accessory "slips" of gastrocnemius muscle
Type 4	Compression of popliteal artery by popliteus muscle, nerve tissue, or fibrous bands
Type 5	Any of the above also involving compression of the popliteal vein

Only a few conditions lead to claudication in young patients. Among these are accelerated atherosclerosis, degenerative disease of a persistent sciatic artery with underlying aplasia or hypoplasia of the femoral and iliac arteries, adventitial popliteal cystic disease, arteritides, and hypercoagulable conditions. Popliteal artery entrapment, however, is more common than any of these, occurring in up to 60% of young men with claudication.[42] Approximately 90% of cases occur in men, and bilateral disease occurs in up to 33% of patients.[43] The overall incidence of the disease is unknown, although studies suggest a range of 0.165% to 3.5% depending on the population investigated.[44,45] Roughly 70% of patients have claudication; 10% will have evidence of limb threat in the form of rest pain or tissue loss.[46]

Pathophysiology of Popliteal Artery Entrapment

The medial head of the gastrocnemius muscle normally migrates from a lateral to medial position during embryogenesis. It is now accepted that formation of the mature popliteal artery can occur before this process is complete, a situation that allows the muscle to pull the artery medially along with it. This is a type I lesion. In a slightly different situation, the artery may prevent the complete migration of the muscle, leading to a compressed, although not medially deviated, artery (type II). The artery may also be entangled in any number of fibromuscular slips or bands (type III). Type IV lesions occur when the popliteus muscle traps the artery, a process thought to occur due to persistence of segment of the axial artery during development. Finally, if the popliteal vein is involved in any of these processes, it is termed type V disease.

Compression in any of these scenarios can lead to problems ranging from mild symptoms that occur with dorsiflexion of the foot to aneurysm formation, distal embolization, or popliteal artery occlusion. Histologically, most patients have no injury to the artery itself; the symptoms are secondary to the temporary occlusion of blood flow. With repeated insult, however, the artery may undergo degenerative changes or thrombose.

Diagnosis of Popliteal Artery Entrapment

The patient may have normal distal pulses unless provocative maneuvers, such as ankle dorsiflexion and plantar flexion, are performed. These positional changes should be undertaken during examination of the pulses. This same principle is applied when using Doppler examinations to diagnose this condition, with the subsequent attenuation of both the waveform and ankle-brachial index during maneuvers. Angiography in both a neutral position and with forced dorsiflexion or plantar flexion of the ankle against resistance has been the gold standard for the diagnosis of popliteal artery entrapment syndrome (Fig. 64-7). If there is no arterial damage, an angiogram performed in the neutral position may appear normal. Some physicians use MRI, MRA, and CT scanning to diagnose popliteal artery entrapment. These techniques are capable of demonstrating both the soft tissue anatomy, as well as providing information about the artery itself. The combination of MRI and MRA is particularly useful when arterial damage is suspected and runoff information is required. In many cases, the MRA may obviate the need for conventional angiography.[47]

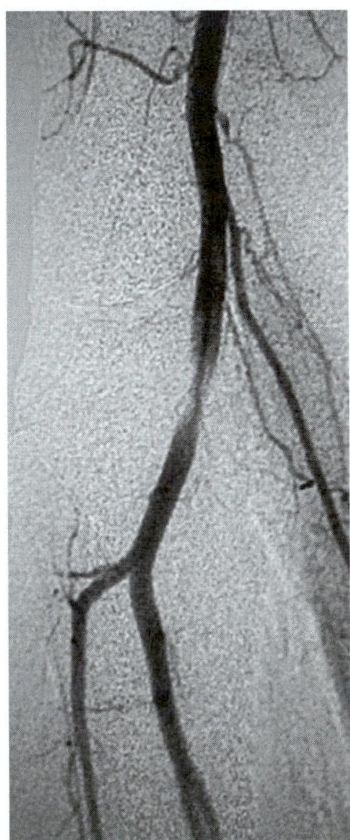

A

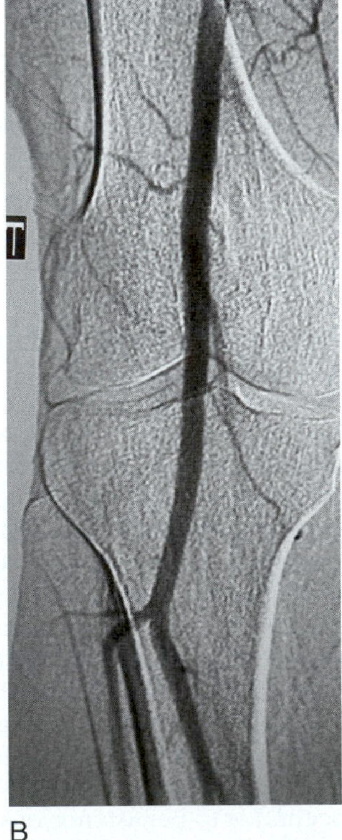

B

FIGURE 64-7. These two angiograms clearly show compression of the popliteal artery with forced dorsiflexion of the foot (**A**) and subsequent filling when the leg is relaxed (**B**). Note the presence of underlying disease in both the affected segment of the artery and in the runoff vessels.

Treatment of Popliteal Artery Entrapment

The symptoms of popliteal artery entrapment should be aggressively treated. Even with relatively minor symptoms, the risk of progressive arterial damage mandates intervention. In the absence of arterial injury, a posterior approach to the popliteal fossa allows identification of the causative lesion, as well as inspection of the artery itself. When the medial head of the gastrocnemius must be divided to relieve the compression, most surgeons recommend reattachment of the muscle to the femoral condyle. However, most of the aberrant fibromuscular bands that are encountered (as well as the popliteus muscle) can be divided with impunity.

When arterial damage has occurred, standard techniques of reconstruction must be employed. It is critical, as with any arterial reconstruction, to appreciate the runoff bed before operation. If thrombosis has occurred, consideration should be given to intra-arterial administration of thrombolytic drugs, particularly if there is evidence of distal propagation of clot.[48] Even when distal bypass is required, patients with popliteal artery entrapment tend to have normal tibial vessels, with better outcomes than are found when treating atherosclerotic disease.

CELIAC COMPRESSION

No arterial compression syndrome has generated as much controversy as that involving the celiac artery. Although it has been demonstrated that both neural tissues and the median arcuate ligament are capable of impinging on the celiac artery at approximately the L1 level, it is not clear why occlusion or stenosis of one mesenteric vessel should lead to symptoms. In fact, there is a syndrome of median arcuate ligament compression of both the celiac and superior mesenteric arteries leading to mesenteric ischemia.[49] Nonetheless, it appears that certain patients do benefit from celiac decompression. Perhaps it is understanding of the pathophysiology that is lacking.

The syndrome typically, though not exclusively, affects women in their 30s and 40s. Patients complain of vague abdominal pains that have often been occurring for some time (even years). The classic "food fear" found with intestinal angina is an inconsistent finding, and there usually has been an extensive medical work-up by the time the patient consults a vascular surgeon.

The diagnosis of celiac compression syndrome is complicated by the fact that close to 40% of healthy asymptomatic adults have some angiographic evidence of celiac artery impingement.[50] Thus even in view of such a finding, it is still a diagnosis of exclusion. Biliary, pancreatic, and gastric disease must be sought by laboratory, radiographic, and endoscopic studies. Duplex ultrasonography of the mesenteric vessels may be useful but probably will not obviate the need for arteriography. The angiographic findings of external impingement of the artery are distinct, with an eccentric narrowing roughly 1 cm from the celiac origin. These findings can be accentuated by taking expiration and inspiration

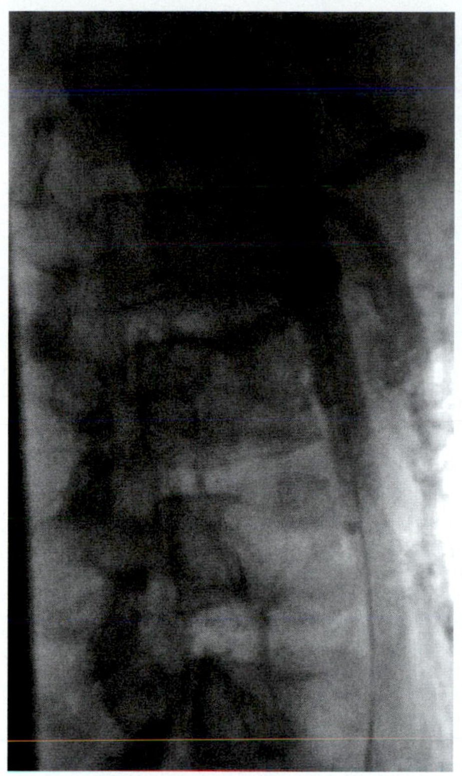

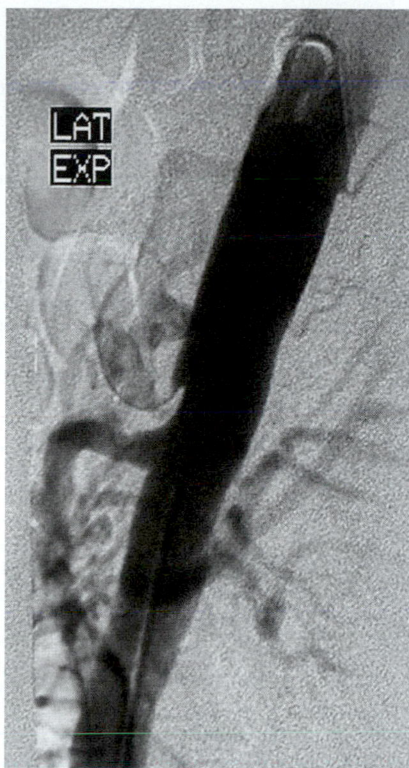

FIGURE 64-8. Lateral angiograms of the celiac axis in both inspiration (**A**) and expiration (**B**) demonstrate the characteristic compression of the artery. This finding is frequently noted in the absence of clinical findings.

films (Fig. 64-8). During the expiratory phase, the stenosis is typically tightest (coinciding with the most prominent bruit heard on physical examination). The diagnosis is made when the clinical findings cannot be otherwise explained and the angiogram is consistent with celiac compression.

Treatment of Celiac Compression

Operative intervention for celiac compression, at its simplest, involves dividing the offending structures and separating all tissue from the celiac trunk until it is free of constriction. If there is no evidence of stenosis, most authorities recommend measuring celiac artery pressures to check for a gradient. If present, the stenosis can be treated by either dilation or bypass, although the former tends to be significantly less demanding. If the lesion is not susceptible to dilation, bypass or reimplantation to the aorta are options.

Results from operative therapy have been mixed, although the series by Reilly and colleagues[51] showed improvement in 53% of patients undergoing decompression alone, 79% of those undergoing dilation, and 71% of patients receiving bypasses. These results are better than most but support operative intervention in correctly selected cases. As more is understood regarding the pathophysiology of this condition, better patient selection hopefully will lead to improved outcomes.

NUTCRACKER SYNDROME

The nutcracker syndrome refers to hematuria and obstruction of the left renal vein secondary to its compression between the aorta and the superior mesenteric artery. There is some suggestion that the syndrome is associated with an abnormal takeoff of the superior mesenteric artery.[52] In its benign form, the syndrome can present with mild hematuria and proteinuria, with spontaneous remission. This is frequently the case in adolescents.[53]

However, in a more dramatic presentation, severe pelvic pain and massive hemorrhage may be encountered. Patients develop varices at the hilum of the left kidney, and their subsequent rupture into the collecting system leads to the hematuria. Diagnosis of the disorder is frequently difficult, but it should always be considered when evaluating hematuria from a left kidney source. This determination is usually made at cytoscopy, and CT angiography, MRA, or magnetic resonance venography can then be used to provide the anatomic information to secure the diagnosis.

Treatment can range from observation to renal autotransplantation or nephrectomy for life-threatening bleeding. Endovascular stenting is becoming the most common intervention, with standard transfemoral approaches to the left renal vein.[54,55] These early reports indicate that the outcomes after treatment are excellent, with permanent compromise in renal function being unusual.

ADDUCTOR CANAL COMPRESSION

This syndrome is similar to popliteal entrapment syndrome, with the abnormal band of tissue taking its origin from the adductor magnus muscle and inserting in such a way as to cross the superficial femoral artery. Although typically of no consequence at rest, exercise leads to compression of the artery within the adductor canal.

Subsequent arterial damage and thrombosis can occur. The incidence is not known, but it is an extremely unusual condition.[56] As in popliteal entrapment, treatment consists of dividing the offending bands so that arterial compression is no longer created, and by restoring arterial continuity if significant damage or thrombosis has occurred.

ILIAC ARTERY COMPRESSION (EXTERNAL ILIAC ENDOFIBROSIS)

This syndrome describes the finding of stenosis of the external iliac artery in high-performance cyclists. It is unusual, although there have been multiple reports published since 1986.[57] Often referred to as *external iliac endofibrosis,* this entity may not represent a true compression syndrome. Although compression of the artery at the inguinal ligament is sometimes thought to be the cause, the histopathologic findings of stenosis secondary to marked intimal thickening are in all likelihood related to flow phenomenon and the peculiar position assumed by these athletes.[58] The changes do not typically lead to occlusion, and it is only at exercise that the symptoms are unmasked. Treatment may be in the form of open endarterectomy or bypass, although current reports suggest that balloon angioplasty may provide a useful, noninvasive approach.[59]

REFERENCES

1. Peet RM, Hendricksen JD, Anderson TP, et al: Thoracic outlet syndrome: Evaluation of the therapeutic exercise program. Mayo Clin Proc 31:281, 1956.
2. Clagett OT: Presidential address: Research and prosearch. J Thorac Cardiovasc Surg 44: 153, 1962.
3. Roos DB: Transaxillary approach for first rib resection to relieve thoracic outlet compression syndrome. Ann Surg 1966;163:354, 1966.
4. Machleder HI: Vascular Disorders of the Upper Extremity, 2nd ed. Mt Kisco, N.Y., Futura Press, 1989.
5. Roos DB: Historical perspectives and anatomic considerations. Thoracic Outlet Syndrome. Semin Thorac Cardiovasc Surg 8:183, 1996.
6. Firsov GI: Cervical ribs and their distinction from under-developed first ribs. Archiv Anatomii Gistologii I Embriologii 67:101, 1974.
7. Juvonen T, Satta J, Laitala P, et al: Anomalies of the thoracic outlet are frequent in the general population. Am J Surg 170:33, 1995.
8. Roos DB: Congenital anomalies associated with thoracic outlet syndrome: Anatomy, symptoms, diagnosis and treatment. Am J Surg 132:771, 1976.
9. Dijkstra PF, Westra D: Angiographic features of compression of the axillary artery by the musculus pectoralis minor and the head of the humerus in the thoracic outlet compression syndrome. Case report. Radiol Clin (Basel) 47:423, 1978.
10. Daskalakis E, Bouhoutsos J: Subclavian and axillary vein compression of musculoskeletal origin. Br J Surg 67:573, 1980.
11. Sanders RJ, Hammond SL: Management of cervical ribs and anomalous first ribs causing neurogenic thoracic outlet syndrome. J Vasc Surg 36:51, 2002.
12. Gilliat RW, LeQuesne PM, Logue V, et al: Wasting of the hand associated with a cervical rib or band. J Neurol Neurosurg Psychiatry 33:615, 1970.
13. Machleder HI: Thoracic outlet syndromes: New concepts from a century of discovery. Cardiovasc Surg 2:137, 1994.
14. Roos DB, Owens JC: Thoracic outlet syndrome. Arch Surg 93:71, 1966.
15. Costigan DA, Wilbourn AJ: The elevated arm stress test; specificity in the diagnosis of thoracic outlet syndrome. Neurology 35:74, 1985.
16. Wilbourn AJ: Thoracic outlet syndrome is overdiagnosed. Muscle Nerve 22:130, 1999.
17. Toomingas A, Nilsson T, Hagberg M, et al: Predictive aspects of the abduction external rotation test among male industrial and office workers. Am J Ind Med 35:32, 1999.
18. Roos DB: The place for scalenectomy and first-rib resection in thoracic outlet syndrome. Surgery 92:1077, 1982.
19. Franklin GM, Fulton-Kehoe D, Bradley C, et al: Outcome of surgery for thoracic outlet syndrome in Washington state workers' compensation. Neurology 54:1252, 2000.
20. Abe M, Katsuaki I, Nishida J: Diagnosis, treatment and complications of thoracic outlet syndrome J Orthop Sci 4:66, 1999.
21. Jordan SE, Machleder HI: Diagnosis of thoracic outlet syndrome using electrophysiologically guided anterior scalene blocks. Ann Vasc Surg 12:260, 1998.
22. Machleder HI, Mill F, Nuwer M, et al: Somatosensory evoked potentials in the assessment of thoracic outlet compression syndrome. J Vasc Surg 6:177, 1987.
23. Aligne C, Barral X: Rehabilitation of patients with thoracic outlet syndrome. Ann Vasc Surg 6:381, 1992.
24. Jordan SE, Ahn SS, Freischlag JA: Selective botulinum chemodenervation of the scalene muscles for treatment of neurogenic thoracic outlet syndrome. Ann Vasc Surg 14:365, 2000.
25. Ohtsuka T, Wolf RK, Dunsker SB: Port-access first-rib resection. Surg Endosc 13:940, 1999.
26. Kunkel JM, Machleder H: Treatment of Paget-Schroetter syndrome. A staged, multidisciplinary approach. Arch Surg 124:1153, 1989.
27. Angle N, Gelabert HA, Farooq MM, et al: Safety and efficacy of early surgical decompression of the thoracic outlet for Paget-Schroetter syndrome. Ann Vasc Surg 15:37, 2001.
28. Meir GH, Pollak JS, Rosenblatt M, et al: Initial experience with venous stents in exertional axillary-subclavian vein thrombosis. J Vasc Surg 24:974, 1996.
29. Sanders RJ, Jackson CGR, Baushero N, et al: Scalene muscle abnormalities in traumatic thoracic outlet syndrome. Am J Surg 159:231, 1990.
30. Sharp WJ, Nowak LR, Zamani T, et al: Long-term follow-up and patient satisfaction after surgery for thoracic outlet syndrome. Ann Vasc Surg 15:32, 2001.
31. Lepantalo M, Lindgren KA, Leino E, et al: Long-term outcome after resection of the first rib for thoracic outlet syndrome. Br J Surg 76:1255, 1989.
32. Green RM, McNamara J, Ouriel K: Long-term follow-up after thoracic outlet decompression: An analysis of factors determining outcome. J Vasc Surg 14:739, 1991.
33. Sanders RJ, Pearce WH: The treatment of thoracic outlet syndrome; a comparison of different operations. J Vasc Surg 10:626, 1989.
34. Axelrod DA, Proctor MC, Geisser ME, et al: Outcomes after surgery for thoracic outlet syndrome. J Vasc Surg 33:1220, 2001.
35. Roos DB: Thoracic outlet nerve compression. In Rutherford RB (ed): Vascular Surgery, 3rd ed. Philadelphia, WB Saunders, 1989, p 858.
36. Green RM, McNamara J, Ouriel K: Long-term follow-up after thoracic outlet decompression: An analysis of factors determining outcome. J Vasc Surg 14:739, 1991.
37. Sessions RT: Recurrent thoracic outlet syndrome: Causes and treatment. South Med J 75:453, 1982.
38. Tilney NL, Griffiths HJG, Edwards EA: Natural history of major venous thrombosis of the upper extremity. Arch Surg 101:792, 1970.
39. Feugier P, Aleksic I, Salari R: Long-term results of venous revascularization for Paget-Schroetter syndrome in athletes. Ann Vasc Surg 15:212, 2001.
40. Stuart TP: A note on a variation in the course of the popliteal artery. J Anat Physiol 13:162, 1879.
41. Love JW, Whelan TJ: Popliteal artery entrapment syndrome. Am J Surg 109:620, 1965.
42. Murray A, Halliday M, Corft RJ: Popliteal artery entrapment syndrome. Br J Surg 173:84, 1991.
43. Di Marzo L, Cavallaro A, Sciacca V, et al: Surgical treatment of popliteal artery entrapment syndrome: a ten-year experience. Eur J Vasc Surg 5:59, 1991.
44. Gibson MHL, Mills JG, Johnson GE, et al: Popliteal artery entrapment syndrome. Ann Surg 144:604, 1977.
45. Bouthoutsos J, Daskalakis E: Muscular abnormalities affecting the popliteal vessels. Br J Surg 68:501, 1981.

46. Persky JM, Kempczinski RF, Fowl RJ: Entrapment of the popliteal artery. Surg Gynecol Obstet 173:84, 1991.
47. McGuiness G, Durham JD, Rutherford RB, et al: Popliteal artery entrapment: Findings at MR imaging. J Vasc Interv Radiol 2:241,1991.
48. Steurer J, Hoffmann U, Schneider E, et al: A new therapeutic approach to popliteal artery entrapment syndrome. Eur J Vasc Endovasc Surg 10:243, 1995.
49. Lawson JD, Ochsner JL: Median arcuate ligament syndrome with severe two-vessel involvement. Arch Surg 119:226, 1984.
50. Stanley JC, Fry WJ: Median arcuate ligament syndrome. Arch Surg 103:252, 1971.
51. Reilly LM, Ammar AD, Stoney RJ, et al: Late results following operative repair for celiac artery compression syndrome. J Vasc Surg 2:79, 1985.
52. Hohenfellner M, Steinbach F, Schultz-Lampel D, et al: The nutcracker syndrome: New aspects of pathophysiology, diagnosis and treatment. J Urol 146:685, 1991.
53. Tanaka H, Waga S: Spontaneous remission of persistent severe hematuria in an adolescent with nutcracker syndrome: Seven years' observation. Clin Exp Nephrol 8:68, 2004.
54. Wei SM, Chen ZD, Zhou M: Intravenous stent placement for treatment of the nutcracker syndrome. J Urol 170:1934, 2003.
55. Segawa N, Azuma H, Iwamoto Y, et al: Expandable metallic stent placement for nutcracker phenomenon. Urology 53:631, 1999.
56. Verta MJ Jr, Vitello J, Fuller J: Adductor canal compression syndrome. Arch Surg 119:345, 1984.
57. Abraham P, Chevalier JM, Loire R: External iliac artery endofibrosis in a young cyclist. Circulation 100:38, 1999.
58. Rousselet MC, Saint-Andre JP, L'Hoste P, et al: Stenotic intimal thickening of the external iliac artery in competition cyclists. Hum Pathol 21:524, 1990.
59. Wijesinghe LD, Coughlin PA, Robertson I, et al: Cyclist's iliac syndrome: Temporary relief by balloon angioplasty. Br J Sports Med 35:70, 2001.

■ ■ ■ chapter 65

Congenital Malformations of the Vasculature

Renu Virmani
Allen P. Burke
Allen J. Taylor

VASCULAR MALFORMATIONS WITHIN THE HEART

Anomalous Venous Connections

An anomalous venous connection abnormally connects a systemic or pulmonary vein to another venous structure or directly to the left or right atrium. The connections arise from failed development of normal embryologic venous communications or persistence, lack of regression of normal embryologic venous communications, or both.

Anomalous Pulmonary Venous Connections

Anomalous pulmonary venous connection refers to the absence of one or more pulmonary venous connections to the left atrium without reference to the subsequent drainage of the anomalously disconnected pulmonary vein(s). *Total anomalous pulmonary venous connection* (TAPVC) refers to the bilateral absence of a connection of both pulmonary veins of each lung to the left atrium. The pulmonary veins connect directly into the right atrium (RA) or into one of its tributaries. TAPVC almost always is associated with some type of atrial septal defect (ASD) in order for life to be sustained beyond the newborn period.[1] *Partial anomalous pulmonary venous connection* (PAPVC) is the presence of connection of one or more—but not all—pulmonary veins to the RA or one of its tributaries. TAPVC is found in about 2% of autopsied cases with congenital heart disease and has a male predominance. PAPVCs constitute about 0.6% of autopsied cases of congenital heart disease.[1] TAPVC is an isolated anomaly in two thirds of patients and is associated with complex congenital heart disease in the remaining third, especially the heterotaxy syndromes (so-called *isomeric TAPVC*).

Embryology

In the human embryo, the lung buds and their pulmonary veins connect to the veins of the foregut, the splanchnic plexus. With growth, a new pulmonary venous channel—the primary pulmonary vein—grows as a bulging of the left atrium. At the same time, the intrapulmonary veins lose their connections with the splanchnic plexus and fuse with the primary pulmonary vein. The intrapulmonary veins eventually form the four pulmonary veins and are absorbed into the left atrium. The failure to sever the connection between the intrapulmonary and splanchnic veins results in the anomalous pulmonary venous connections, which may be total, partial, bilateral, or unilateral. The drainage site of pulmonary veins may be supradiaphragmatic or infradiaphragmatic.

When drainage is supradiaphragmatic, both lungs may drain into a confluence, which may then drain into the left innominate vein and the superior vena cava (SVC), or the supradiaphragmatic drainage may be directly into the left SVC or indirectly, to the SVC via azygos or hemiazygos veins (Fig. 65-1).[1]

Familial occurrence of partial and complete anomalous pulmonary veins has been shown.[2] Familial total anomalous pulmonary venous return is an autosomal dominant trait with reduced penetrance, genetically linked to chromosomal bands 4p13-q12.[3]

Total Anomalous Pulmonary Venous Connection

The level of the anomaly relative to the heart or diaphragm classifies TAPVC. Type I denotes anomalous connection at the supracardiac level; type II, anomalous connection at the cardiac level; type III, anomalous connection at the infracardiac level; and type IV, anomalous connection at two or more of those levels.[4] The common forms of TAPVC are illustrated in Figure 65-2. The frequency from two separate studies is 26% to left innominate vein (LIV) (supracardiac level), 18% to coronary sinus (cardiac level), 8% to RA (cardiac level), 15% to right SVC (supracardiac level), 24% to the portal system (infracardiac level), 5% to multiple sites, and 4% to unknown or other sites.[4] One third of the patients with TAPVC have other major cardiac malformations, especially asplenia/heterotaxy; in the other two thirds, TAPVC exists as an isolated anomaly.

The intrauterine diagnosis of TAPVC above the diaphragm may be suggested by ventricular and great arterial disproportion. However, in the presence of an atrial septal defect or with infradiaphragmatic drainage, right heart dilatation may not occur until late in pregnancy. Total anomalous pulmonary venous drainage in fetal life is definitively excluded only by direct examination of pulmonary venous blood flow entering the left atrium on color or pulsed flow mapping.[5]

The presence of obstructive lesions determines the hemodynamic state, clinical features, and survival in

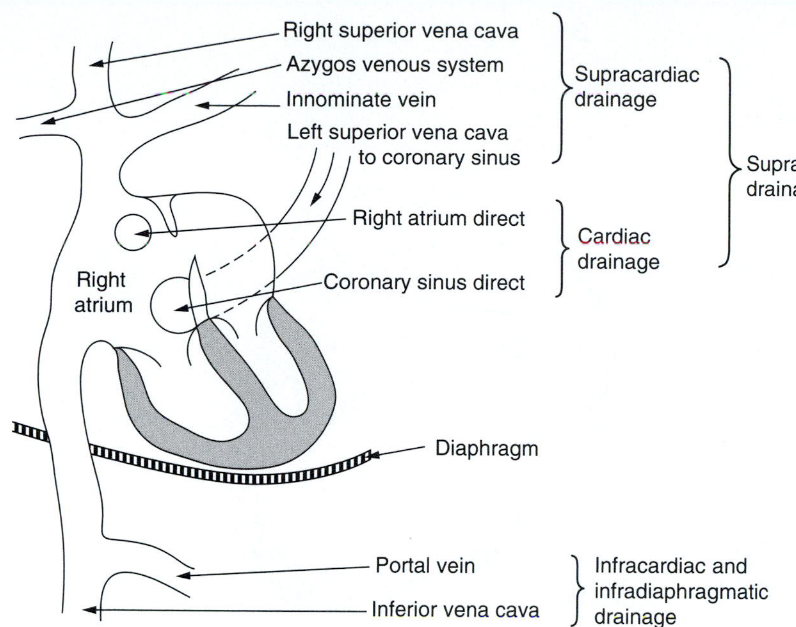

FIGURE 65-1. Possible sites of drainage for anomalous pulmonary venous connections into the venous system. (From Becker AE, Anderson RH: Pathology of Congenital Heart Disease. London, Butterworths, 1981, pp 47, 333.)

infants with TAPVC. The obstruction may be at the interatrial septum and, when small, results in inadequate flow to the left atrium. There may be obstruction in the anomalous venous channel, which may result from intrinsic narrowing of the wall of the channel or by extrinsic compression.[6] The infracardiac TAPVC is almost always associated with venous obstruction. Fifty percent of supracardiac TAPVCs demonstrate pulmonary venous obstruction, at various sites. The most common sites of obstruction are at the level of the left pulmonary artery (left vertical vein) and at the insertion into the SVC (right vertical vein).[7]

The size of the ASD has been shown to relate to longevity in TAPVC; the larger the ASD, the longer the survival. The individual pulmonary-vein size at diagnosis also is a strong, independent predictor of survival in patients with TAPVC.[8]

Associated cardiac anomalies are transposition of the great arteries (TGAs), pulmonary atresia (PA), coarctation of the aorta (COA), and anomalies of systemic veins. There is a high frequency of TAPVC in patients with congenital heart disease and asplenia (heterotaxy syndromes). In a recent autopsy series of TAPVC associated with asplenia, anomalous pulmonary venous connection to a systemic vein was total in 42 (58%) of 72 and partial in 2 (3%) of 72, with obstruction in 24 (55%) of 44.[9]

In TAPVC the RA serves as a mixing chamber for the pulmonary venous blood and the systemic circuits. The physiologic features of TAPVC depend on the distribution of the mixed venous blood between the pulmonary and systemic circuits and the state of the interatrial septum. If the ASD is small, the volume of blood reaching the left atrium is small and the systemic cardiac output is reduced. The right atrial pressure is increased, which is reflected in elevation of pressure in both venous circuits.

In patients with a widely patent foramen ovale or ASD, which allows free communication between the two atria and mixing of the venous blood, the flow of blood depends on the resistance in the pulmonary and systemic arterial circuits. In cases without pulmonary venous obstruction, the resistance at birth is equal; therefore the distribution of blood is equal between the pulmonary and systemic circuits. However, within a few weeks of birth, the pulmonary resistance decreases and a larger proportion of the mixed venous blood returns to the pulmonary circuit, resulting in a nearly three to five times greater pulmonary-to-systemic flow ratio of 3:1 to 5:1 and an equalization of oxygen saturation between the right and the left heart. In the presence of pulmonary venous obstruction, there is elevated pulmonary venous pressure, which results in pulmonary edema, a decrease in pulmonary flow, pulmonary hypertension, right ventricular hypertrophy, and ultimately right heart failure.

The signs and symptoms, therefore, depend on the underlying hemodynamics (i.e., presence or absence of pulmonary venous obstruction and the extent of the mixing of blood between the right and left atrium). If interatrial mixing is inadequate, symptoms occur at birth or shortly thereafter. In TAPVC without pulmonary venous obstruction, the patients usually are asymptomatic at birth; however, at least 50% become symptomatic within 1 month of life but usually not in the first 12 hours of life. Once symptoms appear, however, they are rapidly progressive. Diagnosis may be established by angiography, echocardiography, or T1-weighted spin-echo magnetic resonance.[10]

Infants with TAPVC have an unfavorable prognosis, with only 20% surviving the first year of life. Surgical repair of TAPVC was associated with a high mortality until recently. Overall, early mortality from 14 centers is 18% to 20% for infants younger than 1 month of age. Improvements in surgical technique, as well as preoperative and postoperative management, account for the reduction in mortality and need for reoperation for most types of TAPVC. However, the presence of a small venous

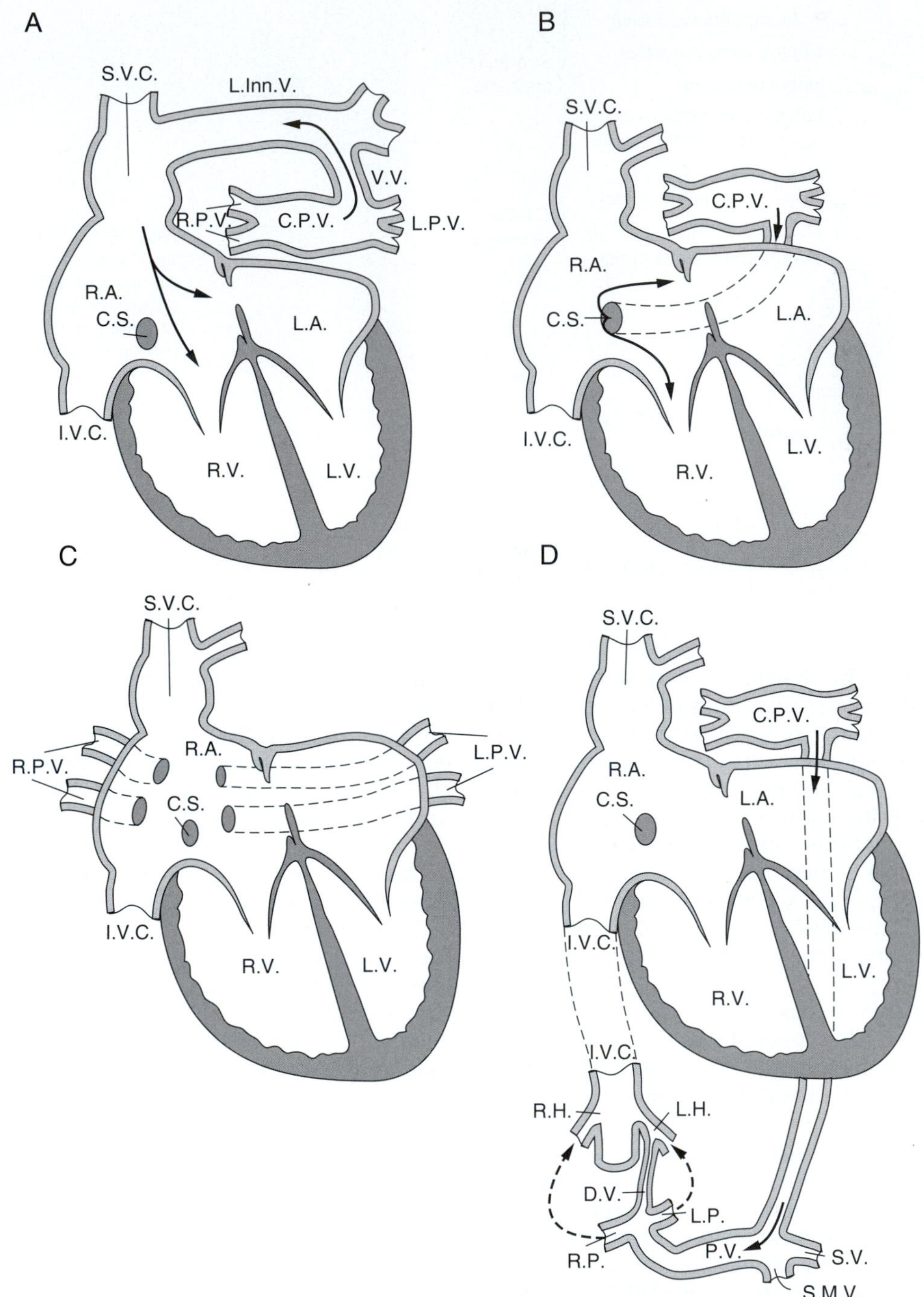

FIGURE 65-2. The most common patterns of circulation in total anomalous pulmonary connection (TAPVC). **A,** TAPVC to the left innominate vein by way of a vertical vein. **B,** TAPVC to coronary sinus. **C,** TAPVC to right atrium. The right and left pulmonary veins usually enter the right atrium separately. **D,** TAPVC to the portal vein. CPV, common pulmonary vein; CS, coronary sinus; DV, ductus venosus; IVC, inferior vena cava; LA, left atrium; LH, left hepatic vein; L Inn V, left innominate vein; LP, left portal vein; LPV, left pulmonary vein; LV, left ventricle; PV, portal vein; RA, right atrium; RH, right hepatic vein; RP, right portal vein; RPV, right pulmonary vein; RV, right ventricle; SMV, superior mesenteric vein; SV, splenic vein; SVC, superior vena cava; vv, vertical vein. (From Lucas RV, Krabill RA: Anomalous venous connections, pulmonary and systemic. In Adams FH, Emmanouilides GC [eds]: Moss' Heart Disease in Infants, Children and Adolescents, 4th ed. Baltimore, Williams & Wilkins, 1989, p 580.)

confluence and diffuse pulmonary vein stenosis remains a risk factor for adverse outcome.[11]

The postoperative prognosis after surgery for TAPVC has improved.[12] Many factors have been implicated in poor survival in patients with TAPVC including the type of anatomic connection, year of operation, sex, age at operation, intra-atrial communication size, pulmonary hypertension, arterial oxygen saturation, and heart volume.[13] The main goal in the surgical repair of total anomalous pulmonary venous drainage is to reestablish a wide patent connection between the common pulmonary vein and the left atrium. If complicated by pulmonary vein stenosis, either at presentation or secondary to the repair, the long-term outcome is compromised.

Early mortality ranges from 7%[14,15] to 35%.[16] Recurrent or iatrogenic pulmonary vein stenosis occurs in about 10% of patients and is treated by balloon angioplasty, endovascular stent placement, or surgery. Overall survival of this subgroup of patients is slightly better than one half.[15] Cardiac arrhythmias can occur in otherwise asymptomatic patients after correction for total anomalous pulmonary venous connection.[17] Long-term significant arrhythmias occur in nearly 50% of patients, including sinus node dysfunction and multiform ventricular ectopic beats.[16]

Supracardiac and infracardiac TAPVC repair include the double-patch technique with left atrial enlargement and side-to-side anastomosis between the pulmonary venous confluence and the left atrium. Left atrial enlargement procedures appear to be associated with higher risk of late arrhythmias.[14] The modified superior approach for the repair of supracardiac total anomalous pulmonary venous drainage can be useful to enhance exposure during surgical repair and may contribute to improved patient outcome.[18]

Partial Anomalous Pulmonary Venous Connection

PAPVC is defined when one or more, but not all, pulmonary veins are connected to the RA or to a systemic vein. Usually, only one lung or part of a lung is involved. The right pulmonary veins are six times more commonly involved than the left pulmonary veins, and the upper lobes of the lung are more commonly involved than the lower. The left-sided pulmonary veins usually connect to the derivatives of the left cardinal system (i.e., the coronary sinus and the left innominate vein [LIV]). The right pulmonary veins connect to the derivatives of the right cardinal system (i.e., the SVC and the inferior vena cava [IVC] or the right atrium). The most common connections are right pulmonary veins to SVC, right pulmonary veins to the right atrium, veins of the right lung to the IVC, and left pulmonary veins to the LIV.

In a recent series of 28 children, 20 patients had one anomalous pulmonary vein (APV) and 8 had more than two APVs. Twenty-five patients (89%) had APVs originating from the right lung, 2 (7%) from the left lung, and 1 (4%) from both lungs. In the 25 patients with APVs originating from the right lung, 9 had APVs draining into the SVC, 13 into the RA, 1 into the IVC, and 2 into both the SVC and RA. In the two patients with APVs originating from the left lung, one had APVs draining into the RA and the other had APVs draining into the innominate vein. One patient had APVs originating from both lungs that connected to the IVC.[19] The precise site of connection can be made with certainty only by selective pulmonary angiography.[19]

The heart usually exhibits mild dilatation and hypertrophy of RA and right ventricle with dilatation of the pulmonary artery. The left-sided chambers are normal. Usually, ASD accompanies PAPVC; conversely, 9% of cases of ASD have PAPVC. In the case of the right pulmonary vein connecting to the SVC, the right upper and middle lobe veins connect to the SVC. The vein of the right lower lobe usually enters the left atrium but may connect to the right atrium. The lower part of the SVC, below the azygos vein and above the right atrium, is dilated approximately twice the normal size. Most cases have associated ASD of the sinus venosus type, but occasionally a secundum or, rarely, a primum ASD may occur (Fig. 65-3).

Generally, the presence of highly saturated blood in the right heart is a key to diagnosis; in some patients, however, a lack of detectable shunting occurs when there is obstruction of anomalous veins due to thromboembolism.[20] Isolated partial anomalous pulmonary venous connection may be missed even when patients present with mild right ventricular enlargement. Imaging from the suprasternal window with color flow and ultrasound contrast echocardiography aid the diagnosis.[21]

Associated cardiovascular defects are common, occurring in up to 80% of patients.[19] Major cardiac anomalies are found in about 20% of cases and include tetralogy of Fallot, ventricular septal defect, single ventricle, coarctation of the aorta, transposition of the great arteries, and hypoplastic left heart syndrome. Indications for surgery for isolated PAPVC include a pulmonary-to-systemic flow ratio of more than 2.[19]

In untreated patients there is paucity of information regarding the prognosis, but overall, if one pulmonary vein is anomalously connected and there is no ASD, the prognosis is excellent. However, in patients with high pulmonary flow, surgical repair is associated with a dramatic reduction in symptoms and a normal longevity. The prognosis may not be so favorable if pulmonary hypertension is present. Correction of partial anomalous pulmonary venous connection to the SVC is often complicated by sinus node dysfunction secondary to the creation of intracaval conduits. An intra-atrial baffle, combined with cavo-atrial anastomosis, lowers the rate of postoperative arrhythmias.[22,23]

When all right pulmonary veins drain the right middle and lower lobes and enter the IVC, either above or below the diaphragm, the pattern of the pulmonary veins is altered, giving a "fir-tree" appearance (see Fig. 65-3). The atrial septum is intact, and this malformation is called *scimitar syndrome.* It is associated with right-lung anomalies, dextrocardia of the heart, hypoplasia of the right pulmonary artery, and anomalous connection between aorta and right lung. The diagnosis of scimitar syndrome is straightforward when the scimitar vein is visible on the chest radiograph; however, a diagnosis is not definitive when this vein is obscured by dextroversion. In such cases pulmonary angiography, CT scan, MRI, and transesophageal echocardiography (TEE) are essential in diagnosis.[24] The hemodynamic status in scimitar syndrome may be noninvasively assessed by means of velocity-encoded cine MRI, with a left-to-right shunt calculated from direct blood flow measurements performed in the ascending aorta, main pulmonary artery, and aberrant pulmonary vein.[25]

In the connection of the left pulmonary veins to the LIV, the veins of the left upper lobe or the whole left lung connect to the LIV via the vertical vein. ASD of the secundum type usually is present, and the septum rarely is intact (see Fig. 65-3). Other sites of PAPVC are the left pulmonary veins draining into the coronary sinus, IVC, right SVC, right atrium, or left subclavian vein. In rare

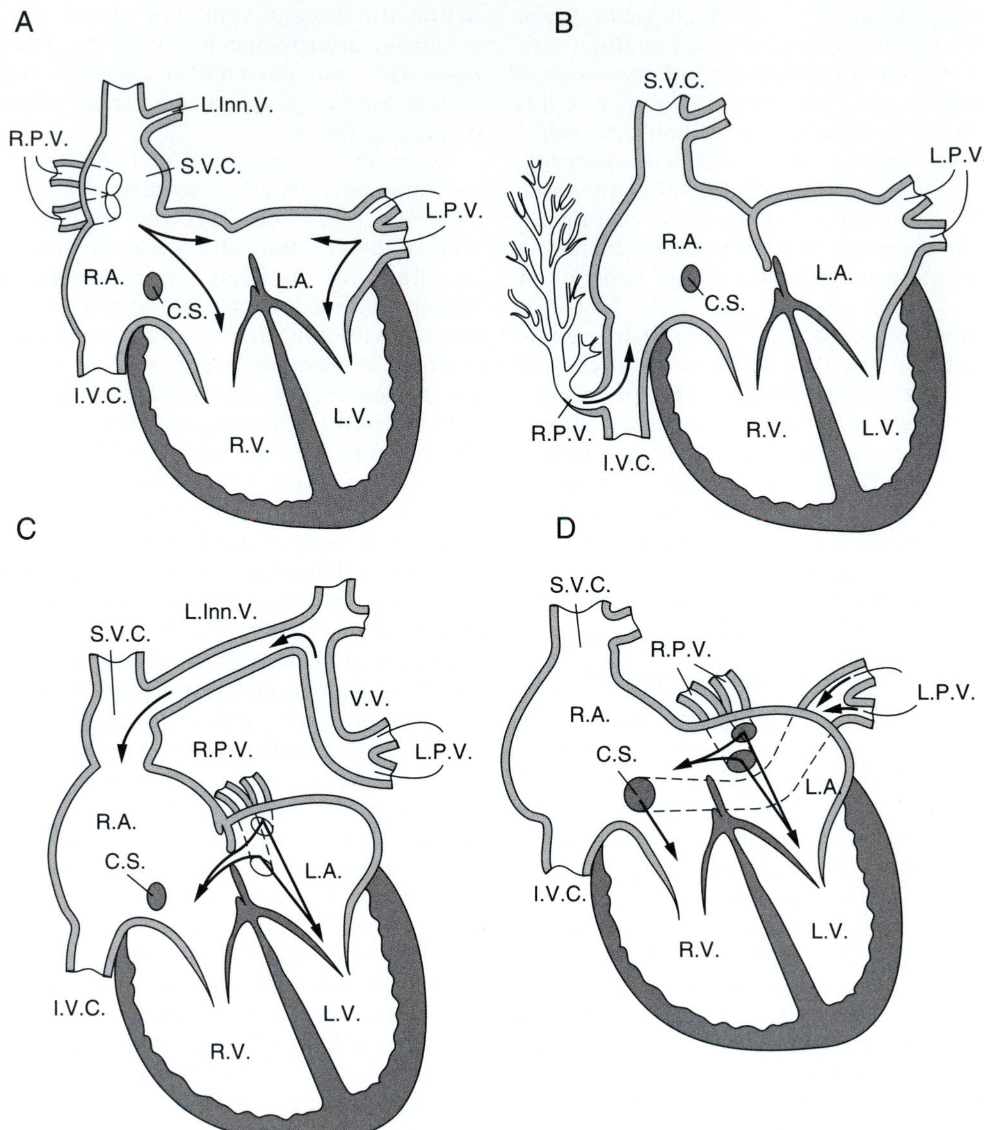

FIGURE 65-3. The most common patterns of circulation in partial anomalous pulmonary connection (PAPVC). **A,** Anomalous connection of the right pulmonary veins to superior vena cava. **B,** Anomalous connections of the right pulmonary veins to the inferior vena cava in the presence of an intact atrial septum. **C,** Anomalous connection of the left pulmonary veins to the left innominate by way of a vertical vein. **D,** Anomalous connection of the left pulmonary veins to coronary sinus. CS, coronary sinus; IVC, inferior vena cava; LA, left atrium; L Inn V, left innominate vein; LPV, left pulmonary vein; LV, left ventricle; RA, right atrium; RPV, right pulmonary vein; RV, right ventricle; SVC, superior vena cava; vv, vertical vein. (From Lucas RV, Krabill RA: Anomalous venous connections, pulmonary and systemic. In Adams FH, Emmanouilides GC [eds]: Moss' Heart Disease in Infants, Children and Adolescents, 4th ed. Baltimore, Williams & Wilkins, 1989, p 580.)

cases, veins of both lungs drain anomalously but a small segment of the pulmonary venous system drains normally. Edwards termed this condition *subtotal anomalous pulmonary venous connection.*[52]

The hemodynamic consequences of PAPVC connection depend on the number of anomalously connected veins, the site of the anomalous connections, the presence or absence of an interatrial communication, the size and location of the interatrial communication, and associated cardiac and extracardiac abnormalities. If there is no interatrial communication, there is no right-to-left shunting and therefore no pulmonary hypertension. If there is an ASD, the hemodynamics and clinical course are those of a large ASD.[1]

The clinicopathologic characteristics of PAPVC diagnosed in adulthood have not been studied in detail until recently. The overall prevalence of a partial anomalous pulmonary venous connection in adults undergoing chest CT is approximately 0.2%. In comparison, PAPVC was found in 0.6% of 801 anatomical dissections. In stark contrast to pediatric PAPVC, the majority of adults have left-sided anomalies, atrial septal defects are uncommon, and most patients are female. The anomalous veins are often incidental; in one series, only 40% of adults with PAPVC had symptoms solely attributable to the defect. Seventy-nine percent had an anomalous left upper lobe vein connecting to a persistent left vertical vein. Seventeen percent had an anomalous right upper lobe vein draining into the superior vena cava, and 3% had an anomalous right lower lobe vein draining into the suprahepatic inferior vena cava. Less than 5% had atrial septal defects. At presentation, chest radiographic findings included abnormal left mediastinal contour, abnormal right mediastinal contour, pulmonary artery enlargement, and cardiomegaly; these findings were reflected in CT findings.[26]

Atresia of Common Pulmonary Veins

In this rare anomaly, the pulmonary veins unite into a blind pouch posterior to the left atrium and have no communication with the left atrium or with any other cardiac chamber or systemic veins.

Physiologically, there is severe obstruction to pulmonary venous flow, and these patients usually become cyanotic and die within a few days of birth.

Cor Triatriatum

Cor triatriatum is a relatively rare cardiac anomaly (0.4% of autopsied cases with congenital heart disease, male-to-female ratio of 1.5:1).[27] In this condition, the pulmonary veins enter an accessory chamber lying posterior to the left atrium and joining the left atrium through a narrow opening. The following broad classification has been suggested by a number of authors.[28,29]

1. Accessory atrial chamber that receives all pulmonary veins and communicates with the left atrium; no other connections (classic cor triatriatum)
2. Accessory atrial chamber that receives part of pulmonary veins and does not communicate with left atrium
3. Subtotal cor triatriatum:
   a. Accessory atrial chamber that receives part of the pulmonary veins and connects to the left atrium
   b. Accessory atrial chamber that receives part of the pulmonary veins and connects to the right atrium

Physiologically, when the blood from the accessory atrial chamber drains into the right atrium, the hemodynamic features are those of TAPVC. A stenotic opening between the accessory atrium and the left atrium, however, results in features of severe pulmonary obstruction. In subtotal cor triatriatum, when obstruction affects only one lung, the result is reflex pulmonary arterial obstruction with decreased flow through that portion of the lung. The rest of the unobstructed lung receives increased flow, but there is no elevation in pulmonary arterial pressure.[29]

The classic cor triatriatum patients have onset of symptoms in the first few years of life. Patients usually have history of breathlessness and frequent respiratory infections. Right-heart failure usually is present, along with signs of pulmonary hypertension. Diagnosis is established noninvasively by echocardiography. On cardiac catheterization, there is a delay between opacification of the accessory left atrial chamber and the opacification of the true left atrium and ventricle. The timing of surgical intervention is tailored to the severity of the stenosis in an individual patient. Surgery has been advocated as early as the neonatal period,[30] and balloon dilatation may be successful in older children.[31] Associated complex congenital heart disease may be found in children, in whom transesophageal echocardiography provides optimal imaging of the defects.[32]

Some patients remain asymptomatic until adulthood[33] or present with sick sinus syndrome in advanced years.[34] The clinical features on presentation in adults can mimic those of mitral stenosis due to the obstructive properties of the membrane[35] and include dyspnea with increased pulmonary capillary wedge pressure at exertion.[36] As with other anomalies of the pulmonary venous system, associated anomalies may occur, including atrioventricular septal defect.[37]

The prognosis of cor triatriatum is related to the size of the orifice in the obstructing membrane. Survival is poor if the opening is smaller than 3 mm. When pulmonary edema and right-heart failure occur, the survival is just a few months. When there is associated atrial fibrillation, mitral valve insufficiency, and deformity, the Maze procedure and mitral valve repair have been advocated in addition to excision of the membrane.[38] There may be associated congenital pulmonary stenosis to complicate the surgical procedure.[39]

Pulmonary vascular changes in cor triatriatum are progressive medial thickening and intimal fibrosis in pulmonary arteries and veins accompanied by lymphangiectasia. In contrast to persistent left-to-right shunts, no plexiform lesions or more advanced stages of pulmonary vascular disease occur, which may explain the reversibility of pulmonary hypertension due to congenital pulmonary venous obstruction.[40]

Congenital Stenosis of Pulmonary Veins

Congenital pulmonary vein stenosis is often associated with other anomalies such as anomalous connections, cor triatriatum, and ventricular septal defects.[41] The isolated form generally comes to clinical attention because of symptoms related to pulmonary hypertension.[42] In its most severe form, congenital pulmonary vein stenosis is a progressive disease with rapid pulmonary hypertension and rare survival beyond the first year of life.[43]

Two types of pulmonary vein stenoses exist: One is localized stenosis of the pulmonary veins at the junction of the left atrium, which may involve one or more pulmonary veins; the other is characterized by narrowing of the lumen of the pulmonary vein, either intrapulmonary or extrapulmonary in location, and is called *hypoplasia of the pulmonary veins.* The latter type is occasionally present in patients with pulmonary artery atresia or hypoplastic left-heart syndrome. Clinically, patients have a history of respiratory symptoms, which may progress to right-heart failure. The localized stenosis of pulmonary veins at the junction of the left atrium is best visualized by echocardiography, whereas the distal stenosis of pulmonary veins is seen angiographically, revealing prolongation of transit time of the dye through the lung.

Because of poor surgical results, balloon angioplasty and stenting currently are being evaluated as noninvasive treatments for pulmonary artery stenosis. In the most severe forms, lung transplantation appears to be an important option.[43]

Anomalous Systemic Venous Connections

Anomalous systemic venous connections, especially persistent left SVC, usually are asymptomatic and are of little functional significance because systemic venous flow to the RA is not impaired. However, if they are not recognized, systemic venous anomalies may be accidentally severed during cardiac surgery. A classification based on embryologic principles includes anomalies of the cardinal venous system, anomalies of the IVC, and anomalies of the valves of the sinus venosus.[28]

Anomalies of the cardinal venous system include persistent left SVC; persistent left SVC connecting to the right or left atrium with and without failure of development of coronary sinus; right SVC connected to the left atrium; and anomalies of the coronary sinus. Anomalies of the IVC include double IVC, left IVC, and many lesser anomalies, which usually are of no clinical significance except that they may present problems to the surgeon.[44,45] Infrahepatic interruption of the IVC with drainage via the enlarged azygos vein to the SVC has been found to occur in 2.9% of congenital heart defects.[28] Anomalies of the valves of the sinus venosus involve the eustachian and thebesian valves and crista terminalis. Minor abnormal persistence results in larger valves and Chiari network. Large outgrowth of the valve of the sinus venosus may result in complete or partial subdivision of the right atrium.

As with anomalous pulmonary veins, anomalous systemic venous return is a hallmark of the heterotaxy syndromes, especially asplenia. In a recent autopsy review of 72 cases of asplenia, the superior vena cava was bilateral in 51 cases (71%) and unilateral in 21 (29%). In nine cases of bilateral SVC, one SVC was partly or totally atretic. Although the IVC was never interrupted, a prominent azygos vein was found in six cases (8%). An intact coronary sinus was rare.[9]

Embryology

The early embryonic vascular plexus forms three sets of paired venous systems, which return venous blood to the sinus venosus at the atrial end of the embryonic heart. The umbilical veins are the most medial veins in the caudal aspect of the embryo and conduct oxygenated blood from the chorionic villi to the sinus venosus. Just lateral to the umbilical veins are the vitelline veins, which conduct caudal venous blood from the yolk sac to the sinus venosus. The third and most lateral veins are the posterior cardinal veins, which also drain the caudal region of the embryo. The anterior cardinal veins drain the cranial region of the embryo into the sinus venosus. After the formation of the posterior cardinal vein, the paired subcardinal veins form to drain the developing midline urogenital system. Next is the formation of the intersubcardinal anastomosis between the subcardinal veins. Hepatocardinal channels form venous connections between the hepatic sinusoids and the proximal portions of the vitelline veins. Normally, the left anterior cardinal vein regresses in the sixth fetal month, leading to the formation of the innominate vein and its connection across the midline to the right SVC. The paired precursors of the IVC coalesce into a single IVC, which may persist as paired IVCs. These are not uncommon but are usually incidental and not functionally significant.

Persistence of the left anterior cardinal vein results in a persistent left SVC, which usually drains via the coronary sinus into the RA and, rarely, directly into the left atrium or via the coronary sinus into the left atrium. Persistent left SVC is found in about 0.3% of all autopsies and up to 5% of autopsied congenital heart disease cases, particularly in conditions with cyanosis.

Cor Triatriatum Dexter

Cor triatriatum dexter is an unusual cardiac abnormality with division between the sinus and primitive atrial portions of the right atrium. Three-dimensional echocardiography is a recently developed technique that defines this entity.[46] Symptoms in adults with isolated cor triatriatum dexter include lifelong exertional cyanosis and dyspnea. A definitive diagnosis of cor triatriatum dexter with associated heart defects is best made by transesophageal echocardiography.[47]

Congenital Coronary Artery Anomalies

The incidence of coronary artery anomalies is between 0.46% and 1.55% in angiographic series and 0.3% in autopsy series. The major anomalies are discussed as follows.

Anomalous Left Main

The most common coronary anomaly resulting in clinical symptoms is an aberrant left main arising in the right coronary sinus of Valsalva. There is a male-to-female ratio of 4:1 to 9:1. Sudden death occurs in up to two thirds of individuals with this anomaly, 75% of which occur during exercise.[48] Most patients are adolescents or young adults, although death may occur as young as 1 month of age. There are often premonitory symptoms of syncope or chest pain, but stress electrocardiograms and stress echocardiograms are often negative.

Pathologically, there are several variants to this anomaly. The common feature is the presence of the left main ostium within the right sinus (see Fig. 65-3). This ostium is typically near the commissure, and in some cases actually lies above the commissure between the right and left sinuses. Often the ostium is somewhat malformed and slitlike, and an ostial ridge is present. The proximal artery lies within the aortic media and traverses between the aorta and pulmonary trunk.

The pathophysiology of sudden death in patients with aberrant left main coronary artery may be related to compression of the left main by the pulmonary trunk and aorta, diastolic compression of the vessel lying within the aortic media, and poor filling during diastole because of ostial ridges or slitlike ostia.

Anomalous Right Coronary Artery

In contrast to anomalous left main coronary artery, anomalous right coronary artery from the left aortic sinus is usually an incidental finding, although up to one third of patients may die suddenly. In the majority of cases (67%), the anomalous vessel courses between the aorta and pulmonary trunk with the remainder usually coursing posterior to the aorta.[48] Almost 50% of sudden deaths are exercise related, and most deaths occur in young and middle-aged adults younger than the age of 35 years.

Grossly, there are two ostia located in the left sinus of Valsalva. The ostium supplying the right coronary artery may have similar features as anomalous left ostia located in the right sinus. Namely, there may be upward displacement, location near the commissure, and slitlike ostia with ostial ridges. The proximal anomalous right coronary generally also courses between the aorta and pulmonary trunk. The pathophysiology of sudden death is similar to that of anomalous left coronary artery, and, like that anomaly, evidence of acute or remote ischemia in the ventricular myocardium is not often found.

Anomalous Left Circumflex Artery

This is the most common anomaly of the origin of a coronary artery, accounting for 28% of anomalies identified by cardiac catheterization and with an incidence of 1 in 300.[49] This anomaly is considered benign. Awareness of this anomaly is important during cardiac surgery to avoid problems with myocardial protection or during prosthetic valve replacement.

Origin from Pulmonary Trunk

The left main coronary artery arises from the pulmonary trunk in 1/50,000 to 1/300,000 autopsies. Most cases are identified in the first year of life, and sudden death occurs in approximately 40% of cases. In a minority of cases (approximately 20%), sufficient myocardial collaterals develop from the normally structured right coronary artery, causing potential survival into adulthood. In these cases, a continuous murmur may be present with other symptoms including angina pectoris, myocardial infarction, dyspnea, and syncope. Sudden death usually occurs at rest but may occur after strenuous activity in older children. Pathologically, the aberrant artery arises in the left pulmonary sinus in 95% of cases. Typically, the artery appears thin walled and veinlike, and the right coronary artery, while normal in location, is tortuous.

Angiographic and Other Imaging in Diagnosis of Anomalous Coronary Arteries

Identifying anomalous right or left main coronary artery from the contralateral coronary sinus angiographically depends on the vessel's course between the aorta and pulmonary trunk. This particular course is angiographically distinct in the right anterior oblique projection when the left main forms a cranial-posterior loop (Fig. 65-4). An alternative method is to perform simultaneous pulmonary and coronary arteriography, or more practically, insert a pulmonary artery catheter as an angiographic marker for the location of the pulmonary vessels and then perform an angiogram of the aberrant coronary artery in the steep anteroposterior (AP) caudal projection.

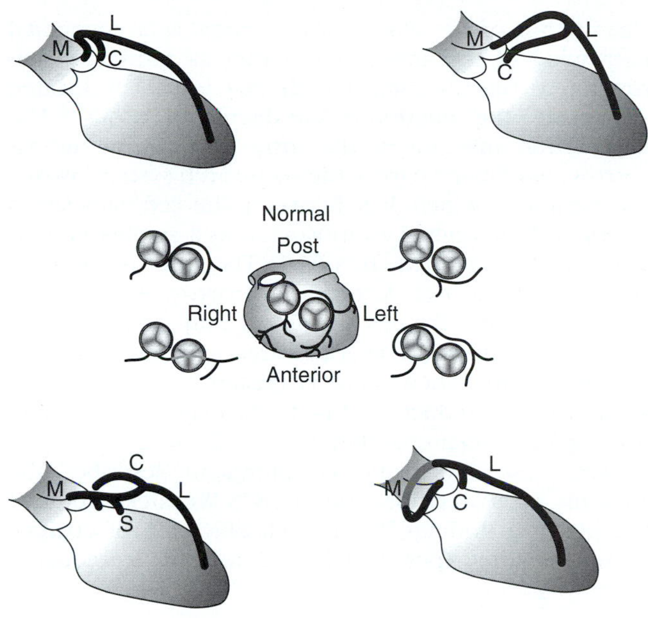

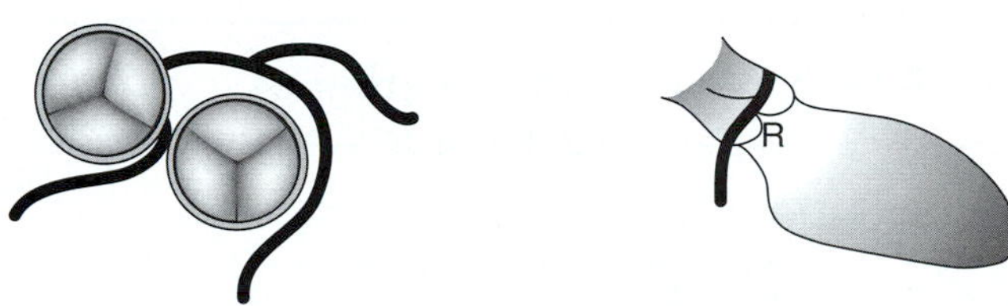

FIGURE 65-4. Angiographic appearance of coronary artery anomalies. The four different angiographic courses of the anomalous left main coronary artery from the right coronary sinus are shown, as is an anomalous right coronary artery from the left coronary sinus. C, circumflex coronary artery; L, left anterior descending; M, left main coronary artery; R, right coronary artery; S, septal perforator branch. (From Taylor AJ, Virmani R: Coronary artery anomalies. In Crawford MH, Dimarco JP, Paulus WJ [eds]: Cardiology. Edinburgh, Mosby, 2004, p 201.)

Standard 2-D echocardiography has recently been used as a screening procedure for coronary anomalies in athletes. An echocardiographic screening study of 3650 athletes found 3 cases of anomalous right (n = 2) and left (n = 1) coronary arteries from the contralateral aortic sinus.[50] However, the specificity of transthoracic echocardiography is insufficient for this test to serve as an accurate screening tool.[51] Alternative noninvasive procedures in the case of inadequate screening echocardiograms include transesophageal echocardiography.

MALFORMATIONS AFFECTING THE GREAT VESSELS

Coarctation of the Aorta

Coarctation of the aorta (COA) occurs as a congenital narrowing of the aortic arch, either as a discrete narrowing or one of some length that is usually located adjacent to the junction of the ductus arteriosus.[52] The obstruction may be in the form of uniform tubular narrowing of some part of the aortic arch system, usually the isthmus (which lies between the left subclavian artery and the ductus arteriosus) or as a shelflike coarctation within the arch (Box 65-1). The latter is the more common of the two lesions. The narrowing may vary in severity but becomes significant only when there is a pressure gradient across the area of narrowing. That usually occurs when there is greater than 50% cross-sectional area reduction, but there may be lesser narrowing for tubular coarctation.

More than 200 years ago, Morgagni described the anatomy of coarctation, and in 1875 Wernicke outlined the physical findings.[53-57] The classification of coarctation into adult (postductal) and infantile (preductal) types by Bonnett[58] is now generally accepted as being inadequate. The first extensive review of 200 autopsy cases (mean age 30 years) was published by Abbot in 1928.[59] All patients were older than 3 years; the oldest was a 92-year-old man and is probably the longest recorded survival. Bicuspid aortic valve was present in 24% of patients with coarctation and bacterial endocarditis in 10%. Reifenstein and coworkers[60] described another 104 autopsy cases; all were older than 3 years. Bicuspid aortic valve was seen twice as frequently [43%], and the incidence of bacterial endocarditis was higher. In the early series, it was believed that when COA occurred as an isolated malformation, it rarely caused death. That concept has changed only since 1950, when several authors reported that isolated COA could cause death in infancy.[61,62]

BOX 65-1 Classification of Coarctation of the Aorta

I. Discrete coarctation of aorta
   A. Coarctation distal to ductus arteriosus
      1. With closed ductus
      2. With patent ductus
   B. Coarctation proximal to ductus arteriosus
      1. With closed ductus
      2. With patent ductus
   C. Coarctation with anomalies of subclavian arteries or aortic arches
      1. Atresia or stenosis of left subclavian artery
      2. Stenosis of right subclavian artery
      3. Anomalous origin of right subclavian artery
         a. Distal to coarctation
         b. Proximal to coarctation
      4. Double aortic arch with stenosis of right and coarctation of the left
   D. Coarctation of unusual locations
      1. Proximal to left subclavian artery
         a. With normal branches
         b. With anomalous origin of right subclavian artery
      2. At multiple sites
      3. Of lower thoracic
II. Tubular hypoplasia (isolated or coexistent with discrete COA)
   A. Involving aorta beyond the origin of innominate to the origin of ductus arteriosus
   B. Involving only part of the segment of the aorta

Modified from Edwards JE: Congenital malformations of the heart and great vessel. H. Malformations of the thoracic aorta. In Gould SE (ed): Pathology of the Heart and Blood Vessels, 3rd ed. Springfield, Ill.: Thomas, 1968, p 391.

Incidence

Isolated COA is the fifth or sixth most common anomaly of all the congenital heart diseases.[56] Among the New England regional study of congenital heart defects, COA accounts for 7.5% of infants younger than 1 year of age.[63] That may be an underestimation, since COA in newborn infants may not be detected because of similar blood pressure in the upper and lower extremities.[64] The male-to-female ratio is 1.74:1.[65] In older patients with isolated COA, the incidence also is higher in males. There is no evidence of a Mendelian pattern of inheritance in the majority of patients with COA.[56] COA is the most common cardiovascular defect found with Turner's syndrome. Noncardiac abnormalities that have been reported with COA are hypospadias, clubfoot, and ocular defects.[65]

Pathology

The severity of luminal narrowing in the region of the coarctation at autopsy reveals 42% severe (pinhole) stenosis, 25% atresia, and 33% moderate narrowing in individuals 2 years of age and older.[60] In cases of COA containing a contraductal shelf, there is an infolding of the aortic media into the lumen located opposite the ductus arteriosus, marked on the adventitial side by a localized indentation like a waist in the aortic wall.[66] The aorta distal to the coarctation shows poststenotic dilatation and the wall of the aorta is thinner, whereas proximally, where the pressure is higher, the wall is thicker. The shelf of the coarctation may be preductal or postductal, but most often it is juxtaductal.[67] Flow patterns in the fetus with various congenital defects determine the development of the aortic isthmus. In a normal fetus the level of blood flow across the aortic isthmus is lower (25% of the combined total ventricular output) than after birth; therefore the aortic isthmus at birth is narrower than the descending thoracic aorta.[67] In congenital heart disease with reduced pulmonary arterial flow (pulmonary stenosis), the diameter of the isthmus is wider than normal because it carries greater flow in the fetus and coarctation is virtually unknown. In lesions interfering with left ventricular outflow (mitral and aortic stenosis), the aortic isthmus is underdeveloped.

When localized juxtaductal coarctation is present, aortic obstruction is not present during fetal life, but when the ductus arteriosus begins to close at birth, obstruction appears after birth.[68] The ductus closes from the pulmonary end; obstruction of the aortic end and a gradient across the coarctation may be delayed.

The ductal tissue itself plays an important role in the mechanism of coarctation formation. Normally, ductal tissue, composed mostly of smooth muscle cells, extends only partially around the circumference of the aorta. In a patient with left-sided obstruction, there is right-to-left flow through the ductus in utero. This results in the migration of ductal tissue into the adjacent aortic wall, resulting in a circumferential distribution.[67] Ho and Anderson,[69] using a serial-section technique, have confirmed that ductal tissue completely surrounds the juxtaductal aorta such that "the ductal and descending aorta form a common channel of structural continuity, and the isthmus enters this channel" rather than the ductus entering the isthmus descending aortic region.[70]

Collateral Circulation

Olney and Stephens[71] and Bahn and colleagues[72] have reported that collateral circulation is poorly developed in infants who die with coarctation (Fig. 65-5). Bahn and colleagues[72] noted that this depends on the location of the coarctation in relation to the ductus arteriosus; if the blood from the ductus enters the aorta proximal to the coarctation (preductal), then collateral circulation develops (Fig. 65-6). If the ductal blood flow enters below the coarctation (postductal), however, there is little stimulation during fetal life for development of collateral circulation. In this situation postnatal closure of the ductus results in obstructive hypertension and hypovolemia, which together result in left ventricular failure.

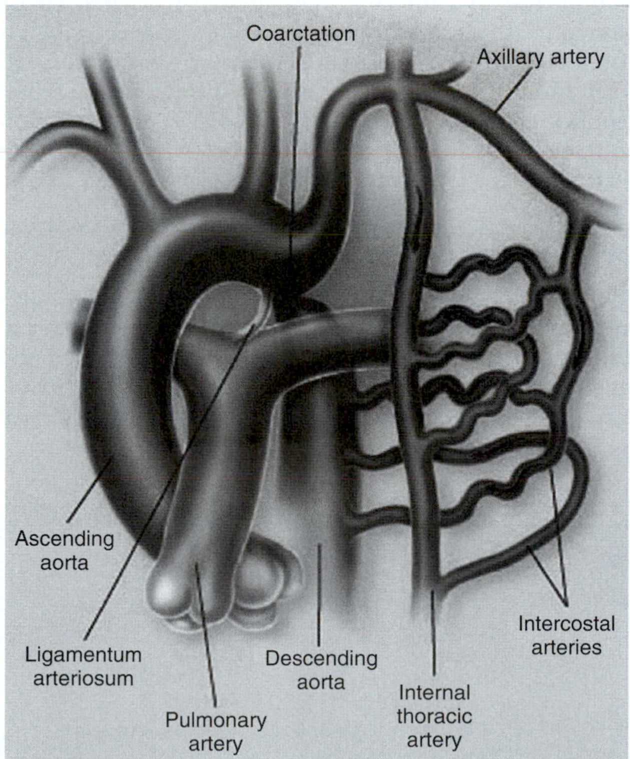

FIGURE 65-5. (See also Color Plate 65-5.) Coarctation of the aorta. Coarctation causes severe obstruction of blood flow in the descending thoracic aorta. The descending aorta and its branches are perfused by collateral channels from the axillary and internal thoracic arteries through the intercostal arteries (*arrows*). (From Brickner ME: Congenital heart disease in adults. N Engl Med 342:256, 2000.)

The collateral circulation in COA between the proximal aorta and the distal aorta usually is present to some extent at birth but develops further as the patient ages. Collateral circulation involves primarily branches of both subclavian arteries, especially the internal mammary, vertebral, costocervical, and thyrocervical trunks, which carry blood to the lower limbs, usually through third and fourth intercostal arteries and the subscapular arteries. The subclavian arterial branches become greatly enlarged and are responsible for the classic signs of coarctation such as rib notching, which extends from the third to the eighth rib, and parascapular pulsations.[52,55,73] Collateral circulation also reaches the lower limbs through the internal mammary to the superior epigastric, which in turn connects with the inferior epigastric and joins the iliac arteries. The anterior spinal artery may provide additional collateral channels through its communication with the vertebral arteries above the coarctation and with intercostals and vertebral arteries below the coarctation.[52,55] The development of good collateral circulation and clinical manifestations vary depending on the presence of stenosis of the left subclavian artery, which is an important source of collateral circulation; rib notching is seen only on the right side. If the right subclavian artery arises as a fourth branch and is distal to the coarctation, it is not a source of collateral flow and rib notching occurs only on the left side.[56]

Today coarctation may be visualized by echocardiography, and with Doppler it is possible to estimate the transcoarctation pressure gradient. Other modalities like CT, MRI, and contrast aortography show the exact location and length of the coarctation. Aortography also permits visualization of the collateral circulation.[74]

Associated Conditions

As stated earlier, COA is commonly associated with bicuspid aortic valve, but the exact incidence remains speculative (27% to 46%).[70,75] Among 250 patients with COA studied by Tawes and associates,[75] bicuspid valve disease was present in 32 (13%). The most common lesion is stenosis and, unusually, incompetence, which occurs on the basis of bicuspid valve with persistent hypertension.[57]

A high incidence (85%) of major cardiac defects is associated with COA in neonates[67]; in infants aged 1 to 11 months, however, the incidence drops to 52%. After 1 year of age, the incidence drops further to 40% (excluding bicuspid valve), as reported by Kirklin and Barratt-Boyes.[57] Infants undergoing operations in the first 3 months of life have a 60% incidence of other congenital cardiac anomalies, compared with 25% of those between 6 and 12 months.[57]

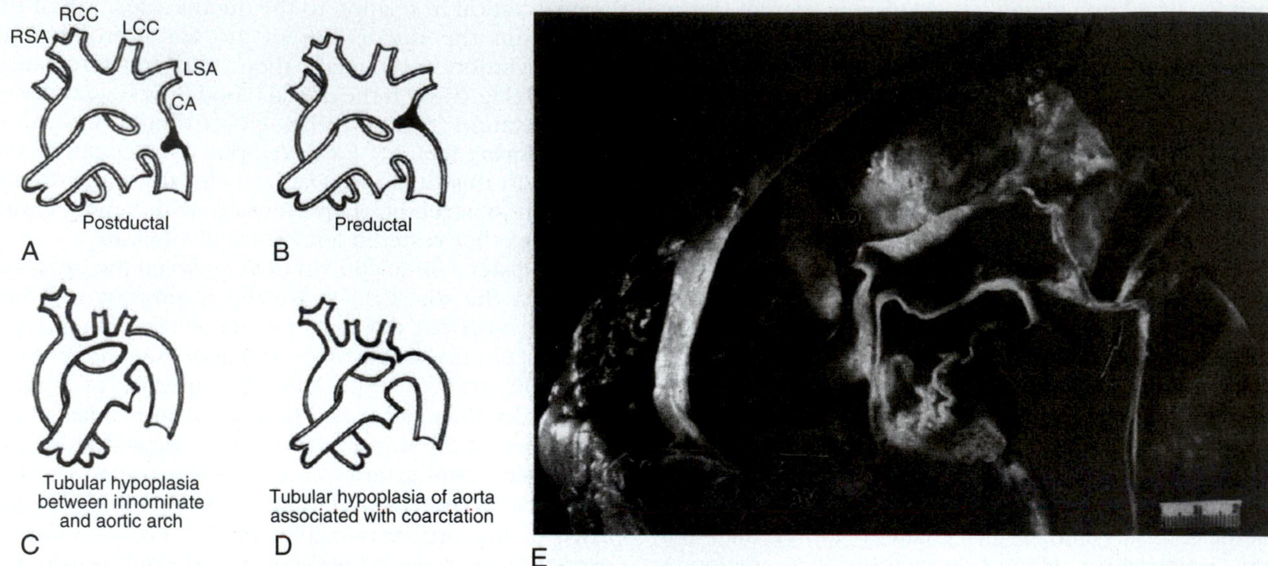

FIGURE 65-6. Coarctation of aorta in the left panel. **A,** Postductal and **B,** preductal, with patent ductus arteriosus. **C,** Tubular hypoplasia of aortic arch between innominate and subclavian artery with patent ductus arteriosus. **D,** Tubular hypoplasia (between common carotid and left subclavian) associated with coarctation of aorta (*arrow*). **E,** Gross photography of heart and aorta from a 76-year-old male with postductal coarctation of the aorta (*arrow*). Note dilated and thinned aorta both proximally and distally to the COA. He also had a heavily calcified congenital bicuspid aortic valve. AO, aorta; AV, aortic valve. (**A-D,** Modified from Moller JH, Amplatz K, Edwards JE: Congenital Heart Disease. Kalamazoo, Mich., Upjohn, 1974, p 46.)

Patent ductus arteriosus is present in virtually all neonates and is considered part of the coarctation complex.[57] Ventricular septal defect (VSD) occurs in 30% to 36% of cases of COA.[55,56] COA in TGA occurs in 10%, and ASD in 6% to 7%.[76] Mitral valve disease, which causes mitral stenosis and regurgitation, is present in less than 10%.[76]

Complications

Aortic rupture usually occurs in the second or third decade and normally involves the ascending aorta, with resultant tamponade. Aortic rupture also may occur distal to the coarctation, where the aorta is thin and dilated (poststenotic dilatation).[57] Some ruptures may be accompanied by dissecting aneurysms.[57] Women with coarctation are at a high risk of aortic dissections during pregnancy.

Cerebrovascular accidents, as reported by Liberthson and colleagues,[76] usually occur in older patients: older than 40 years, 21%; 11 to 39 years, 8%; and patients younger than 11 years, less than 1%. The main cause is usually rupture of a congenital berry aneurysm in the circle of Willis and is secondary to the presence of hypertension.[77] Other causes are atherosclerosis in older patients and emboli from bacterial endocarditis. Infective endocarditis normally involves the bicuspid aortic valve and, rarely, the mitral valve, at the site of VSD or at sites of jet lesion in the aortic wall.

Aortic Arch Anomalies

Malformations of the aortic arch are a complex group of lesions first described in the eighteenth century. A classification of the aortic arch malformations is presented in Box 65-2. Observations of the basic development of the aortic arches and their derivatives, reviewed and summarized by Congdon in 1922,[78] were of little use to clinicians until the 1940s, when Gross pioneered the first surgical repairs of vascular rings.[79] *Vascular ring* is the broad term used to describe an aortic-arch malformation in which the trachea and the esophagus are compressed. The first clinical description of tracheal and esophageal compression by a double aortic arch is credited to Wolman in 1939.[80]

Incidence

The true incidence of aortic-arch malformations and vascular rings is difficult to determine because so many lesions are asymptomatic. Congenital heart defects involving the outflow tract, aortic arch, ductus arteriosus, and pulmonary arteries account for 20% to 30% of

BOX 65-2 Aortic Arch Malformations

I. Vascular rings
    A. Double aortic arch
    B. Right aortic arch
        1. Without retroesophageal component
        2. With retroesophageal component
    C. Left aortic arch
        1. Aberrant right subclavian artery
        2. Ductus arteriosus sling
II. Cervical aorta
III. Complete interruption of the aortic arch

all congenital heart defects.[81] The incidence of vascular rings is thought to be approximately 1% of congenital heart disease. In 1948 Edwards proposed the hypothetic double-aortic-arch model to conceptualize all the known and possible aortic-arch malformations.[82]

Today there is a greater understanding of the embryology, and it has been shown that the final arrangement and morphology of these great arteries requires reciprocal signaling between endothelial cells lining the pharyngeal aortic arteries and their surrounding smooth muscle cells and mesenchyme, derived from neural crest cells (NCCs, Fig. 65-7). The septation of the truncus into the aorta and pulmonary artery is accompanied by migration of the cardiac NCCs into the pharyngeal arches and the heart, and this occurs in the mouse embryo 9 (E9.0) days onward. Following septation, the vessels rotate in a twisted manner to achieve the final connection with the left and right ventricles. The NCCs also contribute to the bilaterally symmetric aortic arches that arise from the aortic sac and undergo extensive remodeling, resulting in the formation of the aorta, ductus arteriosus, proximal subclavian, and carotid and pulmonary arteries. The NCC is remodeled to give rise to segments of the mature aortic arch, which is present from E12.5 days onward.[81] The three paired aortic arch arteries arise sequentially along the AP axis and are therefore not all present simultaneously. The arch arteries traverse the pharyngeal arches before joining the dorsal aorta.[83] The first and second arches involute, while the fifth arch does not form fully; however, the mechanisms involved in the vascularization and regression are unknown. The left and right third arch arteries form the common carotid arteries, and the right fourth arch artery forms the proximal portion of the right subclavian artery. The left sixth arch artery forms the ductus arteriosus, and the right sixth arch artery regresses.[84] Recent work with transgenic mice has shown which factors may be important for the normal development of the arch vessels. For example, disruption of the Forkhead transcription factor Mfh1 causes hypoplasia of the fourth aortic arch artery in mice, resulting in the absence of the transverse aortic arch, resembling the interruption of the aortic arch in man.[85]

Morphology

Aortic arch anomalies (vascular rings) are anomalies of the great arteries that compress the trachea, the esophagus, or both.[86]

Double Aortic Arch

The double aortic arch is the most frequent type of aortic-arch malformation to result in a vascular ring. The ascending aorta arises normally, and as it leaves the pericardium it divides into two branches, a left and a right aortic arch that join posteriorly to form the descending aorta. The left arch passes anteriorly and to the left of the trachea in the usual position and then becomes the descending aorta by the ligamentum arteriosum or the ductus arteriosus. The right aortic arch passes to the right and then posterior to the esophagus to join the left-sided descending aorta, thereby completing the vascular ring.[86] From each arch arises a carotid artery and a subclavian artery (Fig. 65-8).

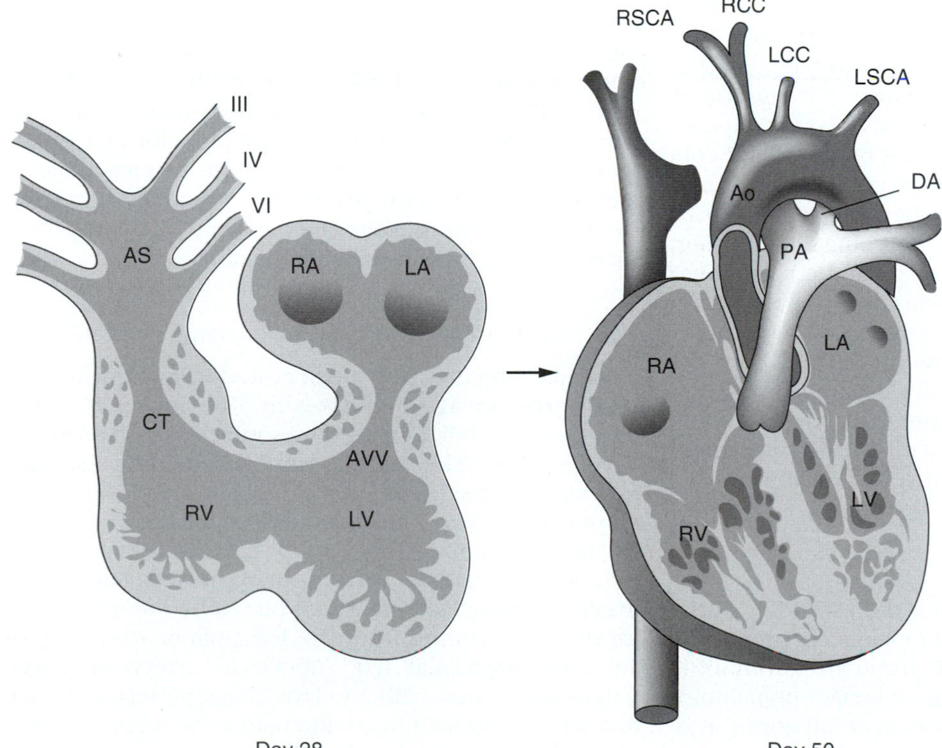

FIGURE 65-7. Schematic of the development of the arch vessels and the outflow tract of the heart. Neural crest cells populate the bilaterally symmetric aortic arch arteries (III, IV, and V) and aortic sac (AS), which together contribute to specific segments of the mature aortic arch. Mesenchymal cells form the cardiac valve from the conotruncal (CT) and atrioventricular valve (AVV) segments. Corresponding days of human embryonic development are indicated. A, atrium; Ao, aorta; DA, ductus arteriosus; LA, left atrium; LCC, left common carotid; LSC, left subclavian artery; LV, left ventricle; PA, pulmonary artery; RCC, right common carotid artery; RSC, right subclavian artery; RV, right ventricle. (From Srivastava D, Olson EN: A genetic blueprint for cardiac development. Nature 407:221, 2000.)

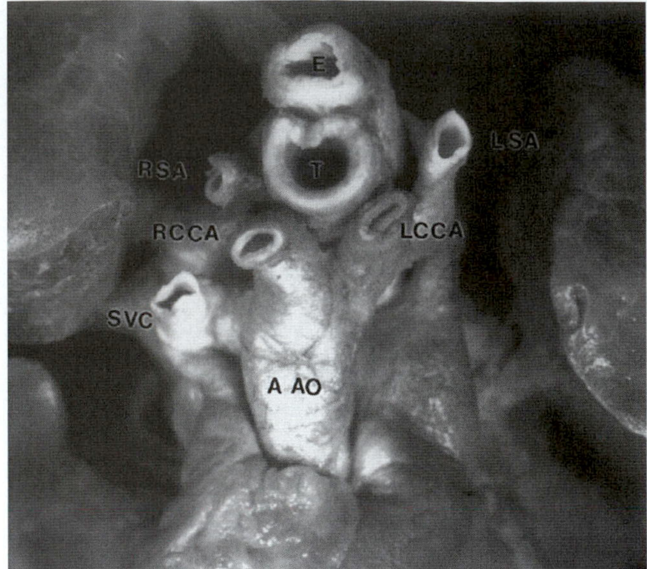

A

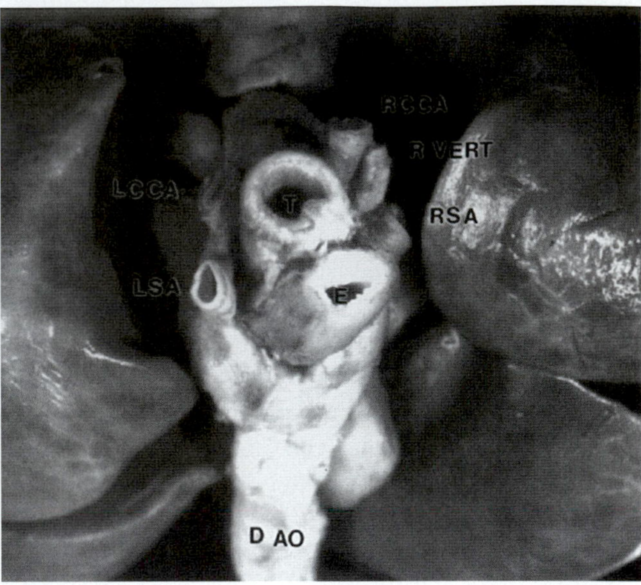

B

FIGURE 65-8. (See also Color Plate 65-8.) **A,** Double aortic arch, anterior/cranial view. The ascending aorta bifurcates into an anterior left branch, supplying the left common carotid artery and the left subclavian artery, and a posterior right branch, supplying the right common carotid and right subclavian arteries. **B,** Double aortic arch, posterior/cranial view. The continuation of the aorta viewed from behind demonstrates the anterior left branch wrapping around the trachea and esophagus, as well as the right posterior branch emerging from under the esophagus. The distal aorta continues as a centrally located structure. A AO, ascending aorta; D AO, descending aorta; E, esophagus; LCCA, left common carotid artery; LSA, left subclavian artery; RCCA, right common carotid artery; RSA, right subclavian artery; Rvert, right vertebral artery; SVC, superior vena cava; T, trachea.

The arches usually are not equal in size: One arch, often the right, is larger. One arch may be represented by a single atretic segment; in that case, the right arch usually persists. It is theoretically possible, using the double-aortic-arch model, that the ductus arteriosus could be bilateral or on the right or left side only. No case of functional double arch with bilateral ductus arteriosus has been reported. The descending aorta may be on the right, left, or, occasionally, in the midline.[82,86-88] Associated cardiac anomalies in most series were low but reportedly as high as 45% in the 1997 series by Kocis and colleagues,[89] and these include tetralogy of Fallot and TGA.[87] Most patients present at the time of diagnosis with many symptoms, the commonest being those arising from the respiratory system. Wheezing is the most common, followed by stridor, pneumonia, upper respiratory tract infection, respiratory distress, cough, and respiratory cyanosis. If such symptoms occur in the newborn or young infant and occur recurrently, it should alert the physician to the possibility of the presence of arch anomalies.[90] Surgical repair is ideal and is usually performed approximately 18 months after the initial diagnosis.

Right Aortic Arch

A right aortic arch is present when the ascending aorta and arch pass anteriorly to the right main stem bronchus. There are two main types of right aortic arch: without a retroesophageal component (mirror-image branching) and with a retroesophageal component. Right aortic arch is said to exist in 0.1% of the population.[91]

Right Aortic Arch without Retroesophageal Component

In the usual right aortic arch, there is mirror-image branching of the arch vessels compared with the normal left arch. The first vessel is a left innominate artery, and the second and third are the right common carotid and right subclavian arteries (Fig. 65-9). The majority of patients have a left ductus arteriosus arising from the left pulmonary artery and inserting into the left subclavian artery. Bilateral ducti are associated with congenital cardiac anomalies, usually tetralogy of Fallot or truncus arteriosus.[88] Right aortic arch without retroesophageal component does not produce a vascular ring (see Fig. 65-9). The abnormality does not produce symptoms but may be picked up radiographically.

Right Aortic Arch with Retroesophageal Component

A vascular ring is usually present in the right aortic arch with retroesophageal component. The right aortic arch extends to the left, behind the esophagus, in the form of a diverticulum. The vascular ring is formed by the right arch and a left-sided ductus arteriosus arising from the left pulmonary artery and extending to the upper descending thoracic aorta. This group of abnormalities also includes anomalous retroesophageal left subclavian artery. The vascular ring is completed by the left ductus arteriosus extending from the left pulmonary artery to the retroesophageal left subclavian artery or aorta. A right aortic arch with a mirror image pattern is associated with congenital heart anomalies, the most common of which are tetralogy of Fallot and truncus arteriosus.[92]

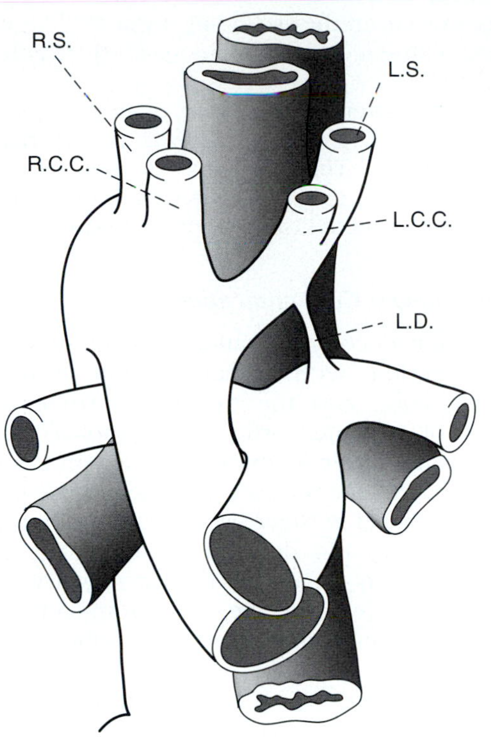

FIGURE 65-9. Right aortic arch with mirror-image branching and left ductus arteriosus. LCC, left common carotid artery; LD, left ductus arteriosus; LS, left subclavian artery; RCC, right common carotid artery; RS, right subclavian artery. (From Bankl H: Congenital Malformations of the Heart and Great Vessels. Synopsis of Pathology, Embryology, and Natural History. Baltimore, Urban & Schwarzenberg, 1977, p 159.)

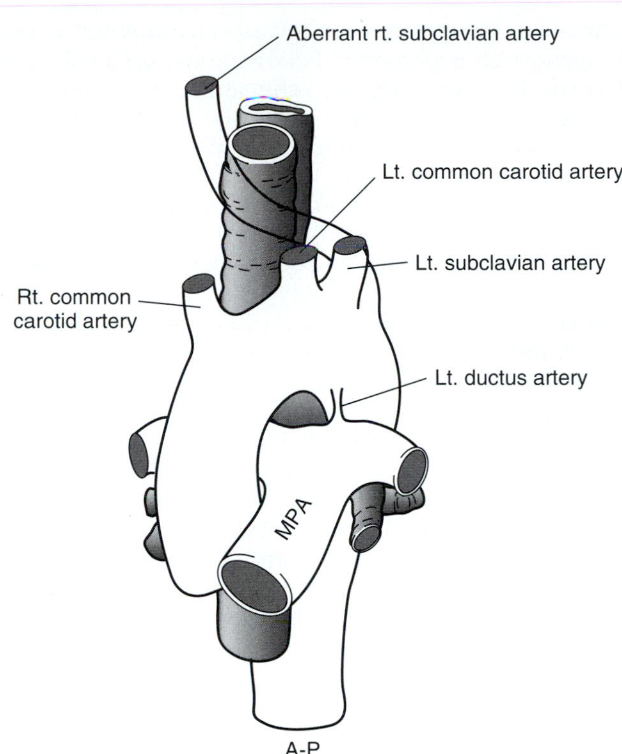

FIGURE 65-10. Aberrant right subclavian artery from an anteroposterior (A-P) view. (From Stewart JR, Kincaid OW, Edwards JE: An Atlas of Vascular Rings and Related Malformations of the Aortic Arch System. Springfield, Ill, Thomas, 1964.)

Left Aortic Arch

A vascular ring is frequently associated with a left aortic arch.

Aberrant Right Subclavian Artery

The most common left arch abnormality is aberrant right subclavian artery. The right subclavian artery arises as the fourth branch of the aortic arch, distal to the left subclavian artery. Aberrant right subclavian artery does not result in a vascular ring unless there is a right ductus arteriosus extending from the right pulmonary artery to the right subclavian (Fig. 65-10). This anomaly is important because of its frequent association with tetralogy of Fallot and the difficulty of using this vessel for the Blalock-Taussig anastomosis.[93] Aberrant right subclavian artery also is associated with COA.[87] Compression of the esophagus by the aberrant right subclavian was once thought to induce dysphagia lusoria.[94] That view is disputed, and the anomaly is generally thought not to be a cause of major symptoms.[88]

Ductus Arteriosus Sling

An aberrant ductus arteriosus extending from the right pulmonary artery between the trachea and the esophagus to the aorta near the origin of an aberrant right subclavian artery has been reported.[95] The patient may have dyspnea and wheezing, which are relieved by surgical division of the vessel.

Cervical Aortic Arch/Interrupted Aortic Arch

Complete interruption of the aortic arch is different from coarctation of the aortic arch in that there is no continuity of the aorta. Interrupted aortic arch is a rare congenital malformation occurring in three per million live births. It is defined as a loss of continuity between the ascending and descending thoracic aorta and has poor prognosis without surgical treatment. Almost all cases have a patent ductus arteriosus and associated intracardiac anomalies such as VSD, subaortic stenosis, and truncus arteriosus. The symptoms of complete interruption of the aortic arch are severe right-to-left shunting. In infants the clinical presentation is severe congestive heart failure. If untreated, 90% of these infants die at a median age of 4 days. Only rare cases in adults have been reported.[96]

Clinical Presentation and Diagnosis

Patients with vascular rings present within the first 6 months of life, and close to 50% have symptoms at birth. Those with associated cardiac defects may not present earlier. The signs and symptoms of tracheal and esophageal compression vary with the severity of compression. Infants may present with stridor, wheeze, and recurrent respiratory infections. They often demonstrate poor feeding and dysphagia for solid foods.[75] The plain-film chest radiograph and barium upper gastrointestinal series are essential for diagnosis.[89] An esophagram is a useful diagnostic tool for demonstrating right and left indentations in the esophagus when a double aortic arch is present.[87] Following the establishment of aortic arch anomaly, an echocardiogram should be obtained to identify any associated cardiac defects. Bronchoscopy is indicated in cases of suspected innominate artery compression. MRI, although available for clarifying the presence of an aortic arch anomaly, is usually unnecessary for diagnosing the anomaly. However, CT and MRI are helpful in the work-up of pulmonary artery sling.[90]

Surgery is indicated when esophageal- and tracheal-compression symptoms are severe. Left thoracotomy is the most common operative approach (85%); however, in the presence of other cardiac congenital anomalies, medial thoracotomy may be indicated. Complications following surgery are reported in 11% of patients, and death is reported in 4%.[90] No late deaths have occurred in isolated vascular rings since 1967.[97,98] On long-term follow-up, 92% of patients are free of respiratory symptoms.[98] When symptoms are of borderline severity, they may disappear as the child grows.[98]

Malformation of the Pulmonary Trunk and Arteries

Isolated pulmonary-artery abnormalities are rare and can be divided into those with anomalous arterial supply to one lung in the presence of separate aortic and pulmonary valves (and without inherent interposition of ductal tissue) and those with lungs receiving normally connected pulmonary arteries.

Origin of Right or Left Pulmonary Artery from Ascending Aorta

When the right pulmonary artery arises from the aorta, it usually arises from the right or posterior aspect of the ascending aorta.[99] The origin usually is within 1 to 3 cm of the aortic valve, and the right pulmonary artery is larger than the left.[99] The pulmonary vascular bed of both lungs may be similar, especially in patients dying within 6 months of birth.[100] In older patients, however, hypertensive vascular disease usually is present and usually is similar in its extent in both lungs.[99] This lesion is seen as an isolated defect in 20% of cases, but most often it is associated with patent ductus arteriosus (50%).[101,102] Occasionally, the lesion coexists with (left) pulmonary-vein stenosis.[99] The pulmonary stenosis may be tubular or membranous.[99]

The origin of the left pulmonary artery from the ascending aorta is rarer than the right pulmonary artery from the aorta and usually is seen in association with right aortic arch.[99] This anomaly is isolated in 40% of cases, and the most commonly associated lesion is tetralogy of Fallot. Also, part of one lung may receive anomalous vascular supply, called *sequestration of the lung*. A distinct form of sequestration, *scimitar syndrome*, involves abnormal arterial supply, as well as venous drainage into the IVC.[103] The more severe type of sequestration occurs when one lung is supplied completely from a systemic source. Only one case has been reported where both the right and the left pulmonary arteries arose from the ascending aorta.[99,104] Much more common is absence of one pulmonary artery, either right or left.[103]

Pulmonary arteries may arise from the pulmonary trunk, but the left artery connects to the right lung and vice versa.[103] This anomaly has been described in truncus arteriosus, as well as when the pulmonary trunk is normally connected to the right ventricle.[103]

Aortopulmonary Communication

Aortopulmonary communication, or window, is a distinct anatomic lesion, with communication between the ascending aorta and the pulmonary trunk and the presence of separate aortic and pulmonary valves.[105] The defect is a true window with no length to the communication between the aorta and the pulmonary trunk. Usually the defect is single, large, and oval; infrequently (<10% of cases) the defect is small.[106] The communication usually is situated in the left lateral wall of the ascending aorta (close to the origin of the left coronary artery) in communication with the right wall of the pulmonary trunk (inferior to the origin of the right pulmonary artery).[106,107] It is not surprising, therefore, that the right or, more rarely, the left coronary arteries may be seen arising from the pulmonary trunk. Rarely, the communication may be more downstream.[106-108] Because the defect usually is large, it is not surprising that pulmonary vascular disease may develop early, similar to that seen in VSDs and patent ductus arteriosus.[105,106]

Aortopulmonary window is associated with other cardiovascular malformations, usually VSDs; tetralogy of Fallot; subaortic stenosis; and, infrequently, right aortic arch, ASD, or patent ductus arteriosus.[106-109]

VASCULAR MALFORMATIONS

Benign vascular malformations are generally classified as either arteriovenous malformations (AVMs) or hemangiomas, although the distinction is not always clear. AVMs are associated with arteriovenous shunting and histologically are characterized by a proliferation of heterogeneous vascular elements including arteries, dysplastic arteries, veins, and arterialized veins. Hemangiomas, on the other hand, are more homogeneous histologically, do not cause significant arteriovenous shunting, and are more likely peripheral lesions. Either proliferation, AVMs, or hemangiomas may be associated with syndromes, especially when multiple.

A third type of vascular lesion, the telangiectasia, is probably not a proliferation of vessels per se but a collection of thin-walled capillaries and venules with a propensity for dilatation. Telangiectasias, while in the collapsed state, are often difficult to identify pathologically. Similar to true AVMs and hemangiomas, they may form part of a syndrome of vascular malformations.

The pathogenesis and true nature of many types of benign vascular lesions is yet unknown. Vascular malformations are diagnosed differently by clinicians, radiologists, and pathologists. Although a precise classification using histologic criteria has been adopted for many vascular tumors, it can be difficult to adapt the classification from one organ system to another. The clinical relevance of the subclassification of vascular tumors is still uncertain for some organs, although the value of precise diagnosis is becoming more evident with currently available imaging techniques and the identification of clinical syndromes.

Arteriovenous Malformation

AVMs represent abnormal vascular communications between arteries and veins that occur without an intervening capillary bed and that result in the formation of a mass. These malformations are also referred to as arteriovenous fistulas, arteriovenous hemangiomas, arteriovenous aneurysms, and racemose or cirsoid aneurysms.

Arteriovenous Malformations of the Central Nervous System, Head, and Neck

Although AVMs are described in almost every organ of the body, approximately 50% are located in the head and neck region, including the CNS.[110-117] Congenital AVMs are often multiple and have a female predominance. Occasionally, there may be familial AVMs in the absence of a defined syndrome.[118] AVMs of the CNS may result in seizures or subarachnoid hemorrhage, and are treated with a combination of surgery, radiosurgery, embolization, and radiation.[118,119] When the malformation results in vein of Galen steal, treatment consists of coil embolization.[120] An associated venous malformation may be within the brain.[121] Presenting symptoms of oral and maxilla AVMs vary but include soft tissue swelling, pain, changes in skin and mucosal color, erythematous and bleeding gingiva, bruit, and paresthesias. The radiologic appearance is not pathognomonic. AVMs of the cranial bones can cause bleeding after dental surgery and are also treated with embolization.[122] Some are thought to be hamartomas[122] and can be associated with other vascular anomalies such as persistent trigeminal artery.[123] Treatment of osseous AVMs of the head and neck include direct transosseous injection of cyanoacrylate.

Arteriovenous Malformations of the Lung

Pulmonary AVMs were first described at autopsy in the nineteenth century, but the first clinical diagnosis based on the triad of cyanosis, clubbing, and polycythemia was made in 1939.[124] Pulmonary AVM causes a shunt of venous blood from the pulmonary arteries to the pulmonary veins, thus decreasing arterial oxygen saturation. Although most patients are asymptomatic, pulmonary AVMs can cause dyspnea from right-to-left shunt. Because of paradoxic emboli, various CNS complications including stroke and brain abscess have been described. A strong association between pulmonary AVMs and hereditary hemorrhagic telangiectasia (HHT) exists. Up to 36% of patients with solitary pulmonary AVMs and 60% of patients with multiple pulmonary AVMs have associated HHT, which is described later.[125,126] Chest radiography and contrast-enhanced CT are essential initial diagnostic tools, but pulmonary angiography is the gold standard by which to establish the presence of shunting. Contrast echocardiography is useful for diagnosis and monitoring after treatment. Most patients should be treated. Therapeutic options include angiographic embolization with metal coil or balloon occlusion and surgical excision.[127] Occasionally a pulmonary AVM receives blood from a systemic artery in addition to a pulmonary artery.[128] Pulmonary AVMs may be single or multiple, small or large enough to involve an entire lung. These can be associated with cerebral AVMs in patients with HHT.[129] They may present during pregnancy with hemoptysis, often heralding HHT, and treatment with embolization is indicated if the patient is symptomatic.[121]

Cyanosis is present since childhood and occasionally since birth. Neurologic symptoms may be due to brain abscesses resulting from a loss of the filtering function of the lung.[130] Decrease in arterial oxygen saturation occurs with pulmonary AVM, and pulmonary angiography demonstrates the malformation with early filling of the left atrium.

The frequency of fatal complications is significant in pulmonary AVM.[125] These include rupture, hemorrhage, endocarditis, and brain abscess. Surgery is indicated with segmental resection whenever possible to preserve the maximum amount of lung tissue, but lobectomy may be necessary.[130]

Arteriovenous Malformations of Other Sites

Other locations for AVMs are the gastrointestinal tract, heart, liver, and kidney. Those of the gastrointestinal tract typically present with bleeding or mucosal ulceration.[131] They may occur anywhere in the gastrointestinal tract, and endoscopically are raised lesions that may show nonspecific histologic alterations.[132] Those of the kidney and pelvis may present with various symptoms and are initially treated with embolization.[133] Multiplicity and early age at onset are signs that the lesion may be part of a syndrome, especially Klippel-Trénaunay syndrome (KTS) or HHT. The physical findings in AVM are closely related to the location and size of the lesion. Patients may present with swelling, pain, or hemorrhage. If located near the skin, the lesion is often a pulsatile mass with a thrill or bruit. There may be erythema or cyanosis distal to the lesion. Cutaneous or mucosal AVMs may ulcerate and bleed, or there may be thrombosis or cellulitis, or both, superficially. Hypertrophy of an extremity can occur if a large shunt is present. Cardiomegaly in infancy is occasionally due to an unsuspected AVM, and large aneurysms, particularly in the brain or liver, may cause neonatal heart failure. CNS AVM may present as repeated episodes of intracranial hemorrhage or as seizure disorders secondary to gliosis or atrophy of the adjacent cortex.

Angiographically, the lesions have multiple anomalous arterial branches and anastomoses with early filling of the venous system. Vessels are dilated, elongated, and tortuous. MRI is also capable of differentiating AVMs from other types of hemangiomas in the CNS, as well as the skin and subcutaneous tissue.[110] AVMs may be present at birth, become apparent soon after birth, or be asymptomatic until adulthood.[113] Unlike capillary hemangiomas in infants, AVMs do not regress but grow with the growth of the child. A specialized form of AVM that occurs in the gastric mucosa is Dieulafoy's disease, making the patient prone to massive upper gastrointestinal hemorrhage. Indications for the treatment of AVM include congestive heart failure, cosmetic deformity, hemorrhage, or ulceration. Coil embolization of hepatic AVMs may improve heart failure, although there is risk of hepatic damage.[134] Other complications of embolization therapy include stroke,[116] skin sloughing, and blindness.[111] The treatment of AVM is tailored to the particular location and size of the lesion. Various therapeutic modalities have been used to treat AVM including radiation, surgery, and embolization techniques. Surgical treatment of AVM involves resection. Isolated ligation of the vessel is not curative, as collateral circulation can reestablish flow to the lesion.[111,116]

AVM can recur if not completely excised.[115] The morbidity of surgery relates to hemorrhage, disseminated intravascular coagulation, and cosmetic deformity.[115] Various materials have been used for embolization including autologous materials such as fat or muscle, hemostatic agents such as gelatin sponges or polyvinyl alcohol, and methyl methacrylate or silicon spheres. More recently, coils and balloons have been used. The amount of shunting and the diameter of shunts determine the size of the embolization particles.

Venous Hemangiomas

Unlike AVMs, vascular malformations composed entirely of veins do not show significant enhancement by radiographic procedures.[134] The imaging characteristics, especially those of MRI, are otherwise similar to those of hemangiomas. Typically, there is a focus of attachment to muscle in those occurring in deep sites. Venous hemangiomas have been reported in various sites including the mediastinum, mesentery, skeletal muscle, and retroperitoneum.[135-140] The cavernous hemangiomas of the blue rubber bleb nevus syndrome are sometimes predominantly venous (see later).

Pathology

The pathologic diagnosis of AVM rests on the presence of communicating arteries and veins in a vascular lesion. In the larger AVM, the gross appearance of the specimen is one of multiple blood-filled spaces, often aneurysmally dilated. Smaller AVMs removed for pathologic examination may require extensive sectioning to demonstrate the lesion, and ultimately the diagnosis may rest on radiological correlation. Microscopically, AVM is marked by the presence of arteries and veins with little intervening tissue. The direct communication between an artery and a vein may be difficult to locate. Vessels are often elongated and dilated, and the structure of the vessel walls in AVM is usually abnormal. Artery walls are thinned or may be hypertrophied, with disruption and loss of elastic lamina and medial smooth muscle. The medial smooth muscle may also form nodules projecting into the vessel lumen. Vein walls become thickened or arterialized with the acquisition of internal elastic lamina. Rarely, the malformation may be composed entirely of veins, representing the so-called *venous hemangioma.* Elastic stains can be helpful, but it is not always possible in AVM to classify a vessel as an artery or a vein.

Cardiac Hemangiomas/Arteriovenous Malformations

Vascular malformations within the heart include coronary artery fistulas (see coronary artery anomalies) and cardiac hemangiomas. Hemangiomas involving the myocardium are a diverse group of lesions that represent either hamartomatous malformations or, less likely, benign neoplasms. The histologic classification includes those composed of multiple dilated thin-walled vessels (cavernous type), smaller vessels resembling capillaries (capillary type), and dysplastic malformed arteries and veins (arteriovenous hemangioma, cirsoid aneurysm). Cardiac hemangiomas often have combined features of cavernous, capillary, and arteriovenous hemangiomas, and many contain fibrous tissue and fat. These features are reminiscent of intramuscular hemangiomas of skeletal muscle.

Intramuscular cardiac hemangioma has a superficial resemblance to AVM, with the presence of heterogeneous vessel types including muscularized arteries, veins, and capillaries. In contrast to capillary hemangioma, they are infiltrative lesions and occur within the myocardium. They are histologically identical to intramuscular hemangiomas within skeletal muscle and may possess, in addition to the vessels, fat and fibrous tissue. Because of the latter features, some intramuscular cardiac hemangiomas are misclassified as lipomas or fibrolipomas.

Most cardiac hemangiomas are discovered incidentally, but patients may present with dyspnea on exertion, arrhythmias, right-sided heart failure, pericarditis, pericardial effusion, and failure to thrive.[141] Patients may have associated vascular syndromes (e.g., Kasabach-Merritt).

Whereas chest roentgenograms are abnormal in the majority of cases, the diagnosis of a cardiac tumor is rarely made on the basis of plain radiographs alone. A characteristic tumor blush on coronary arteriography suggests the diagnosis of a cardiac hemangioma.[142] Echocardiography usually directs the diagnosis toward a cardiac mass. Enhanced-contrast CT scan or MRI establishes the diagnosis of hypervascularized cardiac tumor.

The most frequent locations are the lateral wall of the left ventricle (21%), the anterior wall of the right ventricle (21%), the interventricular septum (17%), and occasionally the right ventricular outflow tract.[143]

Cardiac hemangiomas are often large, and gross appearance depends on the size of the vascular spaces in the tumor. The capillary type is frequently slightly raised from the endocardial surface and appears red to purple. Intramuscular types appear infiltrative. Cavernous hemangiomas are usually large and are also poorly circumscribed.

Capillary/Cavernous Hemangiomas

Capillary hemangiomas are composed of nodules of small capillary-size vessels, each of which is subserved by a "feeder" vessel. This lobular or grouped arrangement of vessels is helpful for distinguishing these benign from malignant vascular proliferations. Mast cells and factor XIII-positive interstitial cells are a consistent feature. *Cavernous hemangiomas* are composed of large dilated vascular spaces. When in the heart, they tend to infiltrate the myocardium. The lining cells are bland and flattened and mitotically inactive, in contrast to angiosarcoma.

Capillary hemangiomas of the retina are associated with the von Hippel-Lindau (VHL) disease. The incidence of VHL disease is approximately 1 in 40,000 live births. The inheritance of VHL disease is autosomal dominant with high penetrance. Retinal capillary hemangioma may be managed by observation, laser photocoagulation, cryotherapy, and plaque radiotherapy. Typical extraocular lesions associated with VHL disease are CNS hemangioma, renal cyst, renal carcinoma, pancreatic cysts and adenoma, pancreatic islet cell tumors, pheochromocytoma, endolymphatic sac tumor of the inner ear, and cystadenoma of the epididymis and the broad ligament.[144] The disease is caused by germline alterations of the VHL gene, which has been cloned recently and identified as a tumor suppressor gene. Histologic features of VHL tumors are characterized by their high degree of vascularization and the presence of a clear cell component. Hypervascularization is induced by overexpression of vascular endothelial growth factor (VEGF).[145]

Another syndrome associated with hemangiomas is the blue rubber bleb nevus syndrome (BRBNS), a developmental disorder originally identified by the presence of distinctive cutaneous blue nevi, especially of the tongue, lips, and neck, and gastrointestinal hemangiomas, with a predominance for the small bowel.[146] More recently, CNS vascular malformations including venous anomalies have been associated with BRBNS.[147,148] Colonoscopy with laser photocoagulation is a noninvasive method of controlling bleeding from colonic hemangiomas, although surgical resection may be necessary to control chronic gastrointestinal blood loss.[149] Histologically, the lesions are typically classified as cavernous hemangiomas,[150] sometimes with a capillary component,[151] although the gastrointestinal lesions often have a predominantly venous component.[152] Virtually all other internal organs including the orbit[153] have been reported as involved in BRBNS, as well as multiple cutaneous sites. There is often a diffuse, mild consumptive coagulopathy.[154]

Telangiectasias

Telangiectasias are localized dilatations of capillaries and venules that are presumed congenital and may form part of an inherited syndrome. Unlike hemangiomas, there is no proliferation of vessels, but rather an idiopathic dilatation of preexisting capillaries and venules. However, the term "hemangioma" has often been used, especially clinically, for these lesions. Most forms of telangiectasias are present in the skin, but internal organs including the brain can be affected. There are generally few or no symptoms attributable to the telangiectasia itself, other than cosmetic problems when it involves the skin or hemorrhagic complications of gastrointestinal hemangiomas. Incidental telangiectasias of the brain are found predominantly in the pons and have only rarely been reported to cause symptoms by bleeding.

Cutaneous Telangiectasias

The most common congenital cutaneous telangiectasia is the nevus flammeus, or ordinary birthmark. Nevus flammeus appears as a mottled macular lesion on the head and neck and usually regresses. The port-wine stain is a specialized form of nevus flammeus that demonstrates no tendency to fade and often becomes elevated, reminiscent of a true hemangioma. Unlike true hemangiomas, telangiectasias appear histologically as congested, normal vessels that are separated by intervening tissue. Indeed, in most cases there is no detectable histopathologic abnormality after processing the tissue for examination.

At least three syndromes are associated with port-wine stains. The Sturge-Weber syndrome is characterized by telangiectasias of the face in the distribution of the trigeminal nerve and ipsilateral vascular malformations of the leptomeninges or retina. Patients afflicted with the full-blown syndrome suffer from seizures, hemiplegia, and mental retardation. KTS (see later) is characterized by port-wine stains of an extremity, usually one leg. The affected leg is hypertrophied, there are severe venous varicosities, and deep veins of phlebography are often absent. A subset of patients with KTS have associated AVMs. Because of the difference in clinical symptoms, the term *Parkes Weber syndrome* is usually applied for these individuals, who may suffer from congestive heart failure.

Hereditary Hemorrhagic Telangiectasia

HHT, or Osler-Weber-Rendu disease, is a disorder characterized by multiple skin and mucosal telangiectasias and pulmonary AVMs. HHT is an autosomal dominant disorder characterized by vascular dysplasia and hemorrhage. A small number of cases is sporadic. The types of vascular malformations seen in patients with HHT are diverse. Underlying the disorder are defects in the genes that code for endoglin and ALK-1, which are TGF-β receptors expressed exclusively on vascular endothelial cells and are involved in angiogenesis.[155] A large number of mutations has been found underlying the syndrome in different families including missense, nonsense, frameshift, and deletion mutations. The disease affects the sexes equally. HHT shows great genetic heterogeneity, and its phenotypes have been classified on the basis of the recently identified mutated genes: endoglin (HHT-1) and activin-like kinase receptor-1 (HHT-2).

HHT affects 1 in 5000 to 8000 individuals and typically manifests as anemia, frequent gastrointestinal and nasal bleeding, and characteristic mucocutaneous telangiectasias. The vascular lesions seen in HHT include AVMs and telangiectasias. The AVMs most commonly involve the pulmonary and cerebral circulations. AVMs may cause serious complications when they are located in the lungs, liver, or brain.[156] The age at presentation is variable, and patients may become symptomatic initially in late adulthood.[157] Idiopathic pulmonary arterial hypertension can occur in a subset of patients with HHT (≈10%).[158]

Telangiectasias are found in the skin or mucosal surfaces of the gastrointestinal, respiratory, and urinary tracts. Nosebleeds and gastrointestinal and urinary tract bleeding are common clinical manifestations. Vascular lesions may also be present in other organs such as liver and brain, where they are usually incidental autopsy findings. Liver involvement is reported in up to 30% of persons affected by HHT. Large AVMs in the liver can lead to significant complications including high-output congestive heart failure, portal hypertension, hepatic encephalopathy, biliary ischemia, and liver failure. Embolization of large AVMs in the liver remains controversial; however, liver transplantation can successfully eradicate these complications.[159] Patients with HHT may present with hepatomegaly or neurologic symptoms. CNS emboli and abscesses may result from paradoxic emboli.[160] The hemorrhagic tendency in patients with HHT appears to increase with age. HHT is strongly associated with pulmonary AVM. In a review of 350 cases of pulmonary AVM, 36% of patients with solitary AVM and 57% of patients with multiple AVMs had HHT.[128] In a review of 91 members of a family with HHT, 15% had pulmonary AVM.[126]

Other Telangiectasia Syndromes

Ataxia telangiectasia is an autosomal dominant inherited disease that is characterized by cerebellar degeneration, immunodeficiency, oculocutaneous telangiectasia, cancer risk, and radiosensitivity. The vascular manifestations are heralded by appearance in childhood of telangiectasias of the bulbar conjunctivae and skin of the face and extremities.[161] The vascular lesions are preceded by ataxia, which occurs in infancy. Ocular telangiectasias often do not appear until several years after the ataxia. The patients generally succumb to an underlying immunological abnormality that results in recurrent infections and the development of lymphoproliferative disorders. The most common type of malignancy is lymphoma, usually of the B-cell type. Leukemias also occur.[162]

Histologic examination of the telangiectasias demonstrates the presence of dilated subpapillary venous channels. The syndrome is generally not associated with vascular malformations.

Currently, the genetic basis is believed related to mutations in the ataxia telangiectasia (ATM) gene. Since the cloning of ATM in 1995,[163] more than 100 ATM mutations occurring in patients with ataxia telangiectasia have been documented. The mutations are broadly distributed throughout the ATM gene.[164] The product of the ATM gene is a 350 kDa protein ATM involved in DNA damage recognition and cell cycle control in response to ionizing radiation damage. Evidence indicates that the ATM gene may also have a more general signaling role.[165] Affected homozygotes are at increased risk for a wide range of malignancies; however, the elevated risk of malignancy is not observed among heterozygotes with ataxia telangiectasia, with the possible exception of breast carcinoma.[166]

Generalized essential telangiectasia is another localized form of telangiectasia that is generally not associated with vascular malformations or significant gastrointestinal hemorrhage, but rather recurrent cutaneous telangiectasis.[167] Another form of telangiectasia that can result in gastrointestinal bleeding is watermelon stomach, or gastric antral vascular ectasia. Watermelon stomach has been increasingly recognized as an important cause of occult gastrointestinal blood loss and anemia. The histological hallmark of watermelon stomach is superficial capillary ectasia of gastric antral mucosa and microvascular thrombosis in the lamina propria. Endoscopic findings of the longitudinal antral folds containing visible columns of tortuous red ectatic vessels (watermelon stripes) are pathognomonic.[168] Watermelon stomach is usually isolated but has been reported in patients with autoimmune diseases, especially scleroderma.[169-171] The precise nature of the vascular defects is unclear, as underlying fibromuscular dysplasia of the gastric arteries has been suggested as a cause for the superficial lesions.[168]

Klippel-Trénaunay Syndrome

KTS is a rare anomaly characterized by cutaneous hemangiomas (nevus flammeus or port-wine stain), soft tissue hypertrophy, and varicosities. Unlike HHT, there is no known underlying defect or specific inheritance pattern; indeed, the condition may be heterogeneous. KTS shows familial clustering, but a clear mode of inheritance has not been established. Autosomal predominant and dominant modes of inheritance have been proposed. Translocations have been identified in two patients with Klippel-Trénaunay-Weber syndrome, t(5;11)(q13.3;p15.1) and t(8;14)(q22.3;q13), but specific gene defects remain to be identified.[172,173] Cutaneous hemangiomas (nevus flammeus) of varying extent and irregular contour are often present in the hypertrophic regions. Associated deep venous system abnormalities have been reported.[174] The association of three physical findings including capillary malformation, varicosities, and hypertrophy of bony and soft tissues was initially described by the two French physicians Klippel and Trénaunay in 1900. KTS differs from Parkes Weber syndrome in that KTS does not incorporate significant hemodynamic arteriovenous fistulas. In a large review of 136 female and 116 male patients with KTS, capillary malformations (port-wine stains) were found in 246 patients (98%), varicosities or venous malformations in 182 (72%), and limb hypertrophy in 170 (67%). All three features of KTS were present in 159 patients (63%), and 93 (37%) had two of the three features. Atypical veins, including lateral veins and persistent sciatic veins, occurred in 182 patients (72%).

Deep vascular malformations may occur in internal viscera, including the gastrointestinal tract (Fig. 65-11), deep soft tissues, other viscera, and bones.[175,176] The clearest indication for operation is a leg-length discrepancy projected to exceed 2 cm at skeletal maturity. Removal of symptomatic varicosities or localized superficial venous malformations in selected patients can yield good results.[177] Skin ulcerations lead to persisting and recurrent bleeding, and persistent hematochezia,

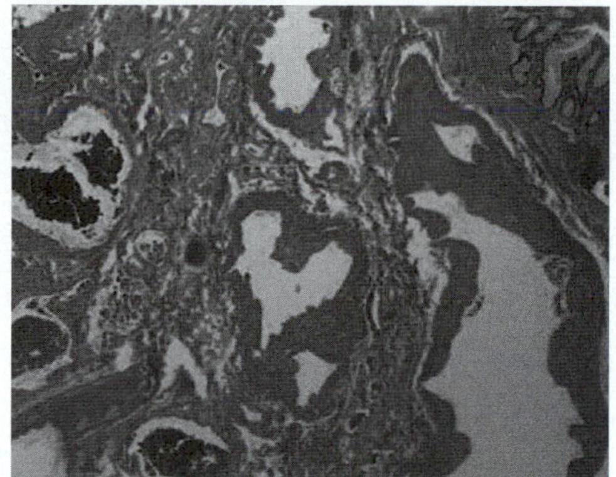

A

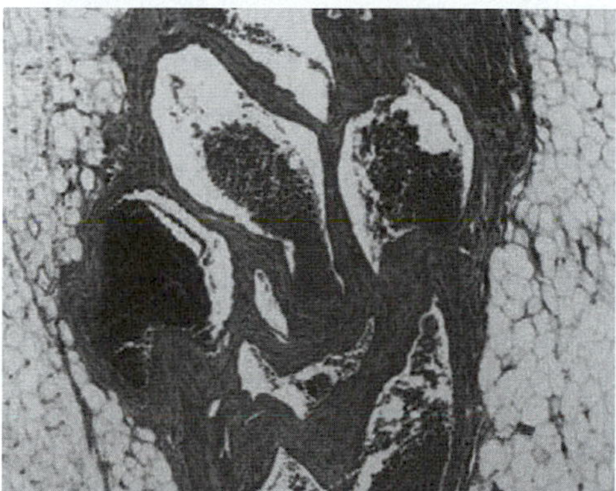

B

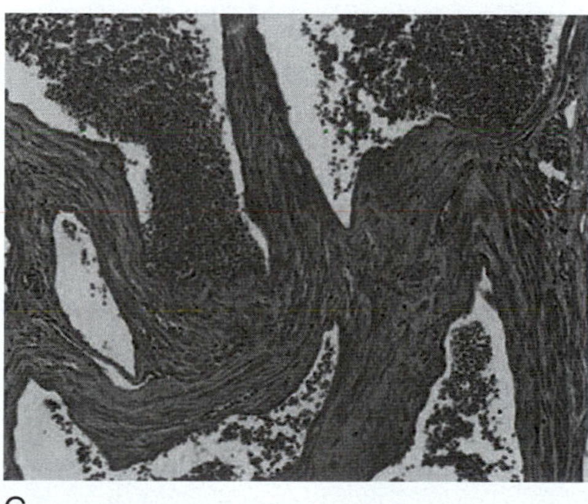

C

FIGURE 65-11. Histologic section of a vascular malformation in the rectosigmoid colon of a 35-year-old patient with known Klippel-Trénaunay syndrome. **A,** A lower magnification demonstrates bowel mucosa (*upper right*) with a vascular malformation filling the submucosa. There is a mixture of thick-walled arteries and veins. **B,** A higher magnification demonstrates an area suggestive of cavernous hemangioma. **C,** The cavernous area shows blood-filled spaces lined by a barely perceptible endothelial cell lining; the nature of the abnormal vessels (venous vs. arterial) cannot be determined on the basis of the lack of developed media.

hematuria, and vaginal and esophageal bleeding may be the result of mucosal vascular malformations.[178] The genitourinary features of KTS have been recently reviewed.[179] The typical oral manifestations of KTS are hemifacial hypertrophy and premature eruption of teeth.[180] The prevalence of cerebral hemihypertrophy in a series of patients with KTS was 18%. When present, cerebral hemihypertrophy was associated with hypertrophy of the leg and a cutaneous hemangioma on the same side as the brain abnormality. Cerebral KTS is not associated with intracranial vascular malformation, unilateral megalencephaly, cerebral atrophy, or hydrocephalus.[181]

FIBROMUSCULAR DYSPLASIA

Fibromuscular dysplasia (FMD) is a generic term for a group of structural abnormalities of one or more layers of medium-sized and large arteries that result in luminal narrowing by fibrous, smooth muscle or fibromuscular tissue with or without associated aneurysms and dissections of the media. Fibromuscular dysplasia is an uncommon angiopathy that occurs in young to middle-aged, predominantly female individuals. The disease consists of a heterogeneous group of histologic changes, which ultimately lead to arterial narrowing. Clinical manifestations reflect the arterial bed involved, most commonly hypertension (renal) and stroke (carotid). Fibromuscular dysplasia is a pathologic diagnosis, but the characteristic changes seen on an angiogram can be used to make the diagnosis in the appropriate clinical setting.

This noninflammatory disease is a common mimic of vasculitis.[182] The process is usually due to congenital malformation of the arterial structure, affecting young Caucasian women and involving most commonly the renal and carotid arteries. Classification is based on the histopathologic localization and pattern of the structural abnormalities, which affects the angiographic appearance. Most often, the initial manifestations are hypertension, stroke, and abdominal pain, depending on the vascular bed involved. The most common lesions become symptomatic as a high-grade stenosis producing renovascular hypertension or as an embolic source for the cerebral circulation. Treatment is reserved for symptomatic lesions. Most simple lesions are effectively treated by catheter-based intervention. Surgical therapy is warranted for more complex lesions. Both produce durable, long-term results.[183]

Although the causes of FMD remain obscure, they may include estrogen exposure, mechanical factors, ischemic factors, environmental toxins such as cigarette smoke, and autoantibodies. There is no doubt an underlying genetic predisposition to the development of FMD. Whites are much more likely to develop FMD than blacks, and many cases are familial, with an autosomal dominant transmission with variable penetrance.

The histologic classification of renal FMD is generally based on the layer of vessel involved. Although this classification is well established in the literature, we, as well as others,[184] have not always found this classification useful and reproducible. A simplified classification, based on the presence of smooth muscle hyperplasia, has been proposed.[184]

Fibromuscular Dysplasia of Renal Arteries

FMD of the renal arteries is a common condition that accounts for approximately 25% of cases of renovascular hypertension and about 2% of all cases of hypertension. It is estimated that about 5% of the overall hypertensive population have renovascular hypertension. Whereas most renovascular lesions are caused by atherosclerosis, stenosis due to fibrous dysplasia is an important disease. In children and young adults, fibromuscular dysplasia of the renal arteries is the most common cause of renovascular hypertension.[185] The renal arteries are by far the most common site of symptomatic FMD, accounting for about 75% of cases. Multivessel FMD, which involves renal as well as other arteries, occurs in approximately 25% of patients with renal FMD.

The potential of FMD involving transplant kidneys and affecting the remaining donor kidney has led to the routine use of digital subtraction and MRA in potential kidney donors.[186-189]

Although the cause of FMD of the renal arteries is unknown, there is an association with the HLA-DRw6 antigen. In one series of patients, this HLA antigen was more common in the 33 fibromuscular dysplasia patients than in the 61 renal transplant donor control subjects (odds ratio = 2.5, P = .03).[190]

Histologic Subtypes

The histologic classification of renal FMD has been established based on the layer of vessel involved (Fig. 65-12).[191] The value of this classification has been questioned.[184] These authors have suggested a simplified classification based on the presence of smooth muscle hyperplasia, which imparts a better prognosis. Classically, FMD has been divided into medial (Fig. 65-13), intimal (Fig. 65-14), and adventitial types (Fig. 65-15). Medial FMD accounts for up to 95% of cases and has been further subdivided into medial fibroplasia, perimedial fibroplasia, and medial hyperplasia.[192] Intimal fibroplasia, medial fibroplasia, and perimedial hyperplasia impart the typical "beading" appearance on angiography.

Medial fibroplasia is characterized by fibromuscular ridges of hyperplastic smooth muscle cells and fibrous tissue, which project into the lumen of the affected artery. Perimedial hyperplasia implies a predominance of fibrous tissue, and the proliferation is primarily in the outer layer of the media. Pure medial hypertrophy is rare and represents a concentric hypertrophy of the medial wall, which is relatively smooth, lacking fibrosis, and causing severe stenosis. Angiographically and grossly, the stenosis is usually subtotal, sometimes tubular and smooth. Intimal hyperplasia, which represents less than 5% of lesions, is characterized by proliferation of fibrous tissue, including smooth muscle cells, within the intima.

There is no lipid deposition or inflammatory cell infiltrate, and the internal elastic lamina is preserved. Endarteritis secondary to inflammatory conditions or trauma may be associated with intimal fibroplasia in muscular arteries that may mimic the histologic picture of intimal fibroplasias. The morphologic appearance may be virtually indistinguishable from that of secondary or reactive intimal fibroplasia seen after endarterectomy or in the initial proliferative stage of atherosclerosis. Intimal fibroplasia may also occur concomitantly with medial fibromuscular dysplasia. In adventitial or periarterial fibroplasia, the primary lesion is a dense collagenous replacement of the loose fibrous tissue of the arterial adventitia. This fibrosis may extend into the surrounding adipose and connective tissues. The media and intima are normal.

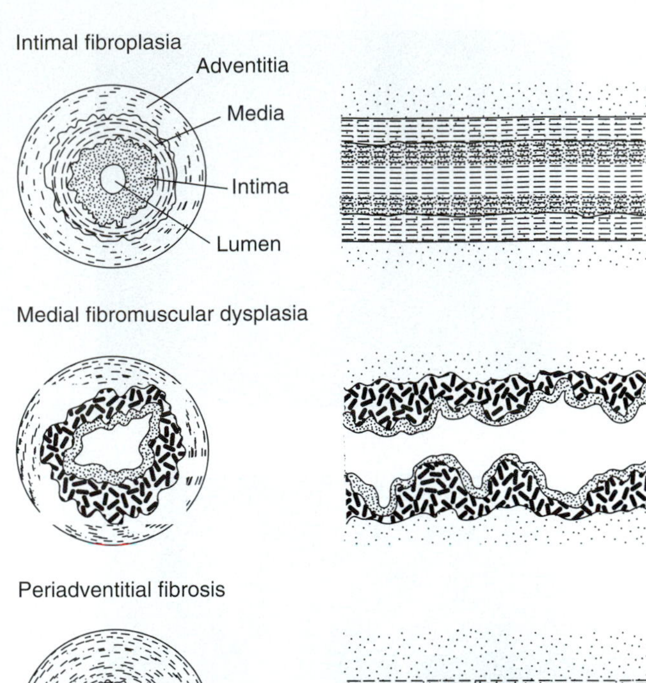

FIGURE 65-12. Schematic showing transverse and longitudinal patterns of involvement of the arteries by the major types of fibromuscular dysplasia. (Modified from Harrison EG Jr, McCormack LJ: Pathologic classification of renal arterial disease in renovascular hypertension. Mayo Clin Proc 46:161, 1971 and Luscher TF, Lie JT, Stanson AW, et al: Arterial fibromuscular dysplasia. Mayo Clin Proc 62:931, 1987.)

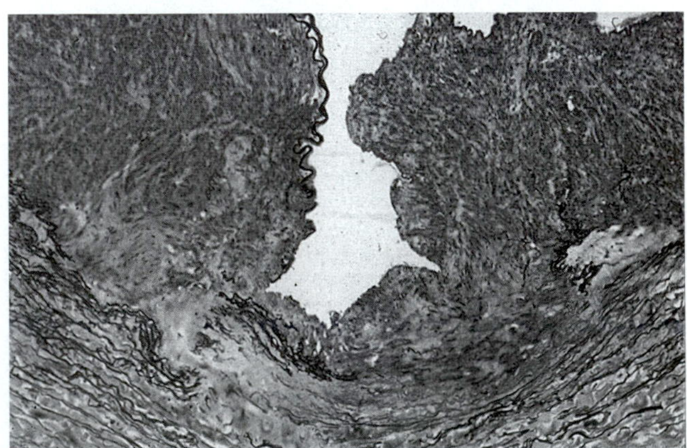

FIGURE 65-13. Arterial dysplasia, medial type. A high magnification demonstrates a gap in the arterial media. A succession of such defects results in the string-of-beads appearance on angiogram. (From Virmani R, Burke AP, Farb A: Arterial dysplasia, aneurysms, and dissections. In Virmani R, Burke AP, Farb A [eds]: Atlas of Cardiovascular Pathology. Philadelphia, WB Saunders, 1996, p 184.)

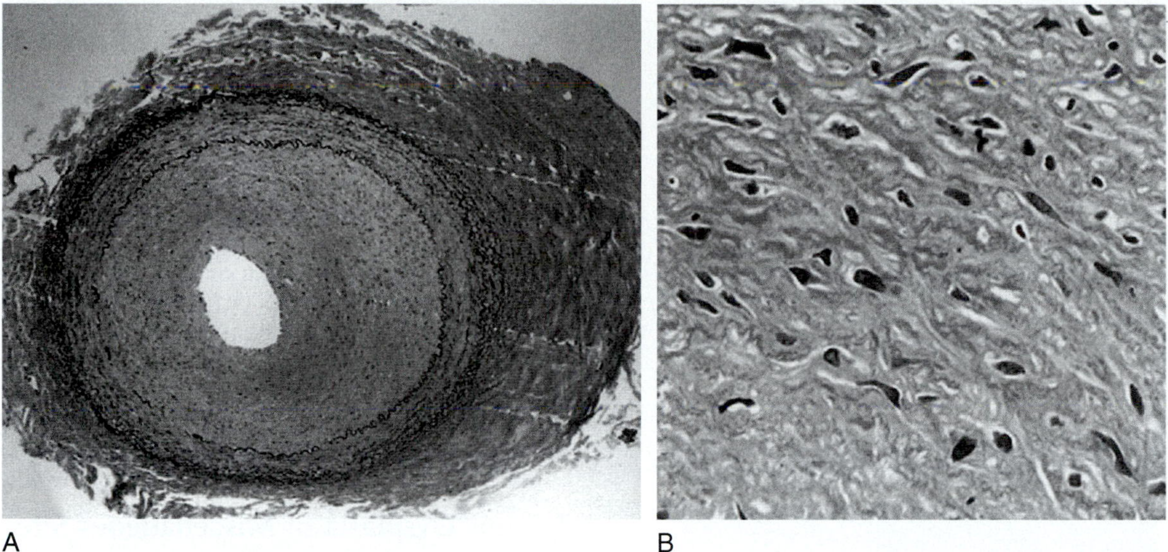

FIGURE 65-14. Fibromuscular dysplasia, primarily intimal. A 55-year-old woman underwent coronary artery bypass graft surgery. Her internal mammary artery (demonstrated histologically) was grossly cordlike, as were other arteries in the mediastinum. **A,** A low magnification shows the marked concentric thickening of the intima, with a relatively normal media. There is also a degree of adventitial scarring. **B,** A higher magnification of the intima shows smooth muscle cells within a proteoglycan matrix.

Patients with renal FMD are often young women. The diagnosis of FMD is usually made on investigation for unexplained hypertension. The right renal artery is more often involved than the left, and cases of bilateral involvement are often associated with extrarenal FMD. The distal two thirds of the artery is typically involved, with frequent extension into the branch arteries. Helical CT angiography, especially the combination of transverse sections and maximum-intensity-projection reconstructions, can reliably reveal renal artery fibromuscular dysplasia.[193] Complications of arterial occlusion and renal infarction may result from arterial dissection, embolization originating in the aneurysm, and aneurysmal thrombosis. Treatment includes medical management of hypertension; surgical vascular reconstruction; percutaneous transluminal angioplasty; and, in cases refractory to treatment, nephrectomy. Although the restenosis rate is as high as in nonostial atherosclerotic lesions of the renal vessels, there remains a considerable higher therapeutic effect.[194] Stents are also used.[195,196] Progression of disease is the rule without mechanical or surgical intervention, although rare cases may reverse with medical treatment.[197]

In a large recent series of 104 unrelated hypertensive patients (94 women) with renal artery fibromuscular dysplasia, 81 had multifocal, 16 had unifocal, and 7 had both types of stenosis. Fifty-four patients had bilateral FMD. The documented prevalence of familial cases was 11% in this series; familial cases all exhibited the multifocal type and were more commonly bilateral.[198]

Fibromuscular Dysplasia of Aortic Arch Vessels

FMD has been described involving the carotid, subclavian, and vertebral arteries.[197,199,200] The internal carotid artery is typically involved at the level of C-1 and C-2 and is usually "typical" medial FMD resulting in a classic string-of-beads angiographic appearance. Heterozygous α_1-antitrypsin deficiency may be a genetic risk factor for the development of FMD of the internal carotid artery.[201] Fibromuscular dysplasia is a rare cause of cerebral ischemia; however, FMD of the internal carotid artery is typically diagnosed after symptoms such as transient ischemic attacks, amaurosis fugax, minor stroke, or nonfocalized ischemic cerebral symptoms. FMD of the arch vessels is increasingly being found incidentally. Surgical intervention in symptomatic cases includes endoluminal graduated dilatation, with rigid dilators up to 4.5 mm, thromboendarterectomy of the bifurcation, venous interposition graft, and venous patching.[202]

Patients with cerebrovascular FMD have a high incidence of berry aneurysms of the circle of Willis, especially the intracranial internal carotid artery and the middle cerebral artery. Aneurysms in these locations are relatively likely to be found in females with other vascular lesions such as FMD or other aneurysms. In contrast, aneurysms of the anterior cerebral artery are more likely sporadic and found in men. The prevalence of intracranial aneurysms in patients with cervical internal carotid artery or vertebral artery (VA) FMD, or both, is approximately 7%, which is not nearly as high as the 21% to 51% prevalence that has been previously reported.[203]

Subclavian and vertebral FMD is less likely to have a characteristic angiographic appearance and has been termed, on the basis of radiologic findings, as "atypical" FMD. FMD involving more distal branches of the aortic arch such as the brachial artery is unusual.[204]

Cerebrovascular FMD and FMD of the subclavian arteries are often asymptomatic and may be an incidental angiographic finding. The overall incidence of this disease, and therefore the proportion of cases that are asymptomatic, are unknown. Symptoms occur if there is stenosis of major cephalic arteries, embolization from thrombosed areas of FMD, and severe narrowing of the

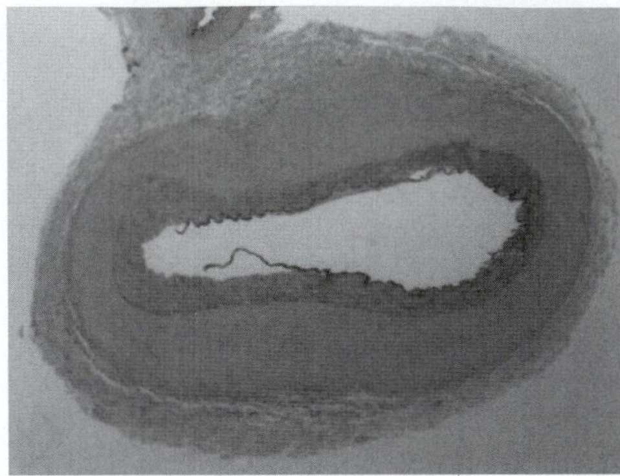

A

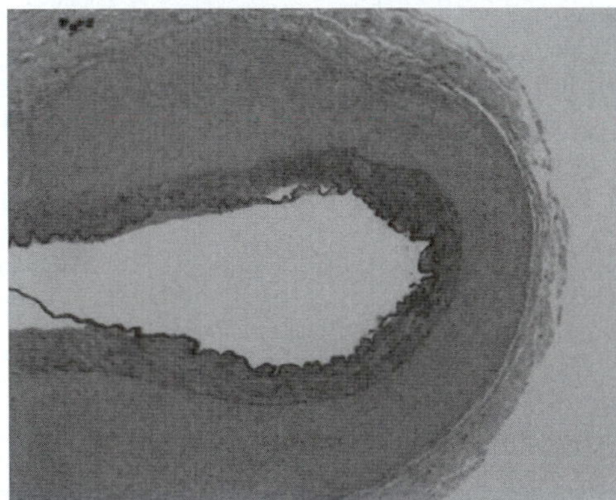

B

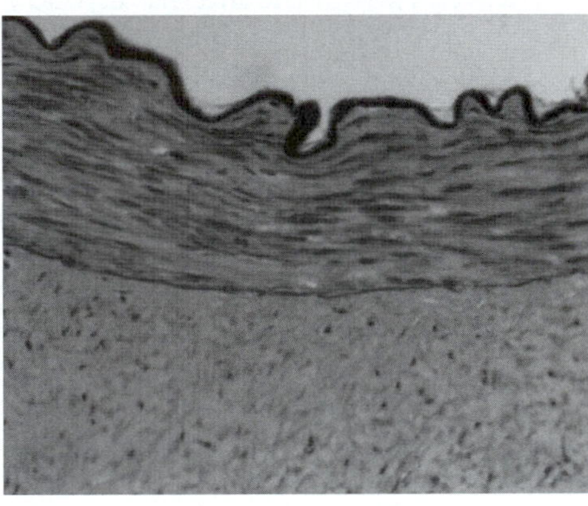

C

FIGURE 65-15. Fibromuscular dysplasia, primarily adventitial. **A,** Low magnification of an artery with normal media and intima but a markedly thickening adventitia. **B,** The adventitial scarring is seen at intermediate magnification. **C,** Normal internal elastic lamina, relatively normal media, and cellular adventitia.

subclavian artery. Symptoms include transient ischemic attacks, strokes, and subarachnoid hemorrhage from associated berry aneurysms of the circle of Willis, the subclavian steal syndrome, and weakness or claudication of the arms. Complications of cerebrovascular FMD include arterial dissections and carotid-cavernous fistulas. FMD of the cerebrovascular circulation and subclavian arteries appears to be more often multifocal and bilateral than isolated renovascular FMD. Patients with subclavian FMD often have systemic FMD, including FMD of the renal arteries.[205]

The natural history of cerebrovascular and subclavian FMD is relatively benign. Patients with ischemic cerebral symptoms and involvement of multiple vessels, however, have a poor prognosis. Treatment of cerebrovascular and subclavian FMD includes percutaneous transluminal angioplasty, graduated intraluminal dilation, surgical resection with end-to-end anastomosis or interposition graft, or bypass grafts. Antiplatelet drugs and other anticoagulants are alternative medical therapies for patients with symptomatic FMD with or without dissections.

Trauma may precipitate dissections in patients with aortic arch dysplasia, especially of the vertebral artery, which may lead to fatal subarachnoid hemorrhages.[206] The dissections may be spontaneous or fatal.[207] They may be treated with a multidisciplinary approach including coils, stents, and surgery.[208]

Fibrous Dysplasia of Miscellaneous Sites

FMD has been described in the visceral arteries[209-211]; iliac,[212] axillary, brachial, and coronary arteries; and aorta.[213] Typical arteries involved in FMD of the visceral arteries are the celiac artery, mesenteric arteries, hepatic artery,[214] and splenic artery. These are often found in association with renal arterial FMD.[211,215] Segmental arterial mediolysis, a rare form of mesenteric arteriopathy that typically results in spontaneous dissections and hemoperitoneum in hypertensive patients, may be a form of mesenteric arterial dysplasia. Symptoms related to stenotic lesions of the visceral arteries are rare due to well-developed collateral vessels. FMD of miscellaneous arteries are prone to similar complications of renal FMD and FMD of the aortic arch, including dissection and embolization.

REFERENCES

1. Burroughs JT, Edwards JE: Total anomalous pulmonary venous connection. Am Heart J 59:913, 1960.
2. Ruggieri M, Abbate M, Parano E, et al: Scimitar vein anomaly with multiple cardiac malformations, craniofacial, and central nervous system abnormalities in a brother and sister: Familial scimitar anomaly or new syndrome? Am J Med Genet 116A:170, 2003.
3. Gelb BD: Molecular genetics of congenital heart disease. Curr Opin Cardiol 12:321, 1997.
4. Darling RC, Rothney WB, Criaig JM: Total pulmonary venous drainage into the right side of the heart: Report of 17 autopsied cases not associated with other major cardiovascular anomalies. Lab Invest 6:44, 1957.
5. Allan LD, Sharland GK: The echocardiographic diagnosis of totally anomalous pulmonary venous connection in the fetus. Heart 85:433, 2001.
6. Elliott LP, Edwards JE: The problem of pulmonary venous obstruction in total anomalous pulmonary venous connection to the left innominate vein. Circulation 25:913, 1962.
7. Brown VE, De Lange M, Dyar DA, et al: Echocardiographic spectrum of supracardiac total anomalous pulmonary venous connection. J Am Soc Echocardiogr 11:289, 1998.
8. Jenkins KJ, Sanders SP, Orav EJ, et al: Individual pulmonary vein size and survival in infants with totally anomalous pulmonary venous connection. J Am Coll Cardiol 22:201, 1993.
9. Rubino M, Van Praagh S, Kadoba K, et al: Systemic and pulmonary venous connections in visceral heterotaxy with asplenia: Diagnostic and surgical considerations based on seventy-two autopsied cases. J Thorac Cardiovasc Surg 110:641, 1995.

10. Masui T, Seelos KC, Kersting-Sommerhoff BA, et al: Abnormalities of the pulmonary veins: Evaluation with MR imaging and comparison with cardiac angiography and echocardiography. Radiology 181:645, 1991.
11. Bando K, Turrentine MW, Ensing GJ, et al: Surgical management of total anomalous pulmonary venous connection: Thirty-year trends. Circulation 94:II12, 1996.
12. Boger AJ, Baak R, Lee PC, et al: Early results and long-term follow-up after corrective surgery for total anomalous pulmonary venous return. Eur J Cardiothorac Surg 16:296, 1999.
13. Raisher BD, Grant JW, Martin TC, et al: Complete repair of total anomalous pulmonary venous connection in infancy. J Thorac Cardiovasc Surg 104:443, 1992.
14. Michielon G, Di Donato RM, Pasquini L, et al: Total anomalous pulmonary venous connection: Long-term appraisal with evolving technical solutions. Eur J Cardiothorac Surg 22:184, 2002.
15. Hyde JA, Stumper O, Barth MJ, et al: Total anomalous pulmonary venous connection: Outcome of surgical correction and management of recurrent venous obstruction. Eur J Cardiothorac Surg 15:735, 1999.
16. Korbmacher B, Buttgen S, Schulte HD, et al: Long-term results after repair of total anomalous pulmonary venous connection. Thorac Cardiovasc Surg 49:101, 2001.
17. Bhan A, Umre MA, Choudhary SK, et al: Cardiac arrhythmias in surgically repaired total anomalous pulmonary venous connection: A follow-up study. Indian Heart J 52:427, 2000.
18. Serraf A, Belli E, Roux D, et al: Modified superior approach for repair of supracardiac and mixed total anomalous pulmonary venous drainage. Ann Thorac Surg 65:1391, 1998.
19. Hijii T, Fukushige J, Hara T: Diagnosis and management of partial anomalous pulmonary venous connection: A review of 28 pediatric cases. Cardiology 89:148, 1998.
20. AboulHosn JA, Criley JM, Stringer WW: Partial anomalous pulmonary venous return: Case report and review of the literature. Catheter Cardiovasc Interv 58:548, 2003.
21. Al-Ahmari S, Chandrasekaran K, Brilakas E, et al: Isolated partial anomalous pulmonary venous connection: Diagnostic value of suprasternal color flow imaging and contrast echocardiography. J Am Soc Echocardiogr 16:884, 2003.
22. Baron O, Roussel JC, Videcoq M, et al: Partial anomalous pulmonary venous connection: Correction by intra-atrial baffle and cavo-atrial anastomosis. J Card Surg 17:166, 2002.
23. Gustafson RA, Warden HE, Murray GF: Partial anomalous pulmonary venous connection to the superior vena cava. Ann Thorac Surg 60:S614, 1995.
24. Idris MT: Diagnostic aid of transesophageal echocardiography in an adult case of scimitar syndrome: Confirmation of the findings at surgery and review of the literature. J Am Soc Echocardiogr 11:387, 1998.
25. Henk CB, Prokesch R, Grampp S, et al: Scimitar syndrome: MR assessment of hemodynamic significance. J Comput Assist Tomogr 21:628, 1997.
26. Haramati LB, Moche IE, Rivera VT, et al: Computed tomography of partial anomalous pulmonary venous connection in adults. J Comput Assist Tomogr 27:743, 2003.
27. Perry LW, Scott LP III. Cor triatriatum: Clinical and pathophysiological features. Clin Proc Child Hosp Dist Columbia 23:294, 1967.
28. Herlong JR, Jaggers JJ, Ungerleider RM: Congenital Heart Surgery Nomenclature and Database Project: Pulmonary venous anomalies. Ann Thorac Surg 69:S56, 2000.
29. Buchholz S, Jenni R: Doppler echocardiographic findings in 2 identical variants of a rare cardiac anomaly, "subtotal" cor triatriatum: A critical review of the literature. J Am Soc Echocardiogr 14:846, 2001.
30. Tueche S: Cor triatriatum dextrum: Surgical treatment in a neonate. Acta Cardiol 58:39, 2003.
31. Huang TC, Lee CL, Lin CC, et al: Use of Inoue balloon dilatation method for treatment of cor triatriatum stenosis in a child. Catheter Cardiovasc Interv 57:252, 2002.
32. Shuler CO, Fyfe DA, Sade R, et al: Transesophageal echocardiographic evaluation of cor triatriatum in children. Am Heart J 129:507, 1995.
33. Chen Q, Guhathakurta S, Vadalapali G, et al: Cor triatriatum in adults: Three new cases and a brief review. Tex Heart Inst J 26:206, 1999.
34. Jeong JW, Tei C, Chang KS, et al: A case of cor triatriatum in an eighty-year-old man: Transesophageal echocardiographic observation of multiple defects. J Am Soc Echocardiogr 10:185, 1997.
35. Slight RD, Nzewi OC, Sivaprakasam R, et al: Cor triatriatum sinister presenting in the adult as mitral stenosis. Heart 89:e26, 2003.
36. Rorie M, Xie GY, Miles H, et al: Diagnosis and surgical correction of cor triatriatum in an adult: Combined use of transesophageal echocardiography and catheterization. Catheter Cardiovasc Interv 51:83, 2000.
37. Goel AK, Saxena A, Kothari SS: Atrioventricular septal defect with cor triatriatum: Case report and review of the literature. Pediatr Cardiol 19:243, 1998.
38. Nakajima H, Kobayashi J, Kurita T, et al: Maze procedure and cor triatriatum repair. Ann Thorac Surg 74:251, 2002.
39. Ito M, Kikuchi S, Hachiro Y, et al: Congenital pulmonary vein stenosis associated with cor triatriatum. Ann Thorac Surg 71:722, 2001.
40. Endo M, Yamaki S, Ohmi M, et al: Pulmonary vascular changes induced by congenital obstruction of pulmonary venous return. Ann Thorac Surg 69:193, 2000.
41. Victor S, Nayak VM: Deringing procedure for congenital pulmonary vein stenosis. Tex Heart Inst J 22:166, 1995.
42. Omasa M, Hasegawa S, Bando T, et al: A case of congenital pulmonary vein stenosis in an adult. Respiration 71:92, 2004.
43. Spray TL, Bridges ND: Surgical management of congenital and acquired pulmonary vein stenosis. Semin Thorac Cardiovasc Surg Pediatr Card Surg Annu 2:177, 1999.
44. Yee ES, Turley K, Hsieh WR, et al: Infant total anomalous pulmonary venous connection: Factors influencing timing of presentation and operative outcome. Circulation 76:III83, 1987.
45. Lincoln CR, Rigby ML, Mercanti C, et al: Surgical risk factors in total anomalous pulmonary venous connection. Am J Cardiol 61:608, 1988.
46. Roldan FJ, Vargas-Barron J, Espinola-Zavaleta N, et al: Cor triatriatum dexter: Transesophageal echocardiographic diagnosis and 3-dimensional reconstruction. J Am Soc Echocardiogr 14:634, 2001.
47. Dobbertin A, Warnes CA, Seward JB: Cor triatriatum dexter in an adult diagnosed by transesophageal echocardiography: A case report. J Am Soc Echocardiogr 8:952, 1995.
48. Taylor AJ, Rogan KM, Virmani R: Sudden cardiac death associated with isolated congenital coronary artery anomalies. J Am Coll Cardiol 20:640, 1992.
49. Yamanaka O, Hobbs RE: Coronary artery anomalies in 126,595 patients undergoing coronary arteriography. Cathet Cardiovasc Diagn 21:28, 1990.
50. Zeppilli P, dello RA, Santini C, et al: In vivo detection of coronary artery anomalies in asymptomatic athletes by echocardiographic screening. Chest 114:89, 1998.
51. Frescura C, Basso C, Thiene G, et al: Anomalous origin of coronary arteries and risk of sudden death: A study based on an autopsy population of congenital heart disease. Hum Pathol 29:689, 1998.
52. Edwards JE: Anomalous pulmonary venous connections. In Gould SE (ed): Pathology of the Heart and Blood Vessels, 3rd ed. Springfield, Ill, Thomas, 1968.
53. Edwards JE: Pathology of left ventricular outflow tract obstruction. Circulation 31:586, 1965.
54. Christenson NA: Coarctation of the aorta: Historical review. Proc Staff Meet Mayo Clin 23:322, 1948.
55. Moller JH, Amplatz K, Edwards JE: Congenital heart disease. Kalamazoo, Mich., Upjohn, 1974, p 46.
56. Gersony WM: Coarctation of the aorta. In Adams FH, Emmanouilides GC (eds): Heart Disease in Infants, Children and Adolescents. Baltimore, Williams & Wilkins, 1989, p 243.
57. Kirklin JW, Barratt-Boyes BG: Coarctation of the aorta and interrupted aortic arch. In Cardiac Surgery. New York, Wiley, 1993, p 1263.
58. Bonnett LM: Sur la lesion dite stenose congenitale de l'aorte dans la region de l'isthme. Rev de Med 23:108, 1903.
59. Abbot ME: Coarctation of the aorta of the adult type II: A statistical study and historical retrospect of 200 recorded cases with autopsy of stenosis or obliteration of the descending aorta in subjects over the age of two years. Am Heart J 3:574, 1928.
60. Reifenstein GH, Levine SA, Gross RE: Coarctation of the aorta: A review of 104 autopsied cases of the "adult type," 2 years of age or older. Am Heart J 33:146, 1947.
61. Calodney MM, Carson MJ: Coarctation of the aorta in early infancy. J Pediat 1:41, 1950.

62. Gross RE: Coarctation of the aorta. Circulation 7:757, 1953.
63. Fyler DC, Rothman KJ, Buckley LP, et al: The determinants of five year survival of infants with critical congenital heart disease. Cardiovasc Clin 11:393, 1981.
64. Edwards JE: Anomalous pulmonary venous connection. In Gould SE (ed): Pathology of the Heart and Blood Vessels. Springfield, Ill, Thomas, 1968, p 455.
65. Campbell M, Polani PE: The aetiology of coarctation of the aorta. Lancet 1:463, 1961.
66. Pellegrino A, Deverall PB, Anderson RH, et al: Aortic coarctation in the first three months of life: An anatomopathological study with respect to treatment. J Thorac Cardiovasc Surg 89:121, 1985.
67. Shinebourne EA, Elseed AM: Relation between fetal flow patterns, coarctation of the aorta, and pulmonary blood flow. Br Heart J 36:492, 1974.
68. Rudolph AM, Heymann MA, Spitznas U: Hemodynamic considerations in the development of narrowing of the aorta. Am J Cardiol 30:514, 1972.
69. Ho SY, Anderson RH: Coarctation, tubular hypoplasia, and the ductus arteriosus. Histological study of 35 specimens. Br Heart J 41:268, 1979.
70. Becker AE, Becker MJ, Edwards JE: Anomalies associated with coarctation of aorta: Particular reference to infancy. Circulation 41:1067, 1970.
71. Olney MB, Stephens HB: Coarctation of the aorta in children: Observations in fourteen cases. J Pediat 37:192, 1950.
72. Bahn RC, Edwards JE, DuShane JW: Coarctation of the aorta in children: Observations in fourteen cases. Pediatrics 8:192, 1951.
73. Edwards JE: Pathologic considerations in coarctation of the aorta. Proc Staff Meet Mayo Clin 23:324, 1948.
74. Brickner ME, Hillis LD, Lange RA: Congenital heart disease in adults: Second of two parts. N Engl J Med 342:334, 2000.
75. Tawes RL Jr, Berry CL, Aberdeen E: Congenital bicuspid aortic valves associated with coarctation of the aorta in children. Br Heart J 31:127, 1969.
76. Liberthson RR, Pennington DG, Jacobs ML, et al: Coarctation of the aorta: Review of 234 patients and clarification of management problems. Am J Cardiol 43:835, 1979.
77. Lucas RV, Krabill RA: Anomalous venous connections, pulmonary and systemic. In Adams FH, Emmanouilides GC (eds): Heart Disease in Infants, Children, and Adolescents. Baltimore, Williams & Wilkins, 1989, p 580.
78. Congdon ED: Transformation of the aortic arch system during the development of the human embryo. Contrib Embryol 14:47, 1922.
79. Gross RE: Surgical relief for tracheal obstruction from a vascular ring. N Engl J Med 233:586, 1945.
80. Wolman LJ: Syndrome of constricting double aortic arch in infancy: Report of a case. J Pediat 14:527, 1939.
81. Creazzo TL, Godt RE, Leatherbury L, et al: Role of cardiac neural crest cells in cardiovascular development. Annu Rev Physiol 60:267, 1998.
82. Edwards JE: Anomalies of the derivatives of the aortic arch system. Med Clin N Am 6:925, 1948.
83. Srivastava D, Olson EN: A genetic blueprint for cardiac development. Nature 407:221, 2000.
84. Conway SJ, Kruzynska-Frejtag A, Kneer PL, et al: What cardiovascular defect does my prenatal mouse mutant have, and why? Genesis 35:1, 2003.
85. Iida K, Koseki H, Kakinuma H, et al: Essential roles of the winged helix transcription factor MFH-1 in aortic arch patterning and skeletogenesis. Development 124:4627, 1997.
86. Kirklin JW, Baratt-Boyes BG: Vascular rings and slings. In Cardiac Surgery. New York, Wiley, 1986, p 1111.
87. Stewart JR, Kincaid OW, Edwards JE: Atlas of Vascular Rings and Related Malformations of the Aortic Arch System. Springfield, Ill., Thomas, 1964.
88. Sissman NJ: Anomalies of the aortic arch complex. In Adams FH, Emmanouilides GC (eds): Heart Disease in Infants, Children, and Adolescents. Baltimore, Williams & Wilkins, 1983, p 199.
89. Kocis KC, Midgley FM, Ruckman RN: Aortic arch complex anomalies: 20-year experience with symptoms, diagnosis, associated cardiac defects, and surgical repair. Pediatr Cardiol 18:127, 1997.
90. Woods RK, Sharp RJ, Holcomb GW III, et al: Vascular anomalies and tracheoesophageal compression: A single institution's 25-year experience. Ann Thorac Surg 72:434, 2001.
91. Moes CA, Freedom RM: Rare types of aortic arch anomalies. Pediatr Cardiol 14:93, 1993.
92. Gil-Jaurena JM, Murtra M, Goncalves A, et al: Aortic coarctation, vascular ring, and right aortic arch with aberrant subclavian artery. Ann Thorac Surg 73:1640, 2002.
93. Taussig HB: Congenital Malformations of the Heart, 2nd ed, vol 2. Cambridge, Mass., Harvard University Press, 1960.
94. Lincoln JC, Deverall PB, Stark J, et al: Vascular anomalies compressing the oesophagus and trachea. Thorax 24:295, 1969.
95. Binet JP, Conso JF, Losay J, et al: Ductus arteriosus sling: Report of a newly recognised anomaly and its surgical correction. Thorax 33:72, 1978.
96. Messner G, Reul GJ, Flamm SD, et al: Interrupted aortic arch in an adult single-stage extra-anatomic repair. Tex Heart Inst J 29:118, 2002.
97. Bankl H: Congenital Malformations of the Heart and Great Vessels. Synopsis of Pathology, Embryology, and Natural History. Munich: Urban & Schwarzenberg, 1977, p 176.
98. Backer CL: Vascular rings, slings, and tracheal rings. Mayo Clin Proc 68:1131, 1993.
99. Kirklin JW, Baratt-Boyes BG: Origin of the right or left pulmonary artery from the ascending aorta. In: Cardiac Surgery. New York, Wiley, 1993, p 1159.
100. Keane JF, Maltz D, Bernhard WF, et al: Anomalous origin of one pulmonary artery from the ascending aorta: Diagnostic, physiological and surgical considerations. Circulation 50:588, 1974.
101. Calder AL, Brandt PW, Barratt-Boyes BG, et al: Variant of tetralogy of Fallot with absent pulmonary valve leaflets and origin of one pulmonary artery from the ascending aorta. Am J Cardiol 46:106, 1980.
102. Penkoske PA, Castaneda AR, Fyler DC, et al: Origin of pulmonary artery branch from ascending aorta: Primary surgical repair in infancy. J Thorac Cardiovasc Surg 85:537, 1983.
103. Becker AE, Anderson RH: Malformations of the pulmonary trunk and arteries. In: Pathology of Congenital Heart Disease. London, Butterworths, 1981, p 339.
104. Beitzke A, Shinebourne EA: Single origin of right and left pulmonary arteries from ascending aorta, with main pulmonary artery from right ventricle. Br Heart J 43:363, 1980.
105. Becker AE, Anderson RH: Aortopulmonary communications. In: Pathology of Congenital Heart Disease. London, Butterworths, 1981, p 345.
106. Kirklin JW, Baratt-Boyes BG: Aortopulmonary window. In: Cardiac Surgery. New York, Wiley, 1993, p 1153.
107. Neufeld HN, Lester RG, Adams P Jr, et al: Aorticopulmonary septal defect. Am J Cardiol 9:12, 1962.
108. Luisi SV, Ashraf MH, Gula G, et al: Anomalous origin of the right coronary artery with aortopulmonary window: Functional and surgical considerations. Thorax 35:446, 1980.
109. Blieden LC, Moller JH: Aorticopulmonary septal defect: An experience with 17 patients. Br Heart J 36:630, 1974.
110. Awad IA, Robinson JR, Mohanty S, et al: Mixed vascular malformations of the brain: Clinical and pathogenetic considerations. Neurosurgery 33:179, 1993.
111. Coleman CC: Diagnosis and treatment of congenital arteriovenous fistulas of the head and neck. Am J Surg 126:424, 1973.
112. Finn MC, Celowack J, Mulliken JB: Congenital vascular lesions: Clinical application of a new classification. J Pediatr Surg 1983; 18:894.
113. Garcia-Gonzalez R, Gonzalez-Palacios J, Maganto-Pavon E: Congenital renal arteriovenous fistula (cirsoid aneurysm). Urology 24:495, 1984.
114. Jellinger K: Vascular malformations of the central nervous system: A morphologic overview. Neurosurg Rev 9:177, 1986.
115. Trout HH III, McAllister HA Jr, Giordano JM, et al: Vascular malformations. Surgery 97:36, 1985.
116. Trout HH: Management of patients with hemangiomas and arteriovenous malformations. Surg Clin N Am 66:333, 1986.
117. Watson WL, McCarthy WD: Blood and lymph vessel tumors: A report of 1,056 cases. Surg Gynecol Obstet 71:569, 1940.
118. Herzig R, Burval S, Vladyka V, et al: Familial occurrence of cerebral arteriovenous malformation in sisters: Case report and review of the literature. Eur J Neurol 7:95, 2000.
119. Irie K, Nagao S, Honma Y, et al: Treatment of arteriovenous malformation of the brain: Preliminary experience. J Clin Neurosci 7:24, 2000.
120. Brunelle F: Arteriovenous malformation of the vein of Galen in children. Pediatr Radiol 27:501, 1997.

121. Yanaka K, Hyodo A, Nose T: Venous malformation serving as the draining vein of an adjoining arteriovenous malformation: Case report and review of the literature. Surg Neurol 56:170, 2001.
122. Kacker A, Heier L, Jones J: Large intraosseous arteriovenous malformation of the maxilla: A case report with review of literature. Int J Pediatr Otorhinolaryngol 52:89, 2000.
123. Nakai Y, Yasuda S, Hyodo A, et al: Infratentorial arteriovenous malformation associated with persistent primitive trigeminal artery: Case report. Neurol Med Chir (Tokyo) 40:572, 2000.
124. Smith HL, Horton BT: Arteriovenous fistula of the lung associated with polycythemia vera: Report of a case in which the diagnosis was made clinically. Am Heart J 18:589, 1939.
125. Burke CM, Safai C, Nelson DP, et al: Pulmonary arteriovenous malformations: A critical update. Am Rev Respir Dis 134:334, 1986.
126. Hodgson C: Hereditary hemorrhagic telangiectasia and pulmonary arteriovenous fistula: Survey of a large family. N Engl J Med 26: 625, 1959.
127. Khurshid I, Downie GH: Pulmonary arteriovenous malformation. Postgrad Med J 78:191, 2002.
128. Bosher LH, Blake A, Byrd BR: An analysis of the pathologic anatomy of pulmonary arteriovenous aneurysms with particular reference to the applicability of local excision. Surgery 45:91, 1959.
129. Tripathy U, Kaul S, Bhosle K, et al: Pulmonary arteriovenous fistula with cerebral arteriovenous malformation without hereditary hemorrhagic telangiectasia: Unusual case report and literature review. J Cardiovasc Surg (Torino) 38:677, 1997.
130. Chow LT, Chow WH, Ma KF: Pulmomary arteriovenous malformation: Progressive enlargement with replacement of the entire right middle lobe in a patient with concomitant mitral stenosis. Med J Aust 158:632, 1993.
131. Aida K, Nakamura H, Kihara Y, et al: Duodenal ulcer and pancreatitis associated with pancreatic arteriovenous malformation. Eur J Gastroenterol Hepatol 14:551, 2002.
132. Hayakawa H, Kusagawa M, Takahashi H, et al: Arteriovenous malformation of the rectum: Report of a case. Surg Today 28:1182, 1998.
133. Game X, Berlizot P, Hassan T, et al: Congenital pelvic arteriovenous malformation in male patients: A rare cause of urological symptoms and role of embolization. Eur Urol 42:407, 2002.
134. Hisamatsu K, Ueeda M, Ando M, et al: Peripheral arterial coil embolization for hepatic arteriovenous malformation in Osler-Weber-Rendu disease; useful for controlling high output heart failure, but harmful to the liver. Intern Med 38:962, 1999.
135. Abe K, Akata S, Ohkubo Y, et al: Venous hemangioma of the mediastinum. Eur Radiol 11:73, 2001.
136. Igarashi J, Hanazaki K: Retroperitoneal venous hemangioma. Am J Gastroenterol 93:2292, 1998.
137. Ichikawa MM, Ishida-Yamamoto A, Hashimoto Y, et al: Venous hemangioma: An immunohistochemical and ultrastructural study. Acta Derm Venereol 77:382, 1997.
138. Itosaka H, Tada M, Sawamura Y, et al: Vanishing tumor of the temporalis muscle: Repeated hemorrhage in an intramuscular venous hemangioma. AJNR Am J Neuroradiol 18:983, 1997.
139. Tada M, Sawamura Y, Abe H, et al: Venous hemangioma of the temporalis muscle. Neurol Med Chir (Tokyo) 36:23, 1996.
140. Hanatate F, Mizuno Y, Murakami T: Venous hemangioma of the mesoappendix: Report of a case and a brief review of the Japanese literature. Surg Today 25:962, 1995.
141. Kojima S, Sumiyoshi M, Suwa S, et al: Cardiac hemangioma: A report of two cases and review of the literature. Heart Vessels 18:153, 2003.
142. Grebenc ML, Rosado de Christenson ML, Burke AP, et al: Primary cardiac and pericardial neoplasms: Radiologic-pathologic correlation. Radiographics 20:1073, 2000.
143. Burke A, Johns JP, Virmani R: Hemangiomas of the heart: A clinicopathologic study of ten cases. Am J Cardiovasc Pathol 3:283, 1990.
144. Singh AD, Shields CL, Shields JA: von Hippel-Lindau disease. Surv Ophthalmol 46:117, 2001.
145. Sano T, Horiguchi H: von Hippel-Lindau disease. Microsc Res Tech 60:159, 2003.
146. Bedocs PM, Gould JW: Blue rubber-bleb nevus syndrome: A case report. Cutis 71:315, 2003.
147. Gabikian P, Clatterbuck RE, Gailloud P, et al: Developmental venous anomalies and sinus pericranii in the blue rubber-bleb nevus syndrome. Case report. J Neurosurg 99:409, 2003.
148. Eiris-Punal J, Picon-Cotos M, Viso-Lorenzo A, et al: Epileptic disorder as the first neurologic manifestation of blue rubber bleb nevus syndrome. J Child Neurol 17:219, 2002.
149. Morris L, Lynch PM, Gleason WA Jr, et al: Blue rubber bleb nevus syndrome: Laser photocoagulation of colonic hemangiomas in a child with microcytic anemia. Pediatr Dermatol 9:91, 1992.
150. Oranje AP: Blue rubber bleb nevus syndrome. Pediatr Dermatol 3:304, 1986.
151. Ishii T, Asuwa N, Suzuki S, et al: Blue rubber bleb naevus syndrome. Virchows Arch A Pathol Anat Histopathol 413:485, 1988.
152. Ertem D, Acar Y, Kotiloglu E, et al: Blue rubber bleb nevus syndrome. Pediatrics 107:418, 2001.
153. McCannel CA, Hoenig J, Umlas J, et al: Orbital lesions in the blue rubber bleb nevus syndrome. Ophthalmology 103:933, 1996.
154. Rodrigues D, Bourroul ML, Ferrer AP, et al: Blue rubber bleb nevus syndrome. Rev Hosp Clin Fac Med Sao Paulo 55:29, 2000.
155. Azuma H: Genetic and molecular pathogenesis of hereditary hemorrhagic telangiectasia. J Med Invest 47:81, 2000.
156. Haitjema T, Westermann CJ, Overtoom TT, et al: Hereditary hemorrhagic telangiectasia (Osler-Weber-Rendu disease): New insights in pathogenesis, complications, and treatment. Arch Intern Med 156:714, 1996.
157. Begbie ME, Wallace GM, Shovlin CL: Hereditary haemorrhagic telangiectasia (Osler-Weber-Rendu syndrome): A view from the 21st century. Postgrad Med J 79:18, 2003.
158. Newman JH, Trembath RC, Morse JA, et al: Genetic basis of pulmonary arterial hypertension: Current understanding and future directions. J Am Coll Cardiol 43:33S, 2004.
159. Larson AM: Liver disease in hereditary hemorrhagic telangiectasia. J Clin Gastroenterol 36:149, 2003.
160. Dong SL, Reynolds SF, Steiner IP: Brain abscess in patients with hereditary hemorrhagic telangiectasia: Case report and literature review. J Emerg Med 20:247, 2001.
161. Woods CG, Taylor AM: Ataxia telangiectasia in the British Isles: The clinical and laboratory features of 70 affected individuals. Q J Med 82:169, 1992.
162. Gatti RA: Ataxia-telangiectasia. Dermatol Clin 13:1, 1995.
163. Uhrhammer N, Bay JO, Bignon YJ: Seventh International Workshop on Ataxia-Telangiectasia. Cancer Res 58:3480, 1998.
164. Concannon P, Gatti RA: Diversity of ATM gene mutations detected in patients with ataxia-telangiectasia. Hum Mutat 10:100, 1997.
165. Lavin MF, Khanna KK: ATM: The protein encoded by the gene mutated in the radiosensitive syndrome ataxia-telangiectasia. Int J Radiat Biol 75:1201, 1999.
166. Yuille MA, Coignet LJ: The ataxia telangiectasia gene in familial and sporadic cancer. Recent Results Cancer Res 154:156, 1998.
167. Checketts SR, Burton PS, Bjorkman DJ, et al: Generalized essential telangiectasia in the presence of gastrointestinal bleeding. J Am Acad Dermatol 37:321, 1997.
168. Novitsky YW, Kercher KW, Czerniach DR, et al: Watermelon stomach: Pathophysiology, diagnosis, and management. J Gastrointest Surg 7:652, 2003.
169. Elkayam O, Oumanski M, Yaron M, et al: Watermelon stomach following and preceding systemic sclerosis. Semin Arthritis Rheum 30:127, 2000.
170. Watson M, Hally RJ, McCue PA, et al: Gastric antral vascular ectasia (watermelon stomach) in patients with systemic sclerosis. Arthritis Rheum 39:341, 1996.
171. Goel A, Christian CL: Gastric antral vascular ectasia (watermelon stomach) in a patient with Sjogren's syndrome. J Rheumatol 30:1090, 2003.
172. Wang Q, Timur AA, Szafranski P, et al: Identification and molecular characterization of de novo translocation t(8;14)(q22.3;q13) associated with a vascular and tissue overgrowth syndrome. Cytogenet Cell Genet 95:183, 2001.
173. Whelan AJ, Watson MS, Porter FD, et al: Klippel-Trénaunay-Weber syndrome associated with a 5:11 balanced translocation. Am J Med Genet 59:492, 1995.
174. Dogan R, Faruk Dogan O, Oc M, et al: A rare vascular malformation, Klippel-Trénaunay syndrome: Report of a case with deep vein agenesis and review of the literature. J Cardiovasc Surg (Torino) 44:95, 2003.

175. Arguedas MR, Shore G, Wilcox CM: Congenital vascular lesions of the gastrointestinal tract: Blue rubber bleb nevus and Klippel-Trénaunay syndromes. South Med J 94:405, 2001.
176. Wilson CL, Song LM, Chua H, et al: Bleeding from cavernous angiomatosis of the rectum in Klippel-Trénaunay syndrome: Report of three cases and literature review. Am J Gastroenterol 96:2783, 2001.
177. Jacob AG, Driscoll DJ, Shaughnessy WJ, et al: Klippel-Trénaunay syndrome: Spectrum and management. Mayo Clin Proc 73:28, 1998.
178. Capraro PA, Fisher J, Hammond DC, et al: Klippel-Trénaunay syndrome. Plast Reconstr Surg 109:2052, 2002.
179. Furness PD III, Barqawi AZ, Bisignani G, et al: Klippel-Trénaunay syndrome: 2 case reports and a review of genitourinary manifestations. J Urol 166:1418, 2001.
180. Mueller-Lessmann V, Behrendt A, Wetzel WE, et al: Orofacial findings in the Klippel-Trénaunay syndrome. Int J Paediatr Dent 11:225, 2001.
181. Torregrosa A, Marti-Bonmati L, Higueras V, et al: Klippel-Trénaunay syndrome: Frequency of cerebral and cerebellar hemihypertrophy on MRI. Neuroradiology 42:420, 2000.
182. Begelman SM, Olin JW: Fibromuscular dysplasia. Curr Opin Rheumatol 12:41, 2000.
183. Curry TK, Messina LM: Fibromuscular dysplasia: When is intervention warranted? Semin Vasc Surg 16:190, 2003.
184. Alimi Y, Mercier C, Pellissier JF, et al: Fibromuscular disease of the renal artery: A new histopathologic classification. Ann Vasc Surg 6:220, 1992.
185. Fenves AZ, Ram CV: Fibromuscular dysplasia of the renal arteries. Curr Hypertens Rep 1:546, 1999.
186. Andreoni KA, Weeks SM, Gerber DA, et al: Incidence of donor renal fibromuscular dysplasia: Does it justify routine angiography? Transplantation 73:1112, 2002.
187. Indudhara R, Kenney, Bueschen AJ, et al: Live donor nephrectomy in patients with fibromuscular dysplasia of the renal arteries. J Urol 162:678, 1999.
188. Williams ME, Shaffer D: ACE inhibitor-induced transplant acute renal failure due to donor fibromuscular dysplasia. Nephrol Dial Transplant 14:760, 1999.
189. Wolters HH, Vowinkel T, Schult M, et al: Fibromuscular dysplasia in a living donor: Early post-operative allograft artery stenosis with successful venous interposition. Nephrol Dial Transplant 17:153, 2002.
190. Sang CN, Whelton PK, Hamper UM, et al: Etiologic factors in renovascular fibromuscular dysplasia. A case-control study. Hypertension 14:472, 1989.
191. Harrison EG, McCormack LJ: Pathologic classification of renal arterial disease in renovascular hypertension. Mayo Clin Proc 46:161, 1971.
192. Hata J, Hosoda Y: Perimedial fibroplasia of the renal artery. Arch Pathol Lab Med 103:220, 1979.
193. Beregi JP, Louvegny S, Gautier C, et al: Fibromuscular dysplasia of the renal arteries: Comparison of helical CT angiography and arteriography. AJR Am J Roentgenol 172:27, 1999.
194. Birrer M, Do DD, Mahler F, et al: Treatment of renal artery fibromuscular dysplasia with balloon angioplasty: A prospective follow-up study. Eur J Vasc Endovasc Surg 23:146, 2002.
195. Bisschops RH, Popma JJ, Meyerovitz MF: Treatment of fibromuscular dysplasia and renal artery aneurysm with use of a stent-graft. J Vasc Interv Radiol 12:757, 2001.
196. Damaraju S, Krajcer Z: Successful Wallstent implantation for extensive iatrogenic renal artery dissection in a patient with fibromuscular dysplasia. J Endovasc Surg 6:297, 1999.
197. Luschner TF, Lie JT, Stanson AW, et al: Arterial fibromuscular dysplasia. Mayo Clin Proc 62:931, 1987.
198. Pannier-Moreau I, Grimbert P, Fiquet-Kempf B, et al: Possible familial origin of multifocal renal artery fibromuscular dysplasia. J Hypertens 15:1797, 1997.
199. Perry MO: Fibromuscular dysplasia. Surg Gynecol Obstet 139:97, 1974.
200. Sato S, Hata J: Fibromuscular dysplasia. Its occurrence with a dissecting aneurysm of the internal carotid artery. Arch Pathol Lab Med 106:332, 1982.
201. Schievink WI, Meyer FB, Parisi JE, et al: Fibromuscular dysplasia of the internal carotid artery associated with alpha1-antitrypsin deficiency. Neurosurgery 43:229, 1998.
202. Van Damme H, Sakalihasan N, Limet R: Fibromuscular dysplasia of the internal carotid artery: Personal experience with 13 cases and literature review. Acta Chir Belg 99:163, 1999.
203. Cloft HJ, Kallmes DF, Kallmes MH, et al: Prevalence of cerebral aneurysms in patients with fibromuscular dysplasia: A reassessment. J Neurosurg 88:436, 1998.
204. Suzuki H, Daida H, Sakurai H, et al: Familial fibromuscular dysplasia of bilateral brachial arteries. Heart 82:251, 1999.
205. Leventer RJ, Kornberg AJ, Coleman LT, et al: Stroke and fibromuscular dysplasia: Confirmation by renal magnetic resonance angiography. Pediatr Neurol 18:172, 1998.
206. Eachempati SR, Sebastian MW, Reed RL II: Posttraumatic bilateral carotid artery and right vertebral artery dissections in a patient with fibromuscular dysplasia: Case report and review of the literature. J Trauma 44:406, 1998.
207. Arunodaya GR, Vani S, Shankar SK, et al: Fibromuscular dysplasia with dissection of basilar artery presenting as "locked-in-syndrome." Neurology 48:1605, 1997.
208. Manninen HI, Koivisto T, Saari T, et al: Dissecting aneurysms of all four cervicocranial arteries in fibromuscular dysplasia: Treatment with self-expanding endovascular stents, coil embolization, and surgical ligation. AJNR Am J Neuroradiol 18:1216, 1997.
209. Kojima A, Shindo S, Kubota K, et al: Successful surgical treatment of a patient with multiple visceral artery aneurysms due to fibromuscular dysplasia. Cardiovasc Surg 10:157, 2002.
210. Safioleas M, Kakisis J, Manti C: Coexistence of hypertrophic cardiomyopathy and fibromuscular dysplasia of the superior mesenteric artery. N Engl J Med 344:1333, 2001.
211. Sandmann W, Schulte KM: Multivisceral fibromuscular dysplasia in childhood: Case report and review of the literature. Ann Vasc Surg 14:496, 2000.
212. Verhelst H, Lauwers G, Schroe H: Fibromuscular dysplasia of the external iliac artery. Acta Chir Belg 99:171, 1999.
213. Suarez WA, Kurczynski TW, Bove EL: An unusual type of combined aortic coarctation due to fibromuscular dysplasia. Cardiol Young 9:323, 1999.
214. Jones HJ, Staud R, Williams RC Jr: Rupture of a hepatic artery aneurysm and renal infarction: 2 complications of fibromuscular dysplasia that mimic vasculitis. J Rheumatol 25:2015, 1998.
215. Ebaugh JL, Chiou AC, Morasch MD, et al: Staged embolization and operative treatment of multiple visceral aneurysms in a patient with fibromuscular dysplasia: A case report. Vasc Surg 35:145, 2001.

chapter 66

Peripheral Vascular Anomalies and Vascular Tumors

Francine Blei

In the 1980s Mulliken and Glowacki[1] proposed functionally dividing vascular lesions into two groups, proliferative nonmalignant vascular lesions and static vascular lesions. Box 66-1 delineates this useful classification. The separation of vascular anomalies into proliferative lesions versus static malformations represents an important distinction, as prognosis and management varies. Early detection, proper evaluation, and appropriate diagnosis are essential, as these entities are medically very different. This chapter expands the topic of peripheral (i.e., not CNS or cardiac) vascular anomalies to include vascular tumors and syndromic vascular entities.

PROLIFERATIVE VASCULAR ANOMALIES AND TUMORS

Hemangiomas are considered the most common tumors of childhood. They are benign growths of endothelial cells with a unique natural history, characterized by a rapid growth phase usually beginning in the first weeks of life and continuing until 9 to 12 months of age (Fig. 66-1). Subsequently, the majority of hemangiomas undergo a spontaneous, gradual but extensive involution. Histologic correlation with the growth phase demonstrates involution and is characterized by increased connective tissue in the dermis and fat in the subcutaneous tissues.[2] An important exception to this growth/ regression pattern is the recently recognized group of rapidly involuting congenital hemangiomas (RICH), which are generally present in full at birth (or even detected prenatally) and may remain static or undergo rapid regression.[3-5] "Congenital nonprogressive hemangiomas" have been shown by North and colleagues[4] to be histologically and immunophenotypically distinct from classical hemangiomas of infancy and are speculated to have a differing pathogenesis. Enjolras and colleagues[6] have coined the term "noninvoluting congenital hemangioma" (NICH) for a subset of discrete cutaneous vascular lesions of intrauterine onset. These lesions were found to have high flow clinically (as assessed by Doppler) and inferred histologically (in that small arteries were seen "shunting" into lobular vessels or abnormal veins).

For unclear reasons, "typical" hemangiomas are most common in females, premature infants, and in the facial region. Waner and colleagues[6a] recently assessed the nonrandom distribution of facial hemangiomas and found two patterns of growth: focal lesions (in 76.3% of the 205 patients assessed) and diffuse lesions in 23.7%. The focal hemangiomas correlated to 22 sites of occurrence, all near lines of mesenchymal or mesenchymal-ectodermal embryonic fusion. The diffuse hemangiomas were in a segmental distribution and were specified as frontonasal (27%), maxillary (35%), or mandibular (38%). There was a threefold increased incidence of ulceration in patients with diffuse hemangiomas compared with that in patients with focal hemangiomas.[7]

Nakayama reviewed 1250 cases of "the strawberry mark" over a 16-year period,[2] classifying hemangiomas into three clinical subgroups—plaque type, tumor type, and subcutaneous type—according to the degree of dermal and subcutaneous components. Histologic correlation with growth phase demonstrated involution associated with increased connective tissue in the dermis and fat in the subcutaneous tissues. Plaquelike hemangiomas regressed the fastest, while the tumor type and giant lesions were the slowest to regress. Additionally, regression of the bulky, subcutaneous component progressed more slowly. Martinez-Perez and colleagues[8] described an important minority (4%) of patients who had hemangiomas that "did not look like strawberries." They divided these patients into four groups—(1) deep

BOX 66-1 Functional Classification of Vascular Anomalies

Proliferative nonmalignant* vascular lesions and tumors
- Hemangiomas of infancy
  - Rapidly involuting congenital hemangiomas of infancy (RICH)
  - Noninvoluting congenital hemangiomas of infancy (NICH)
- Kaposiform hemangioendothelioma
- Tufted angioma
- Pyogenic granuloma
- Kaposi's sarcoma

Static vascular lesions (vascular malformations)
- Simple or combined
- Arteriovenous
- Venous
- Capillary
- Lymphatic

*Mitotic figures absent or rare.

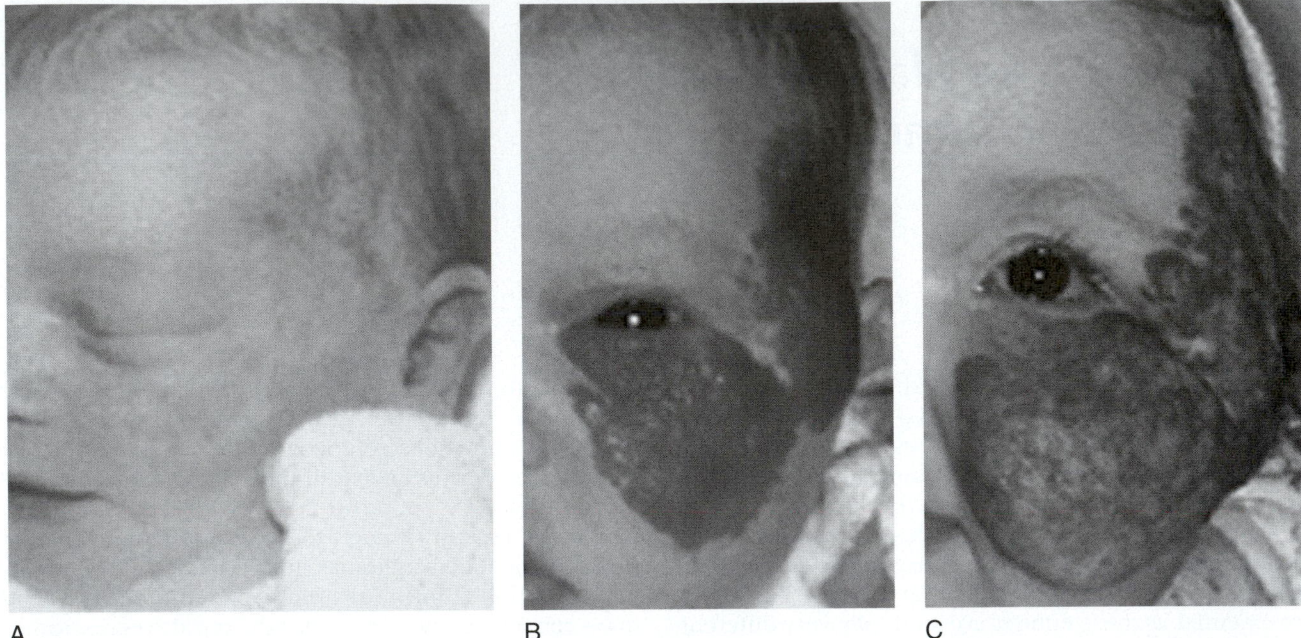

FIGURE 66-1. (See also Color Plate 66-1.) **A-C,** Sequential photos of infant who developed aggressive, proliferative hemangioma with ophthalmologic as well as cosmetic issues. In early phases (*left photograph*), this lesion is not easily differentiated from a capillary malformation.

lesions without a cutaneous component, (2) macular lesions resembling capillary malformations but with the natural history typical of hemangiomas, (3) telangiectatic hemangiomas, and (4) those with a high flow component. These authors concluded that in 90% of cases, hemangioma is a clinical diagnosis when examined by physicians with a trained eye. For cases that are not obvious, serial examinations over time or biopsy for lesions suspicious of malignancy may be necessary.[9]

Most hemangiomas are asymptomatic and therefore require no therapy. Despite this clinical course, hemangiomas nonetheless may be the source of significant psychosocial morbidity (although this has not been well studied),[10,11] and up to 10% of hemangiomas may cause complications requiring medical therapy to catalyze the involution phase. These complications may include obstruction of the upper airway[12]; ophthalmologic disturbances[13,14]; ulceration or bleeding; persistent soft tissue deformity; cerebral vasculopathy[15]; and high-output congestive heart failure.[16] These problems are discussed as follows.

Kasabach-Merritt Phenomenon, Kaposiform Hemangioendothelioma, and Tufted Angioma

Trapping of platelets and other blood elements (Kasabach-Merritt phenomenon) has been known to occur in association with some vascular anomalies since it was first described in 1940.[17] This is an extremely important diagnosis, as early detection and rapid evaluation and treatment (if clinically symptomatic) are essential. Perhaps one of the most surprising observations in the past decade has been that Kasabach-Merritt phenomenon is not associated with common hemangiomas of infancy but with kaposiform hemangioendotheliomas or tufted angiomas. On examination, the lesion is often edematous, smooth, and ecchymotic (Fig. 66-2). Anatomic predilection is for the chest wall and shoulder, groin extending down the leg, retroperitoneum, or face. The gender distribution tends to be equal. Hematologic features include thrombocytopenia, hypofibrinogenemia, elevated fibrin degradation products, and D-dimers. Radiologic hallmarks of kaposiform hemangioendotheliomas are cutaneous thickening, diffuse enhancement with ill-defined margins, small feeding/draining vessels, stranding, and hemosiderin deposits.[18,19] The histologic features of kaposiform hemangioendotheliomas are spindled endothelial cells resembling Kaposi's sarcoma (KS, but not associated with HIV infection), abnormal lymphatic-like vessels, microthrombi, hemosiderin, and decreased mast cells and pericytes (which are often seen in hemangiomas).[18,19] There may be residual tumor after resolution of hematologic abnormalities. Radiologic studies demonstrate persistent vascular tumors. Residua of kaposiform hemangioendothelioma–associated tumors may be "dormant" vascular tumors, rather than "scars." Clinically, as well as histologically, they differ considerably from involuted hemangioma.[20]

Tufted angioma, first described in the late 1980s, is a benign vascular tumor, typified by tufts of capillaries in the dermis.[21] The clinical appearance ranges from erythematous, indurated, annular nodules to plaques, with or without hypertrichosis (Fig. 66-3). Tufted angiomas are frequently tender. They commonly occur on the trunk and extremities, and they may be associ-ated with Kasabach-Merritt phenomenon.[22] Chu and colleagues[23] suggest that kaposiform hemangioendothelioma and tufted angioma may represent a continuum, as they report a case of transformation between both tumors within a single patient. Familial cases of tufted angioma are rare.[24]

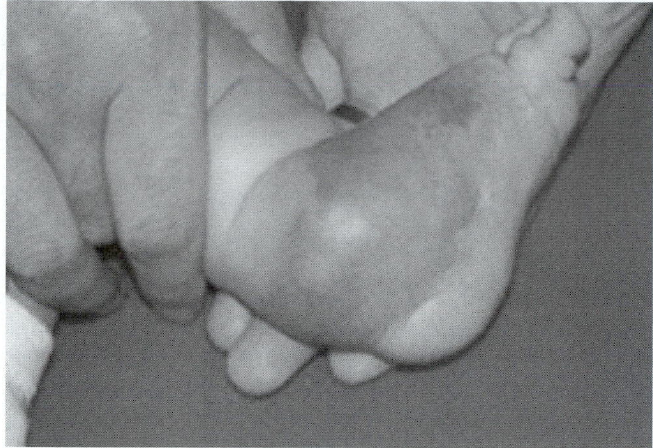
A

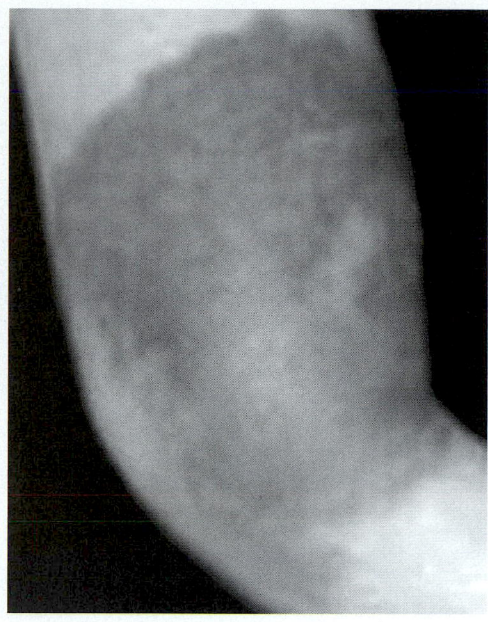
B

FIGURE 66-2. (See also Color Plate 66-2.) Kaposiform hemangioendothelioma presenting as soft tissue at birth (**A**), swelling, and leathery mass (**B**). Both patients developed lymphedema and leg-length discrepancy. Patient on left (**A**) had mild Kasabach-Merritt phenomenon.

Pyogenic Granuloma

Pyogenic granuloma (also termed *lobular capillary hemangioma*) is an acquired vascular lesion of the skin and mucous membranes seen in pediatric patients. The lesions have a cervicofacial propensity but can also be located on the trunk or extremities. The majority occur on the skin, and less frequently the mucous membranes (oral cavity and conjunctivae). These lesions are small and papular and tend to bleed. Treatment includes: (1) excision and linear closure, (2) shave excision, and (3) cauterization. In one series, there were no recurrences in patients treated with excision and linear closure, with more than 40% recurrence in patients treated with shave excision or cauterization.[25]

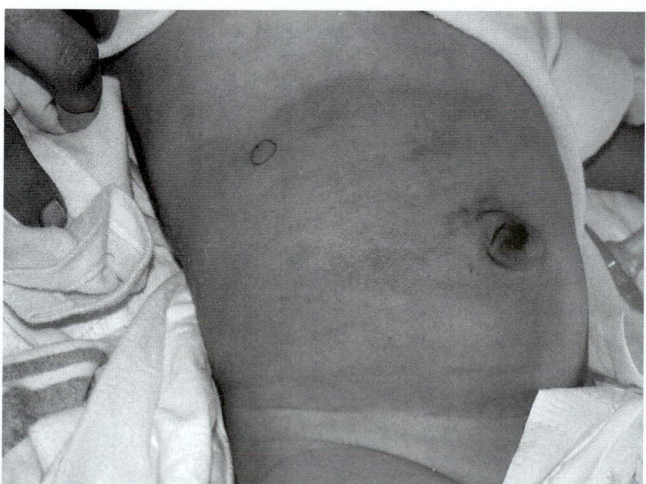

FIGURE 66-3. Tufted angioma on abdominal surface. Patient had Kasabach-Merritt phenomenon. Note site that was biopsied.

Kaposi's Sarcoma

KS is the most common neoplasm in patients with AIDS. It is an unusual vascular neoplasm originally described in 1872. The clinical appearance begins as violaceous macules, which progress to plaques and papules and then nodules. KS is thought to be multifocal rather than metastatic, with multiple lesions occurring simultaneously at different anatomic locations. Histologic features include spindle cells and endothelial cells, with rare mitotic figures. Evidence indicates that KS is monoclonal, although these data are conflicting. A novel human herpes virus, known as KS-associated herpes virus (KSHV), human herpes virus type 8 (HHV8) has been identified in KS tissue, supporting a viral etiology. Growth factors and cytokines are also believed to be involved in KS development. Therapies directed against KS include antiviral agents, antiangiogenic drugs, and immunosuppressive agents. Some researchers believe it is probable that drug combinations targeting several pathogenic mechanisms will be more effective single agents in suppressing KS growth.[26]

VASCULAR MALFORMATIONS

Vascular malformations are present at birth and grow in parallel with the rate of growth of the child, with no propensity to spontaneous involution. They are due to developmental anomalies of the vasculature and may involve one or several types of vessels (arteries, veins, capillaries, or lymphatics). Vascular malformations are properly described according to the affected anomalous vascular channel. They can range from capillary malformations (commonly referred to as *port-wine stains*) (Fig. 66-4) to large, bulky growths that can distort the normal structures of the body and potentially lead to a high output cardiac state (arterial malformations).

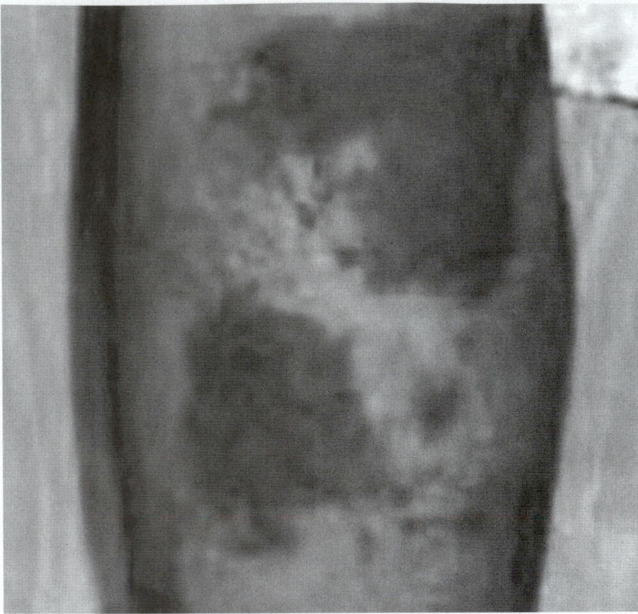

FIGURE 66-4. Capillary malformations.

Studies suggest that capillary malformations may be due to abnormal innervation of discrete capillary beds, causing chronic focal vascular dilatation.[27,28]

Lymphatic malformations may cause focal or generalized lymphedema, depending on the magnitude of aberrant lymphatics. Abnormal growth of lymphatic circulation encompasses overdevelopment (in lymphangiodysplasias, lymphangiomas, and lymphangiomatosis) or underdevelopment of lymphatic vasculature, or both. Disorders of the lymphatic circulation are common, diverse, and often devastating in their functional consequences. Clinical issues common to lymphatic anomalies reflect the tendency of these malformations to develop: (1) local (and systemic) infections/cellulitis (infectious and aseptic); (2) leakage (e.g., superficial blebs, chylous ascites, chylothorax, peritonitis, pleural effusions); (3) malabsorptive syndromes with significant metabolic consequences; (4) craniofacial distortion interfering with swallowing, airway, or significant visceral dysfunction (Fig. 66-5); (5) recurrences or complications after surgery; and (6) swelling of the affected anatomy, with functional limitations.

SYNDROMIC VASCULAR ANOMALIES (Box 66-2)

Dysmorphic syndromes are more commonly associated with *vascular malformations* than with hemangiomas.[29] Klippel-Trénaunay syndrome is one of the most common vascular malformations. This disorder constitutes a triad of vascular malformation (capillary, venous, or lymphatic); ipsilateral limb enlargement; and venous varicosities or developmental anomalies, or both (Fig. 66-6).[132] Males and females are affected in equal proportion, and the lower limb is the most frequent site of the anomaly. In severe cases there may be a bleeding diathesis characterized by a normal to slightly decreased platelet count, decrease in fibrinogen, and increased D-dimers and fibrin degradation products.[105] The Sturge-Weber syndrome includes a capillary malformation in the trigeminal distribution, intracranial dysplasia, seizures, and glaucoma. There are reports of concomitant Sturge-Weber syndrome in Klippel-Trénaunay patients, representing a more extensive vascular anomaly syndrome.[133] Other examples of dysmorphic syndromes associated with vascular malformation are Turner's and Noonan's syndromes, Parkes Weber syndrome, hereditary hemorrhagic telangiectasia (HHT), blue rubber bleb nevus syndrome,[30] Maffucci's syndrome (Fig. 66-7),[31] and Bannayan-Riley-Ruvalcaba syndrome.[32] Syndromes with vascular anomalies of the CNS include von Hippel-Lindau, ataxia-telangiectasia, and tuberous sclerosis.

Dysmorphic syndromes associated with *hemangiomas* are predominantly variations of (1) PHACES syndrome or (2) sacrococcygeal anomalies. The PHACES syndrome includes **P**osterior fossa structural malformations, **H**emangiomas, **A**rterial anomalies, **C**ardiac defects, **E**ye abnormalities, and **S**ternal and other midline

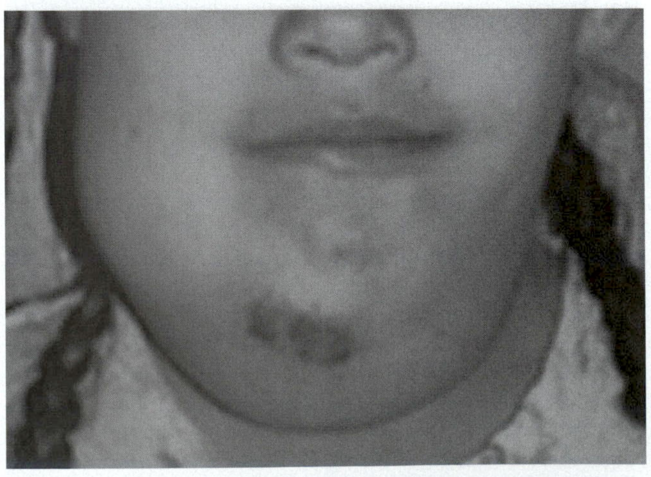

A

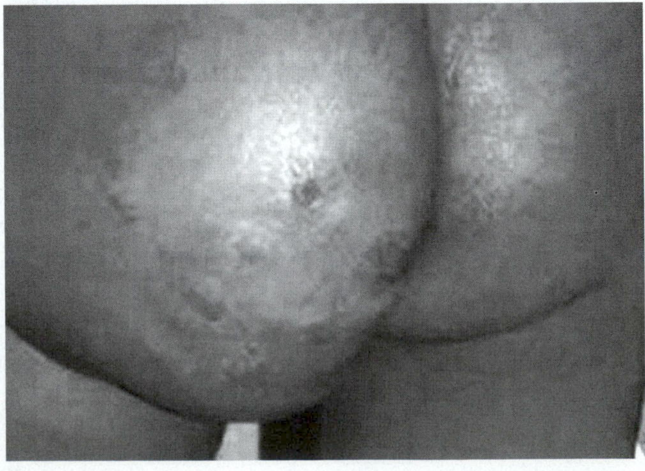

B

FIGURE 66-5. Patient on left (**A**) with extensive lymphatic malformation requiring tracheotomy and patient on right (**B**) with lymphatic malformation of buttocks.

BOX 66-2 Syndromic Vascular Anomalies

- PHACES syndrome
  - Posterior fossa malformations
  - Hemangioma
  - Arterial anomalies
  - Cardiac anomalies
  - Eye anomalies
  - Sternal or other midline deformities
- Klippel-Trénaunay syndrome
  - Cutaneous capillary/venular malformation
  - Limb hypertrophy
  - Deep vessel anomalies
- Parkes Weber syndrome
  - Klippel-Trénaunay syndrome
  - Arteriovenous shunting
- Hereditary hemorrhagic telangiectasia
  - Arteriovenous malformations
  - Telangiectasias
  - Cutaneous tissues
  - Mucous membranes and gastrointestinal tract
  - ± Intracranial, pulmonary, or hepatic arteriovenous malformations
- Maffucci's syndrome[24-26,223]
  - Multifocal enchondromas
  - Cutaneous vascular anomalies
  - Increased malignant potential
- Sturge-Weber syndrome
  - Encephalotrigeminal angiomatosis
  - Cutaneous capillary malformation in trigeminal distribution
  - Ipsilateral glaucoma
  - Seizures
- Blue rubber bleb syndrome[19]
  - Multifocal cutaneous and gastrointestinal vascular malformations
- Bannayan-Riley-Ruvalcaba syndrome[29]
  - Multiple subcutaneous lipomas and vascular malformations
  - Lentigines of the penis and vulva, verrucae, and acanthosis nigricans
  - Macrocephaly with normal ventricular size
  - Mental retardation
  - CNS vascular malformations
  - Intestinal polyposis
  - Skeletal abnormalities
  - Thyroid tumors
- von Hippel-Lindau disease
  - Multisystem angiomatosis, especially CNS (hemangioblastoma)
  - Renal
  - Adrenal
  - Pancreas
  - Increased risk of renal malignancy
- Ataxia-telangiectasia
  - Progressive cerebellar ataxia
  - Oculocutaneous telangiectasis
  - Humoral and cellular immune defects
  - Chromosomal breakage
  - Predisposition to malignancy[224,225]
- Tuberous sclerosis
  - Angiogenic neoplasms of kidney, brain, and skin[226]

deformities (Fig. 66-8).[33,34] Sacral or genitourinary defects, or both, are associated with hemangiomas in the lumbar area.[29,35] In contrast with several heritable vascular malformation syndromes, the hemangiomas observed in syndromic associations do not appear to be inherited.

PRENATAL DIAGNOSIS OF VASCULAR ANOMALIES

With the availability of improved techniques in fetal ultrasound and MRI, prenatally diagnosed vascular anomalies are becoming increasingly recognized. Most parentally diagnosed vascular lesions are vascular malformations. Greenlee[36] observed that many human conceptuses overall die prenatally, and of these, a significant number involve a disorder of the lymphatic system. A number of the vascular lesions detected prenatally are associated with high-risk pregnancies, as they are symptomatic in utero, necessitating prenatal therapy (e.g., maternal steroids or digoxin in the case of high-flow vascular lesions compromising fetal hemodynamic status) in some cases to prevent nonimmune fetal hydrops (Fig. 66-9).[3] There are also reports of maternal steroid therapy for the successful management of fetal hemangiomas.[37]

ETIOLOGY OF HEMANGIOMAS AND VASCULAR MALFORMATIONS

Why do vascular anomalies occur? The simple answer is that they are due to many causes—mechanical, environmental, hormonal, and genetic, although no single etiology is thematic. Within the past decade, research activity has focused on unraveling the potential etiologic factors leading to formation of vascular anomalies. Some authors implicate a *viral etiology* as causal in hemangioma development, describing increased expression of papilloma or cytomegalovirus virus in hemangioma specimens.[38] Other studies have reported lack of expression of human herpes virus 8 in hemangioma tissue.[39,40]

Burton and colleagues[41] implicated *mechanical disruption early in gestation* as a potential etiologic factor in hemangioma development, because in their series, infants born to mothers who had chorionic villous sampling had an increased incidence of hemangiomas. Mechanisms underlying the spontaneous involution of hemangioma have not been well studied.

North and colleagues[42] showed that juvenile hemangiomas and placental vessels share immunoreactivity, suggesting that some hemangiomas may represent ectopic placenta. Initially, hemangiomas were shown to highly express GLUT1, a glucose transporter normally restricted to blood-tissue barrier endothelia (as in brain and placenta).[155] Further studies demonstrated hemangiomas, and placental vessels coexpressed Fc gamma RII, Lewis Y antigen (LeY), and merosin.[43]

Gurtner and colleagues[44] have identified a 15-fold increase in circulating CD34+AC133+ cells and a 2.5-fold increase in KDR/VEGFR2+ cells in children with hemangiomas compared with age-matched controls. Others have identified increased numbers of KDR^+, $CD133^+$,

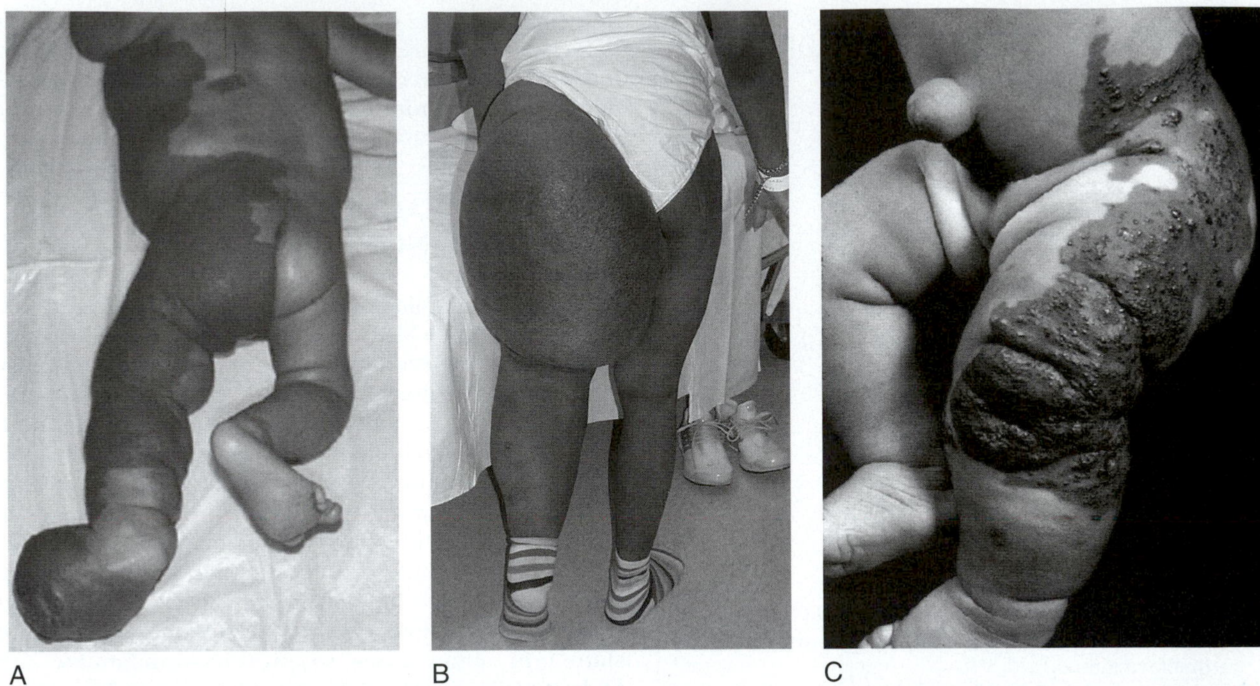

FIGURE 66-6. (See also Color Plate 66-6.) **A,** Patient with Klippel-Trénaunay vascular malformation syndrome, complicated by leg-length discrepancy, asymmetric foot size requiring custom orthotics, lymphopenia, and frequent septic episodes due to abnormal lymphatic communications. **B,** Patient with Klippel-Trénaunay syndrome with associated gigantism, lymphatic dysfunction, frequent infections, gastrointestinal bleeding, severe pain, and thromboses within lesions. **C,** Patient with Klippel-Trénaunay vascular malformation syndrome, with cutaneous capillary malformation and blebs prone to bleeding.

CD34+ endothelial precursor cells, and lymphatic endothelial hyaluronan receptor-1 (LYVE-1) in proliferating hemangioma tissue.[45,46] These studies suggest a potential role for immature endothelial cells in the proliferative growth of hemangiomas.

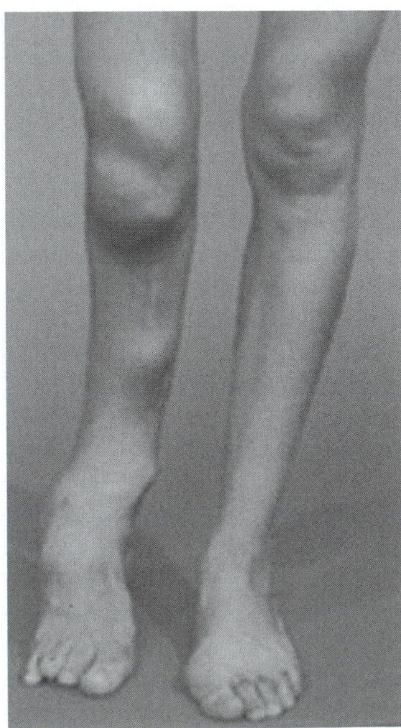

FIGURE 66-7. Patient with Maffucci's syndrome. Note limb-length discrepancy, scars from orthopedic surgery, enchondromas, and vascular masses.

The vast majority of hemangiomas appear to be sporadic. Sporadic hemangiomas generally have a 3:1 predilection for females, more frequently involve the craniofacial regions, and are more common in premature infants. Several authors have noted a more marked female predilection in "complex" hemangiomas, far above the expected 3 to 4:1 female predominance.[33,47] Sasaki and associates[48] reported increased levels of circulating estradiol in patients with hemangiomas. Additionally, increased estrogen receptor expression was detected in hemangioma tissue. Lui and colleagues[49] detected estrogen, progesterone, and androgen receptors in hemangioma tissues. These observations raise the question of the relationship between hormones or genetic factors, or both, in the pathophysiology of these lesions.

Insight into Involution

Apoptosis (programmed cell death) has been studied in hemangioma tissue, demonstrating an inverse relationship between proliferation and apoptosis.[50] These data provide some insight into the pathogenesis of hemangiomas, but the expression of growth factors and enzymes described may be secondary responses to an underlying primary molecular event leading to hemangioma development. Analysis of mRNA from biopsy specimens from three different growth phases showed increased expression of clusterin/apoJ (clust/apoJ), an apoptosis-associated glycoprotein, in the involuting samples.[51] In these studies, clust/apoJ was increased in hemangioma with progression from proliferative to the involuting and involuted phases. The authors suggest that

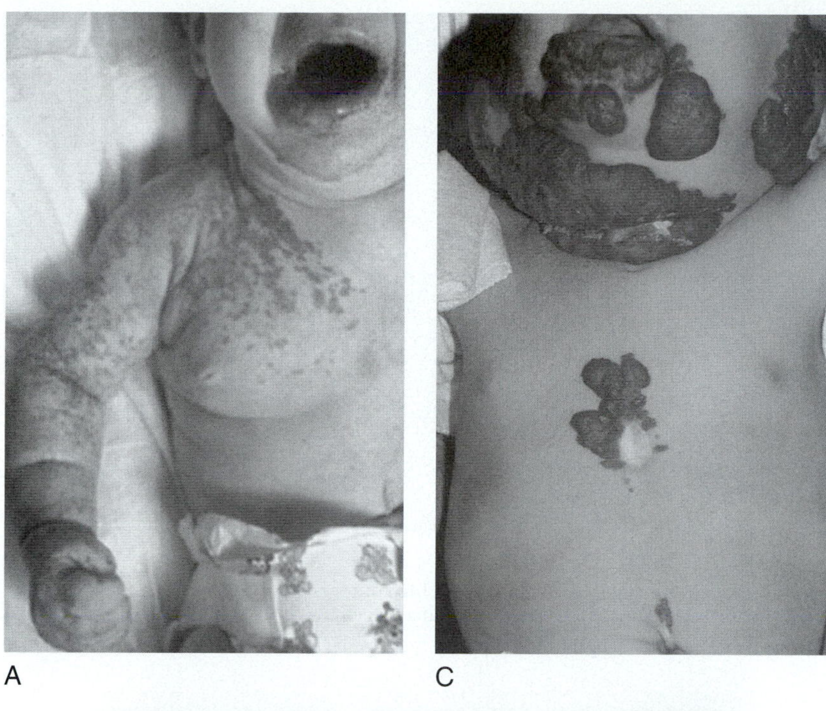

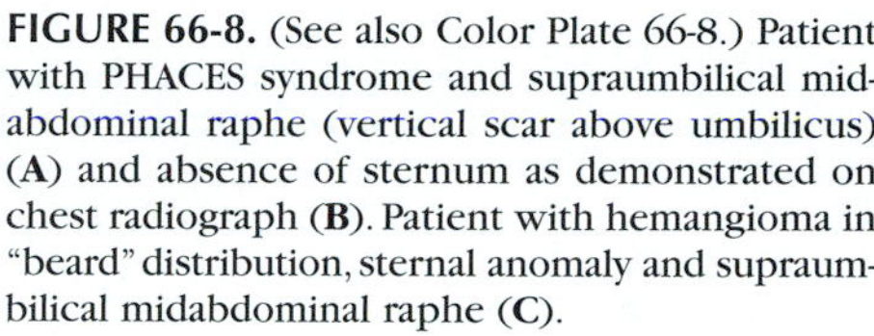

FIGURE 66-8. (See also Color Plate 66-8.) Patient with PHACES syndrome and supraumbilical midabdominal raphe (vertical scar above umbilicus) (**A**) and absence of sternum as demonstrated on chest radiograph (**B**). Patient with hemangioma in "beard" distribution, sternal anomaly and supraumbilical midabdominal raphe (**C**).

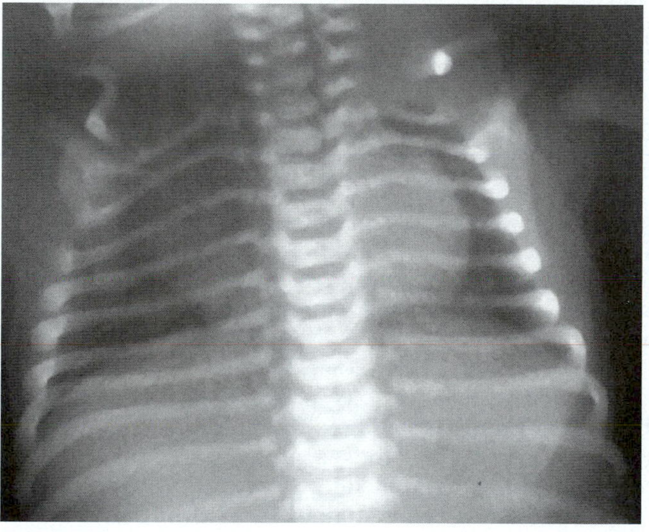

clust/apoJ is involved in apoptosis regulation during spontaneous regression of hemangioma and postulate a role for mast cells (with clust/apoJ-rich granules) in this process. Other studies have demonstrated Ets-1, a transcription factor, is proapoptotic to endothelial cells by modulating the expression of apoptosis-related genes.[52]

Unique Markers for Vascular Anomalies

Growth factors, hormonal influences from other cell types, and mechanical influences are thought to affect the focal abnormal growth of endothelial cells in hemangiomas and perhaps vascular malformations. Takahashi and colleagues[52a] analyzed tissue from proliferating, involuting, and involuted hemangiomas, finding a pattern of expression of markers specific for each phase of growth. Proliferating cell nuclear antigen (PCNA), vascular endothelial growth factor (VEGF), and type IV collagenase (markers of cell growth or the angiogenic phenotype) were detected in the proliferating phase, whereas basic fibroblast growth factor (bFGF) and urokinase (markers associated with angiogenesis, as well as tissue remodeling) were detected in both the proliferating and involution stages, but much less so in the involution phase. Tissue inhibitor of metalloproteinase (TIMP) (a correlate of antiangiogenesis) was observed only in the involution phase.

Martin-Padura and associates[53] demonstrated normal endothelial and basement membrane markers in hemangioma tissue, suggesting abnormal growth in proliferating hemangiomas is related to local release of growth factors rather than an altered endothelial phenotype.[53]

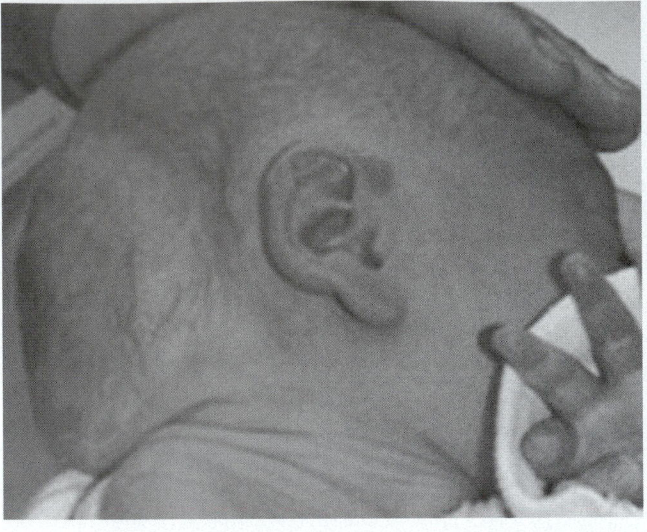
A

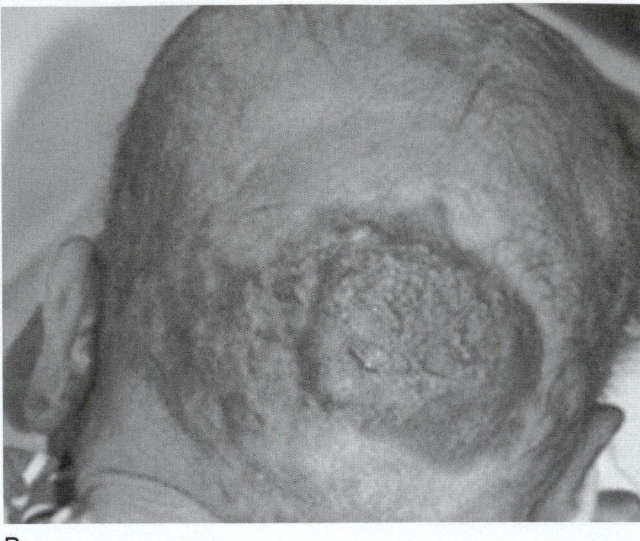
B

FIGURE 66-9. (See also Color Plate 66-9.) Vascular lesion of scalp detected in utero caused high-output failure in the fetus, necessitating prenatal treatment with maternal digoxin. Postnatally, the mass had arterial flow and behaved clinically as a rapidly involuting congenital hemangioma (RICH).

Berard and colleagues[54] demonstrated that cultured stromal cells obtained from hemangioma biopsies demonstrated angiogenic activity as they released VEGF. This study implicates an important role for stromal cells in the proliferation of hemangiomas.[54] These authors also suggest that anti-VEGF drugs may prove useful in the treatment of hemangiomas. Chang and colleagues[55] demonstrated, by in situ hybridization, upregulation of bFGF and VEGF mRNA in proliferative hemangiomas. Dosanjh and colleagues[56] showed that hemangioma cells retained morphologic and protein expression similar to embryonic microvascular cells.

Macrophage-derived angiogenesis factors may contribute to hemangioma proliferation,[57] possibly via increased expression of monocyte chemoattractant protein 1 (MCP-1).[58] Several groups have studied the changes in matrix composition and sensory nerve and other cellular components during phases of growth.[59,60] Huang and colleagues[61] identified increased activity of type 3 iodothyronine deiodinase in large hemangiomas, yielding profound hypothyroidism in patients. Recent data from Boudreau (unpublished) showed increased expression of homeobox D3 in proliferating hemangiomas and increased D10 in involuting lesions. Endothelial cells showed negative immunoreactivity for CD146, an endothelial marker in a study by Li.[62] Arbiser and colleagues examined expression of phosphorylated mitogen-activated protein kinase (MAPK) in various vascular tumors—hemangiomas of infancy, pyogenic granulomas, hemangioendotheliomas, angiosarcoma, Kaposi's sarcoma, and verruga peruana, demonstrating an inverse relationship between MAPK staining and malignancy. There was strong expression in benign endothelial tumors, including capillary hemangioma of infancy and pyogenic granuloma, as well as infectious endothelial tumors (Kaposi's sarcoma and verruca peruana) and decreased expression in angiosarcoma.[63]

PHYSIOLOGIC AND PATHOLOGIC ANGIOGENESIS

Judah Folkman, a pioneer in the field of angiogenesis, commented "we gradually realized that a hemangioma on a baby's face is but a subset of a more general process."[64] The process was angiogenesis, the growth of new blood vessels. Knowledge about the development and proliferation of blood vessels is essential to understanding vascular anomalies.

Although the cardiovascular system is the first to develop embryologically, only recently have the critical pathways for this process become evident.[65] Blood-forming tissue is mesoderm derived. The yolk sac develops blood islands, a precursor common to angioblasts and hematopoietic cells. Vasculogenesis defines the differentiation of angioblasts from mesoderm and the formation of primitive blood vessels from angioblasts.[65] Vascular endothelial growth factor and its receptor, tyrosine kinase flk-1, represent a signaling system crucial for the differentiation of endothelial cells and the development of the vascular system.[65]

Other factors essential to this highly regulated process are: homeobox genes, transcription factors of the ETS family, endothelial-specific receptor tyrosine kinases TIE-1, TIE-2, and their respective ligands, the angiopoietins, other vascular endothelial growth factors and their receptors; and fibroblast growth factors.[66,67] Cell adhesion molecules, mechanical forces, vascular regression and remodeling are involved in the subsequent events of endothelial cell differentiation, apoptosis, and angiogenesis.[68] Mouse endothelioma cells expressing the polyoma middle T oncogene induced hemangiomas in various species, presumably by recruiting nonprolife rating host endothelial cells.[69] TIE-1 and TIE-2 receptor tyrosine kinases are expressed in developing vascular endothelial cells and have been shown in knock-out mouse models to have important but distinct roles in blood vessel formation. These studies have suggested that TIE-1 plays a role in establishing structural integrity of vascular endothelial cells and that TIE-2 is important for vascular network formation.[70] However, there are no animal models to date that effectively replicate the life cycle of an infantile hemangioma, and no animals appear to be afflicted with the vascular malformation syndromes seen in humans.

Adult endothelial cells are normally quiescent; however, they retain the capacity to proliferate when exposed to "angiogenic stimuli" (e.g., hypoxia, growth factors). Physiologic angiogenesis is a tightly regulated process of vascular growth and is normally restricted to ovulation, menstruation, development of the embryo and placenta, and wound healing. In contrast, pathologic angiogenesis is the hallmark of many diseases including the growth of tumors, hemangiomas, proliferative retinopathy, rheumatoid arthritis, and others. Vascular anomalies afford a phenotype of vascular aberration—infantile hemangiomas are the prototype of uniquely orchestrated vascular proliferation (angiogenesis) and involution, whereas vascular malformations represent focal aberrant development of the vasculature. In the past decade, the basic sciences have achieved major advances in unraveling several interrelated mechanisms of vasculogenesis and angiogenesis. Are vascular malformations disorders of vasculogenesis and hemangiomas disorders of angiogenesis?

GENETICS AND VASCULAR MALFORMATIONS

Well-known hereditary vascular syndromes, where genetic mutations and inheritance patterns have been clearly identified, include HHT, von Hippel-Lindau disease and ataxia-telangiectasia. Genetic linkage and mutational analysis for an increasing number of other vascular syndromes is now available (Table 66-1). HHT has been associated with mutations of endoglin, an endothelial cell TGF-β binding protein, or ALK-1, the activin receptor kinase gene. Mutations in one of two different genes, endoglin or ALK-1, can cause HHT. Interestingly, patients with the endoglin mutation appear predisposed to pulmonary arteriovenous malformations, thus a genotype-phenotype relationship occurs. Both ALK-1 and endoglin belong to the transforming growth factor TGF-β receptor family and are expressed primarily on endothelial cells. Marchuk and colleagues[23] provide an excellent review of the potential role of ALK-1 and TGF-β signaling in HHT and cerebral cavernous malformations. Eerola and associates[71] recently reported cases of "atypical" capillary malformation in family members in

TABLE 66-1 CHROMOSOMAL MUTATIONS ASSOCIATED WITH VASCULAR DISORDERS

Primary Disorder	Chromosomal Abnormality	Gene	Associated Process
Hereditary hemorrhagic telangiectasia[23,139]	Type I 9q33-34	Endoglin	TGF-β signaling
	Type II 12q13 (ALK-1)	ALK-1	
Familial cerebral cavernous malformation[140-143]	Type 1 (CCM1) 7q 7p15-p13	KRIT1	Ras-GTPase signal transducer
	Type 2 (CCM2) 3q25.2-q27	MGC4607	Integrin signaling
Familial capillary malformation - arteriovenous malformation[71]	5q	RASA-1 Inactivating mutation	p120-RasGAP signaling
Familial glomus tumor[88]	11q23 (paraganglionic) 1p21-p22 (glomangioma)		Amine precursor uptake and decarboxylation
Familial venous malformation[144,145]	9p	TIE-2 Activating mutation	Vessel stabilization via extracellular interactions
Familial juvenile hemangioma[79]	5q33-q34	VEGFR-2 (FLK-1) VEGFR-3 (FLT-4)	Angiogenesis
Hereditary lymphedema[135]	5q34-q35	VEGFR-3 (FLT-4) Ang-2	Lymphatic development
Lymphedema-distichiasis[146]	16q24.3	FOXC2 Prox-1 Nrp-2	Lymphatic development
Turner's syndrome with lymphedema[147,148]	?T(Y;16)(ql 2?;q24.3)		
Milroy's lymphedema[149]	5q35.3	VEGFR-3 (FLT-4)	
Familial hypotrichosis, lymphedema, and telangiectasia[150]	20q13	SOX18 transcription factor	Hair and blood vessel development; development or maintenance of lymphatic vessels, or both

addition to either arteriovenous malformation, arteriovenous fistula, or Parkes Weber syndrome. Heterozygous inactivating RASA1 mutations were identified in these kindreds.

The gene for hereditary lymphedema has been linked to distal chromosome 5q, an area where vascular endothelial growth factor C receptor (FLT4) has been mapped. The FLT4 gene is a marker for lymphatic endothelium during development, and VEGF-C receptor has been detected in lymphatic vasculature. Distichiasis is the presence of a second row of eyelashes arising from the meibomian glands of the eyelids. This can be inherited alone or as a component of lymphedema-distichiasis syndrome. Mutations in the FOXC2 gene (a forkhead, or Fox-box gene, coding for winged helix transcription factors) have been identified in the lymphedema-distichiasis syndrome.[72] Additionally, Brooks and colleagues[73] identified the same mutation in patients with isolated distichiasis, suggesting that hereditary distichiasis and lymphedema-distichiasis may represent the same disorder with different phenotypic expression. Levinson reported congenital lymphedema among FLT4 mutation families and pubertal among FOXC2 mutation families, with similar male and female penetrance in both groups.[74]

Although most hemangiomas are sporadic, there are published reports of rare kindreds with "familial hemangiomas." In contrast to the generally accepted female-to-male ratio of 3 to 4:1 seen in sporadic hemangiomas, the "hemangioma families" demonstrated a 2:1 ratio. Vascular malformations and hemangiomas may be present in different members of the same family.[75] The vascular lesions appeared to be transmitted in an autosomal dominant fashion with moderate to high penetrance. Genetic linkage analysis within hemangioma kindreds suggests a germline mutation with autosomal dominant segregation and linkage to chromosome 5q31-33 in some of these kindreds.[76,77]

Mutations that are passed through the germline and predispose family members to hemangioma development may also be involved in sporadic hemangiomas. Consistent with this speculation, two recent studies indicate clonality, demonstrating nonrandom x-inactivation and loss of heterozygosity.[78,79] Furthermore, Walters and colleagues[79] recently identified two unique somatic mutations of the vascular endothelial growth factor receptor (VEGFR) genes, VEGFR2 (FLK1/KDR) and VEGFR3 (FLT4) in hemangioma specimens.

CLINICAL ISSUES (Tables 66-2 and 66-3)

Facial Port-Wine Stains

When an infant has a macular vascular stain covering the trigeminal distribution, the diagnosis may not initially be apparent. If the lesion remains static, the diagnosis is capillary malformation, and the child is at risk for Sturge-Weber syndrome (dysmorphogenesis of cephalic neuroectoderm) and must be followed for development of glaucoma, seizures, and developmental delay. The risk of ophthalmologic sequelae appears to be highest in patients with lesions located in the ophthalmic (or V1 trigeminal) cutaneous area.[80] In one study, port-wine stains of the eyelids, bilateral distribution of the birthmark, and unilateral port-wine stains involving all three branches of the trigeminal nerve were associated with a significantly higher likelihood of having eye or CNS complications, or both.[81] Patients with large facial and upper trunk hemangiomas, especially of plaquelike quality, should be evaluated for PHACES syndrome, with (1) cervicofacial MRI evaluation for assessment of structural and vascular abnormalities, (2) cardiac evaluation, (3) ophthalmologic evaluation, (4) thyroid function studies, and (5) thorough examination to assess

TABLE 66-2 HEMANGIOMAS: SIGNIFICANT CLINICAL ISSUES WARRANTING EVALUATION

Clinical Finding	Recommended Evaluation
Hemangiomatosis—multiple, small, cutaneous hemangiomas	Evaluate for parenchymal hemangiomas, especially hepatic/CNS/gastrointestinal
Cutaneous hemangiomas in "beard" distribution	Evaluate for airway hemangioma, especially if presenting with stridor
Facial hemangioma involving significant area of face	Evaluate for PHACES—MRI for orbital hemangioma ± posterior fossa malformation Cardiac, ophthalmologic evaluation Evaluate for midline abnormality—supraumbilical raphe, sternal atresia, cleft palate, thyroid abnormality Evaluate thyroid function MRI evaluation of craniocervical vessels for anomaly
Periocular hemangioma	MRI of orbit Ophthalmologic evaluation
Paraspinal midline vascular lesion	Ultrasound (if less than 6 months of age) or MRI to evaluate for occult spinal dysraphism ± underlying vascular lesion
Thrill or bruit, or both, associated with hemangioma	Cardiac evaluation and echo to rule out diastolic reversal of flow of aorta MRI/Doppler of vascular lesion to evaluate flow characteristics
Large hemangioma, especially hepatic	Ultrasound with Doppler flow MRI Thyroid function studies
Preferential position (e.g., torticollis, flexure contracture)	Consider physical therapy evaluation
Delayed milestones	Consider side effect of corticosteroids (myopathy, weight related) or interferon (especially spastic diplegia)

TABLE 66-3 CLINICAL FINDINGS AND TREATMENT OF HEMANGIOMAS AND VASCULAR MALFORMATIONS

Clinical Finding	Recommended Treatment
Hemangiomas	
Severe ulceration/maceration	Encourage cleansing regimen twice daily Dilute sodium bicarbonate soaks ± Flashlamp-pulsed dye laser ± Oral/intralesional corticosteroids ± Metronidazole cream
Bleeding (not Kasabach-Merritt phenomenon)	Gelfoam (Pharmacia Pfizer, New York)/Surgifoam (Johnson & Johnson, Somerset, NJ) Compression therapy ± Embolization
Hemangioma with ophthalmologic sequelae	Patching therapy as directed by ophthalmologist Topical vs. intralesional vs. oral corticosteroids vs. surgery
Subglottic hemangioma	Oral/local corticosteroids ± KTP laser ± surgery Tracheotomy if required
Kasabach-Merritt phenomenon	Corticosteroids, aminocaproic acid, vincristine, ± chemotherapy, interferon-alfa ± Embolization
High-flow hepatic hemangioma	Corticosteroids ± embolization ± Chemotherapy, ± surgery, ± synthroid Transplantation
Vascular Malformations	
Swelling	If airway consider tracheotomy vs. surgery Massage, compression therapy Look for source of infection and treat
Phlebolith	Anti-inflammatory agent
Limb-length discrepancy	Shoe insert vs. epiphysiodesis vs. serial observation
Shoe-size discrepancy	Wear two different shoe sizes Epiphysiodesis vs. ray resection
Pain	Evaluate for phlebolith or deep venous thrombosis Analgesics Anticoagulation if thrombosis ± Nerve block, ± sclerotherapy (if not thrombosis)
Recurrent infections/swelling	Rotating oral antibiotic prophylaxis
Chylous ascites	Low-fat diet/parenteral nutrition

for clefting or other anomalies (e.g., sternum, palate, midline supraumbilical raphe) (see Fig. 66-8).

Airway Symptoms

Recurrent stridor with progressive worsening of symptoms (in an infant with or without cutaneous hemangiomas) should alert the physician to the possibility of a subglottic hemangioma. Definitive diagnosis is made by bronchoscopy with direct visualization of the airway. Orlow and colleagues[12] reported the increased risk of symptomatic airway hemangiomas in association with a distinctive cutaneous "beard" hemangioma distribution. However, in the absence of cutaneous signs, one should also entertain this diagnosis. Controversies in management of subglottic hemangiomas include surgery (submucous resection); laser (CO_2 vs. potassium titanyl phosphate [KTP]); steroids (intralesional vs. systemic); interferon-alpha (IFN-α) or tracheotomy, or both. CO_2 or KTP laser may be helpful for noncircumferential subglottic hemangiomas.[82] Intralesional photocoagulation with the KTP or Nd:YAG laser has been reported successful in proliferative hemangiomas.[83] There is one reported case of intralesional steroid injection successfully treating a subglottic hemangioma.[84]

Periocular Vascular Anomalies

Periocular lesions present unique management problems. What is visible externally is the "tip of the iceberg." Thus early radiologic evaluation by MRI and ophthalmologic evaluation and follow-up are essential. Vascular lesions put patients at risk for ptosis, amblyopia, strabismus, and anisotropia. Early intervention is essential to minimize ocular sequelae. Periocular hemangiomas belong to the class of hemangiomas that warrant close evaluation and early, active treatment because some have the potential to threaten or permanently compromise vision. Failure to do so can lead to severe and permanent visual disturbances by occluding the visual axis, compressing the globe, or expanding into the retrobulbar space.

Complications such as amblyopia, significant refractive errors, and strabismus are seen in up to 80% of patients with untreated periocular hemangiomas.[85] Therefore all children with periocular hemangiomas warrant serial follow-up by regular serial cycloplegic refractions, performed by someone skilled in retinoscopy of preverbal children. Therapies include patching of the contralateral eye; topical, intralesional, or systemic corticosteroids; IFN-α; and surgery.[13,86] Unique risks of intralesional steroids include central retinal artery occlusion.[87]

Hepatic Hemangiomas

Hepatic hemangiomas represent a special category. Although many hepatic hemangiomas are asymptomatic, a subset carry a high morbidity and mortality rate.They may be solitary or multiple and may be seen in association with cutaneous hemangiomatosis or be an isolated finding. Even if radiologically extensive, the clinical spectrum ranges from asymptomatic to life threatening, with high-output congestive heart failure or profound secondary hypothyroidism (see earlier) and profound hematologic abnormalities. Therapies include steroids, interferon, embolization, antifibrinolytic therapies, surgical resection, and liver transplantation with inconsistent results.[88-90]

Midline Hemangiomas

Midline hemangiomas over the lower spine may be associated with occult spinal dysraphism or anogenitourinary defects (e.g., renal anomalies, bony sacral anomalies, lipomeningocele, imperforate anus).There are reports of clinically asymptomatic patients with midline lumbar hemangiomas associated with tethered spinal cord that were detected by radiological evaluation only.[35,91] Thus radiologic evaluation of the spine (ultrasound for infants younger than 3 months of age, MRI for infants older than 3 months) and genitourinary system (ultrasound) are indicated in patients with cutaneous vascular lesions in this anatomic location.

Hemangiomatosis

The child with multiple hemangiomas may have diffuse neonatal hemangiomatosis (DNH), a dermatosis with a more grave prognosis or benign neonatal hemangiomatosis. A subset of babies with numerous (small) cutaneous hemangiomas is predisposed to parenchymal hemangiomas, especially of the liver (also CNS, eye, pancreas, gastrointestinal tract, lungs, or other organs).[92]

Ulcerating Lesions

Hemangiomas of specific anatomical sites most prone to ulcerate are in mucosal (perineum, lip) or intertriginous areas or at pressure points (e.g., back).[93] Local wound care may be adequate (e.g., metronidazole or other antibiotic cream, Vaseline gauze, hydrocolloid gels). If infected, topical or systemic antibiotics, or both, are indicated. Other required therapies may be intralesional or systemic steroids or flashlamp-pulsed dye laser.[94] Topical Imiquimod and platelet-derived growth factor have been reported as successful therapies for ulcerated hemangiomas.[95,96] Pain management can be achieved with topical and oral analgesics. Simple but helpful measures to comfort the infant with a painful ulcerating hemangioma include twice-daily sitz baths, air drying, and construction of foam rubber cushions with custom-designed cutout areas to relive direct pressure on the painful area.

Coagulation Abnormalities Associated with Vascular Lesions

As noted earlier, bleeding due to Kasabach-Merritt phenomenon (thrombocytopenia, hypofibrinogenemia, and increased fibrinolysis) is often associated with lesions (kaposiform hemangioendothelioma, tufted angioma). In addition to therapy directed toward the primary tumor, antifibrinolytic agents, antiplatelet agents, and heparin are used.[19,97] Bleeding is often a temporary complication of ulcerating hemangiomas. One report described the use of an enuresis blanket to alert parents to significant bleeding.[98] Bedside cauterization with silver nitrate may be sufficient. One case responded to topical aminocaproic acid and Gelfoam.[99] Compression therapy is a useful adjunct for bleeding hemangiomas, as well as those lesions with a large bulky component.[100]

Hemodynamic Sequelae

Rarely, hemangiomas may demonstrate transient high flow, functionally (until they have undergone significant involution) mimicking arteriovenous malformations. Hemangiomas with high flow are most frequently located in the liver. These lesions can lead to significant morbidity, with high output cardiac failure. Nonhepatic hemangiomas, which seem prone to develop a high flow element, include those involving the parotid gland; upper arm; chest wall; scalp; and, rarely, the upper lip. These lesions appear to behave as transiently "arterialized" hemangiomas.[16] During this time, patients may have a failure to thrive–type picture, hyperdynamic precordium, tachycardia, bounding pulses with a widened pulse pressure, and a thrill/bruit over the hemangioma. These findings should alert the treating physician to monitor the hemodynamic status of patients with hemangiomas, by careful physical examination and frequent follow-up evaluation. A minority of patients develop high cardiac output states requiring intervention including diuretics, inotropic agents, or an embolization procedure.

Orthopedic Concerns

Orthopedic issues associated with vascular anomalies involve those relating to limb-dimension discrepancies (including limb length, hypertrophy, atrophy, macrodactyly, polydactyly, and gigantism) and other less common orthopedic problems (including foot and hand deformities and joint abnormalities). Limb-length discrepancies may be associated with quadriceps fatigue, hip and lower back pain, or secondary scoliosis. Serial assessment of limb-length data and bone ages at regular intervals is recommended. Interventions include shoe lifts versus epiphyseodesis (surgical growth plate closure) for more modest discrepancies; however, for discrepancies predicted to be greater than 5 cm, or in patients who have already reached skeletal maturity, limb shortening and lengthening are the only options to equalize limb lengths.[101] Macrodactyly and gigantism may cause functional problems and difficulty with shoe fit. Therapeutic options include custom shoes, ray or digital resection for macrodactyly of the fingers or toes, debulking procedures, and amputation for severe and otherwise unmanageable cases of hypertrophy.[101] These procedures include removal of subcutaneous fat and ray resection removal of one or more metatarsals and the associated phalanges. Patients with vascular anomalies can also develop joint contractures due to a mass effect from the lesion. Physical therapy with stretching exercises may be adequate to relieve symptoms; however, direct sclerotherapy plus or minus surgical excision may be required.[101]

Gynecologic Issues in Patients with Vascular Malformations

Some women with vascular anomalies have such severe menorrhagia that they undergo hysterectomy. Furthermore, pregnancy is not often seen as an option for women with severe vascular anomalies of the lower extremities, due to the exacerbation of leg swelling, pain, and bleeding from the increased pressure of a full uterus. The normal physiologic changes of pregnancy include increased plasma volume and cardiac output, increased venous pressure, leg edema, and venous stasis. Additionally, during pregnancy there is a 5.5 times increased risk of thromboembolism; this risk is augmented in patients with vascular anomalies who already have an increased prothrombotic risk. Increased risk of thrombosis with oral contraceptives limits these patients' choices of contraception. This is also an issue when oral contraceptives are considered to treat dysmenorrhea or other gynecologic problems.[102]

Pregnancy for women with vascular anomalies, especially those in the lower extremities, may cause unique problems due to hormonal changes, as well as compression of venous structures by the enlarging uterus. Preliminary data suggest that the risk of obstetric complications, especially preeclampsia and thrombotic events, is higher in women with vascular anomalies of the lower extremities.[103] It is recommended that management of pregnancy be under the direction of an obstetrician who is aware of these risks. Therapy with daily injections of low molecular weight heparin during pregnancy may prevent some prothrombotic complications.[104] In addition to pregnancy, other hormonal changes, such as those associated with puberty (in males or females) or the menstrual cycle may present an increased risk of thrombosis within vascular lesions, necessitating medical intervention with anticoagulants.[105]

Psychosocial Issues

Despite the benign clinical course of infantile hemangiomas in the majority of patients and tendency of these lesions to naturally involute, families of patients frequently undergo stress related to social interactions and medical care.[11,106] Tanner and colleagues[11] conducted interviews of parents of 25 children (5 months to 8 years of age) with facial hemangiomas. They found great variability in parental emotion regarding the lesion. However, support from extended family appeared to be an important factor in coping.[10] Interactions with strangers were a major stress in the majority of cases. Contact with "stable familiars" (i.e., family members, friends, preschool) appeared to be the least stressful. Many families were dissatisfied with medical care, often due to (1) imprecise treatment plans, which are inherent with the nature of many hemangiomas, and (2) what the parents perceived as insensitivity on the part of physicians. Williams and colleagues[107] assessed the psychological profile of children with hemangiomas and their families in a survey distributed to parents of children with hemangiomas. The results suggested that the families, rather than the infants, experienced emotional and psychological distress.[107]

Contact with other families who are going through or have gone through the same experience enables the families to see "the light at the end of the tunnel" of this curable disorder.[106] In this sense, local "family support groups" organized at some medical centers, as well as national support networks, are increasingly providing the necessary stability for families and patients. The Internet has played an enormous role in assisting the exchange of information, as well as enabling families to connect with one another (Box 66-3). As the field becomes more well known, older patients who had hemangiomas as infants and children are becoming role models, publishing their experiences and speaking at meetings—further enforcing the optimistic outcome. Furthermore, adult patients with vascular malformations are networking with younger patients.

TREATMENT OF HEMANGIOMAS

Observation, Laser, Corticosteroids

"Cautious observation" is recommended for the majority of hemangiomas, providing there is no impending danger associated with the lesion. Various reviews and guidelines for treatment are available in the medical literature.[108-110] Flashlamp pulsed dye laser is a therapeutic option for some cutaneous hemangiomas.[111] The mechanism of action of this treatment appears to be selective photothermolysis, allowing selective destruction of superficial dermal vessels while sparing surrounding tissue.[112] Pulsed dye laser therapy may also be an effective means of treating ulcerated hemangiomas, although this remains controversial.[94] Further information regarding therapy of subglottic hemangiomas is discussed later.

Corticosteroids remain one of the most common treatment modalities for proliferating hemangiomas that have a documented or impending morbidity.[113,114] Steroids are antiangiogenic in a number of in vitro settings. The precise mechanism of action by which steroids catalyze involution of hemangiomas is unknown but may be related to inhibition of the proteolytic activity associated with angiogenesis. Steroids inhibit VEGF expression in human vascular endothelial cells and inhibit proteolytic activity in endothelial cells.[115,116] Other studies have shown an increase in mast cell density, reduced transcription of several cytokines, and an increased

BOX 66-3 Web Resources for Patients and Physicians

Arkansas Children's Hospital Vascular Anomalies Program	http://www.birthmarks.org
Boston Children's Hospital Vascular Anomalies Program	http://web1.tch.harvard.edu
Children's Hospital of Wisconsin	http://www.chw.org/display/PPF/DocID/30282/NAV/1/router.asp
Cincinnati Children's Hospital Vascular Anomalies Program	http://www.cincinnatichildrens.org/svc/prog/vascular
Institute for Reconstructive Plastic Surgery	www.med.nyu.edu/irps
NYU Medical Center Vascular Anomalies Program	
NYU Pediatric Hematology	http://www.med.nyu.edu/pedhematology/
UCSF Vascular Anomalies Program	http://dermatology.medschool.ucsf.edu/clinics/vac.aspx
Support Groups	
About Face	http://www.aboutfaceinternational.org
Forward Face	http://www.forwardface.org
National Organization of Vascular Anomalies	http://www.novanews.org
Hemangioma Newsline	http://www.hnline.org
Klippel-Trénaunay Foundation	http://www.ktfoundation.com/
Klippel-Trénaunay Support Group	http://www.k-t.org
National Foundation for Facial Reconstruction	http://www.nffr.org
Sturge-Weber Foundation	http://www.sturge-weber.com
Vascular Birthmark Foundation	http://www.birthmark.org

expression of the mitochondrial cytochrome b gene in hemangioma tissue biopsy material from an infant with an ulcerated proliferating hemangioma before and after intralesional triamcinolone injection.[117] More recent studies suggest that glucocorticoids may modulate hemangioma growth via upregulation of cytochrome b, clust/apoJ, or IL-6, or a combination.[118] Additionally, steroids may influence capillary vascular tone.

Hemangiomas in different anatomic sites appear to respond differentially to medical therapy (corticosteroids or interferon). Parotid hemangiomas were found to have a diminished response to medical intervention, as determined by physical examination, serial photographs, and radiologic evaluation.[119]

Steroid-related side effects seen in infants with hemangiomas treated with systemic corticosteroids may be short termed or chronic. Side effects include Cushingoid facies, personality changes, gastric irritation, fungal infection (oral thrush or perineal infection), hypertension, myocardial hypertrophy (independent of hypertension), and decreased linear growth or weight.[120,121] Diminished linear growth may correlate with duration of therapy and age at initiation of treatment. No serious long-term complications were reported in either series.

Infants with hemangiomas tend to tolerate the medication; however, they must be closely monitored for side effects during and after therapy. A dosage of 2 to 3 mg/kg/day of prednisolone given in the morning, with an antacid, appears to be adequate for most patients with endangering hemangiomas. Serial office visits are indicated to observe efficacy, as well as to monitor for toxicity. Parents can be reassured that the side effects are generally transient. Growth charts must be kept impeccably to oversee trends in height, weight, and head circumference. Blood pressure and urinary glucose should be monitored. During the course of therapy, inactivated immunizations may be given; however, live virus vaccines must be avoided. Parents should be informed about risks associated with exposure to or development of varicella and the importance of contacting medical personnel should either occur.[120,121]

Developmental assessment should be documented at each visit, as steroid-related myopathy or obesity may interfere with normal developmental milestones. Referral for early intervention and physical therapy can ameliorate these findings. Routine administration of *Pneumocystis carinii* pneumonia prophylaxis is controversial but should be strongly considered for those patients on corticosteroids for a prolonged period. Additionally, children older than 6 months of age should receive the inactivated influenza vaccine in season, and immunization of close family members should be considered.

Other Therapies

In 1989 White and colleagues[122] described the successful use of IFN-α for the treatment of a child with recalcitrant pulmonary hemangiomatosis. Subsequently, a number of case reports and small series have reported the use of this agent for the treatment of hemangiomas of infancy.[123] Unfortunately, an unforeseen neurologic side effect has been associated with this drug. Barlow and colleagues[124] reported spastic diplegia in 5 of 26 patients treated with interferon. In some patients, this finding was reversible. The reason for this toxicity is not known.[125,126] This deleterious effect has also been described with the use of IFN-α 2b.[127] Vincristine has been used for corticosteroid-resistant hemangiomas.[128]

Surgery

The indications for and timing of surgery for hemangiomas remain controversial. Most physicians use steroids as first-line therapy, followed by IFN-α for nonresponders. Some surgeons prefer to defer surgery until the hemangioma has undergone substantial involution, with the rationale that the surgery will be less complex and cosmetically more favorable. Other surgeons advocate early intervention, to possibly prevent medical complications, or to prevent the psychological effects of the hemangioma on the patient and family. In any case, a well-planned strategy of sequential procedures can provide excellent results. Many hemangioma patients require judicious serial debulking of excess tissue.[129] Mulliken and colleagues[3] reported surgical outcome of 25 children with localized hemangioma who underwent circular excision with purse-string closure, with improved cosmetic results compared with more traditional surgical approaches. Liposuction is becoming another therapeutic option for involuted hemangiomas.[130,131]

TREATMENT OF VASCULAR MALFORMATIONS

Because vascular malformation is a more chronic condition and fewer specific therapies are available for it, a more supportive approach is often taken. The general rule is, "if it's not broken, don't fix it." If there are no clinical symptoms, alert observation is often adequate. Patients with venous vascular malformations (Fig. 66-10) often experience painful episodes—this is often in conjunction with a "phlebolith" or local clot. Therapy with ibuprofen usually suffices. Bleeding from cutaneous blebs may respond to laser cauterization. More severe bleeding from the genitourinary tract may require a combined approach with angiography-guided embolization, laser, or sclerotherapy. Large symptomatic thromboses may require anticoagulation, as might the coagulopathy associated with severe cases.[105]

Patients with arterial and venous abnormalities must be cautioned about "triggers." Quiescent vascular anomalies may become more problematic secondary to local trauma, infections, or hormonal fluctuations such as puberty, menstruation, and pregnancy. These changes are usually manifest as increased fullness of the malformation, as well as pain. The etiology of these difficulties is not clearly understood, but in the hormonally mediated settings it is likely related to hormonal stimulation of endothelial cell surface receptors.

Lymphatic malformations are among the most frustrating cases encountered. Evaluation of patients with lymphedema involves physical examination and radiologic studies including lymphoscintigraphy.[134] Therapy is generally supportive and involves sclerotherapy when possible, complete decompressive massage, compression, and pneumatic therapy.[135] Complete decongestion therapy is a protocol designed to prevent infection, along with manual massage and compression bandages to enhance fluid drainage. Studies have shown decreased expression of inflammatory genes after complete decompressive therapy.[136] Lymphatic abnormalities involving the mouth and gastrointestinal tract seem prone to infection; therefore patients with lymphatic malformation in these sites may benefit from rotating prophylactic antibiotic regimens. Macrocystic lymphatic malformations of the head and neck may respond well to sclerotherapy or surgery, or both. Picibanil (OK-432) is a sclerosing agent derived from a low-virulence strain of *Streptococcus pyogenes.* A multicenter, prospective, nonrandomized trial is under way to evaluate the efficacy of Picibanil in the treatment of macrocystic cervicofacial lymphatic malformations.[137] The preliminary results of this study are promising. The pathobiology of lymphatic vascular malformation and the consequences of this pathology are elusive. Despite these shortcomings, there is brisk research in lymphatic development, with preclinical studies demonstrating the therapeutic potential for lymphangiogenesis

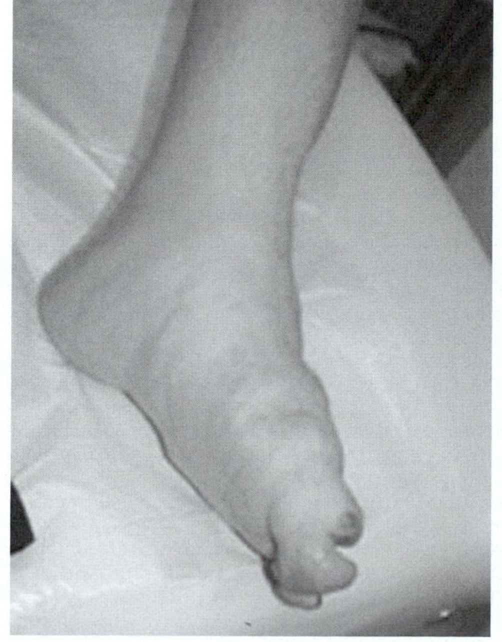

A

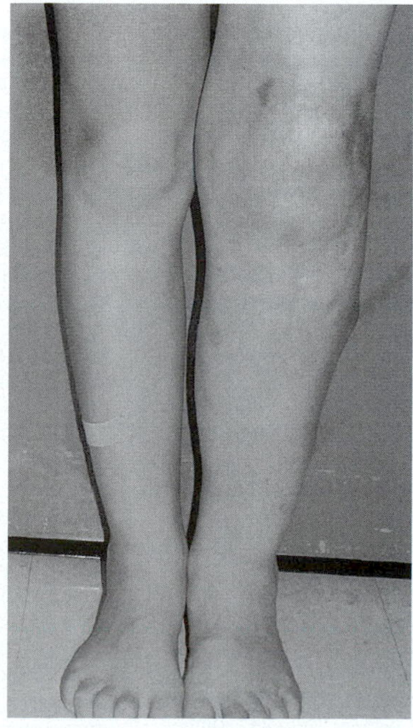

B

FIGURE 66-10. (See also Color Plate 66-10.) Two patients with venous vascular malformations (**A** and **B**) causing foot (**A**) and knee (**B**) pain.

with lymphangiogenic growth factors (e.g., VEGF-C).[135] Functional lymphatic vessels were generated in lymphedema mice using virus-mediated VEGF-C gene therapy, offering promise for therapy congenital of lymphedema patients.[138]

Acknowledgments

The author extends gratitude to the patients with vascular anomalies and their families, as well as the staffs of the Institute for Reconstructive Surgery and the Stephen D. Hassenfeld Children's Center of New York University Medical Center.

REFERENCES

1. Mulliken JB, Glowacki J: Classification of pediatric vascular lesions. Plast Reconstr Surg 1982;70:120, 1982.
2. Nakayama H: Clinical and histological studies of the classification and the natural course of the strawberry mark. J Dermatol 18:277, 1981.
3. Mulliken JB, Rogers GF, Marler JJ: Circular excision of hemangioma and purse-string closure: The smallest possible scar. Plast Reconstr Surg 109:1544, 2002.
4. North PE, Waner M, James CA, et al: Congenital nonprogressive hemangioma: A distinct clinicopathologic entity unlike infantile hemangioma. Arch Dermatol 137:1607, 2001.
5. Boon LM, Enjolras O, Mulliken JB: Congenital hemangioma: Evidence of accelerated involution. J Pediatr 128:329, 1996.
6. Enjolras O, Mulliken JB, Boon LM, et al: Noninvoluting congenital hemangioma: A rare cutaneous vascular anomaly. Plast Reconstr Surg 107:1647, 2001.

6a. Waner M, North PE, Scherer KA, et al: The nonrandom distribution of facial hemangiomas. Arch Dermatol 139:869, 2003.

7. Bubman D, Cesarman E: Pathogenesis of Kaposi's sarcoma. Hematol Oncol Clin North Am 17:717, 2003.
8. Martinez-Perez D, Fein NA, Boon LM, et al: Not all hemangiomas look like strawberries: Uncommon presentations of the most common tumor of infancy. Pediatr Dermatol 12:1, 1995.
9. Boon LM, Fishman SJ, Lund DP, et al: Congenital fibrosarcoma masquerading as congenital hemangioma: Report of two cases. J Pediatr Surg 30:1378, 1995.
10. Kunkel EJ, Zager RP, Hausman CL, et al: An interdisciplinary group for parents of children with hemangiomas. Psychosomatics 35:524, 1994.
11. Tanner JL, Dechert MP, Frieden IJ: Growing up with a facial hemangioma: Parent and child coping and adaptation. Pediatrics 101:446, 1998.
12. Orlow SJ, Isakoff MS, Blei F: Increased risk of symptomatic hemangiomas of the airway in association with cutaneous hemangiomas in a "beard" distribution. J Pediatr 131:643, 1997.
13. Yap EY, Bartley GB, Hohberger GG: Periocular capillary hemangioma: A review for pediatricians and family physicians. Mayo Clin Proc 73:753, 1998.
14. Ceisler EJ, Santos L, Blei F: Periocular hemangiomas: What every physician should know. Pediatr Dermatol 21:1, 2004.
15. Burrows PE, Robertson RL, Mulliken JB, et al: Cerebral vasculopathy and neurologic sequelae in infants with cervicofacial hemangioma: Report of eight patients. Radiology 207:601, 1998.
16. Blei F, Rutkowski M: Transiently arterialized hemangiomas: Relevant clinical and cardiac issues. Lymphatic Res Biol 1:317, 2003.
17. Kasabach H, Merritt K: Capillary hemangioma with extensive purpura. Am J Dis Child 59:1063, 1940.
18. Sarkar M, Mulliken JB, Kozakewich HP, et al: Thrombocytopenic coagulopathy (Kasabach-Merritt phenomenon) is associated with Kaposiform hemangioendothelioma and not with common infantile hemangioma. Plast Reconstr Surg 100:1377, 1997.
19. Enjolras O, Wassef M, Mazoyer E, et al: Infants with Kasabach-Merritt syndrome do not have "true" hemangiomas. J Pediatr 130:631, 1997.
20. Enjolras O, Mulliken JB, Wassef M, et al: Residual lesions after Kasabach-Merritt phenomenon in 41 patients. J Am Acad Dermatol 42:225, 2000.
21. Padilla RS, Orkin M, Rosai J: Acquired "tufted" angioma (progressive capillary hemangioma): A distinctive clinicopathologic entity related to lobular capillary hemangioma. Am J Dermatopathol 9:292, 1987.
22. Wong SN, Tay YK: Tufted angioma: A report of five cases. Pediatr Dermatol 19:388, 2002.
23. Marchuk DA, Srinivasan S, Squire TL, et al: Vascular morphogenesis: Tales of two syndromes. Hum Mol Genet 12 Spec No 1:R97, 2003.
24. Tille JC, Morris MA, Brundler MA, et al: Familial predisposition to tufted angioma: Identification of blood and lymphatic vascular components. Clin Genet 63:393, 2003.
25. Patrice SJ, Wiss K, Mulliken JB: Pyogenic granuloma (lobular capillary hemangioma): A clinicopathologic study of 178 cases. Pediatr Dermatol 8:267, 1991.
26. Krown SE: Therapy of AIDS-associated Kaposi's sarcoma: Targeting pathogenetic mechanisms. Hematol Oncol Clin North Am 17:763, 2003.
27. Smoller BR, Rosen S: Port-wine stains: A disease of altered neural modulation of blood vessels? Arch Dermatol 122:177, 1986.
28. Rosen S, Smoller BR: Port-wine stains: A new hypothesis. J Am Acad Dermatol 17:164, 1987.
29. Burns AJ, Kaplan LC, Mulliken JB: Is there an association between hemangioma and syndromes with dysmorphic features? Pediatrics 88:1257, 1991.
30. Boente MD, Cordisco MR, Frontini MD, et al: Blue rubber bleb nevus (Bean syndrome): Evolution of four cases and clinical response to pharmacologic agents. Pediatr Dermatol 16:222, 1999.
31. Davidson TI, Kissin MW, Bradish CF, et al: Angiosarcoma arising in a patient with Maffucci syndrome. Eur J Surg Oncol 11:381, 1985.
32. Fargnoli MC, Orlow SJ, Semel-Concepcion J, et al: Clinicopathologic findings in the Bannayan-Riley-Ruvalcaba syndrome. Arch Dermatol 132:1214, 1996.
33. Reese V, Frieden IJ, Paller AS, et al: Association of facial hemangiomas with Dandy-Walker and other posterior fossa malformations. J Pediatr 122:379, 1993.
34. Metry DW, Dowd CF, Barkovich AJ, et al: The many faces of PHACE syndrome. J Pediatr 139:117, 2001.
35. Albright AL, Gartner JC, Wiener ES: Lumbar cutaneous hemangiomas as indicators of tethered spinal cords. Pediatrics 83:977, 1989.
36. Greenlee R, Hoyme H, Witte M, et al: Developmental disorders of the lymphatic system. Lymphology 26:156, 1993.
37. Morris J, Abbott J, Burrows P, et al: Antenatal diagnosis of fetal hepatic hemangioma treated with maternal corticosteroids. Obstet Gynecol 94:813, 1999.
38. Cannistra C, Standoli L: [Viral implication in immature angiomas. Etiopathogenic hypothesis and immunohistopathologic study of eleven cases]. Pathol Biol (Paris) 42:150, 1994.
39. Smoller BR, Chang PP, Kamel OW: No role for human herpes virus 8 in the etiology of infantile capillary hemangioma. Mod Pathol 10:675, 1997.
40. Dupin N, Enjolras O, Wassef M, et al: [Absence of HHV-8 virus detected in immature hemangiomas in infants]. Ann Dermatol Venereol 125:98, 1998.
41. Burton BK, Schulz CJ, Angle B, et al: An increased incidence of haemangiomas in infants born following chorionic villus sampling (CVS). Prenat Diagn 15:209, 1995.
42. North PE, Waner M, Mizeracki A, et al: A unique microvascular phenotype shared by juvenile hemangiomas and human placenta. Arch Dermatol 137:559, 2001.
43. Brown CS, Goodwin PC, Sorger PK: Image metrics in the statistical analysis of DNA microarray data. Proc Natl Acad Sci U S A 98:8944, 2001.
44. Kleinman ME, Tepper OM, Capla JM, et al: Increased circulating CD 34+, AC 133+ endothelial progenitor cells in children with hemangiomas. Lymphatic Res Biol 1:301, 2003.
45. Yu Y, Flint AF, Mulliken JB, et al: Endothelial progenitor cells in infantile hemangioma. Blood 103:1373, 2004.
46. Dadras SS, North PE, Bertoncini J, et al: Infantile hemangiomas are arrested in an early developmental vascular differentiation state. Mod Pathol 17:1068, 2004.
47. Enjolras O, Gelbert F: Superficial hemangiomas: Associations and management. Pediatr Dermatol 14:173, 1997.

48. Sasaki GH, Pang CY, Wittliff JL: Pathogenesis and treatment of infant skin strawberry hemangiomas: Clinical and in vitro studies of hormonal effects. Plast Reconstr Surg 73:359, 1984.
49. Lui W, Zhang S, Hu T, et al: Sex hormone receptors of hemangiomas in children. Chin Med J (Engl) 110:349, 1997.
50. Razon MJ, Kraling BM, Mulliken JB, et al: Increased apoptosis coincides with onset of involution in infantile hemangioma. Microcirculation 5:189, 1998.
51. Hasan Q, Ruger BM, Tan ST, et al: Clusterin/apoJ expression during the development of hemangioma. Hum Pathol 31:691, 2000.
52. Teruyama K, Abe M, Nakano T, et al: Role of transcription factor Ets-1 in the apoptosis of human vascular endothelial cells. J Cell Physiol 188:243, 2001.
52a. Takahashi K, Mulliken JB, Kozakewich HP, et al: Cellular markers that distinguish the phases of hemangioma during infancy and childhood. J Clin Invest 93:2357, 1994.
53. Martin-Padura I, De Castellarnau C, Uccini S, et al: Expression of VE (vascular endothelial)-cadherin and other endothelial-specific markers in haemangiomas. J Pathol 175:51, 1995.
54. Berard M, Sordello S, Ortega N, et al: Vascular endothelial growth factor confers a growth advantage in vitro and in vivo to stromal cells cultured from neonatal hemangiomas. Am J Pathol 150:1315, 1997.
55. Chang J, Most D, Bresnick S, et al: Proliferative hemangiomas: Analysis of cytokine gene expression and angiogenesis. Plast Reconstr Surg 103:1, 1999.
56. Dosanjh A, Chang J, Bresnick S, et al: In vitro characteristics of neonatal hemangioma endothelial cells: Similarities and differences between normal neonatal and fetal endothelial cells. J Cutan Pathol 27:441, 2000.
57. Sunderkotter C, Goebeler M, Schulze-Osthoff K, et al: Macrophage-derived angiogenesis factors. Pharmacol Ther 51:195, 1991.
58. Isik FF, Rand RP, Gruss JS, et al: Monocyte chemoattractant protein-1 mRNA expression in hemangiomas and vascular malformations. J Surg Res 61:71, 1996.
59. Kraling BM, Razon MJ, Boon LM, et al: E-selectin is present in proliferating endothelial cells in human hemangiomas. Am J Pathol 148:1181, 1996.
60. Jang YC, Isik FF, Gibran NS: Nerve distribution in hemangiomas depends on the proliferative state of the microvasculature. J Surg Res 93:144, 2000.
61. Huang SA, Tu HM, Harney JW, et al: Severe hypothyroidism caused by type 3 iodothyronine deiodinase in infantile hemangiomas. N Engl J Med 343:185, 2000.
62. Li Q, Yu Y, Bischoff J, et al: Differential expression of CD146 in tissues and endothelial cells derived from infantile haemangioma and normal human skin. J Pathol 201:296, 2003.
63. Arbiser JL, Weiss SW, Arbiser ZK, et al: Differential expression of active mitogen-activated protein kinase in cutaneous endothelial neoplasms: Implications for biologic behavior and response to therapy. J Am Acad Dermatol 44:193, 2001.
64. Folkman J: Toward a new understanding of vascular proliferative disease in children. Pediatrics 74:850, 1984.
65. Risau W, Flamme I: Vasculogenesis. Annu Rev Cell Dev Biol 11:73, 1995.
66. Boudreau N, Andrews C, Srebrow A, et al: Induction of the angiogenic phenotype by Hox D3. J Cell Biol 139:257, 1997.
67. Korpelainen EI, Karkkainen M, Gunji Y, et al: Endothelial receptor tyrosine kinases activate the STAT signaling pathway: Mutant Tie-2 causing venous malformations signals a distinct STAT activation response. Oncogene 18:1, 1999.
68. Shattil SJ, Ginsberg MH: Integrin signaling in vascular biology. J Clin Invest 100:S91, 1997.
69. Williams RL, Risau W, Zerwes HG, et al: Endothelioma cells expressing the polyoma middle T oncogene induce hemangiomas by host cell recruitment. Cell 57:1053, 1989.
70. Sato T: Transcriptional regulation of vascular development. Circ Res 88:127, 2001.
71. Eerola I, Boon LM, Mulliken JB, et al: Capillary malformation–arteriovenous malformation, a new clinical and genetic disorder caused by RASA1 mutations. Am J Hum Genet 73:1240, 2003.
72. Kriederman BM, Myloyde TL, Witte MH, et al: FOXC2 haploinsufficient mice are a model for human autosomal dominant lymphedema-distichiasis syndrome. Hum Mol Genet 12:1179, 2003.
73. Brooks BP, Dagenais SL, Nelson CC, et al: Mutation of the FOXC2 gene in familial distichiasis. J AAPOS 7:354, 2003.
74. Levinson KL, Feingold E, Ferrell RE, et al: Age of onset in hereditary lymphedema. J Pediatr 142:704, 2003.
75. Garzon MC, Enjolras O, Frieden IJ: Vascular tumors and vascular malformations: Evidence for an association. J Am Acad Dermatol 42:275, 2000.
76. Walter JW, Blei F, Anderson JL, et al: Genetic mapping of a novel familial form of infantile hemangioma. Am J Med Genet 82:77, 1999.
77. Blei F, Walter J, Orlow SJ, et al: Familial segregation of hemangiomas and vascular malformations as an autosomal dominant trait. Arch Dermatol 134:718, 1998 [Erratum in Arch Dermatol 134:1425, 1998].
78. Boye E, Yu Y, Paranya G, et al: Clonality and altered behavior of endothelial cells from hemangiomas. J Clin Invest 107:745, 2001.
79. Walter J, North P, Waner M, et al: Somatic mutation of vascular endothelial growth factor receptors in juvenile hemangioma. Genes Chromosomes Cancer 33:295, 2001.
80. Enjolras O, Riche MC, Merland JJ: Facial port-wine stains and Sturge-Weber syndrome. Pediatrics 76:48, 1985.
81. Tallman B, Tan OT, Morelli JG, et al: Location of port-wine stains and the likelihood of ophthalmic and/or central nervous system complications. Pediatrics 87:323, 1991.
82. Kacker A, April M, Ward RF: Use of potassium titanyl phosphate (KTP) laser in management of subglottic hemangiomas. Int J Pediatr Otorhinolaryngol 59:15, 2001.
83. Achauer BM, Celikoz B, VanderKam VM: Intralesional bare fiber laser treatment of hemangioma of infancy. Plast Reconstr Surg 101:1212, 1998.
84. Wang LY, Hung HY, Lee KS: Infantile subglottic hemangioma treated by intralesional steroid injection: report of one case. Acta Paediatr Taiwan 44:35, 2003.
85. Robb RM: Refractive errors associated with hemangiomas of the eyelids and orbit in infancy. Am J Ophthalmology 83:52, 1977.
86. Elsas FJ, Lewis AR: Topical treatment of periocular capillary hemangioma. J Pediatr Ophthalmol Strabismus 31:153, 1994.
87. Shorr N, Seiff SR: Central retinal artery occlusion associated with periocular corticosteroid injection for juvenile hemangioma. Ophthalmic Surg 17:229, 1986.
88. Boon LM, Brouillard P, Irrthum A, et al: A gene for inherited cutaneous venous anomalies ("glomangiomas") localizes to chromosome 1p21-22. Am J Hum Genet 65:125, 1999.
89. Enjolras O, Riche MC, Merland JJ, et al: Management of alarming hemangiomas in infancy: A review of 25 cases. Pediatrics 85:491, 1990.
90. Hurvitz SA, Hurvitz CH, Sloninsky L, et al: Successful treatment with cyclophosphamide of life-threatening diffuse hemangiomatosis involving the liver. J Pediatr Hematol Oncol 22:527, 2000.
91. Goldberg NS, Hebert AA, Esterly NB: Sacral hemangiomas and multiple congenital abnormalities. Arch Dermatol 122:684, 1986.
92. Held JL, Haber RS, Silvers DN, et al: Benign neonatal hemangiomatosis: Review and description of a patient with unusually persistent lesions. Pediatr Dermatol 7:63, 1990.
93. Kim HJ, Colombo M, Frieden IJ: Ulcerated hemangiomas: Clinical characteristics and response to therapy. J Am Acad Dermatol 44:962, 2001.
94. David LR, Malek MM, Argenta LC: Efficacy of pulse dye laser therapy for the treatment of ulcerated haemangiomas: A review of 78 patients. Br J Plast Surg 56:317, 2003.
95. Martinez MI, Sanchez-Carpintero I, North PE, et al: Infantile hemangioma: Clinical resolution with 5% imiquimod cream. Arch Dermatol 138:881, 2002.
96. Sugarman J, Mauro T, Frieden I: Treatment of an ulcerated hemangioma with recombinant platelet-derived growth factor. Arch Dermatol 138:314, 2002.
97. Blei F, Karp N, Rofsky N, et al: Successful multimodal therapy for kaposiform hemangioendothelioma complicated by Kasabach-Merritt phenomenon: Case report and review of the literature. Pediatr Hematol Oncol 15:295, 1998.
98. Mallory SB, Morris P: Bleeding hemangioma detected by enuresis blanket. Pediatr Dermatol 6:139, 1989.
99. Blei F, Chianese J, Kauvar A, et al: Topical amicar and gelfoam as adjunctive therapies for bleeding hemangiomas. Int Pediatr 14:168, 1999.

100. Miller S, Smith R, Shochat S: Compression treatment of hemangiomas. Plast Reconstr Surg 58:573, 1976.
101. Scher D: Orthopaedic issues in patients with vascular anomalies. Lymphatic Res Biol 2:51, 2004.
102. Rebarber A, Roshan D, Roman A, et al: Obstetrical management of patients with Klippel-Trénaunay syndrome: Case series and review of the literature. Obstet Gynecol 104:1205, 2004.
103. Watermeyer SR, Davies N, Goodwin RI: The Klippel-Trénaunay syndrome in pregnancy. BJOG 109:1301, 2002.
104. Ginsberg JS, Greer I, Hirsh J: Use of antithrombotic agents during pregnancy. Chest 119:122S, 2001.
105. Mazoyer E, Enjolras O, Laurian C, et al: Coagulation abnormalities associated with extensive venous malformations of the limbs: Differentiation from Kasabach-Merritt syndrome. Clin Lab Haematol 24:243, 2002.
106. Dieterich-Miller CA, Safford PL: Psychosocial development of children with hemangiomas: Home, school, health care collaboration. Child Health Care 21:84, 1992.
107. Williams EF III, Hochman M, Rodgers BJ, et al: A psychological profile of children with hemangiomas and their families. Arch Facial Plast Surg 5:229, 2003.
108. Frieden IJ, Eichenfield LF, Esterly NB, et al: Guidelines of care for hemangiomas of infancy. American Academy of Dermatology Guidelines/Outcomes Committee. J Am Acad Dermatol 37:631, 1997.
109. Frieden IJ: Which hemangiomas to treat—and how? Arch Dermatol 133:1593, 1997.
110. Werner J, Dunne A, Lippert B, et al: Optimal treatment of vascular birthmarks. Am J Clin Dermatol 4:745, 2003.
111. Eichenfield LF: Vascular lesion laser: Practical techniques or some "light" suggestions. Pediatr Dermatol 16:332, 1999.
112. Anderson RR, Parrish JA: Microvasculature can be selectively damaged using dye lasers: A basic theory and experimental evidence in human skin. Lasers Surg Med 1:263, 1981.
113. Brown SH, Neerhout RC, Fonkalsrud EW: Prednisone therapy in the management of large hemangiomas in infants and children. Surgery 71:168, 1972.
114. Fost NC, Esterly NB: Successful treatment of juvenile hemangiomas with prednisone. J Pediatr 72:351, 1968.
115. Blei F, Wilson EL, Mignatti P, et al: Mechanism of action of angiostatic steroids: Suppression of plasminogen activator activity via stimulation of plasminogen activator inhibitor synthesis. J Cell Physiol 155:568, 1993.
116. Pepper MS, Vassalli JD, Wilks JW, et al: Modulation of bovine microvascular endothelial cell proteolytic properties by inhibitors of angiogenesis. J Cell Biochem 55:419, 1994.
117. Hasan Q, Tan ST, Gush J, et al: Steroid therapy of a proliferating hemangioma: Histochemical and molecular changes. Pediatrics 105:117, 2000.
118. Hasan Q, Tan ST, Xu B, et al: Effects of five commonly used glucocorticoids on haemangioma in vitro. Clin Exp Pharmacol Physiol 30:140, 2003.
119. Blei F, Isakoff M, Deb G: The response of parotid hemangiomas to the use of systemic interferon alpha-2a or corticosteroids. Arch Otolaryngol Head Neck Surg 123:841, 1997.
120. Blei F, Chianese J: Corticosteroid toxicity in infants treated for endangering hemangiomas: Experience and guidelines for monitoring. Int Pediatr 14:146, 199.
121. Boon LM, MacDonald DM, Mulliken JB: Complications of systemic corticosteroid therapy for problematic hemangioma. Plast Reconstr Surg 104:1616, 1999.
122. White CW, Sondheimer HM, Crouch EC, et al: Treatment of pulmonary hemangiomatosis with recombinant interferon alfa-2a. N Engl J Med 320:1197, 1989.
123. Ezekowitz RA, Mulliken JB, Folkman J: Interferon alfa-2a therapy for life-threatening hemangiomas of infancy. N Engl J Med 326:1456, 1992.
124. Barlow CF, Priebe CJ, Mulliken JB, et al: Spastic diplegia as a complication of interferon Alfa-2a treatment of hemangiomas of infancy. J Pediatr 132:527, 1998.
125. Egbert JE, Nelson SC: Neurologic toxicity associated with interferon alfa treatment of capillary hemangioma. J AAPOS 1:190, 1997.
126. Enjolras O: Neurotoxicity of interferon alfa in children treated for hemangiomas. J Am Acad Dermatol 39:1037, 1998.
127. Dubois J, Hershon L, Carmant L, et al: Toxicity profile of interferon alpha-2b in children: A prospective evaluation. J Pediatr 135:782, 1999.
128. Perez J, Pardo J, Gomez C: Vincristine: An effective treatment of corticoid-resistant life-threatening infantile hemangiomas. Acta Oncol 41:197, 2002.
129. Zide BM, Glat PM, Stile FL, et al: Vascular lip enlargement: Part I. Hemangiomas: Tenets of therapy. Plast Reconstr Surg 100:1664, 1997.
130. Berenguer B, De Salamanca JE, Gonzalez B, et al: Large involuted facial hemangioma treated with syringe liposuction. Plast Reconstr Surg 111:314, 2003.
131. Fisher MD, Bridges M, Lin KY: The use of ultrasound-assisted liposuction in the treatment of an involuted hemangioma. J Craniofac Surg 10:500, 1999.
132. Jacob AG, Driscoll DJ, Shaughnessy WJ, et al: Klippel-Trénaunay syndrome: Spectrum and management. Mayo Clin Proc 73:28, 1998.
133. Happle R: Sturge-Weber-Klippel-Trénaunay syndrome: What's in a name? Eur J Dermatol 13:223, 2003.
134. Szuba A, Shin WS, Strauss HW, et al: The third circulation: radionuclide lymphoscintigraphy in the evaluation of lymphedema. J Nucl Med 44:43, 2003.
135. Witte MH, Bernas MJ, Martin CP, et al: Lymphangiogenesis and lymphangiodysplasia: From molecular to clinical lymphology. Microsc Res Tech 55:122, 2001.
136. Foldi E, Sauerwald A, Hennig B: Effect of complex decongestive physiotherapy on gene expression for the inflammatory response in peripheral lymphedema. Lymphology 33:19, 2000.
137. Greinwald JH, Jr., Burke DK, Sato Y, et al: Treatment of lymphangiomas in children: An update of Picibanil (OK-432) sclerotherapy. Otolaryngol Head Neck Surg 121:381, 1999.
138. Karkkainen MJ, Saaristo A, Jussila L, et al: A model for gene therapy of human hereditary lymphedema. Proc Natl Acad Sci U S A 98:12677, 2001.
139. Berg JN, Walter JW, Thisanagayam U, et al: Evidence for loss of heterozygosity of 5q in sporadic haemangiomas: Are somatic mutations involved in haemangioma formation? J Clin Pathol 54:249, 2001.
140. Lucas M, Costa AF, Montori M, et al: Germline mutations in the CCM1 gene, encoding Krit1, cause cerebral cavernous malformations. Ann Neurol 49:529, 2001.
141. Gunel M, Awad IA, Finberg K, et al: A founder mutation as a cause of cerebral cavernous malformation in Hispanic Americans. N Engl J Med 334:946, 1996.
142. Craig HD, Gunel M, Cepeda O, et al: Multilocus linkage identifies two new loci for a mendelian form of stroke, cerebral cavernous malformation, at 7p15-13 and 3q25.2-27. Hum Mol Genet 7:1851, 1998.
143. Liquori CL, Berg MJ, Siegel AM, et al: Mutations in a gene encoding a novel protein containing a phosphotyrosine-binding domain cause type 2 cerebral cavernous malformations. Am J Hum Genet 73:1459, 2003.
144. Vikkula M, Boon LM, Carraway KL III, et al: Vascular dysmorphogenesis caused by an activating mutation in the receptor tyrosine kinase TIE2. Cell 87:1181, 1996.
145. Gallione CJ, Pasyk KA, Boon LM, et al: A gene for familial venous malformations maps to chromosome 9p in a second large kindred. J Med Genet 32:197, 1995.
146. Finegold DN, Kimak MA, Lawrence EC, et al: Truncating mutations in FOXC2 cause multiple lymphedema syndromes. Hum Mol Genet 10:1185, 2001.
147. Schmidt Drury S, Erickson RP, Glover TW: Y;16 translocation breakpoint associated with a partial Turner phenotype identifies a foamy virus insertion. Cytogenet Cell Genet 80:199, 1998.
148. Erickson RP, Hudgins L, Stone JF, et al: A "balanced" Y;16 translocation associated with Turner-like neonatal lymphedema suggests the location of a potential anti-Turner gene on the Y chromosome. Cytogenet Cell Genet 71:163, 1995.
149. Irrthum A, Karkkainen MJ, Devriendt K, et al: Congenital hereditary lymphedema caused by a mutation that inactivates VEGFR3 tyrosine kinase. Am J Hum Genet 67:295, 2000.
150. Irrthum A, Devriendt K, Chitayat D, et al: Mutations in the transcription factor gene SOX18 underlie recessive and dominant forms of hypotrichosis-lymphedema-telangiectasia. Am J Hum Genet 72:1470, 2003.

INDEX

Note: Page numbers followed by b, f, and t indicate boxed material, figures, and tables, respectively.

D

E

F

G

H

J

K

L

M

N

O

R

S

W

X

Y